Disorders Index

Continued

Disorders Index

Expert CONSULT

Activate your access at expertconsult.com

1 REGISTER

- Visit **expertconsult.com.**
- Click **"Register Now."**
- Fill in your **user information.**
- Click **"Create Account."**

2 ACTIVATE YOUR BOOK

- Scratch off your **Activation Code** below and enter it into the **"Add a title"** box.
- **You're done!** Click on the book's title under **"My Titles."**

For technical assistance, email **online.help@elsevier.com** or call **800-401-9962** (inside the US) or **+1-314-995-3200** (outside the US).

Activation Code

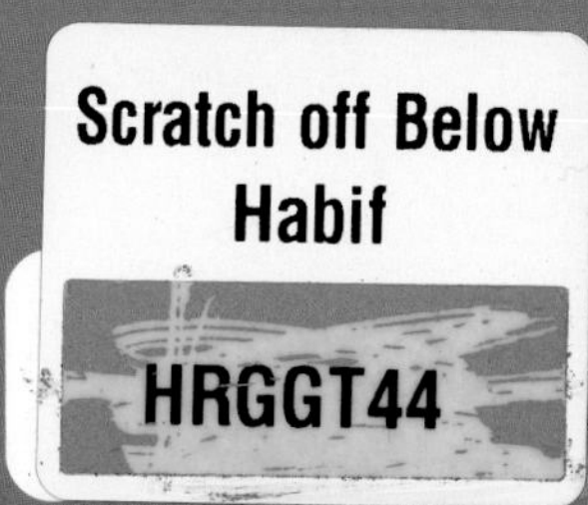

QUICK REFERENCE FORMULARY

(Topical corticosteroids are listed on the inside back cover)

ACNE MEDICATIONS: Retinoids			
Product	**Base**	**Concentration**	**Packaging**
Retin-A (Tretinoin)	Cream Gel	0.025%, 0.05%, 0.1% 0.01%, 0.025%	20, 45 gm 15, 45 gm
Retin-A Micro (Tretinoin)	Gel	0.1%, 0.04%	20, 45, 50 gm pump
Tazorac (Tazarotene)	Gel Cream	0.1%, 0.05% 0.1%, 0.5%	30, 100 gm 30, 60 gm
Differin (Adapalene)	Gel Cream	0.1%, 0.3% 0.1%	45 gm 45 gm
Epiduo	Gel	0.1% adapalene + 2.5% benzoyl peroxide	45 gm

ACNE MEDICATIONS: Topical Antibiotics		
Product	**Antibiotics**	**Packaging**
Aczone	5% dapsone	30, 60 gm gel
Benzaclin	1% clindamycin 5% benzoyl peroxide	25 gm, 50 gm gel, pump
Benzamycin	3% erythromycin 5% benzoyl peroxide	23.3, 46.6 gm gel
Cleocin T	1% clindamycin	30, 60 ml liquid, 30, 60 gm gel, 60 ml lotion
Duac gel	1% clindamycin 5% benzoyl peroxide	45 gm gel
Klaron 10%	10% sodium sulfacetamide	4 oz bottle
Clenia	5% sulfur, 10% sodium sulfacetamide	1 oz emollient cream
Sulfacet-R lotion	5% sulfur, 10% sodium sulfacetamide	25 ml, larger in generic
AVAR cleanser	5% sulfur, 10% sodium sulfacetamide	8 oz pump

ACNE MEDICATIONS: Oral Antibiotics		
Generic	**Preparation**	**Adult dosage (mg unless noted)**
Doxycycline	50, 75, 100, 150 mg	Every day, twice/day
Minocycline	50, 75, 100 mg	Every day, twice/day
Minocycline extended release tablets (Solodyn)	45 mg (90-131 lb), 90 mg (132-199 lb), 135 mg (200-300 lb)	1 tablet every day (1 mg/kg/day)

ANTINEOPLASTIC AGENTS: Topical		
	Product	**Packaging**
Aldara	5% imiquimod	Box of 12 or 24 packets
Carac	0.5% fluorouracil	30 gm tube
Fluoroplex	1% fluorouracil	30 ml solution, 30 gm cream
Efudex	2% or 5% fluorouracil 5% fluorouracil	10 ml liquid 25 gm cream

ANTIPRURITIC CREAMS AND LOTIONS		
Product	**Active ingredient**	**Packaging**
Eucerin itch relief	Menthol 0.15%	6.8 oz spray
Neutrogena anti-itch moisturizer	Camphor 0.1%, dimethicone 0.1%	10.1 oz
PrameGel	1% pramoxine, 0.5% menthol	
Sarna original	0.5% each of camphor, menthol	7.5 oz bottle
Sarna sensitive anti-itch lotion	Pramoxine HCL	7.5 oz
Sarna Ultra anti-itch cream	Menthol 0.5% and pramoxine	2 oz
Zonalon	5% doxepin	45 gm

ATOPIC DERMATITIS: Nonsteroidal Barrier Creams	
Atopiclair	100 gm
Eletone	100 gm
Epiceram	90 gm
Mimyx	140 gm

PSORIASIS: Topical Vitamin D_3 Analogs		
Brand name	**Active ingredient**	**Packaging**
Dovonex cream	Calcipotriene	30, 60, 100 gm tubes
Vectical ointment	Calcitriol	100 gm tube
Taclonex ointment, scalp	Calcipotriene + betamethasone	60 gm, 60 ml

ROSACEA: Topical Medications		
Brand name	**Generic name**	**Packaging**
Avar	5% Sulfur, 10% sodium sulfacetamide	45 gm aqueous gel
Avar Green	5% Sulfur, 10% sodium sulfacetamide	45 gm aqueous gel with green color masks redness
Clenia	5% Sulfur, 10% sodium sulfacetamide	1 oz cream, 6 oz, 12 oz foaming wash
Finacea 15%	Azelaic acid	30 gm gel
Klaron 10%	10% sodium sulfacetamide	4 oz
Generic gel, cream, lotion 0.75%	Metronidazole	45 gm, 45 gm, 120 ml
Metrogel 1%	Metronidazole	45 gm
Noritate cream 1%	Metronidazole	30 gm tube
Sulfacet-R lotion	5% Sulfur, 10% sodium sulfacetamide	25 gm bottle

SKIN BLEACHES AND DEPIGMENTING AGENTS		
Brand name	**Active ingredient**	**Packaging**
Generic	4% Hydroquinone	1 oz, 2 oz jar
TriLuma	4% Hydroquinone, 0.01% fluocinolone acetonide, 0.05% tretinoin	30 gm

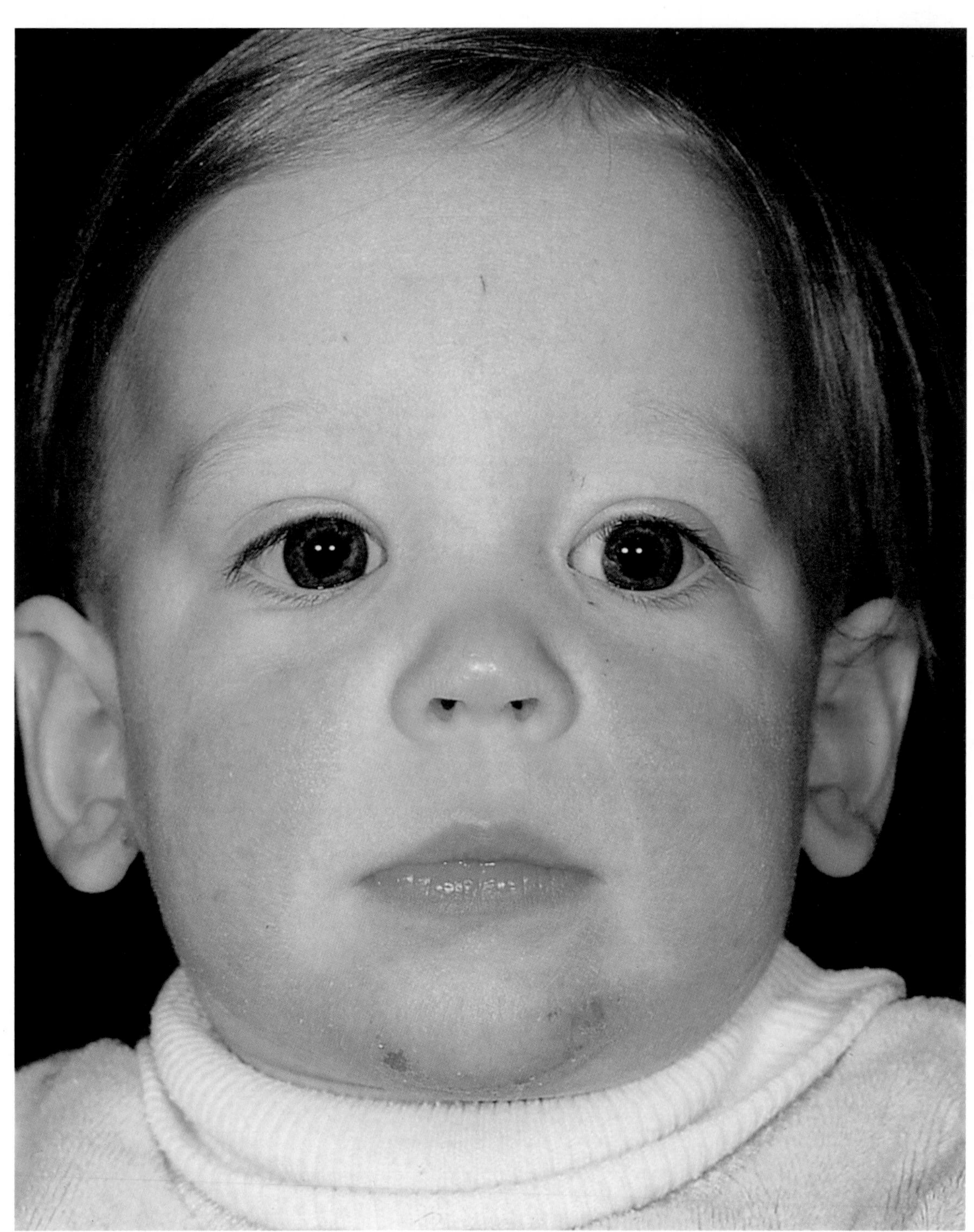

CLINICAL DERMATOLOGY

FIFTH EDITION

A COLOR GUIDE TO DIAGNOSIS AND THERAPY

Thomas P. Habif, MD
Adjunct Professor of Medicine (Dermatology)
Dartmouth Medical School
Hanover, NH, USA

Acquisitions Editor: Claire Bonnett
Development Editors: Sven Pinczewski and Louise Cook
Editorial Assistant: Kirsten Lowson
Project Manager and Layout Design: Jeanne Genz
Cover and Page Designer: Charles Gray
Compositors: Graphic World, Inc.
Gary Clark, CSR; Lyn Watts, Michele Margenau, Victoria Brown
Image Processing: Graphic World, Inc.
Mark Lane, Tom Lane
Illustrators: Graphic World, Inc.
Gwen Gilbert, Trese Gloriod, Patty Bassman
Project Organization: Laura A. McCann
Copyeditor: Beth Welch
Proofreader: Denise L. Davis
Production Assistant: Natalie Jackson
Indexer: Razorsharp Communications
Printer: C&C Offset Printing Company, Ltd.
Medical Photography: Alan N. Binnick, MD;
Thomas P. Habif, MD; Lawrence B. Meyerson, MD
Moral Support: Dorothy, David, and Tommy

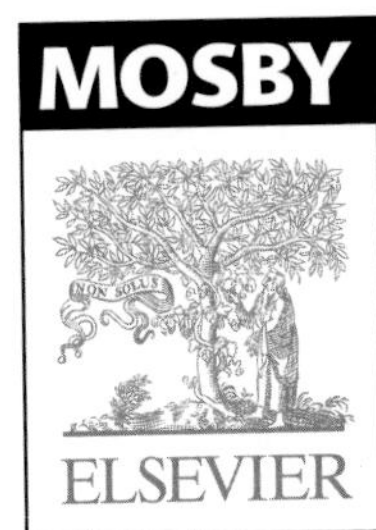

Activate your access to additional online content at **www.expertconsult.com**

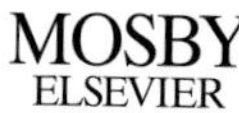

MOSBY is an affiliate of Elsevier Inc

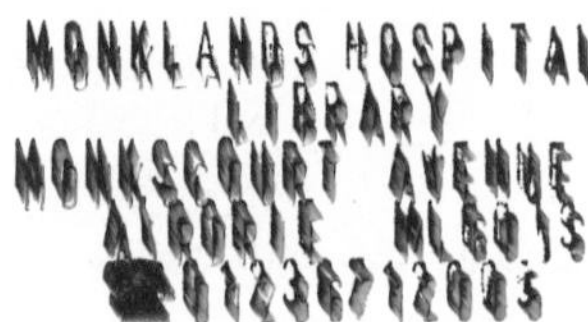

First published 2010
First edition published 1984
Second edition published 1990
Third edition published 1996
Fourth edition published 2004

ISBN: 978-0-7234-3541-9

British Library Cataloguing in Publication Data

Habif, Thomas P.
Clinical dermatology. - 5th ed.
1. Dermatology - Atlases 2. Skin - Diseases - Diagnosis - Atlases 3. Skin - Diseases - Treatment - Atlases
I. Title
616.5

Notice

Medical knowledge is constantly changing. Standard safety precautions must be followed, but as new research and clinical experience broaden our knowledge, changes in treatment and drug therapy may become necessary or appropriate. Readers are advised to check the most current product information provided by the manufacturer of each drug to be administered to verify the recommended dose, the method and duration of administration, and contraindications. It is the responsibility of the practitioner, relying on experience and knowledge of the patient, to determine dosages and the best treatment for each individual patient. Neither the Publisher nor the author assumes any liability for any injury and/or damage to persons or property arising from this publication.

The Publisher's policy is to use paper manufactured from sustainable forests

Printed in China
Last digit is the print number: 9 8 7 6 5 4 3 2 1

Preface

Clinical Dermatology is intended to be a practical resource for the clinician. Over 1500 illustrations are combined with disease descriptions and current and comprehensive therapeutic information. Bold headings are used to facilitate rapid access to information.

RAPID ACCESS TO THE TEXT

1. *Disorders Index:* A list of diseases with page references is located inside the front cover. This is the best place to start if you know the diagnosis.
2. Chapter 1—*Regional Differential Diagnosis Atlas:* New to the fifth edition, this very large section with page references will help you to narrow the differential diagnosis.
3. A list of *topical corticosteroids* can be found on the inside back cover.
4. The complete *Dermatologic Formulary,* previously in the book, can now be found online (using your login details), and we are able to offer updates. However, a *Quick Reference Formulary* to the most commonly used drugs is on pp. ii-iii.

PMID numbers (PubMed identification numbers)

References are no longer placed at the end of the chapter. They have been replaced by PMID numbers (blue letters and numbers) and are embedded in the text. Go to PubMed's home page. Be sure the search box is empty. There should be no limits set on the left-hand limits tab. Type in just the number in the search line and click on Go. You will be taken to the paper and abstract. Classic references and PMID numbers are found in tables and boxes.

Web-based text

The book with extra images and a mannequin-based aid to diagnosis are provided.

Web-based formulary 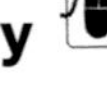

New therapeutic agents often become available. Therefore, the *Dermatologic Formulary* has been moved online. The formulary may be printed and kept as a separate document. The formulary will be updated regularly.

Text organization and content

The classic method of organizing skin diseases is used. Common diseases are covered in depth. Illustrations of classic examples of these disorders and photographs of variations seen at different stages are included. Theoretical information, disease mechanisms, and rare diseases are found in comprehensive textbooks.

HOW TO USE THIS BOOK

Students in the classroom

Students should learn the primary and secondary lesions and look at every page in the *Regional Differential Diagnosis Atlas* at the end of Chapter 1. Select a few familiar diseases from each list and read about them. Obtain an overview of the text. Turn the pages, look at the pictures, and read the captions.

Students in the clinic

You see skin abnormalities every day in the clinic. Try to identify these diseases, or ask for assistance. Study all diseases, especially tumors, with a magnifying glass or an ocular lens. Read about what you see and you will rapidly gain a broad fund of knowledge.

Study Chapters 20 (Benign Skin Tumors), 21 (Premalignant and Malignant Nonmelanoma Skin Tumors), and 22 (Nevi and Malignant Melanoma). Skin growths are common, and it is important to recognize their features.

House officers are responsible for patient management. Read Chapter 2 carefully, and study all aspects of the use of topical steroids. These agents are used to treat a variety of skin conditions. It is tempting to use these agents as a therapeutic trial and ask for a consultation only if therapy fails. Topical steroids mask some diseases, make some diseases worse, and create other diseases. Do not develop bad habits; if you do not know what a disease is, do not treat it.

The diagnosis of skin disease is deceptively easy. Do not make hasty diagnoses. Take a history, study primary lesions and the distribution, and be deliberate and methodical. Ask for help. With time and experience you will feel comfortable managing many common skin diseases.

The non-dermatologist provider

Most skin diseases are treated by non-dermatologist providers. This includes primary care physicians, nurse practitioners and physician assistants. Clinicians involved in direct patient care should read the above guidelines for using this book. Look at the *Regional Differential Diagnosis Atlas* in Chapter 1 as a general guide. Learn a few topical steroids in each potency group. There are a great number of agents in the *Dermatologic Formulary*. Many in each table contain similar ingredients and have the same therapeutic effect. Develop an armamentarium of agents and gain experience in their use.

Inflammatory conditions are often confusing, and sometimes biopsies are of limited value in their diagnosis. Eczema is common, read Chapters 2 and 3. Acne is seen everyday, read Chapter 7. Managing acne effectively will provide a great service to many young patients who are very uncomfortable with their appearance. The clinical diagnosis of pigmented lesions is complicated. Look at Chapters 20, 21, and 23. Don't be afraid to ask for help. A dermatologist can often make a diagnosis without the need for a biopsy.

The dermatologist

Use the *Disorders Index* on the inside front cover to rapidly access the text. Many dermatologists use the pictures as an aid to reassure patients. Examine the patient, make a diagnosis, and then show them an illustration of their disease. Many patients see the similarity and are reassured.

This book is designed to be a practical resource. All of the most current descriptive and therapeutic information that is practical and relevant has been included. All topics are researched on Medline. Details about basic science and complex mechanisms of disease can be found elsewhere. Rare diseases are found in larger textbooks.

IMAGES

The photographs were taken with film and digital cameras. The images for this text come from three main sources. Alan N. Binnick, MD, Adjunct Assistant Professor of Medicine (Dermatology), Dartmouth Medical School, and Lawrence B. Meyerson, Clinical Associate Professor of Dermatology at the University of Texas Southwestern Medical School provided very large collections of images taken with transparency film. I provided film and digital images. Transparency film images are in many ways superior to digital images. Each contributor has over 30 years experience as a dermatologist and a medical photographer. A combination of these three collections with over 23,000 images can be found at www.dermnet.com.

PRODUCTION

Manufacturing an illustrated book is a complicated process. The large number of people involved in this effort is listed on the title page. As my first editor said 25 years ago, "If people ever realized what was involved in making a book, they would not believe that it could ever get done."

The layout and design of each page in this book is done the "old fashioned way," by cutting and pasting images and strips of text by the layout artist. Page layout design is a science and an art. Jeanne Genz has done the page layout for all five editions of this book. This older, slower, non-computerized technique performed by an expert produces pages that are balanced and of maximum clarity. The final "pasted" book is then converted to a digital file and then converted to a pdf file that is sent to the printer who must balance color through a calibration process. The book is printed in China on high-grade glossy paper on a sheet-fed press. Glossy paper retains ink at the surface to enhance definition. Sheet-fed presses print slowly and allow ink to be laid down precisely so that exceptional sharpness and color balance are achieved.

Thomas P. Habif
2009

Contents

20 Benign Skin Tumors 776

21 Premalignant and Malignant Nonmelanoma Skin Tumors 801

22 Nevi and Malignant Melanoma 847

23 Vascular Tumors and Malformations 891

24 Hair Diseases 913

25 Nail Diseases 947

26 Cutaneous Manifestations of Internal Disease 975

ONLINE ONLY CONTENT

27 Dermatologic Surgical Procedures 999

SKIN ANATOMY

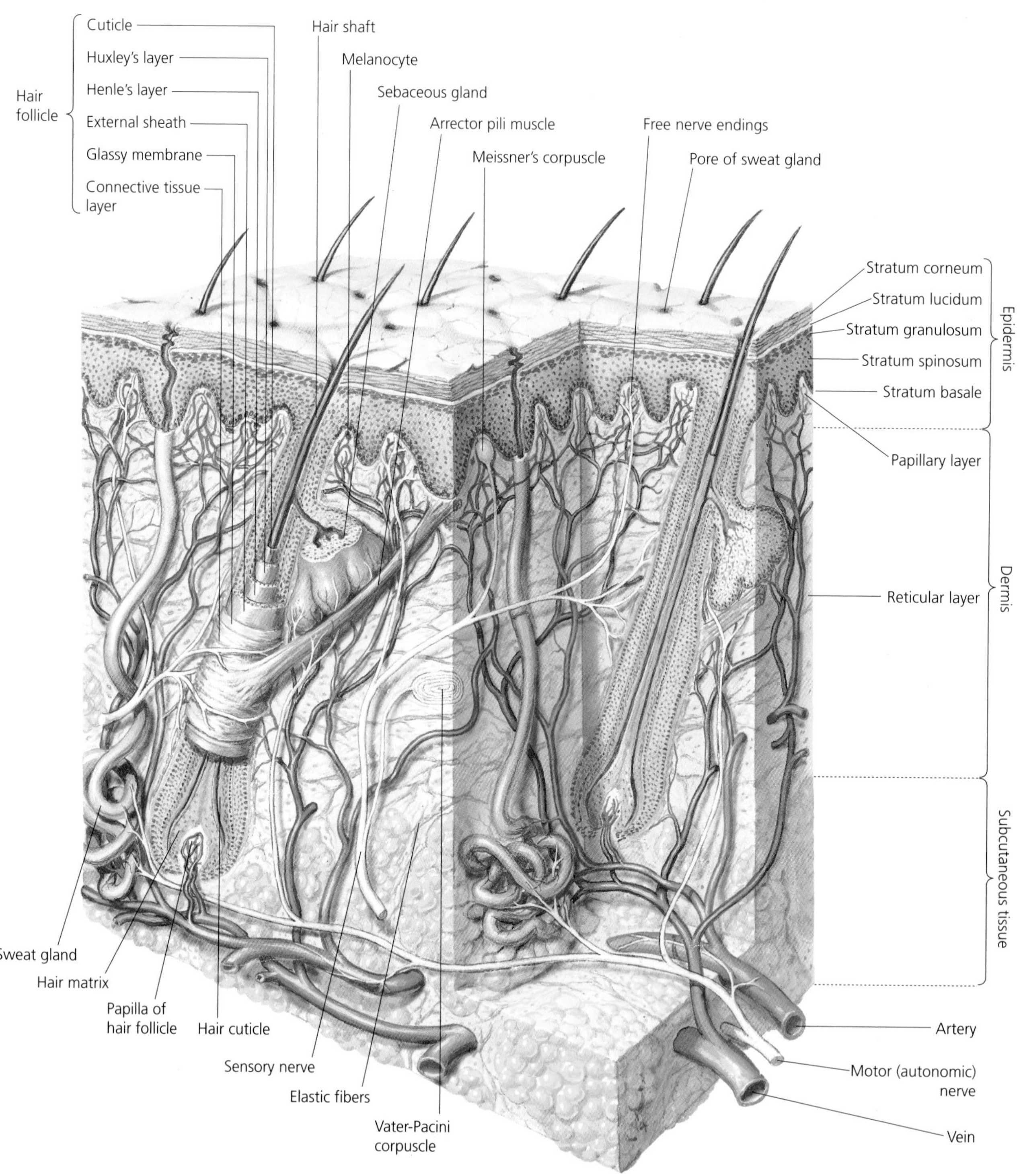

Chapter 1

Principles of Diagnosis and Anatomy

CHAPTER CONTENTS

SKIN ANATOMY

The skin is divided into three layers: the epidermis, the dermis, and the subcutaneous tissue. The skin is thicker on the dorsal and extensor surfaces than on the ventral and flexor surfaces.

Epidermis

The epidermis is the outermost part of the skin; it is stratified squamous epithelium. The thickness of the epidermis ranges from 0.05 mm on the eyelids to 1.5 mm on the palms and soles. The microscopic anatomy of the epidermal-dermal junction is complex; it is discussed in detail in Chapter 16. The innermost layer of the epidermis consists of a single row of columnar cells called basal cells. Basal cells divide to form keratinocytes, which comprise the spinous layer. The cells of the spinous layer are connected to each other by intercellular bridges or spines, which appear histologically as lines between cells. The keratinocytes synthesize insoluble protein, which remains in the cell and eventually becomes a major component of the outer layer (the stratum and corneum). The cells continue to flatten, and their cytoplasm appears granular (stratum granulosum); they finally die as they reach the surface to form the stratum corneum. There are three types of branched cells in the epidermis: the melanocyte, which synthesizes pigment (melanin); the Langerhans cell, which serves as a frontline element in immune reactions of the skin; and the Merkel cell, the function of which is not clearly defined.

Dermis

The dermis varies in thickness from 0.3 mm on the eyelid to 3.0 mm on the back; it is composed of three types of connective tissue: collagen, elastic tissue, and reticular fibers. The dermis is divided into two layers: the thin upper layer, called the papillary layer, is composed of thin, haphazardly arranged collagen fibers; the thicker lower layer, called the reticular layer, extends from the base of the papillary layer to the subcutaneous tissue and is composed of thick collagen fibers that are arranged parallel to the surface of the skin. Histiocytes are wandering macrophages that accumulate hemosiderin, melanin, and debris created by inflammation. Mast cells, located primarily around blood vessels, manufacture and release histamine and heparin.

Dermal nerves and vasculature

The sensations of touch and pressure are received by Meissner's and Vater-Pacini corpuscles. The sensations of pain, itch, and temperature are received by unmyelinated nerve endings in the papillary dermis. A low intensity of stimulation created by inflammation causes itching, whereas a high intensity of stimulation created by inflammation causes pain. Therefore scratching converts the intolerable sensation of itching to the more tolerable sensation of pain and eliminates pruritus.

The autonomic system supplies the motor innervation of the skin. Adrenergic fibers innervate the blood vessels (vasoconstriction), hair erector muscles, and apocrine glands. Autonomic fibers to eccrine sweat glands are cholinergic. The sebaceous gland is regulated by the endocrine system and is not innervated by autonomic fibers. The anatomy of the hair follicle is described in Chapter 24.

DIAGNOSIS OF SKIN DISEASE

What could be easier than the diagnosis of skin disease? The pathology is before your eyes! Why then do nondermatologists have such difficulty interpreting what they see?

There are three reasons. First, there are literally hundreds of cutaneous diseases. Second, a single entity can vary in its appearance. A common seborrheic keratosis, for example, may have a smooth, rough, or eroded surface and a border that is either uniform or as irregular as a melanoma. Third, skin diseases are dynamic and change in morphology. Many diseases undergo an evolutionary process: herpes simplex may begin as a red papule, evolve into a blister, and then become an erosion that heals with scarring. If hundreds of entities can individually vary in appearance and evolve through several stages, then it is necessary to recognize thousands of permutations to diagnose cutaneous entities confidently. What at first glance appeared to be simple to diagnose may later appear to be simply impossible.

Dermatology is a morphologically oriented specialty. As in other specialties, the medical history is important; however, the ability to interpret what is observed is even more important. The diagnosis of skin disease must be approached in an orderly and logical manner. The temptation to make rapid judgments after hasty observation must be controlled.

A methodical approach

The recommended approach to the patient with skin disease is as follows:

- **History.** Obtain a brief history, noting duration, rate of onset, location, symptoms, family history, allergies, occupation, and previous treatment.
- **Distribution.** Determine the extent of the eruption by having the patient disrobe completely.
- **Primary lesion.** Determine the primary lesion. Examine the lesions carefully; a hand lens is a valuable aid for studying skin lesions. Determine the nature of any secondary or special lesions.
- **Differential diagnosis.** Formulate a differential diagnosis.
- **Tests.** Obtain a biopsy and perform laboratory tests, such as skin biopsy, potassium hydroxide examination for fungi, skin scrapings for scabies, Gram stain, fungal and bacterial cultures, cytology (Tzanck test), Wood's light examination, patch tests, dark field examination, and blood tests.

Examination technique

DISTRIBUTION. The skin should be examined methodically. An eye scan over wide areas is inefficient. It is most productive to mentally divide the skin surface into several sections and carefully study each section. For example, when studying the face, examine the area around each eye, the nose, the mouth, the cheeks, and the temples.

During an examination, patients may show small areas of their skin, tell the doctor that the rest of the eruption looks the same, and expect an immediate diagnosis. The rest of the eruption may or may not look the same. Patients with rashes should receive a complete skin examination to determine the distribution and confirm the diagnosis. Decisions about quantities of medication to dispense require visualization of the big picture. Many dermatologists now advocate a complete skin examination for all of their patients. Because of an awareness that some patients are uncomfortable undressing completely when they have a specific request such as treatment of a plantar wart, other dermatologists advocate a case-by-case approach.

PRIMARY LESIONS AND SURFACE CHARACTERISTICS. Lesions should be examined carefully. Standing back and viewing a disease process provides valuable information about the distribution. Close examination with a magnifying device provides much more information. Often the primary lesion is identified and the diagnosis is confirmed at this step. The physician should learn the surface characteristics of all the common entities and gain experience by examining known entities. A flesh-colored papule might be a wart, sebaceous hyperplasia, or a basal cell carcinoma. The surface characteristics of many lesions are illustrated throughout this book.

Approach to treatment

Most skin diseases can be managed successfully with the numerous agents and techniques available. If a diagnosis has not been established, medications should not be prescribed; this applies particularly to prescription of topical steroids. Some physicians are tempted to experiment with various medications and, if the treatment fails, to refer the patient to a specialist. This is not a logical or efficient way to practice medicine.

Primary lesions

Most skin diseases begin with a basic lesion that is referred to as a primary lesion. Identification of the primary lesion is the key to accurate interpretation and description of cutaneous disease. Its presence provides the initial orientation and allows the formulation of a differential diagnosis. Definitions of the primary lesions and their differential diagnoses are listed and illustrated on pp. 3 to 11.

Secondary lesions

Secondary lesions develop during the evolutionary process of skin disease or are created by scratching or infection. They may be the only type of lesion present, in which case the primary disease process must be inferred. The differential diagnoses of secondary lesions are listed and illustrated on pp. 12 to 16.

PRIMARY LESIONS—MACULES

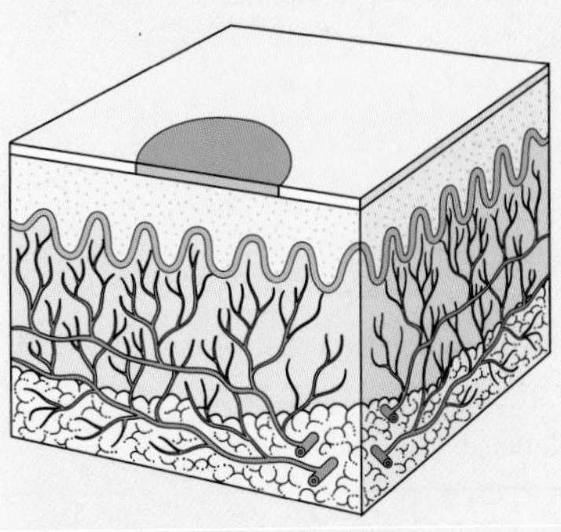

Macule
A circumscribed, flat discoloration that may be brown, blue, red, or hypopigmented

Hypopigmented
Idiopathic guttate hypomelanosis (p. 769)
Nevus anemicus (p. 770)
Piebaldism
Postinflammatory psoriasis
Radiation dermatitis
Tinea versicolor (p. 537)
Tuberous sclerosis (p. 987)
Vitiligo (p. 764)

Brown
Becker's nevus (p. 854)
Café-au-lait spot (p. 983)
Erythrasma (p. 501)
Fixed drug eruption (p. 576)
Freckles (p. 771)
Junction nevus (p. 848)
Lentigo (p. 771)
Lentigo maligna (p. 868)
Melasma (p. 772)
Photoallergic drug eruption (p. 764)
Phototoxic drug eruption (p. 761)
Stasis dermatitis (p. 122)
Tinea nigra palmaris

Blue
Ink (tattoo)
Maculae ceruleae (lice)
Mongolian spot
Ochronosis

Red
Drug eruptions (p. 568)
Juvenile rheumatoid arthritis (Still's disease)
Rheumatic fever
Secondary syphilis (p. 400)
Viral exanthems (p. 558)

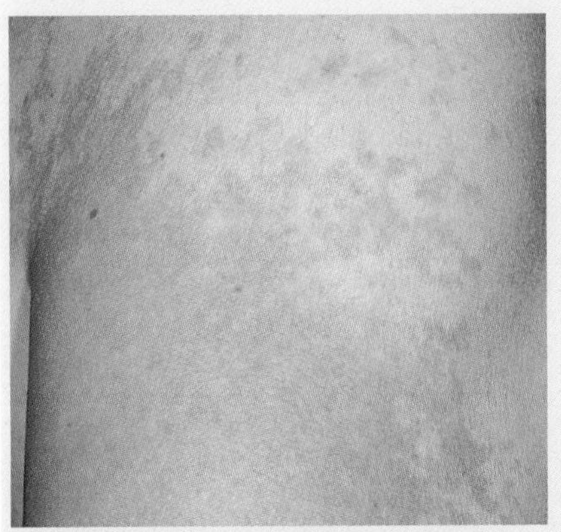

Becker's nevus

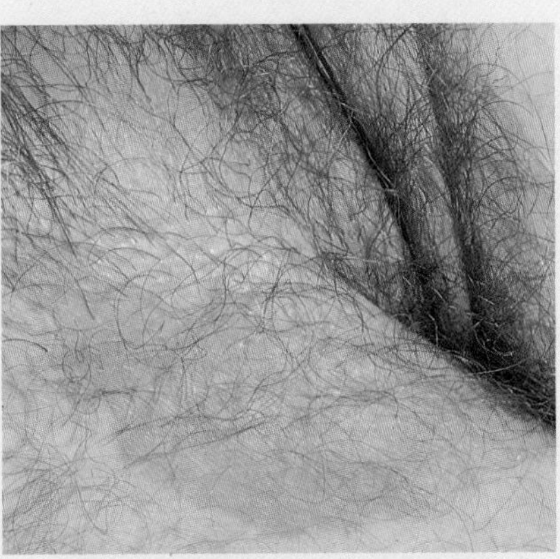

Erythrasma

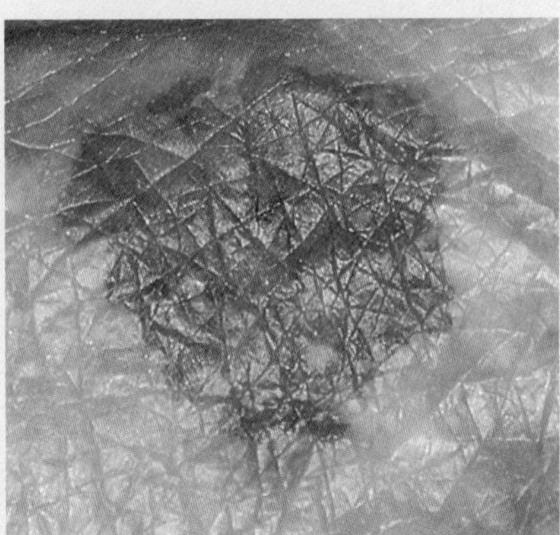

Lentigo

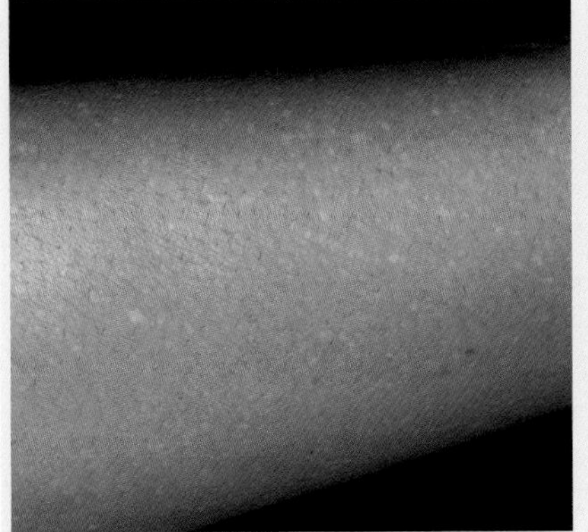

Idiopathic guttate hypomelanosis

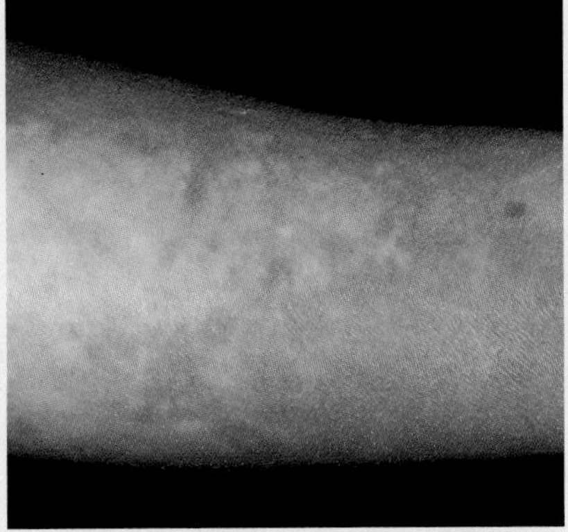

Phototoxic drug eruption

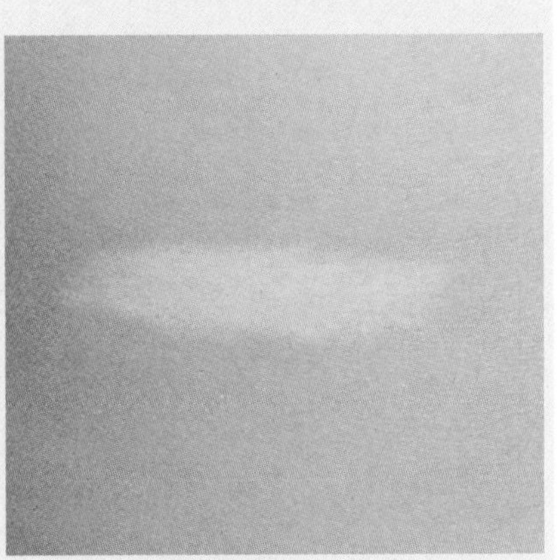

Tuberous sclerosis

PRIMARY SKIN LESIONS—PAPULES

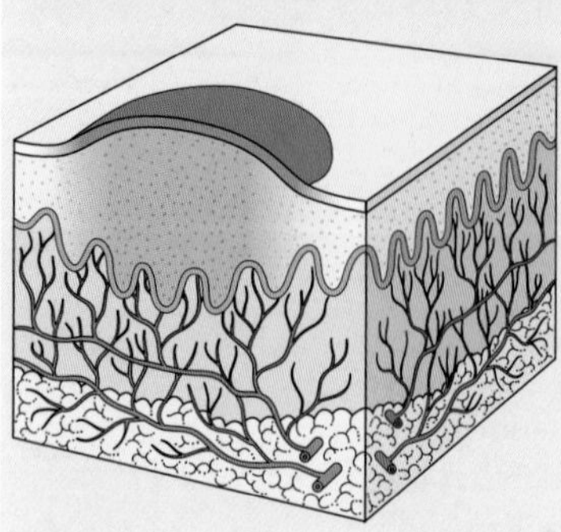

Papule
An elevated solid lesion up to 0.5 cm in diameter; color varies; papules may become confluent and form plaques

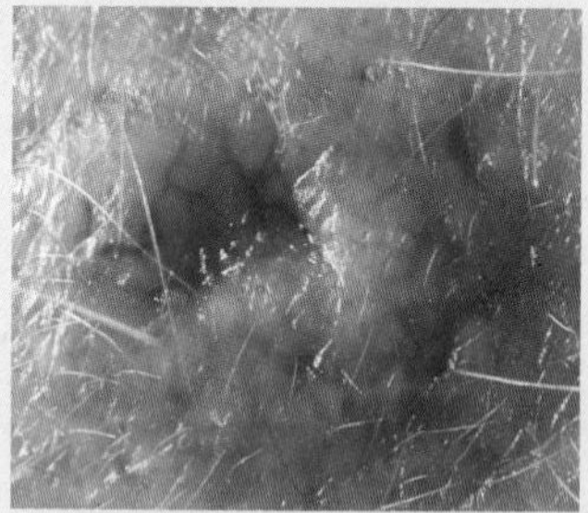

Sebaceous hyperplasia

Flesh colored, yellow, or white
Achrochordon (skin tag) (p. 785)
Adenoma sebaceum (p. 988)
Basal cell epithelioma (p. 804)
Closed comedone (acne) (p. 226)
Flat warts (p. 459)
Granuloma annulare (p. 976)
Lichen nitidus
Lichen sclerosus (p. 327)
Milia (p. 251)
Molluscum contagiosum (p. 465)
Nevi (dermal) (p. 848)
Neurofibroma (p. 984)
Pearly penile papules (p. 423)
Pseudoxanthoma elasticum
Senile sebaceous hyperplasia (p. 799)
Skin tags (achrochordon) (p. 784)
Syringoma (p. 800)

Brown
Dermatofibroma (p. 787)
Melanoma (p. 860)
Nevi (p. 847)
Seborrheic keratosis (p. 776)
Urticaria pigmentosa (p. 212)
Warts (pp. 419, 454)

Red
Acne (p. 219)
Atopic dermatitis (p. 157)
Cat-scratch disease (p. 614)
Cherry angioma (p. 904)
Cholinergic urticaria (p. 197)
Chondrodermatitis nodularis (p. 795)
Eczema (p. 91)
Folliculitis (p. 351)
Insect bites (p. 622)
Keratosis pilaris (p. 168)
Leukocytoclastic vasculitis (p. 727)
Miliaria (p. 263)
Polymorphous light eruption (p. 751)
Psoriasis (p. 264)
Pyogenic granuloma (p. 971)
Scabies (p. 583)
Urticaria (p. 183)

Blue or violaceous
Angiokeratoma (p. 904)
Blue nevus (p. 856)
Lichen planus (p. 320)
Lymphoma
Kaposi's sarcoma (p. 907)
Melanoma (p. 860)
Mycosis fungoides (p. 832)
Venous lake (p. 905)

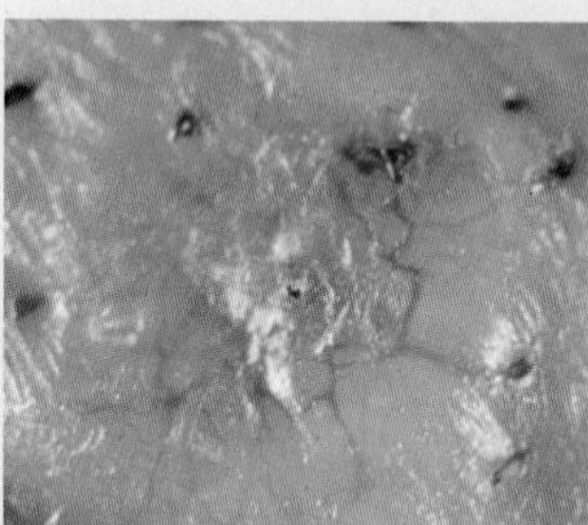

Basal cell epithelioma

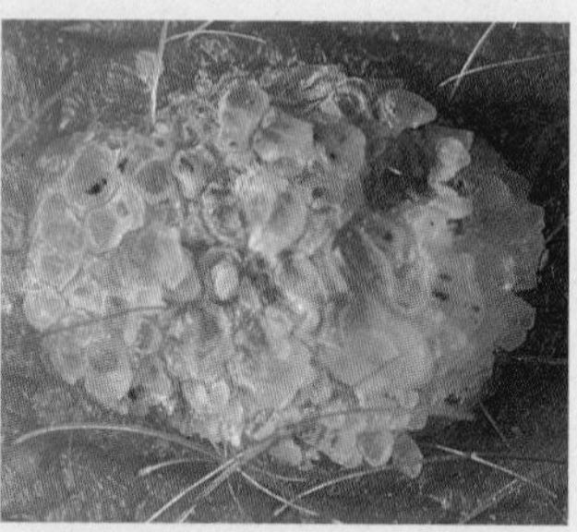

Wart (cylindrical projections)

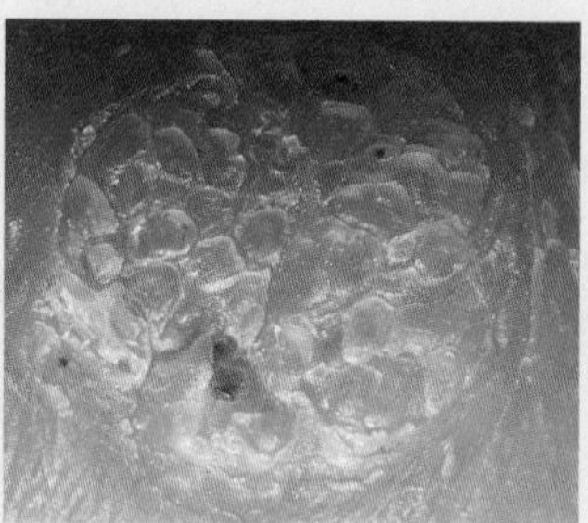

Wart (mosaic surface)

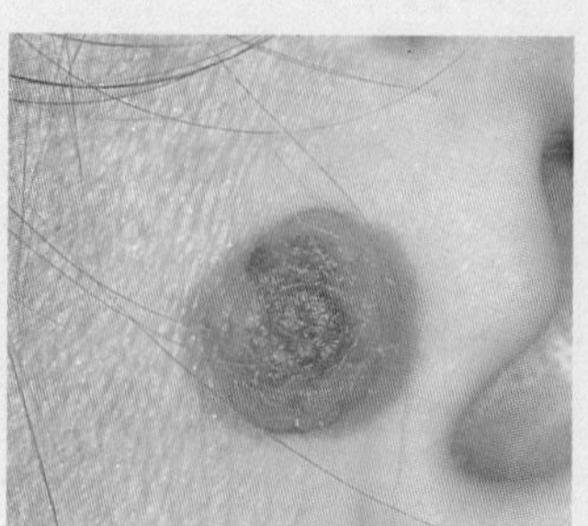

Nevi (dermal)

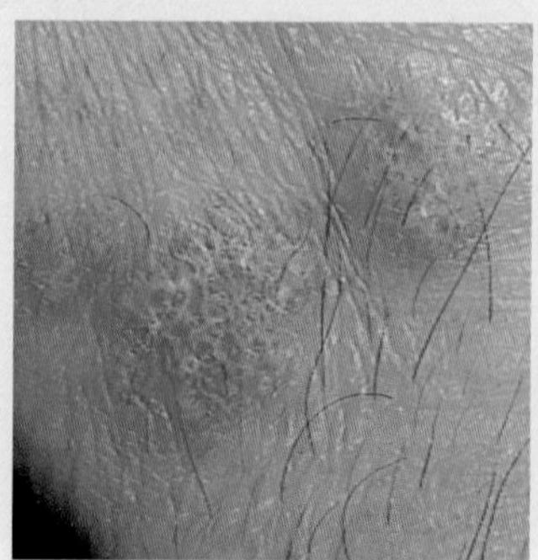

Lichen planus

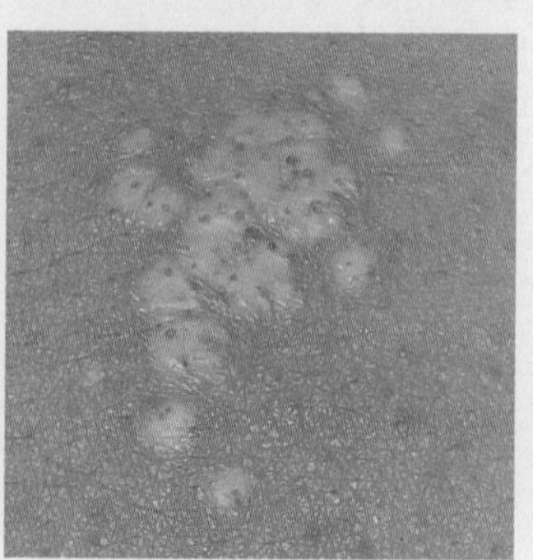

Lichen sclerosus

PRIMARY SKIN LESIONS—PAPULES—cont'd

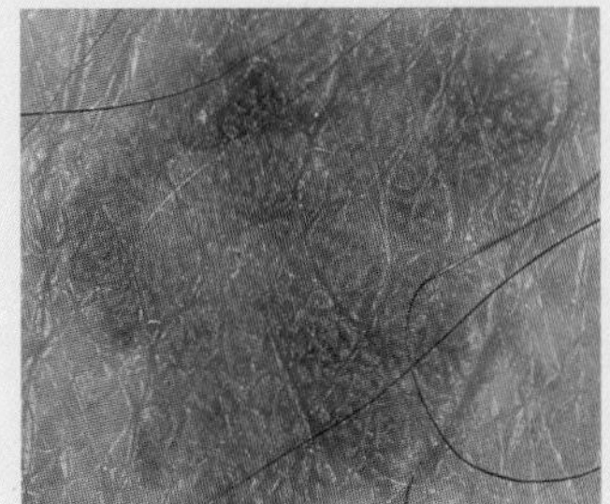
Seborrheic keratosis

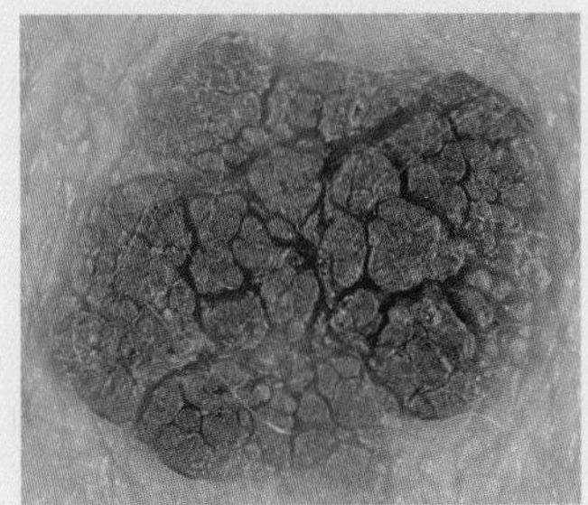
Seborrheic keratosis

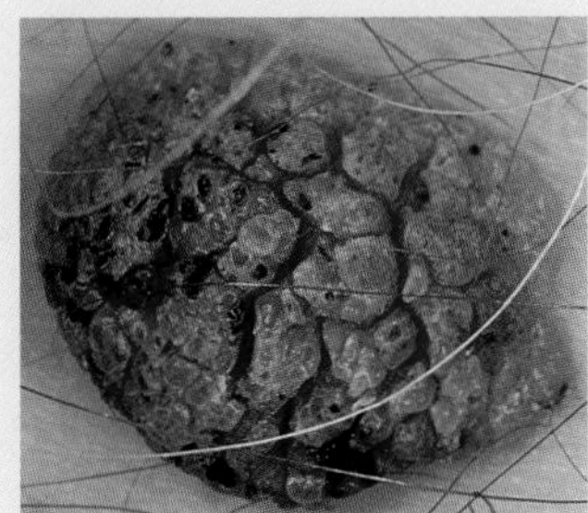
Seborrheic keratosis

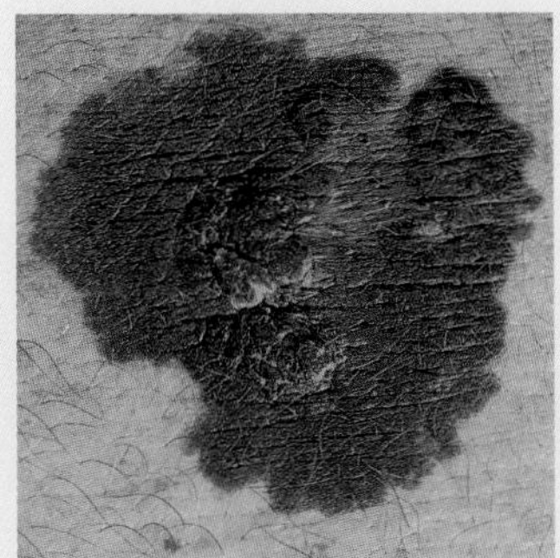
Melanoma

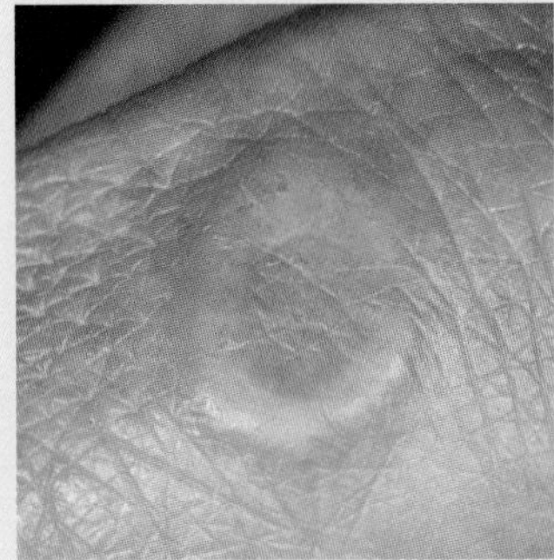
Granuloma annulare

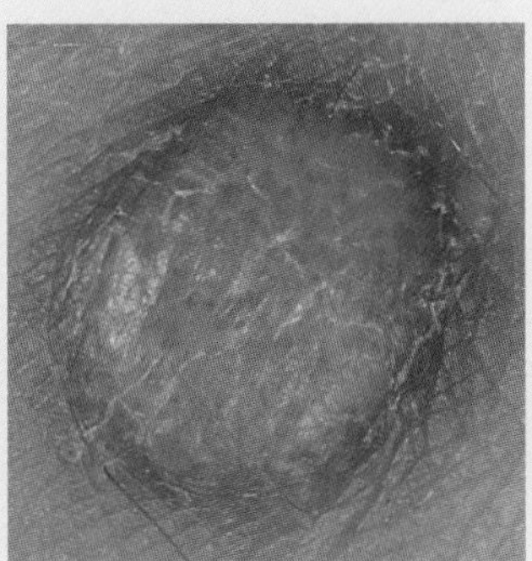
Dermatofibroma

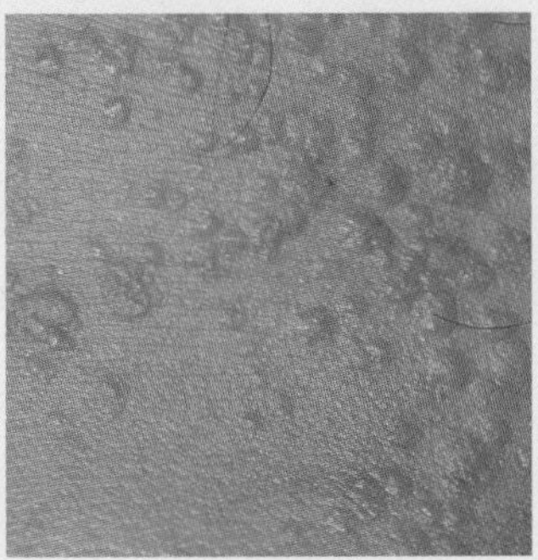
Flat warts

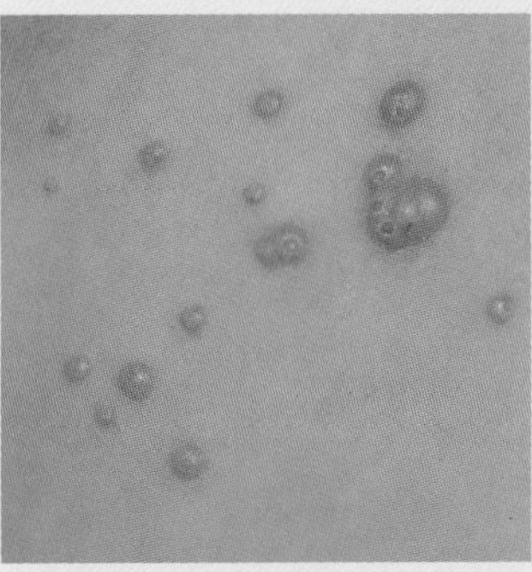
Molluscum contagiosum

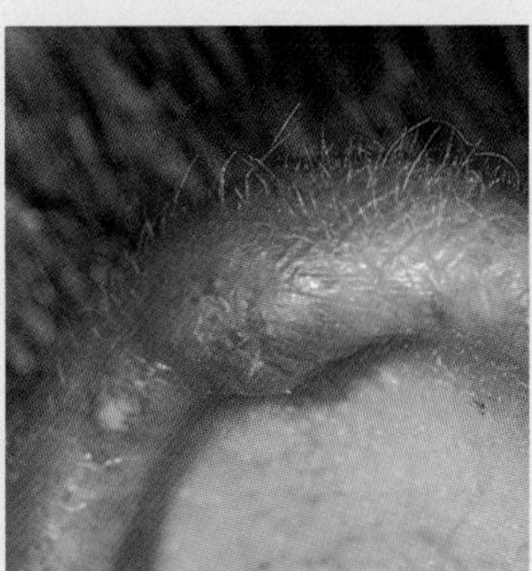
Chondrodermatitis nodularis

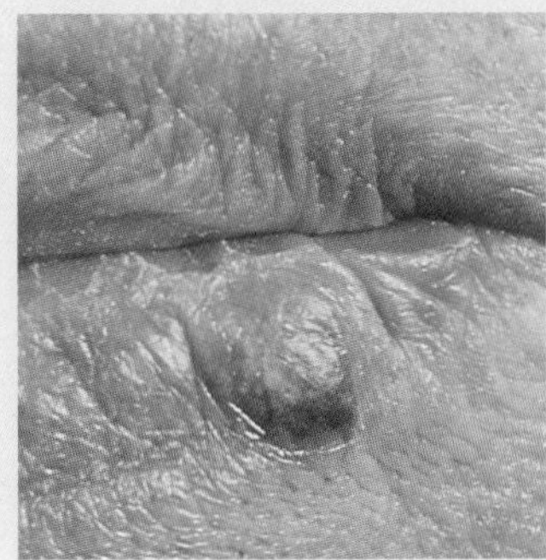
Venous lake

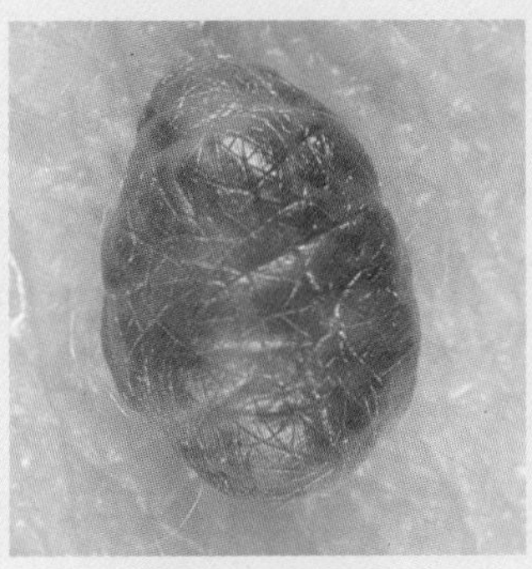
Cherry angioma

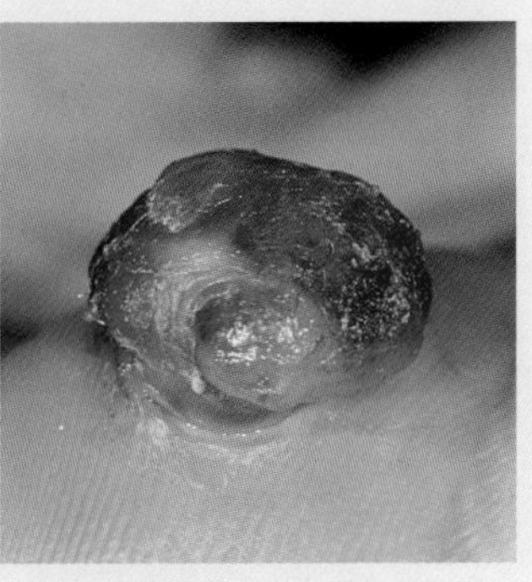
Pyogenic granuloma

PRIMARY SKIN LESIONS—PLAQUES

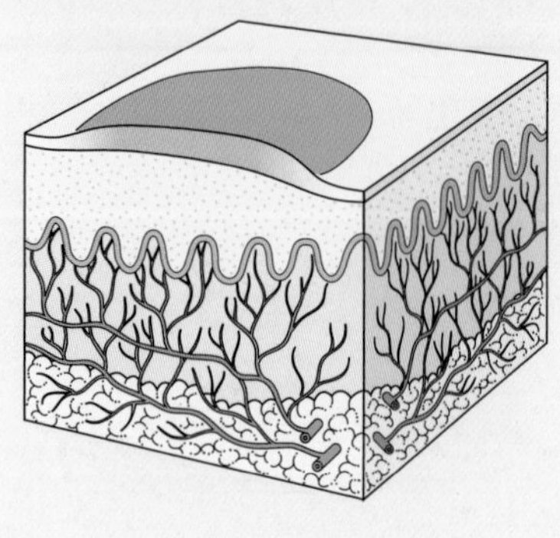

Plaque

A circumscribed, elevated, superficial, solid lesion more than 0.5 cm in diameter, often formed by the confluence of papules

Chronic cutaneous (discoid) lupus erythematosus (p. 682)
Eczema (p. 91)
Cutaneous T-cell lymphoma (p. 832)
Lichen planus (p. 320)
Paget's disease (p. 843)
Papulosquamous (papular and scaling) lesions (p. 264)
Sweet's syndrome (p. 734)
Pityriasis rosea (p. 316)
Psoriasis (p. 264)
Seborrheic dermatitis (p. 312)
Syphilis (secondary) (p. 400)
Tinea corporis (p. 502)
Tinea pedis (p. 495)
Tinea versicolor (p. 537)

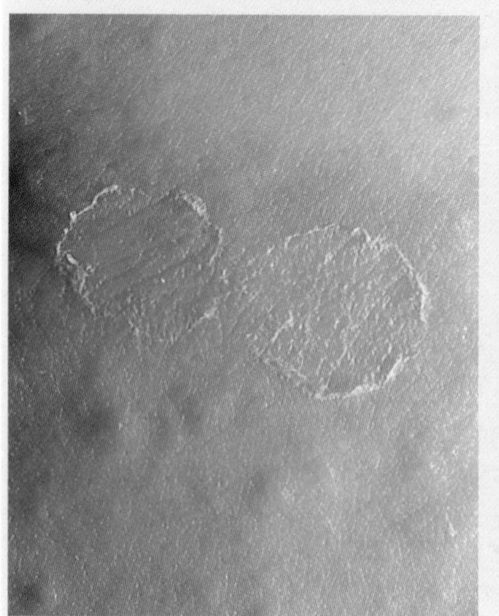
Pityriasis rosea

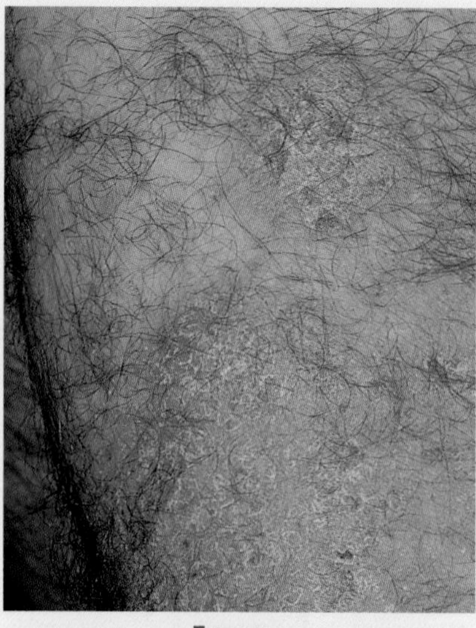
Eczema

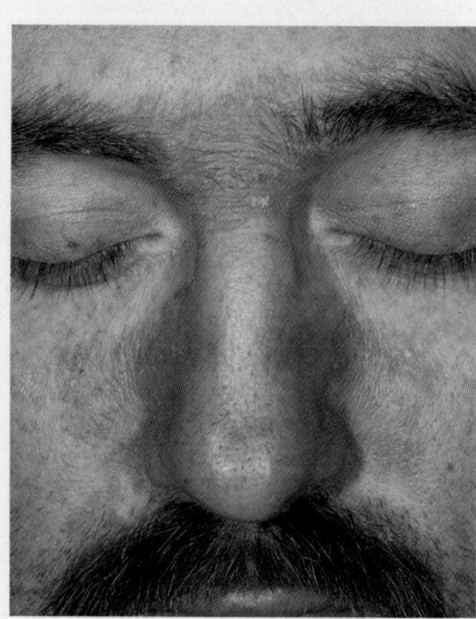
Seborrheic dermatitis

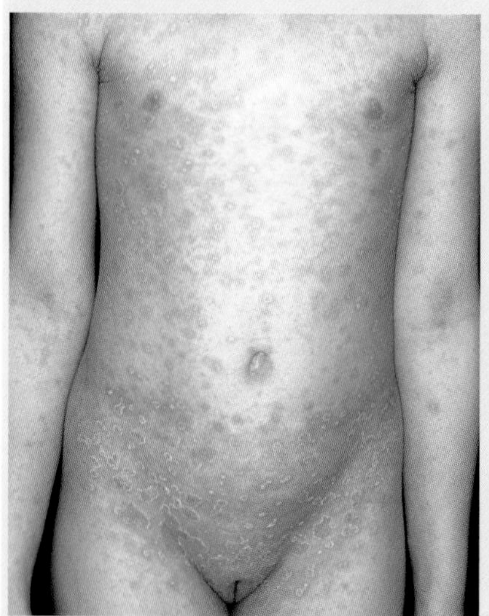
Pityriasis rosea

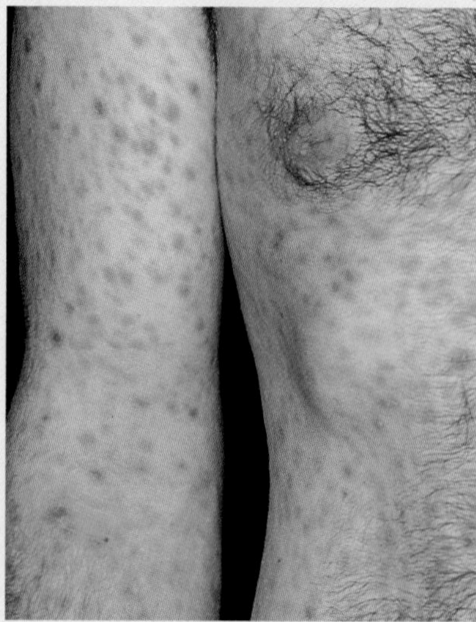
Syphilis (secondary)

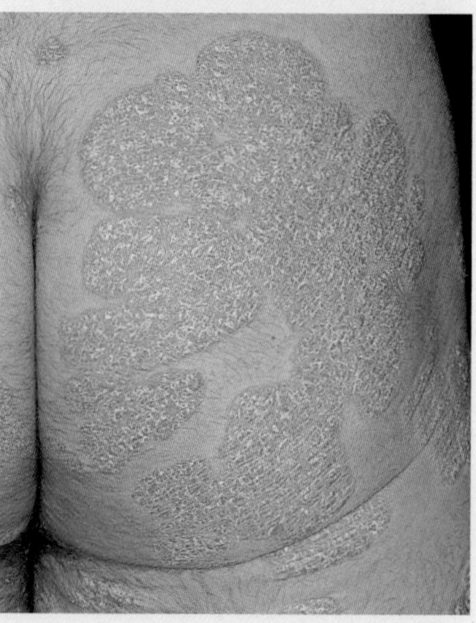
Psoriasis

PRIMARY SKIN LESIONS—PLAQUES—cont'd

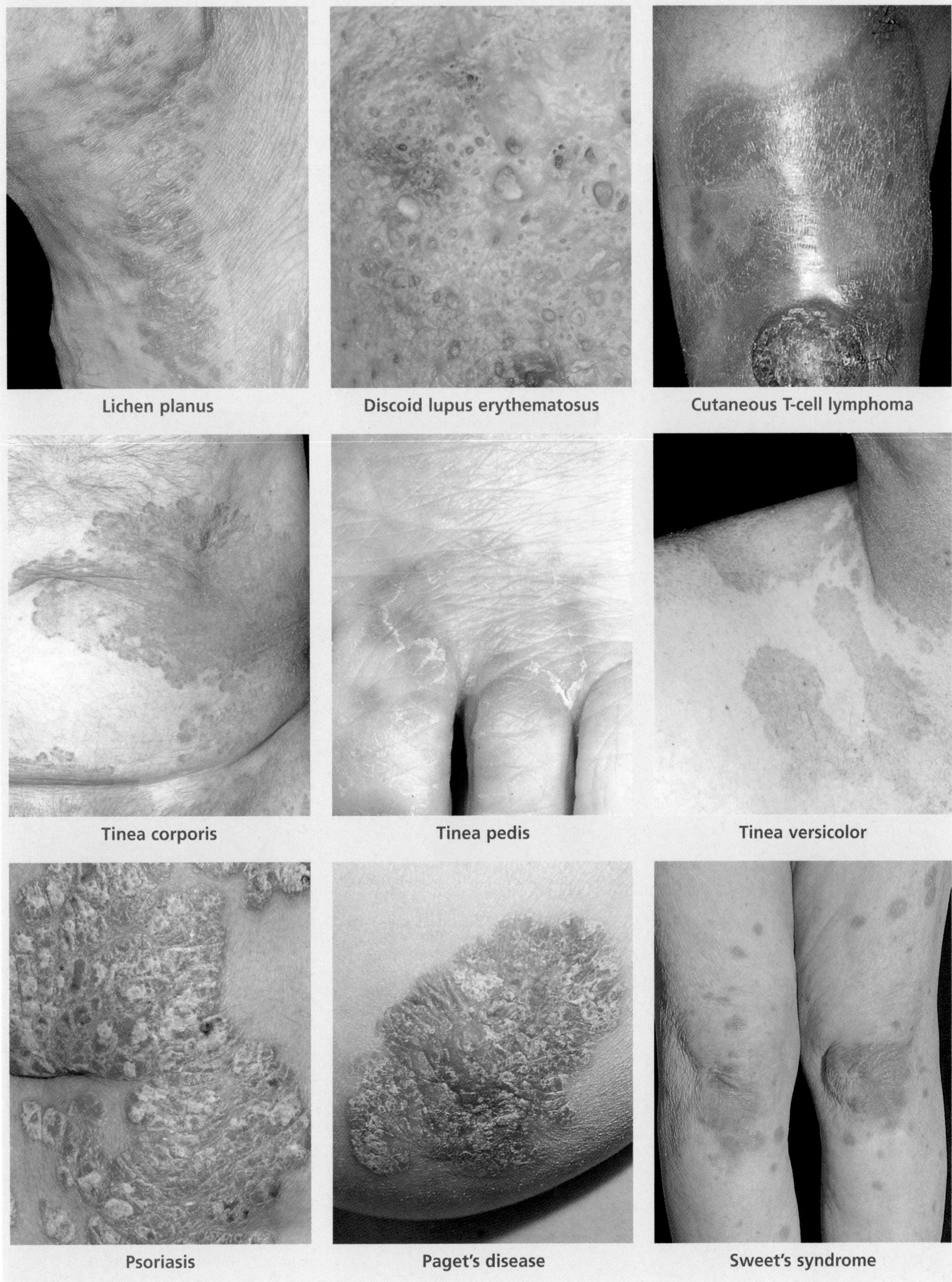

Lichen planus

Discoid lupus erythematosus

Cutaneous T-cell lymphoma

Tinea corporis

Tinea pedis

Tinea versicolor

Psoriasis

Paget's disease

Sweet's syndrome

PRIMARY SKIN LESIONS—NODULES

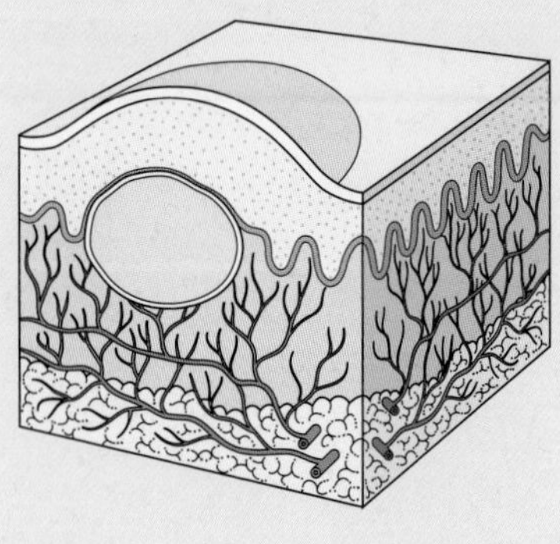

Nodule

A circumscribed, elevated, solid lesion more than 0.5 cm in diameter; a large nodule is referred to as a tumor

Basal cell carcinoma (p. 801)
Cutaneous T-cell lymphoma (p. 832)
Erythema nodosum (p. 720)
Furuncle (p. 356)
Hemangioma (p. 904)
Kaposi's sarcoma (p. 907)
Keratoacanthoma (p. 790)
Lipoma
Lymphoma
Melanoma (p. 860)
Metastatic carcinoma (p. 845)
Neurofibromatosis (p. 983)
Prurigo nodularis (p. 119)
Sporotrichosis
Squamous cell carcinoma (p. 826)
Warts (pp. 419, 454)
Xanthoma (p. 980)

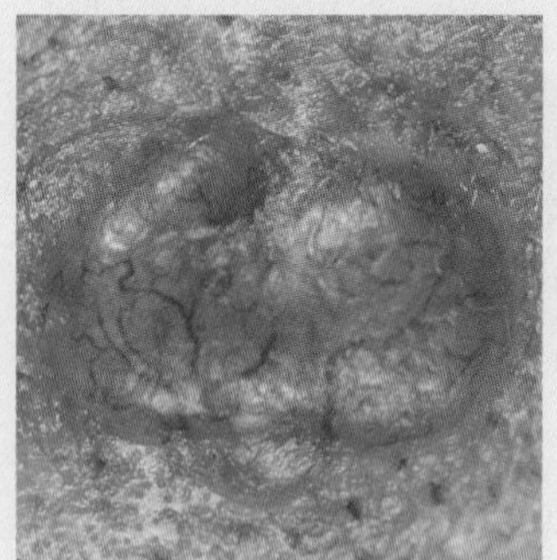

Basal cell carcinoma

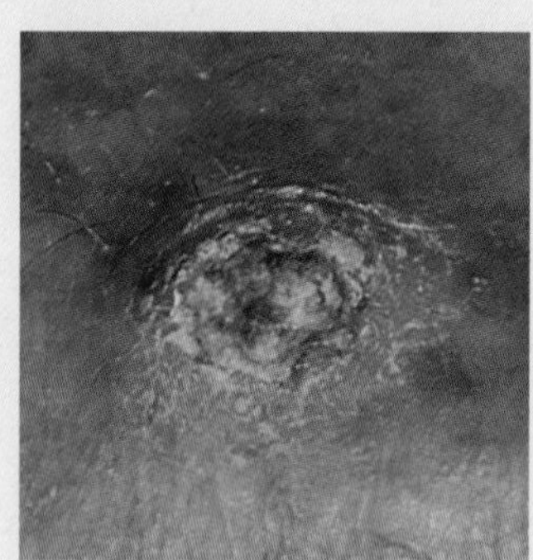

Squamous cell carcinoma

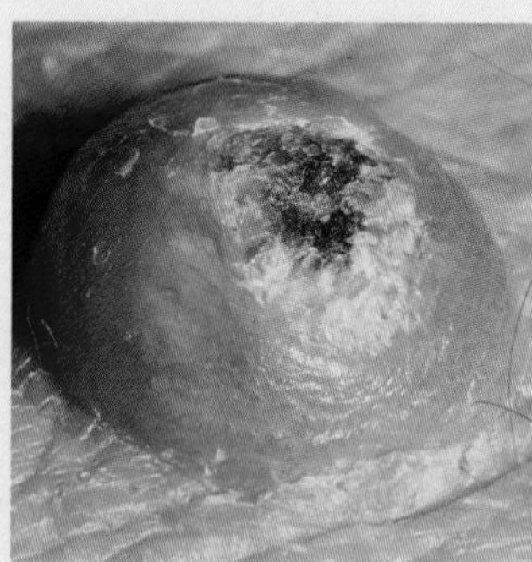

Keratoacanthoma

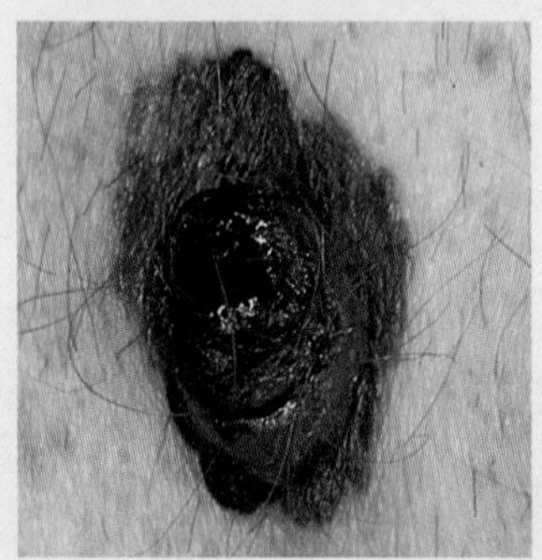

Melanoma

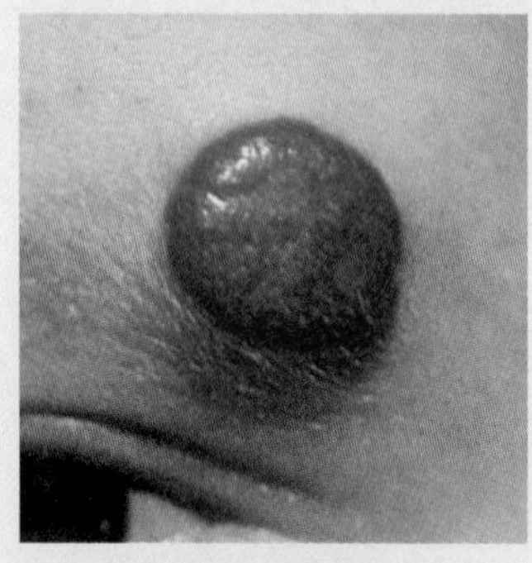

Hemangioma

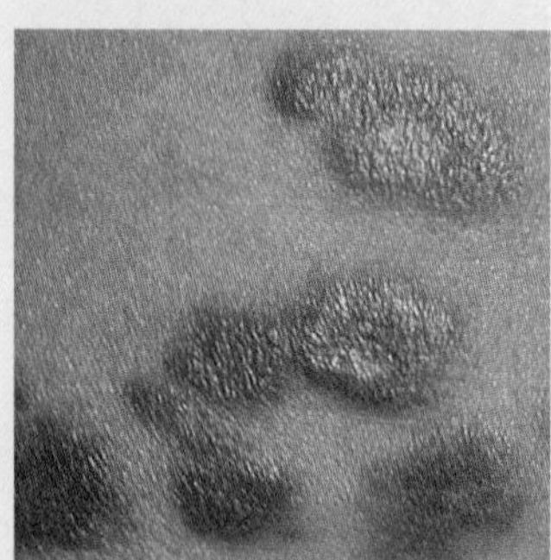

Kaposi's sarcoma

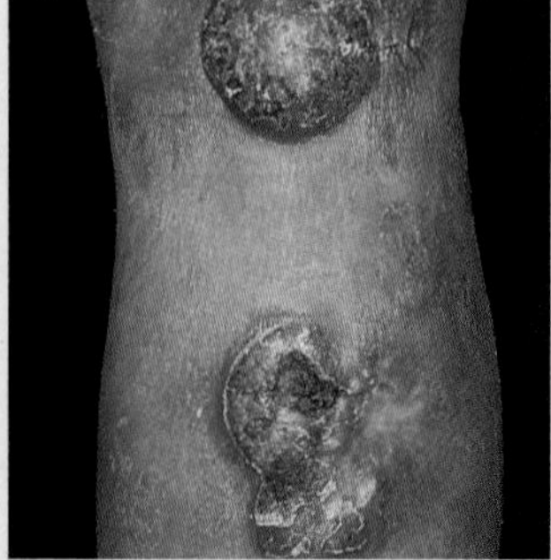

Cutaneous T-cell lymphoma

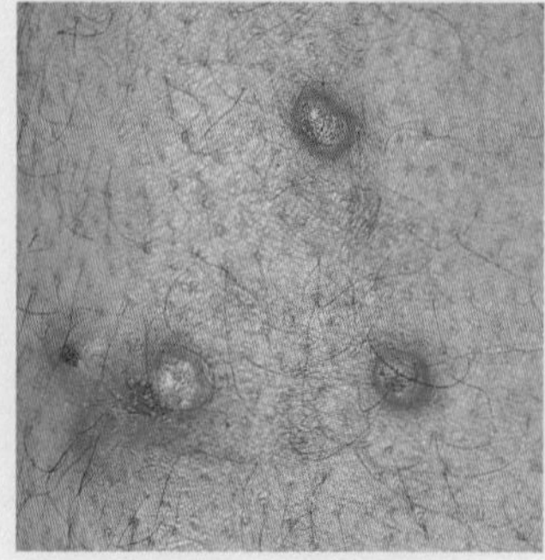

Prurigo nodularis

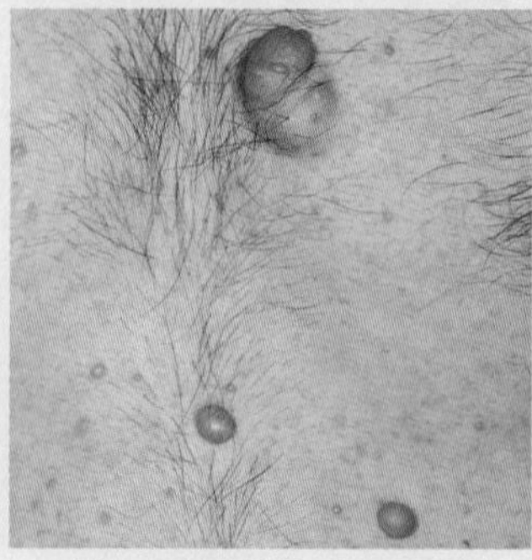

Neurofibromatosis

PRIMARY SKIN LESIONS—PUSTULES

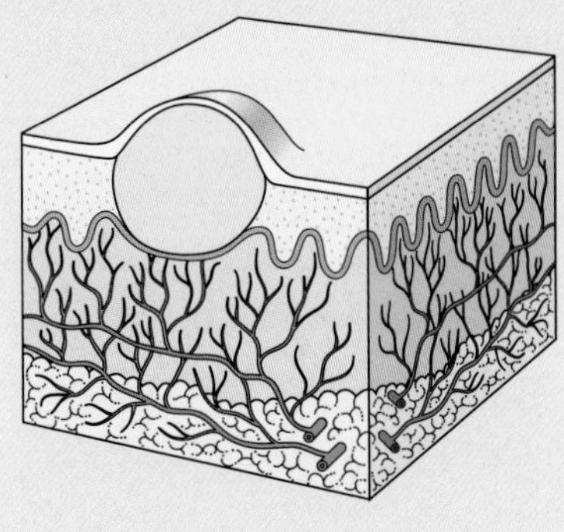

Pustule

A circumscribed collection of leukocytes and free fluid that varies in size

Acne (p. 226)
Candidiasis (p. 523)
Chickenpox (p. 474)
Dermatophyte infection (p. 497)
Dyshidrosis (pompholyx) (p. 109)
Folliculitis (p. 351)
Gonococcemia (p. 416)
Hidradenitis suppurativa (p. 260)
Herpes simplex (p. 467)
Herpes zoster (p. 480)
Impetigo (p. 335)
Keratosis pilaris (p. 168)
Pseudomonas folliculitis (p. 363)
Psoriasis (p. 269)
Pyoderma gangrenosum (p. 737)
Rosacea (p. 256)
Scabies (p. 584)
Varicella (p. 474)

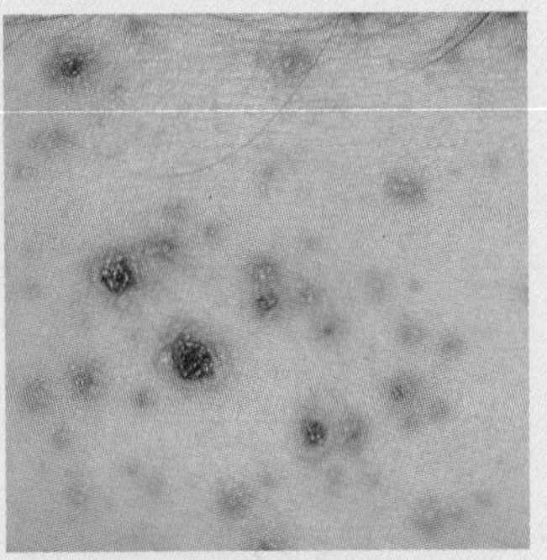

Chickenpox

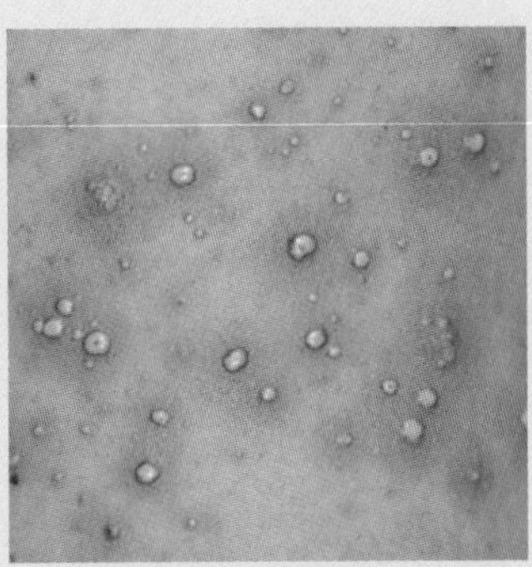

Folliculitis

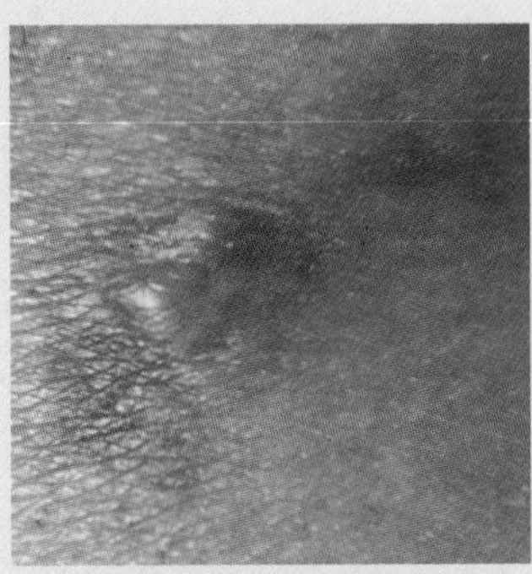

Gonococcemia

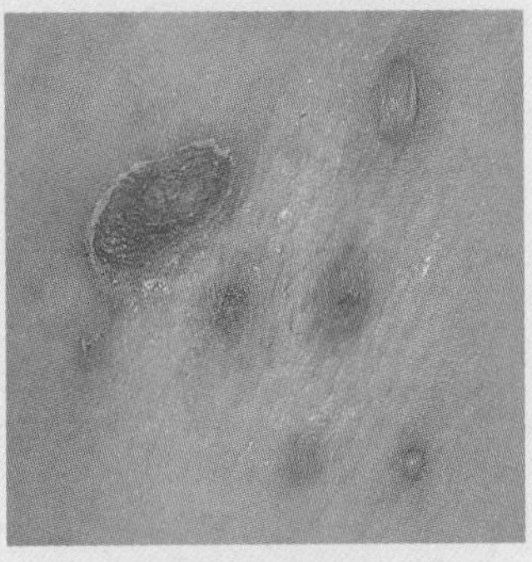

Impetigo

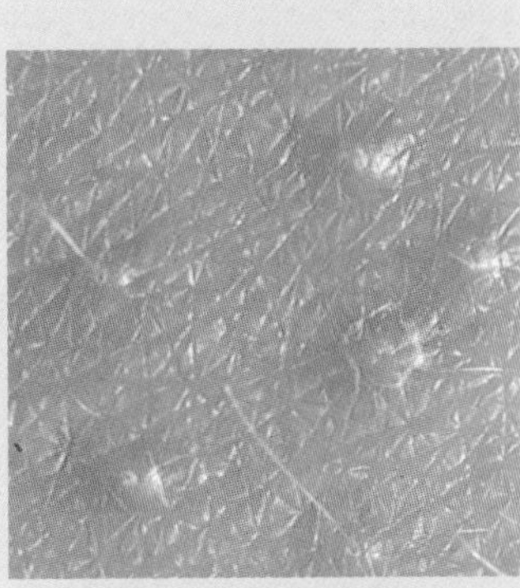

Keratosis pilaris

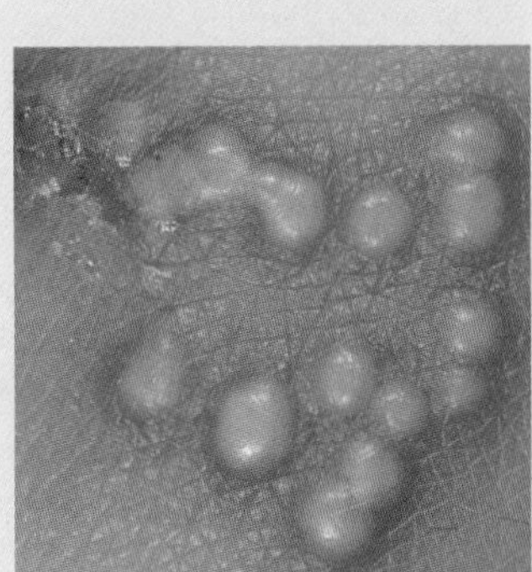

Herpes simplex

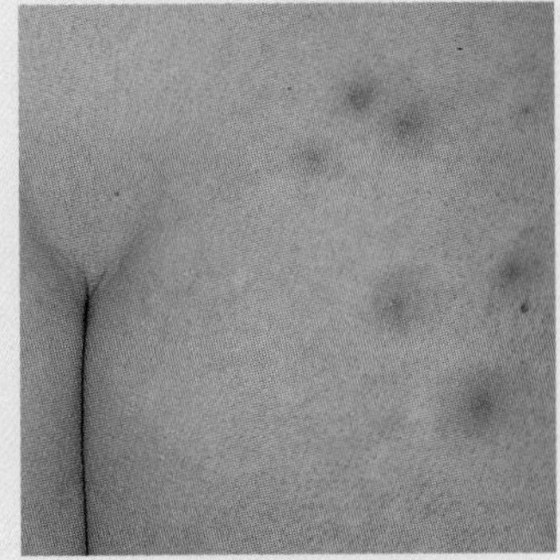

Pseudomonas folliculitis

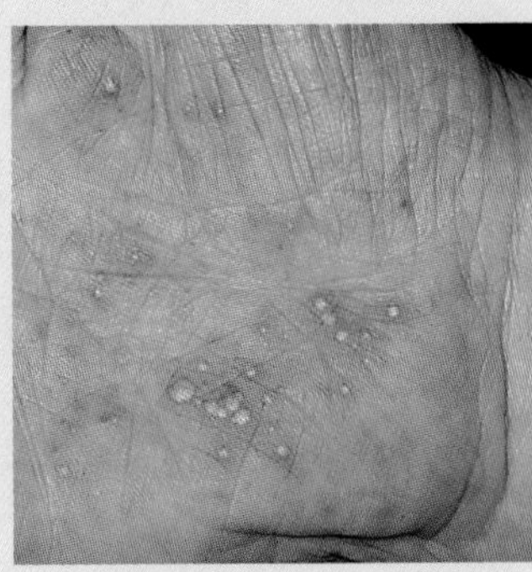

Dyshidrosis (pompholyx)

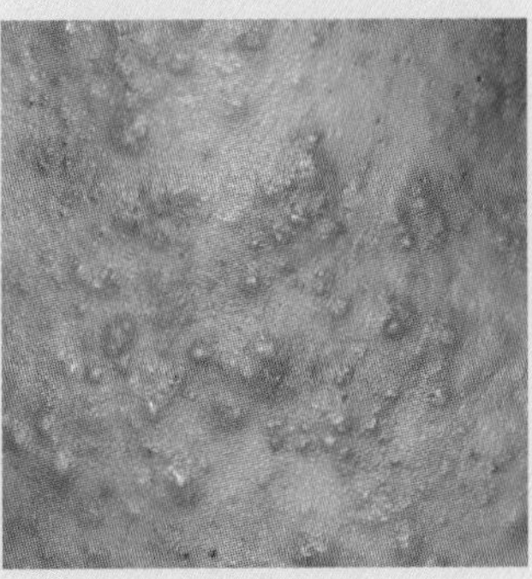

Acne

PRIMARY SKIN LESIONS—VESICLES AND BULLAE

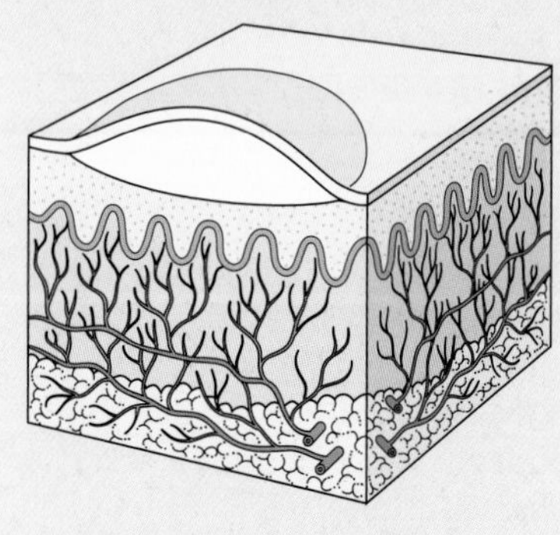

Vesicle

A circumscribed collection of free fluid up to 0.5 cm in diameter

Benign familial chronic pemphigus (p. 662)
Cat-scratch disease (p. 614)
Chickenpox (p. 474)
Dermatitis herpetiformis (p. 643)
Eczema (acute) (p. 93)
Erythema multiforme (p. 713)
Herpes simplex (p. 467)
Herpes zoster (p. 480)
Impetigo (p. 336)
Lichen planus (p. 320)
Pemphigus foliaceus (p. 650)
Porphyria cutanea tarda (p. 756)
Scabies (p. 584)

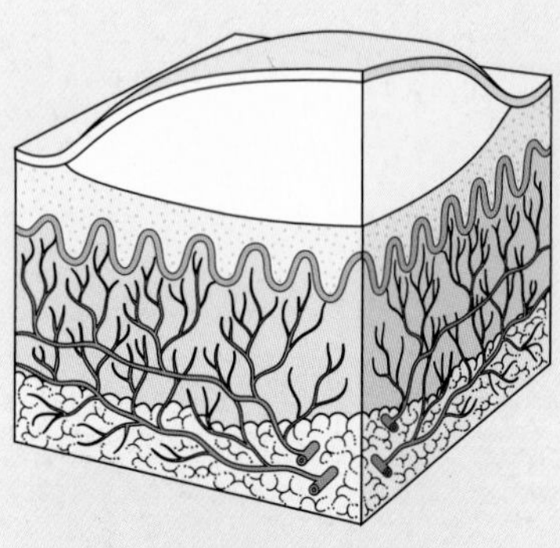

Bulla

A circumscribed collection of free fluid more than 0.5 cm in diameter

Bullae in diabetics (p. 646)
Bullous pemphigoid (p. 655)
Cicatricial pemphigoid (p. 655)
Epidermolysis bullosa acquisita (p. 661)
Fixed drug eruption (p. 576)
Herpes gestationis (p. 660)
Lupus erythematosus (p. 686)
Pemphigus (p. 647)

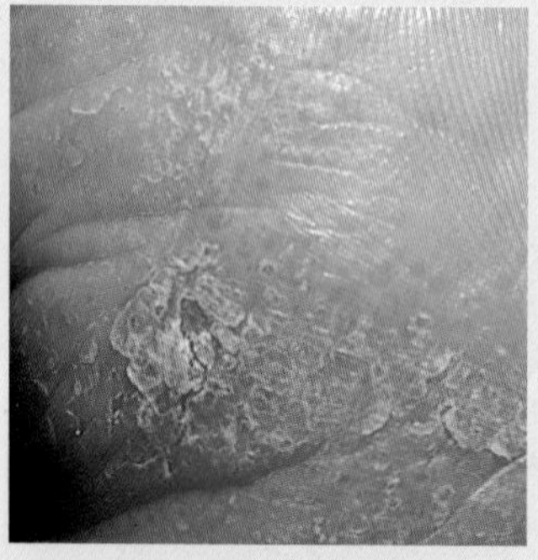

Eczema (acute)

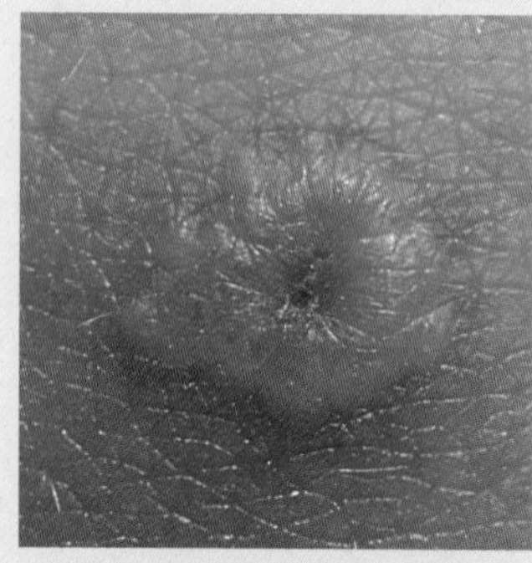

Chickenpox

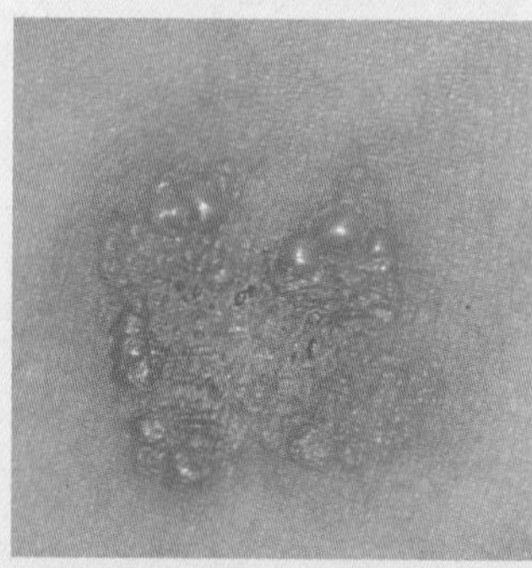

Dermatitis herpetiformis

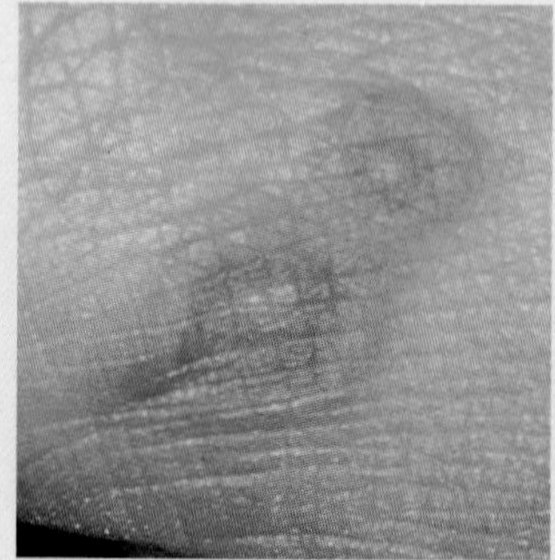

Erythema multiforme

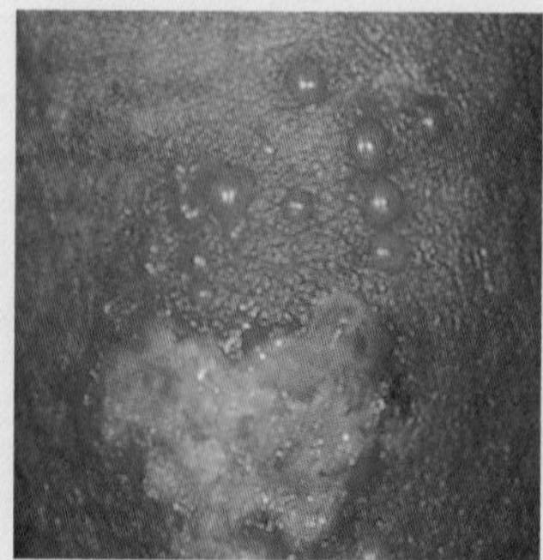

Herpes simplex

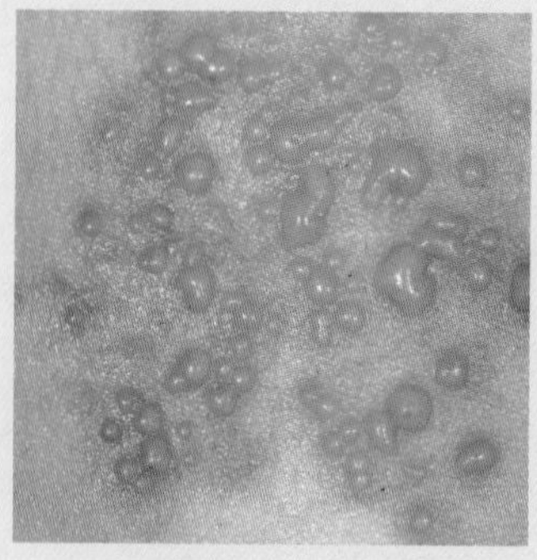

Herpes zoster

PRIMARY SKIN LESIONS—WHEALS (HIVES)

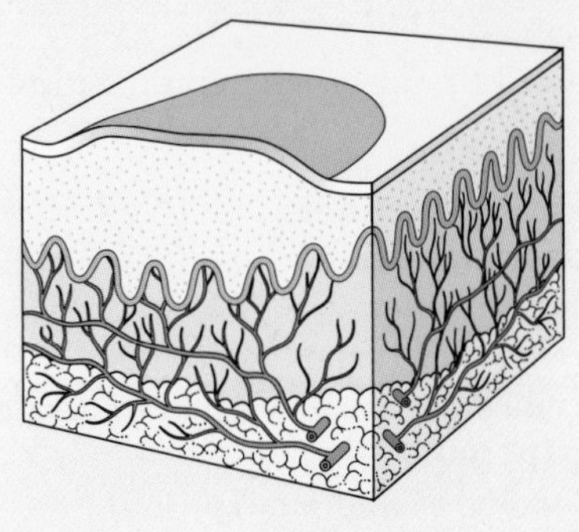

Wheal (hive)

A firm, edematous plaque resulting from infiltration of the dermis with fluid; wheals are transient and may last only a few hours

Angioedema (p. 200)
Bullous pemphigoid (p. 655)
Cholinergic urticaria (p. 197)
Dermographism (p. 194)
Hives (p. 183)
PUPP (p. 207)
Urticaria pigmentosa (mastocytosis) (p. 211)

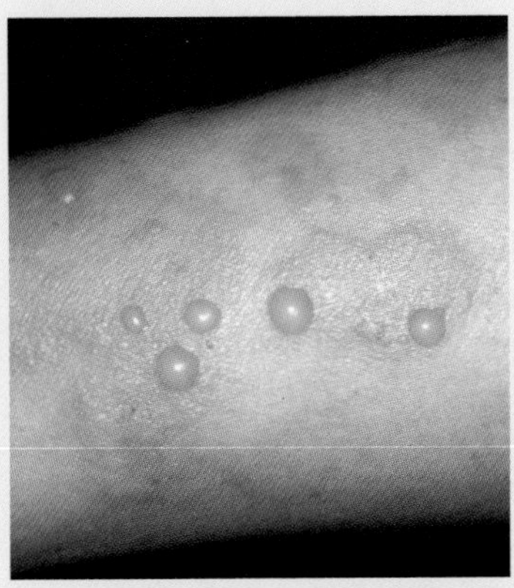

Bullous pemphigoid

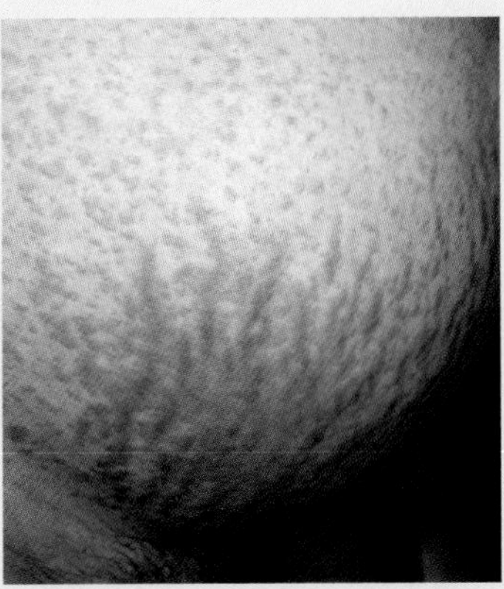

PUPP

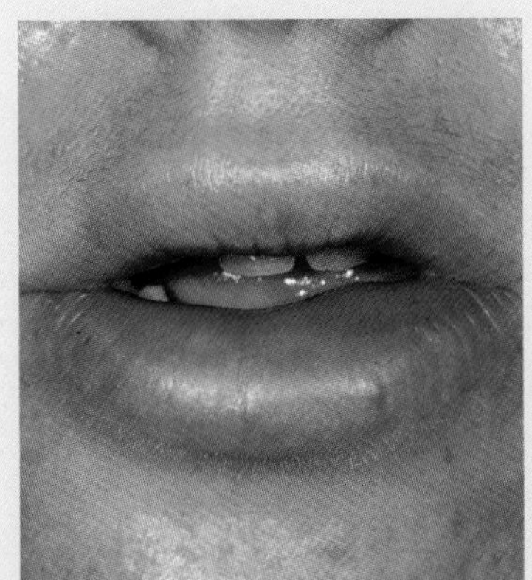

Angioedema

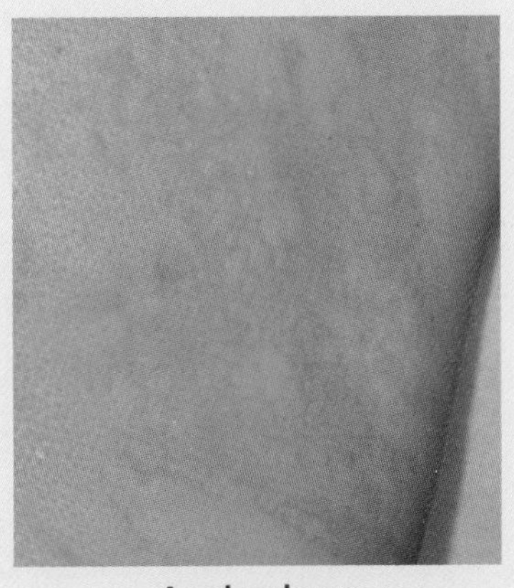

Angioedema

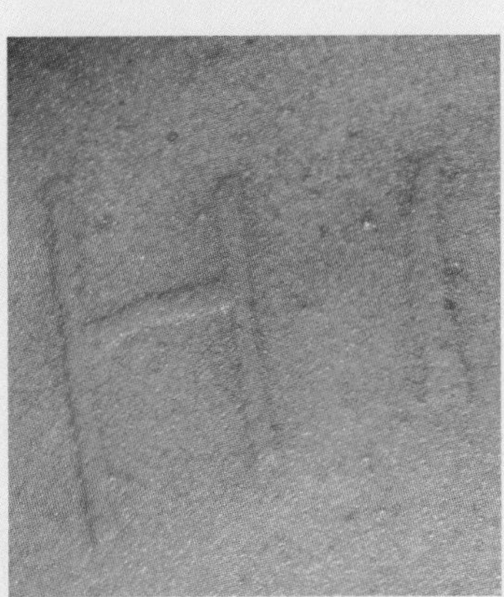

Dermographism

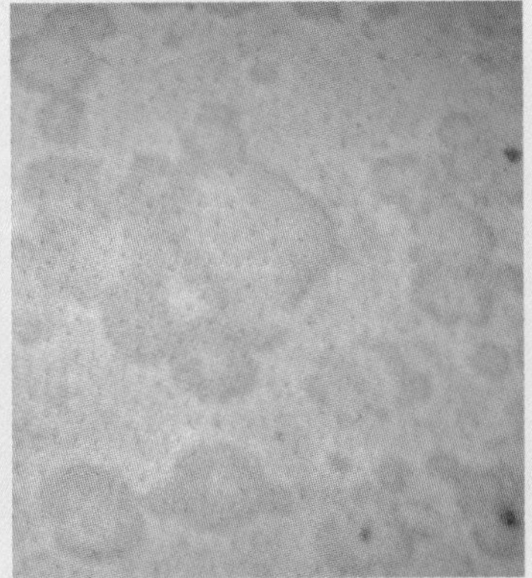

Hives

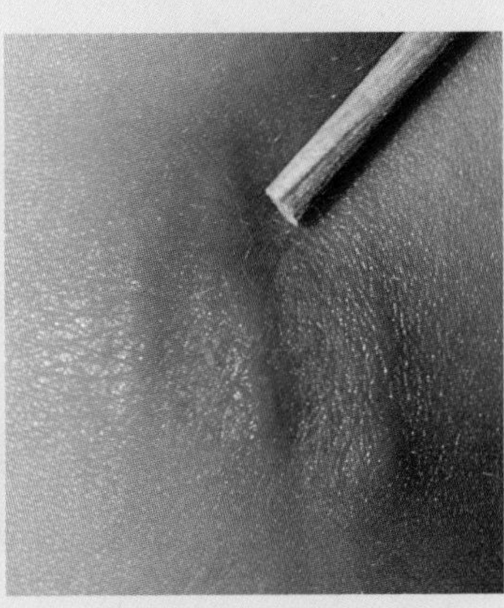

Urticaria pigmentosa

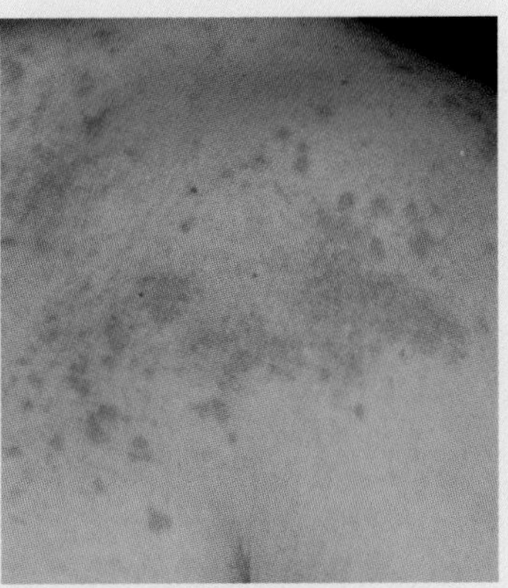

Cholinergic urticaria

SECONDARY SKIN LESIONS—SCALES

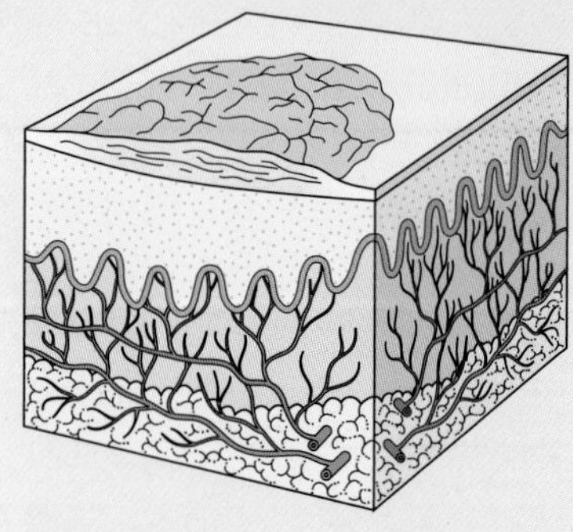

Scales

Excess dead epidermal cells that are produced by abnormal keratinization and shedding

Fine to stratified

Erythema craquelé (p. 110)
Ichthyosis—dominant (quadrangular) (p. 167)
Ichthyosis—sex-linked (quadrangular) (p. 167)
Lupus erythematosus (carpet tack) (p. 682)
Pityriasis rosea (collarette) (p. 316)
Psoriasis (silvery) (p. 265)
Scarlet fever (fine, on trunk) (p. 549)
Seborrheic dermatitis (p. 312)
Syphilis (secondary) (p. 400)
Tinea (dermatophytes) (p. 492)
Tinea versicolor (p. 537)
Xerosis (dry skin) (p. 110)

Scaling in sheets (desquamation)

Kawasaki disease (p. 560)
Scarlet fever (hands and feet) (p. 551)
Staphylococcal scalded skin syndrome (p. 360)
Toxic shock syndrome (p. 566)

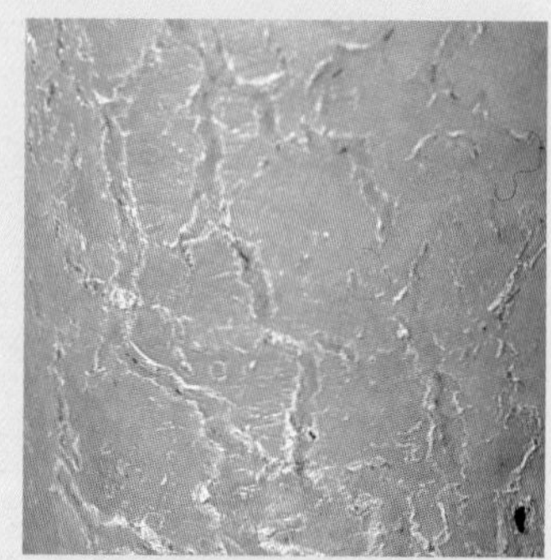

Erythema craquelé (dense scale)

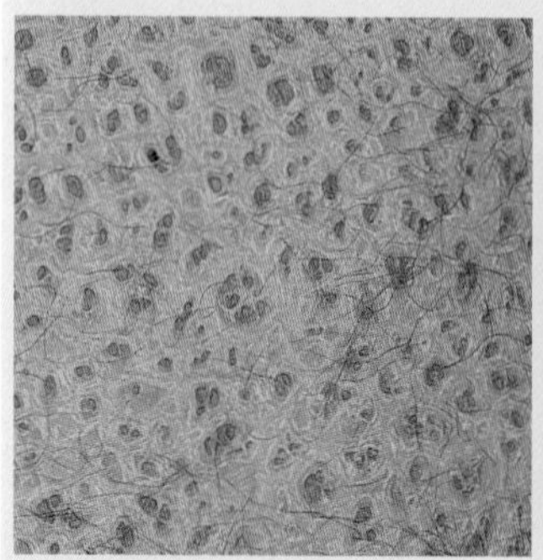

Ichthyosis—sex-linked (quadrangular)

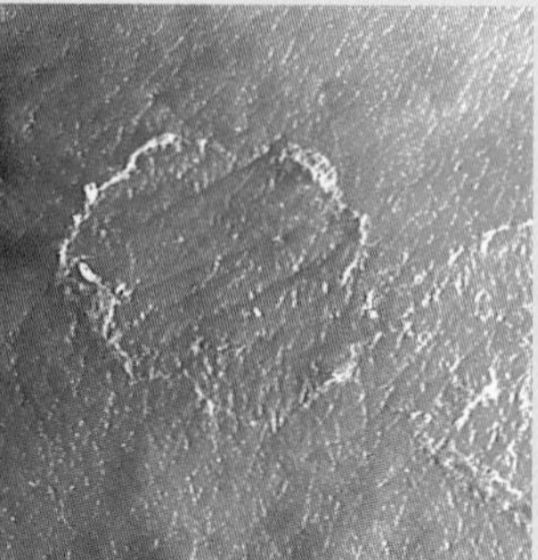

Pityriasis rosea (collarette)

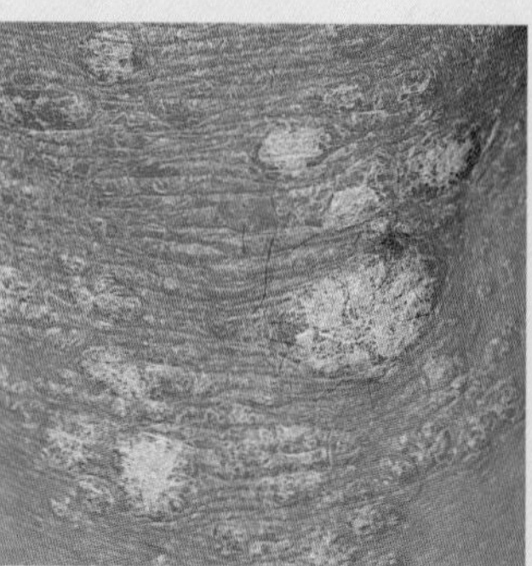

Psoriasis (silvery)

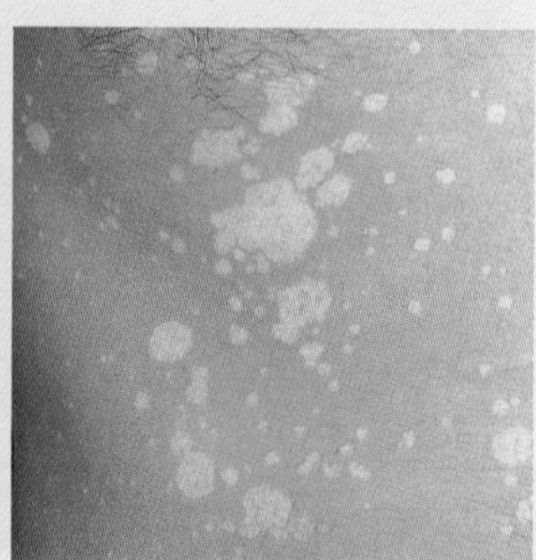

Tinea versicolor (fine)

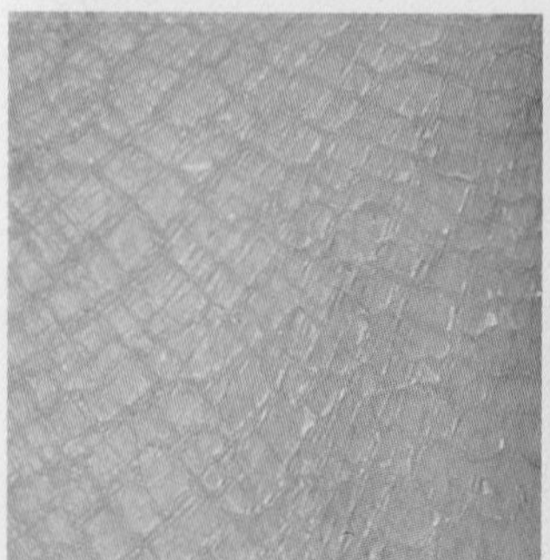

Ichthyosis—dominant (quadrangular)

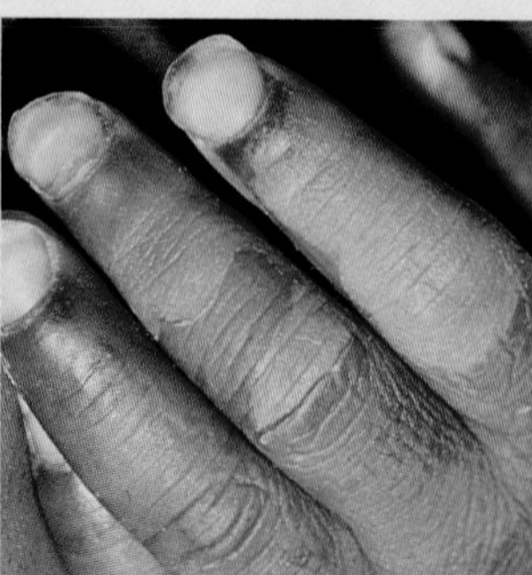

Kawasaki disease (desquamation)

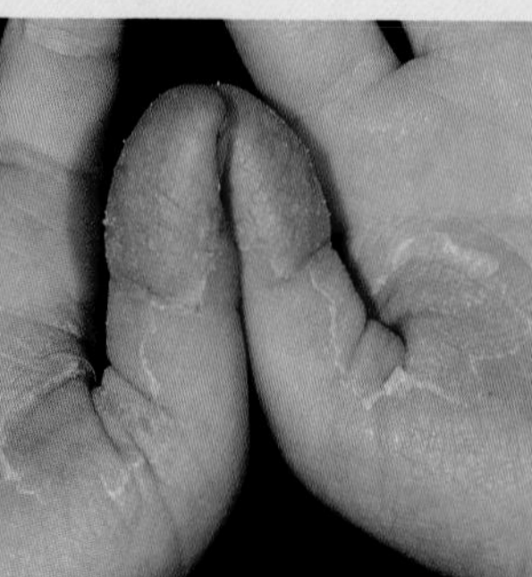

Scarlet fever (desquamation)

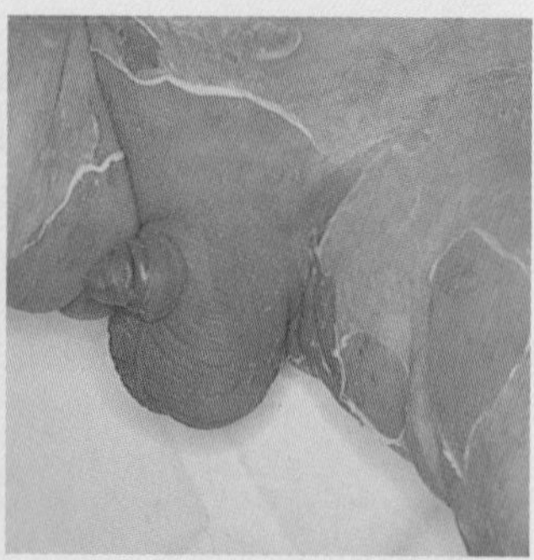

Staphylococcal scalded skin syndrome (desquamation)

SECONDARY SKIN LESIONS—CRUSTS

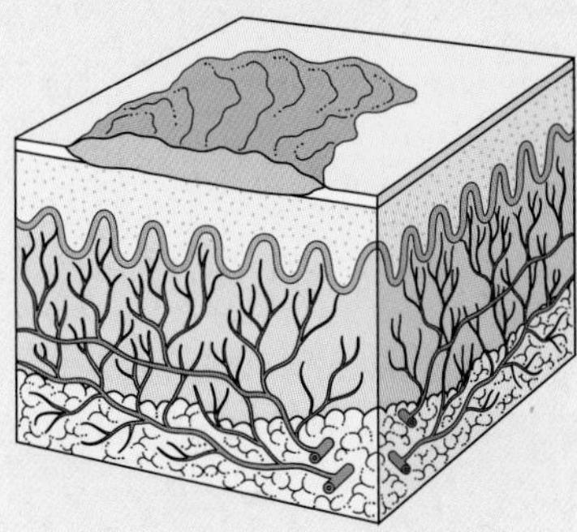

Crust

A collection of dried serum and cellular debris; a scab

Acute eczematous inflammation (p. 93)
Atopic (face) (p. 158)
Impetigo (honey colored) (p. 338)
Pemphigus foliaceus (p. 650)
Tinea capitis (p. 509)

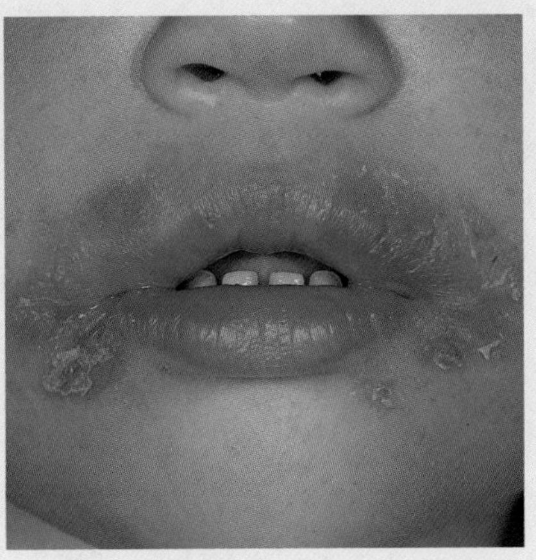

Atopic (lips)

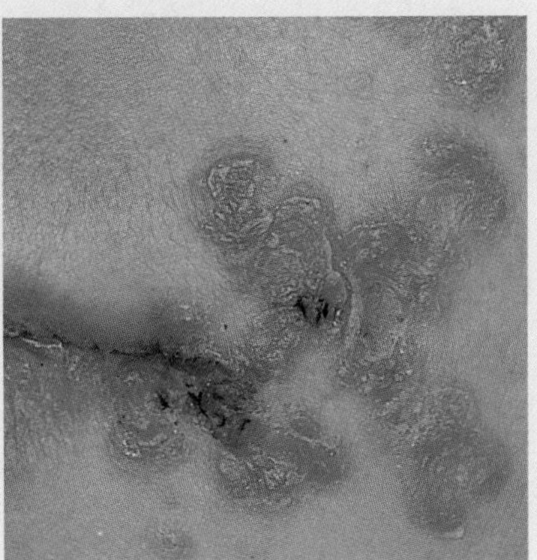

Impetigo (honey colored)

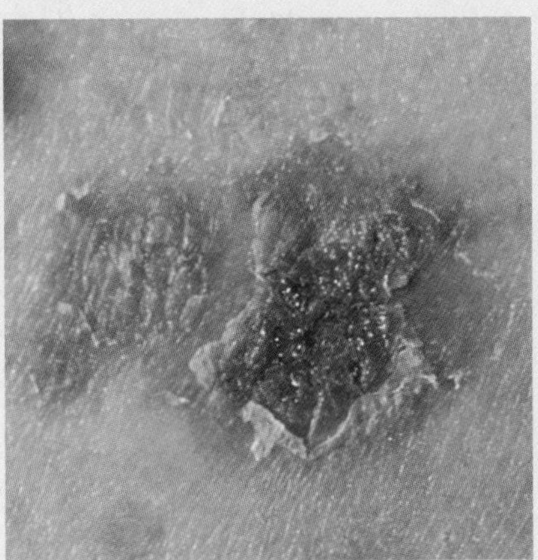

Pemphigus foliaceus

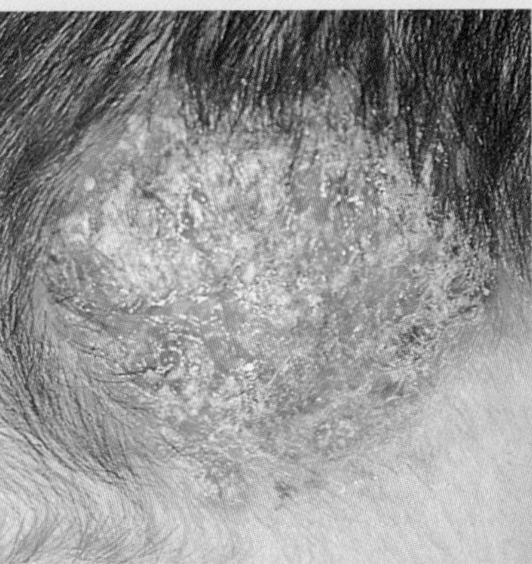

Tinea capitis

SECONDARY SKIN LESIONS—EROSIONS AND ULCERS

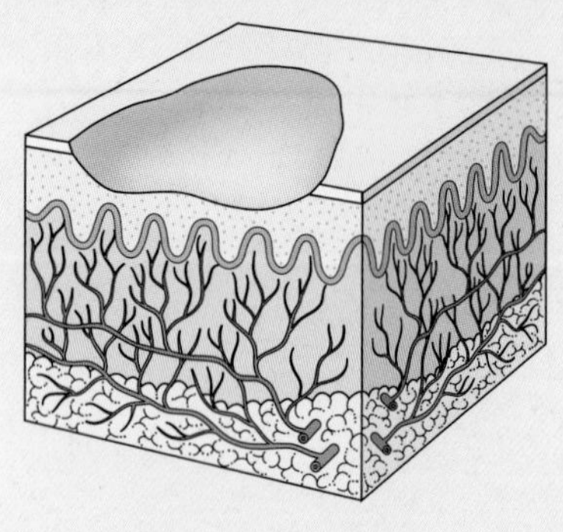

Erosion

A focal loss of epidermis; erosions do not penetrate below the dermoepidermal junction and therefore heal without scarring

Candidiasis (p. 523)
Dermatophyte infection (p. 495)
Eczematous diseases (p. 91)
Herpes simplex (p. 467)
Intertrigo (p. 501)
Neurotic excoriations (p. 120)
Perlèche (p. 536)
Sun-damaged skin (p. 744)
Tinea pedis (p. 495)
Toxic epidermal necrolysis (p. 719)
Vesiculobullous diseases (p. 635)

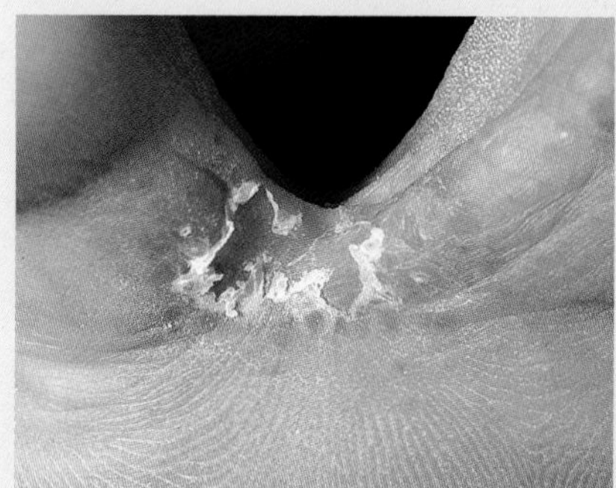

Tinea pedis

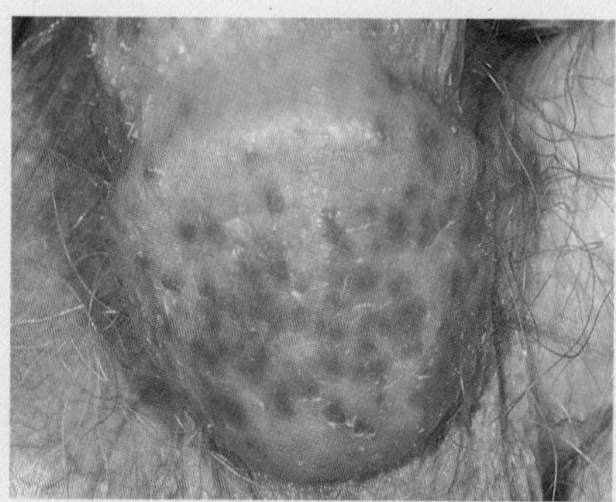

Candidiasis

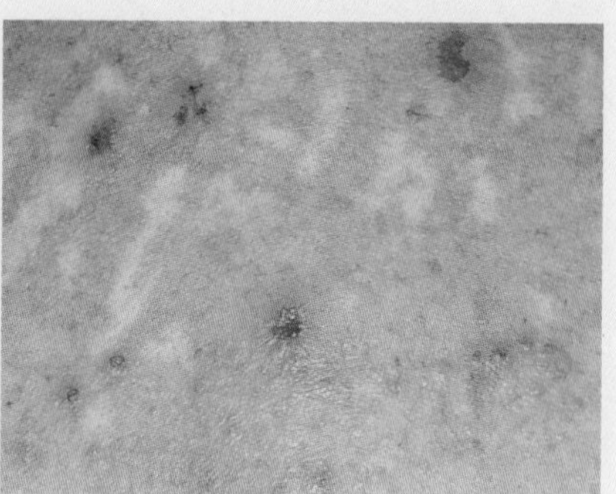

Neurotic excoriations

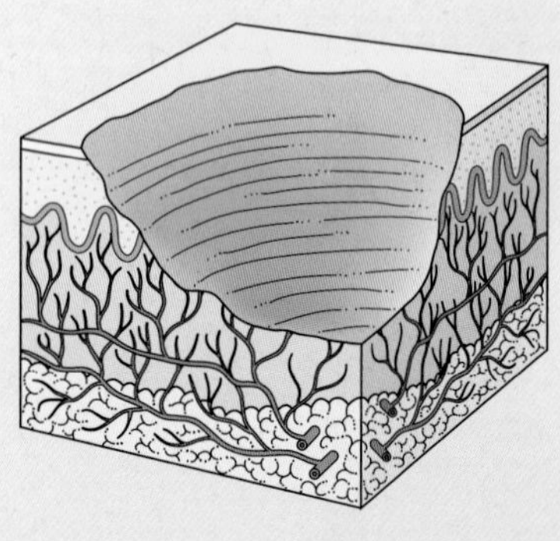

Ulcer

A focal loss of epidermis and dermis; ulcers heal with scarring

Aphthae
Chancroid (p. 410)
Decubitus
Factitial (p. 120)
Ischemic
Necrobiosis lipoidica (p. 975)
Neoplasms (p. 805)
Pyoderma gangrenosum (p. 737)
Radiodermatitis
Syphilis (chancre) (p. 398)
Stasis ulcers (p. 122)

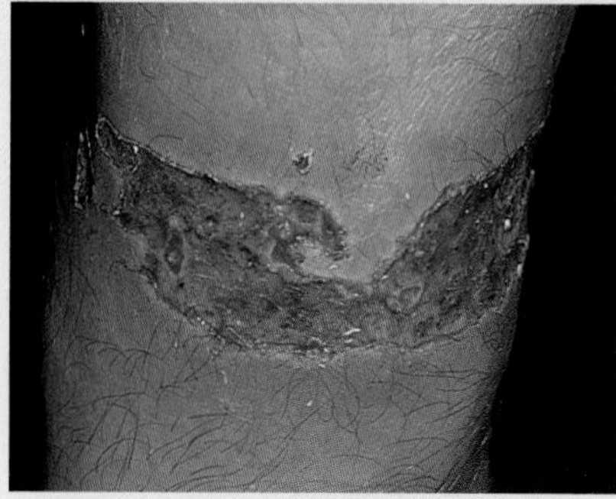

Ulcer

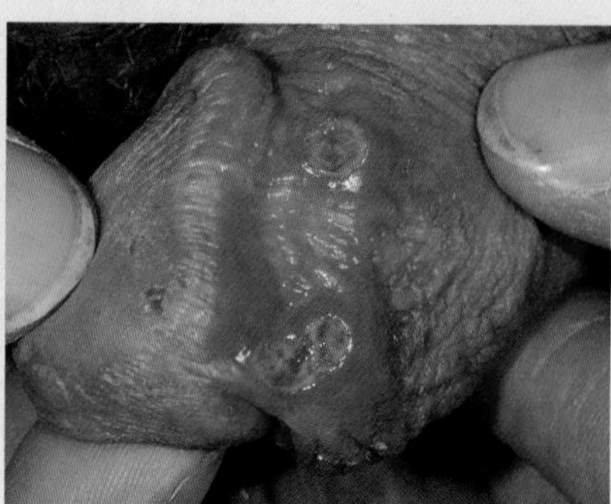

Chancroid

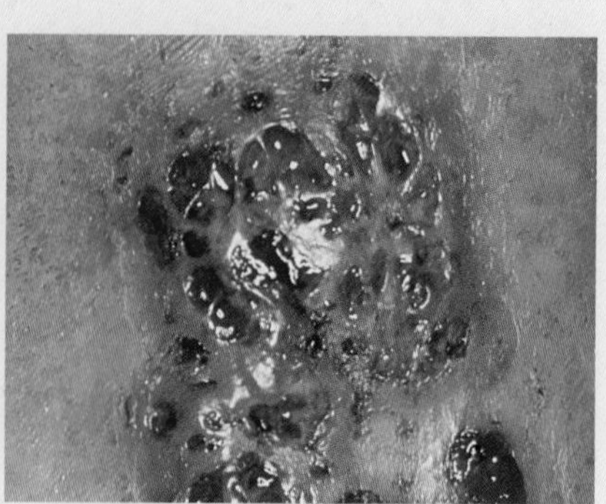

Pyoderma gangrenosum

SECONDARY SKIN LESIONS—FISSURES AND ATROPHY

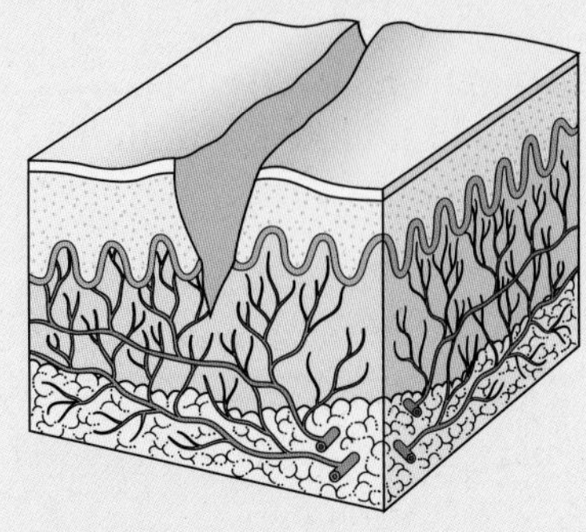

Fissure

A linear loss of epidermis and dermis with sharply defined, nearly vertical walls

Chapping (hands, feet) (pp. 102, 103)
Eczema (fingertip) (p. 106)
Intertrigo (p. 501)
Perlèche (p. 536)

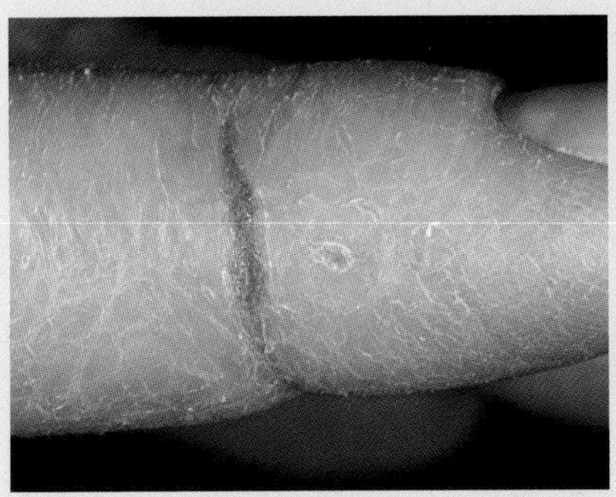

Eczema

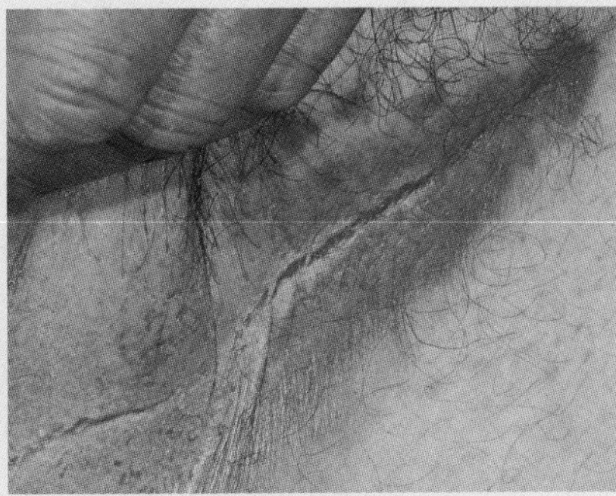

Intertrigo

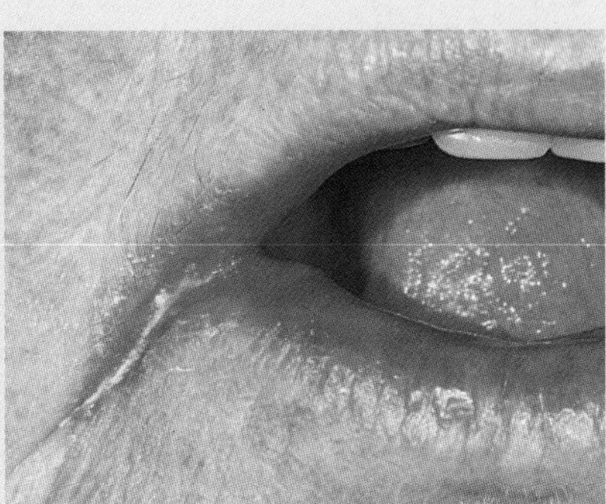

Perlèche

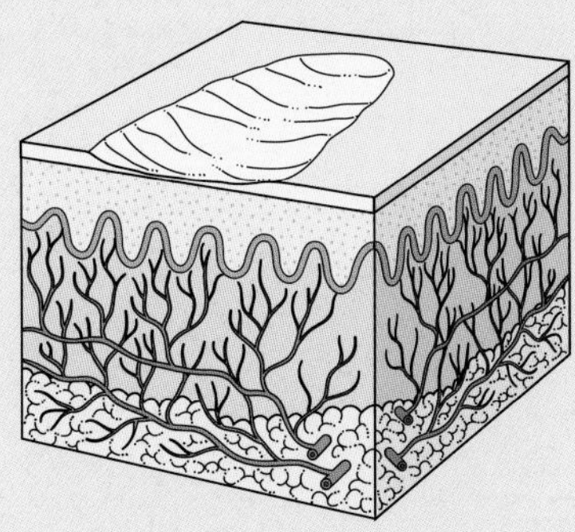

Atrophy

A depression in the skin resulting from thinning of the epidermis or dermis

Chronic cutaneous (discoid) lupus erythematosus (p. 682)
Dermatomyositis (p. 692)
Lichen sclerosus (p. 327)
Morphea (p. 707)
Necrobiosis lipoidica (p. 975)
Radiodermatitis
Striae (p. 88)
Sun-damaged skin (p. 745)
Topical and intralesional steroids (pp. 85, 86)

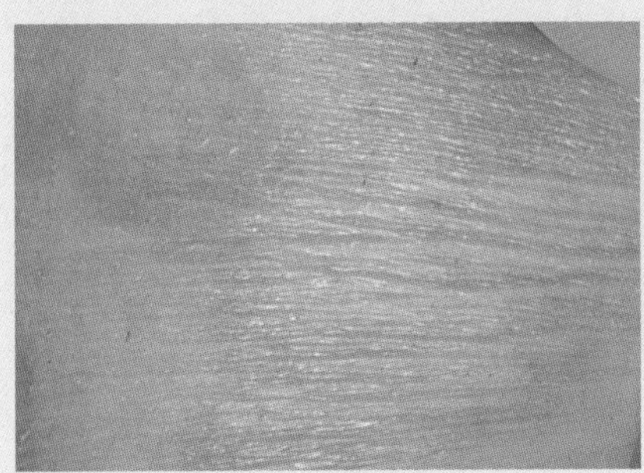

Lichen sclerosus

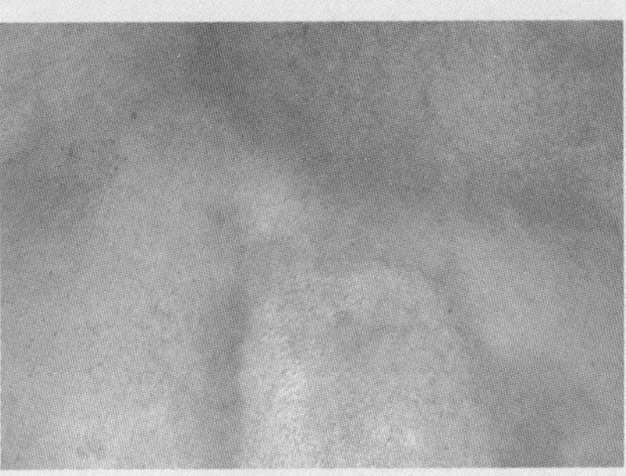

Morphea

Topical and intralesional steroids

SECONDARY SKIN LESIONS—SCARS

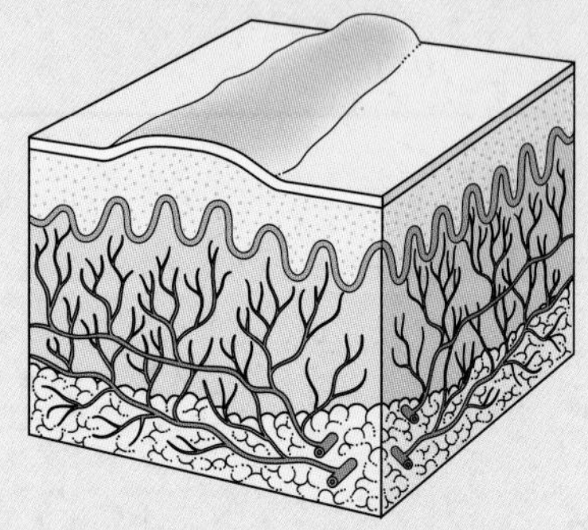

Scar

An abnormal formation of connective tissue implying dermal damage; after injury or surgery scars are initially thick and pink but with time become white and atrophic

Acne (p. 252)
Bullous pemphigoid (p. 655)
Burns
Cicatricial pemphigoid (p. 658)
Herpes zoster (p. 486)
Hidradenitis suppurativa (p. 260)
Keloid (p. 788)
Porphyria (p. 757)
Varicella (p. 474)

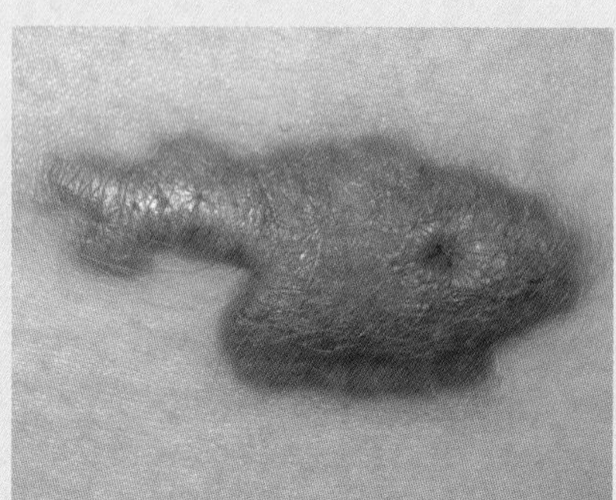

Keloid

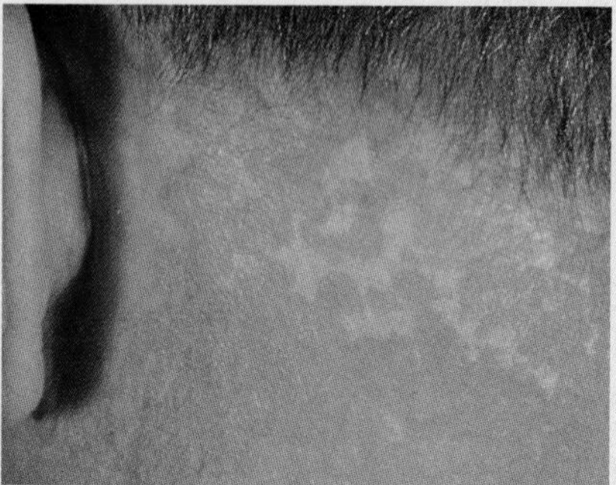

Herpes zoster

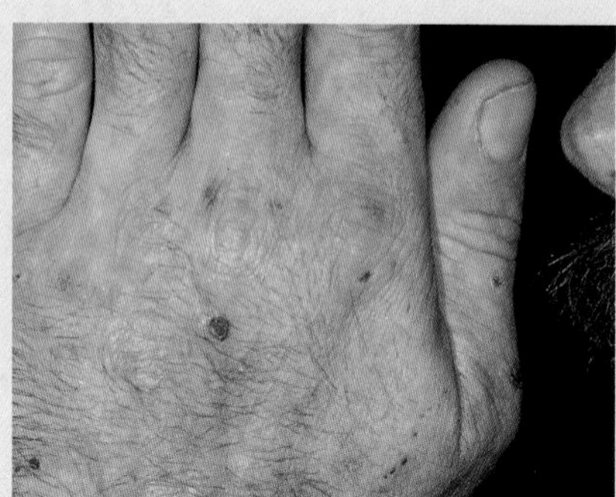

Porphyria

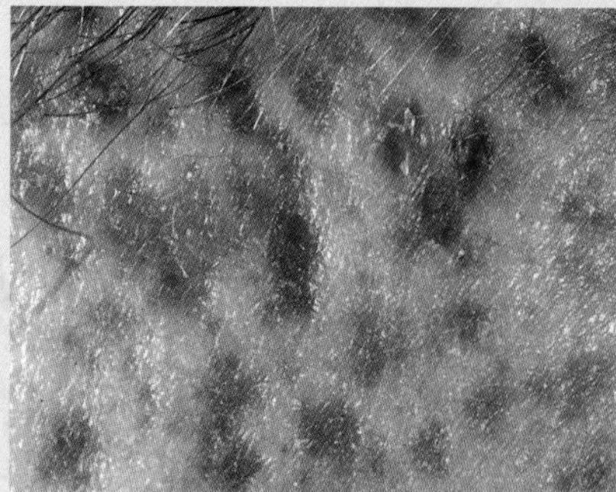

Cystic acne

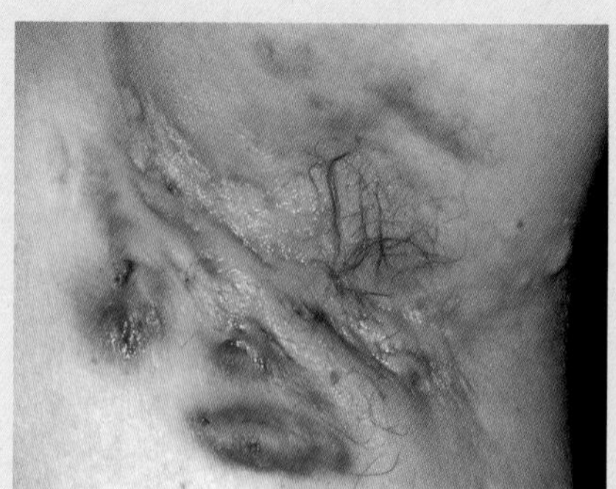

Hidradenitis suppurativa

SPECIAL SKIN LESIONS

Excoriation
An erosion caused by scratching; excoriations are often linear

Comedone
A plug of sebaceous and keratinous material lodged in the opening of a hair follicle; the follicular orifice may be dilated (blackhead) or narrowed (whitehead or closed comedone)

Milia
A small, superficial keratin cyst with no visible opening

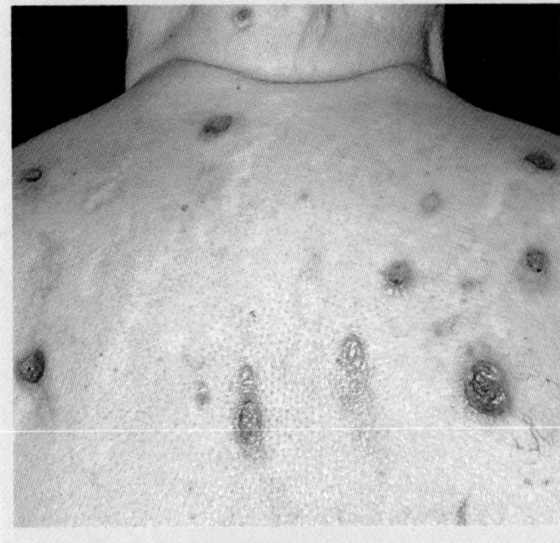
Excoriation

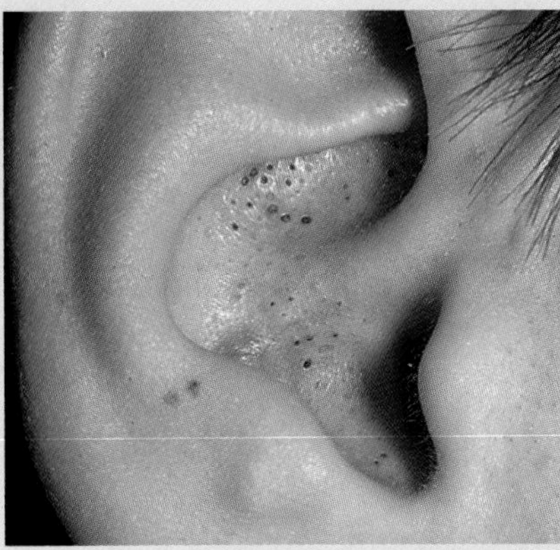
Comedones

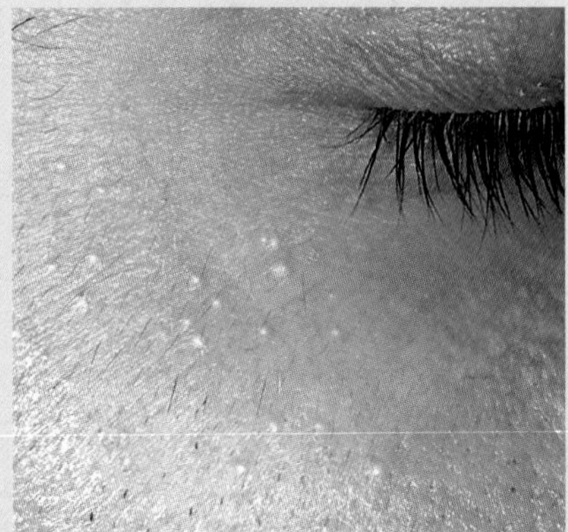
Milia

Cyst
A circumscribed lesion with a wall and a lumen; the lumen may contain fluid or solid matter

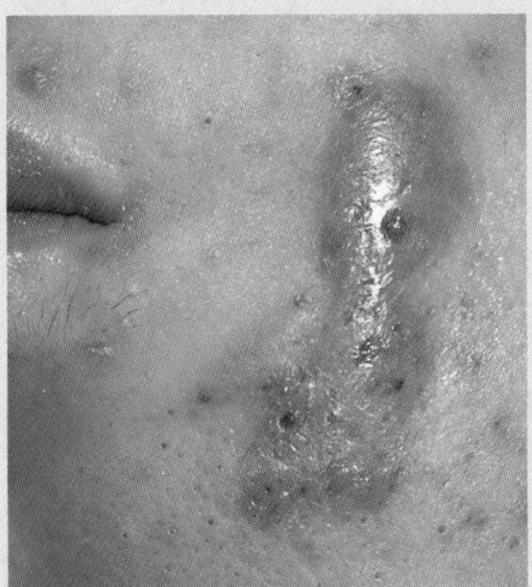
Acne cyst

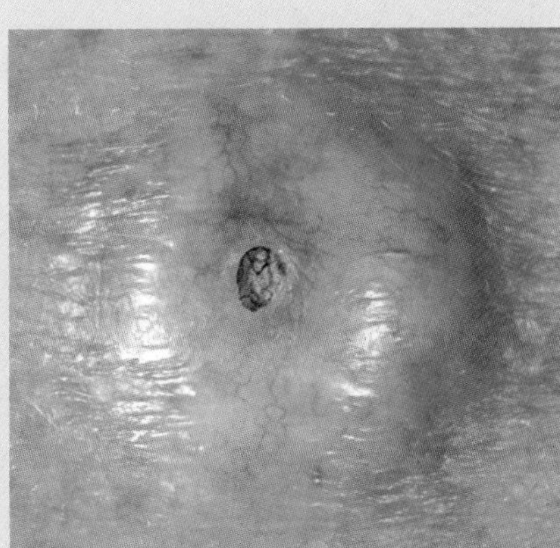
Epidermal cyst

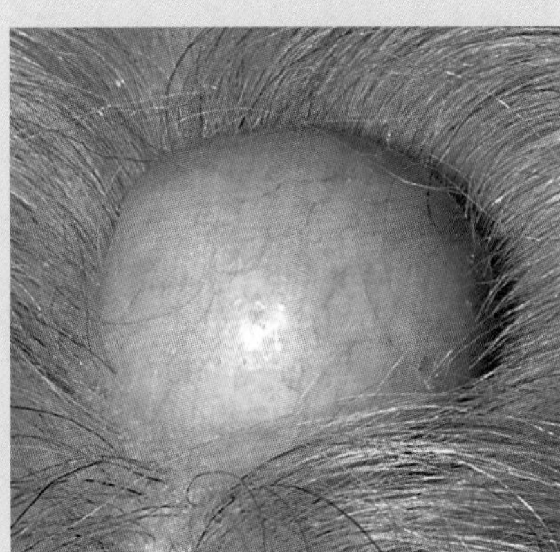
Pilar cyst

SPECIAL SKIN LESIONS—cont'd

Petechiae
A circumscribed deposit of blood less than 0.5 cm in diameter

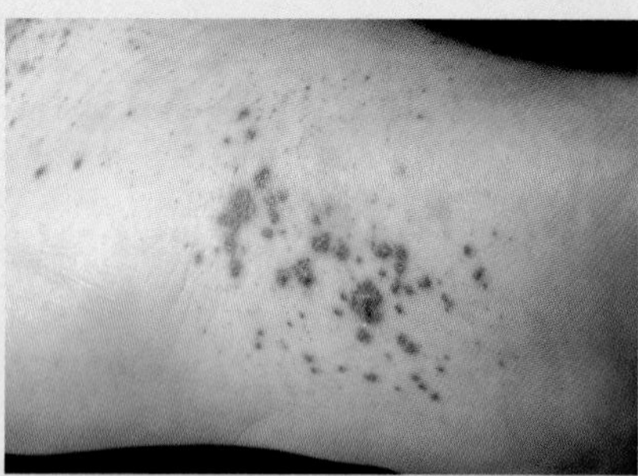
Henoch-Schönlein purpura

Purpura
A circumscribed deposit of blood greater than 0.5 cm in diameter

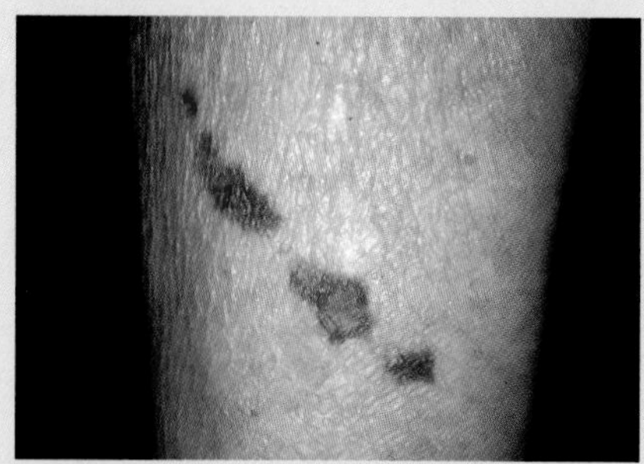
Sun-damaged skin

Burrow
A narrow, elevated, tortuous channel produced by a parasite

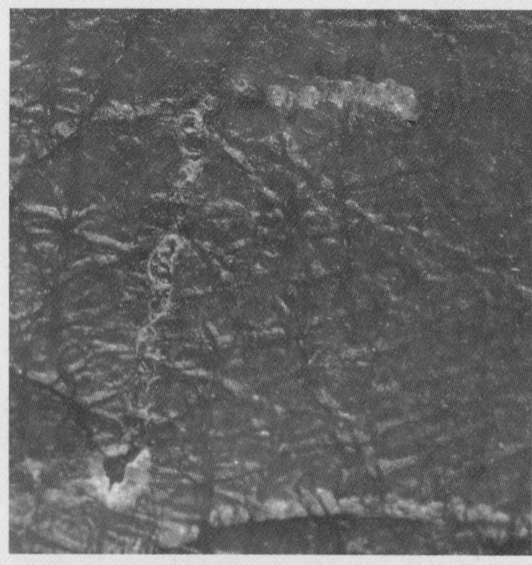
Scabies burrow

Lichenification
An area of thickened epidermis induced by scratching; skin lines are accentuated so the surface looks like a washboard

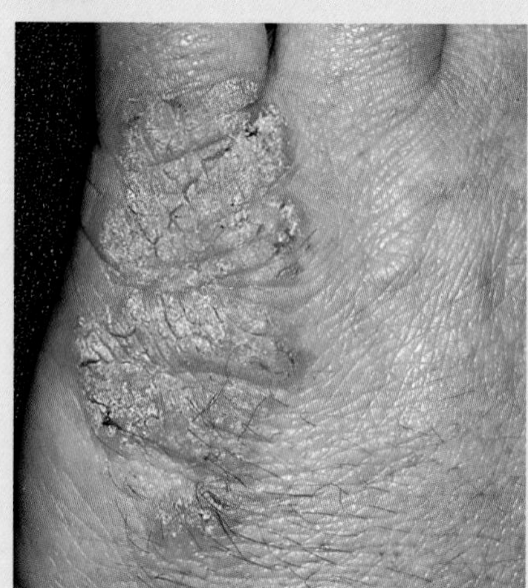
Lichenification

Telangiectasia
Dilated superficial blood vessels

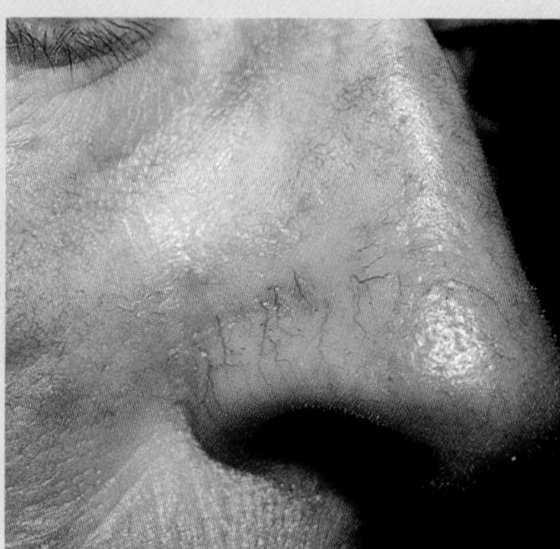
Telangiectasia rosacea

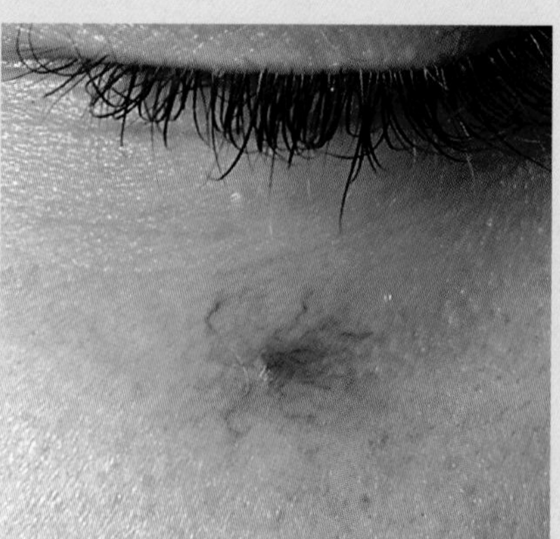
T. spider angioma

REGIONAL DIFFERENTIAL DIAGNOSES ATLAS

Most skin diseases have preferential areas of involvement. Disease locations are illustrated below; diseases are listed alphabetically by location on pp. 20-74. Common diseases that are obvious to most practitioners are not included.

Diseases such as contact dermatitis and herpes zoster that can be found on any skin surface have also been left out of most of the lists.

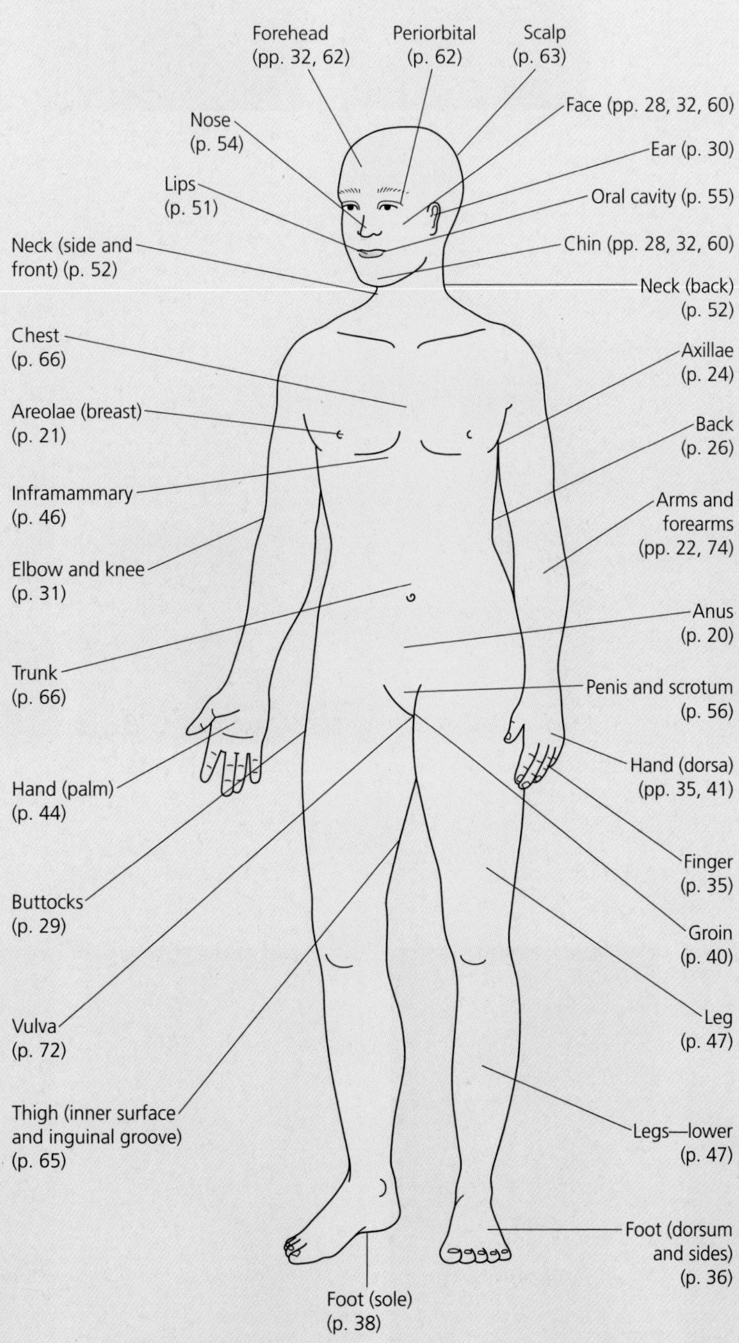

Anus

Allergic contact dermatitis (p. 133)
Anal excoriation (p. 115)
Baboon syndrome (p. 144)
Candidiasis (p. 523)
Extramammary Paget's disease (p. 844)
Gonorrhea (p. 413)
Herpes simplex/zoster (p. 467)
Hidradenitis suppurativa (p. 260)
Inverse psoriasis (p. 274)
Lichen planus (p. 320)
Lichen sclerosus (p. 327)
Lichen simplex chronicus (p. 115)
Streptococcal cellulitis (p. 348)
Syphilis (primary and secondary) (p. 401)
Vitiligo (p. 764)
Warts (p. 422)

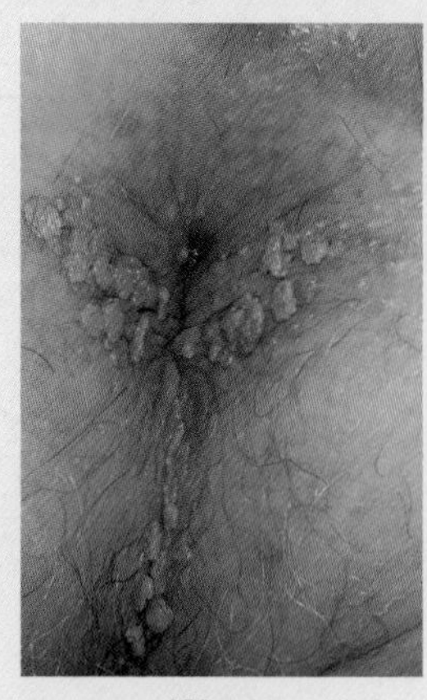
Warts

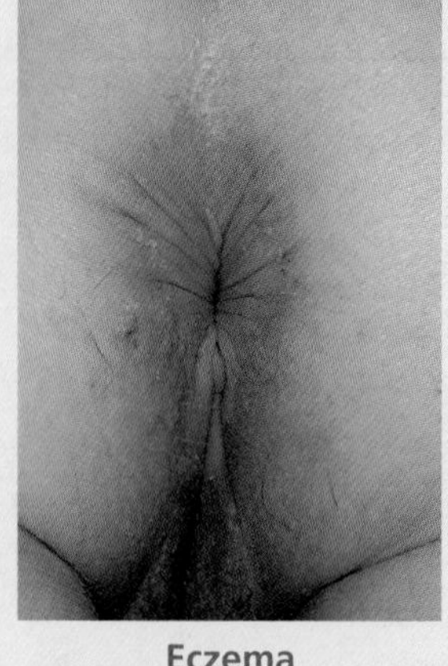
Eczema

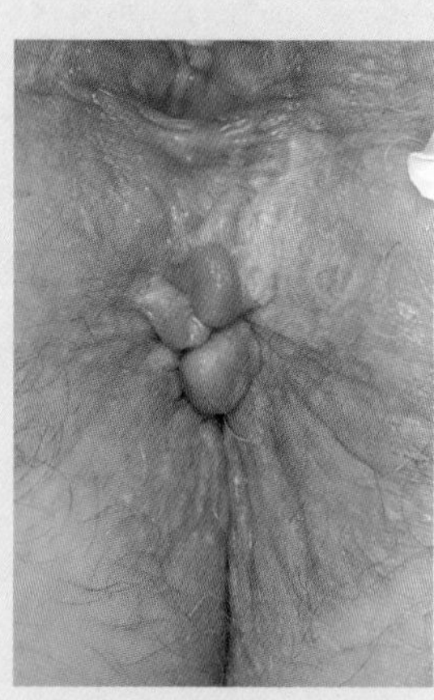
Lichen planus

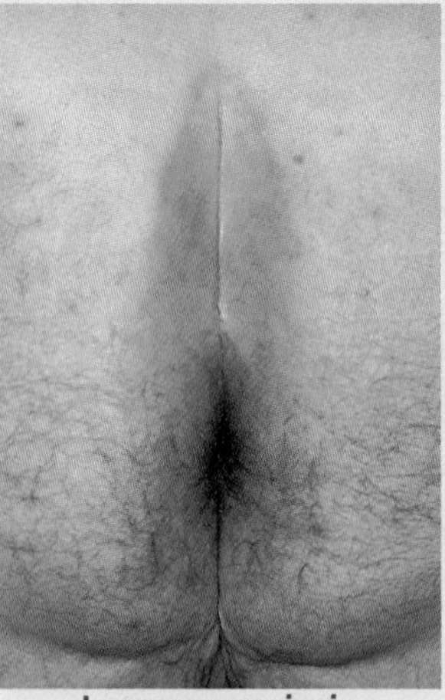
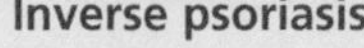
Inverse psoriasis

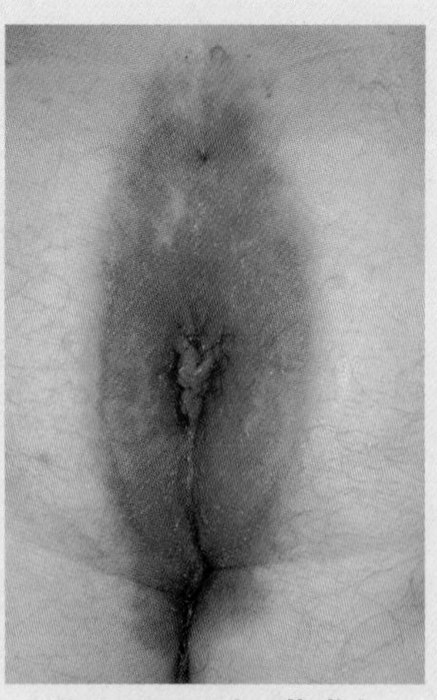
Streptococci cellulitis

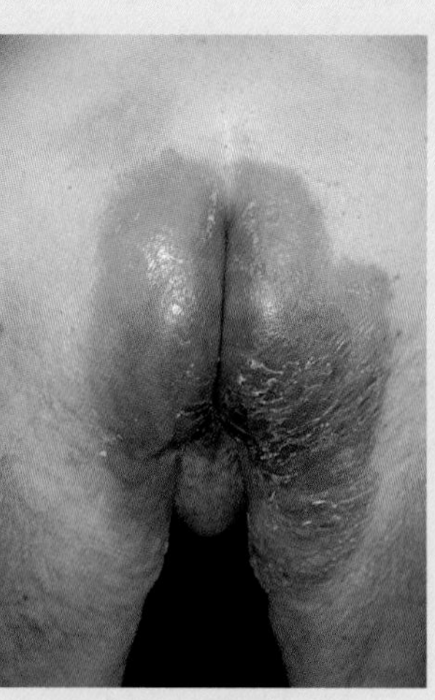
Baboon syndrome

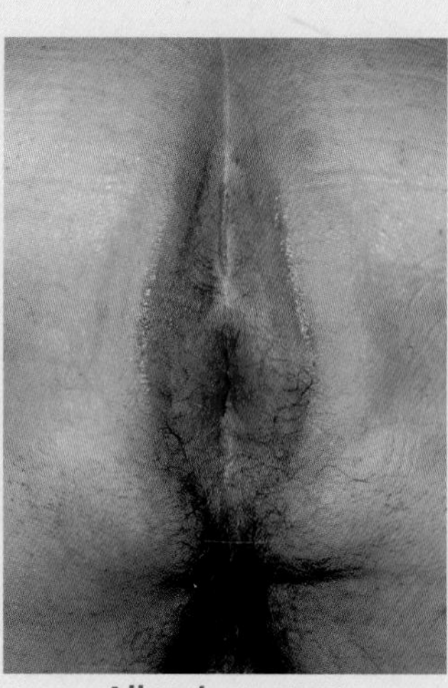
Allergic contact dermatitis

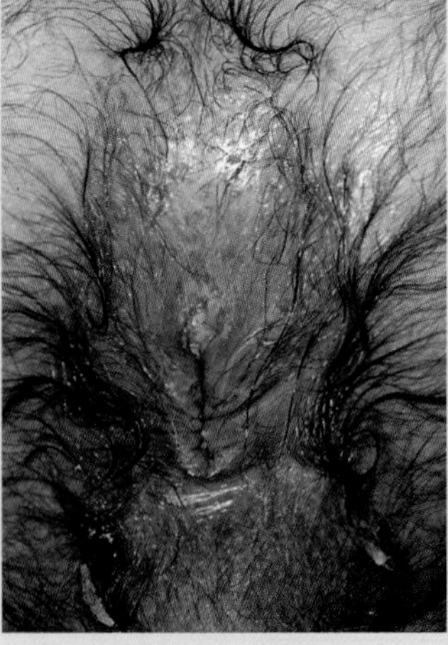
Herpes simplex

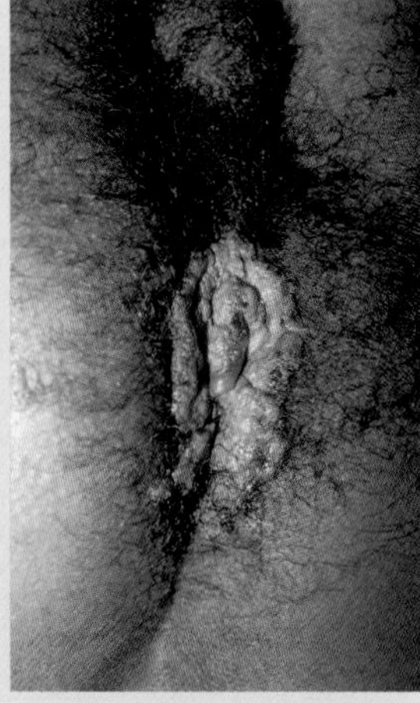
Secondary syphilis

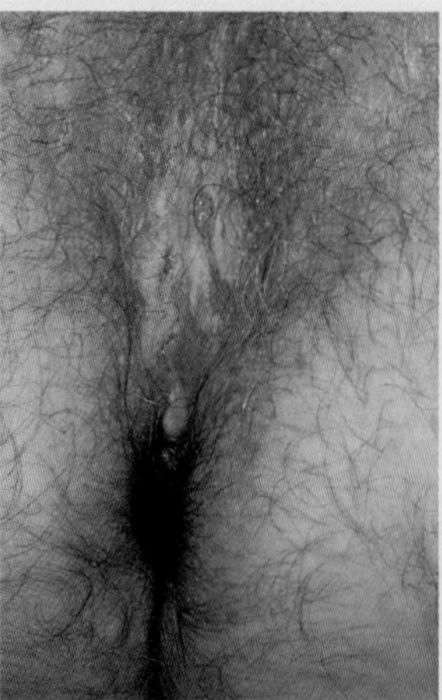
Anal excoriation

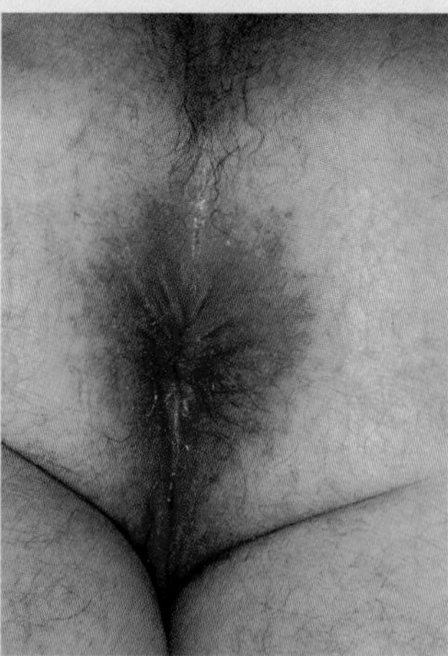
Candidiasis

Areolae (breast)
Acanthosis nigricans (p. 979)
Eczema (pp. 95, 96)
Fordyce spots (p. 224)
Paget's disease (p. 843)
Seborrheic keratosis (p. 776)

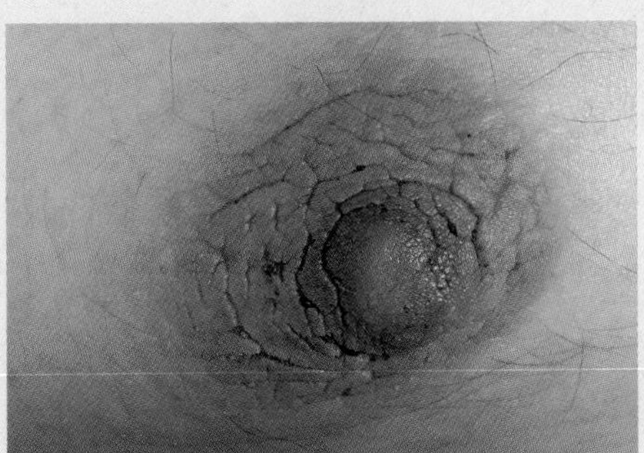
Acanthosis nigricans

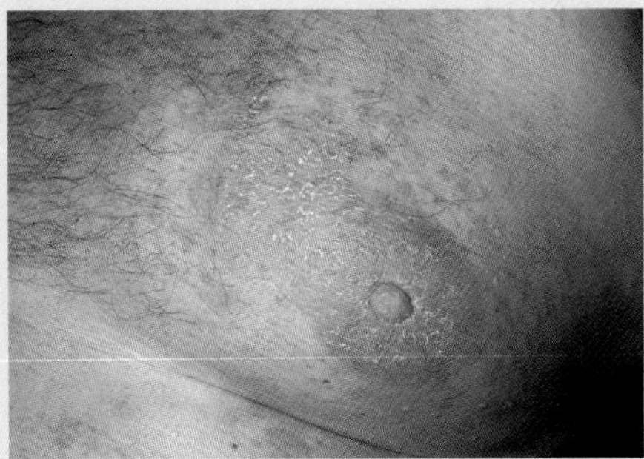
Eczema, subacute

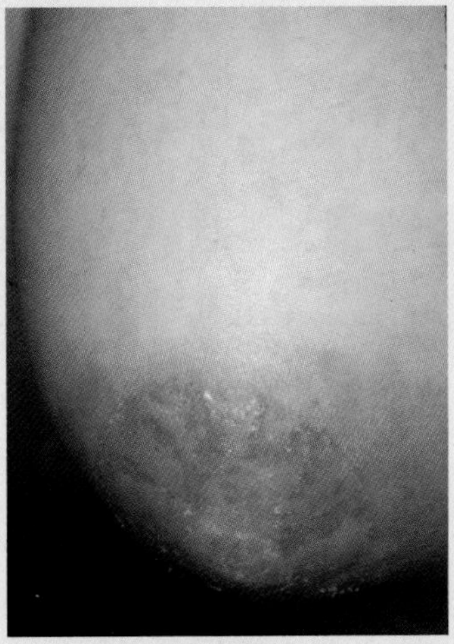
Eczema, subacute

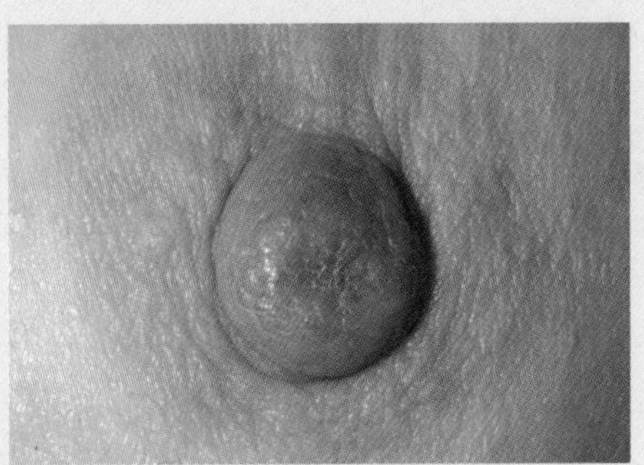
Paget's disease, nipple

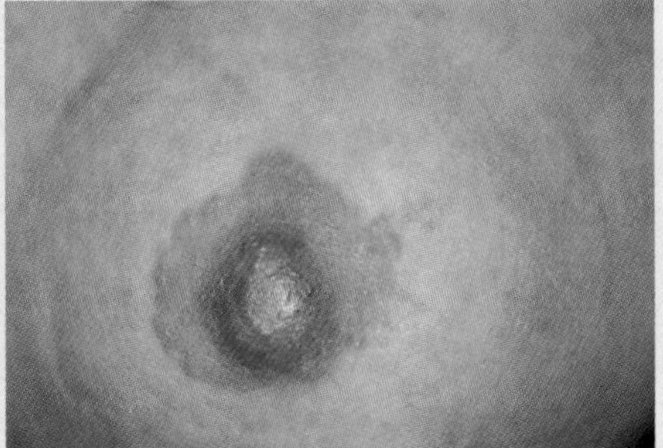
Paget's disease, areola

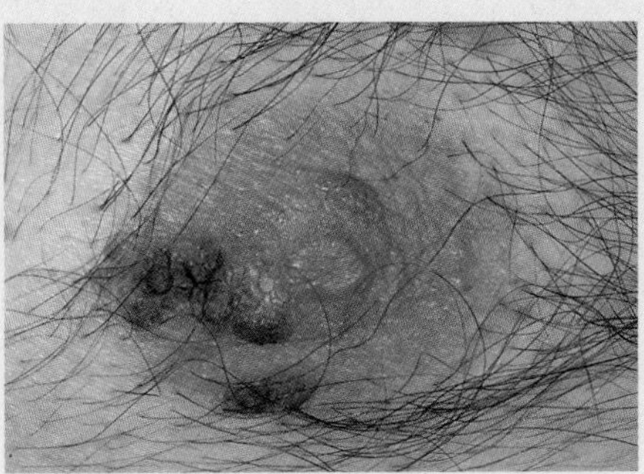
Seborrheic keratosis

Arms and forearms

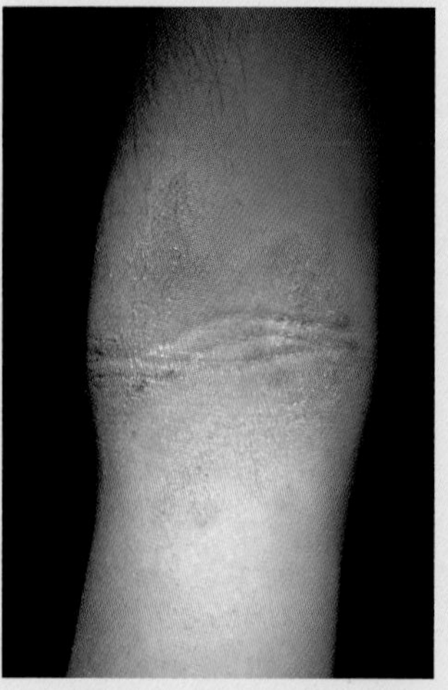
Atopic dermatitis

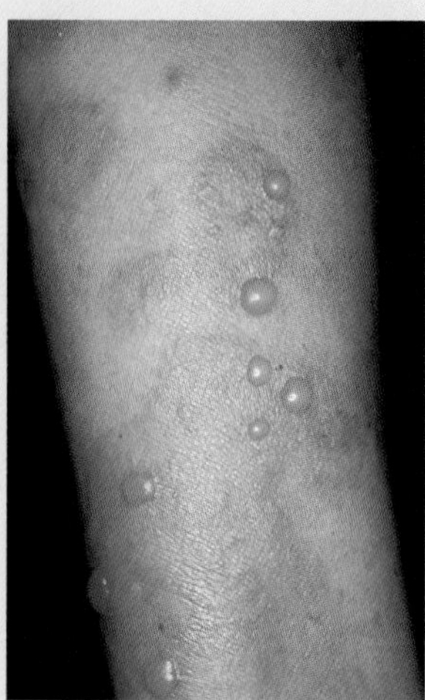
Bullous pemphigoid

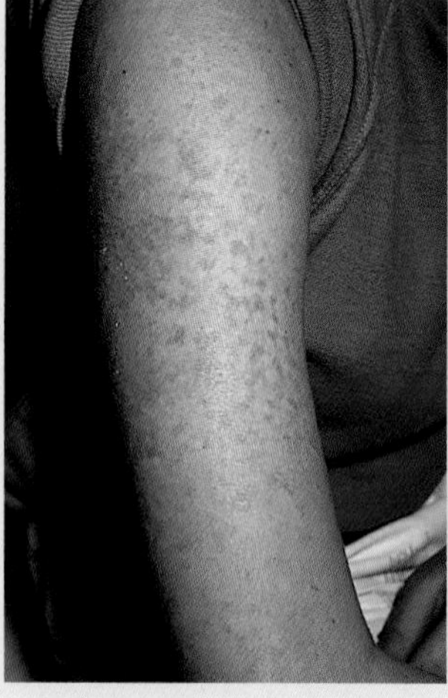
Lupus erythematosus

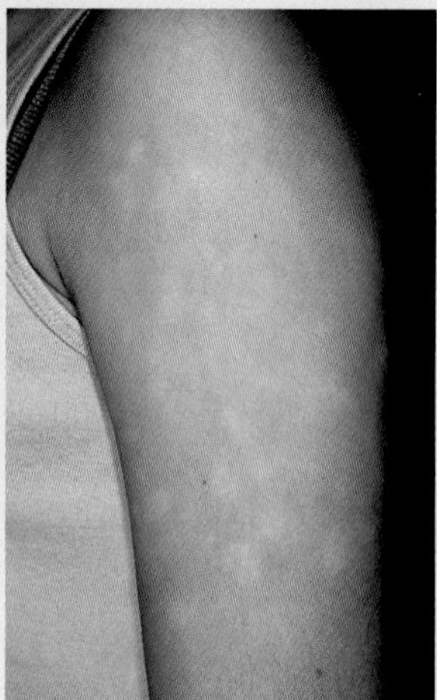
Pityriasis alba

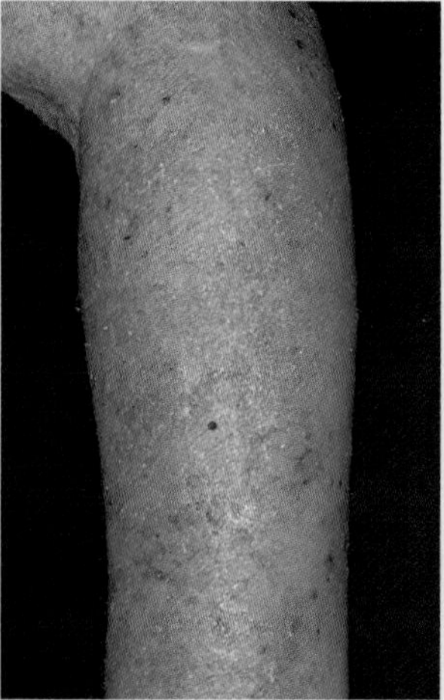
Eczema, subacute

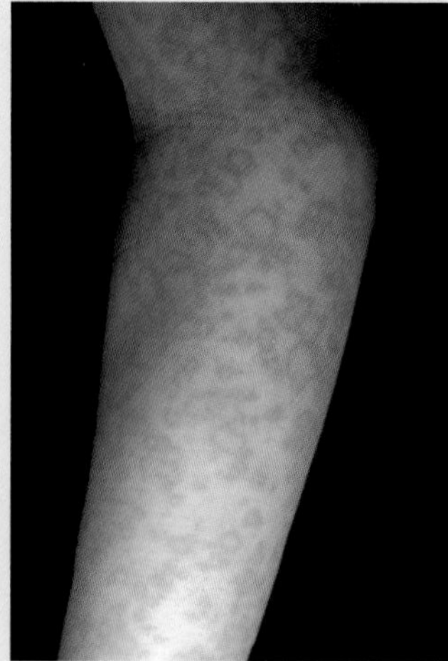
Erythema infectiosum

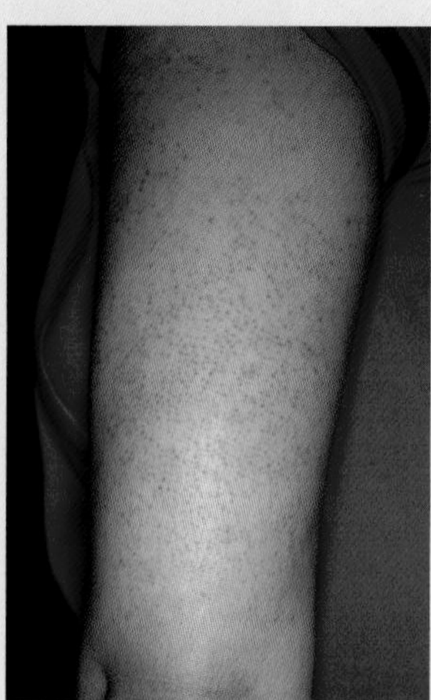
Keratosis pilaris

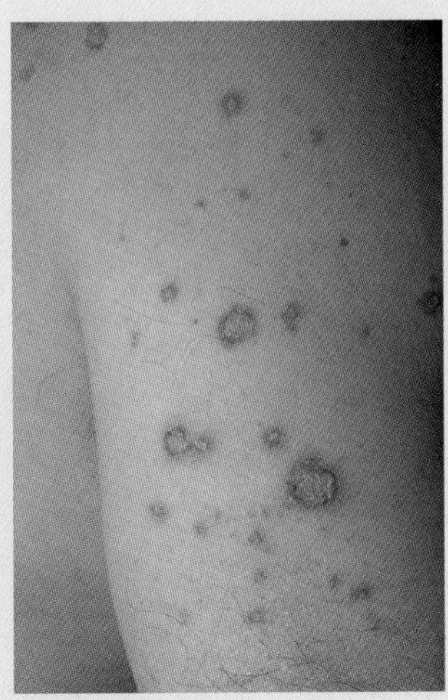
Nummular eczema

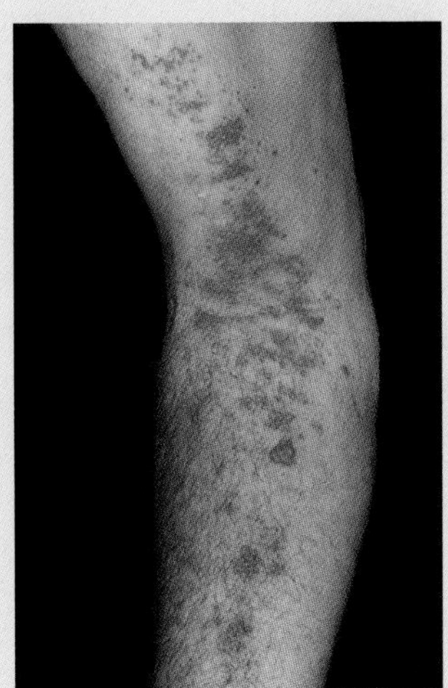
Herpes zoster

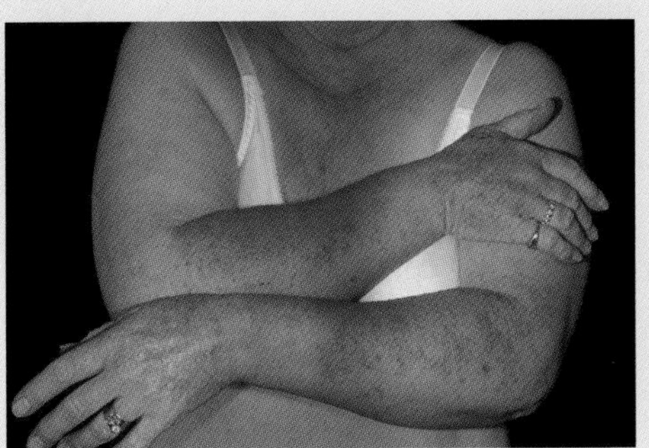
Polymorphous light eruption

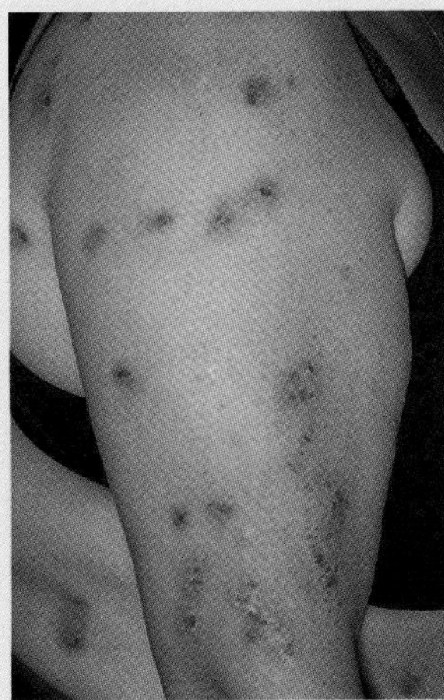
Neurotic excoriations

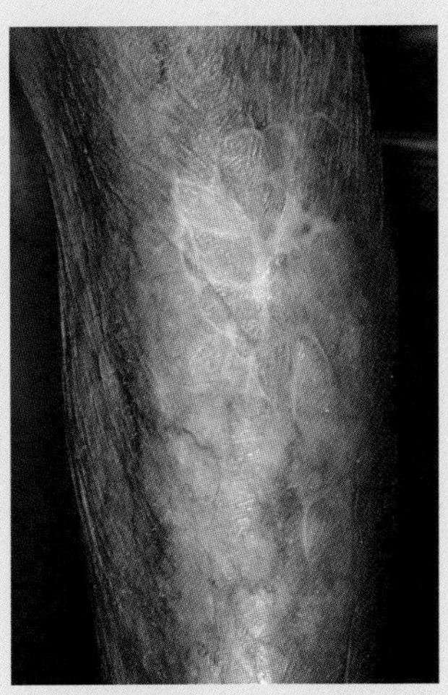
Sun-damaged skin

Axillae

Acanthosis nigricans (p. 978)
Acrochordons (skin tags) (p. 785)
Allergic contact dermatitis (p. 133)
Benign familial chronic pemphigus (p. 663)
Candidiasis (p. 523)
Eczema (p. 91)
Erythrasma (p. 501)
Fordyce spots (p. 224)
Furunculosis (p. 356)
Granular parakeratosis
Hailey-Hailey disease (p. 663)
Hidradenitis suppurativa (p. 260)
Impetigo (p. 336)
Inverse psoriasis (p. 274)
Lice (p. 590)
Lichen planus (p. 322)
Pseudoxanthoma elasticum
Scabies (p. 586)
Striae (p. 88)
Tinea (p. 502)
Trichomycosis axillaris (p. 946)
von Recklinghausen's disease (neurofibromatosis) (p. 983)

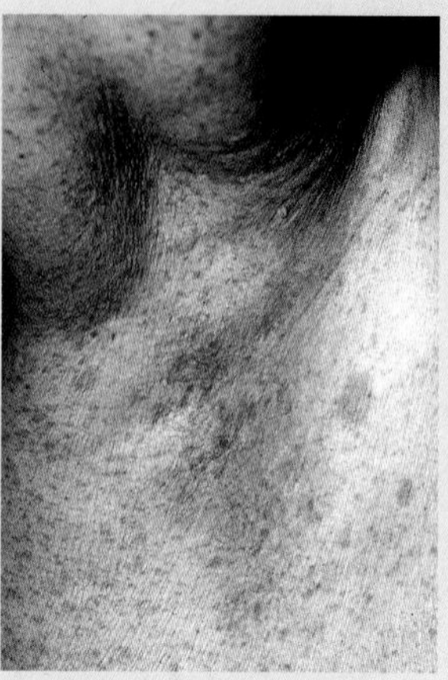
Neurofibromatosis

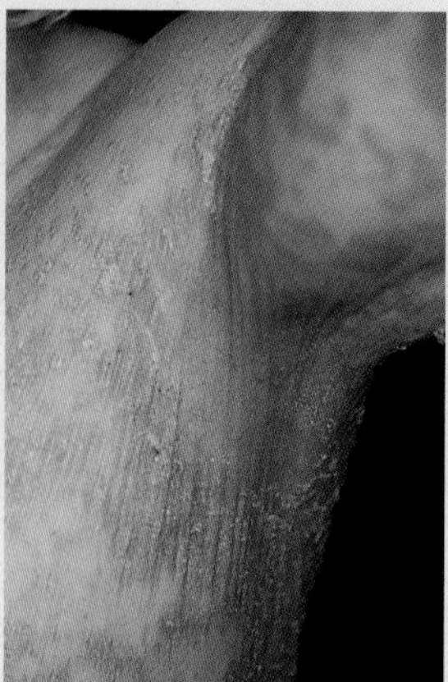
Pustular psoriasis

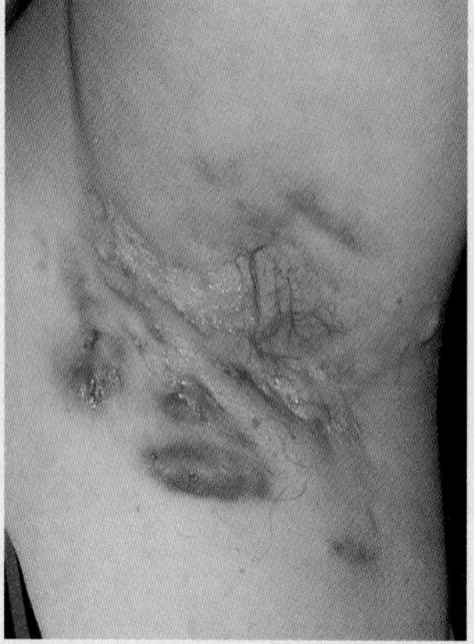
Hidradenitis suppurativa

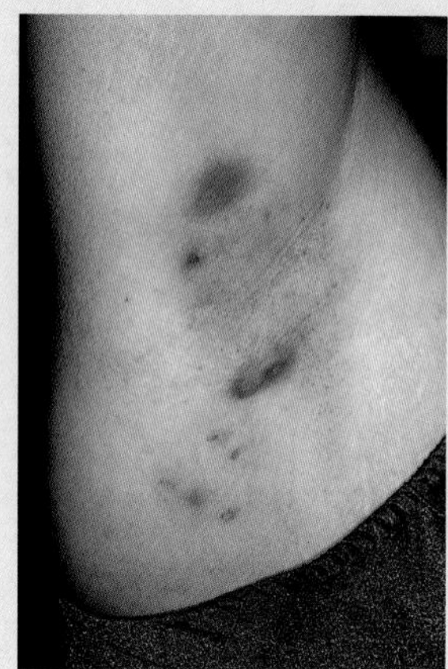
Hidradenitis suppurativa

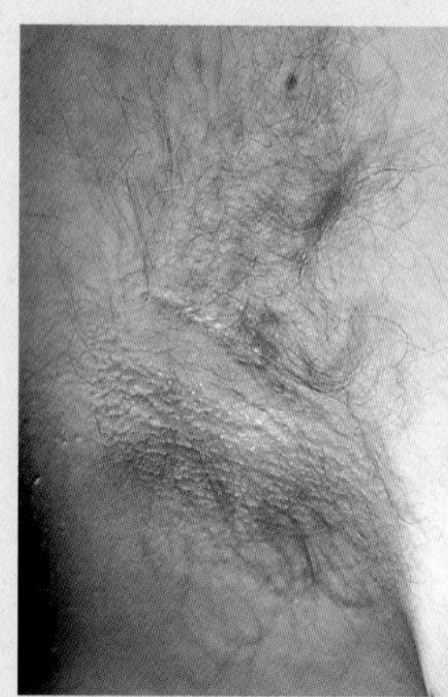
Acanthosis nigricans

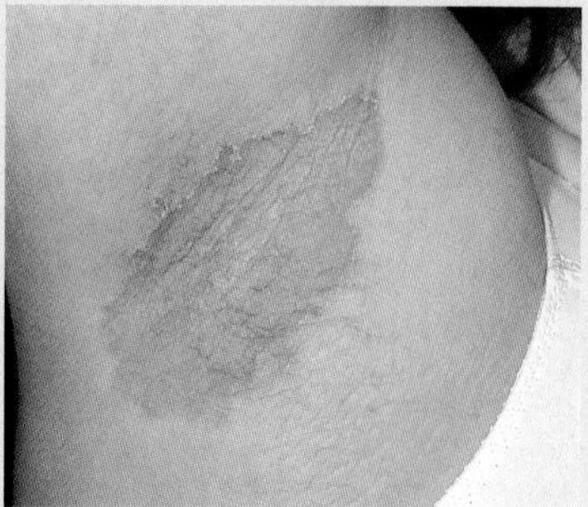
Candidiasis

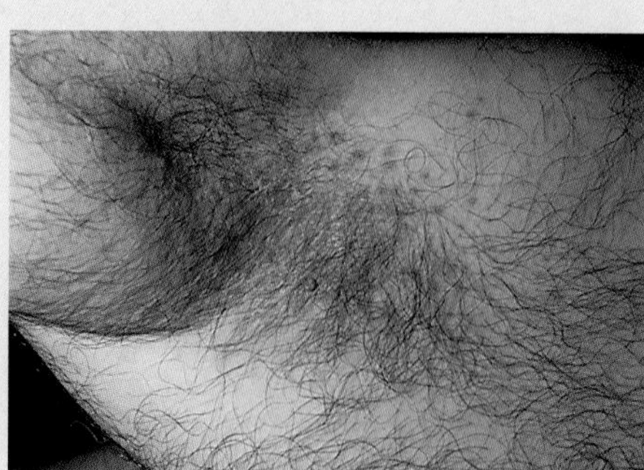
Candidiasis

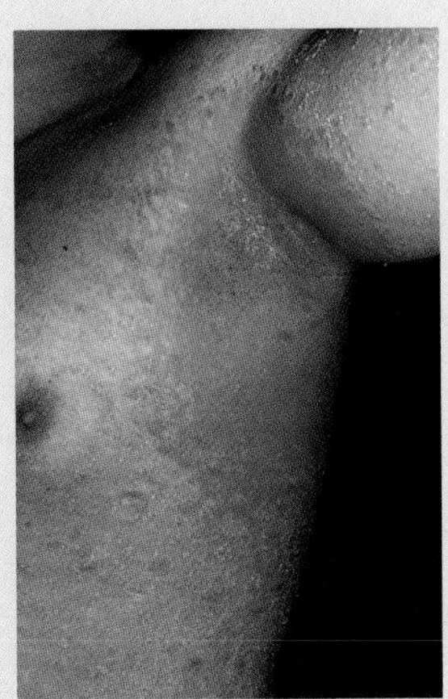
Allergic contact dermatitis

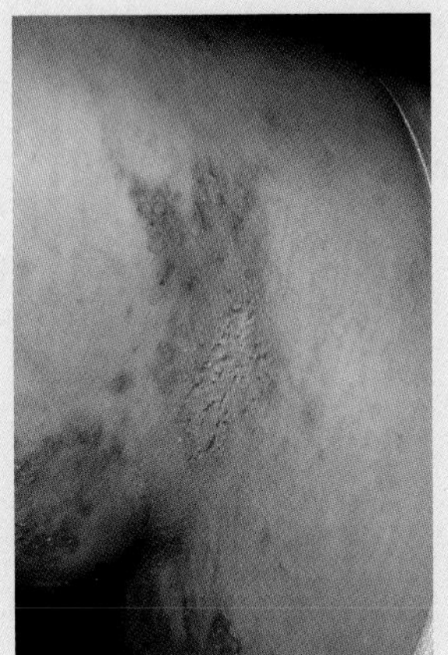
Benign familial chronic pemphigus (Hailey-Hailey disease)

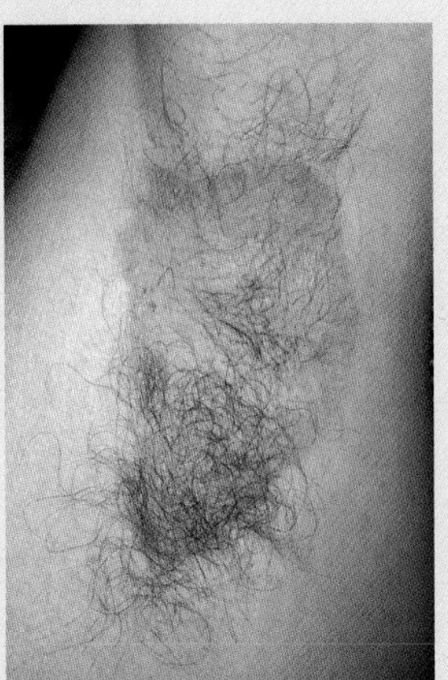
Eczema

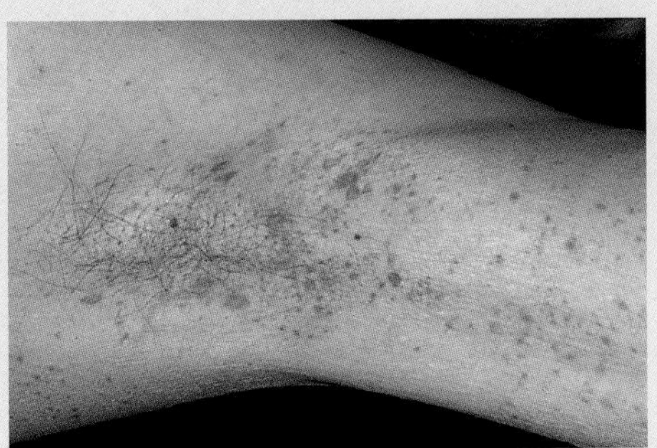
Lichen planus

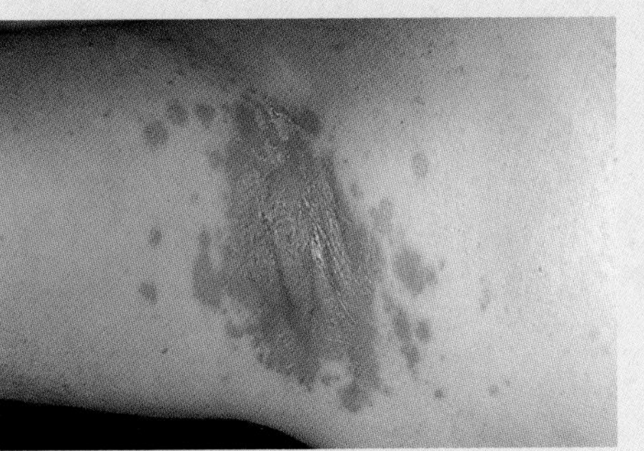
Inverse psoriasis

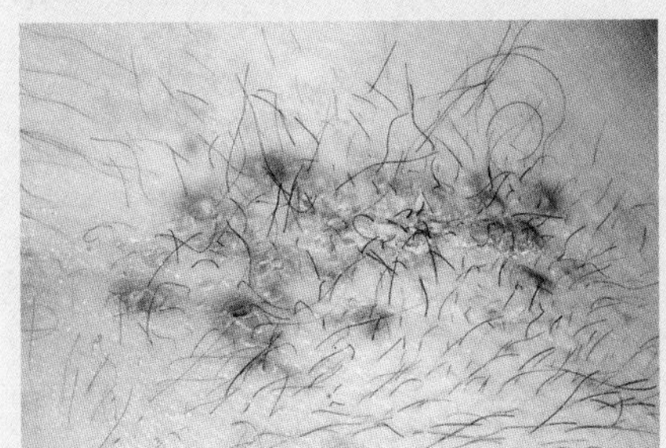
Granular parakeratosis

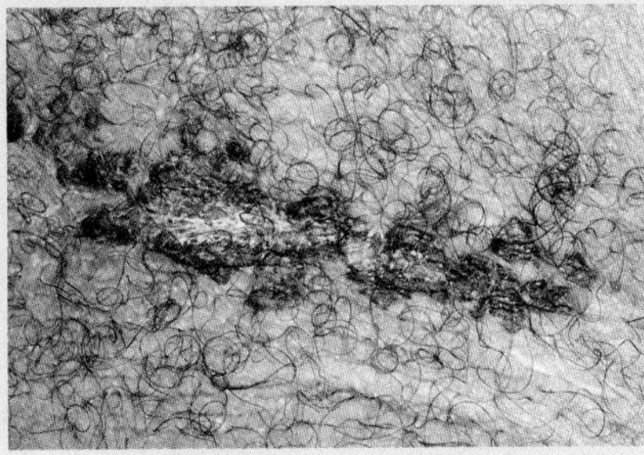
Granular parakeratosis

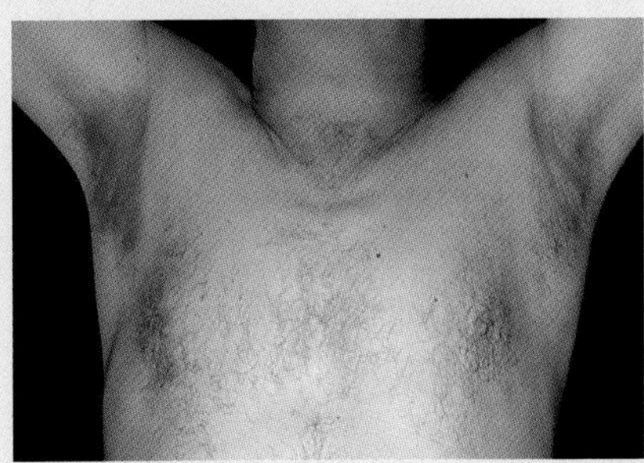
Allergic contact dermatitis

Back

Acne (p. 233)
Amyloidosis
Atrophoderma
Becker's nevus (p. 854)
Cutaneous T-cell lymphoma (p. 832)
Dermatographism (p. 194)
Eczema (p. 112)
Erythrodermic psoriasis (p. 269)
Erythema ab igne (p. 775)
Grover's disease (p. 334)
Keloids—acne scars (p. 786)
Lichen planus (p. 323)
Lichen sclerosus (p. 327)
Lichen simplex chronicus (p. 104)
Lichen spinulosis
Melanoma (p. 860)
Neurotic excoriation (p. 120)
Nevus anemicus (p. 770)
Notalgia paresthetica
Nummular eczema (p. 111)
Pityriasis lichenoides (p. 332)
Pityrosporum folliculitis (p. 540)
Seborrheic keratosis (p. 777)
Striae (p. 88)
Tinea versicolor (p. 537)

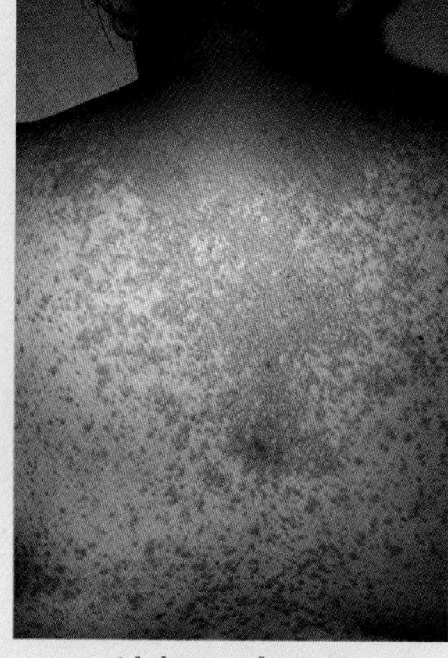
Lichen planus

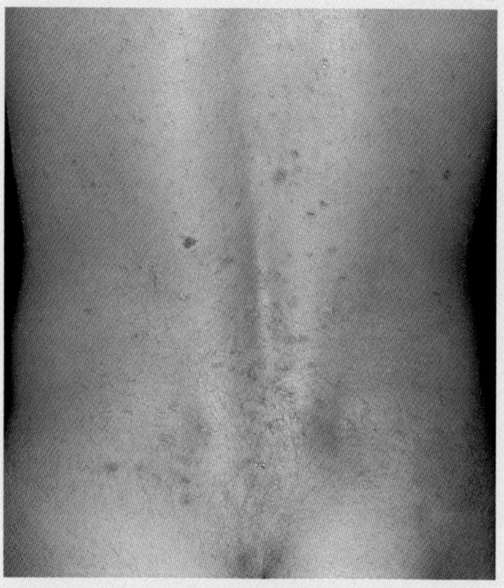
Lichen planus

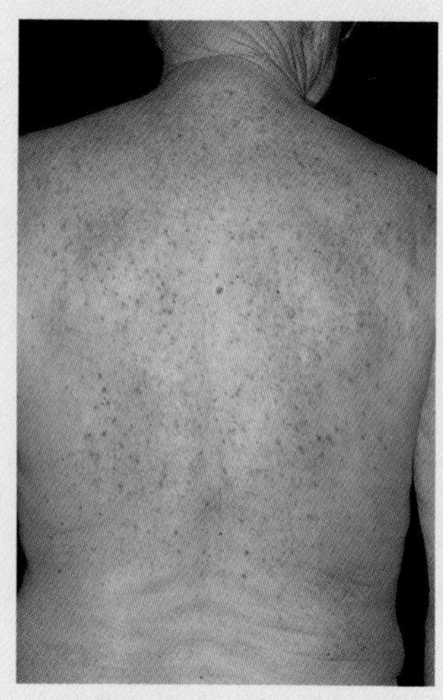
Eczema, subacute

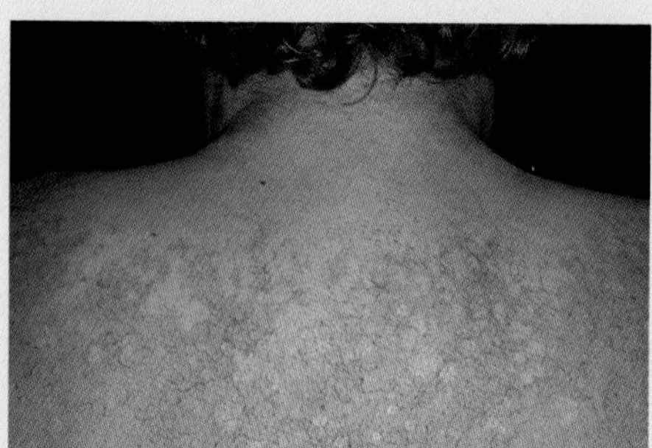
Tinea versicolor

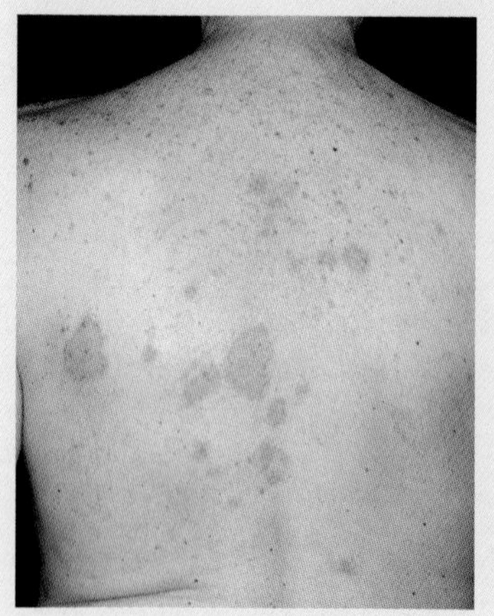
Nummular eczema

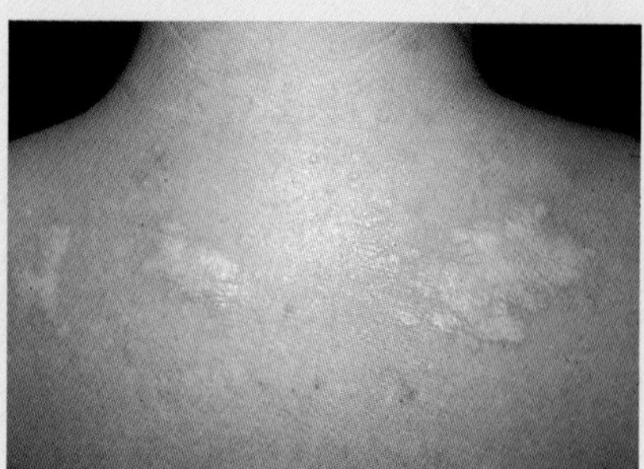
Lichen sclerosus

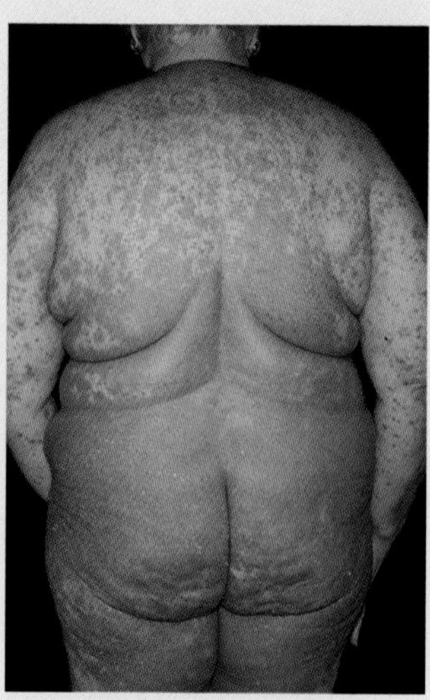
Erythrodermic psoriasis

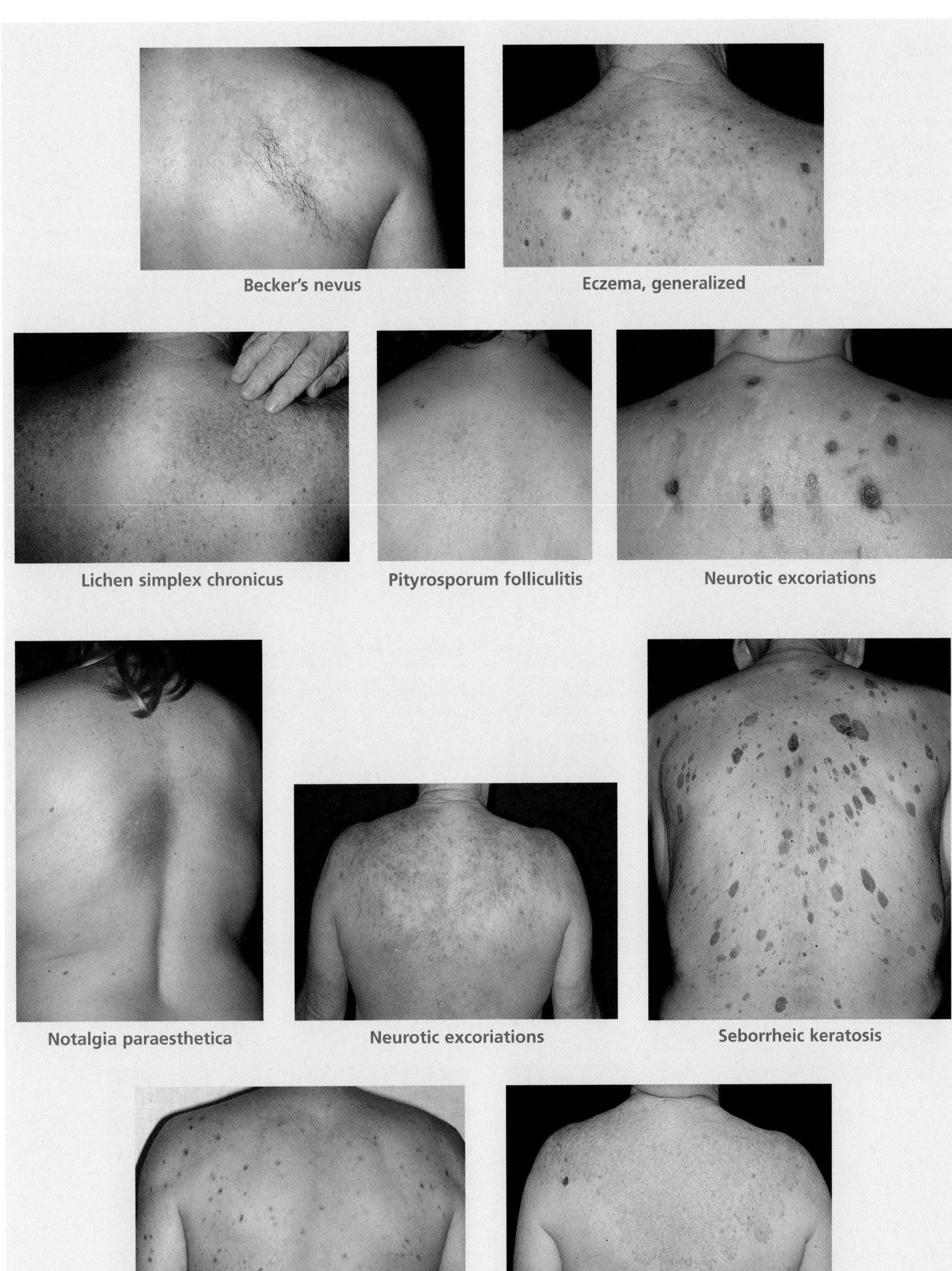

Becker's nevus

Eczema, generalized

Lichen simplex chronicus

Pityrosporum folliculitis

Neurotic excoriations

Notalgia paraesthetica

Neurotic excoriations

Seborrheic keratosis

Pityriasis lichenoides

Tinea

Beard

Alopecia areata (p. 932)
Chronic cutaneous (discoid) lupus erythematosus (p. 682)
Pseudofolliculitis barbae (p. 352)
Seborrheic dermatitis (p. 315)
Sycosis barbae (p. 354)
Tinea barbae (p. 517)

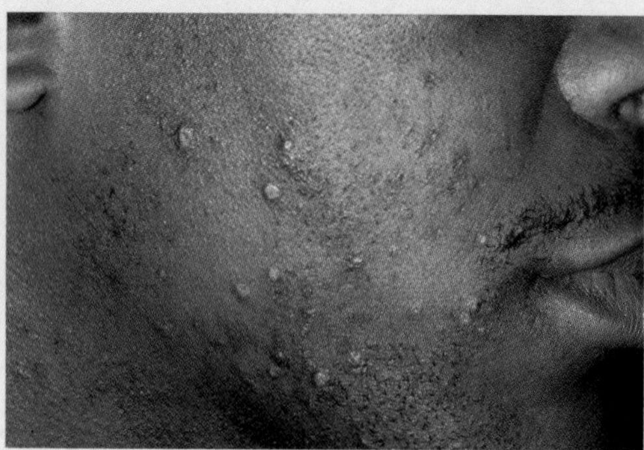

Pseudofolliculitis barbae

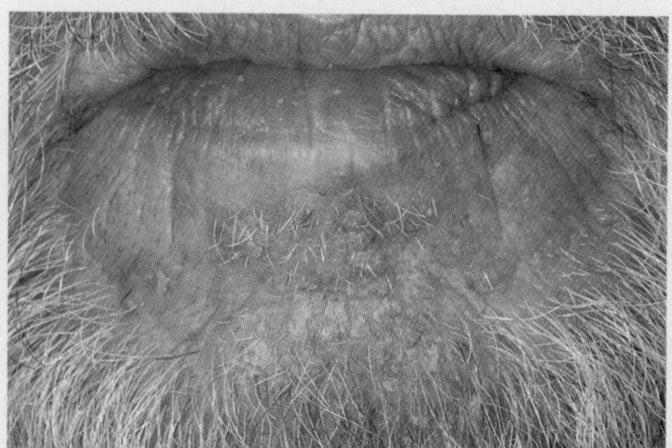

Seborrheic dermatitis

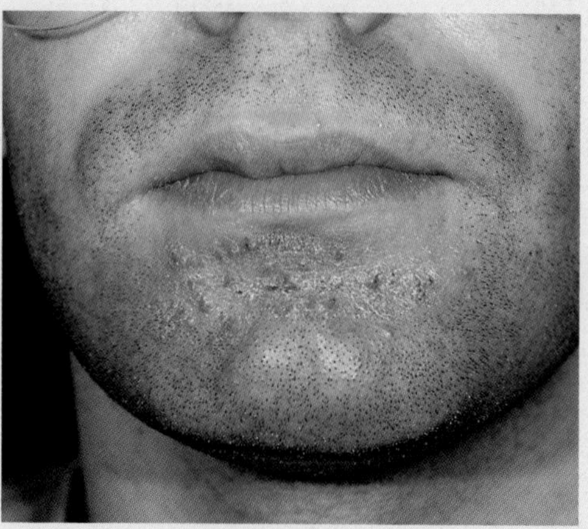

Sycosis barbae

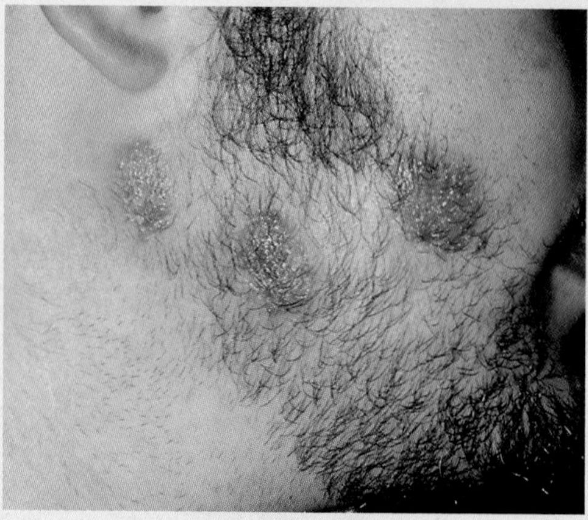

Tinea barbae

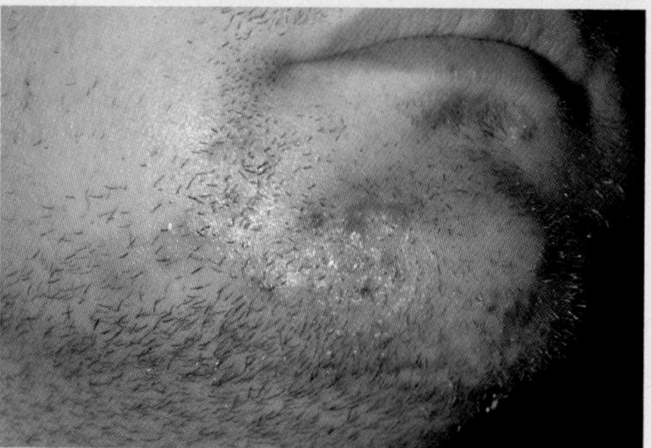

Tinea barbae

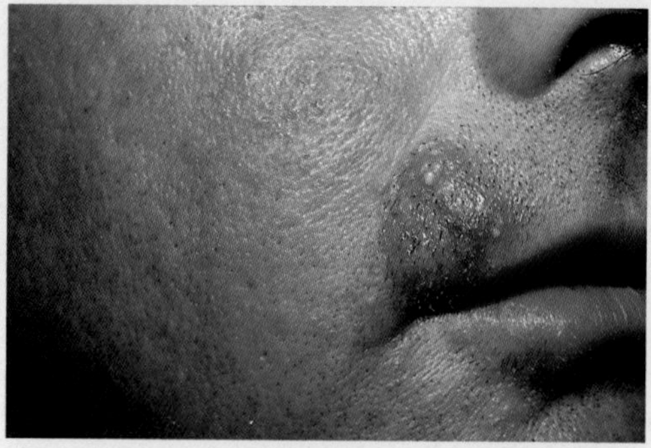

Tinea barbae

Buttocks

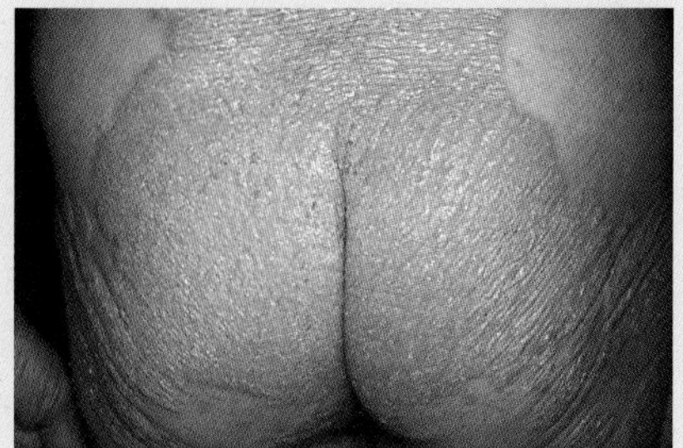
Psoriasis, chronic plaque

Tinea corporis

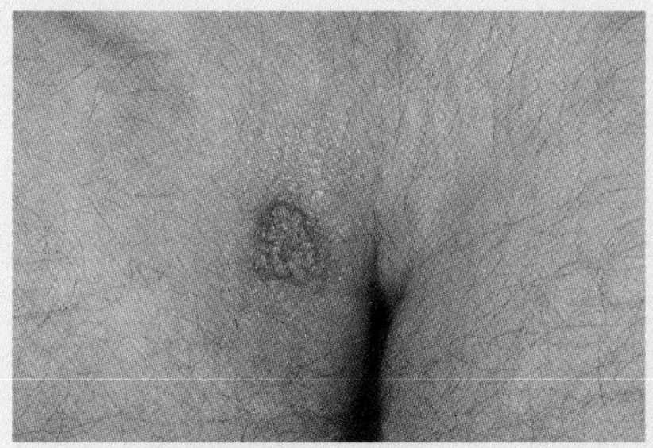
Herpes simplex

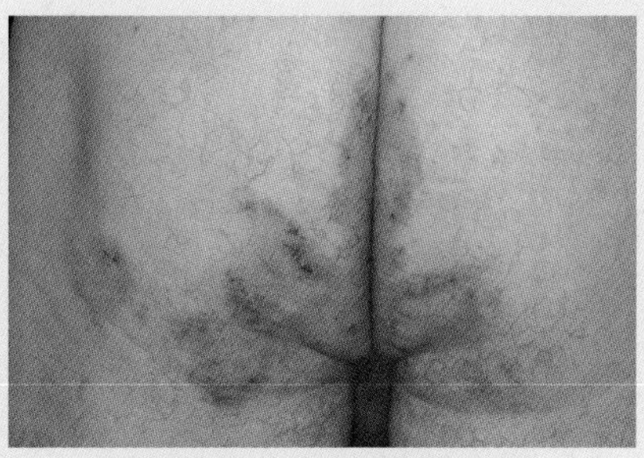
Dermatitis herpetiformis

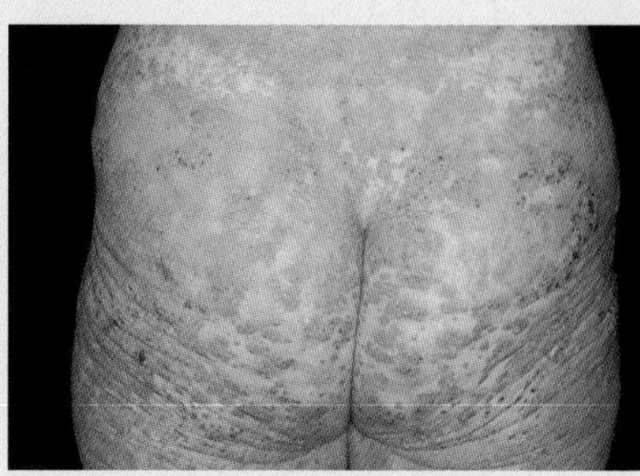
Psoriasis, chronic plaque

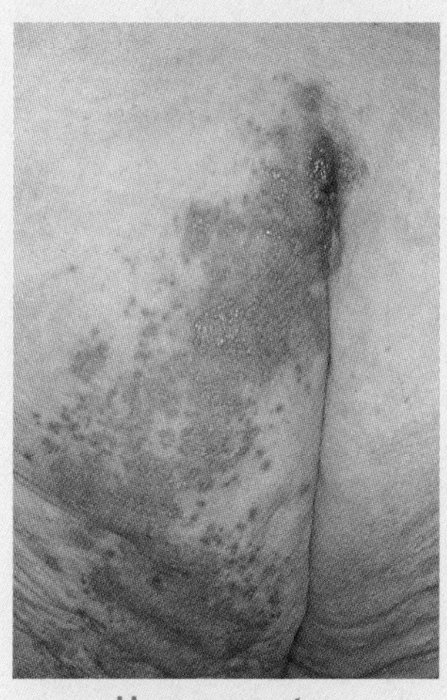
Herpes zoster

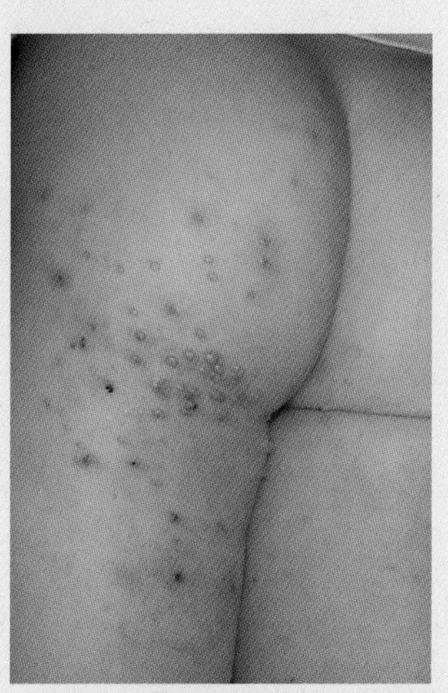
Molluscum contagiosum

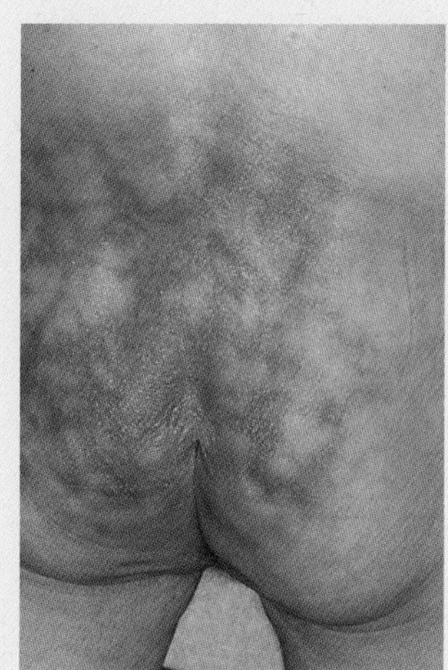
Erythema ab igne

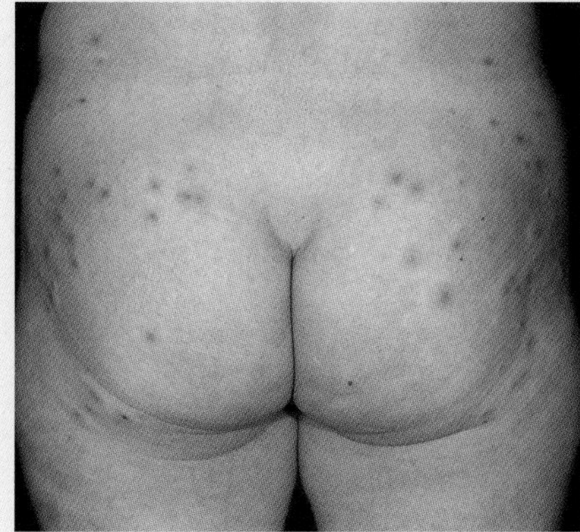
Pseudomonas folliculitis

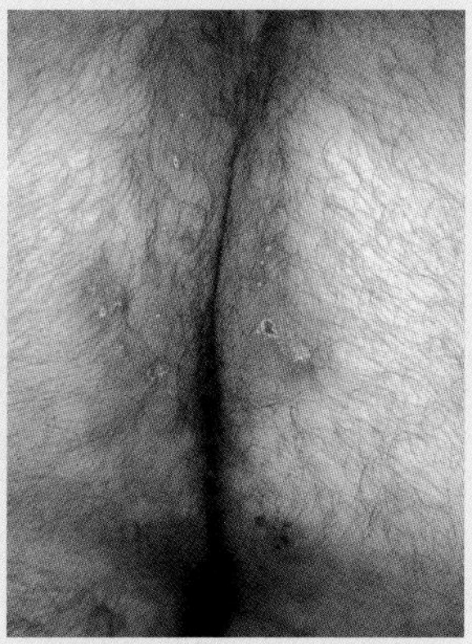
Hidradenitis suppurativa

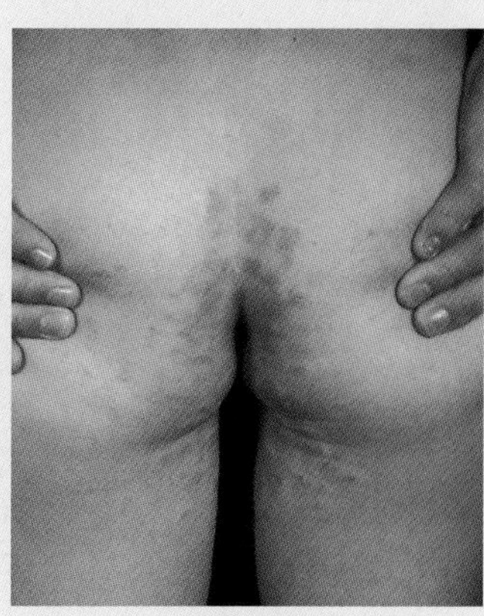
Scabies

Ear

Actinic keratosis (p. 813)
Allergic contact dermatitis (p. 143)
Atypical fibroxanthoma
Basal cell carcinoma (p. 805)
Bowen's disease (p. 822)
Cellulitis (p. 366)
Chondrodermatitis nodularis (p. 795)
Eczema (p. 94)
Epidermal cyst (p. 796)
Hydroa vacciniforme (p. 753)
Keloid (lobe) (p. 788)
Lichen simplex chronicus (p. 99)
Lupus erythematosus (discoid) (p. 682)
Lymphangitis (p. 349)
Melanoma (p. 860)
Psoriasis (p. 274)
Ramsay Hunt syndrome (herpes zoster) (p. 484)
Relapsing polychondritis
Seborrheic dermatitis (p. 312)
Squamous cell carcinoma (p. 826)
Tophi (gout)
Weathering nodules

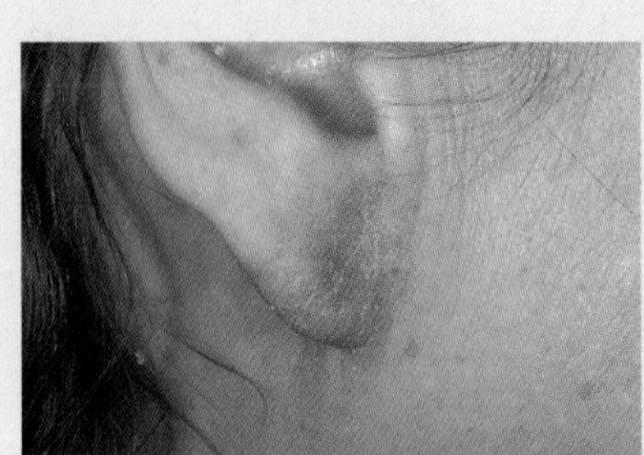
Allergic contact dermatitis

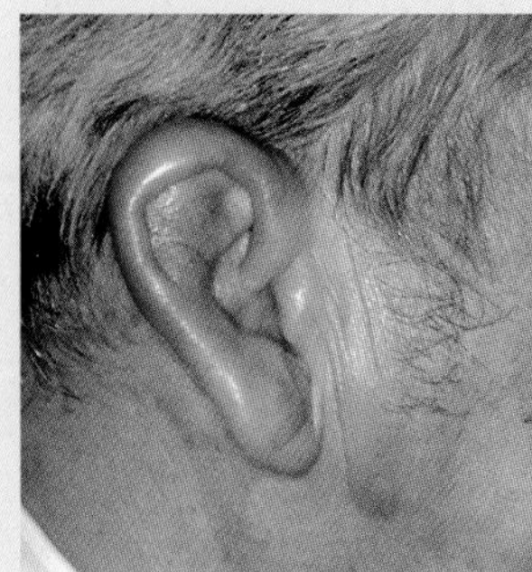
Relapsing polychondritis

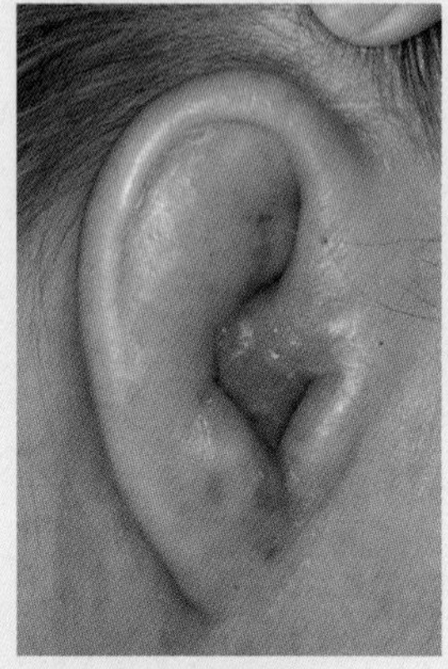
Cellulitis

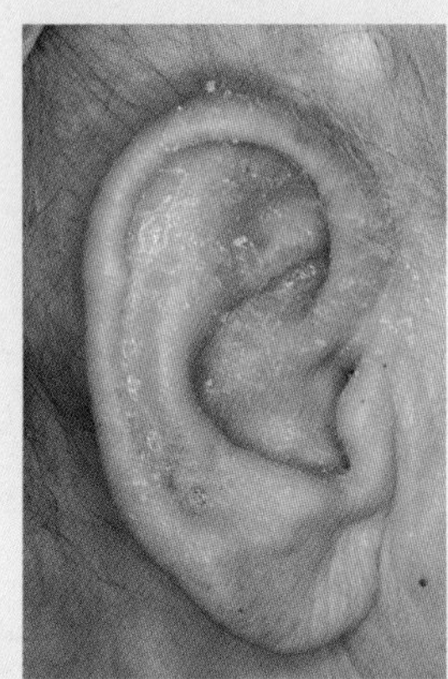
Eczema

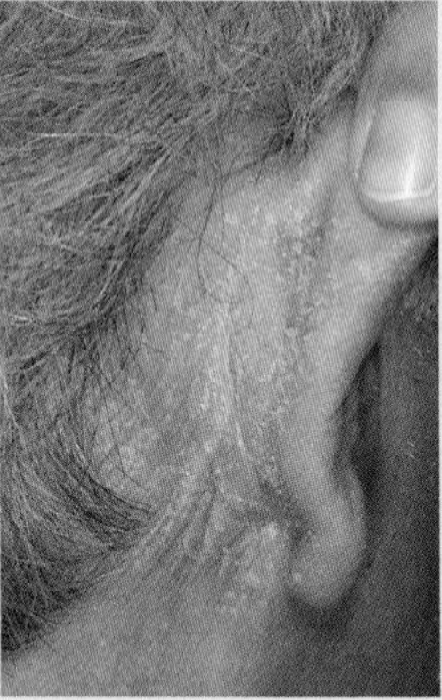
Seborrheic dermatitis

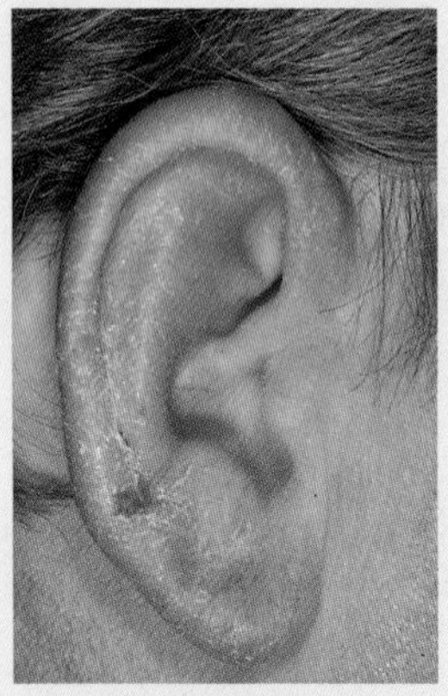
Allergic contact dermatitis

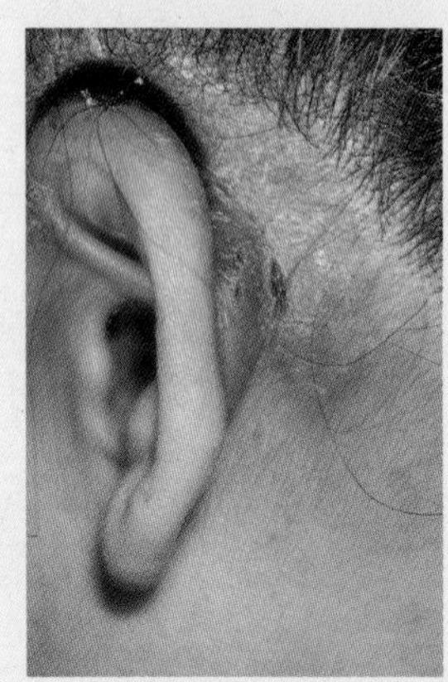
Lichen simplex chronicus

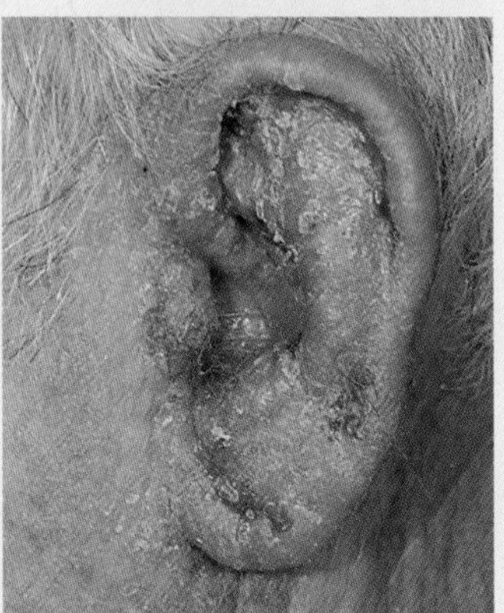
Eczema, impetiginized

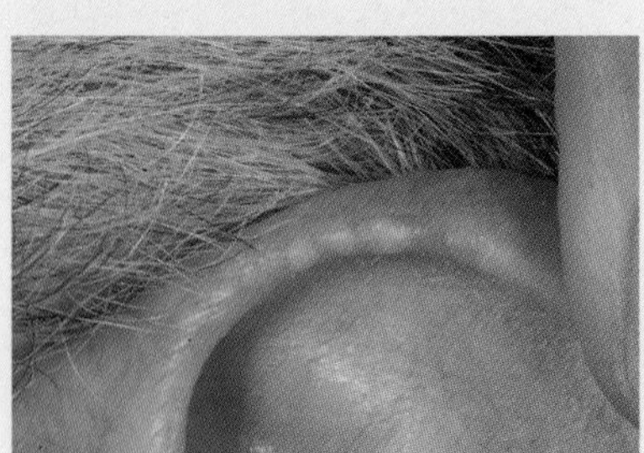
Weathering nodules

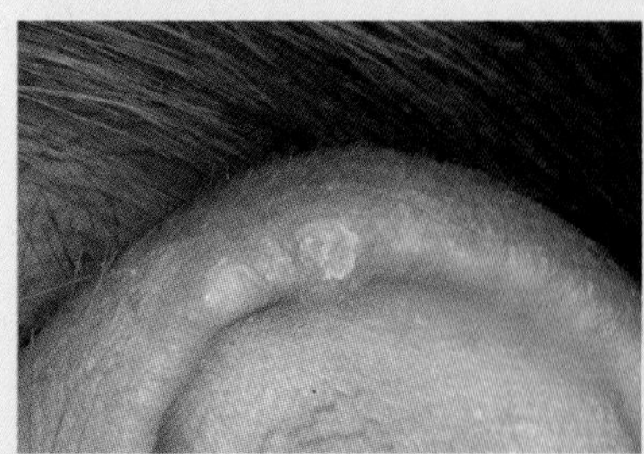
Chondrodermatitis

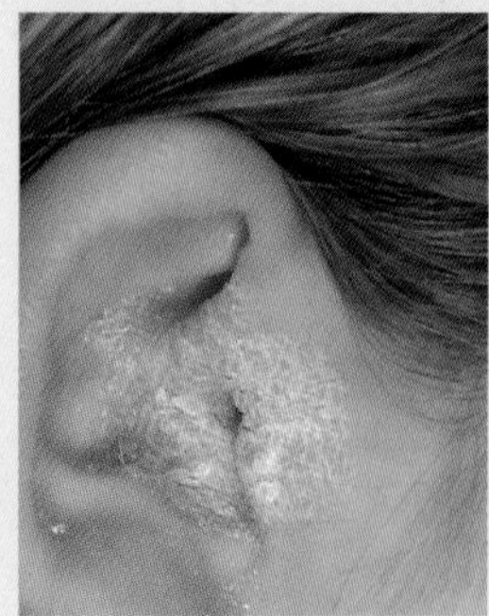
Psoriasis, chronic plaque

Elbows and knees

Atopic dermatitis (p. 161)
Calcinosis cutis/CREST syndrome (p. 704)
Dermatitis herpetiformis (p. 643)
Erythema multiforme (p. 710)
Gout
Granuloma annulare (p. 976)
Lichen simplex chronicus (p. 104)
Nummular eczema (p. 111)
Psoriasis (p. 265)
Rheumatoid nodule
Scabies (p. 586)
Steroid atrophy (p. 86)
Xanthoma (p. 980)

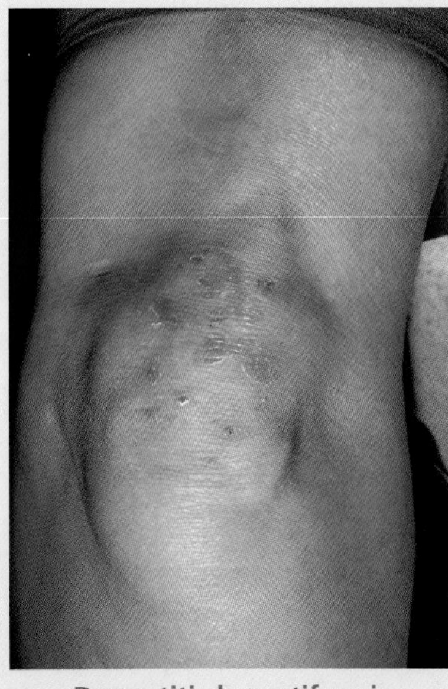
Dermatitis herpetiformis

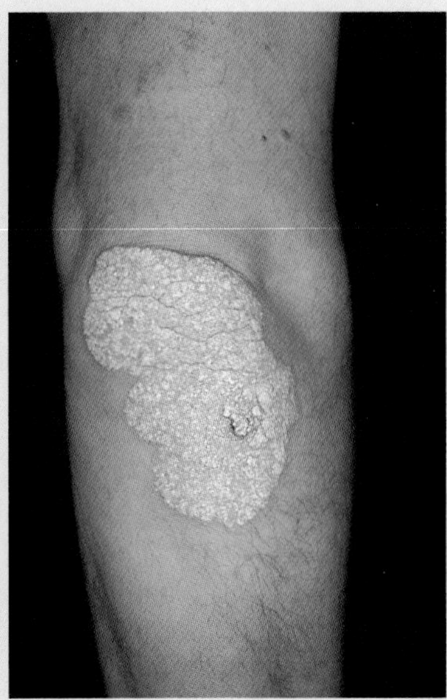
Psoriasis, chronic plaque

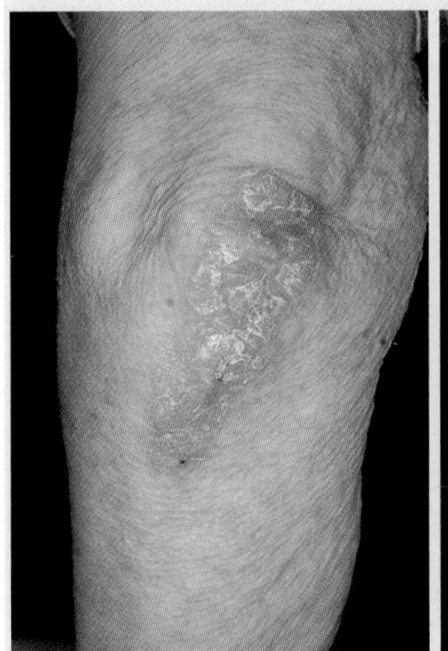
Psoriasis, chronic plaque

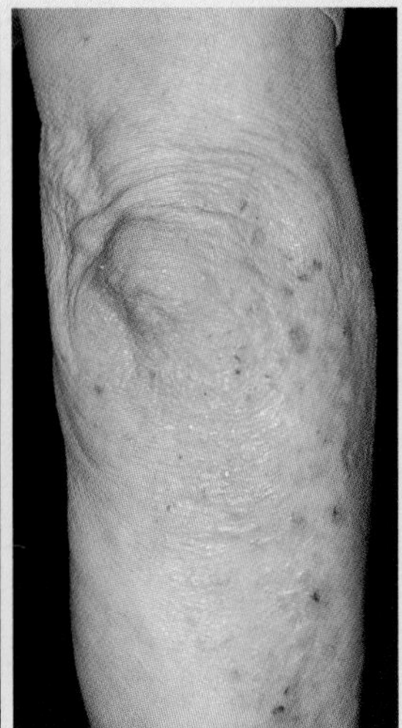
Atopic dermatitis

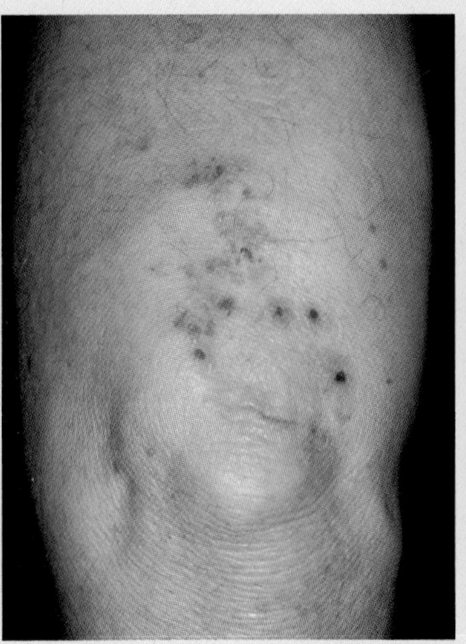
Dermatitis herpetiformis

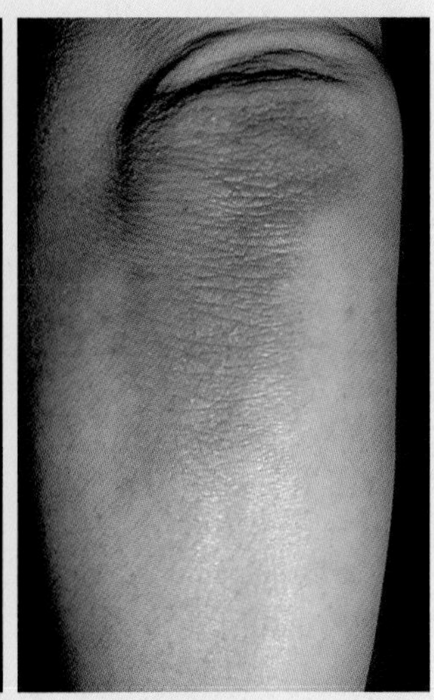
Lichen simplex chronicus

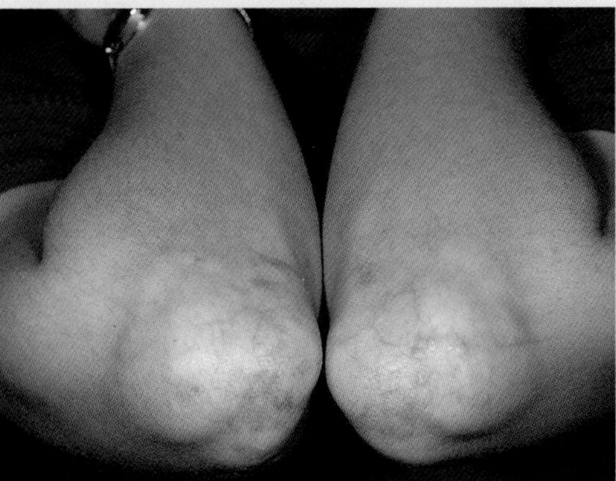
Steroid atrophy

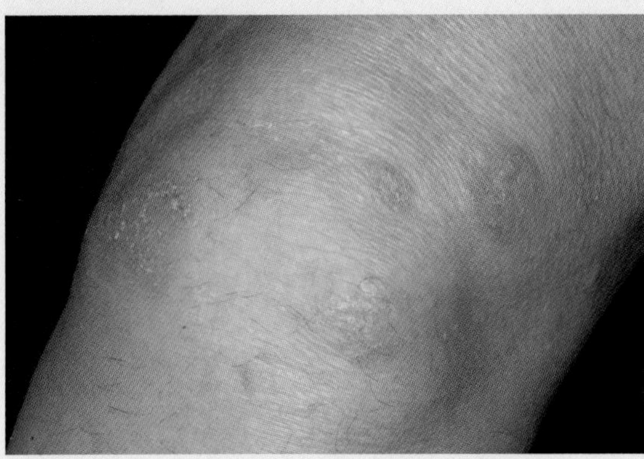
Nummular eczema

Face

Actinic keratosis (p. 813)
Adenoma sebaceum (p. 988)
Allergic contact dermatitis (p. 147)
Alopecia mucinosa
Angioedema (p. 200)
Atopic dermatitis (p. 158)
Basal cell carcinoma (p. 804)
Cowden disease (p. 997)
CREST syndrome (p. 705)
Dermatosis papulosa nigra (p. 786)
Eczema (p. 91)
Erysipelas (p. 342)
Factitial dermatitis (p. 120)
Favre-Racouchot syndrome (senile comedones) (p. 251)
Birt-Hogg-Dubé syndrome (p. 1004)
Herpes simplex (p. 470)
Herpes zoster (p. 482)
Impetigo (p. 337)
Keratoacanthoma (p. 790)
Keratosis pilaris (p. 168)
Lentigo maligna (p. 868)
Lupus erythematosus (p. 687)
Melasma (p. 773)
Molluscum contagiosum (p. 465)
Nevus sebaceous (p. 794)
Pemphigus erythematosus (p. 649)
Perioral dermatitis (p. 253)
Pityriasis alba (white spots) (p. 170)
Post-topical steroid flare (p. 83)
Psoriasis (p. 264)
Rosacea (p. 256)
Scleroderma (p. 700)
Sebaceous hyperplasia (p. 799)
Seborrheic dermatitis (p. 312)
Seborrheic keratosis (p. 780)
Spitz nevus (p. 855)
Squamous cell carcinoma (p. 823)
Steroid rosacea (p. 83)
Stevens-Johnson syndrome (p. 716)
Sweet's syndrome (p. 734)
Sycosis barbae (folliculitis—beard) (p. 354)
Syphilis (p. 400)
Tinea (p. 517)
Trichoepitheliomas (p. 1003)
Varicella (p. 475)
Warts (flat) (p. 459)
Wegener's granulomatosis (p. 724)

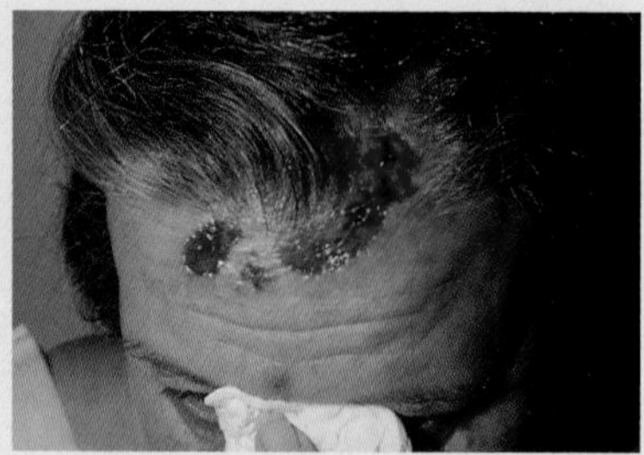
Factitial dermatitis

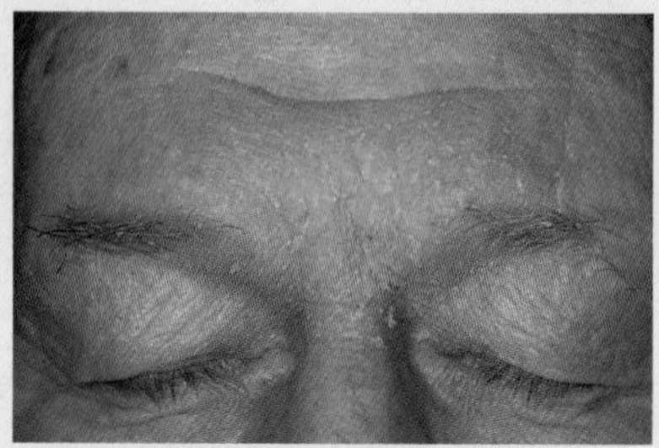
Seborrheic dermatitis

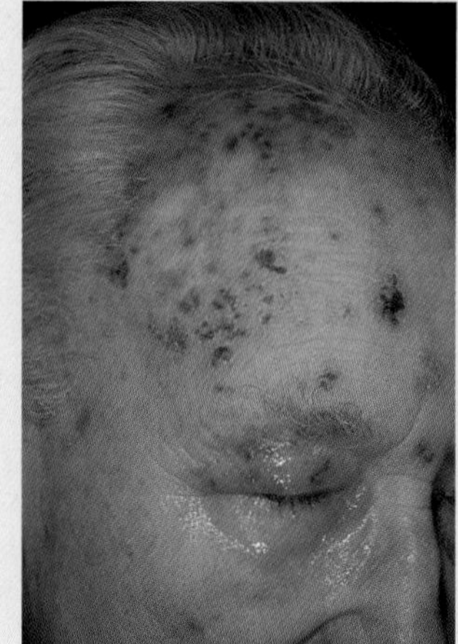
Herpes zoster

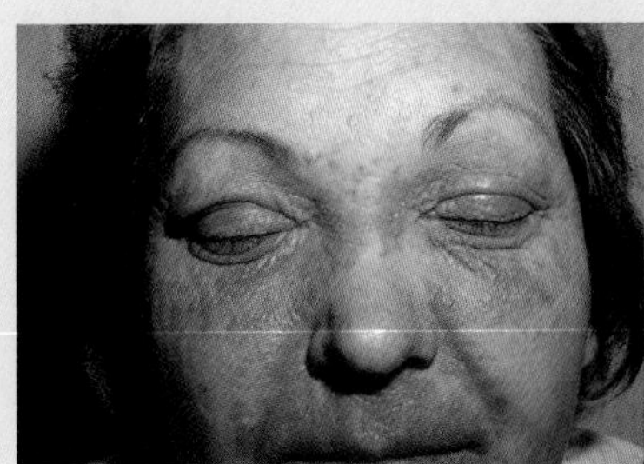
Allergic contact dermatitis

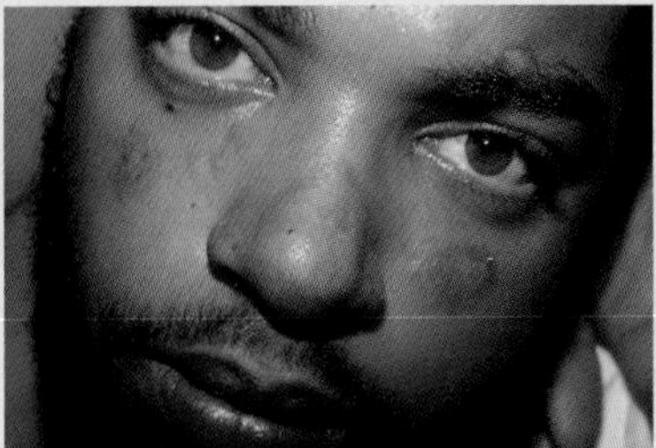
Lupus, chronic cutaneous

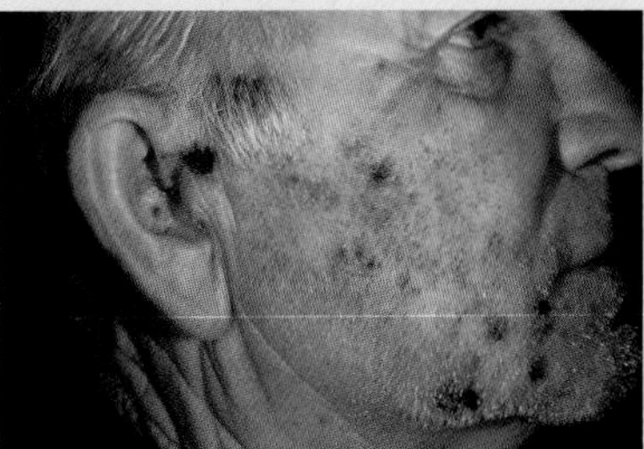
Herpes zoster

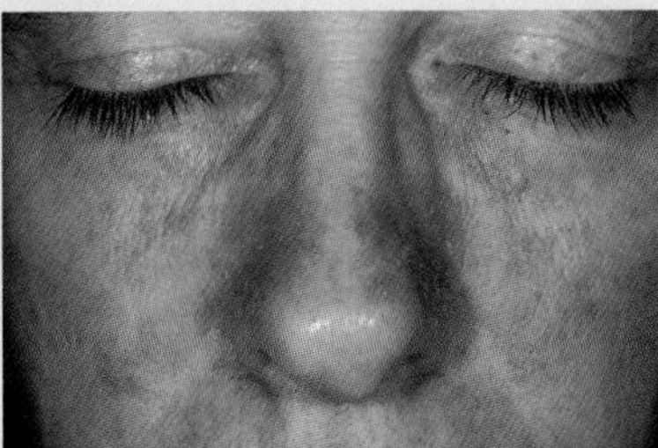
Seborrheic dermatitis

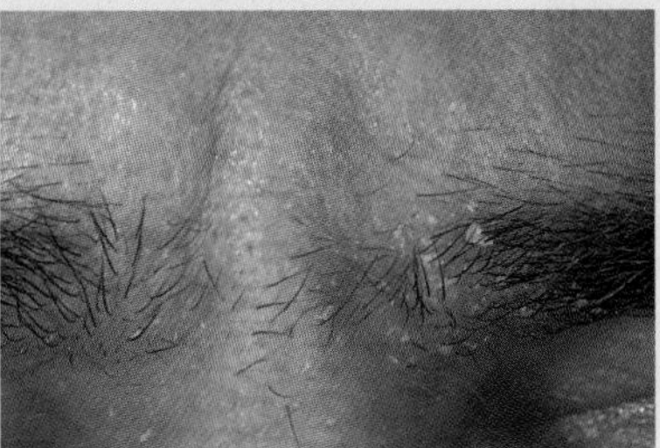
Seborrheic dermatitis

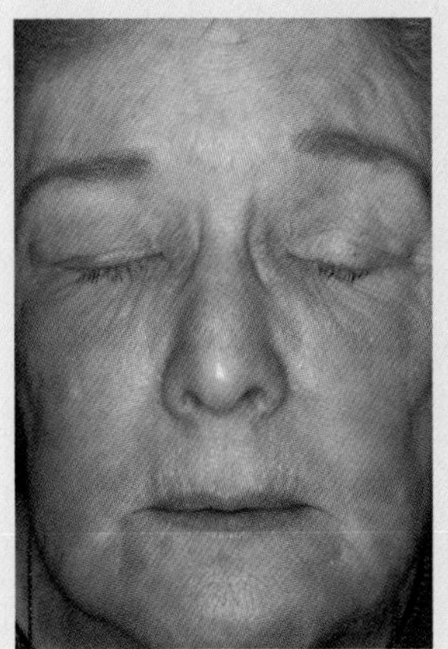
Allergic contact dermatitis

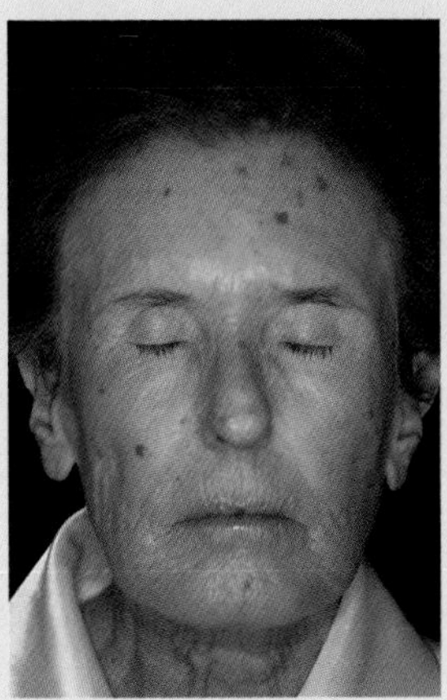
CREST syndrome

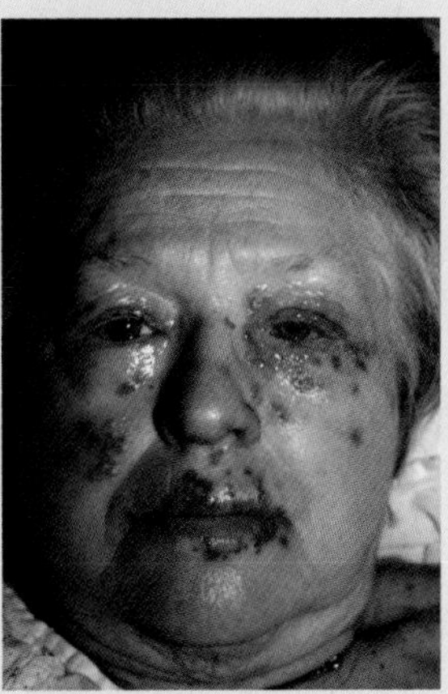
Eczema herpeticum

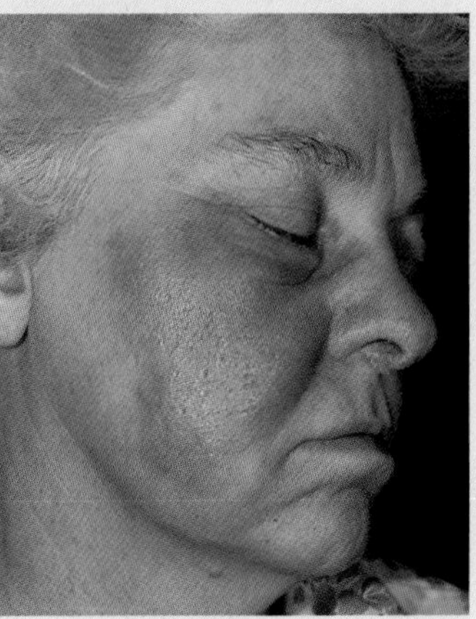
Erysipelas

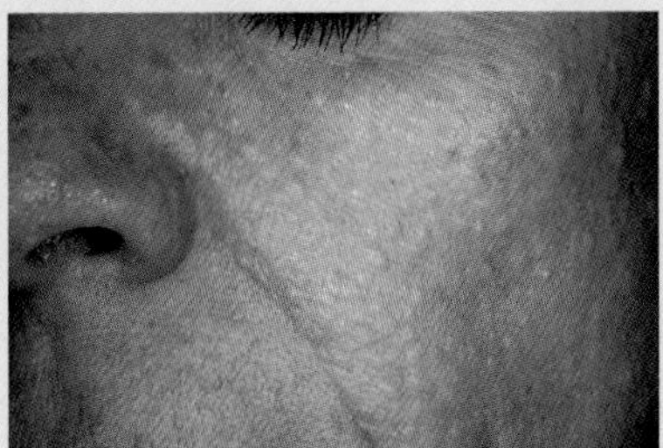
Birt-Hogg-Dubé syndrome

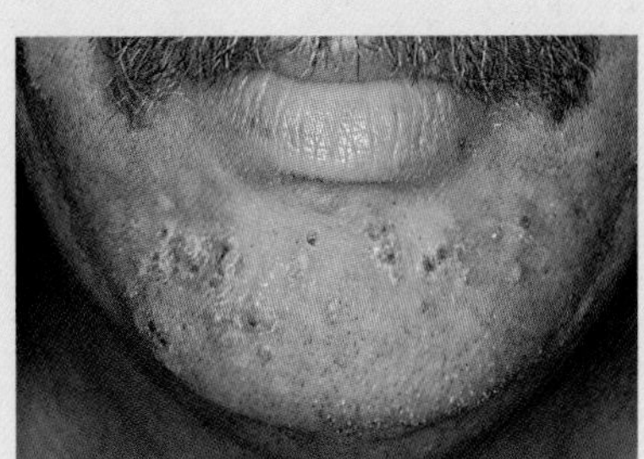
Folliculitis MRSA

Face

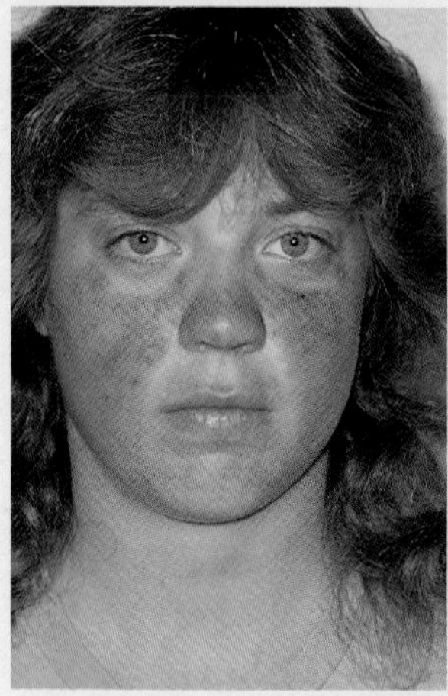

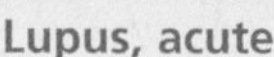

Lupus, acute

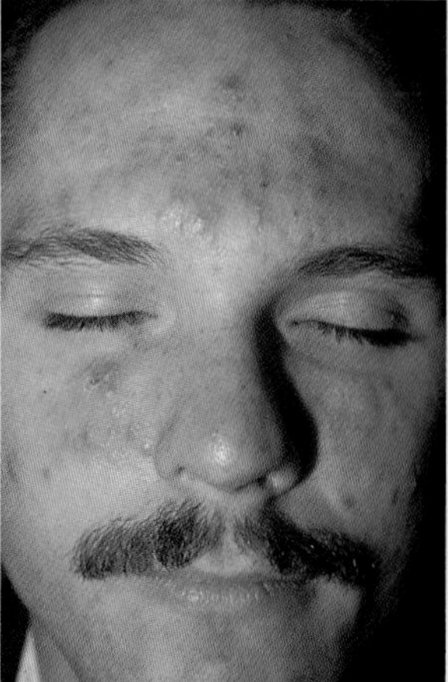

Rosacea

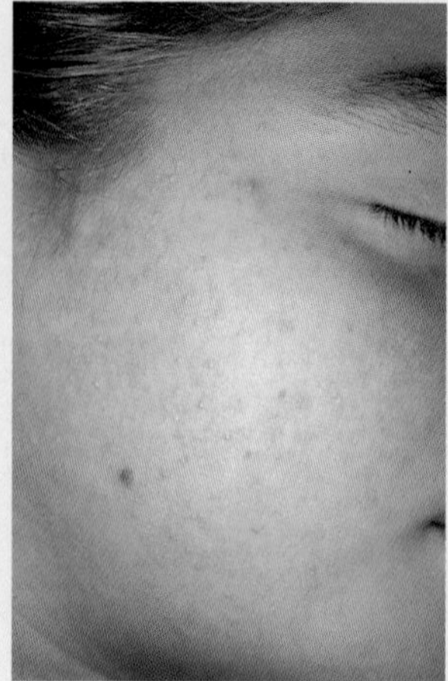

Keratosis pilaris

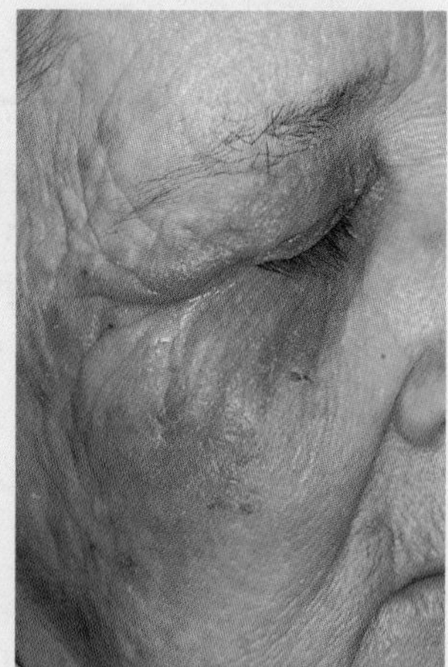

Allergic contact dermatitis

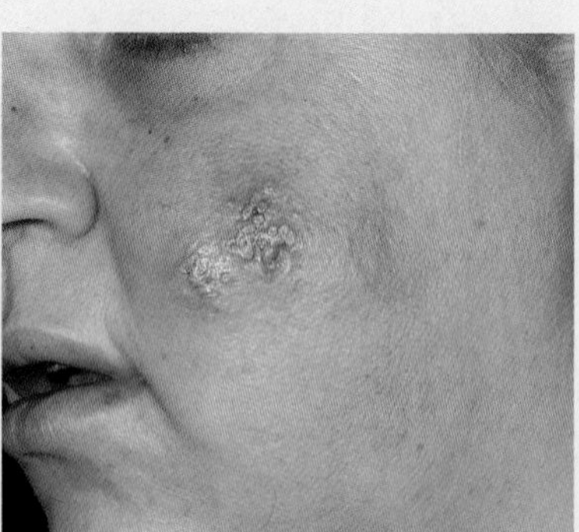

Herpes simplex, Type 1, primary

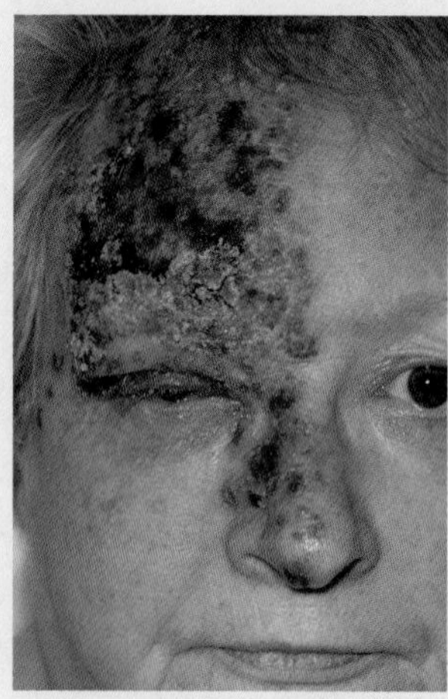

Herpes zoster

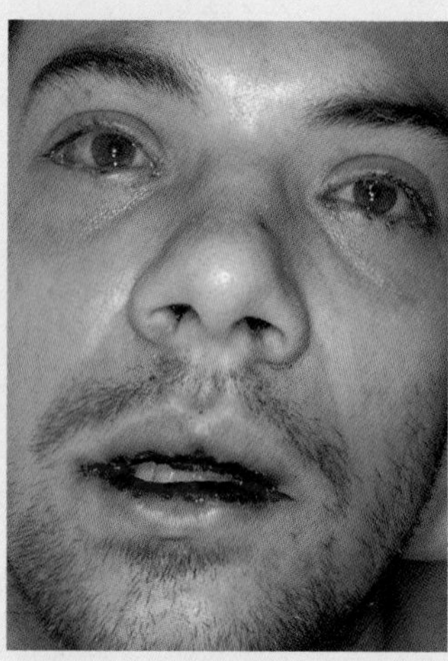

Stevens-Johnson syndrome

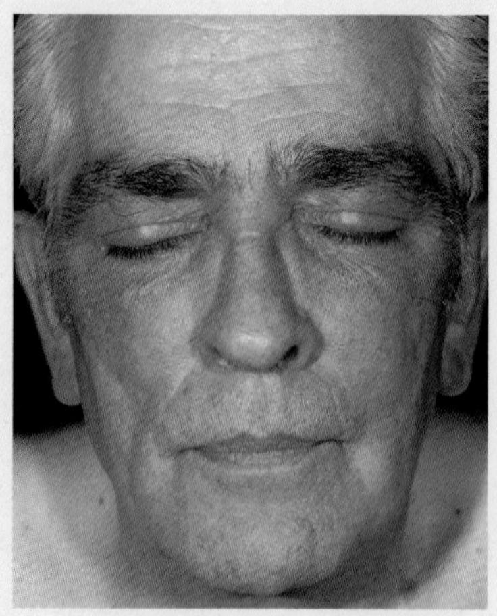

Post-topical steroid flare

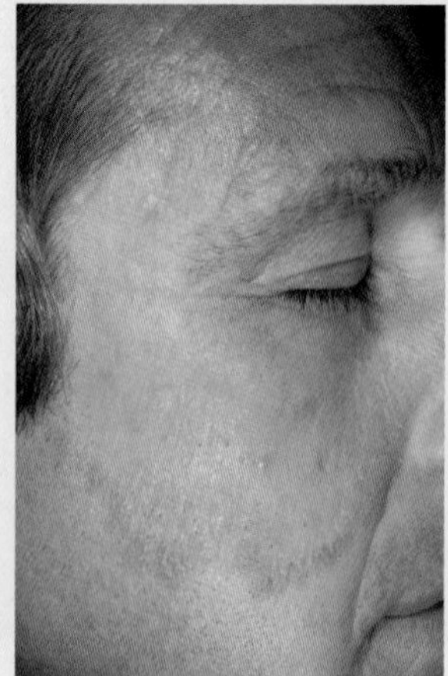

Tinea

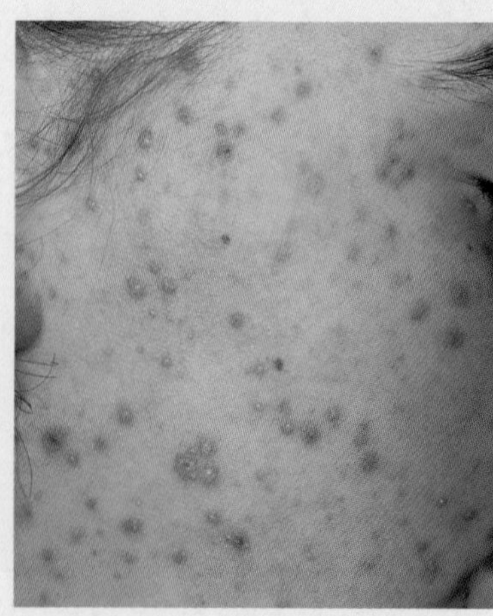

Varicella (chickenpox)

Finger

Atypical Sweet's syndrome (p. 735)
Dermatomyositis (p. 694)
Eczema (p. 106)
Candida (finger webs) (p. 535)
Erysipeloid (p. 359)
Fissure (p. 107)
Gonorrhea (p. 416)
Hand-foot-and-mouth disease (p. 547)
Herpetic whitlow (p. 955)
Id reaction (p. 109)
Mucous cyst (p. 970)
Orf
Pyogenic granuloma (p. 971)

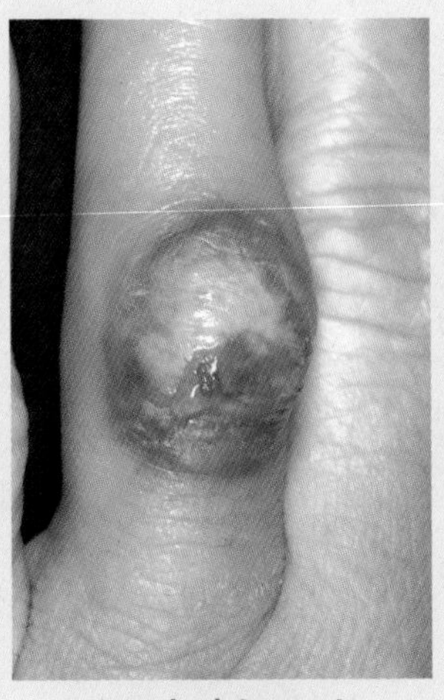
Atypical Sweet's syndrome

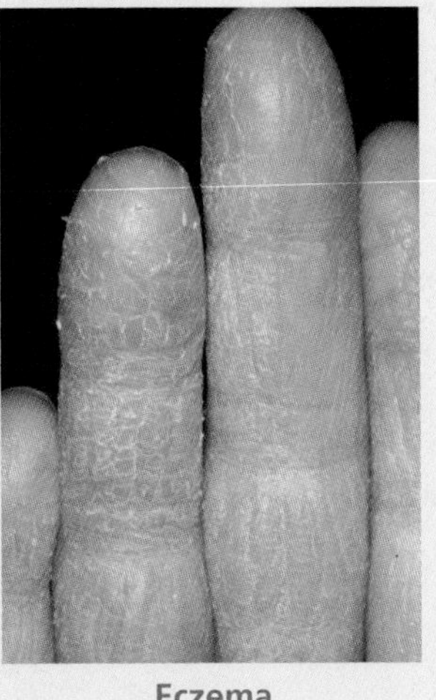
Eczema

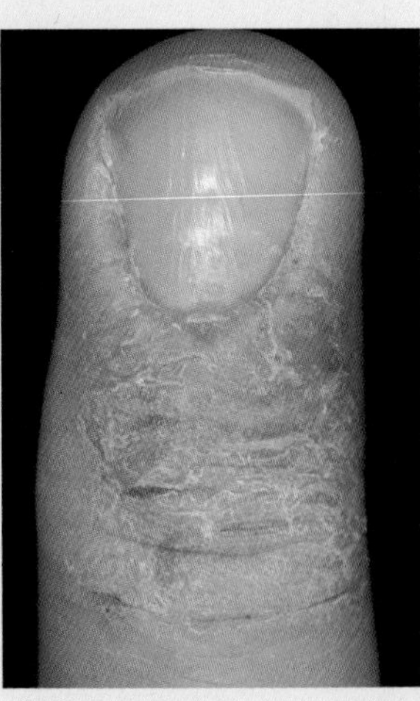
Eczema

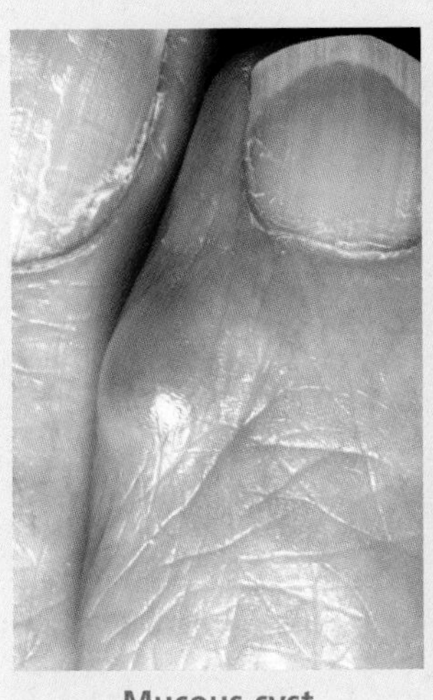
Mucous cyst

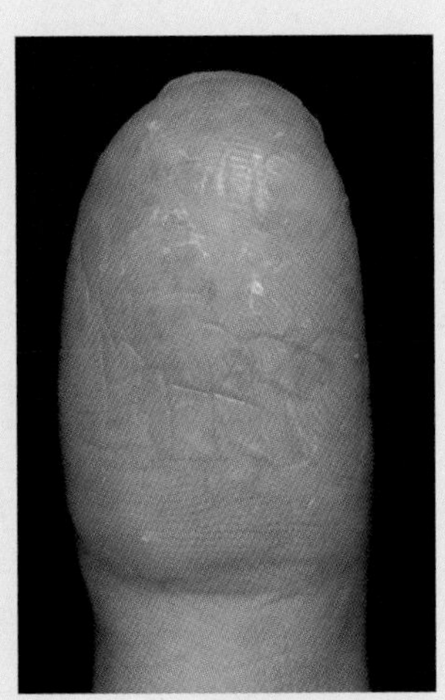
Eczema

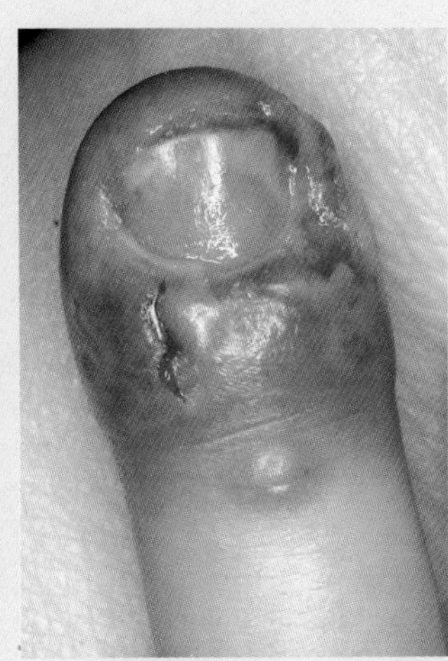
Herpetic whitlow

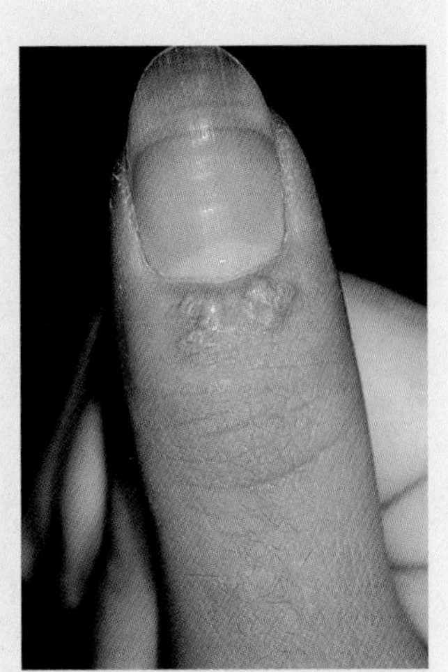
Herpetic whitlow

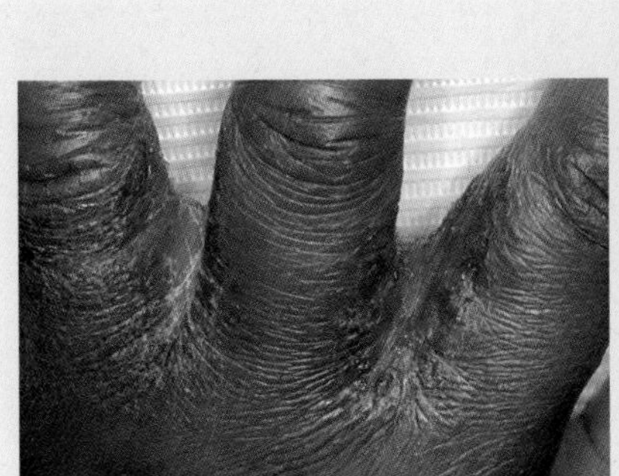
Candida (finger webs)

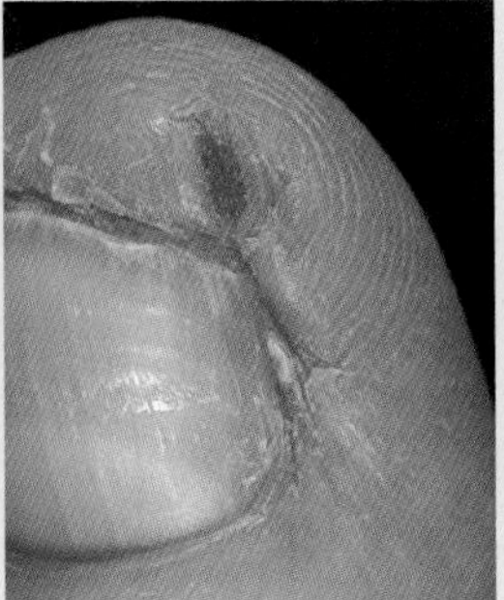
Fissure

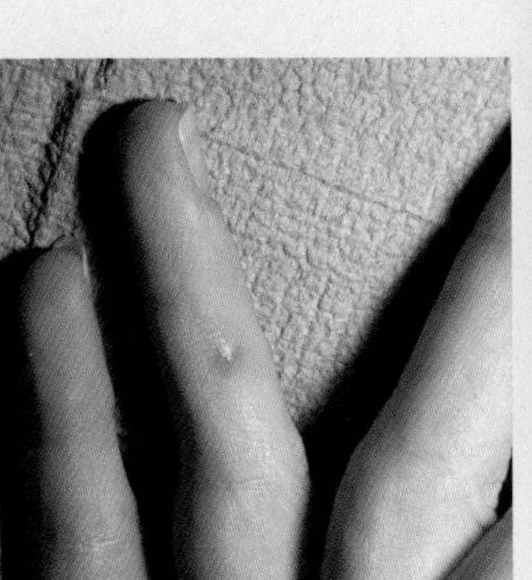
Gonorrhea

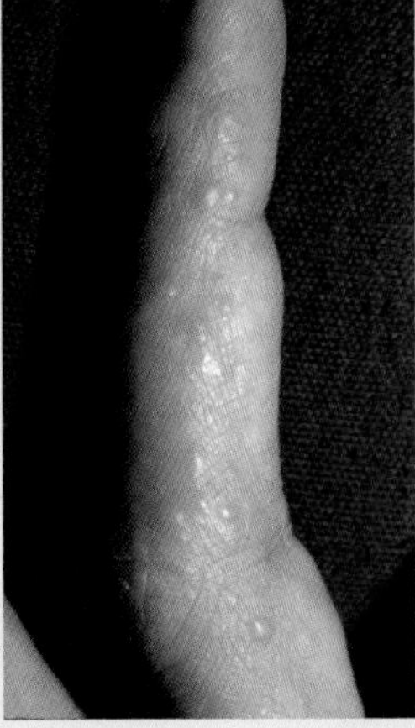
Id reaction

Foot (dorsum and sides)

Actinic keratosis (p. 812)
Atopic dermatitis (p. 165)
Calcaneal petechiae (black heel) (p. 461)
Contact dermatitis (p. 142)
Eczema (p. 96)
Erythema multiforme (p. 713)
Granuloma annulare (p. 976)
Hand-foot-and-mouth disease (p. 548)
Lichen planus (p. 320)
Lichen simplex chronicus (p. 116)
Meningococcemia (p. 371)
Psoriasis (p. 267)
Pyogenic granuloma (pp. 906, 971)
Reiter syndrome (p. 272)
Scabies (p. 586)
Tinea (p. 495)
Vasculitis (p. 728)

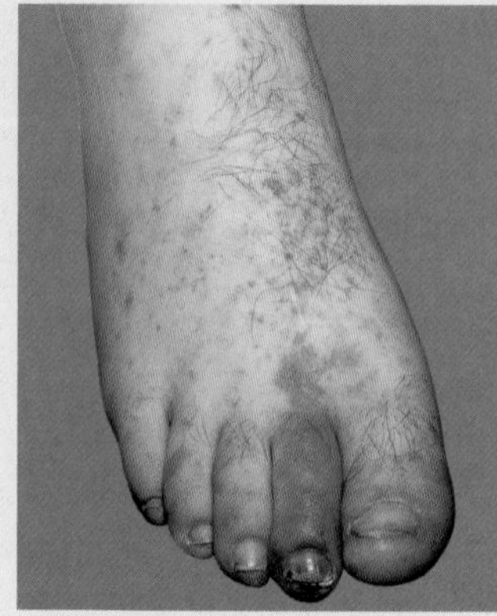

Meningococcemia

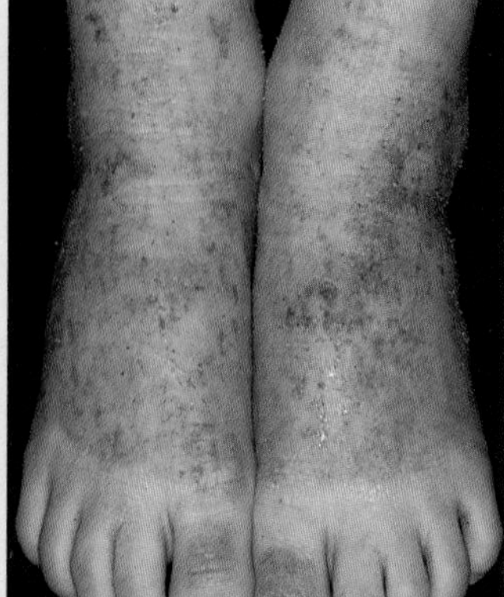

Atopic dermatitis

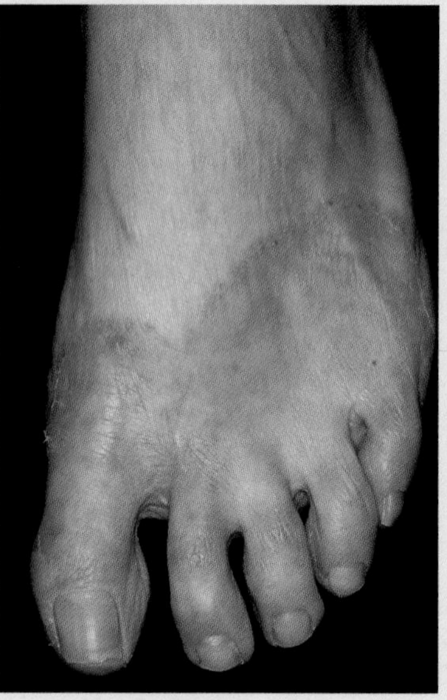

Tinea

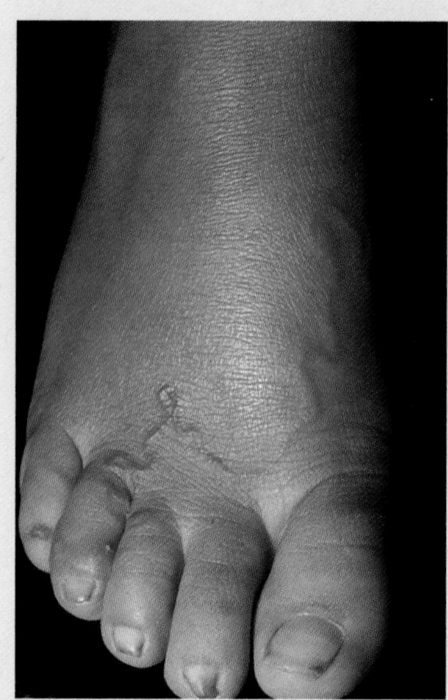

Cutaneous larva migrans

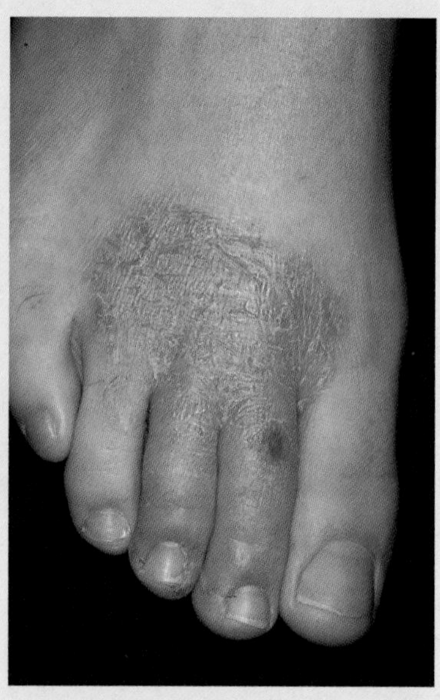

Eczema

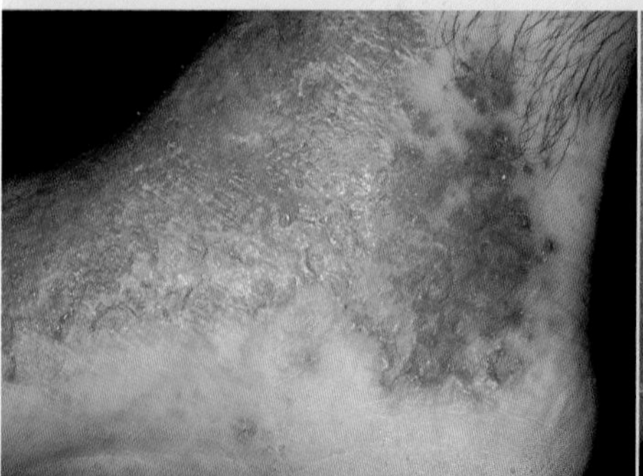

Eczema, impetiginized

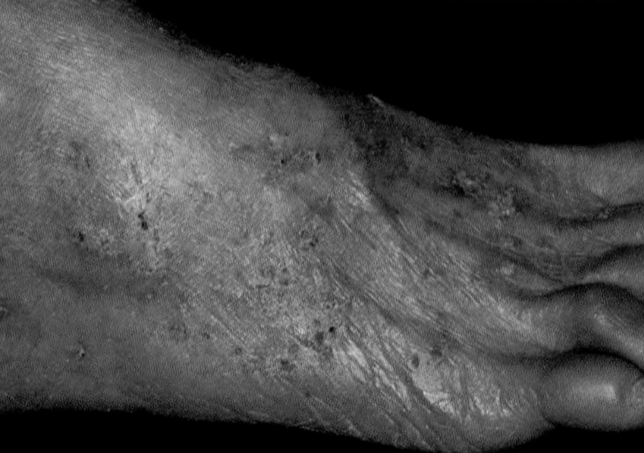

Actinic keratosis

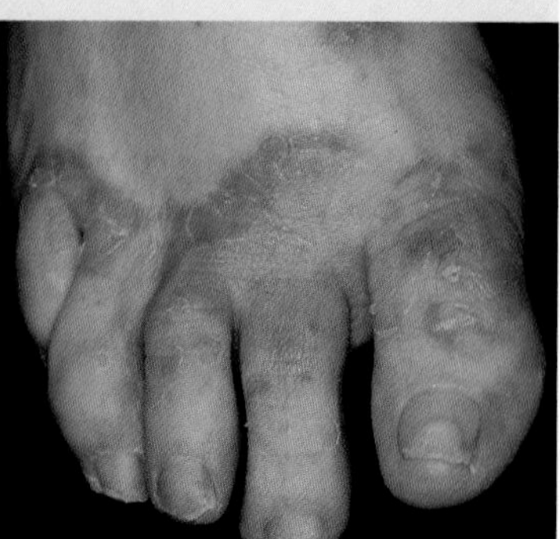

Tinea incognito

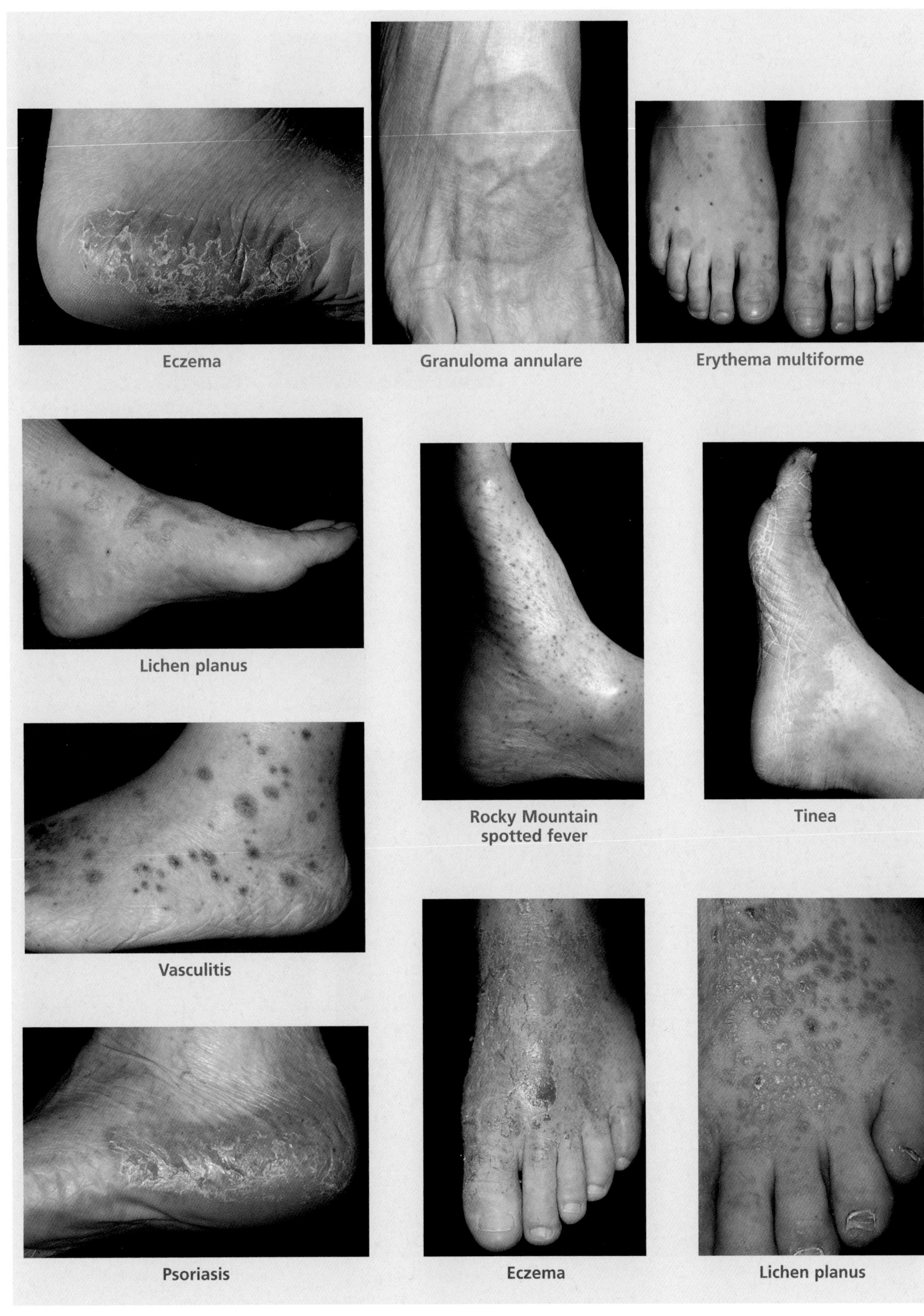
Eczema
Granuloma annulare
Erythema multiforme
Lichen planus
Rocky Mountain spotted fever
Tinea
Vasculitis
Psoriasis
Eczema
Lichen planus

Foot (sole)

Arsenical keratosis (p. 824)
Chapped fissured feet (p. 113)
Corn (clavus) (p. 461)
Cutaneous larva migrans (p. 625)
Eczema (p. 96)
Epidermolysis bullosa (p. 664)
Erythema multiforme (p. 710)
Hand-foot-and-mouth disease (p. 548)
Hyperkeratosis
Keratoderma blennorrhagicum (Reiter syndrome) (p. 272)
Lichen planus (p. 320)
Melanoma (p. 870)
Nevi (p. 848)
Pitted keratolysis (p. 498)
Pityriasis rubra pilaris (p. 309)
Pseudomonas cellulitis (p. 369)
Psoriasis (p. 271)
Pyogenic granuloma (p. 971)
Rocky Mountain spotted fever (p. 611)
Scabies (infants) (p. 584)
Syphilis (secondary) (p. 407)
Tinea (p. 495)
Tinea (bullous) (p. 497)
Verrucous carcinoma (p. 830)
Warts (p. 460)

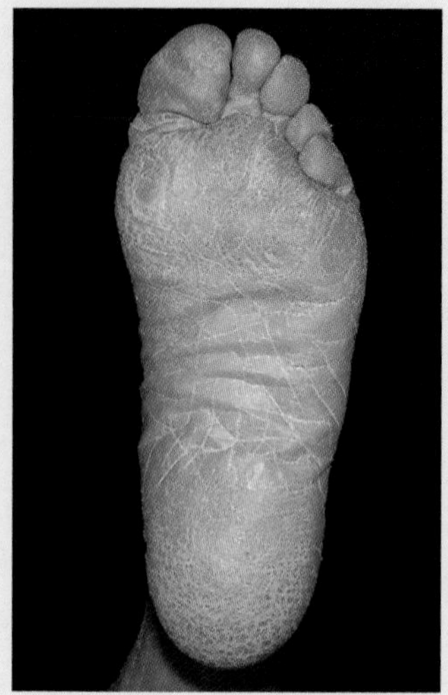

Tinea

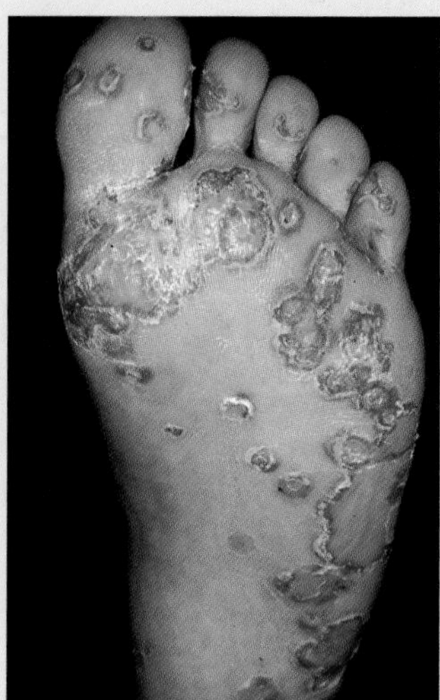

Reiter syndrome

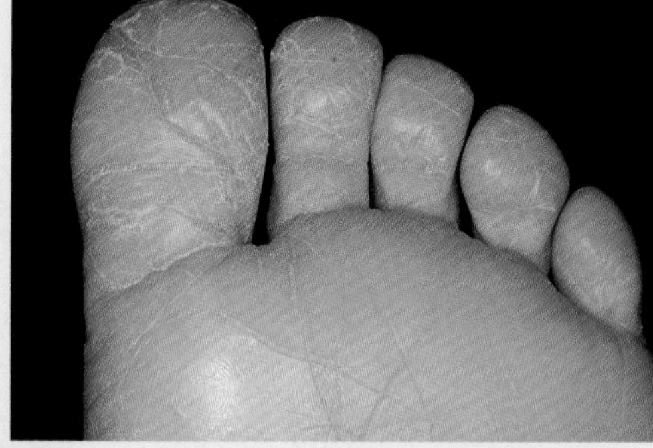

Chapped fissured feet

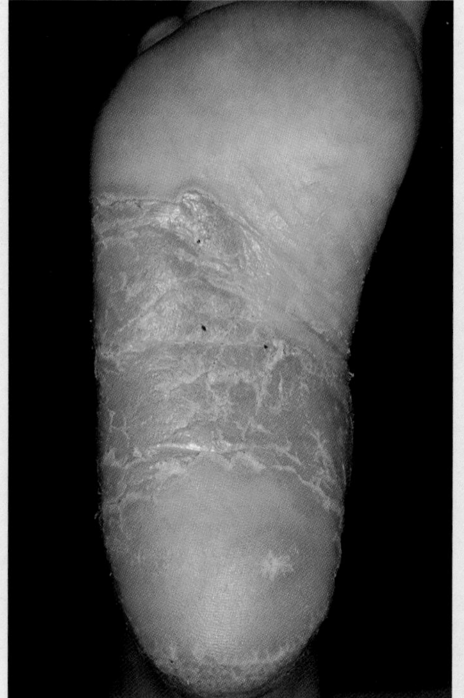

Psoriasis

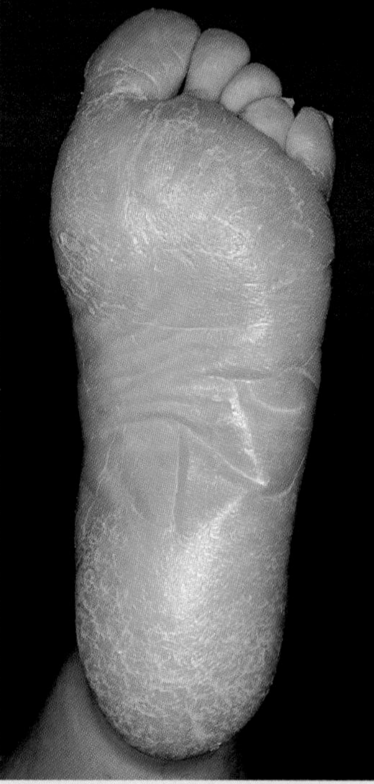

Pityriasis rubra pilaris

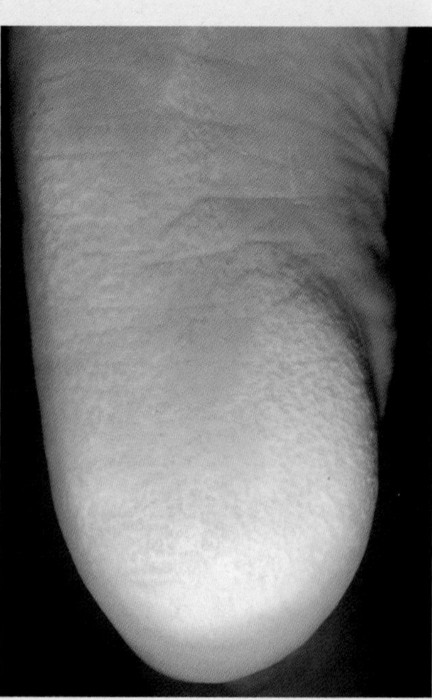

Pitted keratolysis

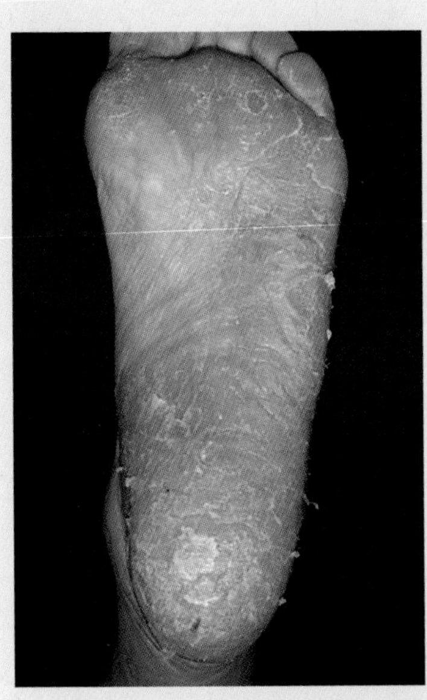

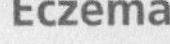
Eczema

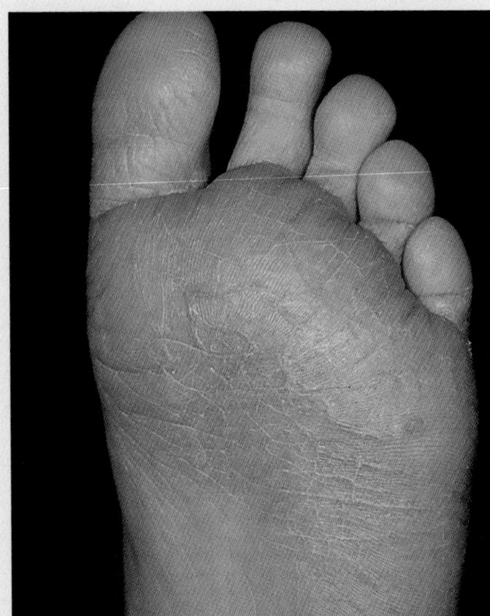
Chapped fissured feet

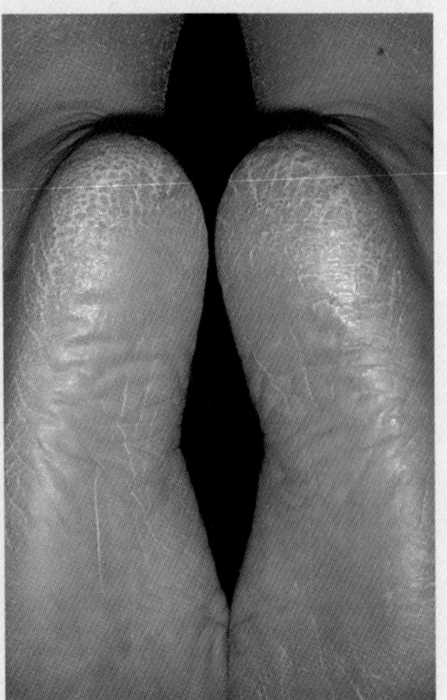
Eczema

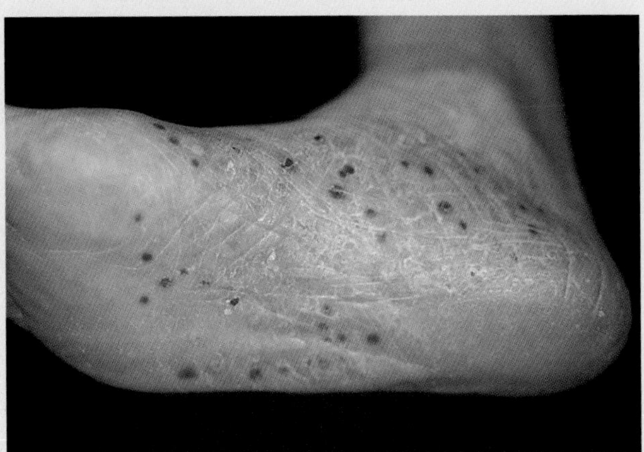
Pustular psoriasis

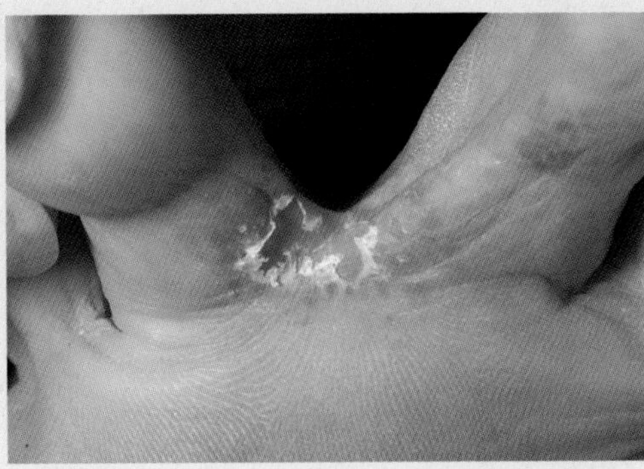
Tinea

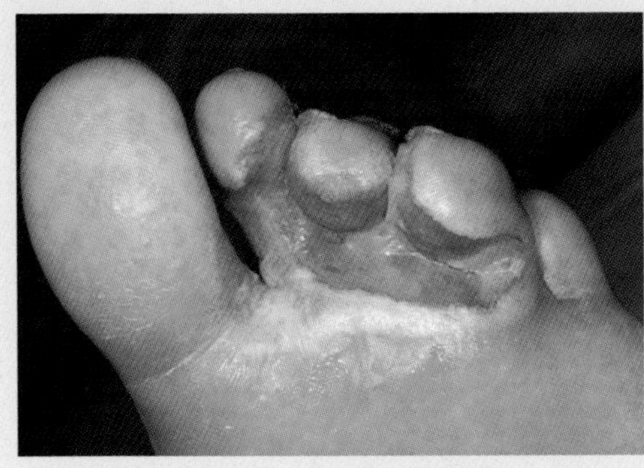
Pseudomonas cellulitis

Groin

Acrochordons (skin tags) (p. 785)
Benign familial chronic pemphigus (p. 663)
Candidiasis (p. 523)
Condyloma (p. 421)
Erythrasma (p. 501)
Extramammary Paget's disease (p. 844)
Hailey-Hailey disease (p. 663)
Hidradenitis suppurativa (p. 260)
Histiocytosis X
Intertrigo (p. 501)
Lichen simplex chronicus (pp. 104, 115)
Molluscum contagiosum (p. 465)
Pemphigus vegetans (p. 648)
Psoriasis (without scale) (p. 274)
Seborrheic keratosis (p. 780)
Striae (topical steroids) (p. 88)
Tinea (p. 499)

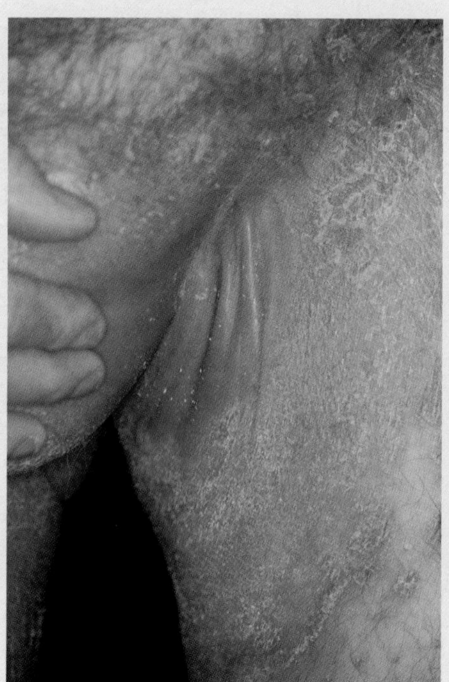

Inverse psoriasis

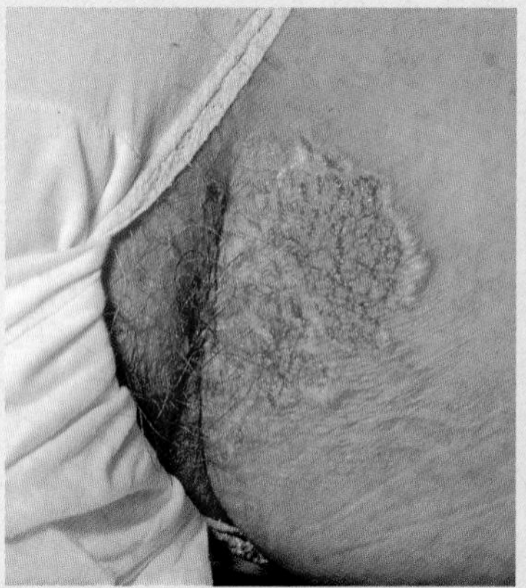

Benign familial chronic pemphigus (Hailey-Hailey disease)

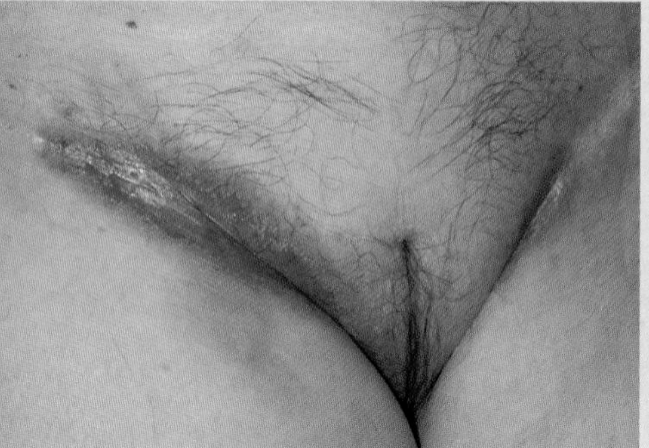

Candidiasis

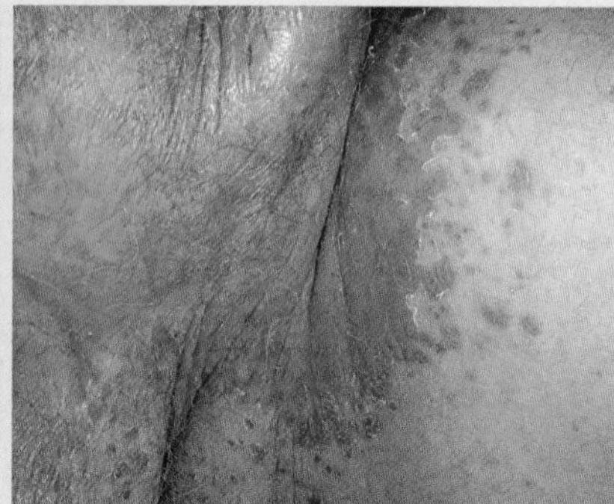

Candidiasis

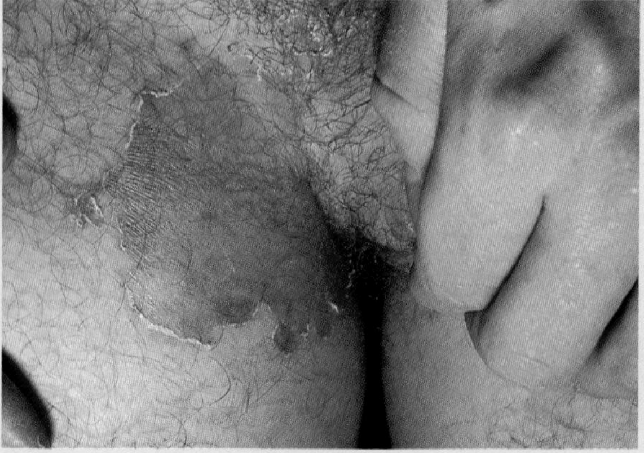

Tinea

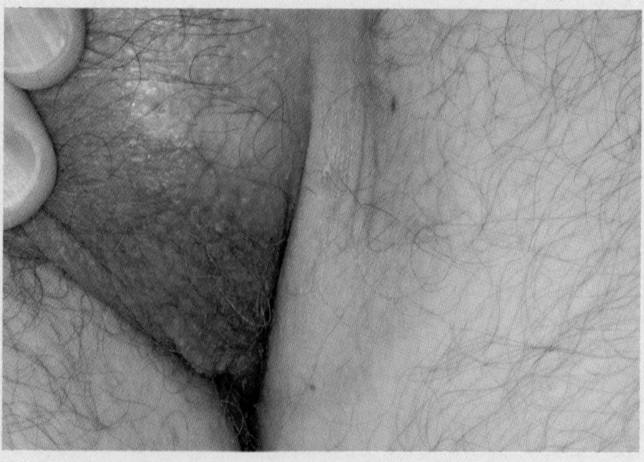

Erythrasma

Hands (dorsa)

Acquired digital fibrokeratoma
Acrosclerosis (p. 702)
Actinic keratosis (p. 812)
Atopic dermatitis (pp. 103, 164)
Atypical mycobacterium (p. 381)
Blue nevus (p. 856)
Calcinosis cutis/CREST syndrome (p. 704)
Cat-scratch disease (p. 614)
Contact dermatitis (p. 141)
Cowden disease (p. 998)
Dermatomyositis (p. 694)
Dyshidrosis (p. 109)
Eczema (p. 100)
Erysipeloid (p. 359)
Erythema multiforme (p. 714)
Gonorrhea (p. 416)
Granuloma annulare (p. 976)
Herpes simplex (p. 472)
Herpes zoster (p. 482)
Id reaction (p. 109)
Impetigo (p. 336)
Keratoacanthoma (p. 790)
Knuckle pads
Lentigo (p. 771)
Leishmaniasis (p. 633)
Lichen planus (p. 321)
Lichen simplex (pp. 104, 115)
Lupus erythematosus (systemic) (p. 688)
Paronychia (acute, chronic) (p. 954)
Pityriasis rubra pilaris (p. 309)
Polymorphous light eruption (p. 751)
Porphyria cutanea tarda (p. 757)
Pseudoporphyria (p. 759)
Psoriasis (p. 271)
Pyogenic granuloma (p. 971)
Scabies (p. 584)
Scleroderma (p. 701)
Seborrheic keratosis (p. 780)
Sporotrichosis
Squamous cell carcinoma (p. 826)
Stucco keratosis (p. 784)
Sweet's syndrome (p. 735)
Swimming pool granuloma (p. 379)
Tinea (p. 506)
Vesicular "id reaction" (p. 109)
Xanthoma (p. 981)

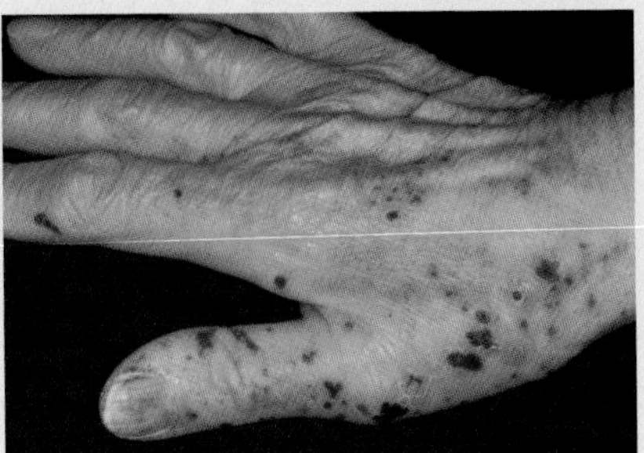
Herpes zoster

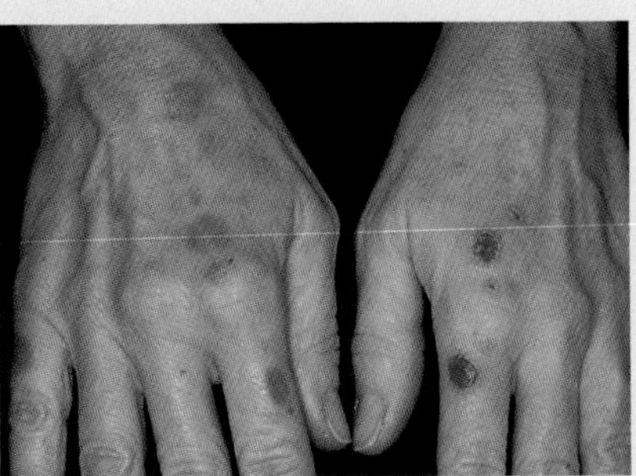
Pseudoporphyria

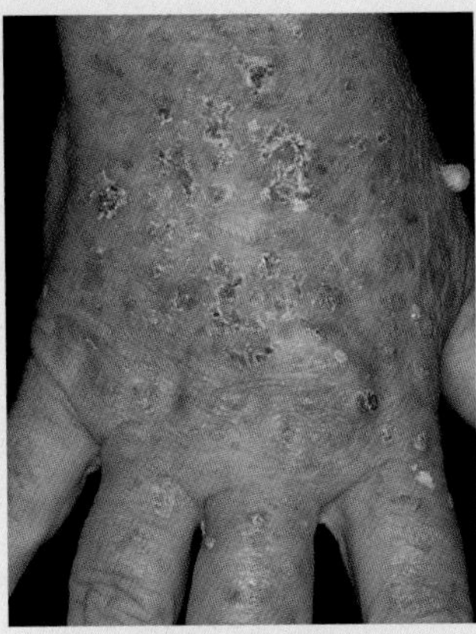
Actinic keratosis

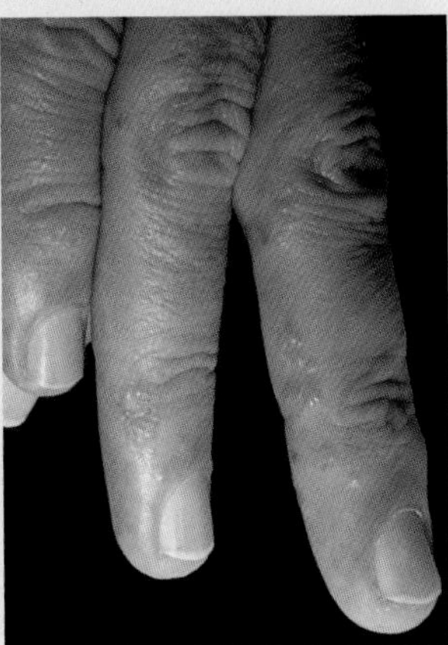
Dyshidrosis

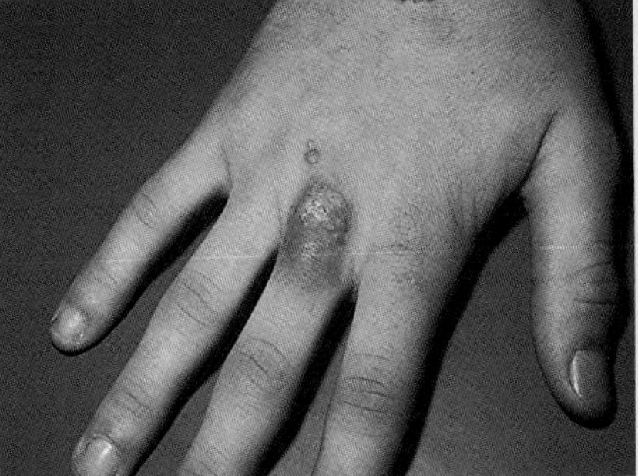
Atypical mycobacterium

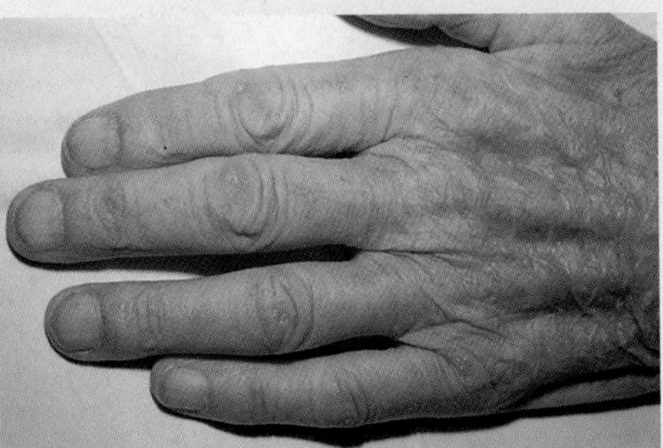
Dermatomyositis

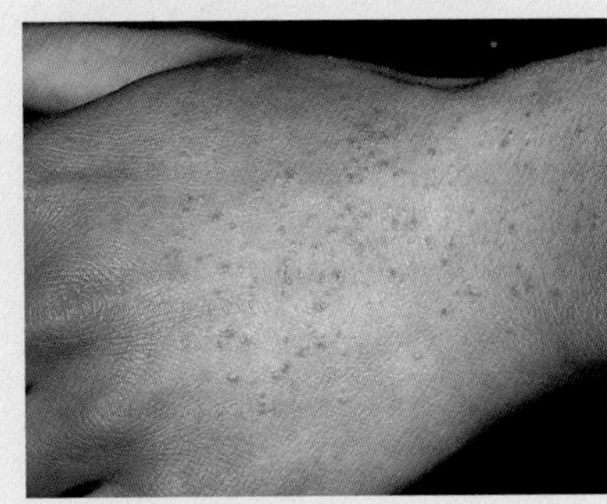
Polymorphous light eruption

Hands (dorsa)

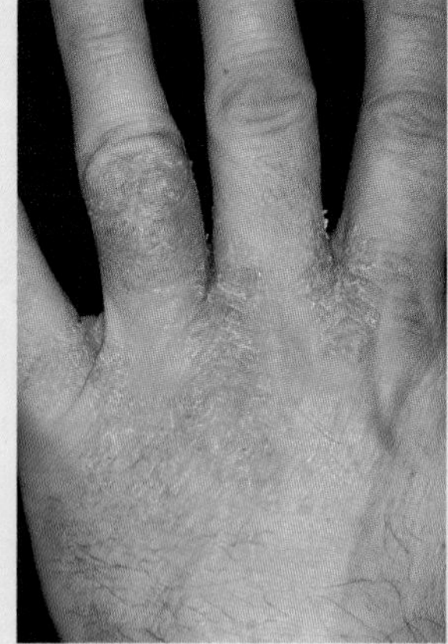
Eczema

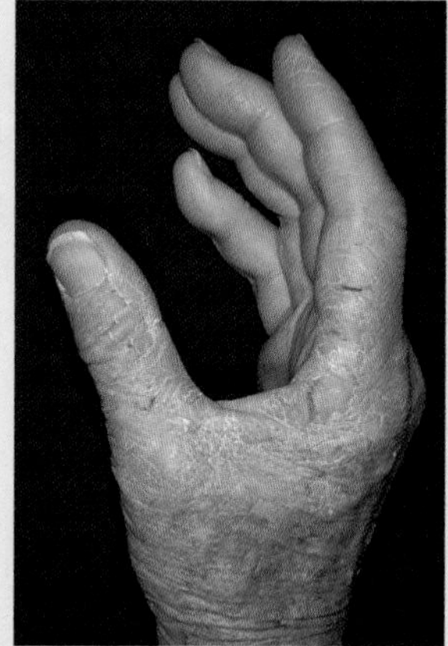
Eczema

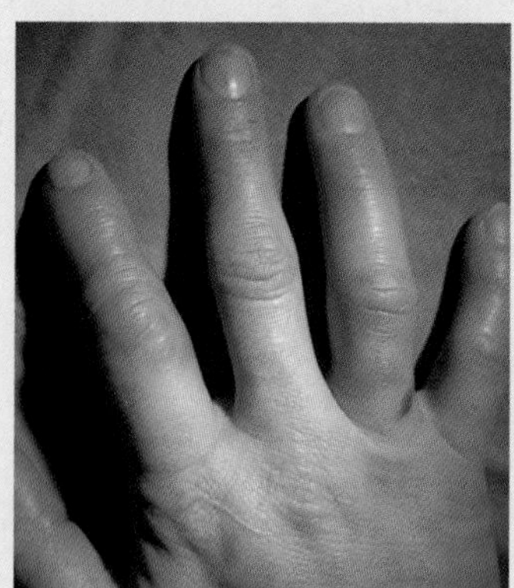
Erysipeloid

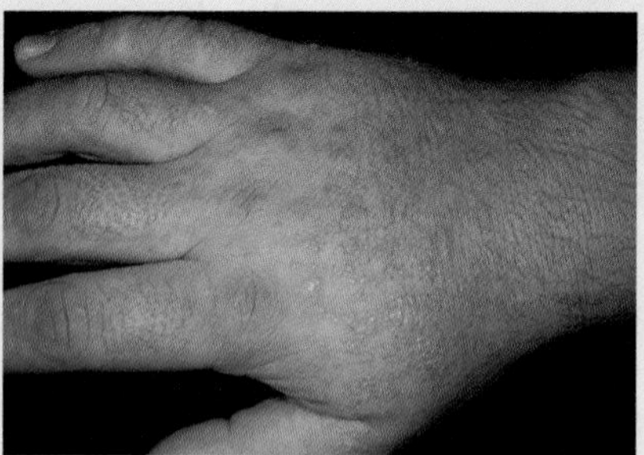
Lichen planus

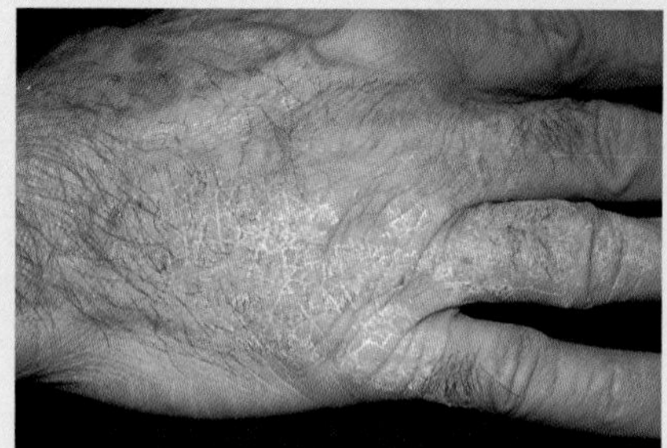
Lichen simplex chronicus

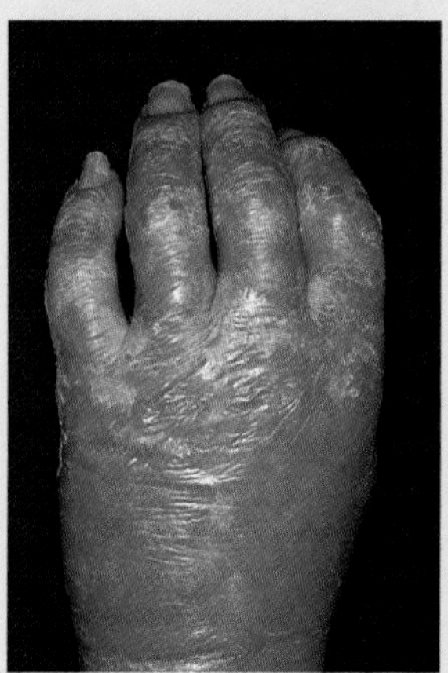
Erythrodermic psoriasis

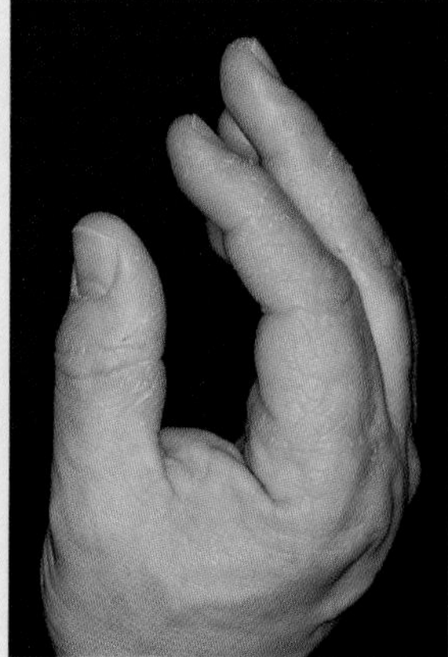
Psoriasis

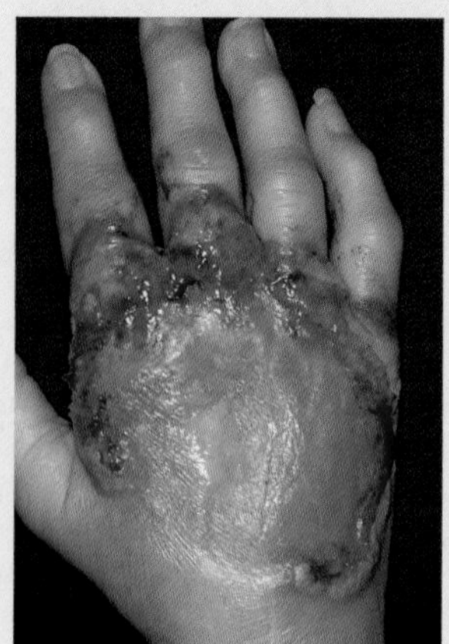
Atypical Sweet's syndrome

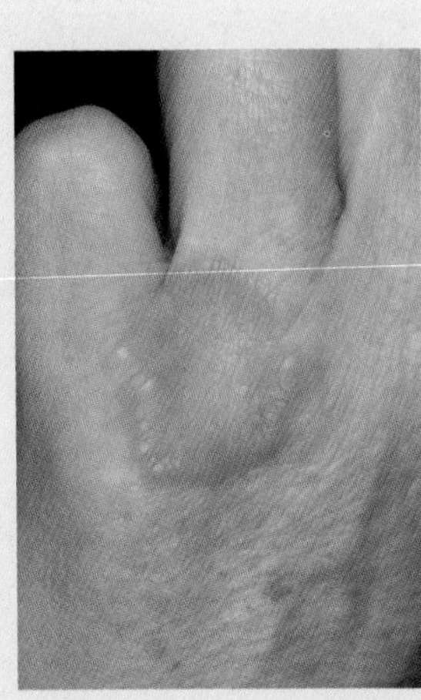
Granuloma annulare

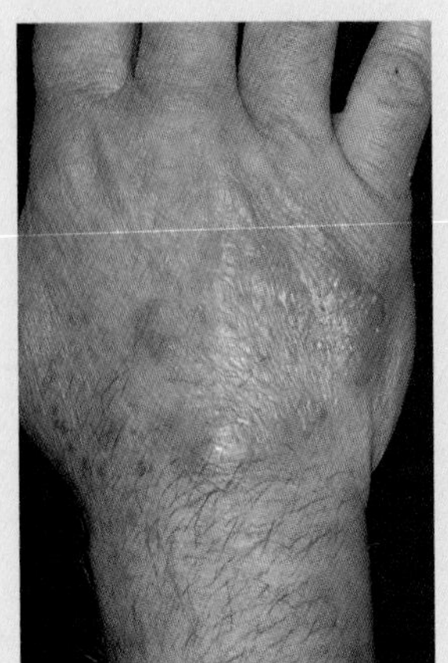
Tinea

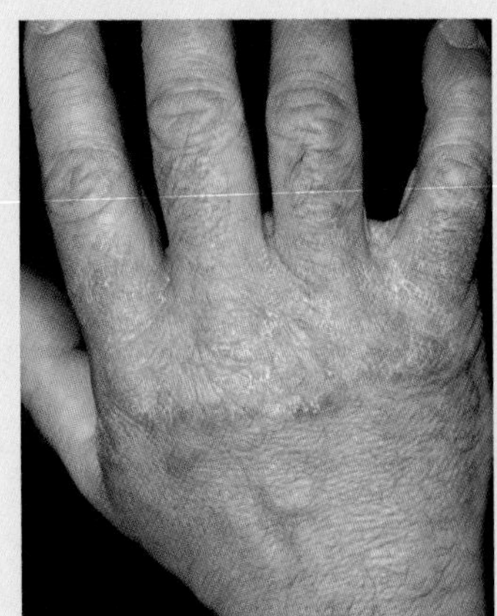
Tinea

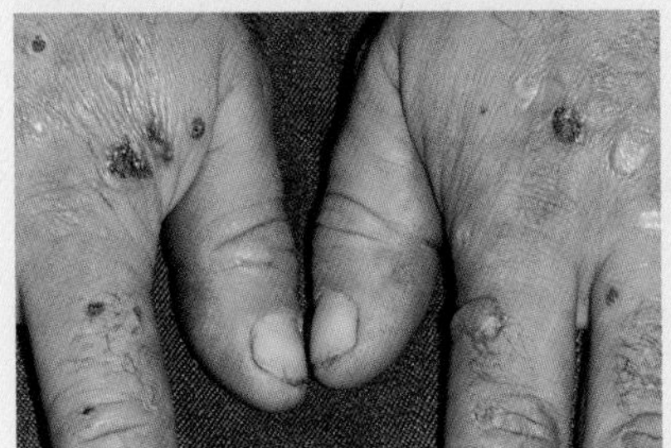
Porphyria cutanea tarda

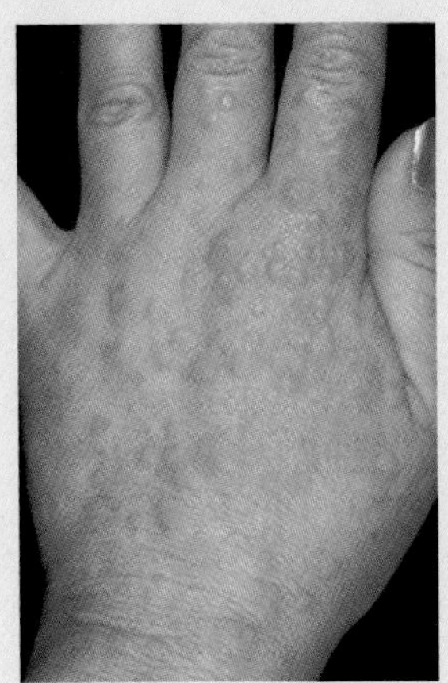
Erythema multiforme

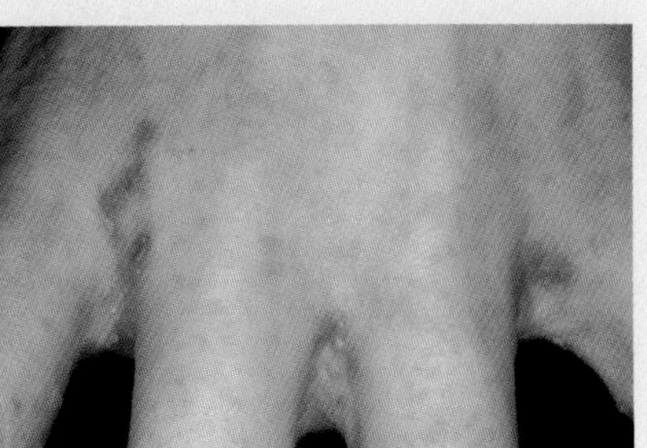
Scabies

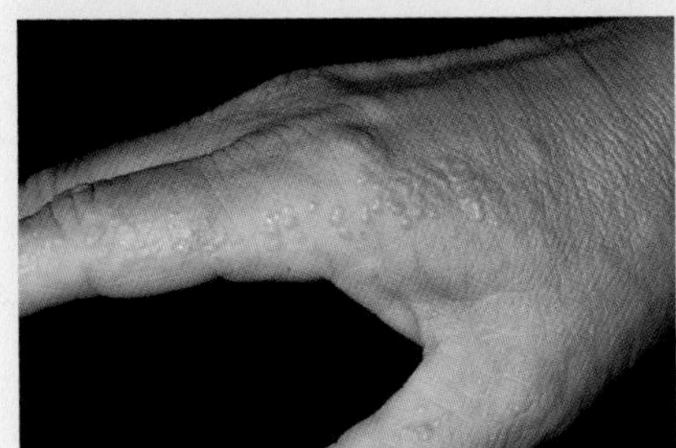
Id reaction

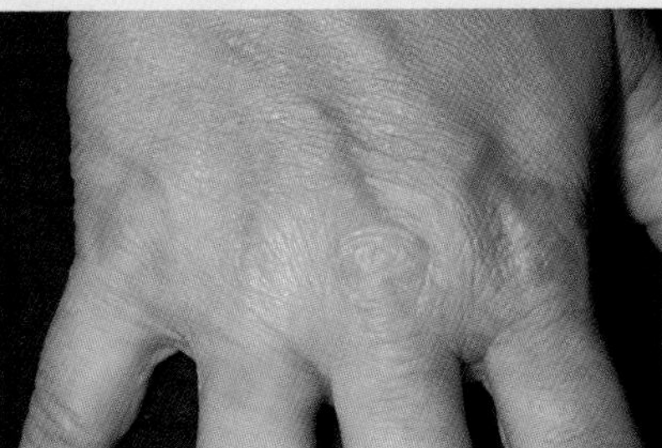
Knuckle pads

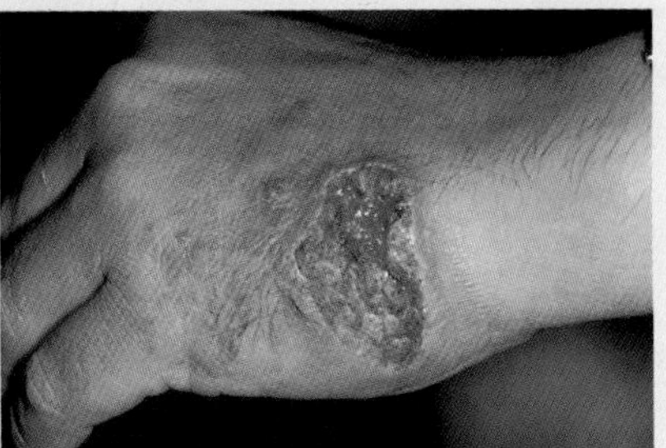
Leishmaniasis

Hands (palms)

Angioedema (p. 200)
Calluses/corns (p. 460)
Contact dermatitis (p. 131)
Cowden disease (p. 996)
Dyshidrosis (pompholyx) (p. 109)
Eczema (p. 96)
Erythema multiforme (p. 713)
Hand-foot-and-mouth disease (p. 547)
Keratoderma
Keratolysis exfoliativa (p. 105)
Lichen planus (vesicles) (p. 322)
Lupus erythematosus (p. 688)
Melanoma (p. 870)
Nevoid basal cell carcinoma syndrome (p. 808)
Pityriasis rubra pilaris (p. 311)
Pompholyx (dyshidrosis) (p. 109)
Psoriasis (p. 271)
Pyogenic granuloma (pp. 906, 971)
Rocky Mountain spotted fever (p. 611)
Scabies (infants) (p. 586)
Syphilis (secondary) (p. 400)
Tinea (p. 507)
Vesicular "id reaction" (p. 109)
Viral exanthem (p. 558)
Warts (p. 457)

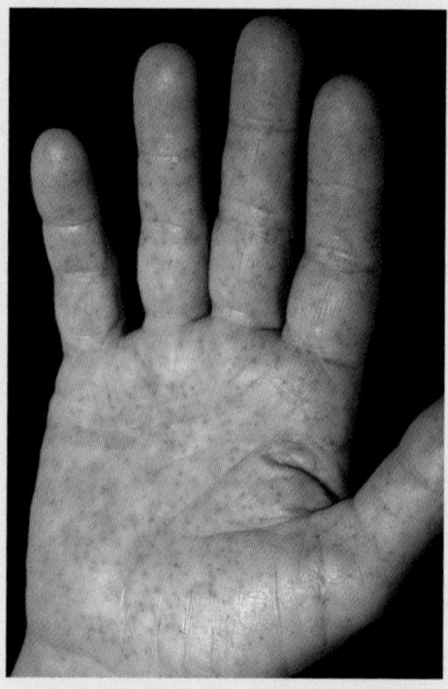

Rocky Mountain spotted fever

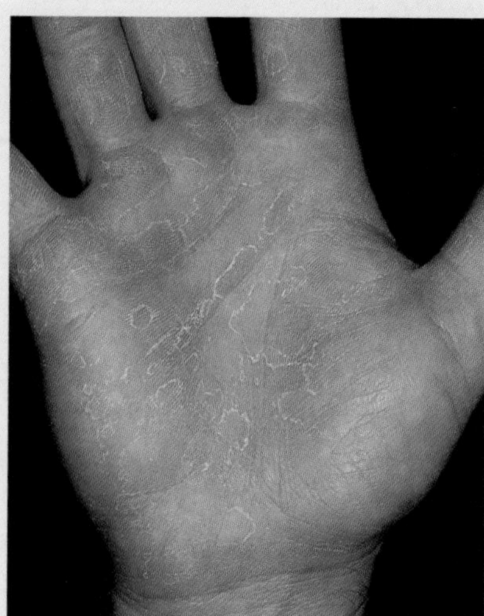

Keratolysis exfoliativa

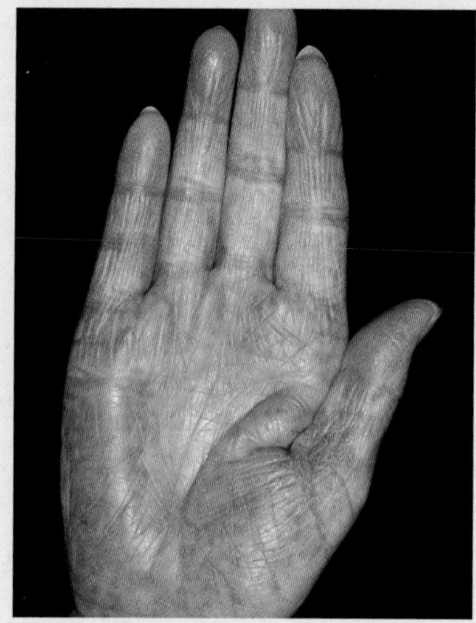

Lupus, acute

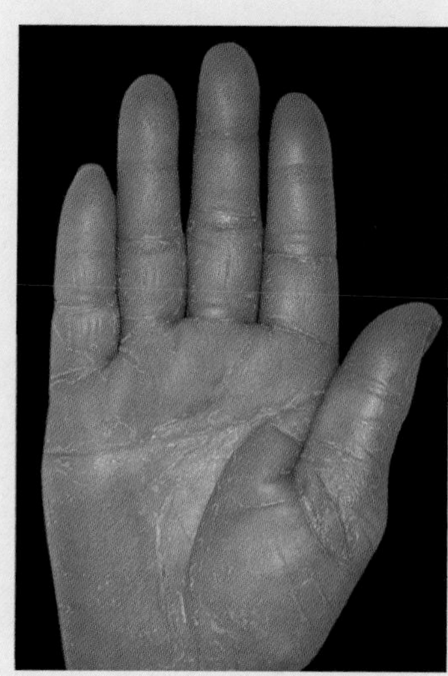

Pityriasis rubra pilaris

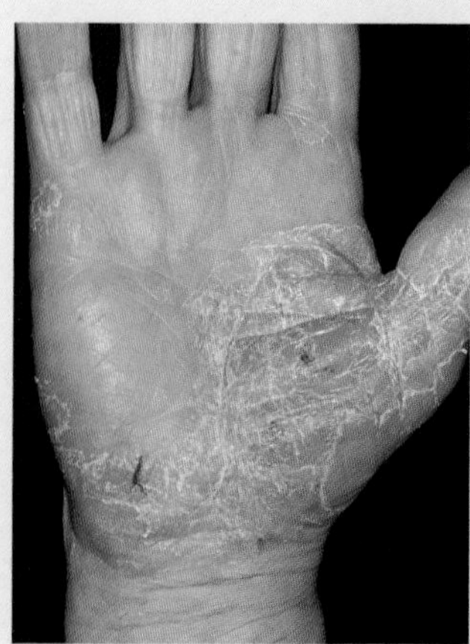

Eczema

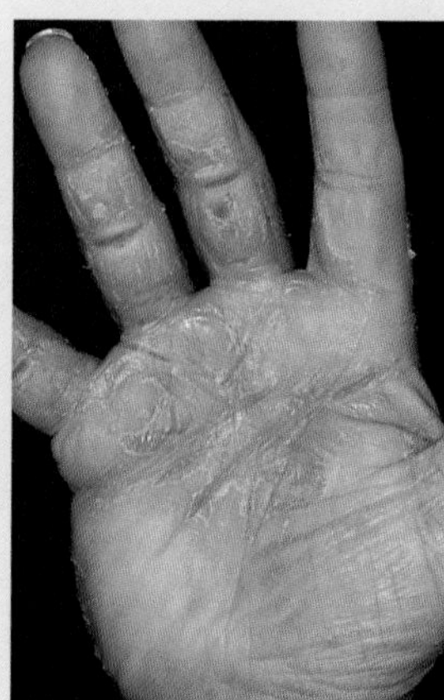

Eczema

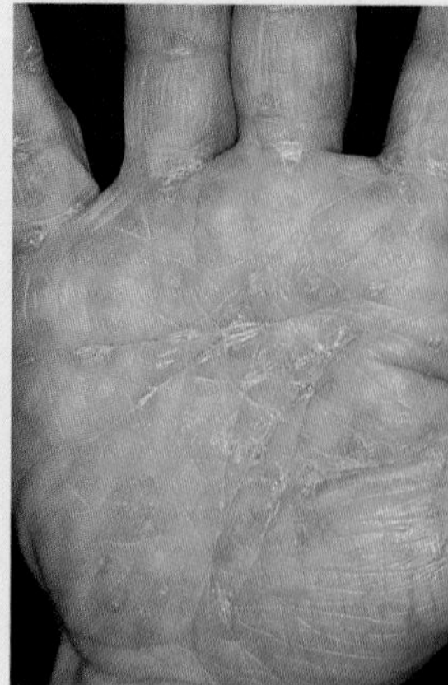

Secondary syphilis

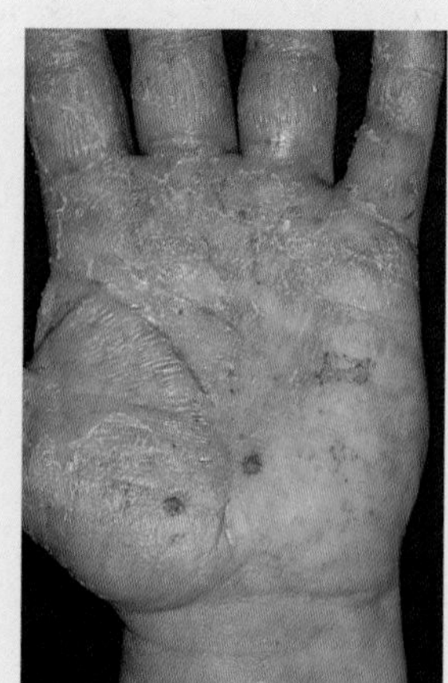

Dyshidrosis

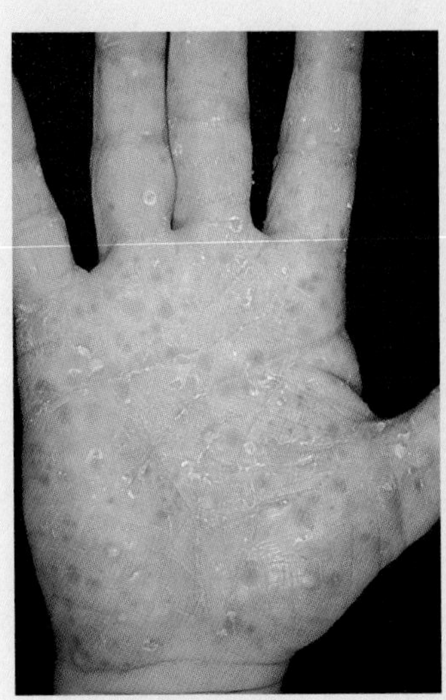
Pustular psoriasis

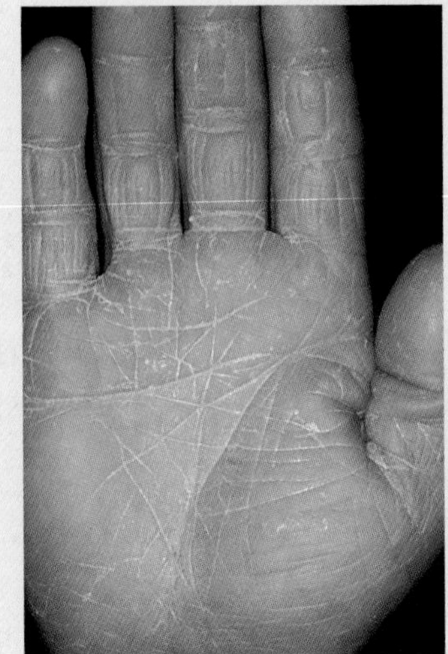
Tinea

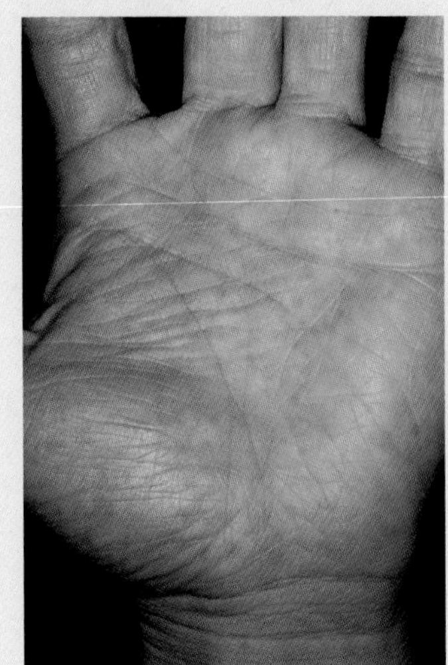
Viral exanthem

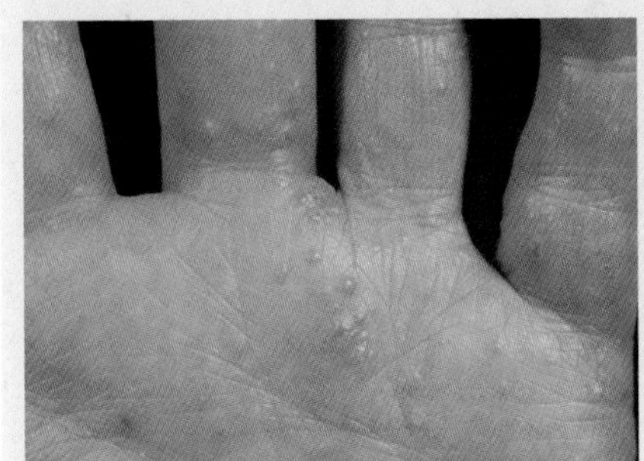
Dyshidrosis

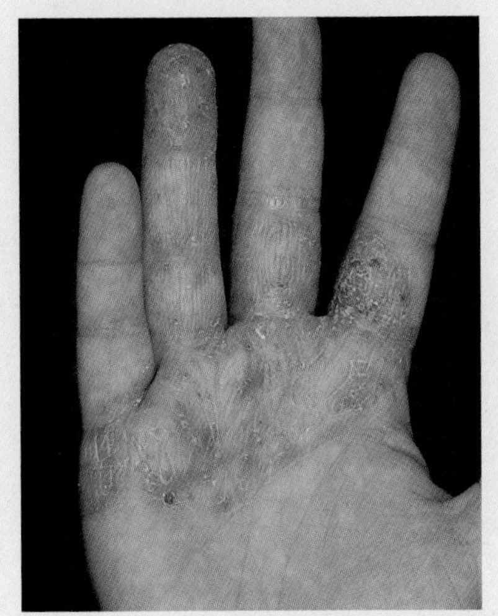
Eczema

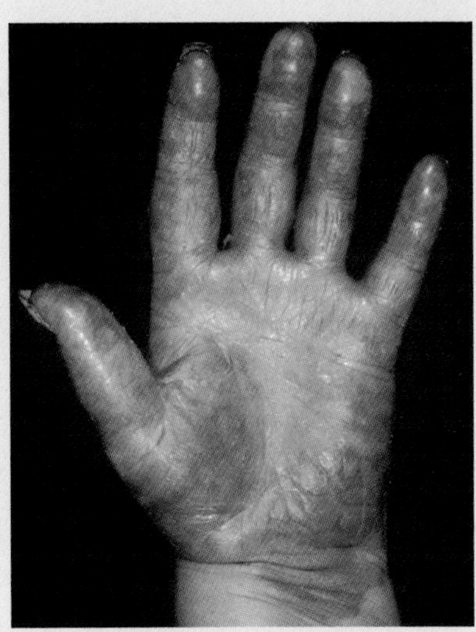
Erythrodermic psoriasis

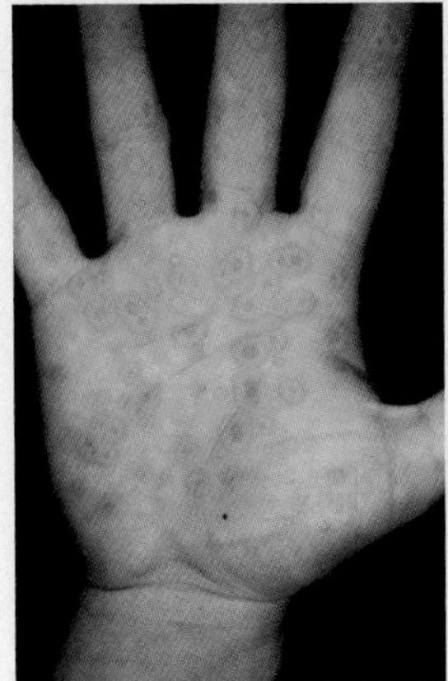
Erythema multiforme

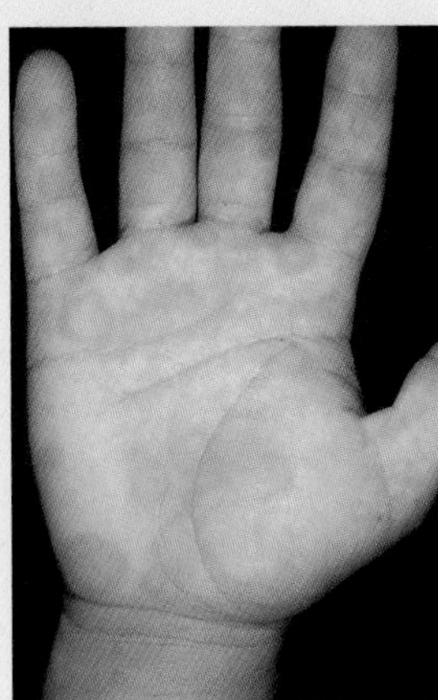
Angioedema

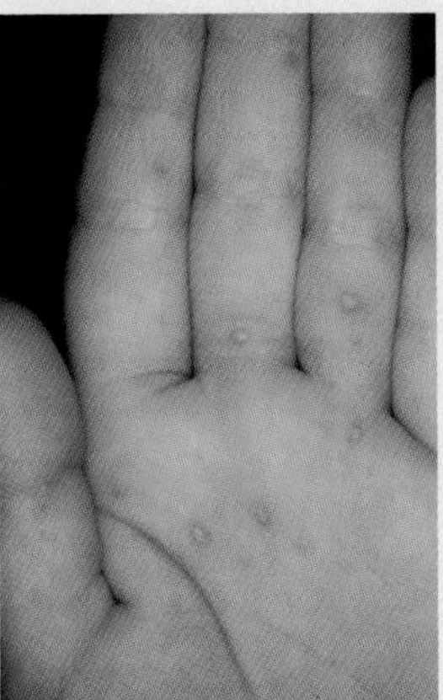
Hand-foot-and-mouth disease

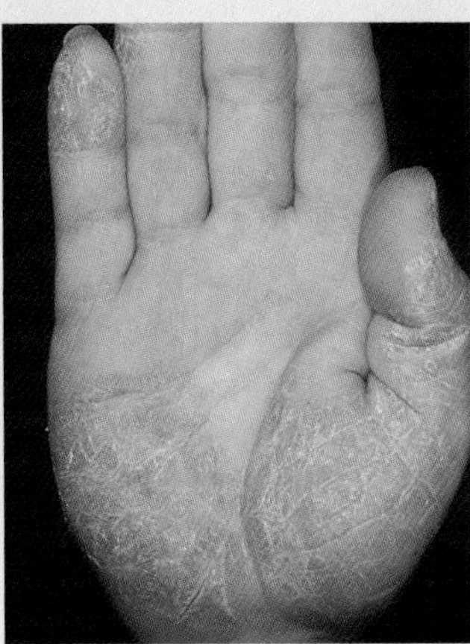
Psoriasis

Inframammary
Acrochordon (skin tags) (p. 785)
Candidiasis (p. 532)
Grover's disease (p. 334)
Hidradenitis suppurativa (p. 260)
Intertrigo (p. 501)
Psoriasis (without scale) (p. 274)
Seborrheic keratosis (p. 780)
Tinea versicolor (p. 537)

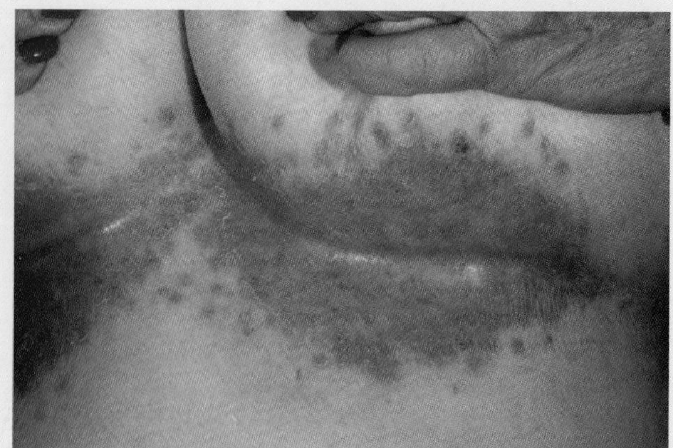

Candidiasis

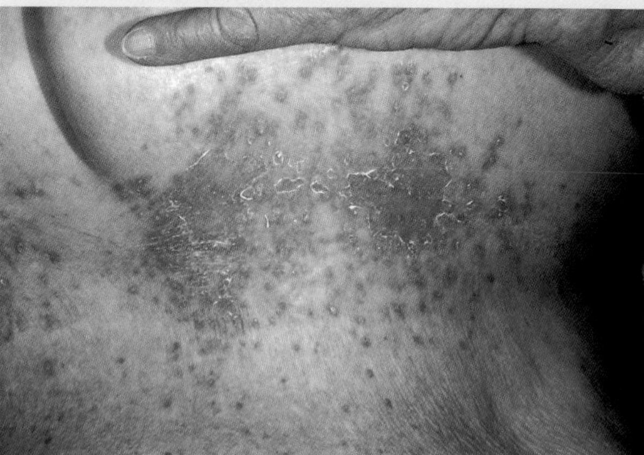

Candidiasis

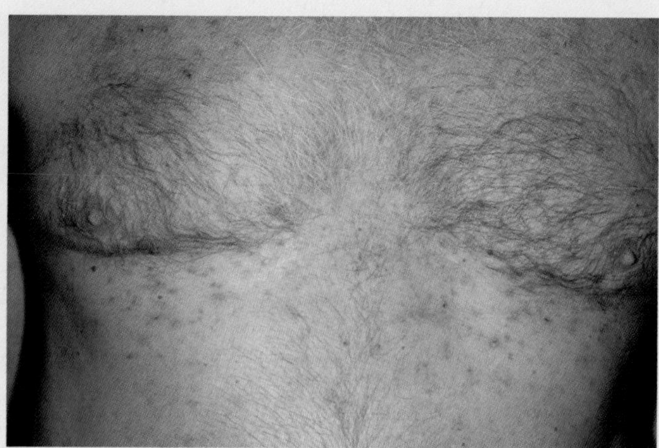

Grover's disease

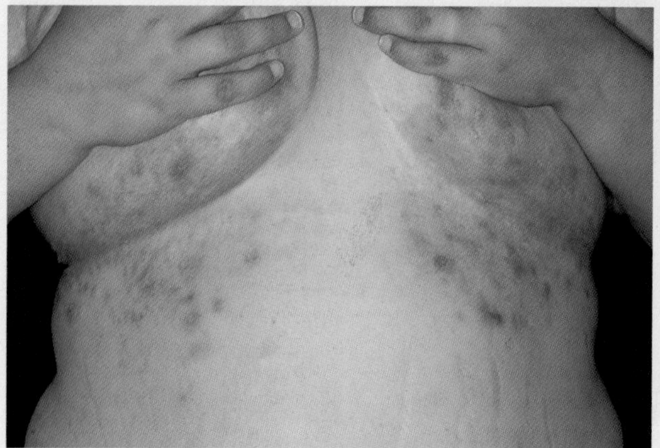

Hidradenitis suppurativa

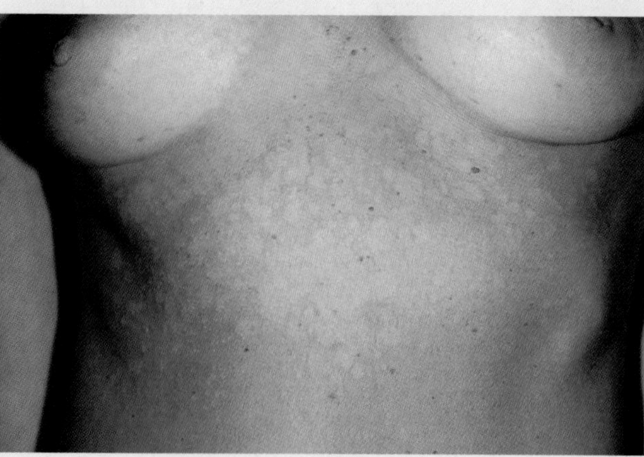

Tinea versicolor

Legs
Atopic dermatitis (p. 165)
Basal cell carcinoma (p. 805)
Bites (p. 621)
Bowen's disease (p. 821)
Churg-Strauss syndrome (p. 723)
Contact dermatitis (p. 146)
Dermatofibroma (p. 787)
Eczema (p. 91)
Ecthyma gangrenosum (p. 370)
Eruptive xanthomas (p. 982)
Kaposi's sarcoma (p. 907)
Livedo reticularis
Lupus panniculus
Majocchi's granuloma (tinea) (p. 504)
Melanoma (p. 860)
Molluscum contagiosum (pp. 428, 465)
Nummular eczema (pp. 104, 111)
Panniculitis
Pityriasis lichenoides (p. 332)
Polyarteritis nodosa (p. 724)
Porokeratosis of Mibelli
Pretibial myxedema
Prurigo nodularis (p. 119)
Psoriasis (p. 267)
Pyoderma gangrenosum (p. 737)
Rhus dermatitis (poison ivy) (p. 138)
Squamous cell carcinoma (p. 825)
Urticarial vasculitis (p. 209)
Vasculitis (p. 724)
Weber-Christian disease
Wegener's granulomatosis (p. 724)

Legs (lower)
Cellulitis (p. 342)
Diabetic bullae (p. 646)
Diabetic dermopathy (shin spots) (p. 974)
Erysipelas (p. 342)
Erythema induratum
Erythema nodosum (p. 720)
Flat warts (p. 459)
Folliculitis (p. 351)
Granuloma annulare (p. 976)
Henoch-Schönlein purpura (p. 732)
Ichthyosis vulgaris (p. 167)
Idiopathic guttate hypomelanosis (p. 769)
Leukocytoclastic vasculitis (p. 727)
Lichen planus (p. 323)
Lichen simplex chronicus (pp. 104, 115)
Myxedema (pretibial)
Necrobiosis lipoidica (p. 975)
Psychogenic parasitosis (p. 121)
Purpura (p. 18)
Schamberg's disease (p. 740)
Stasis dermatitis (p. 122)
Subcutaneous fat necrosis (associated with pancreatitis)
Sweet's syndrome (p. 734)
Tinea (p. 502)
Xerosis (p. 110)

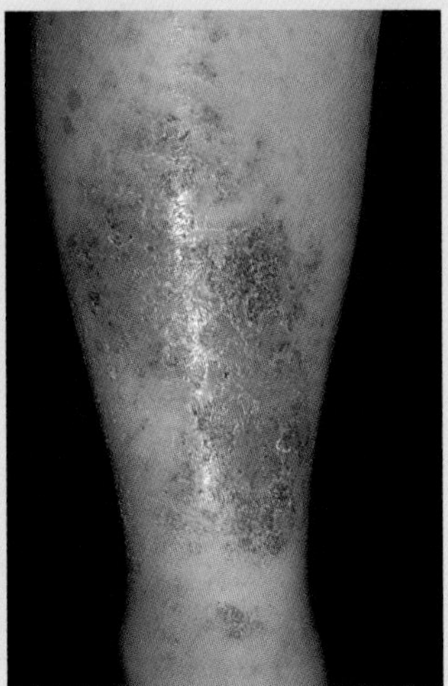

Eczema

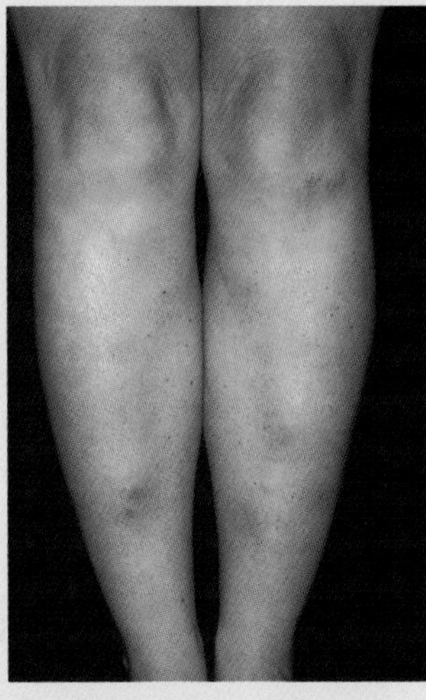

Erythema nodosum

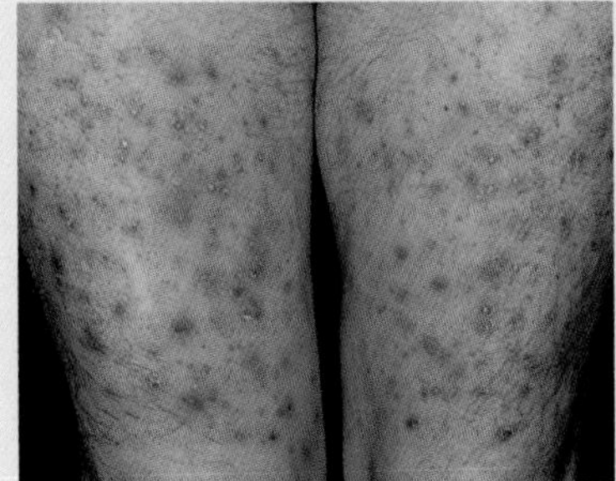

Folliculitis

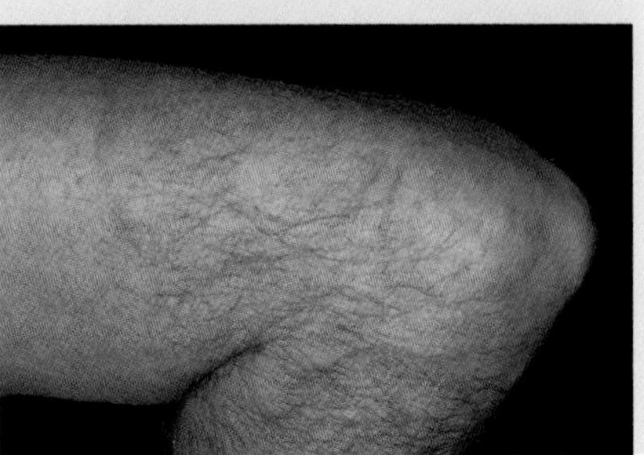

Granuloma annulare

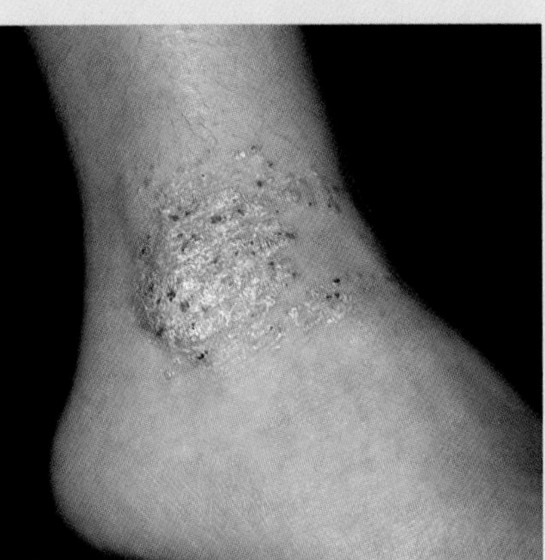

Lichen simplex chronicus

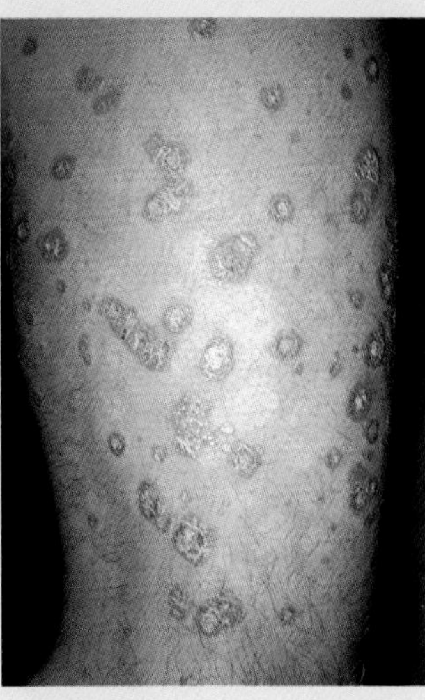

Psoriasis chronic plaque

Legs

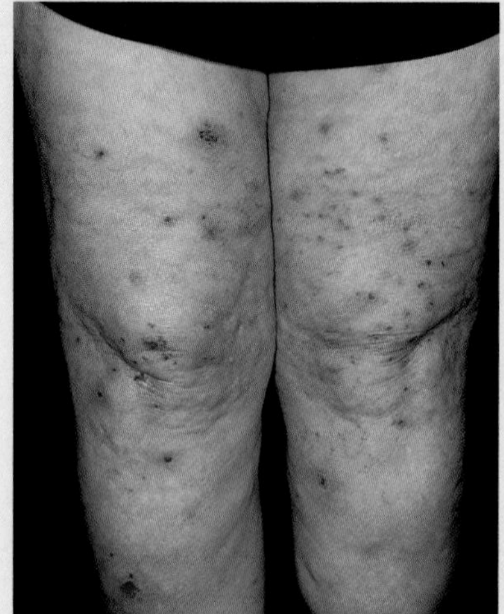
Psychogenic parasitosis

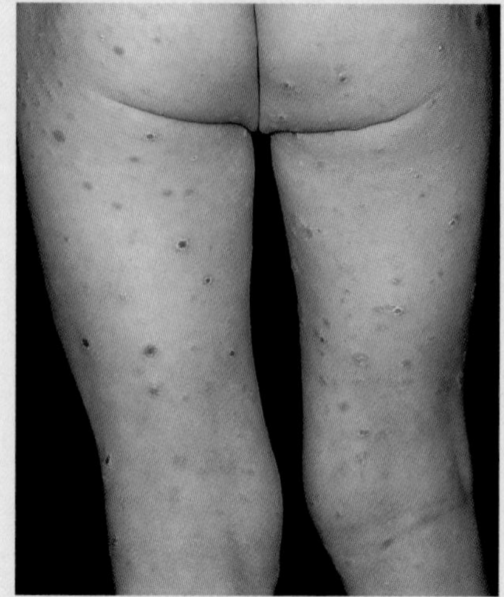
Pityriasis lichenoides

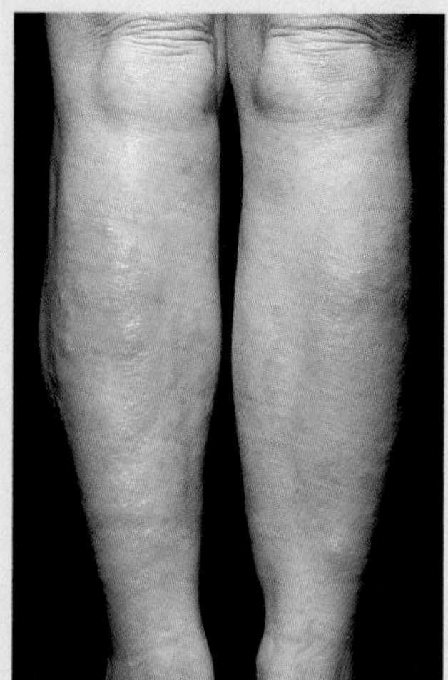
Pretibial myxedema

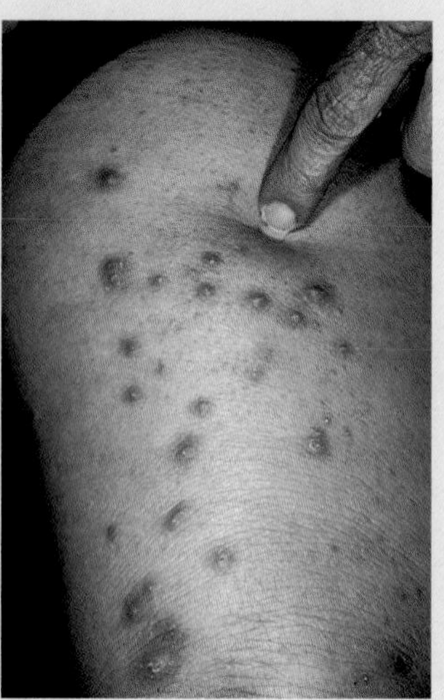
Prurigo nodularis

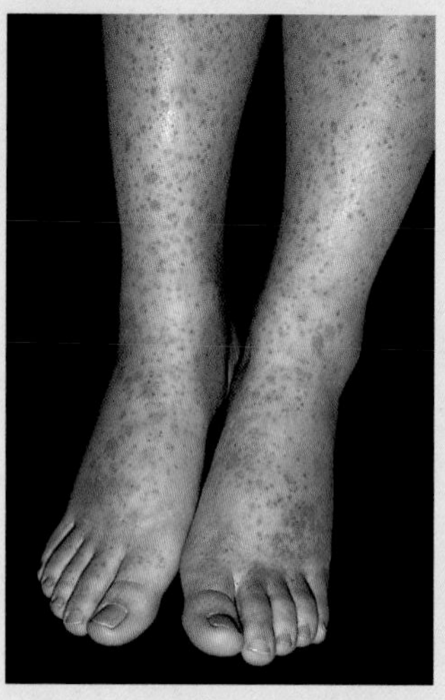
Henoch-Schönlein purpura

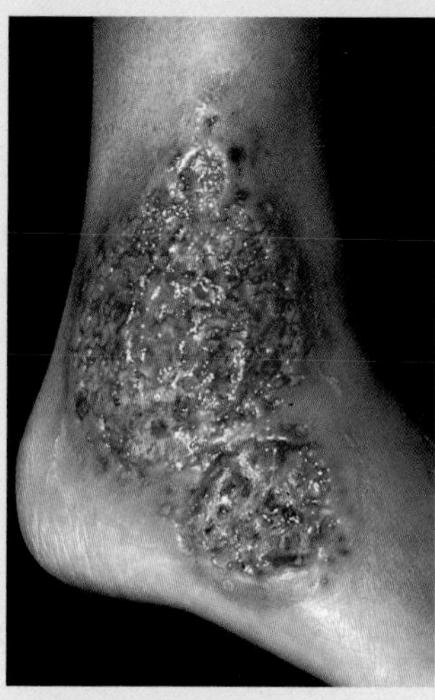
Pyoderma gangrenosum

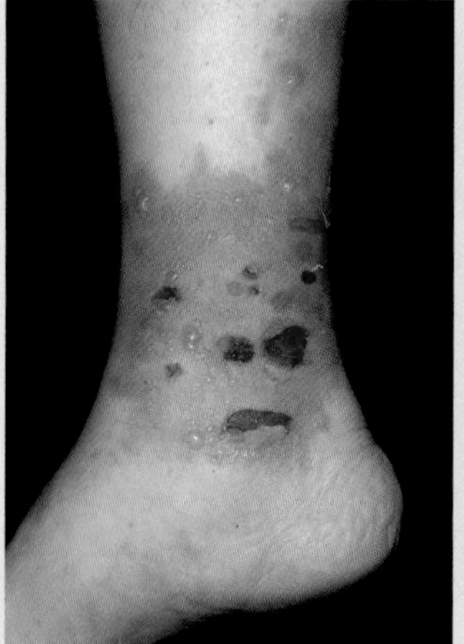
Rhus dermatitis (poison ivy)

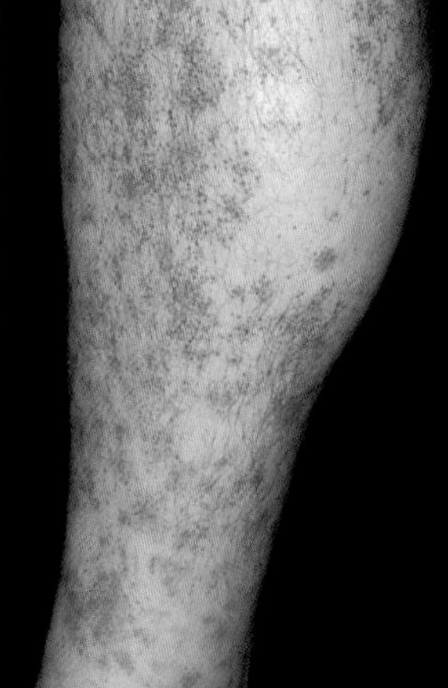
Schamberg's disease

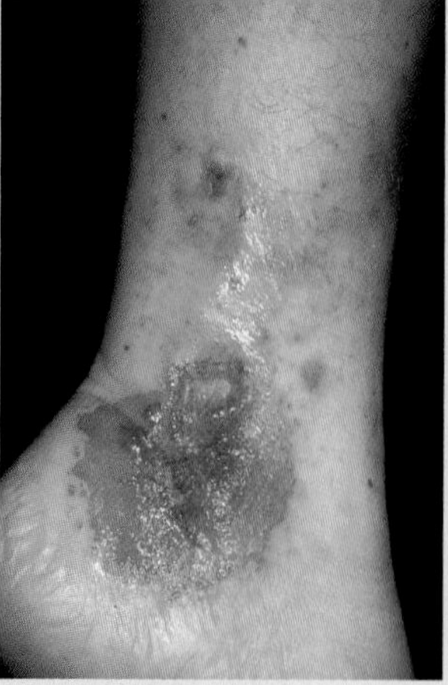
Contact dermatitis, neomycin

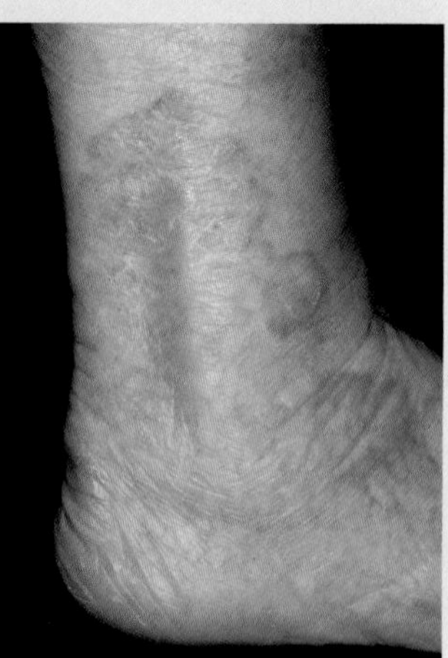
Tinea

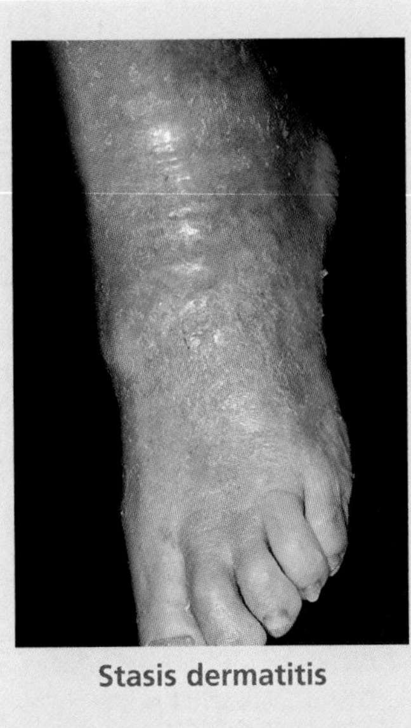
Stasis dermatitis

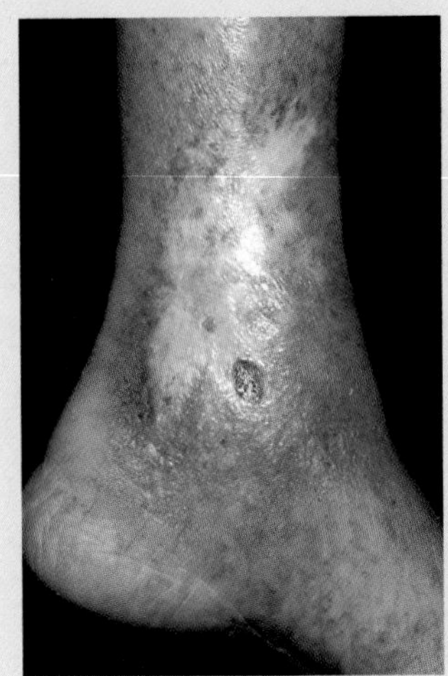
Stasis dermatitis

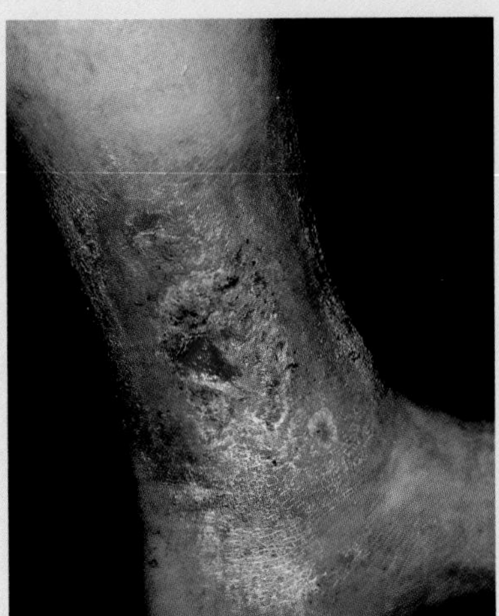
Stasis dermatitis

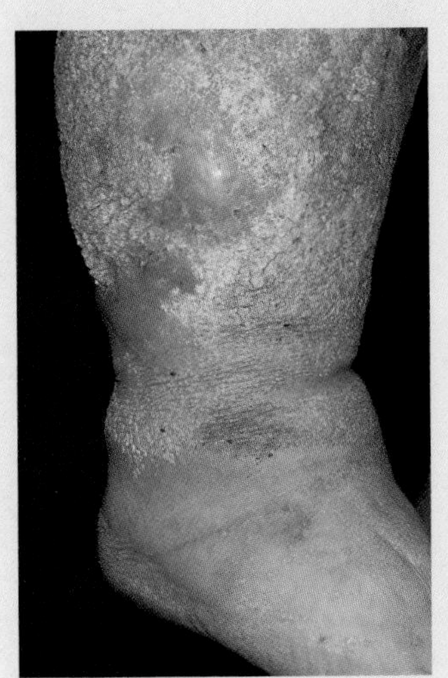
Stasis dermatitis

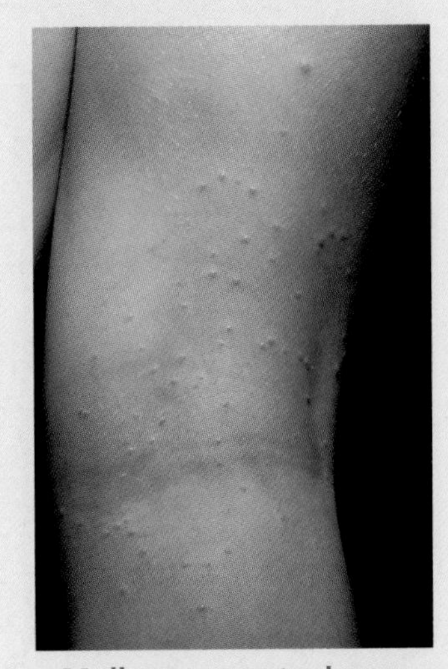
Molluscum contagiosum

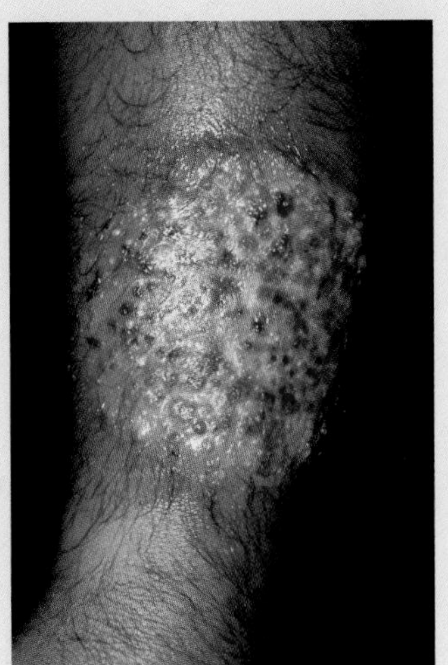
Tinea

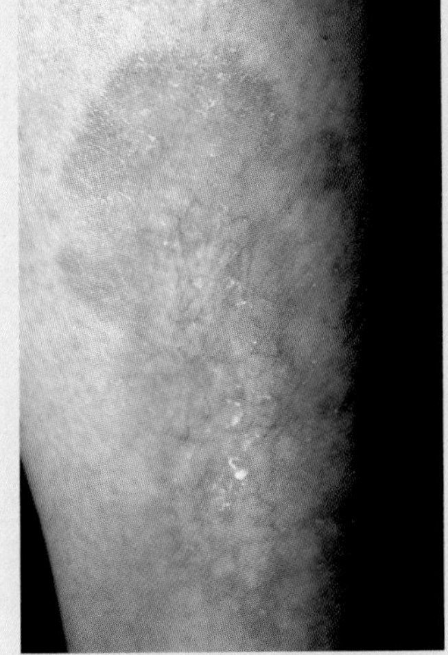
Necrobiosis lipoidica

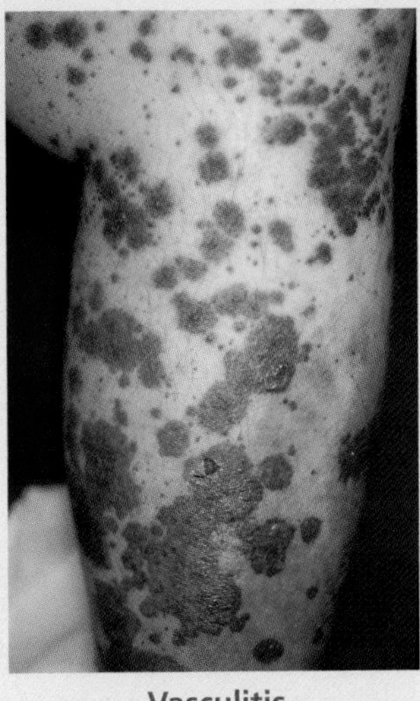
Vasculitis

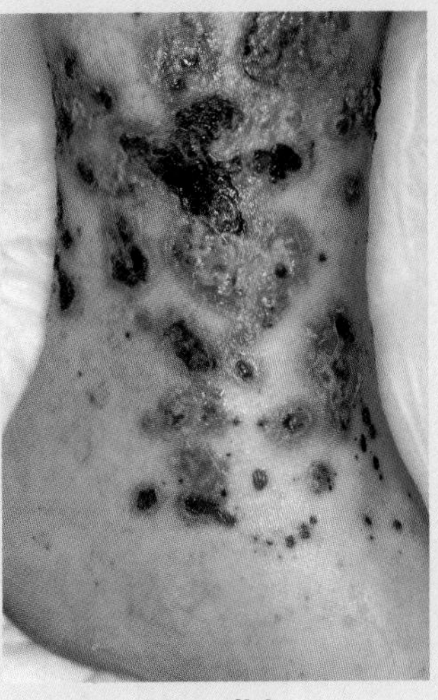
Vasculitis

Legs

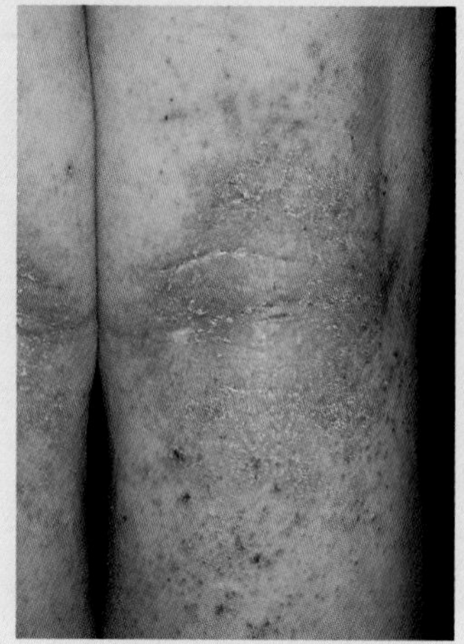
Atopic dermatitis

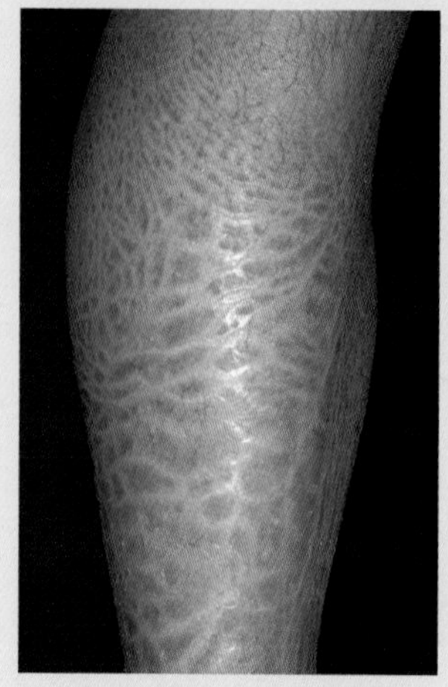
Sex-linked ichthyosis

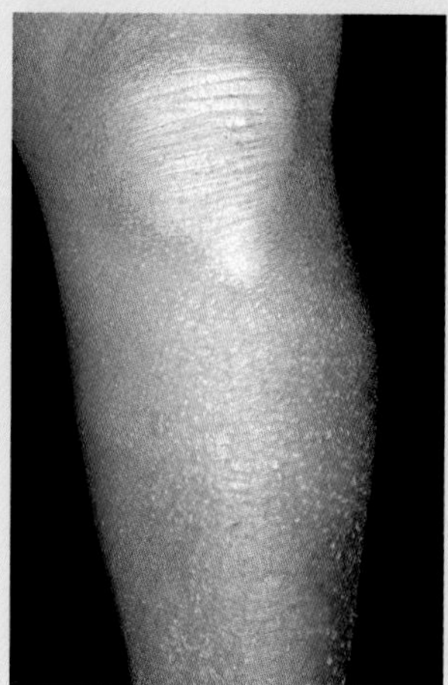
Dominant ichthyosis

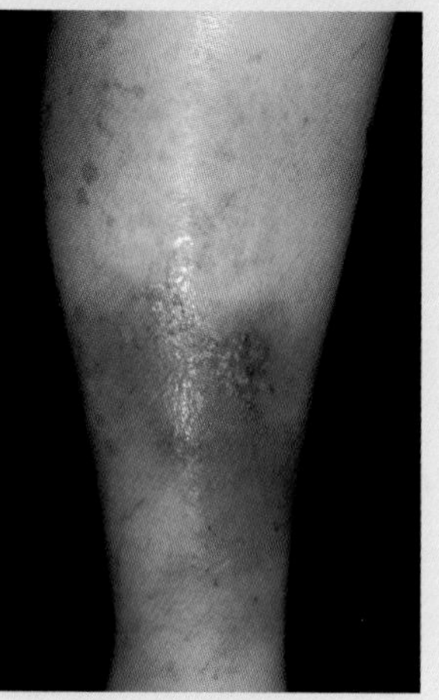
Cellulitis

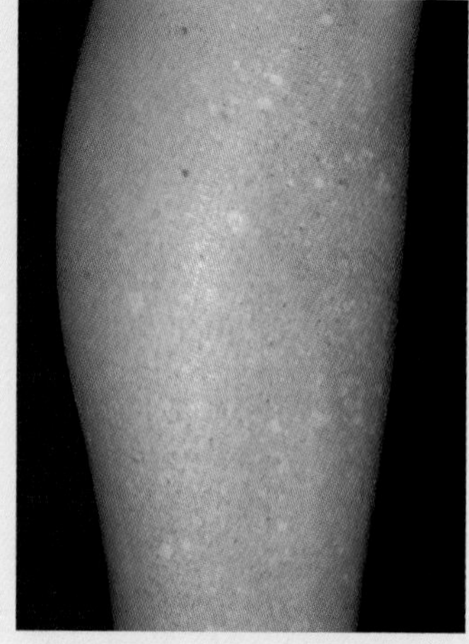
Idiopathic guttate hypomelanosis

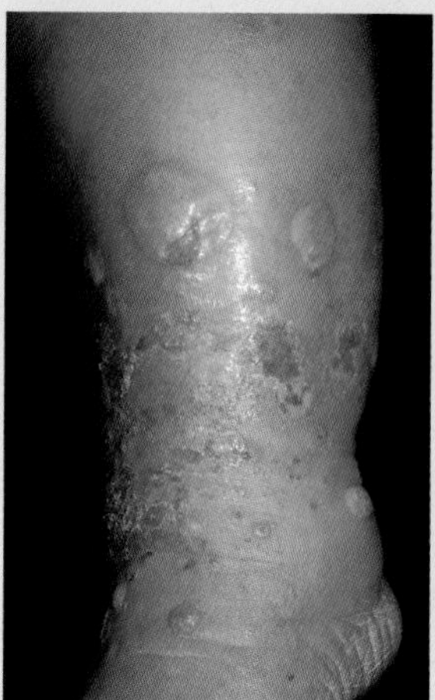
Diabetic bullae

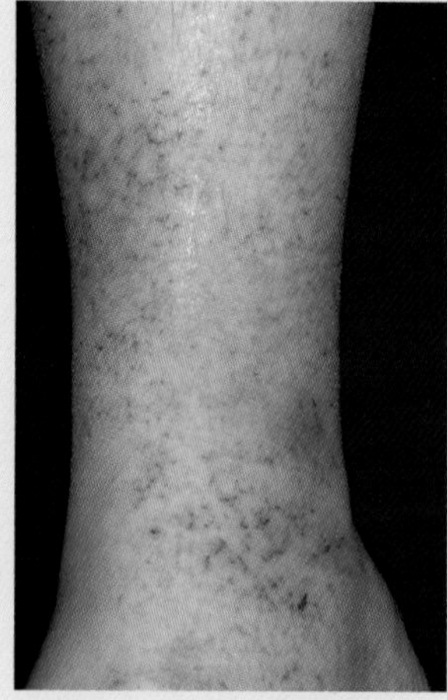
Asteatotic eczema

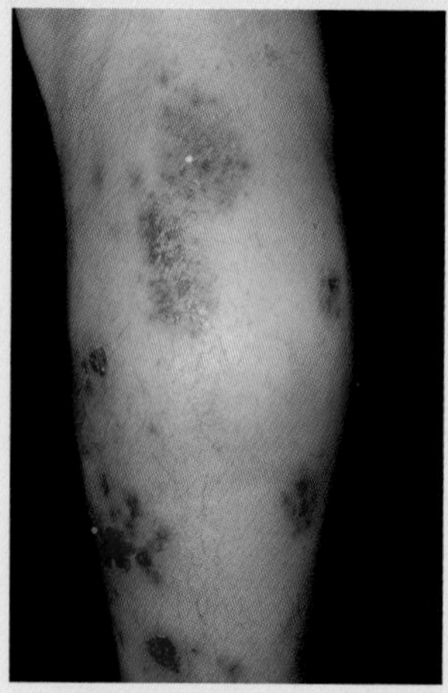
Nummular eczema

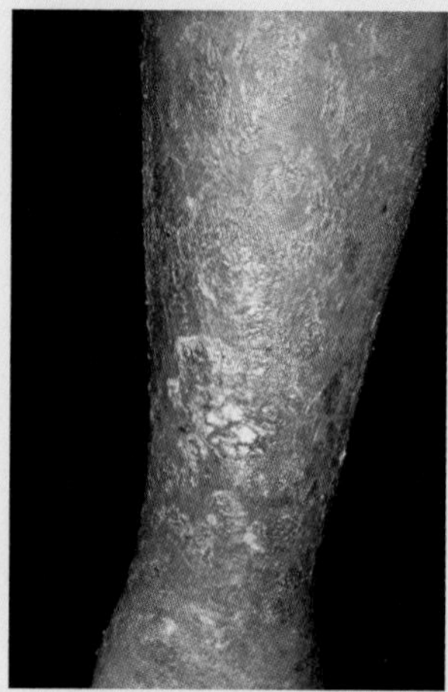
Eczema, subacute

Lips
Actinic cheilitis (p. 818)
Allergic contact dermatitis (p. 132)
Angioedema (p. 200)
Atopic dermatitis (p. 159)
Eczema (p. 95)
Erythema multiforme (p. 713)
Fordyce spots (upper lips) (p. 224)
Herpes simplex (p. 470)
Impetigo (p. 339)
Labial melanotic macule (p. 856)
Leukoplakia (p. 829)
Perlèche (p. 536)
Pyogenic granuloma (pp. 906, 971)
Squamous cell carcinoma (p. 826)
Stevens-Johnson syndrome (p. 716)
Venous lake (p. 905)
Warts (p. 459)

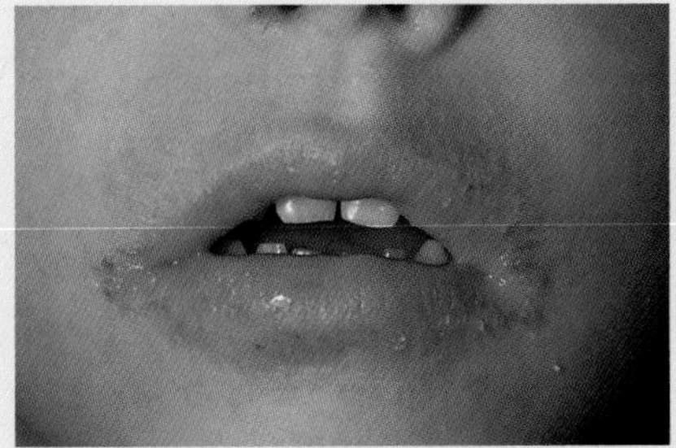
Atopic dermatitis

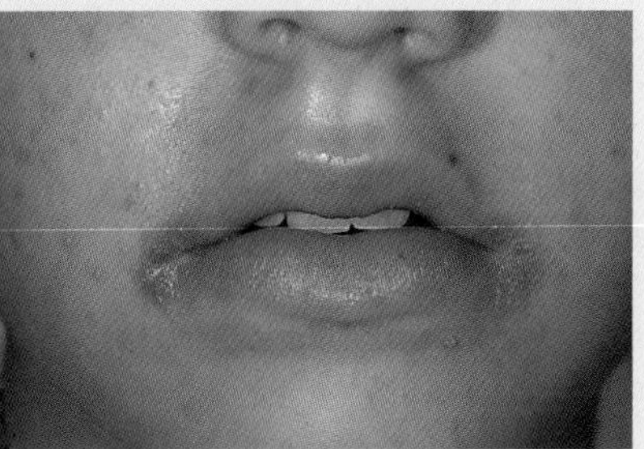
Perlèche, isotretinoin

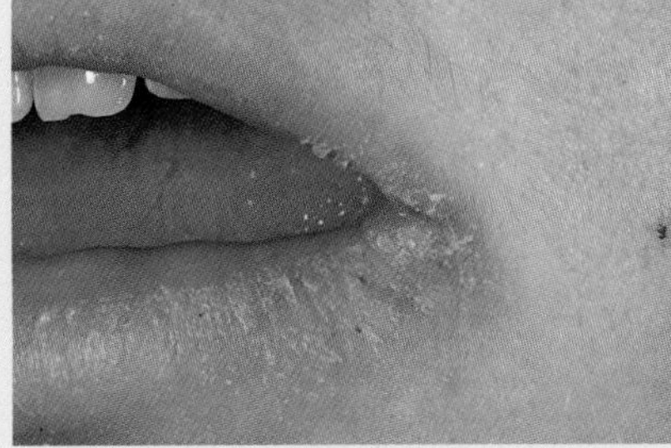
Allergic contact dermatitis

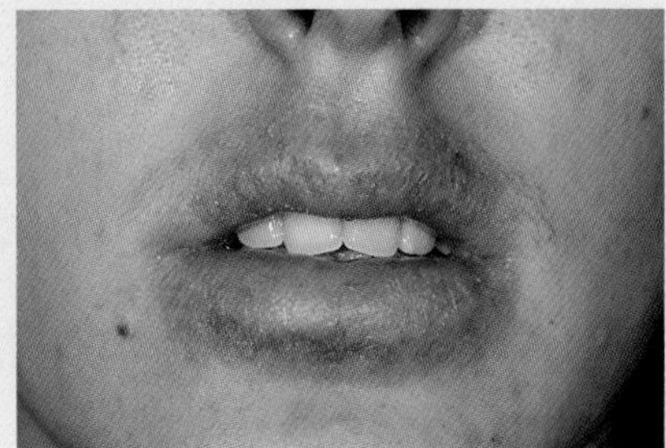
Allergic contact dermatitis

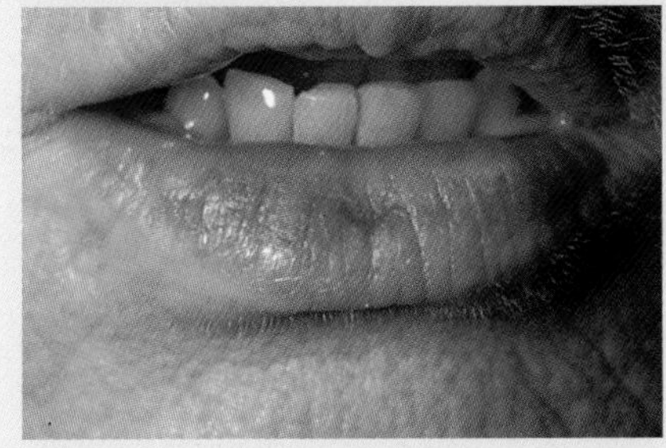
Actinic cheilitis

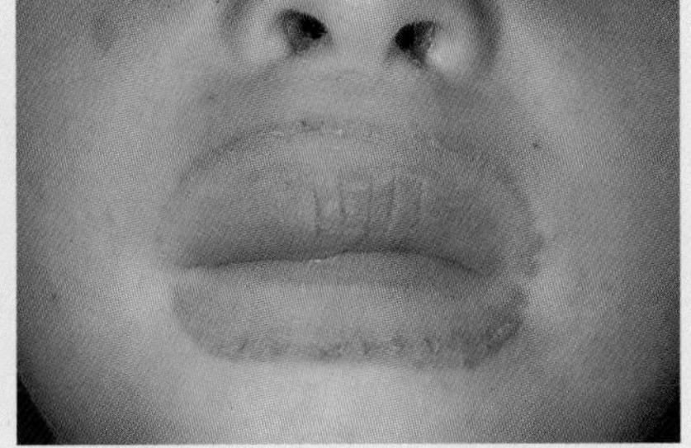
Eczema, lip licking

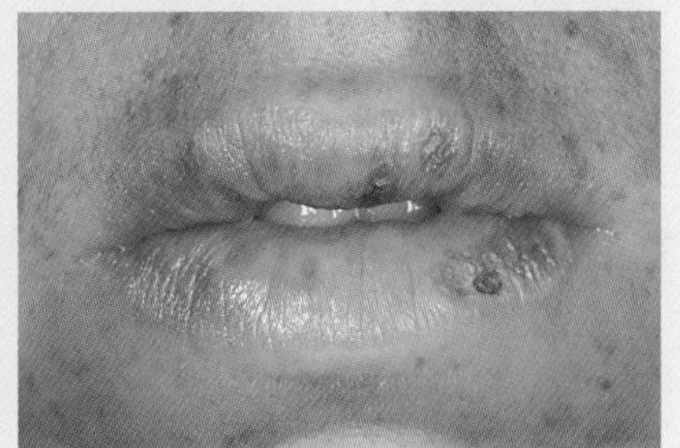
Erythema multiforme

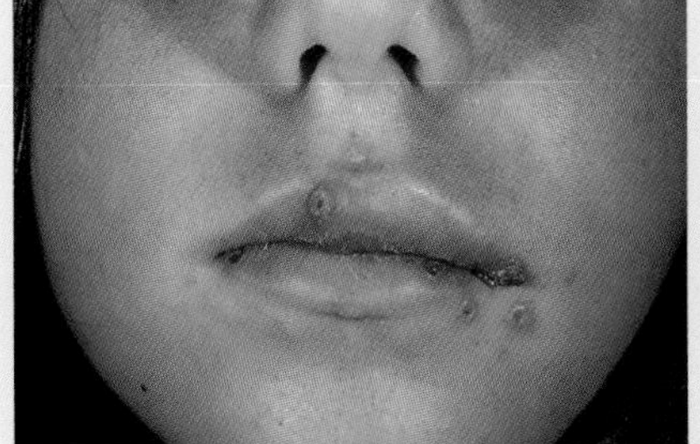
Herpes simplex, Type 1, primary

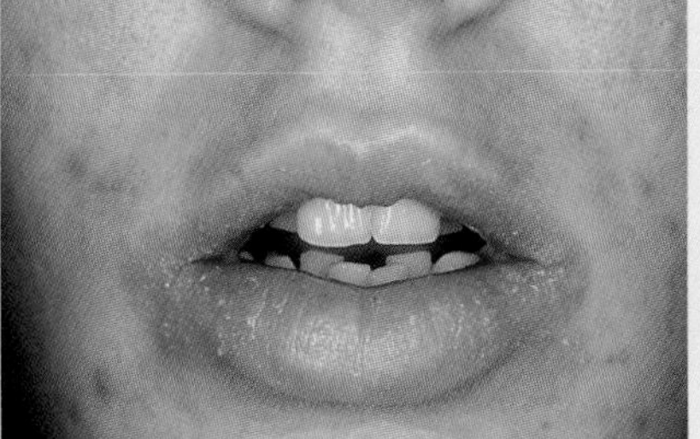
Impetigo

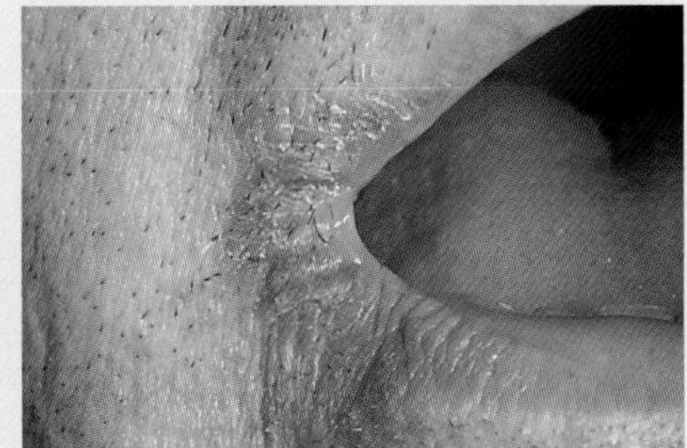
Perlèche

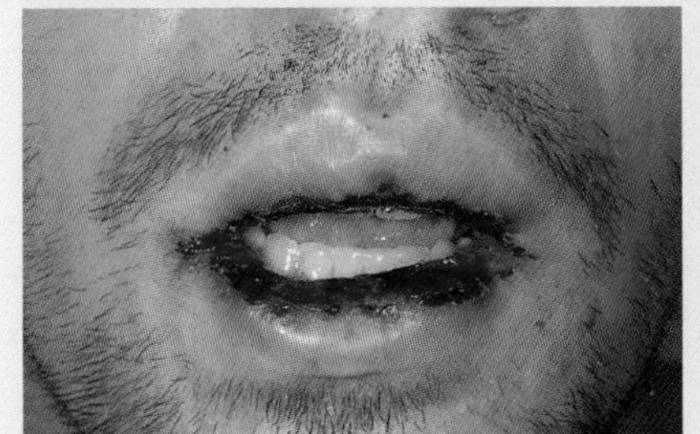
Stevens-Johnson syndrome

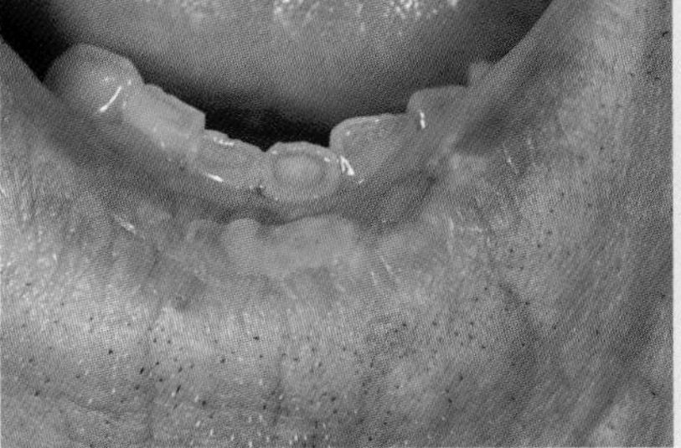
Leukoplakia

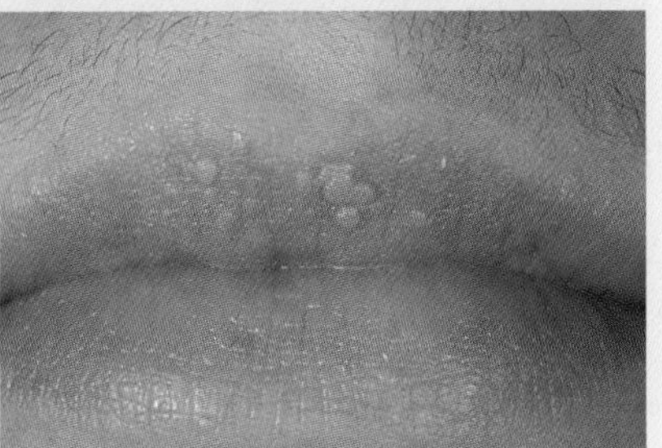
Warts

Neck
Acanthosis nigricans (p. 978)
Acne (p. 226)
Acrochordon (skin tags) (p. 785)
Atopic dermatitis (p. 163)
Berloque dermatitis (p. 763)
Contact dermatitis (p. 147)
Cosmetic fragrance allergy (p. 147)
Dental sinus
Eczema (p. 91)
Elastosis perforans serpiginosa
Epidermal cyst (p. 797)
Folliculitis (p. 351)
Impetigo (p. 338)
Pityriasis rosea (p. 316)
Poikiloderma of Civatte (p. 744)
Pseudofolliculitis (p. 352)
Pseudoxanthoma elasticum
Psoriasis (p. 270)
Sycosis barbae (fungal, bacterial) (p. 354)
Tinea (p. 502)
Warts (p. 458)

Neck (back)
Acne (p. 226)
Acne keloidalis (pp. 355, 944)
Actinic keratosis (p. 812)
Cutis rhomboidalis nuchae (sun-damaged neck) (p. 744)
Epidermal cyst (p. 797)
Folliculitis (p. 351)
Furunculosis (p. 356)
Herpes zoster (p. 479)
Lichen simplex chronicus (pp. 104, 115)
Neurotic excoriations (p. 120)
Salmon patch (p. 903)
Tinea (p. 503)

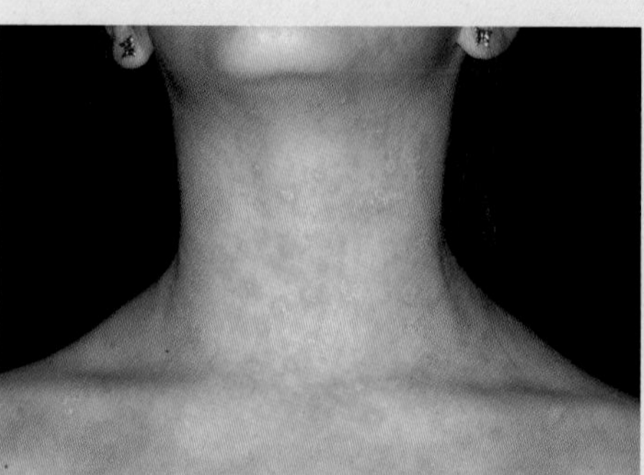
Pityriasis rosea

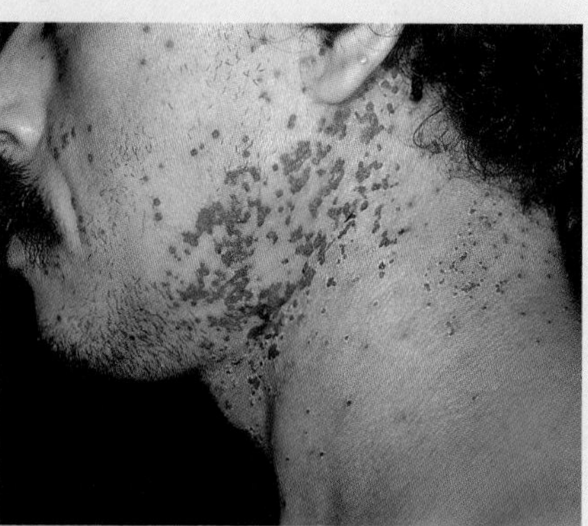
Eczema herpeticum

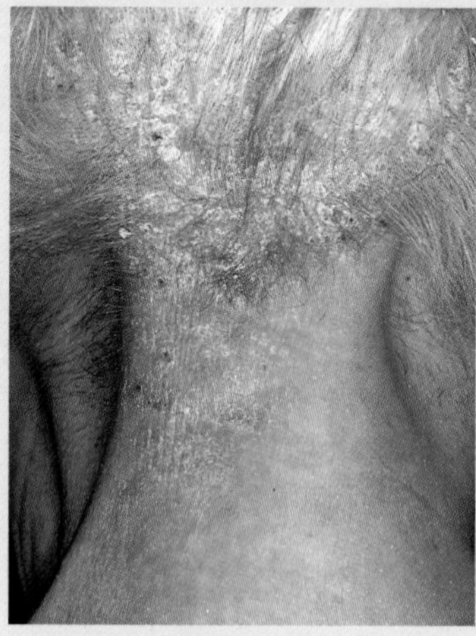
Psoriasis

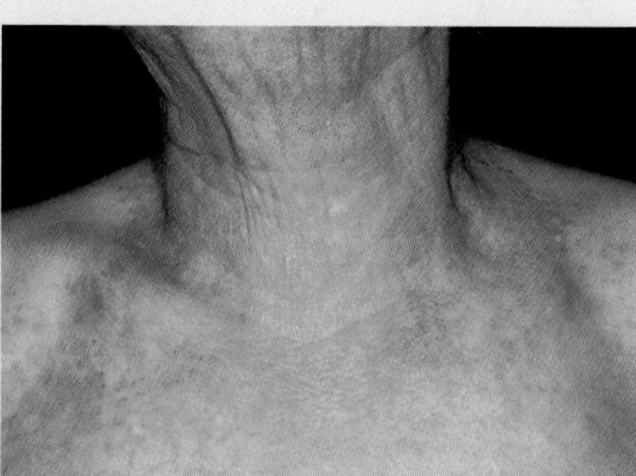
Atopic dermatitis

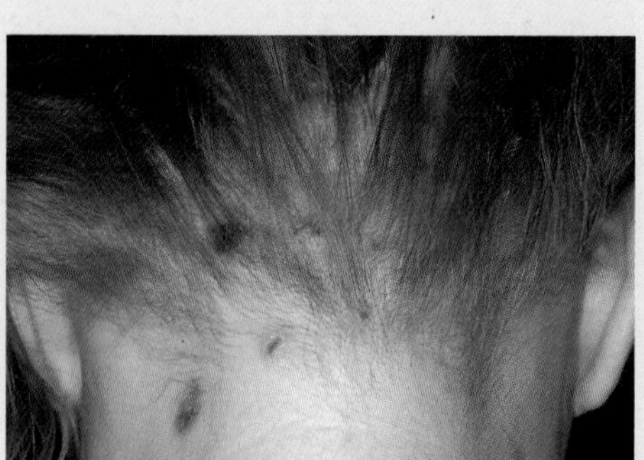
Neurotic excoriations

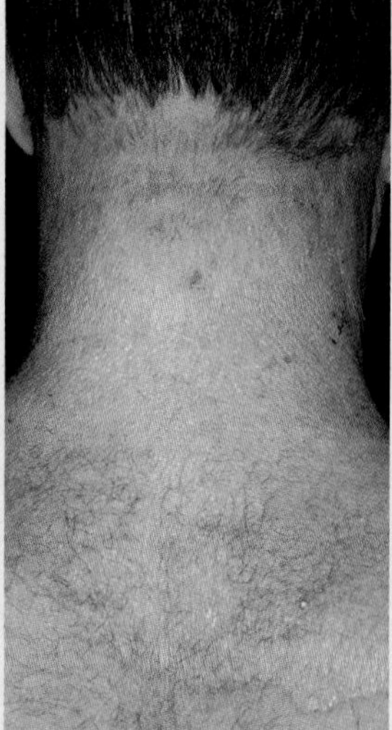
Tinea

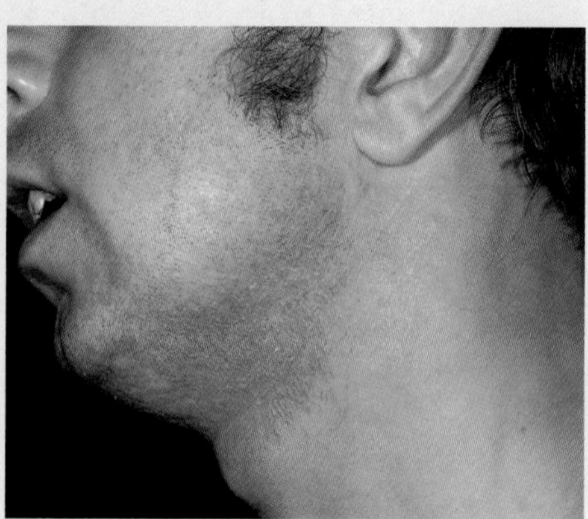
Cosmetic fragrance allergy

Regional differential diagnosis atlas

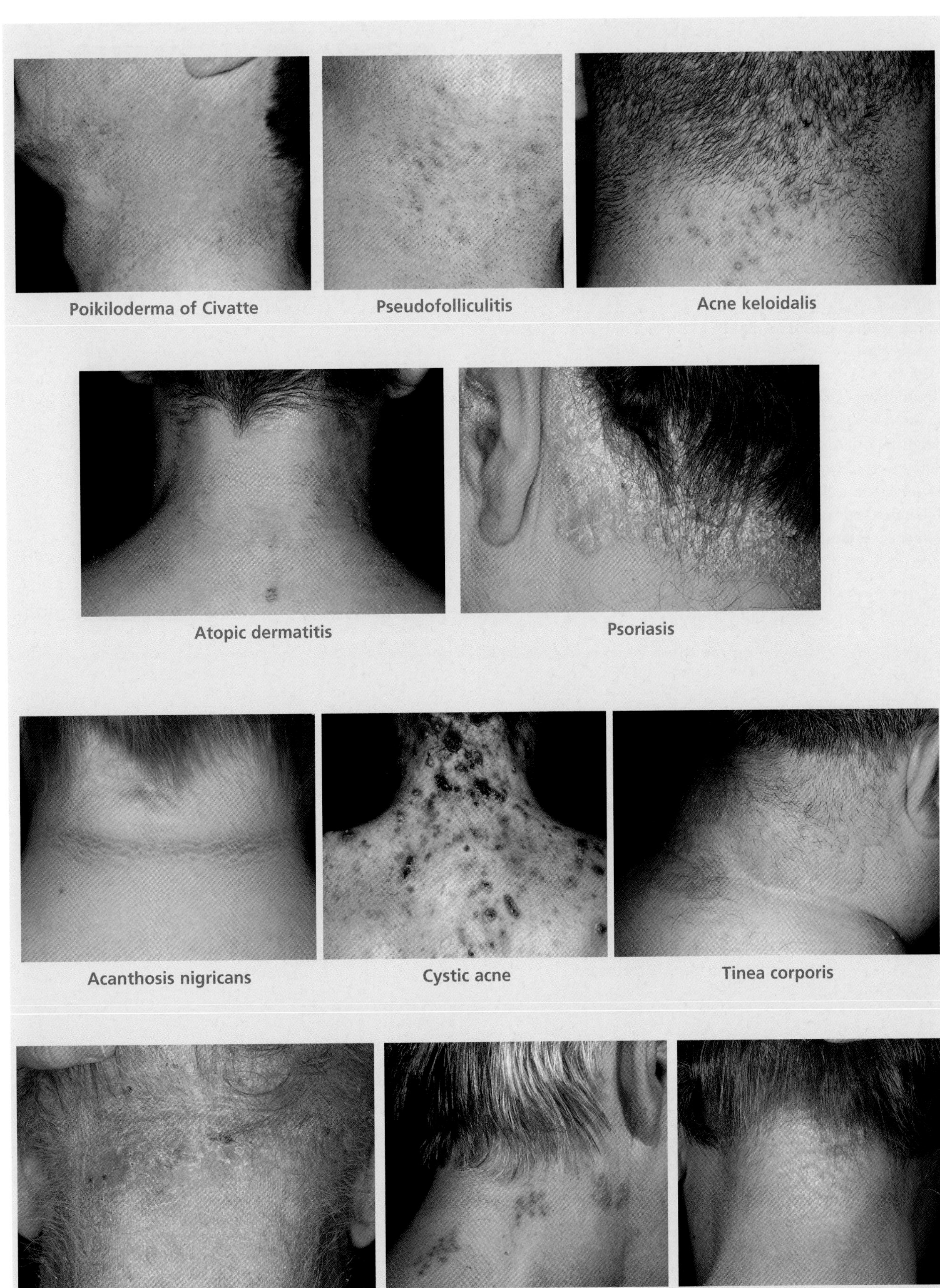

Poikiloderma of Civatte

Pseudofolliculitis

Acne keloidalis

Atopic dermatitis

Psoriasis

Acanthosis nigricans

Cystic acne

Tinea corporis

Eczema

Herpes zoster

Lichen simplex chronicus

Nose

Acne (p. 226)
Actinic keratosis (p. 818)
Adenoma sebaceum (p. 988)
Basal cell carcinoma (p. 805)
Cellulitis (p. 342)
Chronic cutaneous (discoid) lupus erythematosus (p. 682)
Fissure (nostril) (p. 15)
Granulosa rubra nasi
Herpes simplex (p. 471)
Herpes zoster (p. 483)
Impetigo (p. 337)
Lupus erythematosus (p. 682)
Nasal crease
Nevi (p. 848)
Rhinophyma (p. 257)
Rosacea (p. 256)
Seborrheic dermatitis (p. 312)
Squamous cell carcinoma (p. 824)
Staphyloccal folliculitis (p. 351)
Telangiectasias (p. 257)
Wegener's granulomatosis (p. 724)

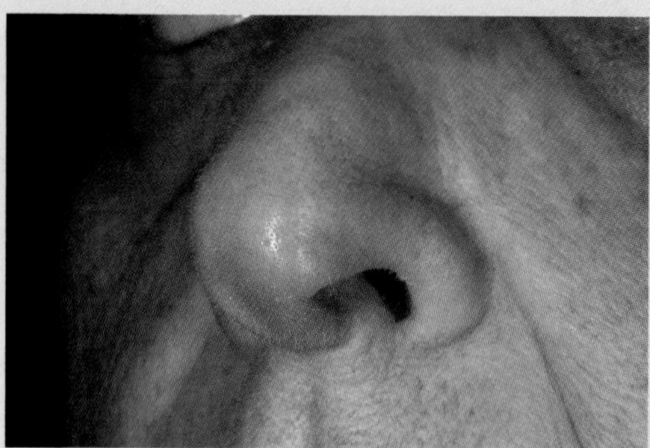

Cellulitis

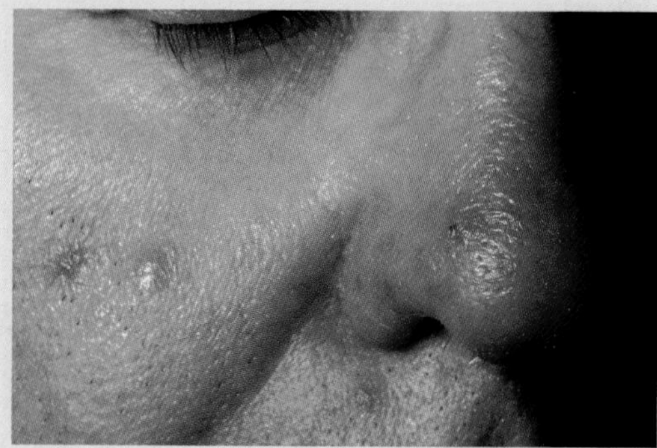

Rosacea

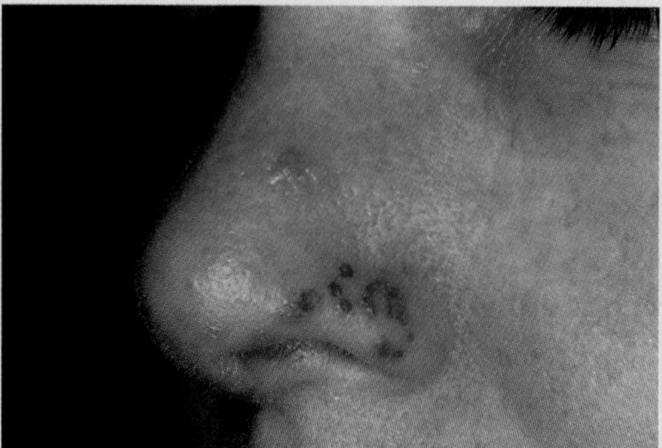

Herpes simplex, Type 1, recurrent

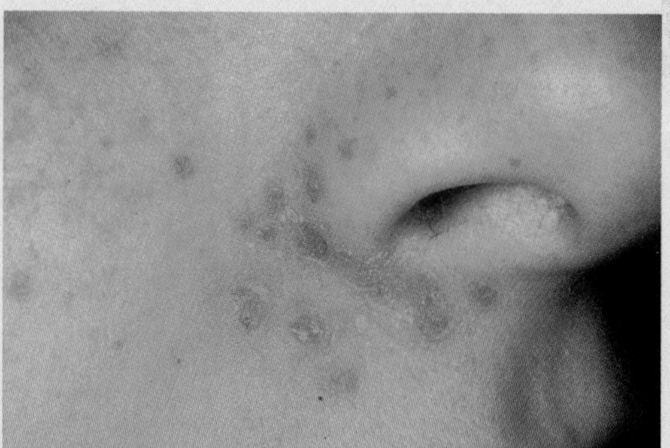

Impetigo

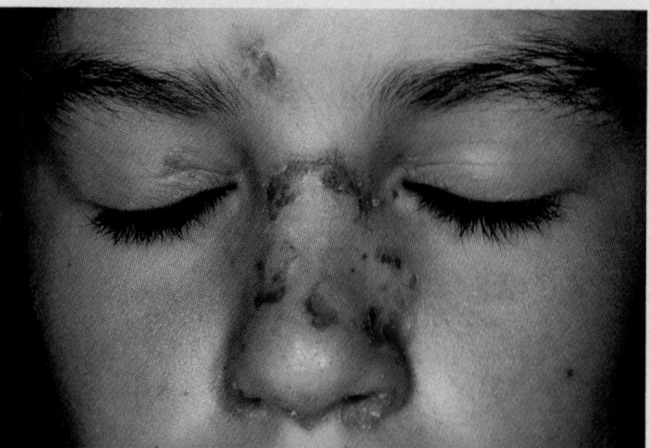

Impetigo

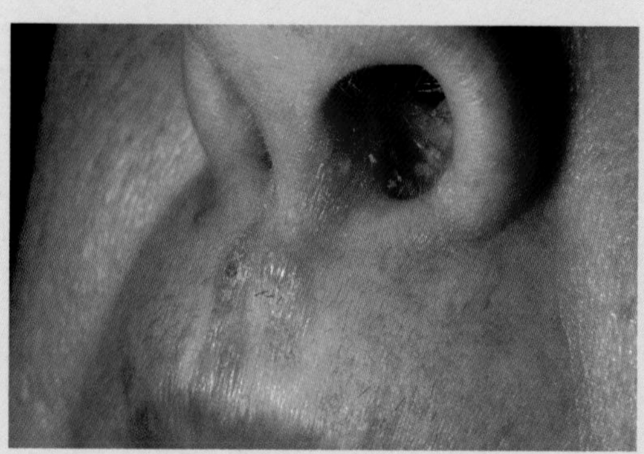

Staphylococcal folliculitis

Oral cavity

Aphthous stomatitis
Candidiasis (p. 529)
Cowden disease (p. 996)
Hairy leukoplakia AIDS (pp. 447, 451)
Hand-foot-and-mouth disease (p. 548)
Herpes simplex, primary (p. 470)
Leukoplakia (p. 829)
Lichen planus (p. 324)
Pemphigus (p. 647)
Secondary syphilis (p. 400)

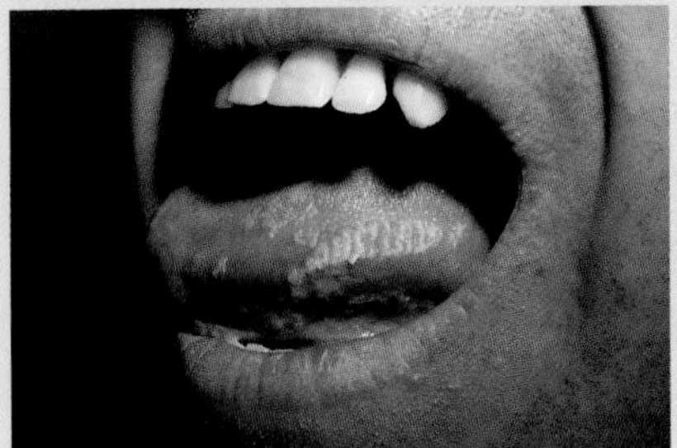
Hairy leukoplakia AIDS

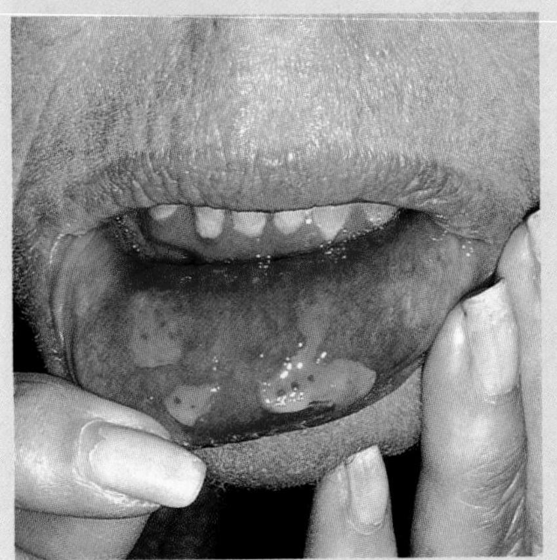
Pemphigus

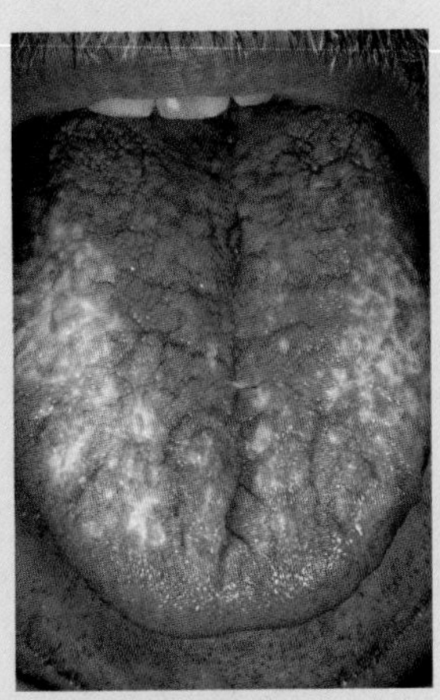
Lichen planus

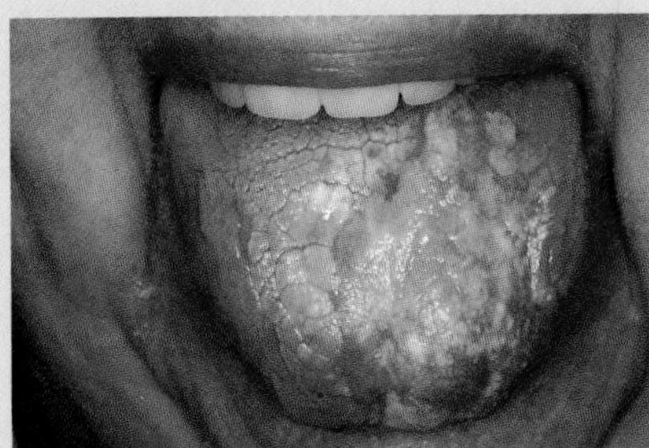
Lichen planus

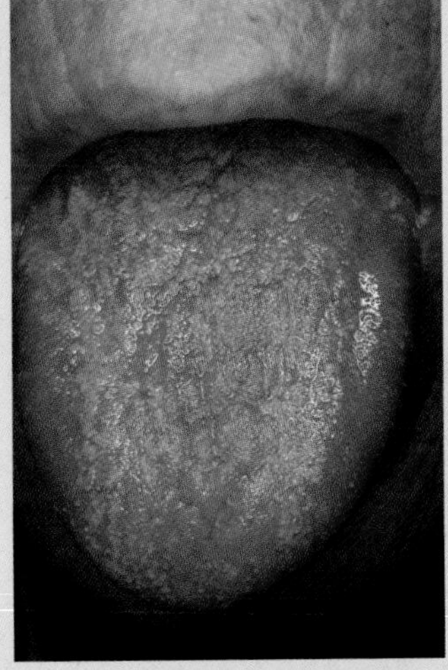
Candidiasis

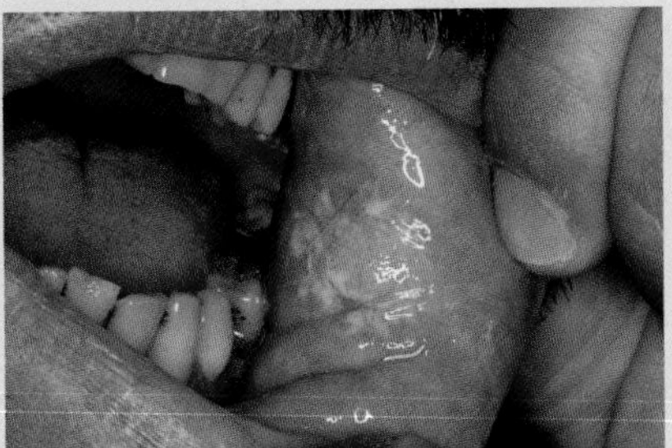
Candidiasis

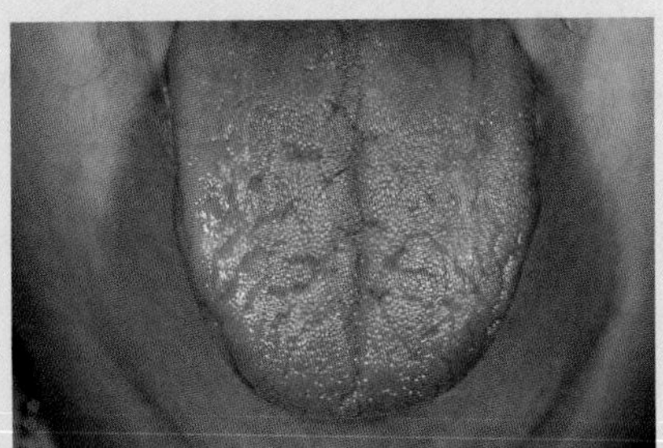
Candidiasis

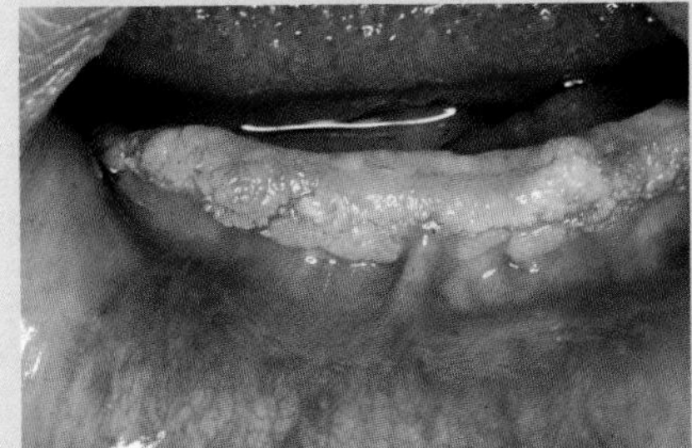
Cowden disease

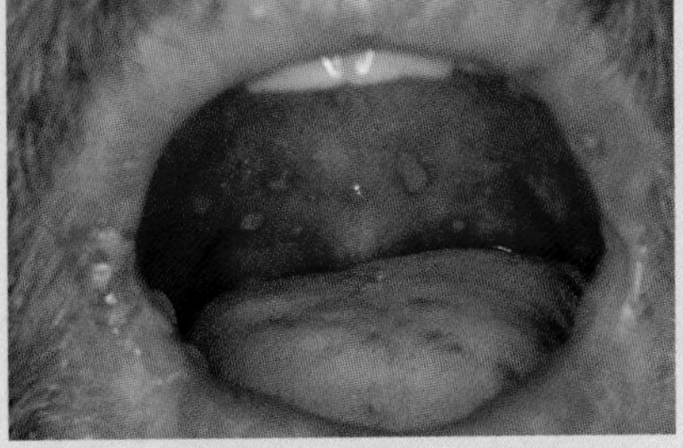
Hand-foot-and-mouth disease

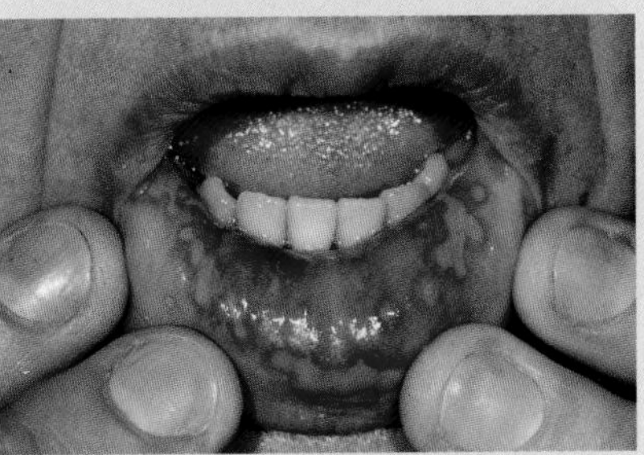
Herpes simplex, primary

Penis

Allergic contact dermatitis (p. 133)
Aphthae (Behçet's syndrome)
Bite (human) (p. 616)
Bowenoid papulosis (p. 427)
Candidiasis (under foreskin) (p. 531)
Chancroid (p. 410)
Condyloma (warts) (p. 421)
Contact dermatitis (condoms) (p. 140)
Eczema (p. 91)
Erythroplasia of Queyrat (Bowen's disease) (p. 823)
Factitious (p. 120)
Fixed drug eruption (p. 577)
Giant condyloma (Buschke-Lowenstein) (p. 830)
Granuloma inguinale (p. 412)
Herpes simplex/zoster (pp. 433, 482)
Lichen nitidus
Lichen planus (p. 325)
Lichen sclerosis (p. 329)
Lymphogranuloma venereum (p. 408)
Molluscum contagiosum (p. 429)
Nevus (p. 848)
Pearly penile papules (p. 423)
Pediculosis (lice) (p. 592)
Penile melanosis
Pseudomonas cellulitis (p. 365)
Psoriasis (p. 273)
Reiter syndrome (p. 273)
Scabies (p. 585)
Sclerosing lymphangitis (nonvenereal)
Seborrheic keratosis (p. 776)
Squamous cell carcinoma (p. 825)
Steroid atrophy (p. 87)
Streptococci cellulitis (p. 348)
Syphilis (chancre) (p. 398)
Warts (p. 421)
Zoon (plasma cell) balanitis

Scrotum

Angiokeratoma (p. 904)
Condyloma (p. 421)
Epidermal cyst (p. 797)
Extramammary Paget's disease (p. 844)
Henoch-Schönlein purpura (p. 733)
Lichen simplex chronicus (pp. 104, 115)
Nevus (p. 848)
Scabies (p. 585)
Seborrheic keratosis (p. 776)

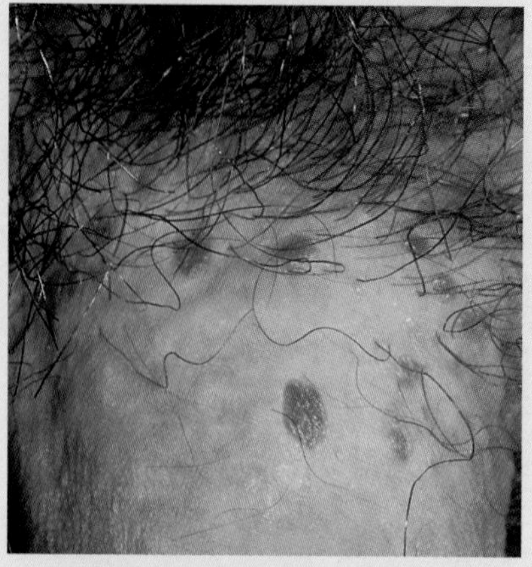
Bowenoid papulosis

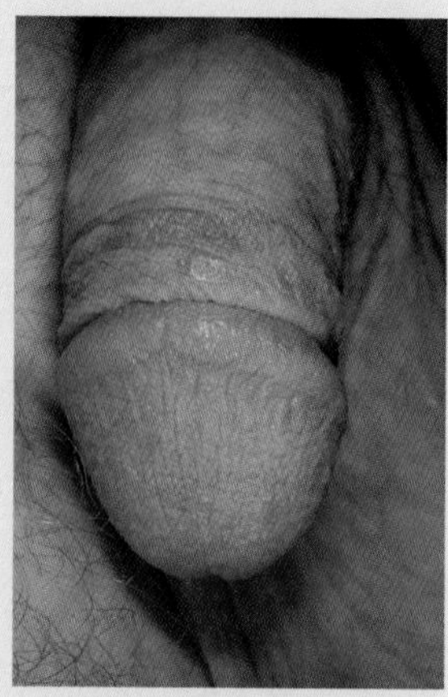
Psoriasis

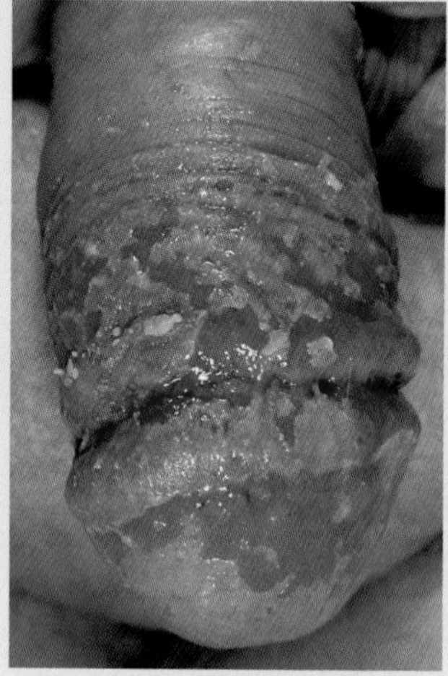
Candidiasis

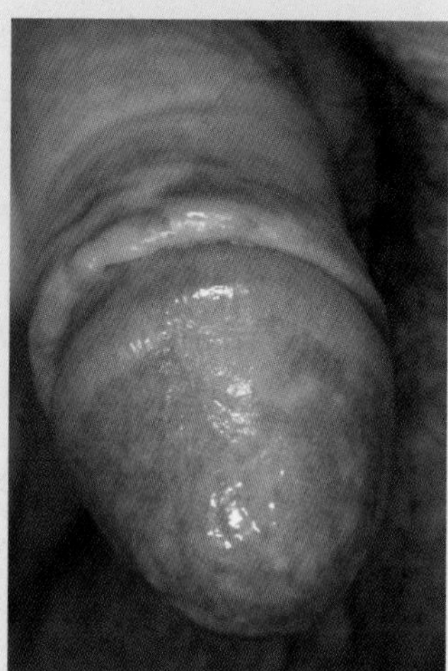
Candidiasis

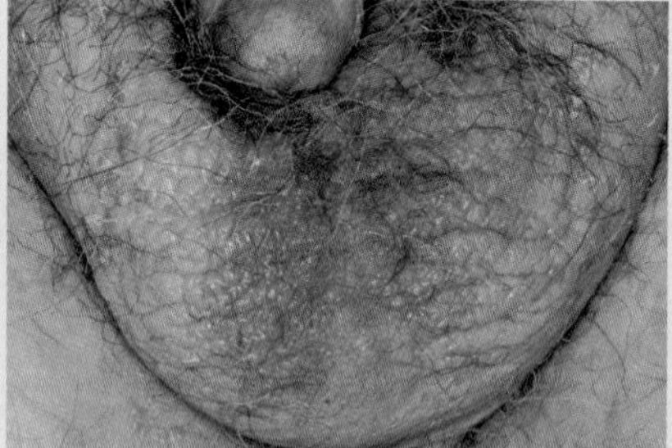
Eczema, lichenified

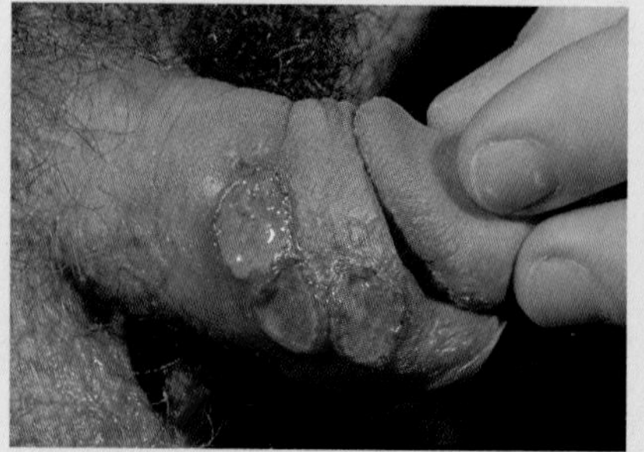
Chancroid

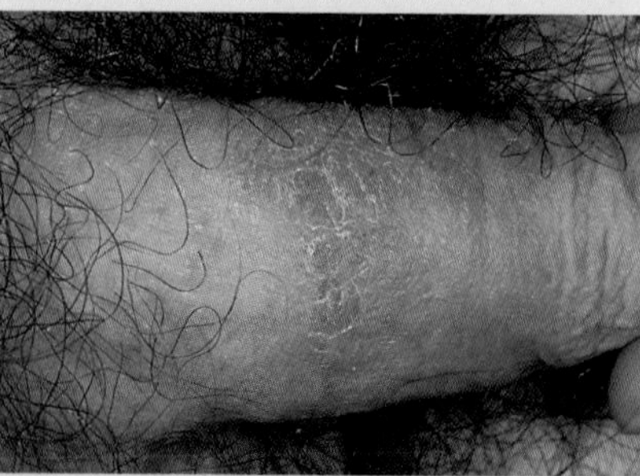
Eczema

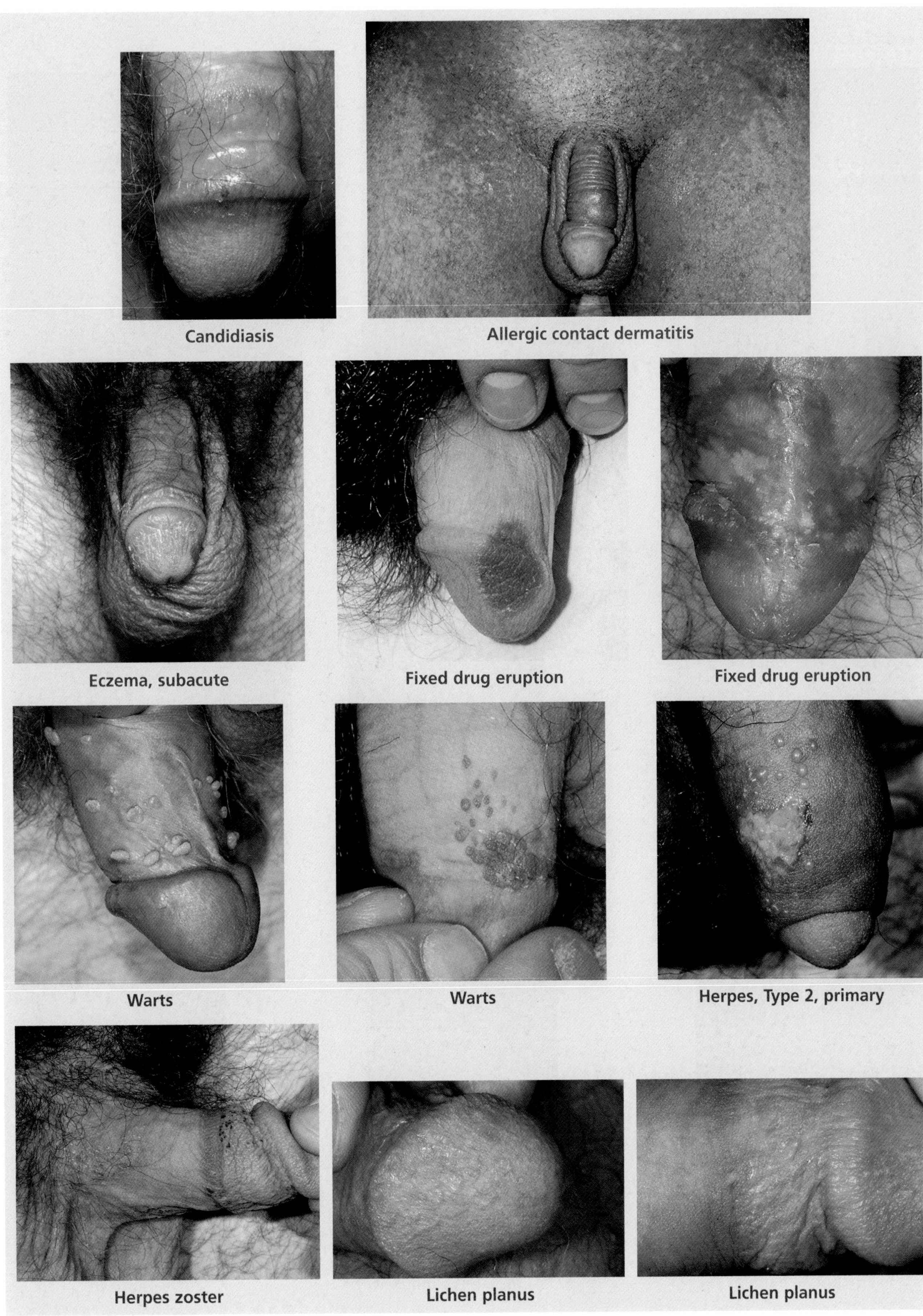

Candidiasis

Allergic contact dermatitis

Eczema, subacute

Fixed drug eruption

Fixed drug eruption

Warts

Warts

Herpes, Type 2, primary

Herpes zoster

Lichen planus

Lichen planus

Penis/Scrotum

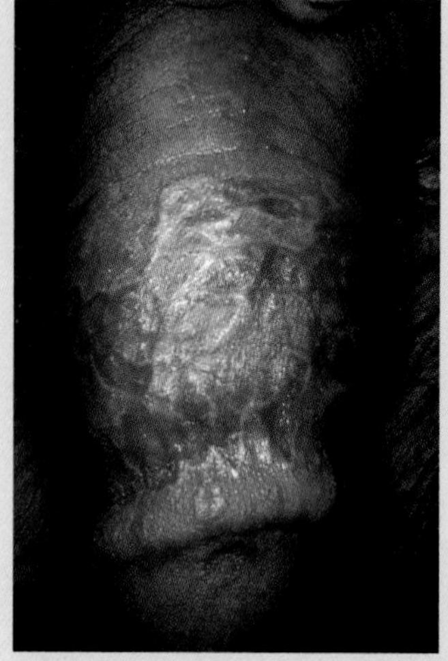

Lichen planus

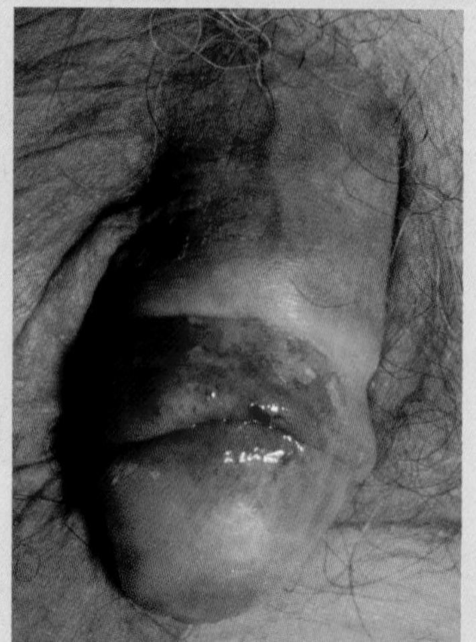

Lichen sclerosis

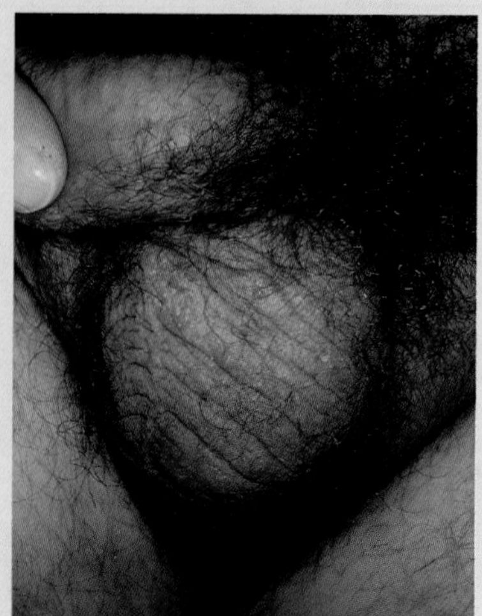

Lichen simplex chronicus

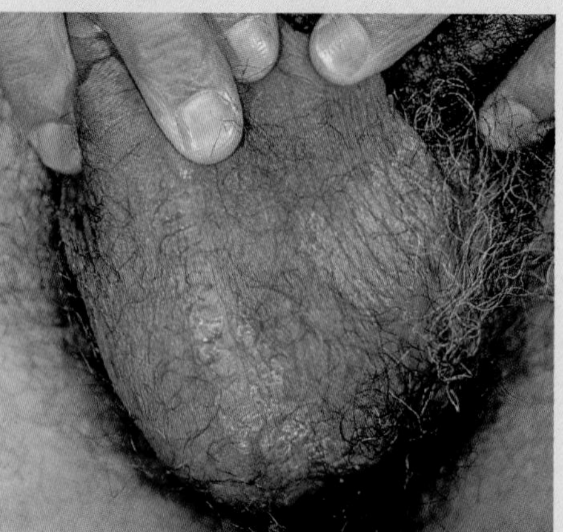

Lichen simplex chronicus

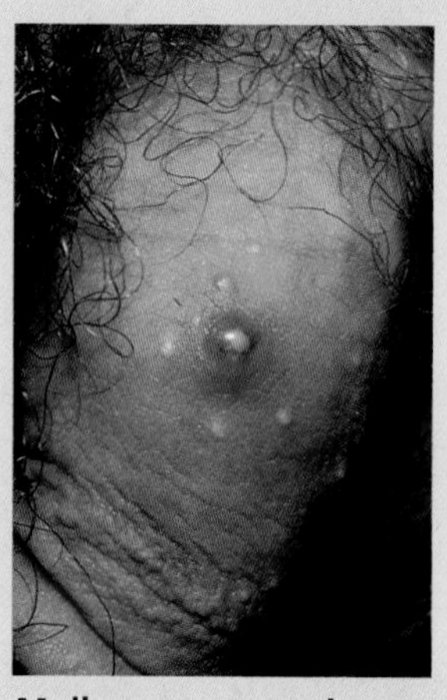

Molluscum contagiosum

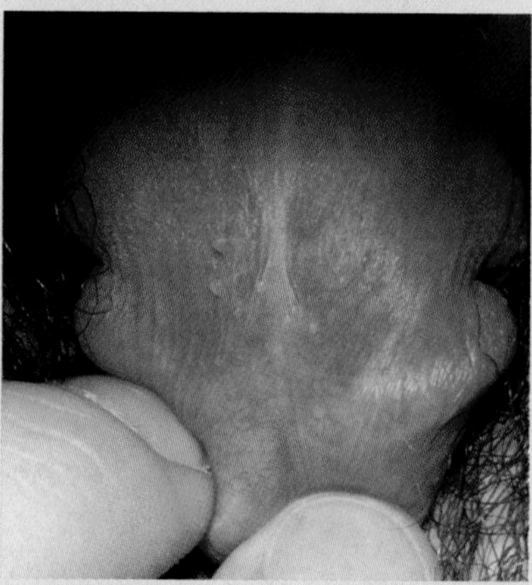

Pearly penile papules

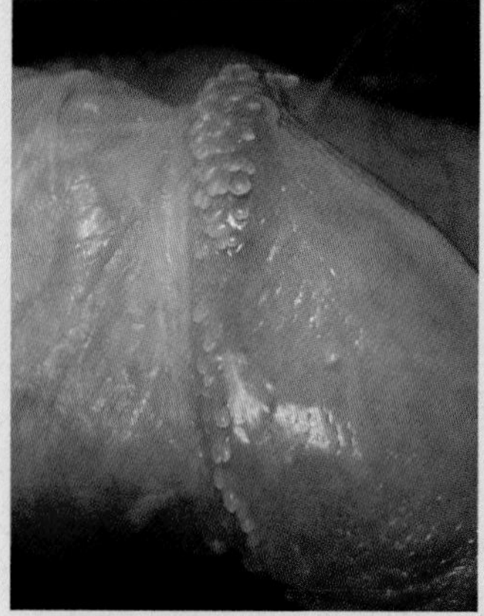

Pearly penile papules

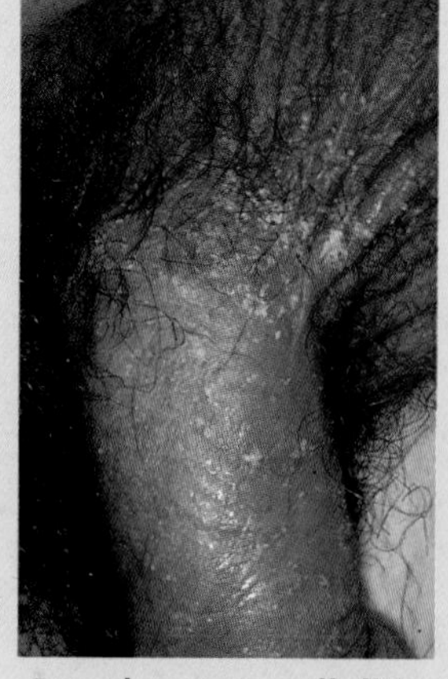

Pseudomonas cellulitis

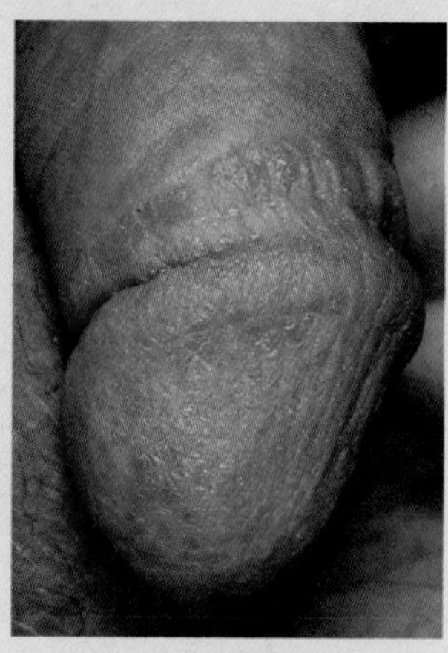

Psoriasis

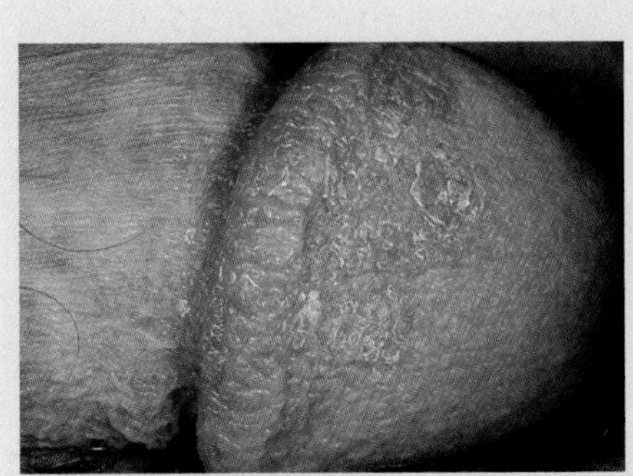
Psoriasis

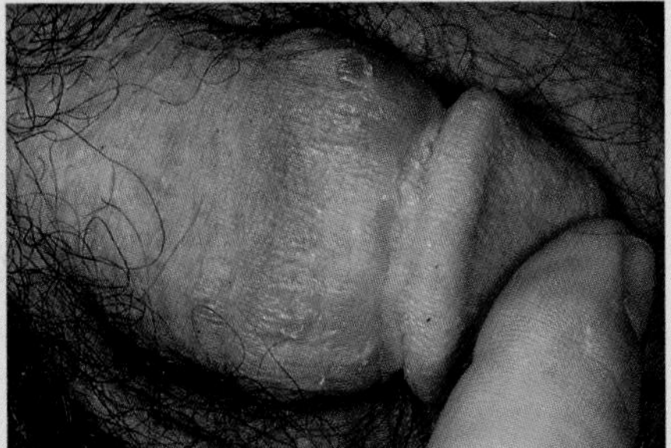
Psoriasis

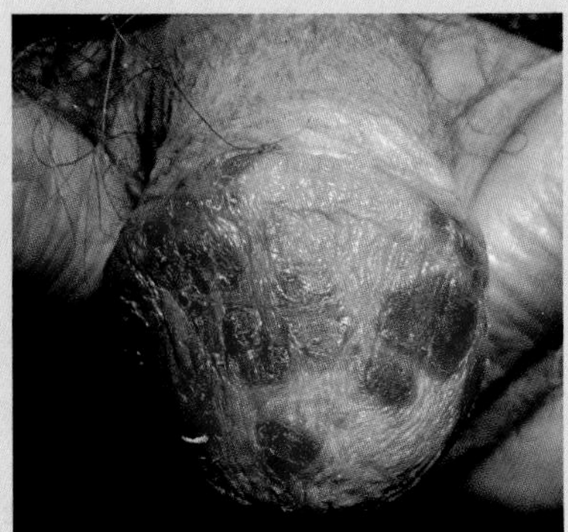
Reiter syndrome

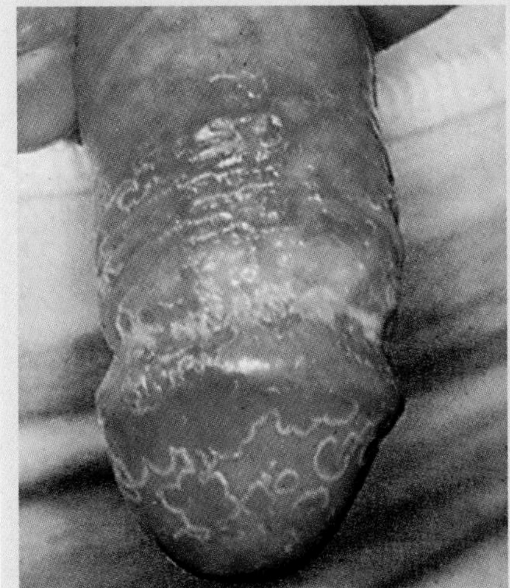
Reiter syndrome

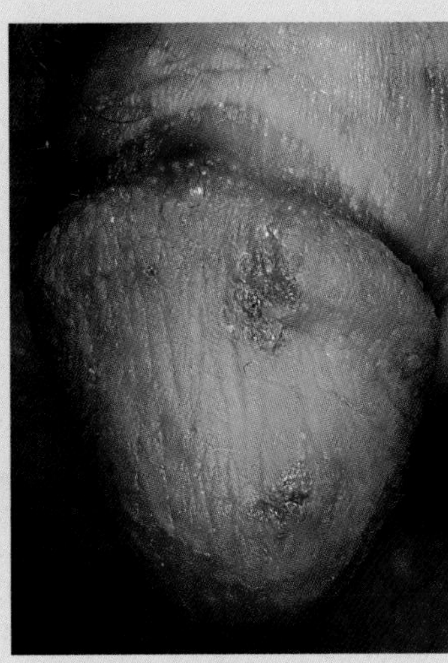
Scabies

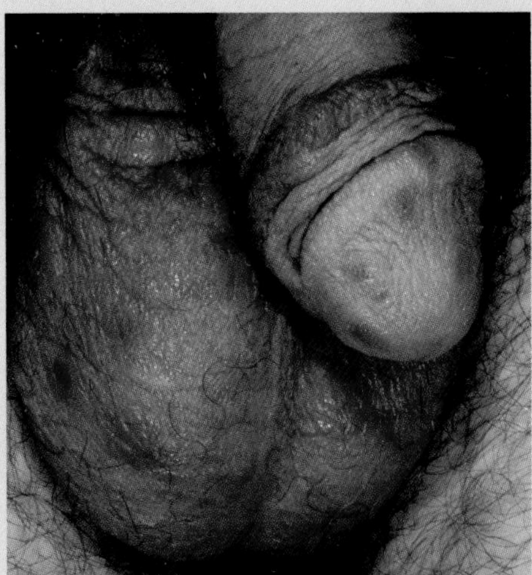
Scabies

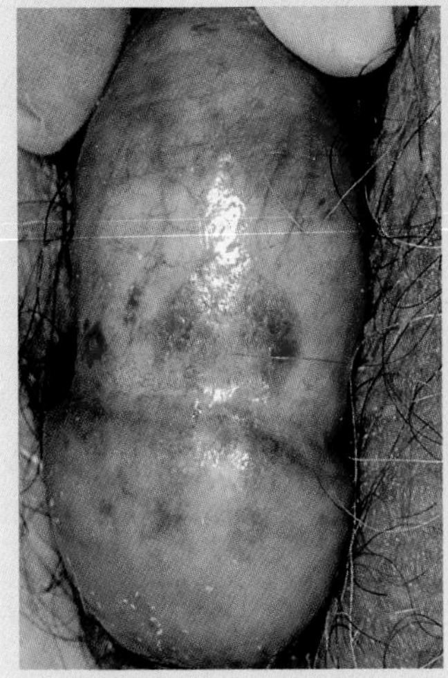
Steroid atrophy

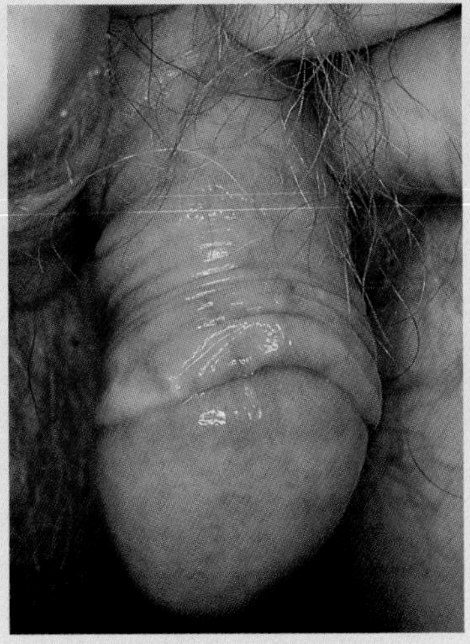
Streptococci cellulitis

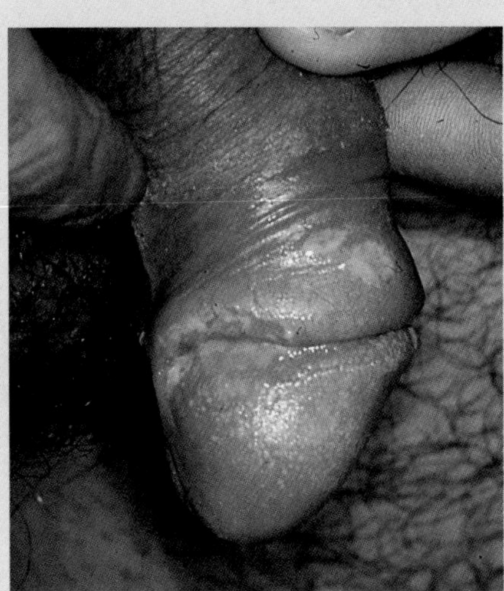
Primary syphilis

Perioral

Acne (p. 227)
Allergic contact dermatitis (p. 133)
Atopic dermatitis (p. 163)
Flat warts (p. 459)
Gram-negative folliculitis (p. 248)
Herpes simplex (p. 467)
Impetigo (p. 338)
Perioral dermatitis (p. 253)
Seborrheic dermatitis (p. 315)
Staphylococcal folliculitis (p. 351)
Sycosis barbae (p. 354)
Tinea incognito (p. 88)

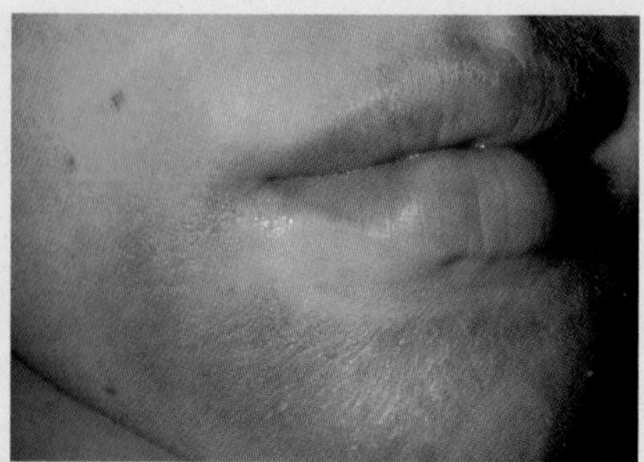
Allergic contact dermatitis

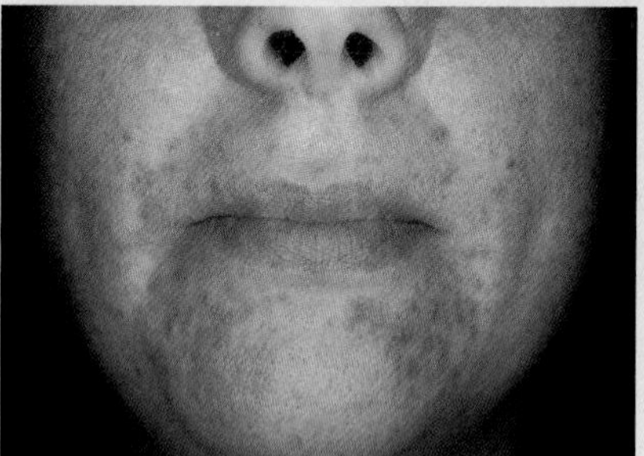
Perioral dermatitis

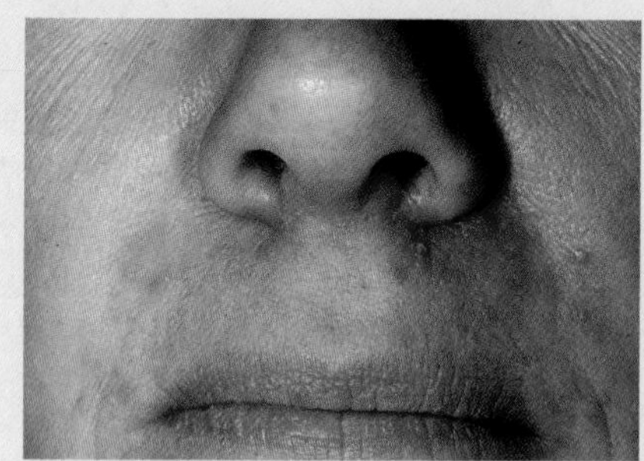
Perioral dermatitis

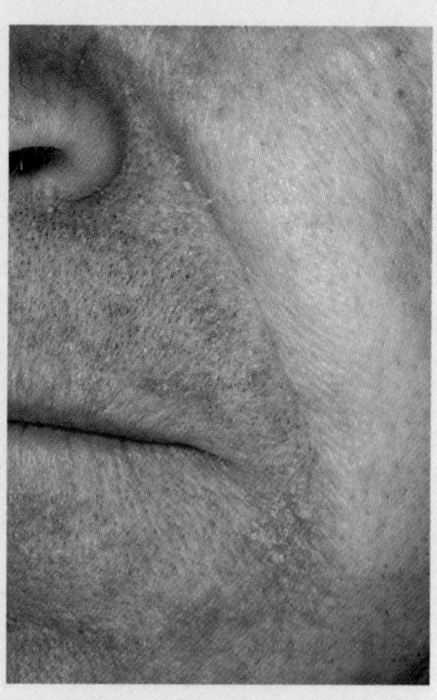
Seborrheic dermatitis

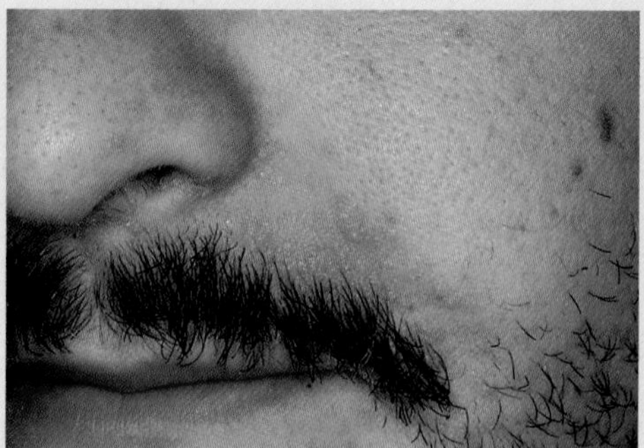
Seborrheic dermatitis

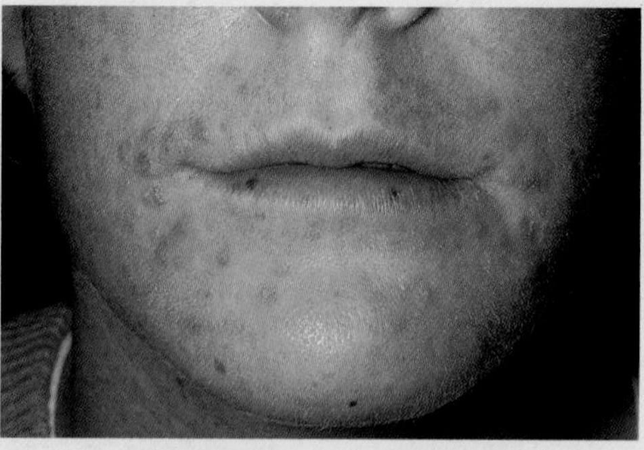
Gram-negative folliculitis

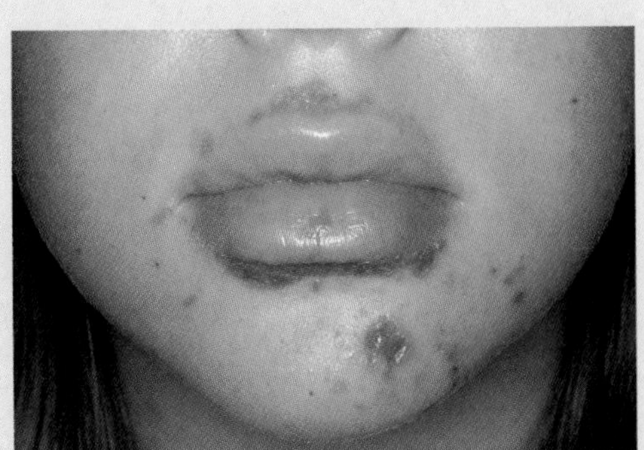
Impetigo

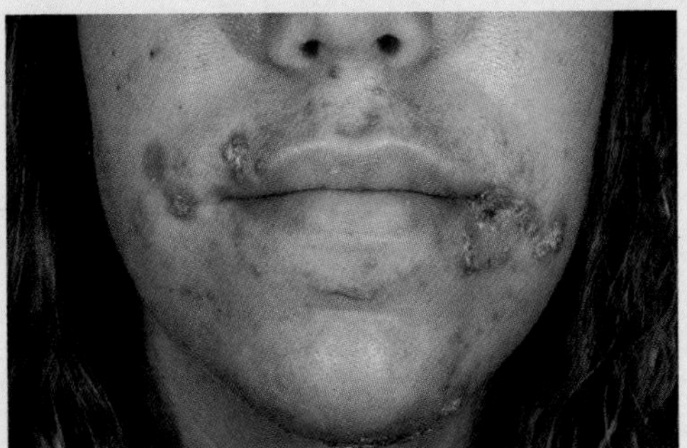
Impetigo

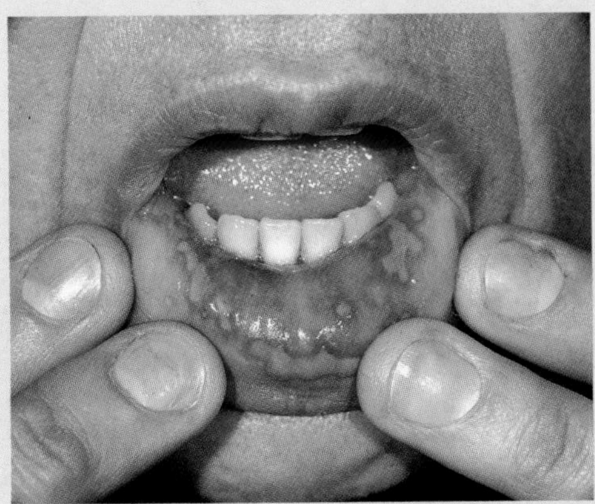
Herpes simplex, Type 1, primary

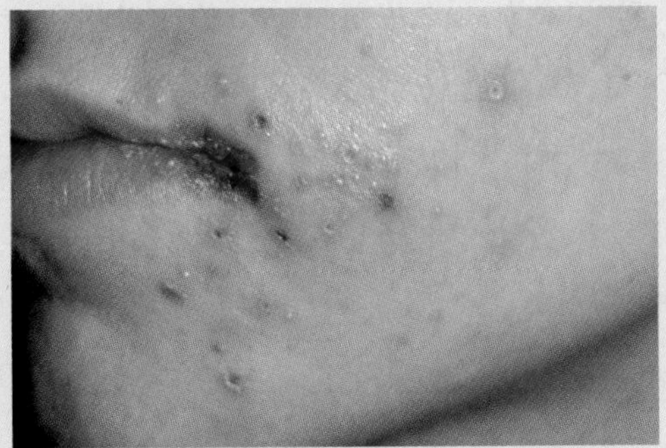
Herpes simplex, Type 1, primary

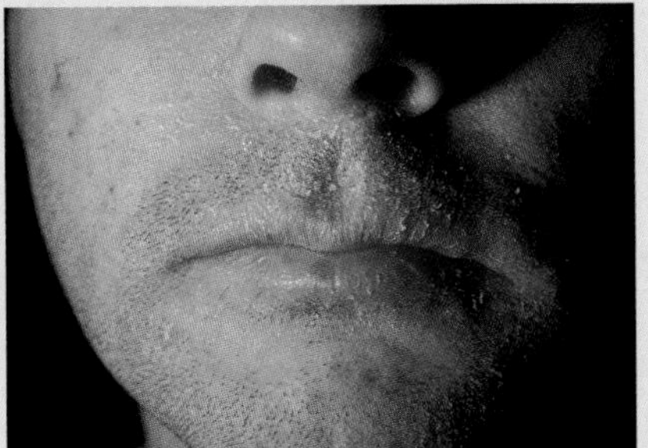
Atopic dermatitis, impetiginized

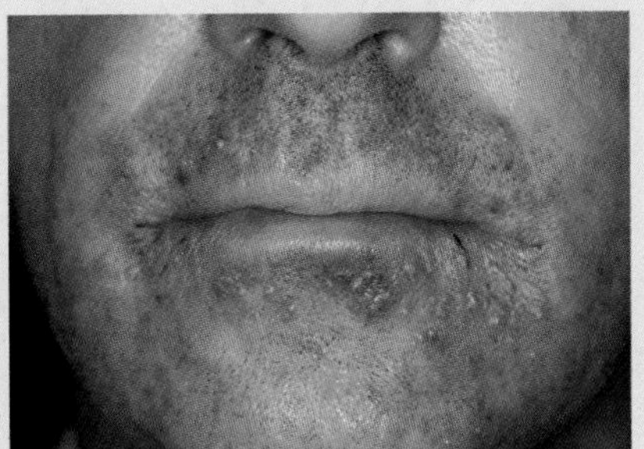
Staphylococcal folliculitis, MRSA

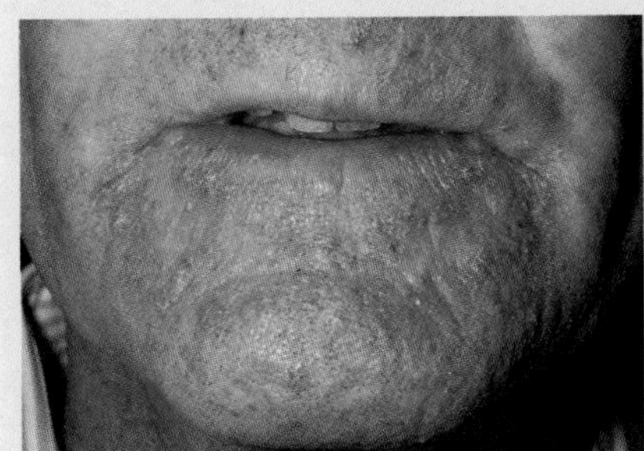
Sycosis barbae

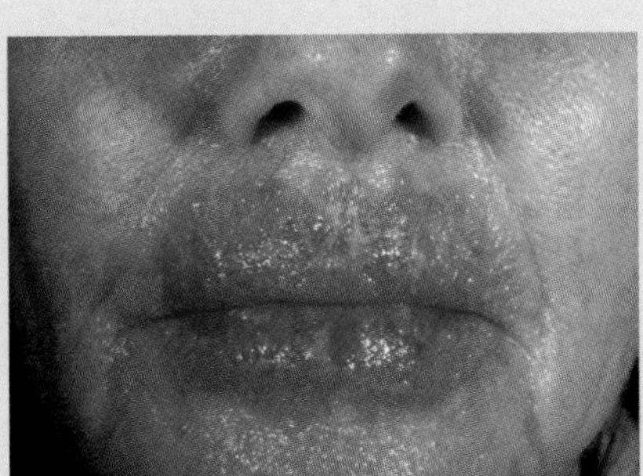
Tinea incognito

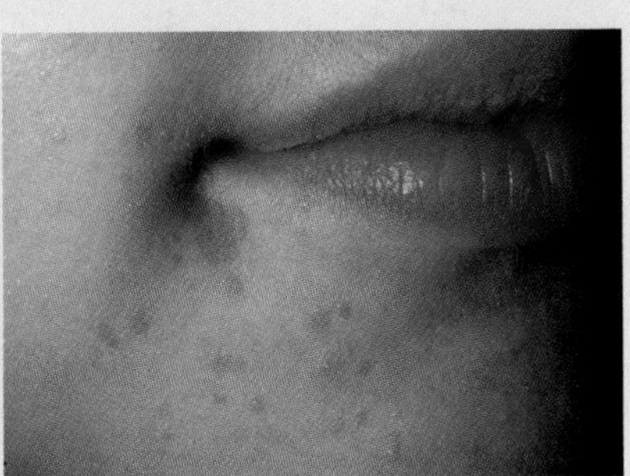
Flat warts

Periorbital

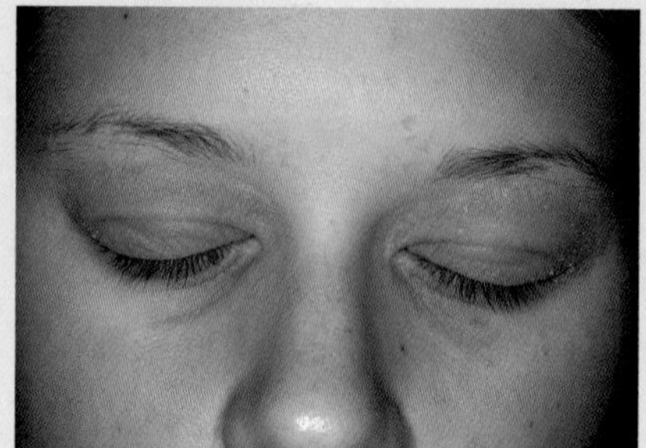
Atopic dermatitis

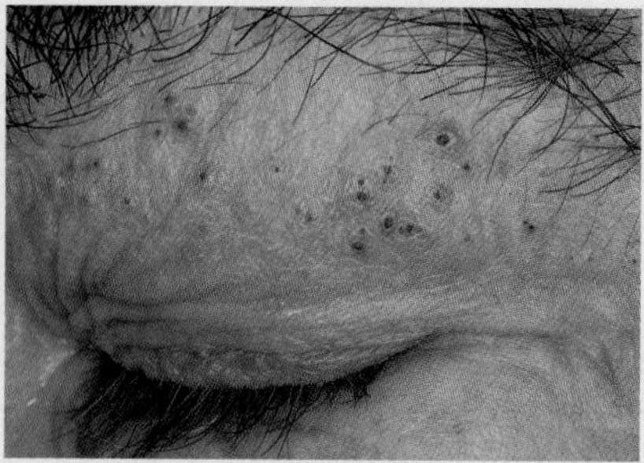
Actinic comedones

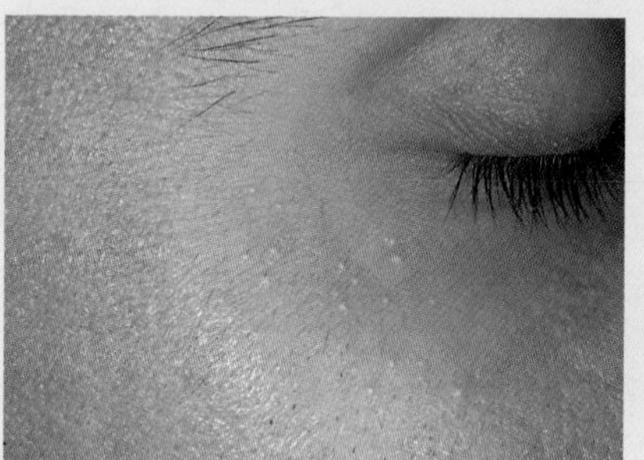
Milia

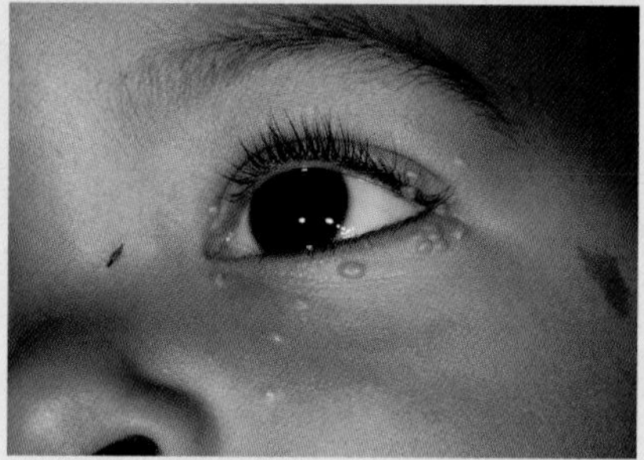
Molluscum contagiosum

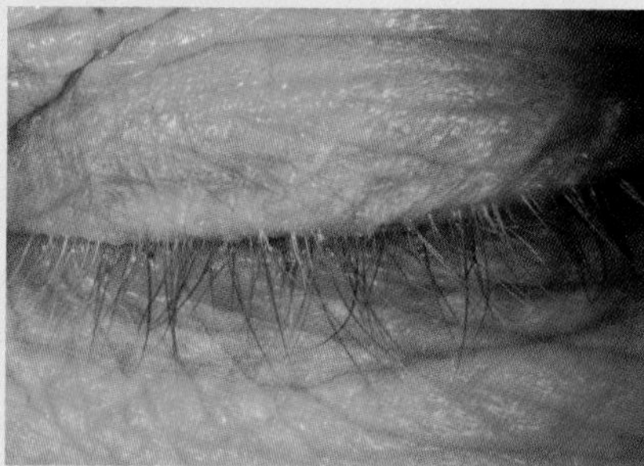
Pediculosis, eyelashes

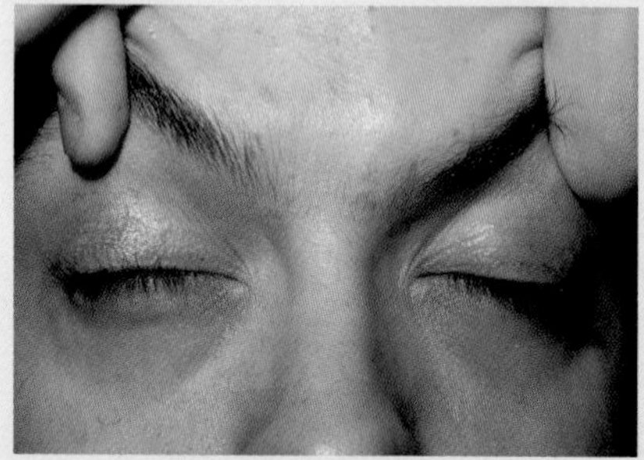
Dermatomyositis

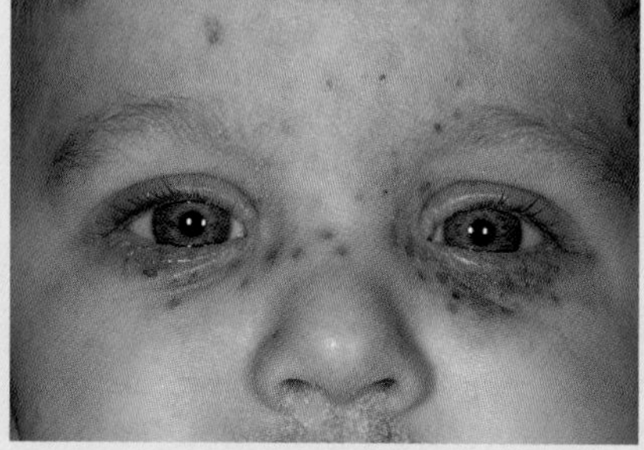
Eczema herpeticum

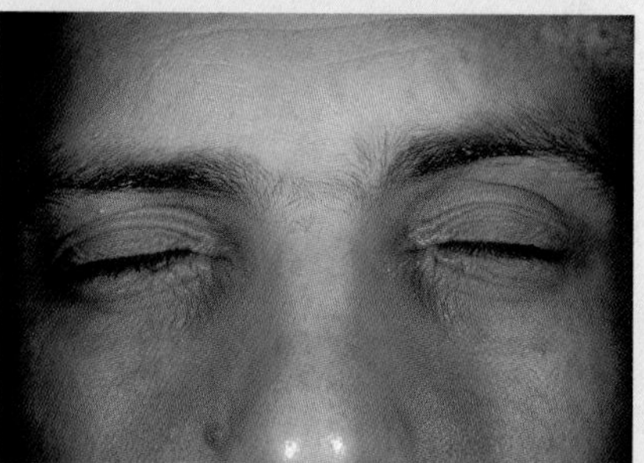
Cosmetic fragrance allergy

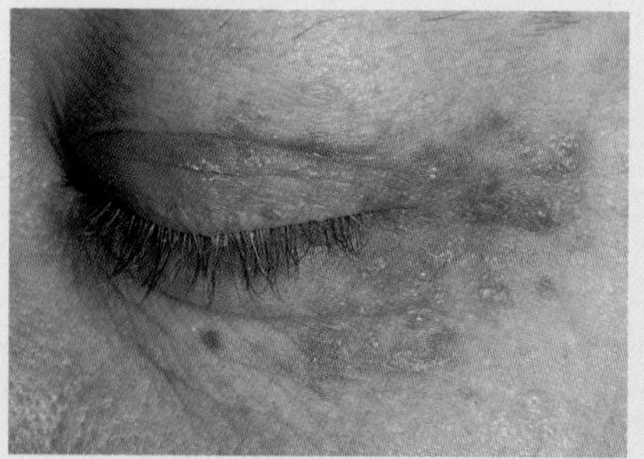
Periorbital dermatitis

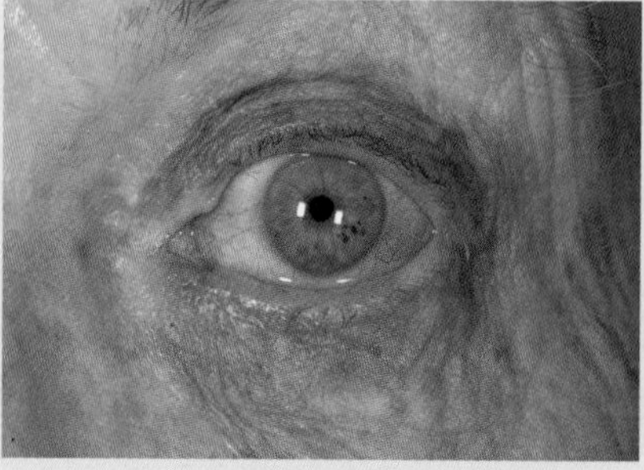
Rosacea

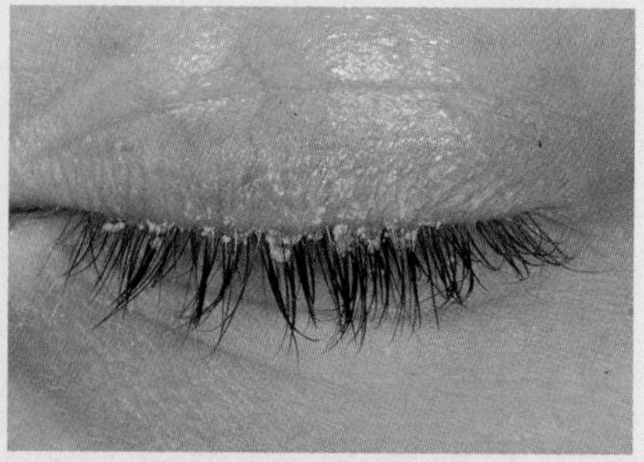
Seborrheic dermatitis

Scalp

Acne necrotica
Actinic keratosis (p. 815)
Alopecia areata (p. 932)
Basal cell carcinoma (p. 801)
Chronic cutaneous (discoid) lupus erythematosus (p. 939)
Contact dermatitis (p. 130)
Dermatomyositis (p. 695)
Dissecting cellulitis (p. 943)
Eczema (p. 99)
Folliculitis (p. 351)
Head lice (p. 591)
Herpes zoster (p. 479)
Kerion (inflammatory tinea) (p. 509)
Lichen planopilaris (p. 940)
Melanoma (p. 860)
Neurotic excoriations (p. 120)
Nevi (p. 848)
Nevus sebaceous (p. 794)
Pediculosis capitis (p. 591)
Pilar cyst (wen) (p. 798)
Prurigo nodularis (p. 119)
Psoriasis (p. 270)
Seborrheic dermatitis (pp. 312, 314)
Seborrheic keratosis (p. 780)
Syphilis (p. 400)
Tinea (p. 509)
Trichotillomania (p. 937)

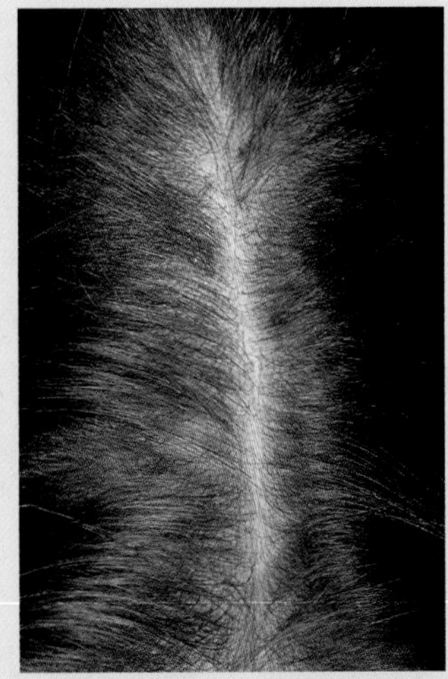
Neurotic excoriations

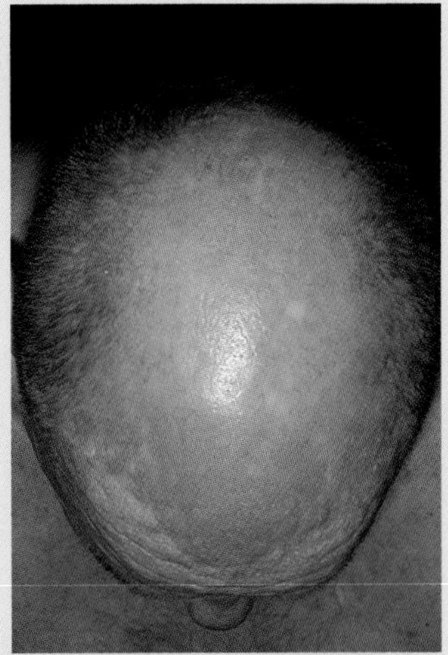
Dermatomyositis

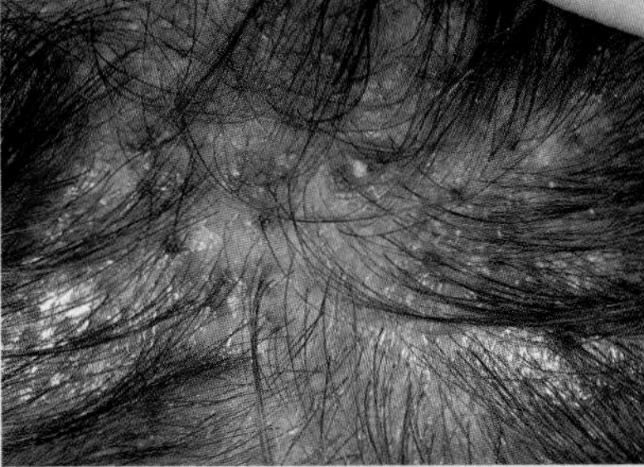
Folliculitis decalvans

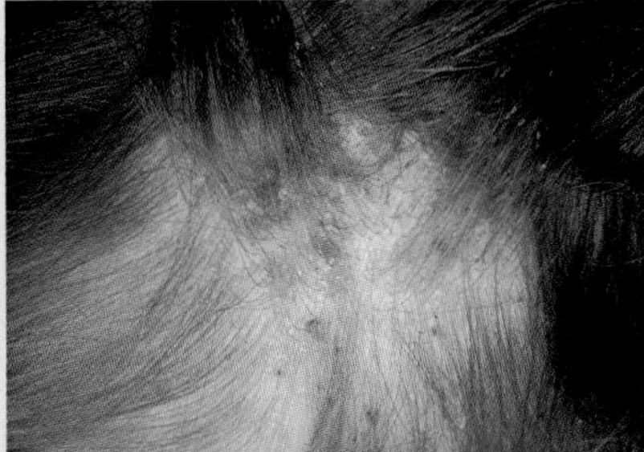
Head lice

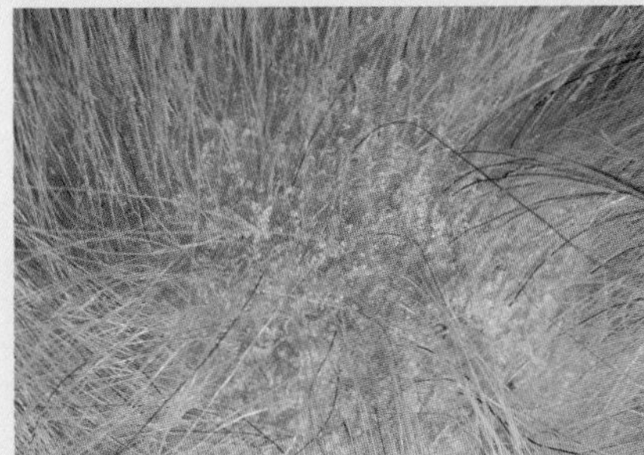
Tinea tonsurans

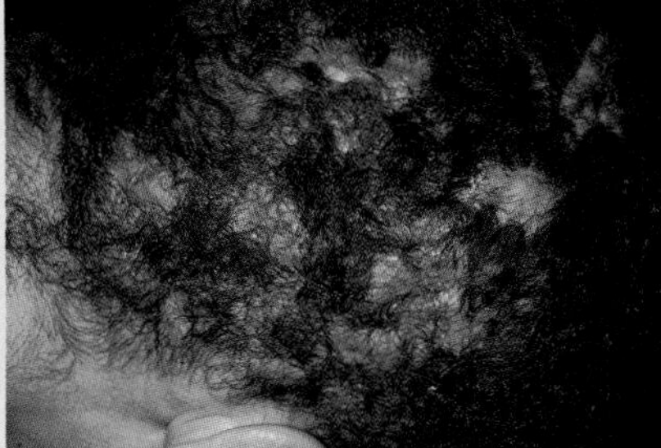
Dissecting cellulitis

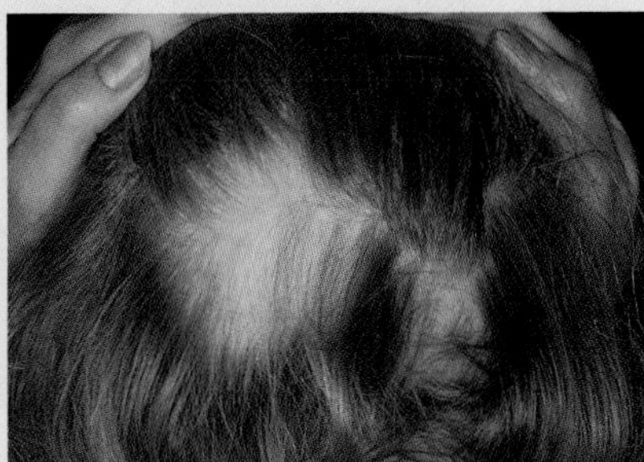
Alopecia areata

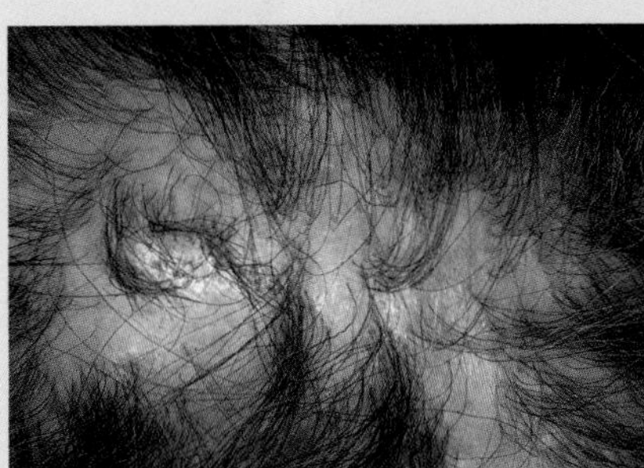
Lichen planopilaris

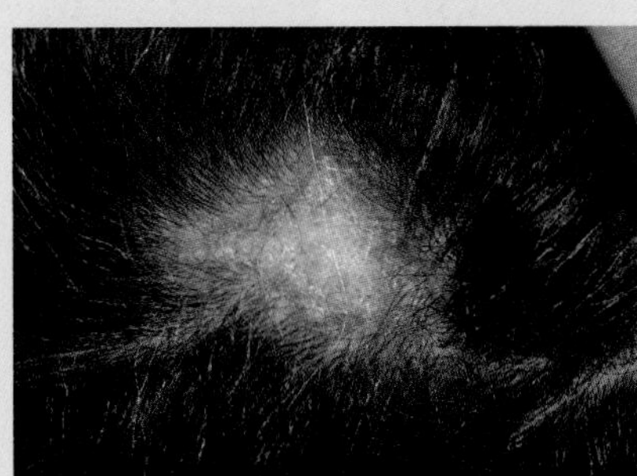
Lupus, chronic cutaneous (discoid)

Scalp

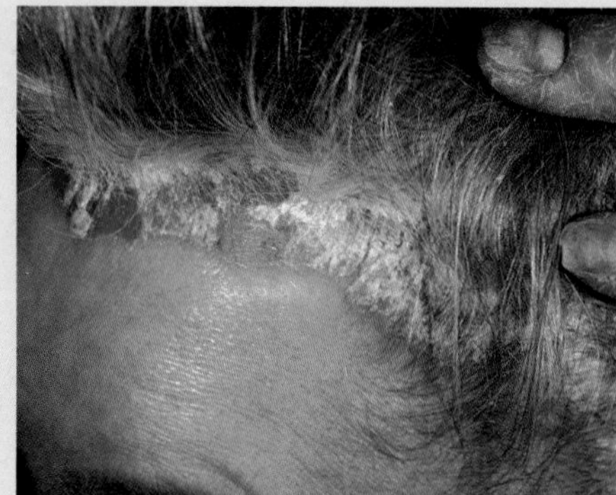

Psoriasis

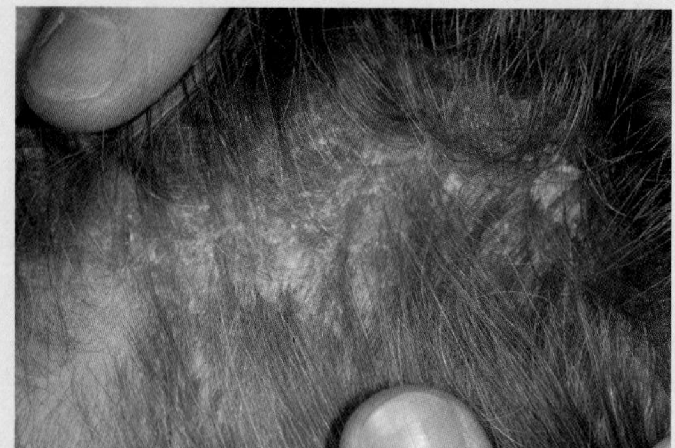

Psoriasis

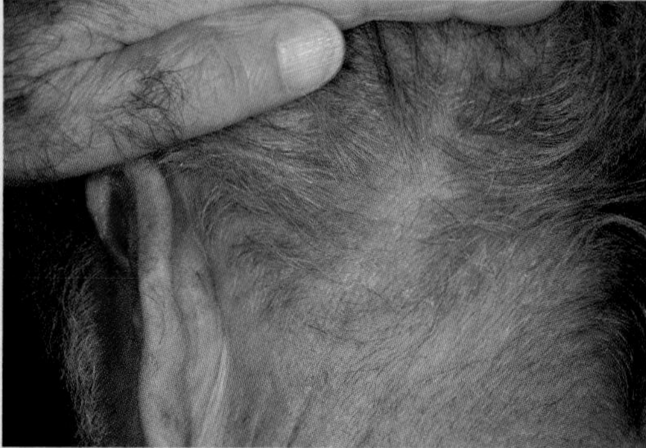

Seborrheic dermatitis

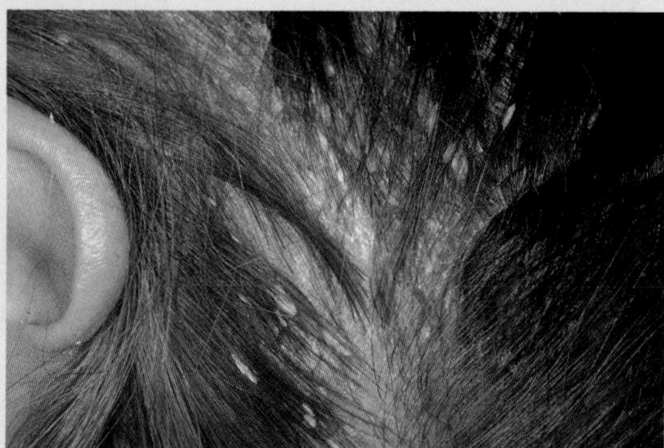

Seborrheic dermatitis

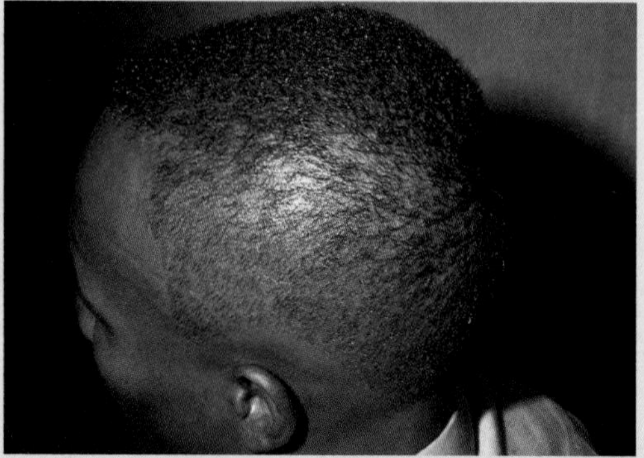

Secondary syphilis

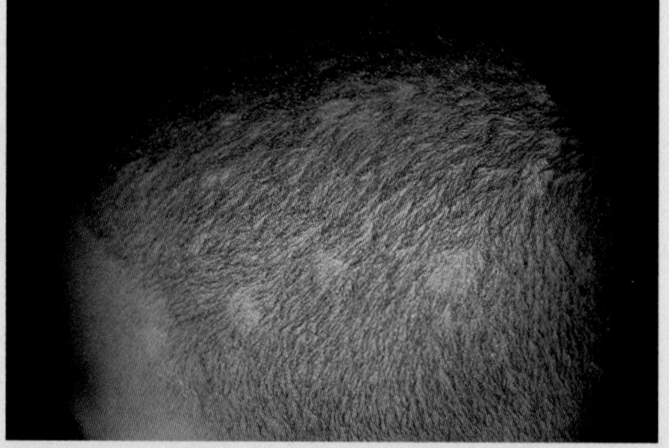

Tinea

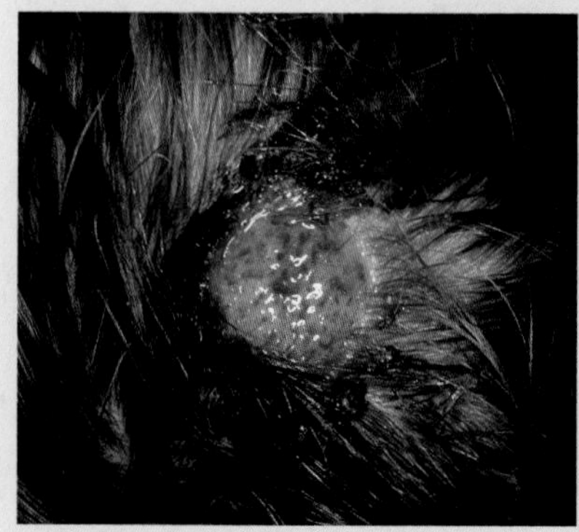

Tinea

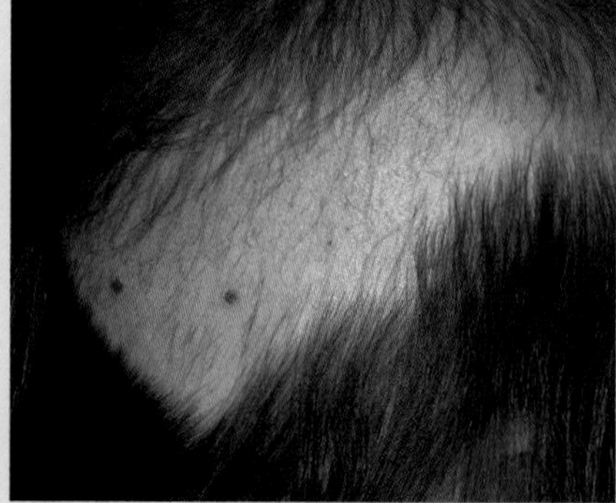

Trichotillomania

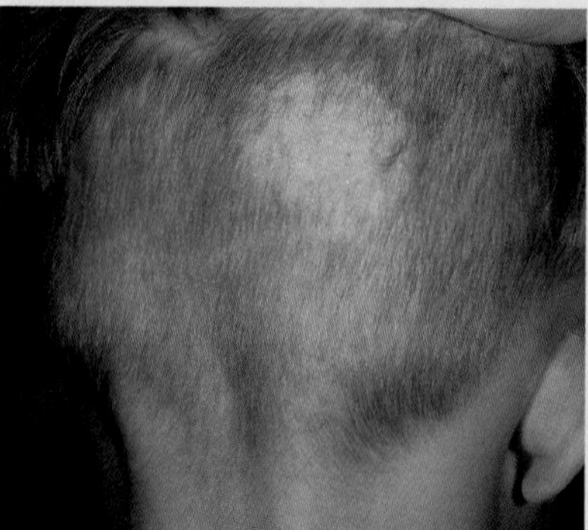

Tinea

Thigh (inner surface and inguinal groove)

Acrochordons (skin tags) (p. 785)
Candidiasis (pp. 499, 531)
Eczema (p. 91)
Erythrasma (p. 501)
Extramammary Paget's disease (p. 844)
Fissures (p. 500)
Granuloma inguinale (p. 412)
Hidradenitis suppurativa (p. 261)
Intertrigo (p. 500)
Keratosis pilaris (anterior) (p. 169)
Lichen sclerosus (p. 328)
Striae (p. 88)
Tinea (p. 499)

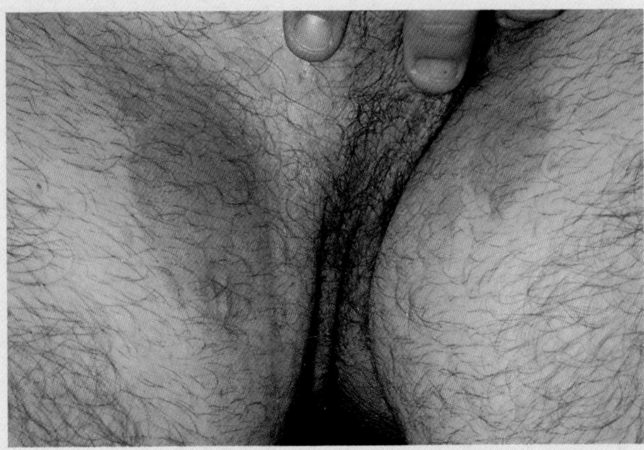

Erythrasma

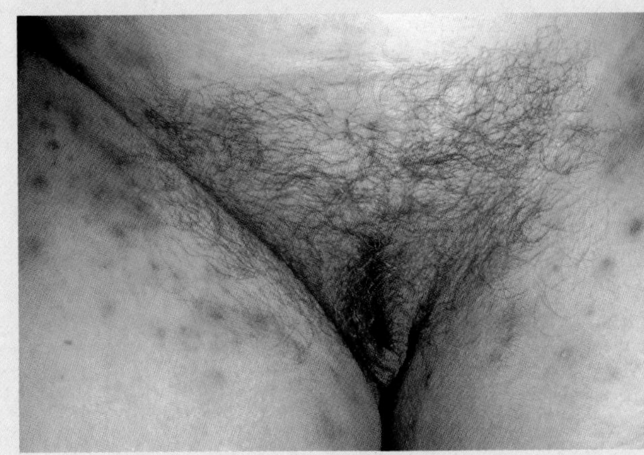

Hidradenitis suppurativa

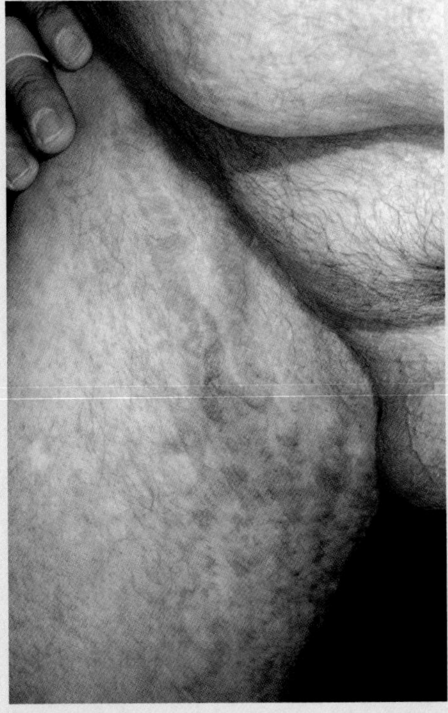

Striae (from strong topical steroids)

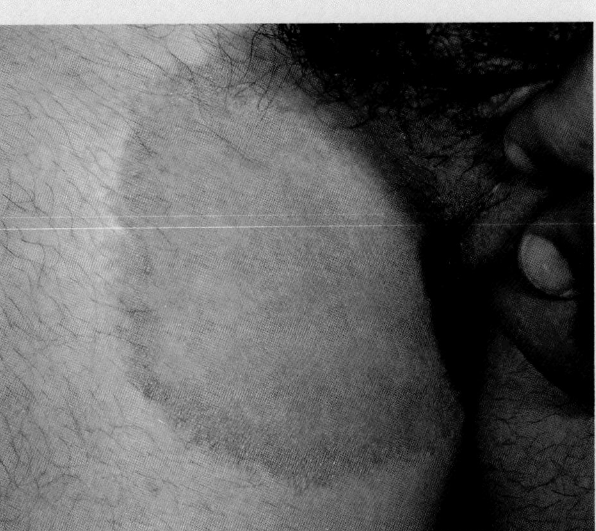

Tinea

Trunk

Accessory nipple
Acne (p. 231)
Actinic keratosis (p. 817)
Anetoderma
Ash-leaf macule (p. 989)
Atopic dermatitis (p. 160)
Chickenpox (p. 475)
CTCL (mycosis fungoides) (p. 832)
Darier's disease
Drug eruption (p. 571)
Eczema (pp. 112, 783)
Epidermal cyst (p. 796)
Eruptive syringoma (p. 800)
Erythema annulare centrifugum
Familial atypical mole syndrome (p. 858)
Fixed drug eruption (p. 576)
Folliculitis (classical and hot tub) (pp. 351, 364)
Granuloma annulare (generalized) (p. 976)
Grover's disease (p. 334)
Hailey-Hailey disease (p. 662)
Halo nevus (p. 885)
Hemangioma (of infancy) (p. 890)
Herpes zoster (p. 479)
Keloids (p. 788)
Leprosy
Lichen planus (p. 320)
Lichen sclerosus (p. 327)
Lupus erythematosus (pp. 684, 685)
Lyme disease (p. 600)
Mastocytosis (p. 211)
Measles (p. 544)
Miliaria (p. 263)
Morphea (p. 708)
Nevus anemicus (p. 770)
Nevus spilus (p. 853)
Parapsoriasis (p. 837)
Pediculosis (lice) (p. 590)
Pemphigus foliaceous (p. 650)
Pityriasis lichenoides (p. 332)
Pityriasis rosea (p. 316)
Pityriasis rubra pilaris (p. 309)
Pityrosporum folliculitis (p. 540)
Poikiloderma vasculare atrophicans (p. 837)
Psoriasis (guttate) (p. 268)
Sarcoid
Scabies (p. 586)
Seborrheic dermatitis (p. 312)
Steatocystoma multiplex
Syphilis (secondary) (p. 401)
Tinea (p. 502)
Tinea versicolor (p. 537)
Unilateral nevoid telangiectasia (p. 912)
Urticaria pigmentosa (p. 212)
Viral exanthem (p. 558)
von Recklinghausen's neurofibromatosis (p. 984)

Chest

Acne (p. 233)
Actinic keratosis (p. 817)
Darier's disease
Eruptive syringoma (p. 800)
Eruptive vellus hair cyst
Keloids (p. 788)
Nevus anemicus (p. 770)
Seborrheic dermatitis (p. 312)
Steatocystoma multiplex
Tinea versicolor (p. 537)
Transient acantholytic dermatitis (Grover's disease) (p. 334)

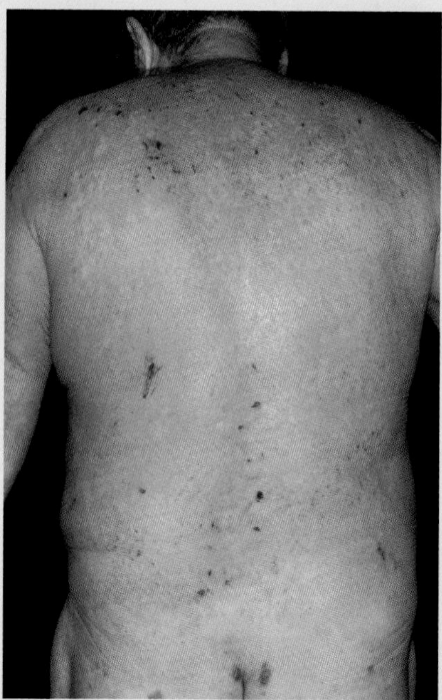

Atopic dermatitis

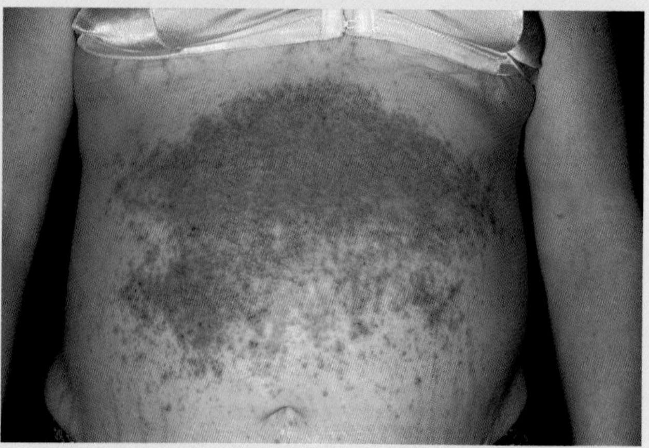

Darier's disease

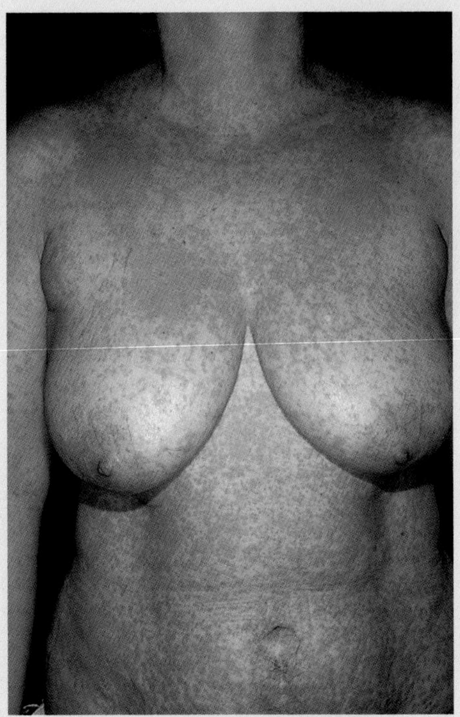
Drug eruption, ampicillin

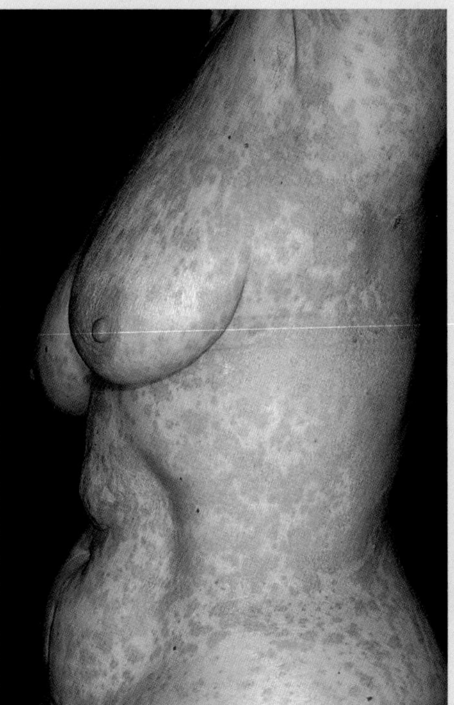
Drug eruption, ampicillin

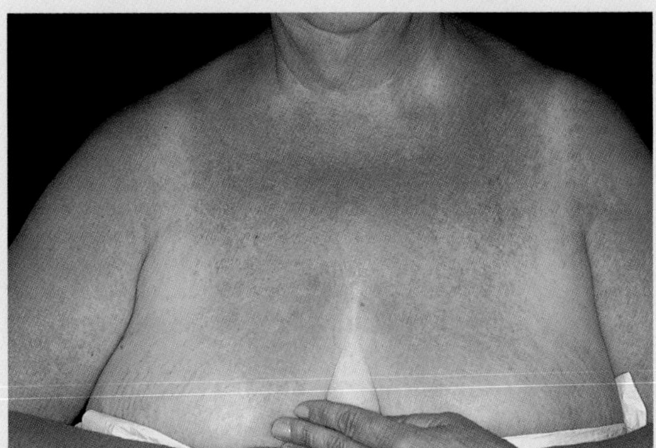
Drug eruption, light induced

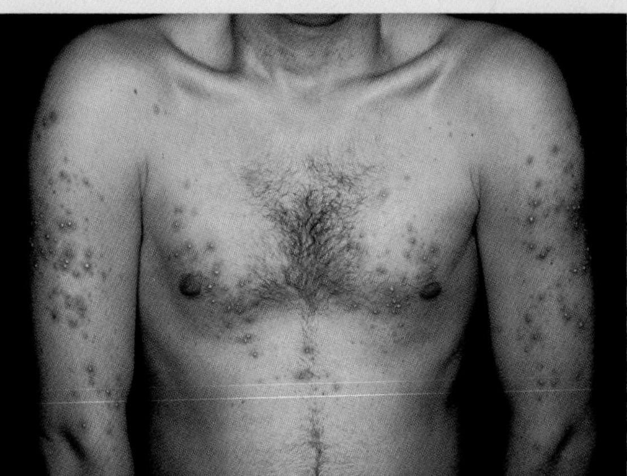
Drug eruption, acute generalized exanthematous pustulosis

Trunk/Chest

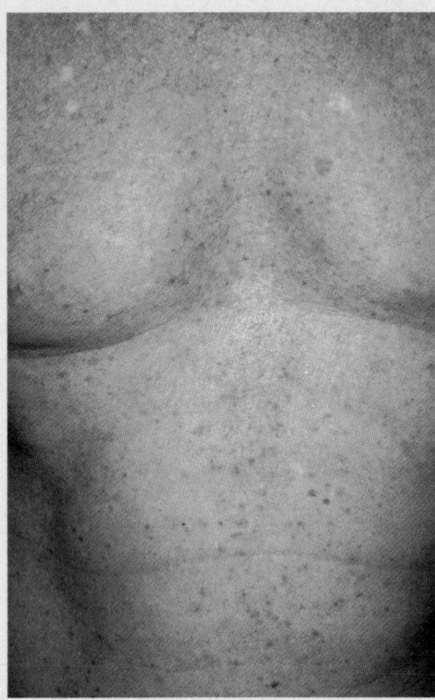

Grover's disease

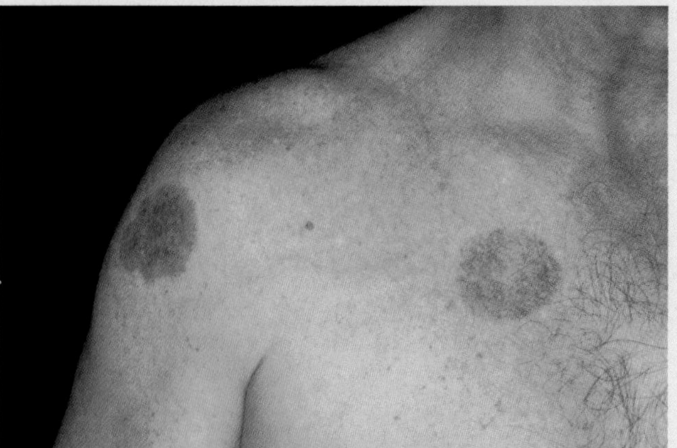

Fixed drug eruption

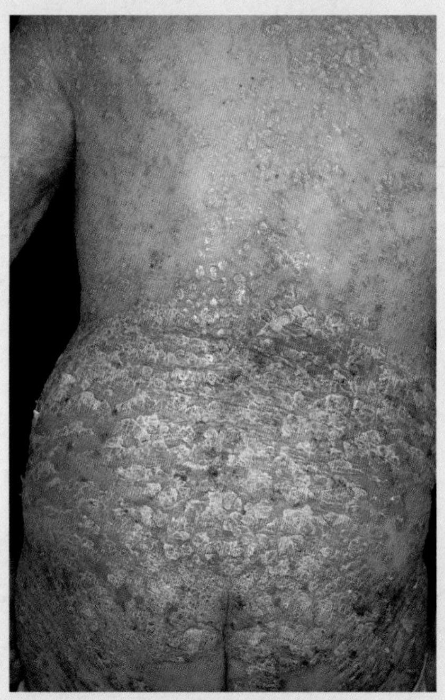

Psoriasis

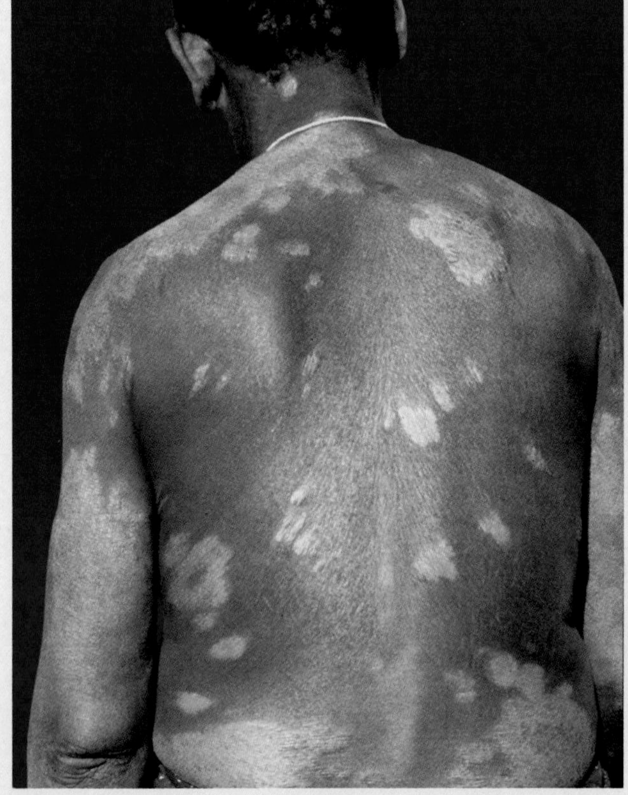

Leprosy

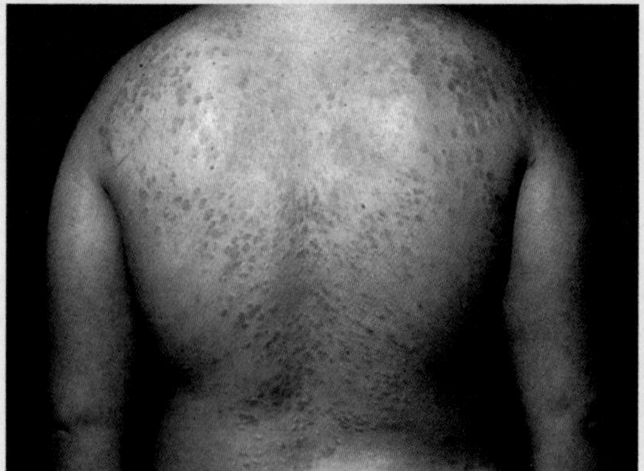

Granuloma annulare

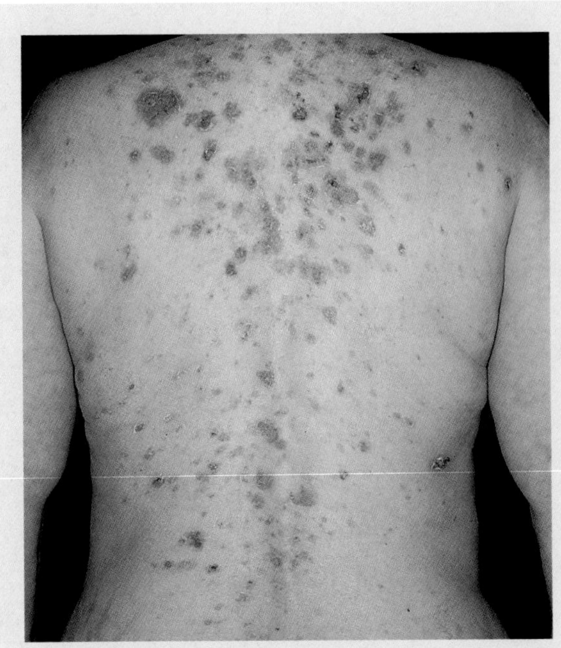
Pemphigus foliaceous

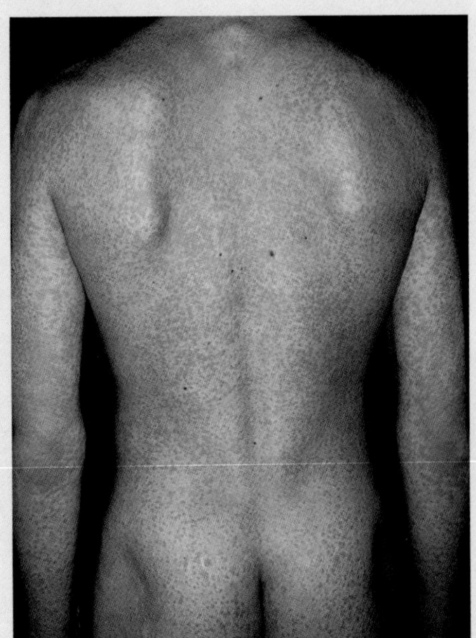
Enterovirus exanthem

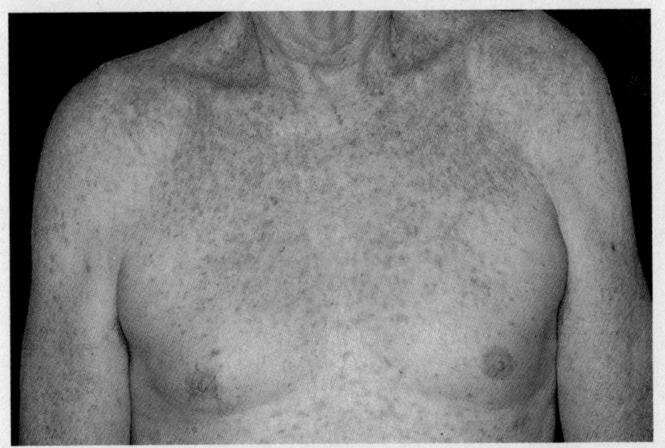
Eczema, generalized

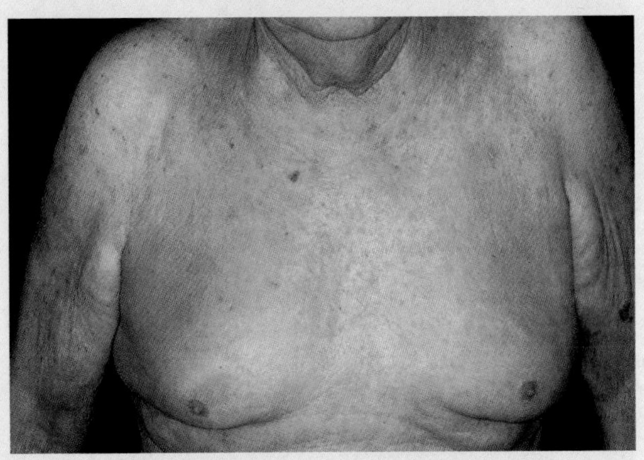
Eczema, generalized

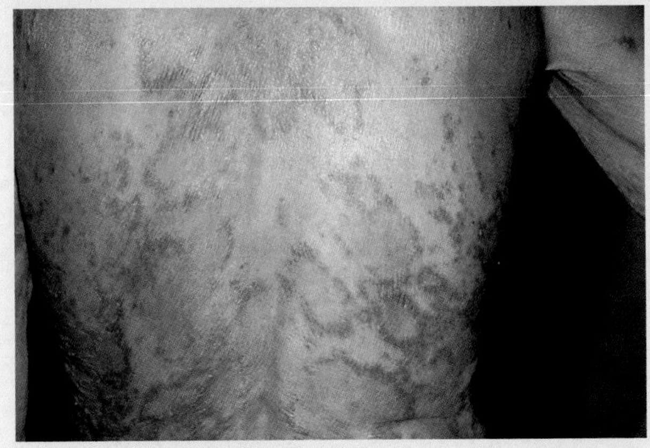
Lupus, subacute

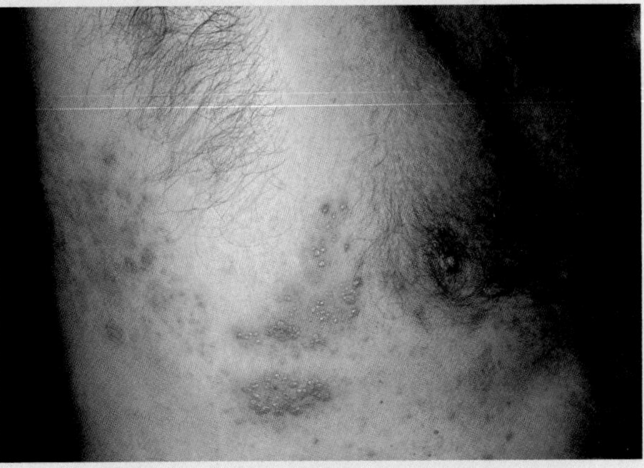
Herpes zoster

Trunk/Chest

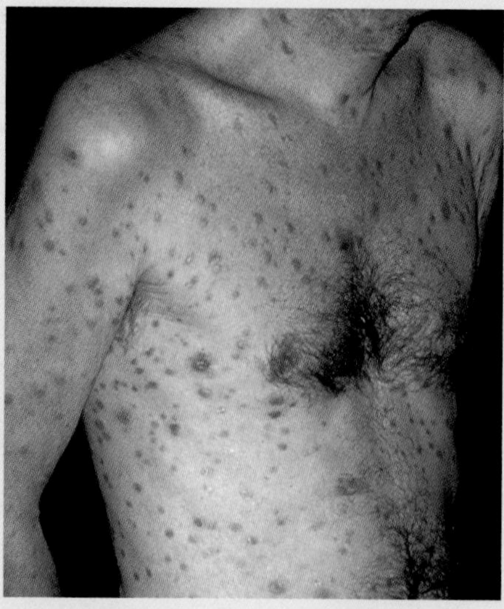
Secondary syphilis

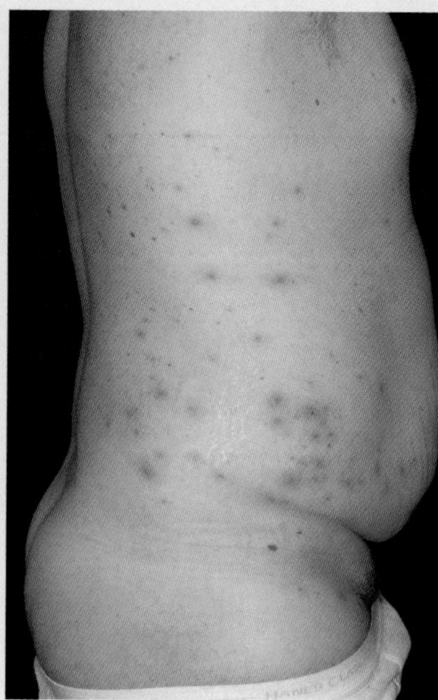
Pseudomonas folliculitis

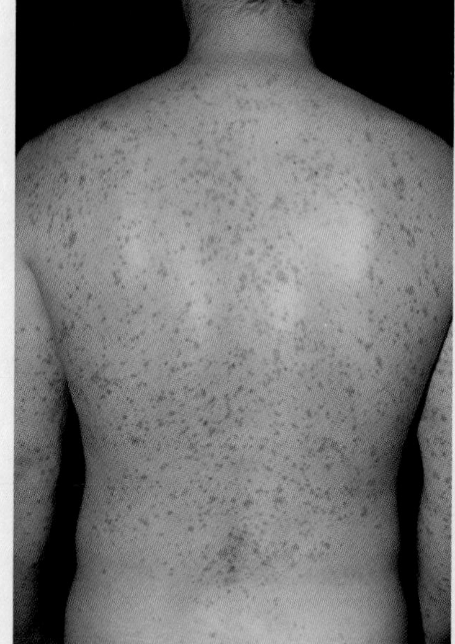
Psoriasis, guttate

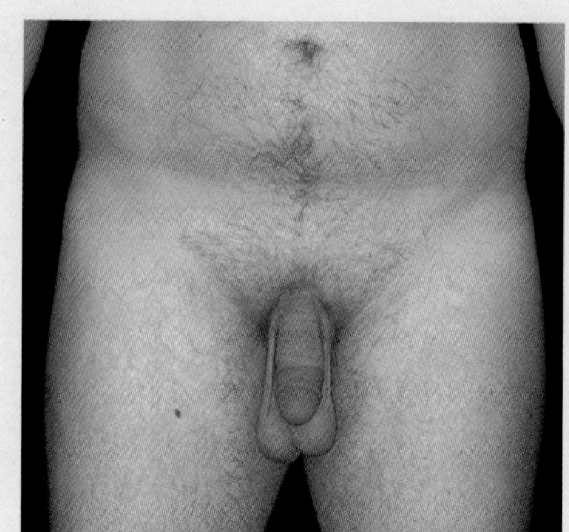
Viral exanthems

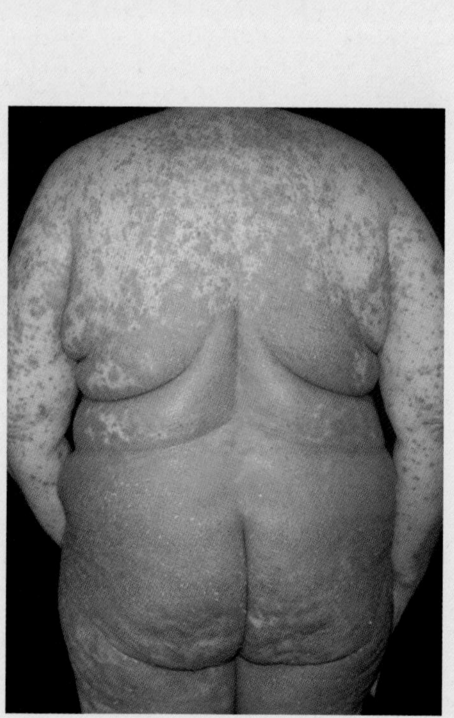
Psoriasis, erythrodermic

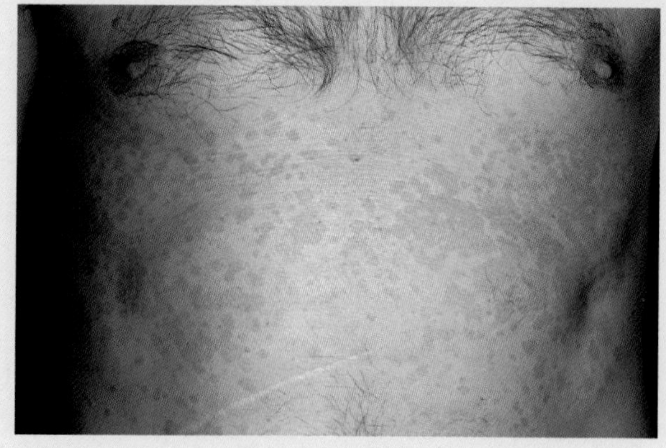
Tinea versicolor

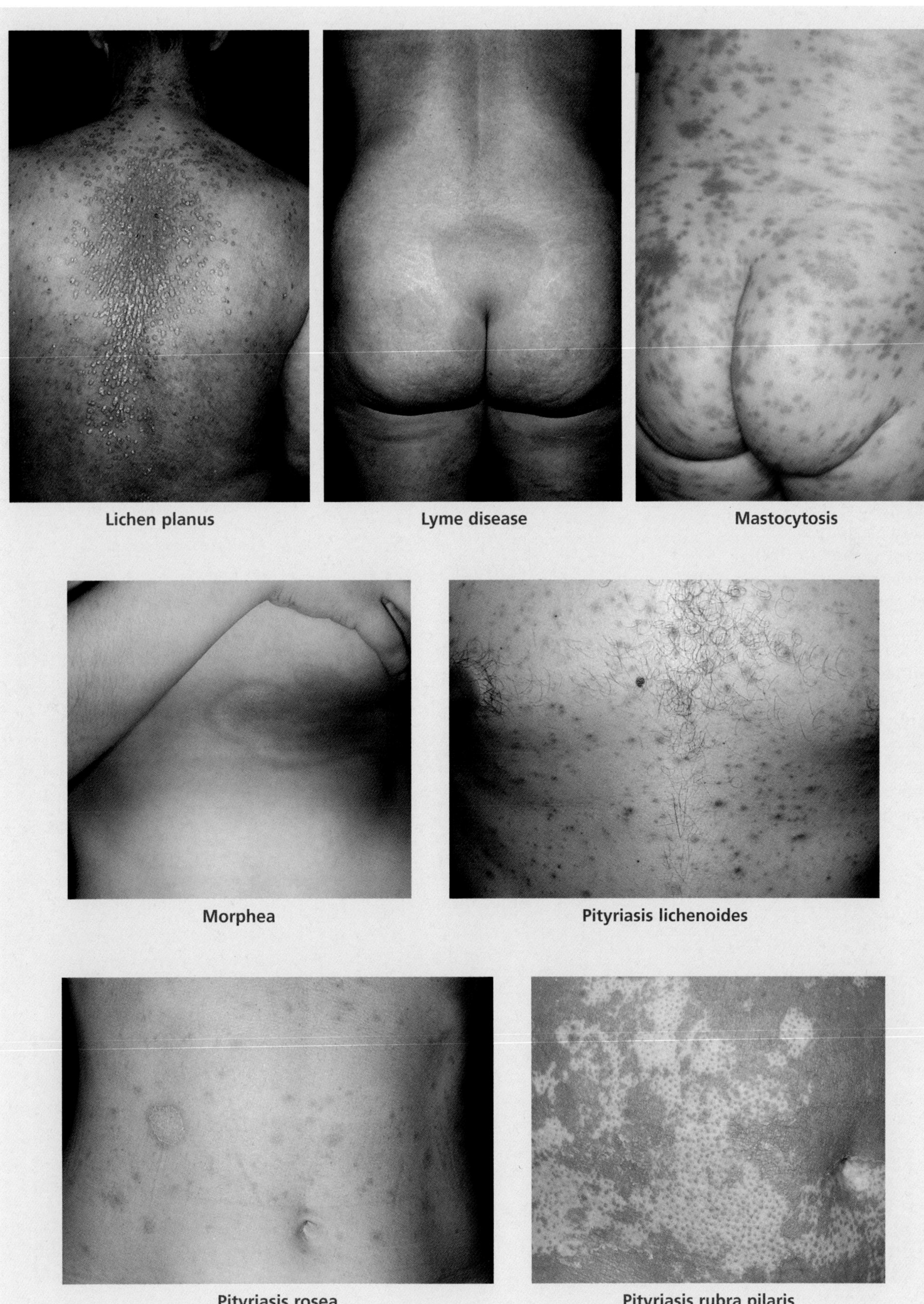

Lichen planus

Lyme disease

Mastocytosis

Morphea

Pityriasis lichenoides

Pityriasis rosea

Pityriasis rubra pilaris

Vulva

Allergic contact dermatitis (p. 133)
Angiokeratoma (p. 904)
Behçet's syndrome
Bowen's disease (p. 821)
Candidiasis (p. 527)
Chancroid (p. 410)
Cicatricial pemphigoid (p. 658)
Eczema (p. 91)
Epidermal cyst (p. 797)
Erythrasma (p. 501)
Extramammary Paget's disease (p. 844)
Fibroepithelial polyp (p. 785)
Folliculitis (p. 351)
Fordyce spots (p. 797)
Furunculosis (p. 356)
Granuloma inguinale (p. 412)
Herpes simplex/zoster (pp. 433, 485)
Hidradenitis suppurativa (p. 261)
Intertrigo (p. 501)
Leukoplakia (p. 829)
Lichen planus (p. 325)
Lichen sclerosus (p. 328)
Lichen simplex chronicus (p. 115)
Melanoma (p. 862)
Molluscum contagiosum (p. 428)
Nevus (p. 848)
Pediculosis (p. 592)
Psoriasis (p. 274)
Squamous cell carcinoma (p. 824)
Stevens-Johnson syndrome (p. 716)
Syphilis (p. 398)
Verrucous carcinoma (p. 830)
Warts (p. 421)

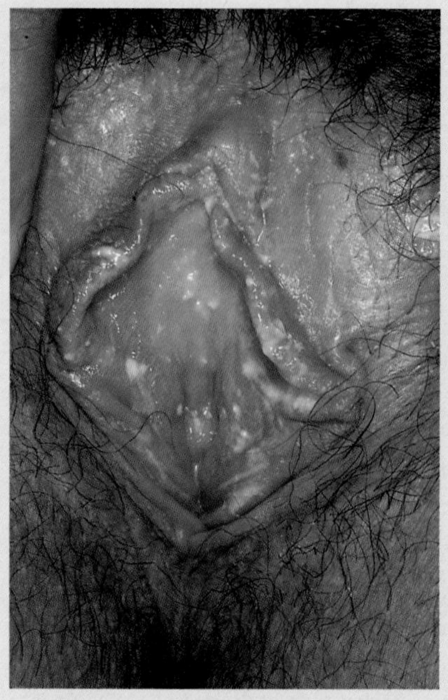

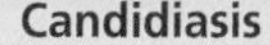

Candidiasis

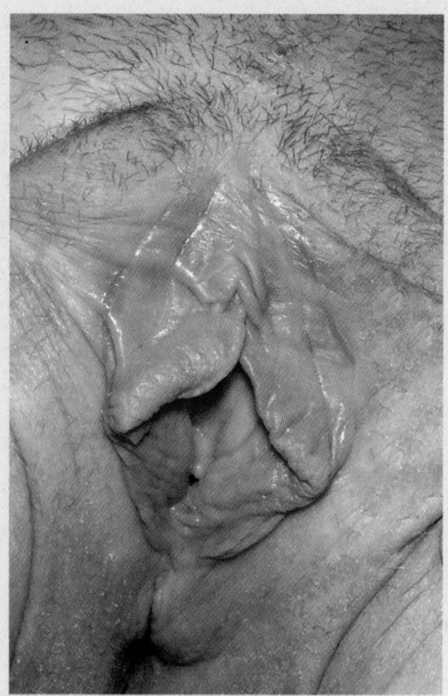

Eczema with fissure

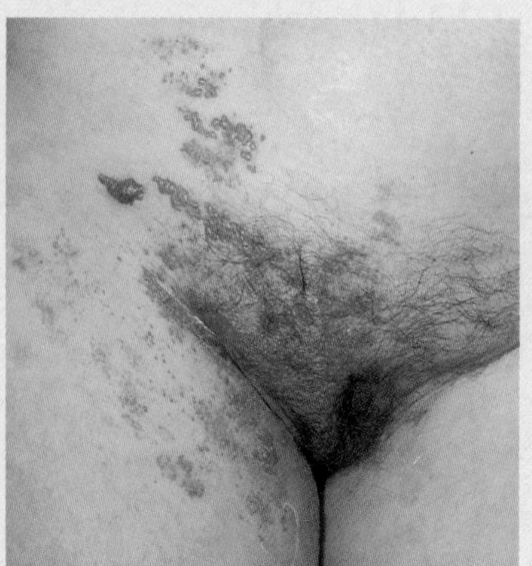

Herpes zoster

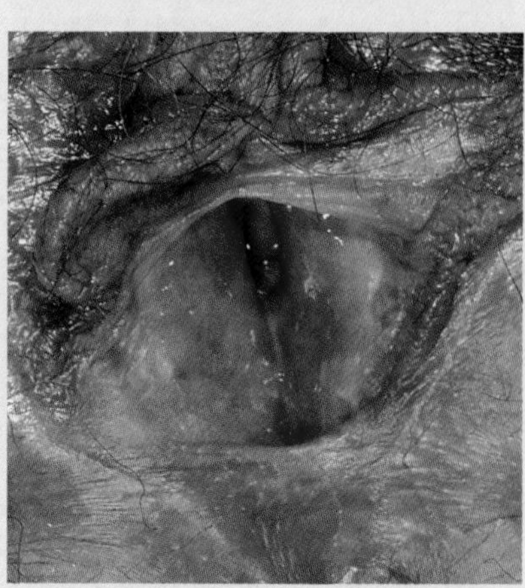

Lichen planus, erosive

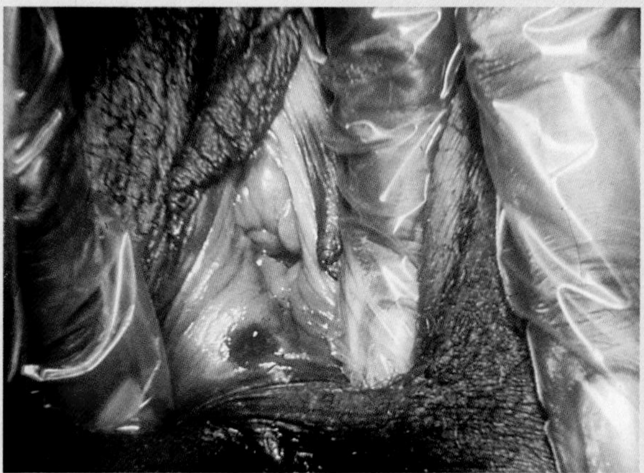

Primary syphilis

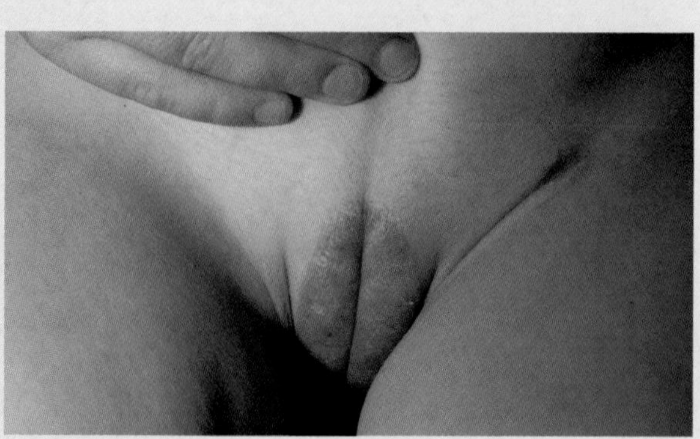

Psoriasis

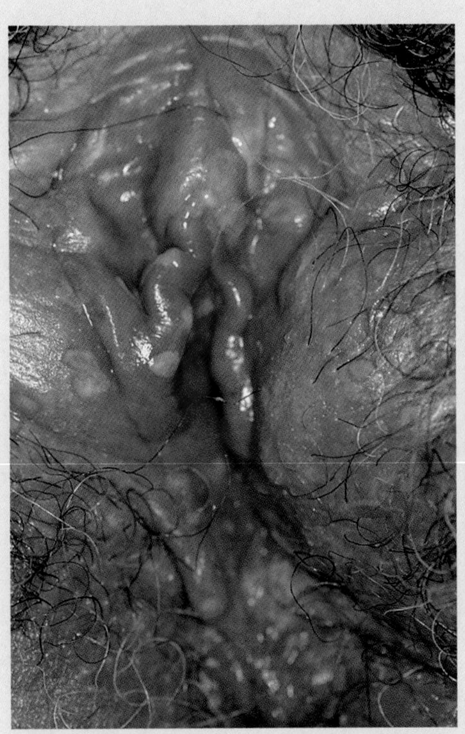
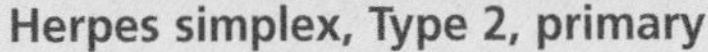

Herpes simplex, Type 2, primary

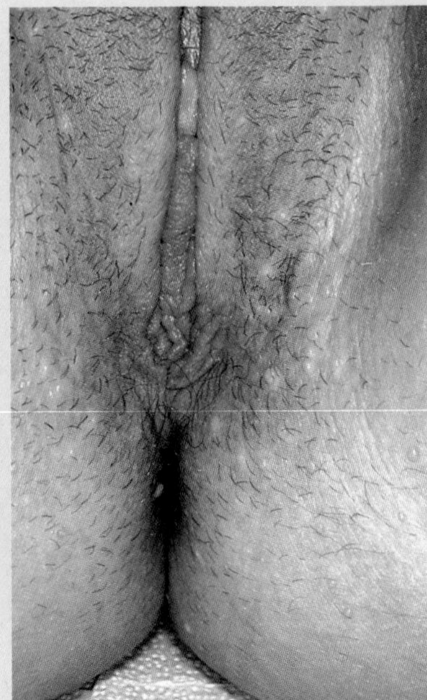

Molluscum contagiosum

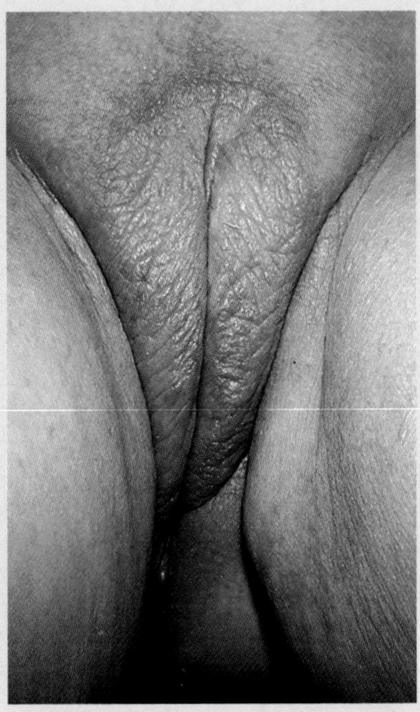

Lichen simplex chronicus

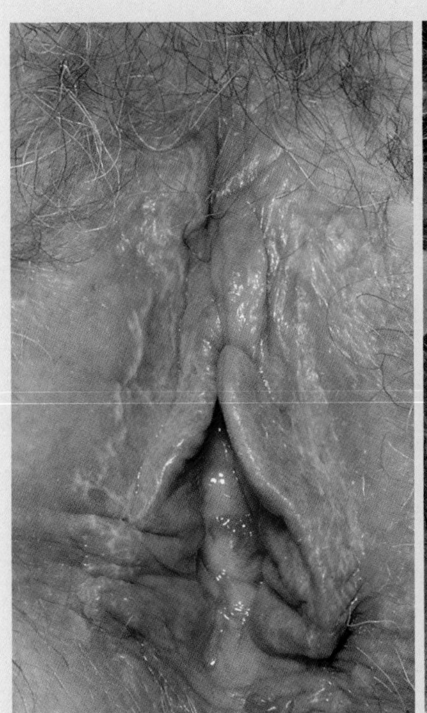

Lichen planus

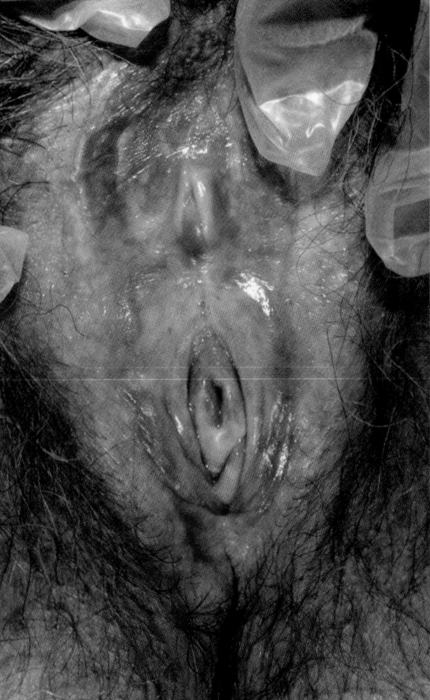

Lichen sclerosus

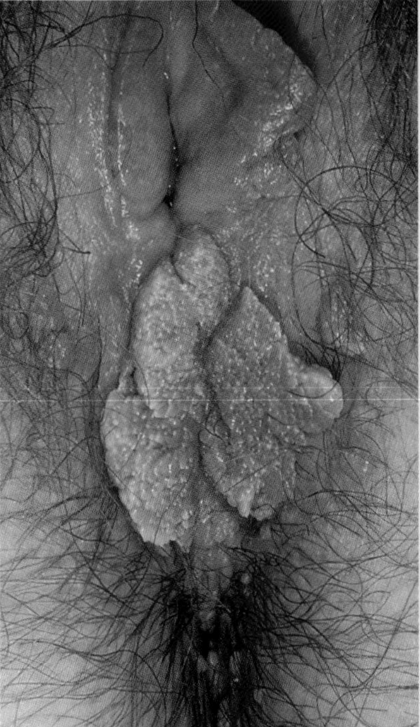

Warts

Wrist

Atopic dermatitis (p. 164)
Lichen planus (p. 323)
Lichen simplex chronicus (pp. 104, 115)
Scabies (p. 586)

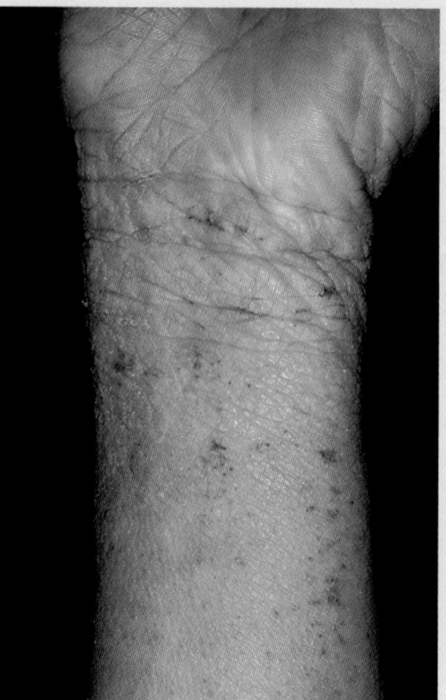

Atopic dermatitis

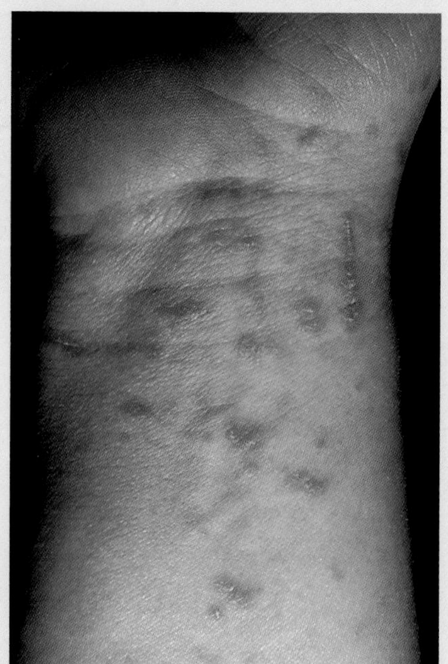

Lichen planus

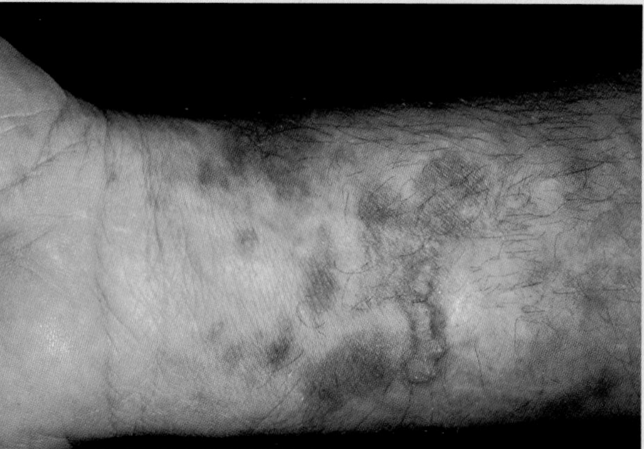

Lichen planus

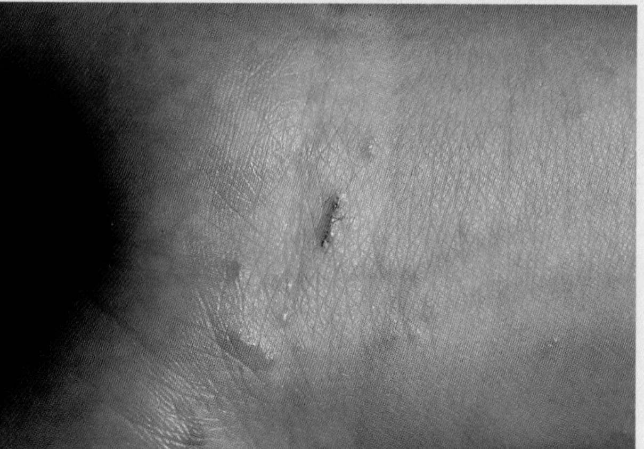

Scabies

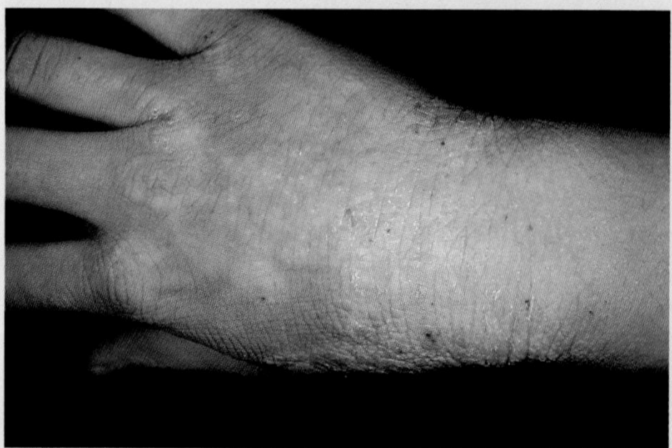

Atopic dermatitis

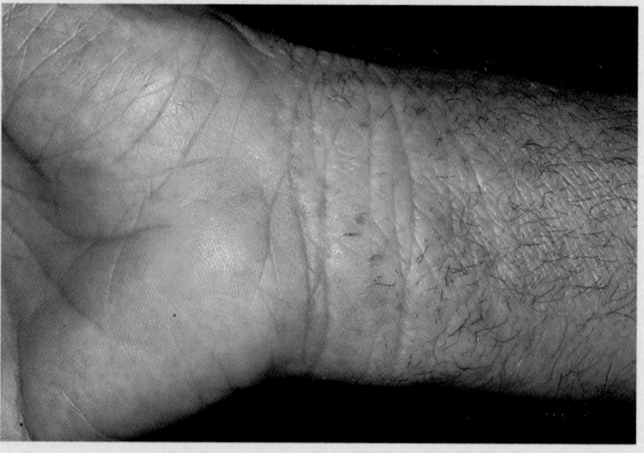

Lichen simplex chronicus, atopic

Chapter 2

Topical Therapy and Topical Corticosteroids

CHAPTER CONTENTS

TOPICAL THERAPY

A wide variety of topical medications are available for treating cutaneous disease (see Formulary). Specific medications are covered in detail in the appropriate chapters, and the basic principles of topical treatment are discussed here.

The skin is an important barrier that must be maintained to function properly. Any insult that removes water, lipids, or protein from the epidermis alters the integrity of this barrier and compromises its function. Restoration of the normal epidermal barrier is accomplished with the use of mild soaps and emollient creams and lotions. There is an old and often-repeated rule: "If it is dry, wet it; if it is wet, dry it."

DRY DISEASES. Dry skin or dry cutaneous lesions have lost water and, in many instances, the epidermal lipids and proteins that help contain epidermal moisture. These substances are replaced with emollient creams and lotions.

WET DISEASES. Exudative inflammatory diseases pour out serum that leaches the complex lipids and proteins from the epidermis. A wet lesion is managed with wet compresses that suppress inflammation and debride crust and serum. Repeated cycles of wetting and drying eventually make the lesion dry. Excessive use of wet dressings causes severe drying and chapping. Once the wet phase of the disease has been controlled, the lipids and proteins must be restored with the use of emollient creams and lotions, and wet compressing should stop.

Emollient creams and lotions

Emollient creams and lotions restore water and lipids to the epidermis (see Formulary). Preparations that contain urea (e.g., Carmol 10, 20, 40; Vanamide) or lactic acid (e.g., Lac-Hydrin, AmLactin) have special lubricating properties and may be the most effective. Creams are thicker and more lubricating than lotions; petroleum jelly and mineral oil contain no water.

Lubricating creams and lotions are most effective if applied to moist skin. After bathing is an ideal time to apply moisturizers. Wet the skin, pat dry, and immediately apply the moisturizer. Emollients should be applied as frequently as necessary to keep the skin soft. Chemicals such as menthol and phenol (e.g., Sarna lotion) are added to lubricating lotions to control pruritus (see Formulary).

Severe dry skin (xerosis)

Dry skin is more severe in the winter months when the humidity is low. "Winter itch" most commonly affects the hands and lower legs. Initially the skin is rough and covered with fine white scales; later, thicker tan or brown scales may appear. The most severely affected skin may be crisscrossed with shallow red fissures. Dry skin may itch or burn. Preparations listed in the Formulary should be used for mild cases; severe dry skin responds to 12% lactate lotion (e.g., Lac-Hydrin, AmLactin).

Wet dressings

Wet dressings, also called compresses, are a valuable aid in the treatment of exudative (wet) skin diseases (see Box 2-1). Their importance in topical therapy cannot be overstated. The technique for wet compress preparation and application is described in the following list.

1. Obtain a clean, soft cloth such as bedsheeting or shirt material. The cloth need not be new or sterilized. Compress material must be washed at least once daily if it is to be used repeatedly.
2. Fold the cloth so there are at least four to eight layers and cut it to fit an area slightly larger than the area to be treated (Figure 2-1).
3. Wet the folded dressings by immersing them in the solution, and wring them out until they are sopping wet (neither running nor just damp).
4. Place the wet compresses on the affected area. Do not pour solution on a wet dressing to keep it wet because this practice increases the concentration of the solution and may cause irritation. Remove the compress and replace it with a new one.
5. Dressings are left in place for 30 minutes to 1 hour. Dressings may be used two to four times a day or continuously. Discontinue the use of wet compresses when the skin becomes dry. Excessive drying causes cracking and fissures.

Wet compresses provide the following benefits:

- *Antibacterial action:* Aluminum acetate, acetic acid, or silver nitrate may be added to the water to provide an antibacterial effect (Table 2-1).
- *Wound debridement:* A wet compress macerates vesicles and crust, helping to debride these materials when the compress is removed.
- *Inflammation suppression:* Compresses have a strong antiinflammatory effect. The evaporative cooling causes constriction of superficial cutaneous vessels, thereby decreasing erythema and the production of serum. Wet compresses control acute inflammatory processes, such as acute poison ivy, faster than either topical applied or orally administered corticosteroids.
- *Drying:* Wet dressings cause the skin to become dry. Wetting something to make it dry seems paradoxical, but the effects of repeated cycles of wetting and drying are observed in lip chapping, caused by lip licking; irritant hand dermatitis, caused by repeated washing; and the soggy sock syndrome in children, caused by perspiration.

The temperature of the compress solution should be cool when an antiinflammatory effect is desired and tepid when the purpose is to debride an infected, crusted lesion. Covering a wet compress with a towel or plastic inhibits evaporation, promotes maceration, and increases skin temperature, which facilitates bacterial growth.

Box 2-1 **Diseases Treated with Wet Compresses**
Acute eczematous inflammation (poison ivy)
Eczematous inflammation with secondary infection (pustules)
Bullous impetigo
Herpes simplex and herpes zoster (vesicular lesions)
Infected exudative lesions of any type
Insect bites
Intertrigo (groin or under breasts)
Nummular eczema (exudative lesions)
Stasis dermatitis (exudative lesions)
Stasis ulcers
Sunburn (blistering stage)
Tinea pedis (vesicular stage or macerated web infections)

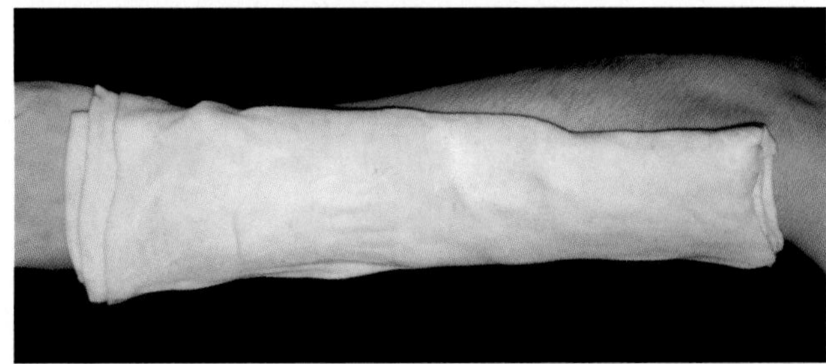

Figure 2-1 Cool wet compresses control acute inflammation.

Table 2-1 Wet Dressing Solutions

Solution	Preparation	Indications
Water	Tap water does not have to be sterilized.	Poison ivy, sunburn, any noninfected exudative or inflamed process
Burow's solution (aluminum acetate) Domeboro astringent powder packets Effervescent tablets	Dissolve one, two, or three packets of Domeboro powder in 16 ounces of water.	Mildly antiseptic; for acute inflammation, poison ivy, insect bites, athlete's foot
Silver nitrate, 0.1-0.5% (prepared by some pharmacists and some hospitals)	Supplied as a 50% aqueous solution; stains skin dark brown and stains metal black.	Bactericidal: for exudative infected lesions (e.g., stasis ulcers and stasis dermatitis)
Acetic acid, 1%-2.5%	Vinegar is 5% acetic acid. Make a 1% solution by adding ½ cup of vinegar (white or brown) to 1 pint of water.	Bactericidal: for certain gram-negative bacteria (e.g., *Pseudomonas aeruginosa*), otitis externa, *Pseudomonas* intertrigo

TOPICAL CORTICOSTEROIDS

Topical corticosteroids are a powerful tool for treating skin disease. Understanding the correct use of these agents will result in the successful management of a variety of skin problems. Many products are available, but all have basically the same antiinflammatory properties, differing only in strength, base, and price.

Strength

POTENCY (GROUPS I THROUGH VII). The antiinflammatory properties of topical corticosteroids result in part from their ability to induce vasoconstriction of the small blood vessels in the upper dermis. This property is used in an assay procedure to determine the strength of each new product. These products are subsequently tabulated in seven groups, with group I the strongest and group VII the weakest (see the Formulary and the inside front matter of this book). The treatment sections of this book recommend topical steroids by group number rather than by generic or brand name because the agents in each group are essentially equivalent in strength.

Lower concentrations of some brands may have the same effect in vasoconstrictor assays as much higher concentrations of the same product. One study showed that there was no difference in vasoconstriction between Kenalog 0.025%, 0.1%, or 0.5% creams.

CHOOSING THE APPROPRIATE STRENGTH. Guidelines for choosing the appropriate strength and brand of topical steroid are presented in Box 2-2 and Figure 2-2. The best results are obtained when preparations of adequate strength are used for a specified length of time. Weaker, "safer" strengths often fail to provide adequate control. Patients who do not respond after 1 to 4 weeks of treatment should be reevaluated.

Box 2-2 **Suggested Strength of Topical Steroids to Initiate Treatment***

Groups I-II	Groups III-V	Groups VI-VII
Psoriasis	Atopic dermatitis	Dermatitis (eyelids)
Lichen planus	Nummular eczema	Dermatitis (diaper area)
Discoid lupus[†]	Asteatotic eczema	Mild dermatitis (face)
Severe hand eczema	Stasis dermatitis	Mild anal inflammation
Poison ivy (severe)	Seborrheic dermatitis	Mild intertrigo
Lichen simplex chronicus	Lichen sclerosis et atrophicus (vulva)	
Hyperkeratotic eczema	Intertrigo (brief course)	
Chapped feet	Tinea (brief course to control inflammation)	
Lichen sclerosis et atrophicus (skin)	Scabies (after scabicide)	
Alopecia areata	Intertrigo (severe cases)	
Nummular eczema (severe)	Anal inflammation (severe cases)	
Atopic dermatitis (resistant adult cases)	Severe dermatitis (face)	

*Stop treatment, change to less potent agent, or use intermittent treatment once inflammation is controlled.
†Use on the face may be justified.

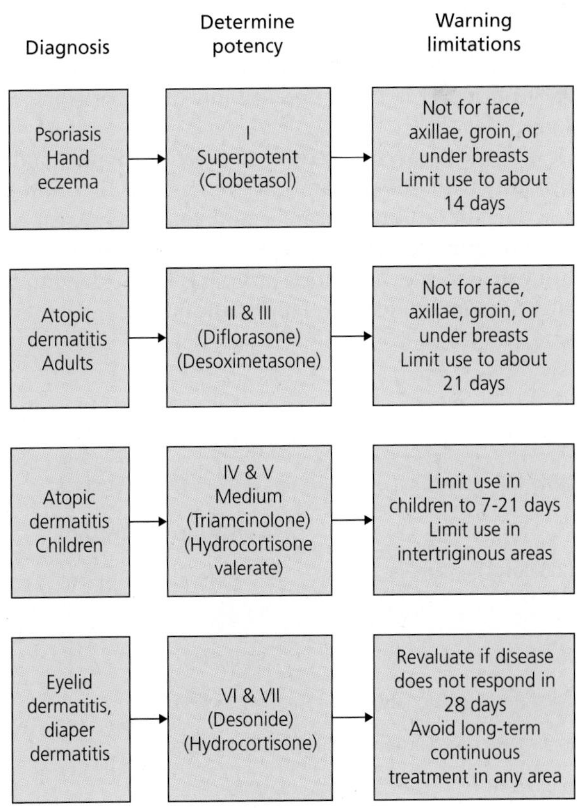

Figure 2-2

MEGAPOTENT TOPICAL STEROIDS (GROUP I)

Clobetasol propionate, halobetasol propionate, betamethasone dipropionate, and diflorasone diacetate are the most potent topical steroids available. Clobetasol and halobetasol are the most potent and betamethasone and diflorasone are equipotent.

In general no more than 45 to 60 grams (gm) of cream or ointment should be used each week (see Table 2-2). Side effects are minimized and efficacy increased when medication is applied once or twice daily for 2 weeks followed by 1 week of rest. This cyclic schedule (pulse dosing) is continued until resolution occurs. Intermittent dosing (e.g., once or twice a week) can lead to a prolonged remission of psoriasis if used after initial clearing. Alternatively, intermittent use of a weaker topical steroid can be used for maintenance. Diflorasone can be used with plastic dressing occlusion; clobetasol, halobetasol, and betamethasone should not be used with occlusive dressings.

Patients must be monitored carefully. Side effects such as atrophy and adrenal suppression are a real possibility, especially with unsupervised use of these medications. Refills should be strictly limited. Add the warning "Not to be applied to face, axillae and groin" to presciptions for treatment of other areas. Explain that prolonged use causes a post steroid flare of erythema and papules on the face and atrophy in the axillae and groin.

CONCENTRATION. The concentration of steroid listed on the tube cannot be used to compare its strength with other steroids. Some steroids are much more powerful than others and need be present only in small concentrations to produce the maximum effect. Nevertheless, it is difficult to convince some patients that clobetasol cream 0.05% (group I) is more potent than hydrocortisone 1% (group VII).

It is unnecessary to learn many steroid brand names. Familiarity with one preparation from groups II, V, and VII gives one the ability to safely and effectively treat any steroid-responsive skin disease. Most of the topical steroids are fluorinated (i.e., a fluorine atom has been added to the hydrocortisone molecule). Fluorination increases potency and the possibility of side effects. Products such as hydrocortisone valerate cream have increased potency without fluorination; however, side effects are possible with this midpotency steroid.

COMPOUNDING. Avoid having the pharmacist prepare or dilute topical steroid creams. The active ingredient may not be dispersed uniformly, resulting in a cream of variable strength. The cost of pharmacist preparation is generally higher because of the additional labor required. High-quality steroid creams, such as triamcinolone acetonide, are available in large quantities at a low cost.

GENERIC VERSUS BRAND NAMES. Many generic topical steroid formulations are available (e.g., clobetasol propionate, betamethasone valerate, betamethasone dipropionate, fluocinolone acetonide, fluocinonide, hydrocortisone, and triamcinolone acetonide). In many states, generic substitutions by the pharmacist are allowed unless the physician writes "no substitution." Vasoconstrictor assays have shown large differences in the activity of generic formulations compared with brand-name equivalents: many are inferior, a few are equivalent, and a few are more potent than brand-name equivalents. Many generic topical steroids have vehicles with different ingredients (e.g., preservatives) than brand-name equivalents.

Vehicle

The vehicle, or base, is the substance in which the active ingredient is dispersed. The base determines the rate at which the active ingredient is absorbed through the skin. Components of some bases may cause irritation or allergy.

CREAMS. The cream base is a mixture of several different organic chemicals (oils) and water, and it usually contains a preservative. Creams have the following characteristics:

- White color and somewhat greasy texture
- Components that may cause irritation, stinging, and allergy

Table 2-2 Restriction on the Use of Group I Topical Steroids*

	Length of therapy	Grams per week	Use under occlusion
Clobetasol propionate	14 days	60	No
Clobetasol scalp solution	14 days	50 ml	No
Clobetasol foam	14 days	50	No
Halobetasol propionate	14 days	60	No
Betamethasone dipropionate	Unrestricted	45	No
Diflorasone diacetate	Unrestricted	Unrestricted	Unrestricted

*Restrictions are listed in the package inserts.

- High versatility (i.e., may be used in nearly any area); therefore creams are the base most often prescribed
- Possible drying effect with continued use; therefore best for acute exudative inflammation
- Most useful for intertriginous areas (e.g., groin, rectal area, and axilla)

OINTMENTS. The ointment base contains a limited number of organic compounds consisting primarily of greases such as petroleum jelly, with little or no water. Many ointments are preservative-free. Ointments have the following characteristics:

- Translucent (look like petroleum jelly)
- Greasy feeling persists on skin surface
- More lubrication, thus desirable for drier lesions
- Greater penetration of medicine than creams and therefore enhanced potency (see inside front matter; triamcinolone cream in group V and triamcinolone ointment in group IV)
- Too occlusive for acute (exudative) eczematous inflammation or intertriginous areas, such as the groin

GELS. Gels are greaseless mixtures of propylene glycol and water; some also contain alcohol. Gels have the following characteristics:

- A clear base, sometimes with a jellylike consistency
- Useful for acute exudative inflammation, such as poison ivy, and in scalp areas where other vehicles mat the hair

SOLUTIONS AND LOTIONS. Solutions may contain water and alcohol, as well as other chemicals. Solutions have the following characteristics:

- Clear or milky appearance
- Most useful for scalp because they penetrate easily through hair, leaving no residue
- May result in stinging and drying when applied to intertriginous areas, such as the groin

FOAMS. A foam preparation of desonide (Verdeso), betamethasone valerate (Luxiq) and clobetasol propionate (Olux-E) is available. Generic foams are now available. Olux contains a superpotent steroid. Treatment beyond 2 consecutive weeks is not recommended, and the total dosage should not exceed 50 gm per week because of the potential for the drug to suppress the hypothalamic-pituitary-adrenal (HPA) axis. Use in children younger than 12 years of age is not recommended. Foams spread between the strands of hair until they reach the scalp, where the foam melts and delivers the active drug. Foams are useful for treatment of scalp dermatoses and in other areas for acute eczematous inflammation such as poison ivy and plaque psoriasis. Foams may cause stinging shortly after they are applied. Emollient foams such as Verdeso and Olux-E do not sting.

Steroid-antibiotic mixtures

LOTRISONE CREAM AND LOTION. Lotrisone cream contains a combination of the antifungal agent clotrimazole and the corticosteroid betamethasone dipropionate. It is indicated for the topical treatment of tinea pedis, tinea cruris, and tinea corporis. This product is used by many physicians as their topical antiinflammatory agent of first choice. Most inflammatory skin disease is not infected or contaminated by fungus. Lotrisone is a marginal drug for cutaneous fungal infections. Brand-name Lotrisone cream is no longer available; it has been replaced by a brand-name lotion.

OTHER ANTIBIOTICS AND CORTICOSTEROID MIXTURES. Mycolog II (nystatin-triamcinolone acetonide) is indicated for the treatment of cutaneous candidiasis. Nystatin does not treat fungi that cause tinea pedis. The majority of steroid-responsive skin diseases can be managed successfully without topical antibiotics.

Amount of cream to dispense

The amount of cream dispensed is very important. Patients do not appreciate being prescribed a $90, 60-gm tube of cream to treat a small area of hand dermatitis. Unrestricted and unsupervised use of potent steroid creams can lead to side effects. Patients rely on the physician's judgment to determine the correct amount of topical medicine. If too small a quantity is prescribed, patients may conclude that the treatment did not work. It is advisable to allow for a sufficient amount of cream, and then to set limits on duration and frequency of application. Many steroids (e.g., triamcinolone, hydrocortisone) are available in generic form. They are purchased in bulk by the pharmacist and can be dispensed in large quantities at considerable savings.

The amount of cream required to cover a certain area can be calculated by remembering that 1 gm of cream covers 100 square centimeters of skin. The entire skin surface of the average-sized adult is covered by 20 to 30 gm of cream.

The fingertip unit and the rule of hand provide the means to assess how much cream to dispense and apply.

FINGERTIP UNIT. A fingertip unit (FTU) is the amount of ointment expressed from a tube with a 5-mm diameter nozzle, applied from the distal skin crease to the tip of the index finger. One FTU weighs approximately 0.5 gm.

THE RULE OF HAND. The hand area can be used to estimate the total area of involvement of a skin disease and to assess the amount of ointment required. The area of one side of the hand is defined as one hand area. One hand area of involved skin requires 0.5 FTU or 0.25 gm of ointment, or four hand areas equal 2 FTUs equal 1 gm. The area of one side of the hand represents approximately 1% of body surface area so it requires 1 FTU (2 hand units) to cover 2% of the body surface. Approximately 282 gm is required for twice-daily applications to the total body surface (except the scalp) for 1 week.

Application

FREQUENCY

TACHYPHYLAXIS. Tachyphylaxis refers to the decrease in responsiveness to a drug as a result of enzyme induction. The term is used in dermatology in reference to acute tolerance to the vasoconstrictive action of topically applied corticosteroids. Experiments have revealed that vasoconstriction decreases progressively when a potent topical steroid is applied to the skin three times a day for 4 days. The vasoconstrictive response returned 4 days after termination of therapy. These experiments support years of complaints by patients about initially dramatic responses to new topical steroids that diminish with constant use. It would therefore seem reasonable to instruct patients to apply creams on an interrupted schedule.

INTERMITTENT DOSING

Group I topical steroids. Optimum dosing schedules for the use of potent topical steroids have not been determined. Studies show that steroid-resistant diseases, such as plaque psoriasis and hand eczema, respond most effectively when clobetasol is applied twice a day for 2 to 3 weeks. Treatment is resumed after 1 week of rest. The schedule of 2 weeks of treatment followed by 1 week of rest is repeated until the lesions have cleared.

Intermittent treatment of healed lesions can lead to prolonged remission. Psoriatic patients with lingering erythema remained clear with applications three times a day on 1 day a week. Twice-weekly applications of clobetasol kept 75% of psoriatic patients and 70% of hand eczema patients in remission.

Short weekly bursts of topical corticosteroids may play a role in keeping an adult's atopic dermatitis under control. Weekly applications of fluticasone ointment (Cutivate), applied once daily for 2 consecutive days each week, maintained the improvements achieved after the initial treatment phase and delayed relapse.

Groups II through VII topical steroids. The optimum frequency of application and duration of treatment for topical steroids have not been determined. Adequate results and acceptable patient compliance occur when the following steps are taken:

1. Apply groups II through VI topical steroids twice each day.
2. Limit the duration of application to 2 to 6 weeks.
3. If adequate control is not achieved, stop treatment for 4 to 7 days and begin another course of treatment.

Excellent control can be achieved with pulse dosing. These are general guidelines; specific instructions and limitations must be established for each individual case.

METHODS

SIMPLE APPLICATION. Creams and ointments should be applied in thin layers and slowly massaged into the site one to four times a day. It is unnecessary to wash before each application. Continue treatment until the lesion is clear. Many patients decrease the frequency of applications or stop entirely when lesions appear to improve quickly. Other patients are so impressed with the efficacy of these agents that they continue treatment after the disease has resolved in order to prevent recurrence; adverse reactions may follow this practice.

Different skin surfaces vary in the ability to absorb topical medicine. The thin eyelid skin heals quickly with group VI or VII steroids, whereas thicker skin on palms and soles offers a greater barrier to the penetration of topical medicine and requires more potent therapy. Intertriginous (skin touches skin) areas (e.g., axilla, groin, rectal area, and underneath the breasts) respond more quickly to creams that are weaker in strength. The apposition of two skin surfaces performs the same function as an occlusive dressing, which greatly enhances penetration. The skin of infants and young children is more receptive to topical medicine and responds quickly to weaker creams. A baby's diaper has the same occlusive effect as covering with a plastic dressing. Penetration of steroid creams is greatly enhanced; therefore only group V, VI, or VII preparations should be used under a diaper. Inflamed skin absorbs topical medicines much more efficiently. This explains why red, inflamed areas generally have such a rapid initial response when treated with weaker topical steroids.

OCCLUSION. Occlusion with a plastic dressing (e.g., Saran Wrap) is an effective method for enhancing absorption of topical steroids. The plastic dressing holds perspiration against the skin surface, which hydrates the top layer of the epidermis, the stratum corneum. Topical medication penetrates a moist stratum corneum from 10 to 100 times more effectively than it penetrates dry skin. Eruptions that are resistant to simple application may heal quickly with the introduction of a plastic dressing. Nearly any area can be occluded; the entire body may be occluded with a vinyl exercise suit, available at most sporting goods stores and Walmart.

Discretion should be used with occlusion. Occlusion of moist areas may encourage the rapid development of infection. Occlusive dressings are used more often with creams than with ointments, but ointments may be covered if the lesions are particularly dry. Weaker, less expensive products (e.g., triamcinolone cream 0.1%) provide excellent results. Large quantities of this medicine may be purchased at a substantial savings.

Method of occlusion. The area should be cleaned with mild soap and water. Antibacterial soaps are unnecessary. The medicine is gently rubbed into the lesions, and the entire area is covered with plastic (e.g., Saran Wrap, Handi-Wrap, plastic bags, or gloves; Figures 2-3 to 2-5). The plastic dressing should be secured with tape so that it is close to the skin and the ends are sealed; an airtight dressing is unnecessary. The plastic may be held in place with an Ace bandage or a sock. The best results are obtained if the dressing remains in place for at least 2 hours. Many patients find that bedtime is the most convenient time to wear a plastic dressing and therefore wear it for 8 hours. More medicine is applied shortly after the dressing is removed and while the skin is still moist.

Dressings should not remain on the area continuously because infection or follicular occlusion may result. If an occluded area suddenly becomes worse or pustules develop, infection, usually with *Staphylococci,* should be suspected (Figure 2-6). Oral anti-staphylococcal antibiotics should be given (e.g., cephalexin [Keflex] 500 mg two to four times a day).

A reasonable occlusion schedule is twice daily for a 2-hour period or for 8 hours at bedtime, with simple application once or twice during the day.

Occluded areas often become dry, and the use of lubricating cream or lotion should be encouraged. Cream or lotion may be applied shortly after medicine is applied, when the plastic dressing is removed, or at other convenient times.

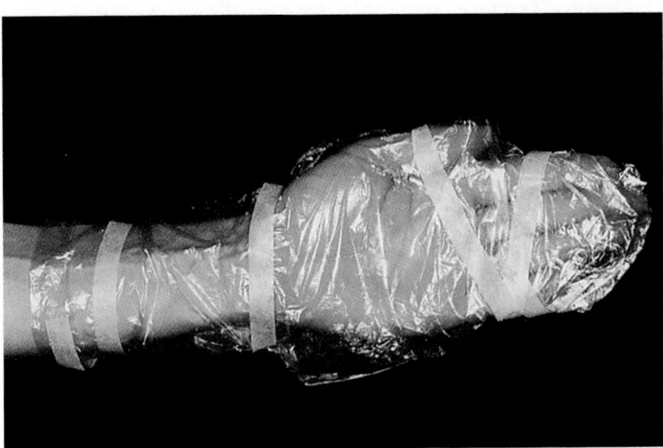

Figure 2-3 Occlusion of the hand. A plastic bag is pulled on and pressed against the skin to expel air. Tape is wound snugly around the bag.

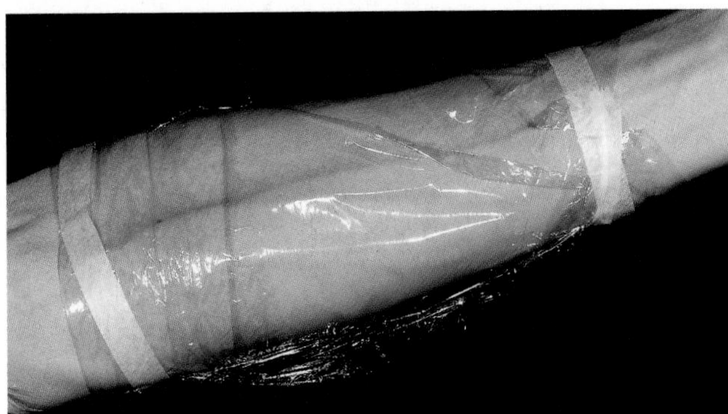

Figure 2-4 Occlusion of the arm. A plastic sheet (e.g., Saran Wrap) is wound about the extremity and secured at both ends with tape. A plastic bag with the bottom cut out may be used as a sleeve and held in place with tape or an Ace bandage.

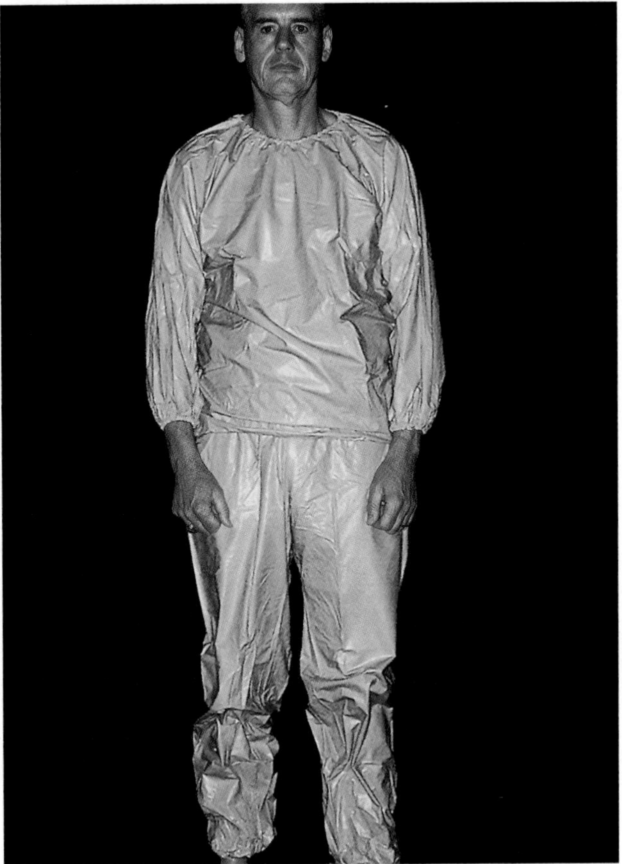

Figure 2-5 Occlusion of the entire body. A vinyl exercise suit is a convenient way to occlude the entire body. This suit is available at Walmart for less than $10.

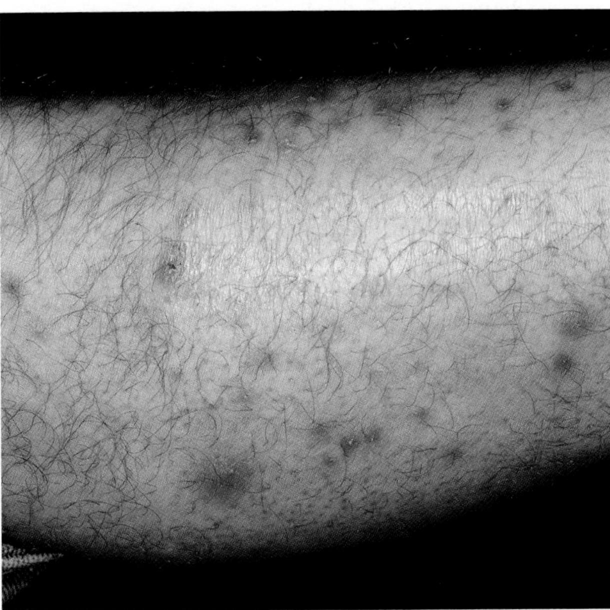

Figure 2-6 Infection following occlusion. Pustules have appeared at the periphery of an eczematous lesion. Plastic dressing had been left in place for 24 hours.

SYSTEMIC ABSORPTION

The possibility of producing systemic side effects from absorption of topical steroids is of concern to all physicians who use these agents. A small number of case reports have documented systemic effects after topical application of glucocorticoids for prolonged periods. Cataracts, retardation of growth, failure to thrive, and Cushing's syndrome have all been reported.

AVOID WEAKER, "SAFE" PREPARATIONS. In an attempt to avoid complications, physicians often choose a weaker steroid preparation than that indicated; these weaker preparations all too frequently fall short of expectations and fail to give the desired antiinflammatory effect. The disease does not improve, but rather becomes worse because of the time wasted using the ineffective cream. Pruritus continues, infection may develop, and the patient becomes frustrated. Treatment of intense inflammation with hydrocortisone cream 0.5% is a waste of time and money. Generally, a topical steroid of adequate strength (see Box 2-2) should be used two to four times daily for a specific length of time, such as 7 to 21 days, in order to obtain rapid control. Even during this short interval, adrenal suppression may result when groups I through III steroids are used to treat wide areas of inflamed skin. This suppression of the hypothalamic-pituitary-adrenal axis is generally reversible in 24 hours and is very unlikely to produce side effects characteristic of long-term systemic use.

CHILDREN. Many physicians worry about systemic absorption and will not use any topical steroids stronger than 1% hydrocortisone on infants. The group V topical steroid fluticasone propionate cream 0.05% (Cutivate) appears to be safe for the treatment of severe eczema for up to 4 weeks in children 3 months of age and older. Children between 3 months and 6 years with moderate to severe atopic dermatitis (≥35% body surface area; mean body surface area treated, 64%) were treated with fluticasone propionate cream 0.05% twice daily for 3 to 4 weeks. *PMID: 11862174* Mean cortisol levels were similar at baseline and at the end of treatment. The relative safety of moderately strong topical steroids and their relative freedom from serious systemic toxicity despite widespread use in the very young have been clearly demonstrated. Patients should be treated for a specific length of time with a medication of appropriate strength. Steroid creams should not be used continually for many weeks, and patients who do not respond in a predictable fashion should be reevaluated.

Group I topical steroids should be avoided in prepubertal children. Use only group VI or VII steroids in the diaper area and for only 3 to 10 days. Monitor growth parameters in children prescribed chronic topical glucocorticoid therapy.

ADULTS. Suppression may occur during short intervals of treatment with group I or II topical steroids, but recovery is rapid when treatment is discontinued. Physicians may prescribe strong agents when appropriate, but the patient must be cautioned that the agent should be used only for the length of time dictated.

Adverse reactions

Because information concerning the potential dangers of potent topical steroids has been so widely disseminated, some physicians have stopped prescribing them. Topical steroids have been used for approximately 50 years with an excellent safety record. They do, however, have the potential to produce a number of adverse reactions. Once these are understood, the most appropriate-strength steroid can be prescribed confidently. Reported adverse reactions to topical steroids are listed in Box 2-3. A brief description of some of the more important adverse reactions is presented in the following pages.

STEROID ROSACEA AND PERIORAL DERMATITIS

Steroid rosacea is a side effect frequently observed in fair-skinned females who initially complain of erythema with or without pustules—the "flusher blusher complexion." In a typical example, the physician prescribes a mild topical steroid, which initially gives pleasing results. Tolerance (tachyphylaxis) occurs, and a new, more potent topical steroid is prescribed to suppress the erythema and pustules that may reappear following the use of the weaker preparation. This progression to more potent creams may continue until group II steroids are applied several times each day. Figure 2-7 shows a middle-aged woman who has applied a group V steroid cream once each day for 5 years. Intense erythema and pustulation occurs each time attempts are made to discontinue topical treatment. The skin may be atrophic and red with a burning sensation.

Box 2-3 **Adverse Reactions to Topical Steroids**

- Rosacea, perioral dermatitis, acne
- Skin atrophy with telangiectasia, stellate pseudoscars (arms), purpura, striae (from anatomic occlusion, e.g., groin)
- Tinea incognito, impetigo incognito, scabies incognito
- Ocular hypertension, glaucoma, cataracts
- Allergic contact dermatitis
- Systemic absorption
- Burning, itching, irritation, dryness caused by vehicle (e.g., propylene glycol)
- Miliaria and folliculitus following occlusion with plastic
- Skin blanching from acute vasoconstriction
- Rebound phenomenon (e.g., psoriasis becomes worse after treatment is stopped)
- Nonhealing leg ulcers; steroids applied to any leg ulcer retard healing process
- Hypopigmentation
- Hypertrichosis of face

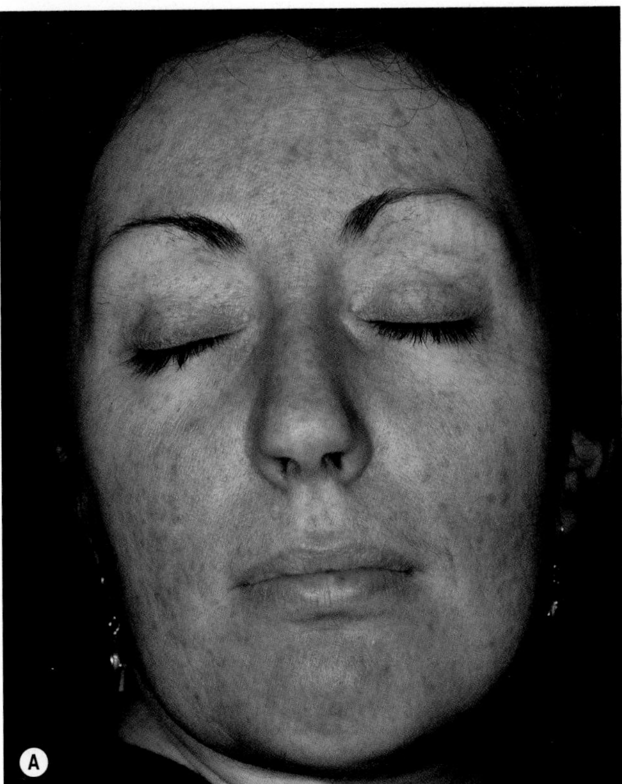

Numerous red papules formed on the cheeks and forehead with constant daily use of a group V topical steroid for more than 5 years.

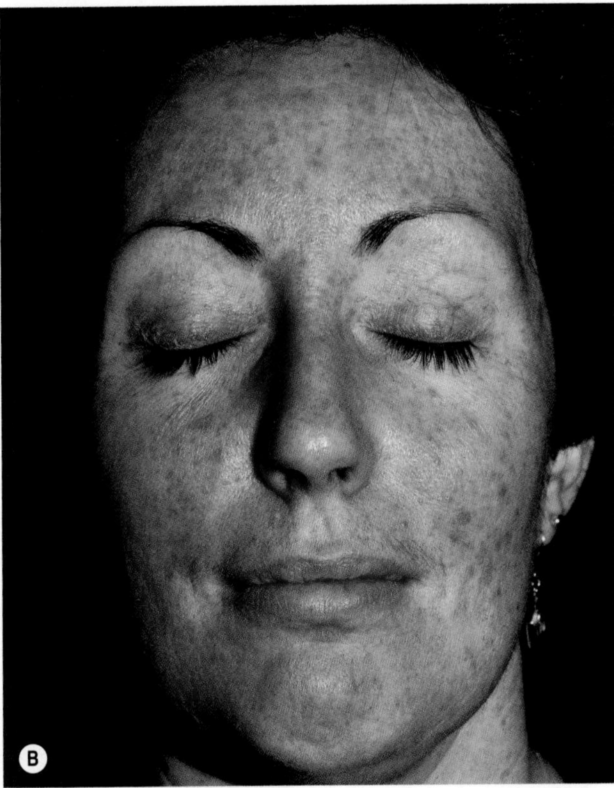

Ten days after discontinuing use of group V topical steroid.

Figure 2-7 Steroid rosacea.

Perioral dermatitis (see Figure 7-52) is sometimes caused by the chronic application of topical steroids to the lower face; pustules, erythema, and scaling occur around the nose, mouth, and chin.

MANAGEMENT. Strong topical steroids must be discontinued. Doxycycline (100 mg once or twice a day) or erythromycin (250 mg four times a day) may reduce the intensity of the rebound erythema and pustulation that predictably occur during the first 10 days (Figures 2-8 to 2-11). Occasionally, cool, wet compresses, with or without 1% hydrocortisone cream, are necessary if the rebound is intense. Thereafter, mild noncomedogenic lubricants (those that do not induce acne may be used for the dryness and desquamation that occur. Erythema and pustules are generally present at a low level for months. Low dosages of doxycycline (50 mg twice a day) or erythromycin (250 mg two or three times a day) may be continued until the eruption clears. The pustules and erythema eventually subside, but some telangiectasia and atrophy may be permanent.

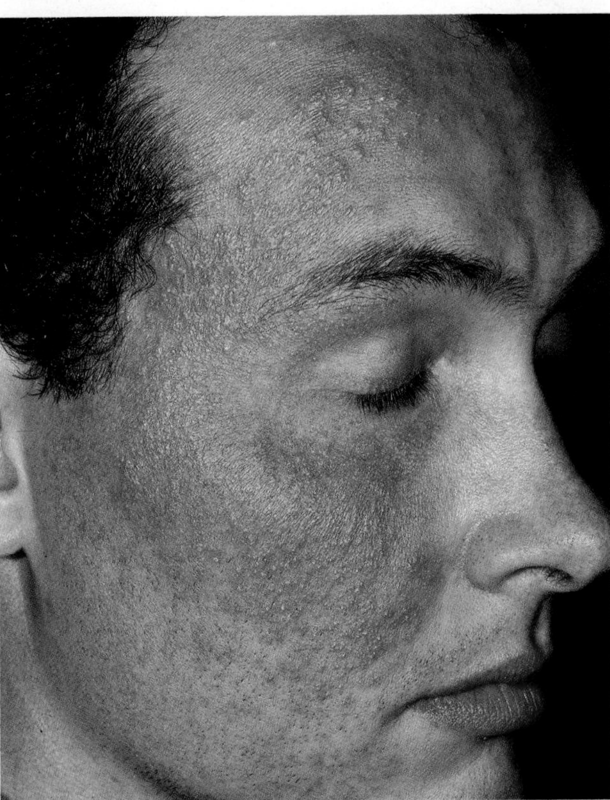

Figure 2-8 Intense erythema and pustulation appeared 10 days after discontinuing use of a group V topical steroid. The cream had been applied every day for 1 year.

STEROID ROSACEA AND PERIORAL DERMATITIS

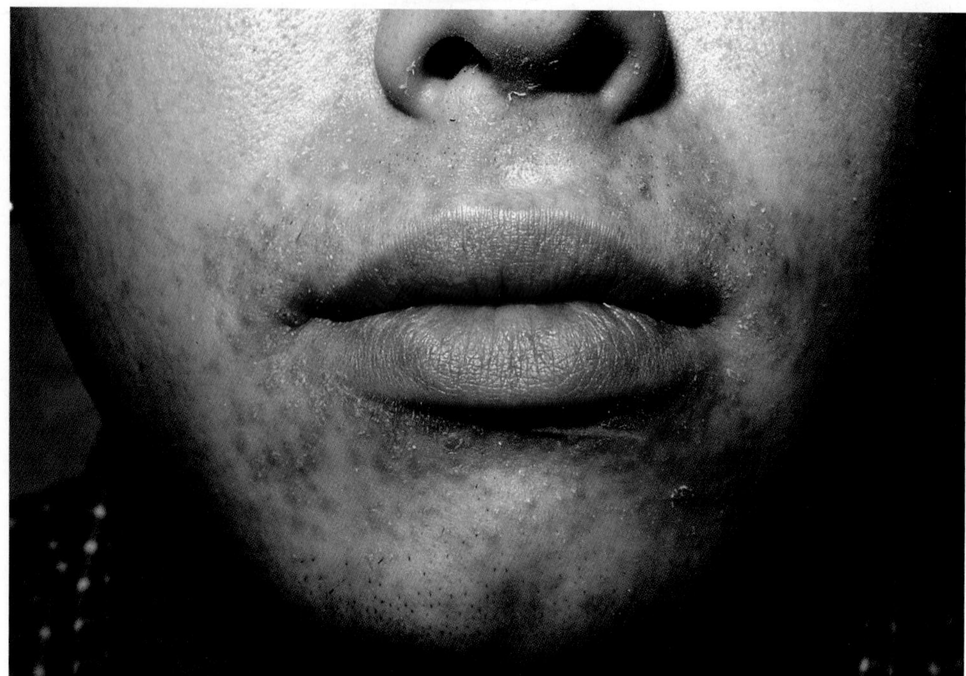

Figure 2-9 Perioral dermatitis. Pustules and erythema have appeared in a perioral distribution following several courses of a group III topical steroid to the lower face. The inflammation flares shortly after the topical steroid is discontinued.

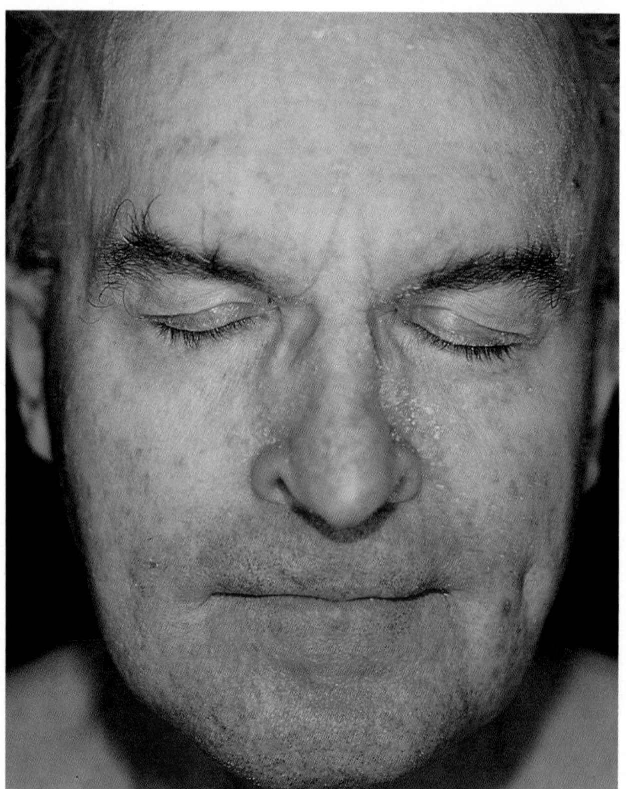

Figure 2-10 Steroid rosacea. A painful, diffuse pustular eruption occurred following daily application for 12 weeks of the group II topical steroid fluocinonide.

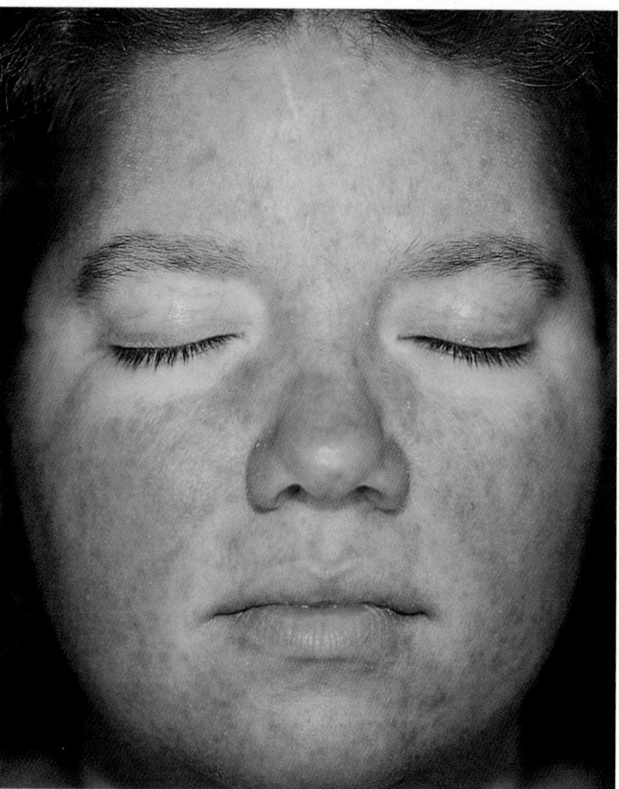

Figure 2-11 Steroid acne. Repeated application to the entire face of a group V topical steroid resulted in this diffuse pustular eruption. The inflammation improved each time the topical steroid was used but flared with increasing intensity each time the medication was stopped.

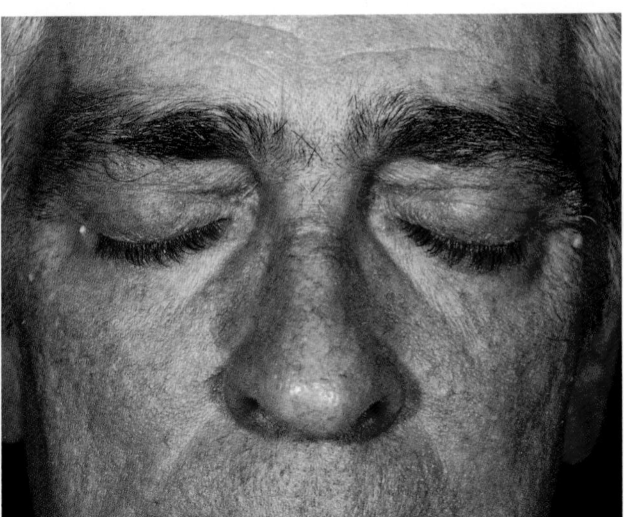

Figure 2-12 Steroid-induced telangiectasia. The patient in Figure 2-14 stopped all topical steroids. One year later he has permanent telangiectasia on the cheeks. His intraocular pressure was elevated but returned to near normal levels 3 months after stopping the fluocinonide.

ATROPHY

Long-term use of strong topical steroids in the same area may result in thinning of the epidermis and regressive changes in the connective tissue in the dermis. The affected areas are often depressed slightly below normal skin and usually reveal telangiectasia, prominence of underlying veins, and hypopigmentation. Purpura and ecchymosis result from minor trauma. The skin becomes lax, wrinkled, and shiny. The face (Figures 2-12 to 2-15), dorsa of the hands (Figure 2-16), extensor surfaces of the forearms and legs, and intertriginous areas are particularly susceptible. In most cases atrophy is reversible and may be expected to disappear in the course of several months. Diseases (such as psoriasis) that respond slowly to strong topical steroids require weeks of therapy; some atrophy may subsequently be anticipated (Figure 2-17).

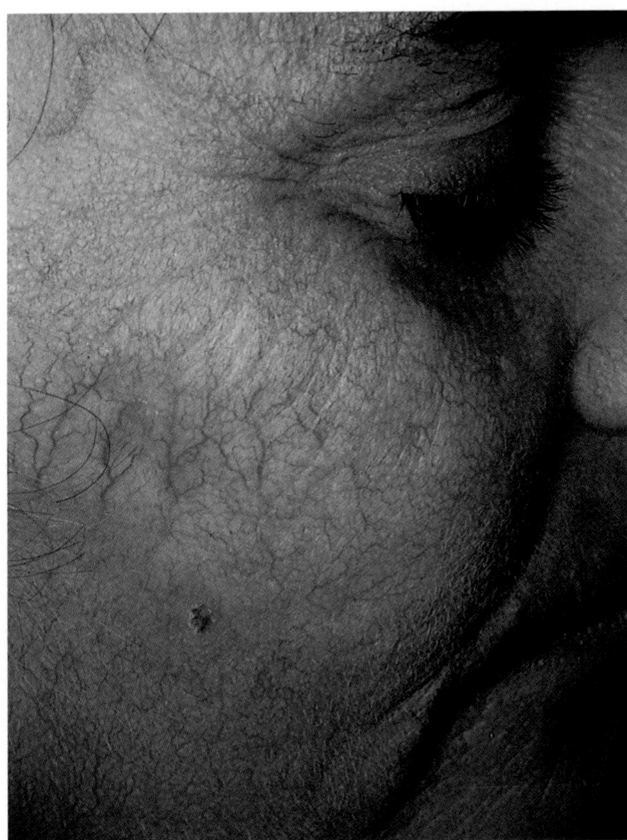

Figure 2-13 Atrophy and telangiectasia after continual use of a group IV topical steroid for 6 months. Atrophy may improve after the topical steroid is discontinued, but telangiectasia often persists.

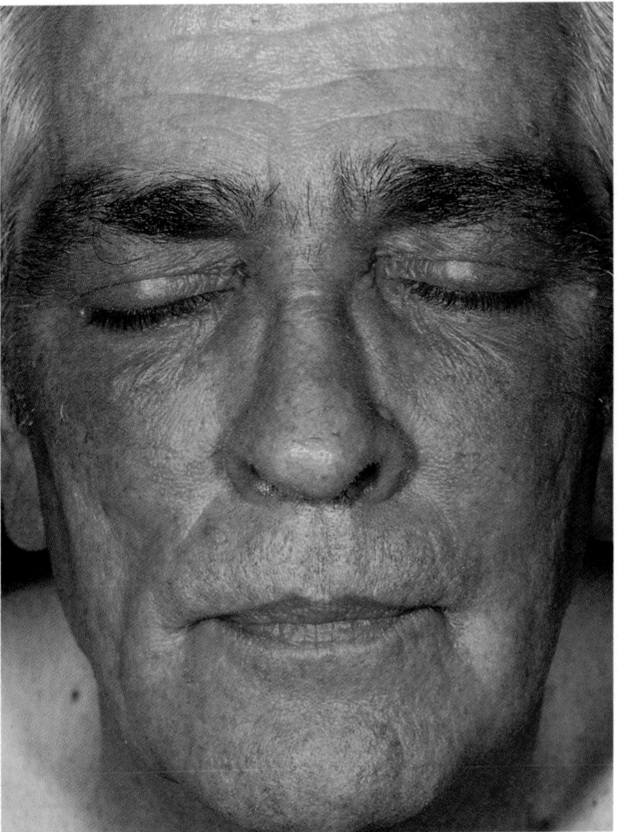

Figure 2-14 Steroid-induced erythema. This patient used the group II topical steroid fluocinonide almost constantly for 12 years. Erythema rather than pustules occurred each time the medication was stopped.

STEROID ATROPHY

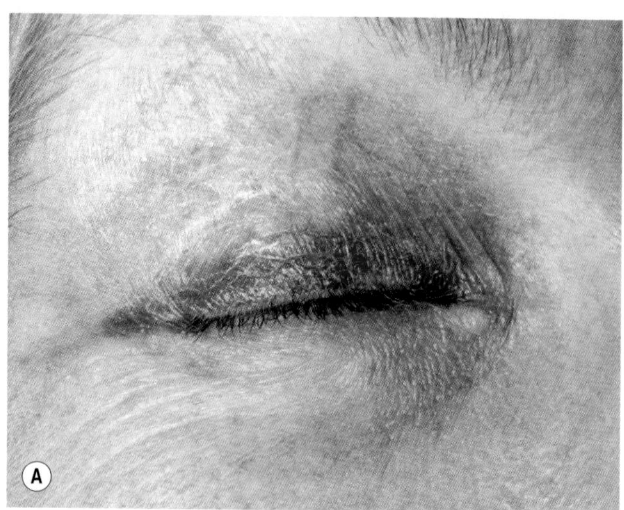

Daily application of the group II topical steroid desoximetasone to the lids resulted in almost complete atrophy of the dermis. The lids bleed spontaneously when touched. The intraocular pressure was elevated. There was marked improvement in the atrophy and intraocular tension 8 weeks after stopping the topical steroid.

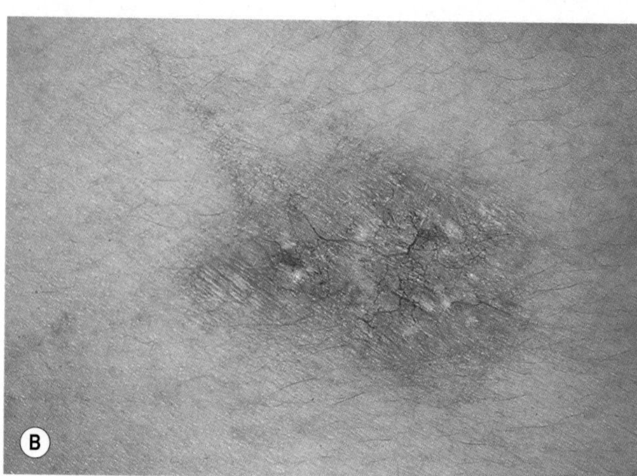

Daily application for months of a group II topical steroid to the skin on the abdomen produced severe atrophy with telangiectasia.

Figure 2-15

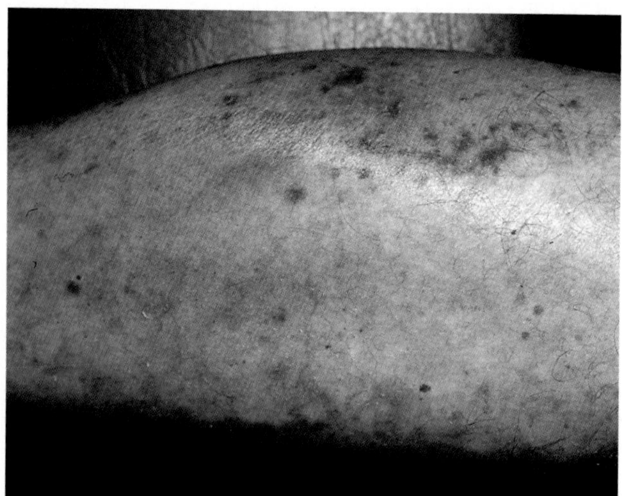

Figure 2-16 Severe steroid atrophy after continual occlusive therapy over several months. Significant improvement in the atrophy occurs after topical steroids are discontinued.

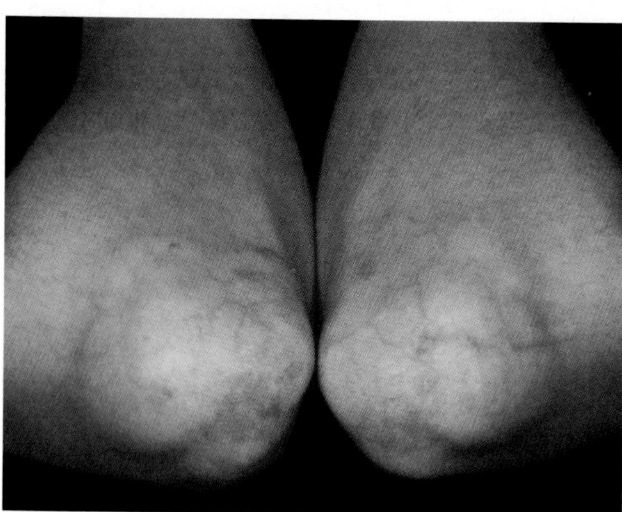

Figure 2-17 Atrophy with prominence of underlying veins and hypopigmentation following use of Cordran tape applied daily for 3 months to treat psoriasis. Note that small plaques of psoriasis persist. Atrophy improves after topical steroids are discontinued, but some hypopigmentation may persist.

OCCLUSION. Occlusion enhances penetration of medicine and accelerates the occurrence of this adverse reaction. Many patients are familiar with this side effect and must be assured that the use of strong topical steroids is perfectly safe when used as directed for 2 to 3 weeks. Patients must also be assured that if some atrophy does appear, it resolves in most cases when therapy is discontinued.

MUCOSAL AREAS. Atrophy under the foreskin (Figure 2-18) and in the rectal and vaginal areas may appear much more quickly than in other areas. The thinner epidermis offers less resistance to the passage of corticosteroids into the dermis. These are intertriginous areas where the apposition of skin surfaces acts in the same manner as a plastic dressing, retaining moisture and greatly facilitating absorption. These delicate tissues become thin and painful, sometimes exhibiting a susceptibility to tear or bleed with scratching or intercourse. The atrophy seems to be more enduring in these areas. Therefore careful instruction about the duration of therapy must be given (e.g., twice a day for 10 days). If the disease does not resolve quickly with topical therapy, reevaluation is necessary.

STEROID INJECTION SITES. Atrophy may appear very rapidly after intralesional injection of corticosteroids (e.g., for treatment of acne cysts or in attempting to promote hair growth in alopecia areata). The side effect of atrophy is used to reduce the size of hypertrophic scars and keloids. When injected into the dermis, 5 mg/ml triamcinolone acetonide (Kenalog) may produce atrophy; 10 mg/ml triamcinolone acetonide almost always produces atrophy. For direct injection into the skin, stronger concentrations should probably be avoided.

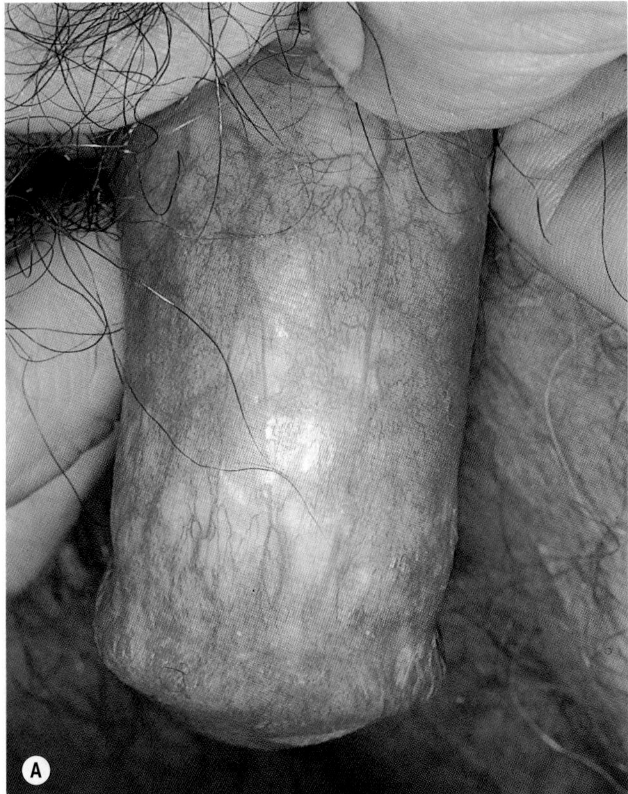

Steroid atrophy under the foreskin. Application of the group V topical steroid triamcinolone acetonide under the foreskin each day for 8 weeks produced severe atrophy and prominent telangiectasia of the shaft of the penis. The foreskin acted like an occlusive dressing to greatly enhance penetration of the steroid. Bleeding occurred with the slightest trauma. There was marked improvement 3 weeks after the medication was stopped.

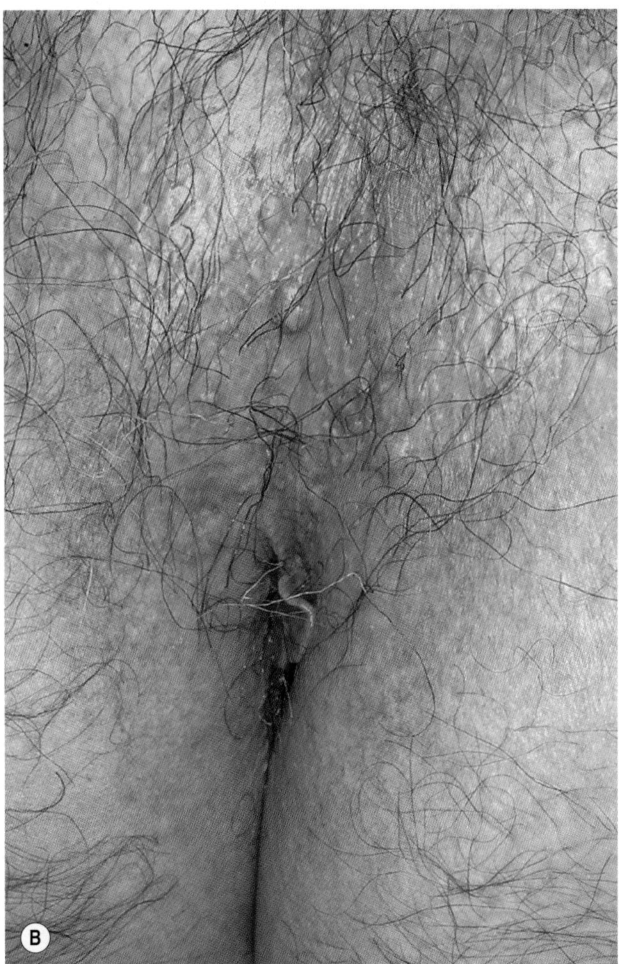

Erythema, atrophy, and pain occurred after the daily application of a group V topical steroid to the anal area for 3 months.

Figure 2-18 Steroid atrophy

LONG-TERM USE. Long-term use (over months) of even weak topical steroids on the upper inner thighs or in the axillae results in striae similar to those on the abdomens of pregnant women (Figure 2-19). These changes are irreversible. Pruritus in the groin area is common, and patients receive considerable relief when prescribed the less potent steroids. Symptoms often recur after treatment is terminated. It is a great temptation to continue topical treatment on an "as needed" basis but every attempt must be made to determine the underlying process and discourage long-term use.

ALTERATION OF INFECTION

Cortisone creams applied to cutaneous infections may alter the usual clinical presentation of those diseases and produce unusual atypical eruptions. Cortisone cream suppresses the inflammation that is attempting to contain the infection and allows unrestricted growth.

TINEA INCOGNITO. Tinea of the groin is characteristically seen as a localized superficial plaque with a well-defined scaly border (Figure 2-20). A group II corticosteroid applied for 3 weeks to this common eruption produced the rash seen in Figure 2-21. The fungus rapidly spreads to involve a much wider area, and the typical sharply defined border is gone. Untreated tinea rarely produces such a florid eruption in temperate climates. This altered clinical picture has been called tinea incognito.

Figure 2-22 shows a young girl who applied a group II cream daily for 6 months to treat "eczema." The large plaques retain some of the characteristics of certain fungal infections by having well-defined edges. The red papules and nodules are atypical and are usually observed exclusively with an unusual form of follicular fungal infection seen on the lower legs.

Boils, folliculitis, rosacea-like eruptions, and diffuse fine scaling resulting from treatment of tinea with topical steroids have been reported. If a rash does not respond after a reasonable length of time or if the appearance changes, the presence of tinea, bacterial infection, or allergic contact dermatitis from some component of the steroid cream should be considered.

INFESTATIONS AND BACTERIAL INFECTIONS. Scabies and impetigo may initially improve as topical steroids suppress inflammation. Consequently, both diseases become worse when the creams are discontinued (or, possibly, continued). Figure 2-23 shows numerous pustules on a leg; this appearance is characteristic of staphylococcal infection after treatment of an exudative, infected plaque of eczema with a group V topical steroid.

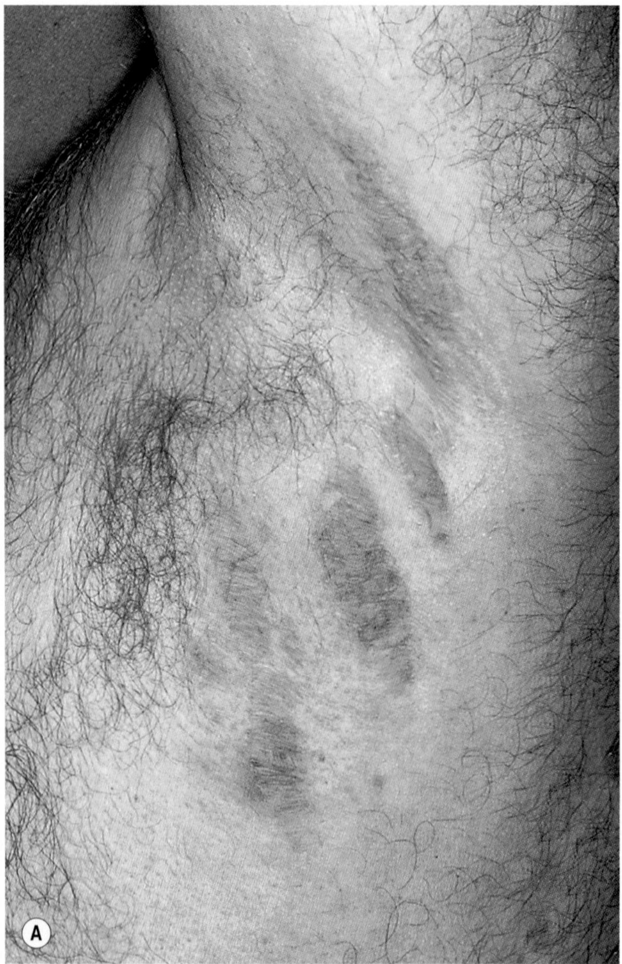

Striae of the axillae appeared after using Lotrisone cream continuously for 3 months.

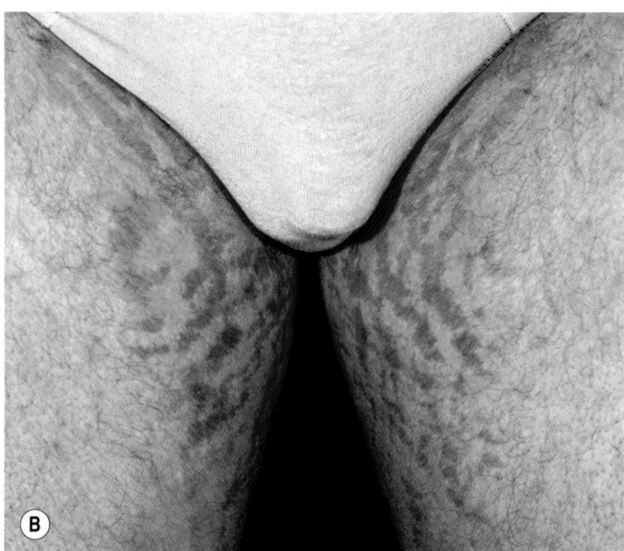

Striae of the groin after long-term use of group V topical steroids for pruritus. These changes are irreversible.

Figure 2-19 Striae, steroid induced.

ALTERATION OF INFECTION BY TOPICAL STEROIDS

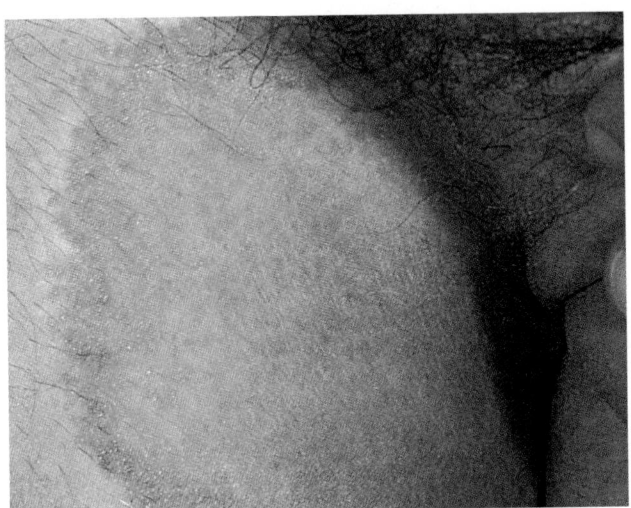

Figure 2-20 Typical presentation of tinea of the groin before treatment. Fungal infections of this type typically have a sharp, scaly border and show little tendency to spread.

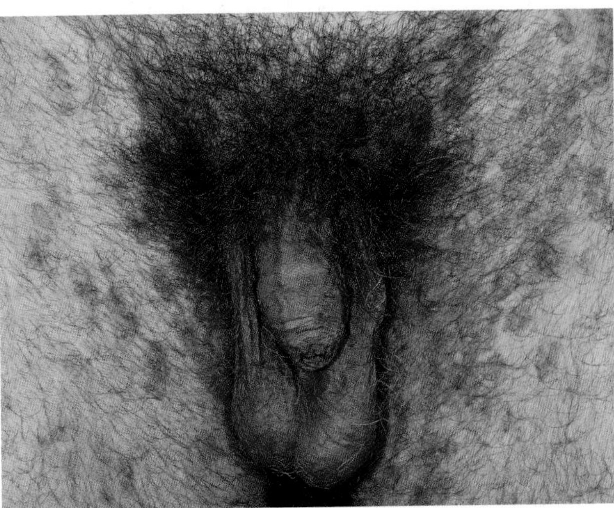

Figure 2-21 Tinea incognito. A bizarre pattern of widespread inflammation created by applying a group II topical steroid twice daily for 3 weeks to an eruption similar to that seen in Figure 2-20. A potassium hydroxide preparation showed numerous fungi.

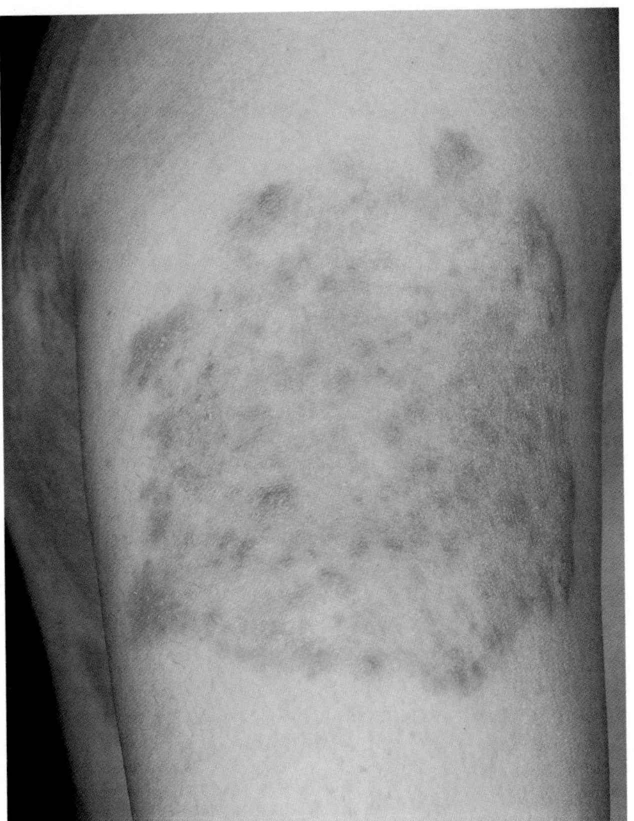

Figure 2-22 Tinea incognito. A plaque of tinea initially diagnosed as eczema was treated for 6 months with a group II topical steroid. Red papules have appeared where only erythema was once present.

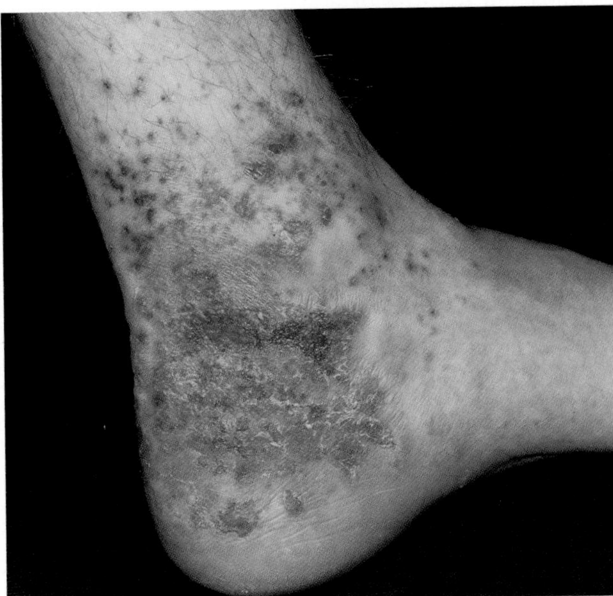

Figure 2-23 Impetiginized eczema with satellite pustules after treatment of exudative, infected eczema with a group V topical steroid.

CONTACT DERMATITIS

Topical steroids are the drugs of choice for allergic and irritant contact dermatitis, but occasionally topical steroids cause such dermatitis. Allergic reactions to various components of steroid creams (e.g., preservatives [parabens], vehicles [lanolin], antibacterials [neomycin], and perfumes) have all been documented. Figure 2-24 shows a patient diagnosed with allergic contact dermatitis to a preservative in a group II steroid gel. The gel was prescribed to treat seborrheic dermatitis. Allergic reactions may not be intense. Inflammation created by a cream component (e.g., a preservative) may be suppressed by the steroid component of the same cream and the eruption simply smolders, neither improving nor worsening, presenting a very confusing picture.

TOPICAL STEROID ALLERGY

Of patch-tested patients with dermatitis, 4% to 5% are allergic to corticosteroids. Patients affected by chronic dermatoses are at high risk for the development of sensitization to corticosteroids. Patients with any condition that does not improve or that deteriorates after administration of a topical steroid may be allergic to a component of the base or to the medication itself. Patients with stasis dermatitis and leg ulceration who are apt to use several topical medications for extended periods are more likely to be allergic to topical steroids. The over-the-counter availability of hydrocortisone makes long-term, unsupervised use possible. Allergy to topical steroids is demonstrated by patch or intradermal testing.

MANAGEMENT. When a patient does not respond as predicted or becomes worse while using topical corticosteroids, all topical treatment should be stopped. If corticosteroid therapy is absolutely necessary, one of the corticosteroids with a low sensitizing potential (e.g., mometasone furoate [Elocon], fluticasone propionate [Cutivate], betamethasone esters) could be used, and then only in an ointment base to avoid other allergens.

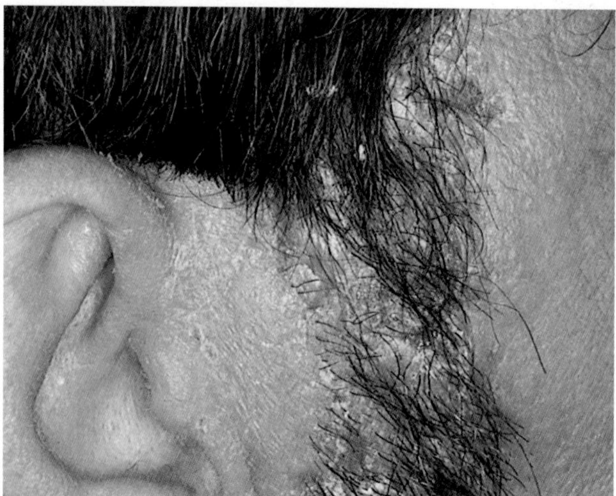

Figure 2-24 Acute contact allergy to a preservative in a group II steroid gel.

PATCH TESTING. Allergy to a component of the vehicle or the steroid molecule may occur. Patch testing for steroid cream allergy is complicated and usually performed by patch-test experts.

Four groups of corticosteroids are recognized, where substances from the same group may cross-react. The groups are: Group A (hydrocortisone type), Group B (triamcinolone acetonides), Group C (betamethasone type, nonesterified), and Group D (hydrocortisone 17-butyrate type). The latter group is subclassified into two groups, group D1 (halogenated and with C16 substitution) and group D2 (the "labile" prodrug esters without the latter characteristics).

Tixocortol pivalate, hydrocortisone 17-butyrate, and budesonide are the screening agents of choice. Patients should be patch tested to screen for corticosteroid allergy. If a corticosteroid sensitivity is detected, a more extensive corticosteroid series should be tested to determine cross-reactivity patterns. Cross-reactivity among topically administered corticosteroids is frequent.

GLAUCOMA

There are isolated case reports of glaucoma occurring after the long-term use of topical steroids around the eyes. Glaucoma induced by the chronic use of steroid-containing eyedrops instilled directly into the conjunctival sac is encountered more frequently by ophthalmologists. The mechanism by which glaucoma develops from topical application is not understood, but presumably, cream applied to the lids seeps over the lid margin and into the conjunctival sac. It also seems possible that enough steroid could be absorbed directly through the lid skin into the conjunctival sac to produce the same results.

Inflammation around the eye is a common problem. Offending agents that cause inflammation may be directly transferred to the eyelids by rubbing with the hand, or they may be applied directly, as with cosmetics. Women who are sensitive to a favorite eye makeup often continue using that makeup on an interrupted basis, not suspecting the obvious source of allergy. Patients have been known to alternate topical steroids with a sensitizing makeup. Unsupervised use of over-the-counter hydrocortisone cream might also induce glaucoma.

No studies have yet determined what quantity or strength of steroid cream is required to produce glaucoma. The patient shown in Figure 2-15 used a group II topical steroid on the eyelids daily for 3 years. Severe atrophy and bleeding with the slightest trauma occurred, and ocular pressure was elevated. Atrophy and glaucoma were gone 3 months after stopping the topical steroid.

It is good practice to restrict the use of topical steroids on the eyelids to a 2- to 3-week period and use only group VI and VII preparations.

Chapter 3

Eczema and Hand Dermatitis

CHAPTER CONTENTS

Eczema (eczematous inflammation) is the most common inflammatory skin disease. Although the term *dermatitis* is often used to refer to an eczematous eruption, the word means inflammation of the skin and is not synonymous with eczematous processes. Recognizing a rash as eczematous rather than psoriasiform or lichenoid, for example, is of fundamental importance if one is to effectively diagnose skin disease. Here, as with other skin diseases, it is important to look carefully at the rash and to determine the primary lesion.

It is essential to recognize the quality and characteristics of the components of eczematous inflammation (erythema, scale, and vesicles) and to determine how these differ from other rashes with similar features. Once familiar with these features, the experienced clinician can recognize a process as eczematous even in the presence of secondary changes produced by scratching, infection, or irritation. With the diagnosis of eczematous inflammation established, a major part of the diagnostic puzzle has been solved.

STAGES OF ECZEMATOUS INFLAMMATION

There are three stages of eczema: *acute, subacute,* and *chronic*. Each represents a stage in the evolution of a dynamic inflammatory process (Table 3-1). Clinically, an eczematous disease may start at any stage and evolve into another. Most eczematous diseases, if left alone (i.e., neither irritated, scratched, nor medicated), resolve in time without complication. This ideal situation is almost never realized; scratching, irritation, or attempts at topical treatment are almost inevitable. Some degree of itching is a cardinal feature of eczematous inflammation.

Table 3-1 Eczematous Inflammation

Stage	Primary and secondary lesions	Symptoms	Etiology and clinical presentation	Treatment
Acute	Vesicles, blisters, intense redness	Intense itch	Contact allergy (poison ivy), severe irritation, id reaction, acute nummular eczema, stasis dermatitis, pompholyx (dyshidrosis), fungal infections	Cold, wet compresses; oral or intramuscular steroids; topical steroids; antihistamines; antibiotics
Subacute	Redness, scaling, fissuring, parched appearance, scalded appearance	Slight to moderate itch, pain, stinging, burning	Contact allergy, irritation, atopic dermatitis, stasis dermatitis, nummular eczema, asteatotic eczema, fingertip eczema, fungal infections	Topical steroids with or without occlusion, lubrication, antihistamines, antibiotics, tar
Chronic	Thickened skin, skin lines accentuated (lichenified skin), excoriations, fissuring	Moderate to intense itch	Atopic dermatitis, habitual scratching, lichen simplex chronicus, chapped fissured feet, nummular eczema, asteatotic eczema, fingertip eczema, hyperkeratotic eczema	Topical steroids (with occlusion for best results), intralesional steroids, antihistamines, antibiotics, lubrication

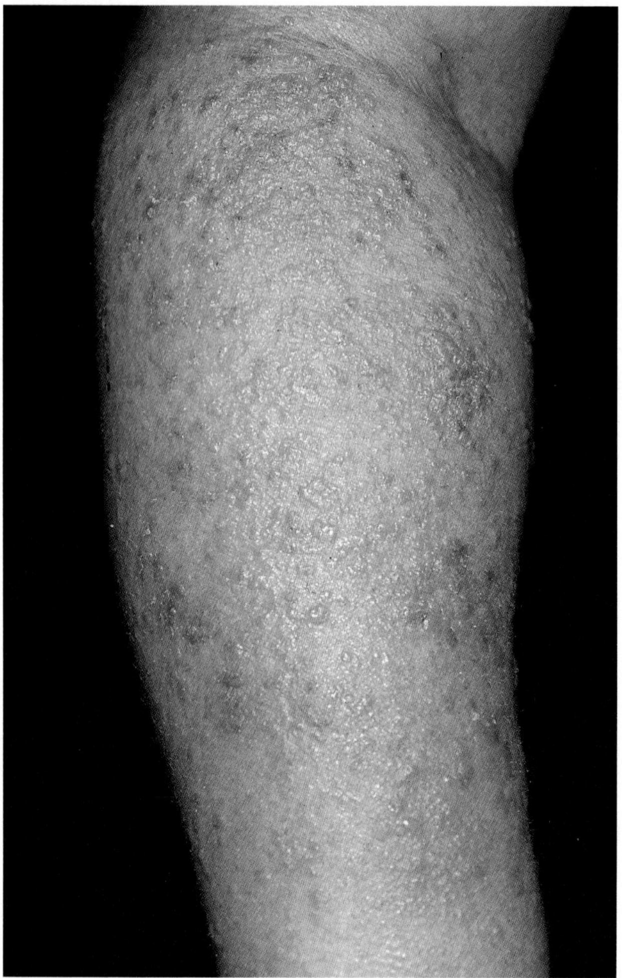

Figure 3-1 Acute eczematous inflammation. Numerous vesicles on a erythematous base. Vesicles may become confluent with time.

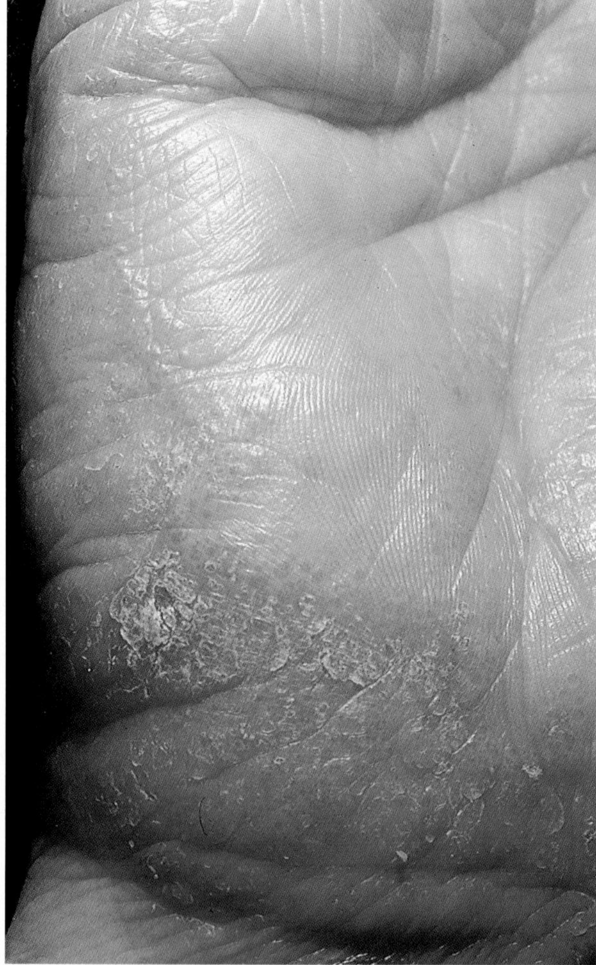

Figure 3-2 Acute eczematous inflammation. Vesicle appeared during a 24-hour period in this patient with chronic hand eczema. Episodes of acute inflammation had occurred several times in the past.

Acute eczematous inflammation

ETIOLOGY. Inflammation is caused by contact with specific allergens such as *Rhus* (poison ivy, oak, or sumac) and chemicals. In the id reaction, vesicular reactions occur at a distant site during or after a fungal infection, stasis dermatitis, or other acute inflammatory processes.

PHYSICAL FINDINGS. The degree of inflammation varies from moderate to intense. A bright red, swollen plaque with a pebbly surface evolves in hours. Close examination of the surface reveals tiny, clear, serum-filled vesicles (Figures 3-1 to 3-3). The eruption may not progress or it may evolve to develop blisters. The vesicles and blisters may be confluent and are often linear. Linear lesions result from dragging the offending agent across the skin with the finger during scratching. The degree of inflammation in cases caused by allergy is directly proportional to the quantity of antigen deposited on the skin. Excoriation predisposes to infection and causes serum, crust, and purulent material to accumulate.

SYMPTOMS. Acute eczema itches intensely. Patients scratch the eruption even while sleeping. A hot shower temporarily relieves itching because the pain produced by hot water is better tolerated than the sensation of itching; however, heat aggravates acute eczema.

COURSE. Lesions may begin to appear from hours to 2 to 3 days after exposure and may continue to appear for 1 week or more. These later occurring, less inflammatory lesions are confusing to the patient, who cannot recall additional exposure. Lesions produced by small amounts of allergen are slower to evolve. They are not produced, as is generally believed, by contact with the serum of ruptured blisters, because the blister fluid does not contain the offending chemical. Acute eczematous inflammation evolves into a subacute stage before resolving.

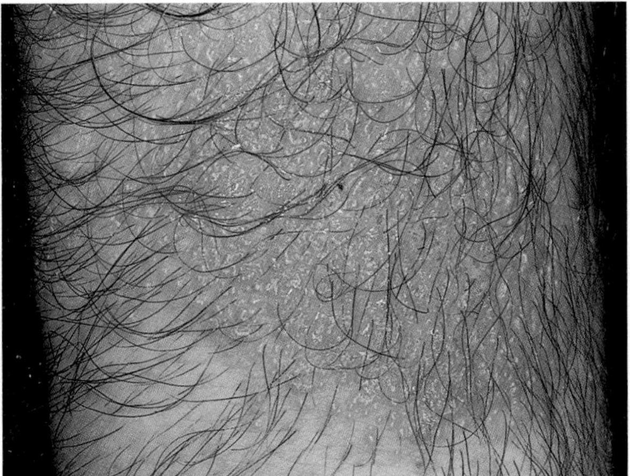

Figure 3-3 Acute eczematous inflammation. Numerous vesicles occurred after exposure to poison ivy.

TREATMENT

Cool, wet dressings. The evaporative cooling produced by wet compresses causes vasoconstriction and rapidly suppresses inflammation and itching. Burow's powder, available in a 12-packet box, may be added to the solution to suppress bacterial growth, but water alone is usually sufficient. A clean cotton cloth is soaked in cool water, folded several times, and placed directly over the affected areas. Evaporative cooling produces vasoconstriction and decreases serum production. Wet compresses should not be held in place and covered with towels or plastic wrap because this prevents evaporation. The wet cloth macerates vesicles and, when removed, mechanically debrides the area and prevents serum and crust from accumulating. Wet compresses should be removed after 30 minutes and replaced with a freshly soaked cloth. It is tempting to leave the drying compress in place and to wet it again by pouring solution onto the cloth. Although evaporative cooling will continue, irritation may occur from the accumulation of scale, crust, and serum and from the increased concentration of aluminum sulfate and calcium acetate, the active ingredients in Burow's powder.

Oral corticosteroids. Oral corticosteroids such as prednisone are useful for controlling intense or widespread inflammation and may be used in addition to wet dressings. Prednisone controls most cases of poison ivy when it is taken in 20-mg doses twice a day for 7 to 14 days (for adults); however, to treat intense or generalized inflammation, prednisone may be started at 30 mg or more twice a day and maintained at that level for 3 to 5 days. Sometimes 21 days of treatment are required for adequate control. The dosage should not be tapered for these relatively short courses because lower dosages may not give the desired antiinflammatory effect. Inflammation may reappear as diffuse erythema and may even be more extensive if the dosage is too low or is tapered too rapidly. Commercially available steroid dose packs taper the dosage and provide treatment for too short a time and so should not be used. Topical corticosteroids are of little use in the acute stage because the cream does not penetrate through the vesicles.

Antihistamines. Antihistamines, such as diphenhydramine (Benadryl) and hydroxyzine (Atarax), do not alter the course of the disease, but they relieve itching and provide enough sedation so patients can sleep. They are given every 4 hours as needed.

Antibiotics. The use of oral antibiotics may greatly hasten resolution of the disease if signs of superficial secondary infection, such as pustules, purulent material, and crusts, are present. *Staphylococcus* is the usual pathogen, and cultures are not routinely necessary. Deep infection (cellulitis) is rare with acute eczema. Cephalexin and dicloxacillin are effective; topical antibiotics are much less effective.

Subacute eczematous inflammation

PHYSICAL FINDINGS. Erythema and scale are present in various patterns, usually with indistinct borders (Figures 3-4 and 3-5). The redness may be faint or intense (Figures 3-6 through 3-9). Psoriasis, superficial fungal infections, and eczematous inflammation may have a similar appearance (Figures 3-10 through 3-12). The borders of the plaques of psoriasis and superficial fungal infections are well-defined. Psoriatic plaques have a deep, rich red color and silvery white scales.

SYMPTOMS. These vary from no itching to intense itching.

COURSE. Subacute eczematous inflammation may be the initial stage or it may follow acute inflammation. Irritation, allergy, or infection can convert a subacute process into an acute process. Subacute inflammation resolves spontaneously without scarring if all sources of irritation and allergy are withdrawn. Excess drying created from washing or continued use of wet dressings causes cracking and fissures. If excoriation is not controlled, the subacute process can be converted to a chronic process. Diseases that have subacute eczematous inflammation as a characteristic are listed in Box 3-1.

Box 3-1 **Diseases Presenting as Subacute Eczematous Inflammation**

Allergic contact dermatitis	Intertrigo
Asteatotic eczema	Irritant contact dermatitis
Atopic dermatitis	Irritant hand eczema
Chapped fissured feet (sweaty sock dermatitis)	Nipple eczema (nursing mothers)
Circumileostomy eczema	Nummular eczema
Diaper dermatitis	Perioral lick eczema
Exposure to chemicals	Statis dermatitis

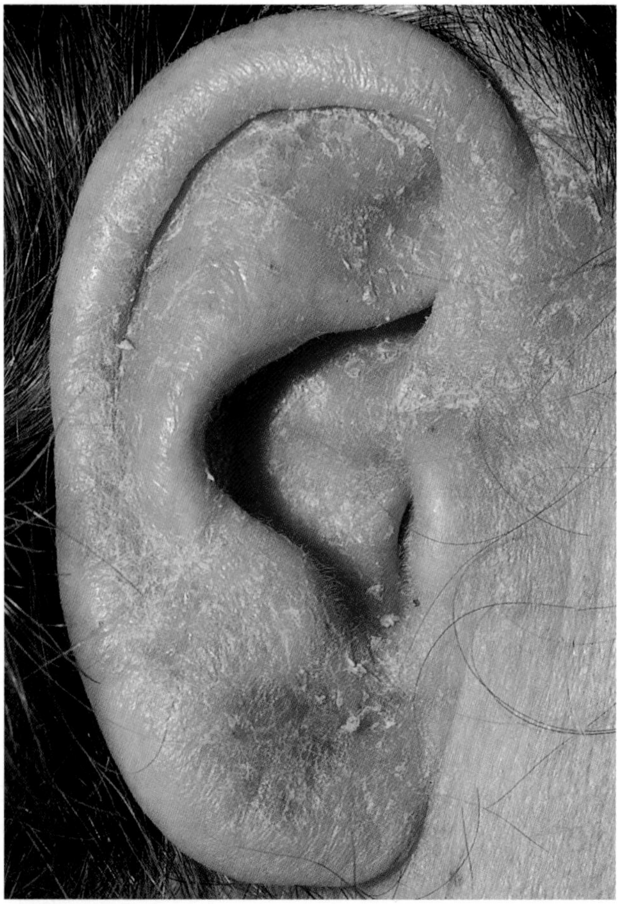

Figure 3-4 Subacute and chronic eczematous inflammation. The skin is dry, red, scaling, and thickened.

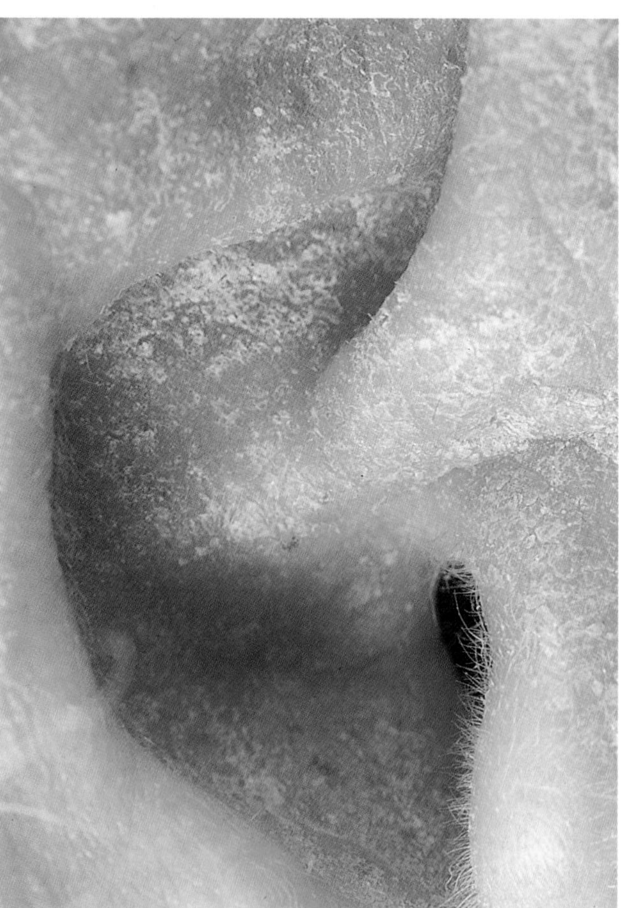

Figure 3-5 Subacute and chronic eczematous inflammation. The ear canal is red, scaling, and thickened from chronic excoriation.

SUBACUTE ECZEMA

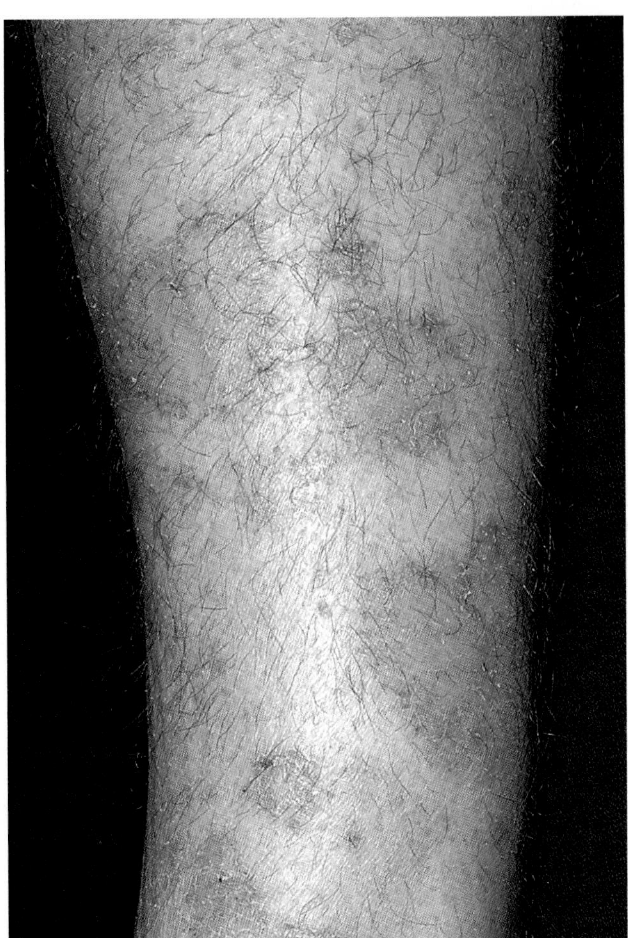

Figure 3-6 Red, scaling, nummular (round) superficial plaques occurred during the winter months from excessive washing.

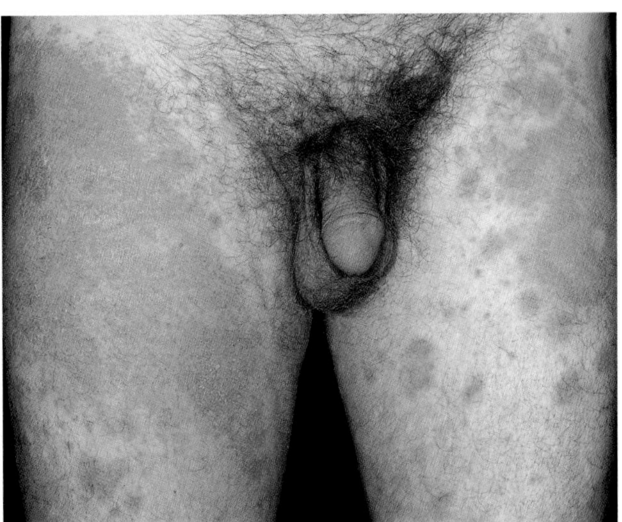

Figure 3-7 Erythema and scaling are present, the surface is dry, and the borders are indistinct.

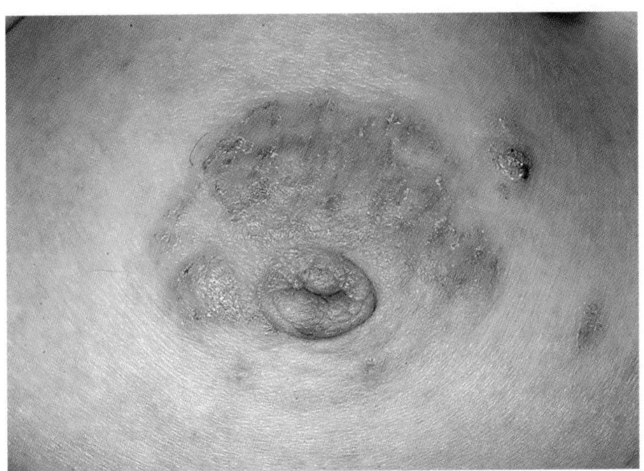

Figure 3-8 The areolae of both breasts are red and scaly. Inflammation of one areola is characteristic of Paget's disease.

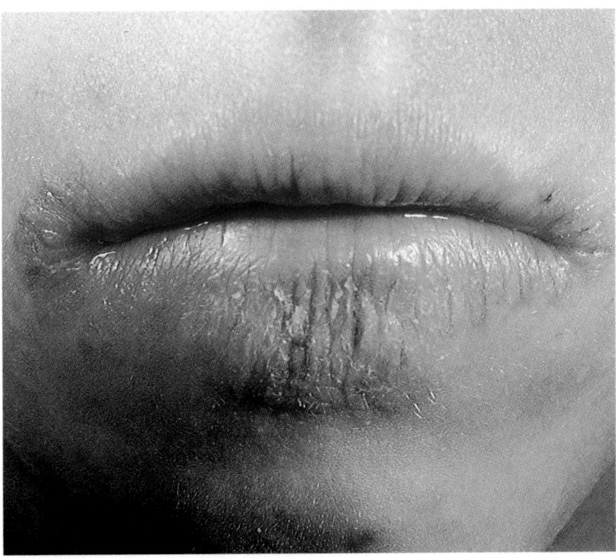

Figure 3-9 Wetting the lip by licking will eventually cause chapping and then eczema.

ECZEMA RESEMBLING PSORIASIS

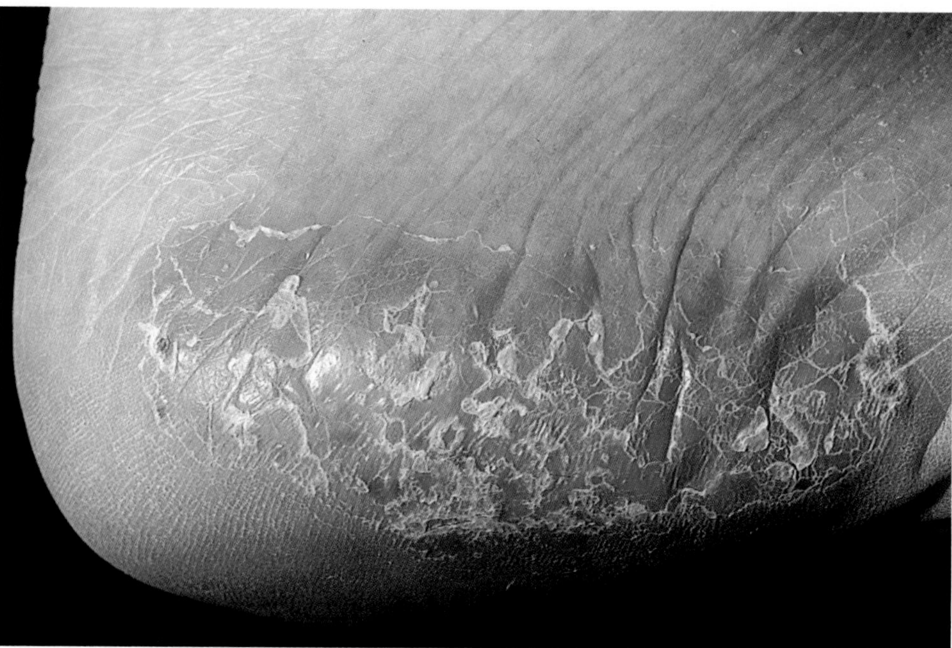

Figure 3-10 Acute and subacute eczematous inflammation. Acute vesicular eczema is evolving into subacute eczema. Vesicles, redness, and scaling are all present in this lesion undergoing transition.

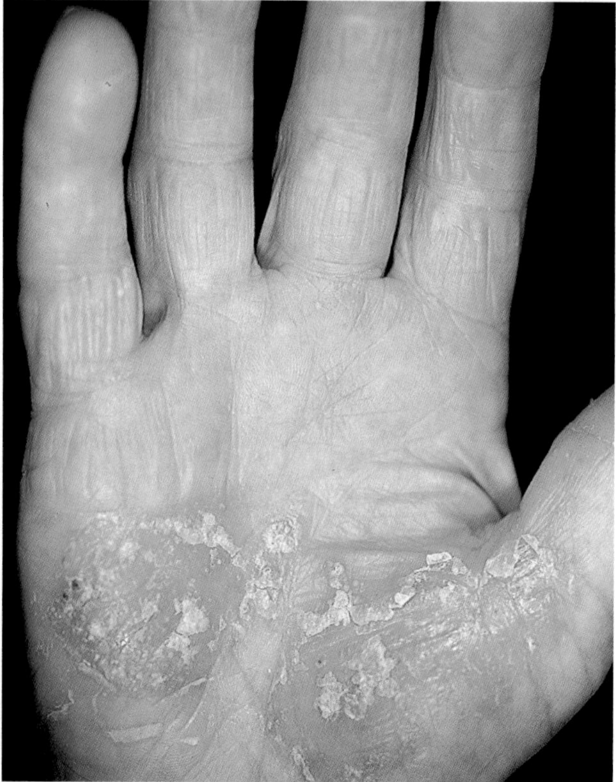

Figure 3-11 Acute vesicular eczema has evolved into subacute eczema with redness and scaling.

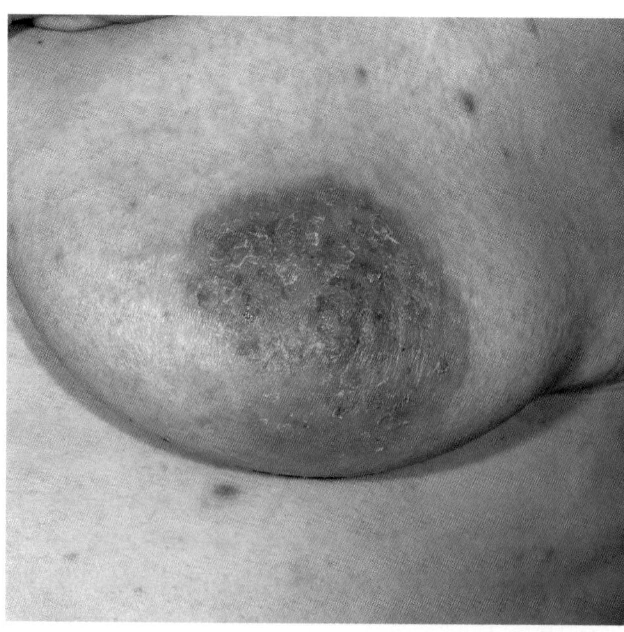

Figure 3-12 Subacute eczematous inflammation. Erythema and scaling in a round or nummular pattern.

TREATMENT. It is important to discontinue wet dressings when acute inflammation evolves into subacute inflammation. Excess drying creates cracking and fissures, which predispose to infection.

Topical corticosteroids. These agents are the treatment of choice (see Chapter 2). Creams may be applied two to four times a day or with occlusion. Ointments may be applied two to four times a day for drier lesions. Subacute inflammation requires group III through V corticosteroids for rapid control. Occlusion with creams hastens resolution, and less expensive, weaker products such as triamcinolone cream 0.1% (Kenalog) give excellent results. *Staphylococcus aureus* colonizes eczematous lesions, but studies show their numbers are significantly reduced following treatment with topical steroids.

Topical macrolide immune suppressants. Tacrolimus ointment (Protopic) and pimecrolimus cream (Elidel) are the first topical macrolide immune suppressants that are not hydrocortisone derivatives. They inhibit the production of inflammatory cytokines in T cells and mast cells and prevent the release of preformed inflammatory mediators from mast cells. Dermal atrophy does not occur. These agents are effective for the treatment of inflammatory skin diseases, such as atopic dermatitis, allergic contact dermatitis, and irritant contact dermatitis. They are approved for use in children 2 years or older. Response to these agents is slower than the response to topical steroids. Topical steroids may be used for several days before the use of these agents to obtain rapid control.

Pimecrolimus (Elidel) cream. Pimecrolimus permeates through skin at a lower rate than tacrolimus, indicating a lower potential for percutaneous absorption. The cream is applied twice a day and may be used on the face. Continuous long-term use of topical calcineurin inhibitors in any age group should be avoided, and application limited to areas of involvement with dermatitis.

Tacrolimus ointment (Protopic). Tacrolimus is effective in the treatment of children (aged 2 years and older) and adults with atopic dermatitis and eczema. The most prominent adverse event is application site burning and erythema. It is available in 0.03% and 0.1% ointment formulations. Some clinicians find the 0.03% concentration to be marginally effective. Continuous long-term use of topical calcineurin inhibitors in any age group should be avoided, and application limited to areas of involvement with dermatitis.

Doxepin cream. A topical form of the antidepressant doxepin (doxepin 5% cream; Zonalon) is effective for the relief of pruritus associated with eczema in adults and children aged over 12 years. The two most common adverse effects are stinging at the site of application and drowsiness. The medication can be applied four times a day as needed.

Lubrication. This is a simple but essential part of therapy. Inflamed skin becomes dry and is more susceptible to further irritation and inflammation. Resolved dry areas may easily relapse into subacute eczema if proper lubrication is neglected. Lubricants are best applied a few hours after topical steroids and should be continued for days or weeks after the inflammation has cleared. Frequent application (one to four times a day) should be encouraged. Applying lubricants directly after the skin has been patted dry following a shower seals in moisture. Lotions or creams with or without the hydrating chemicals urea and lactic acid may be used. Bath oils are very useful if used in amounts sufficient to make the skin feel oily when the patient leaves the tub.

Lotions. Curél, DML, Lubriderm, Cetaphil, or any of the other lotions listed in the Formulary are useful.

Creams. DML, Moisturel, Neutrogena, Nivea, Eucerin, and Acid Mantle or any of the other creams listed in the Formulary are useful.

Mild soaps. Frequent washing with a drying soap, such as Ivory, delays healing. Infrequent washing with mild or superfatted soaps (e.g., Dove, Cetaphil, Basis—see the Formulary) should be encouraged. It is usually not necessary to use hypoallergenic soaps or to avoid perfumed soaps. Although allergy to perfumes occurs, the incidence is low.

Antibiotics. Eczematous plaques that remain bright red during treatment with topical steroids may be infected. Infected subacute eczema should be treated with appropriate systemic antibiotics, which are usually those active against *Staphylococci*. Systemic antibiotics are more effective than topical antibiotics or antibiotic-steroid combination creams.

Tar. Tar ointments, baths, and soaps were among the few effective therapeutic agents available for the treatment of eczema before the introduction of topical steroids. Topical steroids provide rapid and lasting control of eczema in most cases. Some forms of eczema, such as atopic dermatitis and irritant eczema, tend to recur. Topical steroids become less effective with long-term use. Tar is sometimes an effective alternative in this setting. Tar ointments or creams may be used for long-term control or between short courses of topical steroids.

ADULT-ONSET RECALCITRANT ECZEMA AND MALIGNANCY

Generalized eczema or erythroderma may be the presenting sign of cutaneous T-cell lymphoma. Intractable pruritus has been associated with Hodgkin's lymphoma. Unexplained eczema of adult onset may be associated with an underlying lymphoproliferative malignancy. Patients may have widespread erythematous plaques that are poorly responsive to therapy. When a readily identifiable cause (e.g., contactants, drugs, or atopy) is not found, a systematic evaluation should be pursued.

Chronic eczematous inflammation

ETIOLOGY. Chronic eczematous inflammation may be caused by irritation of subacute inflammation, or it may appear as lichen simplex chronicus.

PHYSICAL FINDINGS. Chronic eczematous inflammation is a clinical-pathologic entity and does not indicate simply any long-lasting stage of eczema. If scratching is not controlled, subacute eczematous inflammation can be modified and converted to chronic eczematous inflammation (Figure 3-13). The inflamed area thickens, and surface skin markings may become more prominent. Thick plaques with deep parallel skin marking ("washboard" lesion) are said to be lichenified (Figure 3-14). The border is well-defined but not as sharply defined as it is in psoriasis (Figure 3-15). The sites most commonly involved are those areas that are easily reached and associated with habitual scratching (e.g., dorsal feet, lateral forearms, anus, and occipital scalp), areas where eczema tends to be long-lasting (e.g., the lower legs, as in stasis dermatitis), and the crease areas (antecubital and popliteal fossa, wrists, behind the ears, and ankles) in atopic dermatitis (Figures 3-16 to 3-18).

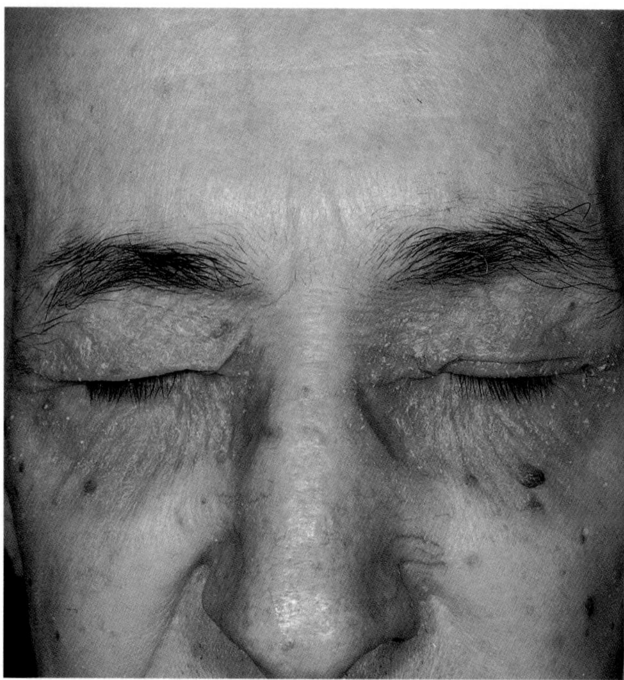

Figure 3-13 Subacute and chronic eczema. Dermatitis of the lids may be allergic, irritant, or atopic in origin. This atopic patient rubs the lids with the back of the hands.

SYMPTOMS. There is moderate to intense itching. Scratching sometimes becomes violent, leading to excoriation and digging, and ceases only when pain has replaced the itch. Patients with chronic inflammation scratch while asleep.

COURSE. Scratching and rubbing become habitual and are often done unconsciously. The disease then becomes self-perpetuating. Scratching leads to thickening of the skin, which itches more than before. It is this habitual manipulation that causes the difficulty in eradicating this disease. Some patients enjoy the feeling of relief that comes from scratching and may actually desire the reappearance of their disease after treatment.

TREATMENT. Chronic eczematous inflammation is resistant to treatment and requires potent steroid therapy.

Topical steroids. Groups II through V topical steroids are used with occlusion each night until the inflammation clears—usually in 1 to 3 weeks; group I topical steroids are used without occlusion. Topical steroid foams (e.g., clobetasol foam) may be very effective. Tacrolimus ointment 0.1% can be used as a primary treatment or used alternately with topical steroids.

Intralesional injection. Intralesional injection (Kenalog, 10 mg/ml) is a very effective mode of therapy. Lesions that have been present for years may completely resolve after one injection or a short series of injections. The medicine is delivered with a 27- or 30-gauge needle, and the entire plaque is infiltrated until it blanches white. Resistant plaques require additional injections given at 3- to 4-week intervals.

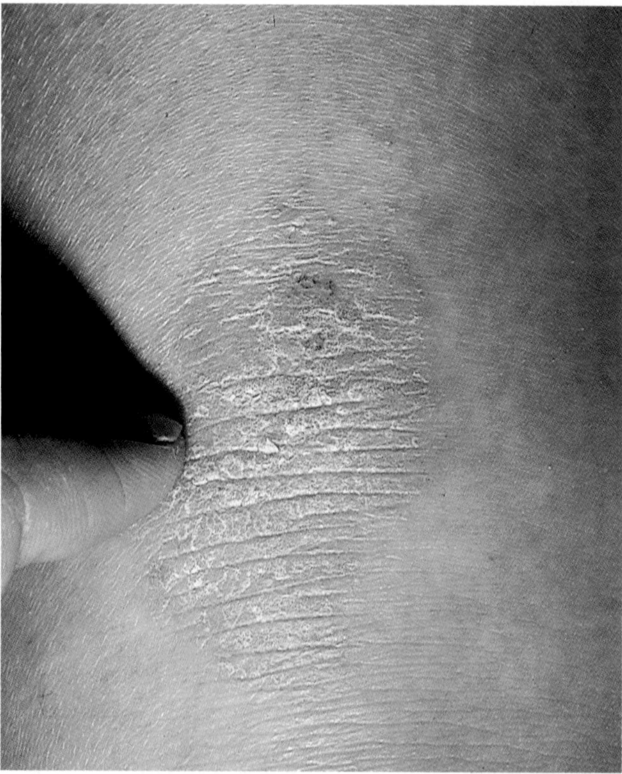

Figure 3-14 Chronic eczematous inflammation. Chronic excoriations thicken the epidermis, which results in accentuated skin lines. Chronic eczema created by picking is called lichen simplex chronicus.

CHRONIC ECZEMATOUS INFLAMMATION

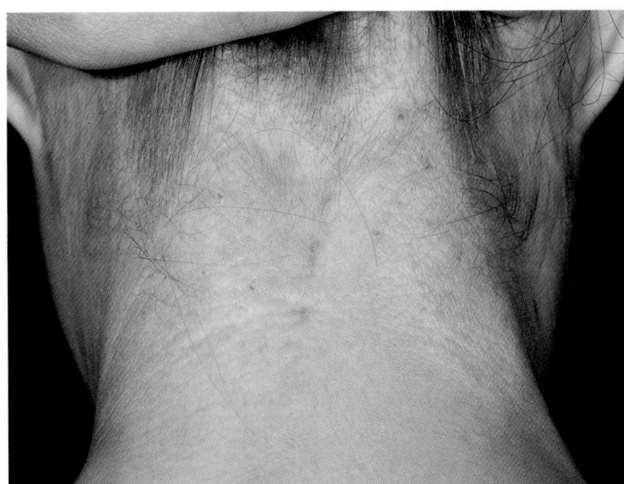

Figure 3-15 Erythema and scaling are present, and the skin lines are accentuated, creating a lichenified or "washboard" lesion.

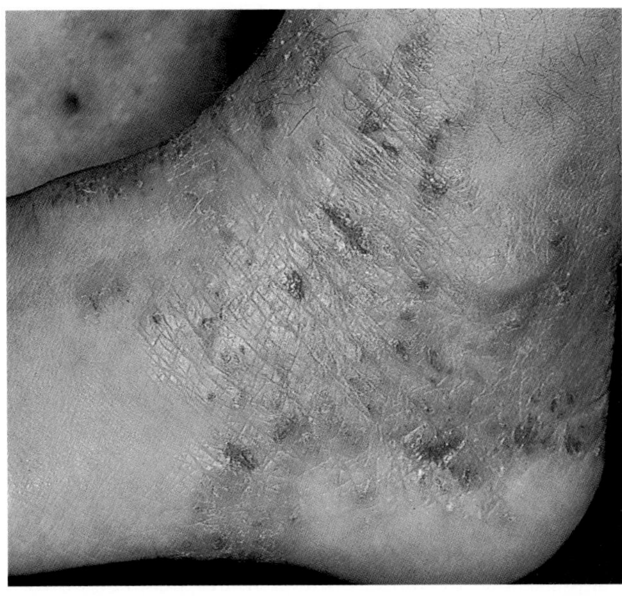

Figure 3-16 Atopic dermatitis. Atopic dermatitis is common in the crease areas. Atopic patients scratch, lichenify the skin, and often create a chronic process.

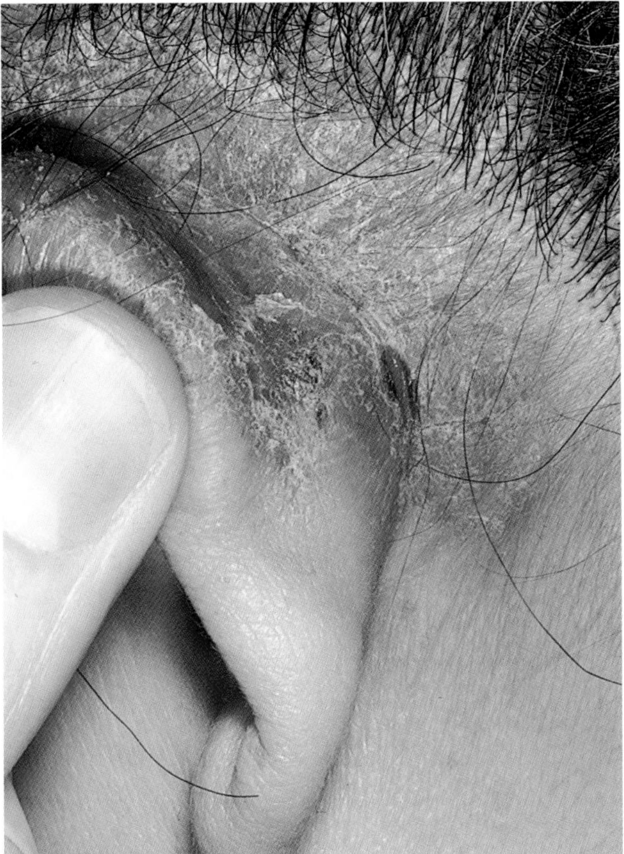

Figure 3-17 Picking and rubbing thickened the skin behind the ear.

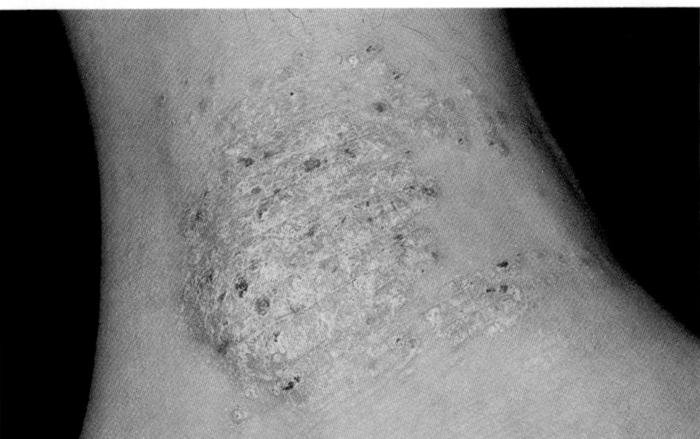

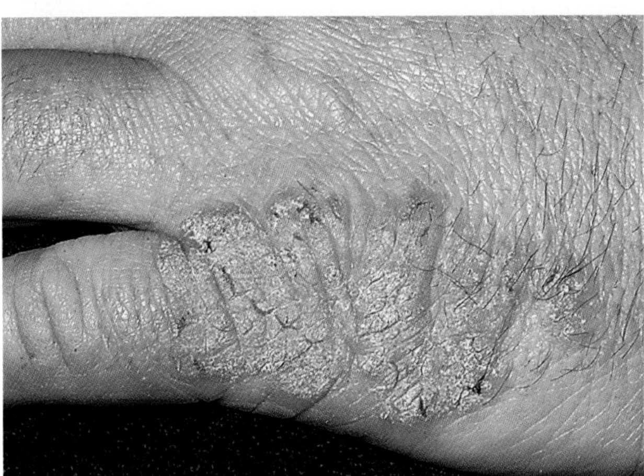

Figure 3-18 A plaque of lichen simplex chronicus created by excoriation is present. Accentuated skin lines and eczematous papules beyond the border help to differentiate this process from psoriasis. f0180

HAND ECZEMA

Inflammation of the hands is one of the most common problems encountered by the dermatologist. Hand dermatitis causes discomfort and embarrassment and, because of its location, interferes significantly with normal daily activities. Hand dermatitis is common in industrial occupations: it can threaten job security if inflammation cannot be controlled. Box 3-2 lists instructions for patients with irritant hand dermatitis.

EPIDEMIOLOGY. A large study provided the following statistics: the prevalence of hand eczema was approximately 5.4% and was twice as common in females as in males. The most common type of hand eczema was irritant contact dermatitis (35%), followed by atopic hand eczema (22%) and allergic contact dermatitis (19%). The most common contact allergies were to nickel, cobalt, fragrance mix, balsam of Peru, and colophony. Of all the occupations studied, cleaners had the highest prevalence at 21.3%. Hand eczema was more common among people reporting occupational exposure. The most harmful exposure was to chemicals, water and detergents, dust, and dry dirt. A change of occupation was reported by 8% and was most common in service workers. Hairdressers had the highest frequency of change. Hand eczema was shown to be a long-lasting disease with a relapsing course; 69% of the patients had consulted a physician, and 21% had been on sick leave at least once because of hand eczema. The mean total sick-leave time was 18.9 weeks; the median was 8 weeks. *PMID: 2145721* The most important predictive factors for hand eczema are listed in Box 3-3.

DIAGNOSIS. The diagnosis and management of hand eczema are a challenge. There is almost no association between clinical pattern and etiology. No distribution of eczema is typically allergic, irritant, or endogenous. Not only are there many patterns of eczematous inflammation (Table 3-2), but also there are other diseases, such as psoriasis, that may appear eczematous. Many patients diagnosed with hand eczema actually have psoriasis. The original primary lesions and their distribution become modified with time by irritants, excoriation, infection, and treatment. All stages of eczematous inflammation may be encountered in hand eczema (Box 3-4).

TREATMENT. Most patients can be managed with skin protection and topical treatments. Skin protection and emollients are important. Topical treatments control the disease but require long-term intermittent use. Systemic treatments provide temporary remission but long-term use of potentially toxic drugs is discouraged. Treatment options are outlined in Box 3-5.

COURSE AND PROGNOSIS. Hand eczema often has a long-lasting and relapsing course. Patients with ongoing hand eczema experience negative psychosocial consequences. There may be far-reaching consequences including long sick-leave periods, sick pension, and changes of occupation.

Box 3-2 **Irritant Hand Dermatitis Instructions for Patients**

1. Wash hands as infrequently as possible. Ideally, soap should be avoided and hands simply washed in lukewarm water.
2. Shampooing must be done with rubber gloves or by someone else.
3. Avoid direct contact with household cleaners and detergents. Wear cotton, plastic, or rubber gloves when doing housework.
4. Do not touch or do anything that causes burning or itching (e.g., wool; wet diapers; peeling potatoes or handling fresh fruits, vegetables, and raw meat).
5. Wear rubber gloves when irritants are encountered. Rubber gloves alone are not sufficient because the lining collects sweat, scales, and debris and can become more irritating than those objects to be avoided. Dermal white cotton gloves should be worn next to the skin under unlined rubber gloves. Several pairs of cotton gloves should be purchased so they can be changed frequently. Try on the rubber gloves over the white cotton gloves at the time of purchase to ensure a comfortable fit.

Box 3-3 **Predictive Factors for Hand Eczema**

History of childhood eczema (most important predictive factor)
Female gender
Occupational exposure
History of asthma and/or hay fever
Service occupation (e.g., professional cleaners)

From Meding B, Swanbeck G: *Contact Dermatitis* 23:154, 1990. *PMID: 2149316*

Box 3-4 **Various Types of Hand Eczema**

Irritant	Recurrent focal palmar peeling
Atopic	Fingertip
Allergic	Hyperkeratotic
Nummular	Pompholyx (dyshidrosis)
Lichen simplex chronicus	Id reaction

Table 3-2 Hand Dermatitis: Differential Diagnosis and Distribution

Location	Redness and scaling	Vesicles	Pustules
Back of hand	Atopic dermatitis Irritant contact dermatitis Lichen simplex chronicus Nummular eczema Psoriasis Tinea	Id reaction Scabies (web spaces)	Bacterial infection Psoriasis Scabies (web spaces) Tinea
Palmar surface	Fingertip eczema Hyperkeratotic eczema Recurrent focal palmar peeling Psoriasis Tinea	Allergic contact dermatitis Pompholyx (dyshidrosis)	Bacterial infection Pompholyx (dyshidrosis) Psoriasis

Box 3-5 **Treatment Options for Hand Eczema**

Skin protection

- Gloves
- Barrier creams
- Bland emollients
- Lifestyle changes
- Workers' education

Topical treatments

- Corticosteroid creams, ointments, emollient foams
- Tacrolimus, pimecrolimus
- Coal tar and derivatives
- Irradiation with UV light
- Irradiation with x-rays

Systemic treatments

- Azathioprine
- Methotrexate (MTX)
- Cyclosporine
- Oral retinoids
- Oral corticosteroids in short treatment courses

Adapted from *Br J Dermatol* 151(2):446-451, 2004.
PMID: 15327553

Irritant contact dermatitis

Irritant hand dermatitis (housewives' eczema, dishpan hands, detergent hands) is the most common type of hand inflammation. Some people can withstand long periods of repeated exposure to various chemicals and maintain normal skin. At the other end of the spectrum, there are those who develop chapping and eczema from simple hand washing. Patients whose hands are easily irritated may have an atopic diathesis.

PATHOPHYSIOLOGY. The stratum corneum is the protective envelope that prevents exogenous material from entering the skin and prevents body water from escaping. The stratum corneum is composed of dead cells, lipids (from sebum and cellular debris), and water-binding organic chemicals. The stratum corneum of the palms is thicker than that of the backs of the hands and is more resistant to irritation. The pH of this surface layer is slightly acidic. Environmental factors or elements that change any component of the stratum corneum interfere with its protective function and expose the skin to irritants. Factors such as cold winter air and low humidity promote water loss. Substances such as organic solvents and alkaline soaps extract water-binding chemicals and lipids. Once enough of these protective elements have been extracted, the skin decompensates and becomes eczematous.

CLINICAL PRESENTATION. The degree of inflammation depends on factors such as strength and concentration of the chemical, individual susceptibility, site of contact, and time of year. Allergy, infection, scratching, and stress modify the picture.

IRRITANT HAND DERMATITIS

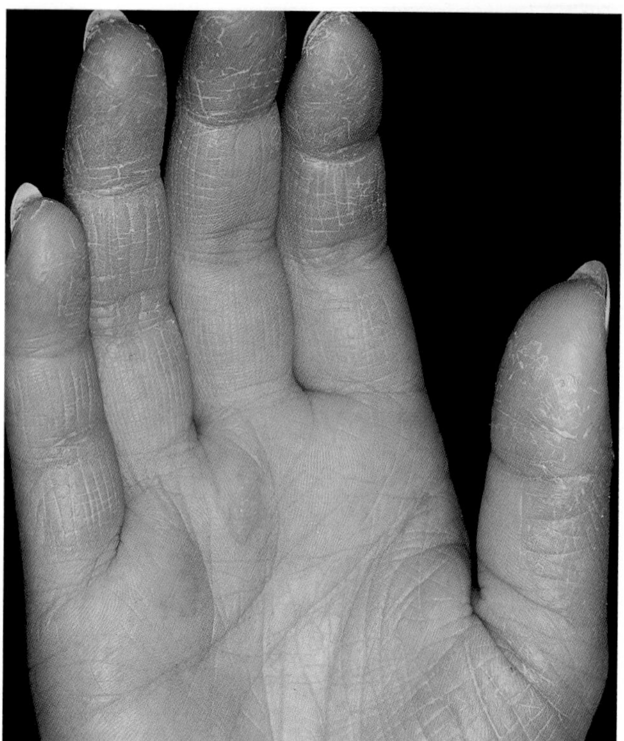

Figure 3-19 Early irritant hand dermatitis with dryness and chapping.

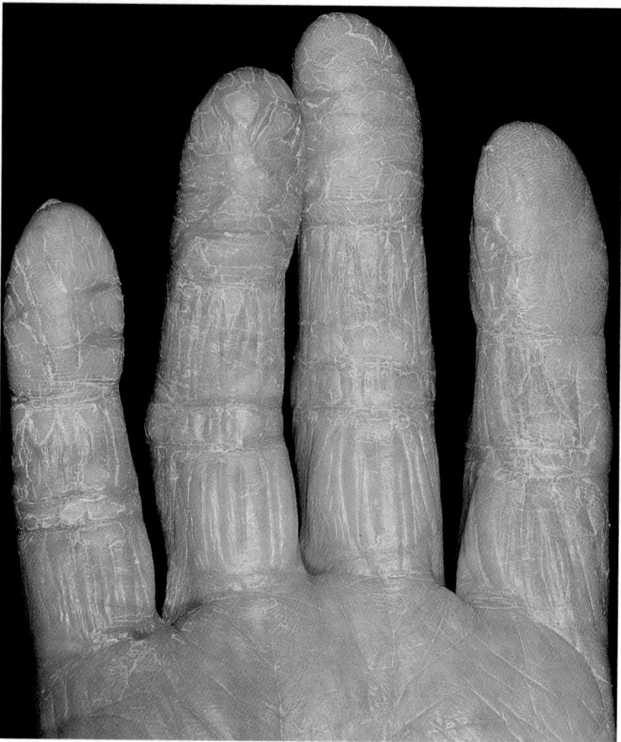

Figure 3-20 Subacute eczematous inflammation with severe drying and splitting of the fingertips.

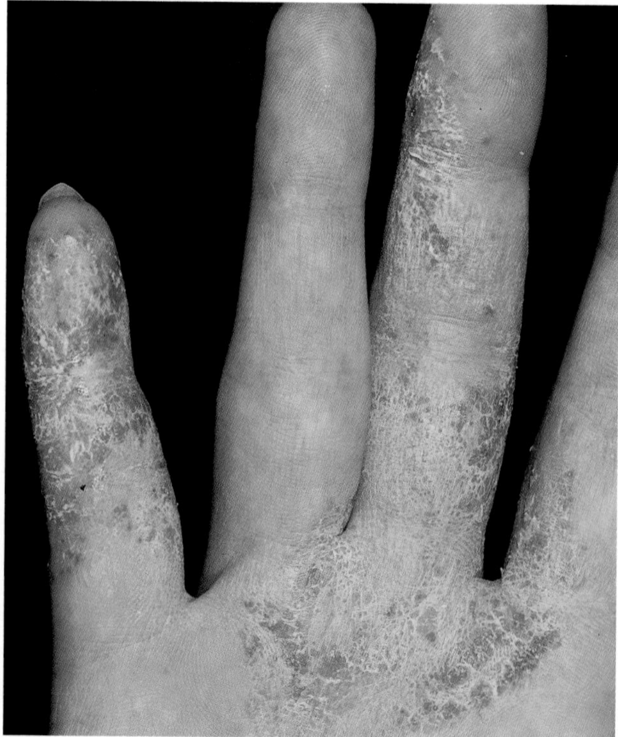

Figure 3-21 Numerous tiny vesicles suddenly appeared on these chronically inflamed fingers.

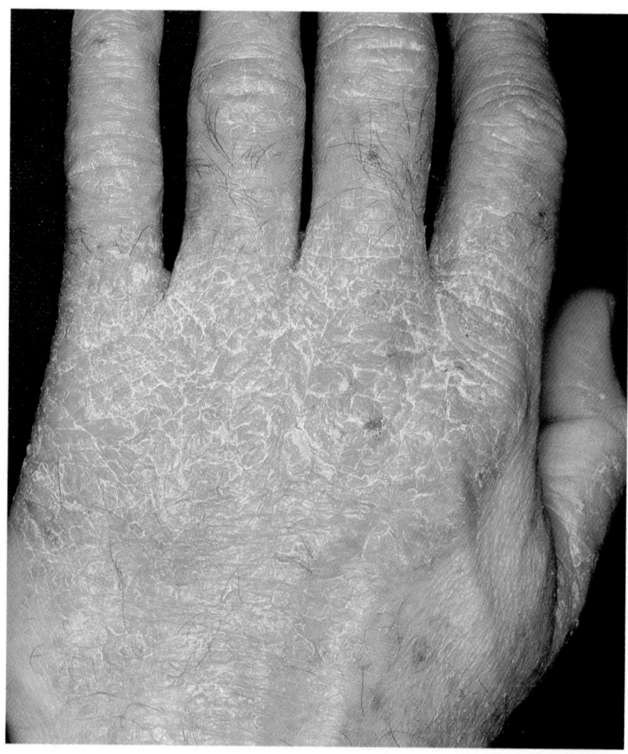

Figure 3-22 Chronic eczematous inflammation. Scratching has thickened the skin. Crusts are signs of infection.

STAGES OF INFLAMMATION. Dryness and chapping are the initial changes (Figure 3-19). Very painful cracks and fissures occur, particularly in joint crease areas and around the fingertips. The backs of the hands become red, swollen, and tender. The palmar surface, especially that of the fingers, becomes red and continues to be dry and cracked. A red, smooth, shiny, delicate surface that splits easily with the slightest trauma may develop. These are subacute eczematous changes (Figure 3-20).

Acute eczematous inflammation occurs with further irritation creating vesicles that ooze and crust. Itching intensifies, and excoriation leads to infection (Figures 3-21 and 3-22).

Necrosis and ulceration followed by scarring occur if the irritating chemical is too caustic.

PATIENTS AT RISK. Individuals at risk include mothers with young children (e.g., from changing diapers), individuals whose jobs require repeated wetting and drying (e.g., surgeons, dentists, dishwashers, bartenders, fishermen), industrial workers whose jobs require contact with chemicals (e.g., cutting oils), and patients with the atopic diathesis.

PREVENTION. One study revealed that hospital staff members who used an emulsion cleanser (e.g., Cetaphil lotion, Duosoft [in Europe]) had significantly less dryness and eczema than those who used a liquid soap. Regular use of emollients prevented irritant dermatitis caused by a detergent.

BARRIER-PROTECTANT CREAMS. Loss of skin barrier function by mechanical or chemical insults may result in water loss and hand eczema. Barrier creams (see Box 3-6) applied at least twice a day on all exposed areas protect the skin and are formulated to be either water-repellent or oil-repellent. The water-repellent types offer little protection against oils or solvents.

TREATMENT. The inflammation is treated as outlined under "Stages of eczematous inflammation." Lubrication and avoidance of further irritation help to prevent recurrence. A program of irritant avoidance should be carefully outlined for each patient (see Box 3-2).

Box 3-6 **Barrier Creams—Applied at Least Twice a Day on All Exposed Areas**

Water repellent

- North 201
- SBS-44
- Kerodex #71

For oil- or solvent-based materials

- Kerodex #51
- SBS-46
- North 222
- Dermashield (both oil- and water-based materials)

General purpose barrier protective creams

- SBR-Lipocream
- TheraSeal

Atopic hand dermatitis

Hand dermatitis may be the most common form of adult atopic dermatitis (see Chapter 5). Hand eczema is significantly more common in people with a history of atopic dermatitis than in others. The following factors predict the occurrence of hand eczema in adults with a history of atopic dermatitis:

- Hand dermatitis before age 15
- Persistent eczema on the body
- Dry or itchy skin in adult life
- Widespread atopic dermatitis in childhood

Many people with atopic dermatitis develop hand eczema independently of exposure to irritants, but such exposure causes additional irritant contact dermatitis.

The backs of the hands, particularly the fingers, are affected (Figure 3-23). The dermatitis begins as a typical irritant reaction with chapping and erythema. Several forms of eczematous dermatitis evolve; erythema, edema, vesiculation, crusting, excoriation, scaling, and lichenification appear and are intensified by scratching. Management for atopic hand eczema is the same as that for irritant hand eczema.

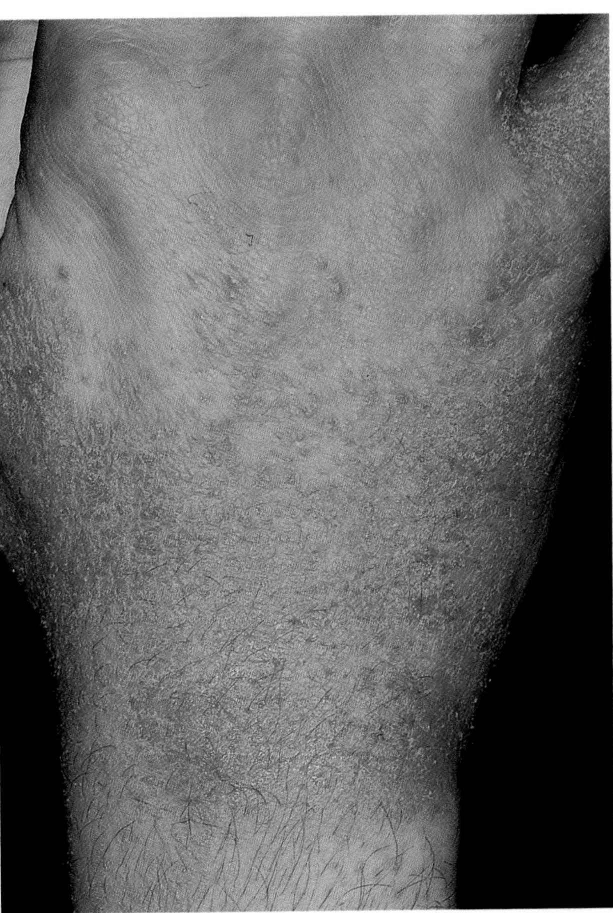

Figure 3-23 Irritant hand dermatitis in a patient with the atopic diathesis. Irritant eczema of the backs of the hands is a common form of adult atopic dermatitis.

Allergic contact dermatitis

Allergic contact dermatitis of the hands is not as common as irritant dermatitis. However, allergy as a possible cause of hand eczema, no matter what the pattern, should always be considered in the differential diagnosis; it may be investigated by patch testing in appropriate cases. The incidence of allergy in hand eczema was demonstrated by patch testing in a study of 220 patients with hand eczema. In 12% of the 220 patients, the diagnosis was established with the aid of a standard screening series now available in a modified form (T.R.U.E. TEST). Another 5% of the cases were diagnosed as a result of testing with additional allergens. The hand eczema in these two groups (17%) changed dramatically after identification and avoidance of the allergens found by patch testing. Table 3-3 lists some possible causes of allergic hand dermatitis.

PHYSICAL FINDINGS. The diagnosis of allergic contact dermatitis is obvious when the area of inflammation corresponds exactly to the area covered by the allergen (e.g., a round patch of eczema under a watch or inflammation in the shape of a sandal strap on the foot). Similar clues may be present with hand eczema, but in many cases allergic and irritant hand eczemas cannot be distinguished by their clinical presentation. Hand inflammation, whatever the source, is increased by further exposure to irritating chemicals, washing, scratching, medication, and infection. Inflammation of the dorsum of the hand is more often irritant or atopic than allergic.

TREATMENT. Allergy may initially appear as acute, subacute, or chronic eczematous inflammation and is managed accordingly.

Table 3-3 Allergic Hand Dermatitis: Some Possible Causes

Allergens	Sources
Nickel	Door knobs, handles on kitchen utensils, scissors, knitting needles, industrial equipment, hairdressing equipment
Potassium dichromate	Cement, leather articles (gloves), industrial machines, oils
Rubber	Gloves, industrial equipment (hoses, belts, cables)
Fragrances	Cosmetics, soaps, lubricants, topical medications
Formaldehyde	Wash-and-wear fabrics, paper, cosmetics, embalming fluid
Lanolin	Topical lubricants and medications, cosmetics

Nummular eczema

Eczema that appears as one or several coin-shaped plaques is called *nummular eczema*. This pattern often occurs on the extremities but may also present as hand eczema. The plaques are usually confined to the backs of the hands (Figure 3-24). The number of lesions may increase, but once they are established they tend to remain the same size. The inflammation is either subacute or chronic and itching is moderate to intense. The cause is unknown. Thick, chronic, scaling plaques of nummular eczema look like psoriasis; treatment for nummular eczema is the same as that for subacute or chronic eczema.

Lichen simplex chronicus

A localized plaque of chronic eczematous inflammation that is created by habitual scratching is called *lichen simplex chronicus* or *localized neurodermatitis*. The back of the wrist is a typical site. The plaque is thick with prominent skin lines (lichenification) and the margins are fairly sharp. Once established, the plaque does not usually increase in area. Lichen simplex chronicus is treated in the same manner as chronic eczematous inflammation.

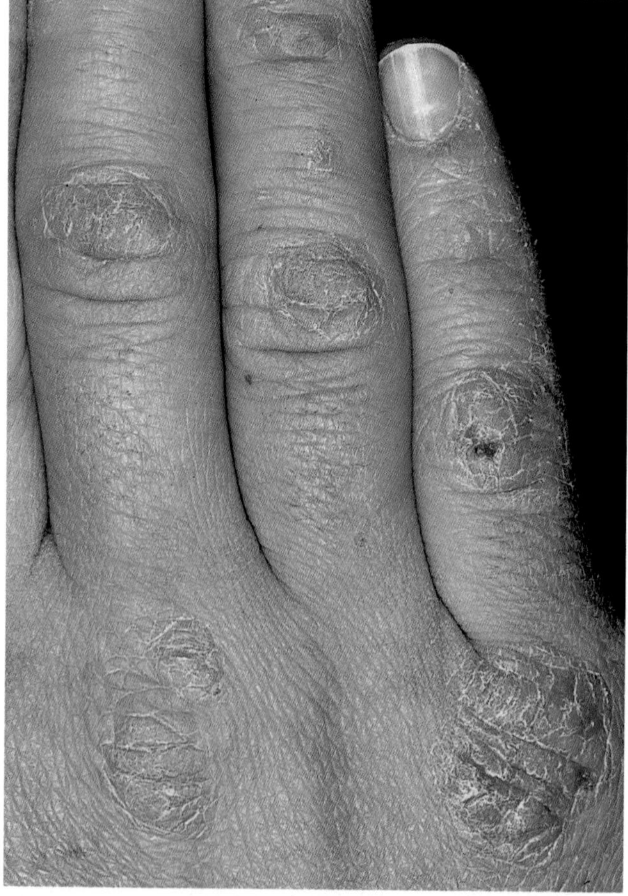

Figure 3-24 Nummular eczema. Eczematous plaques are round (coin-shaped).

Recurrent focal palmar peeling

Keratolysis exfoliativa or recurrent focal palmar peeling is a common, chronic, asymptomatic, noninflammatory, bilateral peeling of the palms of the hands and occasionally soles of the feet; its cause is unknown (Figure 3-25). The eruption is most common during the summer months and is often associated with sweaty palms and soles. Some people experience this phenomenon only once, whereas others have repeated episodes. Scaling starts simultaneously from several points on the palms or soles with 2 or 3 mm of round scales that appear to have originated from a ruptured vesicle; however, these vesicles are never seen. The scaling continues to peel and extend peripherally, forming larger, roughly circular areas that resemble ringworm whereas the central area becomes slightly red and tender. The scaling borders may coalesce. The condition resolves in 1 to 3 weeks and requires no therapy other than lubrication.

Hyperkeratotic eczema

A very thick, chronic form of eczema that occurs on the palms and occasionally the soles is seen almost exclusively in men. One or several plaques of yellow-brown, dense scale increase in thickness and form deep interconnecting cracks over the surface, similar to mud drying in a river bed (Figure 3-26). The dense scale, unlike callus, is moist below the surface and is not easily pared with a blade. Patients discover that the scale is firmly adherent to the epidermis when they attempt to peel off the thick scale, and this exposes tender bleeding areas of the dermis. Hyperkeratotic eczema may result from allergy or excoriation and irritation, but in most cases the cause is not apparent. The disease is chronic and may last for years. Psoriasis and lichen simplex chronicus must be considered in the differential diagnosis. The disease is treated like chronic eczema; although the plaques respond to group II steroid cream and occlusion, recurrences are frequent. Patch testing is indicated for recurrent disease.

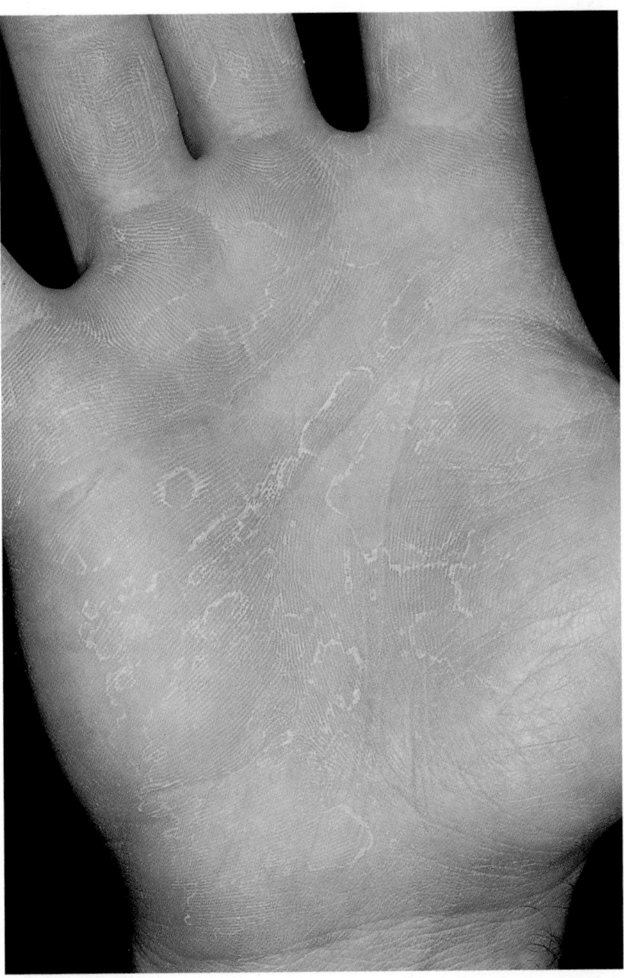

Figure 3-25 Keratolysis exfoliativa. Noninflammatory peeling of the palms that is often associated with sweating. The eruption must be differentiated from tinea of the palms.

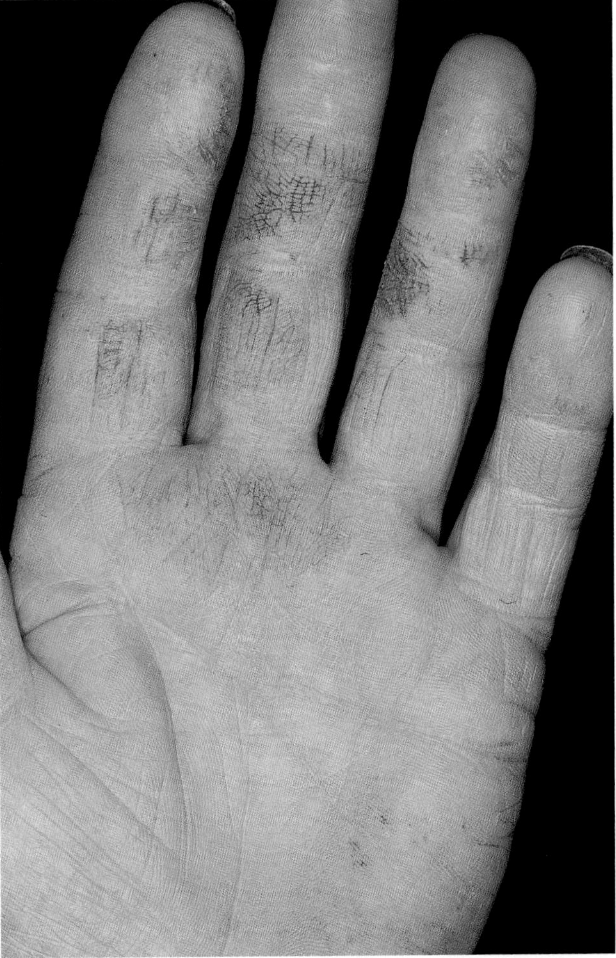

Figure 3-26 Hyperkeratotic eczema. Patches of dense yellow-brown scale occur on the palms. This patient was allergic to a steering wheel.

FINGERTIP ECZEMA

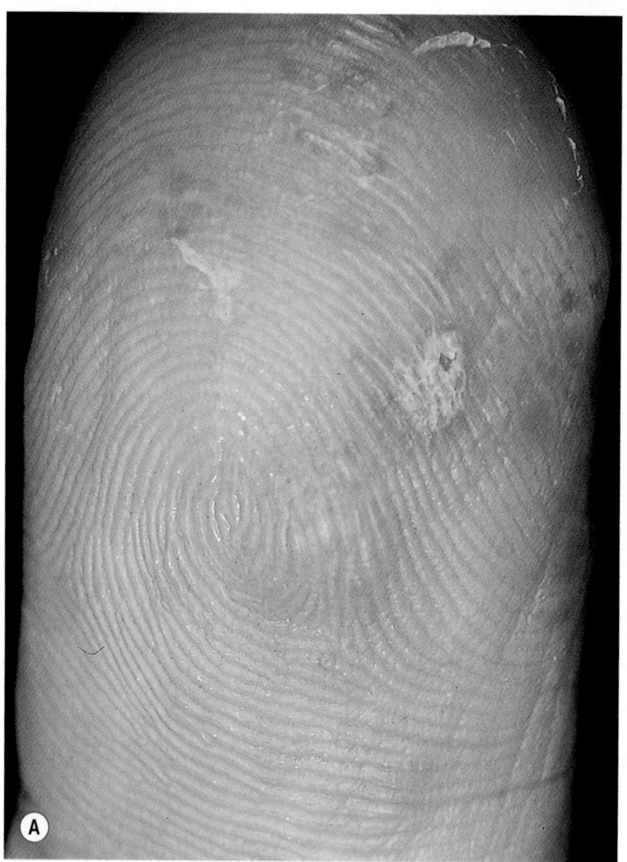

An early stage. The skin is moist. A vesicle is present. Redness and cracking have occurred in the central area.

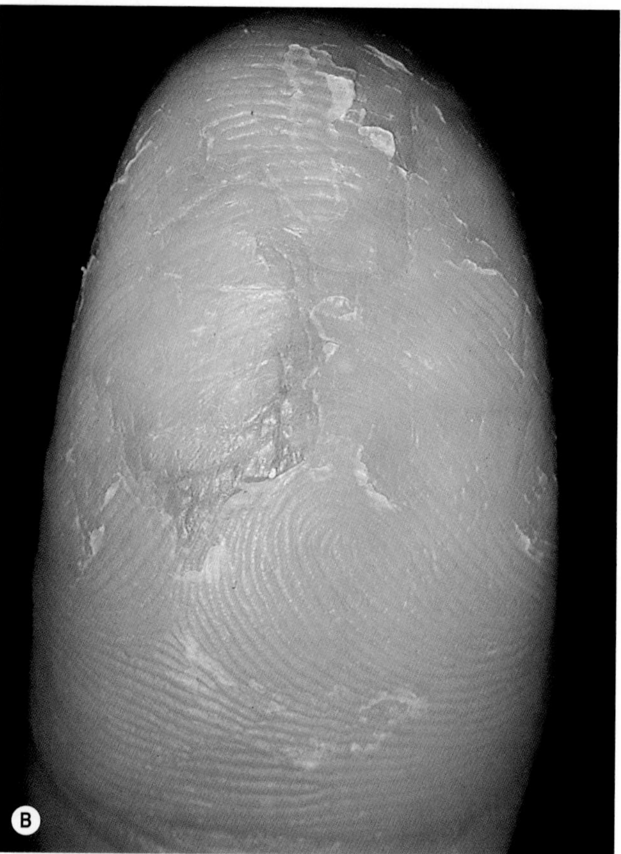

A more advanced stage. Peeling occurs constantly. The skin lines are lost.

Figure 3-27

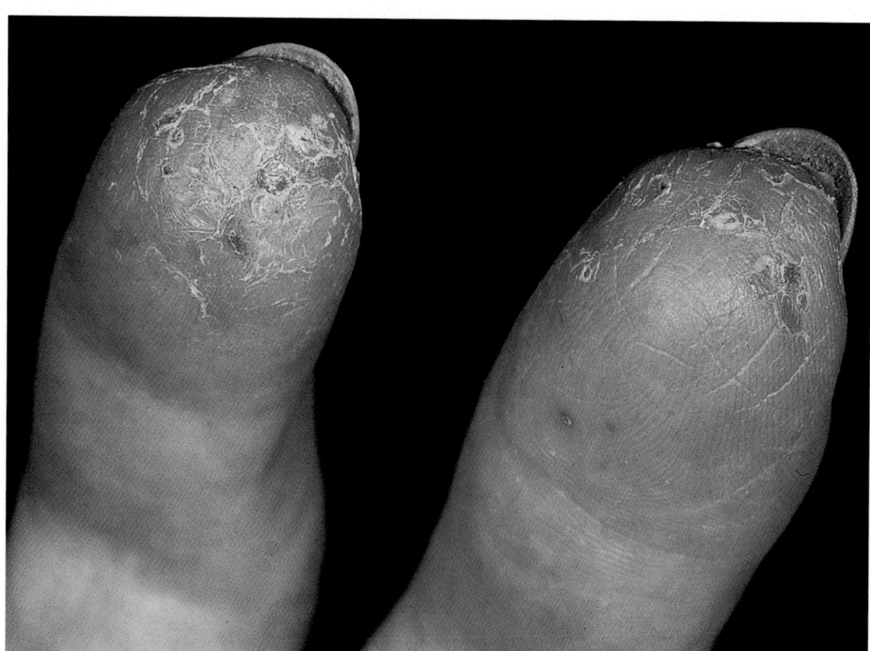

Figure 3-28 Chronic eczema. Excessive washing produced this advanced case with cracking and fissures.

Fingertip eczema

A very dry, chronic form of eczema of the palmar surface of the fingertips may be the result of an allergic reaction (e.g., to plant bulbs or resins) or may occur in children and adults as an isolated phenomenon of unknown cause. One finger or several fingers may be involved. Initially the skin may be moist and then may become dry, cracked, and scaly (Figure 3-27). The skin peels from the fingertips distally, exposing a very dry, red, cracked, fissured, tender, or painful surface without skin lines (Figures 3-27, 3-28, and 3-29). The process usually stops shortly before the distal interphalangeal joint is reached (Figures 3-30 and 3-31). Fingertip eczema may last for months or years and is resistant to treatment. Topical steroids with or without occlusion give only temporary relief. Once allergy and psoriasis have been ruled out, fingertip eczema should be managed the same way as subacute and chronic eczema, by avoiding irritants and lubricating frequently. Elidel or Protopic is sometimes effective; tar creams applied twice each day have at times provided relief.

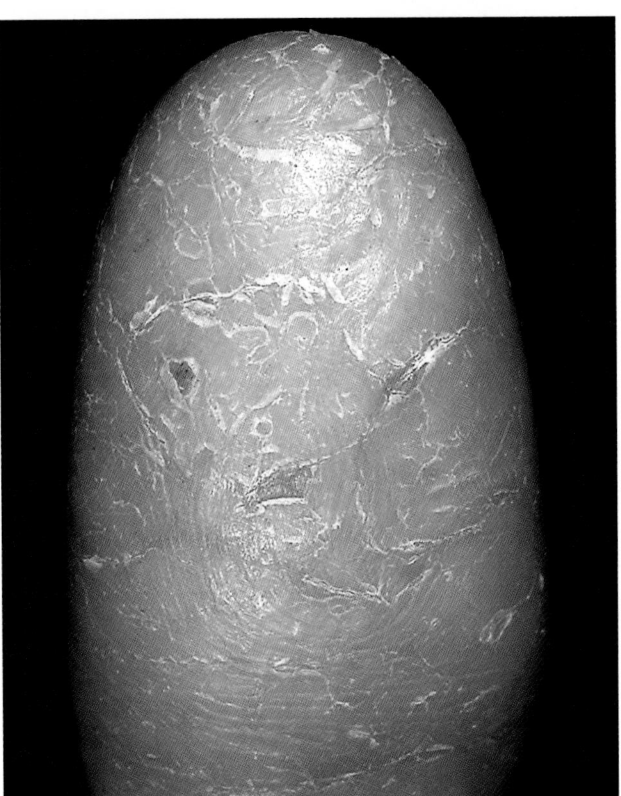

Figure 3-29 Fingertip eczema. Inflammation has been present for months and responded poorly to topical steroids.

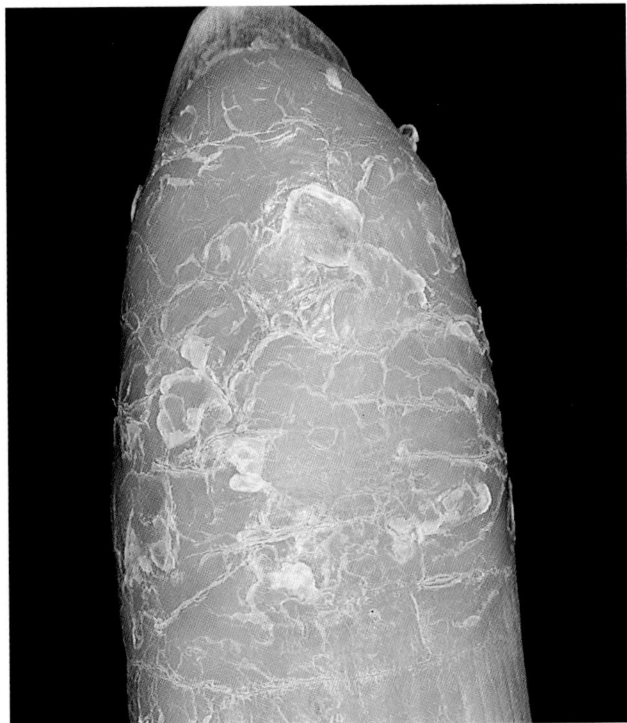

Figure 3-30 Severe chronic inflammation. The skin lines are lost. The dry skin is fragile and cracks easily. Patients are tempted to peel away the dry loose scale.

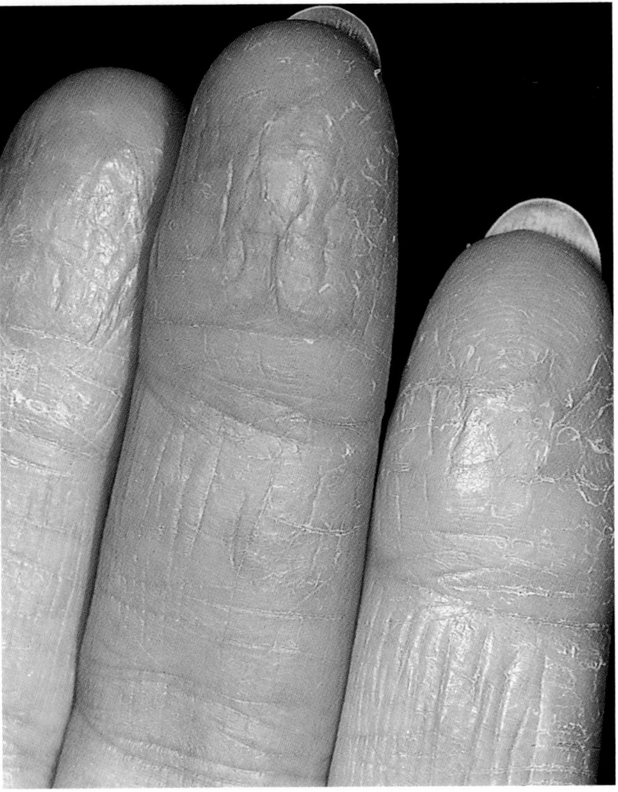

Figure 3-31 The fingers are dry and wrinkled, and the skin is fragile. The skin peels but does not form the thick scale shown in Figures 3-29 and 3-30.

POMPHOLYX (DYSHIDROSIS)

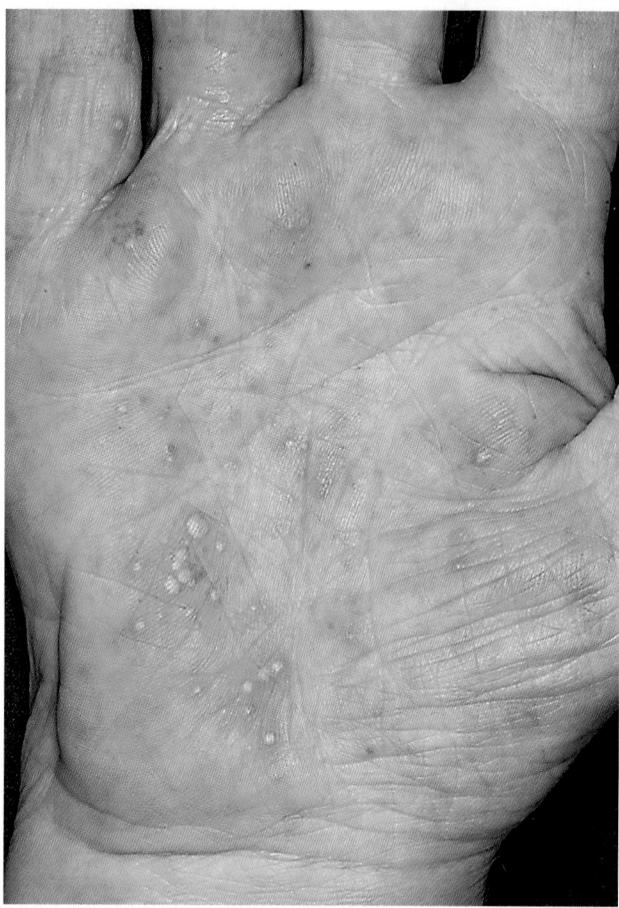

Figure 3-32 Vesicles have evolved into pustules. The eruption has persisted for many weeks.

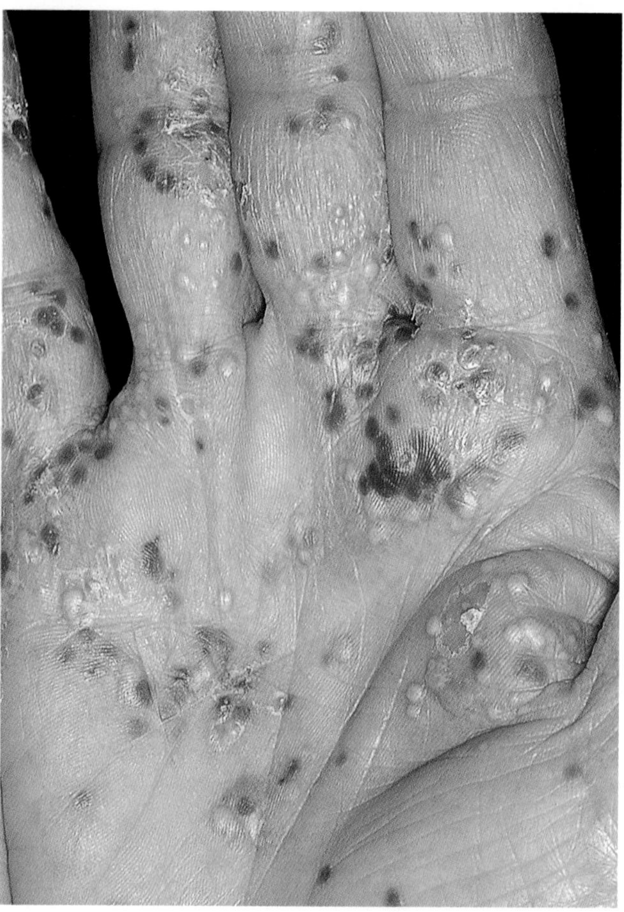

Figure 3-33 Secondary infection resulted in pustules.

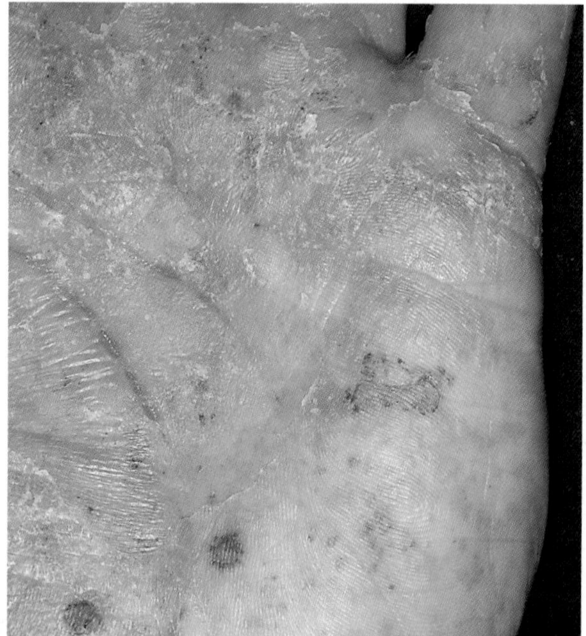

Figure 3-34 The acute process ends as the skin peels, revealing a red, cracked base with brown spots. The brown spots are sites of previous vesiculation.

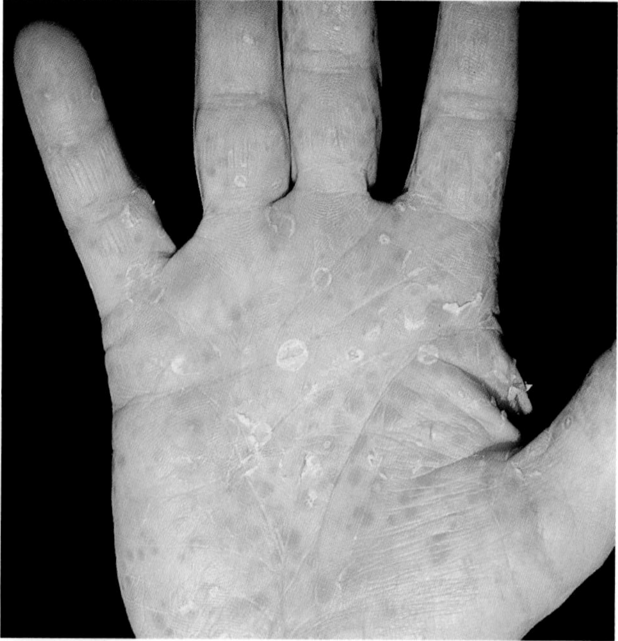

Figure 3-35 A severe form (with large, deep vesicles and blisters) that is indistinguishable from pustular psoriasis of the palms and soles.

Pompholyx

Pompholyx (dyshidrosis) is a distinctive reaction pattern of unknown etiology presenting as symmetric vesicular hand and foot dermatitis (Figure 3-32). Moderate to severe itching precedes the appearance of vesicles on the palms and sides of the fingers (Figure 3-33). The palms may be red and wet with perspiration, hence the name *dyshidrosis*. The vesicles slowly resolve in 3 to 4 weeks and are replaced by 1- to 3-mm rings of scale (Figures 3-34 and 3-35). Chronic eczematous changes with erythema, scaling, and lichenification may follow. Waves of vesiculation may appear indefinitely. Pain rather than itching is the chief complaint. Pustular psoriasis of the palms and soles may resemble pompholyx, but the vesicles of psoriasis rapidly become cloudy with purulent fluid. Pustular psoriasis is chronic and the pustules do not evolve and disappear as rapidly as those of pompholyx. Patients with atopic dermatitis are affected as frequently as others.

ETIOLOGY. A recent study found the following causes of pompholyx in the 120 patients: mycosis (10.0%); allergic contact pompholyx (67.5%), with cosmetic and hygiene products as the main factor (31.7%), followed by metals (16.7%); and internal reactivation from drug, food, or haptenic (nickel) origin (6.7%). The remaining 15.0% of patients were classified as idiopathic patients, but all were atopic. *PMID: 18086998* Ingestion of nickel, cobalt, and chromium can elicit pompholyx in patients who are patch test negative to these metals.

TREATMENT. Topical steroids; cold, wet compresses; and possibly oral antibiotics are used as the initial treatment, but the response is often disappointing. Short courses of oral steroids are sometimes needed to control acute flares. Resistant cases might respond to psoralen plus ultraviolet A (PUVA) therapy. Patients (64%) who flared after oral challenge to metal salt cleared or markedly improved on diets low in the incriminated metal salt, and 78% of those patients remained clear when the diet was rigorously followed (a suggested diet for nickel-sensitive patients with pompholyx appears on p. 144). Attempts to control pompholyx with elimination diets may be worth a trial in difficult cases.

Patients with severe pompholyx who did not respond to conventional therapy or who had debilitating side effects from corticosteroids were treated with low-dose methotrexate (15 to 22.5 mg per week). *PMID: 10188683* This led to significant improvement or clearing, and the need for oral corticosteroid therapy was substantially decreased or eliminated.

Id reaction

Intense inflammatory processes, such as active stasis dermatitis or acute fungal infections of the feet, can be accompanied by an itchy, dyshidrotic-like vesicular eruption ("id reaction"; Figure 3-36). These eruptions are most common on the sides of the fingers but may be generalized. The eruptions resolve as the inflammation that initiated them resolves. The id reaction may be an allergic reaction to fungi or to some antigen created during the inflammatory process. Almost all dyshidrotic eruptions are incorrectly called id reactions. The diagnosis of an id reaction should not be made unless there is an acute inflammatory process at a distant site and the id reaction disappears shortly after the acute inflammation is controlled.

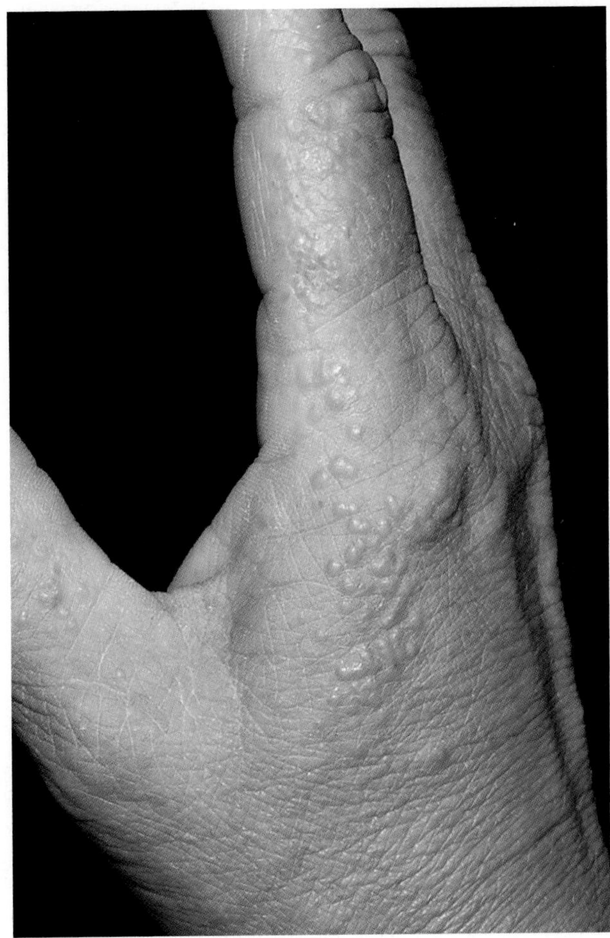

Figure 3-36 Id reaction. An acute vesicular eruption most often seen on the lateral aspects of the fingers.

ECZEMA: VARIOUS PRESENTATIONS

Asteatotic eczema

Asteatotic eczema (eczema craquelé) occurs after excess drying, especially during the winter months and among the elderly. Patients with an atopic diathesis are more likely to develop this distinctive pattern. The eruption can occur on any skin area, but it is most commonly seen on the anterolateral aspects of the lower legs. The lower legs become dry and scaly and show accentuation of the skin lines (xerosis) (Figure 3-37). Red plaques with thin, long, horizontal superficial fissures appear with further drying and scratching (Figure 3-38). Similar patterns of inflammation may appear on the trunk and upper extremities as the winter progresses. A cracked porcelain or "crazy paving" pattern of fissuring develops when short vertical fissures connect with the horizontal fissures. The term *eczema craquelé* is appropriately used to describe this pattern. The severest form of this type of eczema shows an accentuation of the previously described pattern with deep, wide, horizontal fissures that ooze and are often purulent (Figure 3-39). Pain, rather than itching, is the chief complaint with this condition. Scratching or treatment with drying lotions such as calamine aggravates the eczematous inflammation and leads to infection with accumulation of crusts and purulent material.

TREATMENT. The initial stages are treated as subacute eczematous inflammation with group III or IV topical steroid ointments. The severest form may have to be treated as acute eczema. The treatment involves wet compresses and antibiotics to remove crust and suppress infection before group V topical steroids and lubricants are applied. Wet compresses should be used only for a short time (1 or 2 days). Prolonged use of wet compresses results in excessive drying. Lubricating the dry skin during and after topical steroid use is essential. The use of oral steroids should be avoided; the disease flares within 1 or 2 days once they are discontinued.

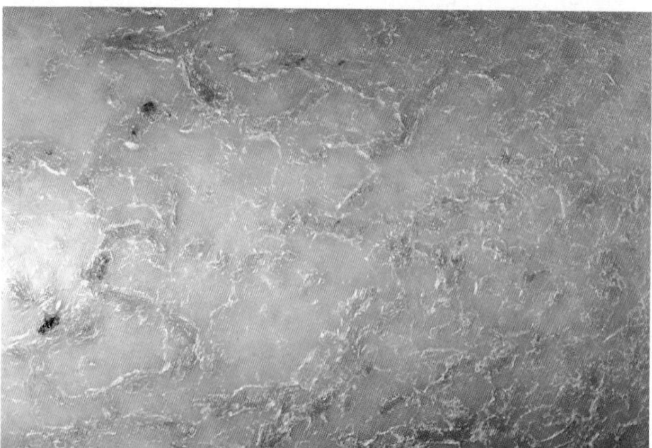

Figure 3-37 Asteatotic eczema (xerosis). The skin is extremely dry, cracked, and scaly. This pattern appears in the winter months when the air is dry.

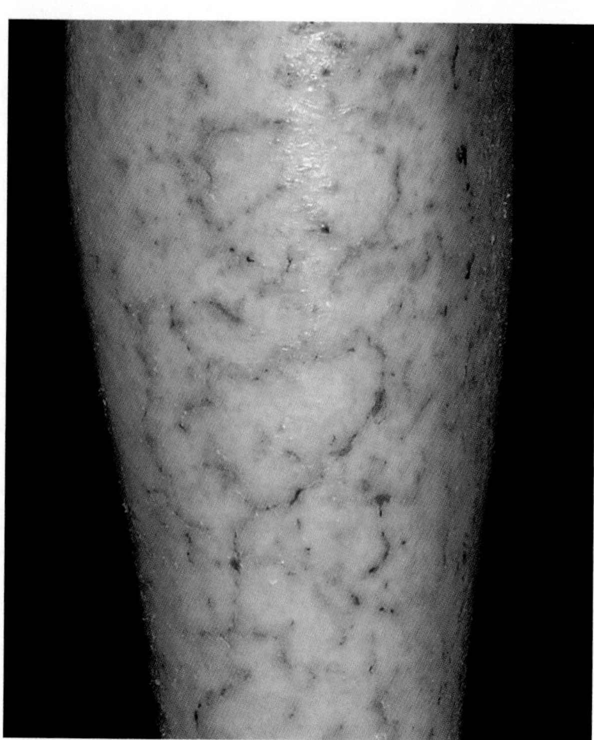

Figure 3-38 Asteatotic eczema (xerosis). Excessive washing of dry skin may result in horizontal, parallel cracks.

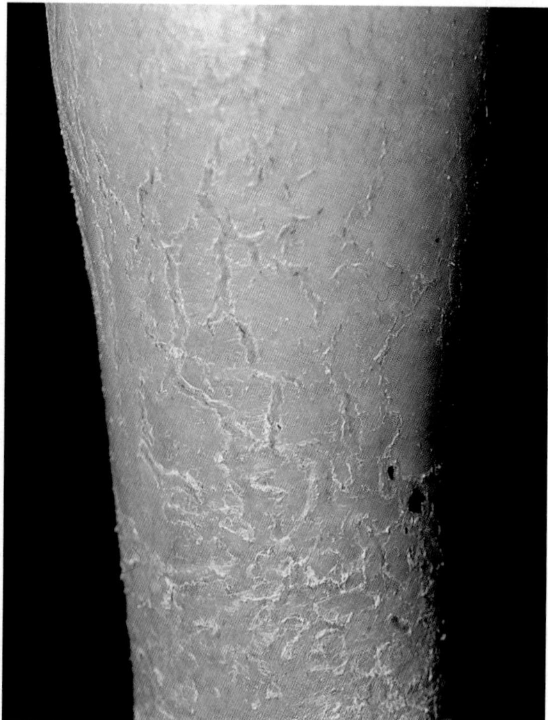

Figure 3-39 Asteatotic eczema (eczema craquelé). Excessive drying on the lower legs may eventually become so severe that long, horizontal, superficial fissures appear. The fissures eventually develop a cracked porcelain or "crazy paving" pattern when short vertical fissures connect with the horizontal fissures.

Nummular eczema

Nummular eczema is a common disease of unknown cause that occurs primarily in the middle-aged and elderly. The typical lesion is a coin-shaped, red plaque that averages 1 to 5 cm in diameter (Figure 3-40). The lesions can itch, and scratching often becomes habitual. In these cases, the term *nummular neurodermatitis* has been used. The plaque may become thicker and vesicles appear on the surface (Figure 3-41); vesicles in ringworm, if present, are at the border. Unlike the thick, silvery scale of psoriasis, this scale is thin and sparse. The erythema in psoriasis is darker. Once the disease is established, lesions may become more numerous, but individual lesions tend to remain in the same area and do not increase in size. The disease is worse in the winter. The back of the hand is the most commonly involved site; usually only one lesion or a few lesions are present (see Figure 3-24). Other frequently involved areas are the extensor aspects of the forearms and lower legs, the flanks, and the hips (Figures 3-42 to 3-44). Lesions in these other sites tend to be more numerous. An extensive form of the disease can occur suddenly in patients with dry skin that is exposed to an irritating medicine or chemical, or in patients who have an active eczematous process at another site, such as stasis dermatitis on the lower legs. The lesions in these cases are round, faintly erythematous, dry, cracked, superficial, and usually confluent.

The course is variable, but it is usually chronic, with some cases resisting all attempts at treatment. Many cases become inactive after several months. Lesions may reappear at previously involved sites in recurrent cases.

TREATMENT. Treatment depends on the stage of activity; all stages of eczematous inflammation may be present simultaneously. The red vesicular lesions are treated as acute, the red scaling plaques as subacute, and the habitually scratched thick plaques as chronic eczematous inflammation. Therefore group I to V topical steroids are intermittently used. Topical steroid foams may be especially effective. Foams with an emollient base such as Verdeso (desonide) or Olux-E (clobetasol) do not sting. Tacrolimus ointment 0.1% used alone or intermittently with topical steroids may be tried.

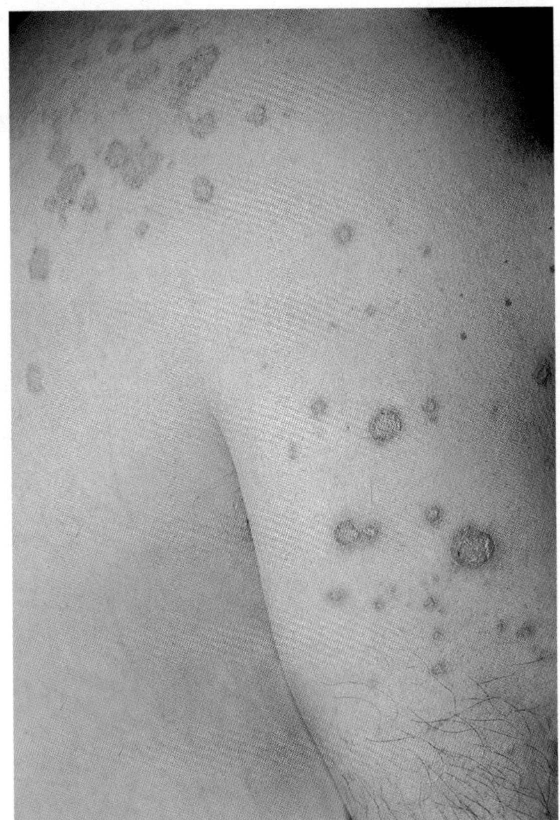

Figure 3-40 Nummular eczema. This form of eczema is of undetermined origin and is not necessarily associated with dry skin or atopy. The round, coin-shaped, eczematous plaques tend to be chronic and resistant to treatment.

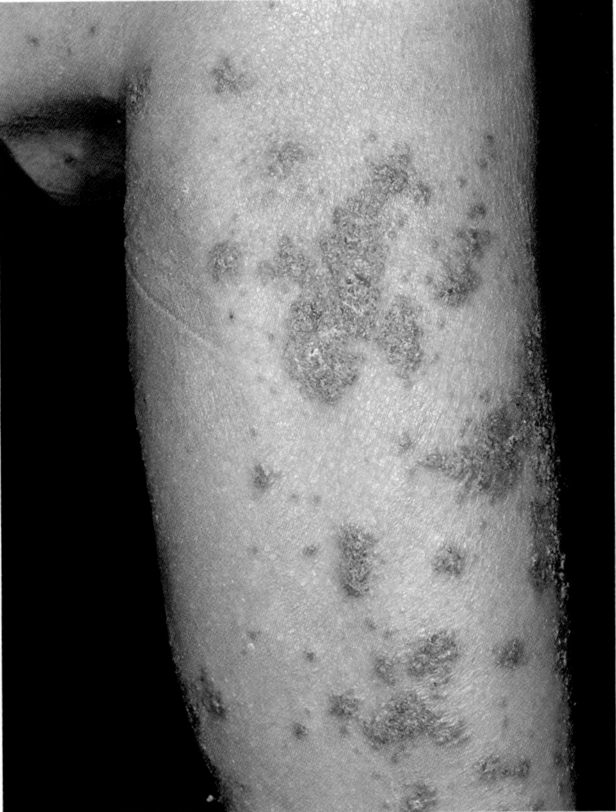

Figure 3-41 Nummular eczema. Round, eczematous plaques formed on the trunk, legs, and arms, and became confluent.

NUMMULAR ECZEMA

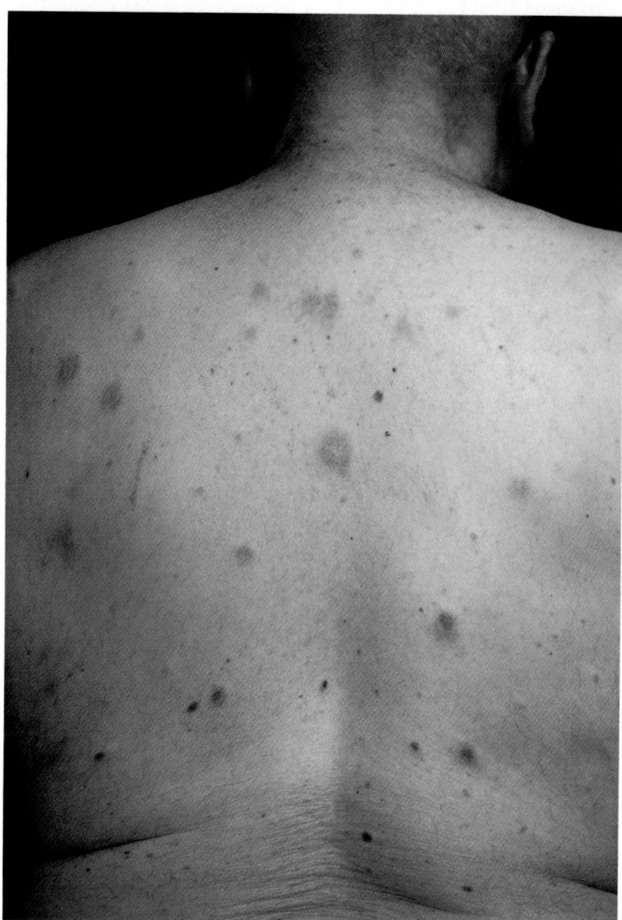

Figure 3-42 Many small round plaques on the trunk may be misdiagnosed as psoriasis or tinea.

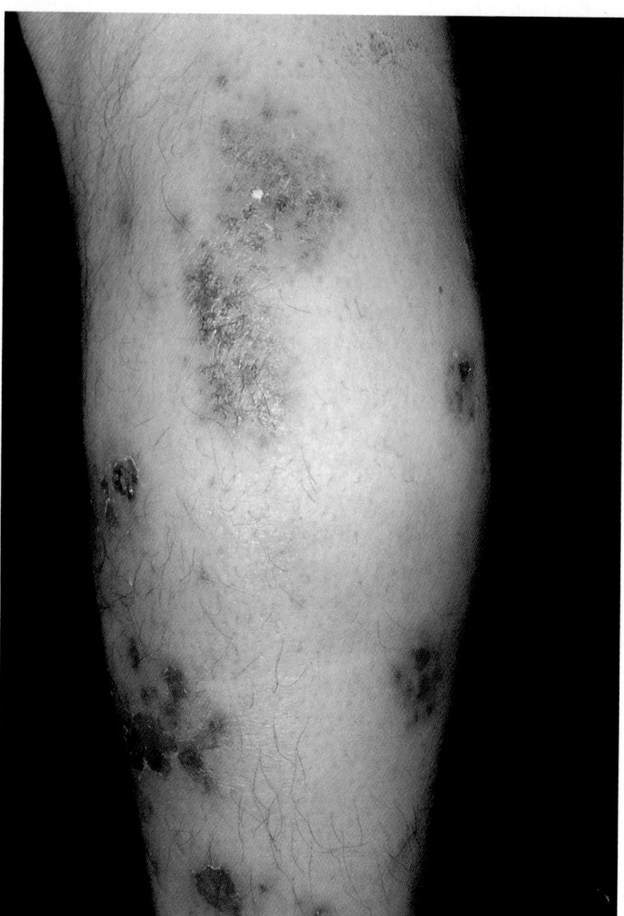

Figure 3-43 Large round plaques are inflamed and may become secondarily infected.

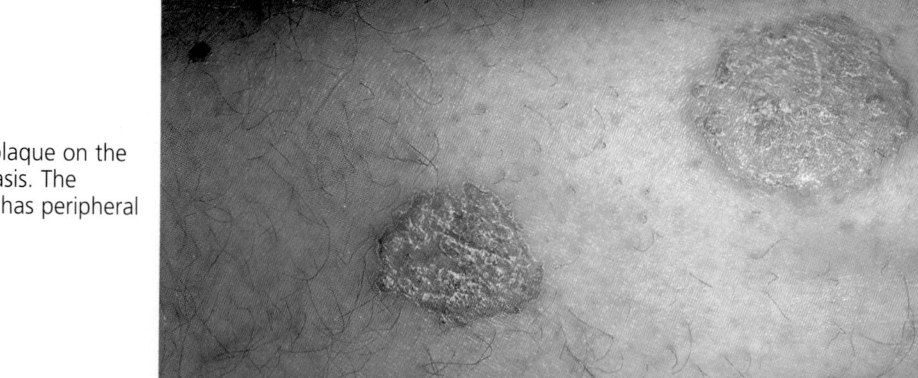

Figure 3-44 The plaque on the left resembles psoriasis. The plaque on the right has peripheral scale like tinea.

CHAPPED FISSURED FEET

CLINICAL PRESENTATION. Chapped fissured feet (sweaty sock dermatitis, peridigital dermatitis, juvenile plantar dermatosis) are seen initially with scaling, erythema, fissuring, and loss of the epidermal ridge pattern. The tendency to severe chapping declines with age and is gone around the age of puberty. The mean age of onset is 7.3 years; the mean age of remission is 14.3 years. Onset is in early fall when the weather becomes cold and heavy socks and impermeable shoes or boots are worn. An artificial intertrigo is created when moist socks are kept in contact with the soles. The skin in pressure areas, toes, and metatarsal regions becomes dry, brittle, and scaly, and then fissured (Figure 3-45). The chapping extends onto the sides of the toes. Eventually, the entire sole may be involved; sometimes the hands are also affected (Figure 3-46).

The eruption lasts throughout the winter, clears without treatment in the late spring, and predictably recurs the next fall. Earlier descriptions referred to this entity as *atopic winter feet* in children, but the name has been changed to include patients who do not have atopic dermatitis. Atopic dermatitis of the feet in children occurs on the dorsal toes and usually not on the plantar surface, and it is itchy. The role of atopy is not yet defined. Children with chapped fissured feet complain of soreness and pain. Affected individuals must be predisposed to chapping because their wearing of moist socks and impermeable boots does not differ from that of unaffected children.

DIFFERENTIAL DIAGNOSIS. The differential diagnosis includes psoriasis, tinea pedis, and allergic contact dermatitis. The erythema in psoriasis is darker and the scales shed; the scales in chapped fissured feet are adherent, and removal of the scales causes bleeding. Tinea of the feet in children is rare. Feet with the rare case of familial *Trichophyton rubrum* are pale brown and have a fine scale. Fissuring is minimal, and there is little seasonal variation. Allergic contact dermatitis to shoes usually affects the dorsal aspect and spares the soles, webs, and sides of the feet. The eruption is bright red and scaly rather than pale red and chapped.

TREATMENT. Treatment is less than satisfactory. Topical steroids and lubrication provide some relief. Group II or III topical steroids are applied twice each day or, preferably, with plastic wrap occlusion at bedtime. Protopic ointment may be effective. PMID: 16681600 Lubricating creams are applied several times each day, especially directly after removing moist socks to seal in moisture. The feet should not be allowed to remain moist inside shoes. Preventive measures include changing into light leather shoes after removing boots at school and changing cotton socks one or two times each day.

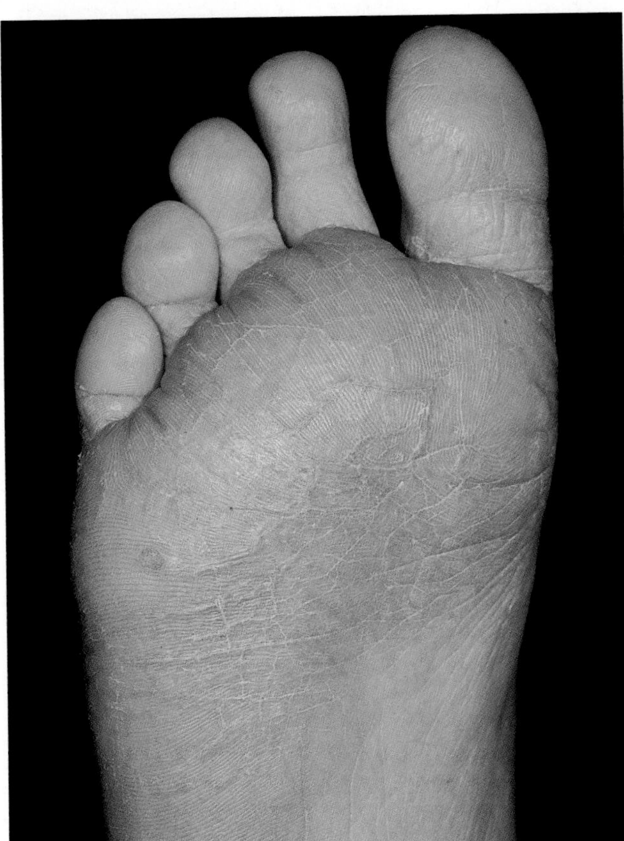

Figure 3-45 Chapped fissured feet. An early stage with erythema and cracking on pressure areas.

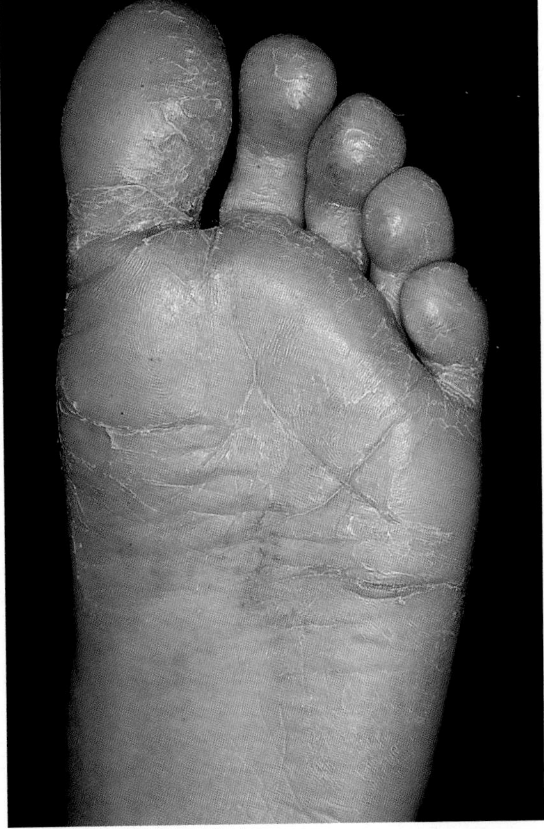

Figure 3-46 An advanced case of chapped fissure feet in which the entire plantar surface is severely dried and fissured.

Table 3-4 Self-Inflicted and Self-Perpetuated Dermatoses

Dermatologic complaint that is a primary psychiatric symptom	Dermatologic features	Possible associated psychiatric disorder	Diagnosis	Treatment
Psychogenic parasitosis (delusions of parasitosis)	Focal erosions and scars Patients convinced they are infested and angry with physicians because "no one believes them"	Delusional disorder, somatic type, or monosymptomatic hypochondriacal psychosis; shared psychotic disorder with another person (folie à deux); major depressive disorder with psychotic features; incipient schizophrenia	Most patients are women over 50	Antipsychotics (pimozide [Orap]) Antidepressants may be used for comorbid depressive disease Anxiolytics and hypnotics may be used in conjunction with antipsychotics in some cases
Factitial dermatitis	Cutaneous lesions are wholly self-inflicted; patient denies their self-inflicted nature Wide range of lesions, blisters, ulcers, burns Bizarre patterns not characteristic of any disease Often a diagnosis of exclusion Adolescents, young adults	Personality disorder, cutaneous lesions are an appeal for help Posttraumatic stress disorder Rule out sexual and child abuse Depression, psychosis, obsessive-compulsive disorder, malingering, and Munchausen's syndrome	Ratio of female to male patients is 4 to 1 Sudden appearance of lesions "Hollow history"; patient cannot describe how lesion evolved	Empathic, supportive approach None in most cases Antipsychotics and antidepressants may be used in posttraumatic stress disorder
Neurotic excoriations and acne excoriée	Possibly initiated by itchy skin disease Repetitive self-excoriation—patient admits self-inflicted nature Linear excoriations in easily reached areas Groups of round or linear scars	Depression, obsessive-compulsive disorder, perfectionistic traits, presence of significant psychosocial stressor in 33-98% of patients Body image problems, including eating disorders, in acne excoriée	Exclude systemic causes of itching Patient admits self-inflicted nature	Empathic, supportive approach Antidepressants, especially SSRIs; antianxiety and antipsychotic drugs may be used as adjunctive therapies where indicated
Lichen simplex chronicus	Created and perpetuated by constant scratching and rubbing Very thick oval plaques Usually just one lesion Severe itching Lasts indefinitely Recurs frequently	No known psychopathology Triggered by stress	Biopsy shows eczematous inflammation or resembles psoriasis	Topical steroids and plastic occlusion Cordran tape Intralesional steroid
Prurigo nodularis	0.5- to 1-cm itchy nodules on arms and legs; lasts for years	Severe pruritus interferes with life activities and sleep	Biopsy shows very thick epidermis and hyperplasia of nerve fibers	Intralesional steroids Cryotherapy Excision Capsaicin cream Calcipotriol ointment

Adapted from Gupta AK, Gupta MA: *Dermatol Clin* 18(4), 2000 PMID: 1105937; Gupta MD, Gupta AK: *J Am Acad Dermatol* 34:1030, 1996. PMID: 8647969.

SSRIs, selective serotonin reuptake inhibitors.

SELF-INFLICTED DERMATOSES

A number of skin disorders are created or perpetuated by manipulation of the skin surface (Table 3-4). Patients may benefit from both dermatologic and psychiatric care. The most common self-inflicted dermatoses are discussed here.

Lichen simplex chronicus

Lichen simplex chronicus (Figures 3-47 through 3-54), or circumscribed neurodermatitis, is an eczematous eruption that is created by habitual scratching of a single localized area. The disease is more common in adults, but may be seen in children. The areas most commonly affected are those that are conveniently reached. These are listed in Box 3-7 in approximate order of frequency. Patients derive great pleasure in the relief that comes with frantically scratching the inflamed site. Loss of this pleasurable sensation or continued subconscious habitual scratching may explain why this eruption frequently recurs.

A typical plaque stays localized and shows little tendency to enlarge with time. Red papules coalesce to form a red, scaly, thick plaque with accentuation of skin lines (*lichenification*). Lichen simplex chronicus is a chronic eczematous disease, but acute changes may result from sensitization with topical medication. Moist scale, serum, crusts, and pustules are signs of infection.

Box 3-7 **Lichen Simplex Chronicus: Areas Most Commonly Affected Listed in Approximate Order of Frequency**
Outer lower portion of lower leg
Scrotum, vulva, anal area, pubis
Wrists and ankles
Upper eyelids
Back (lichen simplex nuchae) and side of neck
Orifice of the ear
Extensor forearms near elbow
Fold behind the ear
Scalp-picker's nodules

Lichen simplex nuchae occur almost exclusively in women who reach for the back of the neck during stressful situations (see Figure 3-51). The disease may spread beyond the initial well-defined plaque. Diffuse dry or moist scale, crust, and erosions extend into the posterior scalp beyond the neck. Secondary infection is common. Nodules, usually less than 1 cm and scattered randomly in the scalp, occur in patients who frequently pick at the scalp; there may be few nodules or many.

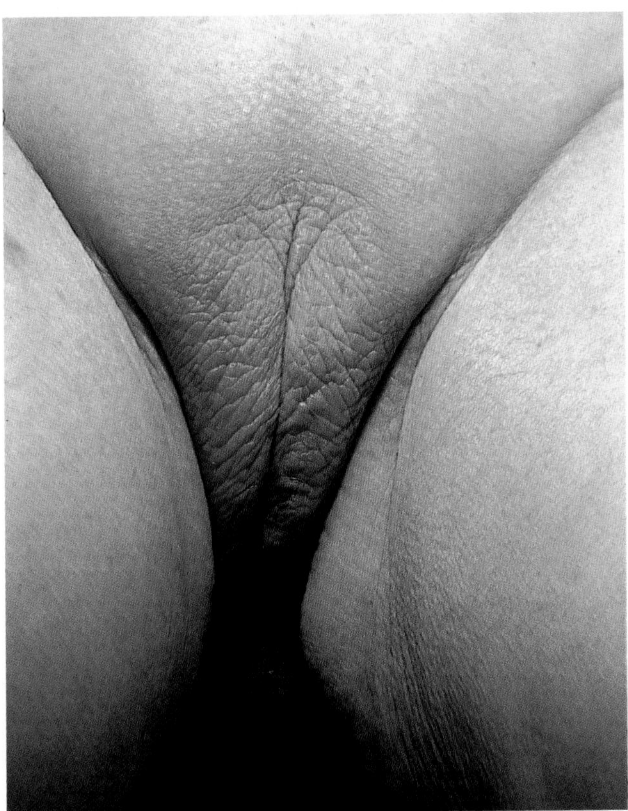

Figure 3-47 Lichen simplex chronicus of the vulva. The skin lines are markedly accentuated from years of rubbing and scratching.

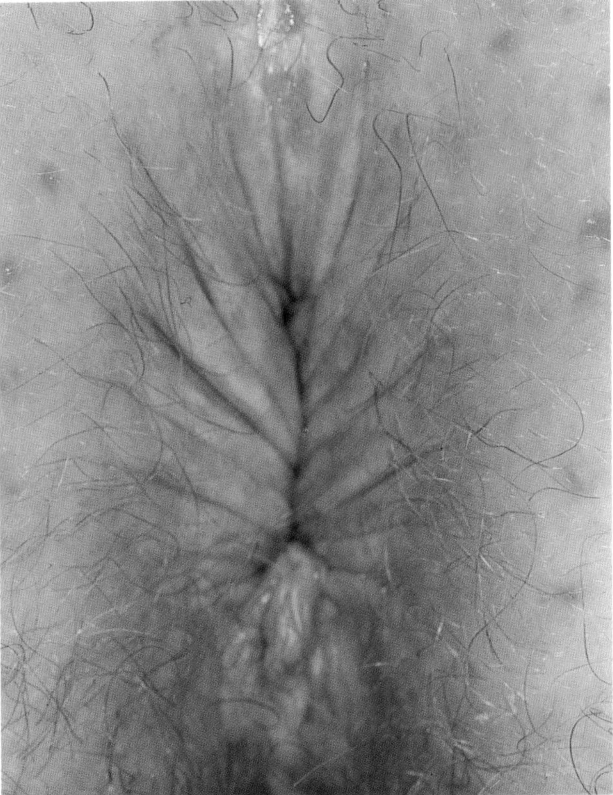

Figure 3-48 Anal excoriations. Scratching has produced focal erosions and thickening of the skin about the anus.

LICHEN SIMPLEX CHRONICUS

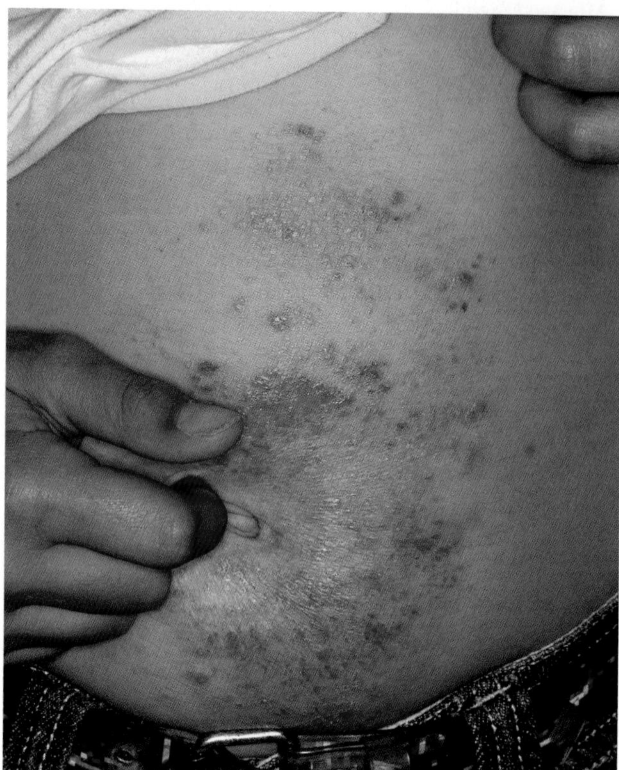

Figure 3-49 The thick plaque had been present for years. Potent topical steroids improved the eruption but the plaque quickly reappeared after renewed habitual scratching.

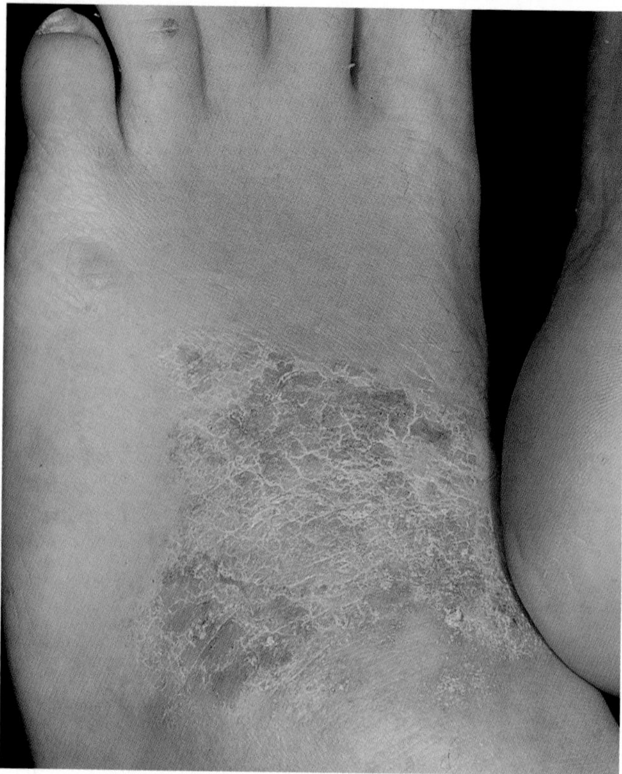

Figure 3-50 This localized plaque of chronic eczematous inflammation was created by rubbing with the opposite heel.

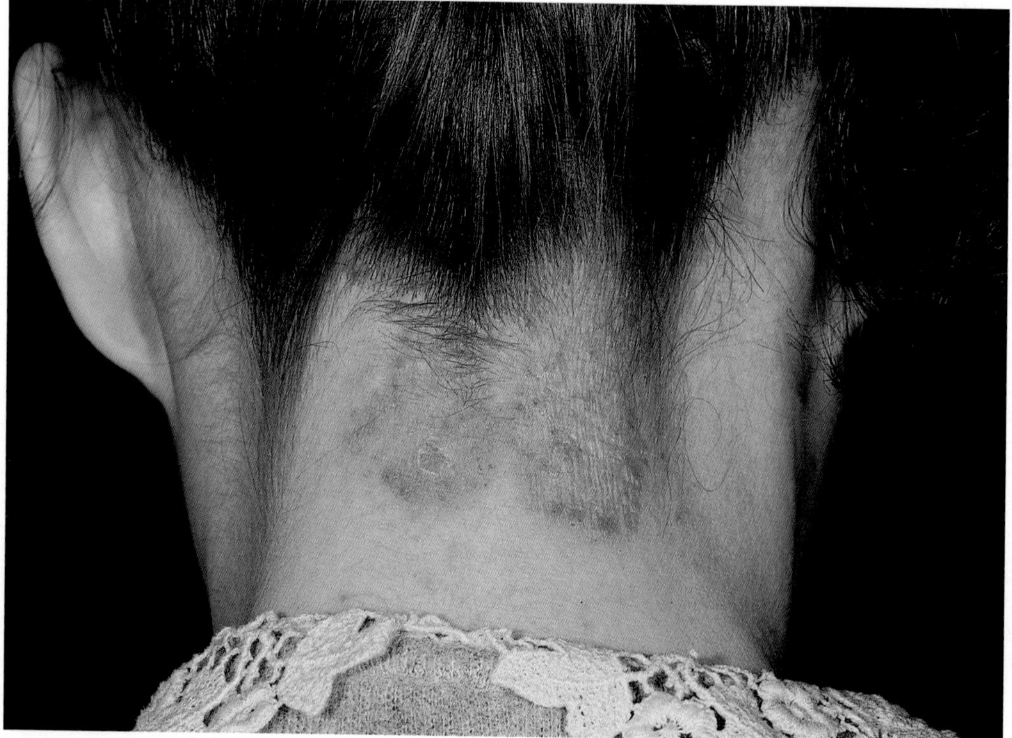

Figure 3-51 Lichen simplex nuchae occurs almost exclusively in women who scratch the back of their neck in stressful situations.

LICHEN SIMPLEX CHRONICUS—SCROTUM

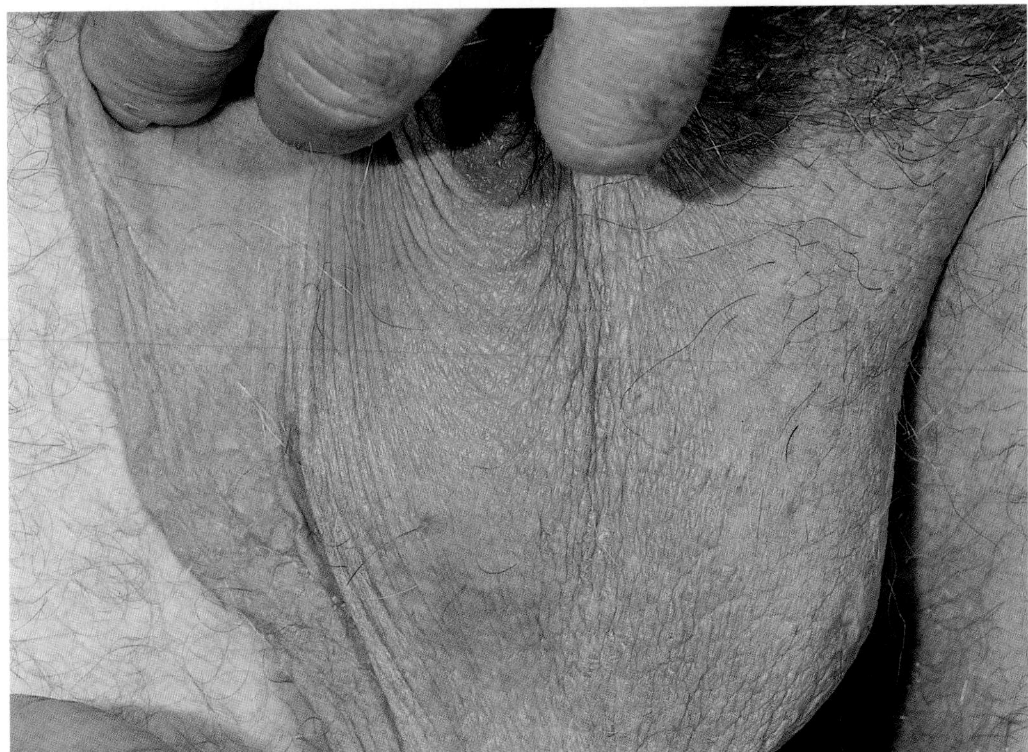

Figure 3-52 The skin is thickened and skin lines are accentuated, unlike the adjacent scrotal skin.

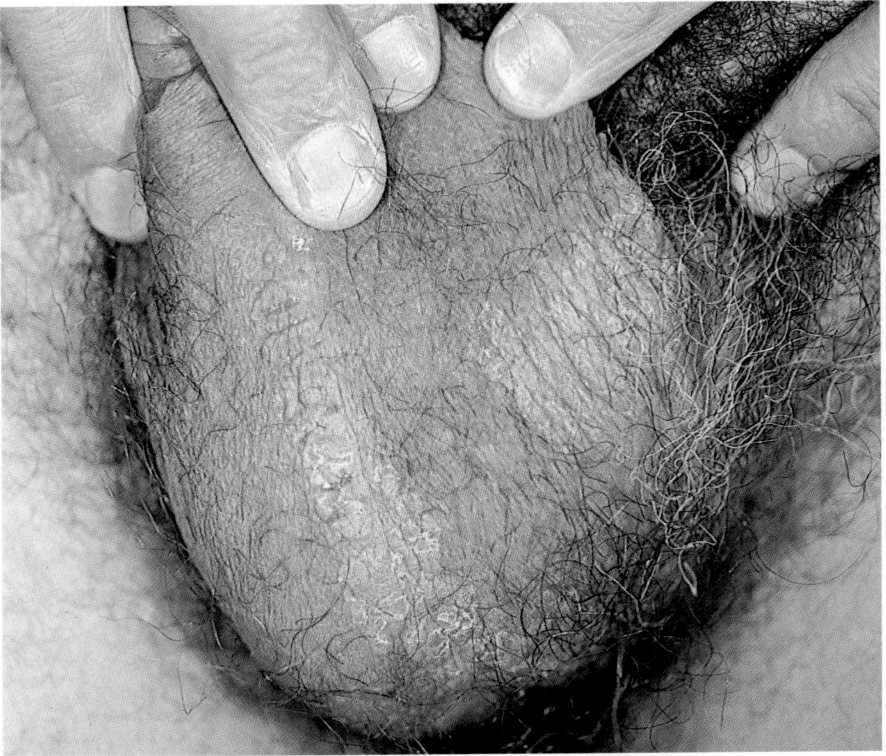

Figure 3-53 Two linear areas are picked and scratched, causing the skin to become very thick. The patient scratches during the day and while asleep.

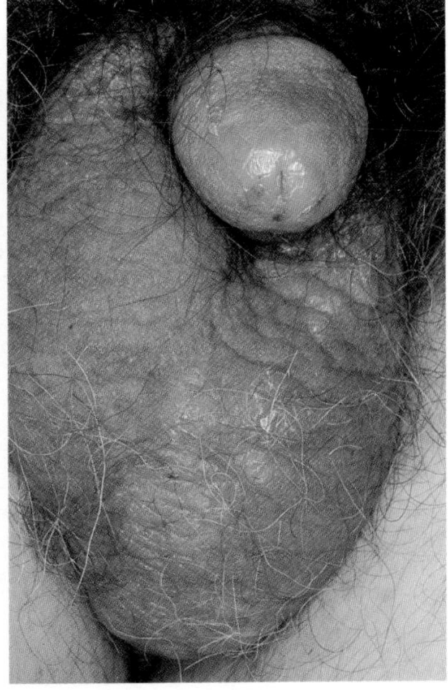

Figure 3-54 The entire anterior part of the scrotum has been lichenified.

CHRONIC VULVAR ITCHING

Women who have chronic vulvar itching usually have eczema. The degree of itching may not correspond to the appearance of the skin. Scratching begins a cycle that makes the skin rough, red, and irritated, producing more itching. Lichen sclerosus, contact dermatits, lichen planus, psoriasis, and Paget's disease are other causes of itching. A 2- to 4-week course of a group I topical steroid is usually very effective.

RED SCROTUM SYNDROME

Lichen simplex of the scrotum is a common finding, and thickened skin with accentuated skin markings is typical. Some patients present with persistent redness of the anterior half of the scrotum that may involve the base of the penis (Figure 3-55). There is persistent itching, burning, or pain. The cause is unknown and it is resistant to treatment. Some men present with erythema of the anterior scrotum and have no symptoms. This is a variant of normal.

TREATMENT. The patient must first understand that the rash will not clear until even minor scratching and rubbing are stopped. Scratching frequently takes place during sleep, and the affected area may have to be covered. Lichen simplex chronicus is chronic eczema and is treated as outlined in the section on eczematous inflammation. Clobetasol foams are very effective and can be used for lesions on the neck, legs, wrists, ankles, and vulva. Treatment of the anal area or the fold behind the ear does not require potent topical steroids as do other forms of lichen simplex; rather, these intertriginous areas respond to group V or VI topical steroids. Lichen simplex nuchae, because of its location, is difficult to treat. Inflammation that extends into the scalp may be treated with a group II steroid gel such as fluocinonide applied twice each day. Moist, secondarily infected areas respond to oral antibiotics and topical steroid solutions (e.g., clobetasol solution). A 2- to 3-week course of prednisone (20 mg twice daily) should be considered when an extensively inflamed scalp does not respond rapidly to topical treatment. Nodules caused by picking at the scalp may be very resistant to treatment, requiring monthly intralesional injections with triamcinolone acetonide (Kenalog 10 mg/ml). Botulinum toxin A injected intradermally into lichenified lesions may block acetylcholine release and control pruritus.

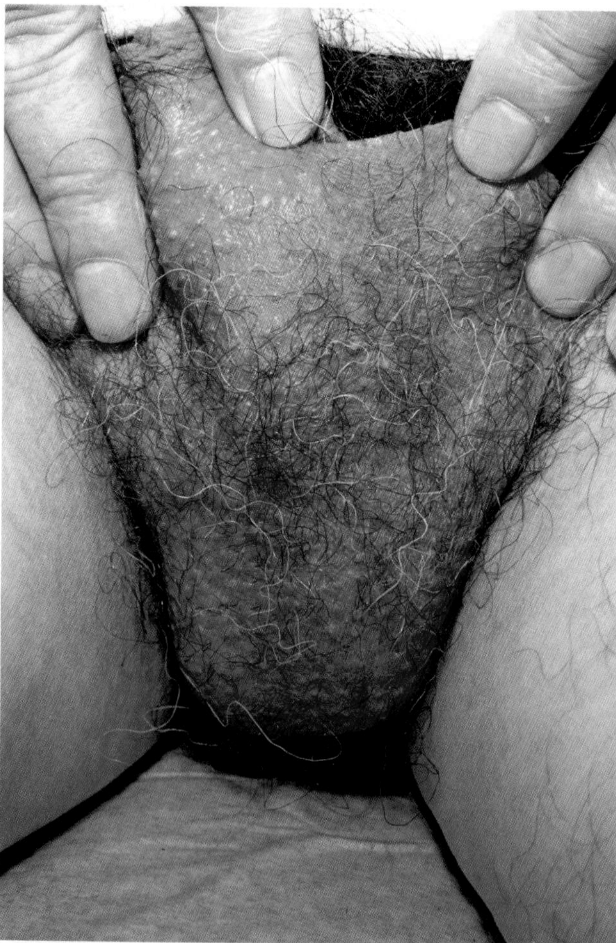

Figure 3-55 Rubbing the anterior part of the scrotum has caused persistent erythema but no lichenification.

Prurigo nodularis

Prurigo nodularis is an uncommon disease of unknown cause that may be considered a nodular form of lichen simplex chronicus. There is intractable pruritus. It resembles picker's nodules of the scalp except that the few to 20 or more nodules are randomly distributed on the extensor aspects of the arms and legs (Figures 3-56 and 3-57). They are created by repeated scratching. The nodules are red or brown, hard, and dome-shaped with a smooth, crusted, or warty surface; they measure 1 to 2 cm in diameter. Hypertrophy of cutaneous papillary dermal nerves is a relatively constant feature. Complaints of pruritus vary. Some patients claim there is no itching and that scratching is only habitual, whereas others complain that the pruritus is intense.

TREATMENT. Prurigo nodularis is resistant to treatment and lasts for years. As with picker's nodules of the scalp, repeated intralesional steroid injections may be effective. Excision of individual nodules is sometimes helpful. Cryotherapy is sometimes successful. Capsaicin 0.025% (Zostrix cream) and capsaicin 0.075% HP (Zostrix-HP cream) interfere with the perception of pruritus and pain by depletion of neuropeptides in small sensory cutaneous nerves. Application of the cream four to six times daily for up to 10 months resulted in cessation of burning and pruritus. Lesions gradually heal. The use of combination or sequential topical calcipotriene with topical steroids has been effective. Naltrexone (50 mg daily), an orally active opiate antagonist, was found to be effective therapy for pruritic symptoms in many diseases. Oral cyclosporine (3 to 5 mg/kg daily) was effective in one study. *PMID: 18445069* Gabapentin has been used in resistant cases. *PMID: 18086601* Depression and dissociative experiences may be associated with this disorder and psychiatric referral may be appropriate.

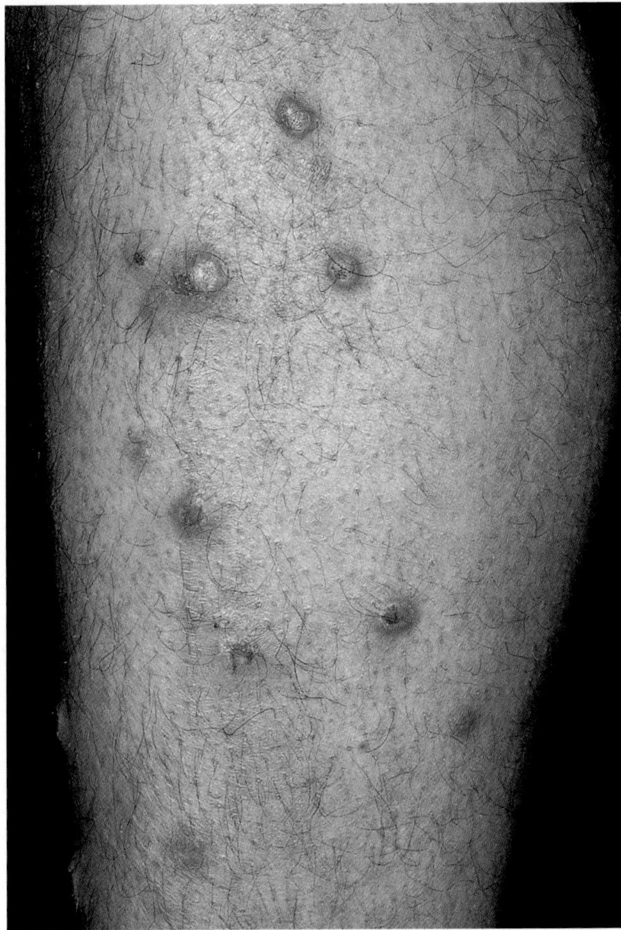

Figure 3-56 Prurigo nodularis. Thick, hard nodules usually present on the extensor surfaces of the forearms and legs from chronic picking.

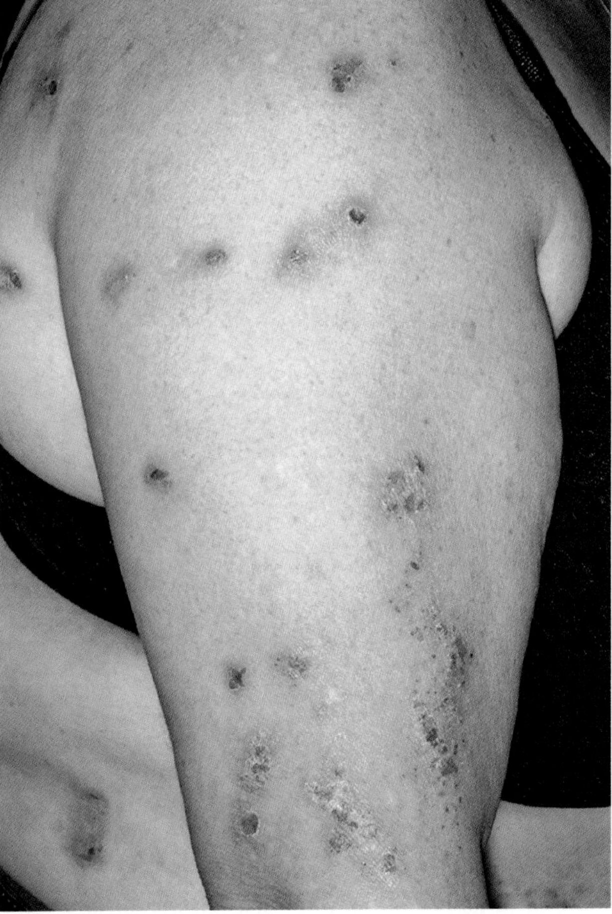

Figure 3-57 Prurigo nodularis. Thick papules and linear excoriations are features of both prurigo nodularis and neurotic excoriations.

Neurotic excoriations

Neurotic excoriations are patient-induced linear excoriations. Patients dig at their skin to relieve itching or to extract imaginary pieces of material that they feel is imbedded in or extruding from the skin. Itching and digging become compulsive rituals. Most patients are aware that they create the lesions. The most consistent psychiatric disorders reported are perfectionistic and compulsive traits; patients manifest repressed aggression and self-destructive behavior. Depression, obsessive-compulsive disorder, anxiety, somatoform disorders, mania, psychosis, and substance abuse have also been associated with itch. Recurrent and intrusive thoughts lead to compulsive skin picking. Obsessive-compulsive disorder is a common comorbid condition. Excoriation is preceded by increased tension and anxiety followed by gratification or relief when excoriating the skin.

CLINICAL APPEARANCE. Repetitive scratching and digging produces few to several hundred excoriations; all lesions are of similar size and shape. They tend to be grouped in areas that are easily reached, such as the extensor surfaces of the arms and legs, abdomen, thighs, and upper parts of the back and shoulders, with the face being the most common site (Figures 3-58 through 3-60). These vary from a few to several hundred and vary in size from a few millimeters to several centimeters. Recurrent picking at crusts delays healing. Groups of white scars surrounded by brown hyperpigmentation are typical; their presence alone can indicate past difficulty.

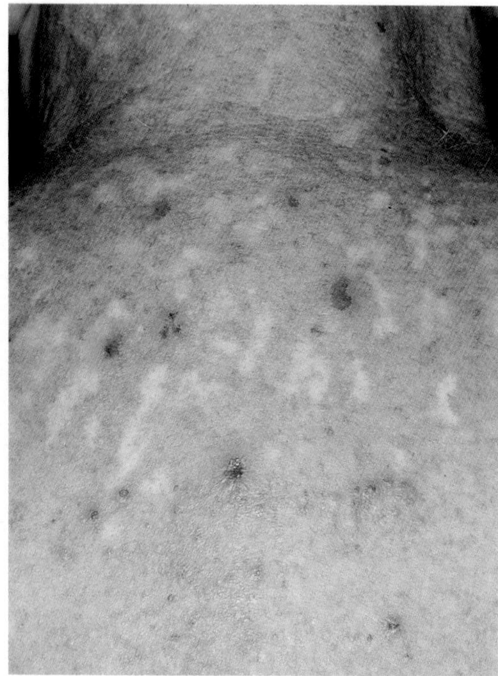

Figure 3-58 Neurotic excoriations. Lesions appear on any area of the trunk and extremities that is easily reached.

TREATMENT. The use of group I topical steroids applied twice a day or group V topical steroids under plastic wrap occlusion combined with systemic antibiotics produces gratifying results. Resistant lesions are treated with monthly intralesional injections with triamcinolone acetonide (Kenalog 10 mg/ml). Frequent lubrication and infrequent washing with only mild soaps should be encouraged once areas are healed. Patients should try to substitute the ritual of applying lubricants for the ritual of digging. An empathic, supportive approach has been reported to be significantly more effective than insight-oriented psychotherapy, which often exacerbates the symptoms. Psychiatric referral is appropriate for patients who fail the supportive approach. Those with depression may be treated with selective serotonin reuptake inhibitors (SSRIs), selective serotonin and norepinephrine reuptake inhibitors (SSNRIs), tricyclic antidepressants (TCAs), doxepin, and psychotherapy. Obsessive-compulsive disorders are treated with SSNRIs, SSRIs, TCAs and behavioral therapy. *PMID: 18318883*

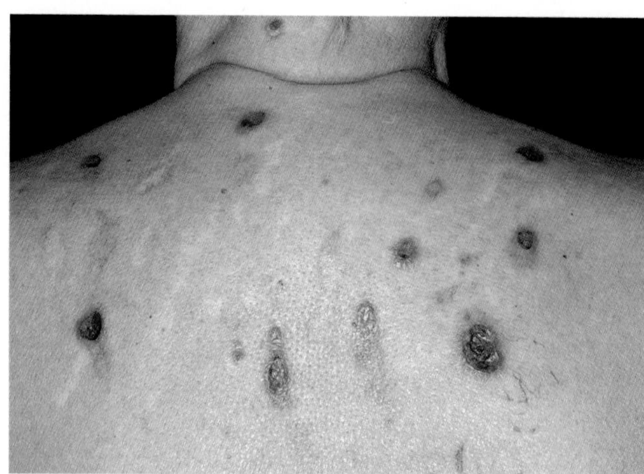

Figure 3-59 Neurotic excoriations. Severe involvement of the upper back. Picking causes shallow erosions and small, round scars. Long, linear scars occur from deep gouging.

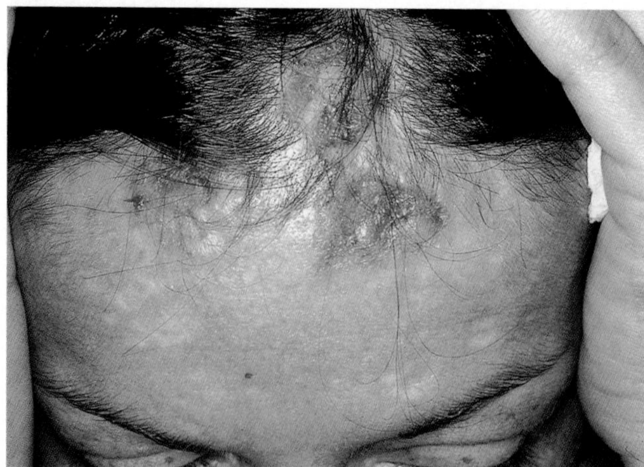

Figure 3-60 Neurotic excoriations. Deep scars occurred after long periods of aggressive picking.

PSYCHOGENIC PARASITOSIS

Patients with psychogenic parasitosis (delusions of parasitosis) believe they are infested with parasites. They move from one physician to another looking for someone who will believe them. A variety of psychiatric disorders may be associated with this disorder, but suggesting psychiatric referral may offend the patient. A supportive, therapeutic relationship is essential.

THE DELUSION. Patients report seeing and feeling parasites. Involvement of the ears, eyes, and nose is common. They present with the "matchbox" sign, in which small bits of excoriated skin, dried blood, debris, or insect parts are brought in matchboxes or other containers as "proof" of infestation. Body fluids thought to contain parasites are brought in jars. Pest control officers may have been hired to rid the house of parasites.

THE SKIN. Excoriations and ulcers and linear scars are common on easily reached areas of the forearms, legs, trunk, and face (Figure 3-61).

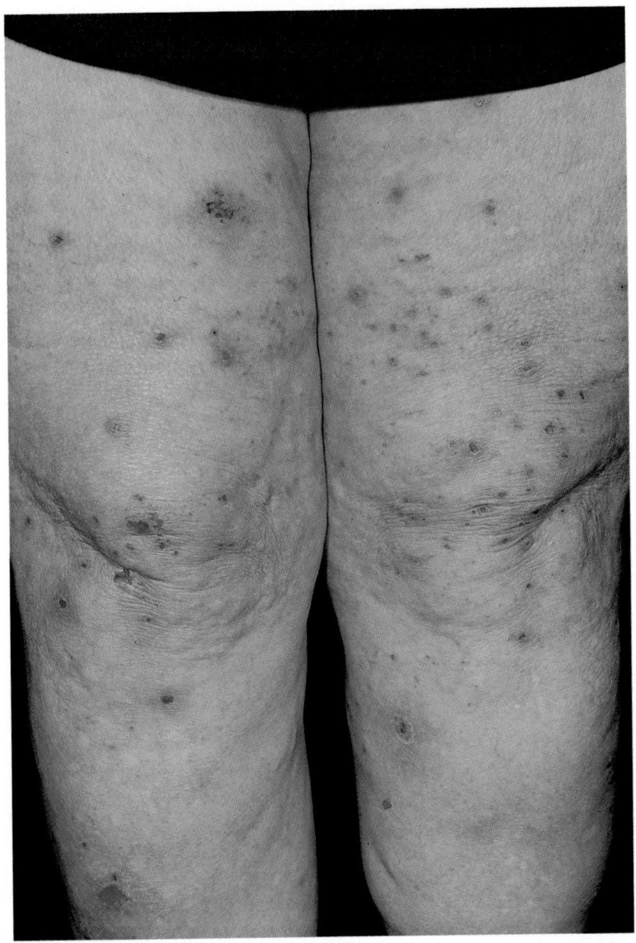

CLASSIFICATION. Classify patients with psychogenic parasitosis into four groups: anxiety/hypochondriasis, anxiety/hypochondriasis with depression, delusional parasitosis, and delusional parasitosis with depression. Patients suffering from anxiety/hypochondriasis may believe that they are infested by parasites but may also express doubt about their infestation, express fears of "going crazy," and agree that parasites may not be present. Patients with anxiety/hypochondriasis and depression may agree to undergo a psychiatric evaluation. Patients who have a true delusion are convinced that they have a parasitic infestation that none of the physicians can find; these patients may have an underlying major depression.

MANAGEMENT. A majority of patients with short-term illness can be cured with suggestion; the remainder have a true delusion. Patients with symptoms for over 3 months are usually not cured by suggestion alone. Listen and show concern; examine the skin with magnification and prepare scrapings; rule out true infestation. Animal and bird mites and scabies may actually be present. Do not suggest that the diagnosis is obvious on the first visit. The second visit can be lengthy. Collect specimens brought in by the patient and set them aside for later evaluation. Conduct a thorough examination and listen for indicators of depression. After two or more visits patients may suggest that this may be "all in my head." At this point, explain that some patients actually see and feel parasites that are not real. Explain that this is an illness that affects sane people. The clinician may sense that the patient doubts the existence of the infestation (i.e., the belief is shakable). The patient is then offered a benzodiazepine to help with anxiety while waiting for the next visit 2 weeks later; a psychiatric referral is suggested at that 2-week follow-up visit.

Patients whose belief is unshakable are considered to have a delusional disorder. Suggest psychiatric referral. Explain that many other patients with similar symptoms have been helped with this treatment and that the medication can be taken as a "therapeutic trial." Antipsychotics (e.g., pimozide, risperidone, olanzapine, quetiapine) are usually prescribed by the psychiatrist.

Figure 3-61 Psychogenic parasitosis. Attempts to pick "bugs" out of the skin produce focal erosions on easily accessed areas such as the arms and legs.

STASIS DERMATITIS AND VENOUS ULCERATION: POSTPHLEBITIC SYNDROMES

Stasis dermatitis

ETIOLOGY. Stasis dermatitis is an eczematous eruption that occurs on the lower legs in some patients with venous insufficiency. The dermatitis may be acute, subacute, or chronic and recurrent, and it may be accompanied by ulceration. Most patients with venous insufficiency do not develop dermatitis, which suggests that genetic or environmental factors may play a role. The reason for its occurrence is unknown. Some have speculated that it represents an allergic response to an epidermal protein antigen created through increased hydrostatic pressure, whereas others believe that the skin has been compromised and is more susceptible to irritation and trauma.

ALLERGY TO TOPICAL AGENTS. Patients with stasis dermatitis have significantly more positive reactions when patch tested with components of previously used topical agents. Topical medications that contain potential sensitizers such as lanolin, benzocaine, parabens, and neomycin should be avoided by patients with stasis disease. Allergy to corticosteroids in topical medication is also possible.

Types of eczematous inflammation

SUBACUTE INFLAMMATION

Subacute inflammation usually begins in the winter months when the legs become dry and scaly. Brown staining of the skin (hemosiderin) may have appeared slowly for months (Figure 3-62). The pigment is iron left after disintegration of red blood cells that leaked out of veins because of increased hydrostatic pressure. Scratching induces first subacute and then chronic eczematous inflammation. Attempts at self-treatment with drying lotions (calamine) or potential sensitizers (e.g., neomycin-containing topical medicines) exacerbate and prolong the inflammation.

ACUTE INFLAMMATION

A red, superficial, itchy plaque may suddenly appear on the lower leg. This acute process may be eczematous inflammation, cellulitis, or both. Weeping and crusts appear (Figure 3-63). A vesicular eruption (id reaction) on the palms, trunk, and/or extremities sometimes accompanies this acute inflammation. The inflammation responds to systemic antibiotics, wet compresses, and group III to V topical steroids. Wet compresses should be discontinued before excessive drying occurs. The id reaction resolves spontaneously as the primary site improves.

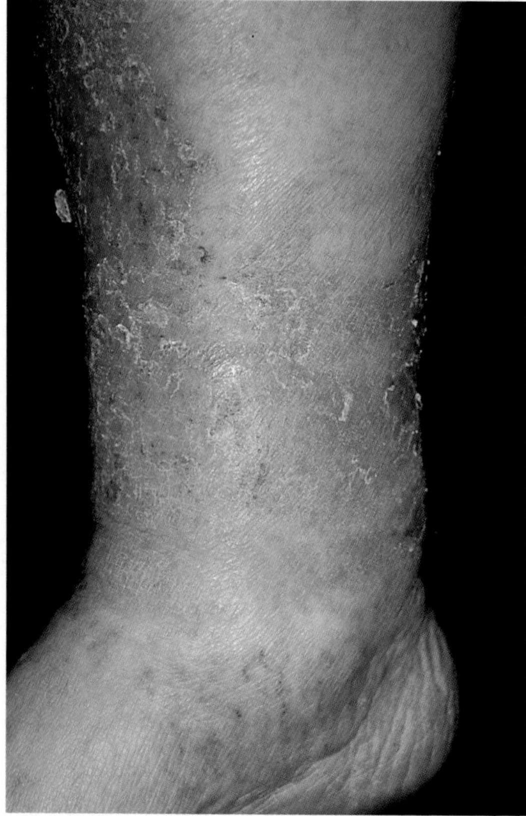

Figure 3-62 Stasis dermatitis in an early stage. Erythema and erosions produced by excoriations are shown.

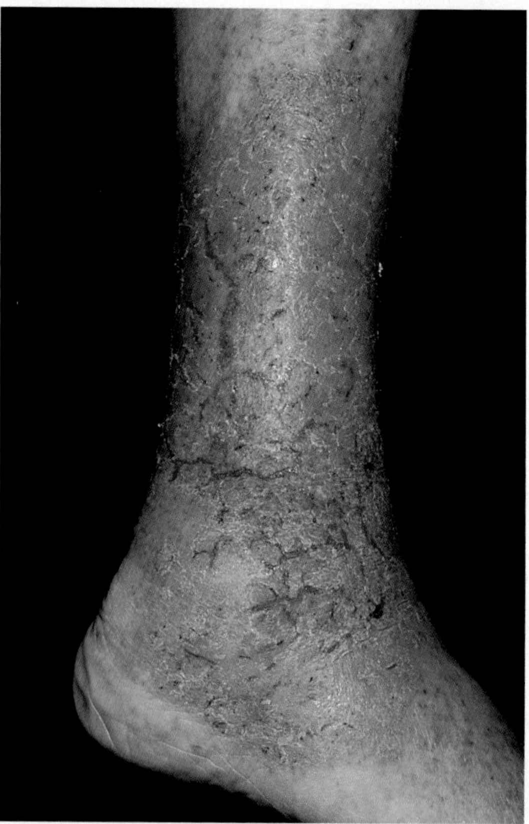

Figure 3-63 Stasis dermatitis (severe inflammation). A red, itchy plaque may suddenly develop acute inflammation and/or cellulitis. Weeping, crusts, and fissuring may be extensive.

CHRONIC INFLAMMATION

Recurrent attacks of inflammation eventually compromise the poorly vascularized area, and the disease becomes chronic and recurrent (Figures 3-64 and 3-65). The typical presentation is a cyanotic red plaque over the medial malleolus. Fibrosis following chronic inflammation leads to permanent skin thickening. The skin surface in these irreversibly changed areas may have a bumpy, cobblestone appearance that results from fibrosis and venous and lymph stasis. The skin remains thickened and diffusely dark brown (postinflammatory hyperpigmentation) during quiescent periods.

TREATMENT OF STASIS DERMATITIS

Topical steroids and wet dressings. The early, dry, superficial stage is managed as subacute eczematous inflammation with group II to V topical steroid creams or ointments and lubricating creams or lotions. Oral antibiotics (usually those active against *Staphylococci*, e.g., cephalexin) hasten resolution if cellulitis is present. Moist exudative inflammation and moist ulcers respond to tepid wet compresses of Burow's solution or just saline or water for 30 to 60 minutes several times a day. Wet dressings suppress inflammation while debriding the ulcer. Adherent crust may be carefully freed with blunt-tipped scissors. Group V topical steroids are applied to eczematous skin at the periphery of the ulcer. Patients must be warned that steroid creams placed on the ulcer stop the healing process. Elevation of the legs encourages healing.

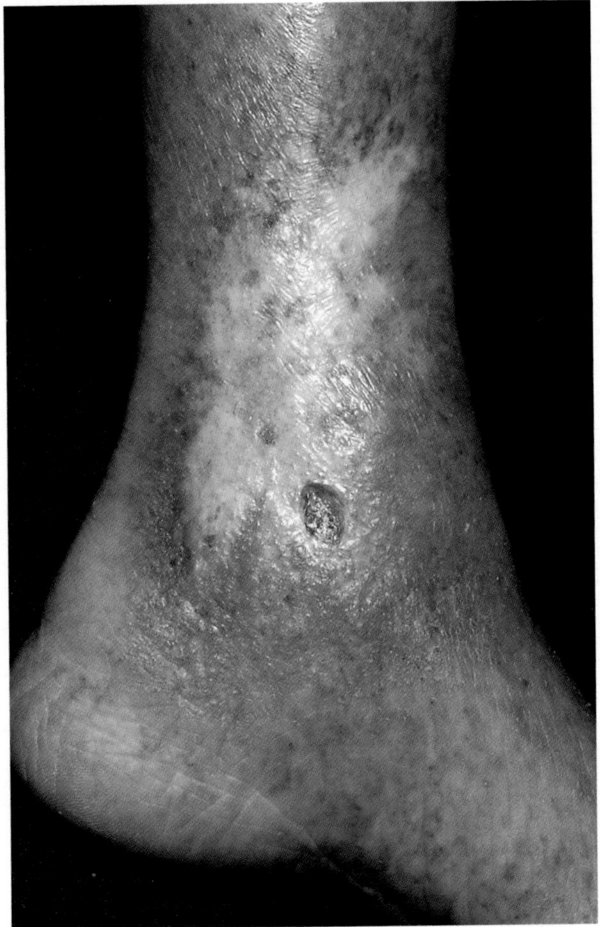

Figure 3-64 Stasis dermatitis. Severe, painful, exudative, weeping, infected eczema with moist crust. Oral antibiotics and cool compresses are initial treatment followed in a few days with group II to V topical steroid creams or ointments.

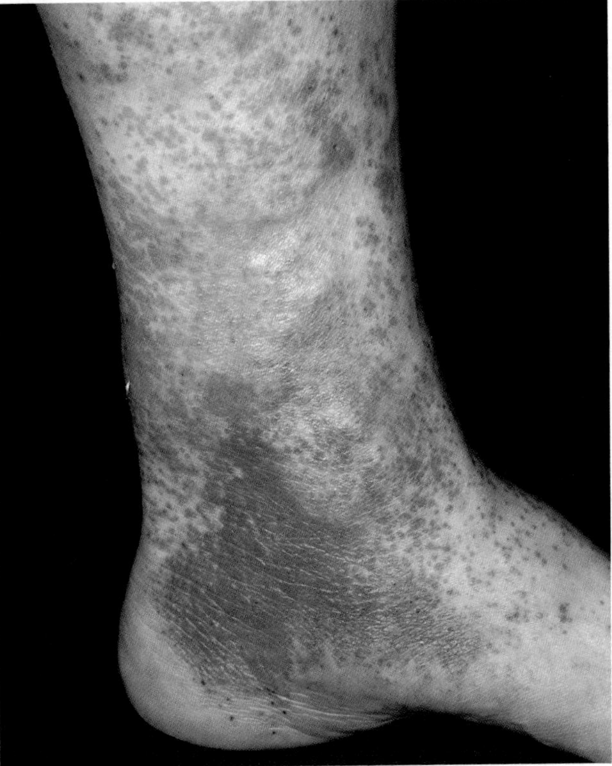

Figure 3-65 Stasis over a period of months to years often results in permanent brown staining of the skin.

Venous leg ulcers

The three main types of lower-extremity ulcers are *venous, arterial,* and *neuropathic* (Table 3-5). Most leg ulcers are venous; foot ulcers are more often caused by arterial insufficiency or neuropathy. Most venous ulcers are located over the medial malleolus and are often larger than other ulcers. Diabetes is a common underlying condition.

DIFFERENTIAL DIAGNOSIS. Many diseases cause leg ulcers (Box 3-8). Biopsy (basal cell carcinomas, squamous cell carcinomas) and culture (fungal, atypical mycobacterial) chronic ulcers that do not respond to conventional therapy. Vasculitis, pyoderma gangrenosum, rheumatoid arthritis, and systemic lupus erythematosus may be associated with lower-extremity ulcers.

PATHOPHYSIOLOGY. The leg has superficial, communicating, and deep veins. The superficial system contains the long (medial) and short (lateral) saphenous veins. Perforator veins connect the superficial veins to the deep venous system. Normally blood flows from the superficial to the deep system. Venous hypertension ("chronic venous insufficiency") occurs if any of the valves dysfunction, a thrombosis blocks the deep system, or there is calf muscle pump failure. Increased pressure causes diffusion of substances, including fibrin, out of capillaries. Fibrotic tissue may predispose the tissue to ulceration.

ETIOLOGY AND LOCATION. Venous insufficiency followed by edema is the fundamental change that predisposes to dermatitis and ulceration. Venous insufficiency occurs when venous return in the deep, perforating, or superficial veins is impaired by vein dilation and valve dysfunction. Deep vein thrombophlebitis, which may have been asymptomatic earlier, is the most frequent precursor of lower leg venous insufficiency. Blood pools in the deep venous system and causes deep venous hypertension and dilation of the perforators that connect the superficial and deep venous systems. Venous hypertension is then transmitted to the superficial venous system. The largest perforators are posterior and superior to the lateral and medial malleoli. These are the same areas where dermatitis and ulceration are most prevalent. Superficial varicosities alone are unlikely to produce venous insufficiency.

Table 3-5 Three Common Types of Leg Ulcers

	Venous	Arterial	Neuropathic
Ulcer location	Medial malleolus; trauma or infection may localize ulcers laterally or more proximally	Distal, over bony prominences; trauma may localize ulcers proximally	Pressure points on feet (e.g., junction of great toe and plantar surface, metatarsal head, heel)
Ulcer appearance	Shallow, irregular borders; base may be initially fibrinous but later develops granulation tissue	Round or punched-out, well-demarcated border; fibrinous yellow base or true necrotic eschar; bone and tendon exposure may be seen	Callus surrounding wound and undermined edges are characteristic; blister, hemorrhage, necrosis, and exposure of underlying structures are commonly seen
Physical examination	Varicose veins, leg edema, atrophie blanche, dermatitis, lipodermatosclerosis, pigmentary changes, purpura	Loss of hair; shiny, atrophic skin; dystrophic toenails; cold feet; femoral bruit; absent or decreased pulses; prolonged capillary refilling time	No sensation to monofilament; bone resorption, claw toes, flat foot, Charcot joints
Frequent symptoms	Pain, odor, and copious drainage from wound; pruritus	Claudication, resting ischemic pain	Foot numbness, burning, paresthesia
Ankle-to-brachial blood pressure ratio (ankle/brachial index [ABI]) measured by Doppler ultrasonography	>0.9	ABI <0.7 suggests arterial disease; calcification of vessels gives falsely high Doppler readings	Normal, unless associated with arterial component
Risk factors	Deep venous thrombosis, significant leg injury, obesity	Diabetes, hypertension, cigarette smoking, hypercholesterolemia	Diabetes, leprosy, frostbite
Complications	Allergic contact dermatitis, cellulitis	Gangrene	Underlying osteomyelitis
Treatment pearl	Compression therapy, leg elevation	Pentoxifylline, vascular surgery assessment if ABI <5	Vigorous surgical debridement, pressure avoidance

From Valencia IC et al: *J Am Acad Dermatol* 44:401, 2001. *PMID: 11209109*

CLINICAL FEATURES. Ulceration is almost inevitable once the skin has been thickened and circulation is compromised. Ulceration may occur spontaneously or after the slightest trauma (Figure 3-66). The ulcer may remain small or may enlarge rapidly without any further trauma. A dull, constant pain that improves with leg elevation is present. Pain from ischemic ulcers is more intense and does not improve with elevation.

Ulcers have a sharp or sloping border and are deep or superficial. Removal of crust and debris reveals a moist base with granulation tissue. The base and surrounding skin are often infected. Healing is slow, taking several weeks or months. After healing, it is not uncommon to see ulcers rapidly recur. The ulcers are replaced with ivory-white sclerotic scars. Despite the pain and the inconvenience of treatment, most patients tolerate this disease well and remain ambulatory.

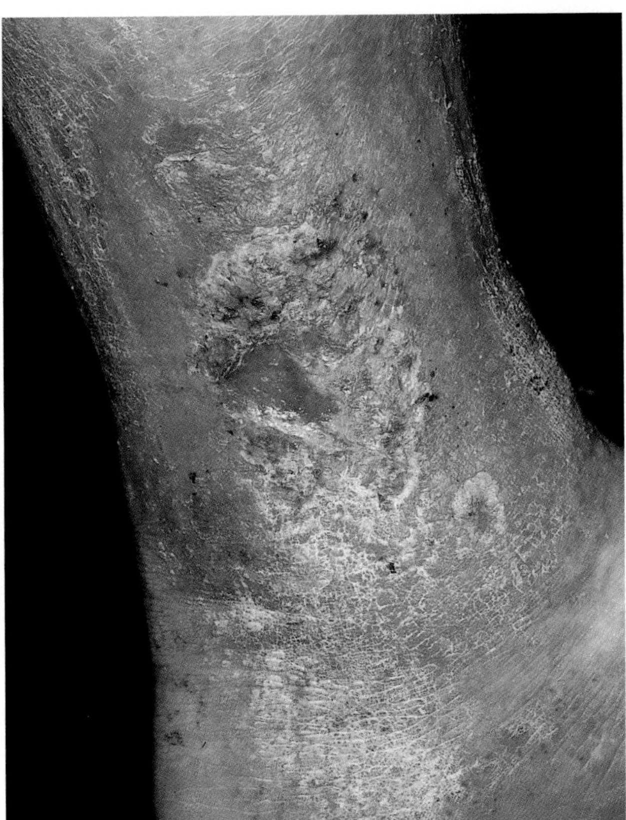

Figure 3-66 The skin is diffusely red, thickened, and bound down by fibrosis. Ulceration occurs with the slightest trauma.

Box 3-8 **Leg Ulcers: Differential Diagnosis**

Venous

Postphlebitic syndrome
Arteriovenous malformation

Arterial

Atherosclerosis
Cholesterol embolism
Thromboangiitis obliterans

Lymphatic (lymphedema)

Neuropathic

Diabetes
Spinal cord lesions
Tabes dorsalis
Vasculitic
Atrophie blanche
Hypersensitivity vasculitis
Lupus erythematosus
Nodular vasculitis
Polyarteritis nodosa
Rheumatoid arthritis
Scleroderma
Wegener's granulomatosis

Hematologic

Sickle cell anemia
Thalassemia

Traumatic

Burns (thermal, radiation)
Cold
Factitial
Pressure

Neoplastic

Basal cell carcinoma
Cutaneous T-cell lymphoma
Metastatic tumors
Sarcoma (e.g., Kaposi's)
Squamous cell carcinoma

Metabolic

Diabetes
Gout

Bacterial infections

Ecthyma gangrenosum
Furuncle
Gram-negative
Mycobacterial
Septic emboli
Syphilis

Fungal infection

Deep fungal
Trichophytin granuloma

Infestations

Spider bites
Protozoal (leishmania)

Panniculitis

Necrobiosis lipoidica
Pancreatic fat necrosis
Weber-Christian disease

Others

Necrobiosis lipoidica
Pyoderma gangrenosum
Sarcoidosis

CHANGES IN SURROUNDING SKIN. Edema is a common finding; it is usually pitting and disappears at night with elevation. Chronic edema, trauma, infection, and inflammation lead to subcutaneous tissue fibrosis, giving the skin a firm, nonpitting, "woody" quality. Fat necrosis may follow thrombosis of small veins, and this may be the most important underlying change that predisposes to ulceration. Recurrent ulceration and fat necrosis is associated with loss of subcutaneous tissue and a decrease in lower leg circumference (lipodermatosclerosis). Advanced disease is represented by an "inverted bottle leg," in which the proximal leg swells from chronic venous obstruction and the lower leg shrinks from chronic ulceration and fat necrosis.

STASIS PAPILLOMATOSIS. Stasis papillomatosis is a condition usually found in chronically congested limbs. Lesions vary from small to large plaques that consist of aggregated brownish or pinkish papules with a smooth or hyperkeratotic surface (Figures 3-67 and 3-68). The lesions most frequently affect the dorsum of the foot, the toes, the extensor aspect of the lower leg, or the area surrounding a venous ulcer. This condition occurs in patients with local lymphatic disturbances; patients with primary lymphedema, chronic venous insufficiency, trauma, and recurrent erysipelas are at greatest risk.

POSTPHLEBITIC SYNDROMES (CLINICAL VARIANTS). Impairment of venous return leads to increased hydrostatic pressure and interstitial fluid accumulation. Six clinical variants (Table 3-6) occur with venous hypertension.

MANAGEMENT OF VENOUS ULCERS

INITIAL EVALUATION AND TREATMENT. Once other causes of lower leg ulcers have been excluded, the area around the ulcer must be prepared for definitive treatment. Ulcers do not heal if edema, infection, or eczematous inflammation is present. The venous system should be investigated. Surgery or sclerotherapy may be needed to control venous reflux.

VARICOSE VEINS. Varicose veins are superficial vessels that are caused by defective venous valves. Perforator vein incompetence may lead to ulceration. Varicose veins cause venous hypertension that leads to edema, cutaneous pigmentation, stasis dermatitis, and ulceration. The goal of therapy is to normalize venous physiology. Deep venous hypertension is managed with compression therapy. Sclerotherapy is used to treat isolated perforator incompetence, even through an ulcer if necessary. Saphenous vein insufficiency is usually managed by surgery.

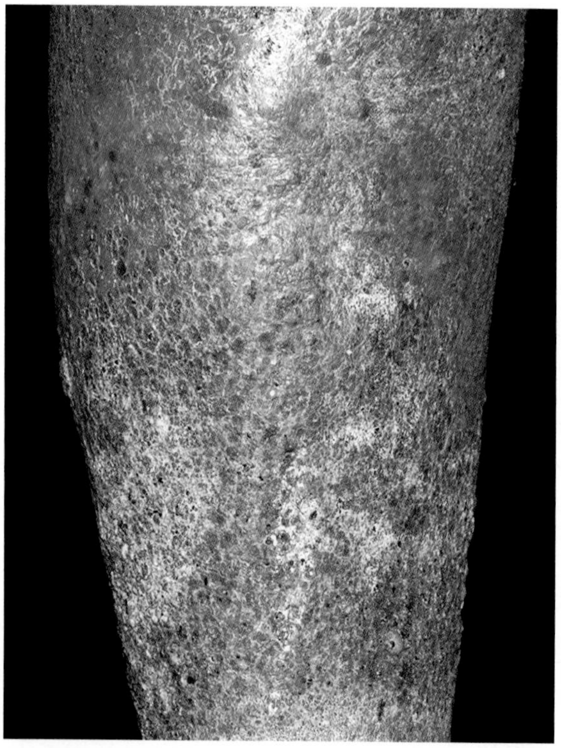

Figure 3-67 Stasis papillomatosis. Chronic inflammation may cause long-standing lymphatic obstruction. This sometimes results in the bizarre appearance of numerous dome-shaped red and blue papules. These changes are irreversible.

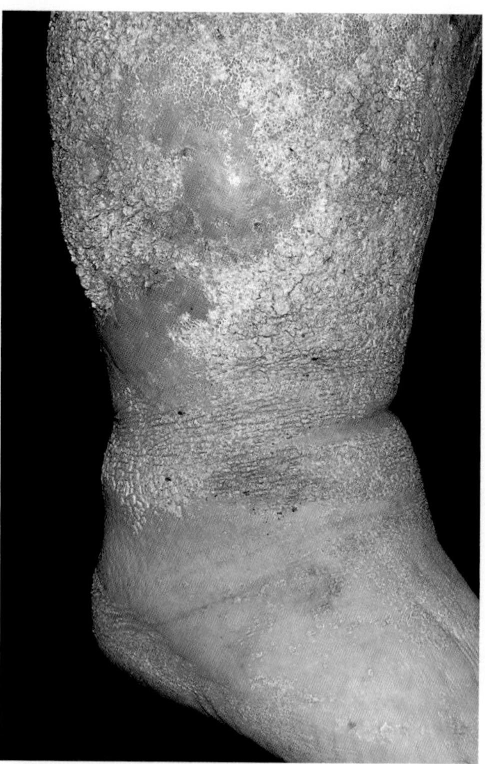

Figure 3-68 Stasis papillomatosis. An extensive case with irrevisible swelling and surface changes.

LABORATORY EVALUATION. Initial evaluation includes complete blood count (CBC), blood glucose level, and sedimentation rate. Consider curet or biopsy of the ulcer for bacterial culture. Biopsy the edge of ulcers that do not heal with conventional therapy to rule out basal cell or squamous cell carcinoma. Radiograph deep ulcers to rule out osteomyelitis.

FUNCTION STUDIES. Doppler, plethysmography, and duplex scanning are used to characterize venous abnormalities in patients with chronic venous insufficiency. Continuous-wave Doppler studies are useful in providing information on the anatomic level of any superficial venous incompetence or obstruction; however, it can be difficult to differentiate superficial from deep venous insufficiency. Plethysmography is a simple test to measure the venous reflux degree and the calf muscle pump efficiency. Image ultrasound associated with pulsated Doppler ultrasound, known as duplex scanning, is a method that provides detailed anatomic information, and is especially useful in identifying which veins are competent. These characteristics enable duplex scanning to substitute for phlebography because duplex scanning is noninvasive and avoids radiological contrasts, showing both anatomic and functional features (reflux or obstruction) of the venous system. It is the examination of choice to assess the superficial, deep, and perforating systems. *PMID: 15941430*

Table 3-6 Venous Ulceration Syndromes (Postphlebitic Syndromes)

Syndrome	Clinical features	Pathophysiology	Management
Dependent edema and ulceration	Pitting edema reversed by elevation Hyperpigmentation	Increased capillary hydrostatic static pressure	Compression bandages Unna's boot Bed rest (short periods) Elevation
Lipodermatosclerosis and ulceration	Induration of skin and subcutaneous tissue Extensive hyperpigmentation Pitting edema Erythema secondary to capillary proliferation	Prolonged high pressure in veins Biopsy shows fibrin deposits around capillaries Fibrin prevents O_2 diffusion to epidermis	Fibrinolytic therapy; stanozol 5 gm twice daily Hyperbaric O_2
Atrophie blanche	White, smooth, flat scars with focal dilated capillaries May be preceded by small painful ulcers	Stasis and platelet sludging causes platelet thrombi Dermal capillary occlusion causes infarction of overlying dermis; heals with white scars	Antiplatelet therapy; aspirin Compression therapy makes ulcers worse Elevation promotes venous return
Ankle blow out syndrome	Multiple small, tortuous veins below and behind malleoli Ulcers usually above and behind medial malleolus in midst of veins Trauma, eczema, bursting of vein causes ulcer	Localized venous valvular incompetence of lower third of leg Exercise makes condition worse	Surgical ligation of localized incompetent veins
Secondary venous varicosity with ulceration	Tortuous saphenous systems	Transmission of hypertension to saphenous system	Compression bandages Hyperbaric O_2
Secondary lymphedema with ulceration	Nonpitting edema	Lymphedema may complicate lipodermatosclerosis syndrome because of involvement of lymphatic channels by fibrotic process	Hyperbaric O_2

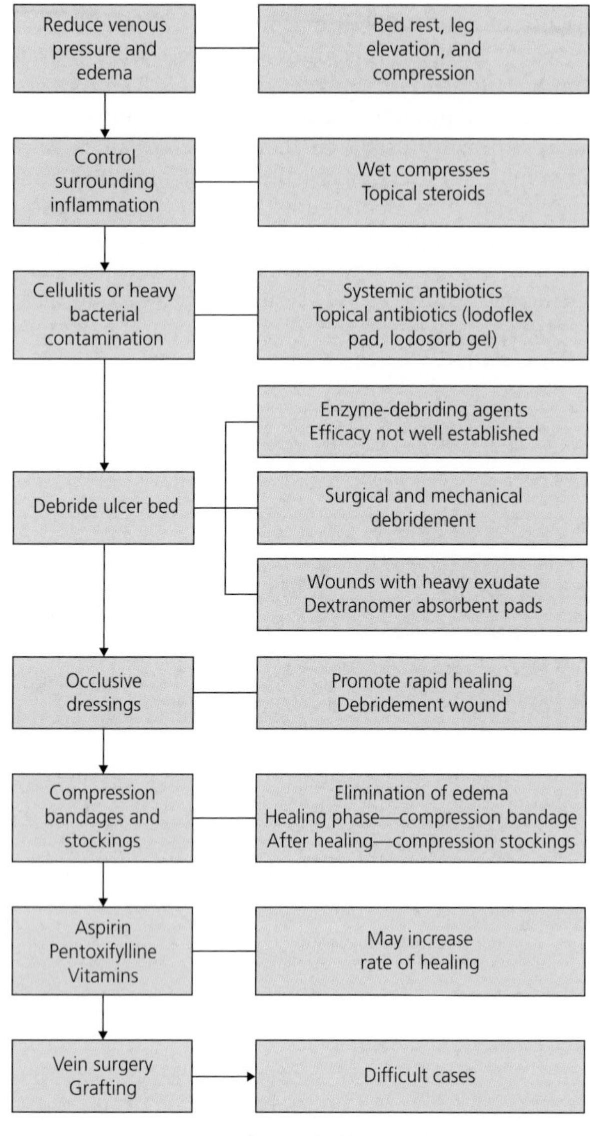

Figure 3-69

TREATMENT. Hospital-based wound care clinics are available for treatment. Venous pressure and leg edema can be reduced with bed rest, leg elevation, and compression. Contributing systemic disease, local infection, and inflammation should be treated (Figure 3-69). Stop cigarette smoking and excessive alcohol intake. Encourage good nutrition. Multivitamin supplements that contain vitamins C and E and zinc may help.

LEG ELEVATION. Venous hypertension must be reversed. Bed rest and leg elevation are effective. Elevation of the legs above the heart level for 30 minutes, three to four times per day, allows swelling to subside. Leg elevation at night is accomplished by raising the foot end of the patient's bed on blocks 15 to 20 cm high.

INFLAMMATION SURROUNDING THE ULCER. Tepid saline or silver nitrate (0.5%) wet compresses rapidly control inflammation. Silver nitrate is preferred when infection is present. Fresh compresses (replaced hourly) should be kept in place almost continuously for 24 to 72 hours. Fluids should not be added to dressings that are in place. Group V topical steroids are applied two to four times each day and may be covered with the compress. Patients with venous ulcers are prone to developing allergic reactions to topical medications in the surrounding compromised skin. Neomycin, paraben preservatives, and lanolin should be avoided. If inflammation persists after appropriate treatment, patch testing should be undertaken.

SYSTEMIC ANTIBIOTICS. Ulcers are typically contaminated with different aerobic and anaerobic bacteria, but routine administration of systemic antibiotics does not increase healing rates. Topical and/or systemic antibiotics may enhance wound healing when heavy bacterial contamination is present. Cellulitis must be treated with systemic antibiotics (see Chapter 9). Stasis dermatitis and cellulitis have a similar appearance and are often confused. Stasis dermatitis may act as a reservoir for infection. Dermatitis is easily treated with short courses of group I to IV topical steroids.

TOPICAL ANTIBIOTICS. Cadexomer-iodine (Iodoflex pad, Iodosorb gel) preparations have antimicrobial properties, debride wounds, and stimulate granulation tissue; other topical antiseptics may be toxic for wounds.

DEBRIDEMENT OF ULCER BED. Once cellulitis and eczematous inflammation have been controlled, the ulcer must be prepared for definitive treatment. Exudate and crust must be removed to expose granulation tissue, the foundation for new epithelium.

Wound debridement. Ulcers should be debrided of necrotic and fibrinous debris. Occlusive dressing, chemical debridement, and surgical and mechanical debridement are three methods that help to remove necrotic tissue and promote granulation tissue.

Occlusive dressings. Occlusive dressings promote rapid healing of leg ulcers. Many products are available; the choice is usually determined by the type of wound and the amount of exudate. These dressings should be used with compression for maximum benefit. Wound care clinics are proficient in the application of these dressings.

Chemical debridement. Enzyme-debriding agents may be considered to remove necrotic tissue. Santyl (collagenase), Panafil (papain), Granulex (trypsin), or Accuzyme is applied one or several times each day. The efficacy of all of these agents is not well established; Elase is ineffective.

Surgical or mechanical debridement. Debridement with sharp surgical instruments must be performed with great care so as not to damage delicate viable tissue. Whirlpool, wound irrigation, wet dressings, and hydrotherapy are all commonly used.

DEFINITIVE TREATMENT

1. Measure the ulcer at each visit.
2. Encourage elevation and periods of exercise and ambulation.
3. Minimize bacteria and necrotic debris.
4. Promote granulation tissue formation.
5. Induce reepithelialization.
6. Reduce edema.
7. Protect from trauma.

COMPRESSION. Compression is the cornerstone of therapy for venous ulcers. Elimination of edema is essential during treatment and after resolution. This is accomplished by applying external compression bandages during the healing phase and graded compression stockings after healing to prevent recurrence. Compression bandages can be applied over occlusive dressing during the healing phase. Some patients may have arterial insufficiency, as well as venous disease. Measure the ankle-brachial pressure index before compression to avoid necrosis or gangrene of the foot.

Compression bandages. Compression therapy and maintenance of a moist wound environment are essential. Compression improves venous hypertension and relieves edema. An external pressure of at least 35 to 40 mm Hg at the ankle is desirable. Many bandage systems are available.

GRADED ELASTIC COMPRESSION STOCKINGS. These stockings exert high pressure at the ankle, with pressure decreasing to the thigh. After healing, compression stockings should be worn to prevent ulcer recurrence. These stockings are put on in the morning soon after the patient gets out of bed. Patients with arthritis who have difficulty putting these stockings on may use the zip-up type. The amount of compression can be specified by the physician (see Table 3-7). Patients with chronic venous insufficiency who have had stasis dermatitis or ulceration require a compression of between 35 and 40 mm Hg. Various lengths can be purchased; an above-the-knee stocking may give the best results but knee-high stockings are most commonly used. The stockings may be difficult for older patients to put on; also, the stockings must be replaced periodically because they may stretch, thereby losing elasticity. Firmly applied Ace bandages are a less effective but convenient alternative.

There are four classes of stockings based on the compression exerted at the ankle.

Nonelastic bandages. Unna's boots (e.g., Dome Paste, Gelocast Bandage, Unna-Flex) are gauze bandages impregnated with zinc oxide paste to create a semirigid "boot" when applied. They protect ulcers from the environment and help control edema and are especially helpful in elderly or noncompliant patients because they can be left in place for 7 to 10 days. Because such a bandage does not eliminate existing edema fluid, it should be applied in the morning after edema has drained. However, when ulcers produce a large amount of exudate, the boot should be changed more often. Unna's boots are not applied over synthetic dressings.

Table 3-7 Compression Stockings (e.g., Jobst, Juzo, Sigvaris)

Class	Ankle pressure (mm Hg)	Indications
I	20-30	Varicose veins, mild edema, or leg fatigue
II	30-40	Moderate leg edema, severe varicosities, and moderate venous insufficiency
III IV	40-50 60	Severe edema or elephantiasis and severe venous insufficiency with secondary postthrombotic edema

Pneumatic compression pumps. Intermittent-compression pumps are considered when a venous ulcer does not respond to treatment with standard compression dressings.

ASPIRIN. Oral enteric-coated aspirin (300 mg) increased the rate of venous ulcer healing.

Pentoxifylline. Pentoxifylline (800 mg three times a day) accelerated the healing rate of venous ulcers and was more effective than the conventional dose (400 mg three times a day).

Vitamins. Patients with signs of malnutrition, such as low serum albumin or transferrin concentrations, may benefit from dietary supplementation. Ascorbic acid (1 to 2 gm/day), zinc sulfate (220 mg three times a day), and vitamin E (200 mg/day) may be used for supplementation. These vitamins are essential for wound healing but should not be prescribed in excessively high dosages.

Grafting. Skin grafts promote healing even if they do not take because they stimulate wound epithelialization. Split-thickness skin grafting is used for large ulcers. Meshed grafts are useful for large ulcers because they allow exudate to escape through the graft interstices. The donor site may be painful and slow to heal, especially in elderly patients. Pinch grafting is useful for smaller wounds. Multiple small pinches or superficial punch biopsies are taken from a donor site (e.g., thigh) and placed dermal side down on the ulcer bed. The tissue-engineered human skin equivalent Apligraf is effective for treating long-standing deep ulcers.

Vein surgery. Ligation or sclerosis of the long and short saphenous systems, with or without communicating vein ligation or sclerosis, is useful only if the deep veins are competent. Superficial vein surgery does not improve the healing rate of venous ulcers.

Chapter 4

Contact Dermatitis and Patch Testing

CHAPTER CONTENTS

- **Irritant contact dermatitis**
- **Allergic contact dermatitis**
  - Phases
  - Cross sensitization
  - Systemically induced allergic contact dermatitis
  - Clinical presentation
  - *Rhus* dermatitis
  - Natural rubber latex allergy
  - Shoe allergy
  - Metal dermatitis
  - Cement dermatitis and burns
  - Patients with leg ulcers
  - Cosmetic and fragrance allergies
- **Diagnosis of contact dermatitis**
  - Patch testing

Contact dermatitis is an eczematous dermatitis caused by exposure to substances in the environment. Those substances act as irritants or allergens and may cause acute, subacute, or chronic eczematous inflammation. To diagnose contact dermatitis one must first recognize that an eruption is eczematous. Contact allergies often have characteristic distribution patterns indicating that the observed eczematous eruption is caused by external rather than internal stimuli. Elimination of the suspected offending agent and appropriate treatment for eczematous inflammation usually serve to manage patients with contact dermatitis effectively. However, in the many cases in which this direct approach fails, patch testing is useful.

It is important to differentiate contact dermatitis resulting from irritation from that caused by allergy. An outline of these differences is listed in Table 4-1.

Table 4-1 Contact Dermatitis: Irritant versus Allergic

	Irritant	Allergic
People at risk	Everyone	Genetically predisposed
Mechanism of response	Nonimmunologic; a physical and chemical alteration of epidermis	Delayed hypersensitivity reaction
Number of exposures	Few to many; depends on individual's ability to maintain an effective epidermal barrier	One or several to cause sensitization
Nature of substance	Organic solvent, soaps	Low-molecular-weight hapten (e.g., metals, formalin, epoxy)
Concentration of substance required	Usually high	May be very low
Mode of onset	Usually gradual as epidermal barrier becomes compromised	Once sensitized, usually rapid; 12 to 48 hours after exposure
Distribution	Borders usually indistinct	May correspond exactly to contactant (e.g., watchband, elastic waistband)
Investigative procedure	Trial of avoidance	Trial of avoidance, patch testing, or both
Management	Protection and reduced incidence of exposure	Complete avoidance

IRRITANT CONTACT DERMATITIS

Irritation of the skin is the most common cause of contact dermatitis. The epidermis is a thin cellular barrier with an outer layer composed of dead cells in a water-protein-lipid matrix. Any process that damages any component of the barrier compromises its function, and a nonimmunologic eczematous response may result. Repeated use of strong alkaline soap or industrial exposure to organic solvents extracts lipids from the skin. Acids may combine with water in the skin and cause dehydration. When the skin is compromised, exposure to even a weak irritant sustains the inflammation. The intensity of the inflammation is related to the concentration of the irritant and the length of exposure. Mild irritants cause dryness, fissuring, and erythema; a mild eczematous reaction may occur with continuous exposure. Continuous exposure to moisture in areas such as the hand, the diaper area, or the skin around a colostomy may eventually cause eczematous inflammation. Strong chemicals may produce an immediate reaction; Figures 4-1 through 4-4 show examples of irritant dermatitis.

Patients vary in their ability to withstand exposure to irritants. Some people cannot tolerate frequent hand washing whereas others may work daily with harsh cleaning solutions without any difficulty.

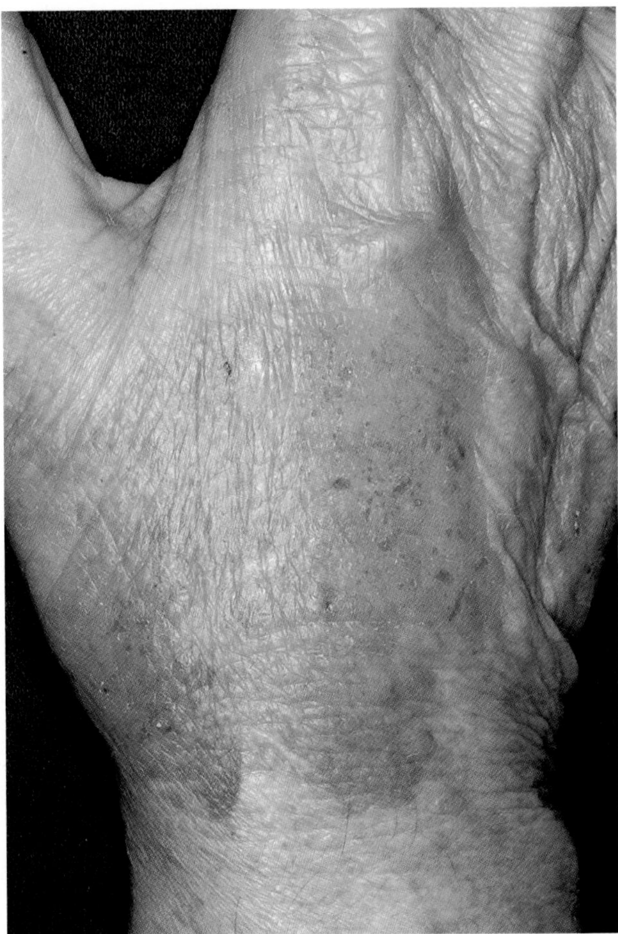

Figure 4-1 Irritant contact dermatitis. Chronic exposure to soap and water has caused subacute eczematous inflammation over the backs of the hands and fingers.

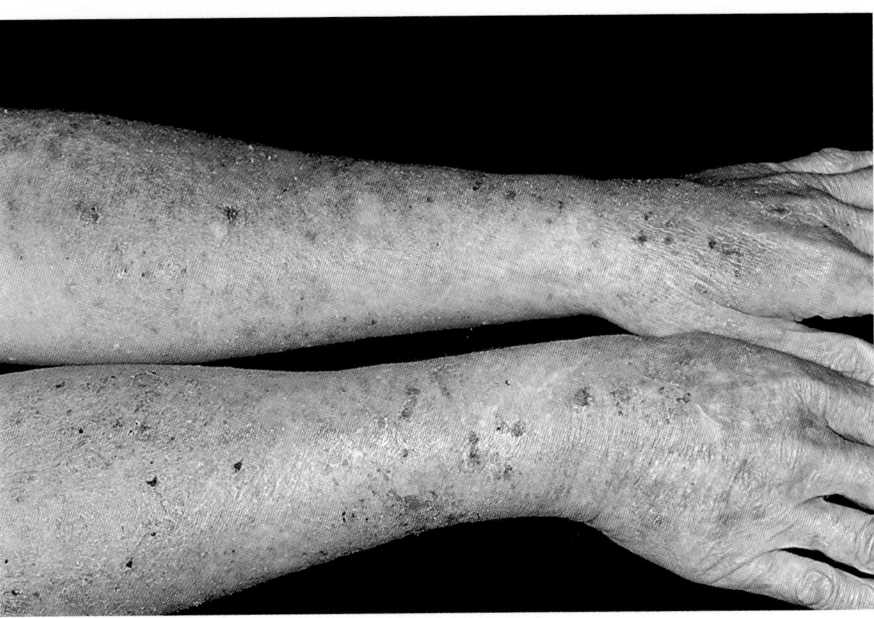

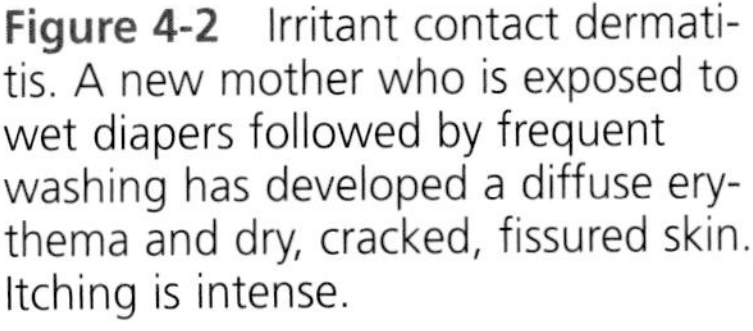

Figure 4-2 Irritant contact dermatitis. A new mother who is exposed to wet diapers followed by frequent washing has developed a diffuse erythema and dry, cracked, fissured skin. Itching is intense.

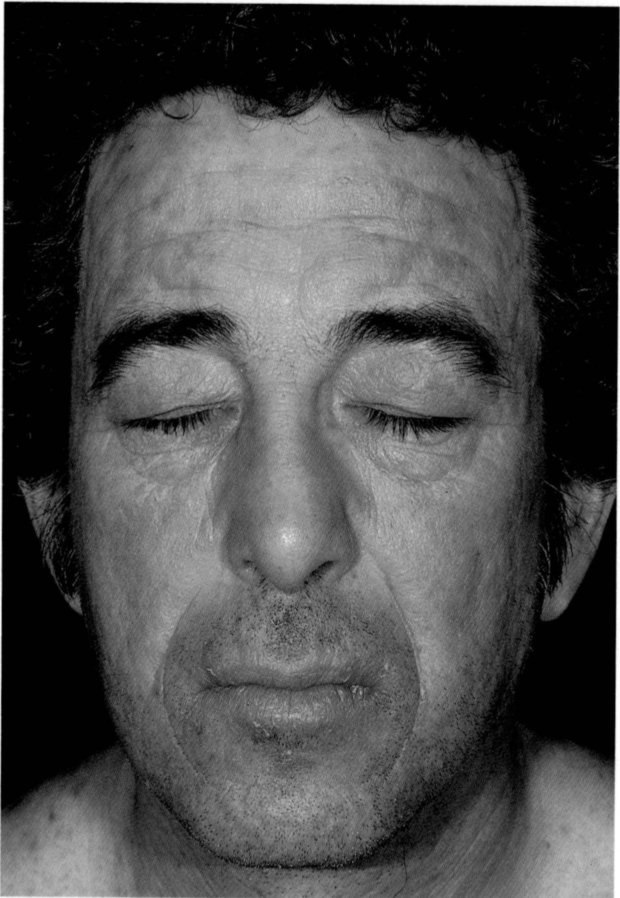

Figure 4-3 Exposure to industrial solvents has resulted in diffuse erythema with dryness and fissuring about the mouth.

MANAGEMENT OF IRRITANT CONTACT DERMATITIS

1. Avoid exposure to irritants by using protective equipment, such as gloves.
2. Topical steroids are used to initially control inflammation but there is some evidence that they may compromise barrier function. Some experts recommend that the use of topical steroids should be avoided.
3. Moisturizers used generously and frequently increase skin hydration, and their lipid component improves the damaged skin barrier. Lipid-rich moisturizers both prevent and treat irritant contact dermatitis.
4. Barrier creams containing dimethicone or perfluoropolyethers, cotton liners, and softened fabrics prevent irritant contact dermatitis.
5. Cool compresses are used for acute inflammation. They suppress vesiculation and decrease inflammation.
6. Hands should be washed in cool or tepid water.
7. Repeated low-level UV exposures may be effective for long-term resistant cases. Grenz-ray therapy is very effective but not generally available.
8. Even after the skin appears normal, it takes approximately 4 months or more for barrier function to normalize.

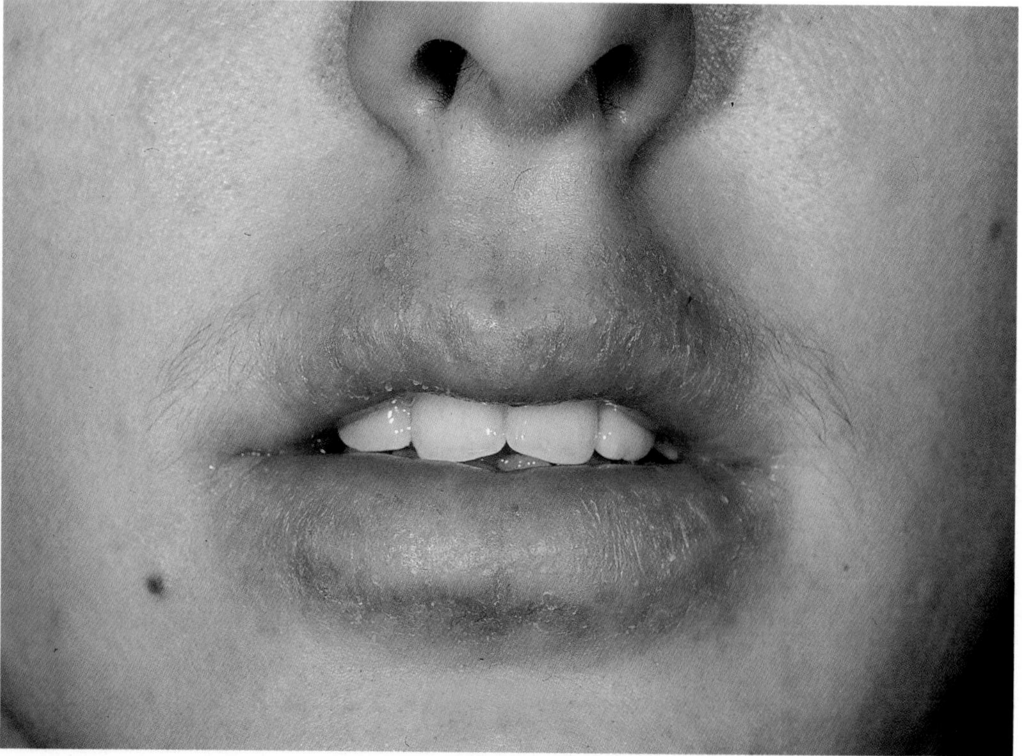

Figure 4-4 Repeated cycles of wetting and drying by lip licking resulted in irritant dermatitis.

ALLERGIC CONTACT DERMATITIS

Allergic contact dermatitis is an inflammatory reaction that follows absorption of antigen applied to the skin and recruitment of previously sensitized, antigen-specific T lymphocytes into the skin. It affects a limited number of individuals. The antigens are usually low-molecular-weight substances that readily penetrate the stratum corneum. Most contact allergens are weak and require repeated exposure before sensitization occurs. Strong antigens, such as poison ivy, require only two exposures for sensitization.

Interaction between antigen and T lymphocytes is mediated by antigen-presenting epidermal cells (Langerhans cells) and is divided into two sequential phases: an initial sensitization phase and an elicitation phase. Langerhans cells are abundant in skin and sparse at mucosal sites.

Phases

SENSITIZATION PHASE

Antigen is applied to the skin surface, penetrates the epidermal barrier (stratum corneum), and is taken up by Langerhans cells in the epidermal basal layer. The antigen is "processed" and displayed on the surface of the Langerhans cell. This cell migrates to the regional lymph nodes and presents the antigen to T lymphocytes. Cytokine-induced proliferation and clonal expansion within the lymph nodes results in T lymphocytes bearing receptors that recognize the specific antigen. These antigen-specific T lymphocytes enter the bloodstream and circulate back to the epidermis.

ELICITATION PHASE

The elicitation phase occurs in sensitized patients with re-exposure to the antigen. Langerhans cells bearing the antigen interact with antigen-specific T lymphocytes that are circulating in the skin. This interaction results in cytokine-induced activation and proliferation of the antigen-specific T lymphocytes and the release of inflammatory mediators. Allergic contact dermatitis develops within 12 to 48 hours of antigen exposure and persists for 3 or 4 weeks.

Cross-sensitization

An allergen, the chemical structure of which is similar to that of the original sensitizing antigen, may cause inflammation because the immune system is unable to differentiate between the original and the chemically related antigen. For example, the skin of patients who are allergic to balsam of Peru, which is present in numerous topical preparations, may become inflamed when exposed to the chemically related benzoin in tincture of benzoin.

Systemically induced allergic contact dermatitis

Systemic contact dermatitis results from the exposure to an allergen by ingestion, inhalation, injection, or percutaneous penetration in a person previously sensitized to the allergen by cutaneous contact. Patients allergic to poison ivy develop diffuse inflammation following the ingestion of raw cashew nuts (Figure 4-5). Cashew nut oil is chemically related to the oleoresin of the poison ivy plant. Persons allergic to balsam of Peru and/or fragrance mix benefit from dietary avoidance of balsams.

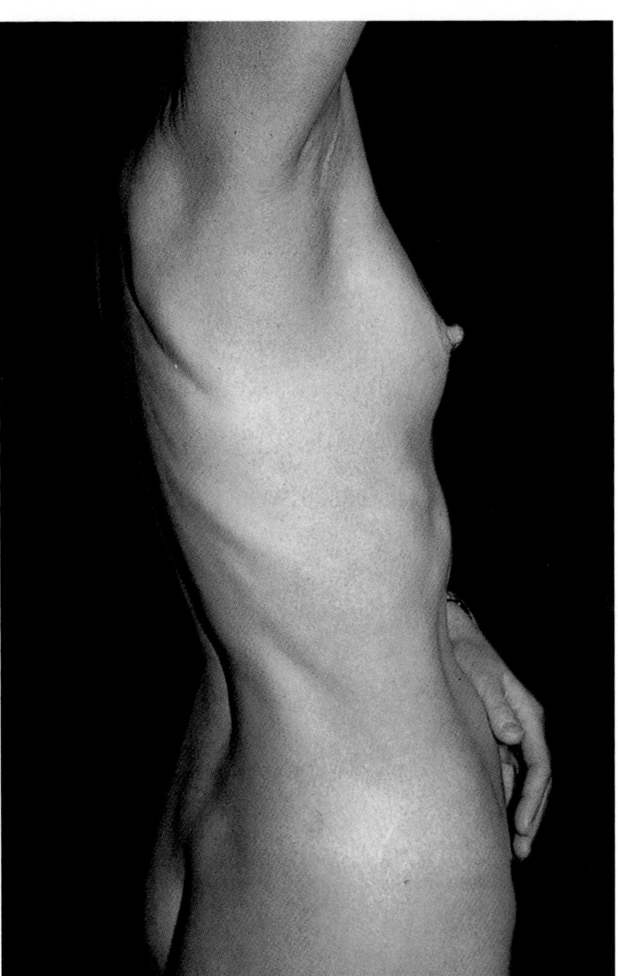

Figure 4-5 Diffuse allergic reaction occurring in a patient allergic to poison ivy who has ingested raw cashew nuts, the oil of which cross-reacts with the oleoresin of poison ivy.

Table 4-2 Contact Dermatitis: Distribution Diagnosis

Location	Material
Scalp and ears	Shampoos, hair dyes, topical medicines, metal earrings, eyeglasses, rubber ear plugs
Face	Cosmetics (preservatives, emulsifiers, fragrances) Acne medications (e.g., benzoyl peroxide), aftershave lotions Respirators, masks, aerosolized mists (machinists), volatile organic substances (e.g., amine hardeners in the plastic industry) Chemicals (hair dyes) applied to scalp spread to face, ears, and neck—spares scalp (scalp is resistant) Airborne allergens (poison ivy from burning leaves, ragweed) Photoallergic reactions—spare upper lip and have sharp cut-off at jawline (sunscreen ingredients—oxybenzone, benzophenone no. 3)
Eyelids	Nail polish (transferred by rubbing), cosmetics, contact lens solution, metal eyelash curlers, make-up sponges (rubber) Lower lids (topical medications) Periocular area (goggles)
Upper and lower eyelids	Cause is usually not allergic (atopic dermatitis, seborrheic dermatitis, psoriasis)
Facial and eyelid accentuation	Airborne contact dermatitis (ragweed, volatile organic substances, fragrances, chemicals in smoke) Products applied to hands and transferred to face (nail enamels)
Mucosal	Most patients allergic to allergens applied intraorally have cheilitis but not stomatitis; individual who reacts to nickel, mercury, palladium, or gold in dental amalgams presents with a systemic contact dermatitis with or without a localized stomatitis
Neck	Necklaces (metals, exotic woods), airborne allergens (ragweed), perfumes, aftershave lotion; cosmetic allergens; textile dermatitis (dyes, formaldehyde resins in clothing)
Trunk	Textile (sparing of axillary and undergarment areas) Azo-aniline dyes (color clothing) Urea formaldehyde resins (wrinkle-resistant clothing) NOTE: *para*-Phenylenediamine (PPD) and formaldehyde are not adequate screens for patch testing for allergy to textile dyes and resins Rubber allergens: Elasticized waist bands, spandex bras NOTE: Standard rubber patch test allergens may be negative; patch test with a portion of elastic band from a garment that has been bleached Generalized reactions Fragrances, preservatives in moisturizing lotions, topical medication, sunscreens; poison ivy; plants (phototoxic reactions); metal belt buckles Laundry detergents rarely cause allergic contact dermatitis
Scattered, generalized dermatitis	"Systemic contact dermatitis"—an individual who has been sensitized topically to an allergen and is subsequently reexposed systemically (drug/chemical introduced intramuscularly, intravenously, orally, rectally, or vaginally), foods, medical or dental devices that contact mucosal surfaces or that have been implanted surgically into body Cinnamic aldehyde and balsam (cosmetics, topical medications, suppositories, dental liquids, and flavorings) or parabens (food preservatives) Contaminants in foodstuffs, such as nickel
Arms	Same as hands; watch and watchband Photosensitive process (rash ends at mid-upper arm) Soap, moisturizing creams

Adapted from Belsito DV: *Dermatol Clin* 17:3, 1999. PMID: 10410868

Table 4-2 Contact Dermatitis: Distribution Diagnosis—cont'd

Location	Material
Fingertips	Hairdressers—glyceryl monothioglycolate in permanent solutions or *p*-phenylenediamine in hair dyes Nurses—glutaraldehyde in disinfectants Dental and orthopedic personnel—glue (methylmethacrylate) Many chemicals penetrate standard gloves
Axillae	Deodorant (axillary vault), clothing (axillary folds)
Hands	Soaps and detergents, foods, spices, poison ivy, industrial solvents and oils, cement, metal (pots, rings), topical medications, rubber gloves in surgeons
Genitals	Poison ivy (transferred by hand), rubber condoms, diaphragms, pessaries
Anal region	Hemorrhoid preparations (benzocaine, Nupercaine)
Lower legs, popliteal fossa, and inner thigh	Topical medication (benzocaine, lanolin, neomycin, parabens) Fragrances, preservatives, and vehicles in moisturizers and cosmetics Dyes in pantyhose (especially blue disperse dyes in darker-colored hose and disperse yellow no. 3 in flesh-colored hose) Textiles
Feet	Shoes—*p-tert*-butylphenol formaldehyde resin (a component of shoe glues), rubber components, and chromate (used to tan leather) Cement spilling into boots

Clinical presentation

SHAPE AND LOCATION. The shape and location of the rash are the most important clues to the cause of the allergen (Table 4-2). The pattern of inflammation may correspond exactly to the shape of the offending substance (Figures 4-6 through 4-9). The diagnosis is obvious when inflammation is confined specifically to the area under a watchband, shoe, or elastic waistband. Plants (e.g., poison ivy) produce linear lesions.

Unfortunately most allergic reactions do not conform precisely to the areas contacting the allergen. The woman allergic to an ingredient in her facial cosmetic typically presents with a patchy facial eczema, rather than with a diffuse dermatitis involving all areas of the face to which the cosmetic was applied. An allergen may be spread to other sites by inadvertent contact. The scalp, palms, and soles are resistant to allergic contact dermatitis and may show only minimal inflammation despite contact with an allergen that produces dermatitis in adjacent areas.

Aeroallergens inflame the exposed skin and spare clothed areas. Clothing allergens cause dermatitis of clothed areas. Table 4-2 lists substances that are common causes of inflammation in specific body regions. Table 4-3 lists substances commonly encountered in specific professions.

The failure of an eczematous dermatitis to respond to standard treatments also suggests that the dermatitis is allergic and not irritant.

INTENSITY AND PATTERNS. The intensity of inflammation depends on the degree of sensitivity and the concentration of the antigen. Strong sensitizers such as the oleoresin of poison ivy may produce intense inflammation in low concentrations whereas weak sensitizers may cause only erythema. The appearance also depends on location and duration. Acute inflammation appears as macular erythema, edema, vesicles, or bullae. Chronic inflammation is characterized by lichenification, scaling, or fissures. Contact allergies may have noneczematous patterns that include the cellulitis-like appearance of dermal contact hypersensitivity, lichenoid variants, contact leukoderma, contact purpura, and erythema multiforme.

DIRECT VERSUS AIRBORNE CONTACT. Acute and chronic dermatitis of exposed parts of the body, especially the face, may be caused by chemicals suspended in the air. Sprays, perfumes, chemical dusts, and plant pollen (e.g., ragweed) are possible sources. Inflammation from airborne sensitizers tends to be more diffuse. Photodermatitis can have the same distribution. Airborne material easily collects on the upper eyelids; this area is particularly susceptible. Volatile substances can collect in clothing.

Table 4-3 Contact Dermatitis: Occupational Exposure

Occupation	Irritants	Allergens
Beauticians	Wet work (shampoos)	Hair tints, permanent solution, shampoos (formaldehyde)
Construction workers	Fuels, lubricants, cement	Cement (chromium, cobalt), epoxy, glues, paints, solvents, rubber, chrome-tanned leather gloves
Chefs, bartenders, bakers	Moist foods, juices, corn, pineapple juice	Orange and lemon peel (oil of limonene), mango, carrot, parsnips, parsley, celery; spices (e.g., capsicum, cinnamon, cloves, nutmeg, vanilla)
Farmers	Milker's eczema (detergents), tractor lubricants and fuels	Malathion, pyrethrum insecticides, fungicides, rubber, ragweed, marsh elder
Forest products industry	Wet work (wood processing)	Poison ivy and oak, plants growing on bark (e.g., lichens, liverworts)
Medical and surgical personnel	Surgical scrubbing	Rubber gloves, glutaraldehyde (germicides), acrylic monomer in cement (orthopedic surgeons), penicillin, chlorpromazine, benzalkonium chloride, neomycin
Printing industry	Alcohols, alkalis, grease	Polyfunctional acrylic monomers, epoxy acrylate oligomers, isocyanate compounds (all used in a new ink-drying method)

ALLERGIC CONTACT DERMATITIS IN CHILDREN

Allergic contact dermatitis may account for as many as 20% of all cases of dermatitis in children. Poison ivy, nickel (jewelry), rubber (shoe dermatitis), balsam of Peru (hand and face dermatitis), formaldehyde (cosmetics and shampoos), and neomycin (topical antibiotic ointments) are the common allergens.

MANAGEMENT OF ALLERGIC CONTACT DERMATITIS

1. Minimize products for topical use.
2. Use ointments instead of creams (creams contain preservatives and are complex mixtures of chemicals).
3. Botanical extracts may be used in "fragrance-free" products.
4. When patch testing, also test the patient's consumer products.
5. Read product labels carefully. Many "dermatologist recommended" products contain sensitizers (e.g., lanolin, fragrance, quaternium-15, parabens, methylchloroisothiazolinone/methylisothiazolinone).

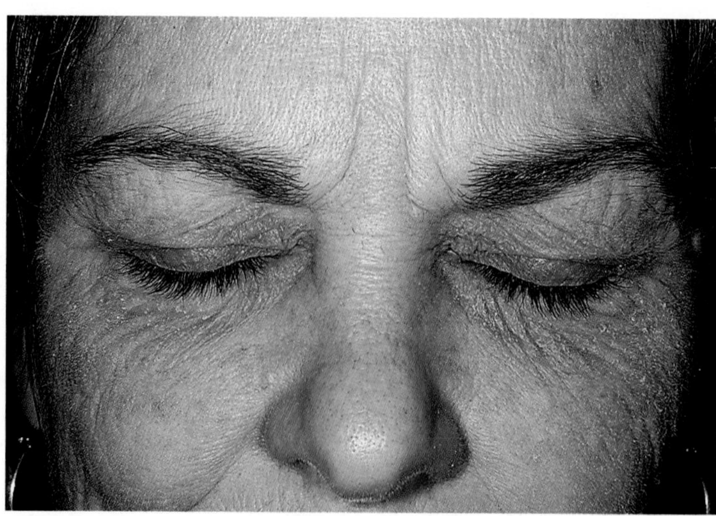

Figure 4-6 Eye cosmetic allergy. Open patch testing with the cosmetic proved the diagnosis. Routine patch testing was positive for fragrance mix.

ALLERGIC CONTACT DERMATITIS

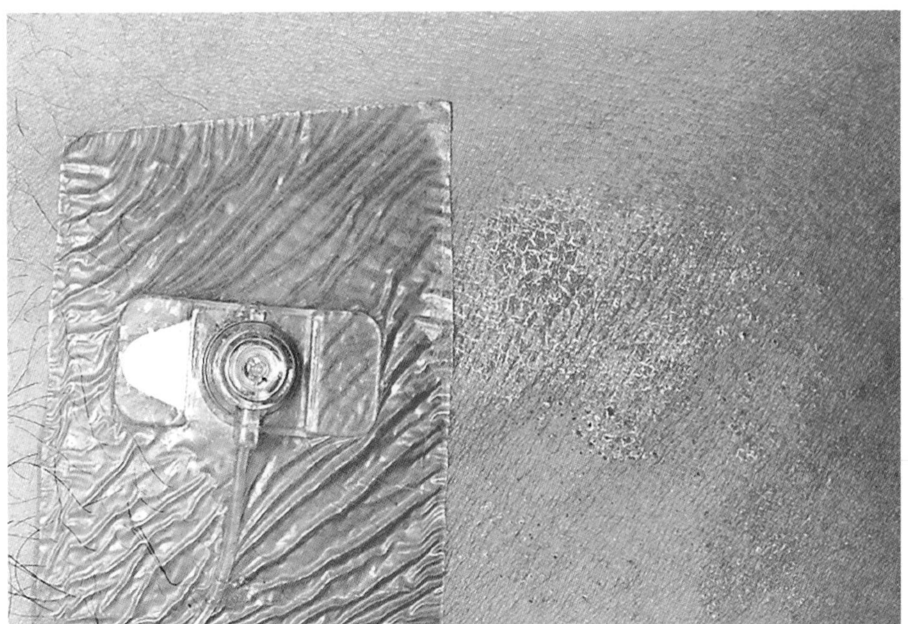

Figure 4-7 Adhesives allergy.

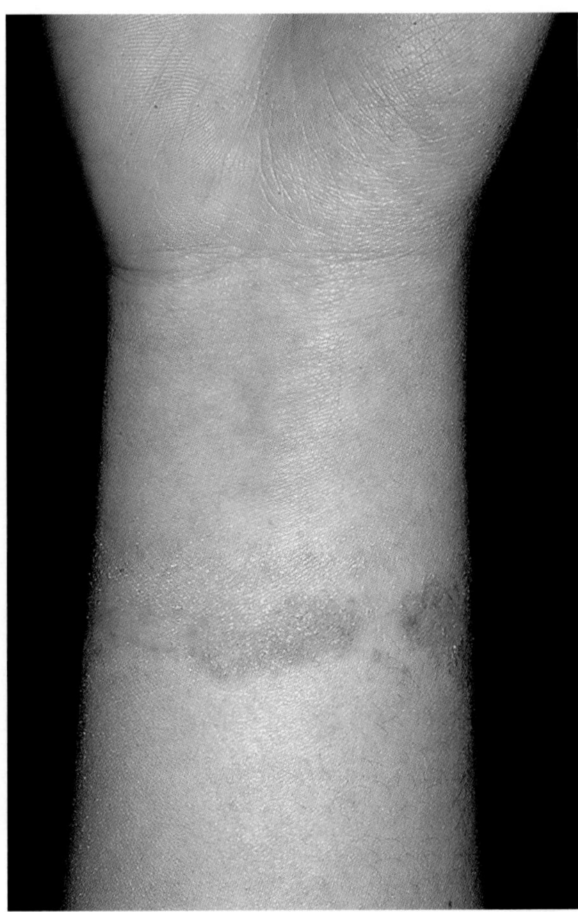

Figure 4-8 Potassium dichromate allergy (leather watch-band).

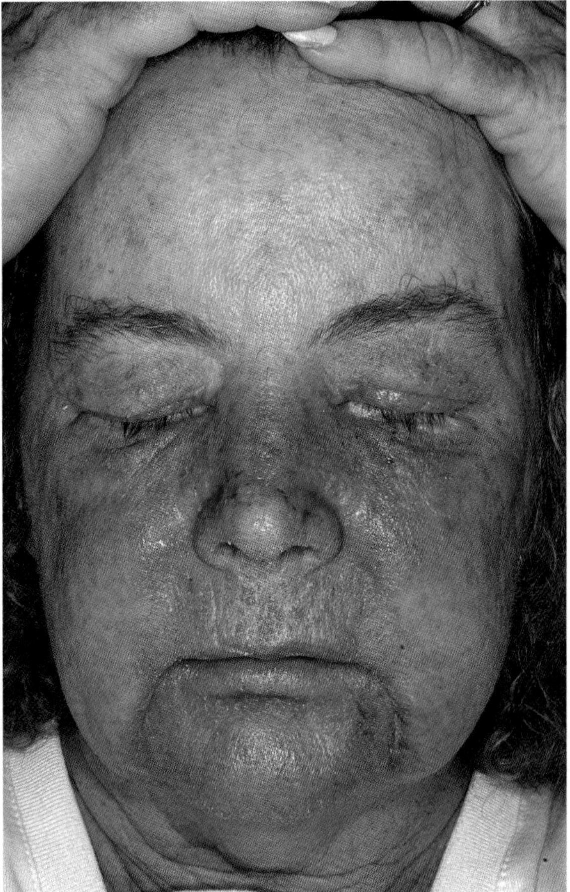

Figure 4-9 Exposure to poison ivy resulted in an intense acute inflammation.

Rhus dermatitis

In the United States poison ivy, poison oak, and poison sumac produce more cases of allergic contact dermatitis than all other contactants combined. The allergens responsible for poison ivy and poison oak allergic contact dermatitis are contained within the resinous sap material termed *urushiol*. Urushiol is composed of a mixture of catechols. All parts of the plant contain the sap. These plants belong to the Anacardiaceae family and the genus *Rhus*. Other plants in that family, such as cashew trees, mango trees, Japanese laquer trees, and ginkgo, contain allergens identical or related to those in poison ivy. Thousands of workers on cashew nut farms in India develop hand dermatitis from direct contact with the irritating resinous oil from cashew nut shells. Poison ivy and poison oak are neither ivy nor oak species.

CLINICAL PRESENTATION. *Rhus* dermatitis occurs from contact with the leaf or internal parts of the stem or root and can be acquired from roots or stems in the fall and winter. The clinical presentation varies with the quantity of oleoresin that contacts the skin, the pattern in which contact was made, individual susceptibility, and regional variations in cutaneous reactivity. Small quantities of oleoresin produce only erythema whereas large quantities cause intense vesiculation (Figures 4-10 through 4-13).

The highly characteristic linear lesions are created when part of the plant is drawn across the skin or from streaking the oleoresin while scratching. Diffuse or unusual patterns of inflammation occur when the oleoresin is acquired from contaminated animal hair or clothing or from smoke while burning the plant. The eruption may appear as quickly as 8 hours after contact or may be delayed for 1 week or more. The appearance of new lesions 1 week after contact may be confusing to the patient, who may attribute new lesions to the spread of the disease by touching active lesions or to contamination with blister fluid. Blister fluid does not contain the oleoresin and, contrary to popular belief, cannot spread the inflammation.

PREVENTION. Washing the skin with any type of soap inactivates and removes all surface oleoresin, thereby preventing further contamination. Washing must be performed immediately after exposure. After 10 minutes, only 50% of urushiol can be removed; after 30 minutes, only 10% can be removed; and after 60 minutes, none can be removed.

BARRIER CREAMS. The organoclay compound 5% quaternium-18 bentonite lotion (Ivy Block) prevents dermatitis in more than 50% of sensitized and exposed patients.

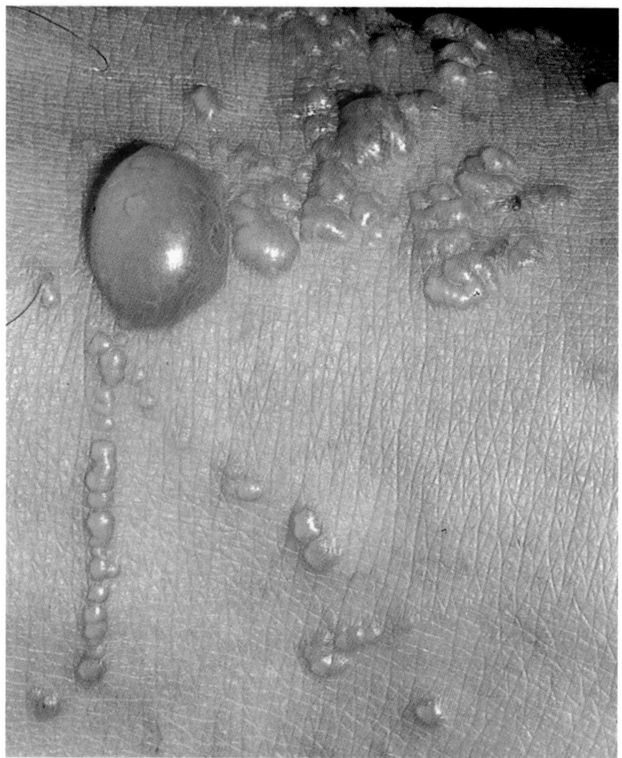

Figure 4-10 Poison ivy. A classic presentation with vesicles and blisters. A line of vesicles (linear lesions) caused by dragging the resin over the surface of the skin with the scratching finger is a highly characteristic sign of plant contact dermatitis.

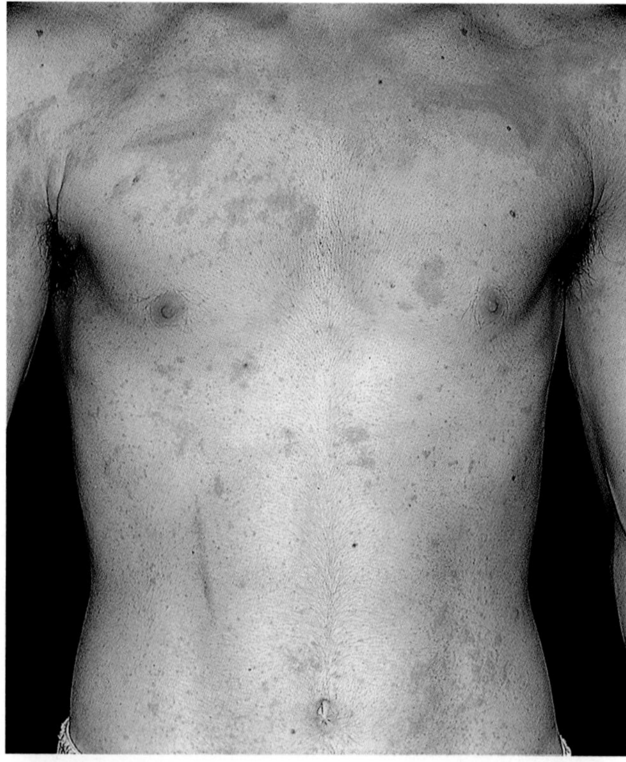

Figure 4-11 Poison ivy dermatitis. Acute inflammation over wide areas. The asymmetric distribution of intense erythema and vesicles suggests the diagnosis of an external insult. Linear lesions are highly characteristic. Inflammation of this intensity usually requires prednisone.

TREATMENT OF INFLAMMATION

Wet compresses. Blisters and intense erythema are treated with cold, wet compresses, and they are highly effective during the acute blistering stage. Cold compresses should be used for 15 to 30 minutes several times a day for 1 to 3 days until blistering and severe itching are controlled. Topical steroids do not penetrate through blisters. Short, cool tub baths with or without colloidal oatmeal (Aveeno) are very soothing and help to control widespread acute inflammation. Calamine lotion controls itching but prolonged use causes excessive drying. Hydroxyzine and diphenhydramine control itching and encourage sleep.

Topical steroids. Mild to moderate erythema may respond to topical steroids. Group I to V creams or gels applied two to four times a day rapidly suppress erythema and itching.

Prednisone. Severe poison ivy is treated with prednisone. A single-dose treatment schedule is shown in Box 4-1. Prednisone, administered in a dosage of 20 mg twice each day for at least 7 days, is an alternative schedule for severe, widespread inflammation. Tapering the dosage after this short course is usually not necessary. Patients who may have trouble adhering to a medication schedule may be treated with triamcinolone acetonide (Kenalog, Aristocort; 40 mg suspension) given intramuscularly. Commercially available steroid dose packs (e.g., Medrol Dosepak) should be avoided because they provide an inadequate amount of medicine and may cause recurrence of rash and pruritus after initial partial amelioration of symptoms during the first days of treatment (rebound dermatitis). Patients who do not initially seem to require medication may become much worse 1 or 2 days after an office visit; they should be advised that prednisone is available if their conditions worsen.

Box 4-1 **Prednisone for Severe Poison Ivy Dermatitis (Adults)**

Day	Dosage (mg/day) 10-mg tablets, taken as a single dose each morning
1-4	60
5-6	50
7-8	40
9-10	30
11-12	20
13-14	10

DIAGNOSIS. The diagnosis is usually obvious. The intense, often linear, vesicular eruption is highly characteristic. Patch testing is not done because the risk of inducing allergic reactions in individuals who have not yet been sensitized is high.

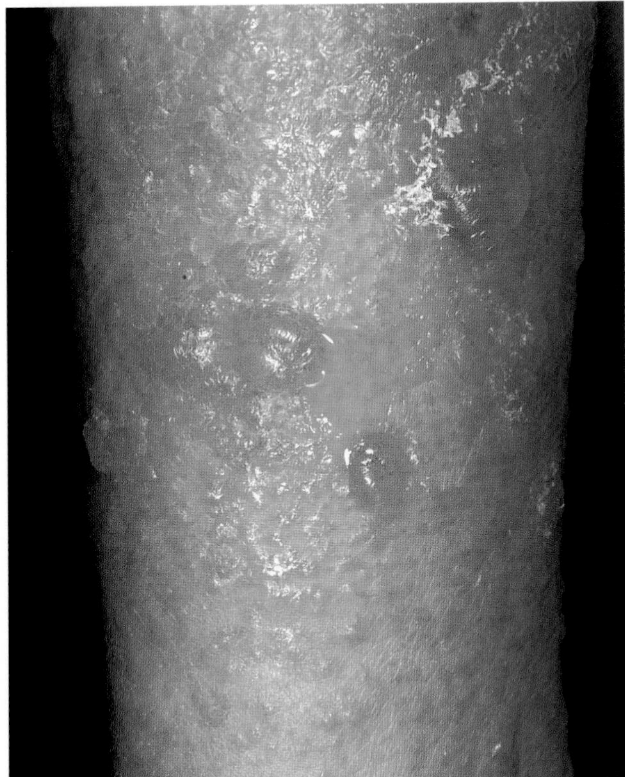

Figure 4-12 Poison ivy dermatitis. Exposure to the plant resulted in intense blistering.

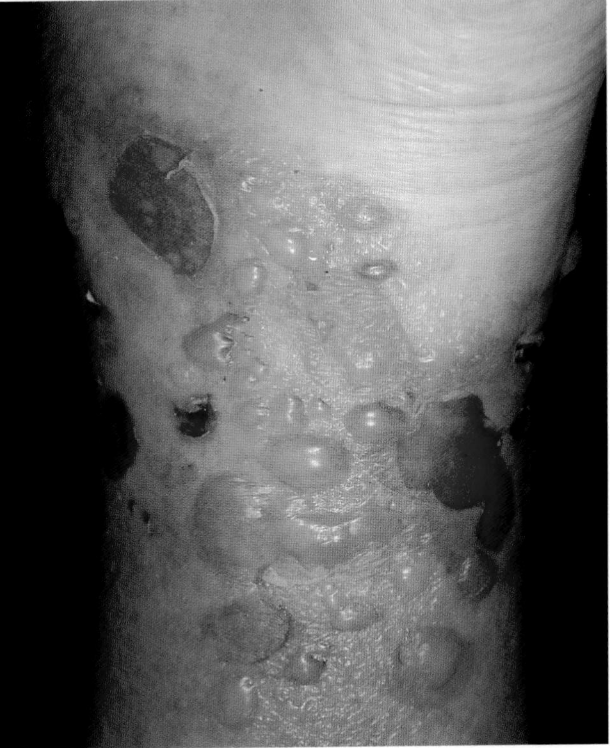

Figure 4-13 Poison ivy dermatitis. The intensity of the reaction was so great that hemorrhage appeared in the blisters.

Natural rubber latex allergy

Allergy to natural rubber latex (NRL) is a national health problem. Groups at highest risk include health care workers, rubber industry workers, and persons who have undergone multiple surgical procedures.

TYPES OF REACTIONS

There are three reactions to NRL products: irritant contact dermatitis, allergic contact dermatitis, and immediate-type hypersensitivity reaction.

IRRITANT CONTACT DERMATITIS. Irritant contact dermatitis is a nonimmune eczematous reaction caused by moisture, heat, and friction under gloves. Reaction severity depends on duration of exposure, degree of skin occlusion, and skin temperature. Symptoms include itching, erythema, and scaling followed by thickened, crusted plaques. The use of a cotton liner under NRL gloves can help.

ALLERGIC CONTACT DERMATITIS (TYPE IV ALLERGY). Latex allergy occurs in up to 10% of operating room nurses. Delayed-type hypersensitivity (type IV) T-cell–mediated sensitization to rubber accelerators (e.g., thiurams, carbamates, mercapto compounds) and antioxidants (not latex proteins) in latex gloves causes an allergic contact dermatitis usually limited to the sites of direct contact (e.g., dorsum of the hand) (Figure 4-14). Glove allergy was caused by thiurams in 72% of cases, carbamates in 25% of cases, and mercapto compounds in 3% of cases. Once sensitized, subsequent challenges from the same allergen will cause an eczematous dermatitis (erythema, scaling, vesiculation). Type IV allergy accounts for about 80% of occupationally acquired rubber allergy. The diagnosis is made by patch testing. The standard patch test screening series (see p. 149) contains the chemicals found in latex products. Patch testing with a thin piece of an NRL product (e.g., glove) may be helpful, but not in patients with suspected type I allergy to NRL. Hand dermatitis and atopy are risk factors for NRL allergy. Allergy to other forms of rubber also occurs (Figures 4-15 and 4-16).

TREATMENT. Once the allergen has been identified by patch testing, alternative rubber articles that use different rubber manufacturing chemicals can be obtained. Patients who have undergone or will require multiple surgical procedures should be offered a latex-safe hospital environment.

Surgeons with rubber sensitivity may use Elastyren or Tactylon hypoallergenic surgical gloves. Unlike latex rubber, these gloves are not vulcanized and therefore contain no metal oxides, sulfur, accelerators, or mercaptobenzothiazole, sensitizers commonly found in rubber products. Allerderm vinyl gloves, for household use, can be used with a cotton liner. Hypoallergenic vinyl gloves for examination are generally available. The unnecessary, "routine" use of latex gloves should be discouraged. Where their use is necessary, only powder-free gloves of low extractable protein content should be used. This should apply not only to all health care settings but also to other settings where glove use is common.

IMMEDIATE-TYPE HYPERSENSITIVITY (TYPE I ALLERGY). This immunoglobulin E (IgE)-mediated reaction requires previous sensitization. Reexposure to the allergen induces the release of histamine and other mediators. Skin exposure causes contact urticaria. Exposure to latex in the air elicits allergic rhinitis, conjunctivitis, asthma, anaphylaxis, and death. Allergic patients are vulnerable in the hospital setting. Latex allergy can present as IgE-mediated anaphylaxis during surgery, barium enema, or dental work. Intraoperative anaphylaxis and death can occur as a result of mucosal latex absorption at the time of surgery or procedure because of exposure to the surgeon's latex gloves. Mucosal exposure can occur from airborne powder particles, used as dry lubricant on gloves. The powder acts as a carrier for the latex proteins in the air. These particles can be dispersed when removing gloves and cause aerosol contamination, resulting in asthma. Patients with type I NRL allergy can have a cross-reaction to certain foods. Anaphylactic reactions (to banana, avocado, tomato, or kiwi) or local irritation when working with such foods has been reported.

DIAGNOSIS. Patients with a history of symptoms from rubber exposure can be screened with a radioallergosorbent test (RAST) to detect latex-specific IgE. If the RAST is positive, no further testing should be done. If negative (RASTs may have a false-negative rate of >30%), a "use" test utilizing a latex glove in a supervised setting may be performed, first with one finger, then an entire hand. If still negative, a skin-prick test should be done with eluted latex protein in solution. Anaphylactic reactions can occur with use and skin-prick tests, so life support equipment must be available. Skin-prick testing and immunoassay should be conducted only by persons experienced both in the techniques and in their interpretation. Skin-prick testing should be avoided in patients with a history of latex anaphylaxis.

TREATMENT. Nonlatex glove alternatives should be provided to health care workers who have type I reactions, and low-allergen, powder-free gloves should be worn by other health care workers at that worksite.

Vinyl gloves may leak and not provide an acceptable barrier for exposure to blood and body fluids. Double-gloving with vinyl gloves may provide greater protection during the performance of mucosal examinations (e.g., oral, rectal, vaginal). Thermoplastic elastomer gloves are more expensive but provide a barrier as effective as NRL gloves.

LATEX/RUBBER ALLERGY

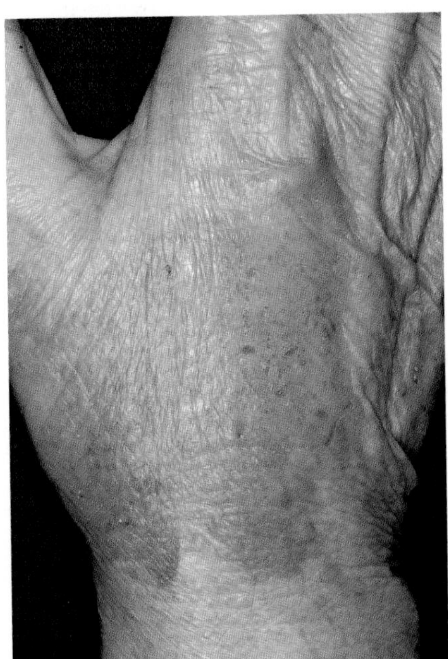

Figure 4-14 Latex glove allergy should be suspected in health care workers who present with eczema on the back of the hands.

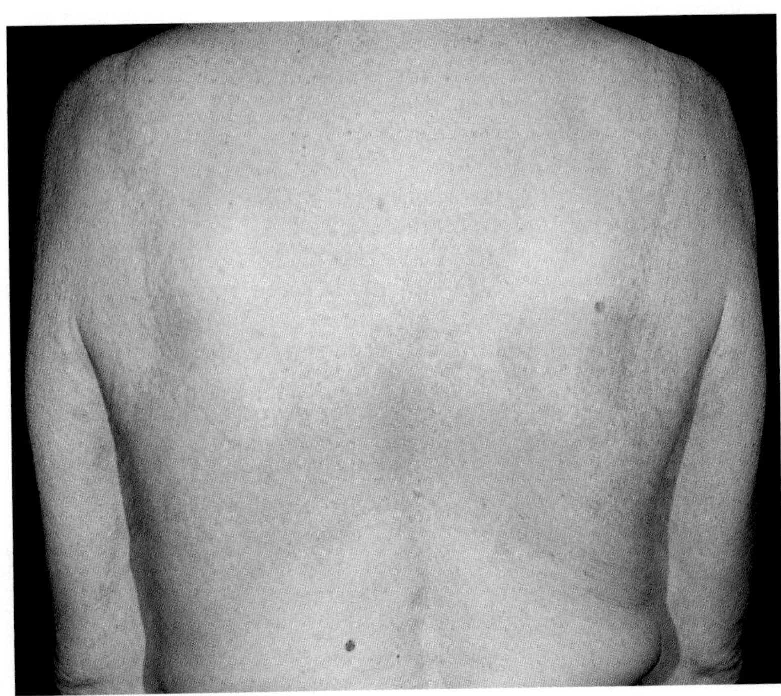

Figure 4-15 Spandex rubber in a bra caused this reaction.

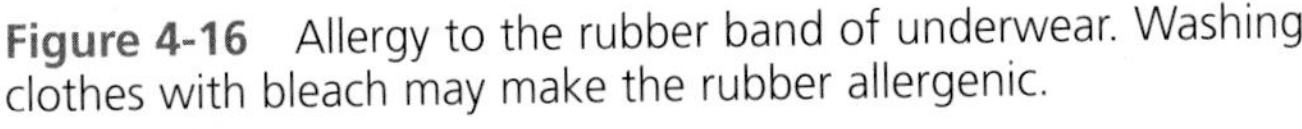

Figure 4-16 Allergy to the rubber band of underwear. Washing clothes with bleach may make the rubber allergenic.

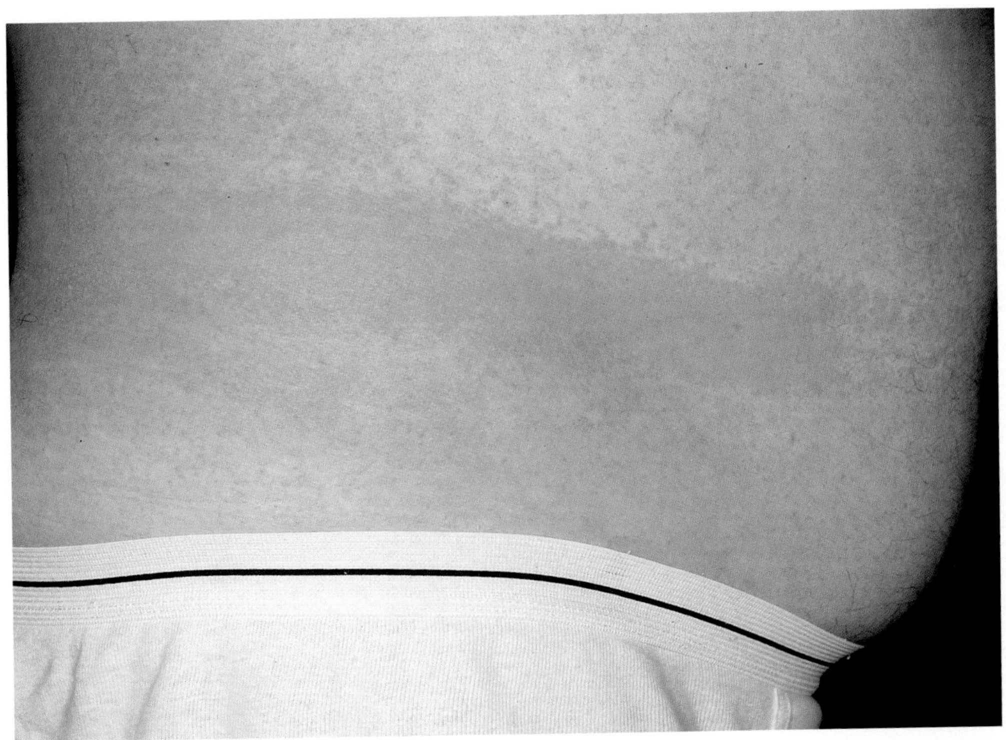

Shoe allergy

All patients with foot dermatitis that does not respond to treatment should be patch tested to exclude shoe allergy. Shoe allergy typically appears as subacute eczematous inflammation with redness and scaling over the dorsa of the feet, particularly the toes (Figures 4-17 and 4-18). The interdigital spaces are spared, in contrast to tinea pedis. Inflammation is usually bilateral, but unilateral involvement does not preclude the diagnosis of allergy. The thick skin of the soles is more resistant to allergens.

DIFFERENTIAL DIAGNOSIS. Fungal infections, psoriasis, and atopic dermatitis are common causes of inflammation of the feet. Shoe allergy should always be considered in the differential diagnosis of inflammation of the feet, particularly in children. Sweaty sock dermatitis, an irritant reaction in children caused by excessive perspiration, presents as diffuse dryness with fissuring on the toes, webs, and soles (see Figure 3-45). These irritated areas may become eczematous and appear as shoe contact dermatitis.

DIAGNOSIS. Patch testing is required to confirm the diagnosis of allergy. The standard patch test series can be used for screening. Special shoe patch testing trays are used by patch testing experts. Pieces of the shoe that cover the inflamed site should also be used for the patch test (Figure 4-18).

1. Cut a 1-inch square piece of material from the shoe and round off the corners.
2. Separate glued surfaces and patch test with all layers.
3. Moisten each layer with water, apply the samples to the upper outer arm, cover with tape, and proceed as described in the section on patch testing.

Rubber (e.g., mercaptobenzothiazole) is the most common allergen, followed by chromate, *p-tert*-butylphenol formaldehyde resin, and colophony. Mercaptobenzothiazole is a rubber component of adhesives used to cement shoe uppers, and potassium bichromate is a leather tanning agent. These chemicals are leached out by sweat.

MANAGEMENT. Patients with shoe allergy must control perspiration. Socks should be changed at least once each day. An absorbent powder such as Z-Sorb applied to the feet may be helpful. Aluminum chloride hexahydrate in a 20% solution (Drysol) applied at bedtime is a highly effective antiperspirant. Most vinyl shoes are acceptable substitutes for rubber-sensitive and chrome-sensitive patients. Inflammation of the soles may be prevented by inserting a barrier such as Dr. Scholl's Air Foam Pads or Johnson's Odor-Eaters. Once perspiration is controlled, it may be possible for sensitized patients to wear both leather shoes and shoes that contain rubber cement. Patients who need special allergy-free shoes should be referred to contact dermatitis clinics at university centers.

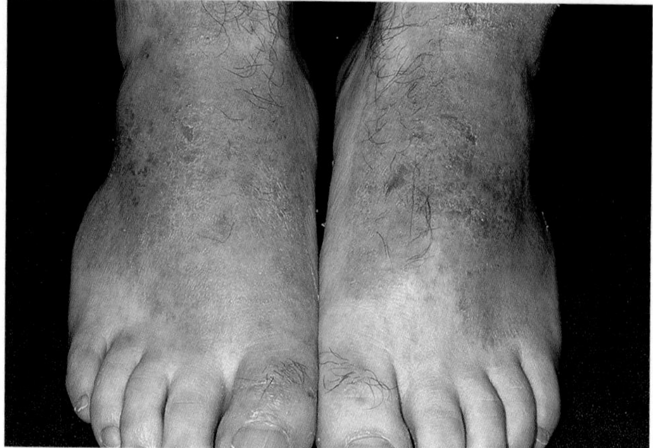

Figure 4-17 Shoe contact dermatitis. Sharply defined plaques formed under a shoe lining impregnated with rubber cement.

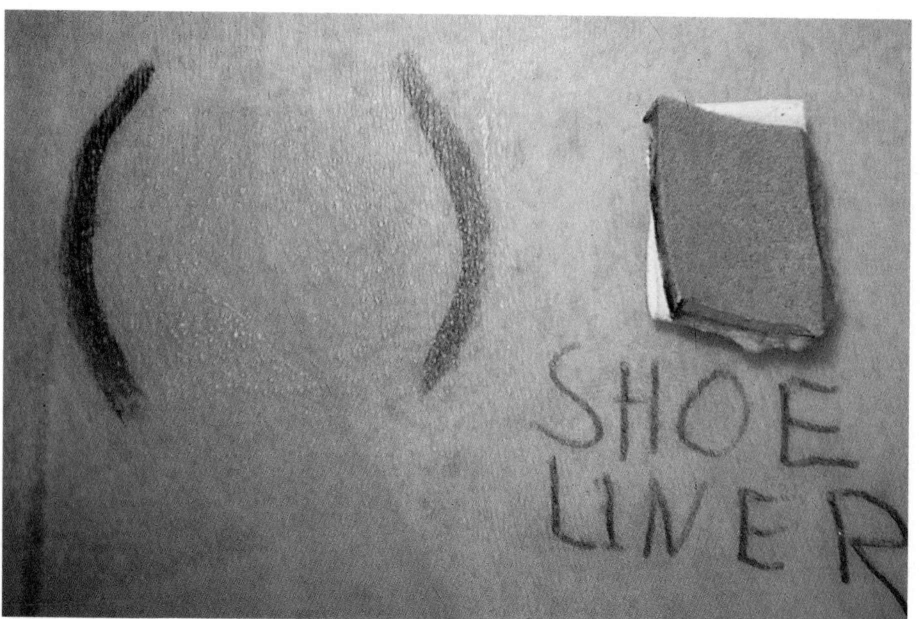

Figure 4-18 Patient in Figure 4-17 was patch tested with a piece of shoe lining. A 2+ positive allergic reaction occurred within 48 hours.

Metal dermatitis

NICKEL

Sensitization to nickel is the leading cause of allergic contact dermatitis worldwide. Women are affected much more frequently than men; men are usually sensitized in an industrial setting. The most common symptom of nickel allergy is a history of reacting to jewelry or to other metal contact on the skin. Allergy to other metals found in jewelry (e.g., palladium, gold) may be the cause of jewelry dermatitis. Ear piercing and the wearing of cheap jewelry are the most common causes of nickel sensitization. Previous sites of inflammation are more reactive than normal skin to rechallenge with nickel.

EARRINGS. Ear or body piercing or wearing clip-on earrings brings metal into direct contact with skin, an ideal setting for sensitization to occur (Figure 4-19). Ears should be pierced with stainless-steel instruments, and stainless-steel or plastic studs should be worn until complete epithelialization takes place. So-called hypoallergenic earrings may sensitize a person to a metal. Some nickel products that contain stainless steel may cause allergic contact dermatitis and others may not. Some gold earrings contain and release nickel. All-plastic earrings with fronts, posts, and backs made of hard nylon are now available.

OTHER SOURCES OF NICKEL. Avoidance is the only way to prevent inflammation. Sources of contact are necklaces, metal in clothing (such as jean buttons and zippers), scissors, door handles, watchbands, bracelets, belt buckles (Figure 4-20), keys carried in pockets, hair and eyelash curlers, hooks, buttons, and coined money (common in cashiers).

Nickel-sensitive persons are not at greater risk of developing discomfort in the oral cavity when wearing an intraoral orthodontic appliance. Modern plastic-to-metal joint replacements rarely cause sensitization to composite metals and are safe for nickel-sensitive patients. Acrylic bone cement has never been implicated in causing dermatitis, although orthopedic surgeons have become sensitized to the methylmethacrylate monomer used in the cement. Surgical skin clips should not be used in nickel-sensitive patients. Cooking with stainless-steel pans does not provide a source of nickel ingestion.

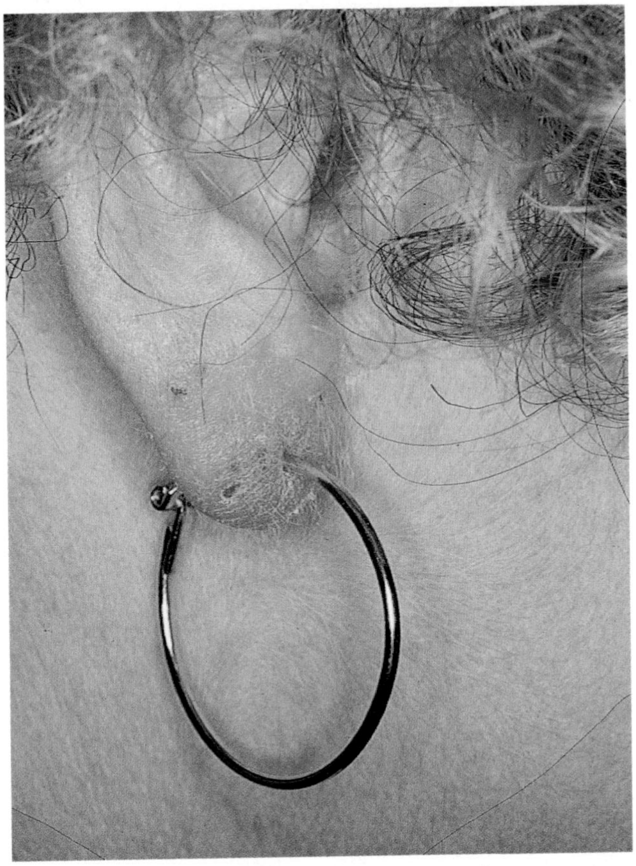

Figure 4-19 Nickel allergy. A classic presentation.

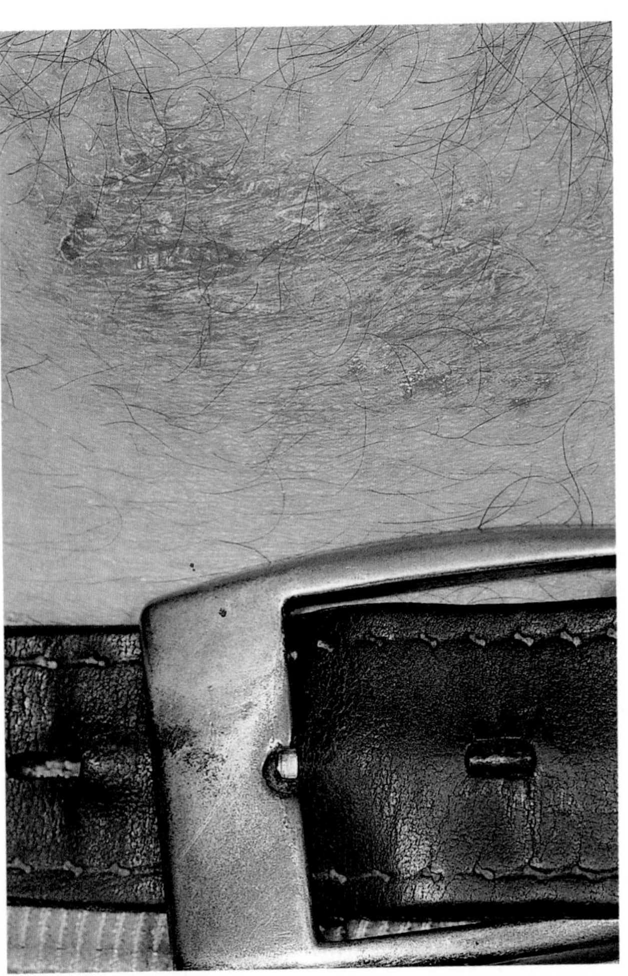

Figure 4-20 Nickel allergy. Belt buckle rubbed against abdomen when the patient bent over.

Box 4-2 **Suggested Diet for Nickel-Sensitive Individuals with Pompholyx**
Permitted foods: All meats, fish (except herring), poultry, eggs, milk, yogurt, butter, margarine, cheese, one medium-sized potato per day, small amounts of the following: cauliflower, cabbage, carrots, cucumber, lettuce, polished rice, flour (except whole grain), fresh fruits (except pears), marmalade/jam, coffee, wine, beer
Prohibited foods: Canned foods, foods cooked in nickel-plated utensils, herring, oysters, asparagus, beans, mushrooms, onions, corn (maize), spinach, tomatoes, peas, whole grain flour, fresh and cooked pears, rhubarb, tea, cocoa and chocolate, baking powder
Foods preferably should be cooked in aluminum or stainless-steel utensils or in utensils that give a negative test for nickel with dimethylgloxime.

DIMETHYLGLYOXIME SPOT TEST. The dimethylglyoxime spot test for nickel involves adding two solutions to a metal surface. If the solution turns pink, the test is positive. All nickel-sensitive patients should be taught how to use the dimethylglyoxime test. This enables them to determine which metallic objects they should avoid. Test kits are available from www.delasco.com and as an ALLEREST Ni test kit in the United States and internationally from Chemotechnique as the Nickel Spot test.

ORAL INGESTION OF NICKEL. Nickel is found in food and water. Some nickel-sensitive patients with periodic vesicular, palmar eczema (pompholyx) may benefit from a low-nickel diet (see Box 4-2). Some cases of so-called endogenous pompholyx-like eruptions in nickel-sensitive persons may be the result of exogenous contact with nickel-plated objects.

Oral ingestion of nickel in a person previously sensitized by contact exposure to nickel may elicit an eczematous reaction and the affected sites usually correspond to those involved in prior contact dermatitis.

Baboon syndrome. The term "baboon syndrome" or *intertriginous drug eruptions* has been used to describe a symmetric eczematous eruption involving the elbows, axillae, eyelids, and sides of the neck accompanied by bright red anogenital lesions. The term derives from the skin lesions, which are compared to the red gluteal region of the baboon. An allergic type IV reaction to systemically administered nickel or other allergens probably underlies lesions of this type (Figure 4-21).

PREVENTION. Diethylenetriaminepentaacetic acid (chelator) cream prevents nickel, chrome, and copper dermatitis.

PATCH TESTING. A positive history of allergic contact dermatitis but negative patch test results to nickel does not rule out nickel allergy. There is individual variation in nickel reactivity to patch testing. Some patients have a negative test reaction on one occasion and a positive test reaction at another time. The shorter the time interval between the previous exposure and reexposure, the stronger the reaction.

MERCURY DENTAL AMALGAM

The mercury amalgam that dentists use to fill decayed teeth does not contain nickel. Allergy to mercury is very rare. Patch testing to mercury is unreliable and rarely done. Gold alloyed with metal other than mercury is used for mercury-sensitive patients. Gold, however, is also a possible cause of allergic contact dermatitis.

CHROMATES

Trivalent chromium (insoluble) and hexavalent chromium (soluble) compounds are sensitizers. Trivalent chromium is found in leather gloves and shoes. Hexavalent chromium is found in cement. Chromate is possibly the most common sensitizer for men in industrialized countries. Sources are cement, photographic processes, metal, and dyes. Cement is the most common cause of chromate allergy and it acts both as an irritant and as a sensitizer.

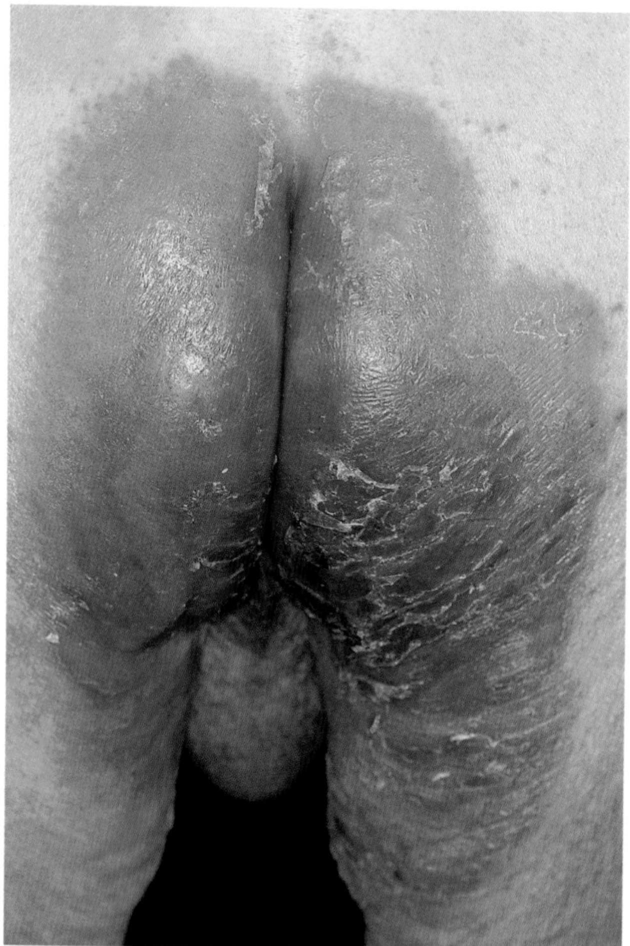

Figure 4-21 Ingestion of nickel in drinking water caused an intertriginous drug reaction called the baboon syndrome.

Cement dermatitis and burns

Most cement workers experience dryness of the skin when first exposed, but most seem to adapt. Severe deep cutaneous alkali (pH 12) burns may occur on the lower legs of men whose skin is in direct contact with wet cement. Initial symptoms are burning and erythema; ulceration develops after 12 hours. The most severe burns occur when cement spills over the boot top and is held next to the skin (Figures 4-22 and 4-23). Chronic pain and scarring may follow severe burns. Industrial workers sensitized to chromates in cement develop eczematous inflammation on the backs of the hands and forearms. The source of contact frequently is not appreciated until these patients do not respond to both topical and systemic steroids. Once the patient is removed from contact with cement, response to treatment is rapid.

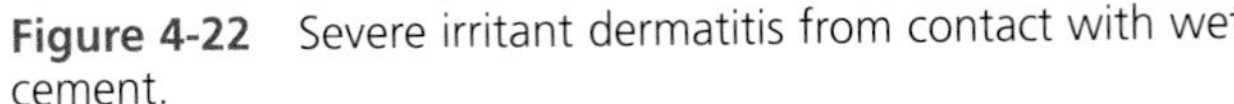

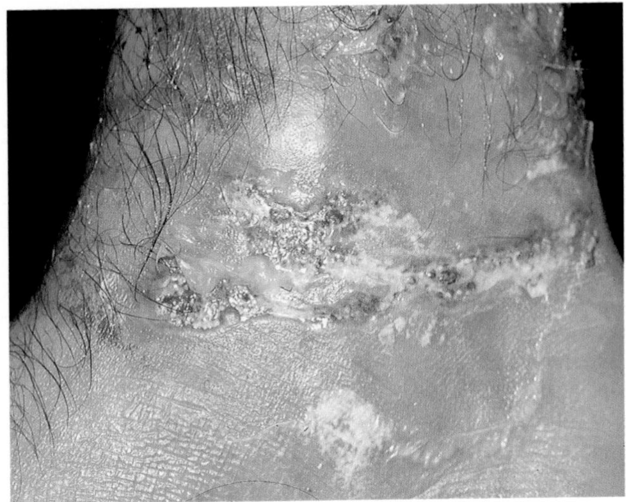

Figure 4-22 Severe irritant dermatitis from contact with wet cement.

Figure 4-23 Deep ulceration occurred after cement poured over the boot tops. This required months of treatment.

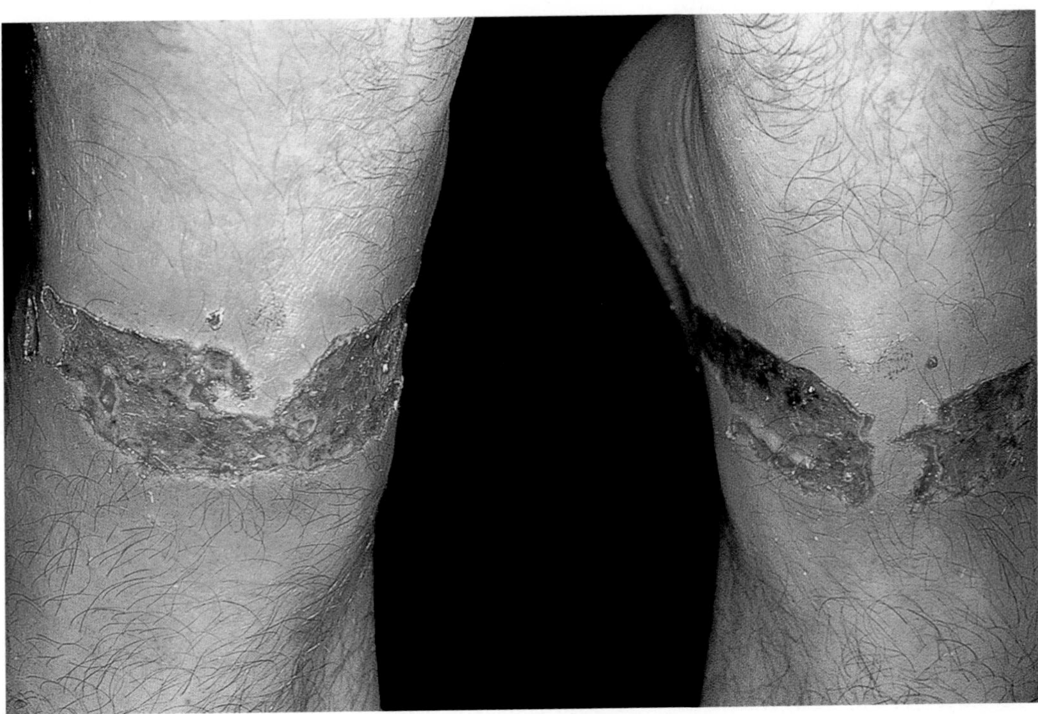

Patients with leg ulcers

Patients with leg ulcers, venous insufficiency, and lower leg edema may have an altered sensitivity to chemicals and are particularly susceptible to contact dermatitis of the lower legs. Topical medicines containing wool alcohols, lanolin, fragrance, parabens, and neomycin and bacitracin should be avoided (Figure 4-24).

Cosmetic and fragrance allergies

Cosmetics are frequently suspected of causing allergic reactions (Figures 4-25 through 4-27). Preservatives, fragrances, and emulsifiers are implicated. Patch testing can be done with suspected products. The Cosmetic, Toiletry, and Fragrance Association (www.ctfa.org) provides information on product formulation and ingredient characteristics of a wide range of products.

The most common cosmetic allergen is fragrance. Fragrances are ubiquitous and are used in a wide range of products other than cosmetics including perfumes, bath additives, deodorants, and household products. Allergy to the fragrance mix was found in 11.7% of patients who were patch tested by the North American Contact Dermatitis Group. Patch testing with balsam of Peru detects approximately 50% of patients with fragrance allergy. Most often when patients react to fragrance, the source of exposure is a skin or hair product with fragrance. Some so-called "fragrance-free" products may contain fragrance chemicals.

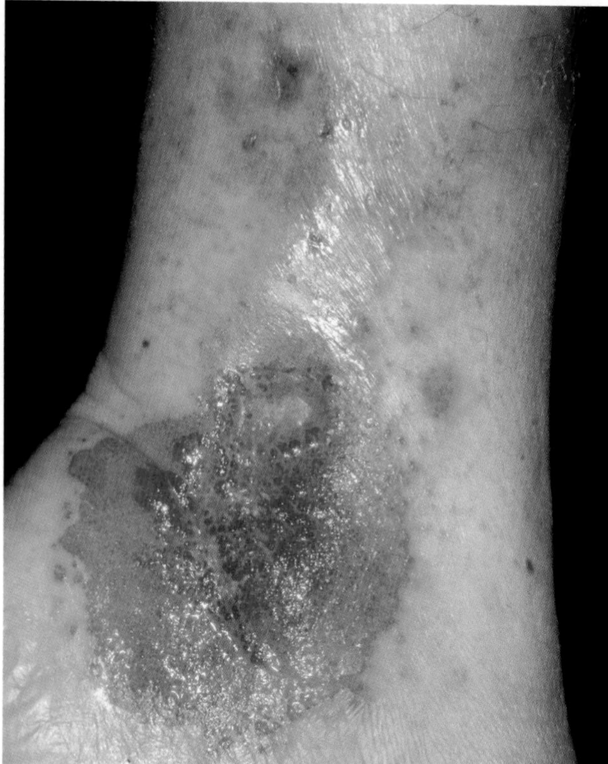

Figure 4-24 Patients routinely apply neomycin ointment to leg ulcers. An allergic contact dermatitis occurred suddenly. The patient had previously used neomycin for years without any ill effects.

BALSAM OF PERU AVOIDANCE DIET

Allergy to fragrance can be associated with systemic contact dermatitis to certain ingested spices and foods and may account for some cases of stomatitis, cheilitis, generalized or resistant palmar dermatitis, and plantar or anogenital dermatitis. Persons allergic to balsam of Peru and/or fragrance mix benefit from dietary avoidance of balsams (see Box 4-3 on foods to avoid if allergic to balsam of Peru or fragrance mix). Patients most likely to benefit from a balsam-restricted diet include those with (1) a chronic dermatitis of at least 1 year's duration that persists despite avoidance of cutaneous contact with known allergens, (2) a dermatitis that symmetrically involves the hands and/or feet, the anogenital area, and/or the skin folds, and (3) a positive patch test to balsam of Peru and/or fragrance mix. Place these patients on a balsam-restricted diet for at least 4 weeks and, if the dermatitis significantly improves, recommend long-term compliance. Subsequently, one food (e.g., tomatoes) can be reintroduced into the diet every several weeks to ascertain whether this particular substance exacerbated the dermatitis.

TOPICAL GLUCOCORTICOSTEROIDS

The medication used to treat eczema can be the cause. Allergic reactions to glucocorticosteroids may occur, and patch testing is required to prove the diagnosis. Patients can cross-react to multiple steroid preparations (see Chapter 2). The use of 3 or 4 screening corticosteroid allergens detects between 68% and 74% of corticosteroid allergies. Testing to an extended corticosteroid series is appropriate when corticosteroid allergy is suggested. *PMID: 17239989*

Box 4-3 **Balsam of Peru Diet (Foods to Avoid) for Selected Patients with Allergy to Balsam of Peru or Fragrance Mix**

- Products that contain citrus fruits* (oranges, lemons, grapefruit, bitter oranges, tangerines, and mandarin oranges), for example, marmalade, juices, and bakery goods
- Flavoring agents such as those found in Danish pastries and other bakery goods, candy, and chewing gum
- Spices* such as cinnamon, cloves, vanilla, curry, allspice, anise, and ginger
- Spicy condiments such as ketchup, chili sauce, barbecue sauce, chutney, and liver paste
- Pickles and pickled vegetables
- Wine, beer, gin, and vermouth
- Perfumed or flavored tea and tobacco, such as mentholated tobacco products
- Chocolate*
- Certain cough medicines and lozenges
- Ice cream
- Cola* and other spiced soft drinks such as Dr. Pepper
- Chili;* pizza, Italian, and Mexican foods with red sauces
- Tomatoes* and tomato-containing products

*Food items most commonly mentioned as causes of flare-up of dermatitis.

COSMETIC AND FRAGRANCE ALLERGIES

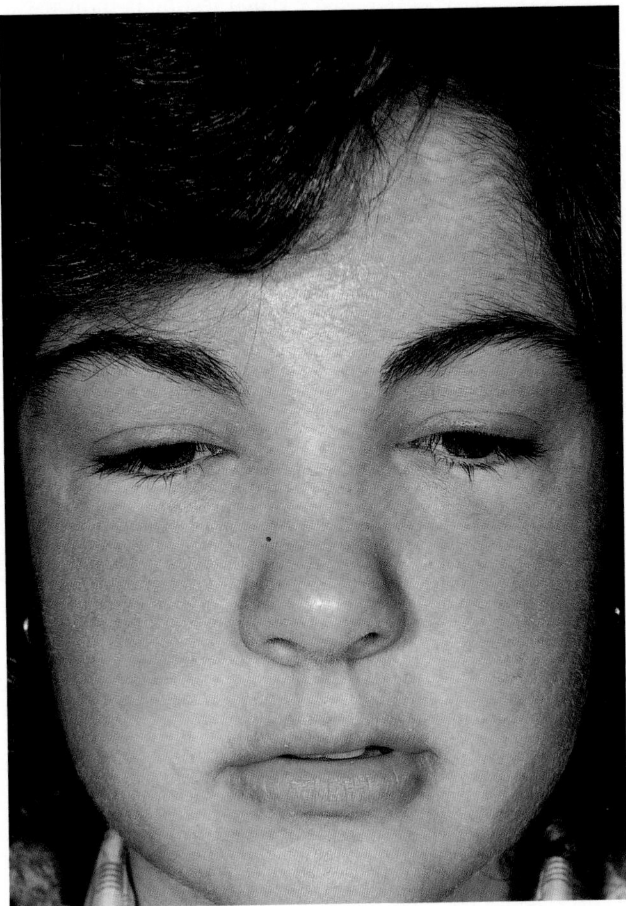

Figure 4-25 A beautician with diffuse erythema of the face. Patch testing showed a positive reaction (Figure 4-30).

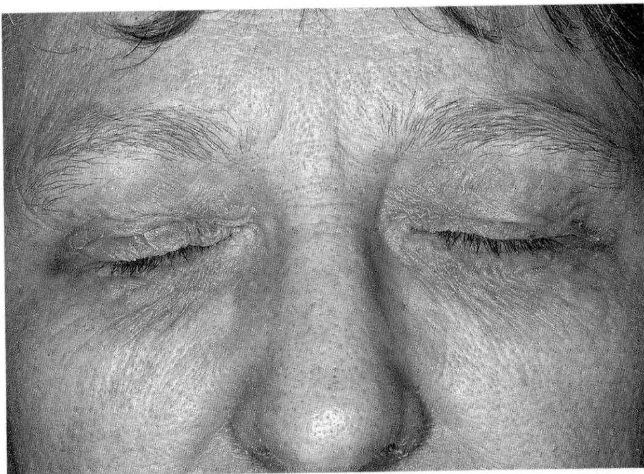

Figure 4-26 This patient purchased many different products in an attempt to find something she could tolerate. Fragrance allergy was later proven by patch testing. Fragrance-free cosmetics caused no inflammation.

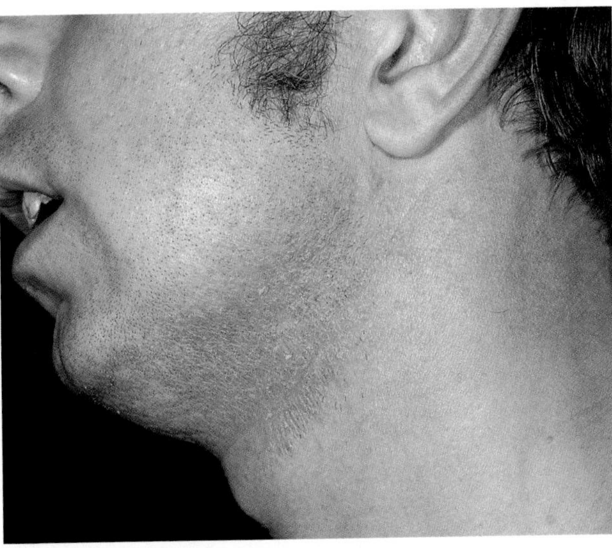

Figure 4-27 Allergic contact dermatitis occurred after application of after-shave lotion.

DIAGNOSIS OF CONTACT DERMATITIS

Determining the allergens responsible for allergic contact dermatitis requires a medical history, physical examination, and, in some instances, patch testing (Figure 4-28). Historical points of interest are date of onset, relationship to work (e.g., improves during weekends or vacations), and types of products used in skin care. The number of different creams, lotions, cosmetics, and topical medications that patients can accumulate is amazing and persistent questioning may eventually uncover the responsible antigen.

Patch testing should not be attempted until the patient has had time to ponder the questions raised by the physician. In many cases all that is required is to avoid the suspected offending material.

Patch testing

Patch testing is indicated for cases in which inflammation persists despite avoidance of the offending agent and appropriate topical therapy. Patch testing is not useful as a diagnostic test for irritant contact dermatitis because irritant dermatitis is a nonimmunologically mediated inflammatory reaction. Not all positive patch test reactions are relevant to the patient's condition, and it is essential that the relevance of positive reactions be determined.

OPEN PATCH TEST. The suspected allergen is applied to the skin of the upper outer arm and left uncovered. Application is repeated twice daily for 2 days and as described in the following section.

USE TEST. The suspected cream or cosmetic is used on a site distant from the original eruption. Suitable areas for testing are the outer arm or the skin of the antecubital fossa. The material is applied twice daily for at least 7 days. The test is stopped if a reaction occurs.

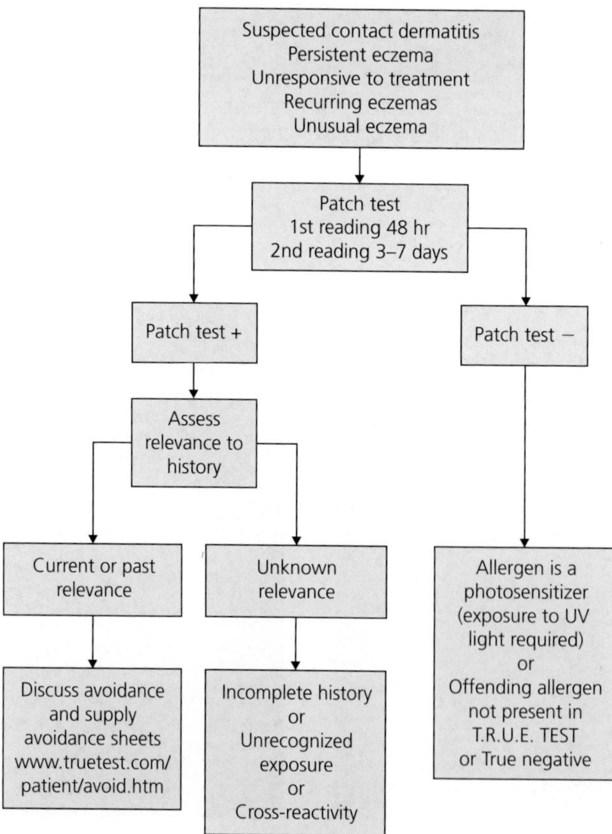

Figure 4-28

CLOSED PATCH TEST. The material is applied to the skin and covered with an adhesive bandage. The adhesive bandage is removed in 48 hours for initial interpretation (Figures 4-29 and 4-30).

Solid objects, such as shoe leather, wood, or rubber materials, or nonirritating materials, such as skin moisturizers, topical medicines, or cosmetics, are well suited to this technique.

Only bland material should be applied directly to the skin surface. Caustic industrial solvents must be diluted. Patch testing with a high concentration of caustic material may lead to skin necrosis. Petrolatum is generally the most suitable vehicle for dispersion of test materials. The concentration required to elicit a response varies with each chemical, and appropriate concentrations for testing can be found in standard textbooks dealing with contact dermatitis. If intense itching occurs, patches should be removed from test sites. A negative patch test with this direct technique does not rule out the diagnosis of allergy. The concentration of material tested may be too weak to elicit a response, or one component of a topical medication (e.g., topical steroids) may suppress the allergic reaction induced by another component of the same cream.

If this technique fails or if the clinical presentation is that of allergic contact dermatitis but a source cannot be uncovered by the history and physical examination, then patch testing with the standard patch test series should be considered.

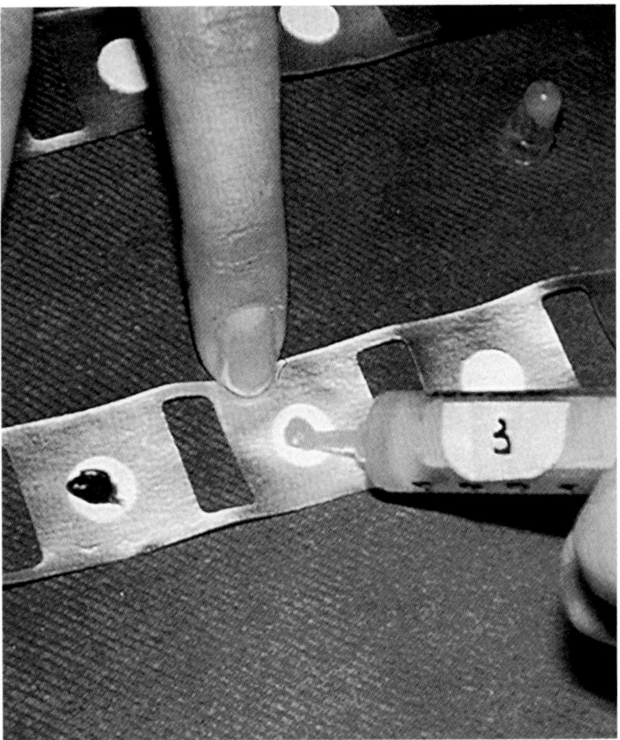

Figure 4-29 Patch testing. Individual allergens are tested on strips obtained from companies that sell individual allergens in syringes.

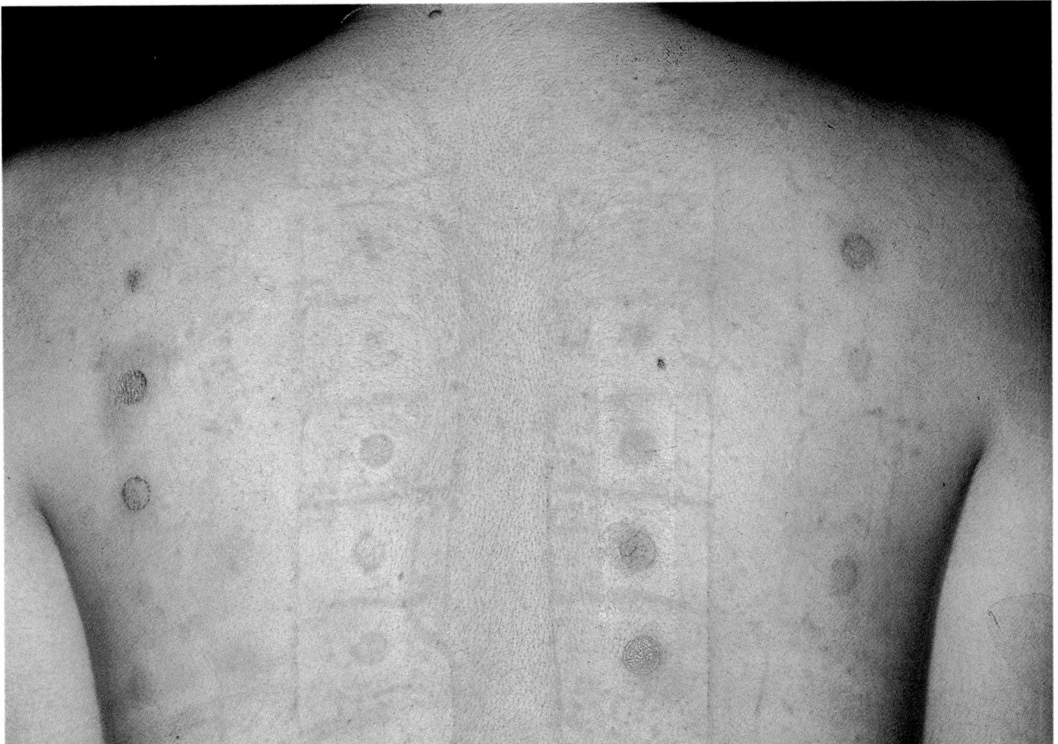

Figure 4-30 The patient in Figure 4-25 was patch tested with several of the preparations used at work. Many positive reactions of varying intensity appeared.

PATCH TEST ALLERGENS

Testing with groups of allergens is generally performed by physicians who frequently see contact dermatitis and have experience with the problems involved in accurately determining the significance of test results. A group of chemicals that have proved to be frequent or important causes of allergic contact dermatitis have been assembled into standard patch test series. The T.R.U.E. test (i.e., thin layer rapid use epicutaneous test) is a ready-to-use patch test for the diagnosis of allergic contact dermatitis. It contains 29 allergens and allergen mixes responsible for as much as 80% of allergic contact dermatitis (Table 4-4). Patch testing experts (usually based at university medical centers) use more allergens beyond those available in this standard series. These additional allergens are available from sources outside the United States. Positive reactions to fragrance mix, balsam of Peru, and the rubber additives thiuram and carba mixes may be missed if the T.R.U.E. test is used alone. TROLAB herbal patch test allergens from Europe are distributed in Canada and in many other countries. Search TROLAB on the web for details. They have a very large number of different allergens available.

TECHNIQUE FOR T.R.U.E. TEST. Each of the three T.R.U.E. test panels employs standardized allergens or allergen mixes fixed in thin, dehydrated gel layers attached to a waterproof backing. Moisture from the skin after application causes the gels to be rehydrated and to release small amounts of allergen onto the patient's skin. After 48 hours, the T.R.U.E. test is removed; reactions are then interpreted sometime between 4 and 7 days after application of the patches (Figures 4-31 and 4-32). The second reading is important for elderly patients, who mount an allergic reaction more slowly than younger patients. More than half of the reactions to neomycin are not evident until 96 hours after application of the patch test.

A number of important allergens are not included in the T.R.U.E. test. Consider referral to contact dermatitis experts at dermatology departments at university centers for further patch testing if T.R.U.E. test does not provide relevant information.

T.R.U.E. TESTING

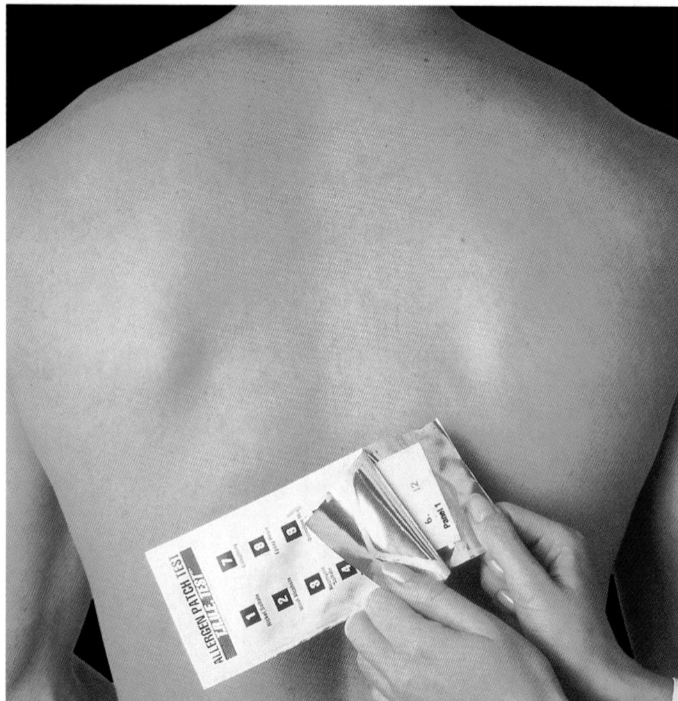

Figure 4-31 There are three T.R.U.E. test panels. The individual packages are opened and applied to the back.

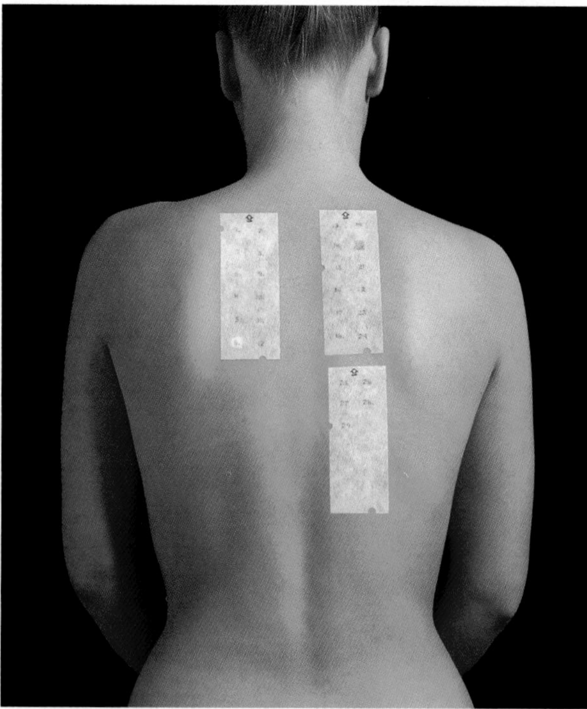

Figure 4-32 The three panels are applied to the back and removed 48 hours later.

Table 4-4 T.R.U.E. Test Allergen Patch Test of 29 Allergens

Component	Occurrence	Reaction frequency (%)*
1. Nickel sulfate	Jewelry, metal, and metal-plated objects	14.2
2. Wool alcohols	Cosmetics and topical medications	3.3
3. Neomycin sulfate	Topical antibiotics	13.1
4. Potassium dichromate	Cutting oils, antirust paints	2.8
5. Caine mix	Topical anesthetics	2.0
6. Fragrance mix	Fragrances, toiletries, scented household products, flavorings	11.7
7. Colophony	Cosmetics, adhesives, industrial products	2.0
8. Paraben mix	Preservative in topical formulations, industrial preparations	1.7
9. Negative control		
10. Balsam of Peru	Fragrances, flavorings, cosmetics	11.8
11. Ethylenediamine dihydrochloride	Topical medications, eye drops, industrial solvents, anticorrosive agents	2.6
12. Cobalt dichloride	Metal-plated objects, paints, cement, metal	9.0
13. *p-tert*-Butylphenol formaldehyde resin	Waterproof glues, leather, construction materials, paper, fabrics	1.8
14. Epoxy resin	Two-part adhesives, surface coatings, paints	1.9
15. Carba mix	Rubber products, glues for leather, pesticides, vinyl	7.3
16. Black rubber mix	All black rubber products, some hair dye	1.5
17. Cl^{+},Me^{-}-Isothiazolinone	Cosmetics and skin care products, topical medications, household cleaning products	2.9
18. Quaternium-15	Preservative in cosmetics and skin care products, household polishes and cleaners, industrial products	9.0
19. Mercaptobenzothiazole	Rubber products, adhesives, industrial products	1.8
20. *p*-Phenylenediamine (PPD)	Dyed textiles, cosmetics, hair dyes, printing ink, photodeveloper	6.0
21. Formaldehyde	Plastics, synthetic resins, glues, textiles, construction material	9.3
22. Mercapto mix	Rubber products, glues for leather and plastics, industrial products	1.8
23. Thimerosal	Preservative in contact lens solutions, cosmetics, nose and ear drops, injectable drugs	10.9
24. Thiuram mix	Rubber products, adhesives, pesticides, drugs	6.9
25. Diazolidinyl Urea	Products for personal care, hygiene, and hair care; cosmetics; cleaning agents; liquid soaps; pet shampoos	-
26. Imidazolidinyl Urea	Products for personal care, hygiene, and hair care; cosmetics; cleaning agents; liquid soaps; moisturizers	-
27. Budesonide	Anti-inflammatory agents; creams, lotions, ointments, and powders; ear, nose, and eye drops; inhalation drugs, tablets, and injectables; rectal suspension (colitis treatments)	-
28. Tixocortol-21-Pivalate	Anti-inflammatory agents/prescription and non-prescription; nasal suspensions for rhinitis; lozenges for pharyngitis; rectal suspension for ulcerative colitis	-
29. Quinolinemix	Paste bandages; prescription and non-prescription preparations as: topical antibiotics and antifungal creams, lotions, ointments; animal food; bacteriostatic and fungistatic cream (e.g., sterosan cream)	-

*These results were obtained with another patch testing system used by the North American Patch Test Group.
Reference manual and allergen avoidance sheets are available online at www.truetest.com. From North American Contact Dermatitis Group: Patch test results, 1996-1998 and 2001-2002 study period, *Dermatitis* 15(4):176-183, 2004. *PMID: 15842061*

PATCH TEST GRADING

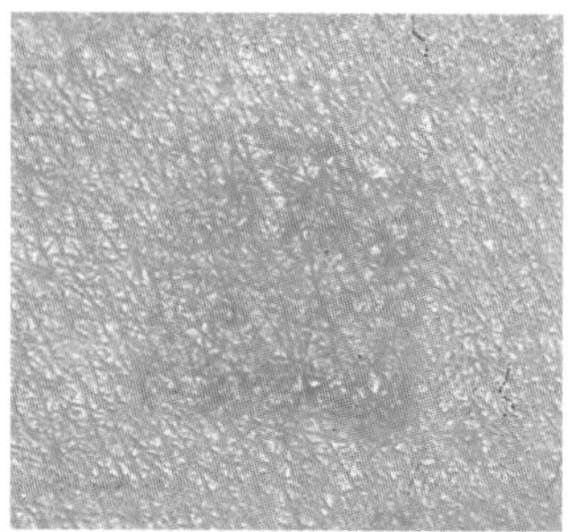

Figure 4-33 A 1+ positive patch test reaction with erythema.

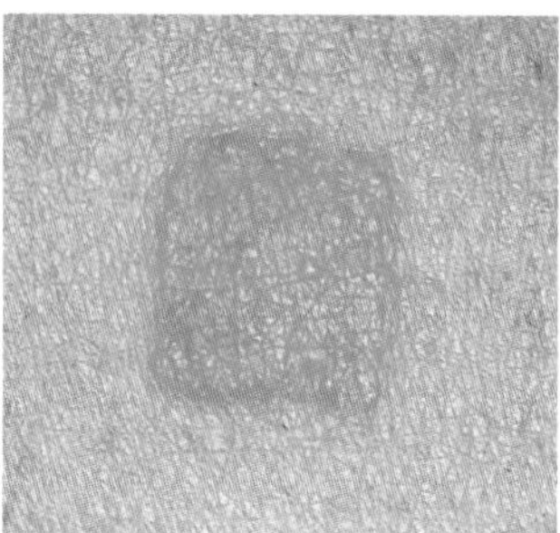

Figure 4-34 A 2+ positive patch test reaction with erythema and vesicles.

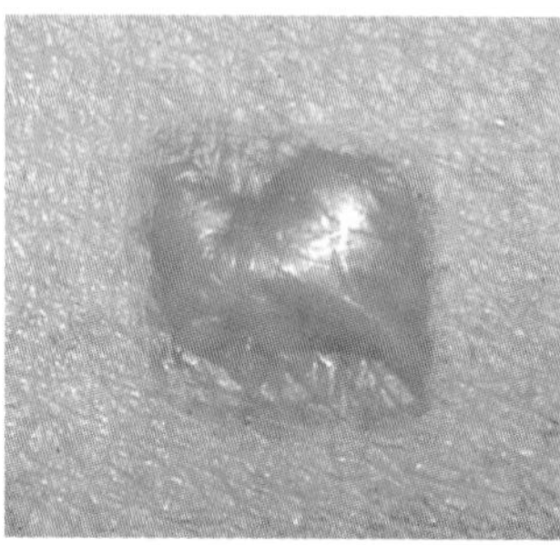

Figure 4-35 A 3+ positive patch test reaction with vesicles and bullae.

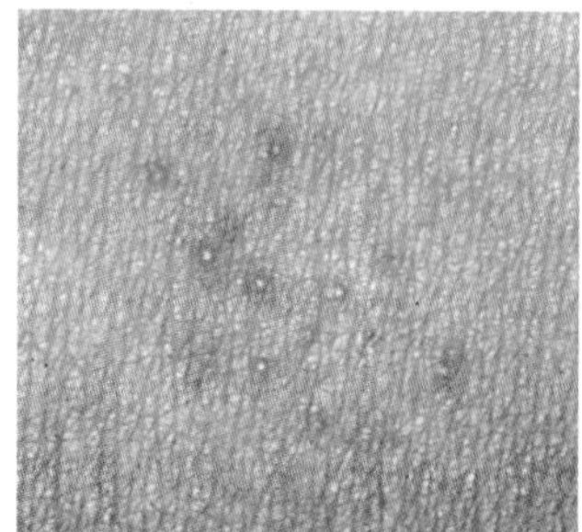

Figure 4-36 This is a pustular irritant reaction. This may happen with allergens such as nickel. This is not a positive test for allergy.

PATCH TEST READING AND INTERPRETATION

The test reactions are graded at each reading as follows:

+ = Weak (nonvesicular) positive reaction: erythema, infiltration, and possibly papules (Figure 4-33)
++ = Strong (edematous or vesicular) positive reaction (Figure 4-34)
+++ = Extreme (spreading, bullous, ulcerative) positive reaction (Figure 4-35)
− = Negative reaction
IR = Irritant reactions of different types (Figure 4-36)
NT = Not tested
Doubtful reaction (macular erythema only)

ALLERGIC VERSUS IRRITANT TEST REACTIONS

It is important to determine whether the test response is caused by allergy or by a nonspecific irritant reaction. Strong allergic reactions are vesicular and may spread beyond the test site. Strong irritant reactions exhibit a deep erythema, resembling a burn. There is no morphologic method of distinguishing a weak irritant patch test from a weak allergic test. Commercially prepared antigens are formulated to minimize irritant reactions. Irritant test responses are caused either by hyperirritability of the skin or by the application of an irritating concentration of a test substance. Irritation is avoided by applying tests only on normal skin that has not been washed or cleaned with alcohol.

WHEN NOT TO PERFORM PATCH TESTING

Avoid testing in the presence of an active, flaring dermatitis that covers more than 25% of the body surface area. Under these conditions, the "angry back reaction" with numerous false-positive tests frequently occurs. Defer testing until 1 or 2 weeks following treatments known to interfere with delayed-type hypersensitivity reactions such as systemic corticosteroids, immunosuppressants (e.g., cyclophosphamide, azathioprine), and ultraviolet B or psoralen plus ultraviolet A (PUVA) phototherapy.

STEROIDS AND PATCH TESTING. Corticosteroids such as prednisone in dosages of 15 mg/day or the equivalent may inhibit patch test reactions. If a patient has been treated with systemic corticosteroids, patch testing should be delayed for at least 2 weeks. The prior application of the group V topical steroid triamcinolone acetonide to skin does not strongly influence patch test reactions. If topical corticosteroids are being used on the back, patch testing should be delayed for 3 days. Allergic contact dermatitis to topical corticosteroids is possible (see Chapter 2).

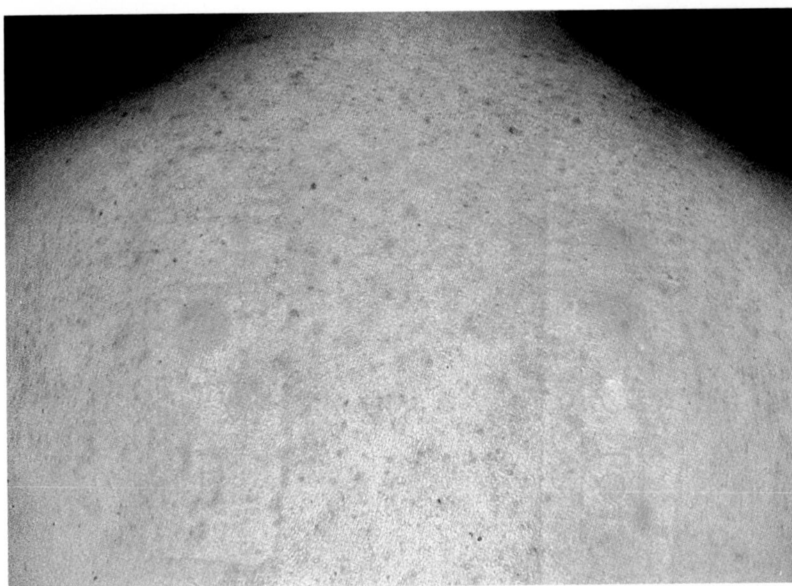

Figure 4-37 The excited skin syndrome. Several tests have become positive, and the severe reactions have stimulated inflammation over the entire back.

THE EXCITED SKIN SYNDROME (ANGRY BACK). "Eczema creates eczema." The excited skin syndrome is a major cause of false-positive patch test reactions. Single or multiple concomitant positive patch test reactions may produce a state of skin hyperreactivity in which other patch test sites, particularly those with minimal irritation, may become reactive. Patients who have multiple strong test reactions should be retested at a later date with one antigen at a time (Figure 4-37). Retesting may show that some of the original tests were false positives. The excited skin syndrome may also be caused by even minimal dermatitis elsewhere.

RELEVANCE OF TEST RESULTS AND MANAGEMENT. A number of possible conclusions may be drawn from the test results:

- The allergen eliciting the positive test is directly responsible for the patient's dermatitis.
- A chemically related or cross-reacting material is responsible for the dermatitis.
- The patient has not recently been in contact with the indicated allergen and, although the patient is allergic to that specific chemical, it is not relevant to the present condition.
- The test is negative but would be positive if a sufficient concentration of the test chemical was used.
- The positive test is an irritant reaction and is irrelevant.

The North American Contact Dermatitis Group (NACDG) patch test results, 2001 to 2002 study period, determined that the top 10 allergens remained the same as those in the 1999 to 2000 study period: nickel sulfate (16.7%), neomycin (11.6%), *Myroxilon pereirae* (balsam of Peru) (11.6%), fragrance mix (10.4%), thimerosal (10.2%), sodium gold thiosulfate (10.2%), quaternium-15 (9.3%), formaldehyde (8.4%), bacitracin (7.9%), and cobalt chloride (7.4%). Of the 4913 patients tested, 69% had at least 1 positive allergic patch test reaction. Of all patients, 15.8% had occupation-related dermatitis, 15.4% were determined to have irritant contact dermatitis, and 11.1% of the 15.4% had a relevant reaction to an occupational irritant. Of all patients tested, 16.7% had a relevant reaction to an allergen not in the NACDG standard series, and 5.5% had a relevant reaction to an occupational allergen not in the standard series. *PMID: 15842061*

CONTACT ALLERGEN SOURCES AND ALTERNATIVES

Review where the allergen is found (including foods), and discuss safe replacements with the patient. Identify potential cross-reacting substances. Visit www.truetest.com.

NEGATIVE TESTS. A number of possibilities exist for a negative test: the eczema may be nonallergic, the responsible chemical may not have been tested, or the result may be a false-negative. Also, a second reading of the test sites after the initial inspection at 48 hours may not have been made. False-negative tests can occur when the concentration of the test allergens is too low to elicit a reaction. Photopatch testing is necessary when the allergen requires photoactivation, as in photoallergic contact dermatitis caused by the sunscreen oxybenzone.

Chapter 5

Atopic Dermatitis

CHAPTER CONTENTS

The term *atopy* was introduced years ago to designate a group of patients who had a personal or family history of one or more of the following diseases: hay fever, asthma, very dry skin, and eczema.

Atopic dermatitis (AD) is a chronic, pruritic eczematous disease that nearly always begins in childhood and follows a remitting/flaring course that may continue throughout life. It develops as a result of a complex interrelationship of environmental, immunologic, genetic, and pharmacologic factors. It may be exacerbated by infection, psychologic stress, seasonal/climate changes, irritants, and allergens. The disease often moderates with age, but patients carry a lifelong skin sensitivity to irritants, and this atopy predisposes them to occupational skin disease.

The disease characteristics vary with age. Infants have facial and patchy or generalized body eczema. Adolescents and adults have eczema in flexural areas and on the hands. The pattern of inheritance is unknown, but available data suggest that it is polygenic.

DIAGNOSTIC CRITERIA. There are no specific cutaneous signs, no known distinctive histologic features, and no characteristic laboratory findings for atopic dermatitis. There are a variety of characteristics that indicate that the patient has atopic dermatitis (see Box 5-1). The diagnosis is made when the patient has three or more of the major features and three or more of the minor features. Each patient is different, with a unique combination of major and minor features.

PREVALENCE. The prevalence of atopic dermatitis has almost tripled in industrialized countries during the past 3 decades. The prevalence is lower in rural as compared with urban areas. Approximately 15% to 30% of children and 2% to 10% of adults are affected. About 45% of cases of atopic dermatitis begin within the first 6 months of life, 60% begin during the first year, and 85% begin before 5 years of age. Up to 70% of children have a remission before adolescence. Atopic dermatitis can start in adults. Genetic factors cannot explain the rapid change in prevalence. Changes in environmental factors and lifestyle, as well as increased recognition of the disease by physicians and families, are contributory factors. Some events in childhood may be of importance (e.g., early infections, early allergen exposure, and early diet).

GENETICS. The concordance rate for atopic dermatitis is higher among monozygotic twins (77%) than among dizygotic twins (15%). Allergic asthma or allergic rhinitis in a parent is a minor factor in the development of atopic dermatitis in the offspring.

Box 5-1 **Criteria for Diagnoses of Atopic Dermatitis**

Major Features (Must Have Three or More)

Pruritus
Typical morphology and distribution
Flexural lichenification in adults
Facial and extensor involvement in infants and children
Dermatitis—chronically or chronically relapsing
Personal or family history of atopy—asthma, allergic rhinitis, atopic dermatitis

Minor Features (Must Have Three or More)

Cataracts (anterior-subcapsular)
Cheilitis
Conjunctivitis—recurrent
Eczema—perifollicular accentuation
Facial pallor/facial erythema
Food intolerance
Hand dermatitis—nonallergic, irritant
Ichthyosis
IgE—elevated
Immediate (type 1) skin test reactivity
Infections (cutaneous)—*Staphylococcus aureus*, herpes simplex
Infraorbital fold (Dennie-Morgan lines)
Itching when sweating
Keratoconus
Keratosis pilaris
Nipple dermatitis
Orbital darkening
Palmar hyperlinearity
Pityriasis alba
White dermographism
Wool intolerance
Xerosis

Data from Roth HL: *Int J Dermatol* 26:139, 1987 *PMID: 3553045*; Hanifin JM, Rajka G: *Acta Derm Venereol (Stockh)* 92(suppl):44, 1980; and Hanifin JM, Lobitz WC Jr: *Arch Dermatol* 113:663, 1977.

COURSE AND PROGNOSIS

Factors associated with a low frequency of healing and increased severity of persistent or recurring dermatitis are listed in order of relative importance in Box 5-2. More than 50% of young children with generalized AD develop asthma and allergic rhinitis by the age of 13. Dermatitis improves in most children.

Seventy percent of atopic patients have a family history of one or more of the major atopic characteristics: asthma, hay fever, or eczematous dermatitis.

MISCONCEPTIONS. There are two common misconceptions about AD. The first is that it is an emotional disorder. It is true that patients with inflammation that lasts for months or years seem to be irritable, but this is a normal response to a frustrating disease. The second misconception is that atopic skin disease is precipitated by an allergic reaction. Atopic individuals frequently have respiratory allergies and, when skin tested, are informed that they are allergic to "everything." Atopic patients may react with a wheal when challenged with a needle during skin testing, but this is a characteristic of atopic skin and is not necessarily a manifestation of allergy. All evidence to date shows that most cases of AD are precipitated by environmental stress on genetically compromised skin and not by interaction with allergens.

Box 5-2 **Atopic Dermatitis: Unfavorable Prognostic Factors***

Persistent dry or itchy skin in adult life
Widespread dermatitis in childhood
Associated allergic rhinitis
Family history of atopic dermatitis
Associated bronchial asthma
Early age at onset
Female gender

*In order of relative importance.
Data from Rystedt I: *Acta Derm Venereol (Stockh)* 65:206, 1985. *PMID: 2411075*

PATHOGENESIS AND IMMUNOLOGY

ELEVATED IgE AND THE INFLAMMATORY RESPONSE. The role of immunoglobulin E (IgE) in AD is unknown. The IgE level is increased in the serum of many patients with AD, but 20% of AD patients have normal serum IgE levels and no allergen reactivity. The levels of IgE do not necessarily correlate with the activity of the disease; therefore elevated serum IgE levels can only be considered supporting evidence for the disease. Total IgE is significantly higher in children with coexistent atopic respiratory disease in all age groups. Most persons with AD have a personal or family history of allergic rhinitis or asthma and increased serum IgE antibodies against airborne or ingested protein antigens. AD usually diminishes during the spring hay fever season, when aeroallergens are at maximum concentrations.

BLOOD EOSINOPHILIA. Eosinophils may be major effector cells in AD. Blood eosinophil counts roughly correlate with disease severity, although many patients with severe disease show normal peripheral blood eosinophil counts. Patients with normal eosinophil counts mainly are those with atopic dermatitis alone; patients with severe atopic dermatitis and concomitant respiratory allergies commonly have increased peripheral blood eosinophils. There is no accumulation of tissue eosinophils; however, degranulation of eosinophils in the dermis releases major basic protein that may induce histamine release from basophils and mast cells and stimulate itching, irritation, and lichenification.

REDUCED CELL-MEDIATED IMMUNITY. Several facts suggest that AD patients have disordered cell-mediated immunity. Patients may develop severe diffuse cutaneous infection with the herpes simplex virus (eczema herpeticum) whether or not their dermatitis is active. Mothers with active herpes labialis should avoid direct contact of their active lesion with their children's skin, as in kissing, especially if the child has dermatitis. The incidence of contact allergy (e.g., reduced sensitivity to poison ivy) may be lower than normal in atopic patients; however, some studies show equal rates of sensitization. Humoral immunity seems to be normal.

AEROALLERGENS. Aeroallergens may play an important role in causing eczematous lesions. Patch testing rates of reactions are the following: house dust, 70%; mites, 70%; cockroaches, 63%; mold mix, 50%; and grass mix, 43%. Patients with AD frequently show positive scratch and intradermal reactions to a number of antigens; avoidance of these antigens rarely improves the dermatitis.

CLINICAL ASPECTS

MAJOR AND MINOR DIAGNOSTIC FEATURES. Box 5-1 (the criteria for diagnosing AD) lists the major and minor diagnostic features for atopic dermatitis and atopy. Each patient has his or her own unique set of features, and there is no precise clinical or laboratory marker for this genetic disease.

ITCHING, THE PRIMARY LESION. "It is not the eruption that is itchy but the itchiness that is eruptive." Atopic dermatitis starts with itching. Abnormally dry skin and a lowered threshold for itching are important features of AD. It is the scratching that creates most of the characteristic patterns of the disease. Most patients with AD make a determined effort to control their scratching, but during sleep conscious control is lost; under warm covers the patient scratches and a rash appears. The itch-scratch cycle is established, and conscious effort is no longer sufficient to control scratching. The act of scratching becomes habitual, and the disease progresses. Atopic skin is associated with a lowered threshold of responsiveness to irritants.

PATTERNS OF INFLAMMATION. Several patterns and types of lesions may be produced by exposure to external stimuli or may be precipitated by scratching. Acute inflammation begins with erythematous papules and erythema. These are associated with excoriations, erosions, and serous exudate. Subacute dermatitis is associated with erythematous, excoriated, scaling papules. Chronic dermatitis is the result of scratching over an extended period, resulting in thickened skin, accentuated skin markings (lichenification), and fibrotic papules. Inflammation resolves slowly, leaving the skin in a dry, scaly, compromised condition called xerosis. There is no single primary lesion in AD. All three types of reactions can coexist in the same individual. These types of lesions are eczematous dermatitis with redness and scaling (Figure 5-1), papules (Figure 5-2), and lichenification (Figure 5-3). Lichenification represents a thickening of the epidermis. It is a highly characteristic lesion, with the normal skin lines accentuated to resemble a washboard. These responses are altered by excoriation and infection.

Although the cutaneous manifestations of the atopic diathesis are varied, they have characteristic age-determined patterns. Knowledge of these patterns is useful; many patients, however, have a nonclassic pattern. AD may terminate after an indefinite period or may progress from infancy to adulthood with little or no relief; 58% of infants with AD were found to have persistent inflammation 15 to 17 years later. AD is arbitrarily divided into three phases.

ATOPIC DERMATITIS PATTERNS OF INFLAMMATION

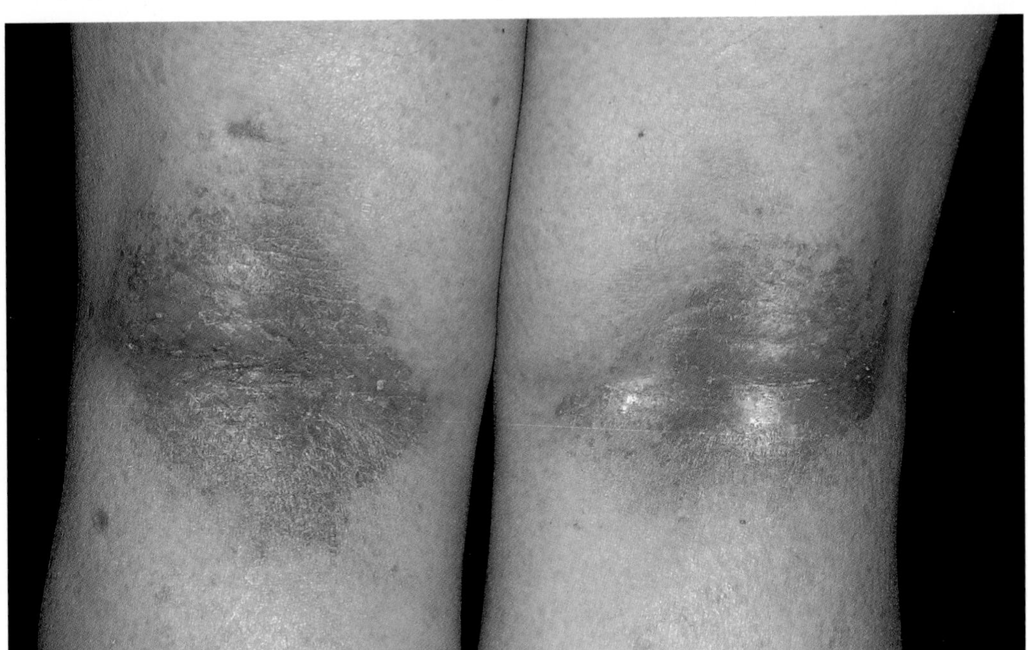

Figure 5-1 Eczematous dermatitis with erythema and scaling in the popliteal fossa.

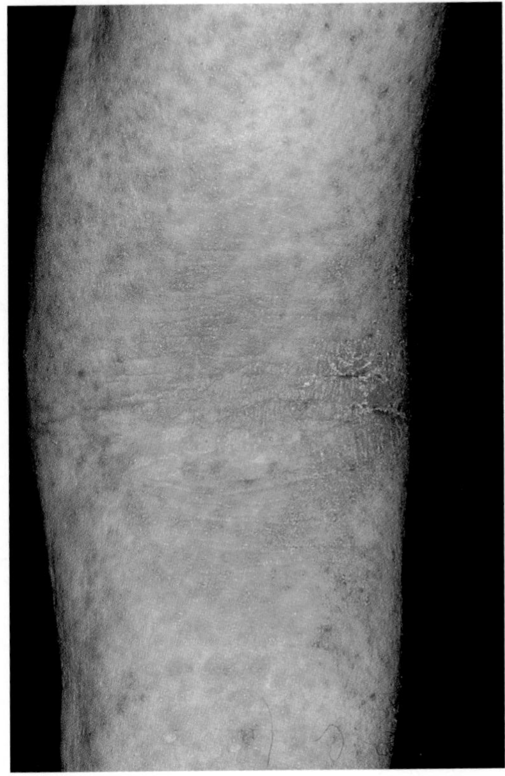

Figure 5-2 Papular lesions are common in the antecubital and popliteal fossae. Papules become confluent and form plaques.

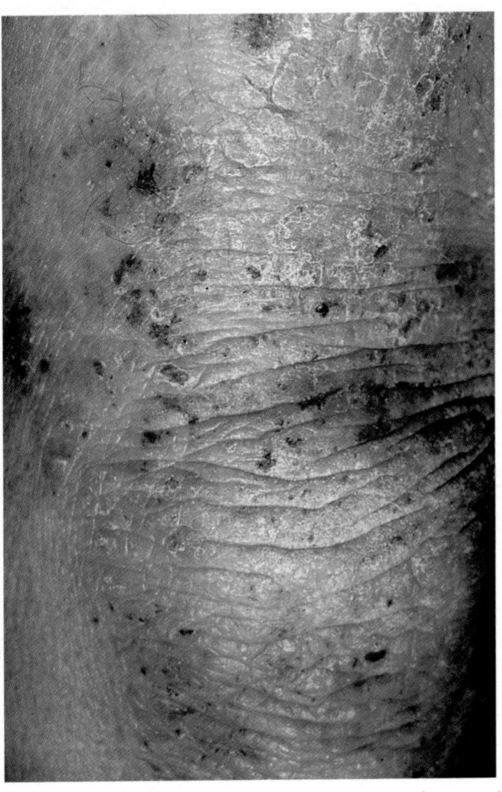

Figure 5-3 Lichenification with accentuation of normal skin lines. This lichenified plaque is surrounded by papules.

Infant phase (birth to 2 years)

Infants are rarely born with atopic eczema, but they typically develop the first signs of inflammation during the third month of life. The most common occurrence is that of a baby who during the winter months develops dry, red, scaling areas confined to the cheeks, but sparing the perioral and paranasal areas (Figures 5-4 through 5-8). This is the same area that becomes flushed with exposure to cold. The chin is often involved and initially may be more inflamed than the cheeks because of the irritation of drooling and subsequent repeated washing. Inflammation may spread to involve the paranasal and perioral area as the winter progresses. Habitual lip licking by an atopic child results in oozing, crusting, and scaling on the lips and perioral skin (Figures 5-9 and 5-10).

Many infants do not excoriate during these early stages, and the rash remains localized and chronic. Repeated scratching or washing creates red, scaling, oozing plaques on the cheeks, a classic presentation of infantile eczema. At this stage the infant is uncomfortable and becomes restless and agitated during sleep.

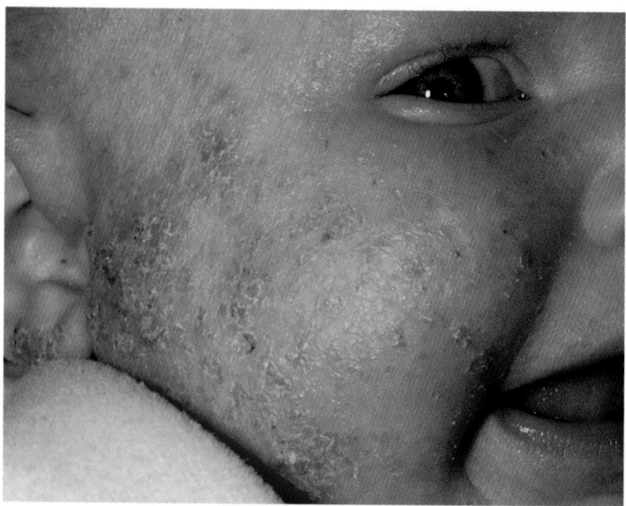

Figure 5-4 Red, scaling plaques confined to the cheeks are one of the first signs of atopic dermatitis in an infant.

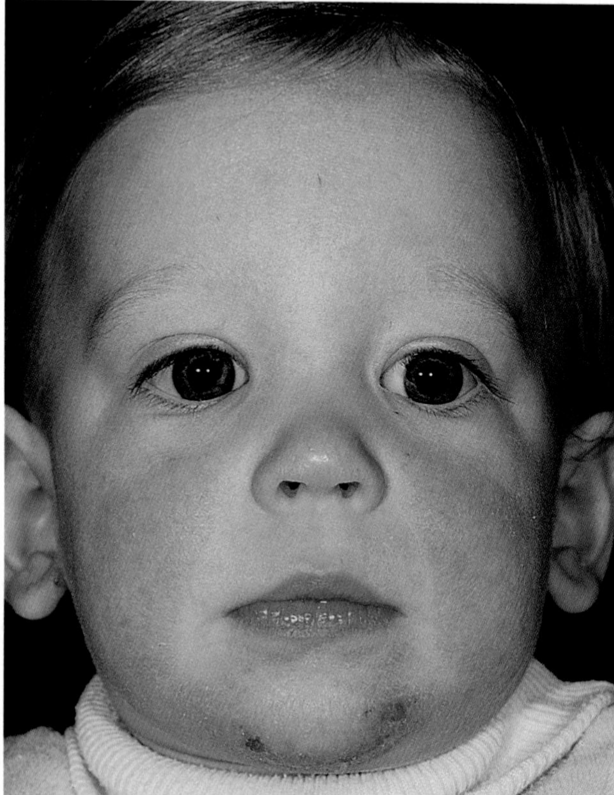

Figure 5-5 Atopic dermatitis. A common appearance in children with erythema and scaling confined to the cheeks and sparing the perioral and paranasal areas.

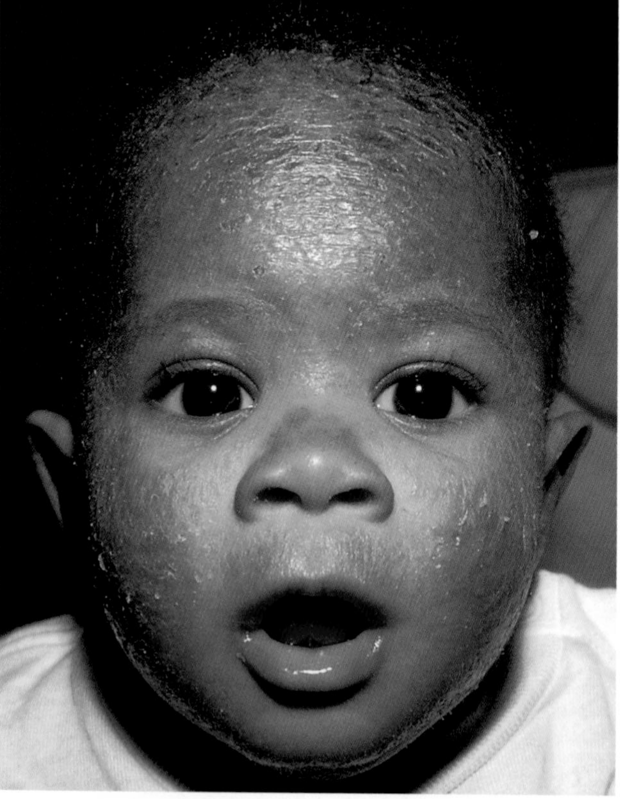

Figure 5-6 Extensive erythema and crusting in this baby with secondarily infected atopic dermatitis of the face.

ATOPIC DERMATITIS—INFANT PHASE

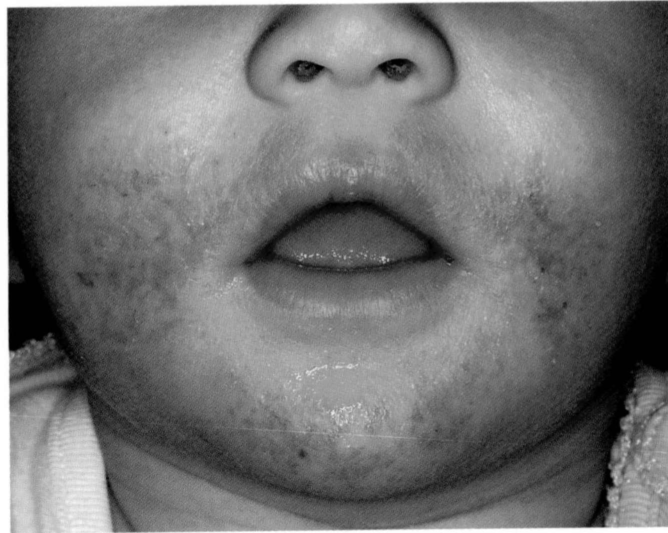

Figure 5-7 Erythema and crusting form after repeated cycles of wetting the skin with saliva and food.

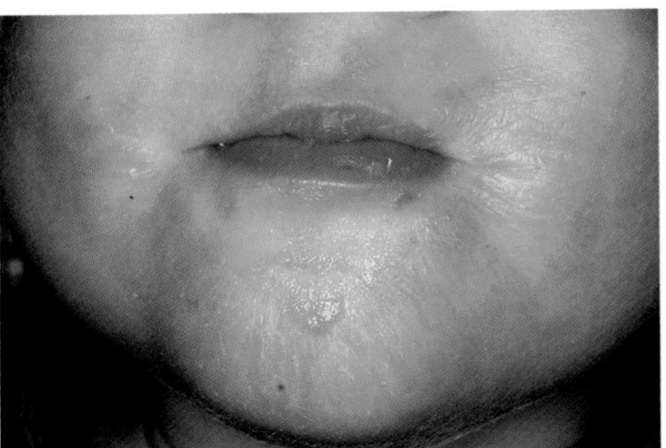

Figure 5-8 Eczematous plaques have become confluent on the lower face

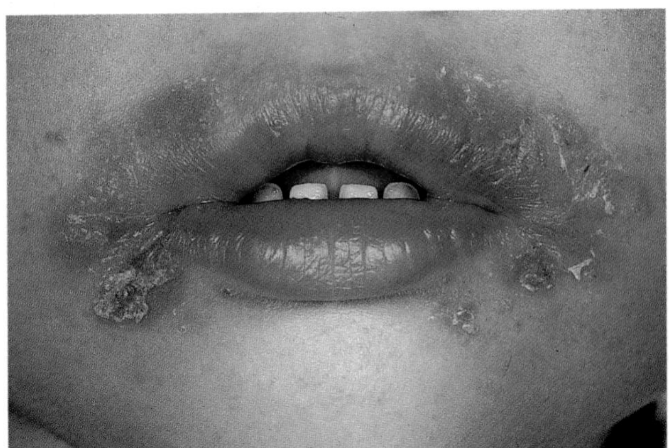

Figure 5-9 Habitual lip licking in an atopic child produces erythema and scaling that may eventually lead to secondary infection.

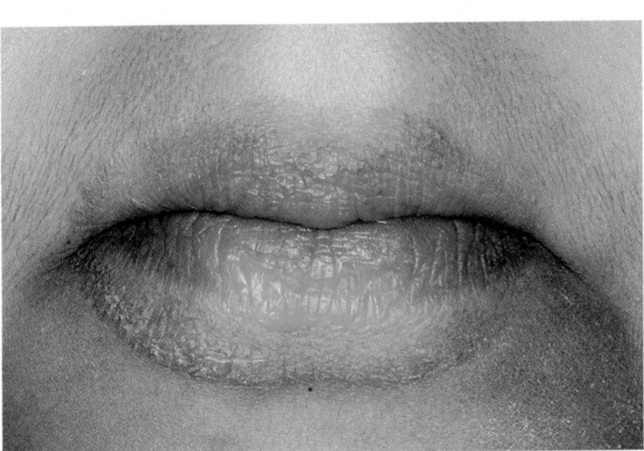

Figure 5-10 Eczema about the mouth has been created by licking with the tongue in a circular pattern. The same presentation is seen in both adults (pictured here) and infants.

A small but significant number of infants have a generalized eruption consisting of papules, redness, scaling, and areas of lichenification. The scalp may be involved, and differentiation from seborrheic dermatitis is sometimes difficult (Figure 5-11). The diaper area is often spared (Figure 5-12). Lichenification may occur in the fossae and crease areas, or it may be confined to a favorite, easily reached spot, such as directly below the diaper, the back of the hand, or the extensor forearm (Figures 5-12 through 5-14). Prolonged AD with increasing discomfort disturbs sleep, and both the parents and the child are distraught.

For years, foods have been suspected as etiologic factors. Food testing and breast-feeding are discussed at the end of this chapter. The course of the disease may be influenced by events such as teething, respiratory tract infections, and adverse emotional stimuli. The disease is chronic, with periods of exacerbation and remission, and resolves in approximately 50% of infants by 18 months; other cases progress to the childhood phase, and a different pattern evolves.

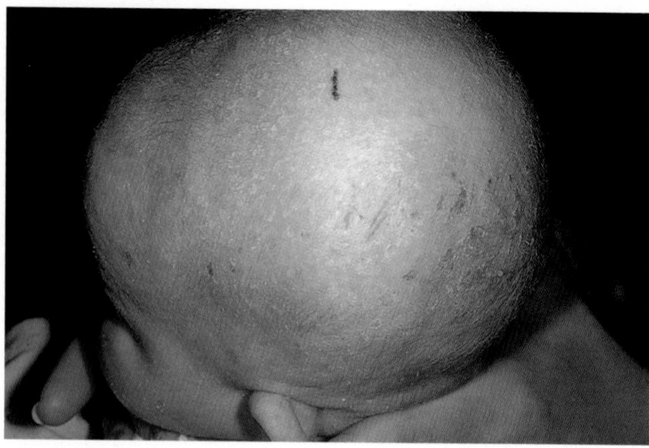

Figure 5-11 Diffuse superficial erythema and scale of the scalp respond rapidly to group VI topical steroids. Hydrocortisone 1% may not be strong enough to control the inflammation.

GROWTH IN ATOPIC ECZEMA. Height is significantly correlated with the surface area of skin affected by eczema. The growth of children with eczema affecting less than 50% of the skin surface area appears to be normal, and impaired growth is confined to those with more extensive disease. Treatment with topical steroids has only marginal additional effect on impaired growth.

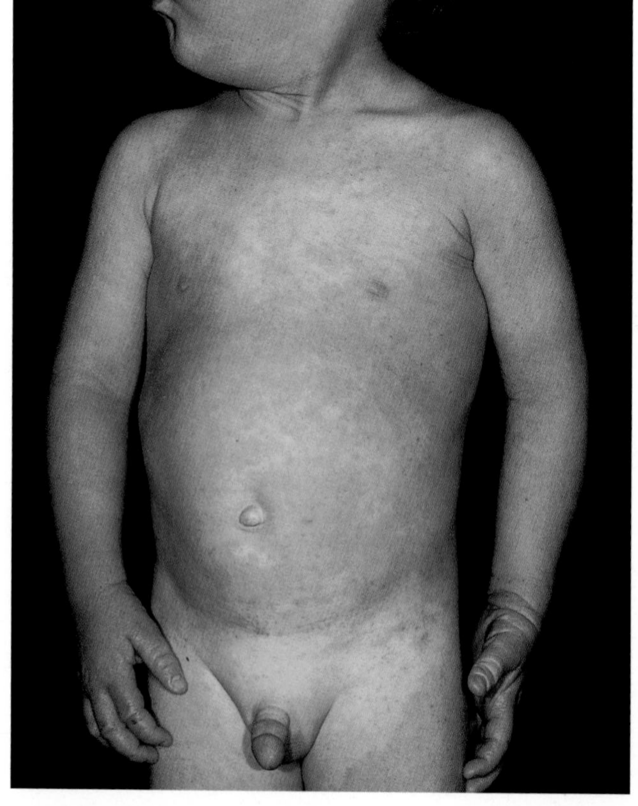

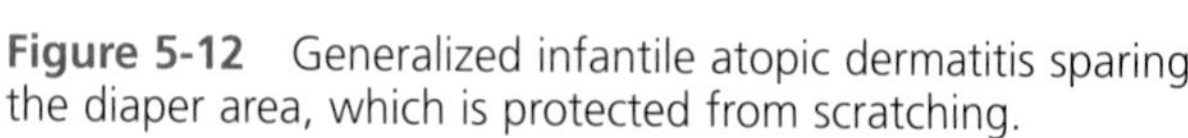

Figure 5-12 Generalized infantile atopic dermatitis sparing the diaper area, which is protected from scratching.

ATOPIC DERMATITIS

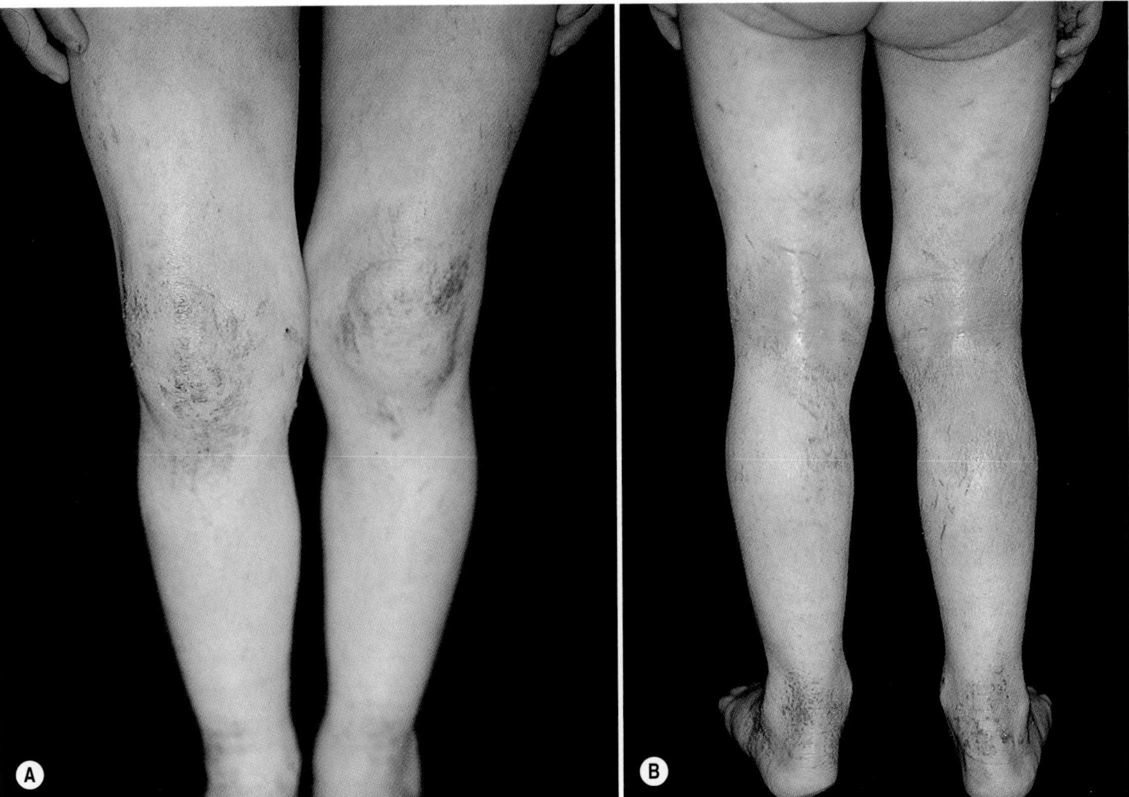

Figure 5-13 **A,** Inflammation in the flexural areas is the most common presentation of atopic dermatitis in children. **B,** Rubbing and scratching the inflamed flexural areas cause thickened (lichenified) skin. These lesions form fissures and are infected with *Staphylococcus aureus*.

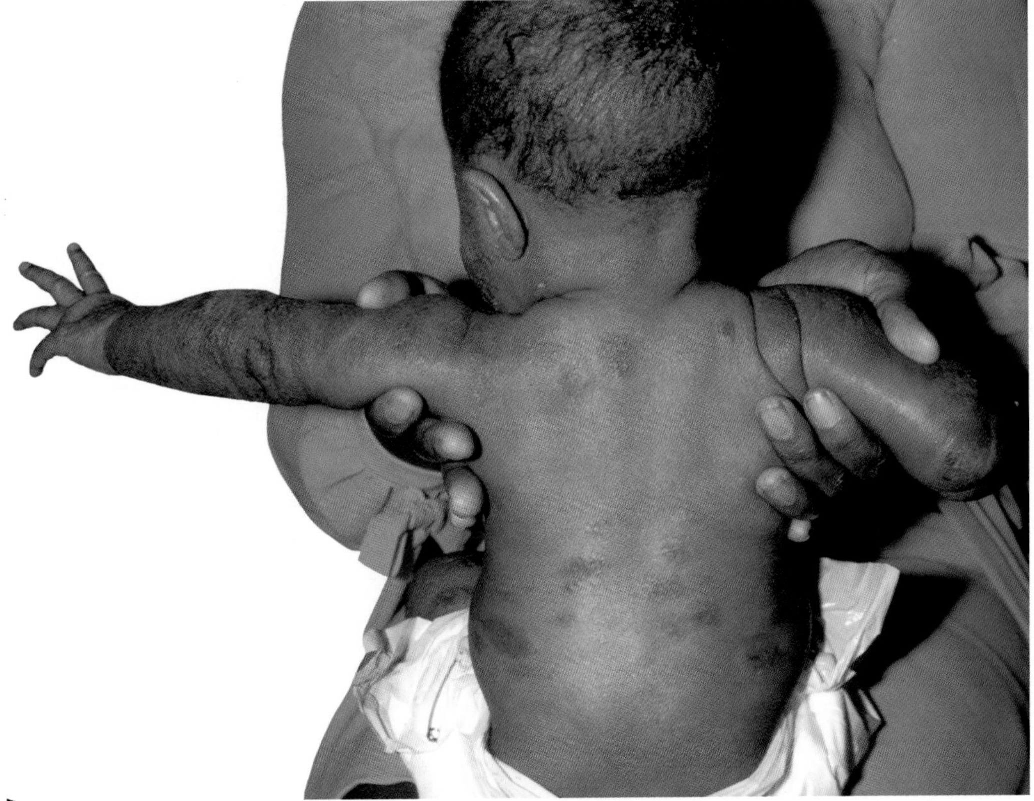

Figure 5-14 Generalized atopic dermatitis.

Childhood phase (2 to 12 years)

The most common and characteristic appearance of AD is inflammation in flexural areas (i.e., the antecubital fossae, neck, wrists, and ankles [Figures 5-15 through 5-18]). These areas of repeated flexion and extension perspire with exertion. The act of perspiring stimulates burning and intense itching and initiates the itch-scratch cycle. Tight clothing that traps heat about the neck or extremities further aggravates the problem. Inflammation typically begins in one of the fossae or around the neck. The rash may remain localized to one or two areas or progress to involve the neck, antecubital and popliteal fossae, wrists, and ankles. The eruption begins with papules that rapidly coalesce into plaques, which become lichenified when scratched. The plaques may be pale and mildly inflamed with little tendency to change (see Figure 5-16); if they have been vigorously scratched, they may be bright red and scaling with erosions. The border may be sharp and well-defined, as it is in psoriasis, or poorly defined with papules extraneous to the lichenified areas. A few patients do not develop lichenification even with repeated scratching. The exudative lesions typical of the infant phase are not as common. Most patients with chronic lesions tolerate their disease and sleep well.

Figure 5-15 Atopic dermatitis. Classic appearance of confluent papules forming plaques in the antecubital fossae.

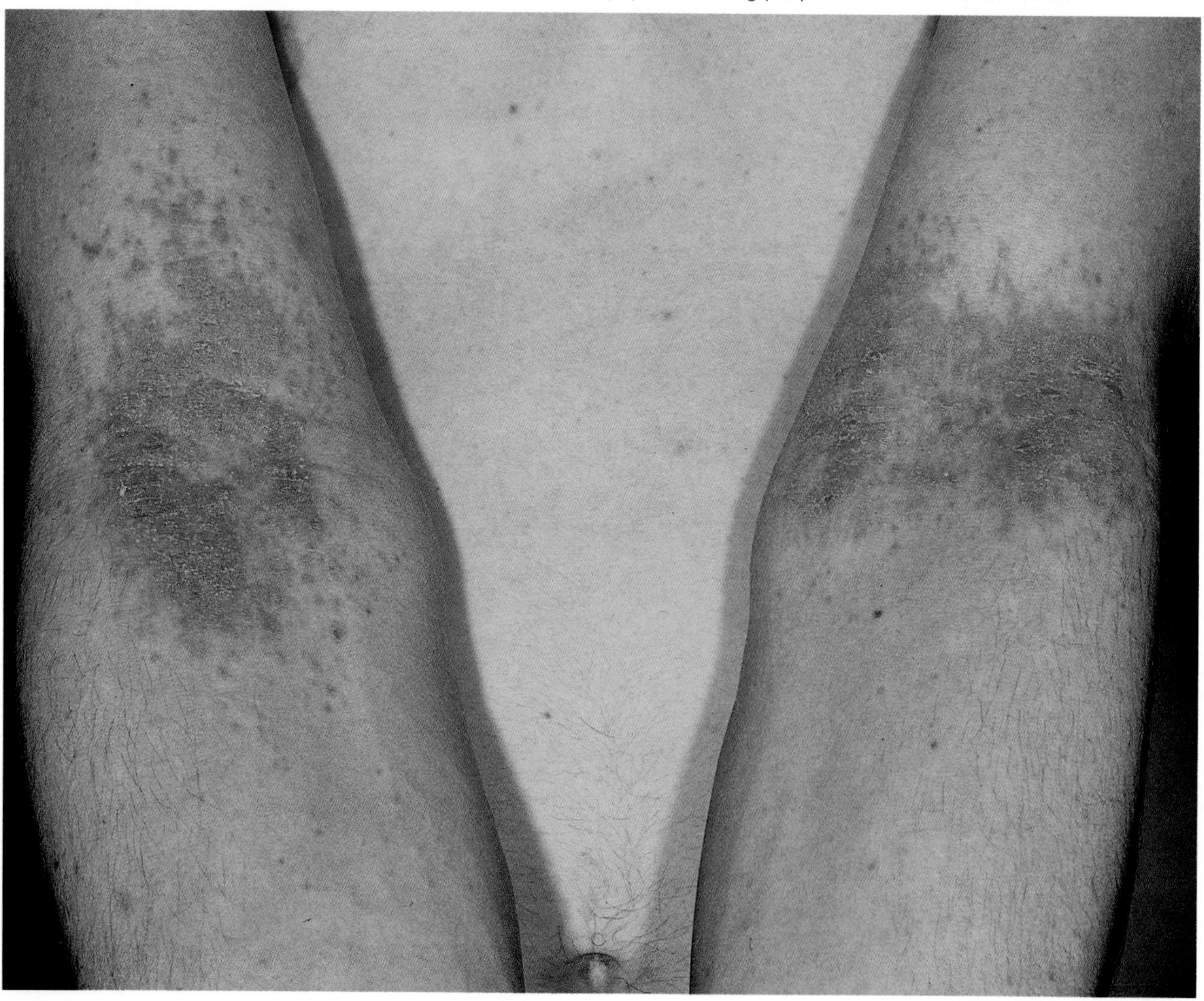

ATOPIC DERMATITIS—CHILDHOOD PHASE

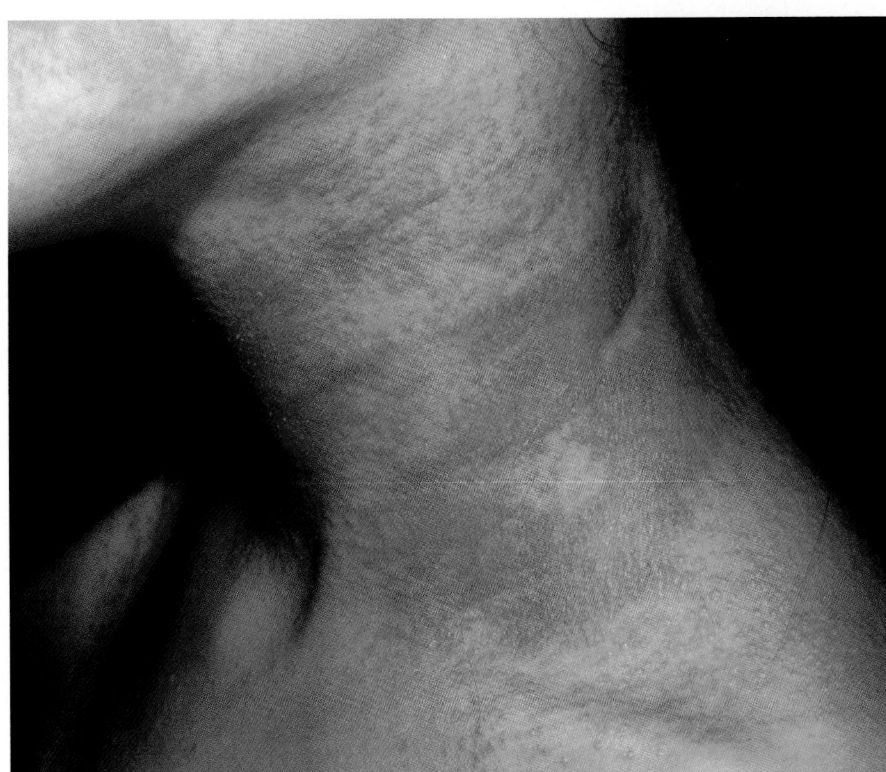

Figure 5-16 Classic appearance of erythema and diffuse scaling about the neck.

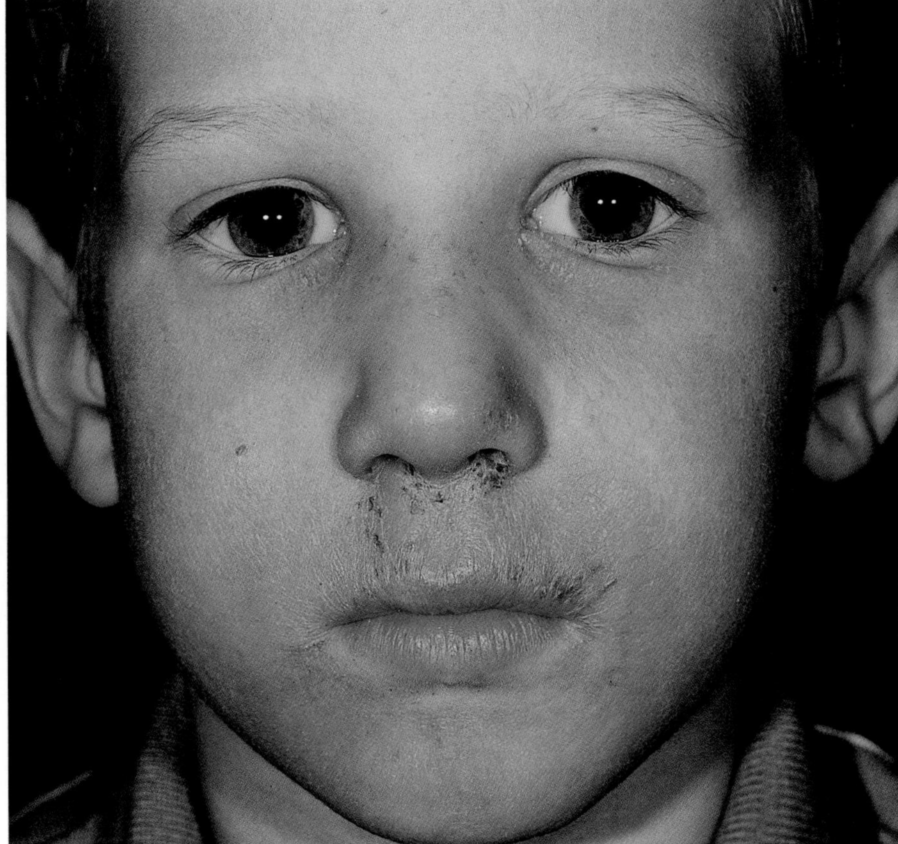

Figure 5-17 Diffuse inflammation on the face of a child. The eczema initially spared the perioral area but has become extensive and confluent with persistent irritation.

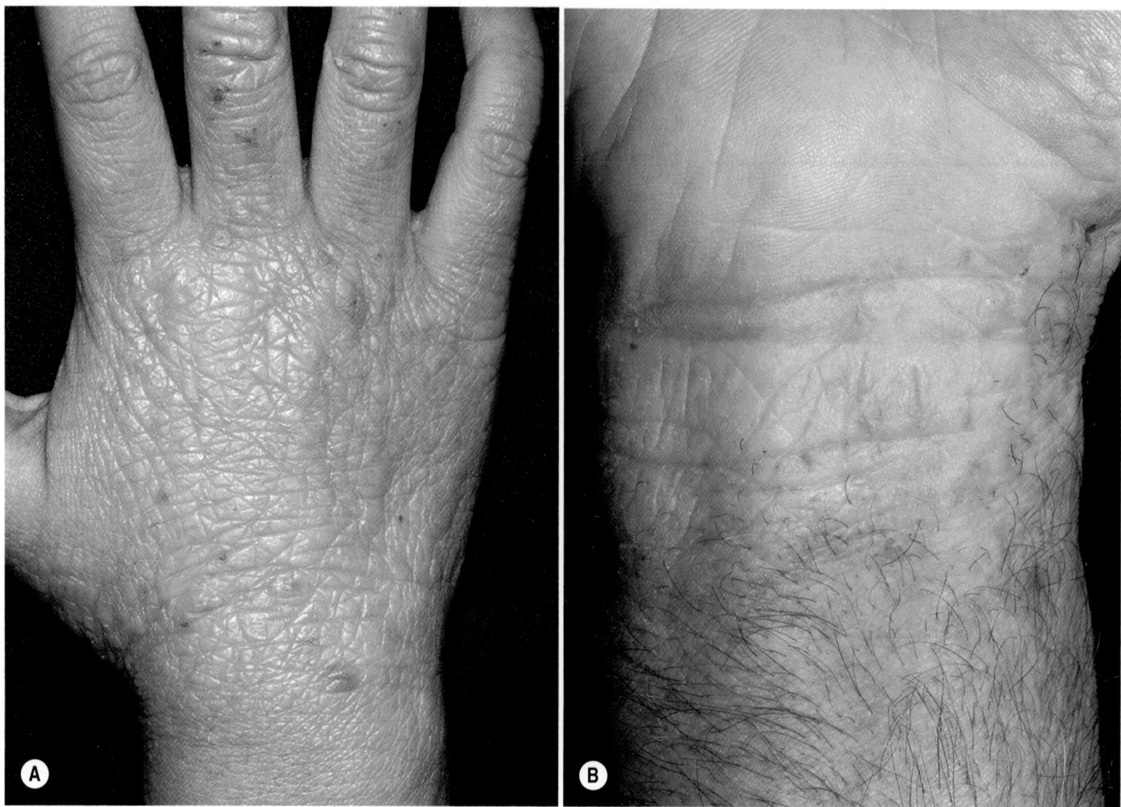

Figure 5-18 **A,** Atopic dermatitis. A chronically inflamed lichenified plaque on the wrist and back of hand. **B,** Eczema of the wrist is classic presentation for atopic dermatitis.

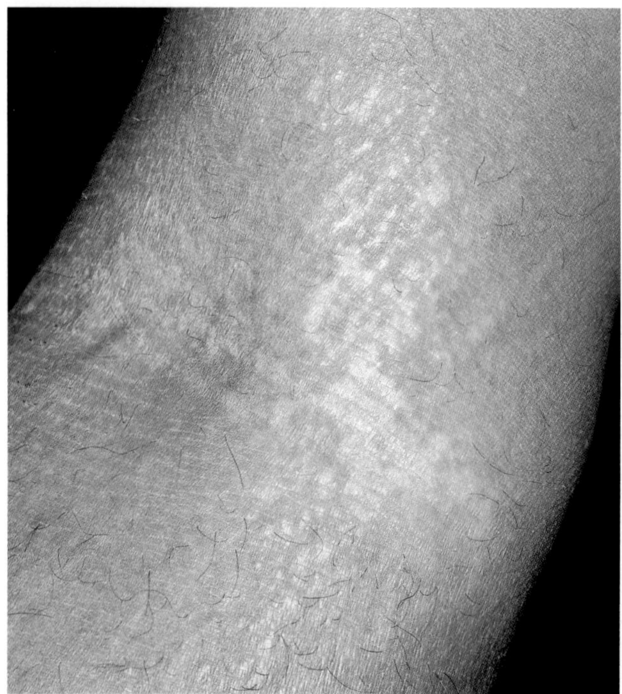

Figure 5-19 Hypopigmentation in the antecubital fossae caused by destruction of melanocytes by chronic scratching.

Constant scratching may lead to destruction of melanocytes, resulting in areas of hypopigmentation that become more obvious when the inflammation subsides. These hypopigmented areas fade with time (Figure 5-19). Additional exacerbating factors such as heat, cold, dry air, or emotional stress may lead to extension of inflammation beyond the confines of the crease areas (Figures 5-20 and 5-21). The inflammation becomes incapacitating. Normal duration of sleep cannot be maintained, and school, work, or job performance deteriorates; these people are miserable. They discover that standing in a hot shower gives considerable temporary relief, but further progression is inevitable with the drying effect produced by repeated wetting and drying. In the more advanced cases, hospitalization is required. Most patients with this pattern of inflammation are in remission by age 30, but in a few patients the disease becomes chronic or improves only to relapse during a change of season or at some other period of transition. Then dermatitis becomes a lifelong ordeal.

SEVERE GENERALIZED ATOPIC DERMATITIS

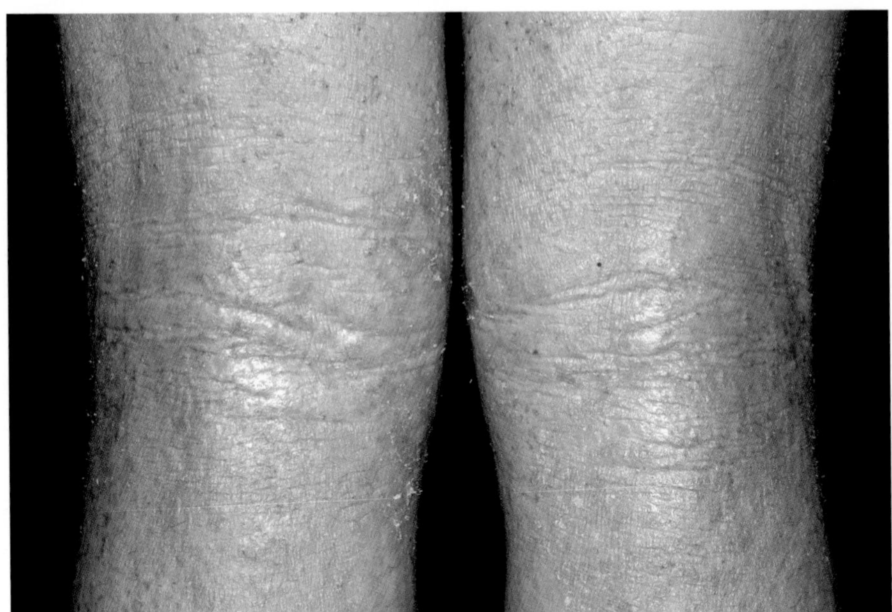

Figure 5-20 Eczema has intensified and spread out of the fossa to involve most of the body. Lesions are highly inflamed and secondarily infected.

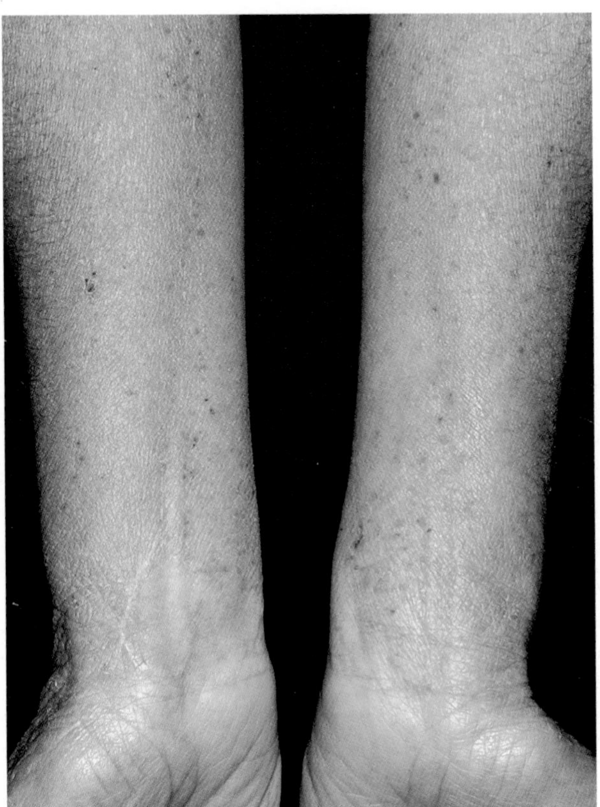

Figure 5-21 The dermatitis has generalized to involve the entire body. Secondary skin infection with *Staphylococcus aureus* is almost always present with this degree of inflammation.

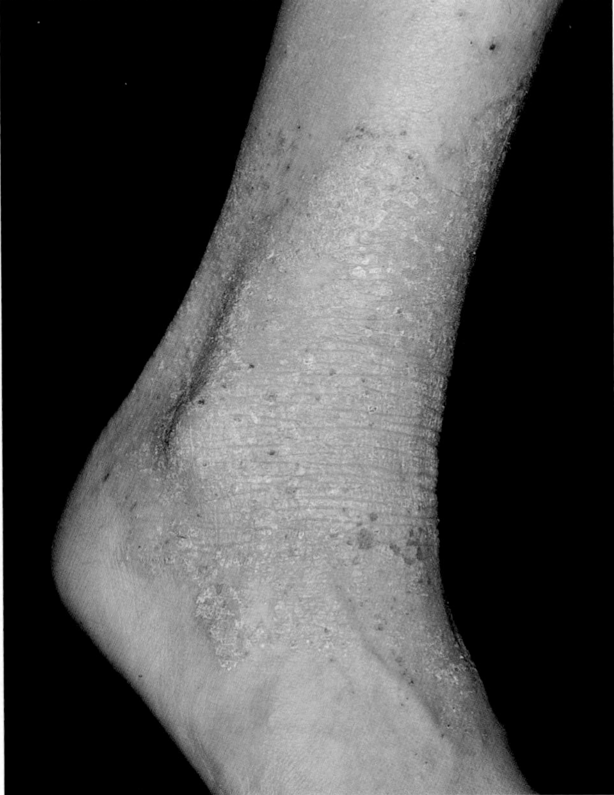

Figure 5-22 Sharply defined lichenified plaque with a silvery scale showing some of the features of psoriasis. Erosions are present.

Adult phase (12 years to adult)

The adult phase of AD begins near the onset of puberty. The reason for the resurgence of inflammation at this time is not understood, but it may be related to hormonal changes or to the stress of early adolescence. Adults may have no history of dermatitis in earlier years, but this is unusual. As in the childhood phase, localized inflammation with lichenification is the most common pattern. One area or several areas may be involved, and there are several characteristic patterns.

INFLAMMATION IN FLEXURAL AREAS. This pattern is commonly seen and is identical to childhood flexural inflammation.

HAND DERMATITIS. Hand dermatitis may be the most common expression of the atopic diathesis in the adult. (See Atopic Hand Dermatitis in Chapter 3.) Adults are exposed to a variety of irritating chemicals in the home and at work, and they wash more frequently than do children. Irritation causes redness and scaling on the dorsal aspect of the hand or about the fingers. Itching develops, and the inevitable scratching results in lichenification or oozing and crusting. A few or all of the fingertip pads may be involved. They may be dry and chronically peeling or red and fissured. The eruption may be painful, chronic, and resistant to treatment. Psoriasis may have an identical presentation.

INFLAMMATION AROUND EYES. The lids are thin, frequently exposed to irritants, and easily traumatized by scratching. Many adults with AD have inflammation localized to the upper lids (Figure 5-23). They may claim to be allergic to something, but elimination of suspected allergens may not solve the problem. Habitual rubbing of the inflamed lids with the back of the hand is typical. If an attempt to control inflammation fails, then patch testing should be considered to eliminate allergic contact dermatitis.

LICHENIFICATION OF THE ANOGENITAL AREA. Lichenification of the anogenital area is probably more common in patients with AD than in others. Intertriginous areas that are warm and moist can become irritated and itch. Lichenification of the vulva (see Figure 3-47), scrotum (see Figure 3-53), and rectum (see Figure 3-48) may develop with habitual scratching. These areas are resistant to treatment, and inflammation may last for years. The patient may delay visiting a physician because of modesty, and the untreated lichenified plaques become very thick. Emotional factors should also be considered with this isolated phenomenon.

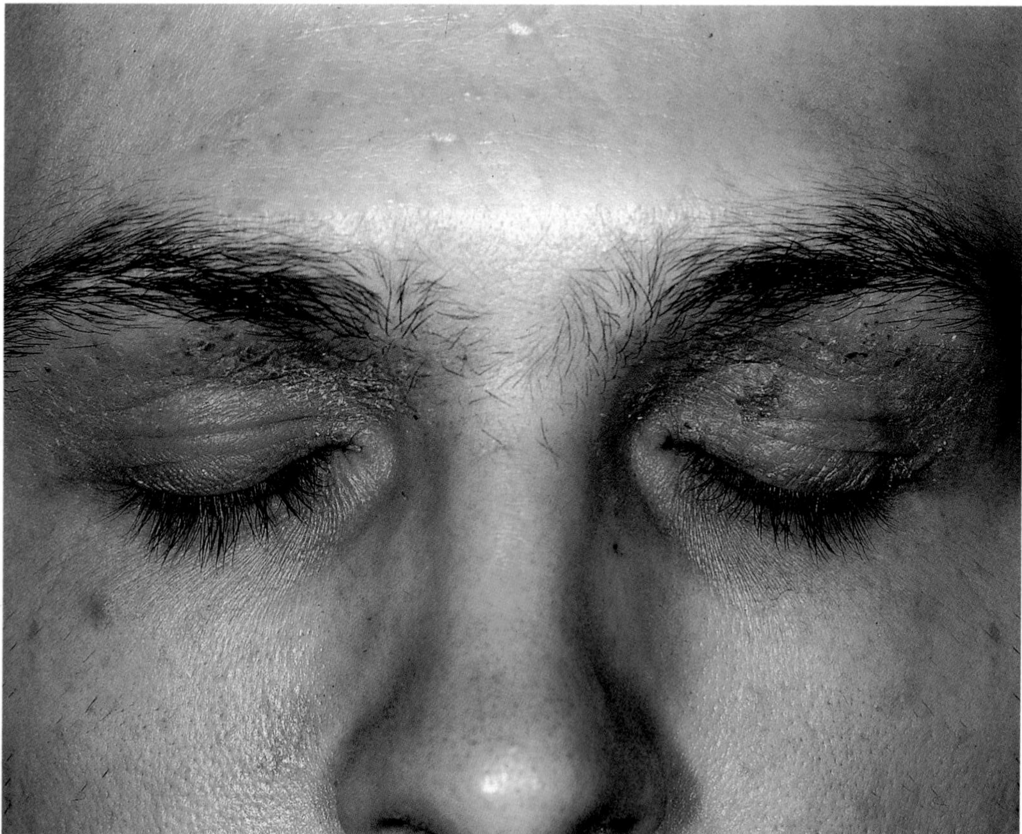

Figure 5-23 Atopic dermatitis of the upper eyelids, an area that is often rubbed with the back of the hand.

ASSOCIATED FEATURES

Dry skin and xerosis

Dry skin is an important feature of the atopic state. It is commonly assumed that patients with AD have inherited dry skin. The dryness may, however, reflect mild eczematous changes, concomitant ichthyosis, or a complex of both of these changes.

Dry skin may appear at any age, and it is not unusual for infants to have dry, scaling skin on the lower legs. Dry skin is sensitive, easily irritated by external stimuli, and, more importantly, itchy. It is the itching that provides the basis for the development of the various patterns of AD. Scratched itchy skin develops eczema; in other words, it is the itch that rashes.

Dry skin is most often located on the extensor surfaces of the legs and arms, but in susceptible individuals it may involve the entire cutaneous surface. Dryness is worse in the winter when humidity is low. Water is lost from the outermost layer of the skin. The skin becomes drier as the winter continues, and scaling skin becomes cracked and fissured. Dry areas that are repeatedly washed reach a point at which the epidermal barrier can no longer maintain its integrity; erythema and eczema occur. Frequent washing and drying may produce redness with horizontal linear splits, particularly on the lower legs of the elderly, giving a cracked or crazed porcelain appearance (see Chapter 3, Figures 3-37, 3-38, and 3-39). Avoid frequent washing. Use mild soaps (e.g, Dove, Cetaphil bar) and routinely apply moisturizing creams or lotions. Moisturizers are effectively bound in the skin if they are applied shortly after patting the skin dry following bathing.

Ichthyosis vulgaris

Ichthyosis is a disorder of keratinization characterized by the development of dry, rectangular scales. There are many forms of ichthyosis. Dominant ichthyosis vulgaris may occur as a distinct entity, or it may be found in patients with AD. Atopic patients with ichthyosis vulgaris often have keratosis pilaris and hyperlinear, exaggerated palm creases. Infants may show only dry, scaling skin during the winter, but with age the changes become more extensive, and small, fine, white, translucent scales appear on the extensor aspects of the arms and legs (Figure 5-24). These scales are smaller and lighter in color than the large, brown polygonal scales of sex-linked ichthyosis vulgaris, which occurs exclusively in males (Figure 5-25). The scaling of the dominant form does not encroach on the axillae and fossae, as is seen in the sex-linked type. Scaling rarely involves the entire cutaneous surface. The condition tends to improve with age. Application of 12% ammonium lactate lotion or cream (Lac-Hydrin, AmLactin) or urea cream is very effective.

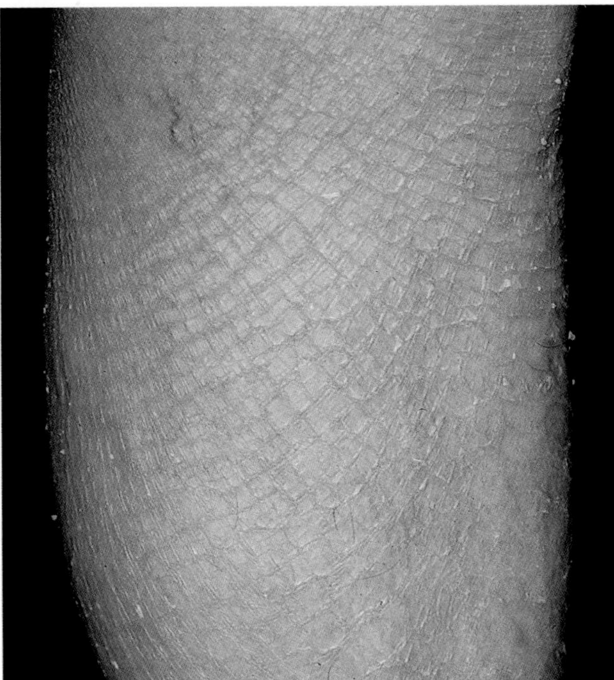

Figure 5-24 Dominant ichthyosis vulgaris. White, translucent, quadrangular scales on the extensor aspects of the arms and legs. This form is significantly associated with atopy.

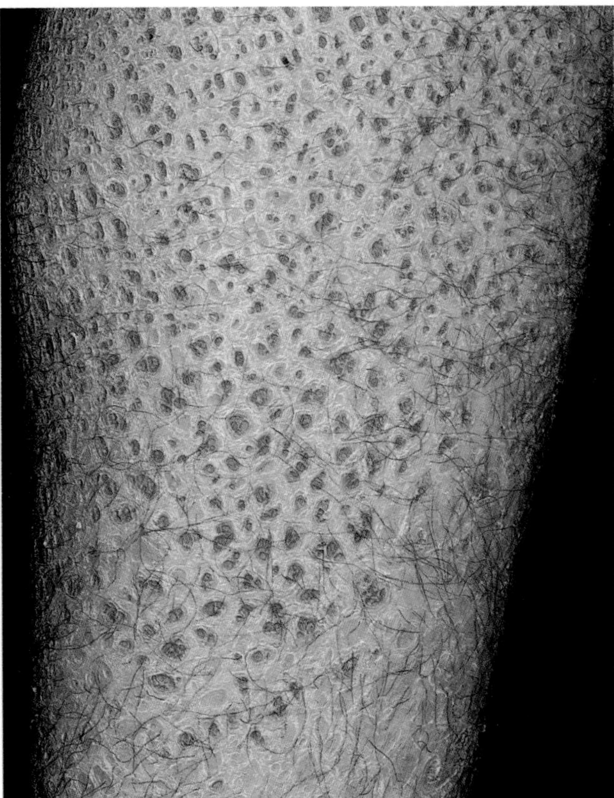

Figure 5-25 Sex-linked ichthyosis vulgaris. Large, brown, quadrangular scales that may encroach on the antecubital and popliteal fossae. Compare this presentation with Figure 5-24. There is no association with atopy.

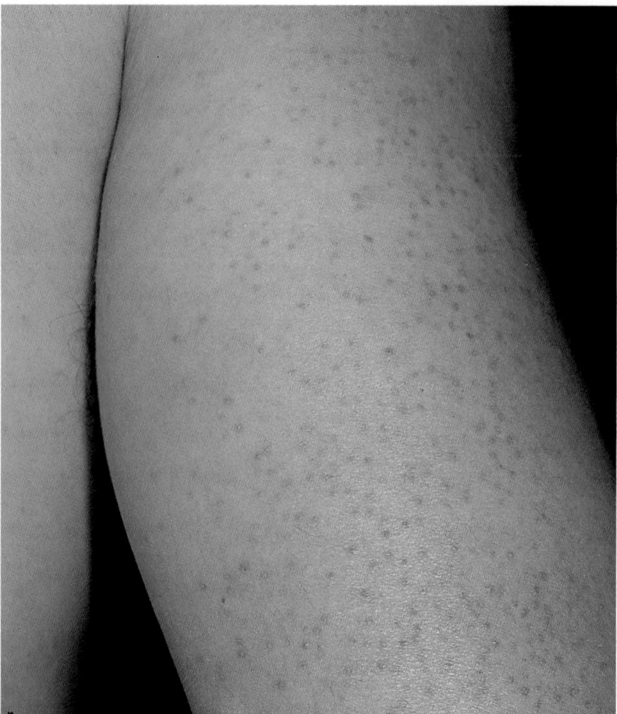

Figure 5-26 Keratosis pilaris. Small, rough, follicular papules or pustules occur most often on the posterolateral aspects of the upper arms and anterior thighs.

Keratosis pilaris

Keratosis pilaris is very common and seems to occur more often and more extensively in patients with AD. Small (1 to 2 mm), rough, follicular papules or pustules may appear at any age and are common in young children (Figure 5-26). The incidence peaks during adolescence, and the problem tends to improve thereafter. Adolescents and adults are disturbed by the appearance.

The posterolateral aspects of the upper arms (Figures 5-26 and 5-27) and anterior thighs are frequently involved, but any area, with the exception of the palms and soles, may be involved. Lesions on the face may be confused with acne, but the uniform small size and association with dry skin and chapping differentiate keratosis pilaris from pustular acne (Figure 5-28). The eruption may be generalized, resembling heat rash or miliaria. Most cases are asymptomatic, but the lesions may be red, inflammatory, and pustular and resemble bacterial folliculitis, particularly on the thighs (Figure 5-29). In the adult generalized form, a red halo appears at the periphery of the keratotic papule. This unusual diffuse pattern in adults persists indefinitely (Figure 5-30). Systemic steroid therapy may greatly accentuate both the lesion and the distribution by creation of numerous follicular pustules.

Treatment with topical retinoids (tretinoin cream or tazarotine cream) may induce improvement, but the irritation is usually unacceptable. Short courses of group V topical steroids reduce the unsightly redness and can be offered when temporary relief is desired before an important event. Application of 12% ammonium lactate lotion (Lac-Hydrin, AmLactin), urea cream (10-40%), or salicylic acid lotion 6% reduces the roughness. Abrasive washing techniques cause further drying.

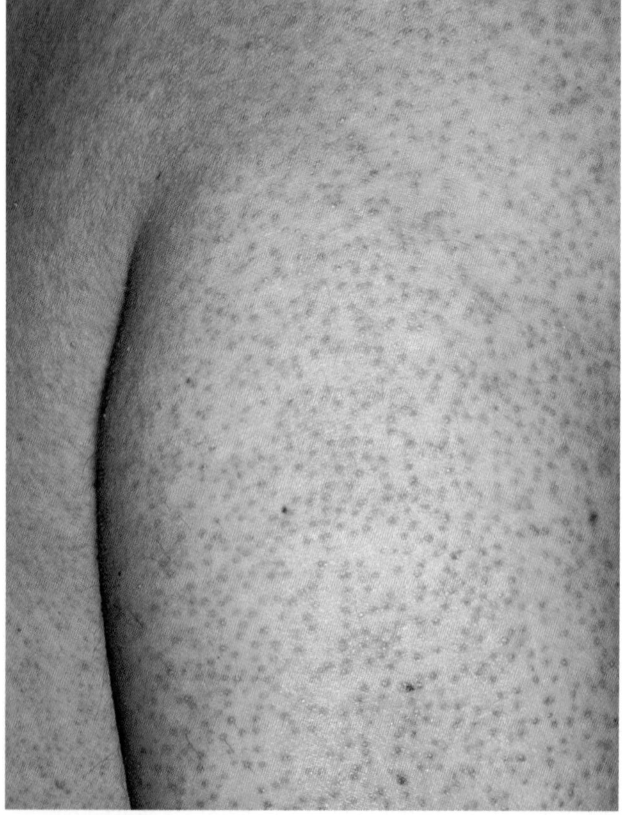

Figure 5-27 Keratosis pilaris. The florid form with a red halo surrounding the follicle can persist in adults.

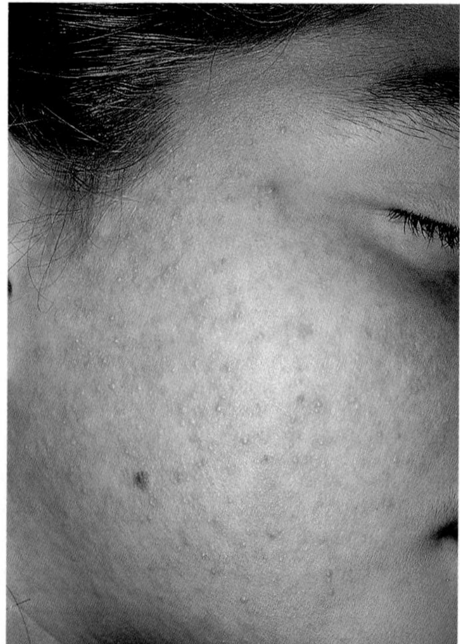

Figure 5-28 Keratosis pilaris. This is common on the face of children and is frequently confused with acne.

KERATOSIS PILARIS

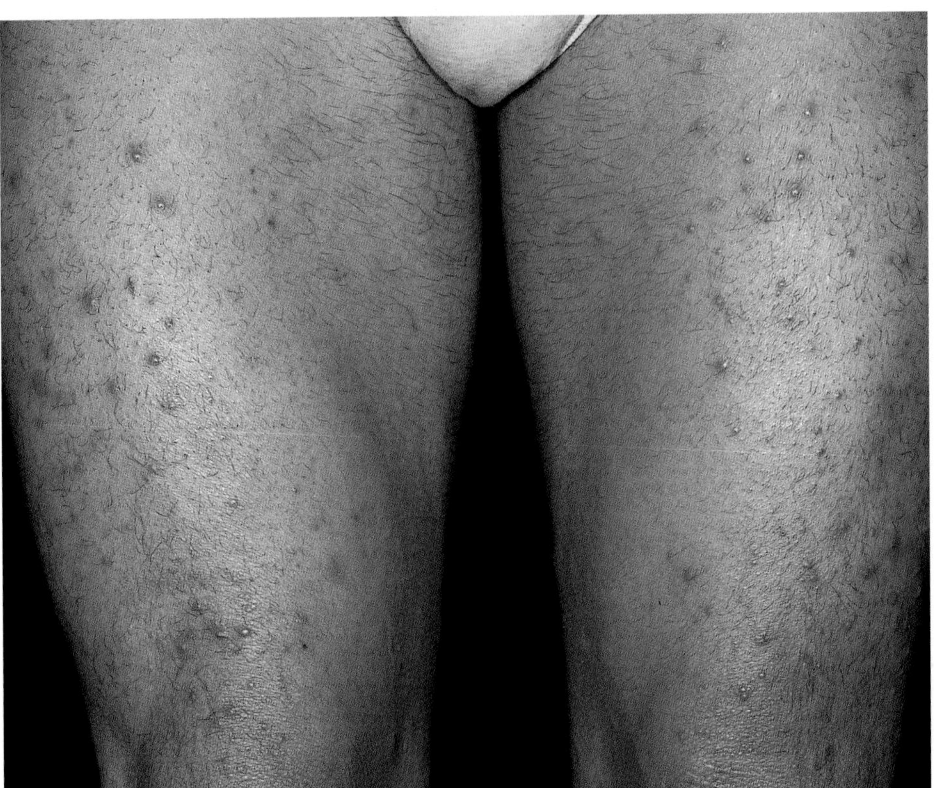

Figure 5-29 Infected lesions in a uniform distribution. Typical bacterial folliculitis has a haphazard distribution.

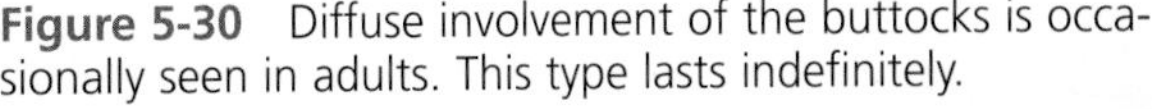

Figure 5-30 Diffuse involvement of the buttocks is occasionally seen in adults. This type lasts indefinitely.

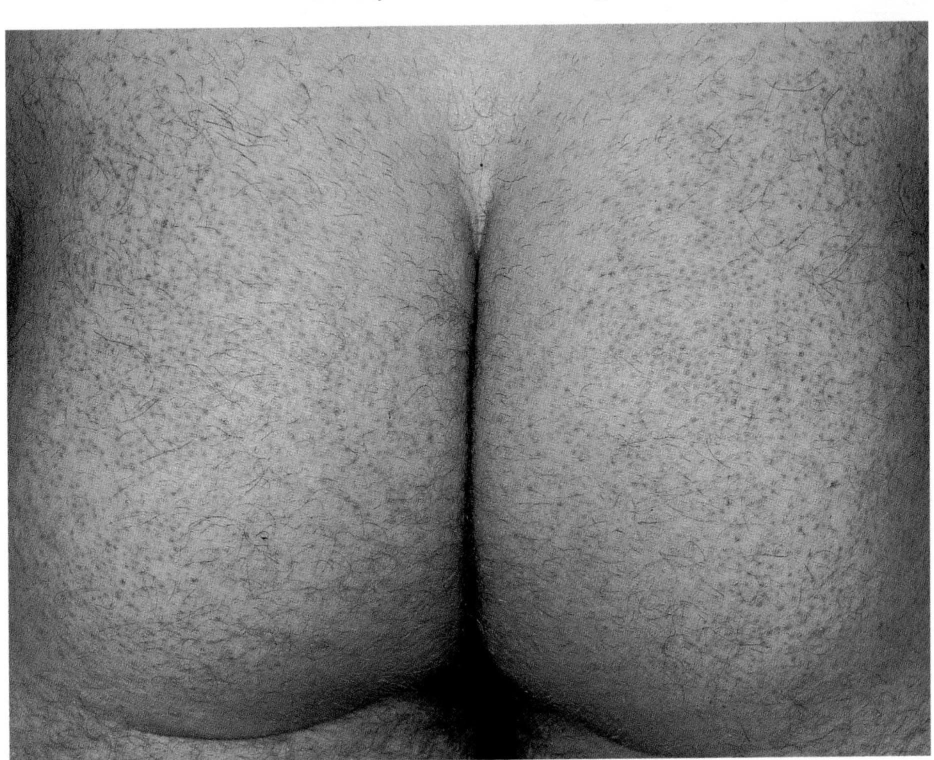

Hyperlinear palmar creases

Atopic patients are frequently found to have an accentuation of the major skin creases of the palms (Figure 5-31). This accentuation may be present in infancy and become more prominent as age and severity of skin inflammation increase. The changes might be initiated by rubbing or scratching. Patients with accentuated skin creases seem to have more extensive inflammation on the body and experience a longer course of disease. Occasionally patients without AD have palm crease accentuation. Moisturizers soften the skin but do not improve crease accentuation.

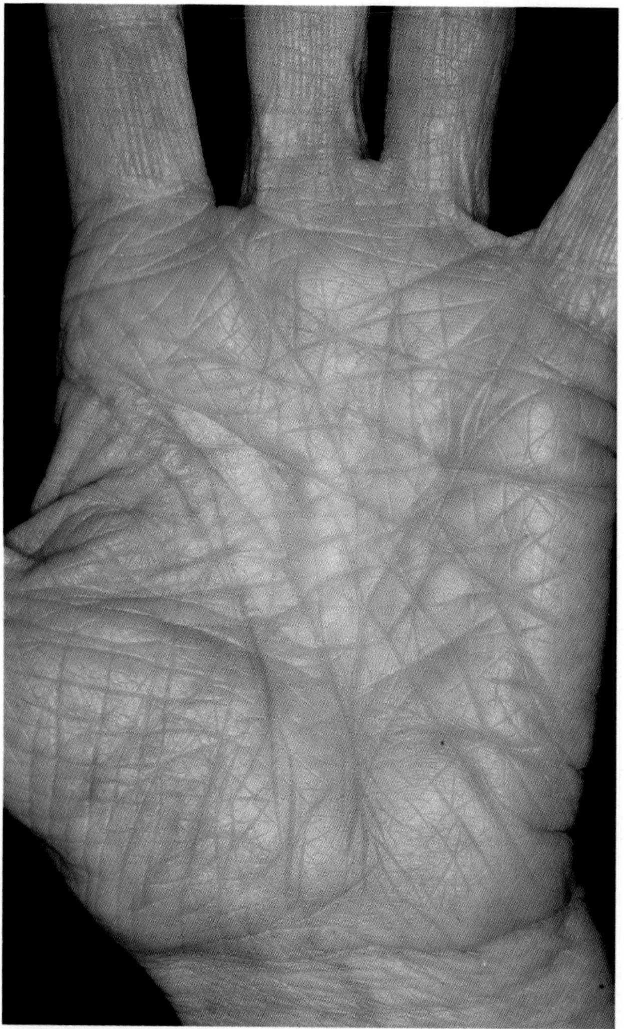

Figure 5-31 Hyperlinear palmar creases. Seen frequently in patients with severe atopic dermatitis.

Pityriasis alba

Pityriasis alba is a common disorder that is characterized by an asymptomatic, hypopigmented, slightly elevated, fine, scaling plaque with indistinct borders. The condition, which affects the face (Figures 5-32 and 5-33), lateral upper arms (Figure 5-34), and thighs (Figure 5-35), appears in young children and usually disappears by early adulthood. The white, round-to-oval areas vary in size, but generally average 2 to 4 cm in diameter (Figure 5-34). Lesions become obvious in the summer months when the areas do not tan.

The loss of pigment is not permanent, as it is in vitiligo. Vitiligo and the fungal infection tinea versicolor both appear to be white, but the margin between normal and hypopigmented skin in vitiligo is distinct. Tinea versicolor is rarely located on the face, and the hypopigmented areas are more numerous and often confluent. A potassium hydroxide examination quickly settles the question. The hypopigmentation usually fades with time. No treatment other than lubrication should be attempted unless the patches become eczematous. Tacrolimus ointment 0.1% applied two times a day for a few weeks may be effective.

Atopic pleats

The appearance of an extra line on the lower eyelid (Dennie-Morgan infraorbital fold) has been considered a distinguishing feature of patients with AD. The line may simply be caused by constant rubbing of the eyes. This extra line may also appear in people who do not have AD, and it is an unreliable sign of the atopic state.

Cataracts

Analysis of a large group of atopic patients showed that the incidence of cataracts was approximately 10%. The reason for their development is not understood. Most are asymptomatic and can only be detected by slit-lamp examination. Data suggest that there is no safe dosage of corticosteroids and that individual susceptibility may determine the threshold for development of cataracts.

PITYRIASIS ALBA

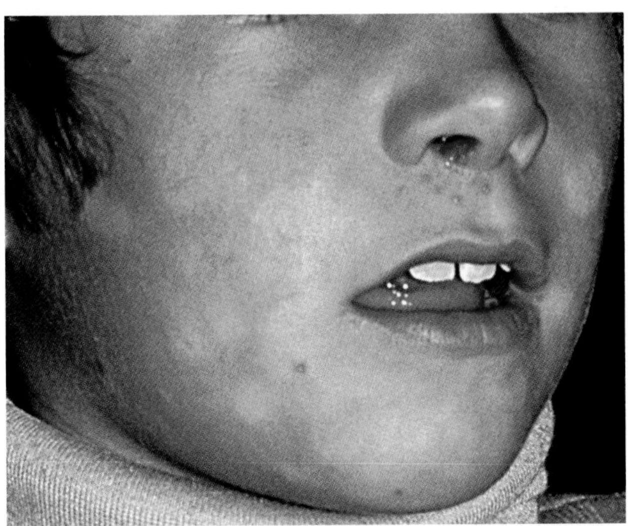

Figure 5-32 Hypopigmented round spots are a common occurrence on the faces of atopic children.

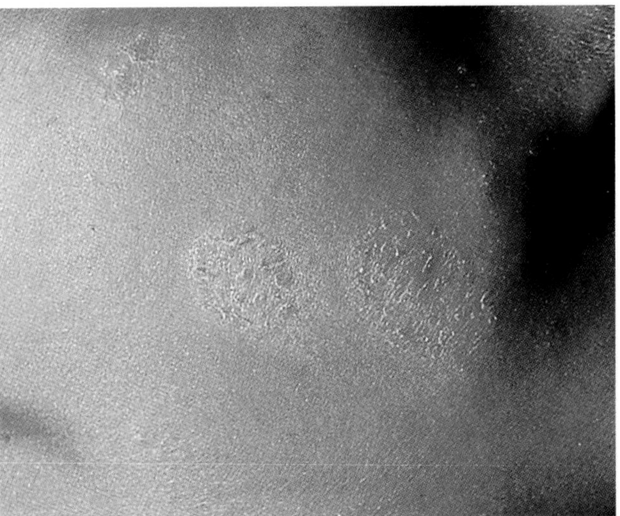

Figure 5-33 The superficial hypopigmented plaques become scaly and inflamed as the dry winter months progress.

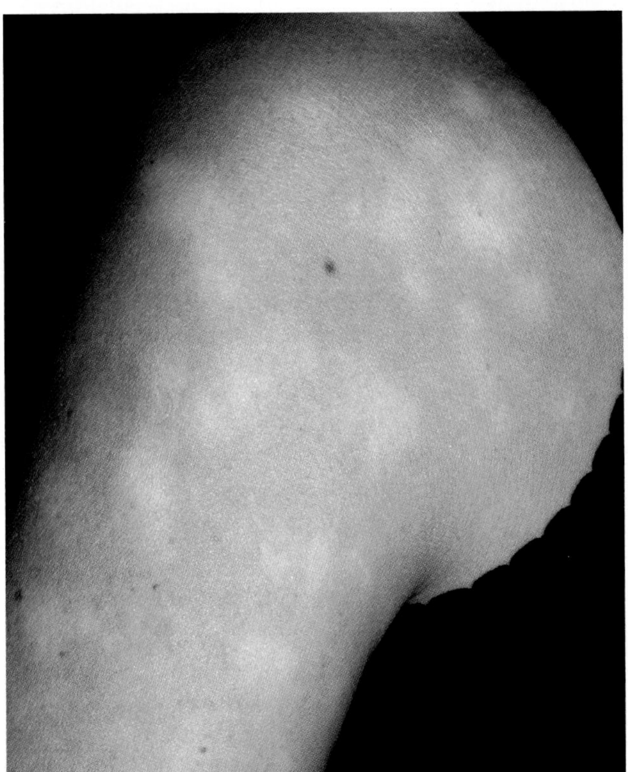

Figure 5-34 Irregular hypopigmented areas are frequently seen in atopic patients and are not to be confused with tinea versicolor or vitiligo.

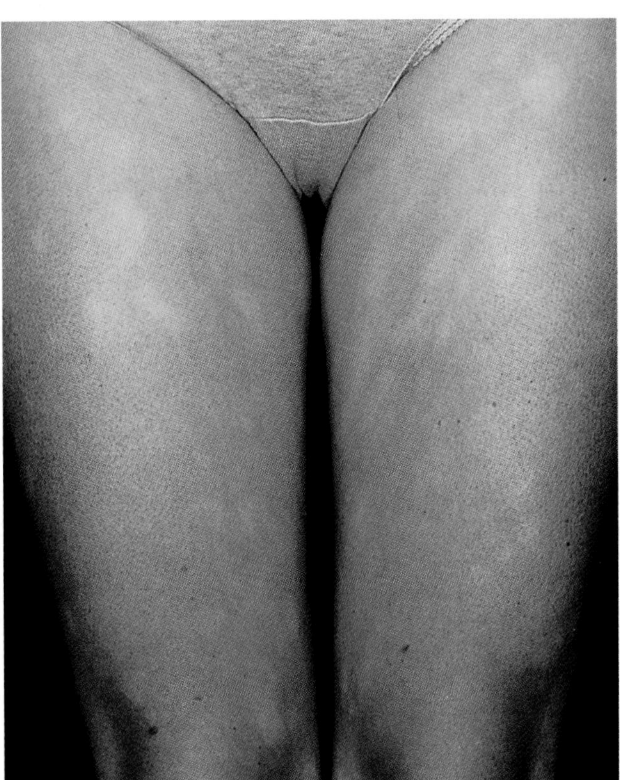

Figure 5-35 Lesions present here are more than are typically seen.

TRIGGERING FACTORS

Factors that promote dryness or increase the desire to scratch worsen AD. Understanding and controlling these aggravating factors are essential to the successful management of AD. A complete patient history is required because there is no standardized test scheme, like that for rhinitis or asthma, to identify specific triggering factors of AD.

Temperature change and sweating

Atopic patients do not tolerate sudden changes in temperature. Sweating induces itching, particularly in the antecubital and popliteal fossae, to a greater extent in atopic patients than in other individuals. Lying under warm blankets, entering a warm room, and experiencing physical stress all intensify the desire to scratch. A sudden lowering of temperature, such as leaving a warm shower, promotes itching. Patients should be discouraged from wearing clothing that tends to trap heat.

Decreased humidity

The beginning of fall heralds the onset of a difficult period for atopic patients. Cold air cannot support much humidity. The moisture-containing outer layer of the skin reaches equilibrium with the atmosphere and consequently holds less moisture. Dry skin is less supple, more fragile, and more easily irritated. Pruritus is established, the rash appears, and the long winter months in the northern states may be a difficult period to endure. Commercially available humidifiers can offer some relief by increasing the humidity in the house to above 50%.

Excessive washing

Repeated washing and drying removes water-binding lipids from the first layer of the skin. Daily baths may be tolerated in the summer months but lead to excessive dryness in the fall and winter.

Contact with irritating substances

Wool, household and industrial chemicals, cosmetics, and some soaps and detergents promote irritation and inflammation in the atopic patient. Cigarette smoke may provoke eczematous lesions on the eyelids. The inflammation is frequently interpreted as an allergic reaction by patients, who claim that they are allergic to almost everything they touch. The complaints reflect an intolerance of irritation. Atopic patients do develop allergic contact dermatitis, but the incidence is lower than normal.

Contact allergy

Contact allergic reactions to topical preparations, including corticosteroids, should be considered in patients who do not respond to therapy. Patch testing (see Chapter 4) may help to identify the offending agent.

Aeroallergens

The house-dust mite is the most important aeroallergen. Many patients with AD have anti-IgE antibodies to house-dust mite antigens, but the role of the house-dust mite in exacerbations of AD is controversial. Inhalation of house-dust antigen and allergen penetration through the skin may occur. Other aeroallergens such as pollens and allergens from pets, molds, or human dander may contribute to atopic dermatitis. Measures for allergen elimination should be undertaken. Hyposensitization may be effective, but there is little experience with this treatment.

Microbic agents

STAPHYLOCOCCUS AUREUS. *S. aureus* is the predominant skin microorganism in AD lesions. It is significantly increased in nonaffected skin. Normally *S. aureus* represents less than 5% of the total skin microflora in persons without atopic dermatitis. Antibiotics given systemically or topically may dramatically improve atopic dermatitis.

Food

Certain foods can provoke exacerbations of AD. Many patients who react to food are not aware of their hypersensitivity. Foods can provoke allergic and nonallergic reactions. The most common offenders are eggs, peanuts, milk, fish, soy, and wheat. Urticaria, an exacerbation of eczema, gastrointestinal or respiratory tract symptoms, or anaphylactic reactions may be signs of a food-induced reaction. Preservatives, colorants, and other low-molecular-weight substances in foods may be offenders, but there are no tests for these substances.

Emotional stress

Stressful situations can have a profound effect on the course of AD. A stable course can quickly degenerate, and localized inflammation may become extensive almost overnight. Patients are well aware of this phenomenon and, regrettably, believe that they are responsible for their disease. This notion may be reinforced by relatives and friends who assure them that their disease "is caused by your nerves." Explaining that AD is an inherited disease that is made worse, rather than caused, by emotional stress is reassuring.

TREATMENT OF ATOPIC DERMATITIS

Treatment goals consist of attempting to eliminate inflammation and infection (see Figure 5-36), preserving and restoring the stratum corneum barrier by using emollients, using antipruritic agents to reduce the self-inflicted damage to the involved skin (Box 5-3), and controlling exacerbating factors (Box 5-4). Most patients can achieve adequate control in less than 3 weeks. The following are possible reasons for failure to respond: poor patient compliance,

Box 5-3 Treating Atopic Dermatitis

Topical Therapy

Topical steroids should be used to treat dermatitis until the skin clears; then steroid application should be discontinued. They are also used when pimecrolimus or tacrolimus fails to adequately control inflammation.

Group V creams or ointments for red, scaling skin

Group I or II creams or ointments for lichenified skin

Parenteral steroids may be used for extensive flares

Prednisone

Topical nonsteroidal antiinflammatory agents may be used without interruption and do not cause atrophy. They are used as initial therapy or following treatment with topical steroids.

Pimecrolimus (Elidel)

Tacrolimus (Protopic)

Tar

Creams (e.g., Fototar)

Bath oil (e.g., Balnetar)

Moisturizers should be applied after showers and after hand washing

Lipid-free lotion cleansers (e.g., Cetaphil)

Antibiotics

Antibiotics may be prescribed to suppress *Staphylococcus aureus;* they may be administered on a short- or long-term basis

Cephalexin (Keflex) 250 mg four times daily

Cefadroxil (Duricef) 500 mg twice daily

Dicloxacillin 250 mg four times daily

Antihistamines

Antihistamines control pruritus and induce sedation and sleep

Hydroxyzine

Doxepin HCl cream 5% (Zonalon)

Treating Severe Cases

Corticosteroids

Oral prednisone

Intramuscular triamcinolone

Cyclosporine

Mycophenate mofetil

Azathioprine

Hospitalization

Home hospitalization (see the box on p. 125)

Topical steroids and rest

Goeckerman regimen (tar plus UVB)

Light Therapy

Combined UVA-UVB

UVA

UVB

UVA1

Narrow-band 311-nm UVB

PUVA

Box 5-4 Controlling Atopic Dermatitis

Protect Skin from the Following Agents

Moisture

Avoid frequent hand washing

Avoid frequent bathing

Avoid lengthy bathing

Use tepid water for baths

Avoid abrasive washcloths

Foods

Avoid prolonged contact (clean food around baby's mouth)

Rough clothing

Avoid wool

Use 100% cotton

Irritants and allergens

Use soaps only in axilla, groin, feet

Avoid perfumes or makeup that burns or itches

Avoid fabric softeners

Scratching

Do not scratch

Pat, firmly press, or grasp the skin

Apply soothing lubricants

Control Environment

Temperature

Maintain cool, stable temperatures

Do not overdress

Limit number of bed blankets

Avoid sweating

Humidity

Humidify the house in winter

Airborne allergens and dust

Do not have rugs in bedrooms

Vacuum drapes and blankets

Use plastic mattress covers

Wet-mop floors

Avoid aerosols

Ventilate cooking odors

Avoid cigarettes

Use artificial plants

Avoid ragweed pollen contact

Minimize animal dander—no cats, dogs, rodents, or birds

Change geographic location; sudden improvement may occur

Control emotional stress

Pleasant work environment

Learn relaxation techniques

Control diet

Diet control is a controversial treatment method (see text for treatment)

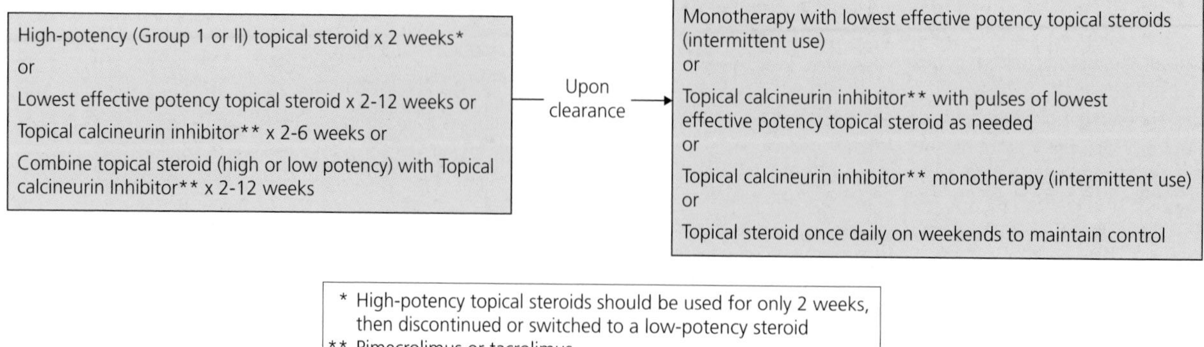

Figure 5-36 (Adapted from Abramovits W, Goldstein AM, Stevenson LC: *Clin Dermatol* 21:381-391, 2003.)

allergic contact dermatitis to a topical medicine, the simultaneous occurrence of asthma or hay fever, inadequate sedation, and continued emotional stress.

Dry skin

Controlling dry skin is essential in treating AD. Explain to patients that bathing dries the skin through the evaporation of water.

However, bathing also hydrates the skin, when moisturizer is applied immediately after bathing before the water has a chance to evaporate (within 3 minutes), thus retaining the hydration and keeping the skin soft and flexible. Pat the skin dry before moisturizer application. Daily bathing is possible if the 3-minute moisturizing rule is followed. Use of unscented moisturizers, such as an ointment like petrolatum or a cream, is ideal, whereas lotions are less effective emollients.

Inflammation and infection

Inflammation is treated with topical steroids and the new topical nonsteroidal antiinflammatory agents (pimecrolimus and tacrolimus; see Atopic Dermatitis: Various Possible Treatment Schedules). The combined optimum use of these agents has not been defined. Some clinicians use topical steroids for rapid control and then switch to pimecrolimus or tacrolimus to complete treatment. Low-grade flare-ups are treated in a similar manner. This combination therapy minimizes the side effects of steroids by reducing their frequency of use. Coadministration of topical steroids and tacrolimus may be of benefit for minimizing the initial local irritation associated with tacrolimus.

TOPICAL STEROIDS AND ANTIBIOTICS. Topical steroids control inflammation. If the crusting or pustulation typically seen with *Staphylococcus aureus* infections is present, antibiotics should be prescribed. Oral antibiotics (e.g., cephalexin, cefadroxil) are more effective than topical antibiotics for controlling infection.

HOW TO USE TOPICAL STEROIDS. Topical steroids are very safe and effective medications when used properly. Hydrocortisone and other low-potency topical steroids (groups VI, VII) provide little relief; inflammation persists, therapy becomes prolonged, and patients and parents become discouraged. Use mid-strength to high-strength (adults) topical steroids as initial treatment. Atopic dermatitis will be rapidly controlled in days. Limit treatment to 2 weeks. Ointment-based medications are preferred for dry skin. Moisturizers may also be used. Introduce patients to pimecrolimus cream (Elidel) or tacrolimus ointment (Protopic). Explain that these drugs are also very safe and do not have the side effects associated with long-term use of topical steroids (e.g., atrophy, striae). Patients will learn what combination of medications and bases works best for them and will feel confident that they can control fluctuations in their disease.

SAFETY IN CHILDREN. The group V topical steroid fluticasone propionate cream 0.05% (Cutivate) appears to be safe for the treatment of severe eczema for up to 4 weeks in children 3 months of age and older. Children between 3 months and 6 years with moderate to severe AD (≥35% body surface area; mean body surface area treated, 64%) were treated with fluticasone propionate cream 0.05% twice daily for 3 to 4 weeks. Mean cortisol levels were similar at baseline and at the end of treatment. Several other group V to VI topical steroids are also appropriate.

MAINTAINING CONTROL. Short weekly bursts of topical corticosteroids may play a role in keeping an adult's AD under control. Weekly applications of fluticasone ointment (Cutivate), applied once daily for 2 consecutive days each week, to known healed and any newly occurring dermatitis sites maintained the improvements achieved after the initial treatment phase and delayed relapse.

TOPICAL NONSTEROIDAL ANTI-INFLAMMATORY AGENTS. Pimecrolimus (Elidel) and tacrolimus (Protopic) are immunosuppressant topical medications that inhibit a calcium-activated phosphatase called calcineurin. The mechanism of action is closely related to that of cyclosporine. They are the first topical immune suppressants that are not hydrocortisone derivatives.

PIMECROLIMUS CREAM 1% (ELIDEL)

INDICATIONS. Pimecrolimus cream 1% is indicated for short-term and intermittent long-term therapy in the treatment of mild to moderate atopic dermatitis in nonimmunocompromised patients 2 years of age and older.

DOSAGE AND ADMINISTRATION. Apply a thin layer to the affected skin twice daily. Pimecrolimus may be used on all skin surfaces, including the head, neck, and intertriginous areas. Pimecrolimus should be used twice daily but not for a long continuous period of time. Advise the patient to stop the medication when signs and symptoms of eczema subside or if symptoms do not improve after 6 weeks of treatment. Treatment should be discontinued when resolution of disease occurs. Pimecrolimus cream should not be used with occlusive dressings.

PREVENTION OF FLARE PROGRESSION STRATEGY. In children and adolescents with a history of mild or moderate AD but free or almost free of signs or symptoms of the disease, early treatment of subsequent atopic dermatitis exacerbations with pimecrolimus cream 1% prevented progression to flares requiring topical steroids, leading to fewer unscheduled visits and reducing corticosteroid exposure. *PMID: 18624866*

In adults with a history of mild or moderate AD but free of active skin lesions, intervention with pimecrolimus cream 1% at the first signs and/or symptoms of a recurrence reduces the number of flares requiring topical steroid use and decreases the number of disease-related office visits.

ABSORPTION. Systemic absorption of pimecrolimus is very low.

ADVERSE EFFECTS. Burning does not occur. Patients should avoid excessive exposure to natural or artificial sunlight (tanning beds or UVA/B treatment) while using tacrolimus because of a possible enhancement of ultraviolet carcinogenicity.

TACROLIMUS OINTMENT (PROTOPIC)

INDICATIONS. Tacrolimus ointment is indicated for short-term and intermittent long-term therapy of patients with moderate to severe AD.

DOSAGE AND ADMINISTRATION. Tacrolimus ointment, both 0.03% and 0.1% for adults and only 0.03% for children aged 2 to 15 years, is indicated as second-line therapy for the short-term and noncontinuous chronic treatment of moderate to severe atopic dermatitis in nonimmunocompromised adults and children who have failed to respond adequately to other topical prescription treatments for atopic dermatitis, or when those treatments are not advisable. Apply a thin layer to the affected areas twice daily. Treatment should continue for 1 week after clearing of signs and symptoms. Continuous long-term use should be avoided. Do not use under occlusive dressings.

PREVENTION OF FLARE PROGRESSION STRATEGY. A 12-month, twice weekly proactive tacrolimus ointment application was an effective treatment in most study patients, preventing, delaying, and reducing the occurrence of AD exacerbations. *PMID: 18592619*

EFFICACY OF TACROLIMUS VERSUS GLUCOCORTICOIDS. Tacrolimus ointment has efficacy similar to a mid-potency steroid such as betamethasone valerate (0.12%) ointment.

TREATING THE FACE. Tacrolimus is safe for treating facial dermatoses because of the lack of atrophy and improved safety for the eye. There was no evidence of increased intraocular pressure when applied to the eyelids.

ABSORPTION. Systemic absorption is minimal even when large areas of skin are treated; blood levels are either undetectable or subtherapeutic. Patients applying large amounts of tacrolimus on severely affected skin may attain significant serum levels of the drug, at least transiently.

ADVERSE EFFECTS. Burning (mild to moderate) at the site of application is the most frequent adverse event, occurring in 31% to 61% of those treated. Burning lasts between 2 minutes and 3 hours and tends to decrease after the first few days of treatment. Tacrolimus ointment is not phototoxic, photosensitizing, or photoallergenic. Patients should avoid excessive exposure to natural or artificial sunlight (tanning beds or UVA/B treatment) while using tacrolimus because of a possible enhancement of ultraviolet carcinogenicity.

Infants

LOCALIZED INFLAMMATION. Topical steroids provide rapid control. Infants with dry, red, scaling plaques on the cheeks respond to group V or VI topical steroids applied twice a day for 7 to 14 days. Elidel cream or Protopic ointment may be used for long-term stability and control.

Flares are treated with topical steroids. Parents are instructed to decrease the frequency of washing, to start lubrication with a bland lubricant during the initial phase of the treatment period, and to continue lubrication long after topical steroids have been discontinued. Antistaphylococcal antibiotics are required only if there is moderate serum and crusting. Cracking about the lips is controlled in a similar fashion, but heavy lubricants (such as petroleum jelly, Aquaphor ointment, or Eucerin) are used after the inflammation has cleared.

GENERALIZED INFLAMMATION. Infants with more generalized inflammation require treatment with a group V to VI topical steroid cream or ointment applied two to three times a day for 10 to 21 days. Secondary infection often accompanies generalized inflammation, and a 3- to 7-day course of an antistaphylococcal antibiotic, such as cephalexin suspension (Keflex), is helpful. Start oral antibiotics 2 days before initiating topical steroid treatment. Sedation with hydroxyzine (10 mg/5 ml) is useful during the initial treatment period. The bedtime dose gives the child a good night's sleep and seems to suppress the unconscious scratching that occurs during disturbed sleep. The parents are grateful; at last they are not up all night with a scratching, crying child.

Potent topical or systemic steroids are potentially hazardous and may be associated with relapse after therapy has been discontinued. Avoidance of certain foods, pets, and house-dust mites is an option; the major drawbacks are the lack of tests to identify triggers or predict response.

Children and adults

LICHENIFIED PLAQUES. Lichenified plaques in older children and adults respond to group II through V topical steroids used with occlusive dressings (Figure 5-37). Occlusive therapy for 10 to 14 days is preferred if the plaques are resistant to treatment or are very thick. Occlusion may be used as soon as infection has been controlled. Adults may be treated with group I topical steroids for 1 to 4 weeks.

DIFFUSE INFLAMMATION. Diffuse inflammation involving the face, trunk, and extremities is treated with group V topical steroids applied two to four times a day. Elidel cream or Protopic ointment can be used as initial treatment for mild to moderate inflammation and for maintenance. A 3- to 7-day course of systemic antistaphylococcal antibiotics is almost invariably required. Start oral antibiotics 2 days before initiating topical steroid treatment. Exudative areas (Figure 5-38) with serum and crust are treated with a Burow's solution compress for 20 minutes three times a day for 2 to 3 days. Dryness and cracking with fissures occur if compressing is prolonged. Resistant cases may be treated with group V topical steroids applied before and after vinyl suit ("psoriasis suit") occlusion. The suit may be worn to bed or worn for 2 hours twice a day. All signs of infection, such as serum and crust, should be clear before initiating occlusive therapy.

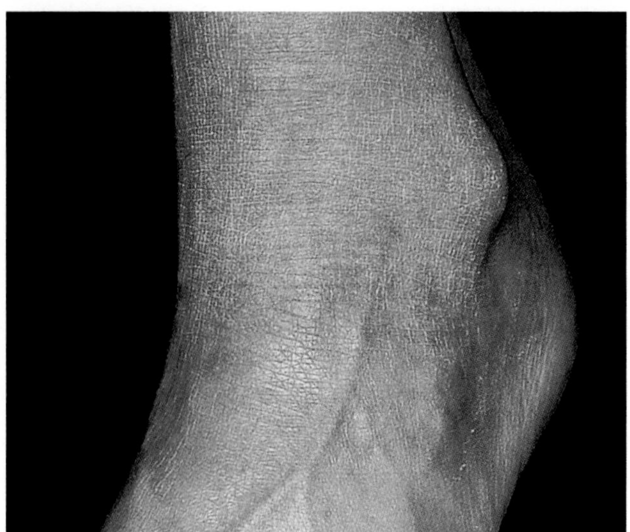

Figure 5-37 Response to treatment. Lichenified plaque shown in Figure 5-21 after 7 days of a group IV topical steroid under occlusive dressing.

SYSTEMIC STEROIDS. Severe AD may be treated with prednisone. A single-dose treatment schedule is shown in Table 5-1. Prednisone, administered in a dosage of 20 mg twice each day for at least 7 days, is an alternative schedule for severe, widespread inflammation; later, taper the dosage over the next 2 or 3 weeks. Patients who may have trouble adhering to a medication schedule may be treated with triamcinolone acetonide (Kenalog, Aristocort; 40 mg suspension) given intramuscularly. Commercially available steroid dose packs (e.g., Medrol Dosepak) should be avoided; they provide an inadequate amount of medicine and result in a recurrence of rash and pruritus after initial partial amelioration of symptoms during the first days of treatment.

Oral and intramuscular steroid therapy has a number of disadvantages. The relapse rate is high, with inflammation returning shortly after the medication is discontinued. Rebound flare upon discontinuation is possible. Enthusiasm for topical therapy diminishes once the patient has experienced the rapid clearing produced by systemic therapy, prompting some patients to request systemic therapy again; this request should be denied. The association of atopic cataracts with systemic steroid therapy has been discussed.

Tar

Tar ointments were the mainstay of therapy before topical steroids were introduced. They were effective and had few side effects but did not work quickly. Tar in a lubricating base such as T-Derm or Fototar applied twice daily is an effective alternative to topical steroids. Intensely inflamed areas should first be controlled with topical steroids. Tar ointments can then be used to complete therapy. Tar can be used as an initial therapy for chronic, superficial plaques.

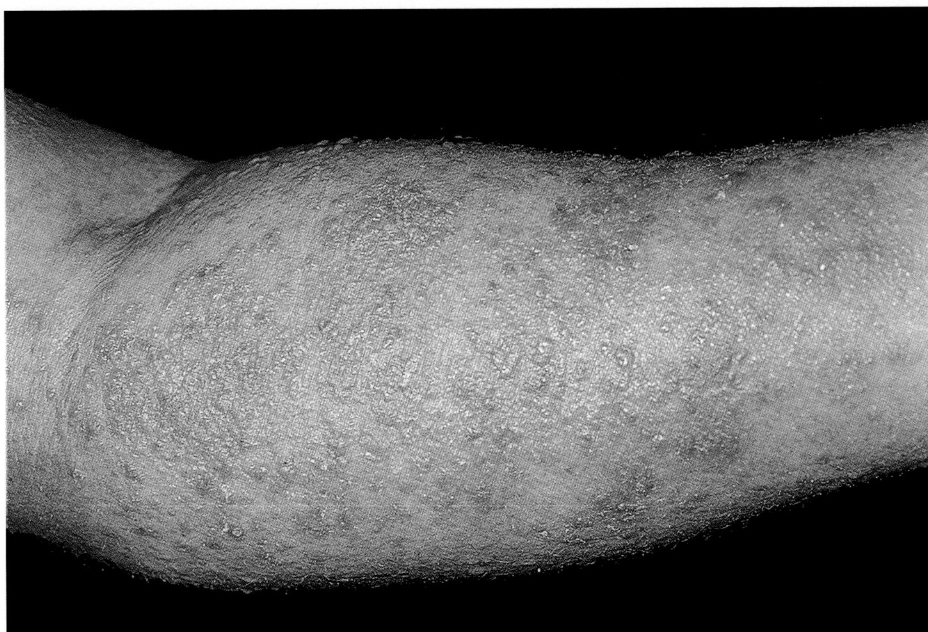

Figure 5-38 Severe generalized atopic dermatitis of this intensity requires prednisone and wet compresses for initial control.

Hospitalization for severely resistant cases

Some patients with severe, generalized inflammation do not respond to or flare soon after a reasonable trial of topical therapy. These patients are candidates for hospitalization. A short stay in the hospital can rapidly help to control a condition that has had a prolonged, unstable course. A program for "home hospitalization" is outlined in Box 5-5.

Table 5-1 Prednisone for Atopic Dermatitis (Adults)

Day	Dosage (mg/day) (10-mg tablets, taken as a single dose each morning)
1-4	60
5-6	50
7-8	40
9-10	30
11-12	20
13-14	10

Box 5-5 **Atopic Dermatitis—Home Hospitalization (Short-Term Intensive Treatment)**

Designate family member or friend as nurse.
All treatment is administered by nurse.
Write orders for home nurse.
Treatment starts Friday night and ends Monday morning.

Orders

1. Complete bed rest with bathroom privileges
2. Semidarkened room
3. No visitors other than nurse
4. Cotton bedclothes; dust-free and animal-free room
5. Temperature 68° to 70° F
6. Humidity 70%
7. Bland diet—no alcohol, spices, or caffeine

Topical Therapy

1. Tepid tub bath with bath oil (e.g., Keri Bath Oil), 20 minutes twice a day
2. Emollient bland cream applied to moist body after patting dry immediately on emergence from tub
3. Body lesions covered with group V steroid cream or ointment twice daily
4. Face lesions covered with group V steroid cream or ointment twice daily
5. Scalp inflammation treated with daily shampoo followed by topical steroid lotion in oil (e.g., Derma-Smoothe F/S)

Systemic Therapy

1. Antibiotics: e.g., cefadroxil 500 mg twice daily; dicloxacillin 250 mg four times daily
2. Sedating antihistamines: e.g., hydroxyzine 10 to 25 mg four times daily; doxepin 10 to 25 mg four times daily; or others
3. Phenothiazines for agitated patients: e.g., chlorpromazine 25 mg four times daily
4. May give a short-acting injectable steroid before hospitalization (e.g., dexamethasone 8 mg IM or betamethasone 6 mg IM)

Modified from Roth HL: *Int J Dermatol* 26:139-149, 1987. *PMID: 3553045*

Lubrication

Restoring moisture to the skin increases the rate of healing and establishes a durable barrier against further drying and irritation. A variety of lotions and creams are available, and most are adequate for rehydration. Petroleum jelly (Vaseline) is especially effective. Some products contain urea; others contain lactic acid. Urea and lactic acid have special hydrating qualities and may be more effective than other moisturizers. Their use should be encouraged, particularly during the winter months. Patients should be cautioned that lotions may sting shortly after application. This may be a property of the base or of a specific ingredient such as lactic acid. If itching or stinging continues with each application, another product should be selected. If inflammation occurs after use of a lubricant, allergic contact dermatitis to a preservative or a perfume should be considered.

Lubricants are most effective when applied after a bath. The patient should gently pat the skin dry with a towel and immediately apply the lubricant to seal in the moisture. Bath oils (e.g., Keri Bath Oil) are an effective method of lubrication, but they can make the tub slippery and dangerous for older patients. In order to be effective, a sufficient amount of oil must be used to create an oily feeling on the skin when leaving the tub. Septic systems may be adversely affected by prolonged use of bath oils. A mild bar soap should be used infrequently. Cetaphil, Dove, Keri, Purpose, Oilatum, and Basis are adequate; Ivory soap is very drying and should be avoided.

Sedation and antihistamines

ORAL ANTIHISTAMINES. Antihistamines generally have offered only marginal therapeutic benefit. Sedating antihistamines may be useful in relieving pruritus at night by helping patients to sleep. The common practice of prescribing antihistamines is based on individual experiences of patients and physicians. There is no objective evidence to support the effectiveness of sedating or nonsedating antihistamines in treating AD or relieving pruritus. Nonsedating agents may be useful for patients with allergic rhinitis, allergic conjunctivitis, allergen-induced asthma, and chronic urticaria; nonsedating antihistamines are very expensive.

TOPICAL ANTIHISTAMINES. Doxepin HCl cream (Zonalon cream) is an antipruritic cream. The mechanism of action is unknown. Doxepin has potent H_1-receptor and H_2-receptor blocking actions. Zonalon cream is indicated for the short-term (up to 8 days) management of moderate pruritus in adults with AD and lichen simplex chronicus. Drowsiness occurs in more than 20% of patients, especially patients receiving treatment to greater than 10% of their body surface area. The most common local adverse effect is burning and/or stinging. A thin film of cream is applied four times each day with intervals of at least 3 hours between applications.

Phototherapy

Phototherapy is effective for mild, moderate, and severe AD. Combined UVA-UVB and UVA or UVB have been shown in the past to be effective. The dosage is considerably lower than that for UVB-treated psoriasis patients. UVA1 irradiation (ranging from 340 to 400 nm) therapy is superior to conventional UVA-UVB phototherapy in patients with severe AD. The optimal dose regarding therapeutic efficacy and possible side effects is still to be determined. A correlation between UVA irradiation and photoaging, skin carcinogenesis, or melanoma induction may exist. Programs to avoid rapid relapses are being investigated. Low-dose UVA1 or narrow-band 311-nm UVB twice weekly for 4 weeks and once weekly for another 4 weeks appears to prevent relapse. Narrow-band UVB (311 nm) as monotherapy is also effective for moderate to severe atopic eczema. Photochemotherapy with methoxsalen plus UVA (PUVA) is effective but many clinicians have abandoned its use for AD because of its risk of long-term carcinogenicity.

ORAL IMMUNOSUPPRESSIVE AGENTS. A few patients remain severely affected by AD despite treatment with systemic steroids and phototherapy. Oral immunosuppressive agents may be considered for these few treatment-resistant cases.

CYCLOSPORINE. Systemic corticosteroids are used more commonly than cyclosporine (CsA) in general practice, but the American Academy of Dermatology guidelines recommend the use of CsA for the treatment of severe AD, on the basis of randomized controlled trials. CsA is not approved by the FDA for treating AD. CsA is an effective and well-tolerated treatment for severe refractory AD in children and adults. CsA can be prescribed on a short-term basis, both in adults and in children. Long-term treatment, up to 1 year, should be considered only in exceptional cases that cannot be controlled by short-term therapy. By starting at a low dose, the therapeutic safety should be further increased. Hence, in severe pediatric AD, CsA microemulsion, when started at a low dose (2.5 mg/kg/day), improves clinical measures of disease. Body-weight–independent dosing with cyclosporine is feasible for short-term treatment. Although the starting dose of 300 mg/day is more effective than 150 mg/day, the 150-mg dose would be preferable for the initiation of therapy because of its excellent renal tolerability. The disease may relapse despite continued treatment or may recur soon after cyclosporine is discontinued. Maintenance therapy may be hampered by side effects in the same way as therapy is hampered by side effects in the treatment of psoriasis. Serum IgE levels and prick test responses are unchanged by cyclosporine.

MYCOPHENOLATE MOFETIL. Mycophenolate mofetil is a highly effective drug for treating moderate-severe AD, with no serious adverse effects. In an open-label pilot study, patients were successfully treated with mycophenolate mofetil, 1 gm, given orally twice daily for 4 weeks. At week 5, the dosage was reduced to 500 mg twice daily and stopped at 8 weeks. *PMID: 11531810*

BIOLOGIC DRUGS. The biologic omalizumab (a recombinant, humanized, monoclonal antibody against IgE) is approved for the treatment of asthma. Its use in the treatment of AD is under investigation.

ALLERGEN (IgE)-MEDIATED DISEASE. Allergic IgE-mediated disease may occur in predisposed individuals. The sequence of sensitization and clinical manifestations begins with eczema and respiratory disease (rhinitis and bronchospasm) in infants and children less than 5 years and is due to food sensitivity (milk, egg, soy, and wheat proteins). Respiratory disease (rhinitis and asthma) then occurs in older children and adults as a result of sensitivity to inhalant allergens (dust mite, mold, and pollen inhalants). Serum testing for IgE antibodies may be useful to establish the diagnosis of an allergic disease and to define the allergens responsible for eliciting signs and symptoms. Detection of IgE antibodies indicates an increased likelihood of allergic disease. Some individuals with clinically insignificant sensitivity to allergens may have measurable levels of IgE antibodies in serum.

Diet restriction and breast-feeding

PREVALENCE OF AD AND FREQUENCY OF FOOD ALLERGY. Food allergy and atopic dermatitis often occur in the same patients. Foods can induce symptoms in a subset of patients with atopic dermatitis. Those at greatest risk are young children in whom eczematous lesions are severe or recalcitrant to therapy. The prevalence of AD is about 10% to 15% of children. Food hypersensitivity affects about 10% to 40% of children with AD.

FOODS. Food hypersensitivity is usually limited to one or two antigens and may be lost after several years. Five foods account for 90% of the positive oral challenges seen in children; in order of frequency they are eggs, peanuts, milk, soy, and wheat. A summary of the role of foods in AD is found in Box 5-6.

A child (especially younger than 7 years) with AD who is unresponsive to routine therapy may have a greater than 50% chance of having food hypersensitivity. A small percentage of children and adults with AD have positive responses to food-challenge tests, resulting in eczematous flares. Significant clinical improvement occurs within 1 or 2 months when an appropriately designed restricted diet is followed. Clinical reactions to food range from mild skin symptoms to life-threatening anaphylactic reactions.

IMMEDIATE-TYPE REACTIONS. Immediate-type clinical reactions to food can easily be identified by history and are associated with a positive skin prick test and specific IgE in serum. Symptoms usually occur within 2 hours of ingesting the food antigen (early-phase reaction). They consist of pruritus, erythema, and edema. A recurrence of pruritus may occur 6 to 8 hours later. This late-phase reaction does not occur in the absence of an early-phase reaction. Urticarial lesions are rarely seen. Many patients complain of nausea, abdominal pain, emesis, or diarrhea. Respiratory symptoms, including stridor, wheezing, nasal congestion, and sneezing, may develop. Anaphylactic reactions are uncommon but possible during food testing.

LATE-PHASE REACTIONS. The evaluation of food allergy in the absence of immediate clinical reactions presents diagnostic difficulties in children with AD. Late-phase clinical reactions are associated with a positive atopy patch test but not all clinicians perform this test.

Box 5-6 **Atopic Dermatitis and Food Allergy**

- The history is not a good method of screening for food allergy.
- The most reliable and practical way of diagnosing food allergy has not been determined.

Testing

- Skin prick test
- Determination of specific IgE antibodies
  Sera are analyzed for total IgE and specific IgE antibody titers (e.g., to cow's milk, hen's egg, wheat, and soy). False-negative IgE findings are uncommon. False-positive findings are common, particularly in the older child.

Exclusion Diets

- A limited trial of an exclusion diet can be recommended for foods that produce positive skin prick tests or are thought to be a possible cause.
- More than 90% of reactions in young children are caused by only five foods: eggs, milk, peanuts, soy, and wheat.

Maternal Diets

- Restricted diets are usually not recommended during pregnancy.
- Nut avoidance during pregnancy and lactation may be of benefit.
- Restricted maternal diet may be necessary in the breast-fed, food-allergic infant if the mother wishes to continue breast-feeding.

Breast-Feeding and Weaning

- Exclusive breast-feeding during the first 3 months of life is protective for atopy and atopic dermatitis during childhood in children with a family history of atopy.
- Food antigens have been identified in breast milk. Infants of mothers who avoid egg whites, cow's milk, fish, peanuts, and soy products during lactation developed less eczema.
- Prolonged breast-feeding should be encouraged in atopic families.
- The introduction of solids during the first 4 months should be avoided.

Older Children and Adults

- Food hypersensivity is rarely a factor.
- Exclusion diets are only rarely helpful.
- Nut and fish allergies are likely to be lifelong.
- Screening tests for IgE of older children ($\geq$6 years) are not very helpful because false-positive reactions are very common and only rarely indicate food hypersensitivity.

SKIN TEST AND IgE. The most reliable and practical way of diagnosing food allergy has not been determined. The history is of marginal value. In the very young child, either skin prick tests or circulating specific IgE (as measured by radioallergosorbent test/Immunocap [RAST/CAP] methods) may be useful as screening tests of IgE-mediated food hypersensitivity. In general, skin prick tests and circulating specific IgE antibodies correlate well. False-negative IgE findings are uncommon. False-positive findings are common, particularly in the older child.

PROVOCATION TESTS. Challenge tests are performed to determine the clinical significance of the positive laboratory tests. The double-blind, placebo-controlled food challenge is recognized as the "gold standard" for food allergy, but this test is not practical for most cases. The test is performed in the hospital with emergency equipment available. An open trial is less accurate but more practical. Patients are given a period of antigen avoidance. Foods that produce positive skin prick tests should be eliminated from the patient's diet for 1 to 2 weeks before the oral food challenge.

RESTRICTED DIETS IN ATOPIC DERMATITIS. If food allergy is thought to be a possibility, a limited trial of an exclusion diet can be recommended, after dietary assessment and advice by a pediatric dietitian. Food hypersensitivity may be a factor in the activity of AD in very young children, and dietary treatment is of value in these patients. More than 90% of reactions in young children are caused by only five foods: eggs, milk, peanuts, soy, and wheat.

EXCLUSION DIETS IN INFANTS. A relationship between the diversity of diet during the first 4 months (delayed introduction of solid foods) and the development of AD occurs. Itch lessens, and the eczema can improve significantly. The diet must be properly supervised by a pediatric dietitian to ensure that it is free of the allergen(s) while also being nutritionally adequate. Eczema develops in fewer children who receive a casein hydrolysate as compared with those receiving soy or cow's milk formula.

PROGNOSIS. Food allergy does not last indefinitely. A gradual reintroduction of the offending foods should be carefully considered after the child is past the third birthday. Milk and soy allergies usually disappear with aging; egg and fish allergies tend to remain.

CONTROLLING AEROALLERGENS. Atopic dermatitis can be elicited by external contact with an aeroallergen. Eczematous skin lesions are found predominantly in the air-exposed areas of the neck, face, and scalp. IgE-mediated sensitization of questionable clinical relevance is routinely demonstrated in patients with atopic eczema by skin prick test or radioallergosorbent test (RAST). A new test, the atopic patch test, which is not in general use, may be the most specific and relevant. The atopic patch test has a higher specificity with regard to clinical relevance of an allergen compared with the skin prick test and RAST. In a large trial, house-dust mite was the most common positive allergen, followed by grass pollen and cat epithelium. Most of the patients were positive only to one allergen, rarely to two or three. A regimen aimed at reducing the presence of house-dust mites can produce clinical improvement in patients with AD who show contact hypersensitivity to mite antigens on skin testing. Reduction of mites with a thorough housecleaning and by covering mattresses may result in dramatic improvement. These home-sanitation programs, which involve cleaning different surfaces, are often recommended by allergists to rhinitis and asthma patients to control aeroallergens such as mites and molds. Allergy Control Products, Inc. (www.allergycontrol.com) offers a full line of supplies to reduce allergen exposure.

Chapter | 6 |

Urticaria and Angioedema

CHAPTER CONTENTS

Urticaria, also referred to as *hives* or *wheals,* is a common and distinctive reaction pattern. Hives may occur at any age; up to 20% of the population will have at least one episode. Hives may be more common in atopic patients. Urticaria is classified as *acute* or *chronic*. The majority of cases are acute, lasting from hours to a few weeks. Angioedema frequently occurs with acute urticaria, which is more common in children and young adults. Chronic urticaria (arbitrarily defined as episodes of urticaria lasting more than 6 weeks) is more common in middle-aged women.

Because most individuals can diagnose urticaria and realize that it is a self-limited condition, they do not seek medical attention.

The cause of acute urticaria is determined in many cases, but the cause of chronic urticaria is determined in only 5% to 20% of cases. Patients with chronic urticaria present a frustrating problem in diagnosis and management. History taking is crucial but tedious, and treatment is usually supportive rather than curative.

These patients are often subjected to detailed and expensive medical evaluations that usually prove unrewarding. Studies demonstrate the value of a complete history and physical examination followed by the judicious use of laboratory studies in evaluating the results of the history and physical examination.

CLINICAL ASPECTS

DEFINITION. A hive or wheal is a circumscribed, erythematous or white, nonpitting, edematous, usually pruritic plaque that changes in size and shape by peripheral extension or regression during the few hours or days that the individual lesion exists. The edematous, central area (wheal) can be pale in comparison to the erythematous surrounding area (flare).

The evolution of urticaria is a dynamic process. New lesions evolve as old ones resolve. Hives result from localized capillary vasodilation, followed by transudation of protein-rich fluid into the surrounding tissue; they resolve when the fluid is slowly reabsorbed. The edema in urticaria is found in the superficial dermis. Lesions of angioedema are less well demarcated. The edema in angioedema is found in the deep dermis or subcutaneous/submucosal locations. The differential diagnosis of hives is found in Box 6-1.

CLINICAL PRESENTATION. Lesions vary in size from the 2- to 4-mm edematous papules of cholinergic urticaria to giant hives, a single lesion of which may cover an extremity. They may be round or oval; when confluent, they become polycyclic (Figures 6-1 to 6-8). A portion of the border either may not form or may be reabsorbed, giving the appearance of incomplete rings (see Figure 6-3). Hives may be uniformly red or white, or the edematous border may be red and the remainder of the surface white. This variation in color is usually present in superficial hives; thicker plaques have a uniform color (Figures 6-1 to 6-6).

Hives may be surrounded by a clear or red halo. Thicker plaques that result from massive transudation of fluid into the dermis and subcutaneous tissue are referred to as angioedema. These thick, firm plaques, like typical hives, may occur on any skin surface, but typically involve the lips, larynx (causing hoarseness or a sore throat), and mucosa of the gastrointestinal (GI) tract (causing abdominal pain) (see Figures 6-7 and 6-8). Bullae or purpura may appear in areas of intense swelling. Purpura and scaling may result as the lesions of urticarial vasculitis clear. Hives usually have a haphazard distribution, but those elicited by physical stimuli have characteristic features and distribution.

SYMPTOMS. Hives itch. The intensity varies, and some patients with a widespread eruption may experience little itching. Pruritus is milder in deep hives (angioedema) because the edema occurs in areas where there are fewer sensory nerve endings than there are near the surface of the skin.

CLINICAL CLASSIFICATION OF URTICARIA/ANGIOEDEMA. The clinical classification of urticaria and angioedema is found in Box 6-2. Urticaria can be provoked by immunologic and nonimmunologic mechanisms, as well as physical stimuli, skin contact, or small vessel vasculitis. Physical and ordinary urticarias may coexist. Angioedema occurs with or without urticaria. Angioedema without urticaria may indicate a C1 esterase inhibitor deficiency. The duration of hives is also an important diagnostic feature (Box 6-3).

Box 6-1 Differential Diagnosis of Urticaria

Bullous pemphigoid (urticarial stage)
Dermatitis herpetiformis
Drug eruptions
Erythema marginatum
Erythema multiforme
Papular urticaria
Pruritic urticarial papules and plaques of pregnancy
Still's disease
Urticaria pigmentosa
Urticarial vasculitis

From Green JJ, Heymann WR: *Adv Dermatol* 17:141-182, 2001. *PMID: 11758115*

Box 6-2 Clinical Classification of Urticaria/Angioedema

Ordinary urticaria (recurrent or episodic urticaria not in the categories below)
Physical urticaria (defined by the triggering stimulus)
- Adrenergic urticaria
- Aquagenic urticaria
- Cholinergic urticaria
- Cold urticaria
- Delayed pressure urticaria
- Dermographism
- Exercise-induced anaphylaxis
- Localized heat urticaria
- Solar urticaria
- Vibratory angioedema

Contact urticaria (induced by biologic or chemical skin contact)
Urticarial vasculitis (defined by vasculitis as shown by skin biopsy specimen)
Angioedema (without wheals)

From Brattan CEH: *J Am Acad Dermatol* 46:645, 2002.

Box 6-3 Duration of Hives

Type of Urticaria	Duration
Ordinary and delayed pressure	4-36 hours
Physical (except delayed pressure)	30 min-2 hours
Contact (may have a delayed phase)	1-2 hours
Urticarial vasculitis	1-7 days

HIVES

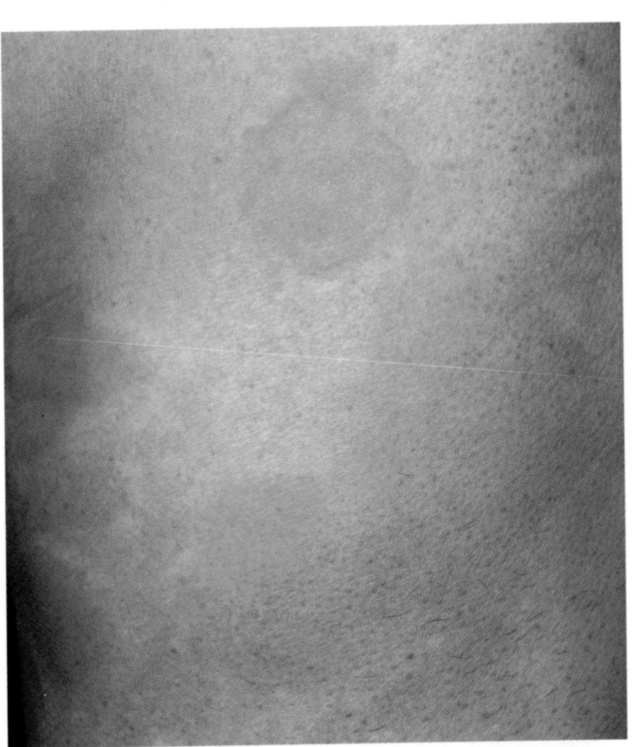

Figure 6-1 The most characteristic presentation is uniformly red edematous plaques surrounded by a faint white halo. These superficial lesions occur from transudation of fluid into the dermis.

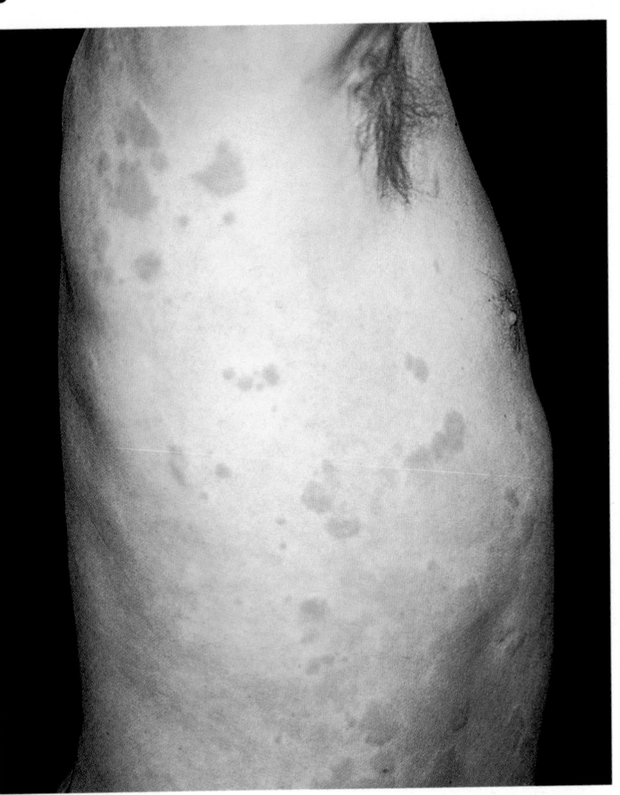

Figure 6-2 Urticarial plaques in different stages of formation.

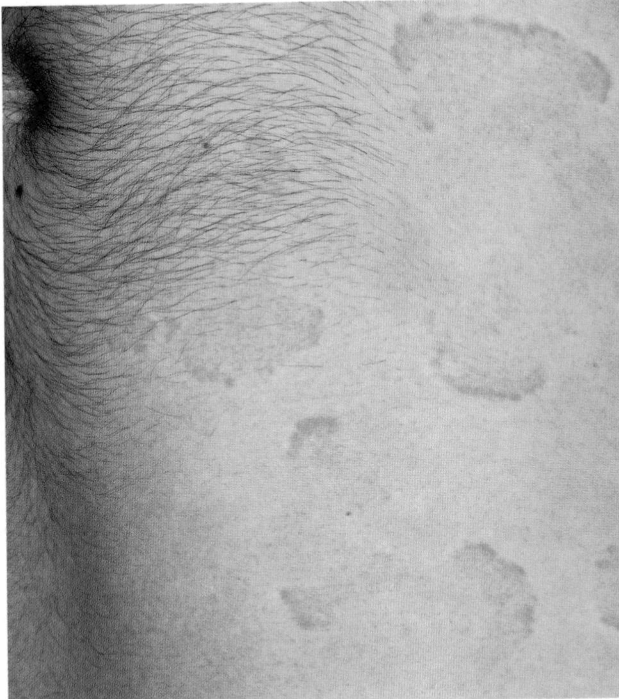

Figure 6-3 Polycyclic pattern.

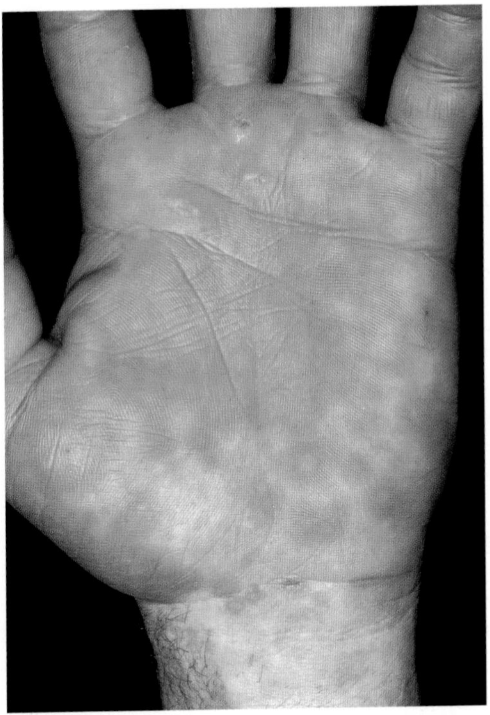

Figure 6-4 The entire palm is affected and is greatly swollen. The lesions resemble those of erythema multiforme.

HIVES

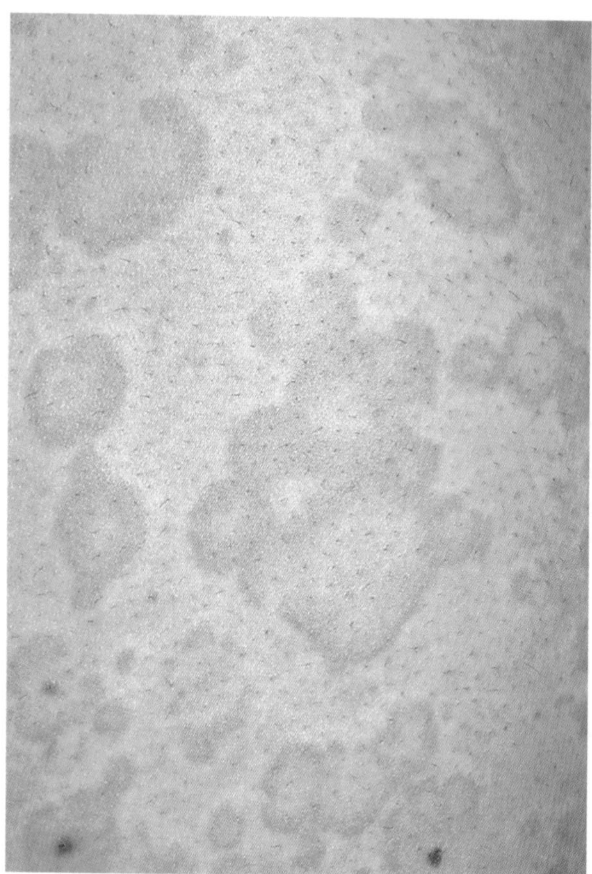

Figure 6-5 Superficial hives vary in color.

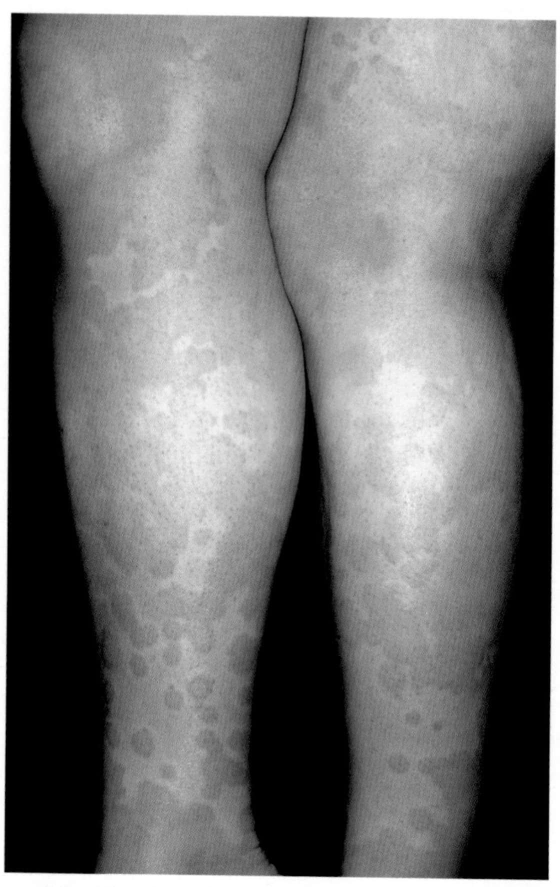

Figure 6-6 Hives have become more extensive and confluent.

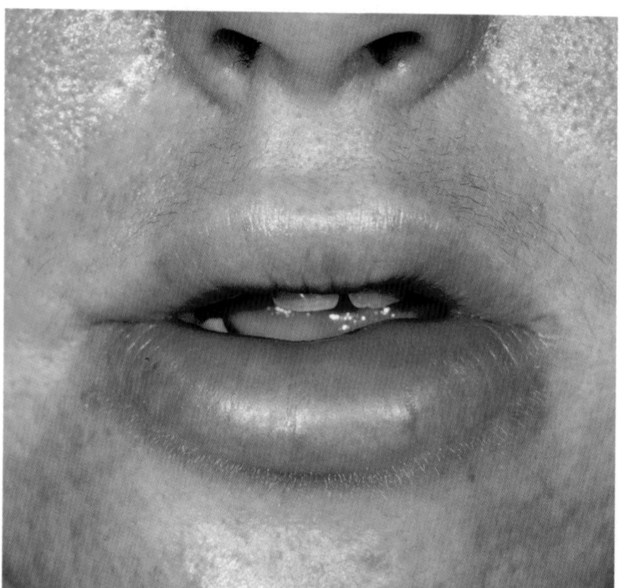

Figure 6-7 Angioedema is a deeper, larger hive than those shown in Figures 6-1 through 6-3. It is caused by transudation of fluid into the dermis and subcutaneous tissue. The lip is a common site.

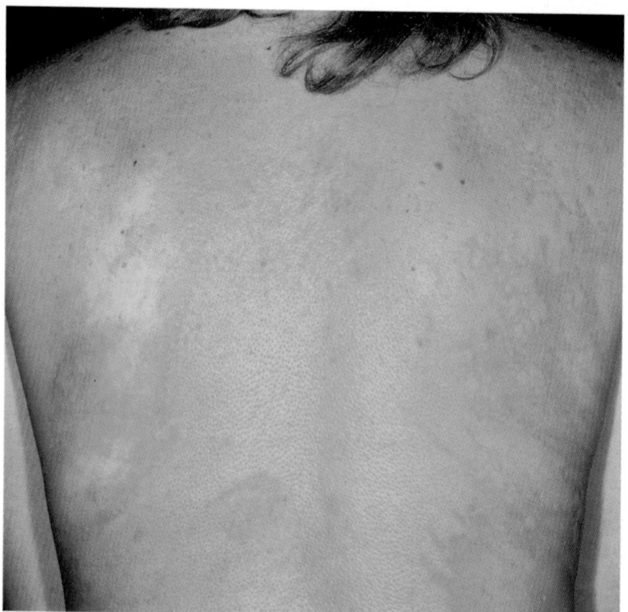

Figure 6-8 Angioedema. Massive swelling of the entire central area of the back.

PATHOPHYSIOLOGY

HISTAMINE

Histamine is the most important mediator of urticaria. Histamine is produced and stored in mast cells. There are several mechanisms for histamine release via mast cell surface receptors. A variety of immunologic, nonimmunologic, physical, and chemical stimuli may be responsible for the degranulation of mast cell granules and the release of histamine into the surrounding tissue and circulation. About one third of patients with chronic urticaria have circulating functional histamine-releasing immunoglobulin G (IgG) autoantibodies that bind to the high-affinity IgE receptor (Fc epsilon RI). Release of mast cell mediators can cause inflammation and accumulation and activation of other cells, including eosinophils, neutrophils, and possibly basophils. Histamine causes endothelial cell contraction, which allows vascular fluid to leak between the cells through the vessel wall, contributing to tissue edema and wheal formation.

When injected into skin, histamine produces the "triple response" of Lewis, the features of which are local erythema (vasodilation), the flare characterized by erythema beyond the border of the local erythema, and a wheal produced from leakage of fluid from the postcapillary venule. Histamine induces vascular changes by a number of mechanisms (Figure 6-9). Blood vessels contain two (and possibly more) receptors for histamine. The two most studied are designated H_1 and H_2.

H_1 RECEPTORS. H_1 receptors, when stimulated by histamine, cause an axon reflex, vasodilation, and pruritus. Acting through H_1 receptors, histamine causes smooth muscle contraction in the respiratory and gastrointestinal tracts and pruritus and sneezing by sensory nerve stimulation. H_1 receptors are blocked by the vast majority of clinically available antihistamines called H_1 antagonists (e.g., chlorpheniramine), which occupy the receptor site and prevent attachment of histamine.

H_2 RECEPTORS. When H_2 receptors are stimulated, vasodilation occurs. H_2 receptors are also present on the mast cell membrane surface and, when stimulated, further inhibit the production of histamine. Activation of H_2 receptors alone increases gastric acid secretion. Cimetidine (Tagamet), ranitidine (Zantac), and famotidine (Pepcid) are H_2 blocking agents (antihistamines). H_2 receptors are present at other sites. Activation of both H_1 and H_2 receptors causes hypotension, tachycardia, flushing, and headache. The H_2 blocking agents are used most often to suppress gastric acid secretion. They are used occasionally, usually in combination with an H_1 blocking agent, to treat urticaria.

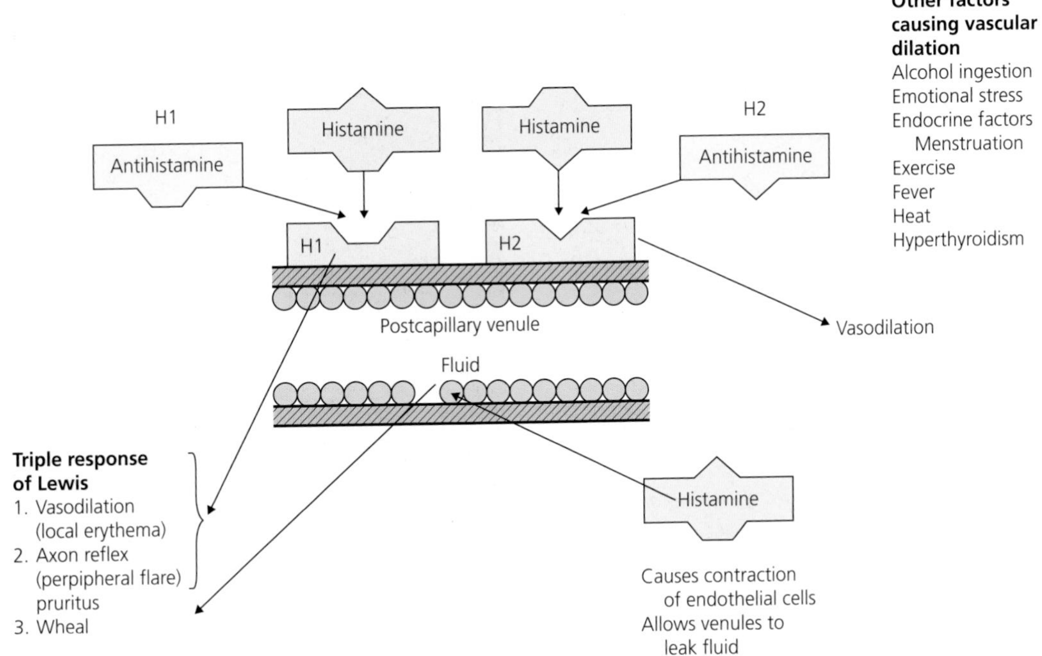

Figure 6-9 Physiology of histamine release.

INITIAL EVALUATION OF ALL PATIENTS WITH URTICARIA

1. Determine by skin examination that the patient actually has urticaria and not bites.
2. Rule out the presence of physical urticaria to avoid an unnecessarily lengthy evaluation. Stroking the arm with the wood end of a cotton-tipped applicator will test for dermographism.
3. Determine whether hives are acute or chronic. The difference in duration has been arbitrarily set at 6 weeks. Acute urticaria involves episodes of urticaria that last less than 6 weeks. Chronic urticaria consists of recurrent episodes of widespread urticaria present for longer than 6 weeks.
4. Review the known causes of urticaria listed in Box 6-4 (Etiologic Classification of Urticaria). Knowledge of the etiologic factors helps to direct the history and physical examination.

ACUTE URTICARIA

If the urticaria has been present for less than 6 weeks, it is considered acute (Figure 6-10). The evaluation and management of acute urticaria are outlined in Box 6-5. A history and physical examination should be performed, and laboratory studies are selected to investigate abnormalities. Histamine release that is induced by allergens (e.g., drugs, foods, or pollens) and mediated by IgE is a common cause of acute urticaria, and particular attention should be paid to these factors during the initial evaluation. There are no routine laboratory studies for the evaluation of acute urticaria. Once all possible causes are eliminated, the patient is treated with antihistamines to suppress the hives and stop the itching. Because urticaria clears spontaneously in most patients, an extensive workup is not advised during the early weeks of a urticarial eruption.

CHILDREN WITH HIVES. Food origin is important in the etiology of infantile urticaria. In one series it accounted for 62% of patients, more often than drug etiology (22%), physical urticaria (8%), and contact urticaria (8%).

ETIOLOGY OF ACUTE URTICARIA

Acute urticaria is IgE-mediated, complement-mediated, or nonimmune-mediated.

IgE-MEDIATED REACTIONS. Type I hypersensitivity reactions are probably responsible for most cases of acute urticaria. Circulating antigens such as foods, drugs, or inhalants interact with cell membrane–bound IgE to release histamine. Food allergies are present in 8% of children less than 3 years of age and in 2% of adults. Food allergies are the most common cause of anaphylaxis. Yellow jackets are the most common cause of insect sting–induced urticaria/anaphylaxis in the United States. Latex-induced urticaria is an IgE-mediated reaction.

COMPLEMENT-MEDIATED, OR IMMUNE-COMPLEX-MEDIATED, ACUTE URTICARIA. Complement-mediated acute urticaria can be precipitated by administration of whole blood, plasma, immunoglobulins, and drugs or by insect stings. Type III hypersensitivity reactions (Arthus reactions) occur with deposition of insoluble immune complexes in vessel walls. The complexes are composed of IgG or IgM with an antigen such as a drug. Urticaria occurs when the trapped complexes activate complement to cleave the anaphylotoxins C5a and C3a from C5 and C3. C5a and C3a are potent releasers of histamine from mast cells. Serum sickness (fevers, urticaria, lymphadenopathy, arthralgias, and myalgias), urticarial vasculitis, and systemic lupus erythematosus are diseases in which hives may occur as a result of immune complex deposition.

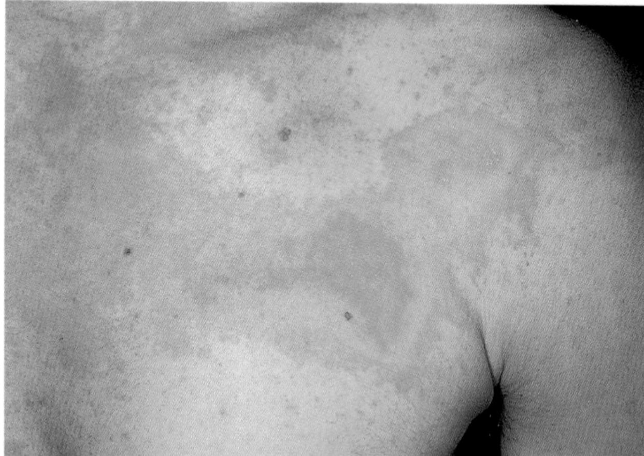

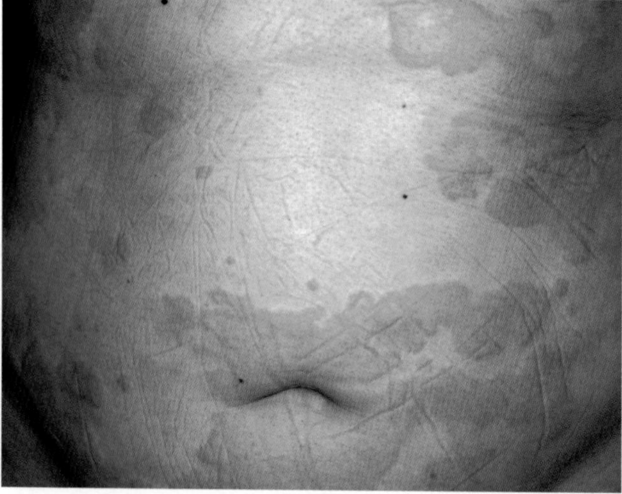

Figure 6-10 Acute urticaria. Wheals vary from a few millimeters to large, continuous plaques that may cover a large area. The plaques have smooth surfaces with curved or polycyclic borders. The degree of erythema varies. Central clearing occurs in expanding lesions.

Box 6-4 Etiologic Classification of Urticaria

Foods

Fish, shellfish, nuts, eggs, chocolate, strawberries, tomatoes, pork, cow's milk, cheese, wheat, yeast

Food additives

Salicylates, dyes such as tartrazine, benzoates, penicillin, aspartame (NutraSweet),* sulfites

Drugs

Penicillin, aspirin, sulfonamides, and drugs that cause a nonimmunologic release of histamine (e.g., morphine, codeine, polymyxin, dextran, curare, quinine)

Infections

Chronic bacterial infections (e.g., sinus, dental, chest, gallbladder, urinary tract), *Campylobacter* enteritis, fungal infections (e.g., dermatophytosis, candidiasis), viral infections (e.g., hepatitis B prodromal reaction, infectious mononucleosis, coxsackie), protozoal and helminth infections (e.g., intestinal worms, malaria)

Inhalants

Pollens, mold spores, animal dander, house dust, aerosols, volatile chemicals

Internal disease

Serum sickness, systemic lupus erythematosus, hyperthyroidism, autoimmune thyroid disease, carcinomas, lymphomas, juvenile rheumatoid arthritis (Still's disease), leukocytoclastic vasculitis, polycythemia vera (acne urticaria-urticarial papule surmounted by a vesicle), rheumatic fever, some blood transfusion reactions

Physical stimuli (physical urticarias)

Dermographism, pressure urticaria, cholinergic urticaria, exercise-induced anaphylactic syndrome, solar urticaria, cold urticaria, heat urticaria, vibratory urticaria, water (aquagenic) urticaria

Nonimmunologic contact urticaria

Plants (e.g., nettles), animals (e.g., caterpillars, jellyfish), medications (e.g., cinnamic aldehyde, compound 48/80, dimethyl sulfoxide)

Immunologic or uncertain mechanism contact urticaria

Ammonium persulfate used in hair bleaches, chemicals, foods, textiles, wood, saliva, cosmetics, perfumes, bacitracin

Skin diseases

Urticaria pigmentosa (mastocytosis), dermatitis herpetiformis, pemphigoid, amyloidosis

Hormones

Pregnancy, premenstrual flare-ups (progesterone)

Genetic, autosomal dominant (all rare)

Hereditary angioedema, cholinergic urticaria with progressive nerve deafness, amyloidosis of the kidney, familial cold urticaria, vibratory urticaria

From Geha R, Buckley CE et al: *J Allergy Clin Immunol* 92:513, 1993.

*Probably does not cause hives.

Box 6-5 Acute Urticaria—Evaluation and Management

History and physical examination

1. Ask the patient if he or she knows what causes the hives. In many instances, the patient will have determined the cause.
2. Take a history. See Box 6-4 for specific etiologies. Drugs are common causes in adults. Viral respiratory tract infections and streptococcal infections are common causes in children.
3. Perform a physical examination.
4. Stroke the arm to test for dermographism.

If the etiology is not determined by history, physical examination, and stroking the arm, order laboratory tests.

Laboratory tests

1. Order CBC with differential, erythrocyte sedimentation rate (ESR), liver function tests (LFTs), and urinalysis.
2. The history and physical examination may provide evidence that warrants additional tests. Consider testing for hepatitis A, B, C; infectious mononucleosis; thyroid function tests; thyroid antibodies; and antinuclear antibodies (ANAs).

Consider allergen testing

1. Skin tests: foods, drugs, aeroallergens, insect venom, natural rubber. Except for penicillin, antibiotics have a high false-positive rate with skin prick testing.
2. Radioallergosorbent tests (RAST) for penicillin, succinylcholine, natural rubber latex.
3. Food testing: Food diaries and elimination diets.
4. Oral challenge testing for food and food additives.

Management

1. Avoid specific allergens.
2. Treat with oral H_1 antagonists.
3. Add H_2 antagonists for resistant cases.
4. Anaphylaxis—subcutaneous epinephrine with or without parenteral H_1 and H_2 antihistamines (e.g., 50 mg of diphenhydramine and 50 mg of ranitidine). Systemic corticosteroids are sometimes useful.
5. Intravenous contrast media reactions—pretreat with H_1 antagonists and corticosteroids.
6. Latex allergic patients—prophylactic administration of corticosteroids before surgery.
7. Insect venom reaction—desensitization, preloaded syringes of epinephrine.

NONIMMUNOLOGIC RELEASE OF HISTAMINE. Pharmacologic mediators, such as acetylcholine, opiates, polymyxin B, and strawberries, react directly with cell membrane–bound mediators to release histamine. Aspirin/NSAIDs cause a nonimmunologic release of histamine. Patients with aspirin/NSAID sensitivity may have a history of allergic rhinitis or asthma. Urticaria may be caused by histamine-containing foods. Fish of the Scombroidea family accumulate histamine during spoilage. The mechanism of radiocontrast-related urticaria/anaphylaxis is unknown. Incidence varies from 3.1% with newer, lower osmolar agents to 12.7% with older, higher osmolar agents. Atopy is a risk factor for urticaria developing after radiocontrast exposure. The physical urticarias may be induced by both direct stimulation of cell membrane receptors and immunologic mechanisms.

CHRONIC URTICARIA

Patients who have a history of hives lasting for 6 or more weeks are classified as having chronic urticaria (CU). The etiology is often unclear. The morphology is similar to that of acute urticaria (Figure 6-11). CU is more common in middle-aged women and is infrequent in children. Individual lesions remain for less than 24 hours, and any skin surface can be affected. Itching is worse at night. Respiratory and gastrointestinal complaints are rare. Angioedema occurs in 50% of cases. Angioedema with chronic urticaria differs from hereditary angioedema in that it rarely affects the larynx. CU patients may experience physical urticaria. Symptoms continue for weeks, months, or years. Pressure urticaria, chronic urticaria, and angioedema frequently occur in the same patient. In one study, delayed pressure urticaria was present in 37% of patients with chronic urticaria. Aspirin/NSAIDs, penicillin, angiotensin-converting enzyme (ACE) inhibitors, opiates, alcohol, febrile illnesses, and stress exacerbate urticaria.

PATHOGENESIS

Chronic urticaria results from the cutaneous mast cell release of histamine. In contrast to acute urticaria, exogenous triggers are not found in most cases. Chronic urticaria in many cases may be an immune-mediated inflammatory disease. Release can be induced by specific immunoglobulin E (IgE), components of complement activation and endogenous peptides, endorphins, and enkephalins. Over 30% of chronic urticaria patients have autoimmune phenomena characterized by positive autologous serum skin tests, antibodies to the alpha subunit of the basophil IgE receptor and to IgE, and thyroid autoimmunity. The evaluation and management of chronic urticaria is outlined in Box 6-6.

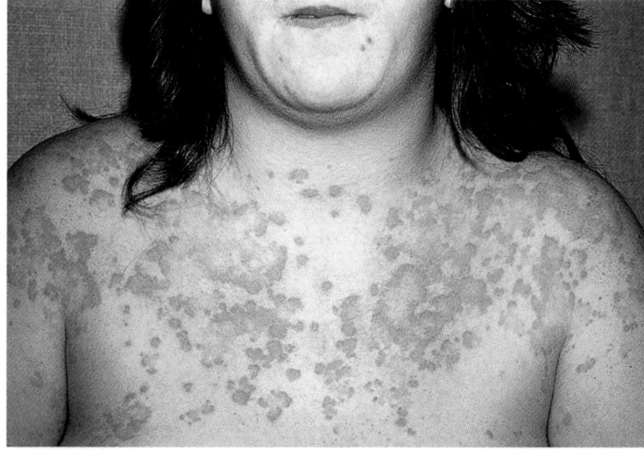

Figure 6-11 Chronic urticaria. Wheals may have the same configuration and intensity as acute urticaria. This patient has red plaques with sharply defined round, oval, and annular borders. The central clearing is highly characteristic of urticaria.

The patient must understand that the course of this disease is unpredictable; it may last for months or years. During the evaluation, the patient should be assured that antihistamines will decrease discomfort. The patient should also be told that although the evaluation may be lengthy and is often unrewarding, in most cases the disease ends spontaneously. Patients who understand the nature of this disease do not become discouraged so easily, nor are they as apt to go from physician to physician seeking a cure.

There are many studies in the literature on chronic urticaria. Most demonstrate that if the cause is not found after investigation of abnormalities elicited during the history and physical examination, there is little chance that it will be determined. It is tempting to order laboratory tests such as antinuclear antibody (ANA) levels and stool examinations for ova and parasites in an effort to be thorough, but results of studies do not support this approach. There are certain tests and procedures that might be considered when the initial evaluation has proved unrewarding.

RULE OUT PHYSICAL URTICARIAS. Unrecognized physical urticarias (see p. 194) may account for approximately 10% of all cases of chronic urticaria. In one large study physical urticarias were present in 71% of patients with chronic urticaria: 22% had immediate dermographism, 37% had delayed pressure urticaria, 11% had cholinergic urticaria, and 2% had cold urticaria.

The presence of physical urticaria should be ruled out by history and appropriate tests (see Table 6-2) before a lengthy evaluation and treatment program is undertaken. Dermographism is the most common type of physical urticaria; it begins suddenly following drug therapy or a viral illness, lasts for months or years, and clears spontaneously. Wheals that appear after the patient's arm is stroked prove the diagnosis.

THYROID AUTOIMMUNE DISEASE. There is a significant association between chronic urticaria and autoimmune thyroid disease (Hashimoto's thyroiditis, Graves' disease, toxic multinodular goiter). Thyroid autoimmunity was found in 12% of 140 consecutively seen patients with chronic urticaria in one series; 88% were women. Most patients with thyroid autoimmunity are asymptomatic and have thyroid function that is normal or only slightly abnormal. Guidelines for evaluation and treatment of thyroid-related urticaria are presented in Box 6-7.

Differential diagnosis

The differential diagnosis of chronic urticaria includes diseases that have lesions that mimic urticaria (Table 6-1). These often have fixed urticarial lesions that have some atypical features, such as duration greater than 24 hours, relative lack of itch, or epithelial changes (e.g., hyperpigmentation or hypopigmentation, vesicles or blisters, or scaling). *PMID: 18426134*

CHANGE OF ENVIRONMENT. Because the environment consists of numerous antigens, patients should con-

Box 6-6 **Chronic Urticaria—Evaluation and Management**

1. CU is a diagnosis of exclusion

Determine that lesions are hives and not insect bites (see Table 6-1 for differential diagnosis). Individual bite lesion lasts longer than 24 hours. Hives last less than 24 hours. Most urticarial plaques are larger than 2 cm. Stroke the patient's arm to rule out dermographism.

2. Take a history

Exact time of onset
Medication
Food and drink
Duration
Acute—days to a few weeks
Chronic—more than 6 weeks
Time of appearance
Time of day
Time of year
  Constant—food, internal disease
  Seasonal—inhalant allergy
Environment
Exposure to pollens, chemicals
  Home—clear while at work or on vacation
  Work—contact or inhalation of chemicals
Appearance after physical stimuli (physical urticaria)
Scratching, pressure, exercise, sun exposure, cold
Associated with arthralgia and fever
Juvenile rheumatoid arthritis, rheumatic fever, serum sickness, systemic lupus erythematosus, urticarial vasculitis, viral hepatitis
Duration of individual lesion
  Less than 1 hour—physical urticarias, typical hives
  Less than 24 hours—typical hives
  More than 25 hours—urticarial vasculitis; scaling and purpura as lesions resolve

3. Physical examination

Stroke the arm to test for dermographism, and rule out other types of physical urticaria.
Size
  Papular—cholinergic urticaria, bites
  Plaque—most cases
Thickness
  Superficial—most cases
  Deep—angioedema
Distribution
  Generalized—ingestants, inhalants, internal disease
  Localized—physical urticarias, contact urticaria
Sources of infection
  Sinus and gum infections
  Cystitis, vaginitis, prostatitis
  Dental examination by dentist
  Fix carious teeth
  Treat periodontal disease
  Internal disease, thyroid examination, gallbladder symptoms
  If the etiology is not determined by history, physical examination, and stroking the arm, then consider ordering laboratory tests.

Laboratory tests

1. Initial screening tests are CBC with differential, erythrocyte sedimentation rate (ESR), liver function tests (LFTs), urinalysis, and studies to confirm findings of history and physical examination.
2. Order screening thyroid function tests and tests for thyroid autoimmunity (thyroid microsomal and thyroglobulin antibodies), especially in women or in those patients with a family history of thyroid disease or other autoimmune diseases.
3. Eosinophilia suggests drug, food, or parasitic causes.
4. Leukocytosis suggests chronic infection.
5. Order ANA and ESR for patients with connective tissue disease symptoms.
6. Sinus radiographs have been advocated.
7. Order oral challenge testing for food additives.
8. Food testing: Use food diaries and elimination diets.
9. Perform lesion biopsy for hives lasting longer than 36 hours (rule out urticarial vasculitis), fever, arthralgias, elevated ESR, petechiae.
10. Order C4 only for patients with angioedema (not for patients with hives).

Management (see also Box 6-8)

1. Second-generation H_1 antihistamines: cetirizine (Zyrtec), loratadine (Claritin), fexofenadine (Allegra). Higher doses than suggested by the manufacturers may be required (e.g., 20-40 mg of cetirizine each day instead of 10 mg). Sedative side effects increase with higher dosages.
2. Add H_2 antagonists if H_1 agents do not provide effective control.
3. Hydroxyzine or doxepin is more sedating and can be added at nighttime. Doxepin can interact with other drugs that are metabolized by the cytochrome P-450 system (e.g., ketoconazole, itraconazole, erythromycin, clarithromycin).
4. Systemic steroids (short courses) may be used to provide temporary relief.
5. Stop vitamins, laxatives, antacids, toothpaste, cigarettes, cosmetics and all toiletries, chewing gum, household cleaning solutions, aerosols.
6. Stop fruits, tomatoes, nuts, eggs, shellfish, chocolate, alcohol, milk, cheese, bread, diet drinks, junk food.
7. Consider a highly restricted diet such as lamb, rice, and salt (rarely effective).
8. Consider empiric treatment with antibiotics. Consider eradication of *H. pylori* in patients with infection.
9. Leukotriene receptor antagonists—zafirlukast (Accolate 10 mg, 20 mg) and montelukast (Singulair 10 mg/day)—may be effective, especially in combination with antihistamines. Leukotriene receptor antagonists may prevent the severe urticaria/angioedema exacerbations that follow the use of NSAIDs in some patients with chronic urticaria.
10. Cyclosporine—patients with severe, unremitting chronic urticaria that responded poorly to antihistamines responded to cyclosporine 4 mg/kg daily in combination with cetirizine 20 mg daily.

Table 6-1 Differential Diagnosis of Chronic Urticaria

Cutaneous lupus erythematosus	Subacute cutaneous lupus erythematosus can present with urticarial-like lesions that burn rather than itch.
Urticarial vasculitis	A small- to medium-vessel leukocytoclastic vasculitis, urticarial wheals; up to 40% have angioedema. Lesions painful or burn, last for several days, heal with dyspigmentation or purpura. UV is a harbinger of more active disease.
Urticaria pigmentosa	Orange to deep brown pigmentation overlying the wheal. Urtication produced by stroking the skin; spares face, scalp, palms, and soles.
Sweet's syndrome	Women 30 to 50 years of age, acute fever, leukocytosis, urticarial-like plaques that may resemble urticaria, but are more persistent. Some lesions are studded with papules.
Fixed drug eruption	Lesions occur in the same spot (or spots) with each exposure to offending agent. Red macule becomes edematous and develops hyperpigmentation.
Bullous pemphigoid	In this autoimmune, subepidermal blistering disease, blisters appear on urticarial plaques.
Muckle-Wells syndrome (urticaria-deafness-amyloidosis syndrome)	Symptoms include recurrent urticarial lesions, fever, arthralgia, arthritis, malaise, conjunctivitis, sensorineural hearing loss, secondary amyloidosis.
Chronic infantile neurologic cutaneous articular syndrome (neonatal onset multisystemic inflammatory disease)	Characteristics include (1) neonatal onset of cutaneous symptoms, (2) chronic meningitis, and (3) joint manifestations with recurrent fever and inflammation.
Schnitzler syndrome	Symptoms include chronic, nonpruritic urticaria, fever, arthralgias or arthritis, bone pain, lymphadenopathy, IgM gammopathy.

Box 6-7 **Guidelines of Evaluation and Treatment of Thyroid-Related Chronic Urticaria**

1. Screen for thyroid autoimmunity by testing for thyroid microsomal and thyroglobulin antibodies, especially in women (female/male ratio was 7:1), or in those patients with a family history of thyroid disease or other autoimmune disorders.
2. The administration of thyroid hormone may alleviate chronic urticaria and/or angioedema in selected patients.

If patients with documented thyroid autoimmunity have been unresponsive to standard therapy for chronic urticaria and/or angioedema, consider the use of levothyroxine if the patients have hypothyroid or euthyroid. An appropriate initial dose is 1.7 mcg/kg per day.

3. The level of thyroid-stimulating hormone should be monitored by weeks 4 to 6 after the initiation of therapy, being kept in the low-normal range, to ensure that the patient is not becoming hyperthyroid.
4. If there has been no response of the chronic urticaria and/or angioedema by week 8 of administration, levothyroxine should be discontinued.
5. After being in remission for at least 1 to 2 months, levothyroxine should be discontinued. Should the chronic urticaria and/or angioedema recur, the hormone may be readministered, with an expectation that most patients will again be responsive to treatment.

From Heymann WR: *J Am Acad Dermatol* 40(2 Pt1):229, 1999.

sider a trial period of 1 or 2 weeks of separation from home and work, preferably with a geographic change.

HIGHLY RESTRICTED DIET. A highly restricted diet may be attempted. Patients are fed lamb, rice, sugar, salt, and water for 5 days. The occurrence of new hives after 3 days suggests that foods have no role. If hives disappear, a new food is reintroduced every other day until hives appear.

TREATMENT OF OCCULT INFECTIONS. Patients occasionally respond to antibiotics even in the absence of clinical infection. Consider eradication of *Helicobacter pylori* in patients with infection.

SKIN BIOPSY. Urticarial reactions display a wide spectrum of changes, ranging from a mild, mixed dermal inflammatory response to true vasculitis. Patients with hives that are characteristic of urticarial vasculitis should have a biopsy taken of the urticarial plaque. These hives burn rather than itch and last longer than 24 hours.

Dermal edema and dilated lymphatic and vascular capillaries occur. Increased numbers of neutrophils and eosinophils occur in patients with acute urticaria and in those with delayed pressure urticaria. Mast cell numbers are higher in the dermis of lesional and uninvolved skin of all patients with urticaria. Mononuclear infiltrates are more pronounced in cold urticaria and chronic urticaria.

TREATMENT OF URTICARIA

Box 6-8 lists the medications used to treat urticaria.

Approach to treatment

FIRST-LINE THERAPY

Nonsedating H_1 antihistamines (e.g., Allegra 180 mg daily) are the first choice for treatment. Older sedating H_1 antihistamines are more effective and so should be used to treat severe urticaria (e.g., 100 to 200 mg of hydroxyzine or diphenhydramine per day). For patients with severe angioedema (involving swelling of the face, tongue, and pharynx), diphenhydramine is particularly effective.

Patients become accustomed to the sedating effects after about a week, but their performance on driving tests remains impaired. H_2-receptor antagonists have very few side effects and may be useful as adjunctive therapy. Leukotriene antagonists are considered safe and are worth trying, but severe disease may require prednisone; many regimens have been suggested.

One approach is to start prednisone at 15 to 20 mg as a single morning dose every other day gradually tapering to 2.5 to 5.0 mg every 3 weeks, depending on the patient's response, and discontinue after 4 to 5 months. Side effects are minimized with the use of dietary discretion and exercise. Some patients require a combination of all of these medications.

Patients who have no response to any of these approaches may respond to immunotherapy with 200 to 300 mg of cyclosporine per day or methotrexate.

ANTIHISTAMINES. For the majority of patients, acute and chronic urticaria may be controlled with antihistamines.

MECHANISM OF ACTION. Antihistamines control urticaria by inhibiting vasodilation and vessel fluid loss. Antihistamines do not block the release of histamine. If histamine has been released before an antihistamine is taken, the receptor sites will be occupied and the antihistamine will have no effect.

Initiation of treatment. Antihistamines are the preferred initial treatment for urticaria and angioedema. Cetirizine, loratadine, or fexofenadine are first-line agents and are given once daily. Higher doses than suggested by the manufacturers may be required; see the box on medications for urticaria (Box 6-8). Patients with daytime and nighttime symptoms can be treated with combination therapy. These patients can be treated with a low-sedating antihistamine in the morning (e.g., loratadine 10 mg, or fexofenadine 180 mg, or cetirizine 10 to 20 mg) and a sedating antihistamine (e.g., hydroxyzine 25 mg) in the evening. Cetirizine can be mildly sedating. Doxepin is an alternative bedtime medication especially for anxious or depressed patients. The initial dose is 10 to 25 mg. Gradually increase the dose up to 75 mg for optimal control. Some patients with chronic urticaria respond when an H_2-receptor antagonist such as cimetidine is added to conventional antihistamines. This may be worth trying in refractory cases.

Side effects. Antihistamines are structurally similar to atropine; therefore they produce atropine-like peripheral and central anticholinergic effects such as dry mouth, blurred vision, constipation, and dizziness. First-generation antihistamines (H_1-receptor antagonists) such as chlorpheniramine, hydroxyzine, and diphenhydramine cross the blood-brain barrier and produce sedation. There is marked individual variation in response and side effects. Antihistamines may produce stimulation in children, especially in those ages 6 through 12.

Long-term administration. Prolonged use of H_1 antagonists does not lead to autoinduction of hepatic metabolism. The efficacy of H_1-receptor blockade does not decrease with prolonged use. Tolerance of adverse central nervous system effects may or may not develop.

H_1 and H_2 antihistamines. The majority of available antihistamines are H_1 antagonists (i.e., they compete for the H_1-receptor sites). Cimetidine, ranitidine, and famotidine are H_2 antagonists that are used primarily for the treatment of gastric hyperacidity. Approximately 85% of histamine receptors in the skin are the H_1 subtype, and 15% are H_2 receptors. The addition of an H_2-receptor antagonist to an H_1-receptor antagonist augments the inhibition of a histamine-induced wheal-and-flare reaction once H_1-receptor blockade has been maximized. It would seem that the combination of H_1 and H_2 antihistamines would provide optimum effects. The results of studies are conflicting but generally show that the combination is not much more effective than an H_1 blocking agent used alone.

First-generation (sedating) H_1 antihistamines. The first-generation H_1 antihistamines are divided into five classes (see Box 6-8). They are lipophilic, cross the blood-brain barrier, and cause sedation, weight gain, and atropine-like complications including dry mouth, blurred vision, constipation, and dysuria. Metabolism occurs via the hepatic cytochrome P-450 (CYP) system. In patients with liver disease, or in patients who are taking CYP 3A4 inhibitors such as erythromycin or ketoconazole, the plasma half-life may be prolonged. The H_1 antagonists suppress the wheal caused by histamine. Antihistamines given during or after the onset of a hive are less effective. They prevent wheals rather than treat them.

Second-generation (low-sedating) H_1 antihistamines. The second-generation antihistamines are not lipophilic and do not readily cross the blood-brain barrier. They cause little sedation and little or no atropine-like activity.

Fexofenadine (Allegra). Fexofenadine in a single dose of 180 mg daily or 60 mg twice daily is the recommended dosage for treating urticaria. Dosage adjustment is not nec-

Box 6-8 **Medications for Urticaria**

Drug	Initial dose (adult)	Maximum dose* (adult)	Liquid formulation	Tablet formulation
H_1-Receptor Antagonists				
Nonsedating*				
Fexofenadine (Allegra)	180 mg daily	180 mg bid	—	30, 60, 180 mg
Desloratadine (Clarinex)	5 mg daily	10 mg daily		5 mg
Loratadine (Claritin)	10 mg daily	20 mg bid	5 mg/5 ml	10 mg
Cetirizine (Zyrtec)	10 mg daily	10 mg bid	5 mg/5 ml	5, 10 mg
Carbinoxamine (Palgic)	4 mg daily	4-8 mg three-four times/day Not for children <3 years of age	4 mg/5 ml	4 mg
Levocetirizine (Xyzal)	5 mg daily	5 mg	2.5 mg/5 ml	5 mg
Sedating				
Hydroxyzine (Atarax)	10 mg four times/day	50 mg four times/day Suspension 25 mg/5 ml	10 mg/5 ml	10, 25, 50, 100 mg
Diphenhydramine (Benadryl)	25 mg bid	50 mg four times/day	Elixir 12.5 mg/5 ml Syrup 6.25 mg/5 ml	25, 50 mg; 12.5-mg chewable tablet
Cyproheptadine (Periactin)	4 mg four times/day	8 mg four times/day	2 mg/5 ml	8 mg
H_2-Receptor Antagonists				
Cimetidine (Tagamet)	400 mg bid	800 mg bid	300 mg/5 ml	200, 300, 400, 800 mg
Ranitidine (Zantac)	150 mg bid	300 mg bid	75 mg/5 ml	150, 300 mg
Famotidine (Pepcid)	20 mg bid	40 mg bid	40 mg/5 ml	20, 40 mg
H_1- and H_2-Receptor Antagonists				
Doxepin (Sinequan)	10 mg four times/day	50 mg four times/day	10 mg/ml	10, 25, 50, 75, 100, 150 mg
Corticosteroids				
Prednisone	20 mg every other day with gradual tapering	Many other dose schedules	5 mg/5 ml	2.5, 5, 10, 20, 50 mg
Methylprednisolone (Medrol)	16 mg every other day with gradual tapering	Many other dose schedules	—	2, 4, 8, 16, 24, 32 mg
Leukotriene Antagonists		—	—	
Zafirlukast (Accolate)	20 mg bid	—	—	10, 20 mg
Montelukast (Singulair)	10 mg daily	—	—	4-mg chewable, 5-mg chewable, 10 mg
Epinephrine	Injection			
Ana-Guard (1:1000)	0.3 ml/dose Sub-Q			
EpiPen (1:1000)	0.3 mg/dose			
EpiPen Jr (1:2000)	Children <12 yr: 0.15 mg/dose			
Immunotherapy				
Cyclosporine	2-3 mg/kg daily	4-6 mg/kg daily	100 mg/ml	25, 50, 100 mg
Methotrexate	2.5 mg PO bid for 3 days of week	5 mg PO bid for 3 days of week	25 mg/ml	2.5 mg

*Higher dosages than recommended by the manufacturer may be required for maximum therapeutic effect.

essary in the elderly or in patients with mild renal or hepatic impairment. Fexofenadine may offer the best combination of effectiveness and safety of all of the low-sedating antihistamines. A dose that is higher than recommended may be required.

Cetirizine (Zyrtec). Cetirizine is a metabolite of the first-generation H_1 antihistamine hydroxyzine. Some patients notice drowsiness after a 10-mg dose. The adult dose is 10 mg daily. A reduced dosage (5 mg daily) is recommended in patients with chronic renal or hepatic impairment. No drug interactions are reported, and there is no cardiotoxicity. A dose higher than recommended may be required.

Loratadine (Claritin). Loratadine is long-acting. A 10-mg dose suppresses whealing for up to 12 hours; suppression lasts longer after a larger dosage. A reduced dosage may be required in patients with chronic liver or renal disease. There are no significant adverse drug interactions. A special form of the medication, Reditabs (10 mg), rapidly disintegrates in the mouth. A dose higher than recommended may be required.

Desloratadine (Clarinex). Desloratadine is an active metabolite of loratadine. A 5-mg dose each day is effective. There is no evidence that it offers any advantage over loratadine.

Tricyclic antihistamines (Doxepin). Tricyclic antidepressants are potent blockers of histamine H_1 and H_2 receptors. The most potent is doxepin. When taken in dosages between 10 and 25 mg three times a day, doxepin is effective for the treatment of chronic idiopathic urticaria. Few side effects occur at this low dosage. Higher dosages may be tolerated if taken in the evening. Doxepin is a good alternative for patients with chronic urticaria who are not controlled with conventional antihistamines and for patients who suffer anxiety and depression associated with chronic urticaria. Lethargy is commonly observed but diminishes with continued use. Dry mouth and constipation are also commonly observed. Doxepin can interact with other drugs that are metabolized by the cytochrome P-450 system (e.g., ketoconazole, itraconazole, erythromycin, clarithromycin).

EPINEPHRINE. Severe urticaria or angioedema requires epinephrine. Epinephrine solutions have a rapid onset of effect but a short duration of action. The dosage for adults is a 1:1000 solution (0.2 to 1.0 ml) given either subcutaneously or intramuscularly; the initial dose is usually 0.3 ml. The epinephrine suspensions provide both a prompt and a prolonged effect (up to 8 hours). For adults, 0.1 to 0.3 ml of the 1:200 suspension is given subcutaneously.

SECOND-LINE AGENTS

ORAL CORTICOSTEROIDS. Many patients with chronic urticaria and angioedema will have little response to even a combination of H_1- and H_2-receptor blockers. Oral corticosteroids should be considered for these refractory cases. Because of toxicity, corticosteroids are reserved for antihistamine failures or the most severe cases. They are reliable and effective. They do not have the potential for drug-free remission. Prednisone 40 mg per day given in a single morning dose or 20 mg twice a day is effective in most cases. Another approach is to prescribe 30 20-mg tablets. The patient receives 5 days each of 60 mg, 40 mg, and 20 mg, and the medication is taken once each morning. Others will respond to prednisone 20 mg every other day with a gradual taper.

LEUKOTRIENE MODIFIERS. Leukotriene modifiers may provide improvement in some cases of antihistamine-resistant chronic urticaria. Excellent safety, absence of required monitoring in the cases of montelukast and zafirlukast, and wide availability make leukotriene modifiers the preferred alternative agent. Montelukast, zafirlukast, and zileuton have been studied. Response may take days to weeks. Randomized controlled trials show zafirlukast and montelukast either singly or in combination with antihistamines are effective but several negative studies have also appeared. Montelukast was demonstrated to be effective for patients with NSAID-exacerbated chronic urticaria. Patients with positive autologous serum skin test (ASST) results may predict better response to leukotriene modifiers. Experience in physical urticarias has also been promising.

DAPSONE. Small studies demonstrate excellent clinical response with dosages that vary from 25 mg/day to 100 mg/day. Response may be fairly rapid, but some patients require several weeks to notice improvement. Monitor for the predictable small decline in hemoglobin level. The drug is generally well tolerated. There is a possibility of sustained remission after stopping the drug. Obtain a G6PD level to avoid more severe hemolytic anemia in G6PD-deficient patients.

CALCINEURIN INHIBITORS. Cyclosporine might be an effective alternative in some chronic urticaria patients unresponsive to conventional treatments and may be considered if leukotriene modifiers and dapsone fail. Patients with severe unremitting disease who respond poorly to antihistamines may respond to 4 mg/kg daily of cyclosporine for 4 weeks. Patients requiring initially high doses of glucocorticosteroids and with a long clinical history are less amenable to cyclosporine treatment.

THIRD-LINE AGENTS

INTRAVENOUS IMMUNOGLOBULIN. Responses ranging from complete and lasting remission to modest transient benefit are reported. Response seems to be rapid. The optimal dose and number of infusions to attempt are unclear. Only case reports and short series of patients are reported.

METHOTREXATE. Methotrexate may be considered in resistant cases of urticaria. Case reports and a small series of patients document benefit within 1 to 2 weeks of starting methotrexate. Because adverse effects may be serious and frequent monitoring is necessary, methotrexate should be reserved for intractable cases in which other alternative agents have failed. Methotrexate 10 to 15 mg weekly or 2.5 mg twice a day for 3 days of the week would be a reasonable starting dose.

TOPICAL MEASURES. Itching is controlled with tepid showering, tepid oatmeal baths (Aveeno), cooling lotions that contain menthol (Sarna lotion), and topical pramoxine lotions (Itch-X). Avoid factors that enhance pruritus (e.g., aspirin, drinking alcohol, or wearing of tight elasticized apparel or coarse woolen fabrics).

PHYSICAL URTICARIAS

Physical urticarias are induced by physical and external stimuli, and they typically affect young adults. More than one type of physical urticaria can occur in an individual. Provocative testing confirms the diagnosis. During the initial examination, the physician should determine whether the hives are elicited by physical stimuli (see Table 6-2). Patients with these distinctive hives may be spared a detailed laboratory evaluation; they simply require an explanation of their condition and its treatment. Unrecognized physical urticarias may account for approximately 20% of all cases of chronic urticaria. A major distinguishing feature of the physical urticarias is that attacks are brief, lasting only 30 to 120 minutes. In typical urticaria, individual lesions last from hours to a few days. The one exception among physical urticarias is pressure urticaria, in which swelling may last for several hours. Most physical urticaria forms persist for about 3 to 5 years or longer.

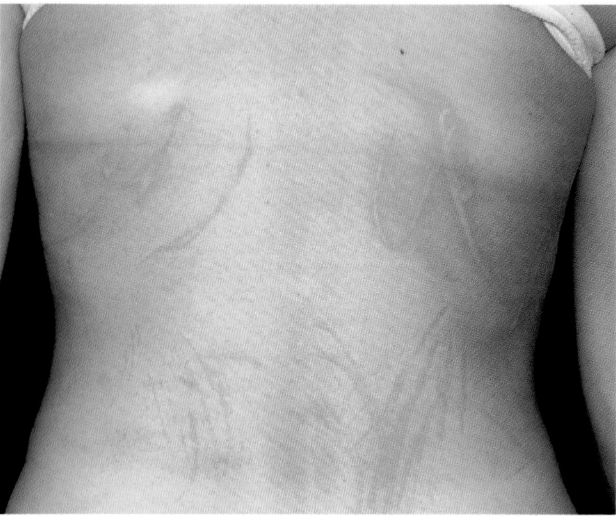

Figure 6-12 This patient has dermographism. Hives are created by rubbing and linear lesions are produced by scratching.

Dermographism

Also known as "skin writing," dermographism is the most common physical urticaria, occurring to some degree in approximately 5% of the population. Scratching, toweling, or other activities that produce minor skin trauma induce itching and wheals. The onset is usually sudden; young patients are affected most commonly. The tendency to be dermographic lasts for weeks to months or years. The condition runs on average a course of 2 to 3 years before resolving spontaneously. It may be preceded by a viral infection, antibiotic therapy (especially penicillin), or emotional upset, but in most cases the cause is unknown. Mucosal involvement and angioedema do not occur. There are no recognized systemic associations (such as atopy or autoimmunity).

The degree of urticarial response varies. A patient will be highly reactive for months and then appear to be in remission, only to have symptoms recur (Figure 6-12). Patients complain of linear, itchy wheals from scratching or wheals at the site of friction from clothing. Delayed dermographism, in which the immediate urticarial response is followed in 1 to 6 hours by a wheal that persists for 24 to 48 hours, is rare.

DIAGNOSIS. A tongue blade drawn firmly across the patient's arm or back produces whealing 2 mm or more in width in approximately 1 to 3 minutes (Darier's sign), an exaggerated triple response (Figure 6-13).

1. A red line occurs in 3 to 15 seconds (capillary dilation).
2. Broadening erythema appears (axon reflex flare from arteriolar dilation).
3. A wheal with surrounding erythema replaces the red line (transudation of fluid through dilated capillaries).

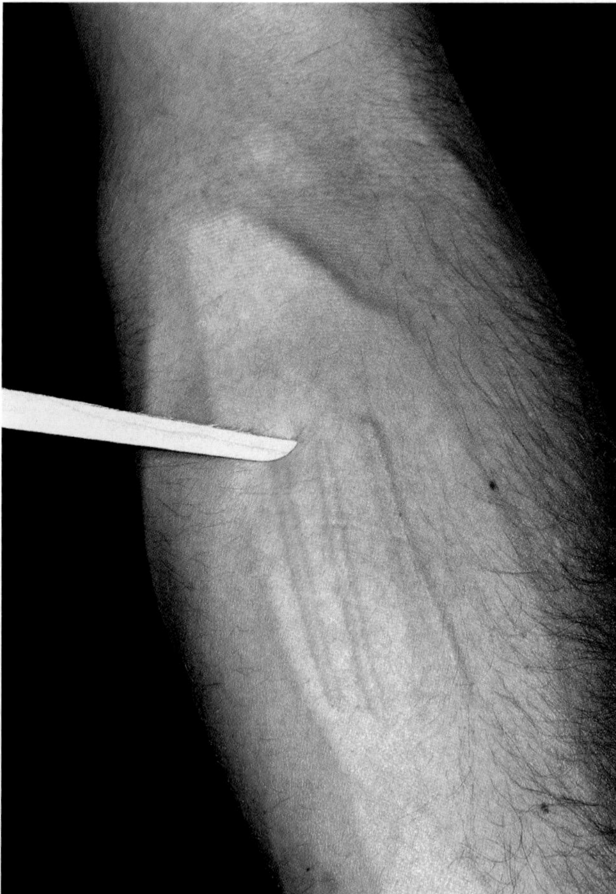

Figure 6-13 Dermographism. A tongue blade drawn firmly across the arm elicits urticaria in susceptible individuals. This simple test should be considered for any patient with acute or chronic urticaria.

Table 6-2 Comparison of the Physical Urticarias

Urticaria	Relative frequency	Precipitant	Time of onset	Duration	Local symptoms	Systemic symptoms	Tests	Mechanism	Treatment
Symptomatic dermographism	Most frequent	Stroking skin	Minutes	2-3 hr	Irregular, pruritic wheals	None	Scratch skin	Passive transfer; IgE; histamine; possible role of adenosine triphosphate; substance P; possible direct pharmacologic mechanism	Continual hydroxyzine regimen or nonsedating antihistamines; combined H_1 and H_2 blockers
Delayed dermographism	Rare	Stroking skin	30 min-8 hr	≤48 hr	Burning; deep swelling	None	Scratch skin; observe early and late	Unknown	Avoidance of precipitants
Pressure urticaria	Frequent	Pressure	3-12 hr	8-24 hr	Diffuse, tender swelling	Flulike symptoms	Apply weight	Unknown	Trial of antihistamines, middle- to low-dose glucocorticosteroids, dapsone
Solar urticaria	Frequent	Various wavelengths of light	2-5 min	15 min-3 hr	Pruritic wheals	Wheezing; dizziness; syncope	Phototest	Passive transfer; reverse passive transfer; IgE; possible histamine	Avoidance of precipitants; antihistamines; sunscreens; hydroxychloroquine
Familial cold urticaria	Rare	Change in skin temperature from cold air	30 min-3 hr	≤48 hr	Burning wheals	Tremor; headache; arthralgia; fever	Expose skin to cold air	Unknown	Avoidance of precipitants
Essential acquired cold urticaria	Frequent	Cold contact	2-5 min	1-2 hr	Pruritic wheals	Wheezing; syncope; drowning	Apply ice-filled copper beaker to arm; immerse arm in cold water	Passive transfer; reverse passive transfer; IgE (IgM); histamine; vasculitis can be induced	Cyproheptadine or other antihistamines; desensitization; avoidance of precipitants, oral doxycycline, or penicillin
Heat urticaria	Rare	Heat contact	2-5 min (rarely delayed)	1 hr	Pruritic wheals	None	Apply hot water-filled cylinder to arm	Possible histamine; possible complement	Antihistamines; desensitization; avoidance of precipitants, hydroxychloroquine
Cholinergic urticaria	Very frequent	General overheating of body	2-20 min	30 min-1 hr	Papular, pruritic wheals	Syncope; diarrhea; vomiting; salivation; headaches	Bathe in hot water; exercise until perspiring; inject methacholine chloride	Passive transfer; possible immunoglobulin; product of sweat gland stimulation; histamine; reduced protease inhibitor	Application of cold water or ice to skin; H_1 antihistamines
Aquagenic urticaria	Rare	Water contact	Several min-30 min	30-45 min	Papular, pruritic wheals	None reported	Apply water compresses to skin	Unknown	Avoidance of precipitants; antihistamines; application of inert oil
Vibratory angioedema	Very rare	Vibrating against skin	2-5 min	1 hr	Angioedema	None reported	Apply body of vibrating mixer to forearm	Unknown	Avoidance of precipitants
Exercise-induced anaphylaxis	Rare	Exercise; some cases ingestion of certain foods	During or after exercise	Minutes to hours	Pruritic wheals	Respiratory distress; hypotension	Exercise testing; immersion tests	Unknown	Antihistamines, epinephrine auto-injector

From Jorizzo JL, Smith EB: *Arch Dermatol* 118:198, 1982; ©1982, American Medical Association.

As a control, the examining physician can perform this test on his or her own arm at the same time.

Unlike urticaria pigmentosa caused by cutaneous mastocytosis (which also manifests dermographism—Darier's sign), there is no increase in skin mast cell numbers.

TREATMENT. Treatment is not necessary unless the patient is highly sensitive and reacts continually to the slightest trauma. Antihistamines are very effective. Nonsedating H_1 antihistamines or hydroxyzine in relatively low dosages (10 to 25 mg daily to four times a day) provides adequate relief. Some patients are severely affected and require continuous suppression. Use the lowest dose possible to stop itching. Many patients adapt to a low dose of hydroxyzine and do not feel sedated.

Pressure urticaria

A deep, itchy, burning, or painful swelling occurring 2 to 6 hours after a pressure stimulus and lasting 8 to 72 hours is characteristic of this common form of physical urticaria. The mean age of onset is the early 30s. The disease is chronic, and the mean duration is 9 years (range: 1 to 40 years). Malaise, fatigue, fever, chills, headache, or generalized arthralgia may occur. Many have moderate to severe disease that is disabling, especially for those who perform manual labor. Pressure urticaria, chronic urticaria, and angioedema frequently occur in the same patient. In one study delayed pressure urticaria was present in 37% of patients with chronic urticaria. This explains the frequency of wheals at local pressure sites in patients with chronic urticaria. It also explains the poor response to H_1 antihistamines in some patients because delayed pressure urticaria is generally poorly responsive to this treatment.

The hands, feet, trunk, buttock, lips, and face are commonly affected. Lesions are induced by standing, walking, wearing tight garments, or prolonged sitting on a hard surface (Figures 6-14 and 6-15).

DIAGNOSIS. Because the swelling occurs hours after the application of pressure, the cause may not be immediately apparent. Repeated deep swelling in the same area is the clue to the diagnosis. Patients with dermographism may have whealing from pressure that occurs immediately, rather than hours later. Tests using weights are used for studies but generally are not performed in clinical practice.

TREATMENT. Protect pressure points. Systemic steroids given in short duration tapers are the most effective treatment for severe, disabling delayed pressure urticaria. Dosages of prednisone greater than 30 mg/day may be required. Antihistamines are usually not helpful but should be tried. Cetirizine (at a dose of 10 mg daily or higher) is reported to be effective. Cetirizine (10 mg PO daily) and theophylline (200 mg PO bid) are more effective than cetirizine alone. *PMID: 16164841*

Dapsone (100 to 150 mg daily) can be very effective. Methotrexate (15 mg/week), montelukast, ketotifen plus nimesulide, sulfasalazine, or topical clobetasol propionate 0.5% are reported effective in single case reports.

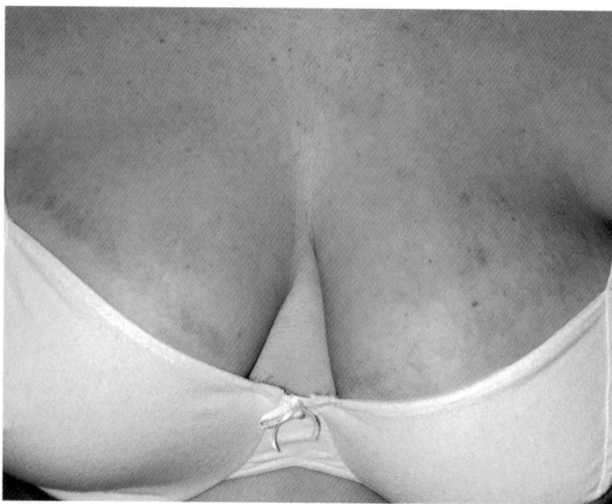

Figure 6-14 Hives form under the edge of the bra from the increased pressure exerted by the edge of the garment.

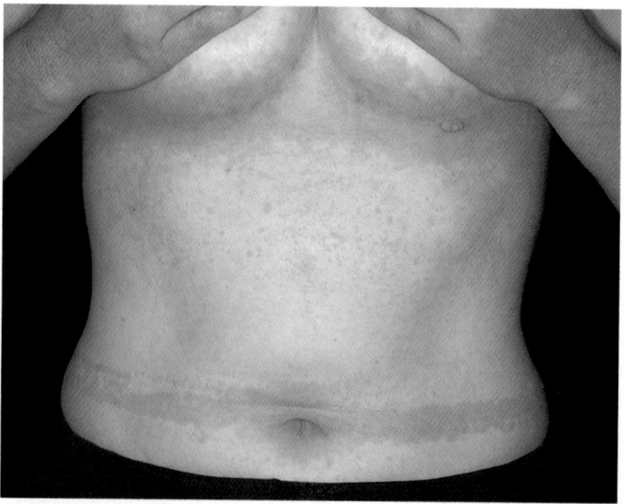

Figure 6-15 Hives form under the edge of the bra and waistband.

Cholinergic urticaria

In its milder form, "heat bumps," cholinergic urticaria is the most common of the physical urticarias. It is primarily seen in adolescents and young adults. The overall prevalence is 11.2%; most of the affected persons are older than 20 years. A very small group is severely afflicted. Most persons have mild symptoms that are restricted to fleeting, pinpoint-size wheals. Most affected people do not seek medical attention. Activation of the cholinergic sympathetic innervation of sweat glands is a possible mechanism.

CLINICAL FEATURES. Round, papular wheals 2 to 4 mm in diameter that are surrounded by a slight to extensive red flare are diagnostic of this most distinctive type of hive (Figures 6-16 and 6-17). Typically, the hives occur during or shortly after exercise. However, their onset may be delayed for approximately 1 hour after stimulation. An attack begins with itching, tingling, burning, warmth, or irritation of the skin. Hives begin within 2 to 20 minutes after the patient experiences a general overheating of the body as a result of exercise, exposure to heat, or emotional stress, and they last for minutes to hours (median: 30 minutes). Cholinergic urticaria may become confluent and resemble typical hives. The incidence of systemic symptoms is very low; however, when they occur, systemic systems include angioedema, hypotension, wheezing, and GI tract complaints.

DIAGNOSIS. The diagnosis is suggested by the history and confirmed by experimentally reproducing the lesions. The most reliable and efficient testing method is to ask the patient to run in place or to use an exercise bicycle for 10 to 15 minutes, and then to observe the patient for 1 hour to detect the typical micropapular hives. Exercise testing should be done in a controlled environment; patients with exercise-induced anaphylaxis may need emergency treatment. Immersion of half the patient in a bath at 43° C can raise the patient's oral temperature by 1° C to 1.5° C and induce characteristic micropapular hives. The immersion test does not induce hives in patients with exercise-induced anaphylaxis.

TREATMENT. Patients can avoid symptoms by limiting strenuous exercise. Showering with hot water may temporarily deplete histamine stores and induce a 24-hour refractory period. Immediate cooling after sweating, such as a cool shower, can abort attacks. Cetirizine (Zyrtec) at twice its recommended dose of 20 mg is very effective. Hydroxyzine (10 to 50 mg) taken 1 hour before exercise attenuates the eruption, but the side effect of drowsiness is often unacceptable. Severely affected unresponsive patients may respond to stanozolol.

CHOLINERGIC URTICARIA

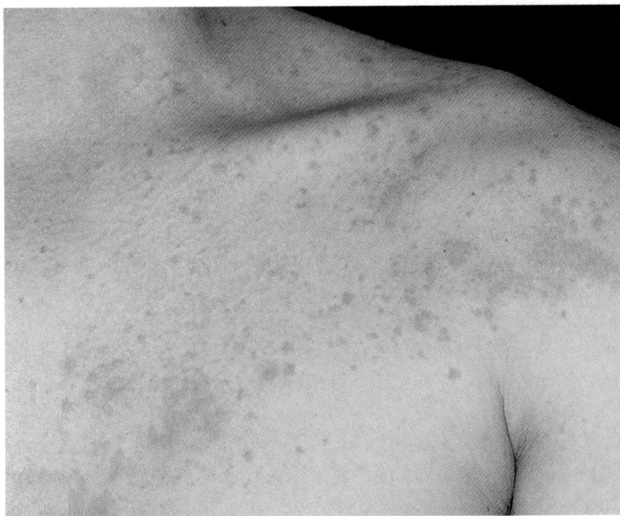

Figure 6-16 Round, red, papular wheals that occur in response to exercise, heat, or emotional stress.

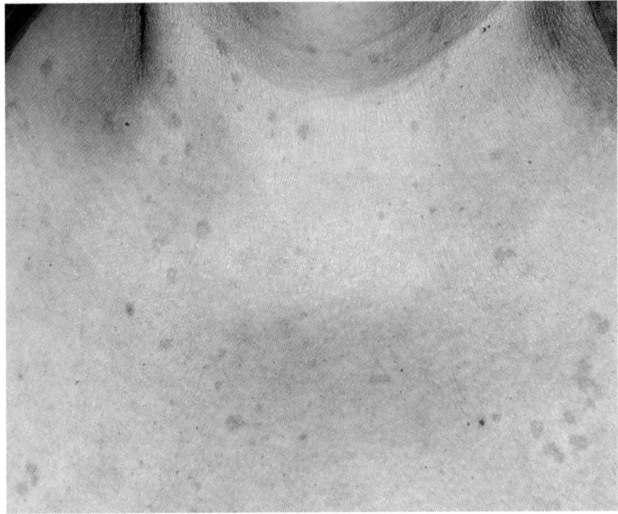

Figure 6-17 Patient had reported small hives after exertion. A test of exertion reproduced the lesions and proved the diagnosis.

Exercise-induced anaphylaxis

Patients develop pruritus, urticaria, respiratory distress, and hypotension after exercise. Symptoms may progress to angioedema, laryngeal edema, bronchospasm, and hypotension, and there is a high frequency of progression to upper airway distress and shock. It is associated with different kinds of exercise, although jogging is the most frequently reported. Exercise acts as a physical stimulus that, through an unknown mechanism, provokes mast cell degranulation and elevated serum histamine levels. In contrast to cholinergic urticaria, the lesions are large and are not produced by hot showers, pyrexia, or anxiety. It is differentiated from cholinergic urticaria by a hot-water immersion test (see Cholinergic urticaria). Exercise-induced anaphylaxis (EIA) or exercise-accentuated anaphylaxis may occur only after ingestion of certain foods such as celery, shellfish, wheat, fruit, milk, and fish (food-dependent EIA). Attacks occur when the patient exercises within 30 minutes after ingestion of the food; eating the food without exercising (and vice versa) causes no symptoms. Patients with wheat-associated EIA have positive skin tests to several wheat fractions. Another precipitating factor includes drug intake; a familial tendency has been reported. The prognosis is not well-defined, but a reduction of attacks occurs in 45% of patients by means of elimination diets and behavioral changes. The differential diagnosis includes exercise-induced asthma, idiopathic anaphylaxis, cardiac arrhythmias, and carcinoid syndrome.

TREATMENT. H_1 antihistamines are recommended as pretreatment and acute therapy. Administration of epinephrine by auto-injector may be required. Exercising with a partner is prudent. Exercise should be stopped if itching, erythema, or whealing occurs. Airway maintenance and cardiovascular support may be required. Prophylactic treatment includes avoidance of exercise, abstention from coprecipitating foods at least 4 hours before exercise, and pretreatment with antihistamines and cromolyn, or the induction of tolerance through regular exercise.

Cold urticaria

Cold urticaria syndromes are a group of disorders characterized by urticaria, angioedema, or anaphylaxis that develops after cold exposure.

PRIMARY ACQUIRED COLD URTICARIA. Primary acquired ("essential") cold urticaria occurs in children and young adults. Local whealing and itching occur within a few minutes of applying a solid or fluid cold stimulus to the skin. The wheal lasts for about a half hour. Dermographism and cholinergic urticaria are found relatively often in patients with cold urticaria. Urticaria may occur in the oropharynx after a cold drink. Systemic symptoms, occasionally severe and anaphylactoid, may occur after extensive exposure such as immersion in cold water. There may be a recent history of a virus infection (*Mycoplasma pneumoniae*). Spontaneous improvement occurs in an average of 2 to 3 years. Hives occur with a sudden drop in air temperature or during exposure to cold water. Many patients have severe reactions with generalized urticaria, angioedema, or both. Swimming in cold water is the most common cause of severe reactions and can result in massive transudation of fluid into the skin, leading to hypotension, fainting, shock, and possibly death. Like dermographism, cold urticaria often begins after infection, drug therapy, or emotional stress.

SECONDARY ACQUIRED COLD URTICARIA. Secondary acquired cold urticaria occurs in about 5% of patients with cold urticaria. Wheals are persistent, may have purpura, and demonstrate vasculitis on skin biopsy. Cryoglobulin, cold agglutinin, or cryofibrinogens are present. Order complete blood count (CBC), erythrocyte sedimentation rate (ESR), antinuclear antibody (ANA), mononucleosis spot test, rapid plasma reagin (RPR), rheumatoid factor, total complement, cryoglobulins, cryofibrinogens, cold agglutinins, and cold hemolysins. Demonstration of a cryoglobulin should prompt a search for chronic hepatitis B or C infection, lymphoreticular malignancy, or glandular fever. The cryoglobulins may be polyclonal (postinfection) or monoclonal (IgG or IgM), and complement activation may be involved.

DIAGNOSIS. The diagnosis is made by inducing a hive with a plastic-wrapped ice cube held against the forearm for 3 to 5 minutes (Figure 6-18). Some patients require up to 20 minutes to elicit a response. A cold-water immersion test, in which the forearm is submerged for 5 to 15 minutes in water at 0° to 8° C, establishes the diagnosis when the results of the ice cube test are equivocal. The patient must be monitored closely because severe reactions are possible.

TREATMENT. Patients must learn to protect themselves from a sudden decrease in temperature. Cyproheptadine, loratadine, cetirizine, doxepin, and other antihistamines may be effective. High dosing with antihistamines, up to four times the daily recommended dose, may be required.

Antibiotic therapy may be effective even if no underlying infection can be detected. Penicillin (e.g., oral phenoxymethylpenicillin 1 milliunit/day for 2 to 4 weeks or doxycycline 200 mg/day for 3 weeks) is recommended.

Solar urticaria

Hives that occur in sun-exposed areas minutes after exposure to the sun and disappear in less than 1 hour are called solar urticaria. This photoallergic disorder is caused by both sunlight and artificial light. It is most common in young adults; females are more often affected. Systemic reactions that include syncope can occur. Previously exposed tanned skin may not react when exposed to ultraviolet light. Hives induced by exposure to ultraviolet light must be distinguished from the much more common sun-related condition of polymorphous light eruption. Lesions of polymorphous light eruption are rarely urticarial. They occur hours after exposure and persist for several days.

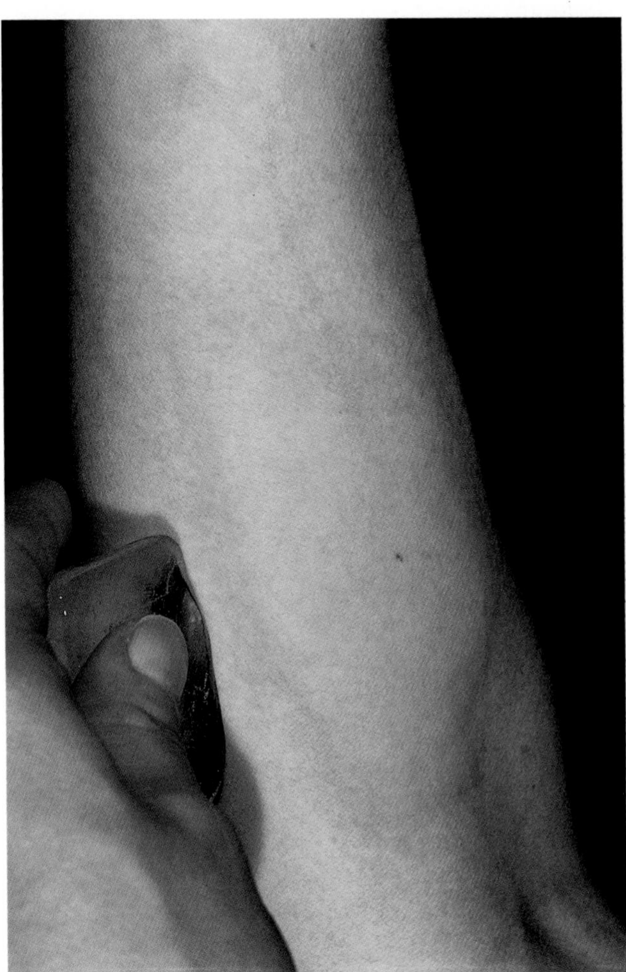

Figure 6-18 Cold urticaria. The hive occurred within minutes of holding an ice cube against the skin.

PATHOGENESIS

Evidence supports an immunologic IgE-mediated mechanism for solar urticaria. There are several different wavelengths that can cause solar urticaria. The disease is classified into six types that correspond to six different wavelengths of light. An individual reacts to a specific wavelength or a narrow band of the light spectrum, usually within the range of 290 to 500 nm. The cause may be an allergic reaction to an antigen formed in the skin by light waves. Those reacting to light wavelengths greater than 400 nm (visible light) develop hives even when exposed through glass. The wavelength responsible for solar urticaria is identified by phototesting. Antihistamines, sunscreens, and graded exposure to increasing amounts of light are effective treatments.

Heat, water, and vibration urticarias

Other physical stimuli such as heat, water of any temperature, or vibration are rare causes of urticaria. Aquagenic urticaria resembles the micropapular hives of cholinergic urticaria. Antihistamine and anticholinergic medication may not prevent the reaction. The mechanism of this phenomenon remains poorly understood.

Aquagenic pruritus

Severe, prickling skin discomfort without skin lesions occurs within 1 to 15 (or more) minutes after contact with water at any temperature and lasts for 10 to 120 minutes (average: 40 minutes). Histamine does not seem to play a key role in the pathogenesis of aquagenic pruritus. Capsaicin cream (Zostrix, Zostrix-HP) applied three times daily for 4 weeks resulted in complete relief of symptoms in the treated areas. Ultraviolet B phototherapy and antihistamines provide some relief. Aquagenic pruritus may be composed of two similar but distinct entities, each of which responds to a different treatment. Some patients with aquagenic pruritus are helped by adding sodium bicarbonate (25 to 200 gm) to the bath water or using the opioid receptor antagonist naltrexone. *PMID: 16502200* Patients with aquagenic pruritus of the elderly responded to emollients. *PMID: 2838535* Polycythemia rubra vera should be ruled out.

ANGIOEDEMA

Angioedema (angioneurotic edema) is a hivelike swelling caused by increased vascular permeability in the subcutaneous tissue of the skin and mucosa and the submucosal layers of the respiratory and GI tracts. A similar reaction occurs in the dermis with hives. Hives and angioedema commonly occur simultaneously and can have the same etiology. All types are listed in Box 6-9 and Table 6-3. The presence of hives is characteristic of several types of angioedema. Absence of hives is characteristic of another group (Box 6-10).

CLINICAL CHARACTERISTICS. The deeper reaction produces a more diffuse swelling than is seen in hives. Itching is usually absent. Symptoms consist of burning and painful swelling. The lips, palms, soles, limbs, trunk, and genitalia are most commonly affected. Involvement of the GI and respiratory tracts produces dysphagia, dyspnea, colicky abdominal pain, and attacks of vomiting and diarrhea. GI symptoms are more common in the hereditary types of angioedema. Angioedema may occur as a result of trauma. Urticaria is rarely seen in hereditary or acquired angioedema.

In 1 report of 17 patients admitted during a 5-year period, 94% had angioedema in the head and neck (3 required urgent tracheotomy or intubation), 35% had recent initiation of angiotensin-converting enzyme inhibitor (ACEI) therapy for hypertension, and 6% demonstrated classic hereditary angioedema. The majority (59%) had unclear etiologies for their symptoms.

Acquired forms of angioedema

IDIOPATHIC ANGIOEDEMA. Most cases of angioedema are idiopathic. Angioedema can occur at any age but is most common in the 40- to 50-year-old age group. Women are most frequently affected. The pattern of recurrence is unpredictable, and episodes can occur for 5 or more years. Involvement of the GI and respiratory tracts occurs, but asphyxiation is not a danger. A daily antihistamine is the initial prophylactic therapy.

Glucocorticoids are effective but the risks of chronic therapy usually outweigh the benefits. Long-term suppression may be needed. Alternate-day therapy is indicated if long-term suppression is required (e.g., prednisone 20 mg every other day), using the lowest dosage of prednisone required to provide adequate control.

ALLERGIC OR IMMUNOGLOBIN E–MEDIATED ANGIOEDEMA. Severe allergic type I immediate hypersensitivity IgE-mediated reactions can cause acute angioedema and urticaria (Figures 6-19 through 6-24 and Table 6-3. IgE antibody on the mast cell surface unites with antigen (food, drug, stinging insect venom, pollen) and precipitates an immediate and massive release of histamine and other mediators from mast cells. Angioedema occurs alone or with the other symptoms of systemic anaphylaxis (i.e., respiratory distress, hypotension). Some forms of cold urticaria are IgE mediated and occur initially as angioedema. Common triggers are listed in Table 6-4. Allergen avoidance is required. Above-normal levels of plasma tryptase and histamine in plasma and urine occur after allergen challenge in patients with immediate hypersensitivity. Order a serum tryptase and a 24-hour urine collection for histamine (see Box 6-12).

Antihistamines and glucocorticoids improve symptoms during an acute episode. Laryngeal edema responds well to epinephrine, which can be given intramuscularly or via an endotracheal tube. Daily antihistamines may decrease the severity of symptoms but often fail to prevent attacks.

Box 6-9 **Syndromes of Angioedema**

- Idiopathic recurrent AE
- Allergic (IgE-mediated) angioedema
- Medication-induced (e.g., ACE inhibitors)
- HAE (hereditary angioedema):
  - Type I: deficiency of C1 INH protein
  - Type II: dysfunctional C1 INH protein
  - Type III: coagulation factor XII gene mutation
- AAE (acquired angioedema):
  - Type I: associated with lymphoproliferative diseases
  - Type II: autoimmune (anti–C1 INH antibody)
- Episodic angioedema with eosinophilia (Gleich's syndrome)
- Thyroid autoimmune disease–associated AE

ACE, angiotensin-converting enzyme; *C1 INH*, C1 esterase inhibitor.

Box 6-10 **Coexistent Urticaria in Syndromes of Angioedema**

Not Associated with Urticaria

- HAE type I
- HAE type II
- Acquired C1 INH* deficiency
- ACE inhibitor–associated AE
- Idiopathic recurrent AE

Associated with Urticaria

- Chronic idiopathic urticaria/AE syndrome
- Allergic (IgE-mediated) AE
- Aspirin or nonsteroidal antiinflammatory drug–induced AE
- ACE inhibitor–associated AE

From *Am J Med* 121(4):282-286, 2008 (review). *PMID: 18374684*
**ACE*, angiotensin-converting enzyme; *AE*, angioedema; *C1 INH*, C1 esterase inhibitor; *Ig, immunoglobulin*.

Table 6-3 Clinical and Laboratory Findings Associated with Angioedema of Various Causes

		LABORATORY FINDINGS				
Type of angioedema	**Clinical findings**	**C4 level**	**Antigenic C1 inhibitor level**	**Functional C1 inhibitor level**	**C1q level**	**C3 level**
Hereditary angioedema	Recurrent angioedema and abdominal attacks without urticaria; attacks are episodic, with intervals between periods of swelling; onset in childhood or young adulthood, with worsening around time of puberty; prolonged attacks (typically 72-96 hr in duration); family history in 75% of patients; attacks do not respond to antihistamines or corticosteroids	Decreased	Decreased (in type I) or normal (in type II)	Decreased	Normal	Normal
Acquired C1 inhibitor deficiency	Attacks similar to those in hereditary angioedema; onset in middle age or later; absence of family history; attacks do not respond to antihistamines or corticosteroids	Decreased	Decreased or normal	Decreased	Decreased	Normal or decreased
Inherited angioedema with normal C1 inhibitor levels	Family history of angioedema; possible preponderance of women among affected persons; may be estrogen-dependent; typically manifested after childhood; face, tongue, and extremities affected more than abdomen; attacks do not respond to antihistamines or corticosteroids	Normal	Normal	Normal	Normal	Normal
ACEI-associated angioedema	History of ACEI use; angioedema tends to affect face and tongue; more common in blacks and smokers than other subgroups; patients can usually tolerate angiotensin-receptor blockers	Normal	Normal	Normal	Normal	Normal
Idiopathic angioedema	Angioedema sometimes accompanied by urticaria; swelling typically lasts up to 48 hr; attacks may occur daily; attacks relieved with antihistamines or corticosteroids	Normal	Normal	Normal	Normal	Normal
Allergic angioedema	Angioedema usually accompanied by urticaria and sometimes anaphylaxis; may be pruritic; associated with exposure to food, venom, latex, drug, or environmental allergen; attacks typically last 24-48 hr; attacks relieved with antihistamines or corticosteroids	Normal	Normal	Normal	Normal	Normal
NSAID-associated angioedema	Angioedema after ingestion of an NSAID; typically accompanied by urticaria; usually class-specific reaction resulting from pharmacologic effect of cyclooxygenase inhibition, but allergic in rare instances	Normal	Normal	Normal	Normal	Normal
Angioedema with urticarial vasculitis	Angioedema usually accompanied by urticaria; skin may show petechiae or purpura after resolution of swelling; often there are other symptoms that are consistent with underlying vasculitis	Decreased	Normal	Normal	Decreased	Decreased

From *New Engl J Med* 359(10):1027-1036, 2008. *PMID: 18768946*

ACEI, angiotensin-converting enzyme inhibitor; *NSAID*, nonsteroidal antiinflammatory drug.

Table 6-4 Common Triggers of Mast Cell-Mediated Angioedema

Medications	Food	Other
Aspirin	Nuts	Venom
NSAIDs	Eggs	Latex
Antihypertensives	Shellfish	
Narcotics	Soy	
Oral contraceptives	Wheat	
	Milk	

From *Am J Med* 121(4):282-286, 2008 (review). *PMID: 18374684*
NSAIDS, Nonsteroidal antiinflammatory drugs.

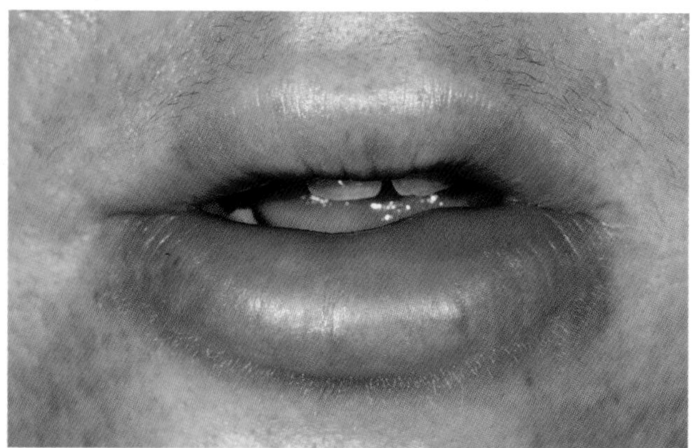

Figure 6-19 Angioedema. Swelling of the lips may be the only manifestation of angioedema.

MEDICATION- AND CHEMICAL-INDUCED ANGIOEDEMA. Contrast dyes used in radiology and drugs may also cause acute angioedema as a result of nonimmunologic mechanisms. Examples include nonsteroidal antiinflammatory drugs, such as aspirin and indomethacin, and ACE-inhibiting drugs.

Prescribe EpiPen or EpiPen Jr for patients who experience severe reactions with insect stings. The epinephrine in EpiPen is packaged in an auto-injector to avoid manual needle insertion.

Advise affected patients to wear a bracelet that identifies the diagnosis; their reactions could be misdiagnosed as symptoms related to alcoholism, stroke, myocardial infarction, or a foreign body in the airway.

ANGIOEDEMA FROM ANGIOTENSIN-CONVERTING ENZYME INHIBITORS. Angiotensin-converting enzyme inhibitors (ACEIs) are widely used for the treatment of mild forms of hypertension. They are the number one cause of acute angioedema in some hospitals. Angioedema occurs in 0.1% to 2.2% of patients receiving an ACE inhibitor and it is a potentially life-threatening adverse effect. The incidence may be higher in black Americans.

The onset usually occurs within hours to 1 week after starting therapy. Angioedema may occur suddenly even though the drug has been well tolerated for months or years; symptoms may regress spontaneously while the patient continues the medication, erroneously prompting an alternative diagnosis. ACE inhibitors seem to facilitate angioedema in predisposed subjects, rather than causing it with an allergic or idiosyncratic mechanism.

Most cases from the short-acting ACEI captopril present with mild angioedema that can be controlled with antihistamines and glucocorticosteroids. In contrast, the angioedema induced by the long-acting ACE inhibitors lisinopril and enalapril has been serious.

The pathology has a special predilection for the tongue, a circumstance that renders orotracheal and nasotracheal intubation difficult; symptoms may progress rapidly despite aggressive medical therapy, necessitating emergency airway procedures. Individuals with a history of idiopathic angioedema probably should not be given ACE inhibitors. C1 inhibitor levels are usually normal.

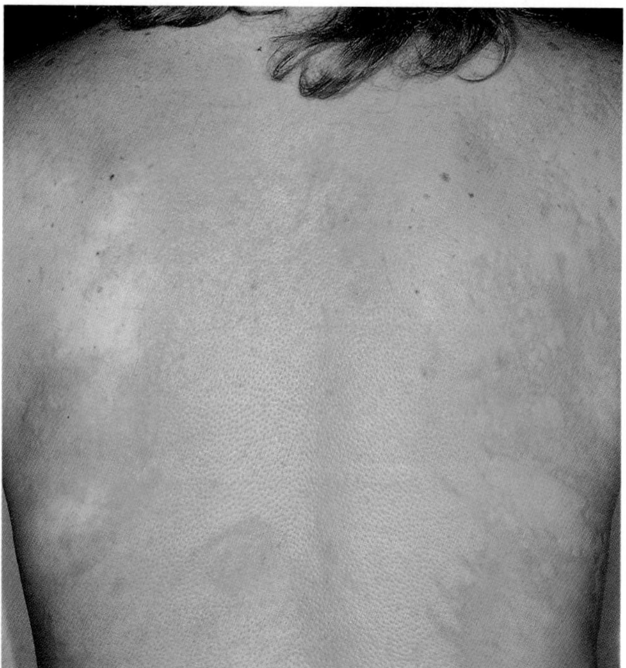

Figure 6-20 Angioedema. An extensive case of unknown etiology.

Treatment includes immediate withdrawal of the ACE inhibitor and acute symptomatic supportive therapy. Angioedema that results from ACEIs is probably not IgE mediated, and antihistamines and steroids may not alleviate the airway obstruction. Alternative therapy with other classes of drugs to manage hypertension and/or heart failure must be chosen. Angiotensin II receptor antagonists have a lower incidence of adverse effects than ACE inhibitors as they do not produce cough and appear much less likely to produce angioedema.

Continuing use of ACE inhibitors, in spite of angioedema, results in a markedly increased rate of angioedema recurrence with serious morbidity.

ANGIOEDEMA

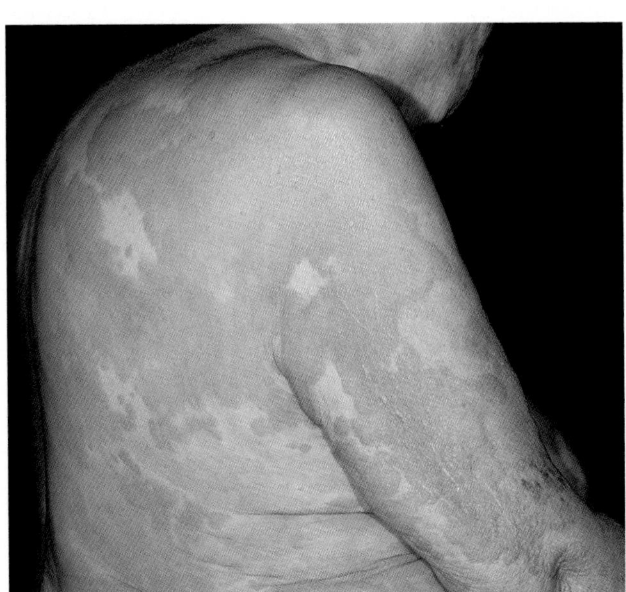

Figure 6-21 Angioedema involving much of the skin surface. The wheals are massive on the back and shoulder.

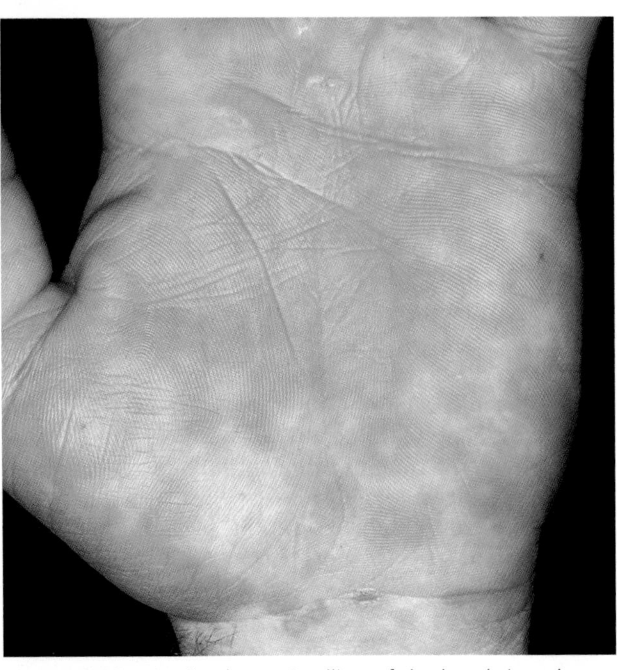

Figure 6-22 Angioedema. Swelling of the hands is a characteristic sign.

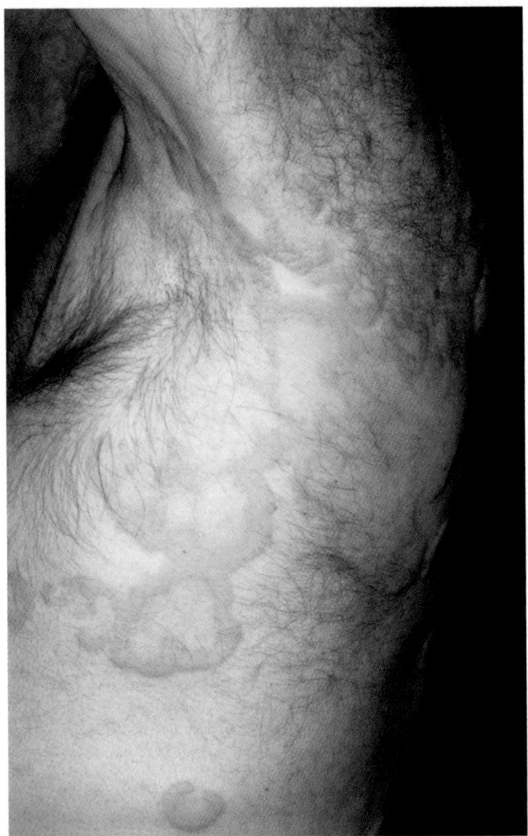

Figure 6-23 Angioedema with massive infiltration of the skin produces very thick wheals.

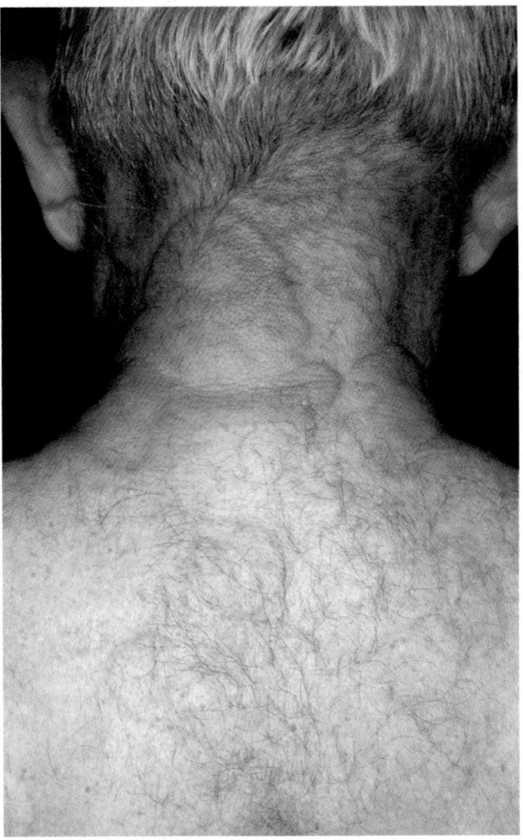

Figure 6-24 Angioedema of the neck and back with thick polycyclic lesions.

ACQUIRED ANGIOEDEMA (C1 INH DEFICIENCY SYNDROMES)

Acquired angioedema (AAE) results from an acquired C1 INH deficiency. Acquired angioedema (AAE) is a rare disease that occurs in two forms: AAE-I and AAE-II. The two types are thought to be autoimmune (see Box 6-9). Type I is associated with lymphoproliferative diseases, including monoclonal gammopathy of unknown significance and high-grade lymphomas, and occurs via consumption of the C1 INH protein by malignant cells. Type II is thought to be caused by the autoantibody to the C1 INH protein. AAE usually presents after the fourth decade of life. The laboratory characteristics of these two rare diseases are shown in Table 6-3. C4, C1q, and C1 INH levels are low. Search for lymphoproliferative disease and other neoplasms. Order serum protein electrophoresis, immunophoresis, peripheral blood lymphocyte immunophenotyping, and CT scans of the chest, abdomen, and pelvis. Initial studies may be negative. Angioedema can precede internal disease by up to 7 years.

Acute attacks are treated with epinephrine and glucocorticoids. High dosages of antihistamines may be effective. C1 INH concentrate and fresh-frozen plasma are the treatments of choice for acute episodes of AAE. These are less efficacious in AAE than in hereditary angioedema (HAE) because of the presence of autoantibody to the protein. Treatment of underlying lymphoproliferative disease is often curative in AAE-I. AAE-II has been treated with immunosuppressives. Androgens such as danazol are useful for frequent attacks.

EPISODIC ANGIOEDEMA-EOSINOPHILIA SYNDROME. This rare, non–life-threatening benign syndrome (also known as cytokine-associated AE syndrome or Gleich's syndrome) consists of periodic attacks of angioedema, urticaria, pruritus, myalgia, oliguria, and fever. During attacks, body weights increase up to 18%, and leukocyte counts reach as high as 108,000/μl (88% eosinophils). Eosinophilia can persist between attacks. Attacks of angioedema last for about 6 to 10 days. Attacks resolve spontaneously or require short courses of corticosteroids to control symptoms and normalize the blood count. There is an increased level of the cytokines granulocyte-macrophage colony-stimulating factor, interleukin-3 (IL-3), IL-5, and IL-6, which implicate CD4+ T lymphocytes in the pathophysiology of this process.

Hereditary angioedema

Hereditary angioedema results from a lack of functional C1 esterase inhibitor. Hereditary angioedema (inherited C1 inhibitor deficiency) is transmitted as an autosomal dominant trait and is due to mutations in the C1 inhibitor (C1 INH) gene. There are two types: type I (85% of cases) and type II (15% of cases). The clinical presentation for both types is the same. Type I is the most common and is characterized by an insufficient production of C1 inhibitor. This affects 85% of all patients with hereditary angioedema. Patients with type 2 have normal or elevated concentrations of C1 inhibitor but the protein is functionally deficient. The disease affects between 1 in 10,000 and 1 in 50,000 persons. In most cases the disease begins in late childhood or early adolescence. Spontaneous occurrences are seen in up to 25% of patients. Many have ancestors who died suddenly from asphyxia. In the past, the mortality rate for attacks involving the upper airways exceeded 25%. Patients live in constant dread of life-threatening laryngeal obstruction.

Persons with hereditary angioedema have one normal and one abnormal C1 inhibitor gene. Under normal circumstances, this defect is clinically silent. Minor trauma, mental stress, and other unknown triggering factors lead to the release of vasoactive peptides that produce episodic swelling. Histamine has no role in this type of edema.

CLINICAL MANIFESTATIONS. Hereditary angioedema of the abdomen or oropharynx can result in death. Attacks may be complicated by incapacitating cutaneous swelling, life-threatening upper airway impediment, and severe GI colic. Patients usually experience attacks by the second decade of life. Delays in diagnosis are common. The diagnosis should be suspected in any patient who presents with recurrent angioedema or abdominal pain in the absence of urticaria. Symptoms begin in childhood, worsen at puberty, and persist throughout life (Box 6-11). There are recurrent episodes of subcutaneous or submucosal edema. Minor trauma and stress frequently precipitate attacks.

Box 6-11 **Diagnostic Features That Should Prompt Investigations for C1 Inhibitor Deficiency**

- Angioedema
  - Recurrent
  - >24 hr
  - Nonpruritic
  - Nonresponsive to antihistamines
- Serpiginous rash
- No urticaria
- Unexplained abdominal pain (recurrent, colicky)
- Family history
- Low C4 level

Angioedema occurs at the following three sites: subcutaneous tissues (face, hands, arms, legs, genitalia, and buttocks); abdominal organs (stomach, intestines, bladder); and the upper airway, which may result in life-threatening laryngeal edema. The extremities are the cutaneous site most commonly reported. Swelling involves the extremities (96%), face (85%), oropharynx (64%), and intestinal mucosa (88%).

SUBCUTANEOUS TISSUES. The swellings are not erythematous, pruritic, or painful. There are no hives. A tingling sensation precedes an attack. Swelling progresses for the first 24 hours and subsides in the next 2 or 3 days. Attacks occur about every 7 to 14 days but may be as often as every 3 days or as infrequent as years apart. Subcutaneous swellings resolve in 1 to 5 days.

ABDOMINAL ORGANS. Swelling of the gastrointestinal mucosa results in nausea, vomiting, diarrhea, and severe pain that can mimic a surgical emergency. Diminished bowel sounds, guarding and rebound tenderness may be misinterpreted and lead to unnecessary abdominal surgery. Abdominal symptoms resolve within 12 to 24 hours.

UPPER AIRWAY. Obstruction of the upper respiratory tract is responsible for the 30% mortality rate.

LABORATORY DIAGNOSIS OF HAE. The diagnosis is suggested by the family and personal history. A laboratory workup confirms the diagnosis (see Box 6-12 and Table 6-3). All patients with hereditary angioedema have a persistently low antigenic C4 level with normal antigenic C1 and C3 levels. Measure C4 levels as a screening test. In rare cases, the C4 level is normal between attacks. If C4 levels are low, then measure antigenic and functional C1 inhibitor levels. This confirms the diagnosis of hereditary angioedema and distinguishes between HAE type I (low antigenic and functional C1 inhibitor levels) and HAE type II (normal antigenic C1 inhibitor level but low functional C1 inhibitor activity). A rare third type (HAE type III) of familial angioedema has been described; in type III HAE, patients have normal antigenic and functional C1 inhibitor levels.

TREATMENT OF HAE. The treatment of C1 inhibitor deficiency is summarized in Table 6-5. Antihistamines, corticosteroids, and adrenergic drugs are of little value. Treatment is graded according to response and the clinical site of swelling. Acute treatment for severe attack is by infusion of C1 inhibitor concentrate and for minor attack attenuated androgens and/or tranexamic acid. Prophylactic treatment is by attenuated androgens and/or tranexamic acid. There are a number of new products in trials.

Box 6-12 **Laboratory Evaluation Angioedema**

	C1 INH quantitative (C1 INH antigen)	C1 INH activity (functional)	C4	C1q	Urine histamine	Tryptase
HAE Type 1	Low	Low	Low	nl	nl	nl
HAE Type 2	nl or high	Low	Low	nl	nl	nl
HAE Type 3	nl	nl	nl	nl	nl	nl
AAE Type 1	Low	Low	Low	Low	nl	nl
AAE Type 2	nl or low	Low	Low	Low	nl	nl
Allergic AE	nl	nl	nl	nl	High*	High*
Idiopathic	nl	nl	nl	nl	nl	nl

Adapted from *Am J Med* 121(4):282-286, 2008 (review). *PMID: 18374684*
C1 INH, C1 esterase inhibitor; *HAE*, hereditary angioedema; *AAE*, acquired angioedema; *AE*, angioedema; *nl*, normal.
*During the acute episode.

Table 6-5 Management of C1 Inhibitors (C1 INH) Deficiency*

Intervention	Therapy	Dosage (adult)	Dosage (children)	Tests
Long-term prophylaxis	Attenuated androgens	Danazol 200 mg once or twice per day; up to 400 mg/day in <20% of cases	Only if indicated (very rare); see text	Every 6 months: liver function tests
		Stanozolol up to 5 mg once or twice per day	Danazol 100-200 mg/day (use lowest effective maintenance dose, consider alternate-day or 2× weekly regimen)	Annual: lipid profile
		Oxandrolone 2.5-20 mg divided dose two to four times per day (use lowest effective maintenance dose, consider alternate-day or 2× weekly regimen)		Biennial: hepatic ultrasound (annual after 10 years of treatment)
	Tranexamic acid	Starting dose 1-1.5 gm two to three times per day, reducing to 0.5 gm once or twice per day	1-2 gm/day; dosage depends on age and size; general guide is 50 mg/kg/day (use lowest effective maintenance dose, consider alternate-day or 2× weekly regimen)	Every 6 months: liver function tests
Short-term prophylaxis (e.g., for dental work)	C1 inhibitor concentrate	500-1500 units up to 24 hr before procedure	<10 years old: 500 units >10 years old: 1000 units up to 24 hr before procedure	
	Attenuated androgens	Danazol 100-600 mg/day for 48 hr before and after procedure	Danazol 300 mg/day for 48 hr before and after procedure	
		Stanozolol 2-6 mg/day for 48 hr before and after procedure		
	Tranexamic acid	1 gm given four times daily for 48 hr before and after procedure	500 mg given four times daily for 48 hr before and after procedure	
Emergency care for acute attacks	C1 inhibitor concentrate	500-1500 units; additional infusion and reassessment if symptoms persist for >2 hr	<10 years old: 500 units >10 years old: 1000 units	Baseline: liver function tests, hepatitis virology
	Attenuated androgens	Danazol up to 1 gm/day		
		Stanozolol up to 16 mg/day		
	Tranexamic acid	1 gm given four times daily for 48 hr		
	Fresh-frozen plasma	2 units (only for use where C1 INH concentrate not available)		Baseline: liver function tests, hepatitis virology
	Pain relief	As appropriate		
Pregnancy	Attenuated androgens	Contraindicated		
	Tranexamic acid	May be used with caution		
	C1 inhibitor concentrate	Emergency care as above; severe cases may require regular replacement		

From *Clin Exp Immunol* 139(3):379-394, 2005 (C1 inhibitor deficiency: consensus document). PMID: 15730382

*The regimen for each affected individual should be guided by the severity of their disease and thus titered to individual need. Includes both genetic Types I and II hereditary angioedema and acquired forms of the disease.

CONTACT URTICARIA SYNDROME

Contact of the skin with various compounds can elicit a wheal-and-flare response. Most patients give a history of relapsing dermatitis or generalized urticarial attacks rather than a localized hive; others complain only of localized sensations of itching, burning, and tingling. This is in contrast to allergic contact dermatitis, which is an eczematous reaction caused by cell-mediated immunity.

Contact urticaria is characterized by a wheal and flare that occur within 30 to 60 minutes after cutaneous exposure to certain agents. Direct contact of the skin with these agents may cause a wheal-and-flare response restricted to the area of contact, generalized urticaria, urticaria and asthma, or urticaria combined with an anaphylactoid reaction. There are nonimmunologic and immunologic forms.

NONIMMUNOLOGIC CONTACT URTICARIA. The nonimmunologic type is the most common and most benign. This form does not require prior sensitization. Nonimmunologic, histamine-releasing substances are produced by certain plants (nettles), animals (caterpillars, jellyfish), and medications (dimethyl sulfoxide [DMSO]). Anaphylaxis may occur after application of bacitracin ointment. Other implicated substances include cobalt chloride, benzoic acid, cinnamic aldehyde, cinnamic acid, and sorbic acid.

IMMUNOLOGIC CONTACT URTICARIA. Immunologic contact urticaria is due to an IgE immediate hypersensitivity reaction. Some patients experience rhinitis, laryngeal edema, and abdominal disturbances. Latex rubber, bacitracin, potato, apple, mechlorethamine, and henna have been implicated.

OTHER PRECIPITATING FACTORS. The mechanism by which wood, plants, foods, cosmetics, and animal hair and dander cause contact urticaria has not been defined. The term protein contact dermatitis is used when an immediate reaction occurs after eczematous skin is exposed to certain types of food (fish, garlic, onion, chives, cucumber, parsley, tomato), animal dander (cow hair and dander), or plant substances. Cooks who complain of burning or stinging when handling certain foods may have contact urticaria syndrome.

DIAGNOSIS. Because there is no standard test battery for routine evaluation of contact urticaria, a careful history concerning the occurrence of immediate reactions, whether localized or generalized, is essential. An open patch test may be performed by applying a drop of the suspected substance to the ventral forearm and observing the site for a wheal 30 to 60 minutes later. Closed tests may be associated with more intense or generalized reactions.

Prick testing (using fresh samples of the food suspected from the patient's history) is an accurate method of investigation for selected cases of hand dermatitis in patients who spend considerable time handling foods (e.g., catering workers, cooks). Seafood is a common allergen. A radioallergosorbent test (RAST) can confirm immunologic contact urticaria.

PRURITIC URTICARIAL PAPULES AND PLAQUES OF PREGNANCY

Pruritic urticarial papules and plaques of pregnancy (PUPPP), or polymorphic eruption of pregnancy, is the most common gestational dermatosis, affecting between 1 in 130 and 1 in 300 pregnancies. It is seen most frequently in primigravidas and begins late in the third trimester of pregnancy (mean onset, 35 weeks) or occasionally in the early postpartum period. The eruption appears suddenly, begins on the abdomen in 90% of patients (Figure 6-25, *A*), and in a few days may spread in a symmetric fashion to involve the buttocks, proximal arms, and backs of the hands (Figure 6-25, *B*). The initial lesions may be confined to striae. The face is not involved. Itching is moderate to intense, but excoriations are rarely seen. The lesions begin as red papules that are often surrounded by a narrow, pale halo. They increase in number and may become confluent, forming edematous urticarial plaques or erythema multiforme–like target lesions that may look like the lesions of herpes gestationis. In other patients, the involved sites acquire broad areas of erythema, and the papules remain discrete. Papulovesicles have been reported. The mean duration is 6 weeks, but the rash is usually not severe for more than 1 week. Unlike urticaria, the eruption remains fixed and increases in intensity, clearing in most cases before or within 1 week after delivery. Recurrence with future pregnancies is unusual. There have been no fetal or maternal complications. Infants do not develop the eruption. Pruritic urticarial papules and plaques of pregnancy are significantly associated with multiple pregnancies, hypertensive disorders, and induction of labor. Perinatal outcome is comparable to that of pregnancies without PUPPP. *PMID: 16753771* It was postulated that abdominal distention or a reaction to it may play a role in the development of PUPPP.

The biopsy reveals a nonspecific perivascular lymphohistiocytic infiltrate. Eosinophils have also been noted in most biopsies. There are no laboratory abnormalities, and direct immunofluorescence of lesional and perilesional skin is negative.

Treatment is supportive. The expectant mother can be assured that pruritus will quickly terminate before or after delivery. Itching can be relieved with group V topical steroids; cool, wet compresses; oatmeal baths; and antihistamines. Antipruritic topical medications (menthol, doxepin) are useful. Prednisone (40 mg/day) may be required if pruritus becomes intolerable. Several patients were treated successfully with UVB therapy.

PUPPP

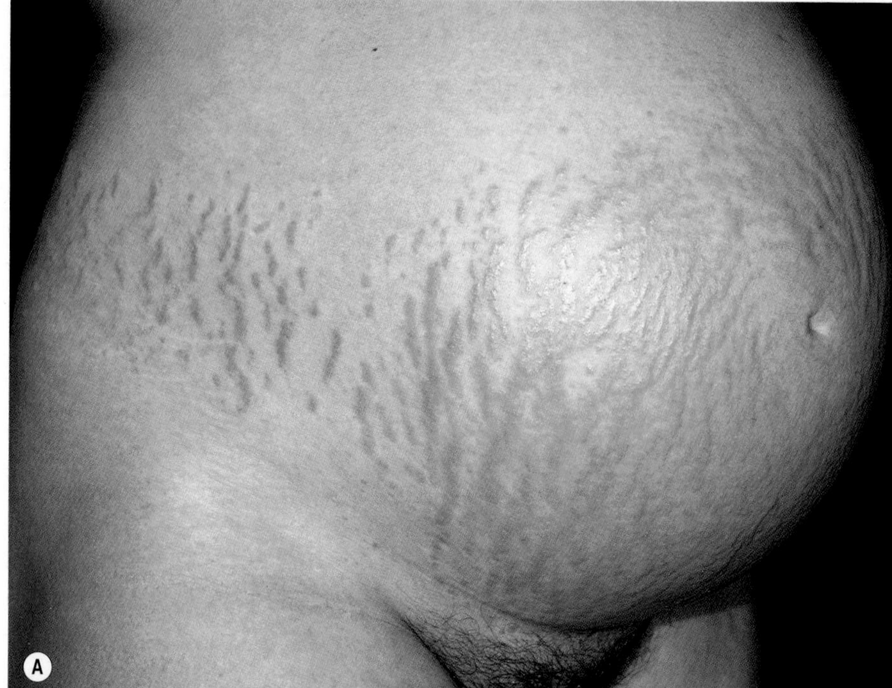

The abdomen is often the initial site of involvement. Initial lesions may be confined to striae.

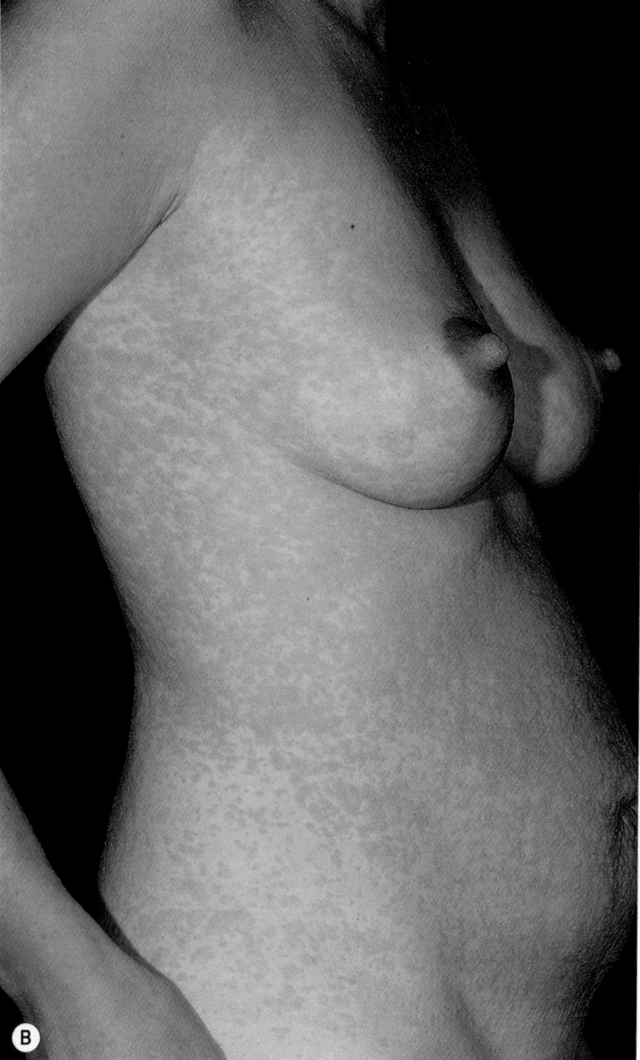

Fully evolved eruption.

Figure 6-25

URTICARIAL VASCULITIS

Urticarial vasculitis (UV) is a subset of vasculitis characterized clinically by urticarial skin lesions and histologically by necrotizing vasculitis.

Immune complexes are thought to lodge in small blood vessels with activation of complement, mast cell degranulation, infiltration by acute inflammatory cells, fibrin deposition, and blood vessel damage.

There is a spectrum of clinical and laboratory features. Many patients have minimal signs or symptoms of systemic disease. Systemic symptoms include angioedema (42%), arthralgias (49%), pulmonary disease (21%), and abdominal pain (17%). Thirty-two percent have hypocomplementemia, 64% have lesions that last more than 24 hours, 32% have painful or burning lesions, and 35% have lesions that resolve with purpura or hyperpigmentation.

CLINICAL FEATURES. Overall, patients with urticarial vasculitis tend to have a benign course. Urticarial plaques in most patients with typical chronic urticaria resolve completely in less than 24 hours and disappear while new plaques appear in other areas. Urticarial vasculitis plaques persist for 1 to 7 days and may have residual changes of purpura, scaling, and hyperpigmentation (Figures 6-26 and 6-27). However, in one study wheals lasted less than 24 hours in 57.4% of patients, and pain or tenderness was reported by 8.6%. Extracutaneous features were present in 81%, hypocomplementemia in 11%, and abnormalities of other laboratory parameters (e.g., raised erythrocyte sedimentation rate, microscopic hematuria) in 76.6%. The le-

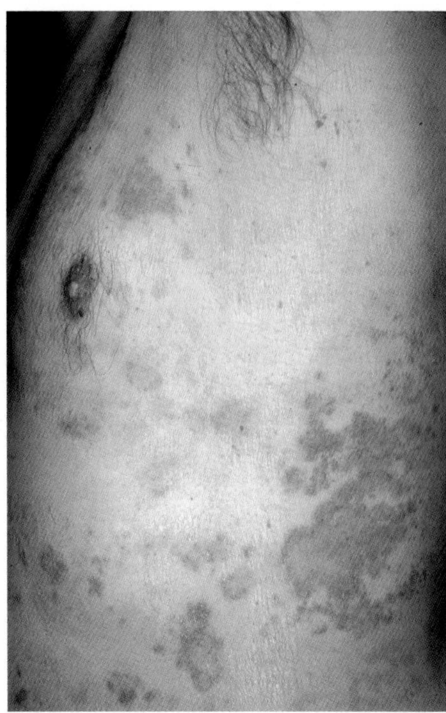

Figure 6-26 Lesions begin as red wheals. Purpura may develop as lesions progress. Lesions may resolve with postinflammatory pigmentation.

Figure 6-27 Urticarial vasculitis. Purpura occurs as the hive resolves.

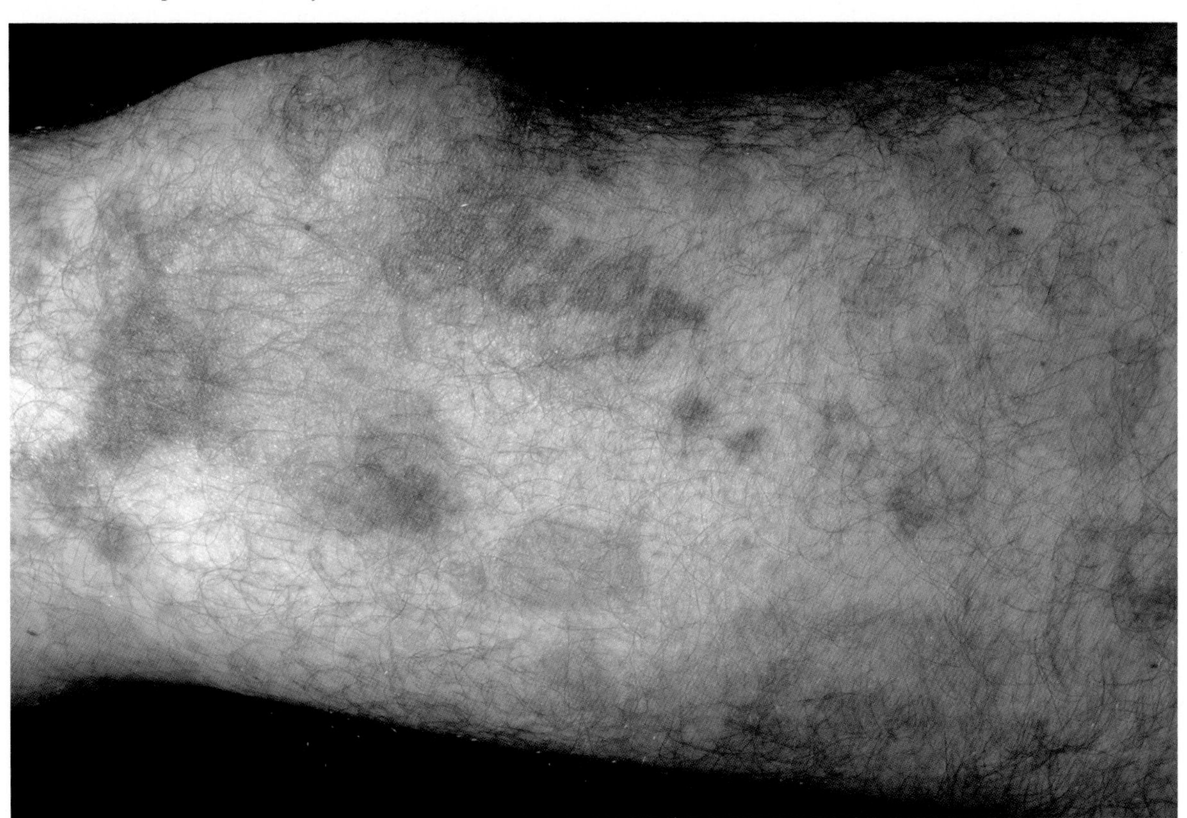

sions are burning and painful rather than itchy. Patients with urticarial vasculitis have been categorized into two subgroups: those with hypocomplementemia and those with normal complement levels.

NORMOCOMPLEMENT UV. Normocomplementemic urticarial vasculitis is usually idiopathic. This most common form has also been described in patients with monoclonal gammopathy, neoplasia, repeated cold exposure, and ultraviolet light sensitivity.

HYPOCOMPLEMENT UV. Patients with hypocomplementemia are more likely to have systemic involvement than patients with normal complement levels. Hypocomplementemic urticarial vasculitis can present as or precede a syndrome that includes obstructive pulmonary disease and uveitis, systemic lupus erythematosus, Sjögren's syndrome, or cryoglobulinemia (which is closely linked with hepatitis B or C virus infection).

LABORATORY TESTS. Order CBC, ESR, blood urea nitrogen (BUN), creatinine, ANA, anti-DNA, anti-Sm, complement assay, anti-C1q antibodies, cryoglobulins, Schirmer's test, and pulmonary function tests.

As with typical cutaneous vasculitis, most patients have an elevated erythrocyte sedimentation rate. Anti-C1q autoantibody develops in disorders characterized by immune complex–mediated injury and appears in most patients with hypocomplementemic urticarial vasculitis syndrome. Patients with more severe involvement have hypocomplementemia (hypocomplementemic urticarial vasculitis syndrome) with depressed CH50, C1q, C4, or C2 levels.

BIOPSY. Biopsy shows a histologic picture that is indistinguishable from that seen in cutaneous necrotizing vasculitis (palpable purpura). Fragmentation of leukocytes and fibrinoid deposition occur in the walls of postcapillary venules, a pattern called leukocytoclastic vasculitis. There is an interstitial neutrophilic infiltrate of the dermis.

IMMUNOFLUORESCENCE. Patients with hypocomplementemia may have an immunofluorescent pattern of immunoglobulins or C3 as determined by routine direct immunofluorescence. Direct immunofluorescence in patients with hypocomplementemia shows deposition of Ig and C3; 87% have fluorescence of the blood vessels, and 70% have fluorescence of the basement membrane zone. Rule out other diseases in which cutaneous vasculitis may present as a urticarial-like eruption (e.g., viral illness, systemic lupus erythematosus, Sjögren's syndrome, and serum sickness).

TREATMENT. Prednisone in dosages exceeding 40 mg/day is effective. Other medications reported to be effective are indomethacin (25 mg three times daily to 50 mg four times daily), colchicine (0.6 mg two or three times daily), dapsone (up to 200 mg/day), low-dose oral methotrexate, and antimalarial drugs. Cinnarizine was effective in a high percentage of the patients. *PMID: 18681869*

SERUM SICKNESS

Serum sickness is a disease produced by exposure to drugs, monoclonal antibody therapy (rituximab), blood products, or animal-derived vaccines. After exposure to these antigens, a strong host-antibody response occurs. These circulating antibodies react with the newly introduced antigen to form precipitating antigen-antibody complexes. This is a type III (immune complex) reaction, or Arthus reaction. These circulating immune complexes are trapped in vessel walls of various organs, where they activate complement. A rise in the level of immune complexes is accompanied by a decrease in serum levels of C3 and C4 and an increase in C3a/C3a desarginine, a split product of C3 whose presence indicates that the complement system has been activated by immune complexes. Inflammatory mediators are released. C3a/C3a des-arginine, a potent anaphylotoxin, induces mast cell degranulation to produce hives.

CLINICAL MANIFESTATIONS. Symptoms appear 8 to 13 days after exposure to the drug or antisera and last for 4 or more days. They include fever, malaise, skin eruptions, arthralgias, nausea, vomiting, occult blood in the stool, and lymphadenopathy. The disease resolves without sequelae in most cases. The skin eruption begins with the onset of other symptoms. A morbilliform rash or urticaria is limited to the trunk or may become generalized. The hands and feet may be involved.

DIAGNOSIS. The white blood count may be as high as 25,000/mm^3. Serum C3 and C4 levels are below normal. Proteinuria occurs in 40% of patients. Direct immunofluorescence of skin lesions less than 24 hours old shows Ig deposits (IgM, IgE, IgA, or C3) in the superficial small blood vessels. Drugs are now the most common cause of serum sickness. Penicillin, sulfa drugs, thiouracils, cholecystographic dyes, hydantoins, aminosalicylic acid, and streptomycin are most often implicated.

TREATMENT. The offending agent must be avoided. Antihistamines such as hydroxyzine control the hives. Prednisone 40 mg/day is used if symptoms are intense.

MASTOCYTOSIS

Mastocytosis is a group of rare diseases characterized by abnormal growth of mast cells in skin, bone marrow, liver, spleen, and lymph nodes. Mast cells store histamine in granules. Histamine is released by scratching the lesions or ingesting certain agents. The most frequent site of organ involvement with all forms of mastocytosis is the skin. In young children, the disease is usually confined to the skin; in adults, mastocytosis is usually systemic. Signs and symptoms result from mast cell mediators and mast cell organ infiltration.

Mast cell degranulation causes episodic flushing, dyspepsia, diarrhea, abdominal pain, musculoskeletal pain, or hypotension.

Pathological examination showing mast cell infiltration confirms the diagnosis. Antihistamines and mast cell–stabilizing agents such as sodium cromolyn provide symptomatic relief. Interferon, cladribine, and imatinib may be helpful. Aggressive disease is managed with chemotherapy or bone marrow transplantation. Familial occurrence is only rarely documented. The cause of mastocytosis is unknown. Several genetic mutations are documented.

Spectrum of disease

Mastocytosis comprises several diseases characterized by an abnormal increase in tissue mast cells. Cutaneous mastocytosis (CM) is the most common form of mastocytosis, affects predominantly children, and presents as a mast cell hyperplasia limited to the skin. Systemic mastocytosis (SM) comprises multiple distinct entities in which mast cells infiltrate the skin and/or other organs. The diagnosis of systemic mastocytosis is based on the presence of one major criterion and one minor criterion or three minor criteria.

CUTANEOUS MASTOCYTOSIS

There are several types of skin mast cell disease. Most cases of pediatric mastocytosis are sporadic and appear during the first 2 years of life, especially on the trunk. Urticaria pigmentosa is the most frequent variant. The prognosis of pediatric mastocytosis is good. There are three main forms of CM defined by the WHO: urticaria pigmentosa (UP), also called maculopapular cutaneous mastocytosis (MPCM); diffuse cutaneous mastocytosis (DCM); and mastocytoma of the skin (Box 6-13). A number of rare subvariants of UP have been described including telangiectasia macularis eruptive persistans (TMEP), a nodular and a plaque form.

A clinical diagnosis is made by typical skin lesions and lack of systemic symptoms. Determine a baseline serum tryptase level. Skin biopsy shows mast cells in the dermis. Immunohistochemical staining with tryptase is more sensitive than metachromatic stains such as Giemsa or toluidine blue. Determine if the patient with cutaneous mastocytosis also has systemic mastocytosis. Figure 6-28 outlines one approach to this diagnostic evaluation. Cutaneous mastocytosis without systemic disease is common in pediatric-onset mastocytosis. Cutaneous mastocytosis is accompanied by systemic disease in most patients who have onset of lesions after age 2.

Box 6-13 **Classification of Cutaneous Mastocytosis**
Solitary or multiple mastocytoma(s)
Urticaria pigmentosa (maculopapular cutaneous mastocytosis)
Diffuse cutaneous mastocytosis
Telangiectasia macularis eruptiva perstans

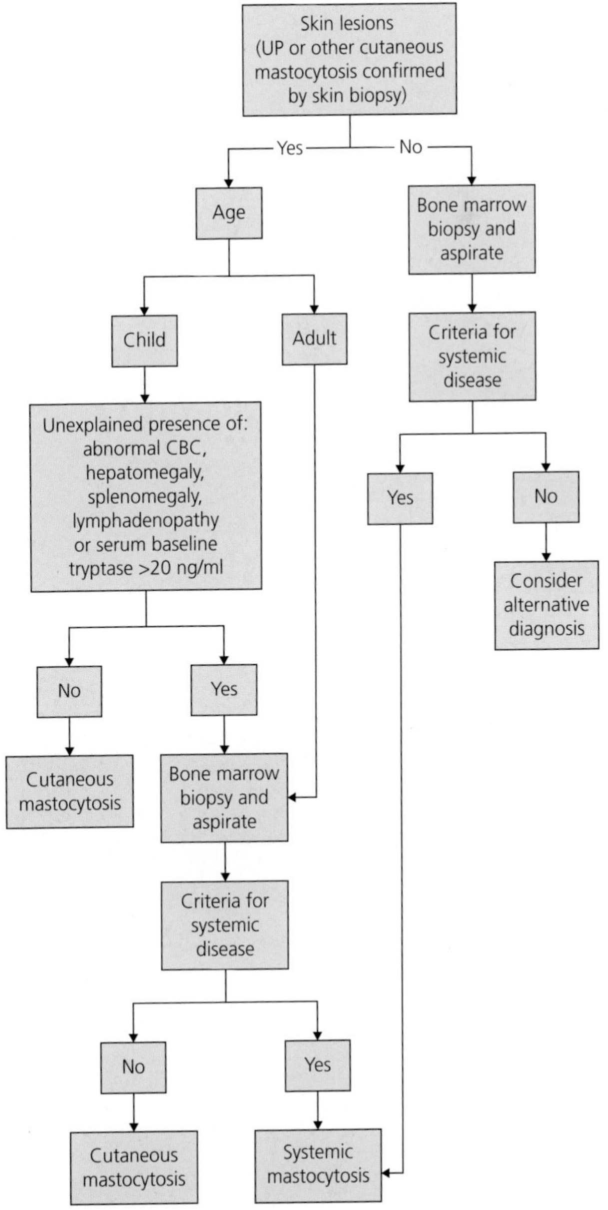

Figure 6-28 (*Annu Rev Med* 55:419-432, 2004. *PMID: 14746529*)

SOLITARY MASTOCYTOMA. A larger solitary collection of mast cells is called a mastocytoma (Figures 6-29 and 6-30). Mastocytoma is the most common type of cutaneous mastocytosis. There are one or multiple lesions. They are reddish brown nodules or plaques that can be several centimeters in diameter. Stroking induces whealing ("Darier's sign"). It is due to cutaneous mast cell degranulation and histamine release. The lesions either are present at birth or develop within a median time of 1 week; most appear within the first 3 months of life. They are rare in adults. Bullae may be seen. Children rarely develop additional mastocytomas more than 2 months after onset of the initial lesions. Most occur on the extremities but not the palms or soles. Lesions may spontaneously involute. If a lesion does not involute, it may be surgically removed. Transition to systemic involvement does not occur.

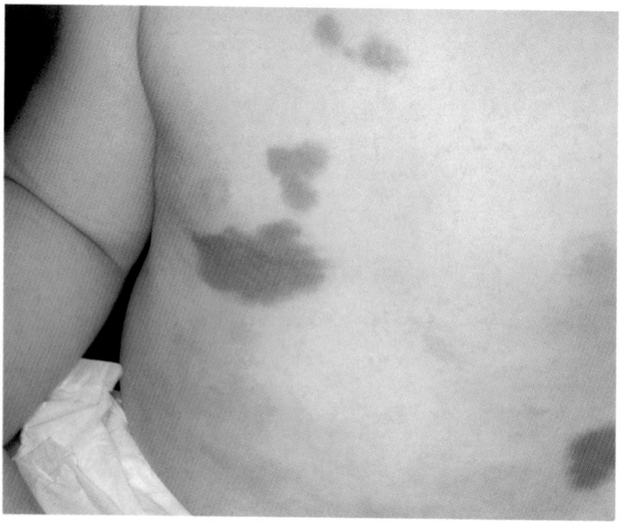

Figure 6-29 These solitary mastocytomas appear as red-brown plaques. They appeared weeks after birth.

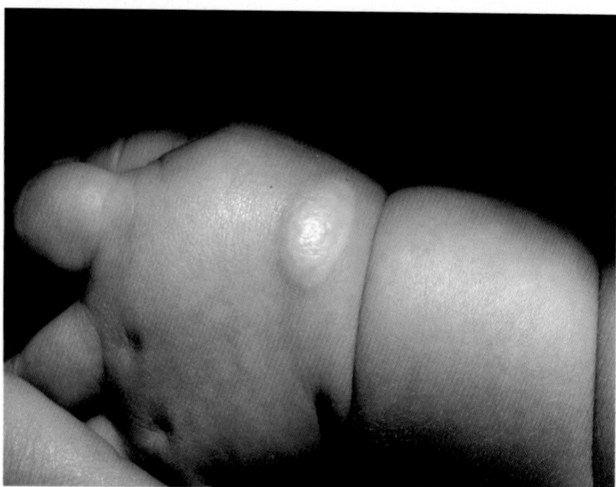

Figure 6-30 A blister formed on this solitary mastocytoma of the hand.

URTICARIA PIGMENTOSA. Urticaria pigmentosa is the second most frequent manifestation of mastocytosis in children. It may be present at birth, may appear in infancy and childhood at a median age of 2.5 months, and is present in 80% of affected individuals within 6 months. Cases gradually improve, and symptoms resolve in about 50% of patients by adolescence. Urticaria pigmentosa that begins after age 10 usually persists and may be associated with systemic disease. After the age of 10 years, the median time of onset for urticaria pigmentosa is 26.5 years. Lesions are well demarcated, red-brown, slightly elevated plaques averaging 0.5 to 1.5 cm in diameter. They occur in small groups on the trunk and are often dismissed as variations of pigmentation (Figures 6-31 through 6-35). Large numbers can occur on any body surface. The palms and soles are spared. Mucous membranes may be involved. Lesions may increase in number for years. Infants may develop bullae and vesicles until the age of 2; bullae are rarely observed after age 2. Bullae heal without scarring. Pruritus, flushing, and dermatographism occur. Darier's sign (the wheal-and-flare reaction that is seen following brisk stroking of the lesions) can be elicited (see Figures 6-31 and 6-34).

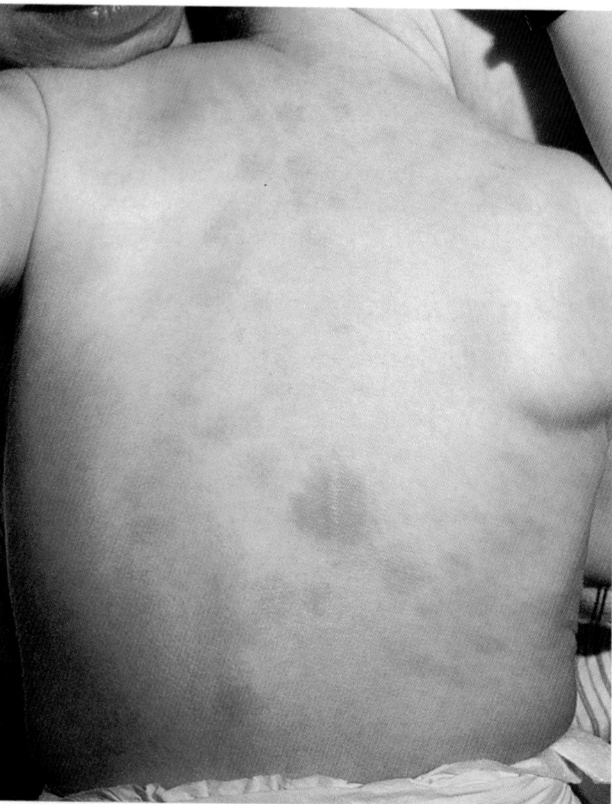

Figure 6-31 Cutaneous mastocytosis (urticaria pigmentosa). Red-brown, slightly elevated plaques averaging 0.5 to 3.5 cm in diameter typically occur in small groups on the trunk. One lesion turned red after being stroked.

URTICARIA PIGMENTOSA

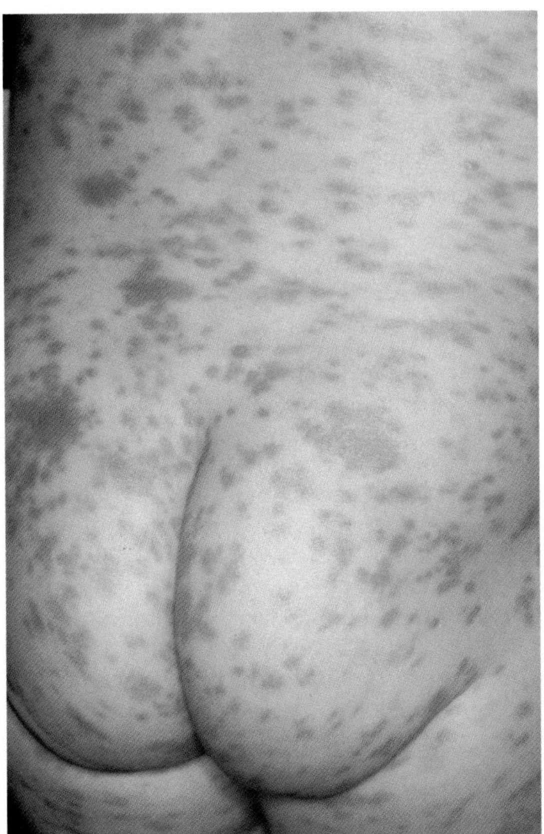

Figure 6-32 Numerous thick plaques began to appear at one month of age. The child scratched constantly.

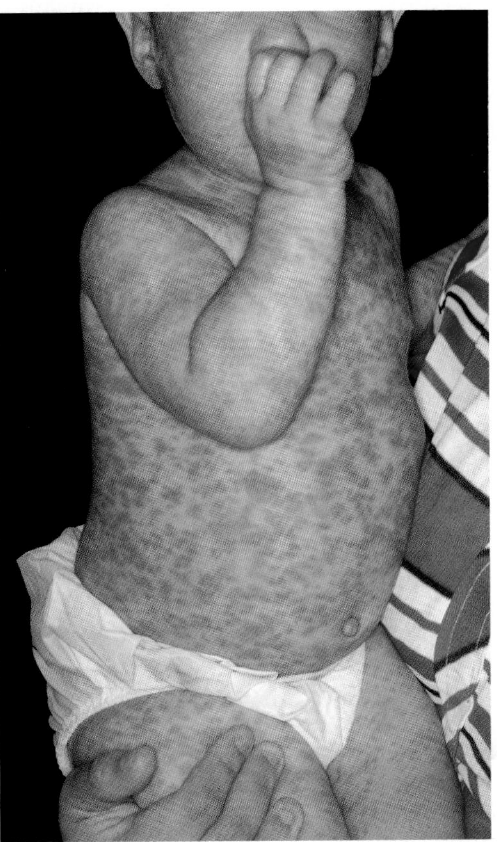

Figure 6-33 Numerous lesions appeared at 2 months and have shown little tendency to resolve. Lesions are well tolerated and the child sleeps without scratching.

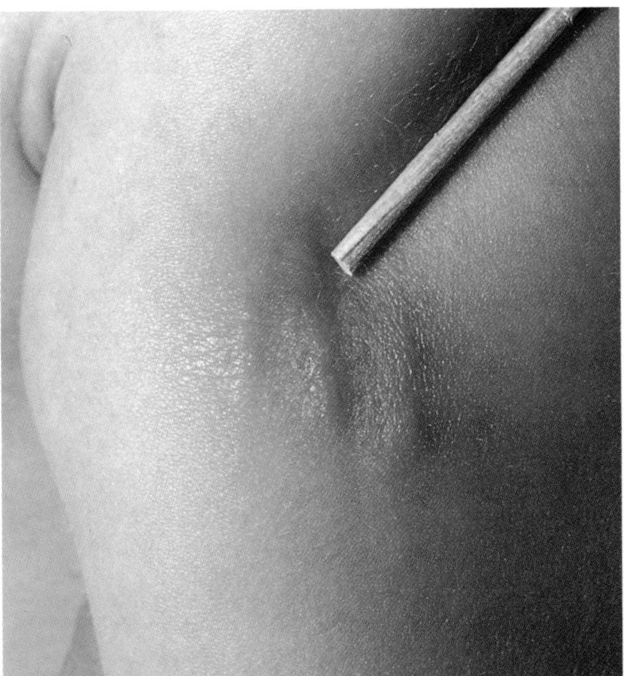

Figure 6-34 Cutaneous mastocytosis (urticaria pigmentosa): Darier's sign. Stroking a lesion with the wooden end of a cotton-tipped applicator produces a wheal that remains confined to the stroked site or enlarges.

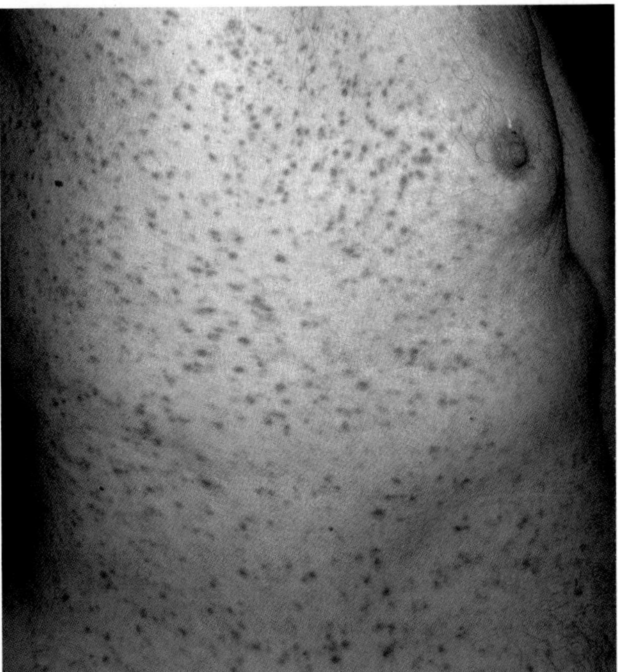

Figure 6-35 Numerous small, slightly elevated, red-brown papules appeared in this adult.

TELANGIECTASIA MACULARIS ERUPTIVA PERSTANS (TMEP). TMEP is the rarest cutaneous form. It is limited to adults and consists of telangiectasias and sparse, widespread mast cell infiltrates that resemble freckles. Pruritus, purpura, and blisters do not occur. The lesions are red-brown, telangiectatic macules with irregular borders. The biopsy in cases of TMEP reveals increased numbers of perivascular mast cells (Figure 6-36).

DIFFUSE CUTANEOUS TYPES. There are two rare, generalized forms of cutaneous disease. Diffuse erythrodermic cutaneous mastocytosis appears either as normal skin or as thickened, reddish brown edematous skin with an orange-peel texture. These pediatric patients have a diffuse infiltration of the entire skin by mast cells. It presents before the age of 3 years. These patients have the highest frequency of systemic mastocytosis. Dermographism with hemorrhagic blisters is common. Diffuse cutaneous mastocytosis usually resolves spontaneously between the ages of 15 months and 5 years. Diffuse generalized infiltration of the skin is called pseudoxanthomatous mastocytosis, or xanthelasmoidea and begins in childhood and persists throughout life.

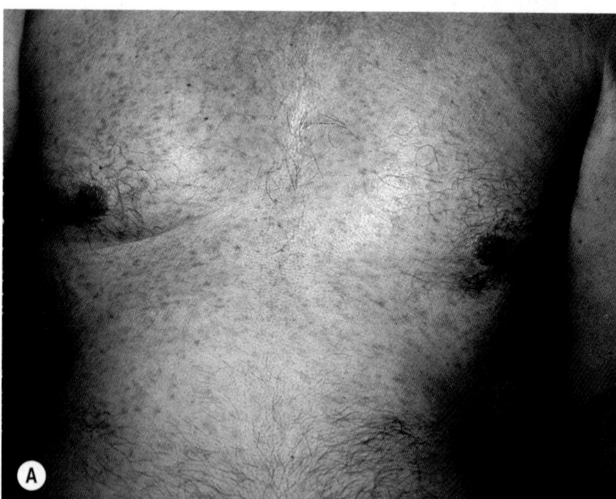

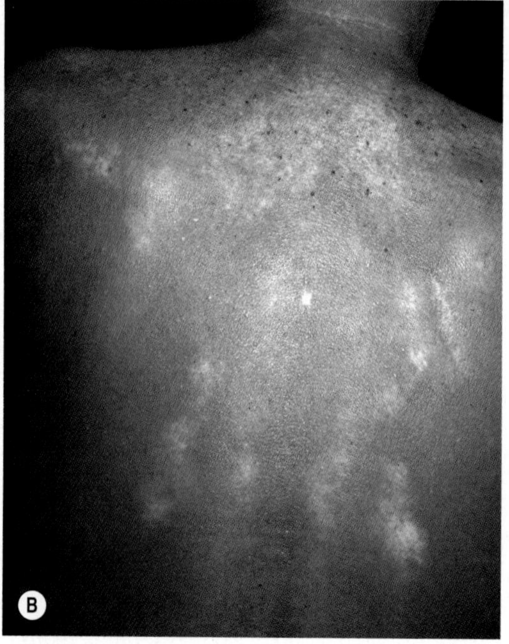

Figure 6-36 **A,** Telangiectasia macularis eruptiva perstans appear in adults as telangiectatic macules. **B,** Diffuse cutaneous mastocytosis began in childhood and has persisted.

SYSTEMIC MASTOCYTOSIS

Systemic mastocytosis can occur at any age but is generally seen in older children and adults. The frequency of skin lesions ranges from 50% to 100%. Systemic mast cell disease occurs in approximately 50% of adult patients with urticaria pigmentosa. There is flushing, syncope, and hypotension. Bone is the most common organ involved after the skin. Bone pain is a presenting symptom. Patients have diffuse or focal bony lesions that may be seen radiographically. Gastrointestinal tract involvement presents with nausea, vomiting, abdominal pain, diarrhea, and weight loss. Infiltration of the liver, spleen, and lymph nodes causes hepatosplenomegaly and lymphadenopathy. Mast cell leukemia occurs in fewer than 2% of patients. It is the most aggressive form of mastocytosis. There is malignant

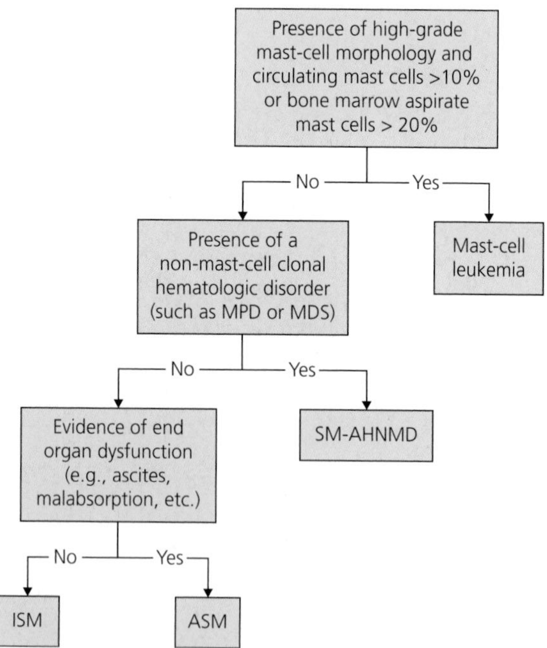

Figure 6-37 Classification to substantiate this diagnosis in patients with one major and one minor criterion, or three minor criteria. *ASM*, aggressive systemic mastocytosis; *ISM*, indolent systemic mastocytosis; *MDS*, myelodysplastic syndrome; *MPD*, myeloproliferative disorder; *SM-AHNMD*, systemic mastocytosis with associated clonal hematological non–mast-cell lineage disease. (*Annu Rev Med* 55:419-432, 2004. *PMID: 14746529*)

transformation in 7% of patients with juvenile-onset systemic disease and in approximately 30% of patients with adult-onset systemic disease.

DIAGNOSIS. The diagnosis is made by bone marrow histologic examination with immunohistochemical studies. Mast cell immunophenotyping, cytogenetic/molecular studies, and serum tryptase levels assist in confirming the diagnosis.

Mastocytosis should be suspected in patients with recurrent anaphylaxis who present with syncopal or near-syncopal episodes without associated hives or angioedema.

DIAGNOSTIC CRITERIA FOR SYSTEMIC MASTOCYTOSIS. The diagnosis of systemic mastocytosis (SM) is made when at least one major and one minor criterion or at least three minor criteria are fulfilled (Box 6-14). An algorithm for classification of systemic mastocytosis to substantiate this diagnosis in patients with one major and one minor criterion or three minor criteria is shown in Figure 6-37. The cutaneous and systemic variants are listed in Table 6-6.

Box 6-14 **WHO Major and Minor Criteria for Diagnosis of Systemic Mastocytosis (SM)***

Major

Multifocal dense infiltrates of mast cells in bone marrow and/or other extracutaneous organs with at least 15 mast cells per aggregate and confirmed by special staining

Minor

1. More than 25% of the mast cells in bone marrow aspirate smears or tissue biopsy sections are spindle shaped and immature, or display atypical morphology
2. Detection of a codon 816 c-Kit point mutation or other kit mutation described in SM in blood, bone marrow, or lesional tissue
3. Mast cells in bone marrow, blood, or other lesional tissue expressing CD25 and/or CD2
4. Baseline serum total tryptase level greater than 20 ng/ml (unless there is an associated clonal myeloid disorder, in which case this parameter is not valid)

*The diagnosis of SM may be made if one major and one minor criteria are present or if at least three minor criteria are present.

Table 6-6 Classification of Mastocytosis (Adapted from World Health Organization Criteria)

Category	Diagnostic features	Prognosis
Cutaneous mastocytosis	Lack of systemic involvement Age of onset generally <2 years	Good
Indolent systemic mastocytosis	Lack of advanced categories of mastocytosis Age of onset generally >2 years Most common category in adult-onset disease	Good
Systemic mastocytosis with associated clonal hematological non–mast cell lineage disease	Commonly associated with myelodysplastic or myeloproliferative disorders Occasionally seen with acute leukemias and lymphomas	Same as associated non–mast cell disorder
Aggressive systemic mastocytosis	Findings of end organ caused by mast cell infiltration, such as: • Bone marrow failure • Liver dysfunction with ascites • Splenomegaly with hypersplenism • Skeletal osteolytes with pathologic fractures • Gastrointestinal involvement with malabsorption and weight loss	Poor
Mast cell leukemia Mast cell sarcoma	Mast cells with high-grade morphology (multilobular or multiple nuclei): >10% mast cells in peripheral blood or >20% mast cells in bone marrow aspirate smears Malignant and destructive soft tissue tumor Mast cells with high-grade morphology	Poor Poor
Extracutaneous mastocytoma	Rare benign tumor consisting of mature mast cells	Good

From *Ann Rev Med* 55:419-432, 2004. *PMID: 14746529*

DIAGNOSIS.

Skin disease. Stroking a lesion with the wooden end of a cotton-tipped applicator induces intense erythema of the entire plaque and a wheal that is usually confined to the stroked site (Darier's sign). This test is highly characteristic and is as reliable as a biopsy for establishing the diagnosis. Metachromatic stains (Giemsa or toluidine blue) stain cytoplasmic mast cell granules in biopsy specimens deep blue. Injecting anesthetic directly into the biopsy site can degranulate mast cells.

Blood and urine studies. Elevated plasma histamine levels have been demonstrated in most children with mastocytosis. High levels occur with diffuse cutaneous mastocytosis. Above-normal levels of histamine in plasma or urine are consistent with the diagnosis of mastocytosis. Measure histamine in urine either in an aliquot from an acidified 24-hour urine collection or in a random urine specimen. Measurements of histamine in urine are subject to interference from histamine-rich foods, including cheese, wine, red meats, spinach, and tomatoes, and are not reliable in patients with urinary tract infections. Histamine levels in blood and urine are suppressed in patients treated with antihistamine drugs. Patients should not have taken antihistamine drugs for 48 hours before testing. Tryptase is a protein component of the secretory granules of mast cells. Measurable levels of tryptase in blood are found 30 to 60 minutes after activation of mast cells and persist for several hours. By comparison, histamine is cleared form the blood within minutes.

Box 6-15 **Triggers That Induce Systemic Mast Cell Degranulation**

Cause	Source
Insect stings, poison	Hymenoptera Jellyfish Snakes
Drugs	Opiate analgesics Codeine Morphine Polymyxin B Vancomycin D-Turbocurarine Succinylcholine Iodinated radiocontrast media Aspirin Nonsteroidal antiinflammatory agents Muscle relaxants Sympathomimetics Others
Temperature changes	Heat, cold
Ingestion of alcohol	
Mechanical irritation	Massage Friction
Infections	Bacterial Viral *Ascaris*
Bacterial toxins	Fish

Adapted from Hartmann K, Metcalfe D: *Hematol Oncol Clin North Am* 14(3):625, 2000. PMID: 10909043

PROGNOSIS.

Early-onset mastocytosis presenting by 3 years of age has a very favorable prognosis. Late-onset disease that presents between 7 and 10 years of age has a greater chance of continuing into adulthood. For approximately 50% of children who have cutaneous mastocytosis, symptoms and lesions will resolve during adolescence. Those whose mastocytosis continues into adulthood will have a 5% to 30% chance of systemic involvement.

MANAGEMENT.

Cutaneous disease. Patients with urticaria pigmentosa and systemic disease may benefit from a combination of H_1 and H_2 histamine antagonists. Oral disodium cromoglycate reduces pruritus and whealing in patients with and without systemic disease. Application of 0.05% betamethasone dipropionate ointment (Diprolene), under plastic-film occlusion for 8 hours daily for 6 weeks, leads to control of pruritus and Darier's sign. Improvement lasts for an average of 1 year. Patients with urticaria pigmentosa may be treated with an intralesional injection of triamcinolone acetonide 40 mg/ml. Control of pruritus, loss of Darier's sign, and cutaneous atrophy occur within 4 weeks and may persist for 1 year. Patients must avoid triggers that induce systemic mast cell degranulation (see Box 6-15).

There is no scientific support for the beneficial effects of diets restricted in biogenic amines and histamine-releasing foods in patients with mastocytosis (Box 6-16). The role of these diets in the treatment of mastocytosis remains hypothetical PMID: 16093574.

Systemic disease treatment. Recommended systemic disease treatment includes H_1 antihistamines for pruritus, H_2 antihistamines for peptic symptoms, and epinephrine (as needed) for episodes of hypotension. Oral cromolyn sodium may control gastrointestinal symptoms. Glucocorticoids are used for frequent hypotensive episodes, and for ascites and diarrhea associated with malabsorption. Psoralen ultraviolet A therapy may provide transient relief of pruritus and fading of skin lesions.

Reduce mast cell burden. Patients with aggressive systemic mastocytosis may benefit from interferon-α, which may restrict the proliferative potential of hematopoietic progenitor cells. Imatinib mesylate is used for certain patients who must undergo mutational analysis of a sample enriched for lesional mast cells.

Box 6-16 **Foods Rich in Histamine and/or Tyramine**

Cheese: Gouda, cheddar, Danish bleu, Emmenthaler, goats' cheese, Gorgonzola, Mascarpone, parmesan, and others
Chocolate
Meat: fermented meat, hare, (dry) sausage, raw ham
Fish: herring, smoked mackerel, smoked fish, shrimp, tinned fish (sardines), tuna fish, anchovy products
Vegetables: eggplant, spinach, sauerkraut
Alcohol: beer and wine
Fermented foods: tamari, marmite, soy sauce, trassi, tempeh

Chapter 7

Acne, Rosacea, and Related Disorders

CHAPTER CONTENTS

ACNE

Acne, a disease of the pilosebaceous unit, appears in males and females who live in westernized societies and are near puberty, and in most cases acne becomes less active as adolescence ends. The intensity and duration of activity vary for each individual.

The disease may be minor, with only a few comedones or papules, or it may occur as the highly inflammatory and diffusely scarring acne conglobata. The most severe forms of acne occur more frequently in males, but the disease tends to be more persistent in females, who may have periodic flare-ups before menstrual periods, which continue until menopause.

An overview of diagnosis and treatment is presented in Figures 7-1 to 7-3 and Table 7-1.

PSYCHOSOCIAL EFFECTS OF ACNE. Acne is too often dismissed as a minor affliction not worthy of treatment. Believing it is a phase of the growing process and that lesions will soon disappear, parents of children with acne postpone seeking medical advice. Permanent scarring of the skin and the psyche can result from such inaction. The disease has implications far beyond the few marks that may appear on the face. Lesions cannot be hidden under clothing; each is prominently displayed and detracts significantly from one's personal appearance and self-esteem. Taunting and ridicule from peers is demoralizing. Appearing in public creates embarrassment and frustration. Because acne is perceived by adolescents to have important negative personal and social consequences, improvement in these areas accompanies medical treatment. Facial appearance then becomes more acceptable to peers, embarrassment diminishes, and patients feel less socially inhibited.

THE PHYSICIAN-PATIENT RELATIONSHIP. Many acne sufferers expect to be disappointed with the results of treatment. They may be sensitive to actual or supposed lack of acceptance on the part of their physicians. Adolescence is usually characterized by the challenge of parental rules, and this transfers to the relationship with the physician. Noncompliance can be decreased by carefully explaining the goals and techniques of treatment and leaving the choice of implementation to the adolescent. Parents who offer to make sure the adolescent follows the treatment plan may encourage noncompliance by placing the treatment within the context of existing parent-child struggles. Greater consideration of adolescents' psychologic situations improves the therapeutic outcome, increases compliance, and leads to a greater confidence in the physician.

POSTADOLESCENT ACNE IN WOMEN. A low-grade, persistent acne is common in professional women. Closed comedones are the dominant lesions, with a few papulopustules. Premenstrual flare-ups are typical. Many of these patients passed through adolescence without acne. One author postulated that chronic stress leads to enhanced secretion of adrenal androgens, resulting in sebaceous hyperplasia and subsequent induction of comedones. A survey was taken of adult premenopausal women treated for mild-to-moderate, nonscarring, inflammatory acne who had undergone standard acne treatments without success or who had a clinical presentation suggesting hyperandrogenism (premenstrual exacerbations, irregular menses, coexisting hirsutism, androgenetic alopecia, seborrhea, or acne distribution on the lower face area, mandibular line, or neck).

The mean duration of acne was 20 years. A mean age at the time of the survey of 37 years and a mean age at onset of 16 years were documented. Acne was reported to be persistent in 80% of the women.

Eighty-three percent reported exacerbation with menses, 67% with stress, and 26% by diet. Pregnancy affected acne in 65% of the women, with 41% reporting improvement and 29% reporting worsening with pregnancy.

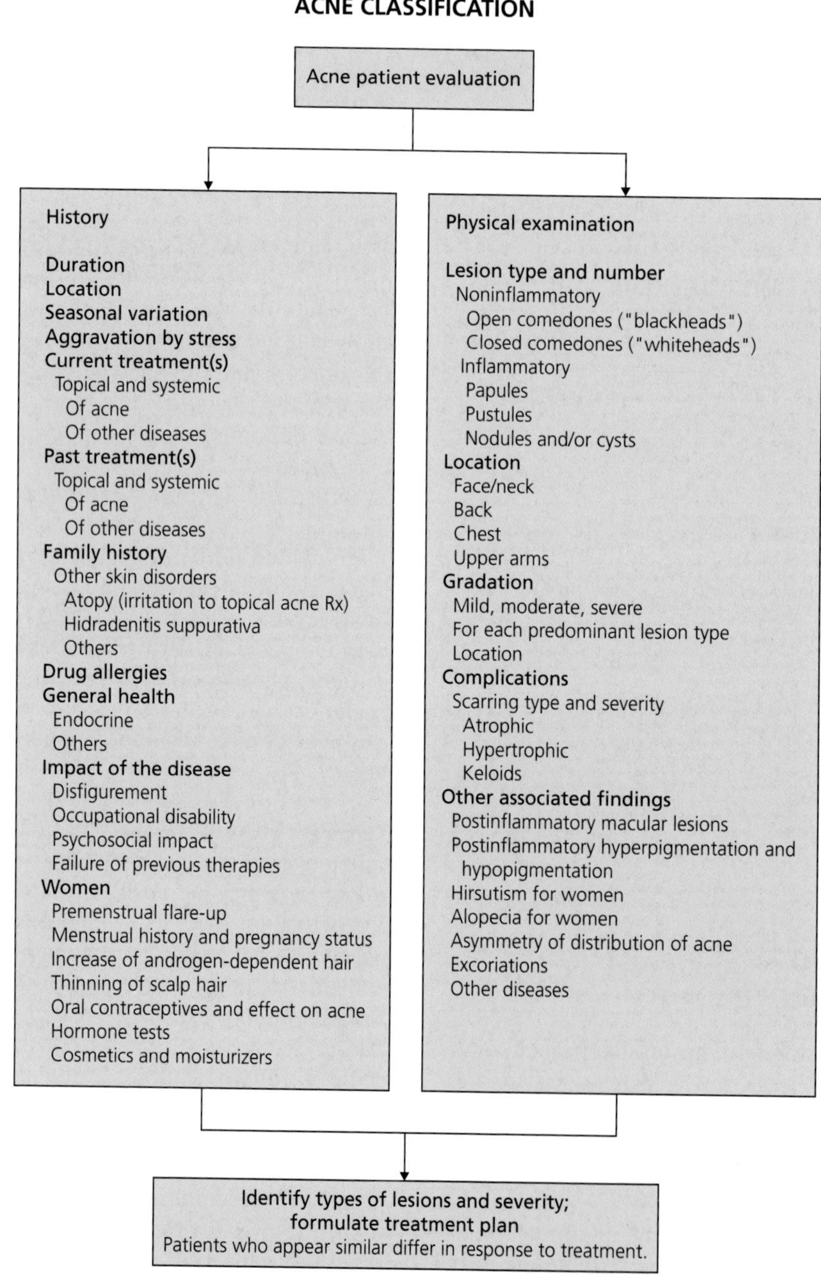

Figure 7-1 Patients who appear similar differ in response to treatment.

Classification

The Consensus Conference on Acne Classification (1990) proposed that acne grading be accomplished by the use of a pattern-diagnosis system, which includes a total evaluation of lesions and their complications such as drainage, hemorrhage, and pain (Figure 7-1). It takes into account the total impact of the disease, which is influenced by the disfigurement it causes. Degree of severity is also determined by occupational disability, psychosocial impact, and the failure of response to previous treatment.

ACNE LESIONS. Acne lesions are divided into inflammatory and noninflammatory lesions (Figure 7-2). Noninflammatory lesions consist of open and closed comedones. Inflammatory acne lesions are characterized by the presence of one or more of the following types of lesions: papules, pustules, and nodules (cysts). Papules are less than 5 mm in diameter. Pustules have a visible central core of purulent material. Nodules are greater than 5 mm in diameter. Nodules may become suppurative or hemorrhagic. Suppurative nodular lesions have been referred to as cysts because of their resemblance to inflamed epidermal cysts. Recurring rupture and reepithelialization of cysts leads to epithelial-lined sinus tracts, often accompanied by disfiguring scars.

For inflammatory acne lesions, the Consensus Panel proposes that lesions be classified as papulopustular and/or nodular. A severity grade based on a lesion count approximation is assigned as mild, moderate, or severe. Other factors in assessing severity include ongoing scarring, persistent purulent and/or serosanguineous drainage from lesions, and the presence of sinus tracts.

TYPE OF LESIONS

Noninflammatory lesions

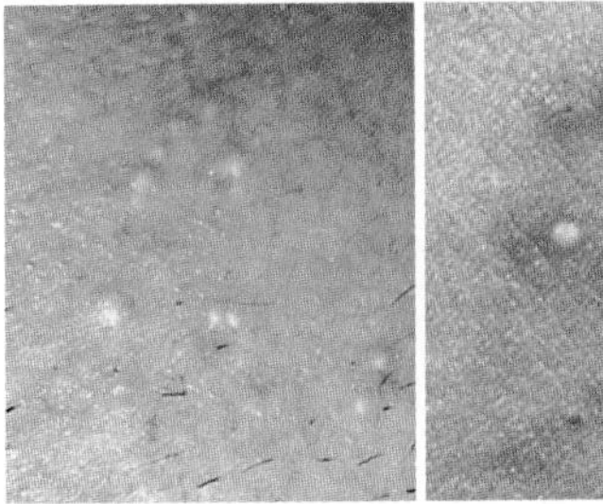

Closed comedones Open comedones

Inflammatory lesions

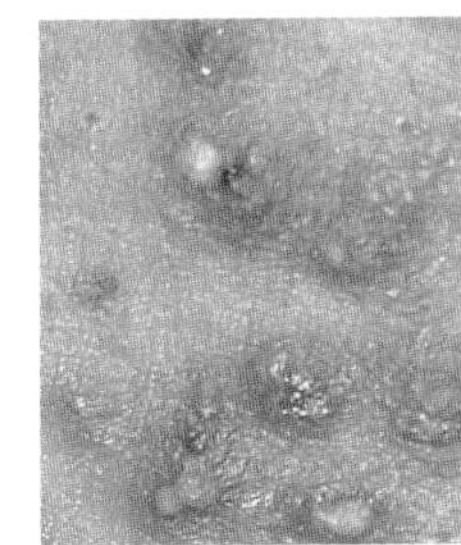

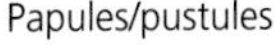

Papules/pustules

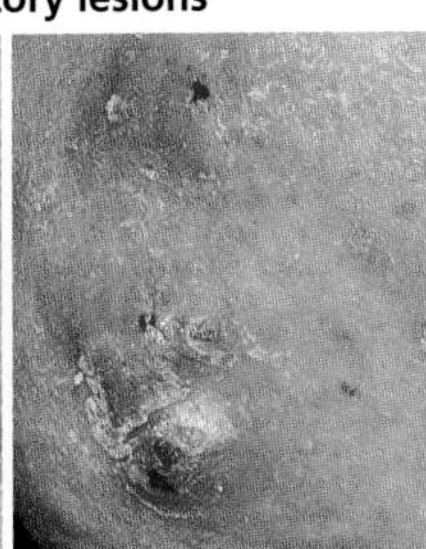

Nodules

ACNE CLASSIFICATION AND GRADING

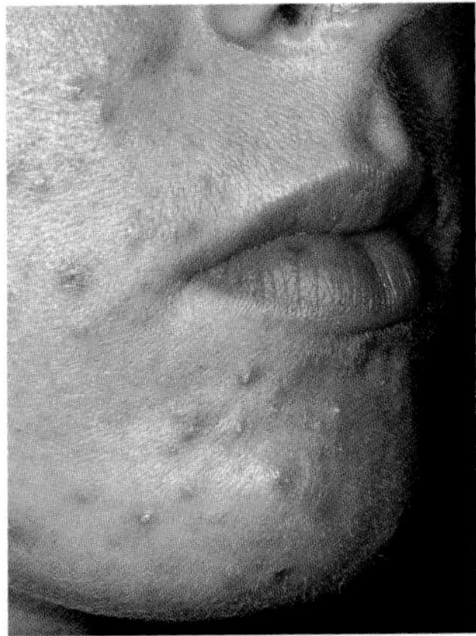

Mild
Papules/pustules +/++
Nodules 0

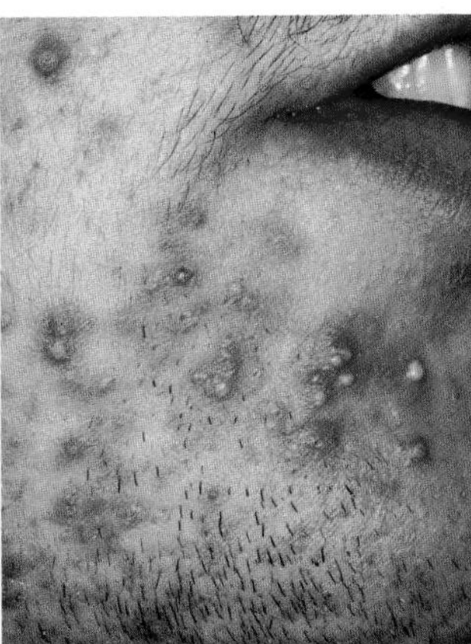

Moderate
Papules/pustules ++/+++
Nodules +/++

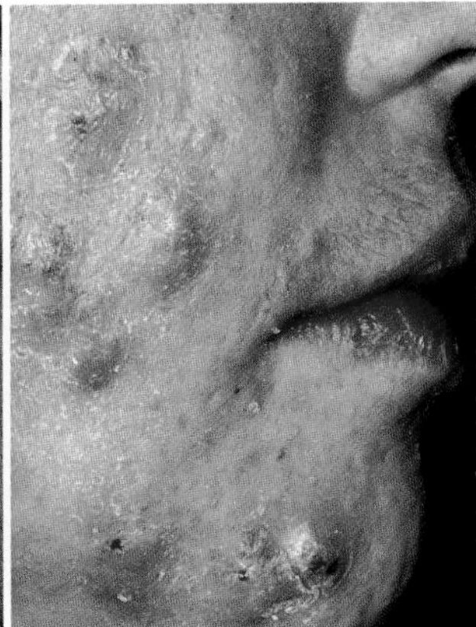

Severe
Papules/pustules +++/++++
Nodules +++

Figure 7-2 Acne classification of lesions.

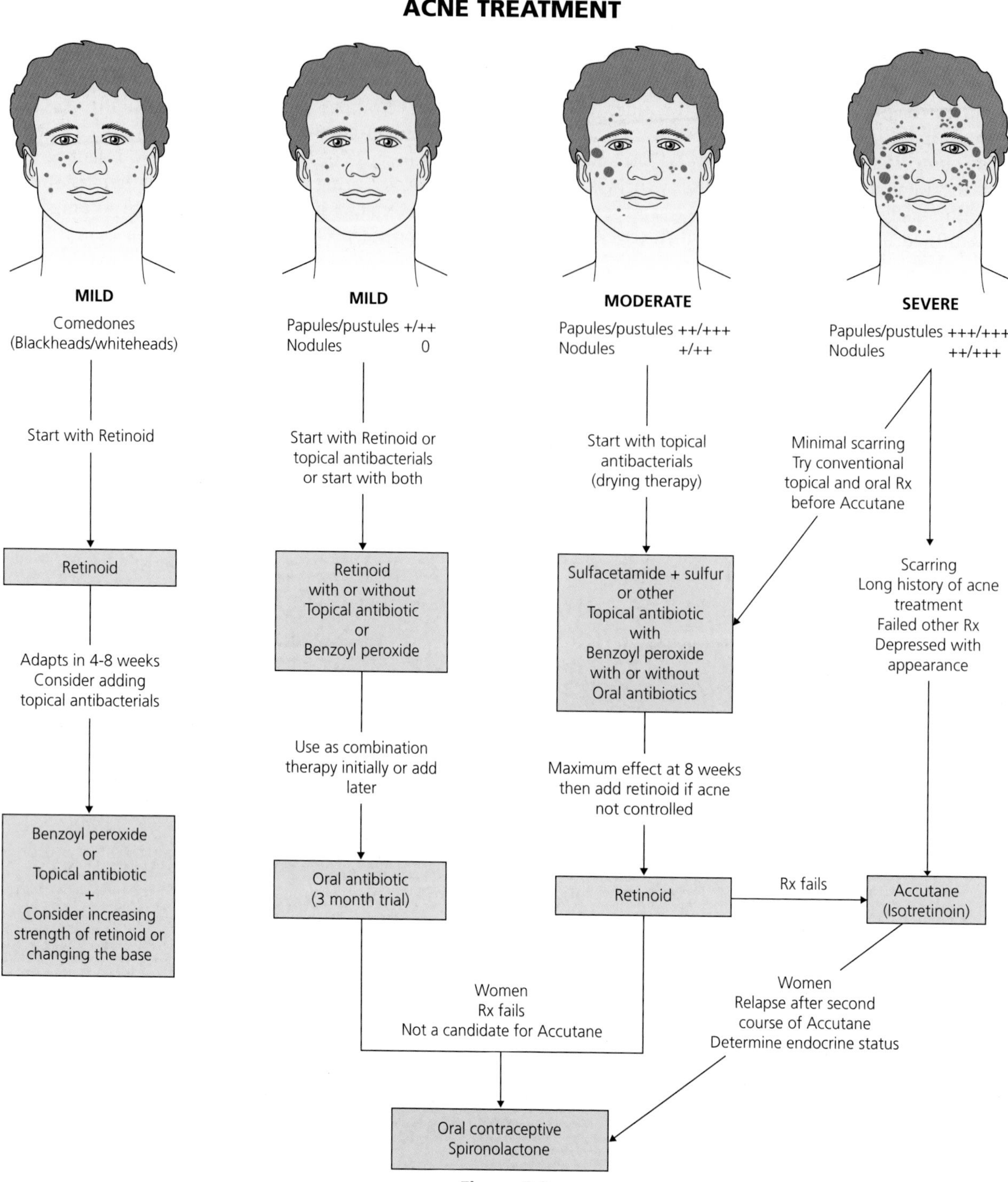
ACNE TREATMENT
MILD
Comedones
(Blackheads/whiteheads)
Start with Retinoid
Retinoid
Adapts in 4-8 weeks
Consider adding
topical antibacterials
Benzoyl peroxide
or
Topical antibiotic
+
Consider increasing
strength of retinoid or
changing the base
MILD
Papules/pustules +/++
Nodules 0
Start with Retinoid or
topical antibacterials
or start with both
Retinoid
with or without
Topical antibiotic
or
Benzoyl peroxide
Use as combination
therapy initially or add
later
Oral antibiotic
(3 month trial)
MODERATE
Papules/pustules ++/+++
Nodules +/++
Start with topical
antibacterials
(drying therapy)
Sulfacetamide + sulfur
or other
Topical antibiotic
with
Benzoyl peroxide
with or without
Oral antibiotics
Maximum effect at 8 weeks
then add retinoid if acne
not controlled
Retinoid
SEVERE
Papules/pustules +++/++++
Nodules ++/+++
Minimal scarring
Try conventional
topical and oral Rx
before Accutane
Scarring
Long history of acne
treatment
Failed other Rx
Depressed with
appearance
Rx fails
Accutane
(Isotretinoin)
Women
Rx fails
Not a candidate for Accutane
Women
Relapse after second
course of Accutane
Determine endocrine status
Oral contraceptive
Spironolactone

Figure 7-3

Table 7-1 Drug Treatment for Acne

Agent (class)	Mechanism of action	Dosage	Notes
Topical retinoids			
Tretinoin	Comedolysis, induction of orthokeratosis, and inhibition of inflammation	Apply every night; gel: 0.025%; cream: 0.025%, 0.05%, 0.1%; microsponge gel: 0.04%, 0.1%	First-line treatment for all acne. Retinoids as a class are known to cause local skin irritation. Acne exacerbation may occur in early weeks of treatment. Pregnancy category C.
Adapalene	Comedolysis, induction of orthokeratosis, and inhibition of inflammation	Apply every night; gel: 0.1% or 0.3%; cream: 0.1%	Alternative first-line treatment for all acne. Retinoids as a class are known to cause local skin irritation. Acne exacerbation may occur in early weeks of treatment. Pregnancy category C.
Tazarotene	Comedolysis, induction of orthokeratosis, and inhibition of inflammation	Apply every night; gel: 0.1%; cream: 0.1%	Second-line treatment for all types of acne because of greater expense, irritation, and lab animal teratogenicity compared with tretinoin and adapalene. Retinoids as a class are known to cause local skin irritation. Acne exacerbation may occur in early weeks of treatment. Pregnancy category X.
Salicylic acid (has retinoid properties)	Keratolysis, mild comedolysis	Apply daily to bid; OTC cleanser: 2%; solutions: 0.5-2%	Nonprescription products useful for mild comedonal acne, adult acne, and keratosis pilaris, mainly in patients with retinoid-intolerant skin. May cause mild local skin irritation. Not recommended for use during pregnancy.
Topical antibacterials, antibiotics, and antiinflammatory drugs			
Benzoyl peroxide	Potent bactericidal against *P. acnes*, keratolysis, and comedolysis	Potent bactericidal against *P. acnes*, keratolysis, and comedolysis: 2.5%, 4%, 5%, 8%, 10% and others	First-line topical therapy for all acne; reduces comedones and inflammatory lesions, no known resistant bacteria. May cause local skin irritation (5%); contact sensitization (1-2.5%); bleaching of skin, hair, fabrics, and carpeting; tumor promotion in lab animals. Use lower concentrations (2.5-4%) for sensitive skin. Pregnancy category C.
Clindamycin phosphate	Antibacterial against *P. acnes*, indirect suppression of inflammation	Apply daily to bid;* solution: 1%; pledgets: 1%; gel: 1%; lotion: 1%	Short-to-intermediate–term therapy for mild-to-moderate inflammatory acne. May cause local skin irritation, promotion of antibiotic-resistant bacteria; pseudomembranous enterocolitis has been reported rarely. Pregnancy category B.
Erythromycin	Antibacterial against *P. acnes*, indirect suppression of inflammation	Apply daily to bid; solution: 2%; pledgets: 2%; gel: 2%	Short-to-intermediate–term therapy for mild-to-moderate inflammatory acne. May cause local skin irritation, promotion of antibiotic-resistant bacteria. Pregnancy category B.
Dapsone	Antibacterial against *P. acnes*, indirect suppression of inflammation	Apply daily to bid; gel: 5%	Short-to-intermediate–term therapy for mild-to-moderate inflammatory acne. May cause local skin irritation. Pregnancy category C.
Sulfur-sulfacetamide sodium	Antibacterial against *P. acnes*, indirect suppression of inflammation; sulfur is a mild keratolytic agent	Apply daily to bid; various OTC and prescription lotions and cleansers: 2-10%	Adjunctive therapy for mild-to-moderate teenage and adult acne. May cause local skin irritation and contact reactions in sulfonamide-sensitive patients; has unpleasant odor. Pregnancy category C.
Azelaic acid (topical antibiotic, mild anticomedonal drug)	Modest antibacterial activity against *P. acnes*, modulates keratin formation	Apply bid; cream: 20%; gel: 15%	Adjunctive therapy for mild-to-moderate acne, especially when hyperpigmentation is present, because of ability to cause hypopigmentation as a side effect. May cause local skin irritation, mainly burning and stinging. Pregnancy category B.
Combination topical antibacterials			
Clindamycin-benzoyl peroxide	Potent bactericidal effect against *P. acnes*, mild keratolytic agent	Apply daily to bid; gel with clindamycin: 1%; benzoyl peroxide: 5%	More effective than individual components alone; benzoyl peroxide prevents bacterial resistance to clindamycin. See side effects of individual agents above. Pregnancy category C.
Erythromycin-benzoyl peroxide	Potent bactericidal effect against *P. acnes*, mild keratolytic agent	Apply daily to bid; gel with erythromycin: 3%; benzoyl peroxide: 5%	Topical antibacterial and keratolytic combination for all acne; more effective than individual components alone, and benzoyl peroxide prevents bacterial resistance to erythromycin. See side effects of individual agents above. Pregnancy category C.

Continued

Table 7-1 Drug Treatment for Acne—cont'd

Agent (class)	Mechanism of action	Dosage	Notes
Oral antibiotic drugs			
Tetracycline	Antibacterial against *P. acnes,* indirect suppression of inflammation	250 mg PO four times/day, 500 mg PO bid	First-line oral therapy for moderate-to-severe inflammatory acne. May cause phototoxicity, vaginal yeast infection, dyspepsia, rare liver toxicity, staining of teeth in fetuses and children, reduced efficacy of oral contraceptives. Requires empty stomach; cannot be taken with dairy products. Pregnancy category D. Not for acne treatment in children under age 12.
Doxycycline	Antibacterial against *P. acnes,* indirect suppression of inflammation	20, 40, 50, 75, or 100 mg PO bid; 75-100 mg PO daily	Modestly priced alternative to tetracycline. May cause dose-related phototoxicity (requires sun protection), vaginal yeast infection, dyspepsia. May be taken with food. Pregnancy category D. Not for acne treatment in children under age 12.
Minocycline	Antibacterial against *P. acnes,* indirect suppression of inflammation	50, 75, or 100 mg PO bid; or extended-release form 45, 90, or 135 mg daily	Second-line alternative to tetracycline because of higher cost. May cause dizziness, vertigo, discolored teeth, blue-gray skin staining, rare hepatotoxicity and lupus-like syndrome. May be taken with food. Extended-release form is most expensive. Pregnancy category D. Not for acne treatment in children under age 12.
Erythromycin	Antibacterial against *P. acnes,* indirect suppression of inflammation	1-1.2 gm/day PO in divided doses	Alternative to tetracycline for moderate-to-severe inflammatory acne. Often causes gastric upset or diarrhea. Useful in pediatric age group. Pregnancy category B.
Azithromycin	Antibacterial against *P. acnes,* indirect suppression of inflammation	500 mg PO on day 1; 250 mg/day PO on days 2-5, several other schedules are reported in the literature	Second-line therapy for moderate-to-severe inflammatory acne because of higher cost. May cause gastric upset or diarrhea, rare cholestatic jaundice and angioedema. Useful in pediatric age group. Pregnancy category B.
Ampicillin or amoxicillin	Antibacterial against *P. acnes,* indirect suppression of inflammation	500 mg bid PO bid	Second-line therapy for moderate inflammatory acne. Pregnancy category B.
Sulfamethoxazole-trimethoprim	Antibacterial against *P. acnes,* indirect suppression of inflammation	1 DS tablet bid	Second-line therapy for severe inflammatory acne. May cause gastric distress, skin rashes, rare Stevens-Johnson syndrome. Useful when isotretinoin is contraindicated. Pregnancy category C. Pediatric use approved after age 2 months.
Oral contraceptive drugs and hormonal therapy			
Norethindrone acetate-ethinyl estradiol (oral contraceptive)	Regulation of androgens by preventing cyclical progesterone surge	1 pill PO daily for 21 days, skip 7 days, then repeat cycle	First-line treatment of moderate-to-severe acne in women with laboratory evidence of hyperandrogenism. May cause skin rashes, nausea, vomiting, migraine headaches, mood disorders, hypertension, menstrual irregularities, venous thrombosis, jaundice. Not for use in children or women who are pregnant or lactating.
Norgestimate-ethinyl estradiol (oral contraceptive)	Regulation of androgens by preventing cyclical progesterone surge	1 pill PO daily for 21 days, skip or take null pill for 7 days, repeat cycle	First-line treatment of moderate-to-severe acne in women with laboratory evidence of hyperandrogenism. May cause skin rashes, nausea, vomiting, migraine headaches, mood disorders, hypertension, menstrual irregularities, venous thrombosis, jaundice. Not for use in children or women who are pregnant or lactating.
Spironolactone (oral antiandrogen)	Spironolactone (oral antiandrogen)	50-100 mg bid PO	Off-label use for moderate-to-severe acne in women with laboratory evidence of hyperandrogenism. May cause breast tenderness, frequent menses, hypotension, hyperkalemia, feminization of male fetuses. Pregnancy category C.

Table 7-1 Drug Treatment for Acne—cont'd

Agent (class)	Mechanism of action	Dosage	Notes
Prednisone (oral corticosteroid)	Antiinflammatory, suppression of adrenal androgen production	High dose: 40 mg PO daily, tapering to zero over 2-4 weeks; low dose: 5 mg PO daily	High dose: useful for temporary control of severe nodular acne, acne conglobata, and acne fulminans. Low dose: useful for longer-term adrenal suppression in rare cases. May cause gastric distress, fluid retention, increased blood glucose level, hypertension, impaired wound healing, mood swings, growth disturbances, cataracts, glaucoma. Pregnancy category C.
Oral retinoid drug			
Isotretinoin (oral retinoid)	Modulation of epidermal proliferation, induction of orthokeratosis, comedolysis, inhibition of inflammation, and inhibition of sebum secretion	0.5-2 mg/kg/day PO, daily or divided bid, for 20-wk total course	Treatment of choice for severe, recalcitrant, nodular acne; prolonged remissions (1-3 yr) are seen in about 80% of cases. Side effects include dry skin, chapped lips, dry eyes, nosebleeds, hair loss, major birth defects, hyperlipidemias, transient liver enzyme elevations, musculoskeletal pain, hyperostosis, decreased bone mineral density, diminution of night vision, and psychiatric effects (controversial), including mood swings, depression, suicide risk, and aggressive or violent behavior. Pregnancy category X. All prescribers, patients, wholesalers, and dispensing pharmacies must be registered in the FDA-approved iPLEDGE program (www.ipledgeprogram.com).

Adapted from Bershad SV: In the clinic. Acne, *Ann Intern Med* 149(1), 2008. PMID: 18591631
bid, Twice daily; *DS*, double strength; *OTC*, over-the-counter; *PO*, orally.

Etiology and pathogenesis

Figure 7-4 illustrates the mechanism of action of therapeutic agents, and Figure 7-5 illustrates the evolution of the different acne lesions. Acne is a disease involving the pilosebaceous unit and is most frequent and intense in areas where sebaceous glands are largest and most numerous. Acne begins in predisposed individuals when sebum production increases. *Propionibacterium acnes* proliferates in sebum, and the follicular epithelial lining becomes altered and forms plugs called comedones. One study suggests that anxiety and anger are significant factors for patients who have severe acne.

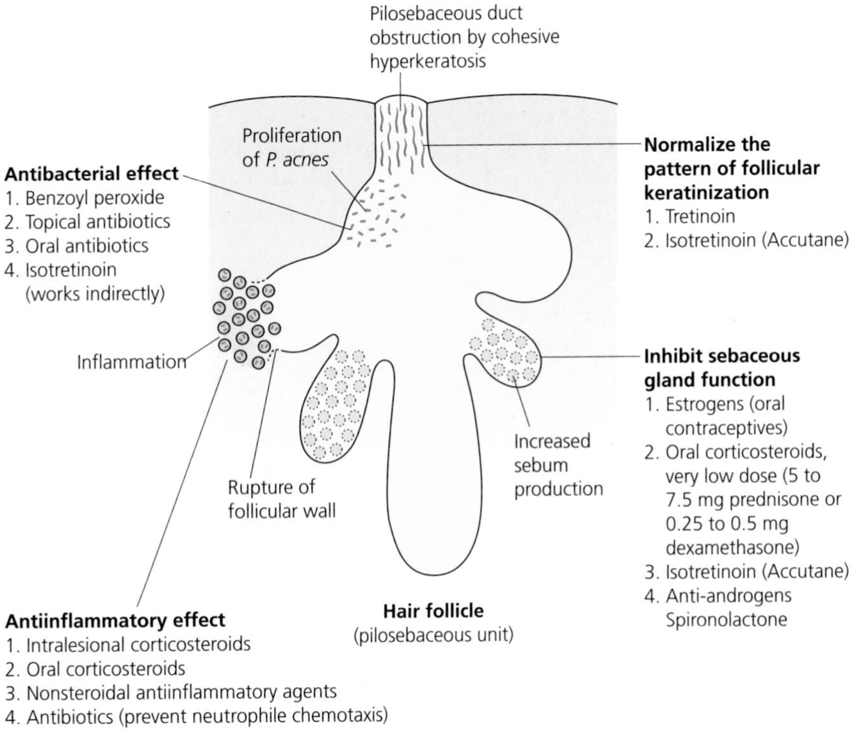

Figure 7-4 Mode of action of therapeutic agents.

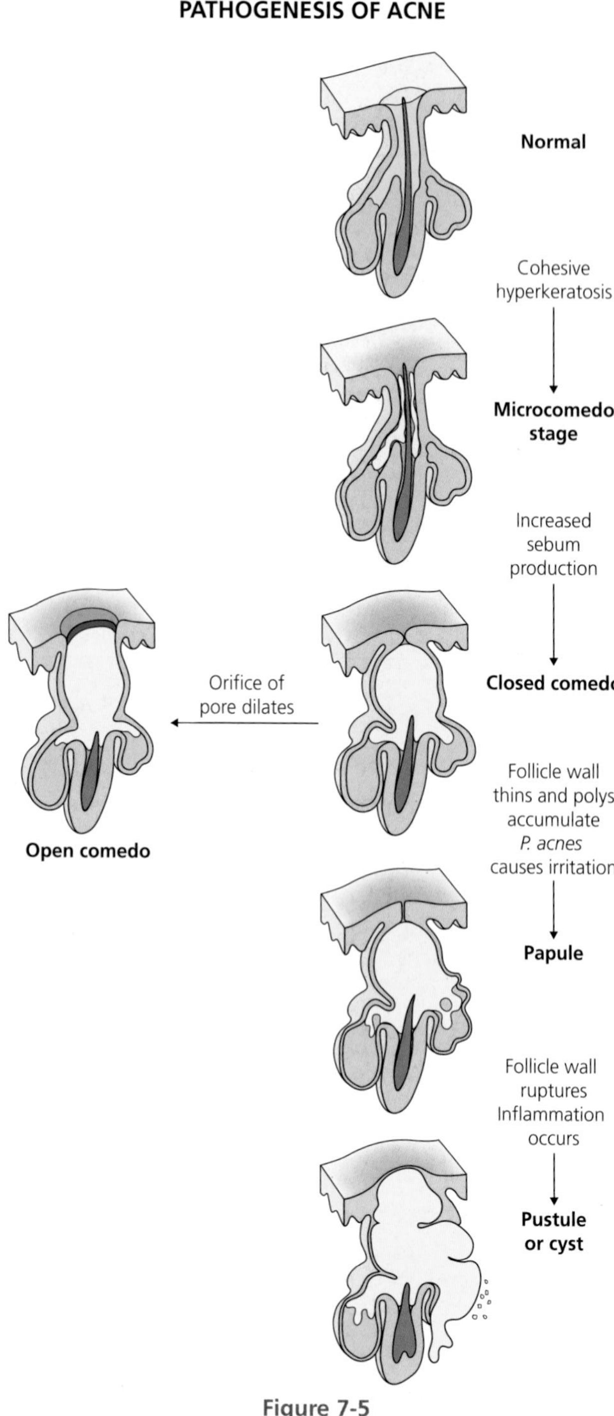

Figure 7-5

SEBACEOUS GLANDS. Sebum is the pathogenic factor in acne; it is irritating and comedogenic, especially when *P. acnes* proliferates and modifies its components. Most patients with acne have a higher-than-normal sebum level.

Sebaceous glands are located throughout the entire body except the palms, soles, dorsa of the feet, and lower lip. They are largest and most numerous on the face, chest, back, and upper outer arms. Clusters of glands appear as relatively large, visible, white globules on the buccal mucosa (Fordyce spots), the vermilion border of the upper lip (Figure 7-6), the female areolae (Montgomery's tubercles), the labia minora, the prepuce, and around the anus.

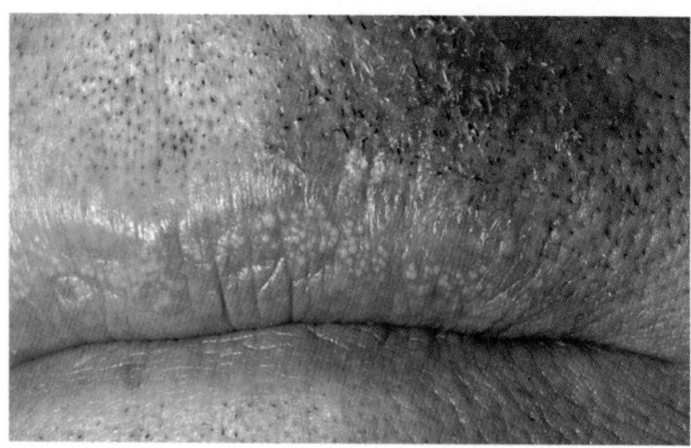

Figure 7-6 Cluster of sebaceous glands (tiny, white-yellow spots) that are normally present on the vermilion border of the upper lip.

Sebaceous glands are large in newborn infants, but regress shortly after birth. They remain relatively small in infancy and most of childhood, but enlarge and become more active in prepuberty. Hormones influence sebaceous gland secretion. Testosterone is converted to dihydrotestosterone in the skin and acts directly on the sebaceous gland to increase its size and metabolic rate. Estrogens, through a less well-defined mechanism, decrease sebaceous gland secretion. Sebaceous gland cells produce a complex mixture of oily material. Sebaceous cells mature, die, fragment, and then extrude into the sebaceous duct, where they combine with the desquamating cells of the lower hair follicle and finally arrive at the skin surface as sebum.

PILOSEBACEOUS DUCT OBSTRUCTION. The early acne lesion results from blockage in the follicular canal. Increased amounts of keratin result from hormonal changes and sebum modified by the resident bacterial flora *P. acnes*. The increased number of cornified cells remain adherent to the follicular canal (retention keratosis) directly above the opening of the sebaceous gland duct to form a plug (microcomedo). Factors causing increased sebaceous secretion (puberty, hormonal imbalances) influence the eventual size of the follicular plug. The plug enlarges behind a very small follicular orifice at the skin surface and becomes visible as a closed comedone (firm, white papule). An open comedone (blackhead) occurs if the follicular orifice dilates. Further increase in the size of a blackhead continues to dilate the pore, but usually does not result in inflammation. The small-pore, closed comedone is the precursor of inflammatory acne papules, pustules, and cysts.

BACTERIAL COLONIZATION AND INFLAMMATION. *P. acnes*, an anaerobic diphtheroid, is a normal skin resident and the principal component of the microbic flora of the pilosebaceous follicle. The bacteria are thought to play a significant role in acne. *P. acnes* generates components that create inflammation, such as lipases, proteases, hyaluronidase, and chemotactic factors. Lipases hydrolyze sebum triglycerides to form free fatty acids, which are comedogenic and primary irritants. Chemotactic factors attract neutrophils to the follicular wall. Neutrophils elaborate hydrolases that weaken the wall. The wall thins, becomes inflamed (red papule), and ruptures, releasing part of the comedone into the dermis. An intense, foreign-body, inflammatory reaction results in the formation of the acne pustule or cyst. Other bacterial substances possibly mediate inflammation by stimulation of immune mechanisms.

Approach to acne therapy

INITIAL VISIT

HISTORY. Many patients are embarrassed to ask for help. Any feeling of apathy or indifference on the part of the physician will be sensed, resulting in a loss of esteem and enthusiasm for the treatment. A careful history should be taken. Inquiring about many details reassures the patient that this is a disease to be taken seriously and managed carefully. Previous treatment should be documented—types of cleansers and lubricants, family history, and history of cyclic menstrual flare-ups. The potential for irritation can be determined by responses to drying therapy with over-the-counter benzoyl peroxide. This experience facilitates the choice of which strength and base of benzoyl peroxide, tretinoin, or other topical agents to prescribe.

PATHOGENESIS AND COURSE. Acne is an inherited disease. It is not possible to predict which members of a family will inherit it. The severity of acne in persons developing the disease is not necessarily related to the severity of acne in their parents. Acne does not end at age 19 but can persist into a person's forties. Many women have their first episode after age 25. Several myths should be discussed. Acne is not caused by dirt. The pigment in blackheads is not dirt and may not be melanin as was once suspected. Excessive washing is unnecessary and interferes with most treatment programs. Gentle manipulation of pustules is tolerated; aggressive pressure and excoriation produces permanent scarring. The erythema and pigmentation that follows resolution of acne lesions in some patients may take many months to fade.

Patients should not have inappropriate expectations. In most cases, acne can be controlled, but not cured. Stress is an important exacerbating factor.

ACNE AND DIET. In Western cultures, acne affects up to 95% of adolescents and persists into middle age in 12% of women and 3% of men. Two non-Westernized populations—the Kitavan Islanders of Papua, New Guinea, and the Ache hunter-gatherers of Paraguay—do not have acne. They eat fruit, fish, game, and tubers but no cereals or refined sugars.

This suggests that high-glycemic carbohydrates (bread, bagels, doughnuts, crackers, candy, cake, chips), those that substantially boost blood glucose levels, trigger a series of hormonal changes that cause acne. Elevated blood glucose levels lead to increased insulin production. This affects other hormones that can cause excess oil in the skin. Therefore low-glycemic diets, including fruits and vegetables, might offer a new treatment option for people with acne and some studies support this. Milk has also been implicated as possibly increasing acne severity.

COSMETICS AND CLEANSERS. Moderate use of non-greasy lubricants and water-based cosmetics is usually well tolerated, but a gradual decrease in the use of cosmetics is encouraged as acne improves. Cream-based cleansers should be avoided.

ORAL CONTRACEPTIVES. If women patients are taking oral contraceptives, a change in estrogen and progestin combinations may be all that is necessary.

INITIAL EVALUATION

TYPE OF LESIONS. An overview of diagnosis and treatment is presented in the beginning of this chapter (see Figures 7-1 to 7-3). The types of lesions present are determined (i.e., comedones, papules, pustules, nodules, or cysts). The degree of severity (mild, moderate, severe) is also determined.

DEGREE OF SKIN SENSITIVITY. The degree of skin sensitivity can be determined by inquiring about experiences with topical medicines and soaps. Degree of pigmentation and hair color are not the sole determinants of skin sensitivity. Atopic patients with dry skin and a history of eczema generally do not tolerate aggressive drying therapy.

SELECTION OF THERAPY. Therapy appropriate to the type of acne is selected. (For initial orientation, refer to Figure 7-3.) If antibiotics are selected for initial therapy, it is best to start with "therapeutic dosages" (see section on Oral Antibiotics, p. 237).

COURSE OF TREATMENT. A program can be established for most patients after three visits, but some difficult cases require continual supervision. For maximum effect treatment must be continual and prolonged. Patients who had only a few lesions that quickly cleared may be given a trial period without treatment 6 to 8 weeks after clearing. In an attempt to suppress further activity, those patients who have numerous lesions should remain on continual topical treatment for several months. The patient's propensity to scar must be ascertained. Patients vary in their tendency to develop scars. Some demonstrate little scarring even after significant inflammation, whereas others develop a scar from nearly every inflammatory papular or pustular lesion. This latter group requires aggressive therapy to prevent further damage. The early use of isotretinoin may be justified in these patients.

Acne treatment

The following treatment programs are offered only as a guide. Modifications must be made for each individual (see Figure 7-3).

COMEDONAL ACNE

CLINICAL PRESENTATION. The earliest type of acne is usually noninflammatory comedones ("blackheads" and "whiteheads") (Figures 7-7 through 7-9). It develops in the preteenage or early teenage years and is caused by increased sebum production and abnormal desquamation of epithelial cells. There are no inflammatory lesions because colonization with *P. acnes* has not yet occurred.

TREATMENT. Closed comedone acne (whiteheads) responds slowly. A large mass of sebaceous material is impacted behind a very small follicular orifice. The orifice may enlarge during treatment, making extraction by acne surgery possible. Comedones may remain unchanged for months or evolve into a pustule or cyst.

Retinoids (Tazorac, Retin-A, Differin, Azelex) are applied at bedtime. The base and strength are selected according to skin sensitivity. Tazorac may be the most effective and most irritating. Start with a low concentration of the cream or gel (available in 0.05% and 0.1%) and increase the concentration if irritation does not occur. Retin-A and Differin are equally effective. Start with Retin-A cream (0.025%, 0.05%, 0.1%) or gel (0.01% and 0.025%) or with Retin-A Micro (0.04 and 0.1) or Differin (gel, cream, solution, pads). Azelex is less potent but is less irritating. It also has antibacterial activity. Medications are used more frequently if tolerated. Add benzoyl peroxide or topical antibiotics or combination medicines (e.g., BenzaClin) later to discourage *P. acne* and the formation of inflammatory lesions. The response to treatment is slow and discouraging. Several months of treatment are required. Large open comedones (blackheads) are expressed; many are difficult to remove. Several weeks of treatment facilitates easier extraction. Topical therapy may have to be continued for extended periods.

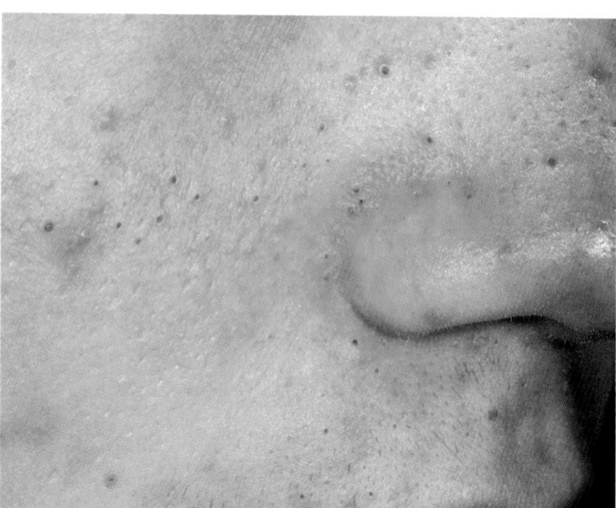

Figure 7-7 Comedones (blackheads) are occasionally inflamed.

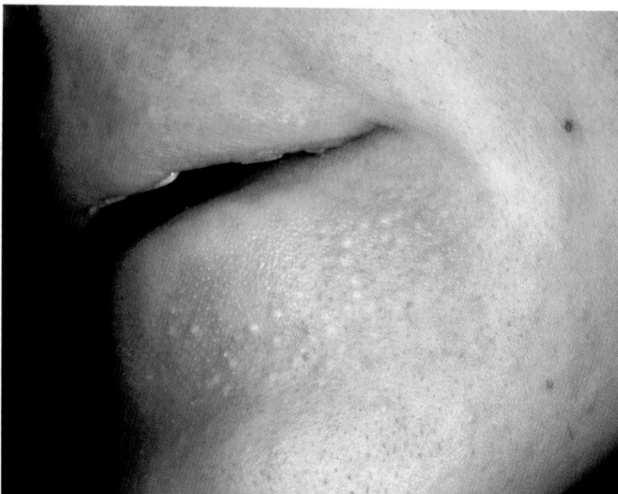

Figure 7-8 The appearance of closed comedones can be accentuated by stretching the skin.

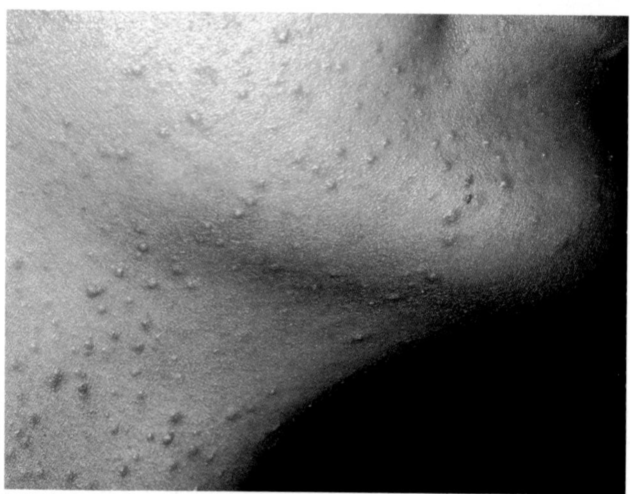

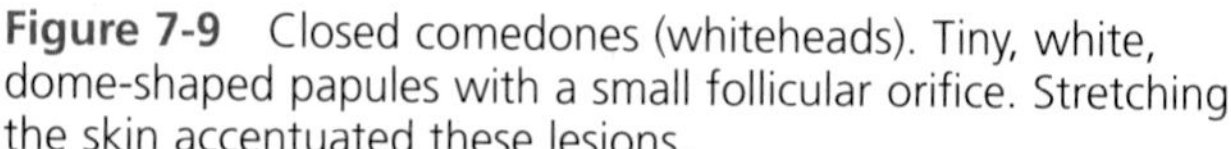

Figure 7-9 Closed comedones (whiteheads). Tiny, white, dome-shaped papules with a small follicular orifice. Stretching the skin accentuated these lesions.

MILD INFLAMMATORY ACNE

CLINICAL PRESENTATION. Mild pustular and papular inflammatory acne is defined as fewer than 20 pustules. Inflammatory lesions occur in comedones after proliferation of *P. acnes*. Papules or pustules with a minimum of comedones may develop after comedonal acne (Figures 7-10 and 7-11).

TREATMENT. Benzoyl peroxide, a topical antibiotic, or combination medicine (e.g., BenzaClin, Duac) and a retinoid are initially applied on alternate evenings. The lowest concentrations are initially used. After the initial adjustment period, the retinoid is used each night and benzoyl peroxide or antibiotic each morning. The strength of the medications is increased if tolerated. Oral antibiotics are introduced if the number of pustules does not decrease. Topical therapy may have to be continued for extended periods.

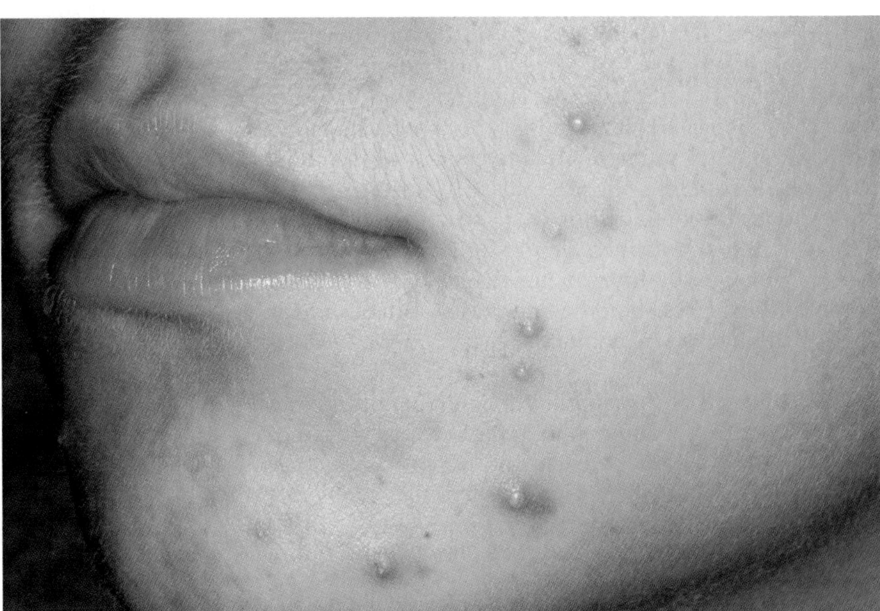

Figure 7-10 Mild acne with papules, pustules, and comedones.

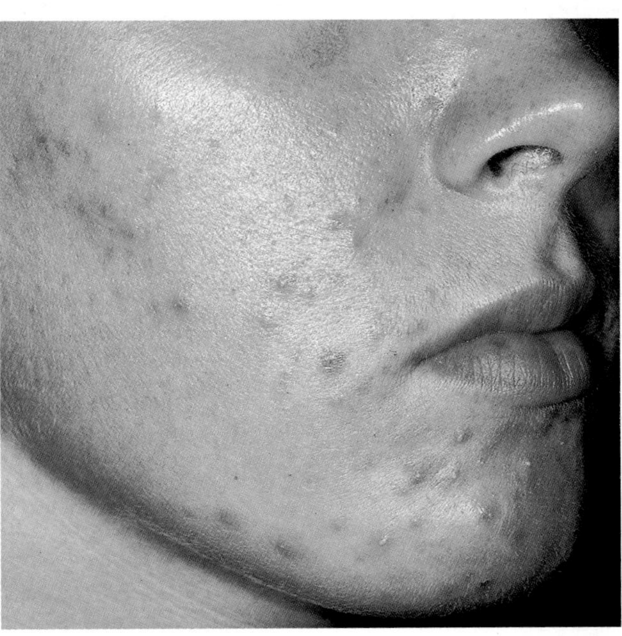

Figure 7-11 Papular and pustular acne (mild). Several papules are localized on the cheeks.

MODERATE-TO-SEVERE INFLAMMATORY ACNE

CLINICAL PRESENTATION. Patients who have moderate-to-severe acne (more than 20 pustules) are temporarily disfigured (Figures 7-12 through 7-16).

Their disease may have been gradually worsening or may be virulent at the onset. The explosive onset of pustules can sometimes be precipitated by stress. There may be few to negligible visible comedones. Affected areas should not be irritated during the initial stages of therapy.

TREATMENT. Many dermatologists will begin with a topical retinoid and combine it with a topical antibiotic. Others will treat with twice-daily application of a topical antibiotic, benzoyl peroxide, or combination medicine (e.g., BenzaClin, Duac) or the combination of benzoyl peroxide and sulfacetamide/sulfur. This drying agent program can be very effective. Patients using drying agents should adjust the frequency of application to induce a mild, continuous peel. Response to treatment may occur in 2 to 4 weeks. Oral antibiotics (tetracycline or doxycycline) are used for patients with more than 10 pustules. Treatment should be continued until no new lesions develop (2 to 4 months) and then should be slowly tapered. If there are any signs of irritation, the frequency and strength of topical medicines should be decreased. Irritation, particularly around the mandibular areas and neck, worsens pustular acne.

A retinoid can be introduced if the number of pustules and the degree of inflammation have decreased. Start minocycline at full dosage if there is no response to tetracycline or doxycycline after 3 months. Pustules are gently incised and expressed. Injecting each pustule with a very small amount of triamcinolone acetonide (Kenalog 2.5 to 5.0 mg/ml) can give immediate and very gratifying results.

Those who have responded well may begin to taper and eventually discontinue oral antibiotics.

Some patients respond very well to lower dosages of oral antibiotics and require tetracycline 250 mg/day or even every other day for control. Those patients may be safely maintained on low-dose oral antibiotics for extended periods. Patients who do not respond to conventional therapy may have lesions that are colonized by gram-negative organisms. Cultures of pustules and cysts are obtained and an appropriate antibiotic such as ampicillin is started. The response may be dramatic.

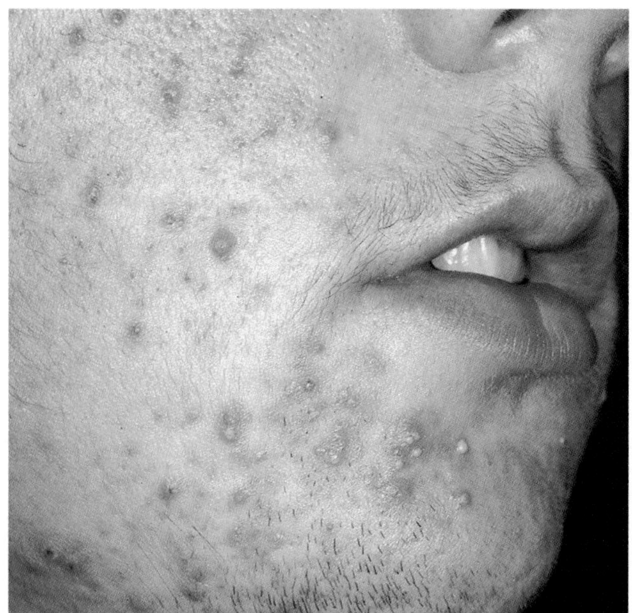

Figure 7-12 Papular and pustular acne (moderate). Many pustules are present, and several have become confluent on the chin area.

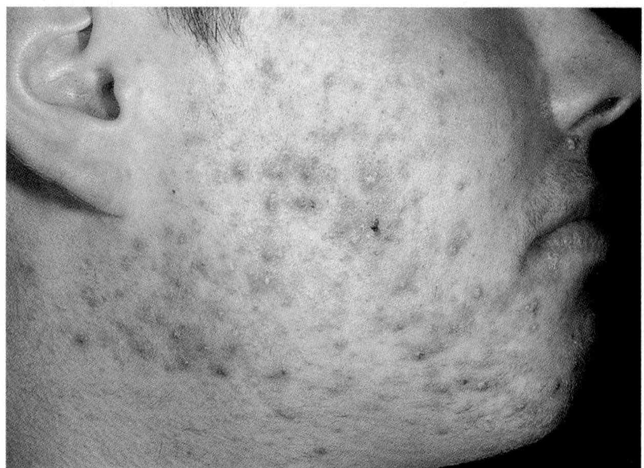

Figure 7-13 Papules, nodules, and cysts cover the entire face. Scarring is extensive.

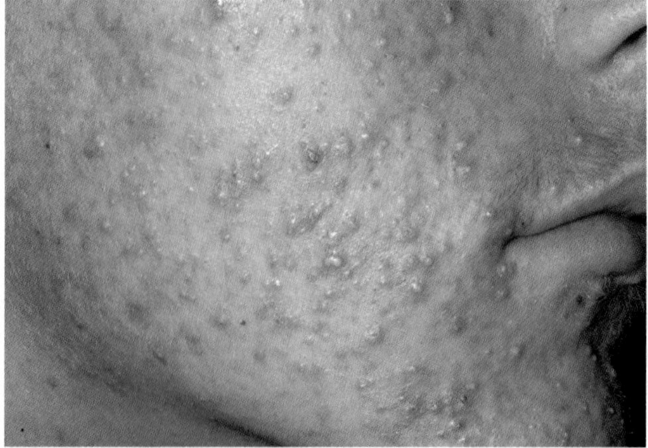

Figure 7-14 All forms of conventional therapy failed to control these numerous pustules. Isotretinoin cleared the acne.

MODERATE-TO-SEVERE INFLAMMATORY ACNE

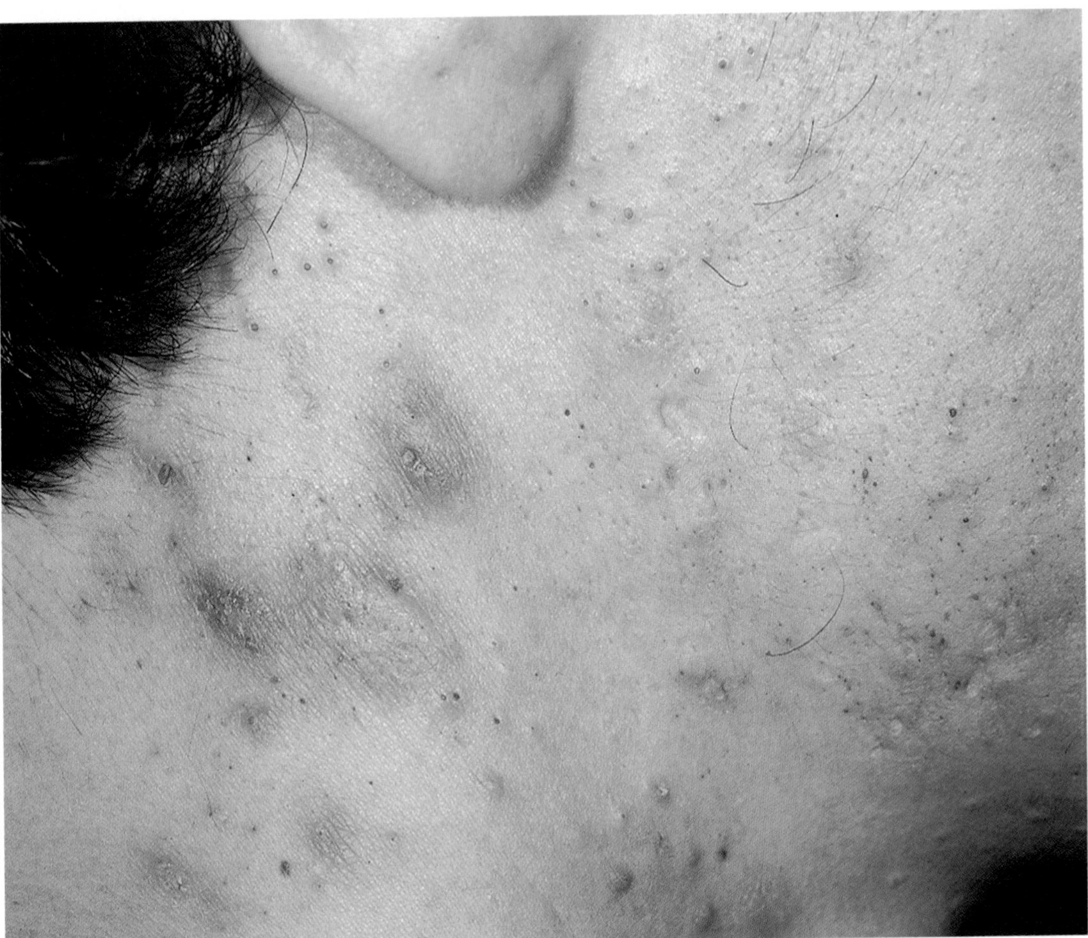

Figure 7-15 Localized nodular and cystic acne. Cystic and nodular lesions appeared in this patient, who has chronic comedo and pustular acne.

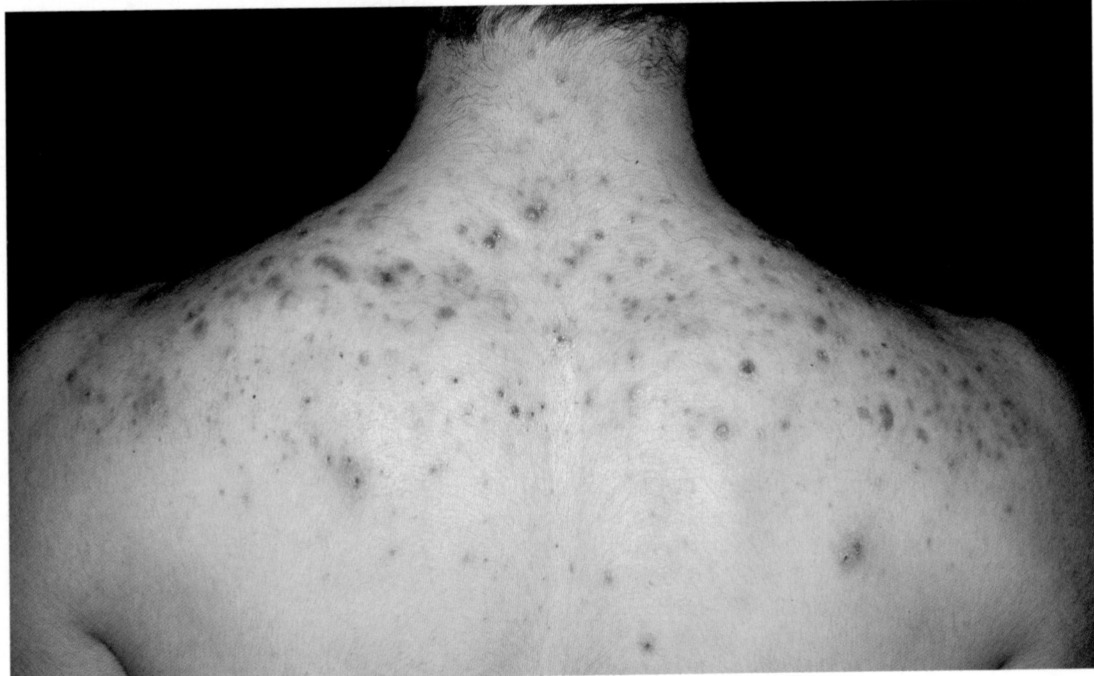

Figure 7-16 Severe inflammatory acne with papules, cysts, and scarring.

SEVERE: NODULOCYSTIC ACNE

CLINICAL PRESENTATION. Nodulocystic acne includes localized cystic acne (few cysts on face, chest, or back), diffuse cystic acne (wide areas of face, chest, and back) (Figures 7-18 through 7-27), pyoderma faciale (inflamed cysts localized on the face in females) (Figure 7-17), and acne conglobata (highly inflammatory, with cysts that communicate under the skin, abscesses, and burrowing sinus tracts) (Figures 7-28 and 7-29).

CYSTIC ACNE

Cystic acne is a serious and sometimes devastating disease that requires aggressive treatment. The face, chest, back, and upper arms may be permanently mutilated by numerous atrophic or hypertrophic scars. Patients sometimes delay seeking help, hoping that improvement will occur spontaneously; consequently, the disease may be quite advanced when first viewed by the physician.

Patients are often embarrassed by and preoccupied with their disease. They may experience anxiety, depression, insecurity, psychic suffering, and social isolation. The physical appearance may be so unattractive that teenagers refuse to attend school and adults fear going to work. Patients report difficulty securing employment when afflicted and problems being accepted in the working environment. Patients with a few inflamed cysts can be treated with a program similar to that outlined for moderate-to-severe inflammatory acne. Oral antibiotics, conventional topical therapy, and periodic intralesional Kenalog injections may keep this problem under adequate control.

Extensive cystic acne requires a different approach. There are three less common variants of cystic acne—pyoderma faciale, acne fulminans, acne conglobata.

PYODERMA FACIALE. Pyoderma faciale is a distinctive variant of cystic acne that remains confined to the face (see Figure 7-17). It is a disease of adult women ranging in age from the teens to the forties. They experience the rapid onset of large, sore, erythematous-to-purple cysts, predominantly on the central portion of the cheeks. Erythema may be intense. Purulent drainage from cysts occurs spontaneously or with minor trauma. Comedones are absent and scarring occurs in most cases. A traumatic emotional experience has been associated with some cases. Many patients do not have a history of acne.

Cultures help to differentiate this condition from gram-negative acne. Highly inflamed lesions can be managed by starting isotretinoin and oral corticosteroids. A study reported effective management with the following: Treatment was begun with prednisolone (1.0 mg/kg daily for 1 to 2 weeks). Isotretinoin was then added (0.2 to 0.5 mg/kg/day [rarely, 1.0 mg/kg in resistant cases]), with a slow tapering of the corticosteroid over the following 2 to 3 weeks. Isotretinoin was continued until all inflammatory lesions resolved. This required 3 to 4 months. None of the patients had a recurrence. This group of patients were "flusher and blushers," and it was suggested that pyoderma faciale is a type of rosacea. The investigators proposed the term rosacea fulminans.

ACNE FULMINANS

Acne fulminans is a rare ulcerative form of acne of unknown etiology with an acute onset and systemic symptoms. It most commonly affects adolescent white boys. A genetic predisposition is suspected. An ulcerative, necrotic acne with systemic symptoms develops rapidly. There are arthralgias or severe muscle pain, or both, that accompany the acne flare. Painful bone lesions occur in approximately 40% of patients. Weight loss, fever, leukocytosis, and elevated erythrocyte sedimentation rate (ESR) are common findings.

Antibiotic therapy is not effective. Oral corticosteroids (e.g., prednisolone 0.5 to 1.0 mg/kg) are the primary therapy. They quickly control the skin lesions and systemic symptoms. Isotretinoin (0.5 mg/kg) is started simultaneously and, as in the therapy of severe cystic acne, is continued for 5 months. Start with a low dosage of isotretinoin. High dosages may precipitate inflamed lesions with granulation tissue. The duration of steroid therapy is often at least 2 months. The bone lesions have a good prognosis; chronic sequelae are rare.

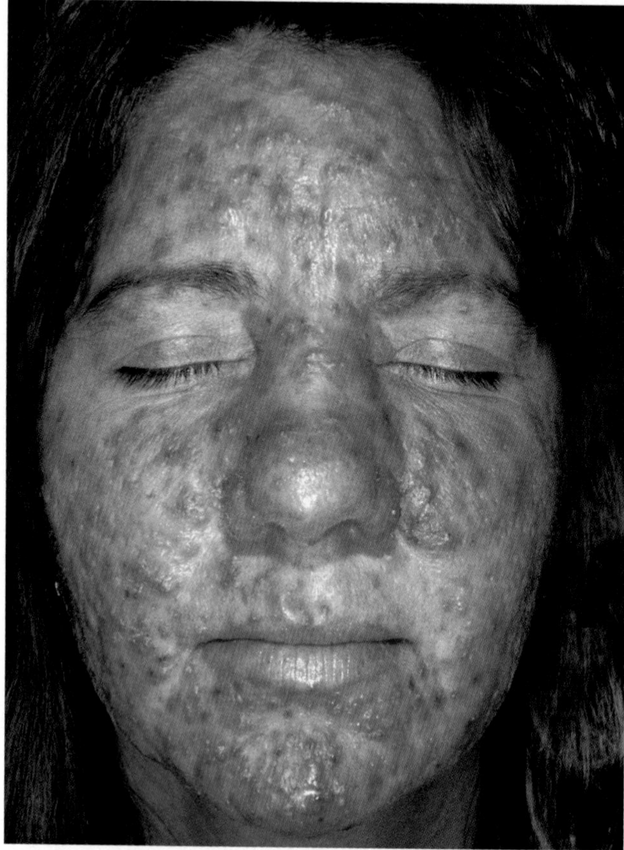

Figure 7-17 Pyoderma faciale (rosacea fulminans). Rapid onset of numerous lesions cleared after treatment with prednisone and isotretinoin.

NODULOCYSTIC ACNE

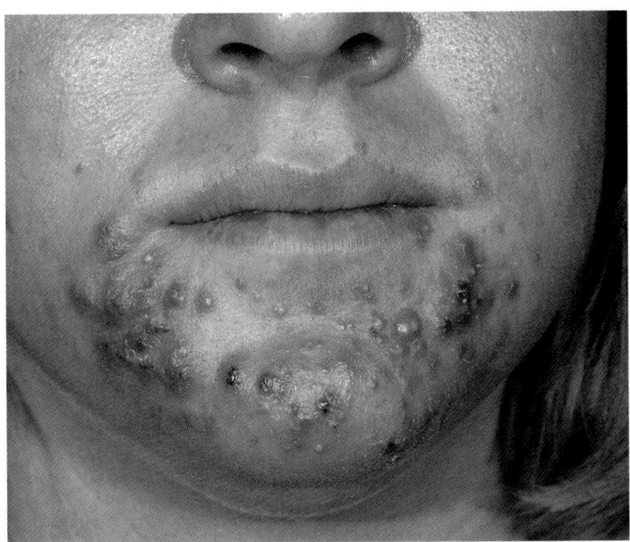

Figure 7-18 Numerous cystic acne lesions became confluent. The eruption was confined the chin.

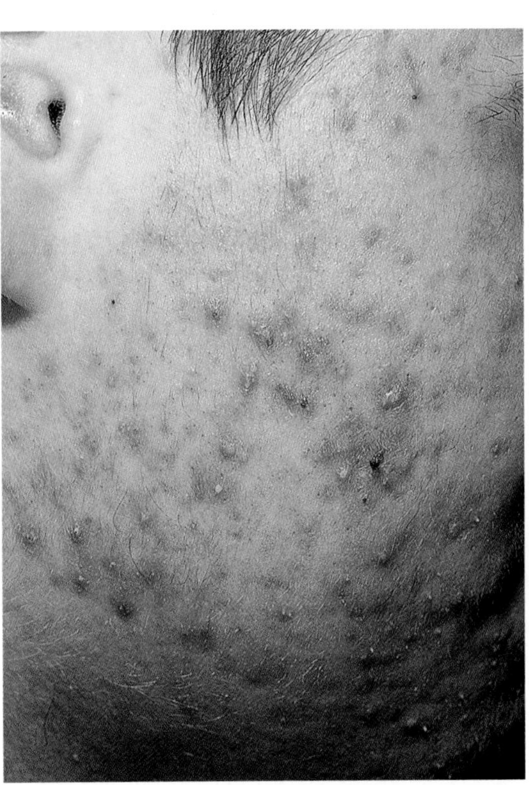

Figure 7-19 Nodular and cystic acne (severe).

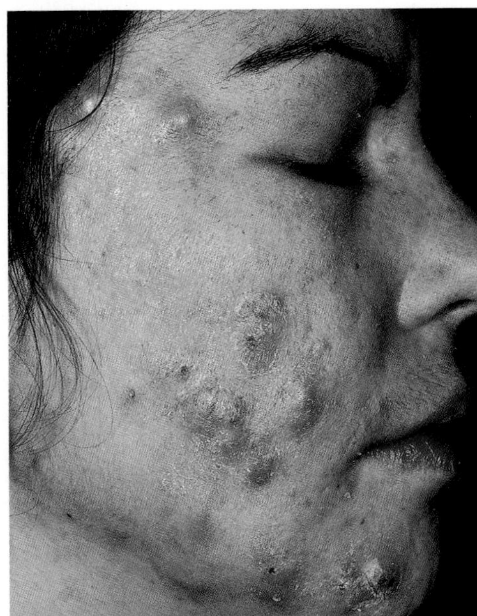

Figure 7-20 Cystic acne. The lesions in this patient are primarily cystic. Only a few pustules and comedones are present.

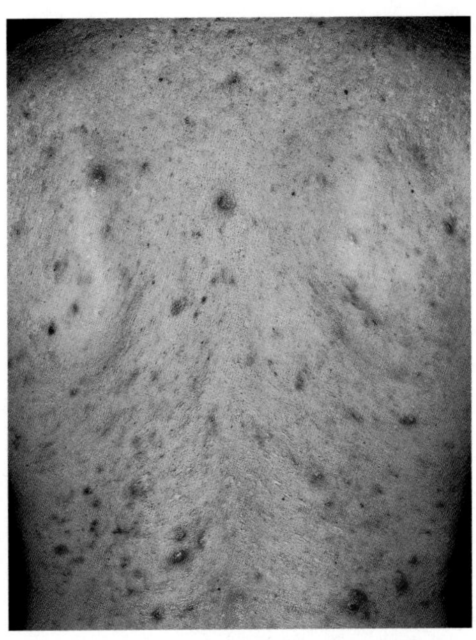

Figure 7-21 Nodular and cystic acne. Years of activity have left numerous scars over the entire back. Several active cysts are present.

NODULOCYSTIC ACNE

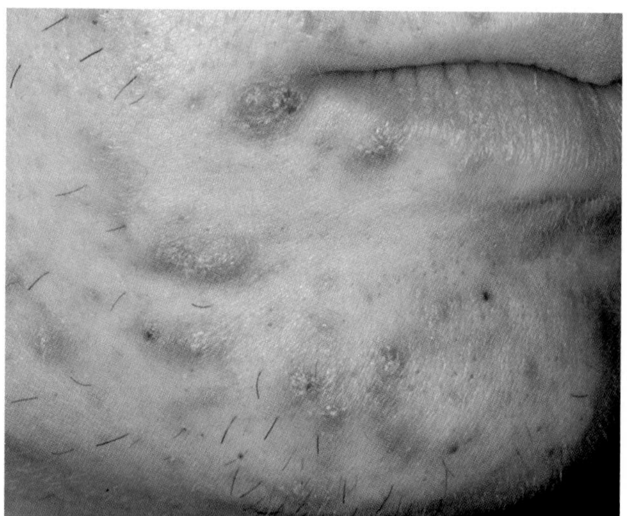

Figure 7-22 Cysts are the only lesions present.

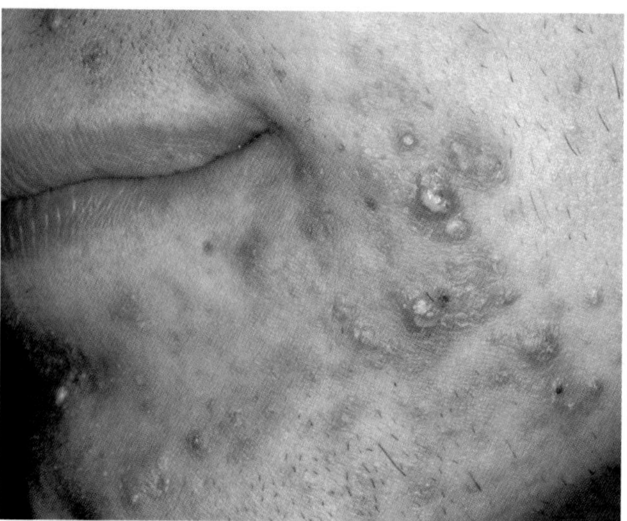

Figure 7-23 Cysts and pustules are present.

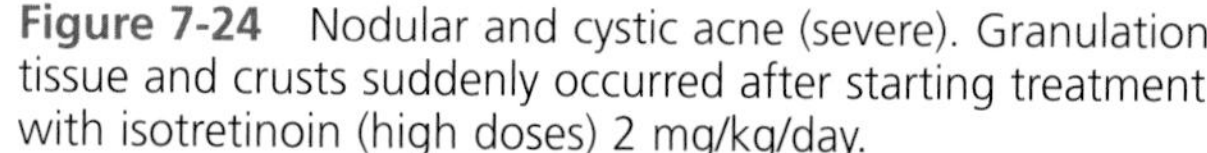

Figure 7-24 Nodular and cystic acne (severe). Granulation tissue and crusts suddenly occurred after starting treatment with isotretinoin (high doses) 2 mg/kg/day.

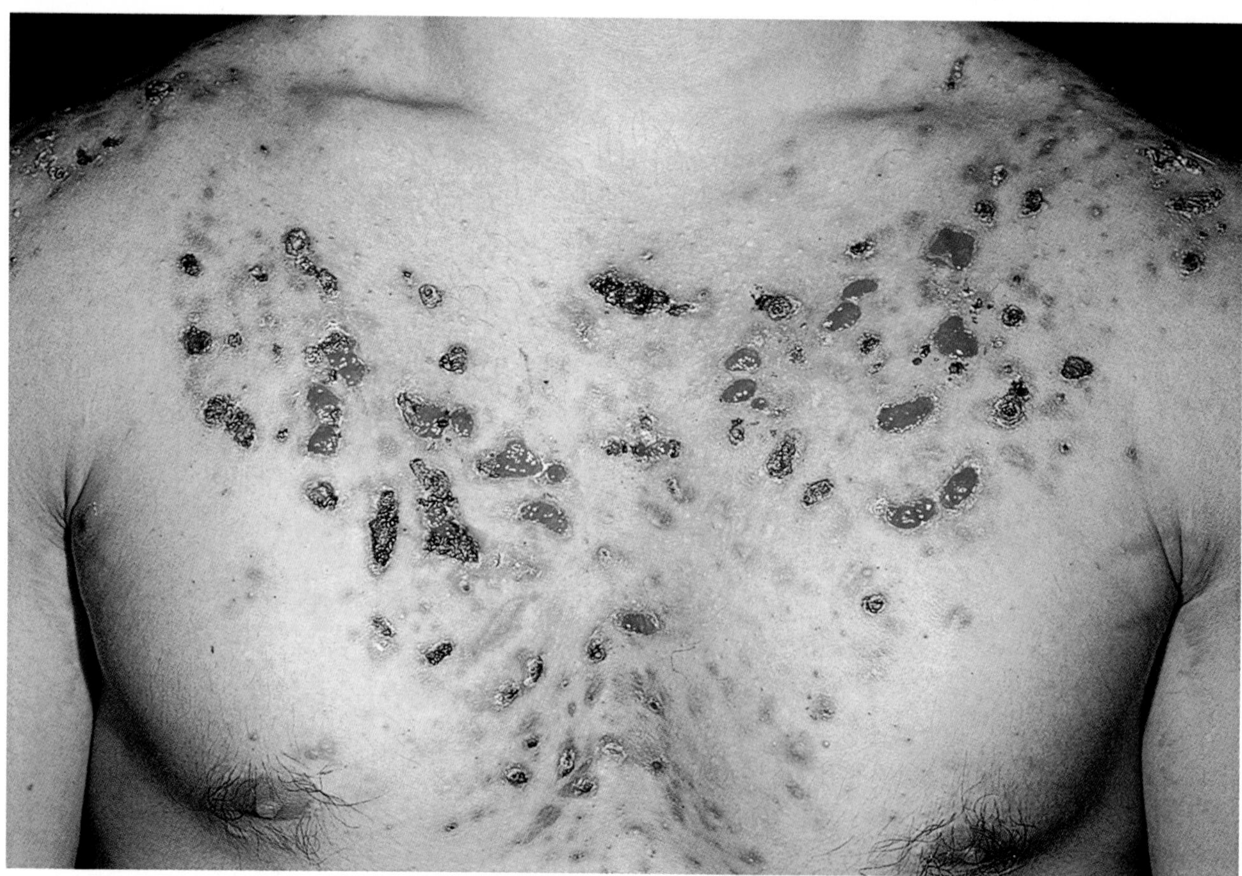

NODULOCYSTIC ACNE

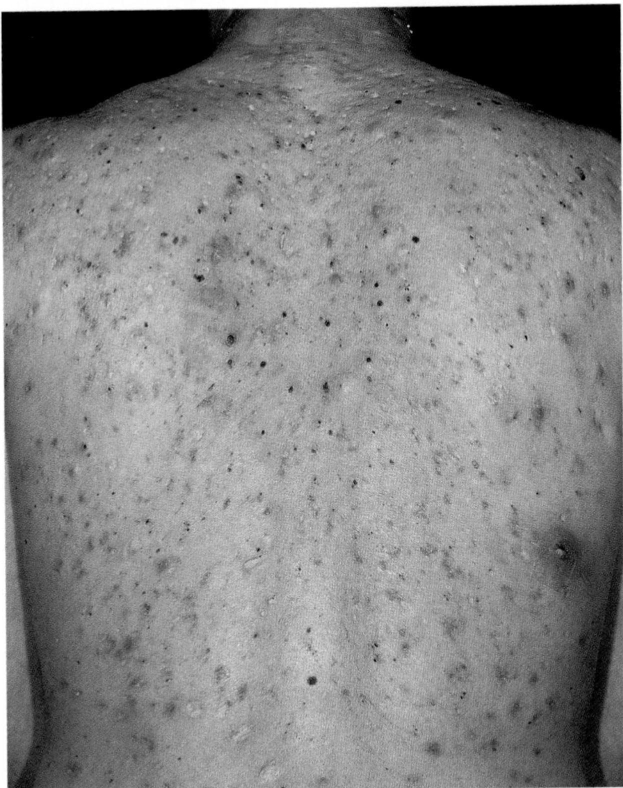

Figure 7-25 Follicular occlusion triad syndrome. Acne conglobata is part of the rare follicular occlusion triad syndrome of acne conglobata, hidradenitis suppurativa, and dissecting cellulitis of the scalp. Note the huge blackheads.

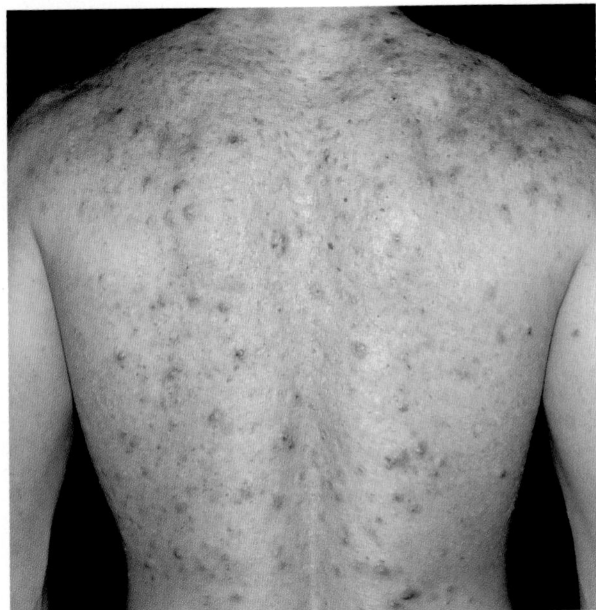

Figure 7-26 Cysts may be localized to the upper back or extend to the waist.

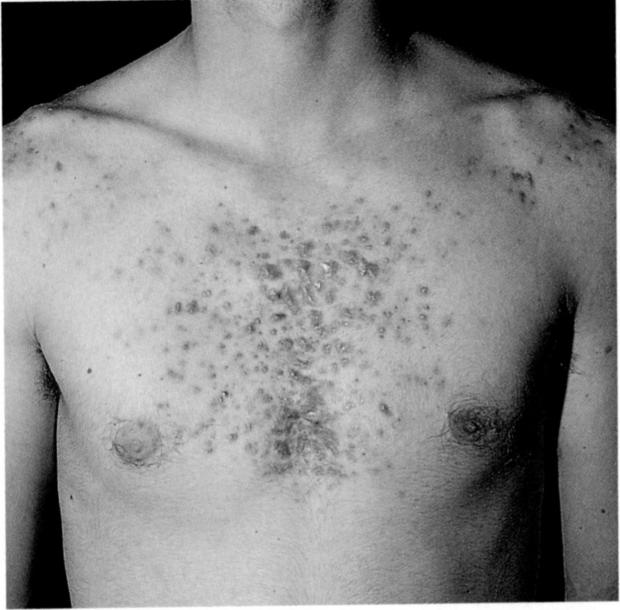

Figure 7-27 Nodular and cystic acne (severe), six months after stopping isotretinoin. There are numerous atrophic and hypertrophic scars with postinflammatory pigmentation.

ACNE CONGLOBATA

Acne conglobata is a chronic, highly inflammatory form of cystic acne in which involved areas contain a mixture of double comedones (two blackheads that communicate under the skin), papules, pustules, communicating cysts, abscesses, and draining sinus tracts (see Figures 7-28 and 7-29). The disease may linger for years, ending with deep atrophic or keloidal scarring. Acne conglobata is part of the rare follicular occlusion triad syndrome of acne conglobata, hidradenitis suppurativa, and dissecting cellulitis of the scalp (see Figure 7-25). Musculoskeletal symptoms have been reported in some of these patients; 85% were black. There is no fever or weight loss as is seen in acne fulminans.

TREATMENT OF NODULOCYSTIC ACNE

The patient is assured that effective treatment is available. Patients should be told that they will be observed closely and, if the disease becomes very active, they will be seen at least weekly until the condition is adequately controlled. A primary therapeutic goal is to avoid scarring by terminating the intense inflammation quickly; prednisone is sometimes required. Cysts with thin roofs are incised and drained. Deeper cysts are injected with triamcinolone acetonide (Kenalog 2.5 to 10 mg/ml).

Patients who show little tendency to scar can be treated as patients with moderate-to-severe inflammatory acne. Most patients will require the rapid introduction of isotretinoin. Start with low dosages of isotretinoin (0.5 mg/kg or lower) to avoid exacerbation of lesions that may have granulation tissue. The simultaneous use of tetracyclines (tetracycline, doxycycline, or minocycline) and isotretinoin is avoided, because a higher incidence of pseudotumor cerebri may occur with this combination. For highly active cases, prednisone (adult dosage is 20 to 30 mg two times a day) is used.

Intralesional triamcinolone acetonide injections and incision and drainage of cysts are important in the early weeks of management. Patients taking isotretinoin are usually not treated with other oral or topical agents.

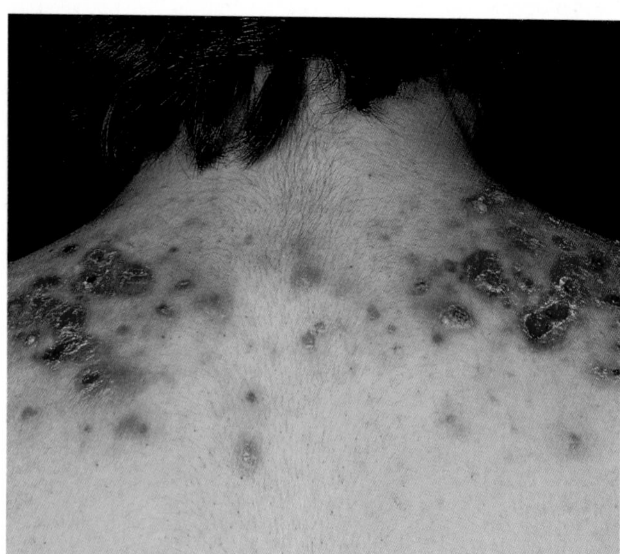

Figure 7-28 Acne conglobata. Abscesses and ulcerated cysts are found over most of the upper shoulder area.

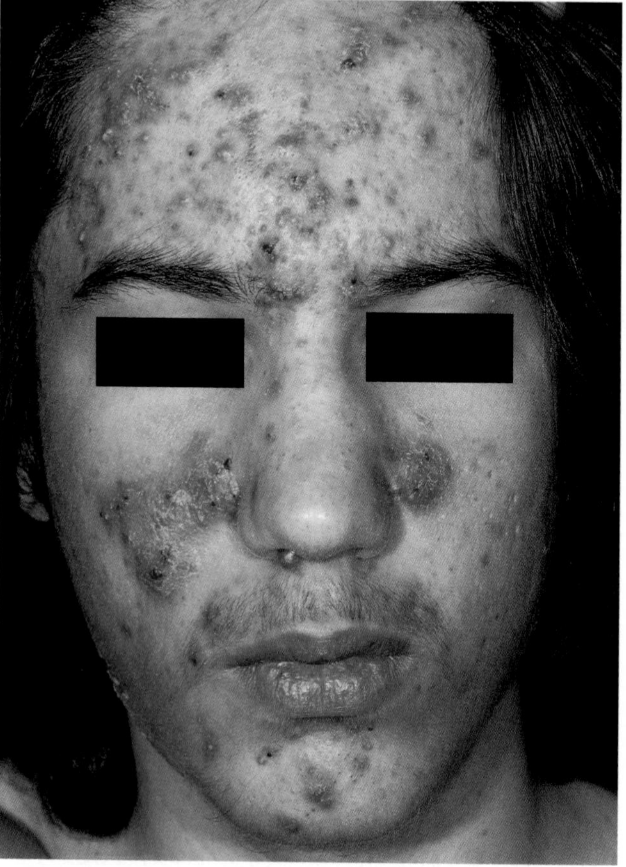

Figure 7-29 Acne conglobata. Large communicating cysts are present on the cheeks; scarring is extensive.

Therapeutic agents for treatment of acne

There are four pathogenetic factors responsible for the development of acne. These are hyperkeratinization (plugging) of the pilosebaceous follicles, increased testosterone levels (producing hyperseborrhea), bacterial colonization with *P. acnes,* and inflammation. Topical agents influence at least one of these factors. More than 50% of patients present with comedones and papulopustular acne. These patients are initially treated with topical treatment. Combination regimens that include an antibiotic and a retinoid to reduce follicular plugging are the mainstay of topical treatment. Pustular acne may respond quickly to drying therapy with a combination of benzoyl peroxide and sulfacetamide and sulfur lotion. Systemic therapy with antibiotics or isotretinoin is used when scarring occurs or for cystic acne.

Topical and oral agents act at various stages (see Figure 7-5) in the evolution of an acne lesion and may be used alone or in combination to enhance efficacy. Topical agents should be applied to the entire affected area to treat existing lesions and to prevent the development of new ones. Potent topical steroid creams produce no short-term improvement in patients with moderate acne.

RETINOIDS

Retinoids reverse the abnormal pattern of keratinization seen in acne vulgaris. Agents that act in a comedolytic and anticomedogenic manner to reduce follicular plugging are the retinoids tretinoin, adapalene and tazarotene, azelaic acid, and isotretinoin. Azelaic acid has strong antibacterial potency without inducing bacterial resistance, similar to benzoyl peroxide. Adapalene has antiinflammatory activity. Retinoids may cause an increase in facial dryness and erythema.

Mechanism of action. Retinoids initiate increased cell turnover in both normal follicles and comedones and reduce the cohesion between keratinized cells. They act specifically on microcomedones (the precursor lesion of all forms of acne), causing fragmentation and expulsion of the microplug, expulsion of comedones, and conversion of closed comedones to open comedones. New comedone formation is prevented by continued use. Inflammation may occur during this process, temporarily making acne worse. Continual topical application leads to thinning of the stratum corneum, making the skin more susceptible to sunburn, sun damage, and irritation from wind, cold, or dryness. Irritants such as astringents, alcohol, and acne soaps will not be tolerated as they were previously. The incidence of contact allergy is very low. Because of the direct action of retinoids on the microcomedone, many clinicians believe retinoids are appropriate for all forms of acne.

Combination therapy—synergism. Retinoids enhance the penetration of other topical agents such as topical antibiotics and benzoyl peroxide. The enhanced penetration results in a synergistic effect with greater overall drug efficacy and a faster response to treatment.

Application techniques. The skin should be washed gently with a mild soap (e.g., Purpose, Basis) no more than two to three times each day, using the hands rather than a washcloth. Special acne or abrasive soaps should be avoided. To minimize possible irritation, the skin should be allowed to dry completely by waiting 20 to 30 minutes before applying retinoids. The retinoid is applied in a thin layer once daily. Medication is applied to the entire area, not just to individual lesions. A pea-sized amount is enough for a full facial application. Patients with sensitive skin or those living in cold, dry climates may start with an application every other or every third day. The frequency of application can be gradually increased to as often as twice each day if tolerated. The corners of the nose, the mouth, and the eyes should be avoided; these areas are the most sensitive and the most easily irritated. Retinoids are applied to the chin less frequently during the initial stages of therapy; the chin is sensitive and is usually the first area to become red and scaly. Sunscreens should be worn during the summer months if exposure is anticipated.

Response to treatment

One to 4 weeks: During the first few weeks, patients may experience redness, burning, or peeling. Those with excessive irritation should use less frequent applications (i.e., every other or every third day). Most patients adapt to treatment within 4 weeks and return to daily applications. Those tolerating daily applications may be advanced to a higher dosage or to the more potent solution.

Three to 6 weeks: New papules and pustules may appear because comedones become irritated during the process of being dislodged. Patients unaware of this phenomenon may discontinue treatment. Some patients never get worse and sometimes begin to improve dramatically by the fifth or sixth week.

After 6 weeks: Most patients improve by the ninth to twelfth week and exhibit continuous improvement thereafter. Some patients never adapt to retinoids and experience continuous irritation or continue to worsen. An alternate treatment should be selected if adaptation has not occurred by 6 to 8 weeks. Some patients adapt but never improve. Retinoids may be continued for months to prevent appearance of new lesions.

TRETINOIN. Tretinoin (Retin-A) is effective for noninflammatory acne consisting of open and closed comedones. It is available in various preparations: Retin-A gel (0.025% and 0.01%) and Retin-A Micro gel (0.04% and 0.1%) and Retin-A cream (0.1%, 0.05%, and 0.025%).

TAZAROTENE. Tazarotene (Tazorac) is a newer retinoid. It is available as a gel (0.05%, 0.1%) and cream (0.05%, 0.1%). Tazarotene 0.1% gel (once daily) is more effective than tretinoin 0.025% gel (once-daily) in reducing the numbers of papules and open comedones, and achieves a more rapid reduction in pustules in mild-to-moderate facial acne. Alternate-day tazarotene 0.1% gel is as effective as once-daily adapalene 0.1% gel. The tolerability of tazarotene gel is comparable to that of tretinoin 0.025% gel, tretinoin 0.1% gel microsphere (Retin-A Micro), and adapalene 0.3% gel. Tolerability of tazarotene is better when initiating therapy with an alternate-day regimen.

A short contact method may be effective. Apply the gel for just a few minutes; then wash it off.

ADAPALENE. Adapalene (Differin) is available as a gel or cream. It has tretinoin-like activity in the terminal differentiation process of the hair follicle. Adapalene has antiinflammatory activity. Adapalene gel 0.1% is as effective as 0.025% tretinoin gel for mild-to-moderate acne. It is better tolerated than tretinoin gel. It does not cause sun sensitivity. Differin gel 0.3% is now available

AZELAIC ACID. Azelaic acid cream (Azelex) is a naturally occurring compound that has antikeratinizing, antibacterial, and antiinflammatory properties. It is effective for noninflammatory and inflammatory acne. It is an effective monotherapy in mild-to-moderate forms of acne, with an overall efficacy comparable to that of tretinoin (0.05%), benzoyl peroxide (5%), and topical erythromycin (2%). Its efficacy can be enhanced when it is used in combination with other topical medications such as benzoyl peroxide 4% gel, clindamycin 1% gel, tretinoin 0.025% cream, and erythromycin 3%/benzoyl peroxide 5% gel. Azelaic acid cream may be combined with oral antibiotics for the treatment of moderate-to-severe acne and may be used for maintenance therapy when antibiotics are stopped. It does not cause sun sensitivity or significant local irritation. It does not induce resistance in *P. acnes*.

BENZOYL PEROXIDE

The primary effect of benzoyl peroxide is antibacterial; therefore it is most effective for inflammatory acne consisting of papules, pustules, and cysts, although many patients with comedone acne respond to it. Benzoyl peroxide is less effective than vitamin A acid at disrupting the microcomedo. Benzoyl peroxide and isotretinoin significantly reduce noninflamed lesions in 4 weeks. In one study, benzoyl peroxide had a more rapid effect on inflamed lesions with significant reductions at 4 weeks, whereas the use of isotretinoin showed a significant improvement at 12 weeks.

Benzoyl peroxide is available over-the-counter and by prescription. Some examples of benzoyl peroxide preparations are water-based gel (Benzac AC 2.5%, 5%, and 10%), alcohol-based gel (Benzagel 5% and 10%), and acetone-based gel (Persa-Gel 5% and 10%) (see the Formulary). Water-based gels are less irritating, but alcohol-based gels, if tolerated, might be more effective. Benzoyl peroxide is also available in a soap base in strengths from 2.5% to 10%.

BENZOYL PEROXIDE/ANTIBIOTIC FORMULATIONS. The combinations of erythromycin/benzoyl peroxide (Benzamycin) and clindamycin/benzoyl peroxide (BenzaClin, Duac) are superior for inflammatory and noninflammatory acne versus either ingredient used alone. The clindamycin/benzoyl peroxide combination gel has an advantage over erythromycin/benzoyl peroxide gel because the former does not require refrigeration. The two products have similar efficacy.

Benzoyl peroxide produces a drying effect that varies from mild desquamation to scaliness, peeling, and cracking. Patients should be reassured that drying does not cause wrinkles. Benzoyl peroxide causes a significant reduction in the concentration of free fatty acids via its antibacterial effect on *P. acnes*. This activity is presumably caused by the release of free radical oxygen, which is capable of oxidizing bacterial proteins. Benzoyl peroxide seems to reduce the size of the sebaceous gland, but whether sebum secretion is suppressed is still unknown. Patients should be warned that benzoyl peroxide is a bleaching agent that can ruin clothing.

PRINCIPLES OF TREATMENT. Benzoyl peroxide should be applied in a thin layer to the entire affected area. Most patients experience mild erythema and scaling during the first few days of treatment, even with the lowest concentrations, but adapt in a week or two. It was previously believed that vigorous peeling was necessary for maximum therapeutic effect; although many patients improved with this technique, others became worse. An adequate therapeutic result can be obtained by starting with daily applications of the 2.5% or 5% gel and gradually increasing or decreasing the frequency of applications and strength until mild dryness and peeling occur.

ALLERGIC REACTION. Approximately 2% of patients develop allergic contact dermatitis from benzoyl peroxide and must discontinue its use. The sudden appearance of diffuse erythema and vesiculation suggests contact allergy to benzoyl peroxide.

DRYING AND PEELING AGENTS

The oldest technique for treating acne is to use agents that induce a continuous mild drying and peeling of the skin. In selected patients, especially those with pustular acne, this technique may provide fast and effective results. Prescription and over-the-counter products used for this purpose contain sulfur, salicylic acid, resorcinol, and benzoyl peroxide. Before the use of tretinoin and antibiotics, this approach secured very acceptable results for many patients.

The goal is to establish a mild continuous peel by varying the frequency of application and strength of the agent. Treatment is stopped temporarily if dryness becomes severe. The drying and peeling technique can be recommended to patients who are reluctant to visit the physician or to parents inquiring about children who are beginning to develop acne. If improvement is negligible after an 8-week trial, the patient should consider evaluation by a physician. Two effective agents are benzoyl peroxide and sulfacetamide 10%, sulfur 5% lotion (Sulfacet-R). One is used in the morning and the other in the evening or as often as tolerated.

TOPICAL ANTIBIOTICS

Topical antibiotics are useful for mild pustular and comedone acne. They can be prescribed initially or as adjunctive therapy after the patient has adapted to tretinoin or benzoyl peroxide. Clinical trials have demonstrated that application twice a day is as effective as oral tetracycline 250 mg taken twice daily or minocycline 50 mg taken twice daily. Most solutions are alcohol-based and may produce some degree of irritation. Cleocin T lotion does not contain propylene glycol and for some patients may be less irritating. Clindamycin (Cleocin T pads, solution, and lotion) is a commonly used topical antibiotic. Dapsone gel 5% (Aczone) has antibiotic and anti-inflammatory properties.

ORAL ANTIBIOTICS

Antibiotics have been used for approximately 4 decades for the treatment of papular, pustular, and cystic acne (see Table 7-1).

MECHANISM OF ACTION AND DOSAGE. The major effect of antibiotics is believed to ensue from their ability to decrease follicular populations of *P. acnes*. The role of *P. acnes* in the pathogenesis of acne is not completely understood. Neutrophil chemotactic factors are secreted during bacterial growth, and these may play an important role in initiating the inflammatory process. Because several antibiotics used to treat acne can inhibit neutrophil chemotaxis in vitro, they are thought to act as an antiinflammatory agent. Subminimal inhibitory concentrations of minocycline were shown to have an antiinflammatory effect by inhibiting the production of neutrophil chemotactic factors in comedonal bacteria. Antibiotic-resistant strains of *P. acnes* have been discovered.

ANTIBIOTIC-RESISTANT PROPIONIBACTERIA AND LONG-TERM THERAPY. *P. acnes* is sensitive to several antibiotics but the prevalence of *P. acnes* resistant to antibiotics is increasing. Resistance genes are easily transferred among different bacteria. After treatment with both systemic and oral antibiotics, *P. acnes* develops resistance in more than 50% of cases, and it is estimated that one in four acne patients harbors strains resistant to tetracycline, erythromycin, and clindamycin. Resistance to minocycline is rare. Carriage of resistant strains results in therapeutic failure of some but not all antibiotic regimens. In many patients with acne, continued treatment with antibiotics can be inappropriate or ineffective. It is important to recognize therapeutic failure and alter treatment accordingly. The use of long-term rotational antibiotics is outdated and will only exacerbate antibiotic resistance.

LONG-TERM TREATMENT. Patients may express concern about long-term use of oral antibiotics but experience has shown that this is a safe practice. Routine laboratory monitoring of patients who receive long-term oral antibiotics for acne rarely detects an adverse drug reaction and does not justify the cost of such testing. Laboratory monitoring should be limited to patients who may be at higher risk for an adverse drug reaction.

DOSAGE AND DURATION. Better clinical results and a lower rate of relapse after stopping antibiotics are achieved by starting at higher dosages and tapering only after control is achieved. Typical starting dosages are tetracycline 500 mg twice daily, doxycycline 100 mg once daily or twice daily, minocycline 100 mg twice daily, and amoxicillin 500 mg twice daily. Antibiotics are prescribed in divided doses; there is better compliance with twice-a-day dosing. Antibiotics must be taken for weeks to be effective and are used for many weeks or months to achieve maximum benefit. Attempts to control acne with short courses of antibiotics, as is often tried to prevent premenstrual flare-ups of acne, are usually not effective.

TETRACYCLINE. Tetracycline is widely prescribed for acne. One major disadvantage is the requirement that tetracycline not be taken with food (particularly dairy products), certain antacids, and iron, all of which interfere with the intestinal absorption of the drug. Failure to adhere to these restrictions accounts for many of the reported therapeutic failures of tetracycline.

Dosing. Efficacy and compliance are obtained by starting tetracycline administration at 500 mg twice each day and continuing this dosage until a significant decrease in the number of inflamed lesions occurs, usually in 3 to 6 weeks. Thereafter the dosage may be decreased to 250 mg twice each day, or oral therapy may be discontinued in favor of topical antibiotics. Patients who do not respond after 6 weeks of adequate dosages of oral tetracycline should be introduced to an alternative treatment. For unknown reasons a significant number of patients who take tetracycline exactly as directed do not respond to high dosages, whereas others respond very favorably to 250 mg once a day or once every other day and experience flare-ups when attempts are made to discontinue treatment.

Adverse effects. The incidence of photosensitivity to tetracycline is low, but it increases when higher dosages are used. All females should be warned about the increased incidence of *Candida albicans* vaginitis. The package labeling of oral contraceptives warns that reduced efficacy and increased incidence of breakthrough bleeding may occur with tetracycline and other antibiotics. Although this association has not been proven, it is prudent to inform patients of this potential risk. Pseudotumor cerebri, a self-limited disorder in which the regulation of intracranial pressure is impaired, is a rare complication of tetracycline treatment. Increased intracranial pressure causes papilledema and severe headaches. Increased intraocular pressure can lead to progressive visual impairment and eventually blindness.

DOXYCYCLINE. Doxycycline is a safe and effective medication. It is commonly prescribed for acne. Studies of doxycycline (50 and 100 mg) showed no significant difference between its clinical efficacy and that of minocycline in treating acne. Doxycycline is less expensive than minocycline. The incidence of photosensitivity is low but increases with increasing dose levels (Figure 7-30).

Dosing. Start at 100 mg once daily or twice daily and decrease the dosage once control is obtained. Doxycycline can be taken with food.

MINOCYCLINE. Minocycline (50-mg and 100-mg capsules and scored tablets; 45-mg, 90-mg, and 135-mg extended-release tablets) is a tetracycline derivative that has proved valuable in cases of pustular acne that have not responded to conventional oral antibiotic therapy. Minocycline is expensive; generic forms are available. One study comparing minocycline (50 mg three times a day) with tetracycline (250 mg four times a day) revealed that minocycline resulted in significant improvement in patients who did not respond to tetracycline. Patients who responded to tetracycline had significantly advanced improvement when switched to minocycline. The inhibitory effect on gastrointestinal absorption with food and milk is significantly greater for tetracycline than for minocycline. Food causes a 13% inhibition of absorption with minocycline and a 46% inhibition with tetracycline, milk a 27% inhibition with minocycline and a 65% inhibition with tetracycline. The simpler regimen and early onset of clinical improvement are likely to result in better patient compliance. Therefore there is justification for the use of minocycline as first-line oral therapy.

Dosing. The usual initial dosage is 50 to 100 mg twice each day. The dosage is tapered when a significant decrease in the number of lesions is observed, usually in 3 to 6 weeks. Solodyn is an extended-release minocycline. It is a once-daily tablet prescribed on the basis of the patient's weight to achieve a dose of approximately 1 mg/kg. The 45-mg tablet is for patients in the 45 to 59 kg (99 to 131 lb) range. The 90-mg tablet is for patients weighing 60 to 90 kg (132 to 199 lb), and the 135-mg tablet is for patients weighing 91 to 136 kg (200 to 300 lb).

Adverse effects. Minocycline is highly lipid-soluble and readily penetrates the cerebrospinal fluid, causing dose-related ataxia, vertigo, nausea, and vomiting in some patients. In susceptible individuals, central nervous system (CNS) side effects occur with the first few doses of medication. If CNS adverse reactions persist after the dosage is decreased or after the capsules are taken with food, alternative therapy is indicated. Penetration of the blood-brain barrier may cause pseudotumor cerebri. Pseudotumor cerebri syndrome associated with minocycline therapy is reported in daily doses of 50 to 200 mg. The duration of treatment ranged from less than 1 week to 1 year. Symptoms were headache (75%), transient visual disturbances (41%), diplopia (41%), pulsatile tinnitus (17%), and nausea and vomiting (25%). Cases of drug hepatitis and lupus-like reactions have been reported. Warn patients to report any symptoms.

A blue-gray pigmentation of the skin, oral mucosa, nails, sclera, bone, and thyroid gland has been found in some patients, usually those taking high dosages of minocycline for extended periods (Figures 7-31 and 7-32). Skin

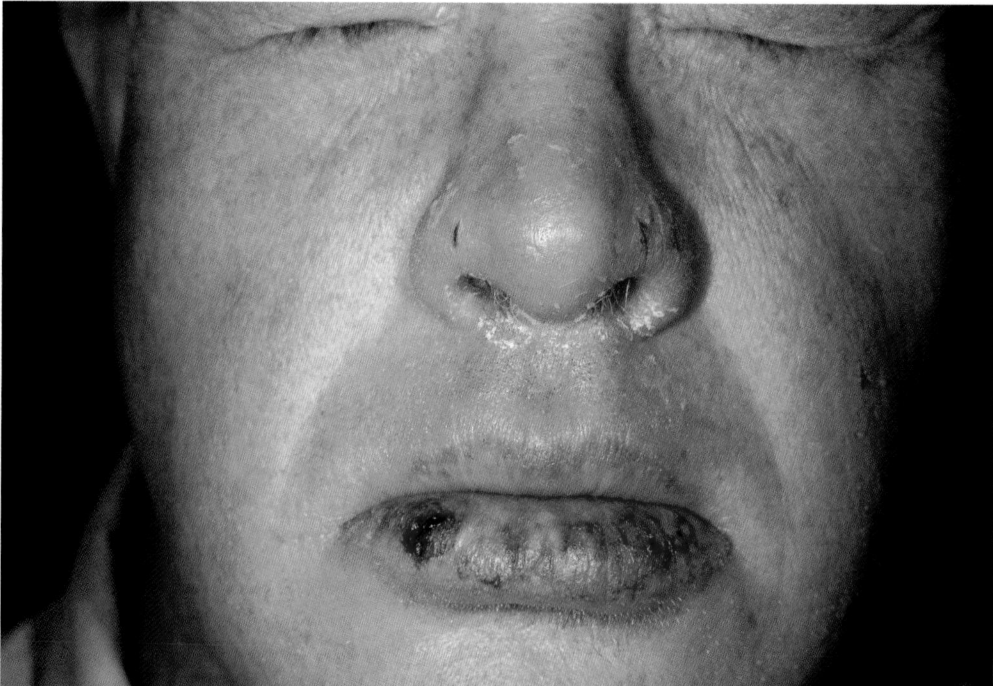

Figure 7-30 A severe sunburn reaction occurred with tingling and burning in this patient who continued to take doxycycline.

pigmentation has been reported in depressed acne scars, at sites of cutaneous inflammation, as macules resembling bruises on the lower legs, and as a generalized discoloration suggesting an off-color suntan. Pigmentation may persist for long periods after minocycline has been discontinued. The consequences of these deposits are unknown. Tooth staining (lasting for years) located on the incisal one half to three fourths of the crown has been reported in adults, usually after years of minocycline therapy. In contrast, tooth staining produced by tetracycline occurs on the gingival third of the teeth in children treated before age 7. Autoimmune hepatitis, serum sickness–like reactions, and drug-induced lupus have been reported in rare instances. p-ANCA may be a serological marker for developing autoimmune disease in patients receiving minocycline. *PMID: 17408394*

CLINDAMYCIN. Clindamycin (75-mg and 150-mg capsules) is a highly effective oral antibiotic for the control of acne. Its use has been curtailed in recent years because of its association with severe pseudomembranous colitis caused by *Clostridium difficile,* which fortunately responds in most cases to oral or intravenous antibiotics. Clindamycin is effective in dosages ranging from 75 to 300 mg twice daily.

AMPICILLIN OR AMOXICILLIN. Long-term use of oral antibiotics for treatment of acne may result in the appearance of cysts and pustules that yield gram-negative organisms when cultured. Ampicillin (250-mg and 500-mg capsules) is effective for this so-called gram-negative acne. Ampicillin is often effective for the treatment of conventional mild-to-moderate inflammatory acne and is a safe alternative for patients who do not respond to tetracycline. Ampicillin may be prescribed for acne during pregnancy or during lactation. A dosage of 500 mg twice each day is maintained until satisfactory control is achieved. The dosage is then decreased. Some patients experience a flare-up of activity at lower dosages and must resume taking 500 mg twice each day.

CEPHALOSPORINS. There are several anecdotal reports extolling the efficacy of cephalosporins. These drugs may be considered for antibiotic-resistant pustular acne.

TRIMETHOPRIM AND SULFAMETHOXAZOLE. Trimethoprim and sulfamethoxazole (Bactrim, Septra) or trimethoprim is useful for treating gram-negative acne and acne that is resistant to tetracycline. The adult dosage is 160 mg of trimethoprim combined with 800 mg of sulfamethoxazole once or twice daily.

TRIMETHOPRIM. Trimethoprim 300 mg twice daily may be considered if other antibiotics fail.

MACROLIDE ANTIBIOTICS. Erythromycin (e.g., E-Mycin 250 mg or 333 mg; Eryc 250 mg; E.E.S. 400 mg) is not first-line drug treatment as it was in the past. Erythromycin-resistant *P. acnes* is a significant problem. Some patients may still, however, respond to erythromycin or related drugs such as azithromycin (Zithromax). Azithromycin has a very long half-life and is given in a single 250-mg or 500-mg dose three times a week. Many other schedules have been tried. Three monthly pulses of azithromycin 500 mg for 3 consecutive days was effective. *PMID: 18608737*

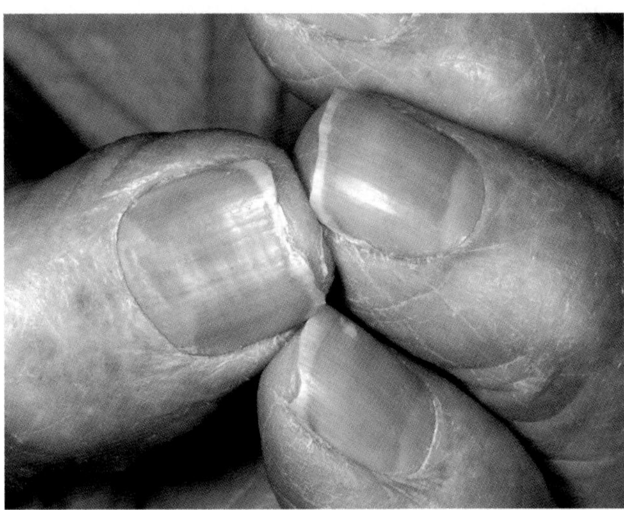

Figure 7-31 A blue pigmentation appeared in the nails after taking minocycline for 2 years. The pigmentation has persisted.

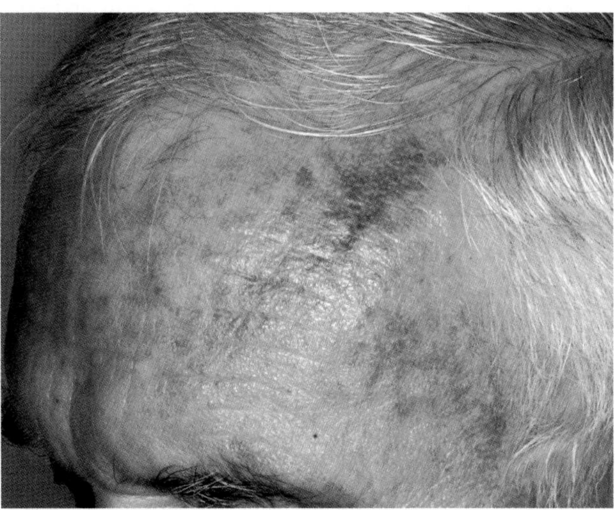

Figure 7-32 Blue pigmentation appeared on the forehead after taking minocycline for rosacea for 3 years.

HORMONAL TREATMENT

Acne can be the presenting sign of the overproduction of androgens. Polycystic ovary syndrome, anovulation, Cushing's disease, and androgen-secreting tumors cause acne and hirsutism.

ANDROGENS. Androgens are produced in response to pituitary hormones (luteinizing hormone, adrenocorticotropic hormone [ACTH]). Testosterone is produced by the testes and, to a lesser extent, by the ovaries. Dehydroepiandrosterone (DHEAS) is produced in the adrenal glands and converted to testosterone. Testosterone is converted at target tissues by 5-alpha-reductase to dihydrotestosterone (DHT). Testosterone and DHT bind to the same androgen receptor on sebocytes. DHT has 10 times the affinity for the receptor than does testosterone. Acne is seen only in the presence of DHT. A combination of the effects of circulating androgens and the effects of their metabolism at the hair follicle modulates sebum production and acne severity. Androgens (free testosterone [fT], dehydroepiandrosterone sulfate [DHEAS]) are the most important hormones in the pathogenesis of acne. Plasma-free testosterone is the active fraction of testosterone and determines plasma androgenicity.

PATIENT POPULATION. There is a group of women with treatment-resistant, late-onset, or persistent acne. Some of these women have signs suggesting hyperandrogenism, such as hirsutism, irregular menses, or menstrual dysfunction, but others are normal. Levels of serum androgens may or may not be elevated.

OVULATION ABNORMALITIES. Ovulation disturbances have been found in 58.3% of women with acne, with a prevalence of anovulation in juvenile acne and of luteal insufficiency in late-onset/persistent acne. Women affected by late-onset or persistent acne have a high incidence of polycystic ovary disease. Polycystic ovaries are not necessarily associated with menstrual disorders, obesity, or hirsutism. The presence of polycystic ovaries in acne patients does not correlate with acne severity, infertility, menstrual disturbance, hirsutism, or biochemical endocrinologic abnormalities.

WHEN TO ORDER HORMONE TESTS. Most women with acne have normal serum androgen concentrations and do not require serum evaluation. Women presenting with rapid onset (1 to 4 months) of acne, hirsutism, androgenetic alopecia, or signs of virilization, such as low voice, increased muscle mass, increased libido, or clitoromegaly, require screening to rule out a tumor. Total testosterone levels of greater than 200 ng/dl (7 nmol/L) suggest a possible tumor, usually ovarian in origin. Serum testosterone levels of 170 ng/dl (6 nmol/L) can be seen in polycystic ovarian disease, and imaging can confirm this diagnosis. Adrenal tumor (rare) should be suspected if the plasma DHEAS level is greater than 800 mcg/dl (normal value, 350 mcg/dl). A second indication for hormone evaluation is when there is obesity, acanthosis nigricans, or concern about diabetes or Cushing's syndrome. Insulin resistance is common in hyperandrogenemic women with polycystic ovary syndrome.

Box 7-1 **Women Best Suited for Hormonal Treatment**

Most likely to respond to hormonal treatment

Increased facial oiliness (seborrhea)
Premenstrual acne flare-ups
Inflammatory acne on mandibular line and neck

Other indications

Acne onset as adult
Acne worsening as adult
Treatment failures with intolerance to standard therapies
Treatment failure with Accutane
History of irregular menses
History of ovarian cysts
Hirsutism by history or examination
Androgenetic alopecia

Adapted from Shaw JC: *Dermatol Clin* 19:169, 2001. *PMID: 11155581*

TESTS TO ORDER. Tests include total testosterone and fT, DHEAS, ACTH stimulation, prolactin, luteinizing hormone, follicle-stimulating hormone, lipid profiles, and glucose tolerance tests. fT and DHEAS are the most practical ways of evaluating hormonal influences in the female. DHEAS is the best index of adrenal androgen activity.

TREATMENT INDICATIONS. Antiandrogenic therapy is reserved for women with acne who have clinical signs of androgen excess and for those in whom other treatments have failed (Box 7-1). Women who have had incomplete responses to systemic antibiotics may be treated with oral contraceptives, spironolactone, or both. The majority of patients with acne do not have serum androgen abnormalities. The profound sebum suppression produced by isotretinoin has to a large extent eliminated the need for antiandrogenic therapy. Patients with abnormal serum androgen levels can be managed as outlined in Table 7-2.

TREATMENT OPTIONS. Acne hormonal treatment is accomplished by androgen receptor blockade or suppression of androgen production. There are three options for treating acne systemically with hormone manipulation. Estrogens (oral contraceptives) suppress ovarian androgens, antiandrogens (spironolactone, cyproterone acetate) act at the peripheral level (hair follicle, sebaceous gland), and glucocorticoids (prednisone, dexamethasone) suppress adrenal androgen. Five alpha-reductase inhibitors are not commonly used to treat acne. The recommended treatment is shown in Table 7-2.

ORAL CONTRACEPTIVES. Ovarian hypersecretion of androgens can be suppressed with oral contraceptives. Most oral contraceptives (Table 7-3) contain combinations

Table 7-2 Hormonal Treatment of Acne

Drug	Indication (also see Table 7-1)	Mechanism of action	Dose
Oral contraceptives	Failed antibiotics No response to dexamethasone or prednisone fT* elevated	Inhibit ovarian androgen secretion	(See Table 7-3)
Spironolactone	Failed antibiotics	Androgen receptor blockade	25-200 mg/day usually taken in two divided doses
Dexamethasone or prednisone	DHEAS elevated DHEAS normal but fails prescription with antibiotics or Accutane Not responsive to oral contraceptives or spironolactone	Inhibits adrenal androgen secretion	0.25-0.5 mg in evening 5-10 mg daily or every other day, in evenings

DHEAS, Dehydroepiandrosterone sulfate; *fT*, free testosterone.

of estrogens and progestational agents. Oral contraceptives with estrogen (e.g., ethinyl estradiol) and progestins of low androgenic activity are the most useful. Most synthetic progesterones have some degree of androgenic activity, which is undesirable in patients who already have signs of androgen excess.

Combination oral contraceptives reduce cutaneous androgen effect by suppressing gonadotropin release (luteinizing hormone), which results in suppression of ovarian androgen production. Oral contraceptives also regulate menstrual cycles in oligomenorrheic women and reduce side effects of androgen receptor blockers.

In many instances, acne flares after the use of oral contraceptives are discontinued. Selection of an appropriate agent may provide the benefit of effective acne therapy for women who have chosen an oral contraceptive for birth control. Women in their thirties and forties without risk factors such as smoking or a family history of premature cardiovascular disease can safely use low-dose oral contraceptives to reduce ovarian androgen secretion.

Indications. Oral contraceptives are useful for acne patients who need birth control, have late-onset acne, and experience menstrual flares. Oral contraceptives are usually combined with topical and systemic retinoids, topical benzoyl peroxide, and topical or systemic antibiotics.

Specific medications. Oral contraceptives are effective in reducing inflammatory and noninflammatory facial acne lesions. Norgestimate/ethinyl estradiol (Ortho Tri-Cyclen), norethindrone acetate/ethinyl estradiol (Estrostep), and drospirenone/ethinyl estradiol (YAZ) are approved by the FDA for the treatment of acne. Levonorgestrel/ethinyl estradiol (Alesse) is also effective (Table 7-2). After 6 to 9 months of use, there is a reduction in inflammatory lesion counts of 30% to 60%, with improvement occurring in 50% to 90% of patients. Any oral contraceptive that contains estrogen is likely to have similar positive effects. The effects on acne of injectable progestins and patch systems have not been evaluated, and progesterone-only contraceptives may make acne worse.

Oral contraceptive side effects. There is an increased risk of venous thromboembolism, stroke, and myocardial infarction. These risks are increased in patients who smoke cigarettes or who have a history of hypertension, diabetes, or migraine. Oral contraceptives may slightly increase the risk of developing breast cancer but have some protective effects against ovarian and endometrial cancer. The most common side effects are mood changes, breast tenderness, nausea, and breakthrough bleeding.

Antibiotics and oral contraceptives. Available scientific and pharmacokinetic data do not support the hypothesis that antibiotics (with the exception of rifampin) lower the contraceptive efficacy of oral contraceptives. The American College of Obstetricians and Gynecologists has stated that tetracycline, doxycycline, ampicillin, and metronidazole do not affect oral contraceptive steroid levels. In a legal action, a court stated there was no evidence of causation between the use of antibiotics and decreased effectiveness of oral contraceptives. The evidence suggests that backup contraception is not necessary for women who reliably use oral contraceptives during oral antibiotic use.

Table 7-3 Oral Contraceptives—FDA Approved for Treating Acne

Brand name	Estrogen	Progestin
Estrostep	Ethinyl estradiol 20, 30, 35 mcg	Norethindrone 1 mg
Ortho Tri-Cyclen	Ethinyl estradiol 35 mcg	Norgestimate 0.18, 0.125, 0.25 mg
YAZ	Ethinyl estradiol 20 mcg	Drospirenone 3 ng

SPIRONOLACTONE. Spironolactone (SPL) is an androgen receptor blocker that has antiandrogenic properties and is used to treat acne, hirsutism, and androgenic alopecia. Men do not tolerate the high incidence of endocrine side effects; therefore it is only used in women. SPL decreases steroid production in adrenal and gonadal tissue. In women, total serum testosterone concentration decreases and dehydroepiandrosterone sulfate level either is decreased or remains unchanged. Free testosterone levels are unchanged or decreased. SPL acts as an antiandrogen peripherally by competitively blocking receptors for dihydrotestosterone in the sebaceous glands.

Indications. Treatment failures are common in adult women. Spironolactone is very successful in treating many adult women with acne.

Spironolactone can be used with antibiotics or oral contraceptives or as a single drug therapy. Therefore it can be used when the source of androgen is either adrenal or ovarian or when screening for serum androgens is normal. Cyproterone acetate has similar effects (available outside the United States). A formulation of cyproterone acetate, in combination with 50 or 35 mg of estradiol, is available outside the United States. These drugs (Diane and Dianette) serve as an oral contraceptive and as an inhibitor of androgen receptors.

Acne. Spironolactone causes a significant reduction in sebum secretion and a decrease in the lesion counts of patients. Studies show that SPL at a dosage of 200 mg/day suppresses sebum production by 75% and can reduce lesion counts by up to 75% over a 4-month period. Indications for its use are listed in Box 7-2. Spironolactone can be used in low doses (50 to 100 mg/day) as a single drug or as an adjunct to standard acne therapies. Clearing of acne occurred in 33% of patients treated with low doses of spironolactone; 33% had marked improvement, 27.4% showed partial improvement, and 7% showed no improvement. The treatment regimen was well tolerated, with 57.5% reporting no adverse effects. The incidence of side effects increases with higher doses. In another study, spironolactone 50 mg twice daily was given on days 5 through 21 of the menstrual cycle. The most common adverse effect was metrorrhagia, which appears to be well tolerated. The incidence of metrorrhagia can be significantly decreased by adding birth control pills to patients' regimens.

Spironolactone with and without oral contraceptives. A total of 27 women (ages 18 to 43) with either severe papular or nodulocystic facial acne were treated with a combined oral contraceptive containing 30 mcg of ethinyl estradiol and 3 mg of drospirenone (Yasmin) and with spironolactone 100 mg taken daily. No significant elevation of serum potassium level was found. Both medications were given as a single morning dose. Eighty-five percent of the subjects were entirely clear of acne lesions or had excellent improvement at the end of the 6-month study. PMID: 17964689 The dosing was different in another study. From the fifth day of the menstrual cycle each patient was given 100 mg/day of spironolactone divided into morning and evening doses, each dose 50 mg, for 16 days. Patients did not take oral contraceptives. The results of both studies were similar. PMID: 15752283

Adverse reactions. Side effects are dose-related. The incidence is low, and the severity is generally mild and most women tolerate treatment. Menstrual irregularities (80%) such as amenorrhea, increased or decreased flow, midcycle bleeding, and shortened length of cycle occur.

Box 7-2 **Guidelines for Treatment of Acne with Spironolactone (Aldactone 25-, 50-, 100-mg Tablets)**

A. Indications

1. Adult women with inflammatory facial acne
2. Hormonal influence suggested by
   a. Premenstrual flares
   b. Onset after age 25 years
   c. Distribution on the lower face, including the mandibular line and chin
   d. Increase in oiliness on the face
   e. Coexistent facial hirsutism
3. Inadequate response or intolerance to standard treatment with topical therapies, systemic antibiotics, or isotretinoin
4. Presence of coexisting symptoms such as irregular menses, premenstrual weight gain, or other symptoms of premenstrual syndrome

B. Pretreatment evaluation

1. Evaluation of serum androgens generally is not required because most women with acne have normal serum levels. In the clinical setting of new onset of acne with other signs of virilization, evaluation by an endocrinologist may be required.
2. Determination of adequate birth control measures
3. Discussion of potential side effects with oral spironolactone
4. Obtaining baseline blood pressure

C. Guidelines for starting treatment

1. Begin with 1 or 2 mg/kg/day (50-100 mg/day) as a single daily dose to minimize side effects. It is not known whether twice-daily dosing has an advantage over a single daily dose.
2. Check serum potassium levels and blood pressure in 1 month. Obtaining a CBC is optional because hematologic abnormalities occur only rarely.
3. Topical therapies and systemic antibiotics may be continued while spironolactone treatment is initiated. Tapering of the standard therapies may then be possible as a beneficial response to spironolactone is noted.
4. Oral contraceptives, if not contraindicated, may be given concomitantly at the start of treatment with spironolactone, or they can be considered if menstrual irregularities develop.
5. If no clinical response is seen in 1 to 3 months, consider increasing the dosage to 150 or 200 mg/day as tolerated. Good clinical responses can be followed by a reduction of the dosage to the lowest effective daily dose.
6. If adverse effects develop, consider lowering the dose; consider adding an oral contraceptive for menstrual irregularities.
7. Effective treatment of hirsutism usually requires longer treatment periods and higher dosages than those used to obtain clinical benefit in the treatment of acne.

From Shaw JC: *J Am Acad Dermatol* 24:236, 1991.
PMID: 1826112

Oral contraceptives reduce the incidence and severity of menstrual irregularities. Breast tenderness or enlargement and decreased libido are infrequent. Other effects include mild hyperkalemia, headache, dizziness, drowsiness, confusion, nausea, vomiting, anorexia, and diarrhea. There are no documented cases of spironolactone-related tumors in human beings. The safety of spironolactone use during pregnancy is unknown.

CORTICOSTEROIDS. Corticosteroids can be considered in recalcitrant cases of acne not responsive to oral contraceptives or spironolactone and for patients with elevated DHEAS level. Corticosteroids can be used alone or in combination with oral contraceptives and antiandrogens. An elevated DHEAS level indicates adrenal androgen overproduction. Either dexamethasone (0.25 to 0.5 mg at bedtime) or prednisone (5 to 7.5 mg at bedtime daily or every other day) is [illegible]bed. Low-dose steroids administered at bedtime prevent [illegible] pituitary from producing extra ACTH and thereby reduce the production of adrenal androgens. Dexamethasone may be the more rational choice for adrenal suppression with its longer duration of action. The drug is given at bedtime so that effective levels will be present during the early morning hours when ACTH secretion is most active. The initial dosage should be dexamethasone 0.25 mg or prednisone 2.5 mg, and the dosage should be increased to dexamethasone 0.5 mg or prednisone 5.0 to 7.5 mg if the DHEAS level has not been decreased after 3 to 4 weeks of treatment. Therapy is continued for 6 to 12 months, but the benefits may persist beyond that. This low dosage produces a clinical improvement and suppresses DHEAS levels. At these dosages, few patients experience shutdown of the adrenal-pituitary axis or other adverse effects of the drug. ACTH stimulation tests or early morning cortisol levels may be performed every few months to make sure that there is no adrenal suppression. Not all patients respond.

CYPROTERONE. The antiandrogen cyproterone acetate (CPA) is available outside the United States. It is the most widely used hormonal antiandrogen. Cyproterone is a potent androgen receptor blocker, has progestin activity, and is used as the progestin in oral contraceptives outside the United States. Low doses (2 mg/day) as part of oral contraceptives (Dianette, Diane) are highly effective in improving acne.

ISOTRETINOIN

Isotretinoin (Accutane, Amnesteen, Sotret 10-, 20-, 30-, 40-mg capsules; 13-*cis*-retinoic acid), an oral retinoid related to vitamin A, is a very effective agent for control of acne and in the induction of long-term remissions, but it is not suitable for all types of acne. Isotretinoin affects all major etiologic factors implicated in acne. It dramatically reduces sebum excretion, follicular keratinization, and ductal and surface *P. acnes* counts. These effects are maintained during treatment and persist at variable levels after therapy. A full list of indications and guidelines for treatment are found in Box 7-3. A number of side effects occur during treatment. Isotretinoin is a potent teratogen; pregnancy must be avoided during treatment. Isotretinoin is not mutagenic; female patients should be assured that they may safely get pregnant but should wait for at least 1 month after stopping isotretinoin. Age is not a limiting factor in patient selection.

Box 7-3 **Guidelines for the Treatment of Acne with Isotretinoin (10-, 20-, 30-, 40-mg Capsules)**

Indications

Severe, recalcitrant cystic acne
Severe, recalcitrant nodular and inflammatory acne
Moderate acne unresponsive to conventional therapy
Patients who scar
Excessive oiliness
Severely depressed or dysmorphic patients

Unusual variants

Acne fulminans
Gram-negative folliculitis
Pyoderma faciale

Dosage

Total cumulative dose determines remission rate

Cumulative dose 120 to 150 mg/kg

88% of patients have a stable, complete remission when treated in this dosage range
No therapeutic benefit from doses >150 mg/kg
0.5 to 1.0 mg/kg/day for 4 months—typical course of prescription
Optimal long-term benefit: 1.0 mg/kg/day for initial course of prescription
1.0 mg/kg/day × 120 days = 120 mg/kg

Treat with 1 mg/kg/day especially in

Young patients
Males
Severe acne
Truncal acne

Treat with 0.5 mg/kg/day in

Older patients, especially men
Double dosage at end of 2 months if no response

Duration

Usually 85% clear in 4 months at 0.5 to 1.0 mg/kg/day; 15% require longer prescription
May treat at lower dosage for longer period to arrive at the optimum total cumulative dosage

Relapse

39% relapse (usually within 3 years, most within 18 months)
23% require antibiotics
16% require additional isotretinoin

Additional courses of isotretinoin

Appears to be safe
Response is predictable
Some patients require three to five courses
Cumulative dosage for each course should not exceed 150 mg/kg

Adapted from Layton AM, Cunliffe WJ: *J Am Acad Dermatol* 27: S2, 1992 *PMID: 1460120*; and Lehucher-Ceyrac D, Weber-Buisset MJ: *Dermatology* 186:123, 1993. *PMID: 8428040*

INDICATIONS

Severe, recalcitrant cystic or nodular and inflammatory acne. A few patients with severe disease respond to oral antibiotics and vigorous drying therapy with a combination of agents such as benzoyl peroxide and sulfacetamide/sulfur lotion. Those who do not respond after a short trial of this conventional therapy should be treated with isotretinoin to minimize scarring.

Moderate acne unresponsive to conventional therapy. Moderate acne usually responds to antibiotics (e.g., tetracycline or doxycycline) plus topical agents. Change to a different antibiotic (e.g., minocycline 100 mg twice daily) if response is poor after 3 months. Change to isotretinoin if response is unsatisfactory after two consecutive 3-month courses of antibiotics. Patients who have a relapse during or after two courses of antibiotics are also candidates for isotretinoin.

Patients who scar. Any patient who scars should be considered for isotretinoin therapy. Acne scars leave a permanent mark on the skin and psyche.

Excessive oiliness. Excessive oiliness is disturbing and can last for years. Antibiotics and topical therapy may provide some relief, but isotretinoin's effect is dramatic. Relief may last for months or years; some patients require a second or third course of treatment. Some patients respond to a long-term low-dose regimen such as 10 mg every other or every third day.

Severely depressed or dysmorphophobic patients. Some patients, even with minor acne, are depressed. Those who do not respond to conventional therapy are candidates for isotretinoin. They respond well to isotretinoin, although some may relapse quickly and require repeat courses.

Sebaceous hyperplasia. Patients with numerous facial lesions of sebaceous hyperplasia may experience a dramatic clearing with a low dosage of isotretinoin. A typical patient is age 40 to 50 and has more than 50 lesions on the forehead and cheeks. Start with 10 mg daily and lower the dosage once control is achieved. Many patients are maintained on 10 mg every other or every third day. Lesions reappear weeks or months after stopping treatment.

DOSAGE. The severity of the side effects of isotretinoin is proportional to the daily dose. Start with lower dosages and progressively increase the dosage in accordance with the tolerance (Table 7-4). Treatment is usually begun at 0.5 mg/kg a day and increased to 1.0 mg/kg a day.

The cumulative dose may be more important than the duration of therapy. A cumulative dose of greater than 120 mg/kg is associated with significantly better long-term remission. This dosage level can be achieved by either 1 mg/kg/day for 4 months or a smaller dosage for a longer period. Six months of treatment with low-dose isotretinoin (20 mg/day) was found to be effective in the treatment of moderate acne, with a low incidence of severe side effects and at a lower cost than higher doses. *PMID: 16546586* The therapeutic benefit from a total cumulative dose of more than 150 mg/kg is virtually nonexistent. Analysis of 9 years of experience demonstrated that 1 mg/kg/day of isotretinoin for 4 months resulted in the longest remissions. Relapse rates in patients receiving 0.5 mg/kg/day were approximately 40% and patients receiving 1.0 mg/kg/day had approximately 20% relapse rates. Younger patients, males, and patients with truncal acne derive maximum benefit from the higher dosages. In these patients, dosages less than 0.5 mg/kg/day for a standard 4-month course are associated with a high relapse rate. Treat older patients with facial acne with a dosage of 0.5 mg/kg/day. Double the dosage if there is no response at the end of 2 months. Intermittent dosing may be useful for patients older than 25 with mild-to-moderate facial acne that is unresponsive to conventional antibiotic therapy or that relapses rapidly after conventional antibiotic therapy. Treat with isotretinoin, 0.5 mg/kg/day, for 1 week in every 4 weeks for a total of 6 months. Very-low-dose isotretinoin may be a useful therapeutic option in rare patients who continue to suffer with acne into their 60s and 70s. Isotretinoin 0.25 mg/kg/day for 6 months is well tolerated and effective. Side effects in all patients depend on the dosage and can be controlled through reduction.

DURATION OF THERAPY. A standard course of isotretinoin therapy is 16 to 20 weeks. Approximately 85% of patients are clear at the end of 16 weeks; 15% require longer treatment. Side effects are related to the dosage. Treat for a longer duration at a lower dosage if mucocutaneous side effects become troublesome. Patients with large, closed comedones may respond slowly and relapse early with inflammatory papules. Another ill-defined group responds slowly and requires up to 9 months until the condition begins to clear. Intermittent isoretinoin (0.5 mg/kg/day) given for the first 10 days of each month for 6 months was effective and patients experienced fewer side effects than those treated with the conventional program. *PMID: 17710426*

Table 7-4 Dosage of Isotretinoin by Body Weight

Body weight		Total mg/day		
Kilograms	Pounds	0.5 mg/kg	1 mg/kg	2 mg/kg
40	88	20	40	80
50	110	25	50	100
60	132	30	60	120
70	154	35	70	140
80	176	40	80	160
90	198	45	90	180
100	220	50	100	200

RELAPSE AND REPEAT COURSES OF ISOTRETINOIN. Approximately 40% of patients relapse and require oral antibiotics or additional isotretinoin. Relapse usually occurs within the first 3 years after isotretinoin is stopped, most often during the first 18 months after therapy. Some patients require multiple courses of therapy. The response to repeat therapy is consistently successful, and side effects are similar to those of previous courses. Repeat courses of isotretinoin seem to be safe.

The following conditions were statistically associated with acne relapse: male gender; younger than 16 years of age and living in an urban area; and receiving isotretinoin cumulative doses greater than 2450 mg and undergoing isotretinoin treatment longer than 121 days. *PMID: 17970803*

ISOTRETINOIN THERAPY. Patients are seen every 4 weeks. Isotretinoin is given in two divided doses daily, preferably with meals. Many patients experience a moderate to severe flare of acne during the initial weeks of treatment. This adverse reaction can be minimized by starting at 10 to 20 mg twice each day and gradually increasing the dosage during the first 4 to 6 weeks. Treatment is discontinued at the end of 16 to 20 weeks, and the patient is observed for 2 to 5 months. Those with persistently severe acne may receive a second course of treatment after the posttreatment observation period.

Response to therapy. At dosages of 1 mg/kg/day, sebum production decreases to approximately 10% of pretreatment values and the sebaceous glands decrease in size. Maximum inhibition is reached by the third or fourth week. Within a week, patients normally notice drying and chapping of facial skin and skin oiliness disappears quickly. These effects persist for an indefinite period when therapy is discontinued.

During the first month, there is usually a reduction in superficial lesions such as papules and pustules. New cysts evolve and disappear quickly. A significant reduction in the number of cysts normally takes at least 8 weeks. Facial lesions respond faster than trunk lesions.

Table 7-5 Laboratory Tests with Isotretinoin

Test	Comments
Pregnancy	See iPLEDGE program guidelines*
Triglyceride level†	Performed during pretreatment, after 2-3 weeks of treatment, and then at 4-week intervals. If levels exceed 350-400 mg/dl, repeat measurement of blood lipids at 2-3-week intervals. Stop if value exceeds 700-800 mg/dl to reduce risk of pancreatitis.
Complete blood cell count	Performed before treatment and after 4-6 weeks of treatment.
Liver function†	Performed before treatment and after 4-6 weeks of treatment.

*www.ipledgeprogram.com
†Liver and lipid abnormalities rarely necessitate dosage reduction.

RESISTANT PATIENTS. Younger patients (14 to 19 years of age) and those who have severe acne relapse more often. Truncal acne relapses more often than facial acne. A return of the reduced sebum excretion rate to within 10% of the pretreatment level is a poor prognostic factor. Patients with microcystic acne (whiteheads) and women with gynecoendocrinologic problems are resistant to treatment. Women who do not clear after a total cumulative dose of 150 mg/kg need laboratory and clinical evaluation of their endocrinologic status. They may benefit from antiandrogen therapy.

PSYCHOSOCIAL IMPLICATIONS. Patients successfully treated with isotretinoin have significant posttreatment gains in social assertiveness and self-esteem. There is also a significant reduction in anxiety and depression.

Patients with minimal facial acne but with symptoms of dysmorphophobia (inappropriate depression and/or anxiety response to mild acne) are often treated with long-term antibiotic therapy with no perceived improvement. These patients respond to isotretinoin in that they are satisfied with the cosmetic results achieved. The incidence of relapse is greater than that of other acne patients and often requires additional therapy in the form of antibiotics or further isotretinoin.

LABORATORY STUDIES. Pregnancy tests, triglyceride tests, complete blood cell counts, and liver function tests are performed on patients taking isotretinoin (Table 7-5); pregnancy tests are performed at each 4-week follow-up.

SIDE EFFECTS. Side effects occur frequently, are dose-dependent, and are reversible shortly after discontinuing treatment. Patients with side effects can be managed at a lower dosage for a period long enough to reach the 120 mg/kg cumulative dose level. Explain to patients that the long-term benefit is related to the cumulative dosage, not to the duration of therapy.

The incidence of side effects was documented in a large study (Table 7-6). Patients in that study stopped isotretinoin for the following reasons: mucous/skin effects (2.5%), elevated triglyceride levels (2.0%), musculoskeletal effects (1.3%), headaches (1.1%), elevated liver enzyme levels (0.6%), amenorrhea (0.4%), and other symptoms (0.5%).

Teratogenicity

Pregnancy prevention program. Isotretinoin is a potent teratogen primarily involving craniofacial, cardiac, thymic, and central nervous system structures. A number of physicians inadvertently prescribed isotretinoin to pregnant women, which resulted in birth defects.

Women should be educated about the risks to the fetus and the need for adequate contraception. Some physicians will not prescribe isotretinoin to women of child-bearing age unless they are taking oral contraceptives. Others withhold isotretinoin if abortion is not an option. Isotretinoin

Table 7-6 Frequency of Mucocutaneous and Musculoskeletal Events in 404 Subjects*

Event	Frequency, no.
Cheilitis	96
Dry skin	87
Pruritus	23
Dry mouth	29
Dry nose	40
Epistaxis	33
Conjunctivitis	40
Musculoskeletal symptoms	42
Rash	16
Hair thinning	6
Peeling	6

*Mean initial isotretinoin dose was 1 mg/kg. Most commonly used initial dosage regimen for males is 80 or 120 mg/day, and 80 or 140 mg/day for females.
From McElwee NE et al: *Arch Dermatol* 127:341, 1991.
PMID: 1825596

is not mutagenic, nor is it stored in tissue. It is recommended that contraception be continued for 1 month after stopping isotretinoin. Patients can be reassured that conception is safe after this 1-month period. One study showed that from the fourth month of treatment onward, a statistically significant increase in the mean sperm density, sperm morphology, and motility were not affected. One year after treatment there was no evidence of any negative influence of 6 months of treatment with isotretinoin on spermatogenesis.

iPledge. The iPLEDGE program in the United States is a computer-based risk management program designed to eliminate fetal exposure to isotretinoin through a special restricted distribution program. The program requires registration of health care professionals prescribing isotretinoin, pharmacies dispensing isotretinoin, and male and female patients prescribed isotretinoin. The program can be very time-consuming and frustrating. Many providers have stopped prescibing this valuable medication because of the complexities of the iPLEDGE program.

Plasma lipid abnormalities. Isotretinoin therapy induces an elevation of plasma triglyceride levels. In one study of patients (ages 14 to 40 years) treated for 20 weeks with 1 mg/kg/day, the maximum mean triglyceride levels increased 46.3 mg/dl in men and 52.3 mg/dl in women. In that study, 2 of 53 patients had a triglyceride elevation greater than 500 mg/dl, and 8 had elevations of 200 to 500 mg/dl. Triglyceride levels increase after 6 weeks of therapy and continue to increase while therapy continues. Age, gender, and weighted dose do not appear to be risk factors for triglyceride elevations. Overweight subjects are 6 times more likely to develop significant elevations in serum triglyceride levels, and subjects with elevated baseline triglyceride levels are 4.3 times more likely to develop significant elevations. Plasma lipid and lipoprotein levels return to baseline by 8 weeks after treatment.

Bony changes. Asymptomatic hyperostoses (spurs) of the spine and extremities can be documented radiographically in some patients but do not seem to be of concern with a standard course of isotretinoin therapy. This toxicity is common and related to dose and to duration of treatment and age. It increases with age. Approximately 10% of patients who are treated for acne with standard courses develop detectable changes. With higher doses, changes are more prominent. After long-term treatment (5 years), they can be found in most patients. Premature epiphyseal closure is rare. It has occurred at the higher doses and decreases with age, occurring only in children. Studies verified that there are no lasting changes in calcium homeostasis or bone mineralization as a result of a single course of isotretinoin for acne.

Cheilitis. Cheilitis is the most common side effect, occurring in virtually all patients. Application of emollients should be started with the initiation of therapy to minimize drying.

OTHER EFFECTS. Approximately 40% of patients develop an elevated sedimentation rate during treatment. Isotretinoin does not specifically affect skeletal or myocardial muscles, although 28% of patients complain of musculoskeletal symptoms. Isotretinoin contains preservative parabens; those patients with a proven allergy to parabens cannot receive isotretinoin. Exuberant granulation tissue may occur at the sites of healing acne lesions and is more likely to develop in patients who have preexisting crusted, draining, or ulcerated lesions. Granulation tissue can be controlled with intralesional steroid injections or silver nitrate sticks. Severe dry skin or eczema commonly occurs on the backs of the hands. Routine use of moisturizers and infrequent washing is recommended. Group V topical steroids treat the eczema.

Depression. In 1998 the manufacturers of isotretinoin, in conjunction with the FDA, announced a new warning: "Psychiatric disorders: isotretinoin may cause depression, psychosis and rarely, suicidal ideation, suicide attempts and suicide. Discontinuation of isotretinoin therapy may be insufficient; further evaluation may be necessary. No mechanism of action has been established for these events." The product labeling now states, "Of the patients reporting depression, some reported that the depression subsided with discontinuation of therapy and recurred with reinstitution of therapy." There are conflicting studies in the medical literature.

PREDNISONE

Prednisone has a limited but definite place in the management of acne. Nodulocystic acne can be resistant to all forms of conventional topical and antibiotic therapy. Nodulocystic acne can be destructive, producing widespread disfigurement through scarring. Intervention with powerful antiinflammatory agents should not be postponed in the case of rapidly advancing disease. Deep cysts improve only slowly with isotretinoin, and much permanent damage can be done while waiting for an effect.

PREDNISONE THERAPY. The dosage and duration of prednisone treatment are determined by the patient's response. The following program has been successful for treating extensive, rapidly advancing, painful cystic acne: Prednisone should be started at 40 to 60 mg per day given in divided doses twice daily. This dosage is maintained until the majority of lesions are significantly improved. Dosage is tapered. The dosage is lowered to 30 mg given as a single dose in the morning. The dosage can be tapered by 5 mg each week until 20 mg is reached, at which point prednisone can be further tapered to 30 mg every other day and withdrawn in 5-mg increments every 4 days. Patients with acne severe enough to require prednisone usually require isotretinoin for lasting control. Both drugs can be started simultaneously.

INTRALESIONAL CORTICOSTEROIDS

Individual nodulocystic and large pustular lesions can be effectively treated with a single injection of triamcinolone acetonide delivered with a 27- or 30-gauge needle. Commercial preparations include Kenalog (10 mg/ml) and TAC 3 (3 mg/ml). The 10 mg/ml suspension can be used at full strength or diluted with 1% lidocaine or physiologic saline. Saline is preferred because injections of Xylocaine mixtures are painful. A 2.5 to 5.0 mg/ml concentration is usually an adequate injection for suppressing inflammation. Some patients with cystic acne have a remarkable improvement with just intralesional corticosteroids. Inject once a month for two or three months.

INTRALESIONAL CORTICOSTEROID THERAPY. The bottle of steroid solution needs to be shaken thoroughly to disperse the white suspension. The syringe should be shaken immediately before injection. The needle is inserted through the thinnest portion of the cyst roof and 0.1 to 0.3 ml of solution is deposited into the cyst cavity. This quantity momentarily blanches most cysts. Atrophy may occur if steroids are injected into the base of the cyst. Patients should be assured that if skin depression does occur, in most cases it is temporary and gradually resolves in 4 to 6 months. Multiple cysts can be injected in the course of one session. Intralesional injection is used specifically to supplement other programs.

It is comforting for patients to know that if a large, painful cyst appears, fast relief is available with this relatively painless procedure. Occasionally, intralesional steroid injections may be given for small papules and pustules when rapid resolution is desired. Prolonged, continual use of intralesional steroids has resulted in adrenal suppression.

Other types of acne

GRAM-NEGATIVE ACNE

Patients with a long history of treatment with oral antibiotics for acne may have an increased carriage rate of gram-negative rods in the anterior nares. There are three presentations. The most common is the sudden development of superficial pustules around the nose and extending to the chin and cheeks. Others present with the sudden development of crops of pustules. Some patients develop deep nodular and cystic lesions. Cultures of these lesions and the anterior nares reveal *Escherichia aerogenes, Proteus mirabilis, Klebsiella pneumoniae, Escherichia coli, Serratia marcescens*, and other gram-negative organisms. Selection of the appropriate antibiotic is made after antibiotic culture and sensitivities.

Ampicillin or trimethoprim and sulfamethoxazole (Bactrim, Septra) are generally the appropriate drugs. Gram-negative acne responds quickly to the proper antibiotic, usually within 2 weeks. A quick relapse is common when antibiotics are stopped, even if given for 6 months. Elimination of the gram-negative organisms is difficult. Isotretinoin (1 mg/kg/day for 20 weeks) is successful for resistant cases of gram-negative acne.

STEROID ACNE

In predisposed individuals, sudden onset of follicular pustules and papules may occur 2 to 5 weeks after starting oral corticosteroids. The lesions of steroid acne (Figure 7-33) differ from those of acne vulgaris by being of uniform size and symmetric distribution, usually on the neck, chest, and back. They are 1- to 3-mm, flesh-colored or pink-to-red, dome-shaped papules and pustules. Comedones may form later. There is no scarring. Steroid-induced acne is rare before puberty and in the elderly. There is no residual scarring. This drug eruption is not a contraindication to continued or future use of oral corticosteroids. Topical therapy with benzoyl peroxide and/or sulfacetamide/sulfur lotion (Sulfacet-R, Plexion TS, Rosula) is effective. The eruption clears when steroids are stopped.

NEONATAL ACNE

Acneiform lesions (Figure 7-34) confined to the nose and cheeks may be present at birth or may develop in early infancy. The lesions clear without treatment as the large sebaceous glands stimulated by maternal androgens become smaller and less active.

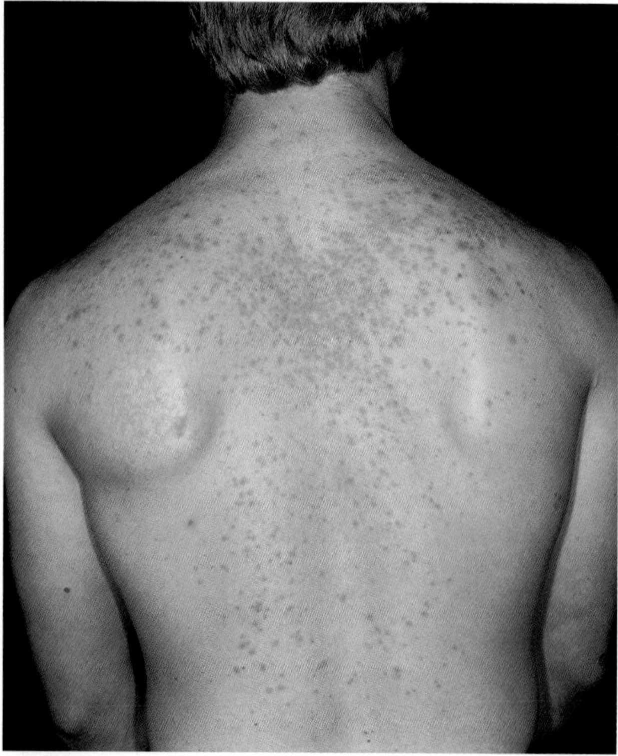

Figure 7-33 Steroid acne. Numerous papules and pustules are of uniform size and symmetrically distributed.

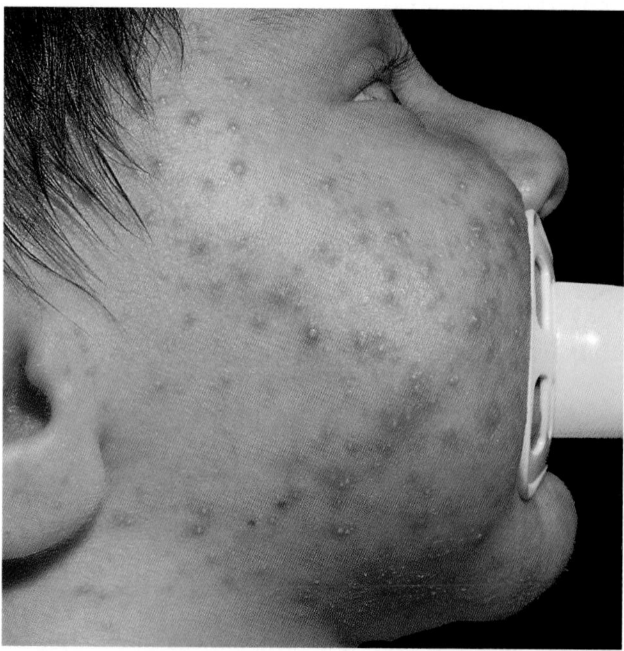

Figure 7-34 Neonatal acne. Small papules and pustules commonly occur on the cheeks and nose of infants.

INFANTILE ACNE

Infantile acne is uncommon. The age at onset is 6 to 16 months. There is a male predominance. The acne is mild, moderate, or severe. It is predominantly inflammatory. A mixed pattern is present in 17% of cases and nodular in 7%. Treatment is similar to that of adult acne, with the exclusion of the use of tetracyclines. Patients with mild acne respond to topical treatment (benzoyl peroxide and retinoids). Most infants with moderate acne respond to oral erythromycin 125 mg twice daily and to topical therapy. Patients with erythromycin-resistant *P. acnes* require oral antibiotics such as trimethoprim 100 mg twice daily. Most patients are able to stop oral antibiotics within 18 months. In 38% of children, long-term oral antibiotics (>24 months) is required. The time for clearance of the acne is 6 to 40 months (median, 18 months). Oral isotretinoin may be used in severe cases. Scarring is possible.

OCCUPATIONAL ACNE

An extensive, diffuse eruption of large comedones and pustules (Figure 7-35) may occur in some individuals who are exposed to certain industrial chemicals. These include chlorinated hydrocarbons and other industrial solvents, coal tar derivatives, and oils. Lesions occur on the extremities and trunk where clothing saturated with chemicals has been in prolonged close contact with the skin. Patients predisposed to this form of acne must avoid exposure by wearing protective clothing or finding other work. Treatment is the same as that for inflammatory acne.

ACNE MECHANICA

Mechanical pressure may induce an acneiform eruption (Figure 7-36). Common causes include forehead guards and chin straps on sports helmets and orthopedic braces.

ACNE COSMETICA

Closed and open comedones, papules, and pustules may develop in postadolescent women who regularly apply layers of cosmetics. This may be the patient's first experience with acne. Trials with specific cosmetics on women have revealed that some formulations cause acne, some have no effect, and some may possibly result in decreasing the number of comedones. Until specific formulations are tested and their comedogenic potential is known, patients

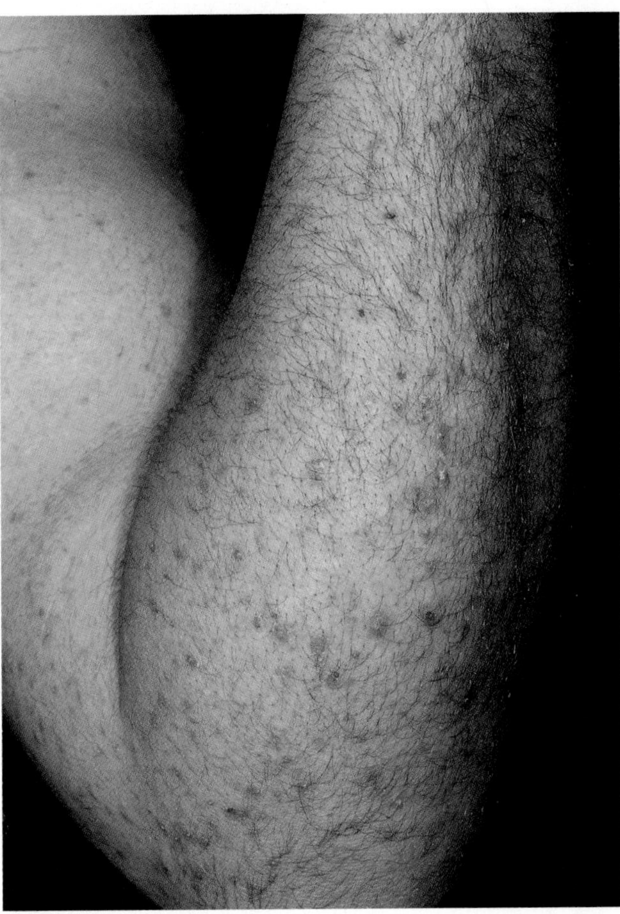

Figure 7-35 Comedones, papules, and pustules occur in areas exposed to oils and industrial solvents.

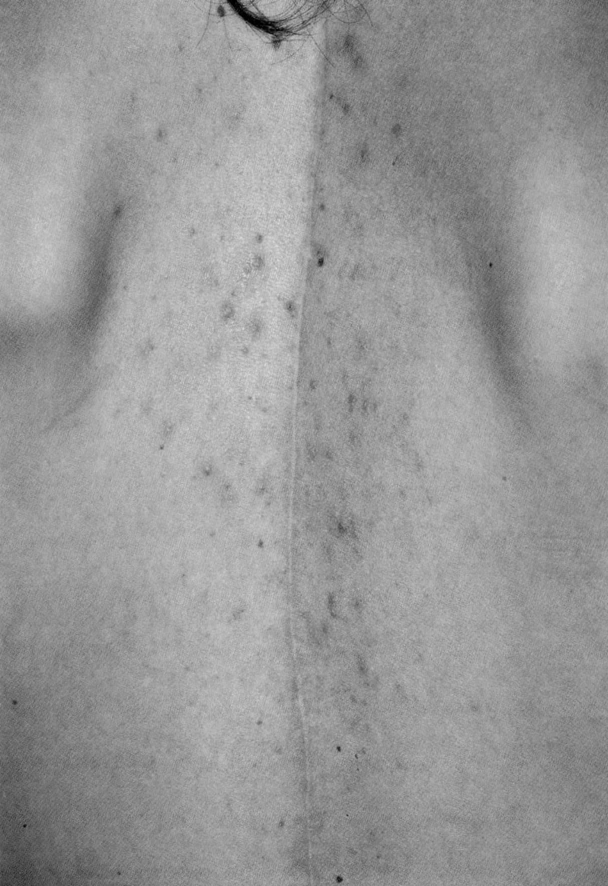

Figure 7-36 Acne mechanica. Comedones, papules, and pustules occurred after a few weeks of wearing a back brace.

should be advised to use light, water-based cosmetics and to avoid cosmetic programs that advocate applying multiple layers of cream-based cleansers and coverups. Many patients are under the false impression that "facials" performed in beauty salons are therapeutic and deep clean pores. The various creams and cosmetics used during a facial are tolerated by most people, but acne can be precipitated by this practice.

One alternative to cosmetics is the use of tinted acne preparations (e.g., Sulfacet-R) (see the Formulary). These are generally very well received by patients.

EXCORIATED ACNE

Most acne patients attempt to drain comedones and pustules with moderate finger pressure. Occasionally, a young woman with little or no acne develops several deep, linear erosions on the face (Figures 7-37 through 7-40). The skin has been picked vigorously with the fingernail and eventually forms a crust. These broad, red erosions with adherent crusts are obvious signs of manipulation and can easily be differentiated from resolving papules and pustules. This inappropriate attempt to eradicate lesions causes scarring and brown hyperpigmentation. Women may deny or be oblivious to their manipulation. It should be explained that such lesions can occur only with manipulation, and that the lesions may be unconsciously created during sleep. Once confronted, many women are capable of exercising adequate restraint. Those unable to refrain from excoriation may benefit from psychiatric care. One patient improved on olanzapine 2.5 mg for 6 months.

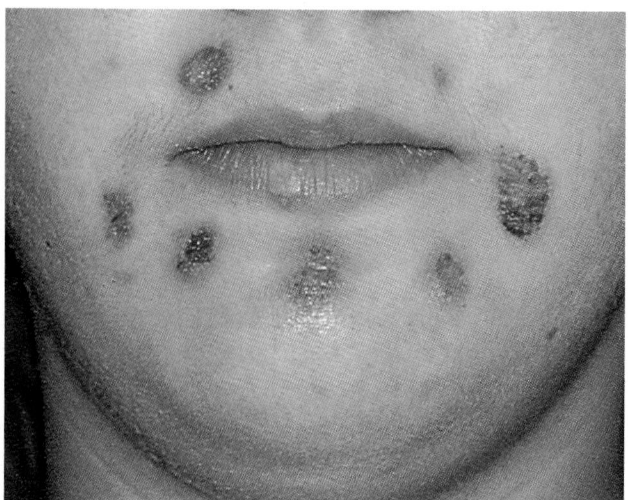

Figure 7-38 Acne excoriée des jeunes filles. Erosions and ulcers are created by inappropriate attempts to drain acne lesions.

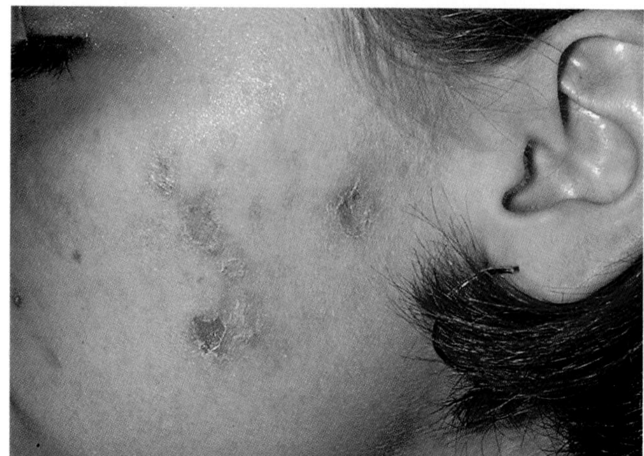

Figure 7-39 Excoriating the face has left this person with thick hyperpigmented scares.

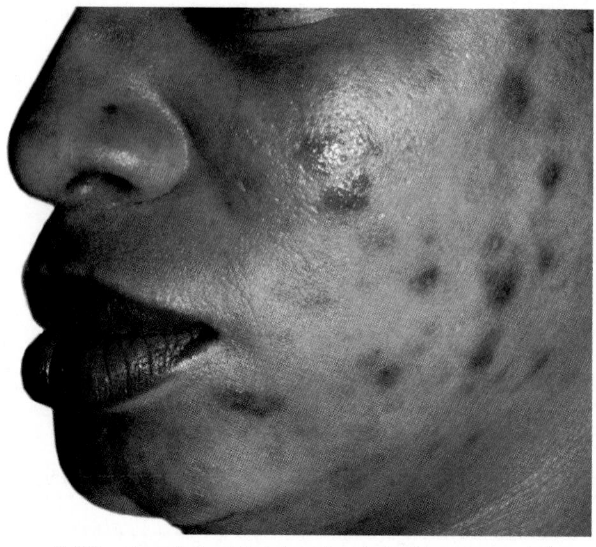

Figure 7-37 Excoriating the face has left this person with thick hyperpigmented scars.

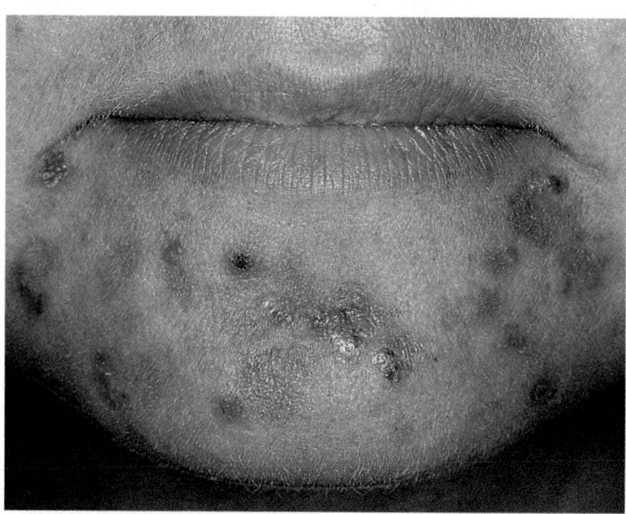

Figure 7-40 Acne excoriée des jeunes filles. Erosions and ulcers are created by inappropriate attempts to drain acne lesions.

SENILE COMEDONES

Excessive exposure to sunlight in predisposed individuals causes large open and closed comedones around the eyes and on the temples (Figures 7-41 and 7-42). Inflammation rarely occurs, and comedones can easily be expressed with acne surgery techniques. Topical retinoids (Retin-A, Tazorac) may be used to loosen impacted comedones and continued to discourage recurrence. Once cleared, the comedones may not return for months or years and retinoids may be discontinued. Lesions that recur can be effectively treated with a 2-mm curette. The skin is held taut, and the comedone is lifted out with a quick flick of the wrist. It is important to go deep enough to remove the entire lesion. Bleeding is controlled with Monsel's solution; electrocautery causes scars and should be avoided.

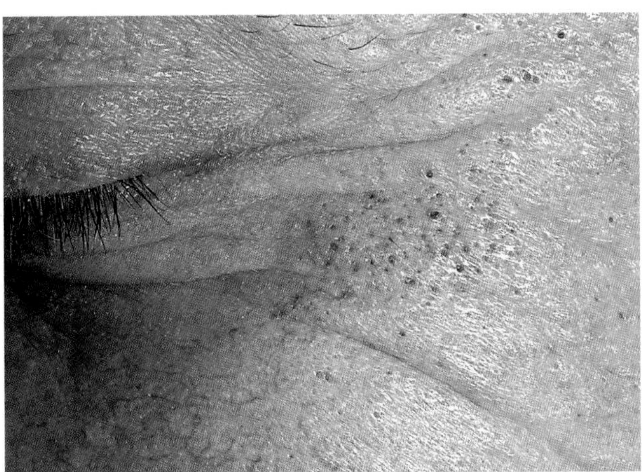

Figure 7-41 Senile comedones. Small comedones are the initial finding.

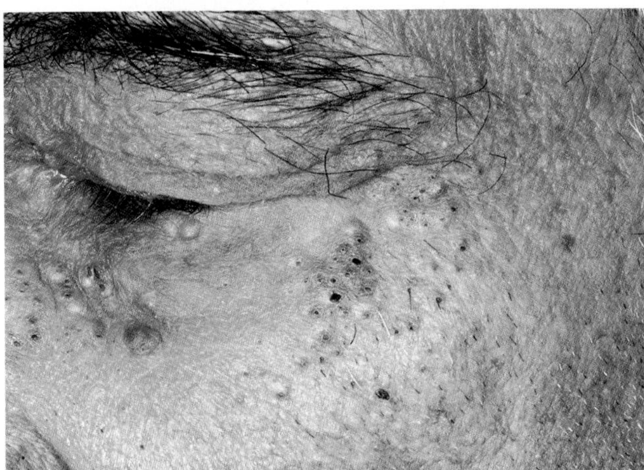

Figure 7-42 Senile comedones. Small or large comedones may appear around the eyes and temples in middle-aged and older individuals. Sunlight is a predisposing factor.

SOLID FACIAL EDEMA

Solid, persistent, inflammatory edema of the face may occur in rare instances in patients with acne and last for years. The edema is often resistant to conventional treatment, including isotretinoin. The therapeutic combination of oral isotretinoin (0.5 mg/kg body weight daily) and ketotifen (2 mg daily) led to complete resolution of all facial lesions in one reported case. Surgical treatment of this problem has been reported.

The pathogenesis of persistent edema remains mysterious but may be related to chronic inflammation that results in obstruction of lymph vessels or fibrosis induced by mast cells.

MILIA

Milia are tiny, white, pea-shaped cysts that commonly occur on the face, especially around the eyes (Figure 7-43). A distinction is made between primary and secondary milia. Primary milia arise spontaneously, most often on the eyelids and cheeks. They are derived from the lowest portion of the infundibulum of the vellus hairs. They are small cysts that differ from epidermal cysts only in size.

Secondary milia may represent retention cysts following injury to the skin. Milia may occur spontaneously or after habitual rubbing of the eyelids. They are seen in blistering dermatoses (such as epidermolysis bullosa, porphyria cutanea tarda, and bullous pemphigoid), after dermabrasion or topical treatment with fluorouracil, in areas of chronic corticosteroid-induced atrophy, and after burns and radiation therapy. Secondary milia are morphologically and histologically identical to primary milia. These tiny structures annoy patients, and drainage is frequently requested.

Milia have no opening on the surface and cannot be expressed like blackheads. A no. 11 pointed surgical blade tip is inserted with the sharp edge up and advanced laterally approximately 1 mm. Apply pressure with the Schamberg extractor to remove the soft, white material. Other treatments are laser ablation or electrodesiccation.

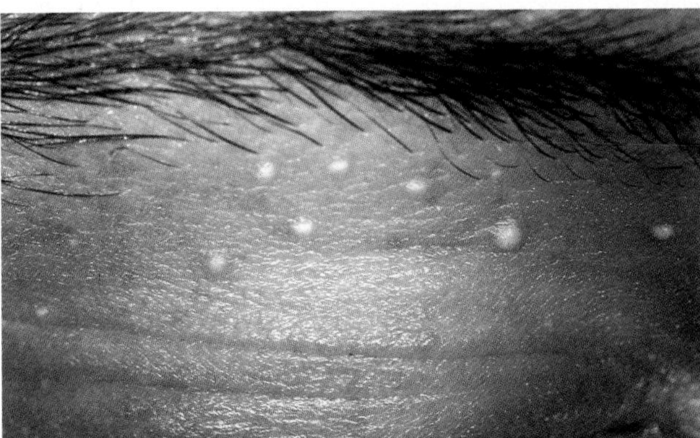

Figure 7-43 Milia. Tiny, white, dome-shaped cysts that occur about the eyes and cheeks. There is no obvious follicular opening like that seen in closed comedones.

ACNE SURGERY

Acne surgery is the manual removal of comedones and the drainage of pustules and cysts. When done correctly, acne surgery speeds resolution and rapidly enhances cosmetic appearance. Three instruments are used: the round loop comedone extractor; the oval loop acne extractor, or the Schamberg extractor; and the no. 11 pointed-tip scalpel blade.

COMEDONES

Removal of open comedones (blackheads) enhances the patient's appearance and discourages self-manipulation. By use of either type of extractor, most comedones can easily be expressed with uniform, smooth pressure. Lesions that offer resistance are loosened and sometimes disengaged by inserting the point of a no. 11 blade into the blackhead and elevating. The orifice of the closed comedone must be enlarged before pressure can be applied. Following the angle of the follicle, the scalpel point is inserted with the sharp edge up approximately 1 mm into the tiny orifice. The blade is drawn slightly forward and up, then pressure is applied with the extractor to remove the sometimes surprisingly large quantity of soft, white material. Macrocomedones (whiteheads, microcystic acne) can also be treated with light cautery.

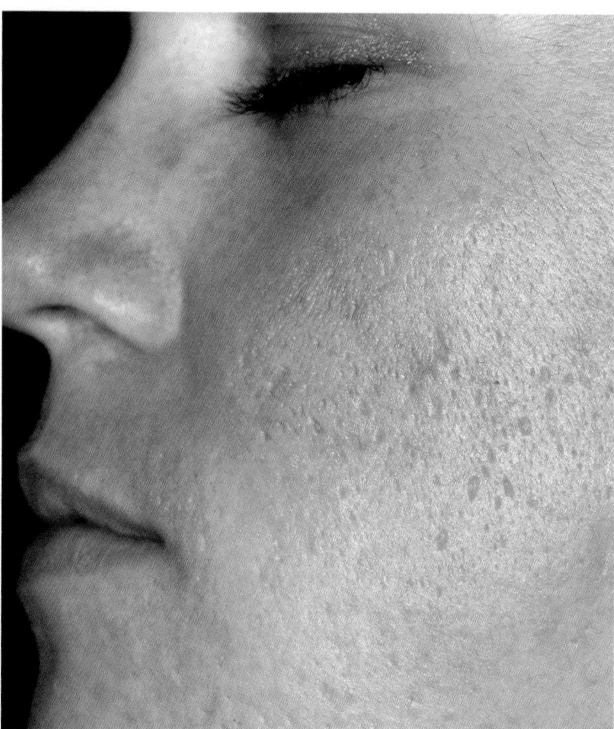

Figure 7-44Pitted acne scars. The dermatologic and plastic surgeons have a number of techniques (e.g., dermabrasion, punch grafting, laser resurfacing) for treating this difficult problem.

PUSTULES AND CYSTS

After the head of the white pustule is nicked with the no. 11 blade, pustules are easily drained by pressing the material with the acne extractor. Cysts are preferably managed by intralesional injection because incision and drainage may cause scarring. Pustules and cysts that have a thin, effaced roof in which fluid contents are easily felt are drained through a small incision by manual pressure. To prevent scarring, a short incision (approximately 3 mm) should be made. After drainage, a no. 1 curette may be inserted through the incision on the cyst to dislodge chunks of necrotic tissue.

SCAR REVISION

Many patients are very self-conscious about the pitted and craterlike scars (Figures 7-44 and 7-45) that remain as a permanent record of previous inflammation. Some people will endure any procedure and spare no expense to rid themselves of the most minute scar. Three scar types: icepick, rolling, and boxcar can form. *PMID: 11423843* Treatments include punch excision, punch elevation, subcutaneous incision (subcision), scar excision, and laser skin resurfacing. A dermatologic or plastic surgeon is best equipped to perform such procedures.

Generally, it is advisable to wait until disease activity has been low or absent for several months. Scars improve as they atrophy. The color contrast is often the most troublesome aspect of acne. Inflamed lesions may leave a flat or depressed red scar that is so obvious patients mistake the mark for an active lesion. The color will fade and approach skin tones in 4 to 12 months.

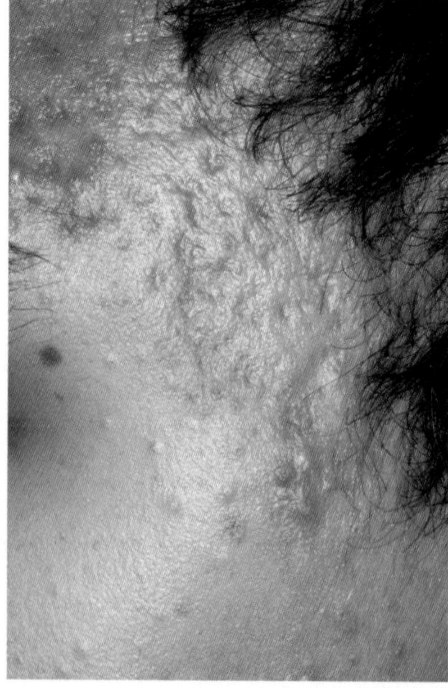

Figure 7-45 Craterlike scars are disfiguring and difficult to revise.

PERIORAL DERMATITIS

Perioral dermatitis is a distinctive eruption. It occurs in young women and resembles acne. Papules and pustules on an erythematous and sometimes scaling base are confined to the chin and nasolabial folds while sparing a clear zone around the vermilion border (Figures 7-46 and 7-47). There are varying degrees of involvement. Patients may develop a few pustules on the chin and nasolabial folds. These cases resemble acne. Pustules on the cheeks adjacent to the nostrils are highly characteristic initially (Figures 7-48 and 7-49), and sometimes the disease remains confined to this area. Pustules and papules may also be seen lateral to the eyes (Figure 7-50).

Perioral dermatitis has been reported in children and is a unique skin disorder of childhood. The age ranges from 7 months to 13 years. Boys and girls, blacks and whites are equally affected. There are perioral, perinasal, and periorbital flesh-colored or erythematous inflamed papules and micronodules. Pustules are rare. The disease waxes and wanes for weeks and months.

Prolonged use of fluorinated steroid creams (Figures 7-51 and 7-52) was thought to be the primary cause when this entity was described more than 35 years ago. However, in recent years, most women have denied using such creams. Perioral dermatitis occurs in an area where drying agents are poorly tolerated; topical preparations such as

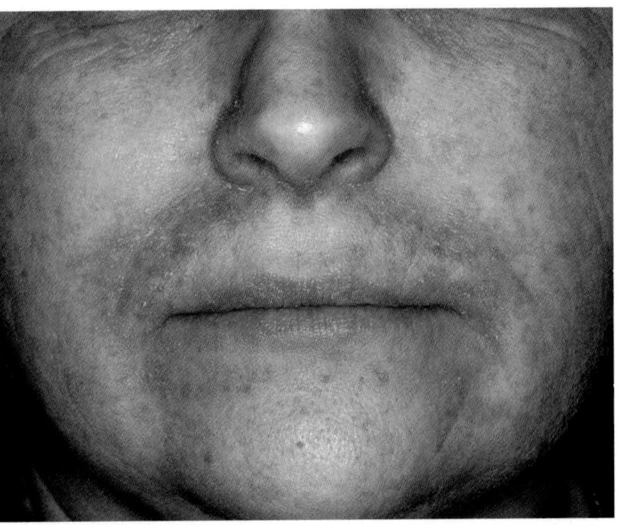

Figure 7-46 Perioral dermatitis. Classic presentation with relative sparing of the skin around the mouth.

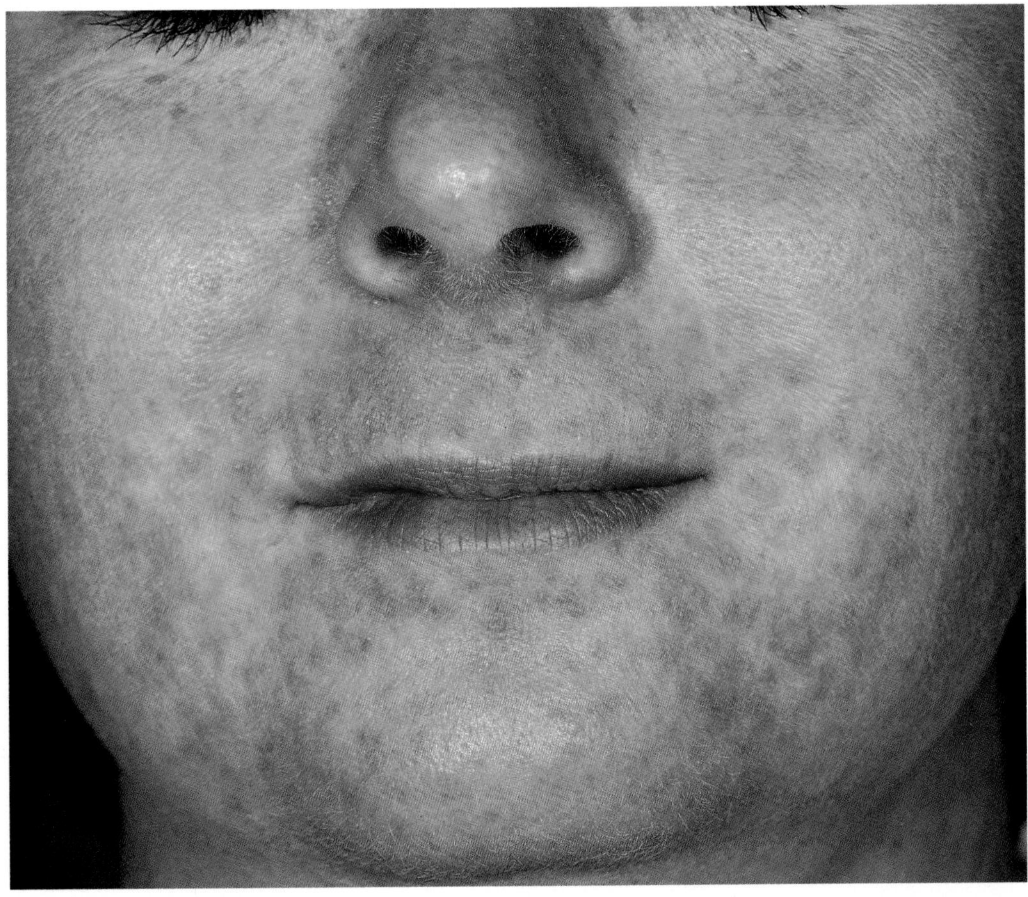

Figure 7-47 Perioral dermatitis. A florid case with numerous tiny papules and pustules located around the mouth.

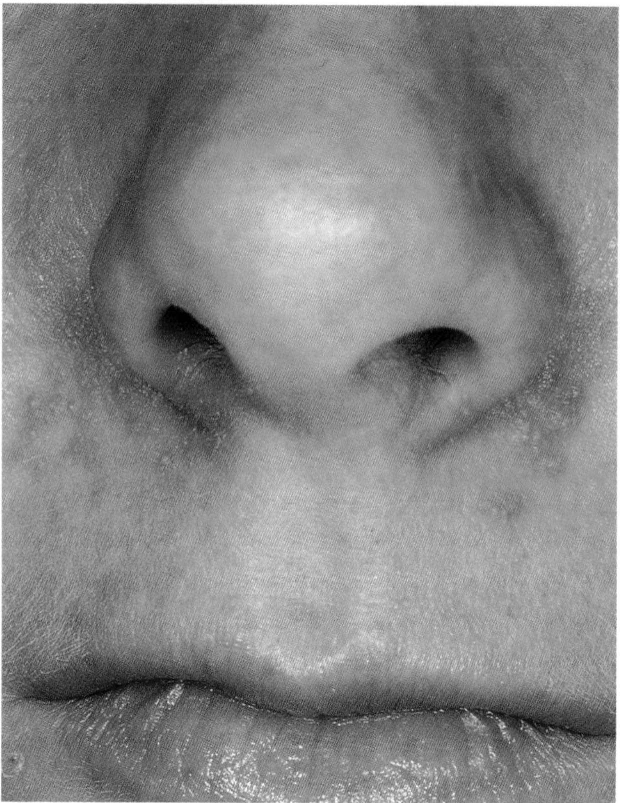

Figure 7-48 Perioral dermatitis. Pinpoint pustules next to the nostrils may be the first sign or the only manifestation of the disease.

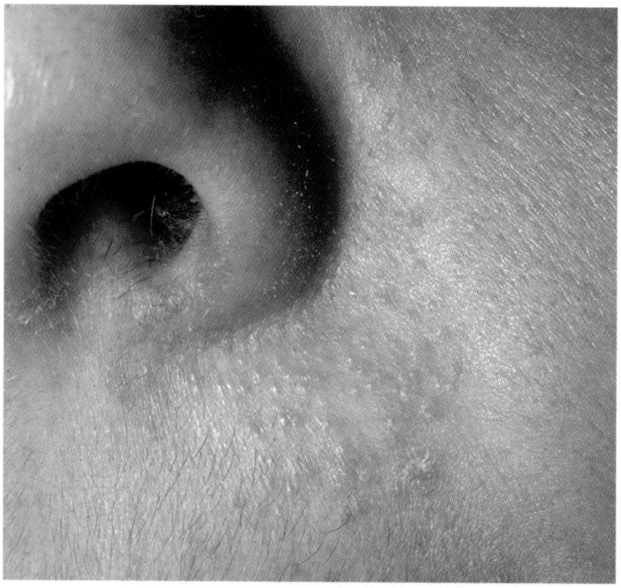

Figure 7-49 Pinpoint papules in a cluster next to the nostrils. These lesions resist topical therapy and often require short courses of oral antibiotics (e.g., tetracycline, doxycycline, minocycline, azithromycin) for control.

benzoyl peroxide, tretinoin, and alcohol-based antibiotic lotions aggravate the eruption.

The pathogenesis is unknown. A group of authors proposed that the dermatitis is a cutaneous intolerance reaction linked to constitutionally dry skin and often accompanied by a history of mild atopic dermatitis. It is precipitated by the habitual, regular, and abundant use of moisturizing creams. This results in persistent hydration of the horny layer, impairment of barrier function, and proliferation of the skin flora. Another study showed that application of foundation in addition to moisturizer and night cream resulted in a 13-fold increased risk for perioral dermatitis. The combination of moisturizer and foundation was associated with a lesser but significantly increased risk. Moisturizer alone was not associated with an increased risk. These findings suggest that cosmetic preparations play a vital role in the etiology of perioral dermatitis, perhaps by an occlusive mechanism.

TREATMENT. Perioral dermatitis uniformly responds in 2 to 4 weeks to 1 gm per day of tetracycline or erythromycin. Doxycycline 100 mg once or twice daily is also effective. Once cleared, the dosage may be stopped or tapered and discontinued in 4 to 5 weeks. Patients with renewed activity should have an additional course of antibiotics. Long-term maintenance therapy with oral antibiotics is sometimes required. Topical antibiotics are frequently prescribed but are not very effective. The twice-daily topical application of 1% metronidazole cream (MetroGel) reduces the number of papules, but oral antibiotics are more effective. Short courses of group VII nonfluorinated steroids, such as hydrocortisone, may occasionally be required to suppress erythema and scaling. Stronger steroids should be avoided. Pimecrolimus cream rapidly improves clinical symptoms and is most effective in corticosteroid-induced perioral dermatitis. *PMID: 18462835* Encourage patients to discontinue or limit the use of moisturizing creams and cosmetics.

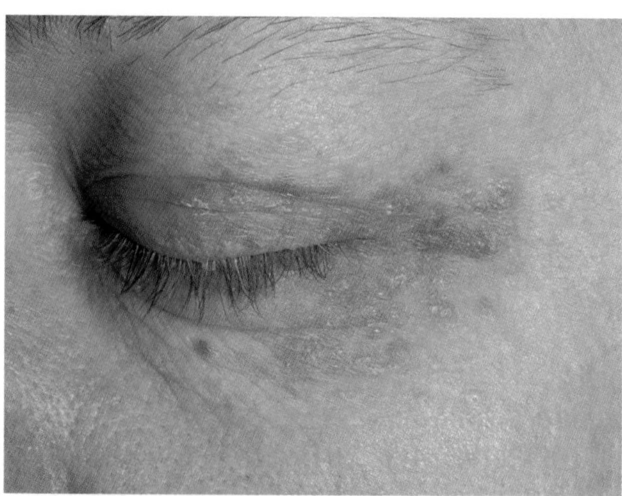

Figure 7-50 Grouped red papules may be found on the lateral portions of the lower lids.

PERIORAL DERMATITIS

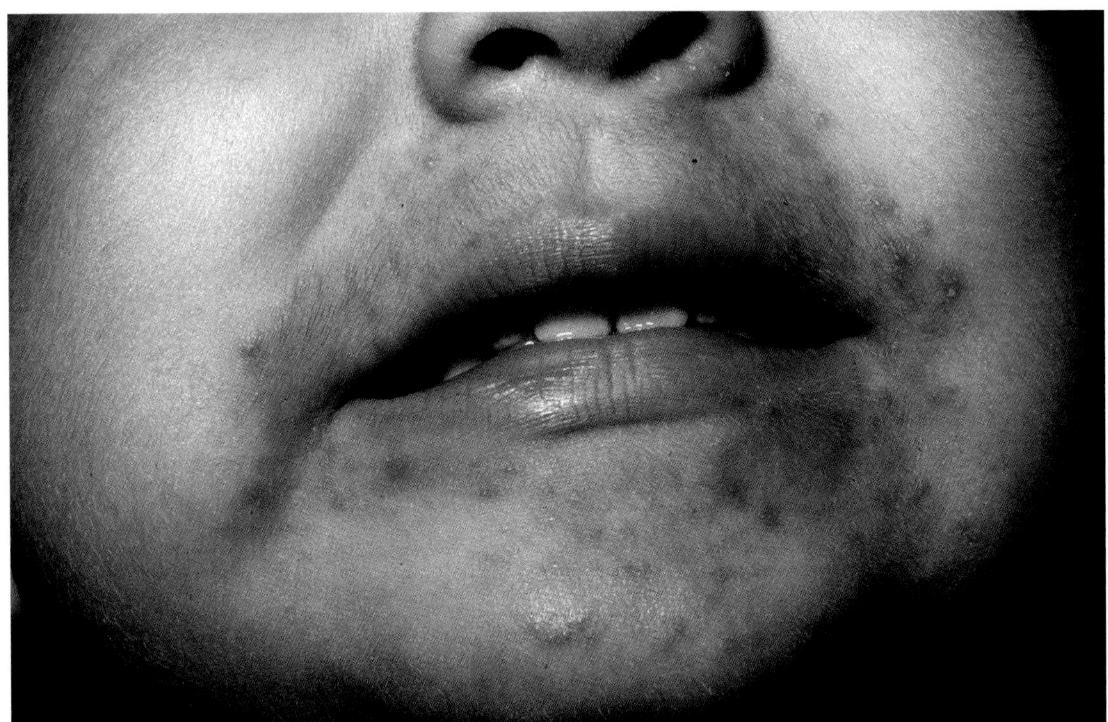

Figure 7-51 Perioral dermatitis in this infant was misdiagnosed as eczema and treated with topical steroids.

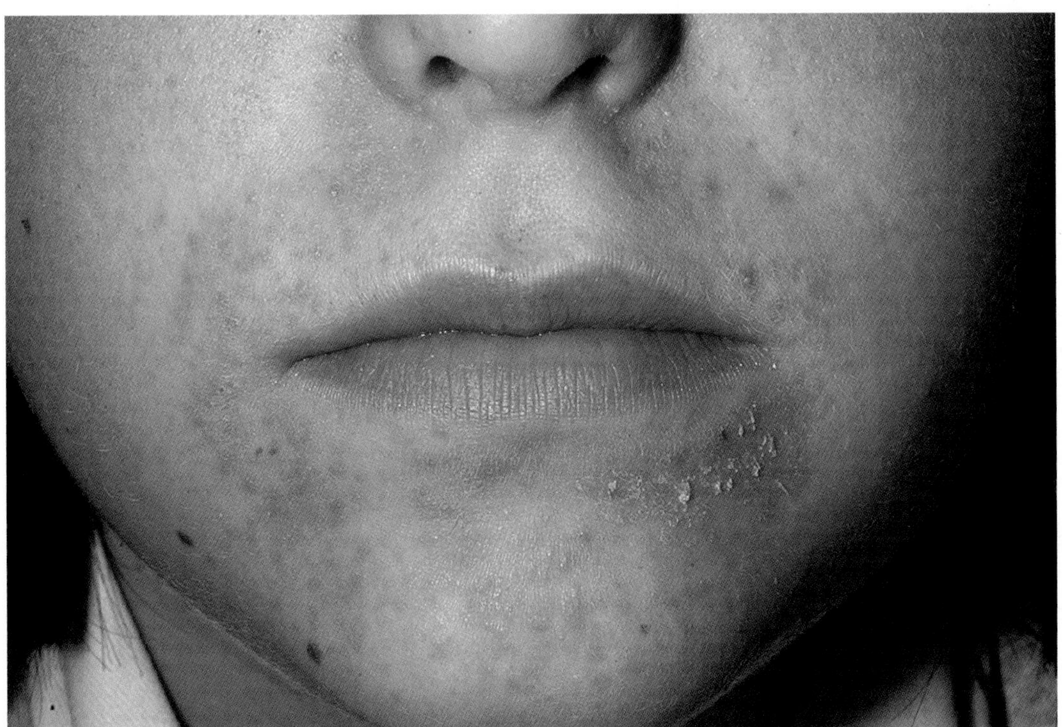

Figure 7-52 Perioral dermatitis. Self-treatment with a group I topical steroid once or twice a week for months resulted in the appearance of papules, pustules, scaling, and swelling. The flaring persisted for 8 weeks after stopping the steroid cream and did not respond to oral antibiotics.

ROSACEA (ACNE ROSACEA)

W.C. Fields drank excessively and had clusters of papules and pustules on red, swollen, telangiectatic skin of the cheeks and forehead. The red, bulbous nose completed the full-blown syndrome of active rosacea. Many patients with rosacea are defensive about their appearance and must explain to unbelieving friends that they do not imbibe. Rosacea with the same distribution and eye changes occurs in children but is rare. The etiology is unknown. Alcohol may accentuate erythema, but does not cause the disease. Sun exposure may precipitate acute episodes, but solar skin damage is not a necessary prerequisite for its development. Coffee and other caffeine-containing products once topped the list of forbidden foods in the arbitrarily conceived elimination diets previously recommended as a major part of the management of rosacea. It is the heat of coffee, not its caffeine content, that leads to flushing. Hot drinks of any type should be avoided. A significant increase in the hair follicle mite, *Demodex folliculorum,* is found in rosacea.

Mite counts before and after a 1-month course of oral tetracycline showed no significant difference. Increased mites may play a part in the pathogenesis of rosacea by provoking inflammatory or allergic reactions, by causing mechanical blockage of follicles, or by acting as vectors for microorganisms.

Skin Manifestations

Rosacea occurs after the age of 30 and is most common in people of Celtic origin. The resemblance to acne is at times striking. A classification system has been established (Box 7-4). The cardinal features are erythema and edema, papules and pustules, and telangiectasia (Figures 7-53 through 7-55). One or all of these features may be present. The disease is chronic, lasting for years, with episodes of activity followed by quiescent periods of variable length. Eruptions appear on the forehead, cheeks, nose, and occasionally about the eyes. Most patients have some erythema, with less than 10 papules and pustules at any one time. At the other end of the spectrum are those with numerous pustules, telangiectasia, diffuse erythema, oily skin, and edema, particularly of the cheeks and nose (Figure 7-56).

Granuloma formation occurs in some patients (granulomatous rosacea). It is characterized by hard papules or nodules that may be severe and lead to scarring. Chronic, deep inflammation of the nose leads to an irreversible hypertrophy called rhinophyma (Figure 7-57).

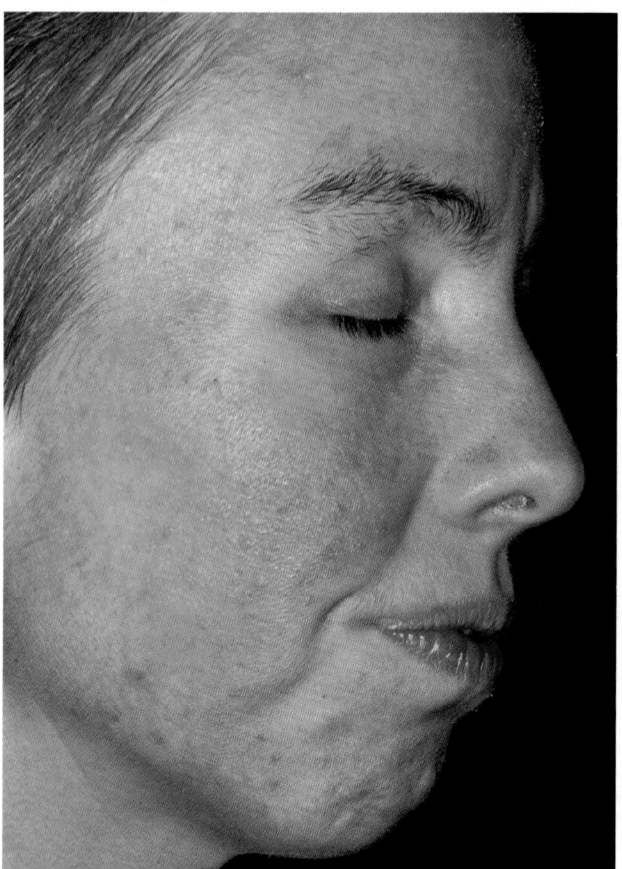

Figure 7-53 Rosacea. Persistent erythema, with a few pustules.

Box 7-4 **Guidelines for the Diagnosis of Rosacea**
Primary features (presence of one or more of the following)
Flushing (transient erythema)
Nontransient erythema
Papules and pustules
Telangiectasia
Secondary features (one or more of the following)
Burning or stinging
Plaque
Dry appearance
Edema
Ocular manifestations
Peripheral location
Phymatous changes

Adapted from Wilkin J et al: *J Am Acad Dermatol* 46:584, 2002. *PMID: 11907512*

ROSACEA

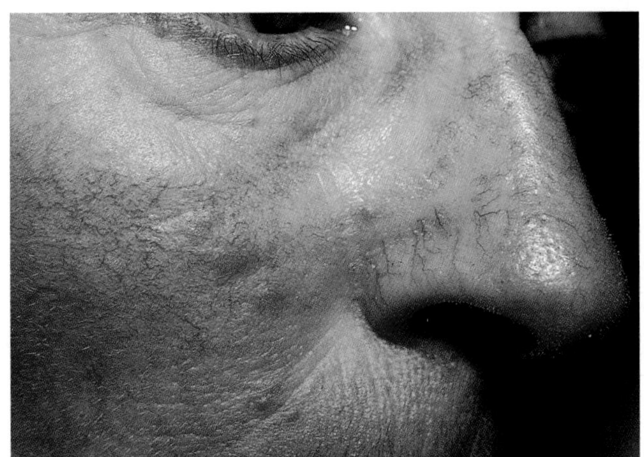

Figure 7-54 Rosacea. Telangiectasia is extensive. There were no papules or pustules. Oral or topical antibiotics will not affect telangiectasia. Laser surgery may provide a very satisfactory result.

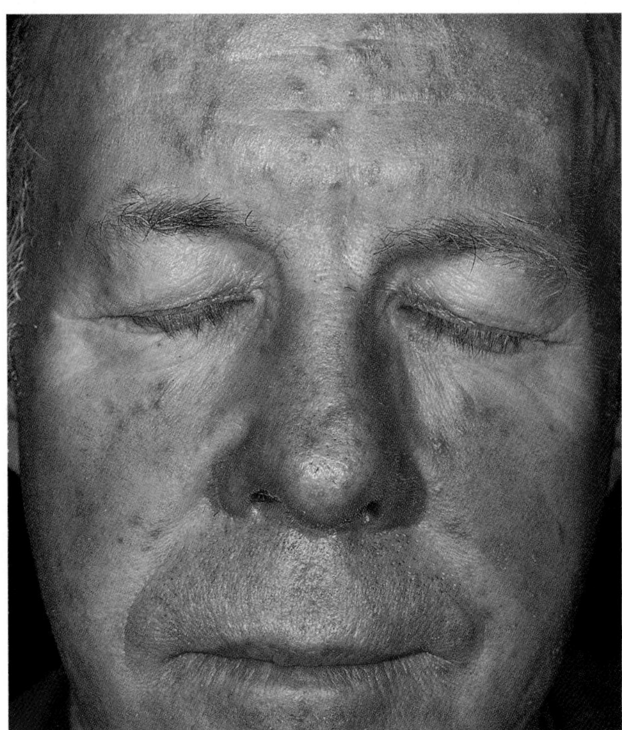

Figure 7-55 Rosacea. Pustules and erythema occur on the forehead, cheeks, and nose.

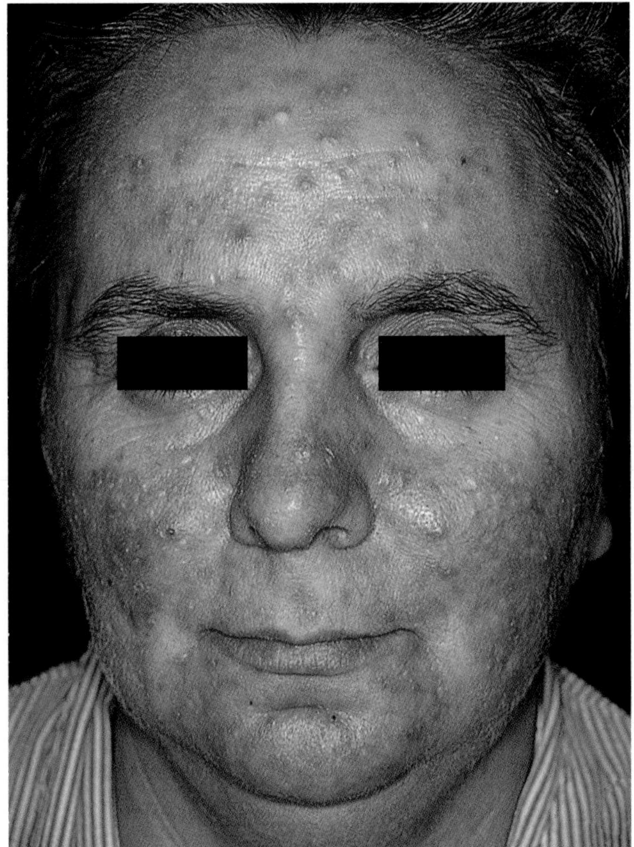

Figure 7-56 Severe rosacea. Oral antibiotics failed. Prednisone followed by isotretinoin cleared the eruption.

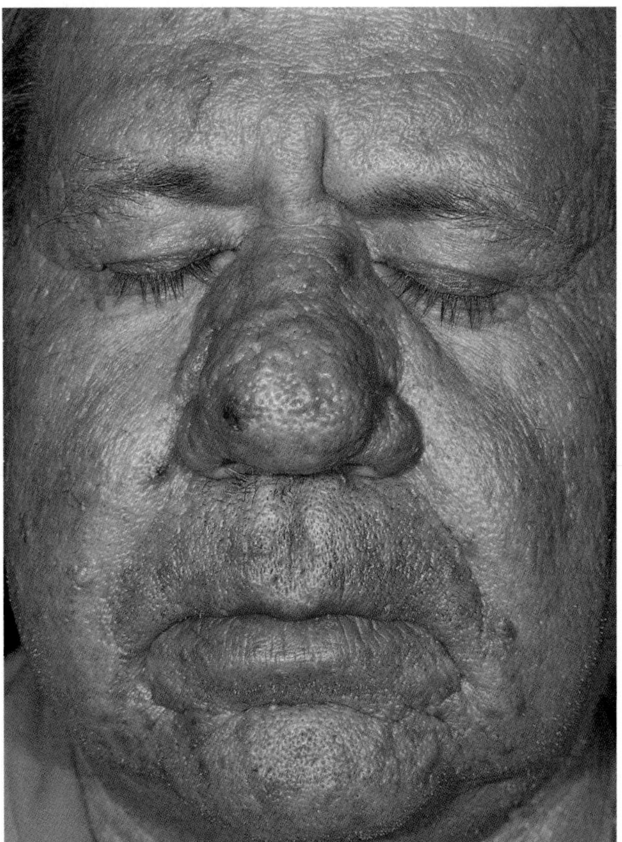

Figure 7-57 Rosacea and rhinophyma. Chronic rosacea of the nose has caused irreversible hypertrophy (rhinophyma).

TREATMENT

Oral antibiotics and isotretinoin. Both the skin and eye manifestations of rosacea respond to doxycycline (100 to 200 mg/day) or tetracycline or erythromycin (1 gm/day in divided doses). A 40-mg controlled-release formulation of doxycycline (Oracea) is reported effective when taken once each day. Some patients are not controlled with this subantimicrobial, antiinflammatory dosage of medication and need conventional dosages. Resistant cases can be treated with 100 to 200 mg/day of minocycline or with 200 mg of metronidazole twice daily. Azithromycin 500 mg on Monday, Wednesday, and Saturday in the first month; 250 mg on Monday, Wednesday, and Saturday in the second month; and 250 mg on Tuesday and Saturday in the third month were as effective as doxycycline. *PMID: 18289334* Medication is stopped when the pustules have cleared. The response after treatment is unpredictable. Some patients clear in 2 to 4 weeks and stay in remission for weeks or months. Others flare and require long-term suppression with oral antibiotics. Treatment should be tapered to the minimum dosage that provides adequate control. Patients who remain clear should periodically be given a trial without medication. However, many patients promptly revert to the low-dose oral regimen. Isotretinoin, 0.5 mg/kg/day for 20 weeks, was effective in treating severe, refractory rosacea; 85% had no relapse at the end of 1 year. Patients resistant to conventional treatment were treated with oral isotretinoin, 10 mg/day, for 16 weeks. Papular and pustular lesions, telangiectasia, and erythema were significantly reduced at the end of 16 weeks.

TOPICAL THERAPY

Patients with mild, moderate, or severe rosacea may respond to 0.75% metronidazole (MetroGel) applied twice each day or 1% metronidazole applied once each day. Topical metronidazole may be used for initial treatment for mild cases or for maintenance after stopping oral antibiotics. The acne medications benzoyl peroxide 5%/erythromycin 3% gel, benzoyl peroxide 5%/clindamycin 1% gel, and benzoyl peroxide alone are effective. Clindamycin in a lotion base is less effective. Sulfacetamide/sulfur lotion (Sulfacet-R, Plexion TS, Rosula) controls pustules. They are effective alone or when used with oral antibiotics. Azelaic acid 20% cream or 15% gel applied once or twice each day is effective and well tolerated in the treatment of papulopustular rosacea. Pimecrolimus 1% cream is effective for steroid-induced rosacea. *PMID: 18363758* Oxymetazoline (Afrin nasal spray), a potent vasoconstrictor applied once each day to two patients with flushing and persistent erythema, provided a durable improvement in the erythema, a marked decrease of erythematous flares, and relief from stinging and burning. *PMID: 18025359*

General management guidelines. Sunscreens are important for this sun-aggravated disease. Special cosmetics can conceal the redness (e.g., green-tinted makeup). Avoid overly strenuous exercise, alcohol, hot beverages, and hot meals. Do not use abrasive cleansers.

Patients with rhinophyma may benefit from specialized procedures performed by plastic or dermatologic surgeons. These include electrosurgery, carbon dioxide laser, and surgery. Unsightly telangiectatic vessels can be eliminated with careful electrocautery or laser.

Ocular rosacea

Ocular rosacea is a common disease. It is widely underdiagnosed by providers. Manifestations of this disease range from minor to severe (Box 7-5). Symptoms frequently go undiagnosed because they are too nonspecific. The prevalence in patients with rosacea is as high as 58%, with approximately 20% of those patients developing ocular symptoms before the skin lesions. The diagnosis should be considered when a patient's eyes have one or more of the signs and symptoms listed in Box 7-5.

A common presentation is a patient with mild conjunctivitis with soreness, foreign body sensation, and burning, grittiness, and lacrimation. Patients with ocular rosacea have been reported to have subnormal tear production (dry eyes), and they frequently have complaints of burning that are out of proportion to the clinical signs of disease. The reported signs are conjunctival hyperemia (86%), telangiectasia of the lid (63%), blepharitis (47%) (Figure 7-58), superficial punctate keratopathy (41%), chalazion (22%), corneal vascularization and infiltrate (16%), and corneal vascularization and thinning (10%). Visual acuity less than 20/400 may result from long-standing disease. Conjunctival epithelium is infiltrated by chronic inflammatory cells. Doxycycline, 100 mg daily, will improve ocular disease and increase the tear breakup time.

TREATMENT. Artificial tears, eyelid hygiene (i.e., cleaning the lids with warm water twice daily), and metronidazole gel applied to lid margins are used to treat mild ocular rosacea. Doxycycline 100 mg daily improves dryness, itching, blurred vision, and photosensitivity.

Box 7-5 **Ocular Rosacea: Signs and Symptoms**
Watery or bloodshot appearance (interpalpebral conjunctival hyperemia)
Foreign body sensation
Burning or stinging
Dryness
Itching
Light sensitivity
Blurred vision
Telangiectases of conjunctiva and lid margin
Lid and periocular erythema
Blepharitis, conjunctivitis, and irregularity of eyelid margins
Chalazion
Hordeolum (stye)
Decreased visual acuity
Punctate keratitis
Corneal infiltrates/ulcers
Marginal keratitis

Adapted from Wilkin J et al: *J Am Acad Dermatol* 46:584, 2002. *PMID: 11907512*

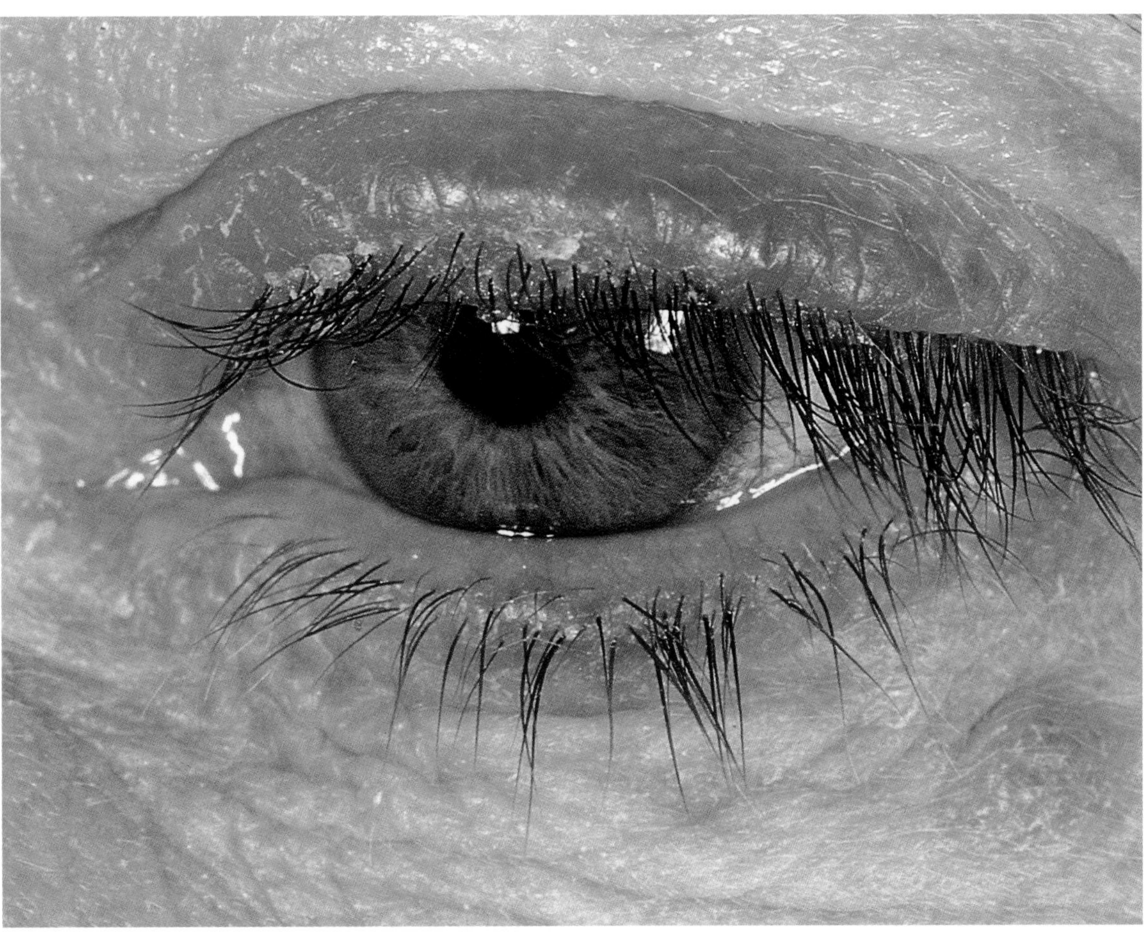

Figure 7-58 Ocular rosacea. The patient has conjunctivitis, soreness, and blepharitis.

HIDRADENITIS SUPPURATIVA

Hidradenitis suppurativa (acne inversa) is a chronic suppurative and scarring disease of the skin and subcutaneous tissue occurring in the axillae, the anogenital regions, and under the female breast (Figures 7-59 through 7-64). Those patients who gain weight will often develop lesions between newly formed folds of fat. There is great variation in clinical severity. Many cases, especially of the thighs and vulva, are mild and misdiagnosed as recurrent furunculosis. The disease is worse in the obese. Inflammatory arthropathy may occur in patients with hidradenitis suppurativa and acne conglobata.

Clinical presentation

A hallmark of hidradenitis is the double comedone—a blackhead with two or sometimes several surface openings that communicate under the skin (Figures 7-62 and 7-64). This distinctive lesion may be present for years before other symptoms appear. Unlike acne, once the disease begins it becomes progressive and self-perpetuating. Extensive, deep, dermal inflammation results in large, painful abscesses (Figures 7-59 and 7-63). The healing process permanently alters the dermis. Cordlike bands of scar tissue crisscross the axillae and groin (Figure 7-59). Reepithelialization leads to meandering, epithelial-lined sinus tracts in which foreign material and bacteria become trapped. A sinus tract may be small and misinterpreted as a cystic lesion. The course varies among individuals from an occasional cyst in the axillae to diffuse abscess formation in the inguinal region.

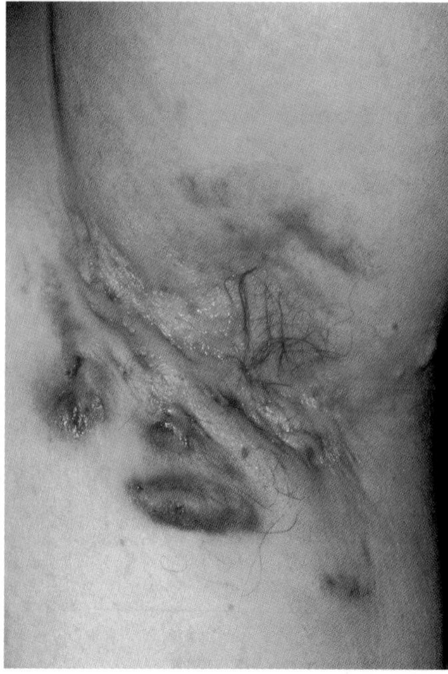

Figure 7-59 Years of inflammation in the axillae has resulted in several band-like scars.

Pathogenesis

Lesions begin with follicular hyperkeratosis and comedo formation and progress to rupture of the follicular infundibulum, with inflammation of the surrounding dermis. A granulomatous infiltrate forms with further local inflammation causing abscess formation and apocrinitis as the inflammation spreads. Early lesions show follicular occlusion with sparing of apocrine glands.

The disease does not appear until after puberty, and most cases develop in the second and third decades of life. Studies show clustering in families. A familial form with autosomal dominant inheritance has been described. As with acne, there may be an excessive rate of conversion of androgens within the gland to a more active androgen metabolite or an exaggerated response of the gland to a given hormonal stimulus.

Hidradenitis is part of the rare follicular occlusion triad syndrome of acne conglobata, hidradenitis suppurativa, and dissecting cellulitis of the scalp.

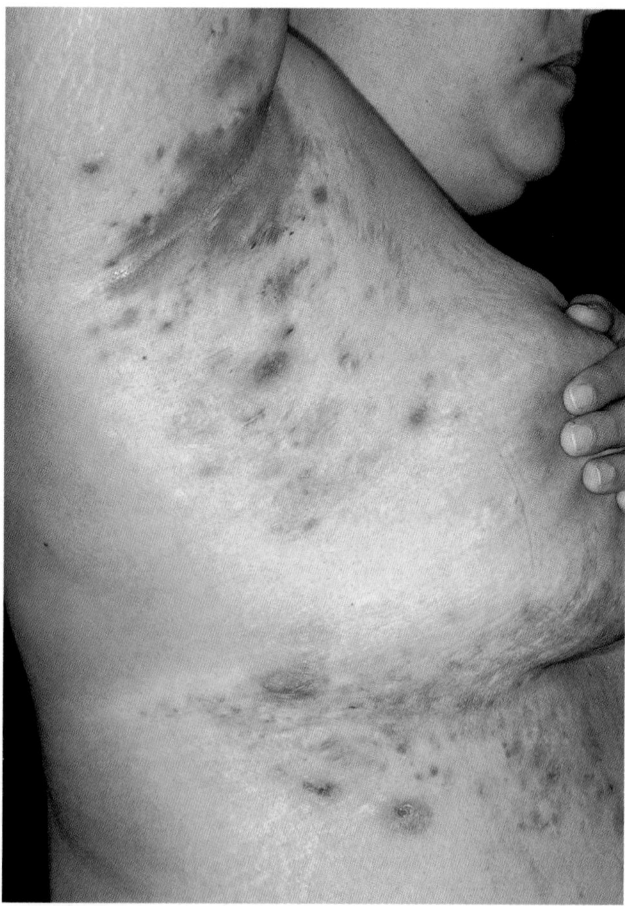

Figure 7-60 Hidradenitis suppurativa. An extensive case with cysts and postinflammatory hyperpigmentation.

HIDRADENITIS

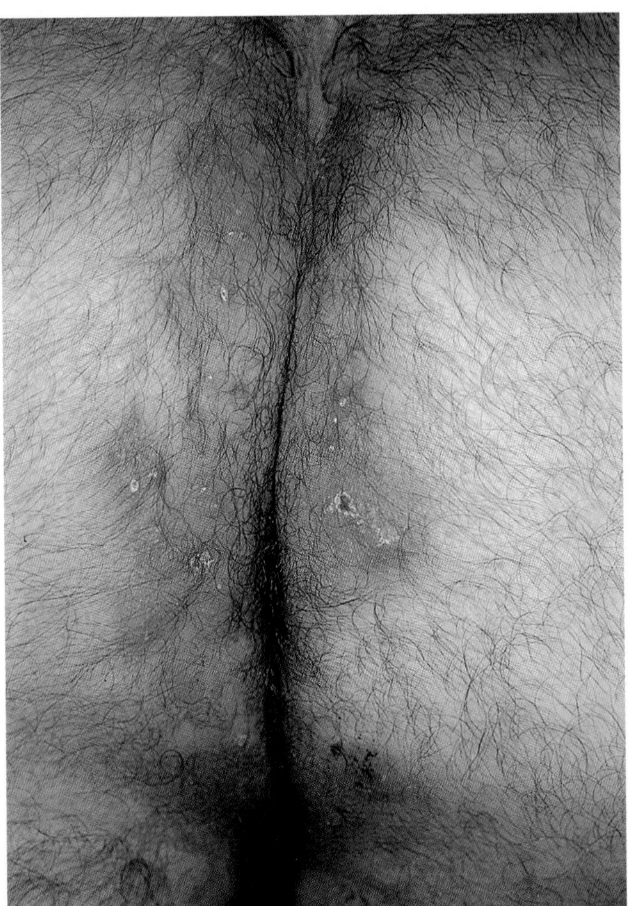

Figure 7-61 Hidradenitis suppurativa on buttocks. Extensive confluent cysts.

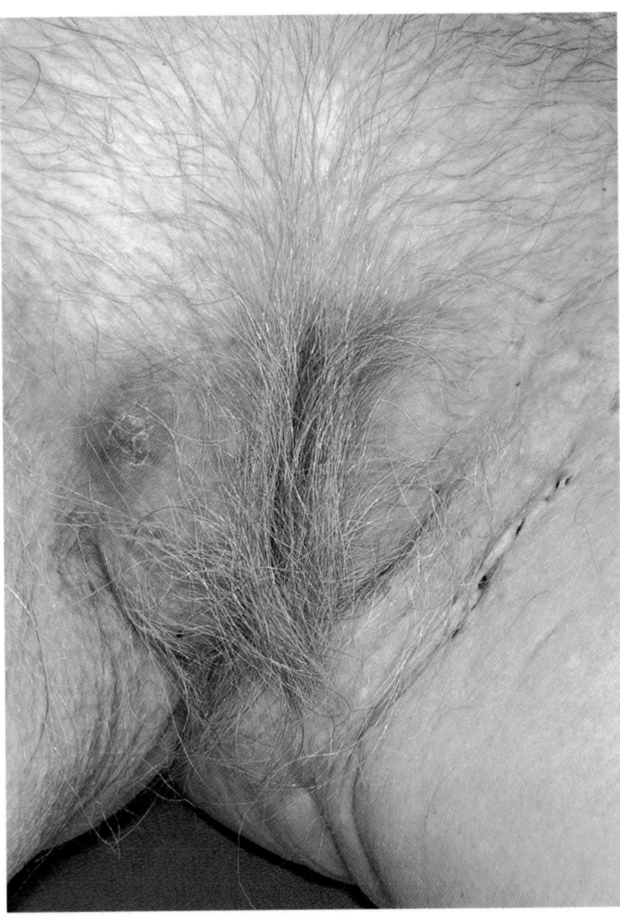

Figure 7-62 Hidradenitis suppurativa. Linear scars and comedones are present in the right groin.

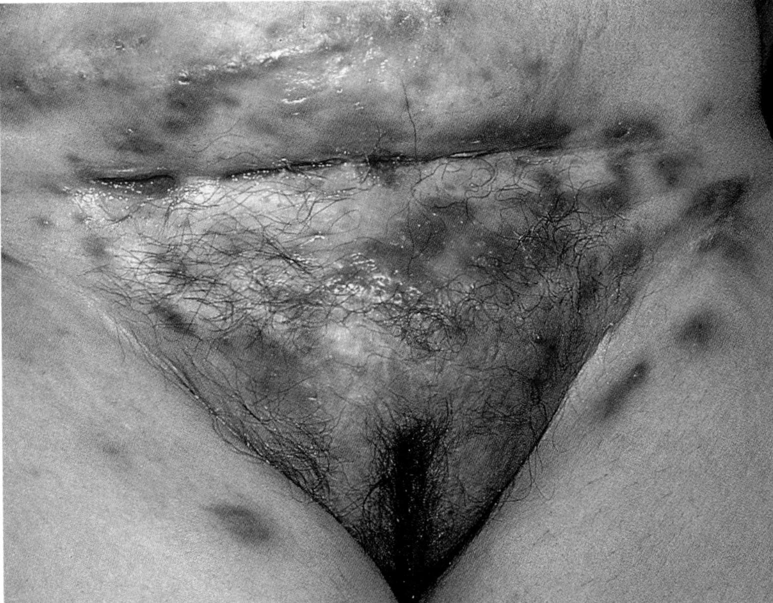

Figure 7-63 The disease may remain localized or involve large areas of the groin or anal area. The inflammation in this case is severe.

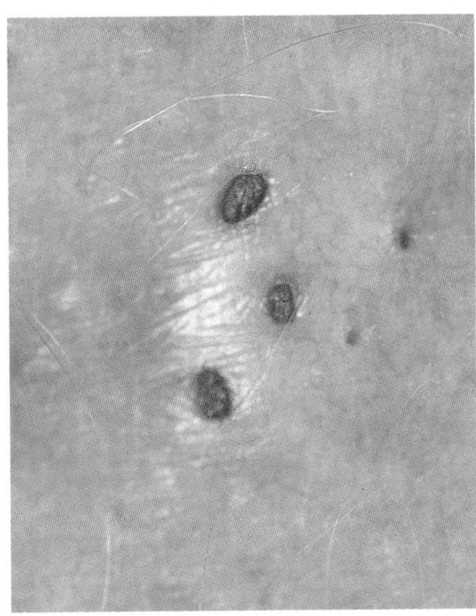

Figure 7-64 A hallmark of hidradenitis is the double and triple comedone, a blackhead with two or sometimes several surface openings that communicate under the skin.

Management

Antiperspirants, shaving, chemical depilatories, and talcum powder are probably not responsible for the initiation of the disease. Tretinoin cream (0.05%) may prevent duct occlusion, but it is irritating and must be used only as tolerated. Large cysts should be incised and drained, whereas smaller cysts respond to intralesional injections of triamcinolone acetonide (Kenalog 2.5 to 10 mg/ml). Weight loss helps to reduce activity.

Actively discharging lesions should be cultured. Repeated bacteriologic assessment is advisable in all cases. The laboratory should be instructed to look specifically for sensitivity to erythromycin and tetracycline in particular. Oral contraceptives do not seem to work nearly as well as they do with acne.

Cigarette smoking has been identified as a major triggering factor. Smoking cessation should be encouraged. It is unknown whether this improves the course of the disease.

ANTIBIOTICS

Antibiotics are the mainstay of treatment, especially for the early stages of the disease. Long-term oral antibiotics such as tetracycline (500 mg twice daily), erythromycin (500 mg twice daily), doxycycline (100 mg twice daily), or minocycline (100 mg twice daily) may prevent disease activation. High dosages are effective for active disease. Lower doses may be effective for maintenance once control is established. A 10-week course of 300 mg of clindamycin twice daily and 300 mg of rifampicin twice daily resulted in remissions of up to 1 to 4 years. *PMID: 16634904* The major side effect is diarrhea.

ISOTRETINOIN

Isotretinoin (1 mg/kg/day for 20 weeks) may be effective in selected cases. The response is variable and unpredictable, and complete suppression or prolonged remission is uncommon. Early cases with only inflammatory cystic lesions in which undermining sinus tracts have not developed have the best chance of being controlled, but severe cases have also responded.

Monotherapy with isotretinoin has a limited therapeutic effect. Retrospective data of patients treated with isotretinoin for 4 to 6 months were analyzed. In 23.5% of the patients, the condition completely cleared during initial therapy and 16.2% maintained their improvement. Treatment was more successful in the milder forms of the disease.

TUMOR NECROSIS FACTOR-α BLOCKERS

There are several reports infliximab is an effective treatment in severe hidradenitis suppurativa. Others show that variable and partial responses are not sustained and that consecutive courses of infliximab provide initial improvement with variable results but show decreased efficacy over long-term treatment. *PMID: 18627370*

Other treatments. Dapsone is reported effective and particularly useful for women of child-bearing age. *PMID: 16971313* Cyclosporin was effective in a single case. *PMID: 16309527* Seven patients (five women and two men) were treated with finasteride at a dose of 5 mg/day as monotherapy was effective. Two women complained of breast enlargement. *PMID: 16019620*

ELECTROSURGERY

A surgical method of excision of the areas with nodules and sinuses, up to the level of subcutaneous fat tissue, and leaving the surgical defect for secondary healing is effective for localized disease. Early intervention increases the success rate. The skin above the lesion is grasped with the forceps and slightly elevated. A loop electrode in the cut and coagulation mode is used to excise all the elevated skin and the subcutaneous tissue to the level of subcutaneous fat tissue. The defect is left for secondary healing; suturing is not performed. The defect is closed with a bandage, using mupirocin cream, and then changed twice daily. In contrast to wide excision, excision with electrosurgery provides a small tissue defect. Lesions heal leaving slightly depressed scars. *PMID: 18093196*

SURGERY

Surgical excision is at times the only solution. Residual lesions, particularly indolent sinus tracts, are a source of recurrent inflammation. Local excision is often followed by recurrence.

Early radical excision is the treatment of choice for some cases. Primary closure results in a recurrence rate in up to 70% of patients. There were no recurrence, no serious complications, and no revision operations in patients treated aggressively by radical excision of all hair-bearing areas and reconstructed with a graft or a flap. *PMID: 15789789*

MILIARIA

Miliaria, or heat rash, is a common phenomenon occurring in predisposed individuals during periods of exertion or heat exposure. Eccrine sweat duct occlusion is the initial event. The duct ruptures, leaks sweat into the surrounding tissues, and induces an inflammatory response. Occlusion occurs at three different levels to produce three distinct forms of miliaria. The papular and vesicular lesions that resemble pustules of folliculitis have one major distinguishing feature: They are not follicular and therefore do not have a penetrating hair shaft. Follicular pustules are likely to be infectious, whereas nonfollicular papules, vesicles, and pustules, such as those seen in miliaria, are usually noninfectious.

Miliaria crystallina

In miliaria crystallina (Figure 7-65), occlusion of the eccrine duct at the skin surface results in accumulation of sweat under the stratum corneum. The sweat-filled vesicle is so near the skin surface that it appears as a clear dew drop. There is little or no erythema and the lesions are asymptomatic. The vesicles appear individually or in clusters and are most frequently seen in infants or bedridden, overheated patients. Rupture of a vesicle produces a drop of clear fluid. A cool water compress and proper ventilation are all that is necessary to treat this self-limited process.

Miliaria rubra

Miliaria rubra (prickly heat, heat rash) (Figure 7-66), the most common of the sweat-retention diseases, results from occlusion of the intraepidermal section of the eccrine sweat duct. Papules and vesicles surrounded by a red halo or diffuse erythema develop as the inflammatory response develops. Instead of itching, the eruption is accompanied by a stinging or "prickling" sensation. The eruption occurs underneath clothing or in areas prone to sweating after exertion or overheating; the palms and soles are spared. The disease is usually self-limited, but some patients never adapt to hot climates and must therefore make a geographic change to aid their condition.

Treatment consists of removing the patient to a cool, air-conditioned area. Frequent application of a mild anti-inflammatory lotion (e.g., desonide lotion) relieves symptoms and shortens the duration of inflammation.

Miliaria profunda

Miliaria profunda is observed in the tropics in patients who have had several bouts of miliaria rubra. Occlusion of the dermal section of the eccrine duct is followed by a white papular eruption. Anhydrous lanolin and isotretinoin are described as effective treatment.

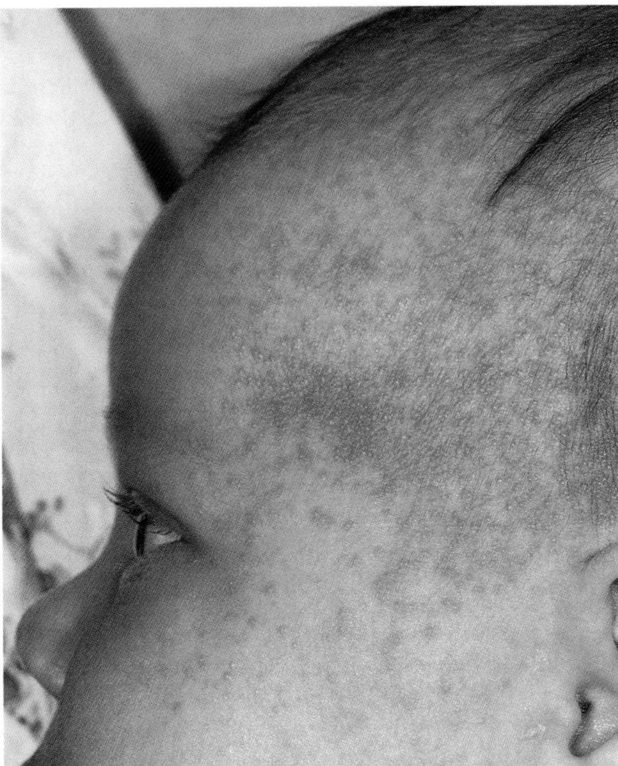

Figure 7-65 Miliaria crystallina. Eccrine sweat duct occlusion at the skin surface results in a cluster of vesicles filled with clear fluid.

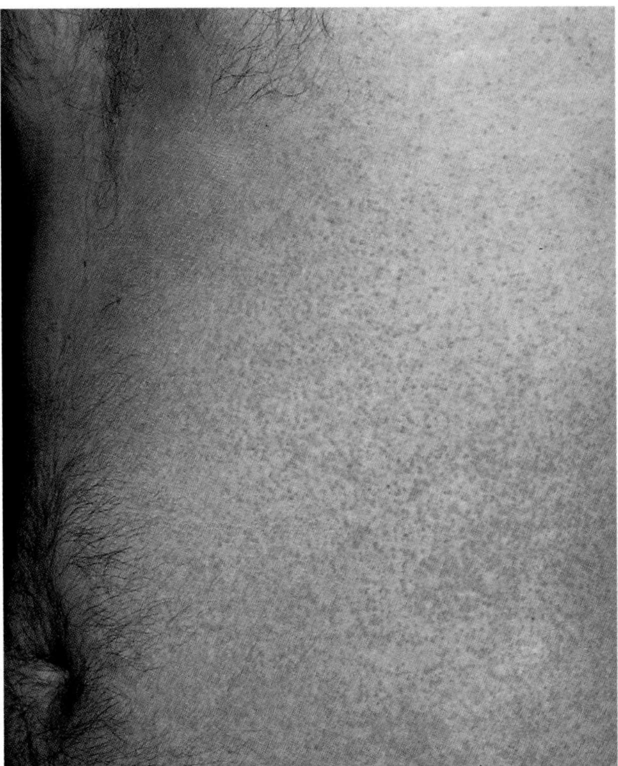

Figure 7-66 Miliaria (prickly heat). A diffuse eruption of tiny papules and vesicles occurs after exertion or overheating.

Chapter 8

Psoriasis and Other Papulosquamous Diseases

CHAPTER CONTENTS

Papulosquamous diseases are a group of disorders characterized by scaly papules and plaques. These entities have little in common except the clinical characteristics of their primary lesion. A complete list of diseases characterized by scaly plaques appears in the section on primary lesions in Chapter 1. The major papulosquamous diseases are described here.

PSORIASIS

Psoriasis occurs in 1% to 3% of the population. The disease is transmitted genetically, most likely with a dominant mode with variable penetrance; the origin is unknown. The disease is lifelong and characterized by chronic, recurrent exacerbations and remissions that are emotionally and physically debilitating.

There may be many millions of people with the potential to develop psoriasis, with only the correct combination of environmental factors needed to precipitate the disease. Stress, for example, may precipitate an episode. Environmental influences may modify the course and severity of disease. Extent and severity of the disease vary widely. Psoriasis frequently begins in childhood, when the first episode may be stimulated by streptococcal pharyngitis (as in guttate psoriasis).

Pathogenesis

Psoriasis is a genetic disease of dysregulated inflammation. The mechanism of inheritance is not completely defined.

Psoriasis is an immune-mediated skin and/or joint inflammatory disease in which intralesional inflammation primes basal stem keratinocytes to hyperproliferate. The efficacy of immunosuppressive drugs such as methotrexate, cyclosporine, and tumor necrosis factor (TNF)-blocking biologics in treating psoriasis suggests that psoriasis involves immunologic mechanisms. Resolution of psoriasis is associated with decreased lesional infiltration of T cells, dermal dendritic cells, Langerhans cells, and neutrophils, and decreased expression of TNF-α-, interferon-γ-, and IL-12/23-dependent genes. Environmental factors also play a role in the pathogenesis of psoriasis, including drugs, skin trauma (Koebner phenomenon), infection, and stress.

"THE HEARTBREAK OF PSORIASIS." Psoriasis for most patients is more emotionally than physically disabling. Psoriasis erodes the self-image and forces the victim into a life of concealment and self-consciousness. Patients may avoid activities, including sunbathing, the very activity that can clear the disease, for fear of being discovered. Therefore even when a patient has only a few asymptomatic, chronic plaques, the disease is more serious than it appears.

Clinical manifestations

The lesions of psoriasis are distinctive. They begin as red, scaling papules that coalesce to form round-to-oval plaques, which can easily be distinguished from the surrounding normal skin (Figure 8-1). The scale is adherent and silvery white, and reveals bleeding points when removed (Auspitz sign). Scale may become extremely dense, especially on the scalp. Scale forms but is macerated and dispersed in intertriginous areas; therefore the psoriatic plaques of skin folds appear as smooth, red plaques with a macerated surface. The most common site for an intertriginous plaque is the intergluteal fold; this is referred to as gluteal pinking (Figure 8-2). The deep, rich red color is another characteristic feature and remains constant in all areas.

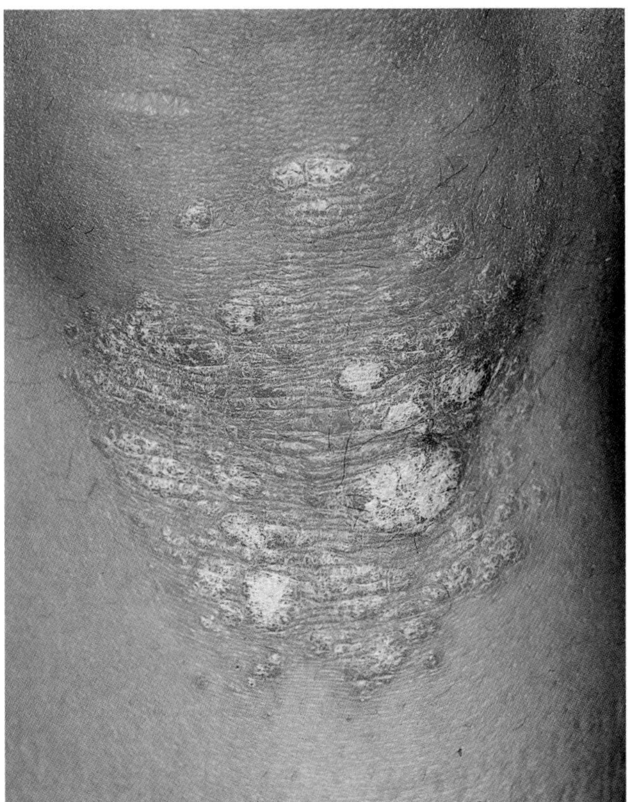

Figure 8-1 Psoriasis. Typical oval plaque with well-defined borders and silvery scale.

Psoriasis can develop at the site of physical trauma (scratching, sunburn, or surgery), the so-called isomorphic or Koebner phenomenon (Figure 8-3; see also Figures 8-8 and 8-10). Pruritus is highly variable. Although psoriasis can affect any cutaneous surface, certain areas are favored and should be examined in all patients in whom the diagnosis of psoriasis is suspected. Those areas are the elbows, knees, scalp, gluteal cleft, fingernails, and toenails.

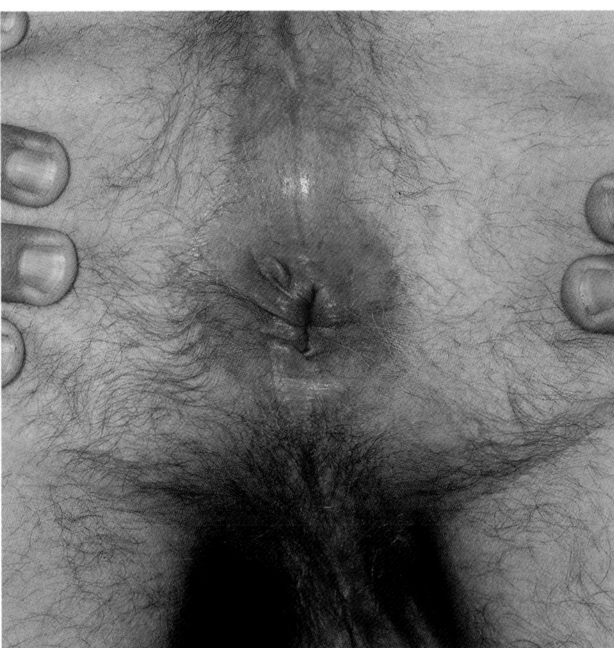

Figure 8-2 Psoriasis. Gluteal pinking, a common lesion in patients with psoriasis. Intertriginous psoriatic plaques retain the rich red color typical of skin lesions but do not retain scale.

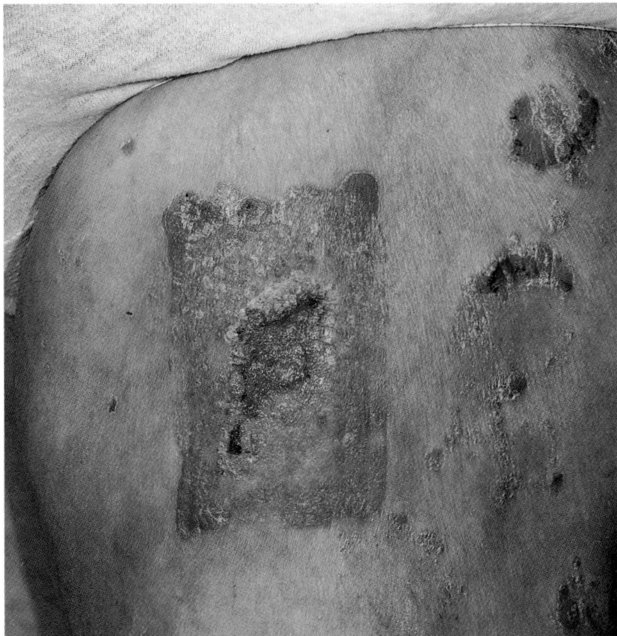

Figure 8-3 Psoriasis. Koebner phenomenon. Psoriasis has appeared on the donor site of the skin graft.

The disease affects the extensor more than the flexor surfaces and usually spares the palms, soles, and face. Most patients have chronic localized disease, but there are several other presentations. Localized plaques may be confused with eczema or seborrheic dermatitis, and the guttate form with many small lesions can resemble secondary syphilis or pityriasis rosea.

DRUGS THAT PRECIPITATE OR EXACERBATE PSORIASIS

LITHIUM. Exacerbation of preexisting psoriasis during lithium treatment is well documented, but preexisting psoriasis is not a general contraindication to lithium treatment. The disease does not worsen in many lithium-treated patients. Lithium dosage reduction or more intensive psoriasis treatment is indicated when lithium must be continued.

BETA-BLOCKING AGENTS. Beta-blockers may worsen psoriasis and should be carefully evaluated in the management of these patients.

ANTIMALARIAL AGENTS. Exfoliative dermatitis and exacerbation of psoriasis are reported in psoriatic patients treated with antimalarials, but the incidence is low. Antimalarials are not contraindicated in psoriasis patients who need prophylactic treatment for malaria.

SYSTEMIC STEROIDS. Systemic steroids rapidly clear psoriasis; unfortunately, in many instances the disease worsens, occasionally evolving into pustular psoriasis when corticosteroids are withdrawn. For this reason systemic corticosteroids have been abandoned as a routine treatment for psoriasis.

Box 8-1 **Medical Comorbidities Associated with Psoriasis**

Autoimmune diseases	Crohn's disease and ulcerative colitis are 3.8 to 7.5 times more likely to occur in patients with psoriasis. Psoriasis occurs more commonly in families of patients with multiple sclerosis (MS).
Cardiovascular disease	There is an increased risk of cardiovascular disease in patients with psoriasis. Patients with psoriasis are more frequently overweight, have an increased incidence of diabetes, have an increased incidence of hypertension, and have an atherogenic lipoprotein profile at the onset of psoriasis with significantly higher very-low-density lipoprotein cholesterol levels and high-density lipoprotein levels. Patients with psoriasis have a higher than normal incidence of myocardial infarction. Treatment with systemic agents may decrease the cardiovascular mortality.
Metabolic syndrome	The combination of obesity, impaired glucose regulation, hypertriglyceridemia, reduced high-density lipoprotein, and hypertension is known as metabolic syndrome. The prevalence of metabolic syndrome in hospitalized patients with psoriasis is significantly elevated.
Lymphoma and nonmelanoma skin cancer	There may be a 1.34- to 3-fold increased relative risk of developing any type of lymphoma. Medications with a known risk of lymphoma might be a potential confounding factor. Caucasians who have received more than 250 psoralen plus UVA (PUVA) treatments have a 14-fold higher risk of cutaneous squamous cell carcinoma.
Depression/suicide	The prevalence of depression in patients with psoriasis may be as high as 60%. Some patients will contemplate suicide. Treatments may decrease depression.
Psychologic and emotional burden of psoriasis	There are elevated rates of poor self-esteem, sexual dysfunction, and anxiety.
Smoking	The Utah Psoriasis Initiative revealed that 37% of patients with psoriasis were smokers versus 13% smokers in the general population. Among patients with psoriasis who smoke, 78% started smoking before the onset of their psoriasis and 22% of patients started after the onset.
Alcohol	The prevalence of psoriasis is increased among patients who abuse alcohol. Whether increased alcohol intake in patients with psoriasis is a factor in the pathogenesis or whether having a chronic disorder such as psoriasis leads to greater intake of alcohol is not known.
Obesity	The Utah Psoriasis Initiative revealed that patients with psoriasis had a significantly higher body mass index (BMI) than control subjects in the general Utah population.
Quality of life	Psoriasis causes psychosocial morbidity and decrement in occupational function. The impact may be large even in patients with small areas of involvement. Psoriasis of the palms and soles tends to have more impact than far more extensive involvement on the trunk. Therefore patients with these types of psoriasis may be considered candidates for systemic treatment.

Adapted from Guidelines of care for the management of psoriasis and psoriatic arthritis: Section 1. Overview of psoriasis and guidelines of care for the treatment of psoriasis with biologics, *J Am Acad Dermatol* 58(5):826-850, 2008. *PMID: 18423260*

Comorbidities associated with psoriasis

The concurrence of multiple diseases or disorders in association with a given disease (i.e., comorbidity) has been observed in psoriasis. Patients with psoriasis are at a higher risk for comorbidities such as arthritis, heart disease, diabetes, cancer, and hypertension than is the general population (Box 8-1).

Comorbidities tend to increase with age. Nearly half of psoriasis patients aged over 65 years have at least three comorbidities and two thirds have two or more comorbidities.

Clinical presentations

Variations in the morphology of psoriasis

- Chronic plaque psoriasis
- Guttate psoriasis (acute eruptive psoriasis)
- Pustular psoriasis
- Erythrodermic psoriasis
- Light-sensitive psoriasis
- HIV-induced psoriasis
- Keratoderma blennorrhagicum (Reiter syndrome)

Variations in the location of psoriasis

- Scalp psoriasis
- Psoriasis of the palms and soles
- Pustular psoriasis of the palms and soles
- Pustular psoriasis of the digits
- Psoriasis inversus (psoriasis of flexural areas)
- Psoriasis of the penis and Reiter syndrome
- Nail psoriasis
- Psoriatic arthritis

Chronic plaque psoriasis

Chronic, noninflammatory, well-defined plaques are the most common presentation of psoriasis. The plaques are irregular, round to oval, with a predilection for extensor surfaces such as the elbows and knees. Plaques have a silvery surface scale and tend to be symmetrically distributed. They can appear anywhere on the skin surface. Plaques enlarge and then tend to remain stable for months or years (Figure 8-4, *A* and *B*). Smaller plaques or papules may coalesce into larger lesions. Numerous lesions may cover almost the entire body surface. A temporary brown, white, or red macule remains when the plaque subsides.

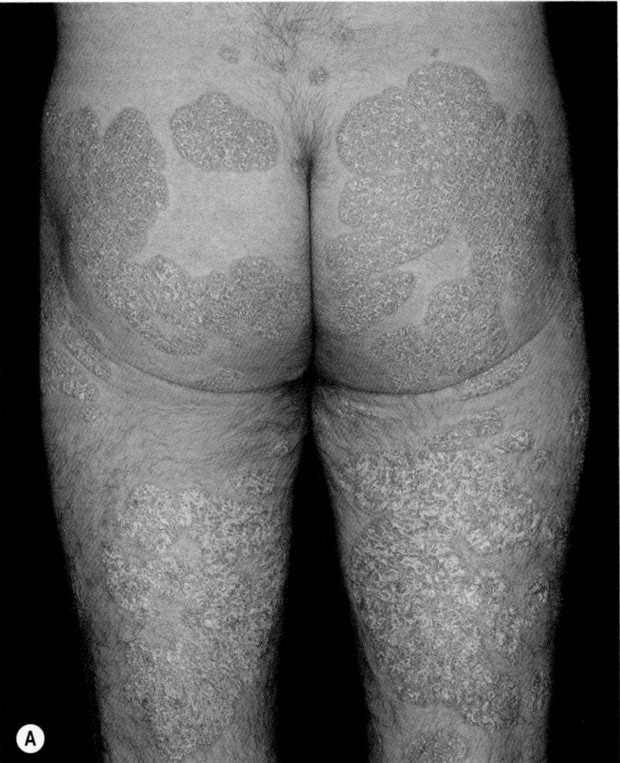

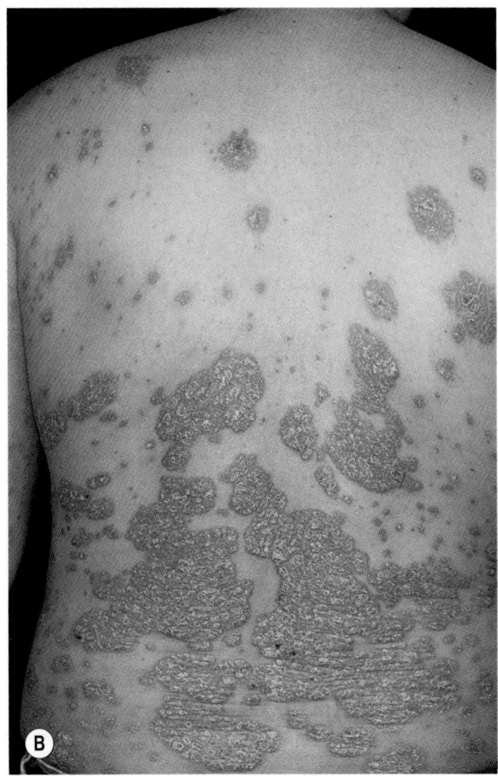

Figure 8-4 **A,** Chronic plaque psoriasis. Noninflamed plaques tend to remain fixed in position for months. **B,** Plaques are more inflamed than on the patient in **A.**

Guttate psoriasis

More than 30% of psoriatic patients have their first episode before age 20; in many instances, an episode of guttate psoriasis is the first indication of the patient's propensity for the disease. Streptococcal pharyngitis or a viral upper respiratory tract infection may precede the eruption by 1 or 2 weeks. Scaling papules suddenly appear on the trunk and extremities, not including the palms and soles (Figure 8-5, *A-D*). Their number ranges from a few to many, and their size may be that of a pinpoint up to 1 cm. Lesions increase in diameter with time. The scalp and face may also be involved. Pruritus is variable. Guttate psoriasis may resolve spontaneously in weeks or months; it responds more readily to treatment than does chronic plaque psoriasis. Throat cultures should be taken to rule out streptococcal infection. There is a high incidence of positive antistreptolysin O titers in this group.

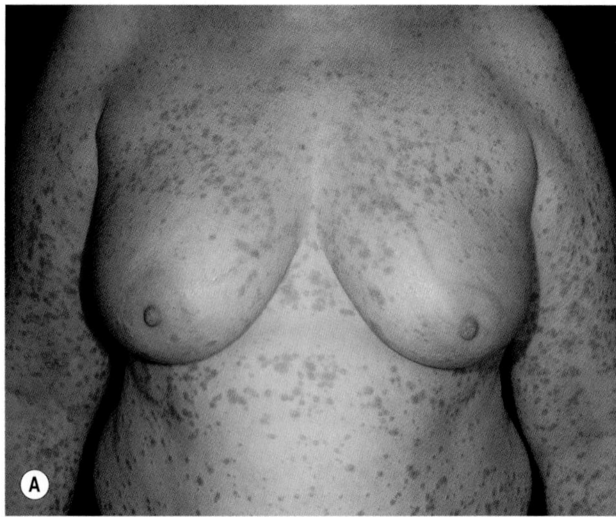

Numerous plaques appeared without a history of streptococcal infection.

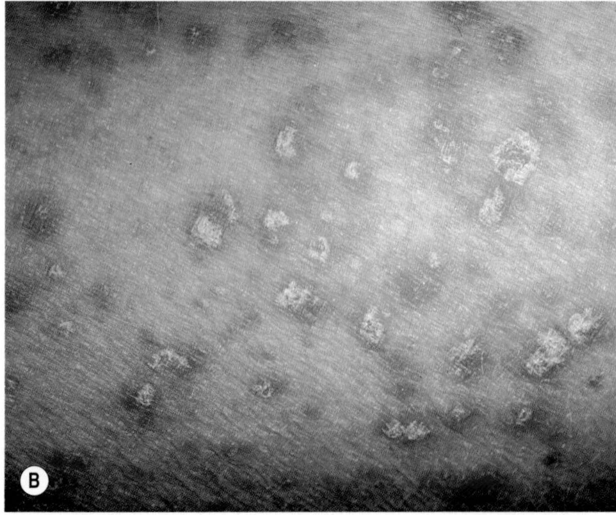

Plaques have increased in size with time.

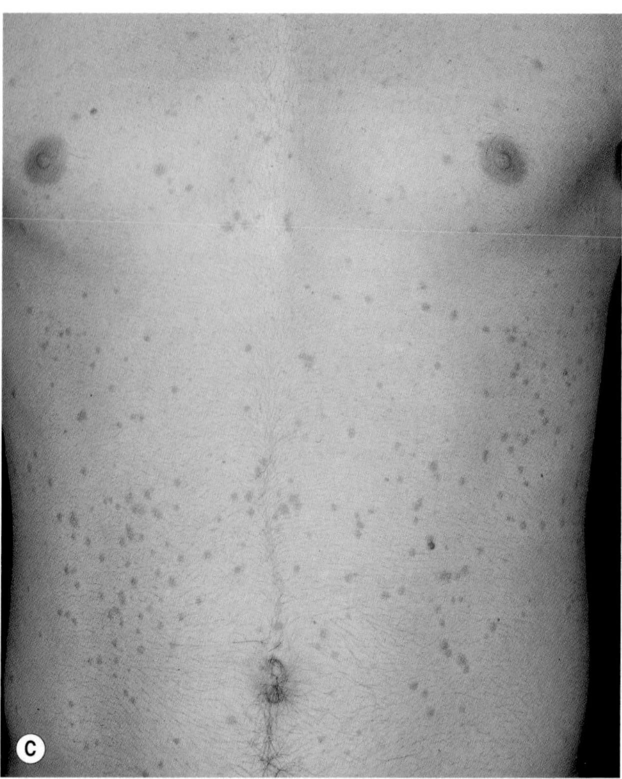

Numerous, uniformly small lesions may abruptly occur following streptococcal pharyngitis.

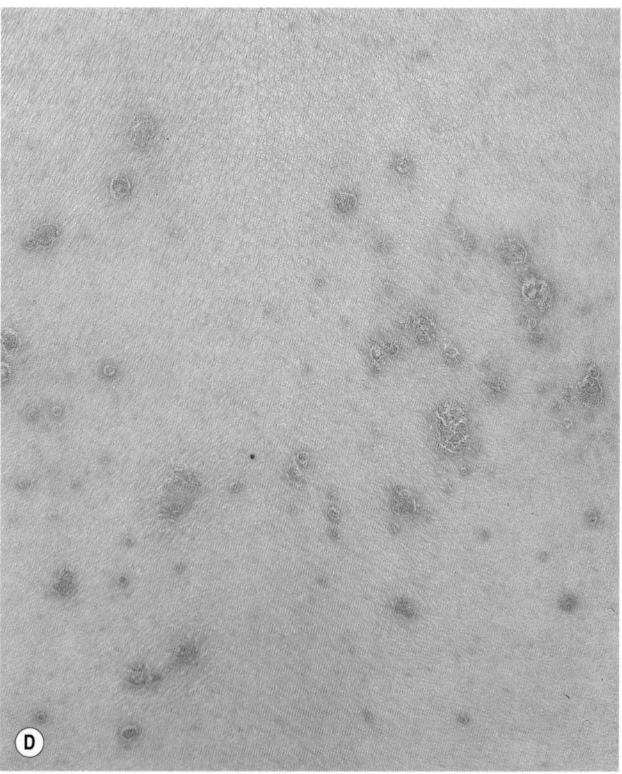

Pinpoint to 1-cm lesions develop typical psoriatic scale soon after appearance.

Figure 8-5 Guttate psoriasis.

Generalized pustular psoriasis

This rare form of psoriasis (also called von Zumbusch's psoriasis) is a serious and sometimes fatal disease. Erythema suddenly appears in the flexural areas and migrates to other body surfaces. Numerous tiny, sterile pustules evolve from an erythematous base and coalesce into lakes of pus (Figure 8-6). The superficial, upper epidermal pustules are easily ruptured. The patient is toxic and febrile, and has leukocytosis. Topical medications such as tar and anthralin may precipitate episodes in patients with unstable or labile psoriasis. Withdrawal of both topical and systemic steroids has precipitated flares. Relapses are common. Wet dressings and group V topical steroids provide initial control. Systemic therapy may be necessary for severe cases. Acitretin yields rapid control. Methotrexate and cyclosporine are also effective.

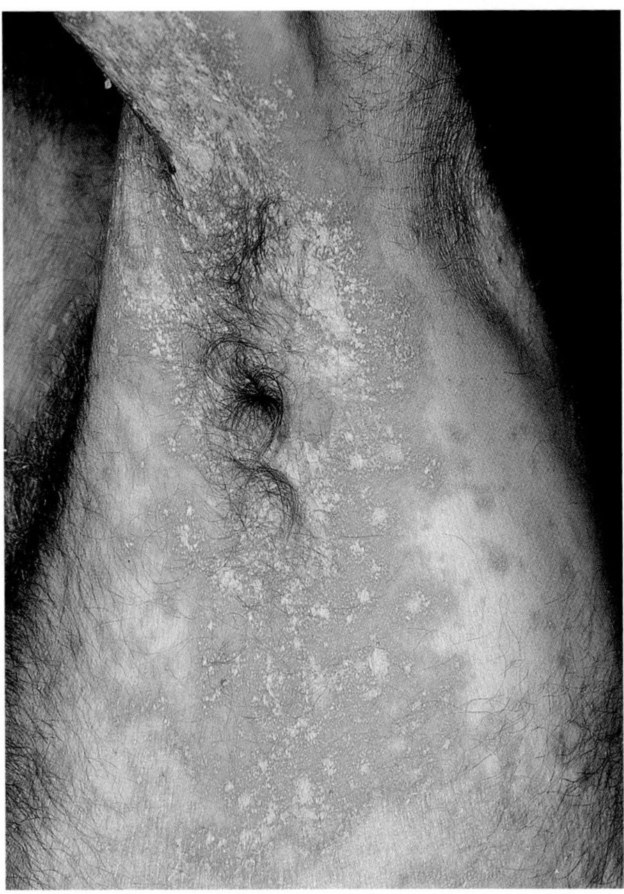

Figure 8-6 Generalized pustular psoriasis. An erythematous plaque has evolved into numerous sterile pustules, which have coalesced in many areas.

Erythrodermic psoriasis

Generalized erythrodermic psoriasis, like generalized pustular psoriasis, is a severe, unstable, highly labile disease that may appear as the initial manifestation of psoriasis but usually occurs in patients with previous chronic disease (Figure 8-7). Precipitating factors include the administration of systemic corticosteroids; the excessive use of topical steroids; overzealous, irritating topical therapy; phototherapy complications; severe emotional stress; and preceding illness, such as an infection. Treatment includes bed rest, initial avoidance of all UV light, Burow's solution compresses, colloidal oatmeal baths, the liberal use of emollients, increased protein and fluid intake, antihistamines for pruritus, avoidance of potent topical steroids, and, in severe cases, hospitalization. Methotrexate, cyclosporine, or acitretin is used if rapid control is not obtained with topical therapy. Tar and anthralin may exacerbate the disease and should be avoided.

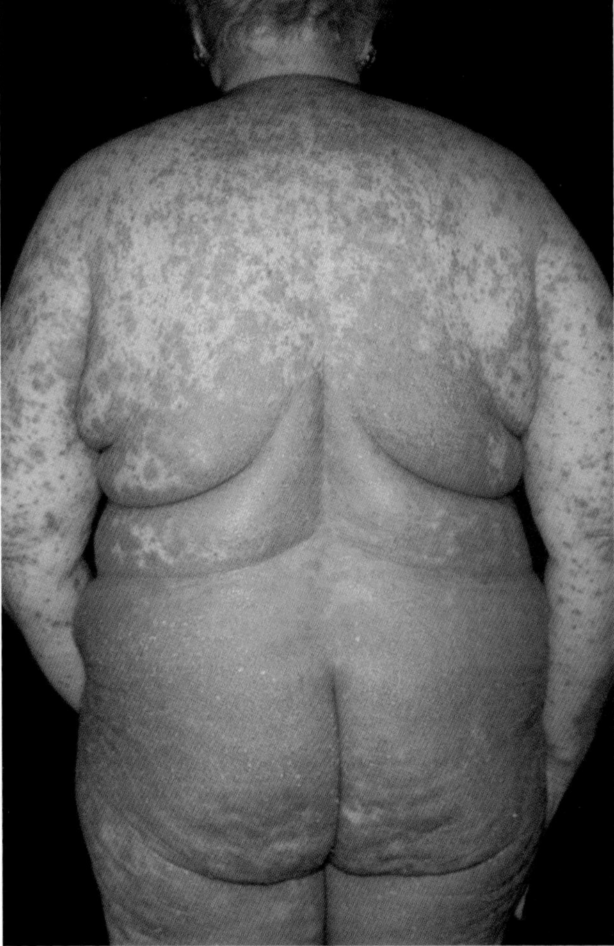

Figure 8-7 Psoriatic erythroderma. Generalized erythema occurred shortly after this patient discontinued use of methotrexate.

Light-sensitive psoriasis

Psoriatic patients wait for sunny summer months when, in most cases, the disease responds predictably to ultraviolet light. However, too much of a good thing can be dangerous, especially for the patient who gets sunburned in an anxious attempt to clear the disease rapidly. As a result of the Koebner phenomenon, guttate lesions or a painful, diffusely inflamed plaque forms in the burned areas (Figure 8-8). Plaques subsequently converge onto the clear, previously protected sites. Some patients do not tolerate ultraviolet light of any intensity.

Psoriasis of the scalp

The scalp is a favored site for psoriasis and may be the only site affected. Plaques are similar to those of the skin except that the scale is more readily retained; it is anchored by hair. Extension of the plaques onto the forehead is relatively common (Figure 8-9). A dense, tight-feeling scale can cover the entire scalp. Even in the most severe cases, the hair is not permanently lost. A distinct scaling eruption of the scalp observed in children is described in this chapter in the section concerning seborrheic dermatitis.

Psoriasis of the palms and soles

The palms and soles may be involved as part of a generalized eruption, or they may be the only locations involved in the manifestation of the disease. There are several presentations. Superficial red plaques with thick brown scale may be indistinguishable from chronic eczema (Figure 8-10). Smooth, deep red plaques are similar to those found in the flexural area (Figure 8-11).

Pustular psoriasis of the palms and soles

Deep pustules first appear on the middle portion of the palms and insteps of the soles; they may either remain localized or spread (Figure 8-12, *A* and *B*). The pustules do not rupture but turn dark brown and scaly as they reach the surface. The surrounding skin becomes pink, smooth, and tender. A thick crust may later cover the affected area. The course is chronic, lasting for years while the patient endures periods of partial remission followed by exacerbations so painful that mobility is affected. There is a considerably higher prevalence of smoking in these patients. Acitretin, methotrexate, psoralen ultraviolet light A (PUVA), narrow-band UVB light (NB-UVB), and intermittent courses of topical steroids under plastic occlusions are therapeutic alternatives.

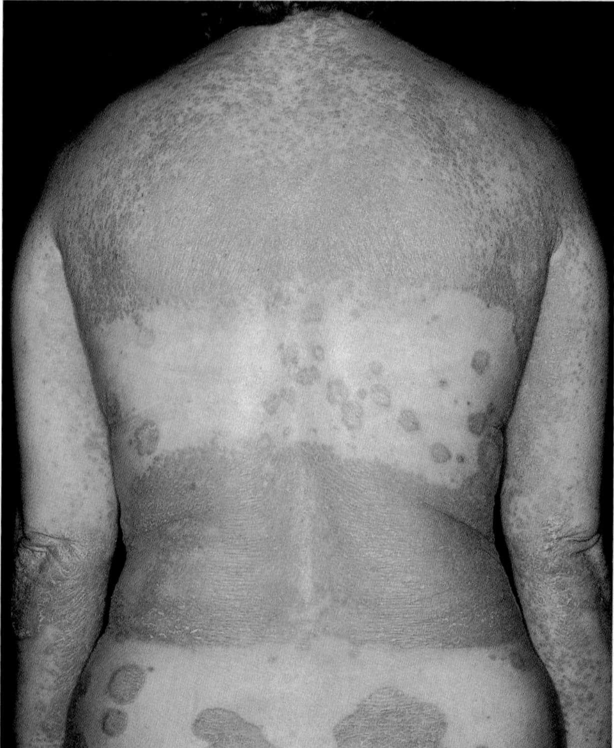

Figure 8-8 Light-induced psoriasis. Overexposure to sunlight precipitated this diffuse flare of psoriasis. The mid back was protected by a wide halter strap.

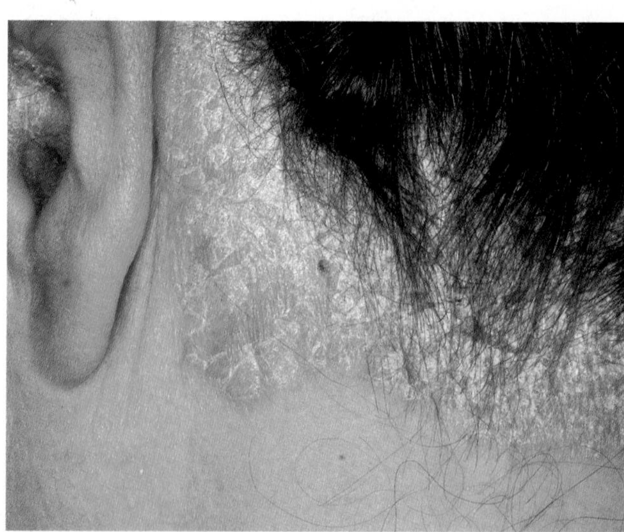

Figure 8-9 Psoriasis of the scalp. Plaques typically form in the scalp and along the hair margin. Occasionally plaques occur on the face.

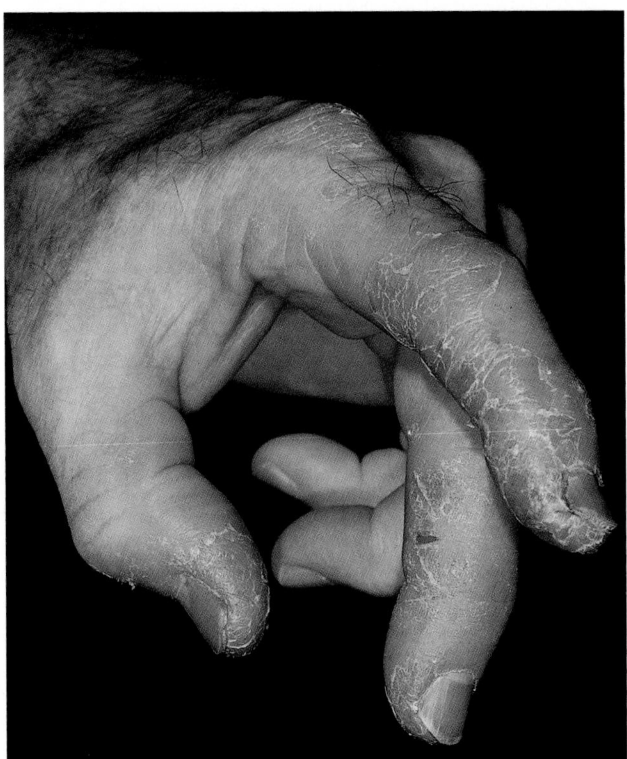

Figure 8-10 Psoriasis of the fingertips. The eruption appears eczematous, but the rich red hue is typical of psoriasis. This eruption occurred as a Koebner phenomenon in a surgeon.

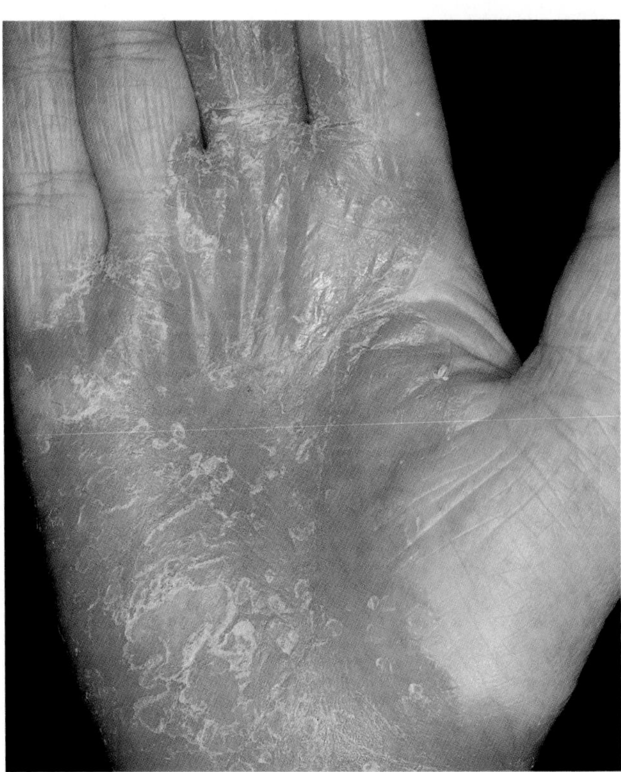

Figure 8-11 Psoriasis of the hand. Deep red, smooth plaque in a patient with typical lesions on the body.

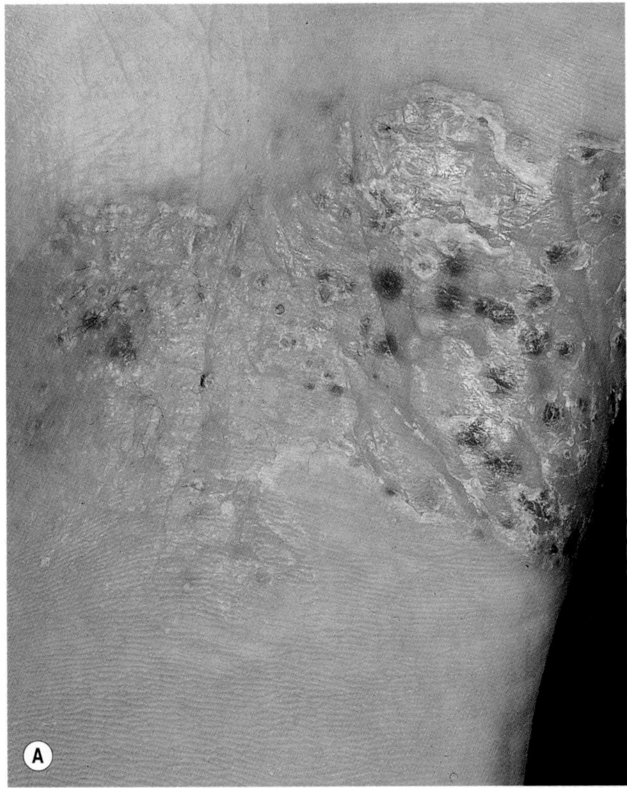

An early case in a typical location.

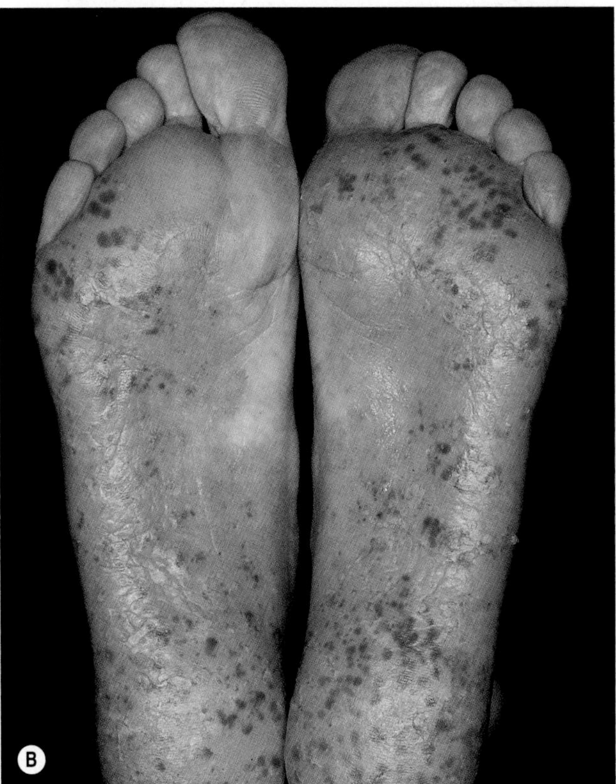

This is a chronic disease in which the soles may remain inflamed for years.

Figure 8-12 Pustular psoriasis of the soles.

Keratoderma blennorrhagicum (Reiter syndrome)

Reiter syndrome appears to be a reactive immune response that is usually triggered in a genetically susceptible individual (60% to 90% of patients are HLA-B27 positive) by any of several different infections, especially those that cause dysentery or urethritis, such as *Yersinia enterocolitica* and *Y. pseudotuberculosis*. Psoriasiform skin lesions develop in patients with Reiter syndrome (urethritis and/or cervicitis, peripheral arthritis of more than 1 month's duration) usually 1 to 2 months after the onset of arthritis; conjunctivitis develops in 25% of patients. The distinctive lesions, keratoderma blennorrhagica, typically appear on the soles (Figure 8-13, *A*) and extend onto the toes (Figure 8-13, *B*) but also occur on the legs, scalp, and hands. Nail dystrophy, thickening, and destruction occur. The plaques are psoriasiform with a distinctive circular, scaly border (Figure 8-14). The scaly, scalloped-edged plaques develop from coalescence of expanding papulovesicular plaques with thickened yellow, heaped-up scale. Similar lesions occur on the penis. Skin and joint symptoms have responded to methotrexate, acitretin, and ketoconazole.

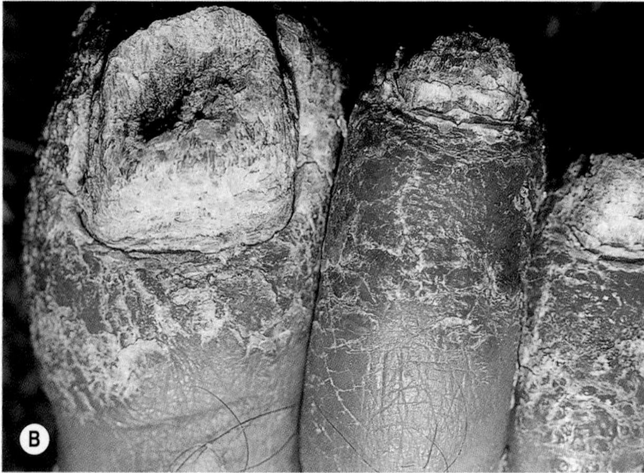

Figure 8-13 Keratoderma blenorrhagicum (Reiter syndrome). **A,** The palms and soles are commonly involved. There are keratoic papules, plaques, and pustules that coalesce to form circular borders like those seen on the penis (see Figure 8-16). **B,** Psoriasiform plaques develop from coalescence of expanding papulovesicular plaques and are typically found on the soles and toes.

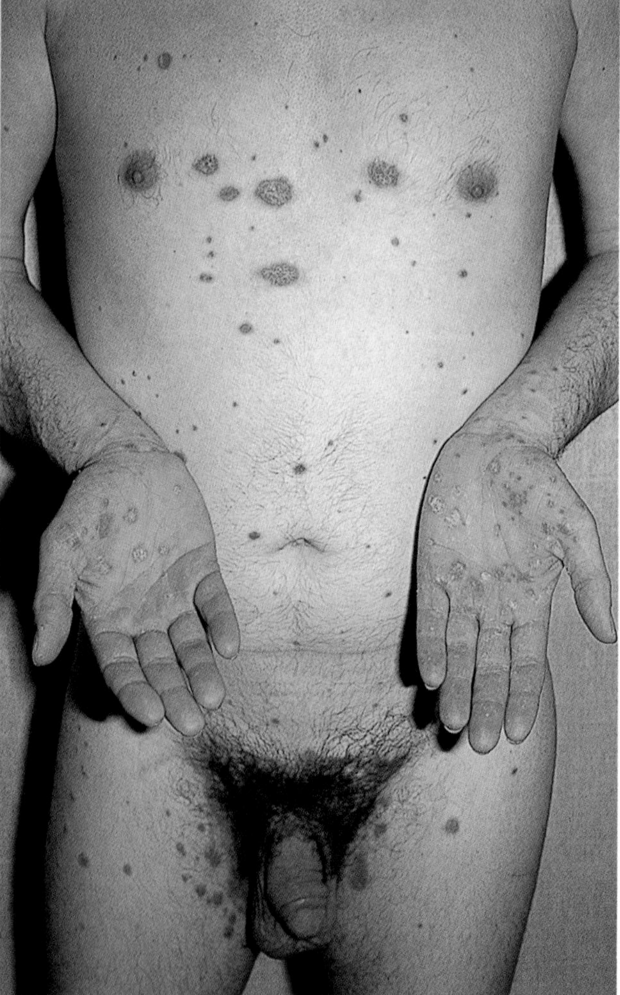

Figure 8-14 Patients with Reiter syndrome develop psoriasiform skin lesions (keratoderma blenorrhagica) with a distinctive circular, scaly border. These distinctive lesions occur most frequently on the soles and toes.

Psoriasis of the penis and Reiter syndrome

Typical psoriatic scaling plaques with white scale can appear on the body and circumcised penis (Figure 8-15). Scale does not form when the penis is covered by a foreskin. A highly characteristic psoriasiform lesion, balanitis circinata, occurs in Reiter syndrome when erosions covered by scale and crust on the corona and glans coalesce to form a distinctive winding pattern (Figure 8-16). A biopsy helps confirm the diagnosis. A potassium hydroxide examination excludes *Candida*.

Pustular psoriasis of the digits

This severe localized variant of psoriasis, also known as acrodermatitis continua, may remain localized to one finger for years. Vesicles rupture, resulting in a tender, diffusely eroded, and fissured surface that continually exudes serum. The loosely adherent, moist crust is easily shed, but recurs (Figure 8-17). Localized pustular psoriasis is very resistant to therapy.

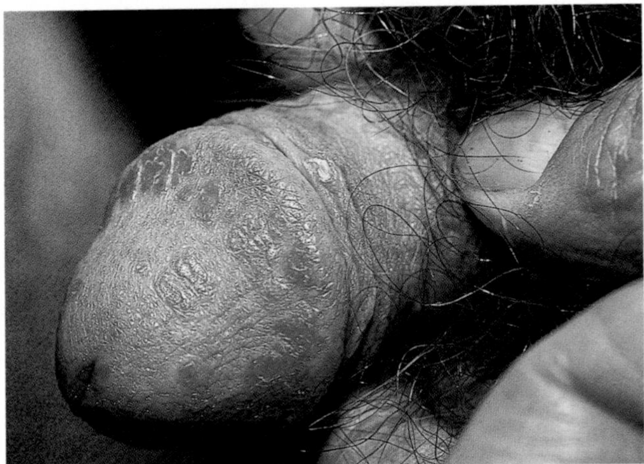

Figure 8-15 Psoriasis. Typical psoriatic scaling plaques with white scale can appear on the circumcised penis. Scale does not form when the penis is covered by a foreskin.

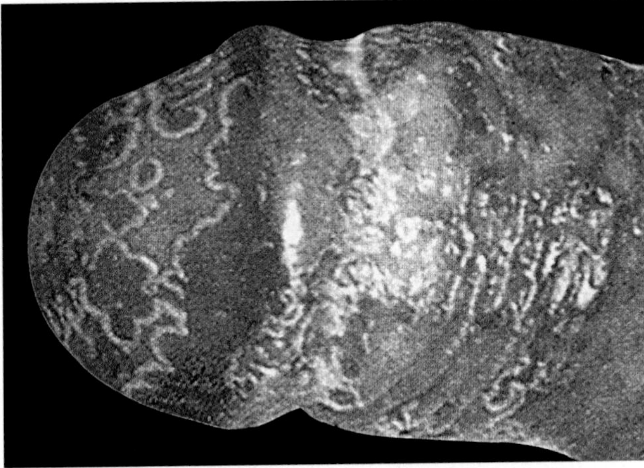

Figure 8-16 Reiter syndrome. Balanitis circinata, a highly characteristic psoriasiform lesion, occurs in Reiter syndrome when erosions covered by scale and crust on the corona and glans coalesce to form a distinctive winding pattern.

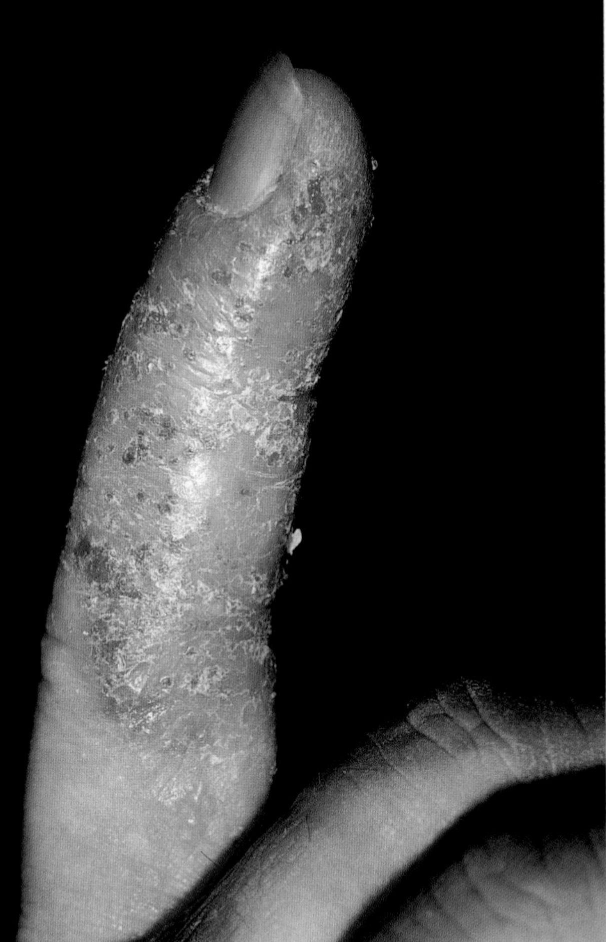

Figure 8-17 Pustular psoriasis of the digits. The eruption has remained localized in this one finger for years.

Psoriasis inversus (psoriasis of the flexural or intertriginous areas)

The gluteal fold, axillae, groin, submammary folds, retroauricular fold, and the glans of the uncircumcised penis may be affected. The deep red, smooth, glistening plaques may extend to and stop at the junction of the skin folds, as with intertrigo or *Candida* infections. The surface is moist and contains macerated white debris. Infection, friction, and heat may induce flexural psoriasis, a Koebner phenomenon. Cracking and fissures are common at the base of the crease, particularly in the groin, gluteal cleft, and superior and posterior auricular folds (Figures 8-18, 8-19, and 8-20). As with typical psoriatic plaques, the margin is distinct. Pustules beyond the plaque border suggest secondary yeast infection. Infants and young children may develop flexural psoriasis of the groin that extends onto the diaper area.

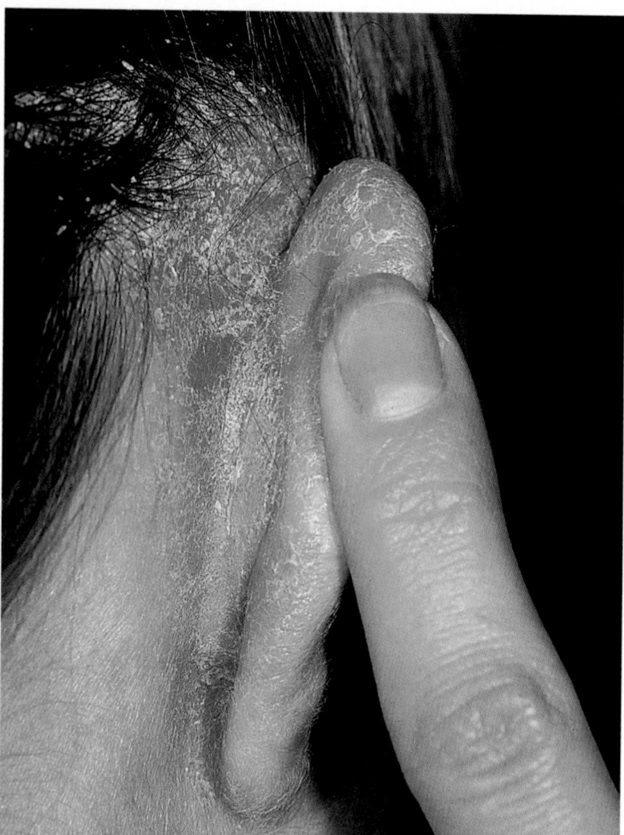

Figure 8-18 Psoriasis of the posterior auricular fold.

Human immunodeficiency virus (HIV)–induced psoriasis

Psoriasis may be the first or one of the first signs of acquired immunodeficiency syndrome (AIDS). Psoriasis in the setting of HIV disease may be mild, moderate, or severe. It can be atypical and unusually severe with involvement of the groin, axilla, scalp, palms, and soles. An explosive onset with erythroderma or pustular lesions that rapidly become confluent should lead one to suspect AIDS. The disease is difficult to treat. PUVA, ultraviolet light B, and topical steroids are immunosuppressive and should be avoided. It is not clear that use of methotrexate adversely affects the natural course of HIV disease. Acitretin is the drug of choice for severe disease. Zidovudine is effective and cleared an acitretin-resistant case.

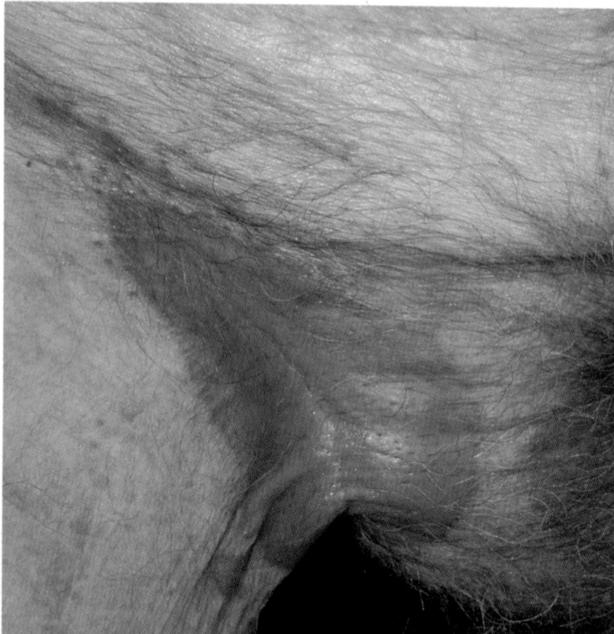

Figure 8-19 Inverse psoriasis. Plaques are red and symmetrical. The differential diagnosis includes candida infection and intertrigo.

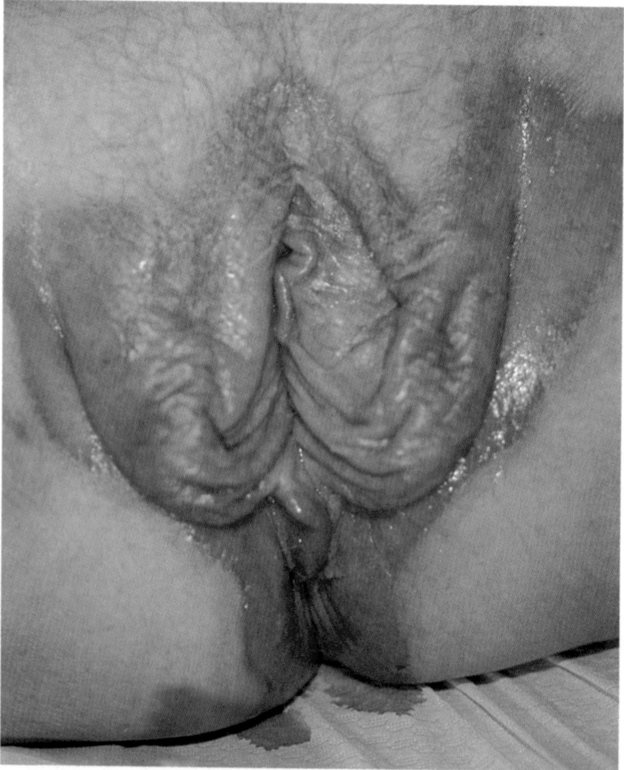

Figure 8-20 Inverse psoriasis. Many clinicians would make the diagnosis of candida infection. The patient's past history of psoriasis suggested the diagnosis.

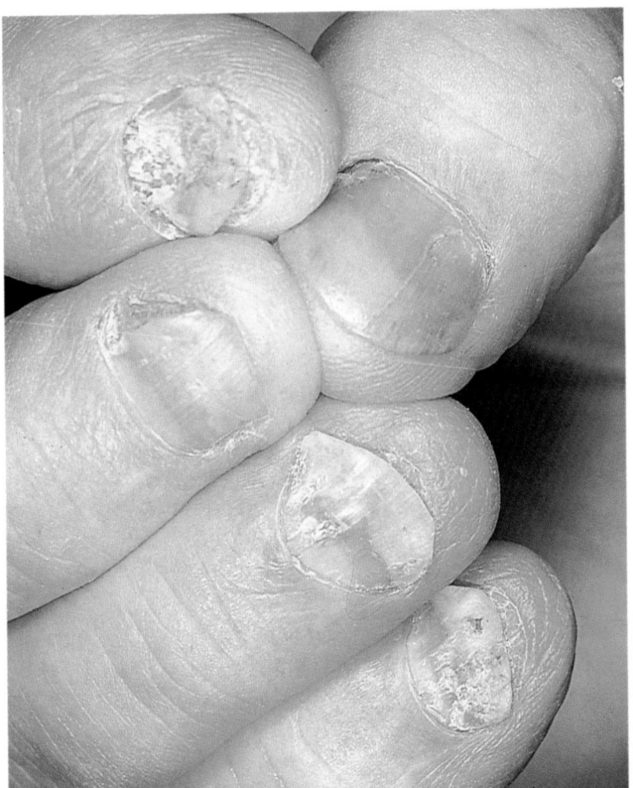

Figure 8-21 Separation of the nail, or onycholysis, is accompanied by yellow discoloration. Scaly debris elevates the nail plate. The debris is commonly mistaken for nail fungus infection.

Psoriasis of the nails

Nail changes are characteristic of psoriasis and the nails of patients should be examined (see Chapter 25). These changes offer supporting evidence for the diagnosis of psoriasis when skin changes are equivocal or absent.

Onycholysis. Psoriasis of the nail bed causes separation of the nail from the nail bed. Unlike the uniform separation caused by pressure on the tips of long nails, the nail detaches in an irregular manner. The nail plate turns yellow, simulating a fungal infection.

Subungual debris. This is analogous to fungal infection; the nail bed scale is retained, forcing the distal nail to separate from the nail bed (see Figure 8-21).

Pitting. Nail pitting is the best known and possibly the most frequent psoriatic nail abnormality (Figures 8-22 and 8-23). Nail plate cells are shed in much the same way as psoriatic scale is shed, leaving a variable number of tiny, punched-out depressions on the nail plate surface. They emerge from under the cuticle and grow out with the nail. Many other cutaneous diseases may cause pitting (e.g., eczema, fungal infections, and alopecia areata), or it may occur as an isolated finding as a normal variation.

Oil spot lesion. Psoriasis of the nail bed may cause localized separation of the nail plate. Cellular debris and serum accumulate in this space. The brown-yellow color observed through the nail plate looks like a spot of oil (see Figure 8-23).

Nail deformity. Extensive involvement of the nail matrix results in a nail losing its structural integrity, resulting in fragmentation and crumbling.

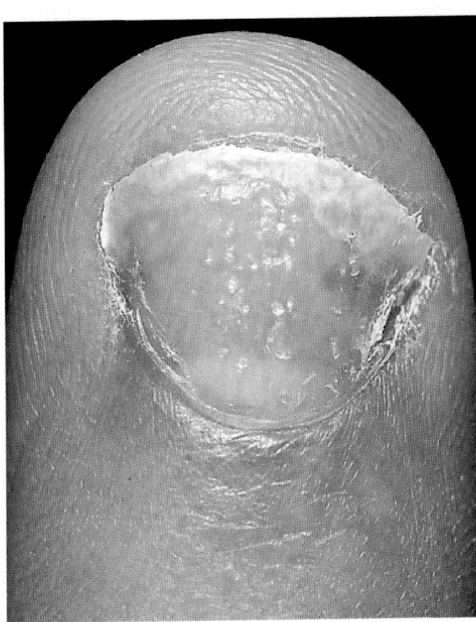

Figure 8-22 Pitting psoriasis of the proximal nail matrix results in loss of parakeratotic cells from the surface of the nail plate. This is a process analogous to the shedding of psoriatic skin scale.

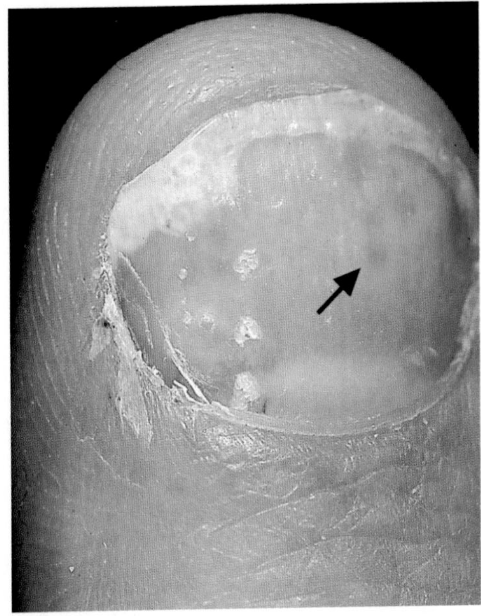

Figure 8-23 Oil spot lesion. A translucent yellow-red discoloration resembles a drop of oil beneath the nail plate. It occurs from psoriasis of the nail bed, which causes serum to be trapped under the nail plate.

Psoriatic arthritis

Psoriatic arthritis (PsA) is a chronic inflammatory arthropathy of the peripheral joints, spine, and entheses; it is associated with psoriasis in which rheumatoid factor and anti-cyclic citrullinated peptide (anti-CCP) measurements are usually negative. It may precede, accompany, or, more often, follow the skin manifestations. Onset may occur at any age, but peak occurrence is between ages 20 and 40; women and men are equally affected. Symmetric polyarthritis with joint pain and joint swelling often indicates erosive progressive disease. Unlike in rheumatoid arthritis, the distal interphalangeal joints are regularly involved. The presence of inflammatory arthritis in patients with psoriasis varies between 5% and 42%. Approximately 15% of patients with PsA have an onset of arthritis before the onset of psoriasis. The prevalence of psoriatic arthritis is higher among patients with more severe cutaneous disease. Nail involvement occurs in more than 80% of patients with psoriatic arthritis, compared with 30% of patients with uncomplicated psoriasis. The prevalence of nail psoriasis is highest among patients with psoriatic arthritis who have arthritic involvement of their fingers, but the presence of nail disease does not have predictive value in determining if a patient is at risk for psoriatic arthritis. Cases of arthritis have been reported to develop following trauma. Patients with psoriatic arthritis who become pregnant improve or even remit in 80% of cases. Despite active treatment and a reduction in joint inflammation and the rate of damage, psoriatic arthritis may be a progressively deforming arthritis.

Defining PsA

The spondylarthritis (SpA) family of diseases includes PsA, rheumatoid arthritis (RA), ankylosing spondylitis (AS), reactive arthritis, and enteropathic arthritis. PsA is characterized by infrequent seropositivity for rheumatoid factor (RF) and anti-cyclic citrullinated peptide (anti-CCP), and an association with HLA-B27 alleles, particularly in those patients with axial involvement.

Other features can include enthesitis, dactylitis, iritis, peripheral arthritis (oligoarticular asymmetric and polyarticular symmetric), spondylitis, and a variable clinical course. The heterogeneity in clinical presentation and course makes PsA difficult to classify and differentiate from other forms of SpA and inflammatory arthropathies.

Dactylitis presents as the "sausage digit"—diffuse swelling of the entire digit. Enthesitis—inflammation at the site of ligamentous and tendinous insertion—is characteristic of all the HLA-B27-associated spondyloarthropathies.

CLINICAL FEATURES. There are five recognized presentations of psoriatic arthritis (Figure 8-24).

The most common pattern is an asymmetric arthritis involving one or more joints of the fingers and toes (Figure 8-25). Usually one or more proximal interphalangeal (PIP), distal interphalangeal (DIP), metatarsophalangeal, or metacarpophalangeal joints are involved. During the acute phase, the joint is red, warm, and painful. Continued inflammation promotes soft tissue swelling on either side of the joint ("sausage finger") and restricts mobility. HLA-DR7 is significantly increased in this group with peripheral arthritis.

MOLL AND WRIGHT CLASSIFICATION. The Moll and Wright classification was developed more than 30 years ago and is still used today to divide PsA into five clinical subtypes (see Table 8-1). These patterns are often mixed and not well-defined.

Table 8-1 Moll and Wright Clinical Subtypes for Psoriatic Arthritis*

Type	Percentage of all psoriatic arthritis	Features
Oligoarticular, asymmetric arthritis (one or more joints)	30-50	Joints of fingers and toes ("sausage finger") are involved.
Polyarticular, symmetric arthritis (RA-like)	30-50	Clinically resembles rheumatoid arthritis, rheumatoid factor negative. The small joints of the hands and feet, wrists, ankles, knees, and elbows may be involved.
Distal interphalangeal joint predominant	25	Mild, chronic, not disabling, and associated with nail disease. Involves hands and feet. This is the most characteristic presentation of arthritis with psoriasis.
Destructive polyarthritis (arthritis mutilans)	5	The most severe form of psoriatic arthritis involves osteolysis of any of the small bones of the hands and feet. Gross deformity and subluxation are attributed to this condition. Severe osteolysis leads to digital telescoping, producing the "opera glass" deformity. This deformity may be seen in rheumatoid arthritis.
Ankylosing spondylitis and sacroiliitis	30-35	Occurs as an isolated phenomenon or in association with peripheral joint disease. Association of HLA-B27 and spondylitis. The strongest association is in males with sacroiliitis. Asymptomatic sacroiliitis occurs in as many as one third of cases of psoriasis. It is usually asymmetric and may be associated with spondylitis.

*To meet the Moll and Wright 1973 classification criteria for psoriatic arthritis, a patient with psoriasis and inflammatory arthritis who is seronegative for rheumatoid arthritis (RA) must present with one of the above five clinical subtypes. Criteria specificity is 98% and sensitivity is 91%.

PSORIATIC ARTHRITIS

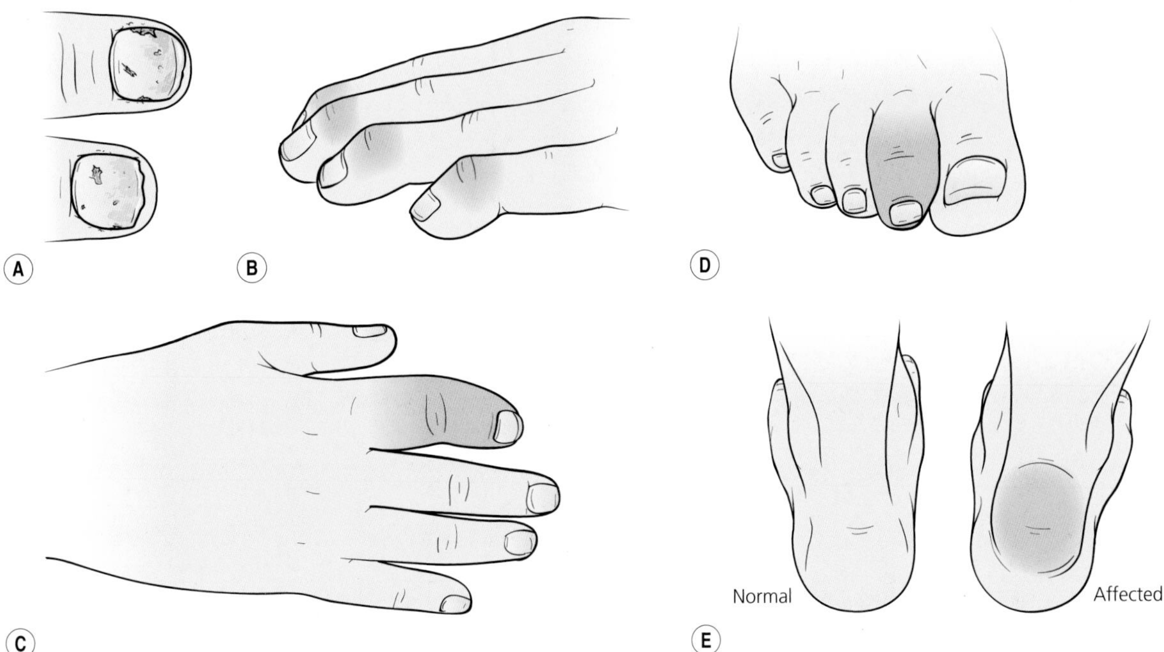

Figure 8-24 Signs and symptoms of psoriatic arthritis. **A,** Pitting, onycholysis, brown nail bed stain. **B** and **C,** Swollen finger joints. **D,** Sausage finger and sausage toe (dactylitis). **E,** Swollen heal at the Achilles tendon (enthesitis).

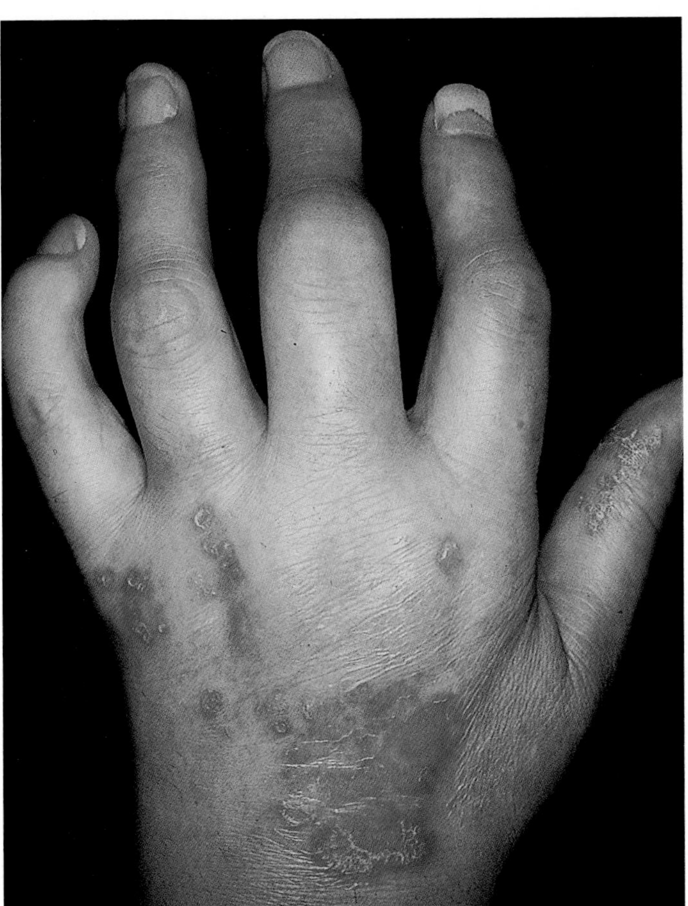

Figure 8-25 Psoriatic arthritis. Asymmetric arthritis pattern.

Table 8-2 CASPAR Criteria for Psoriatic Arthritis*

Inflammatory articular disease (joint, spine, or entheseal) plus the following:

Clinical finding	Score
Psoriasis	Current (2), history of (1), family history of (1); patient-reported history in a first- or second-degree relative
Nail dystrophy	(1) Including onycholysis, pitting, and hyperkeratosis
Negative rheumatoid factor	(1)
Dactylitis	Current (1), history of (1); defined as swelling of an entire digit, or a history of dactylitis recorded by a rheumatologist
Radiographic evidence	Juxtaarticular new bone formation, appearing as ill-defined ossification near joint margins (but excluding osteophyte formation) on plain radiographs of the hand (1)

*To meet the Classification Criteria for Psoriatic Arthritis (CASPAR, 2006), a patient must have inflammatory articular disease and 3 points from the remaining categories; the assigned scores are in parentheses. Criteria specificity is 98.7% and sensitivity is 91.4%.

Table 8-3 Differentiating Psoriatic Arthritis from Rheumatoid Arthritis

	Psoriatic arthritis	Rheumatoid arthritis	Inflammatory osteoarthritis	Gout
Distal interphalangeal joint involvement	Common	Uncommon	Common	Uncommon
Symmetry	Less common	Common	Uncommon	Uncommon
Erythema of joint	Common	Uncommon	Uncommon	Common
Stiffness	In morning and/or with immobility	In morning and/or with immobility	With activity	Uncommon
Tenderness	Mild	Severe	Mild	Severe
Back involvement	Common	Uncommon	Uncommon	Uncommon
Skin lesions	Always	Uncommon	Uncommon	Uncommon
Nail lesions	Common	Uncommon	Uncommon	Uncommon
Dactylitis	Common	Uncommon	Uncommon	Uncommon
Enthesitis	Common	Uncommon	Uncommon	Uncommon
Rheumatoid nodules	Never	Common	Uncommon	Uncommon
Rheumatoid factor	Uncommon	Common	Uncommon	Uncommon
Radiological changes				
Osteopenia	Less common	Common	Uncommon	Uncommon
Periostitis	Common	Rare	Uncommon	Uncommon
Pencil-in-cup change	Common	Rare	Uncommon	Uncommon
Ankylosis	Common	Rare	Uncommon	Uncommon
Sacroiliitis	50%, asymmetric	Rare	Uncommon	Uncommon
Quality of life	Reduced	Reduced	Reduced	?
Function	Reduced	Reduced	Reduced	?
HLA association	CW6, B27	DR4	No	B14
Female to male ratio	1:1	3:1	Hand/foot more common in female patients	1:3.6

Adapted from Clinical, radiological, and functional assessment in psoriatic arthritis: is it different from other inflammatory joint diseases? *Ann Rheum Dis* 65(suppl 3):iii22-24, 2006 (review). No abstract available. *PMID: 17038466*

CLASSIFICATION CRITERIA FOR PSORIATIC ARTHRITIS (CASPAR). A new Classification Criteria for Psoriatic Arthritis (CASPAR) was published by the Classification Criteria for Psoriatic Arthritis Study Group (Table 8-2). These criteria were established for patients with long-standing disease duration (mean, 12.5 years). Classification criteria are not yet validated for early disease.

Differentiating PsA and RA

PsA affects men and women equally; RA affects women more commonly (Table 8-3). RA affects metacarpophalangeal and proximal interphalangeal joints; PsA affects the DIP joints in at least 50% of patients. RA tends to have a symmetric distribution, PsA an asymmetric distribution. PsA often affects all joints of the same digit, leading to a "ray" distribution. Patients with PsA are less tender than patients with RA. The spine is not affected in RA; 50% of PsA patients have spinal involvement manifested as sacroiliitis and/or syndesmophytes. Enthesitis and dactylitis are features of PsA. Skin psoriasis is a defining feature of PsA. It occurs in 2% to 3% of patients with RA, the same frequency as in the general population. Nail lesions are more common in patients with PsA than in patients with just cutaneous psoriasis. *PMID: 17038466*

Differentiating PsA from osteoarthritis (OA) and gout

The presence of DIP involvement requires differentiation between PsA and OA (see Table 8-3). PsA is inflammatory; OA is usually not. Gout is often associated with periarticular inflammation, which is not seen in PsA.

Differentiating psoriatic arthritis from other spondyloarthropathies. The spondylitis seen in PsA is not as severe as with ankylosing spondylitis (AS). Patients with PsA have better mobility and less grade 4 sacroiliitis than patients with AS (Table 8-4). Peripheral arthritis is more common among patients with PsA. Only 2% of patients with PsA have isolated spinal involvement, whereas 10% of patients diagnosed with AS have psoriasis.

Laboratory. PsA patients have normal acute phase reactants, 4.6% are rheumatoid factor positive, and 7.6% are anti-cyclic citrullinated peptide (anti-CCP) antibodies positive. Erythrocyte sedimentation rate (ESR) is the best laboratory guide to disease activity.

Imaging. The (CASPAR) study identified juxtaarticular bone formation as the only radiological differentiation between RA and PsA. PsA patients have less severe radiological changes compared with patients with AS. PsA shows narrowing of joint space, joint erosions, and bony proliferation. Magnetic resonance imaging and ultrasonography detect enthesitis (inflammation at the point of insertion of skeletal muscle to bone).

Table 8-4 Differentiating Psoriatic Arthritis from Other Spondyloarthropathies

Feature	Psoriatic arthritis	Ankylosing spondylitis	Reactive arthritis	Inflammatory bowel disease
Male to female ratio	1:1	3:1	8:1	1:1
Age at onset (years)	35-45	20	20	Any
Peripheral distribution	96% Any	25% Axial Lower limbs	90% Lower limbs	Common Lower limbs
Dactylitis	35%	Uncommon	Common	Uncommon
Enthesitis	Common	Common	Common	Uncommon
Sacroiliitis	50%	100%	80%	20%
Syndesmophytes	Classic and paramarginal	Classic	Classic and paramarginal	Classic
HLA-B	50%	>90%	80%	40%
Psoriasis	Always	Uncommon	Uncommon	Uncommon
Other skin lesions	Nail changes	Uncommon	Keratodermia blennorrhagica	Erythema nodosum, pyoderma gangrenosum
Quality of life	Reduced	Reduced	Likely reduced	Reduced
Function	Reduced	Reduced	Reduced	Reduced

Adapted from Clinical, radiological, and functional assessment in psoriatic arthritis: is it different from other inflammatory joint diseases? *Ann Rheum Dis* 65(suppl 3):iii22-24, 2006 (review). *PMID: 17038466*

TREATMENT OF PSORIATIC ARTHRITIS. Management is similar to that of other chronic inflammatory joint diseases. Nonsteroidal antiinflammatory agents are the mainstay of therapy and usually provide adequate control, but they do not induce remissions. They are first-line agents for mild PsA. Intraarticular injections with corticosteroids may be effective. Neither treatment is capable of inhibiting the development of structural joint damage. Methotrexate controls advanced joint and skin diseases. Sulfasalazine, leflunomide, and cyclosporine are also effective. Anti–tumor necrosis factor-α (TNF-α) therapy (etanercept, infliximab) may be very effective.

Methotrexate. Methotrexate is an effective second-line agent for psoriatic arthritis. It is frequently used as the primary DMARD (disease-modifying antirheumatic drug) in PsA, because of its efficacy in treating both skin and joint involvement in patients with psoriatic disease. Methotrexate is not expensive. Pain and function improve dramatically 2 to 6 weeks after starting methotrexate therapy with 5 mg every 12 hours in three consecutive doses once a week. Lower dosages may not be effective. Methotrexate may also be given as a single dose or divided into two doses taken 12 hours apart. The amount is increased to 25 to 30 mg/week, until control is obtained, and then tapered to a maintenance dose of around 5 to 15 mg/week.

The risk of liver toxicity in patients undergoing long-term, low-dose methotrexate therapy for psoriatic arthritis is substantial, and that risk increases with the total cumulative dose and with heavy consumption of alcohol. Liver biopsies should be done periodically to monitor for liver toxicity (see methotrexate treatment section in this chapter).

Etanercept (Enbrel), adalimumab (Humira), infliximab (Remicade). These anti–tumor necrosis factor (anti-TNF) agents bind and inhibit the activity of TNF. They are highly effective for psoriatic arthritis. The cost is very high. Guidelines for use are discussed under Treatment of Psoriasis. These agents are often combined with DMARDs, particularly methotrexate.

Hydroxychloroquine is inadequately effective for psoriatic arthritis. Systemic corticosteroids are usually avoided because of possible rebound of the skin disease on withdrawal.

Cyclosporine at daily doses usually ranging from 1.5 to 5.0 mg/kg provides impressive relief from arthralgias and improvement of joint function. Although mild-to-moderate relapses occur, rebound phenomena are not observed after discontinuation of treatment. Renal toxicity limits its use.

Treatment of psoriasis

Many topical and systemic agents are available. None of the topical medications are predictably effective. All require lengthy treatment to give relief that is often temporary. Compliance is a problem. Patients become discouraged with moderately effective expensive topical treatment that lasts weeks or months. Limited disease can be managed with topical therapy (Table 8-5). One intralesional steroid injection can heal a small plaque and keep it in remission for months. This is an ideal treatment for patients with a few small plaques. Topical steroid creams and ointments, calcipotriene (Dovonex), tazarotene (Tazorac), anthralin, and tar are the mainstays of topical treatment. These agents are used with or without ultraviolet light exposure. Effective programs can be designed for patients who do not have access to a therapeutic light source and for patients who have limited disease. Without light, tar is moderately effective, but persistent use of calcipotriol, tazarotene, or anthralin can clear the disease and offers the patient substantial remission periods. Topical steroids work quickly, but total eradication of the plaques is difficult to accomplish; remission times are short, and the creams become less effective with continued use.

Patients with psoriasis covering more than 20% of the body need special treatment programs (Table 8-6).

DETERMINING DEGREE OF INFLAMMATION. The most common form of psoriasis is the localized chronic plaque disease involving the skin and scalp. It must be determined whether the plaque is inflamed before instituting therapy (Figure 8-26). Red, sore plaques can be irritated by tar, calcipotriol, and anthralin. Irritation can induce further activity. Inflammation should be suppressed with topical steroids and/or antibiotics before initiating other treatments.

DETERMINING THE END OF TREATMENT. The plaque is effectively treated when induration has disappeared. Residual erythema, hypopigmentation, or brown hyperpigmentation is common when the plaque clears; patients frequently mistake the residual color for disease and continue treatment. If the plaque cannot be felt by drawing the finger over the skin surface, treatment may be stopped.

CONTROL STRESS. A study demonstrated a positive correlation between the severity of psoriatic symptoms and psychologic distress. Stress reduction techniques may be appropriate for certain patients.

DURATION OF REMISSION. Among topical monotherapy, anthralin and tazarotene induce longer remissions than calcipotriene and corticosteroids; among systemic agents, longer remissions occur with acitretin than cyclosporine or methotrexate, but compared with the remission rate of phototherapeutic modalities, the remission rates are much less (see Tables 8-5 and 8-6). Traditional Goeckerman therapy, conducted in a day treatment setting, is more likely to induce prolonged remissions than simple UVB phototherapy, "home Goeckerman therapy" using liquor carbonis detergens (LCD), or heliotherapy. PUVA phototherapy also induces prolonged remissions.

Some treatments are better suited for rapid clearing; others are better suited to be maintenance treatment. The optimum management involves the sequential use of therapeutic agents involving three steps, namely, the clearing phase, the transitional phase, and the maintenance phase.

Table 8-5 Therapeutic Options for Persons with Psoriasis on Less than 20% of the Body

Treatment	Advantages	Disadvantages	Comments
Topical steroids	Rapid response, controls inflammation and itching, best for intertriginous areas and face, convenient, not messy	Temporary relief (tolerance occurs), less effective with continued use, atrophy and telangiectasia occur with continued use, brief remissions, very expensive	Best results occur with pulse dosing (e.g., 2 weeks of medication and 1 week of lubrication only); plastic occlusion is very effective but is not used in intertriginous areas
Calcipotriol (Dovonex)	Well tolerated, long remissions possible	Burning, skin irritation, expensive	Best for moderate plaque psoriasis; newer combination product is more effective (calcipotriene hydrate and betamethasone dipropionate)
Tazarotene (Tazorac)	Effective, long remissions possible	Irritating, expensive	Topical steroids can control irritation and enhance effectiveness
Anthralin	Convenient short-contact programs, long remissions, effective for scalp	Purple-brown staining, irritating, careful application (only to plaque) required	Used on chronic (not inflamed) plaques; best results occur when used with UVB light
Tar	New preparations are pleasant	Only moderately effective in a few patients	Most effective when combined with UVB
UVB and lubricating agents or tar	Insurance may cover part or all of treatment, effective for 70% of patients, no need for topical steroids	Expensive, office-based therapy	Used only on plaque and guttate psoriasis, travel and time required
Tape or occlusive dressing	Convenient, no mess	Expensive, only for limited disease	May be used to occlude topical steroids
Intralesional steroids	Convenient, rapidly effective, long remissions	Only for limited areas, atrophy and telangiectasia occur at injection site	Ideal for chronic scalp and body plaques when small and few in number

Table 8-6 Therapeutic Options for Persons with Psoriasis on More than 20% of the Body

Treatment	Advantages	Disadvantages
UVB and narrow-band ultraviolet B light (NB-UVB)	Effective and safe	Requires many office visits
PUVA	Allows patient to be ambulatory; effective	Many treatments needed; many office visits required, carcinogenic
Methotrexate	"Gold standard" for efficacy; helps arthritis	Hepatotoxicity; liver biopsy periodically required
Acitretin (Soriatane)	Effective for palmar-plantar-pustular, erythrodermic, and pustular types of psoriasis; fast, effective; helps arthritis	Teratogenic; many annoying side effects
Cyclosporine	Fast, effective; helps arthritis	Nephrotoxic; immunosuppressive; expensive
Biologic therapies: adalimumab (Humira), etanercept (Enbrel), infliximab (Remicade); many others in development	No multiorgan adverse effects; very effective; potential for interaction with other drugs is very low	Very expensive; no long-term experience; give by injection or intravenously

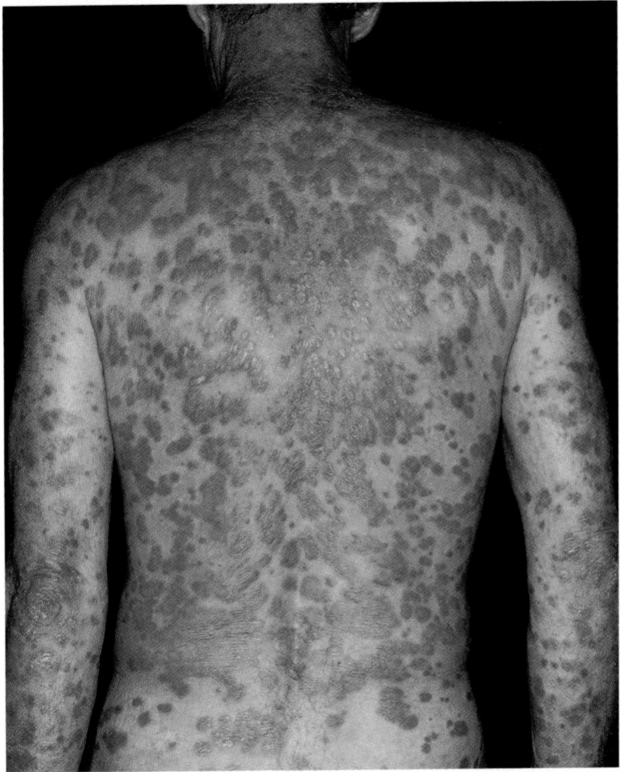

Figure 8-26 Erythrodermic psoriasis. This highly inflamed form of psoriasis responds well to acitretin as monotherapy.

Topical therapy

CALCIPOTRIENE (DOVONEX)

Calcipotriene (Dovonex) 0.005% is a vitamin D_3 analog that inhibits epidermal cell proliferation and enhances cell differentiation. It is effective and safe and well tolerated for the short- and long-term treatment of psoriasis. Up to 100 gm/week can be used. Dovonex ointment has been discontinued. Dovonex cream and Dovonex scalp solution will continue to be available. Calcipotriene is more effective than the group II corticosteroid ointments fluocinonide 0.05% and anthralin. Tachyphylaxis (tolerance) does not occur with calcipotriene. Calcipotriene solution is used for scalp psoriasis. It is not as effective as betamethasone valerate, but it does not have the corticosteroid side effects of atrophy. It is valuable for long-term scalp treatment programs.

Calcipotriene is not as effective as group I corticosteroids, but regimens using calcipotriene and group I corticosteroids are superior over either agent alone. Most patients now use the following regimen: Calcipotriene is applied in the morning and a group I corticosteroid is applied in the evening for 2 weeks. Then a maintenance regimen is begun using group I corticosteroids twice daily on weekends and calcipotriene twice daily on weekdays. Application for 6 to 8 weeks gives a 60% to 70% improvement in plaque-type psoriasis. Remission is maintained with long-term use of this program. Application of calcipotriene twice a day is much more effective than once a day application. Calcipotriene treatment can produce a mild irritant contact dermatitis at the site of application. The face and intertriginous areas are prone to this side effect.

Calcipotriene is not very effective at improving the response to UVB or narrowband UVB. UVB does not inactivate calcipotriene. Hypercalcemia is reported with excessive quantities of calcipotriene applied over large surface areas. Parameters of calcium metabolism do not change when less than 100 gm per week is used.

CALCITROL (VECTICAL)

This new ointment formulation is another vitamin D_3 analog. It has similar properties to Dovonex and may be used in the same manner. It is limited to 200 grams/week and is a pregnancy category C drug. Use with caution in patients receiving medications known to increase serum calcium levels, such as thiazide diuretics. Caution should also be exercised in patients receiving calcium supplements or high doses of vitamin D.

Calcipotriene hydrate and betamethasone dipropionate. The two-compound ointment containing calcipotriene 50 mcg/gm plus betamethasone dipropionate 0.5 mg/gm (Dovobet, Daivobet, Taclonex) combines a vitamin D analog and a corticosteroid. It is applied once each day and is indicated for the topical treatment of psoriasis in adults 18 years of age and older. The ointment can be used acutely for 4 to 8 weeks to bring psoriasis under control. After this, control of the disease can be maintained with once-daily application as needed.

The maximum weekly dose should not exceed 100 gm. Treatment of more than 30% body surface area is not recommended. Taclonex ointment should not be applied to the face, axillae, or groin. Some patients fail to respond to the treatment. It is well-tolerated in repetitive use as required for up to 52 weeks. It is very expensive.

RETINOIDS

Tazarotene (0.05%, 0.1%) is available as a gel and cream. Irritation develops in most patients. The stronger formulation is more effective but more irritating.

Topical steroids can control irritation and enhance effectiveness. Groups I, II, and IV topical steroids are all effective when used in combination with tazarotene. The retinoid may prevent corticosteroid atrophy. Treatment consists of application of tazarotene once a day and a topical steroid approximately 12 hours later.

Remission of psoriasis was maintained for at least 5 months with a regimen of tazarotene gel 0.1% applied Mondays, Wednesdays, and Fridays and clobetasol ointment applied Tuesdays and Thursdays.

Some clinicians believe that a short-contact regimen is effective. Tazarotene is applied for 5 minutes and then washed off. This regimen minimizes irritation but maintains efficacy.

Patients treated with UVB and tazarotene responded more favorably than patients treated with UVB alone. Tazarotene thins the stratum corneum of the epidermis, allowing patients to burn more easily. UV doses are reduced by at least one third if tazarotene is added to a course of phototherapy. Tazarotene remained chemically stable when used in conjunction with UVB or UVA phototherapy.

TOPICAL STEROIDS

Topical steroids (see Chapter 2) give fast but temporary relief. They are most useful for reducing inflammation and controlling itching. Initially, when the patient is introduced to topical steroids, the results are most gratifying. However, tachyphylaxis, or tolerance, occurs, and the medication becomes less effective with continued use. Patients remember the initial response and continue topical steroids in anticipation of continued effectiveness. Long-term use of topical steroids results in atrophy and telangiectasia. Topical steroids are useful for treating inflamed and intertriginous plaques.

A group I through V steroid applied one to four times a day in a cream or ointment base is required for best results. Plastic occlusion of topical steroids is much more effective than simple application. Augmented betamethasone dipropionate and clobetasol are extremely potent, and occlusion is not used with these drugs. Group V topical steroids applied once or twice a day should be used in the intertriginous areas and on the face. Some plaques resolve completely, but most remain only partially reduced with continued application. Continual application for more than 3 weeks should be discouraged. Remissions are usually brief and the plaques may return shortly after treatment is terminated. Topical steroid creams applied under an occlusive plastic dressing promote more rapid clearing, but remissions are not extended.

The rapid appearance of atrophy and telangiectasia occurs when the group I topical steroids are occluded. Topical steroid solutions are useful for scalp psoriasis. Intralesional injection of small plaques with triamcinolone acetonide (Kenalog 5 to 10 mg/ml) almost invariably clears the lesion and accords long-term remission. Atrophy may occur with the 10 mg/ml concentration.

Betamethasone valerate foam (Luxiq) and clobetasol propionate foam (Olux, Olux-E) are available in 50-gm and 100-gm containers. Luxiq is also available in 150-gm containers. The foam becomes a liquid upon contact with the skin. Clobetasol is available as a spray (Clobex). These formulations are very effective and preferred by many patients to creams, ointments, and solutions for treating scalp lesions and plaque psoriasis on the trunk and extremities. Transient stinging occurs in some patients. The foam emollient formulations are very well tolerated. Moisturizers can be applied soon after application of the foam.

INTRALESIONAL STEROIDS

Patients with a few, small, chronic psoriatic plaques of the scalp or body can be effectively treated with a single intralesional injection of triamcinolone acetonide (Kenalog 5 to 10 mg/ml). The 10 mg/ml solution may be diluted with saline. Most injected plaques clear completely and remain in remission for months. Atrophy and telangiectasias may appear at the injection site. The face and intertriginous areas are avoided.

ANTHRALIN

Anthralin is used only for chronic plaques. For years anthralin has been used effectively in the hospital to treat psoriasis. The principal objections were to the mess, long treatment times, and staining. Maximum patient compliance can be achieved with the new, short-treatment time schedules and commercially available preparations. There are several effective treatment programs. Psoriasis clears faster when UVB radiation is used in combination with anthralin.

PREPARATIONS AND USE. Anthralin is commercially available in concentrations of 0.1%, 0.25%, 0.5%, and 1.0% (3% outside of the United States). Patients must be cautioned about irritation and staining. Psoriatec is a 1% anthralin cream formulation designed to reduce the risk of staining and irritation.

Hands should be washed carefully after application, with care to avoid eye contact. Care must also be taken to protect normal skin, and anthralin should not be applied to intertriginous areas or to the face. Ointment is removed by showering with soap. Lubricants are applied to avoid dryness and to remove the last traces of anthralin. If irritation occurs, anthralin should be discontinued, and the patient should be treated with group II through V topical steroids until improvement is noted.

Skin stains fade in a matter of weeks, but purple clothing stains are permanent (Figure 8-27). Anthralin is also used for scalp psoriasis. Triethanolamine, applied when anthralin is removed, prevents irritation and staining of the skin. Hypochlorite detergents have been used successfully to remove anthralin stains from materials, and mild acid soaps wash off anthralin skin stains.

Short-contact therapy. Apply the medication and wash it off in 20 minutes. Contact time can be increased to an hour; longer times are probably no more effective and become inconvenient. The goal is to maintain a daily schedule using the highest concentration of anthralin that can be tolerated without inducing inflammation.

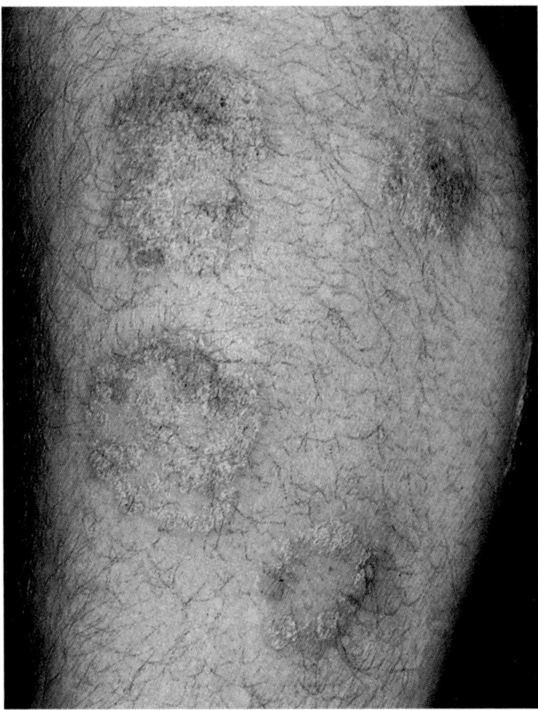

Figure 8-27 Psoriatic plaques under treatment with anthralin. As with all forms of treatment, plaques first clear in the center.

ULTRAVIOLET LIGHT B

The most effective topical programs use ultraviolet light in combination with lubricating agents, tar, or tazarotene. The addition of tazarotene to a regimen of UVB phototherapy results in faster and more effective clearing. Several studies have indicated that the duration of remission is shortened when UVB is administered with topical corticosteroids. When UVB phototherapy is used in conjunction with short-contact anthralin therapy, studies have shown little additional benefit from the combination in comparison to UVB alone, and patients disliked using anthralin. When calcipotriene is used in conjunction with UVB, there is slightly more clearing with the combination of treatments compared with UVB alone.

Ultraviolet light in intensities high enough to be effective can be obtained from natural sunlight or commercially available light cabinets. Inexpensive single-bulb tanning lights and long-wave ultraviolet light (UVA) tanning salon lights are sometimes effective. Most dermatologists have phototherapy units; many patients are best treated in that setting. There is a significant positive correlation between patients' responses to sunbathing and their responses to short-wave ultraviolet light (UVB) phototherapy. Sunlight nonresponders have a 70% chance of failure with UVB phototherapy; sunlight responders have an 80% chance that clearance treatment will succeed.

Tar and light. This regimen combines the daily application of tar with UVB exposure; it is safe and highly effective, and possibly produces the longest remissions. A tar concentrate such as Balnetar can be added to the bath water as a substitute for tar ointments and lotions. Tar-solution soaks are useful for psoriasis of the palms and soles. The feet can be soaked for 1 hour each day in a basin of warm water and one or two capfuls of Balnetar.

ULTRAVIOLET LIGHT B AND LUBRICATING AGENTS. Tar enhances the effectiveness of ultraviolet light, but studies suggest that application of lubricants before UVB exposure provides results similar to those achieved with tar and UVB. Optimum, long-term management may be achieved by continuing UVB phototherapy after initial clearing (average—six treatments per month). Treatment with UVB and lubricating agents is just as effective as UVB and topical steroids; therefore costly topical steroids can be avoided during light therapy. If not removed before phototherapy, preparations containing tar or thickly applied petrolatum or emollients can block UVB.

ULTRAVIOLET LIGHT B AND SYSTEMIC AGENTS. The combination of UVB phototherapy with systemic agents can be very effective. Combining methotrexate and UVB results in clearing of extensive psoriasis. Patients with extensive psoriasis were treated with a 3-week course of methotrexate followed by a combination of UVB therapy and methotrexate. When lesions cleared to less than 5% of body involvement, the methotrexate was stopped, and UVB therapy alone was used as maintenance therapy. This protocol achieved clearance of disease in all patients in a mean of 7 weeks. The combination therapy of methotrexate and UVB allows for clearing of psoriasis at relatively low doses of UVB and methotrexate and thus may reduce the long-term cumulative toxicity of both agents. Similarly, the combination of acitretin with UVB results in more rapid and more effective clearing than monotherapy with either agent alone.

NARROW-BAND ULTRAVIOLET LIGHT B (NB-UVB). The spectrum of UV light most effective for the treatment of psoriasis is in a narrow range (approximately 311 nm). Treatment with these narrow-band bulbs is superior to treatment with broadband UVB. Compared with NB-UVB, PUVA achieves clearance in more patients with fewer treatment sessions and results in longer remissions.

PHOTOCHEMOTHERAPY

The treatment known as PUVA is so designated because of the use of a class of drugs called psoralens (P), along with exposure to long-wave ultraviolet light (UVA). Oxsoralen-Ultra capsules are an encapsulated liquid formulation of methoxsalen (available in 10-mg capsules). Patients ingest a prescribed dose of methoxsalen approximately 2 hours before being exposed to a carefully measured amount of UVA in a uniquely designed enclosure. A major advantage of PUVA is that it controls severe psoriasis with relatively few maintenance treatments, and it can be done on an outpatient basis. Light does not penetrate hair: scalp psoriasis must be treated with conventional therapy.

Indications. PUVA is an effective method of controlling, not curing, psoriasis. Patients should be selected only by physicians who are experienced in the treatment of all forms of psoriasis. PUVA is indicated for the symptomatic control of severe, recalcitrant, and disabling plaque psoriasis that is not adequately responsive to other forms of therapy. Erythrodermic and pustular psoriasis are best treated with acitretin. Pustular psoriasis of the palms and soles responds best to PUVA-acitretin. Because of the concerns about long-term toxicity, PUVA is most appropriate for severe psoriasis in patients older than 50 years of age. The American Academy of Pediatrics has disapproved the use of PUVA therapy in children.

Psoriatic arthropathy of the nonspondylitic type may respond to PUVA with improvement in erythema, tenderness, and inflammation of the peripheral joints.

Treatment regimen. The treatment regimen is divided into two phases: the clearance phase, in which continual treatment is given until clearing occurs; followed by the maintenance phase, in which treatments are given less frequently but in numbers sufficient to prevent a flare-up of the disease.

Response to treatment. After the initial clearing phase, patients require a mean of 30 treatments per year during the first $1^{1}/_{2}$ year. Most patients who are clear after the initial 2- to 3-month maintenance period remain clear for at least 6 to 12 months. Disease control lasts longer after PUVA than after UVB therapy. Continued use of PUVA after initial clearing affords good disease control for prolonged periods. The recurrence rate is higher in patients who do not continue maintenance treatment; however, long-term maintenance results in high cumulative doses of energy.

PUVA COMBINED WITH OTHER MODALITIES. Combining PUVA with other modalities (UVB, calcipotriene, tazarotene, acitretin, and methotrexate) reduces the number of PUVA treatments required to maintain remission, results in fewer adverse effects from treatment, increases efficacy, and reduces cost.

PUVA plus acitretin. Combination therapy of psoriasis with acitretin and phototherapy (psoralen-ultraviolet A [PUVA] or ultraviolet B [UVB]) offers multiple advantages over use of either modality alone.

LONG-TERM SIDE EFFECTS. Most long-term side effects of PUVA are dose-dependent. Methods should be sought to control disease using the minimum amount of PUVA therapy. These include the use of appropriate dosage regimens, the avoidance of maintenance therapy as far as possible, and the use of combination therapies.

Skin tumors. PUVA promotes skin aging, actinic keratoses, and squamous cell carcinoma (SCC), especially in patients previously treated with arsenic or ionizing radiation and in patients with a history of skin cancer. The risk of cutaneous SCC from PUVA is dose-related. There is a strong, dose-dependent increase in the risk of genital tumors associated with exposure to PUVA and ultraviolet B radiation. Men should use genital protection when they are exposed to PUVA and to other forms of ultraviolet radiation for therapeutic, recreational, or cosmetic reasons.

Approximately 15 years after the first treatment with PUVA, the risk of malignant melanoma increases, especially among patients who receive 250 treatments or more (Table 8-7).

Table 8-7 PUVA Cancer Risks

Malignant melanoma	Squamous cell carcinoma	Basal cell cancer
15 years after first PUVA Rx, risk increases in patients with >250 treatments	Persistent, dose-related increase in risk	No increased risk within a decade of beginning treatment
Number of patients small	11-fold increase in patients treated with more than 260 PUVA sessions	

From Morison W et al: *Arch Dermatol* 134(5):595, 1998.
PMID: 9606329

Lentigines. Lentigines develop in many patients after long-term treatment with PUVA. These small black macules occur in PUVA-exposed sites.

Cataracts. Concern has been expressed that PUVA therapy may cause cataracts, but the incidence seems to be very low if eye protection is used. During the first day of PUVA treatment, patients should wear UVA-blocking, plastic, wraparound glasses when they are outdoors from the time they ingest the drug until bedtime. While indoors or in dim light, either wraparound glasses or clear UVA-blocking glasses should be worn. During the second day, either plastic wraparound or clear UVA-blocking glasses should be worn the entire day.

SHORT-TERM SIDE EFFECTS. Short-term side effects include dark tanning, pruritus, nausea, and severe sunburn.

Nausea. Nausea is the most common side effect. It develops shortly after methoxsalen is taken. Nausea is prevented by dividing the psoralen dose over 15 minutes and taking it with food; 1500 mg of ginger ingested 20 minutes before the psoralen may also prevent nausea. PUVA treatments later in the day are less likely to result in nausea than those administered in the morning.

Phototoxicity. Avoid sun exposure on the days of treatment to prevent burns. PUVA burns begin 24 hours after exposure and peak at 48 hours. PUVA is not administered 2 days in a row because the second treatment might be given to a patient who is not aware that a burn will occur from the first day's treatment.

TAPE OR OCCLUSIVE DRESSINGS

One study showed that adhesive occlusive dressings applied and changed every week were therapeutically superior to a group V topical steroid and comparable to UVB therapy. Complete clearing occurred in 47% of the cases in an average of 5 weeks; another 41% improved. Waterproof tape with low-moisture vapor transmission applied continually for 1 week gave similar results. Two or more applications were required. This treatment may be appropriate for treating localized chronic plaques. Actiderm and DuoDERM are self-adhesive patches that are applied alone or over topical steroids and changed every 1 to 7 days.

TREATING THE SCALP

The scalp is difficult to treat because hair interferes with the application of medicine and shields the skin from ultraviolet light. Symptoms of tenderness and itching vary considerably. The goal is to provide symptomatic and cosmetic relief. It is unnecessary and impractical to attempt to keep the scalp constantly clear.

REMOVING SCALE. Scale must be removed first to facilitate penetration of medicine. Superficial scale can be removed with shampoos that contain tar and salicylic acid (e.g., T/Gel). Thicker scale is removed by applying Baker's P & S or 10% liquor carbonis detergens (LCD) in Nivea oil to the scalp and washing 6 to 8 hours later with shampoo or Dawn dishwashing liquid. Combing during the shampoo helps dislodge scale.

Baker's P & S liquid (phenol, sodium chloride, and liquid paraffin) applied to the scalp at bedtime and washed out in the morning is moderately effective in reducing scale. Baker's liquid is pleasant and well tolerated for extended periods.

LCD (10%), a tar extract of crude oil tar, is mixed with Nivea oil by the pharmacist. The unpleasant mixture is liberally massaged into the scalp at bedtime. Warming the mixture before application enhances scale penetration. A shower cap protects pillows and also encourages scale penetration. An impressive amount of scale is removed in the first few days. Nightly applications are continued until the scalp is acceptably clear.

MILD TO MODERATE SCALP INVOLVEMENT. When used at least every other day, tar shampoos (see the Formulary) may be effective in controlling moderate scaling. Corticosteroid solutions are expensive, but a few drops can cover a wide area. Steroid gels (e.g., fluocinonide gel, clobetasol gel, desoximetasone gel), which have a keratolytic base and penetrate hair, are effective for localized plaques. Derma-Smoothe/FS lotion (peanut oil, fluocinolone acetonide 0.01%) is an effective topical steroid that can be applied to the entire scalp and occluded with a shower cap. The scalp is dampened before application. The oil base penetrates and loosens scale. Treatment is repeated each night for 1 to 3 weeks until itching and erythema are controlled.

Betamethasone valerate foam (Luxiq) and clobetasol foam (Olux) are available in 50-gm and 100-gm containers. Luxiq is also available in a 150-gm continers. The foam becomes a liquid upon contact with the skin. This formulation is effective and pleasant, and easily penetrates through hair. Temporary stinging may occur during application.

Small plaques are effectively treated with intralesional steroid injections of triamcinolone acetonide (Kenalog 10 mg/ml). Remissions following use of intralesional steroids are much longer than those following topical steroids.

Ketoconazole cream is sometimes useful. Oral ketoconazole (400 mg daily) may be effective in some cases. The possibility of drug toxicity limits its usefulness.

TREATMENT OF DIFFUSE AND THICK SCALP PSORIASIS. Calcipotriene 0.005% and betamethasone dipropionate 0.064% topical suspension (Taclonex Scalp, Dovobet, Xamiol) is a topical suspension for the treatment of moderate-to-severe psoriasis of the scalp in adults. Apply the suspension to affected areas once daily for 2 weeks or until cleared. Treatment may be continued for up to 8 weeks. The maximum weekly dose should not exceed 100 gm. Patients should shake the bottle before using the product.

The following medications can be used, all of which use oil or ointment-based preparations for scale penetration. They are applied at bedtime and washed out each morning with strong detergents such as Dawn dishwashing liquid. Topical steroid solutions can be applied during the day.

Tar and oil. Ten percent LCD in Nivea oil applied to the scalp, covered with a shower cap and washed out each morning, removes scale and suppresses inflammation. This must be prepared by a compounding pharmacist.

Anthralin. Anthralin ointment applied each evening and removed in the morning is another method for treating resistant scalp psoriasis. A short-contact method similar to that previously described for anthralin is used. Apply 0.5% anthralin ointment and wash completely 10 to 20 minutes after application. Dritho-Scalp is packaged in a tube with a long nozzle for hair penetration.

Systemic therapy

Topical treatment has its limits. Many patients do not respond to the most vigorous topical programs, or the disease may be so extensive that topical treatment is not practical.

Moderate-to-severe psoriasis, variably defined as patients with 20% or more involvement of body surface area or patients unresponsive to topical therapy, can be treated with several modalities including phototherapy, photochemotherapy (PUVA), retinoids, methotrexate, or biologic agents.

A number of systemic drugs are available, some of which have potentially serious side effects. Methotrexate is highly effective, relatively safe, and well tolerated, but the need for periodic liver biopsies discourages some patients and physicians. Photochemotherapy (PUVA) is effective and relatively safe. Acitretin is used to potentiate the effects of PUVA and as a monotherapy for plaque, pustular, and erythrodermic forms of psoriasis. Acitretin has many annoying side effects. Hydrea is not hepatotoxic, but it is rarely used because it is effective in only a few patients. Cyclosporine is rapidly effective, but long-term use may be associated with loss of kidney function. Biologic drugs are safe and effective and are rapidly becoming the preferred systemic therapy for psoriasis.

ROTATIONAL THERAPY

A rotational approach to therapy has been suggested (Figure 8-28). Rotation of available therapies (UVB plus tar, PUVA, methotrexate, acitretin, cyclosporine, and biologic therapy) for moderate-to-severe psoriasis may minimize long-term toxicity and allow effective treatments to be maintained for many years. Patients may receive each form of therapy for 1 to 2 years and then switch to the next form

ROTATIONAL THERAPY

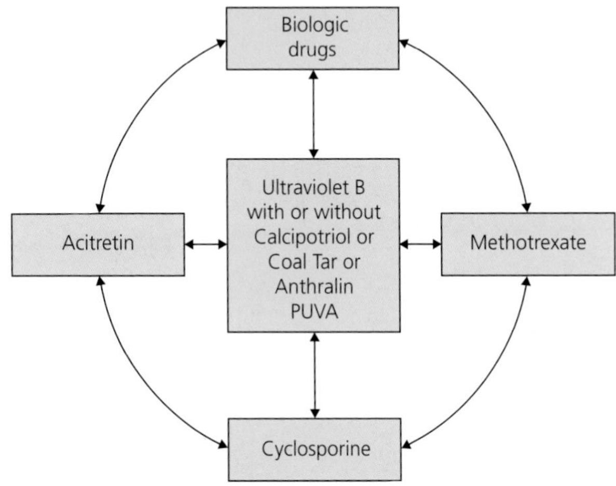

For moderate-to-severe psoriasis to minimize toxic effects from any one therapy. A reasonable sequence would start with phototherapy (PUVA or ultraviolet B), followed by methotrexate, then the other form of radiation, then another oral agent, and so on. Patients who do not tolerate radiation therapy rotate oral agents.

Figure 8-28

of treatment. By rotating each of the treatments at these intervals, it may be 4 or 5 years before the patient needs to return to the first therapy, thereby minimizing the cumulative toxicity by long periods off each treatment.

The physician and patient must make the final decision about which therapeutic modality is appropriate based on the unique features of each individual case.

A reasonable sequence would start with phototherapy (narrow band ultraviolet B), followed by a biologic drug. Patients who do not respond or can not afford biologics can be rotated to methotrexate.

METHOTREXATE (See Boxes 8-2 to 8-10)

INDICATIONS. Methotrexate (MTX) has been used to treat psoriasis for over 40 years. It is the "gold standard" for the treatment of severe psoriasis and is particularly effective in controlling erythrodermic and generalized pustular psoriasis. It induces remissions in the majority of treated patients and maintains remissions for long periods with continued therapy. MTX is also effective for psoriatic arthritis. It is relatively safe and well tolerated, but the need for periodic liver biopsies discourages many patients and physicians from using it.

MECHANISM OF ACTION. MTX is a folic acid antagonist that inhibits dihydrofolate reductase. DNA synthesis is inhibited as the concentrations of thymidine and purines fall after treatment with MTX. MTX suppresses psoriatic epidermal cell reproduction and has antiinflammatory and immunomodulatory effects. Methotrexate is immunosuppressive; use should be avoided in patients with active infections.

DOSING. The oral triple-dose regimen used to be the most common method used. A dose is taken at 12-hour intervals during a 36-hour period once each week. The single weekly dose is now the preferred regimen. An initial test dose of 2.5 to 5 mg is given, and complete blood cell counts and liver function tests (LFTs) are obtained 1 week later. If this dose was well tolerated, start with one 2.5-mg tablet at 12-hour intervals for three doses. The next week the dosage is increased by one to two tablets. In the following weeks, titrate up or down by a 2.5-mg tablet to the most effective and best-tolerated dosage. Most patients are controlled and tolerate 15 mg/week. Once the desired degree of clearing is obtained, the dosage is decreased by one tablet per week every few weeks to arrive at a maintenance regimen (i.e., 2.5 to 5.0 mg/week). The goal is not necessarily 100% clearance, but to reach 80% improvement. This is safer than pushing higher, more toxic dosages to obtain 100% clearance.

Discontinue the drug for several months of rest; the summer months are a good time to attempt this, when sunlight may control the disease. Gradually tapering to withdraw MTX seems to present fewer problems of rebound than does a sudden discontinuance of the drug.

MONITORING. Bone marrow toxicity is the most serious short-term side effect; hepatotoxicity is the most common long-term adverse effect. MTX is excreted mainly via the kidney. Older individuals tend to have reduced renal function and require lower dosages of MTX.

Leukocyte and platelet counts are depressed maximally approximately 7 to 10 days after treatment. A drop in these counts below normal levels necessitates reducing or stopping therapy. LFTs are obtained at least 1 week after the last dose of the drug. MTX causes transient elevations in LFTs for 1 to 3 days after its administration, so a false-positive elevation might be seen if the patient is tested too soon.

SIDE EFFECTS. Short-term side effects include nausea, anorexia, fatigue, oral ulcerations and stomatitis, mild leukopenia, thrombocytopenia, and macrocytic anemia. These are dose-related and rapidly reversible and related to renal and hematologic function. Switching among triple dosing, weekly oral dosing, and intramuscular dosing may decrease these reactions. Hepatic fibrosis or cirrhosis can develop with long-term treatment. Extensive alcohol intake, daily dosing, prior liver disease, and cumulative MTX intake predispose patients to fibrosis and cirrhosis. Male and female patients should discontinue MTX for 3 to 4 months before attempting conception.

FOLIC AND FOLINIC ACID SUPPLEMENTS. Folates may reduce adverse effects and toxicities without affecting efficacy. Nausea, vomiting, diarrhea, alopecia, hepatotoxicity, and bone marrow suppression that results in leukopenia, thrombocytopenia, or pancytopenia may be prevented. Folic acid 1 mg once each day is commonly prescribed as a first-line supplement to patients receiving methotrexate for the treatment of psoriasis. It can be given every day,

Box 8-2 **Recommendations for Methotrexate**

- **Indication:** Severe, recalcitrant, disabling psoriasis that is not adequately responsive to other forms of therapy
- **Dosing:** Methotrexate is administered as a weekly single oral dose or an oral triple dose.

  Doses can be increased gradually until an optimal response is achieved. Total dose should not ordinarily exceed 30 mg per week. Doses should be reduced to the lowest possible amount of drug needed to achieve adequate control of psoriasis with concomitant topical therapy.

  A test dose of 2.5-5 mg is recommended.
- **Duration of Dosing**

  Treatment can be continued for as long as is necessary provided there are no signs of liver or bone marrow toxicity with adequate monitoring.

  Folic acid supplementation 1-5 mg daily by mouth reduces the frequency of side effects.
- **Therapeutic Results**

  In the only placebo-controlled trial of methotrexate for psoriasis, 36% of patients treated with 7.5 mg orally per week, increased as needed up to 25 mg per week, reached PASI 75 after 16 weeks.
- **Absolute Contraindications**

  Pregnancy

  Nursing mothers

  Alcoholism

  Alcoholic liver disease or other chronic liver disease

  Immunodeficiency syndromes

  Bone marrow hypoplasia, leukopenia, thrombocytopenia, or significant anemia

  Hypersensitivity to methotrexate
- **Relative Contraindications**

  Abnormalities in renal function

  Abnormalities in liver function

  Active infection

  Obesity

  Diabetes mellitus
- **Toxicity**

  Elevated LFTs

  - Minor elevations of LFTs are common. If elevation exceeds 2× normal, must check more frequently; if exceeds 3× normal, consider dose reduction; if exceeds 5× normal, discontinue.

  Anemia, aplastic anemia, leukopenia, thrombocytopenia

  Interstitial pneumonitis

  Ulcerative stomatitis

  Nausea, vomiting, diarrhea

  Malaise or fatigue

  Chills and fever

  Dizziness

  Decreased resistance to infection

  Gastrointestinal ulceration and bleeding

  Photosensitivity ("radiation recall")

  Alopecia
- **Drug Interactions**

  Hepatotoxic drugs such as barbiturates

  Acitretin has been used successfully in combination with methotrexate despite the potential for hepatotoxicity from both medications.

  Drugs that interfere with renal secretion of methotrexate such as sulfamethoxazole, NSAIDs, and penicillin

  Folic acid antagonists such as trimethoprim
- **Liver Biopsy**

  Low-risk patients—at baseline, not necessary

  - First biopsy: 3.5-4 gm; subsequent biopsies to be considered after 1.5 gm

  High-risk patients including history of diabetes, obesity, abnormal LFTs, excessive EtOH ingestion, chronic liver disease, family history of heritable liver disease

  - Consider baseline biopsy or at 6 months with subsequent biopsies after 1-1.5 gm

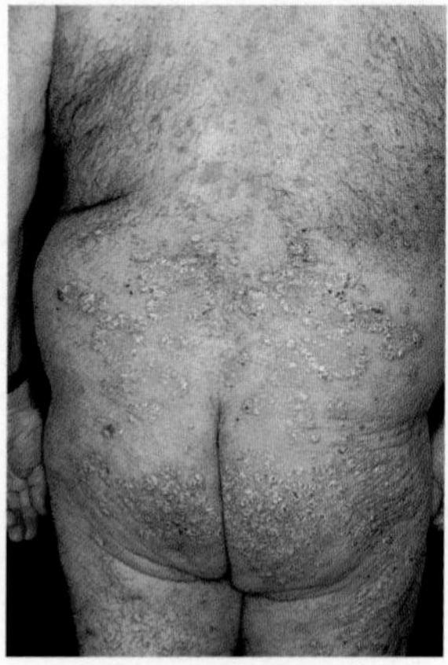

Extensive chronic plaque psoriasis

From Journal of the American Academy of Dermatology (in Press). Guidelines of Care for the Management of Psoriasis and Psoriatic Arthritis. Section 4: Guidelines of Care for the Management and Treatment of Psoriasis with Traditional Systemic Agents.

Box 8-2 Recommendations for Methotrexate—cont'd

- **Baseline Monitoring**
  History and physical examination
  CBC and platelet count
  BUN, creatinine, and LFTs
  Liver biopsy only indicated in patients with a history of significant liver disease
  Pregnancy test and test for HIV in selected patients
  Consider PPD
  Consider chest x-ray if patient has underlying pulmonary disease
- **Ongoing Monitoring**
  CBC and platelet count at varying intervals (initially every 2-4 weeks for first few months and then every 1-3 months depending upon dosage adjustments, symptoms, and previous CBC results)
  LFTs at monthly intervals, BUN, creatinine every 2-3 months depending on dosage adjustments, symptoms, and previous blood results
  Pregnancy test if indicated
  Consider liver biopsy in high-risk patients including history of diabetes, obesity, abnormal LFTs, excessive EtOH ingestion, chronic liver disease, family history of heritable liver disease.
  For those without risk factors, consider liver biopsy in patients with cumulative doses of more than 3.5-4 gm of methotrexate.
  For patients without risk factors, consider repeat liver biopsies after each subsequent 1.5-gm dosage, based on LFTs, risk factors such as diabetes and obesity, or in consultation with a hepatologist.
  The amino-terminal peptide of procollagen III is used in Europe (but is generally not available in the United States) as a test for hepatic fibrosis, reducing the need for frequent liver biopsies.
- **Pregnancy:** Category X; males and females considering conception should stop taking methotrexate for 3 months before attempting to conceive. Should pregnancy ensue before this time, consider genetic counseling.
- **Nursing:** Mothers receiving methotrexate should not breast-feed.
- **Pediatric Use:** Methotrexate is approved for the treatment of juvenile rheumatoid arthritis. Low-dose methotrexate has been used effectively and safely in children for a variety of dermatologic and rheumatologic disorders.
- **Psoriatic Arthritis:** Although there are only two small controlled trials evaluating methotrexate for psoriatic arthritis that are inadequately powered to assess clinical benefit, methotrexate is often used as the primary agent to treat psoriatic arthritis.

Box 8-3 Relative Contraindications for the Use of Methotrexate

- Abnormalities in renal function may require a marked reduction in the dose as 85% of methotrexate is renally excreted.
- Significant abnormalities in liver function—LFTs should be followed and all elevations require careful monitoring.
- Hepatitis, active or recurrent
- Excessive current alcohol consumption—While there are little data to support specific limits on alcohol consumption, some physicians require patients to completely refrain from alcohol while others allow daily alcohol intake. A history of alcoholism is particularly worrisome if there is baseline liver damage.
- Concomitant use of hepatotoxic drugs—More frequent monitoring of liver function tests should be considered.
- Active infectious disease, particularly chronic infections that are likely to be worsened by immunosuppressive effects of methotrexate such as active untreated tuberculosis or acquired immunodeficiency syndrome. Methotrexate should be withheld during acute infections.
- Current use of other immunosuppressive agents
- Conception should be avoided during methotrexate treatment and afterwards for at least 3 months in the male or four ovulatory cycles in the female.
- Recent vaccination with a live vaccine
- Obesity (body mass index greater than 30 kg/m^2)
- Diabetes mellitus
- Unreliable patient

From Journal of the American Academy of Dermatology (in Press). Guidelines of Care for the Management of Psoriasis and Psoriatic Arthritis. Section 4: Guidelines of Care for the Management and Treatment of Psoriasis with Traditional Systemic Agents.

Box 8-4 Risk Factors for Hematologic Toxicity from Methotrexate

- Renal insufficiency
- Advanced age
- Lack of folate supplementation
- Medication errors
- Drug interactions
- Hypoalbuminemia
- Excess alcohol intake
- Multiple concurrent medications

From Journal of the American Academy of Dermatology (in Press). Guidelines of Care for the Management of Psoriasis and Psoriatic Arthritis. Section 4: Guidelines of Care for the Management and Treatment of Psoriasis with Traditional Systemic Agents.

Box 8-5 Indications for Methotrexate in Psoriasis

Severe psoriasis that may be life-ruining physically, emotionally, or economically.

1. Patients with moderate to severe psoriasis
2. Psoriatic erythroderma
3. Psoriatic arthritis, moderate to severe
4. Acute pustular psoriasis, von Zumbusch type
5. More than 20% involvement of body surface
6. Localized pustular psoriasis
7. Psoriatic that affects certain areas of body so that normal function and employment are prevented
8. Lack of response to phototherapy, PUVA, and retinoids

From Roenigk H et al: *J Am Acad Dermatol* 1998; 38(3):478.

including the day of methotrexate administration. Folinic acid is more expensive. Consider using folinic acid if folic acid is not ameliorating laboratory abnormalities (LFT elevations) and symptoms of MTX toxicity. Dosing folinic acid too closely (within 24 hours) to the administration of methotrexate may hinder efficacy. Folinic acid (leucovorin) is prescribed as 5 mg (oral) every 12 h × three doses only. The first dose is given 24 h after the last dose of weekly MTX. This regimen is repeated each week. *PMID: 16198787*

Box 8-6 **Monitoring for Hepatotoxicity in Patients with No Risk Factors for Hepatotoxicity**

- No baseline liver biopsy
- Monitor liver function tests monthly for the first 6 months and then every 1-3 months thereafter:
  - For elevations less than twofold upper limit of normal: repeat in 2-4 weeks.
  - For elevations more than twofold but less than threefold upper limit of normal: closely monitor, repeat in 2-4 weeks, and decrease dose as needed.
  - For persistent elevations in 5/9 AST levels over a 12-month period or if there is a decline in the serum albumin level below the normal range with normal nutritional status, in a patient with well-controlled disease, a liver biopsy should be performed.
- Consider liver biopsy after 3.5-4.0-gm total cumulative dosage.

  or
- Consider switching to another agent or discontinuing therapy after 3.5-4.0-gm total cumulative dosage.

  or
- Consider continuing to follow above guidelines without biopsy.

From Journal of the American Academy of Dermatology (in Press). Guidelines of Care for the Management of Psoriasis and Psoriatic Arthritis. Section 4: Guidelines of Care for the Management and Treatment of Psoriasis with Traditional Systemic Agents.

Box 8-7 **Monitoring for Hepatotoxicity in Patients with Risk Factors for Hepatotoxicity**

- Consider the use of a different systemic agent.
- Consider delayed baseline liver biopsy (after 2-6 months of therapy to establish medications' efficacy and tolerability).
- Repeat liver biopsies after approximately 1-1.5 gm of methotrexate.

From Journal of the American Academy of Dermatology (in Press). Guidelines of Care for the Management of Psoriasis and Psoriatic Arthritis. Section 4: Guidelines of Care for the Management and Treatment of Psoriasis with Traditional Systemic Agents.

Box 8-8 **Duration of Methotrexate Treatment to Achieve a Cumulative Dose of 1.5 gm**

Weekly dose (mg)	Months to 1.5 gm
7.5	50
15.0	25
22.5	17

From Journal of the American Academy of Dermatology (in Press). Guidelines of Care for the Management of Psoriasis and Psoriatic Arthritis. Section 4: Guidelines of Care for the Management and Treatment of Psoriasis with Traditional Systemic Agents.

Box 8-9 **Medications That May Increase Methotrexate Toxicity**

Nonsteroidal anti-inflammatory drugs	Antibiotics	Others
Salicylates	Trimethoprim/ sulfamethoxazole	Barbiturates
Naproxen	Sulfonamides	Colchicine
Ibuprofen	Penicillins	Dipyramidole
Indomethocin	Minocycline	Ethanol
Phenylbutazone	Ciprofloxacin	Phenytoin
		Sulfonylureas
		Furosemide
		Thiazide diuretics

From Journal of the American Academy of Dermatology (in Press). Guidelines of Care for the Management of Psoriasis and Psoriatic Arthritis. Section 4: Guidelines of Care for the Management and Treatment of Psoriasis with Traditional Systemic Agents.

Box 8-10 **Risk Factors for Hepatotoxicity from Methotrexate**

- History of or current excessive alcohol consumption (Methotrexate toxicity is associated with a history of total lifetime alcohol intake before methotrexate therapy. The exact amount of alcohol that leads to risk is unknown and differs from person to person.)
- Persistent abnormal liver chemistry studies
- History of liver disease including chronic hepatitis B or C
- Family history of inheritable liver disease
- Diabetes mellitus
- Obesity
- History of significant exposure to hepatotoxic drugs or chemicals
- Lack of folate supplementation
- Hyperlipidemia

From Journal of the American Academy of Dermatology (in Press). Guidelines of Care for the Management of Psoriasis and Psoriatic Arthritis. Section 4: Guidelines of Care for the Management and Treatment of Psoriasis with Traditional Systemic Agents.

LIVER FIBROSIS, CIRRHOSIS, AND BIOPSY INTERVAL. Methotrexate is liver toxic and is avoided if possible in patients with liver disease or in those with risk factors for liver disease. Active alcoholics must not take methotrexate. Patients who are obese or diabetic can have an increased risk of cirrhosis. Patients receiving long-term methotrexate therapy should be followed up with liver biopsies.

LIVER BIOPSY. Guidelines for obtaining a liver biopsy are listed in Boxes 8-2, 8-6, and 8-7.

Data suggest that at 1.5 gm of cumulative drug usage, cirrhosis can occur in approximately 3% of patients. Cumulative doses of 4 gm or more have led to an incidence as high as 25%. MTX-induced cirrhosis may be of a "low aggressive" type.

The management of abnormal liver biopsy findings is found in Box 8-11. Cirrhosis is more common in patients with psoriasis than in patients with rheumatoid arthritis. Therefore rheumatologists do not require routine liver biopsies.

LUNG TOXICITY. Methotrexate-induced lung injury can be sudden and severe. The presenting symptom is usually a new onset of cough and shortness of breath. It is most often a subacute process, in which symptoms are commonly present for several weeks before diagnosis. Approximately 50% of the cases are diagnosed within 32 weeks from initiation of MTX treatment. A patient who recovers from MTX lung injury should not be retreated. Earlier recognition and drug withdrawal may avoid the serious and sometimes fatal outcome.

The strongest predictors of lung injury were older age, diabetes, rheumatoid pleuropulmonary involvement, previous use of disease-modifying antirheumatic drugs, and hypoalbuminemia.

RECALL OF SUNBURN. Patients taking methotrexate with a previous history of radiation burns or sunburns may experience a flare-up of symptoms in the areas that had been burned. This reaction is distinct from true photosensitivity.

PREGNANCY. Methotrexate is teratogenic and not prescribed for pregnant women. The drug may temporarily affect fertility in males. There are reports of normal infants born to the partners of males who had been treated with methotrexate around the time of conception. Although the risk to the fetus may be low, it has been suggested that methotrexate be discontinued several months before conception.

DRUG INTERACTIONS. Drug interactions are most likely to be a problem in patients with low renal function. Neutropenia is a major problem; life-threatening bone marrow toxicity can occur. Blood counts should be monitored after changes in therapy, especially in patients with impaired renal function, such as the elderly. Nonsteroidal antiinflammatory drugs can reduce renal clearance of methotrexate, resulting in toxic levels. Methotrexate can increase serum levels of some agents (e.g., naproxen). Patients with psoriatic arthritis can be safely treated with ketoprofen, fluorobiprofen, and piroxicam. Avoid trimethoprim-sulfamethoxazole. It is commonly associated with severe methotrexate toxicity. It competes with methotrexate for renal tubular secretion. Plasma prothrombin times should be monitored for patients receiving warfarin anticoagulants.

Box 8-11 **Classification of Liver Biopsy Findings and Management**

Finding	Management
Grade I: Normal; fatty infiltration, mild; nuclear variability, mild; portal inflammation, mild	Continue MTX.
Grade II: Fatty infiltration, moderate to severe; nuclear variability, moderate to severe; portal tract expansion, portal tract inflammation, and necrosis, moderate to severe	Continue MTX.
Grade IIIA: Fibrosis, mild (portal fibrosis here denotes formation of fibrotic septa extending into the lobules; slight enlargement of portal tracts without disruption of limiting plates or septum formation does not classify the biopsy specimen as grade III)	Continue MTX. Repeat biopsy after approximately 6 months of MTX therapy. Consider alternative prescription.
Grade IIIB: Fibrosis, moderate to severe	Stop MTX. Exceptional circumstances, however, may require continued methotrexate therapy, with thorough follow-up liver biopsies.
Grade IV: Cirrhosis (regenerating nodules, as well as bridging of portal tracts, must be demonstrated)	Stop MTX. Exceptional circumstances, however, may require continued methotrexate therapy, with thorough follow-up liver biopsies.

Adapted from Roenigk H et al: *J Am Acad Dermatol* 38(3):478, 1998. PMID: 9520032

RETINOIDS

ACITRETIN. Acitretin (Soriatane) is an oral retinoid and one of the safest systemic psoriasis therapies. As monotherapy, acitretin is most effective in treating pustular and erythrodermic psoriasis. Monotherapy is less effective for plaque psoriasis. Acitretin in combination with PUVA or UVB is more effective for plaque psoriasis than monotherapy. Efficacy and side effects vary among patients. Acitretin is started at a low dose (10 to 25 mg/day) and increased to find the proper balance between efficacy and tolerance of side effects (Box 8-12).

Indications. Pustular and erythrodermic psoriasis are very responsive to acitretin (Figure 8-29). Plaque psoriasis is less responsive to monotherapy; higher, more toxic doses are often required for control. Improvement is gradual, taking more than 3 months to reach optimum dose.

Dosing strategy. Therapeutic and toxic responses to acitretin vary greatly. Some patients are very retinoid-responsive. A single "correct" dose cannot be recommended. Dose escalation is the optimum strategy for establishing the dosage. Start with a low dose of acitretin (10 to 25 mg/day) and escalate as needed to enhance efficacy while minimizing side effects. Start with 25 mg/day for most patients. This regimen allows gradual onset of "tolerance" to side effects and avoids use of higher doses than needed.

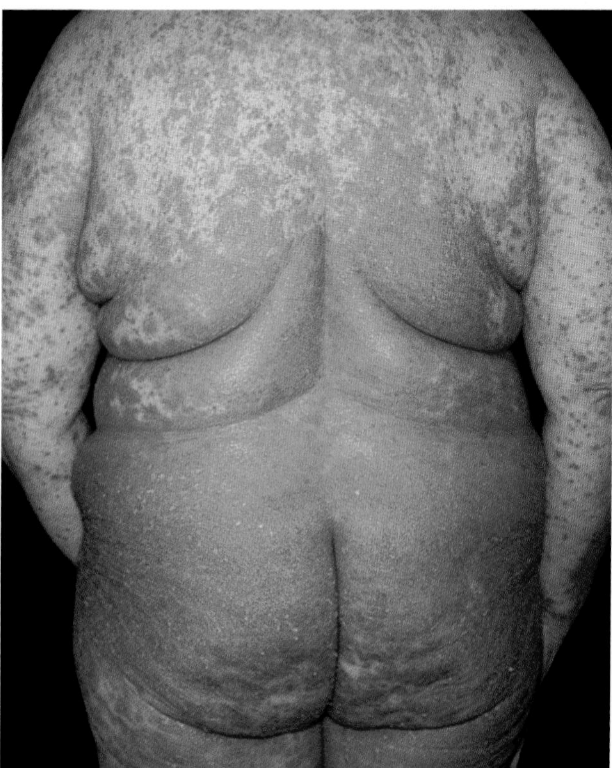

Figure 8-29 Erythrodermic psoriasis is very responsive to acitretin.

Acitretin and ultraviolet light B and PUVA. Compared with either acitretin or UV light monotherapy alone, combination regimens enhance efficacy and limit treatment frequency, duration, and cumulative doses. Lower doses of acitretin are usually effective when used in combination with phototherapy. Acitretin can often be used at the dose range of 10 to 25 mg daily. This results in faster and more complete responses to PUVA and to UVB. Significantly lower ultraviolet doses are required when retinoids are added to a phototherapy regimen.

Laboratory changes. The monitoring schedule is listed in Box 8-13. Elevation of serum lipid level, particularly triglycerides, can be prevented by concomitant administration of gemfibrozil (Lopid) or atorvastatin calcium (Lipitor). Elevation of liver function tests can occur.

Side effects. Acitretin is teratogenic. In the presence of ethanol, acitretin is esterified to etretinate. Etretinate persists in tissue for years. Therefore acitretin is not prescribed to women of child-bearing potential who may become pregnant within 3 years. In doses of 50 mg per day or higher, mucocutaneous side effects are common and include cheilitis, conjunctivitis, hair loss, failure to develop normal nail plates, dry skin, and "sticky skin." Periungual pyogenic granulomas can develop. Headache is a possible sign of pseudotumor cerebri. High doses for long-term treatment may produce calcification of ligaments and skeletal hyperostoses. These are often asymptomatic.

ISOTRETINOIN

Isotretinoin is highly effective for pustular psoriasis and is beneficial when combined with PUVA or UVB for plaque psoriasis.

Box 8-12 **Summary of Studies on Acitretin Therapy for Psoriasis**

- Acitretin monotherapy is very effective for pustular and erythrodermic psoriasis. Combination regimens with UVB or PUVA are preferred for plaque psoriasis; in these cases, it is even more advantageous to start with lower doses of acitretin (10-25 mg/day).
- Optimum dose range for monotherapy is 25-50 mg/day.
- Improvement occurs gradually, requiring up to 3-6 months for peak response.
- Overall rate of complete remission is generally <50%.
- Higher doses (50-75 mg/day) result in more rapid, and possibly more complete, responses but are associated with significantly increased side effects.
- Mucocutaneous side effects, hepatotoxicity, and alterations in serum lipid profile are dose-dependent.
- Initial flare involving increased surface area of psoriatic lesions despite decreased erythema and scaling may occur, lasting 1-2 months after initiation of therapy.

Box 8-13 **Recommendations for Acitretin**

- **Indication:** FDA approved for adults with severe plaque-type psoriasis
- **Dosing:** 10-50 mg/day given as a single dose
  Lower doses (25 mg/day or less) often used to minimize side effects, especially in combination regimens.
  When acitretin is added to UV, light dose should be reduced by 30-50%.
- **Short-Term Results**
  Efficacy rates are not well-defined but are high, based on studies of high dosages that are poorly tolerated.
  Efficacy rates when used in combination with phototherapy are higher.
- **Long-Term Results**
  Not reported
- **Contraindications**
  Acitretin is a potent teratogen and must be avoided in women who become pregnant.
  Severely impaired liver or kidney function
  Chronic abnormally elevated blood lipid values
- **Toxicity**
  Cheilitis
  Alopecia
  Xerosis, pruritus
  Xerophthalmia, night blindness
  Dry mouth
  Paronychia
  Paresthesias
  Headache, pseudotumor cerebri
  Nausea, abdominal pain
  Joint pain
  Myalgia
  Hypertriglyceridemia
  Abnormal LFTs

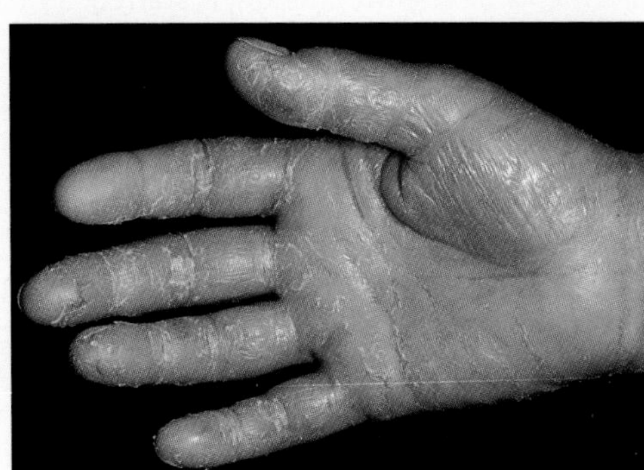

Erythrodermic psoriasis

- **Drug Interactions**
  Etretinate can be formed with concurrent ingestion of acitretin and ethanol.
  Acitretin may potentiate glucose lowering effect of glibenclamide.
  May interfere with the contraceptive effect of microdosed progestin minipill.
  In patients taking methotrexate and etretinate, hepatitis has occurred. Although this is a listed contraindication, its safe usage has also been reported.
  May reduce protein binding of phenytoin.
  Acitretin and tetracyclines can both increase intracranial pressure. Their combined use should be avoided.
  Concomitant administration of vitamin A and other oral retinoids with acitretin should be avoided.
- **Baseline Monitoring**
  History and physical examination
  Lipid profile, CBC, LFTs, renal function tests
  Pregnancy test if indicated
- **Ongoing Monitoring**
  LFTs, lipid profile at 2-wk intervals for the first 8 weeks, then every 6-12 wk
  CBC, renal function tests every 3 months
  Pregnancy test if indicated
- **Pregnancy:** Category X
- **Nursing:** Mothers receiving acitretin should not breast-feed.
- **Pediatric Use:** The safety and efficacy of acitretin in children with psoriasis are not established. High-dose, long-term oral retinoid use has been associated with ossification of interosseous ligaments and tendons of the extremities, skeletal hyperostoses, decreases in bone mineral density, and premature epiphyseal closure.
- **Psoriatic Arthritis:** Generally thought to be ineffective for psoriatic arthritis

From Journal of the American Academy of Dermatology (in Press). Guidelines of Care for the Management of Psoriasis and Psoriatic Arthritis. Section 4: Guidelines of Care for the Management and Treatment of Psoriasis with Traditional Systemic Agents.

CYCLOSPORINE (See Boxes 8-14 to 8-17)

Cyclosporine (CS) at dosages of 2.5 to 5.0 mg/kg/day administered to reliable, carefully selected patients who are closely monitored for both clinical and laboratory parameters produces fast and favorable results for severe plaque psoriasis. Cyclosporine is indicated for the treatment of severe, recalcitrant, plaque psoriasis in adults who are immunocompetent. Cyclosporine microemulsion (Neoral) is available in soft gelatin capsules (25 mg, 100 mg) and oral solution (50-ml bottle to 100 mg/ml). The Cyclosporine Consensus Conference Report provides the guidelines for using this medication.

BASELINE MONITORING. The key to monitoring is to obtain accurate baseline values before therapy is started.

KIDNEY FUNCTION AND CREATININE. Renal changes are functional and anatomic. They are caused by changes in renal blood flow patterns and cytotoxic effects on renal cells. Anatomic changes that include interstitial fibrosis, tubular atrophy, and arteriopathy occur. They occur in nearly all patients treated for at least 1 year. More severe effects occur with increasing age, decreased renal function, and hypertension at baseline. Some loss in renal function occurs in many patients; it is usually mild and reversible.

Elevated creatinine levels usually occur in the first 16 weeks of treatment and stabilize after that. Biweekly measurements are suggested for at least the first 12 weeks of therapy. If the serum creatinine level increases by more than 30% above the baseline, another determination is done within 2 weeks. If the second level confirms the increase, the dosage should be decreased by at least 1 mg/kg/day, and the level rechecked in 1 month. If the level decreases to less than 30% above the baseline, treatment can be continued. If the level remains greater than 30% above the baseline, therapy should be stopped and not resumed until the level returns to within 10% of the baseline. Routine measurements of glomerular filtration rate and creatinine clearance are not necessary. Routine kidney biopsies are not done.

HYPERTENSION. Hypertension develops in 8% to 30% of patients. Antihypertensive therapy can control the blood pressure elevation. The best response is achieved with calcium channel antagonists such as nifedipine, isradipine, or felodipine. Angiotensin-converting enzyme inhibitors are not as effective, and beta-blockers may occasionally worsen psoriasis. Decreased renal function and hypertension are somewhat reversible with a decrease in dose or discontinuation of cyclosporine, but there is irreversible kidney damage

Box 8-14 **Recommendations for Cyclosporine**

- **Indication:** Adult, non-immunocompromised patients with severe, recalcitrant psoriasis
  Severe is defined by the FDA as extensive or disabling plaque psoriasis.
  Recalcitrant is defined by the FDA as those patients who have failed to respond to at least one systemic therapy or in patients for whom other systemic therapies are contraindicated, or cannot be tolerated.
  Some guidelines suggest use of cyclosporine in moderate to severe psoriasis.
  Efficacy observed in erythrodermic psoriasis, generalized pustular psoriasis, and plamoplantar psoriasis.
- **Dosing:** 2.5-5.0 mg/kg/day in two divided doses
  Dose adjustments downward (by 0.5-1.0 mg/kg) when clearance is achieved or when hypertension or decreased renal function tests are observed
- **Duration of Dosing**
  Optimally used as interventional therapy; may be repeated at intervals after a rest period
  U.S. approval: 1-year continuous treatment; non-U.S. approval: 2 years of continuous treatment
- **Short-Term Results**
  At 3 and 5 mg/kg/day, 36% and 65%, respectively, achieved clear or almost clear after 8 weeks
  Dose dependent; after 8-16 weeks, 50-70% of patients achieved PASI 75
- **Long-Term Results**
  Not recommended because of toxicities
  Rapid relapse after abrupt discontinuation of cyclosporine
- **Contraindications**
  Concomitant PUVA or UVB therapy, methotrexate or other immunosuppressive agents, coal tar, prior PUVA or radiation therapy
  Abnormal renal function
  Uncontrolled hypertension
  Malignancy
  Hypersensitivity to cyclosporine
  Avoid live vaccines
  Caution with major infection and poorly controlled diabetes

From Journal of the American Academy of Dermatology (in Press). Guidelines of Care for the Management of Psoriasis and Psoriatic Arthritis. Section 4: Guidelines of Care for the Management and Treatment of Psoriasis with Traditional Systemic Agents.

Box 8-14 Recommendations for Cyclosporine—cont'd

- **Toxicity**
  Renal impairment
  - Acute
  - Chronic (increasing glomerular fibrosis with increasing duration of treatment with higher dosages)

  Hypertension
  Malignancies
  - Cutaneous
  - Lymphoproliferative

  Headache, tremor, paresthesia
  Hypertrichosis
  Gingival hyperplasia
  Worsening acne
  Nausea/vomiting/diarrhea
  Myalgias
  Flulike symptoms
  Lethargy
  Hypertriglyceridemia
  Hypomagnesemia
  Hyperkalemia
  Hyperbilirubinemia
  Increased risk of infection
  May increase risk of cancer

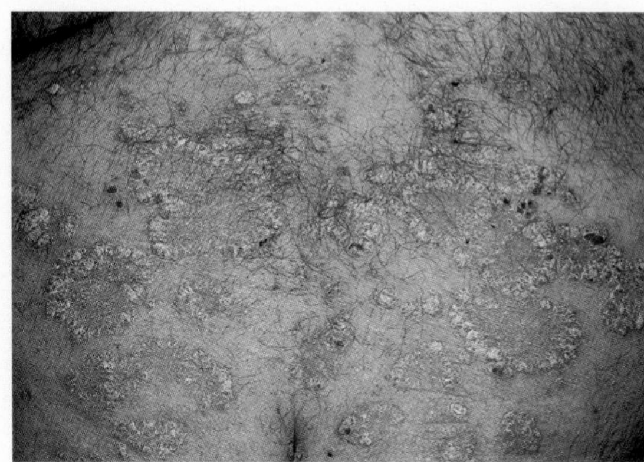

Severe plaque psoriasis

- **Drug Interactions (see Box 8-15)**
  Inducers/inhibitors of cytochrome P-450 3A4
  St. John's wort decreases cyclosporine concentration.
  Cyclosporine may reduce clearance of digoxin, colchicine, prednisolone, statins (increased risk of rhabdomyolysis).
  Potassium-sparing diuretics cause hyperkalemia.
  Thiazide diuretics increase nephrotoxicity.
  Killed vaccines may have decreased efficacy.
  Live vaccination is contraindicated.
  Grapefruit juice
  NSAIDs
- **Baseline Monitoring**
  History and physical examination
  Blood pressure × 2
  BUN and Cr × 2
  Urinalysis
  Consider PPD
  LFTs, CBC, lipid profile, magnesium, uric acid, and potassium
  Pregnancy test if indicated

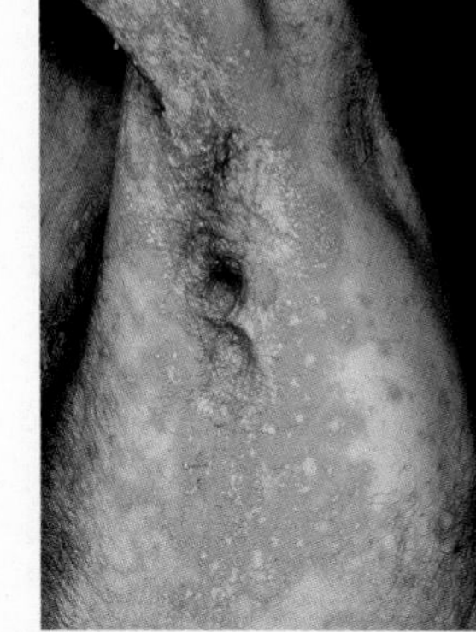

Generalized pustular psoriasis

- **Ongoing Monitoring**
  Every other week during initial 3 months, thereafter at 1-month intervals: blood pressure, BUN, and Cr
  Monthly CBC, LFTs, lipid profile, magnesium, uric acid, and potassium; pregnancy testing if indicated
- **Pregnancy:** Category C; lower birth weight and shorter duration of pregnancy reported in transplant patients. Appears not to be teratogenic in transplant patients.
- **Nursing:** Mothers receiving cyclosporine should not breast-feed.
- **Pediatric Use:** Transplant recipients as young as 1 year old have been treated with no unusual adverse events. While the safety and efficacy of cyclosporine for children <18 years with psoriasis have not been established, it may be considered in this patient population with severe psoriasis.
- **Psoriatic Arthritis:** There are studies demonstrating the efficacy of cyclosporine for psoriatic arthritis.

in many patients. In a few patients hypertension remains after the discontinuation of cyclosporine. A decrease in dosage of 25% to 50% is recommended if hypertension develops.

LIVER FUNCTION. Serum bilirubin level usually is increased. Isolated elevations of bilirubin level should not cause alarm. Only in the presence of other consistent and significant abnormalities of liver function does the patient need referral for further evaluation. The safety of cyclosporine in patients with chronic active hepatitis is unknown.

OTHER CHEMISTRIES. Uric acid level may increase and rarely requires anti-gout therapy. Serum magnesium level may decline; if blood levels are below the normal range, replacement with magnesium tablets is indicated. Cholesterol and triglyceride levels may increase.

OTHER SIDE EFFECTS. Side effects occur in proportion to the dose. Malaise or fatigue, nausea, headaches, and general achiness may occur. Hand tremors, paresthesias, or sensitivity to hot and cold in the fingers and toes tend to occur at higher doses. These symptoms tend to resolve as therapy proceeds. Hypertrichosis may occur. Patients who develop gingival hyperplasia are sent to a dentist. Increased uric acid levels may precipitate gout. Elevations of triglyceride levels (>750 mg/dl) occur in 15% of patients; elevations of cholesterol levels (>300 mg/dl) occur in less than 3%. Most laboratory abnormalities are reversible when cyclosporine is stopped.

DOSAGE. The starting dose depends on the clinical state. There are two approaches to determine the starting dosage. The speed of improvement and the success rate are proportional to the dosage.

Low-dose approach. Start at 2.5 mg/kg/day, and wait at least 1 month before considering increasing the dosage. This approach with slow increments in dosages is for patients with stable, generalized psoriasis or for patients in whom the severity lies between moderate and severe. Increase the dosage by 0.5 to 1.0 mg/kg/day increments every 2 weeks, up to a maximum of 5 mg/kg/day if needed. Higher doses are rarely necessary.

High-dose approach. Start at 5 mg/kg/day dose when rapid improvement is critical. Patients with severe, inflammatory flares, patients with recalcitrant cases that have failed to respond to other modalities, or distressed patients in a crisis situation are candidates for the high-dose approach. High doses are usually well tolerated for short-term use. As soon as there is a response, the dosage is decreased by 0.5 to 1 mg/kg/day, but no more than one step in the decrement of dosage per week, until the minimum effective maintenance dosage is defined.

Intermittent short courses. A new therapeutic strategy to manage moderate-to-severe plaque psoriasis with cyclosporine is the use of intermittent short courses of treatment. It is effective and well tolerated and reduces the risk of side effects. Cyclosporine is initially given at a dose of 2.5 mg/kg/day in two divided doses. This dosage could be increased by increments of 0.5 to 1.0 mg/kg/day each week up to a maximum of 5 mg/kg/day. Treatment is continued until clearance of psoriasis, defined as 90% or more reduction in the area affected, occurs or for a maximum of 12 weeks. Cyclosporine is stopped abruptly. On relapse,

Box 8-15 **Medications That May Interfere with Cyclosporine**

Medications that increase cyclosporine levels:
- Antifungals: ketoconazole, itraconazole, fluconazole, vorinconazole
- Diuretics: furosemide, thiazides, carbonic anhydrase inhibitors
- Calcium antagonists: diltiazem, nicardipine, verapamil
- Corticosteroids: high-dose methylprednisolone
- Antiemetics: metoclopramide
- Antibiotics: macrolides, fluoroquinolones
- Antiarrhythmics: amiodarone
- Antimalarials: hydroxychloquine, chloroquine
- Anti-HIV drugs: ritonavir, indinavir, saquinavir, nelfinavir
- SSRIs: fluoxetine, sertraline

Medications that decrease cyclosporine levels:
- Antibiotics: nafcillin, rifabutin, rifampin, rifapentine
- Antiepileptics: carbamazepine, phenytoin, phenobarbital, valproic acid
- Somatostatin analogs: octreotide
- Tuberculostatics: rifampicin
- Retinoids: bexarotene
- St. John's wort: *Hypericum perforatum*
- Others: octreotide, ticlopidine, bosentan

Medications that may increase the risk of renal toxicity:
- NSAIDs: diclofenac, naproxen, sulindac, indomethacin
- Antifungals: amphotericin B, ketoconazole
- Antibiotics: ciprofloxacin, vancomycin, gentamycin, tobramycin, trimethoprim
- Alkylating agents: melphalan
- Others: H_2-histamine antagonists, tacrolimus

Medications whose levels increase when taken concomitantly with cyclosporine:
- Calcium channel blockers: diltiazem, nicardipine, verapimil
- Erectile dysfunction drugs: sildenafil, tadalafil, vardenafil
- Statins: atorvastatin, lovastatin, simvastatin
- Benzodiazepines: midazolam, triazolam
- Others: prednisolone, digoxin, colchicine, diclofenac, bosentan

It is strongly recommended that an up-to-date pharmaceutical reference be consulted whenever concomitant medication is used during cyclosporine therapy.

From Journal of the American Academy of Dermatology (in Press). Guidelines of Care for the Management of Psoriasis and Psoriatic Arthritis. Section 4: Guidelines of Care for the Management and Treatment of Psoriasis with Traditional Systemic Agents.

patients are given another course of cyclosporine, commencing at the optimum dose from the previous treatment period. Intermittent short courses for up to 2 years appear safe and well tolerated.

RESPONSE TO TREATMENT. Clearance is usually maintained as long as the clearing dose is held constant. Relapse may occur during attempts to adjust to a maintenance dose.

CONTRAINDICATIONS. Vaccination with live vaccines should be avoided; other vaccinations may be less effective during cyclosporine treatment. Patients with prostate or cervical cancer that has been completely eradicated may take cyclosporine.

DRUG INTERACTIONS. Patients taking drugs that are also metabolized by the cytochrome P-450 complex must be cautioned that the concurrent use of cyclosporine may raise or lower blood levels of the interacting drug.

COMBINATION THERAPY. Topical agents (superpotent corticosteroids, tazarotene, calcipotriene) can be used to treat resistant plaques. Topical medication can also be used to maintain clearing. Common programs of treatment include the morning application of a superpotent corticosteroid and an evening application of either tazarotene or calcipotriene to each new erupting lesion. Other agents that can be considered to keep the acute and/or the cumulative dose of cyclosporine as low as possible are listed in Box 8-16. There is not much experience with these combination therapies. The combination of PUVA or UVB and cyclosporine is rarely used because of the concern about the higher incidence of skin cancer in immunosuppressed patients. The use of cyclosporine with acitretin is well tolerated. Switching from cyclosporine to acitretin may be a useful way of withdrawing cyclosporine treatment.

ROTATIONAL THERAPY

Rotational therapy is a standard approach to limit side effects associated with long-term use of single agents. This involves rotating between UVB, PUVA, methotrexate, retinoids, biologic agents, and cyclosporine at intervals of approximately 1 to 2 years. The use of cyclosporine immediately before or especially after PUVA should be avoided because of the possible synergistic effects in the production of skin cancers.

Box 8-16 **Possible Combination Therapies for Psoriasis**

Cyclosporine plus topical agents

- Corticosteroids
- Anthralin
- Calcipotriene
- Tazarotene

Cyclosporine plus systemic drugs

- Acitretin
- Methotrexate
- Hydroxyurea
- Thioguanine
- Sulfasalazine
- Mycophenolic acid

Adapted from Lebwohl M et al: *J Am Acad Dermatol* 39(3):464, 1998. *PMID: 9738783*

Box 8-17 **Cyclosporine/Neoral Dosage**

Capsules (25 mg, 100 mg)
Oral solution (50-ml bottle: 100 mg/ml)
Starting dose: 2.5-5 mg/kg/day in one or two divided doses
Adjust by 0.5-1 mg/kg/day each week as needed

OTHER SYSTEMIC DRUGS FOR PSORIASIS

Several other drugs have been used to treat patients who experience toxicity or fail to respond to retinoids, methotrexate, or cyclosporine. Experience with all of these medications is limited. Guidelines for these drugs are listed in Boxes 8-17 to 8-25, pp. 298-305.

Text continued on p. 306

Box 8-18 Recommendations for Mycophenolate Mofetil

- **Indication**
  There is no FDA-approved use for psoriasis.
- **Dosing**
  1.0-1.5 gm orally two times per day
- **Short-Term Results**
  47% mean reduction in PASI at 12 weeks in 23 patients with psoriasis treated with 1.0-1.5 gm bid.
  47% mean reduction in PASI at 6 weeks in 11 psoriasis patients treated with 1 gm bid for 3 weeks and then 0.5 gm bid for 3 more weeks.
- **Long-Term Results:** No data
- **Contraindications**
  Hypersensitivity to mycophenolate mofetil, mycophenolic acid
- **Toxicity**
  GI side effects (diarrhea, nausea/vomiting, abdominal cramps). These occur early and decrease with continued use.
  Hematologic (leukopenia is most common; anemia, thrombocytopenia)
  Genitourinary (urgency, frequency, dysuria, sterile pyuria)
  Increased incidence of viral, bacterial, and mycobacterial infections
  Progressive multifocal leukoencephalopathy
  Hypercholesterolemia, hypophosphatemia, hyperkalemia, hypokalemia
  Fever and myalgias
  Headache, insomnia
  Peripheral edema
  Hypertension
  Patients taking mycophenolate mofetil should not be given live attenuated virus vaccines.
- **Drug Interactions**
  Antacids containing aluminum and magnesium
  Calcium and iron
  Cholestyramine
  Antibiotics including cephalosporins, fluoroquinolones, macrolides, penems, penicillins, sulfonamides inhibit enterohepatic recirculation and decrease mycophenolate mofetil levels.
  High-dose salicylates
  Phenytoin
  Xanthine bronchodilators
  Probenecid
  Acyclovir, ganciclovir, valganciclovir
- **Baseline Monitoring**
  History and physical examination
  CBC, platelet counts
  Chemistry screen, LFTs
  Pregnancy test if indicated
- **Ongoing Monitoring**
  CBC, platelet count weekly ×1 month; then every 2 weeks for 2 months; then monthly thereafter
  Monthly chemistry panel and LFTs
  Biannual physical examination focusing on lymph node exam and skin cancer exam (SCCs in particular)
  Pregnancy testing if indicated
- **Pregnancy/Nursing:** Pregnancy category D
  Pregnancy and breast-feeding should be avoided during treatment and patients (including males) must use adequate contraceptive precautions.
- **Pediatric Use:** No data
- **Psoriatic Arthritis:** Case reports suggest improvement.

From Journal of the American Academy of Dermatology (in Press). Guidelines of Care for the Management of Psoriasis and Psoriatic Arthritis. Section 4: Guidelines of Care for the Management and Treatment of Psoriasis with Traditional Systemic Agents.

Box 8-19 **Recommendations for Tacrolimus**

- **Indication**
  There is no FDA-approved use for psoriasis.
- **Dosing for Psoriasis**
  0.05-0.15 mg/kg
- **Duration of Dosing**
  Unknown
- **Short-Term Results**
  Efficacy rates are poorly characterized. Patients dosed at 0.05 mg/kg showed no difference from placebo at 3 wk. When dosed at 0.10-0.15 mg/kg, by 9 wk there was a statistically significant improvement in PASI compared to placebo.
- **Long-Term Results**
  Not reported
- **Contraindications**
  Patients with hypersensitivity to tacrolimus or its metabolites
- **Side effect profile similar to cyclosporine:**
  Most common side effects include tremor, headache, nausea, diarrhea, hypertension, and abnormal renal function tests.
  Less common side effects include hyperglycemia, hyperkalemia, elevated LFTs, anemia, leukocytosis, dyspnea, fever, arthralgias, edema, diabetes, insomnia, paresthesias.
- **Drug Interactions**
  Are numerous drug interactions as tacrolimus is metabolized by cytochrome P450 system.
  Do not give tacrolimus and cyclosporine together.
- **Baseline Monitoring**
  History and physical examination
  CBC/diff, renal and LFTs
  Pregnancy test if indicated
- **Ongoing Monitoring—proper frequency is not established**
  Blood pressure
  Serum chemistry
  Renal function
  Liver function
  Pregnancy testing if indicated
- **Pregnancy:** Category C
- **Nursing:** Tacrolimus should not be used by nursing mothers.
- **Pediatric Use:** No data
- **Psoriatic Arthritis:** Case reports suggest improvement.

From Journal of the American Academy of Dermatology (in Press). Guidelines of Care for the Management of Psoriasis and Psoriatic Arthritis. Section 4: Guidelines of Care for the Management and Treatment of Psoriasis with Traditional Systemic Agents.

Box 8-20 **Recommendations for Hydroxyurea**

- **Indication**
  There is no FDA-approved use for psoriasis.
- **Dosing**
  Initial dose of 500 mg PO bid increasing to 3 gm/day as tolerated
  Weekly dose of 3-4.5 gm/week has also been utilized.
- **Short-Term Results**
  Efficacy rates vary widely.
  One study showed that 55% of 31 patients had at least a 70% score (mean treatment time of 36 weeks), while another study comparing hydroxyurea to methotrexate showed a 48% reduction in PASI score after 12 weeks of hydroxyurea.
- **Long-Term Results**
  One study found that 60% of 85 patients treated for a mean of 16 months had a complete or almost complete clearance.
- **Contraindications**
  Marked bone marrow depression, including leukopenia, thrombocytopenia, or anemia
- **Toxicity**
  Bone marrow suppression
  Gastrointestinal symptoms (stomatitis, anorexia, nausea, vomiting, diarrhea, and constipation)
  Dermatologic reactions (rash, ulceration, dermatomyositis-like skin changes, alopecia)
  Dysuria rare
  Neurologic disturbances limited to headache, dizziness, disorientation, hallucinations, and convulsions rarely seen
  Temporary impairment of renal tubular function accompanied by elevations in serum uric acid, BUN, and creatinine
  Fever, chills, malaise, edema, asthenia
  Elevation of hepatic enzymes
  Pulmonary fibrosis rare
  Fatal and nonfatal pancreatitis and hepatotoxicity and severe peripheral neuropathy have been reported in HIV-infected patients who received hydroxyurea in combination with antiretroviral agents.
- **Drug Interactions**
  Concurrent use of hydroxyurea and other myelosuppressive agents or radiation therapy may increase the likelihood of bone marrow depression.
  Hydroxyurea may raise the serum uric acid level; dosage adjustment of uricosuric medication may be necessary.
- **Baseline Monitoring**
  History and physical examination
  Complete blood count at baseline and weekly until stable dose is achieved
  Pregnancy test if indicated
- **Ongoing Monitoring**
  Complete blood count at monthly intervals
  Biannual physical examination focusing on lymph node exam and skin cancer exam (SCCs in particular)
  Pregnancy testing if indicated
- **Pregnancy/Nursing: Pregnancy category D**
  Pregnancy and breast-feeding should be avoided during treatment and patients (including males) must use adequate contraception.
- Pediatric Use: No data
- Psoriatic Arthritis: No data

From Journal of the American Academy of Dermatology (in Press). Guidelines of Care for the Management of Psoriasis and Psoriatic Arthritis. Section 4: Guidelines of Care for the Management and Treatment of Psoriasis with Traditional Systemic Agents.

Box 8-21 **Recommendations for 6-Thioguanine**

- **Indication**
  There is no FDA-approved use for psoriasis.
- **Dosing**
  Start at 80 mg two times per week. Increase by 20 mg every 2-4 weeks.
  Maximum dose is 160 mg three times per week.
- **Short-Term Results**
  Open-label trial of 14 patients treated with pulse dosing followed by maintenance dosage (120 mg twice a week to 160 mg three times per week). Of 11 patients who became longer term responders, 6/11 showed a response after 2-4 weeks.
- **Long-Term Results**
  76 patients followed for over 1 month. At 24 months, 58% were effectively maintained. Has been safely used up to 145 months.
  Another study showed 14/18 patients had 90% improvement.
- **Contraindications**
  Preexisting liver disease
  Immunosuppression
  Anemia, leukopenia, and/or thrombocytopenia
- **Toxicity**
  Myelosuppression
  Liver toxicity from hepatic veno-occlusive disease
  Increased ALT and AST
  Hyperuricemia
  Photodermatitis
  Taste changes
  Gastroesophageal reflux, gastric ulcers
  Headache
  Nausea/vomiting
  Aphthous ulcers
  Fatigue
  Nonmelanoma skin cancer
  Multiple warts, herpes zoster
- **Drug Interactions**
  Aminosalicylate derivatives (olsalazine, mesalazine, or sulfasalazine) may inhibit TPMT.
- **Baseline Monitoring**
  History and physical examination
  CBC, platelet count, chemistry screen, LFTs, hepatitis B and C, PPD
  Pregnancy test if indicated
- **Ongoing Monitoring**
  CBC and platelet count every 2-4 weeks; serum chemistry every 3 months
  Biannual physical examination focusing on lymph node exam and skin cancer exam (SCCs in particular)
  Pregnancy testing if indicated
- **Pregnancy/Nursing:** Pregnancy category D
  Pregnancy and breast-feeding should be avoided during treatment, and patients (including males) must use adequate contraception.
- **Pediatric Use:** No data

From Journal of the American Academy of Dermatology (in Press). Guidelines of Care for the Management of Psoriasis and Psoriatic Arthritis. Section 4: Guidelines of Care for the Management and Treatment of Psoriasis with Traditional Systemic Agents.

Box 8-22 Recommendations for Azathioprine

- **Indication:**
  There is no FDA-approved use for psoriasis.
- **Dosing**
  Thiopurine methyltransferase (TPMT) levels are generally used to guide dosing.
  One suggested daily schedule guided by results of TPMT values:
  - TPMT <5.0 units, do not use azathioprine
  - TPMT 5-13.7 units, 0.5 mg/kg maximum dose
  - TPMT 13.7-19.0 units, 1.5 mg/kg maximum dose
  - TPMT >19.0 units, 2.5 mg/kg maximum dose

  Alternatively, start at 0.5 mg/kg, and monitor for cytopenia. If no cytopenia, can increase dose by 0.5 mg/kg/day after 6-8 wk if necessary and increase by 0.5 mg/kg/day every 4 wk thereafter as needed. Generally dosed at 75-150 mg/day.
- **Efficacy**
  In one study 19/29 patients had >75% improvement, but in another smaller study 5/10 patients had >25% improvement.
- **Contraindications**
  Absolute
  - Allergy to azathioprine?
  - Pregnancy or attempting pregnancy?
  - Clinically significant active infection?

  Relative
  - Concurrent use of allopurinol?
  - Prior treatment with cyclophosphamide or chlorambucil?
- **Toxicity**
  Bone marrow suppression
  Malignancies
  - Cutaneous (SCCs)
  - Lymphoproliferative

  Increased risk of infections
  GI: nausea, vomiting, diarrhea
  Hypersensitivity syndrome
  Pancreatitis
  Hepatitis
- **Drug Interactions**
  Allopurinol—increased risk of pancytopenia (if using concurrently, lower azathioprine dose by 75%)
  Captopril—may increase risk of anemia and leukopenia
  Warfarin—may need an increased dose of warfarin
  Pancuronium—may need an increased dose of this for adequate paralysis
  Co-trimoxazole—increased risk of hematologic toxicity
  Rifampicin—decreases azathioprine efficacy, also hepatotoxic
  Clozapine—increased risk of agranulocytosis
- **Baseline Monitoring**
  History and physical examination
  LFTs, CBC differential, serum chemistry profile, urinalysis, PPD, hepatitis B and C screen
  Pregnancy test if indicated
- **Ongoing Monitoring**
  CBC/diff two times a month for the first 2 months, monthly for the next 2 months, every 2 months thereafter
  LFTs monthly for the first 3 months, then every 2 months thereafter
  Biannual physical examination focusing on lymph node exam and skin cancer exam (SCCs in particular)
  Pregnancy testing if indicated
- **Pregnancy/Nursing:** Pregnancy category D
  Pregnancy and breast-feeding should be avoided during treatment with azathioprine, and patients (including males) must use adequate contraception.
- **Pediatric Use:** No data
- **Psoriatic Arthritis:** A small observational cohort study suggests that azathioprine may be of value in psoriatic arthritis.

From Journal of the American Academy of Dermatology (in Press). Guidelines of Care for the Management of Psoriasis and Psoriatic Arthritis. Section 4: Guidelines of Care for the Management and Treatment of Psoriasis with Traditional Systemic Agents.

Box 8-23 **Recommendations for Fumaric Acid Esters**

- **Indications**
  There is no FDA-approved use for psoriasis in the U.S. Fumaric acid esters are approved in Europe.
- **Dosing**
  Starting dose: 1 tablet of FUMADERM. Increase over the next 8 weeks to a maximum of 6 tablets daily.
- **Short-Term Results**
  Multicenter, randomized, double-blind, placebo-controlled trial of 100 patients showed that after 16 weeks fumarate-treated patients reached a mean PASI 50 compared to placebo patients whose PASI was essentially changed.
  Randomized, double-blind, controlled trial of 143 patients given either fumarates plus calcipotriol or fumarates alone found that patients given combination therapy reached PASI 50 in 3 wk vs. those treated with fumarates alone reaching PASI 50 in 9 wk.
- **Long-Term Results**
  Case series of patients treated up to 14 years suggest no increased risk for infections or malignancies. Large, long-term follow-up studies are necessary to confirm these observations.
- **Contraindications**
  Severe liver disease
  Severe or chronic gastrointestinal disease
  Severe or chronic kidney disease
  Malignancy or a history of malignancy
  Leukopenia and other hematologic abnormalities
  Pregnancy
  Breast-feeding
- **Toxicity**
  Gastrointestinal (abdominal cramps, nausea, diarrhea, fullness, and flatulence)
  Flushing
  Malaise
  Fatigue
  Lymphopenia, leukopenia, eosinophilia
  Hepatotoxicity and elevated LFTs
  Increased cholesterol, triglycerides
  Increased serum creatinine and potassium, and proteinuria
  Rare case reports of renal disease but none in the controlled trials
- **Drug Interactions**
  Other fumaric acid derivatives, methotrexate, cyclosporine, immunosuppressive drugs, and cytostatic drugs may potentiate toxicity.
  Drugs known to cause renal dysfunction
- **Baseline Monitoring**
  History and physical examination
  CBC, platelet counts
  Chemistry screen
  Urinalysis
- **Ongoing Monitoring**
  CBC, platelet count every other week for the first 2 months; monthly until month 6, and bimonthly thereafter
  Serum chemistry and urinalysis every 2 weeks for the first month; then monthly for the first 6 months, and bimonthly thereafter
- **Pregnancy:** Not recommended in pregnancy (no FDA pregnancy category because it is not approved in the U.S.)
- **Nursing:** There are no data and therefore mothers receiving fumaric acid esters should not breast-feed.
- **Pediatric Use:** No data
- **Psoriatic Arthritis:** One small double-blind, placebo-controlled trial suggested minimal efficacy as evidenced by decreased joint pain and sedimentation rate.

From Journal of the American Academy of Dermatology (in Press). Guidelines of Care for the Management of Psoriasis and Psoriatic Arthritis. Section 4: Guidelines of Care for the Management and Treatment of Psoriasis with Traditional Systemic Agents.

Box 8-24 Recommendations for Sulfasalazine

- **Indication**
  There is no FDA-approved use for psoriasis.
- **Dosing for Psoriasis**
  In psoriasis, initial dose of 500 mg PO bid increased to maximum of 3-4 gm/day as tolerated
- **Duration of Dosing**
  As long as needed. There are no known cumulative toxicities.
- **Short-Term Results**
  Efficacy rates not well characterized. In the only randomized, controlled trial, 8 wk of 3-4 gm/day sulfasalazine led to moderate improvement (global improvement of 30-59%) in 7/17 assessable sulfasalazine patients compared to 1/27 assessable placebo patients).
- **Long-Term Results**
  Not reported
- **Contraindications**
  Patients with intestinal or urinary obstruction; patients with porphyria; patients hypersensitive to sulfasalazine, its metabolites, sulfonamides, or salicylates
- **Toxicity**
  Anorexia, headache, gastrointestinal symptoms (including nausea, vomiting, and gastric distress), and oligospermia can occur in up to one third of patients.
  Less frequent reactions include skin rash, pruritus, urticaria, fever, hemolytic anemia, and cyanosis, which may occur in one in 1/30 patients or less.
- **Drug Interactions**
  Reduced absorption of folic acid and digoxin
- **Baseline Monitoring**
  History and physical examination
  CBC/diff and LFTs
  Pregnancy test if indicated
- **Ongoing Monitoring**
  CBC/diff and LFTs every other week for the first 3 months. During the second 3 months, CBC/diff and LFTs monthly and thereafter once every 3 months. Urinalysis and renal function tests should be done periodically.
  Pregnancy testing if indicated
- **Pregnancy:** Category B
- **Nursing:** Sulfonamides are excreted in the milk. In the newborn, they compete with bilirubin for binding sites on the plasma proteins and may thus cause kernicterus.
- **Pediatric Use:** No data
- **Psoriatic Arthritis:** In the largest trial of sulfasalazine for psoriatic arthritis, after 36 weeks of treatment with 2 gm/day, 58% of patients given sulfasalazine compared to 45% of patients given placebo achieved PsARC.

From Journal of the American Academy of Dermatology (in Press). Guidelines of Care for the Management of Psoriasis and Psoriatic Arthritis. Section 4: Guidelines of Care for the Management and Treatment of Psoriasis with Traditional Systemic Agents.

Box 8-25 **Recommendations for Leflunomide**

- **Indication**
  There is no FDA-approved use for psoriasis.
- **Dosing**
  Loading dose of 100 mg/day for 3 days followed by 20 mg/day long term
- **Short-Term Results**
  In the only randomized, controlled trial of 190 patients, 24 wk of leflunomide, dosed as described previously, led to a PASI 75 of 17% vs. placebo response of 8% (p = .048).
- **Long-Term Results**
  Not reported
- **Contraindications**
  Patients with hypersensitivity to leflunomide or its metabolites
- **Toxicity**
  Most common side effects include nausea, diarrhea, loss of appetite, weight loss, headache, dizziness.
  Less frequent adverse reactions may include severe liver injury, including fatal outcome. Most cases of severe liver injury occur within 6 months of therapy and in patients with multiple risk factors for hepatotoxicity.
  There are rare reports of pancytopenia, agranulocytosis, and thrombocytopenia in patients receiving leflunomide. This occurs in patients who have been treated with methotrexate or other immunosuppressive agents, or who had recently discontinued these.
- **Drug Interactions**
  Coadministration of leflunomide with methotrexate demonstrates no pharmacokinetic interaction between the two drugs but can lead to an increased risk of hepatotoxicity.
  When leflunomide is given with rifampin, leflunomide levels are increased.
- **Baseline Monitoring**
  History and physical examination
  CBC/differential and LFTs
  Pregnancy test if indicated
- **Ongoing Monitoring**
  Monthly CBC with differential and liver function tests for the first 6 months and then every 6-8 weeks
  Pregnancy testing if indicated
- **Pregnancy:** Category X
- **Nursing:** Leflunomide should not be used by nursing mothers.
- **Pediatric Use:** No data
- **Psoriatic Arthritis:** In the only randomized, controlled study of 190 patients with psoriasis and psoriatic arthritis, 59% of patients treated with leflunomide vs. 30% of placebo patients were responders by the PsARC.

From Journal of the American Academy of Dermatology (in Press). Guidelines of Care for the Management of Psoriasis and Psoriatic Arthritis. Section 4: Guidelines of Care for the Management and Treatment of Psoriasis with Traditional Systemic Agents.

Biologic therapy for psoriasis

Psoriasis is driven by activated memory T cells. Many biologic agents are available to selectively target the immune system. Biologic agents are proteins that can be synthesized using recombinant DNA techniques (genetic engineering). Biologic agents bind to specific cells and proteins and do not have multiorgan adverse effects as seen with acitretin, cyclosporine, and methotrexate. The potential for interaction with other drugs is very low. There are risks from immunosuppression. PMID: 18423260

GENERAL RECOMMENDATIONS. Obtain laboratory tests. These include a chemistry screen with liver function tests, complete blood cell count including platelet count, a hepatitis panel, and tuberculosis testing, all obtained at baseline and with variable frequencies thereafter. Periodically reevaluate patients for infection and malignancy. Treatment is contraindicated in patients with active, serious infections. If patients develop serious infections (usually defined as an infection that requires antibiotic therapy) while being treated with a biologic agent, hold the biologic agent until the infection has resolved.

VACCINES

Consider giving pneumococcal, hepatitis A and B, influenza, and tetanus-diphtheria vaccines before initiation of immunosuppressive therapy. Once immunosuppressive therapy has begun, patients must avoid vaccination with live vaccines (including varicella; mumps, measles, and rubella; oral typhoid; yellow fever) and live-attenuated vaccines (including intranasal influenza and the herpes zoster vaccine). Studies show adequate but attenuated immune responses to killed virus vaccines such as influenza vaccination and pneumococcal vaccine.

Box 8-26 **General Recommendations for Tumor Necrosis Factor (TNF) Inhibitors**

- Contraindicated in patients with active, serious infections
- Tuberculosis testing (purified protein derivative [PPD]) before treatment (risk of reactivation)
- No live vaccines; inactive or recombinant vaccines tolerated but immune response of these vaccines could be compromised
- Not for patients with multiple sclerosis or first-degree relatives of patients with multiple sclerosis
- Onset and worsening of congestive heart failure are reported
- Hepatitis B reactivation reported; screen patients at risk

Adapted from: Guidelines of care for the management of psoriasis and psoriatic arthritis: Section 1. Overview of psoriasis and guidelines of care for the treatment of psoriasis with biologics. *J Am Acad Dermatol* 58(5):826-850, 2008. PMID: 18423260

TNF-α INHIBITORS FOR THE TREATMENT OF PSORIASIS

TNF-α inhibitors are effective for the treatment of psoriasis and are the most commonly prescribed biologic agents for psoriasis. General recommendations are listed in Box 8-26.

ADALIMUMAB. Adalimumab (Humira) is approved for psoriasis, juvenile rheumatoid arthritis, ankylosing spondylitis, psoriatic arthritis, adult rheumatoid arthritis, and Crohn's disease. Rebound does not typically occur when adalimumab is discontinued; however, clearance is better maintained with continuous use and there is loss of efficacy after restart of adalimumab. Recommendations for adalimumab are listed in Box 8-27.

ETANERCEPT. Etanercept is approved for moderate-to-severe plaque psoriasis, psoriatic arthritis, rheumatoid arthritis, juvenile rheumatoid arthritis, and ankylosing spondylitis. The dosing of etanercept differs in psoriasis than for

Box 8-27 **Recommendations for Adalimumab**

- **Indications:** Moderate-to-severe psoriatic arthritis, moderate-to-severe psoriasis, adult and juvenile rheumatoid arthritis (as young as age 4 years)
- **Dosing for Psoriasis:** 80 mg the first week, 40 mg the second week, followed by 40 mg every other week given subcutaneously
- **Short-Term Results:** 80% of patients achieved PASI-75 at 12 weeks
- **Long-Term Results:** 68% of patients achieved PASI-75 at 60 weeks
- Small percentage of patients lose efficacy with continued use

Toxicities

- Moderately painful injection site reactions are noted in up to 15% of patients. These reactions usually resolve spontaneously within the first 2 months of therapy.
- Rare reports of serious infections (e.g., tuberculosis and opportunistic infections) and malignancies
- There are rare reports of drug-induced, reversible side effects including lupus without renal or CNS complications, cytopenia, MS, and exacerbation of and new onset of CHF.

Baseline Monitoring

- PPD required
- LFT, CBC, and hepatitis profile

Ongoing Monitoring

- Periodic history and physical examination are recommended while on treatment.
- Consider a yearly PPD, and periodic CBC and LFT.
- Pregnancy category B

From Menter A et al: *J Am Acad Dermatol* 60(4):643-659, 2009. PMID 18423260

CBC, Complete blood cell count; *CHF*, congestive heart failure; *CNS*, central nervous system; *LFT*, liver function test; *MS*, multiple sclerosis; *PASI-75*, 75% improvement in the Psoriasis Area and Severity Index score; *PPD*, purified protein derivative.

its other indications. In rheumatoid and psoriatic arthritis, TNF-α inhibitors including etanercept are often used in combination with methotrexate. In psoriasis, all clinical studies have been performed with etanercept as monotherapy. Rebound does not typically occur when etanercept is discontinued. Loss of efficacy over time may occur. This is possibly related to the development of antibodies. Recommendations for etanercept are listed in Box 8-28.

PEDIATRIC PSORIASIS. In a study of etanercept treatment for children and adolescents (ages 4 to 17 years) with plaque psoriasis who were dosed once weekly with 0.8 mg/kg of etanercept (up to a maximum of 50 mg), 57% of patients receiving etanercept achieved PASI-75 (75% improvement in the Psoriasis Area and Severity Index score) as compared with 11% of those receiving placebo ($P < .001$).

Box 8-28 **Recommendations for Etanercept**

- **Indication:** Moderate-to-severe psoriasis, moderate-to-severe psoriatic arthritis, adult and juvenile rheumatoid arthritis (as young as 4 years)
- **Dosing:** 50 mg twice/week given subcutaneously for 3 months followed by 50 mg once/week
- **Short-Term Results:** 49% of patients given 50 mg twice/week achieved a PASI-75 at 12 weeks; 34% of patients given 25 mg twice/week achieved a PASI-75 at 12 weeks.
- **Step-Down Results:** 54% of patients whose dose was decreased from 50 mg twice/week to 25 mg twice/week achieved a PASI-75 at 24 weeks; 45% of patients whose dose remained at 25 mg twice/week achieved a PASI-75 at 24 weeks.

Toxicity

- Mildly pruritic injection site reactions may occur in up to 37% of patients. Mean duration of reactions is 3 to 5 days; these reactions generally occur in the first month and subsequently decrease. The needle cover of the prefilled etanercept syringe contains latex so this formulation should not be used in latex-sensitive patients.
- Rare cases of serious infections (e.g., tuberculosis) and malignancies
- There are also rare cases of drug-induced, reversible side effects including lupus without renal or CNS complications, cytopenia, MS, and exacerbation and new onset of CHF.

Baseline Monitoring

- PPD required
- LFT and CBC

Ongoing Monitoring

- Periodic history and physical examination are recommended while on treatment.
- Consider yearly PPD, and periodic CBC and LFT.
- Pregnancy category B
- Contraindications: Sepsis

From Menter A et al: *J Am Acad Dermatol* 58(5):826-850, 2008. *PMID 18423260*

CBC, Complete blood cell count; *CHF,* congestive heart failure; *CNS,* central nervous system; *LFT,* liver function test; *MS,* multiple sclerosis; *PASI-75,* 75% improvement in the Psoriasis Area and Severity Index score; *PPD,* purified protein derivative.

INFLIXIMAB

Infliximab (Remicade) is approved for psoriasis and psoriatic arthritis. Patients are less likely to develop antibodies against infliximab if they are continuously treated with infliximab rather than on an as-needed basis, and clinical responses are better maintained with continuous therapy. Response to infliximab is rapid. Loss of efficacy over time may occur. Some dermatologists prescribe low-dose methotrexate concurrently with the goal of decreasing the formation of antibodies against infliximab and, hence, maintaining clinical efficacy. Recommendations for infliximab are listed in Box 8-29.

Box 8-29 **Recommendations for Infliximab**

- **Indication:** Severe psoriasis, moderate-to-severe psoriatic arthritis, adult rheumatoid arthritis, ankylosing spondylitis, ulcerative colitis, and Crohn's disease
- **Dosing:** 5 mg/kg dose infusion schedule at weeks 0, 2, and 6 and then every 6-8 weeks; dose and interval of infusions may be adjusted as needed
- **Short-Term Response:** 80% of patients achieved a PASI-75 at week 10; 50% PASI-75 improvement noted by week 2
- **Long-Term Response:** 61% of patients achieved a PASI-75 at week 50

Toxicity

- Infusion reactions and serum sickness can occur, more commonly in patients who have developed antibodies. Infusion-related reactions occur in 16% of patients treated. Most are mild, consisting of pruritus or urticaria. Some patients will have moderate reactions consisting of chest pain, hypertension, and shortness of breath and only rarely will severe reactions with hypotension and anaphylaxis occur. Infusion reaction risk tends to correlate with the development of human antichimeric antibodies and can usually be managed by slowing the rate of infusion or stopping treatment entirely. Patients who are concurrently treated with an immunosuppressive agent, such as methotrexate or azathioprine, or at regularly dosed intervals are likely to have a lowered incidence of infusion reactions.
- The incidence of infusion reactions may be reduced by concurrent administration of methotrexate.
- Rare cases of serious infections (e.g., tuberculosis) and malignancies including hepatosplenic T-cell lymphoma (in children). There are rare reports of drug-induced, reversible side effects including lupus without renal or CNS complications, cytopenia, MS, and exacerbation of and new onset of CHF.

Baseline Monitoring

- PPD required
- LFT, CBC, and hepatitis profile

Ongoing Monitoring

- Periodic history and physical examination are recommended while on treatment.
- Consider a yearly PPD, and periodic CBC and LFT.
- Pregnancy category B
- Contraindications: Infliximab at doses >5 mg/kg should not be given to patients with New York Heart Association functional class III or IV CHF.

From Menter A et al: *J Am Acad Dermatol* 58(5):826-850, 2008. *PMID 18423260*

CBC, Complete blood cell count; *CHF,* congestive heart failure; *CNS,* central nervous system; *LFT,* liver function test; *MS,* multiple sclerosis; *PASI-75,* 75% improvement in the Psoriasis Area and Severity Index score; *PPD,* purified protein derivative.

BIOLOGICS THAT TARGET PATHOGENIC T CELLS

ALEFECEPT. (Amevive) inhibits the activation and reduces the number of memory-effector T lymphocytes. Some patients do not respond Patients who do respond can achieve additional benefit from successive 12-week treatment courses. There is no way to predict which patients will improve. Caution should be exercised in patients who are at risk for or have a history of malignancy or infection, especially clinically significant infections. Alefecept is pregnancy category B. Recommendations for Alefecept are listed in Box 8-30.

BIOLOGICS THAT TARGET CYTOKINES INTERLEUKIN (IL)-12 AND IL-23

Psoriasis results in part from the activation and migration of T cells into the epidermis and the release of inflammatory mediators, which leads to hyperproliferation of skin cells. The cytokines interleukin (IL)-12 and IL-23 are produced by activated antigen-presenting cells and have a role in the differentiation and proliferation of type 1 T-helper cells. There is evidence of high levels of IL-12 and IL-23 expression in psoriatic lesions.

Box 8-30 **Recommendations for Alefecept**

- **Indication:** Moderate-to-severe psoriasis in adults
- **Dosing:** 15 mg every week given as an intramuscular injection for 12 weeks, with a 12-week follow-up nontreatment period

Short-Term Results

- 21% of patients achieved a PASI-75 at week 14.

Long-Term Results

- Associated with long remissions in a subset of responders
- Prior response to Alefecept is a likely marker of future treatment response; thus patients responding to the first course of therapy may be treated long-term with repeated 12-week courses of Alefecept, at a minimum of 24-week intervals.

Toxicity

Excellent safety profile in clinical trials

Baseline Monitoring

CD4 count

Ongoing Monitoring

Biweekly CD4 count required; hold dose for counts <250
Pregnancy category: B
Contraindications: HIV infection

From Menter A et al: *J Am Acad Dermatol* 58(5):826-850, 2008. *PMID 18423260*
PASI-75, 75% improvement in the Psoriasis Area and Severity Index score.

USTEKINUMAB. Ustekinumab is a human monoclonal antibody that targets interleukin-12 (IL-12) and IL-23. It binds to the p40 subunit, common to both IL-12 and IL-23, which prevents these cytokines from binding to the cell surface of T cells, thereby disrupting the inflammatory cascade implicated in psoriasis.

Ustekinumab seems to be as effective as the anti-TNF antibodies during induction therapy and data indicate a stable clinical response over time, with no rebound after withdrawal of the drug and a re-treatment PASI 75 response of approximately 85%. There is evidence that ustekinumab is effective in psoriatic arthritis. Recommendations for ustekinumab are listed in Box 8-31.

Box 8-31 **Recommendations for Ustekinumab (STELARA)**

- **Indication:** Moderate to severe plaque psoriasis in adults
- **Dosing:** 45 mg for people who weigh 100 kg or less, and 90 mg for people who weigh over 100 kg. An initial dose is administered subcutaneously at week 0, followed by another dose at week 4, and then a further dose every 12 weeks. No dose adjustment is needed for patients over age 65. It is not recommended for children below age 18 due to a lack of data.
- **Short-Term Response:** At week 12, a PASI 75 response was achieved by 67% of patients receiving 45 mg ustekinumab, 66% of patients receiving 90 mg ustekinumab. *PMID: 1848673*
- **Long-Term Response:** Maintenance of PASI-75 was significantly superior with continuous ustekinumab treatment compared with treatment withdrawal; at week 76, 84% of patients re-randomized to maintenance treatment achieved a PASI-75 response compared with 19% of patients re-randomized to placebo.
- **Increasing Dose:** Consider increasing dose to once every 8 weeks with ustekinumab 90 mg in patients who do not achieve PASI-75 at 28 weeks. *PMID 18486740*

Toxicity

- The most common adverse reactions (> 10%) are nasopharyngitis and upper respiratory tract infection. Most were considered mild and did not necessitate drug discontinuation.
- Contraindications include clinically important active infection.
- In trials, rates of serious adverse events, including serious infections, malignancies and cardiovascular events, were low and consistent with the expected background rates.

Baseline Monitoring

- PPD and consider chest x-ray
- LFT, CBC, and hepatitis profile

Ongoing Monitoring

- Consider yearly PPD and periodic CBC and LFT
- Periodic history and physical examination

Adapted from product monograph, Janssen-Ortho Inc. Toronto, Ontario, December 12, 2008.

PITYRIASIS RUBRA PILARIS

Pityriasis rubra pilaris (PRP) is a rare, chronic disease of unknown etiology with a unique combination of features. PRP often has a devastating impact on the lives of patients. Descriptions of its histopathologic features are not uniform. Finding a successful therapy can be challenging. PRP may occur at any age, but most cases occur in the first and fifth or sixth decades of life.

GRIFFITHS CLASSIFICATION

Griffiths divides PRP into five types (Table 8-8): types I and II represent the classic and atypical forms of adult PRP; types III, IV, and V are seen in juveniles. The classic types (types I and III) show a wide distribution of follicular papules and plaques with extensive coalescence, sparing islands of normal-appearing skin. Type IV PRP is seen mainly in children, with circumscribed lesions restricted to the elbows and knees and frequent palmoplantar hyperkeratosis. The atypical forms (type II in adults and type V in juveniles) show an ichthyosiform dermatitis and palmoplantar hyperkeratosis. A severe form of PRP may be unmasked, precipitated, or otherwise associated with HIV infection (type VI). It is characterized by a triad of nodulocystic acne, lichen spinulosus, and a PRP-like eruption.

CLINICAL MANIFESTATIONS

Classic adult PRP begins insidiously, usually in the fifth or sixth decade of life, with a small, indolent, red scaling plaque on the face or upper body. The plaque slowly enlarges over days and weeks, the palms and soles begin to thicken, and bright red-orange follicular papules appear on the dorsal aspects of the proximal phalanges, elbows, knees, and trunk as the disease evolves and progresses into a grotesque generalized eruption (Figures 8-30, 8-31, and 8-32). The follicular keratotic papules coalesce on many areas of the trunk to produce a complex pattern of discrete papules and sharply bordered, red plaques with islands of normal skin ("skip spots") (Figures 8-30 and 8-31). The eruption may spread to involve almost the entire cutaneous surface. Scaling is coarse on the lower half of the body and fine and powdery on the upper half. Ectropion is present with extensive facial involvement. The nails show distal yellow-brown discoloration, subungual hyperkeratosis, nail thickening, and splinter hemorrhages. Psoriatic nails show onycholysis (particularly marginal), oil spots, small pits, and larger indentations of the nail plate.

There is little or no itching. The patient is impaired by the thick, tight scales of the scalp, face, and palms and the painful fissures that develop on the soles. The diffuse, red, tight-scaling face destroys the self-image, and these patients remain isolated. The eruption lasts for months and years; 80% are clear within 3 years.

Table 8-8 Griffiths Classification of Pityriasis Rubra Pilaris

Type	% of all cases	Lesion distribution	Typical features	Other distinguishing features	Course and duration
I. Classic adult	50	Generalized	Erythroderma; islands of sparing, salmon-colored palmoplantar keratoderma	Follicular hyperkeratosis; cephalocaudal spread	Acute onset; 80% have a remission in 3 years
II. Atypical adult	5	Generalized	Ichthyosiform lesions; more persistent and psoriasiform, especially on the legs	Areas of eczematous change; alopecia	20 years or more
III. Classic juvenile	10	Generalized	Similar to type I; generalized coalescent hyperkeratotic follicular papules and plaques with islands of spared skin	Cephalocaudal spread	Onset is in first 2 years of life; remission within an average of 1-2 years
IV. Circumscribed juvenile	25	Localized	Focal hyperkeratotic follicular papules and erythema and plaques on elbows, knees, palms, soles	Prepubertal children; disseminated small papules or plaques on face, trunk, or extremities	Acute form resolves in 6 months; an intermediate form resolves in 1 year; chronic form persists over 1 year amd can progress to an erythrodermic form (types I or III)
V. Atypical juvenile	5	Generalized	Follicular hyperkeratosis; generalized ichthyosiform dermatitis	Scleroderma-like changes of palms and soles; most cases of familial PRP belong to this group	Appears in first year of life; runs a chronic, intractable course
VI. HIV-associated PRP	On the increase	Face and upper trunk	Nodulocystic and pustular acneiform lesions; lichen spinulosus–type lesions (elongated follicular plugs)	Resistant to standard treatments; may respond to antiretroviral therapies	Refractory

PITYRIASIS RUBRA PILARIS

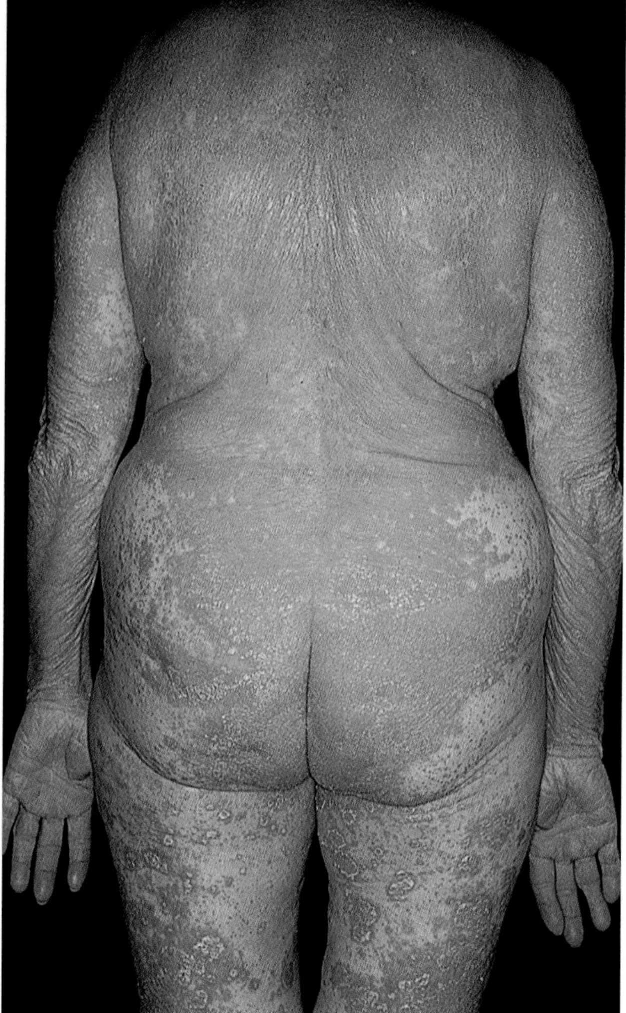

Figure 8-30 Red-orange scaling plaques with sharp borders have expanded to involve the entire body. The areas of uninvolved skin or islands of sparing, "skip spots," are characteristic.

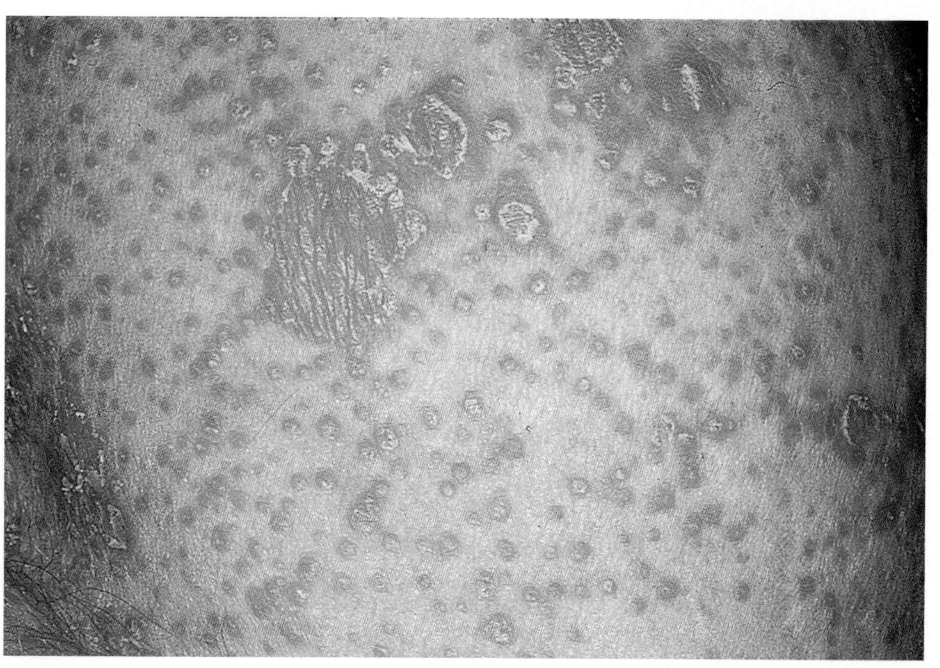

Figure 8-31 The classic presentation. Bright red follicular papules merge to form large, bright red-orange plaques.

CHILDHOOD PITYRIASIS RUBRA PILARIS. Childhood PRP begins on the scalp and face and simulates seborrheic dermatitis. The disease becomes more widespread and follicular keratotic papules develop. The childhood form tends to recur for years, which is not characteristic of the adult form. The circumscribed form is characterized by red-orange plaques, usually on the elbows and knees, consisting of sharply demarcated areas of follicular hyperkeratosis and erythema. The 3-year remission rate is 32%.

DIAGNOSIS

The distinctive clinical picture is the most valuable diagnostic feature. The disease looks like psoriasis when localized to the scalp, elbows, and knees. The biopsy shows thick scale and dense, keratotic, follicular plugs; an increased granular cell layer; and acantholysis. Many other features are reported.

TREATMENT

Etanercept and infliximab are reported effective in single case articles. Frequent use of lubricants such as Lac-Hydrin (12% lactic acid) and Eucerin, Aquaphor, or Vaseline keeps the skin supple. Vanamide (40% urea cream) applied to the feet and covered with a plastic bag at bedtime is an effective approach for removing scale. Application of heavy moisturizers, such as equal parts Aquaphor and Unibase, followed by occlusion with a plastic suit for several hours also makes the skin supple. Dovonex (calcipotriene) may be effective. Systemic retinoids and methotrexate are the first-line treatments for generalized PRP.

RETINOIDS. Retinoids are effective systemic agents. Isotretinoin provides symptomatic improvement of erythema, pruritus, scaling, ectropion, and keratoderma in 4 weeks, while significant improvement or clearing takes 16 to 24 weeks. Remission or maintained improvement persists after stopping therapy in many patients. Dosages in the range of 0.5 to 2.0 mg/kg/day are used for up to 6 months. Acitretin with or without light therapy may be superior to isotretinoin in the treatment of adult-onset disease.

Initial oral retinoids plus concurrent or later low-dose weekly methotrexate resulted in 25% to 75% improvement of PRP in 17 of 24 patients after 16 weeks of therapy.

Megadose vitamin A (1 million units/day) given for 5 to 14 days clears the skin in days in some reports but has been less effective in others. Tazarotene gel applied twice daily might be useful for localized PRP.

METHOTREXATE. Daily methotrexate (2.5 mg/day) is more effective than the standard weekly regimen used for psoriasis and may be more effective than retinoids. Improvement may be noted in the second or third week, and there may be marked improvement in 10 to 12 weeks, at which time the dose can be tapered.

Cyclosporine should be considered in the treatment of classical adult-type PRP. Penicillin, stanozolol, and the Goeckerman regimen (UVB and crude coal tar) are probably not effective. Patients with PRP are photosensitive and the majority flare with either psoralens and ultraviolet A (PUVA) or ultraviolet B therapy.

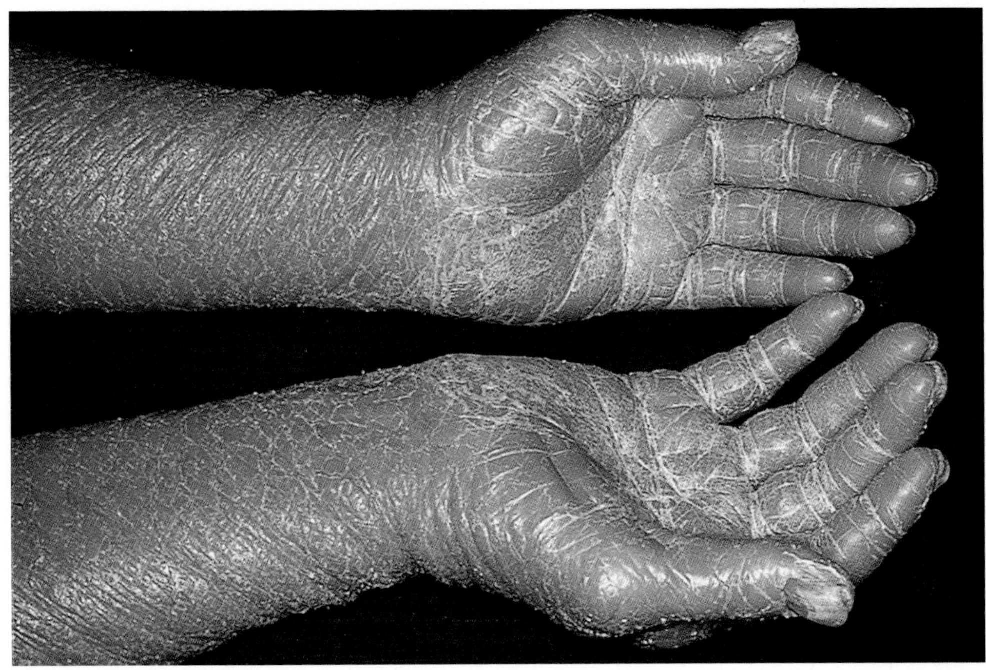

Figure 8-32 Pityriasis rubra pilaris. The entire surface of the palms and soles becomes thick (hyperkeratotic) and yellow.

SEBORRHEIC DERMATITIS

Seborrheic dermatitis is a common, chronic, inflammatory disease with a characteristic pattern for different age groups. The yeast *Malassezia ovalis* probably is a causative factor, but both genetic and environmental factors seem to influence the onset and course of the disease. Many adult patients have an oily complexion, the so-called seborrheic diathesis. In adults, seborrheic dermatitis tends to persist, but it undergoes periods of remission and exacerbation. The extent of involvement among patients varies widely. Most cases can be adequately controlled.

Infants (cradle cap)

Infants commonly develop a greasy adherent scale on the vertex of the scalp. Minor amounts of scale are easily removed by frequent shampooing with products containing sulfur, salicylic acid, or both (e.g., Sebulex shampoo, T/Gel shampoo). Scale may accumulate and become thick and adherent over much of the scalp and may be accompanied by inflammation (Figure 8-33). Secondary infection can occur.

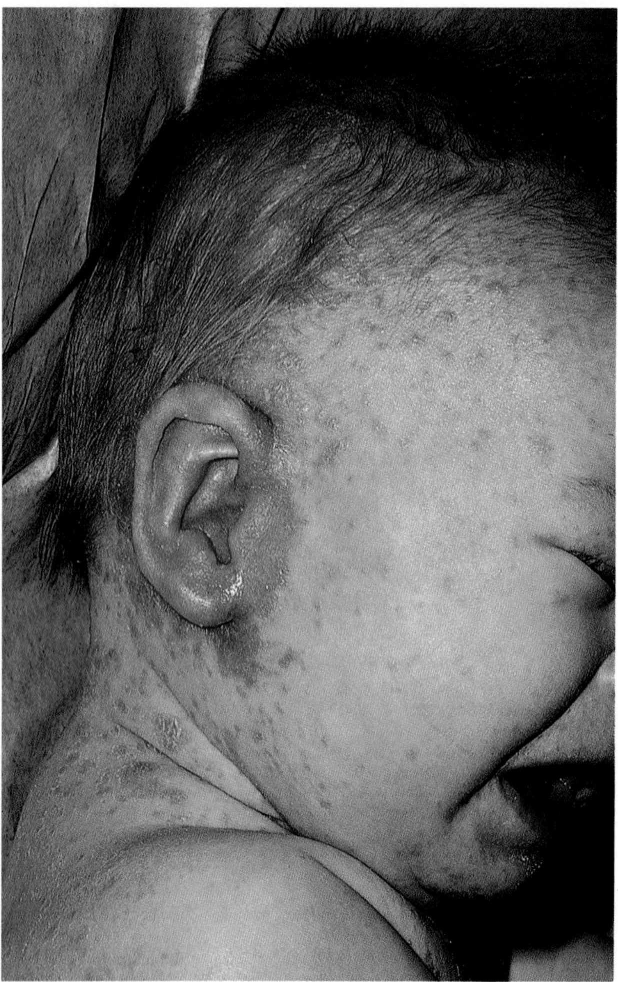

Figure 8-33 Seborrheic dermatitis (cradle cap). Diffuse inflammation with secondary infection. Much of the scale from this child's scalp was removed with shampoos.

TREATMENT. Patients with serum and crust are treated with oral antistaphylococcal antibiotics. Once infection is controlled, erythema and scaling can be suppressed with group VI or VII topical steroid creams or lotions. Dense, thick, adherent scale is removed by applying warm mineral oil, olive oil, or Derma-Smoothe/FS lotion (peanut oil, mineral oil, fluocinolone acetonide 0.01%) to the scalp and washing several hours later. Remissions possibly can be prolonged with frequent use of salicylic acid or tar shampoos (see the Formulary). Carmol scalp solution (sulfacetamide) may also be effective. It is applied once or twice each day. Ketoconazole is another option for the treatment of infantile seborrheic dermatis, to avoid the side effects of topical corticosteroid in long-term use and on large surface areas of treatment. The efficacy of 2% ketoconazole cream and 1% hydrocortisone cream in the treatment of infantile seborrheic dermatitis is similar to either medication used alone.

Young children (tinea amiantacea and blepharitis)

Tinea amiantacea is a characteristic eruption of unknown etiology. Mothers of afflicted children often recall the child experiencing episodes of cradle cap during infancy. Some authors believe that tinea amiantacea is a form of eczema or psoriasis. One patch or several patches of dense scale appear anywhere on the scalp and may persist for months before the parent notices temporary hair loss or the distinctive large, oval, yellow-white plates of scale firmly adhered to the scalp and hair (Figure 8-34). Characteristically, the scale binds to the hair and is drawn up with the growing hair. Patches of dense scale range from 2 to 10 cm. The scale suggests fungal scalp disease, which explains the designation tinea. Amiantacea, meaning asbestos, refers to the platelike quality of the scale, which resembles genuine asbestos.

TREATMENT. Warm 10% liquor carbonis detergens (LCD) in Nivea oil (prescription is for 8 oz; it must be prepared by the pharmacist) is applied to the scalp at bedtime and removed by shampooing each morning with Dawn dishwashing liquid. Derma-Smoothe/FS lotion (peanut oil, mineral oil, fluocinolone acetonide 0.01%) is an effective topical steroid that can be applied to the entire scalp and occluded with a shower cap. The scalp is dampened before application. Treatments are repeated each night for 1 to 3 weeks until itching and erythema are controlled. The scale is completely removed in 1 to 3 weeks, and tar shampoos such as T/Gel or Tarsum are used for maintenance. Periodic recurrences are similarly treated.

White scale adherent to the eyelashes and lid margins with variable amounts of erythema is characteristic of seborrheic blepharitis (Figure 8-35). The disease produces some discomfort and is unbecoming. The disease persists for years and is resistant to treatment. Scale may be suppressed by frequent washing with zinc- or tar-containing antidandruff shampoos (see the Formulary). Although topical steroid creams and lotions suppress this disease, prolonged use of

SEBORRHEIC DERMATITIS

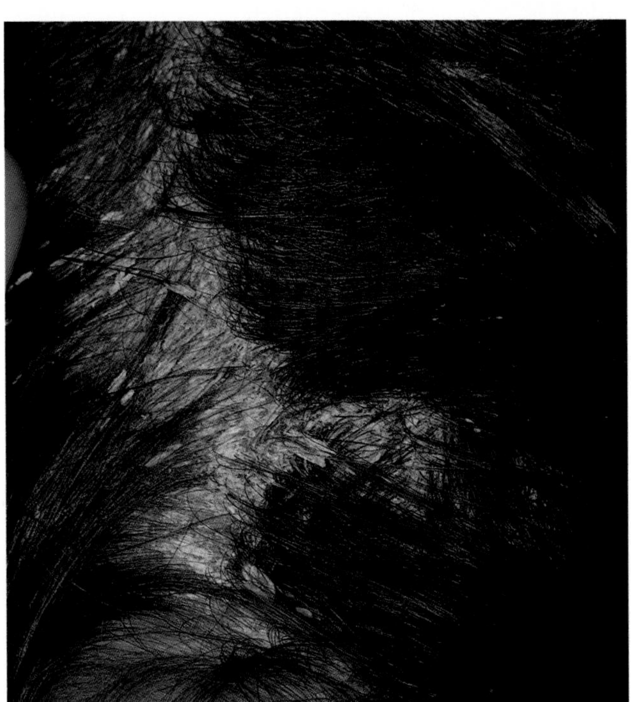

Figure 8-34 Seborrheic dermatitis (tinea amiantacea). The scalp contains dense patches of scale. Large plates of yellow-white scale firmly adhere to the hair shafts.

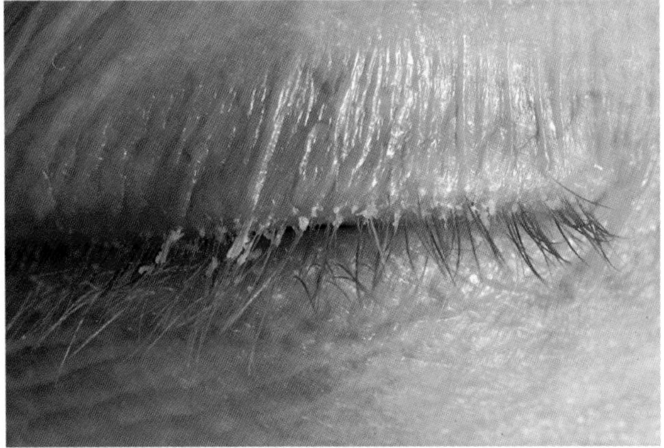

Figure 8-35 Seborrheic dermatitis (blepharitis). Scale accumulates and adheres to the lashes. A few drops of baby shampoo mixed in a cap of warm water can be used as a cleanser. Sulfacetamide ointment may control inflammation and scale.

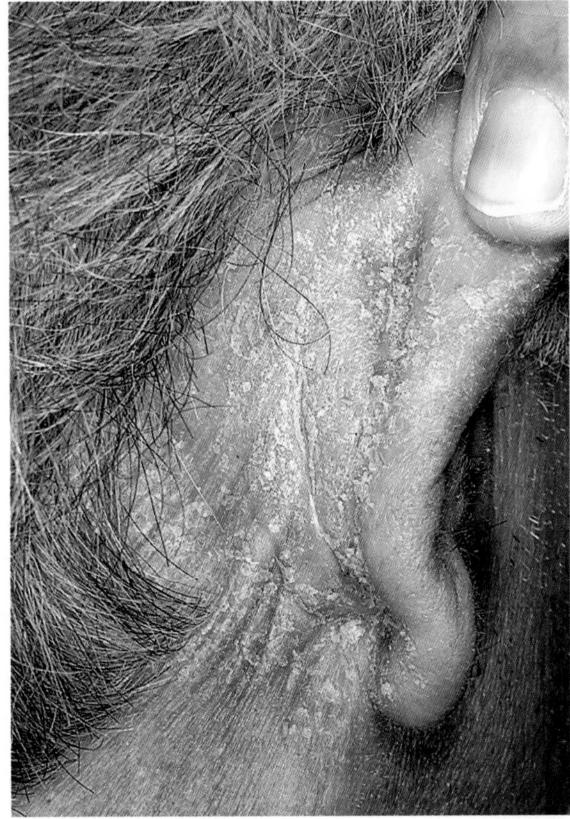

Figure 8-36 Seborrheic dermatitis of the postauricular skin.

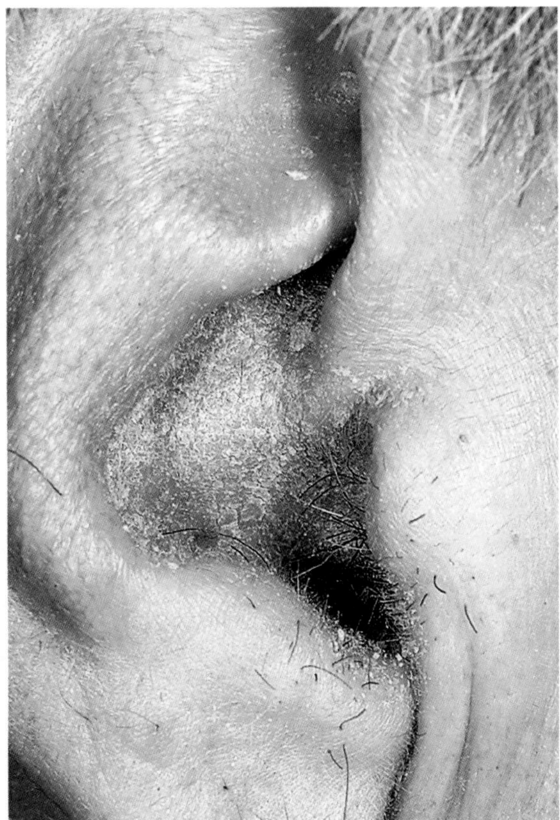

Figure 8-37 Seborrheic dermatitis of the ear canal.

such preparations around the eyes may cause glaucoma and must be avoided. Ketoconazole (Nizoral cream) applied once a day is worth a trial in resistant cases.

Adolescents and adults (classic seborrheic dermatitis)

Most individuals periodically experience fine, dry, white scalp scaling with minor itching; this is dandruff. They tend to attribute this condition to a dry scalp and consequently avoid hair washing. Avoidance of washing allows scale to accumulate and inflammation may occur. Patients with minor amounts of dandruff should be encouraged to wash every day or every other day with antidandruff shampoos (see the Formulary). Fine, dry, white or yellow scale may occur on an inflamed base. The distribution of scaling and inflammation may be more diffuse and occur in the seborrheic areas: scalp and scalp margins, eyebrows, base of eyelashes, nasolabial folds, external ear canals (Figures 8-36 and 8-37), posterior auricular fold, and presternal area (Figure 8-38).

The axillae, inframammary folds, groin, and umbilicus are affected less frequently. Scaling of the ears may be misjudged as eczema or fungus infection. Its presence in association with characteristic scaling in other typical areas assists in supporting the diagnosis. Scaling may appear when a beard is grown and disappear when it is shaved (Figures 8-39 and 8-40). Once established, the disease tends to persist to a variable degree. Older patients, particularly those who are bedridden or those with neurologic problems such as Parkinson's disease, tend to have a more chronic and extensive form of the disease. Occasionally the scalp scale may be diffuse, thick, and adherent. Differentiation from psoriasis may be impossible.

Patients should be reassured that seborrheic dermatitis does not cause permanent hair loss. Tinea capitis caused by *Trichophyton tonsurans* has a dry, white, diffuse scale in the adult that does not fluoresce under Wood's light. Fungal culture and potassium hydroxide examination are indicated for atypical or resistant cases of scalp scaling.

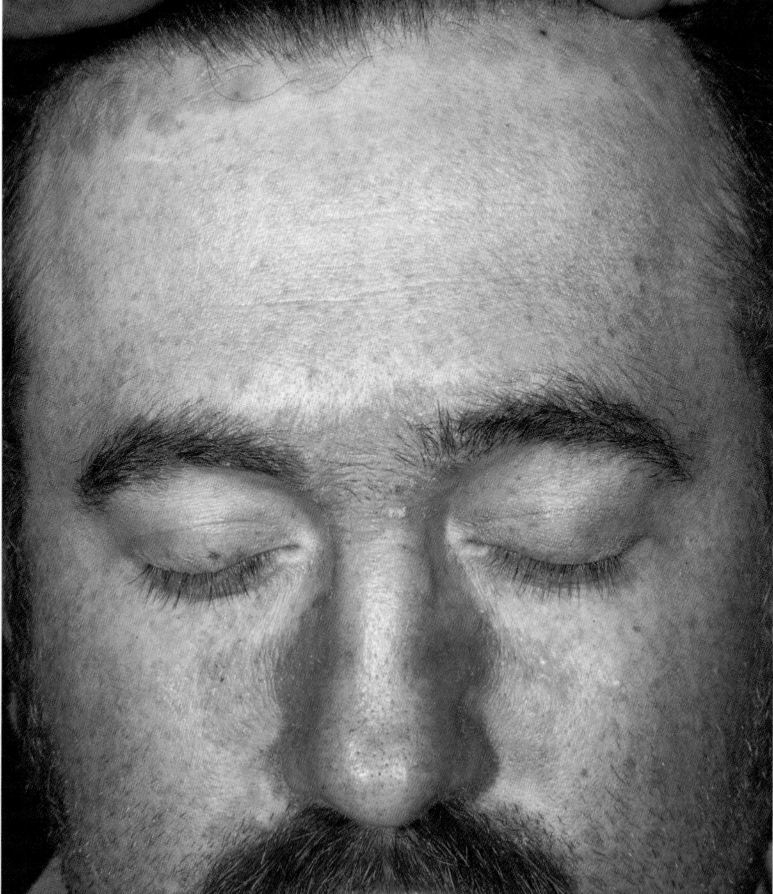

Figure 8-38 Seborrheic dermatitis in an adult with extensive involvement in all of the characteristic sites.

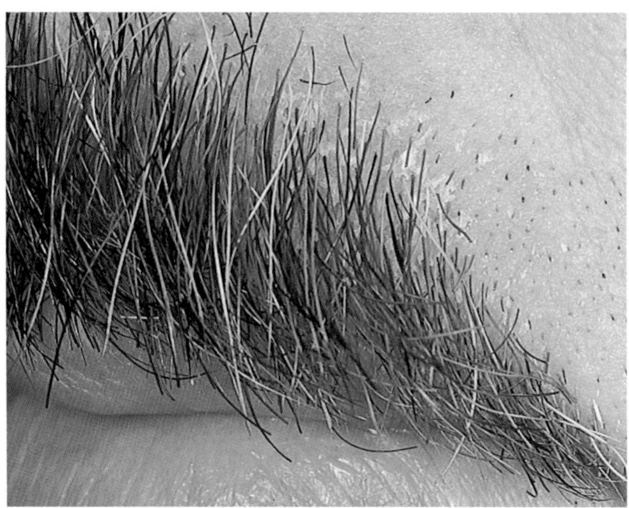

Figure 8-39 Seborrheic dermatitis will appear in predisposed individuals if facial hair is grown.

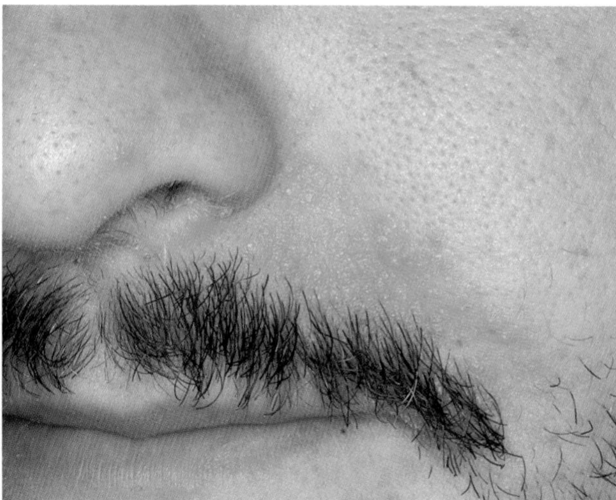

Figure 8-40 Seborrheic dermatitis has extended from the mustache to the base of the nasolabial fold.

Acquired immunodeficiency syndrome

Seborrheic dermatitis is one of the most common cutaneous manifestations of AIDS. The onset usually occurs before the development of AIDS symptoms. The severity of the seborrheic dermatitis correlates with the degree of clinical deterioration.

TREATMENT OF SEBORRHEIC DERMATITIS

SHAMPOOS. Treatment consists of frequent washing of all affected areas, including the face and chest, with an antiseborrheic shampoo. Zinc soaps (Head & Shoulders shampoo, ZNP bar soap), selenium lotions (Head & Shoulders intensive care, Selsun), ciclopirox 1% shampoo, tar (Tarsum, T/Gel), or Sal acid (T/Sal) suppresses activity and maintains remission.

TOPICAL STEROIDS. Inflamed areas respond quickly to group V through VII topical steroid creams. Steroid lotions may be applied to the scalp twice daily. Patients must be cautioned that topical steroids should not be used as maintenance therapy.

Derma-Smoothe/FS lotion (peanut oil, mineral oil, fluocinolone acetonide 0.01%) is an effective topical steroid that can be applied to the entire scalp and occluded with a shower cap. The scalp is dampened before application. Treatments are repeated each night for 1 to 3 weeks until itching and erythema are controlled. The scale is completely removed in 1 to 3 weeks, and tar shampoos such as T/Gel or Tarsum are used for maintenance. Periodic recurrences are similarly treated.

Both pimecrolimus 1% cream and ketoconazole are effective in treating seborrheic dermatitis. The relapse of facial seborrheic dermatitis is observed between 3 to 8 weeks after the discontinuation of pimecrolimus. A rosaceiform dermatitis may occur as a complication of treatment of facial seborrheic dermatitis with 1% pimecrolimus cream.

ANTIYEAST MEDICATIONS. Ketoconazole (Nizoral cream) or ciclopirox olamine (Loprox cream or gel) applied once or twice a day is effective against even the most difficult and diffuse cases. Patients with widespread disease involving the face, ears, chest, and upper back can now be treated effectively by using ketoconazole or ciclopirox to clear the scale and erythema. Curiously, minor seborrheic dermatitis of the face may not respond as well and may require the addition of group V through VII topical steroids or pimecrolimus cream for control.

ORAL ANTIFUNGALS. Oral intraconazole, initially 200 mg/day for 1 week, followed by a maintenance therapy of a single dose of 200 mg every 2 weeks was beneficial in patients with moderate-to-severe seborrheic dermatitis. Maintenance therapy led to only slight further improvement. *PMID: 18669136* Fluconazole 300 mg in a single dose per week for 2 weeks provides marginal and statistically insignificant benefit for the therapy of seborrheic dermatitis (SD). *PMID: 17645378*

Dense, diffuse scalp scaling is treated with Derma-Smoothe/FS lotion (peanut oil, mineral oil, fluocinolone acetonide 0.01%) or 10% LCD in Nivea oil as previously described for treating young children. Adults may apply oil preparations at bedtime and cover with a shower cap. Treatment is repeated each night until the scalp is clear, in approximately 1 to 3 weeks. Shampoo is then used for maintenance.

OTHER TOPICALS. Sulfacetamide (Carmol scalp treatment lotion) applied once or twice each day can be very effective for active disease, especially if pustules are present. Metronidazole 0.75% or 1% gel had a comparable efficacy with that of ketoconazole 2% cream in the treatment of facial seborrheic dermatitis. *PMID: 17309456*

PITYRIASIS ROSEA

Pityriasis rosea (PR) is a common, benign, usually asymptomatic, distinctive, self-limiting skin eruption of unknown etiology. There is some evidence that human herpesvirus 6 (HHV-6) may be involved. Small epidemics have occurred in fraternity houses and military bases. Temporal case clustering exists. *PMID: 15967925* The incidence in men and women varies in different studies. More than 75% of patients are between the ages of 10 and 35 years, with a mean age of 23 years and an age range of 4 months to 78 years. Two percent of patients have a recurrence. The incidence of disease is higher during the colder months. Twenty percent of patients have a recent history of acute infection with fatigue, headache, sore throat, lymphadenitis, and fever; the disease may be more common in atopic patients. Upper respiratory tract infection before the appearance of skin lesions was reported in 68.8%. In pregnancy, PR may foreshadow premature delivery with neonatal hypotonia and even fetal demise, especially if it develops within 15 weeks' gestation. *PMID: 18489054*

DIFFERENTIAL DIAGNOSIS. Pityriasis rosea has several unique features, but variant patterns do exist; these may create confusion between pityriasis rosea and secondary syphilis, guttate psoriasis, viral exanthems, tinea, nummular eczema, and drug eruptions.

CLINICAL MANIFESTATIONS. Typically, the herald patch, a single 2- to 10-cm round-to-oval lesion, abruptly appears in 17% of patients. It may occur anywhere, but is most frequently located on the trunk or proximal extremities. The herald patch retains the same features as the subsequent oval lesions. At this stage, many patients are convinced that they have ringworm.

Within a few days to several weeks (average, 7 to 14 days) the disease enters the eruptive phase. Smaller lesions appear and reach their maximum number in 1 to 2 weeks (Figure 8-41). They are typically limited to the trunk and proximal extremities, but in extensive cases they develop on the arms, legs, and face (Figure 8-42). An inverse distribution involving mainly the extremities is seen in 6% of cases. Lesions are typically benign and are concentrated in the lower abdominal area (Figure 8-43). Individual lesions are salmon pink in whites and hyperpigmented in blacks. Many of the earliest lesions are papular, but in most cases the typical 1- to 2-cm oval plaques appear (Figure 8-44). A fine, wrinkled, tissue-like scale remains attached within the border of the plaque, giving the characteristic ring of scale, called collarette scale (Figure 8-45). The long axis of the oval plaques is oriented along skin lines. Numerous lesions on the back, oriented along skin lines, give the appearance of drooping pine-tree branches, which explains the designation "Christmas-tree distribution." The number of lesions varies from a few to hundreds.

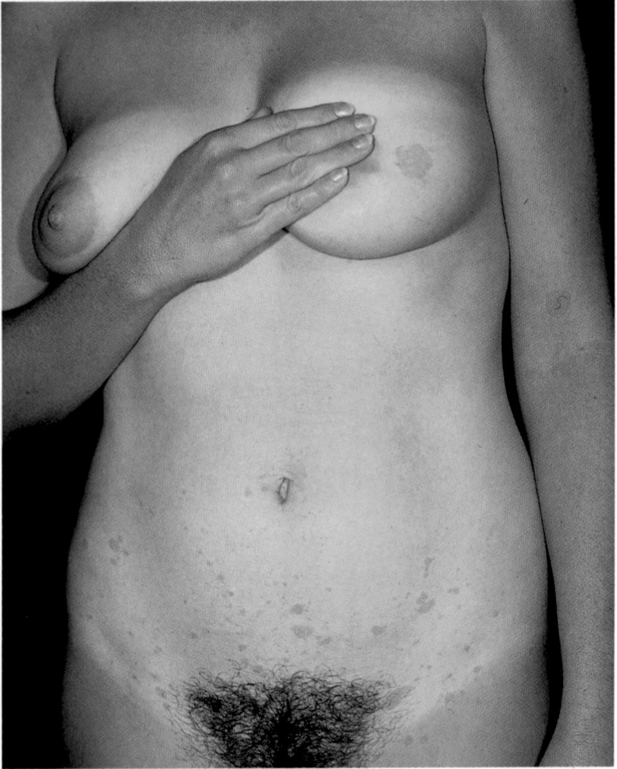

Figure 8-41 Pityriasis rosea. A herald patch is present on the breast. Subsequent lesions commonly begin in the lower abdominal region.

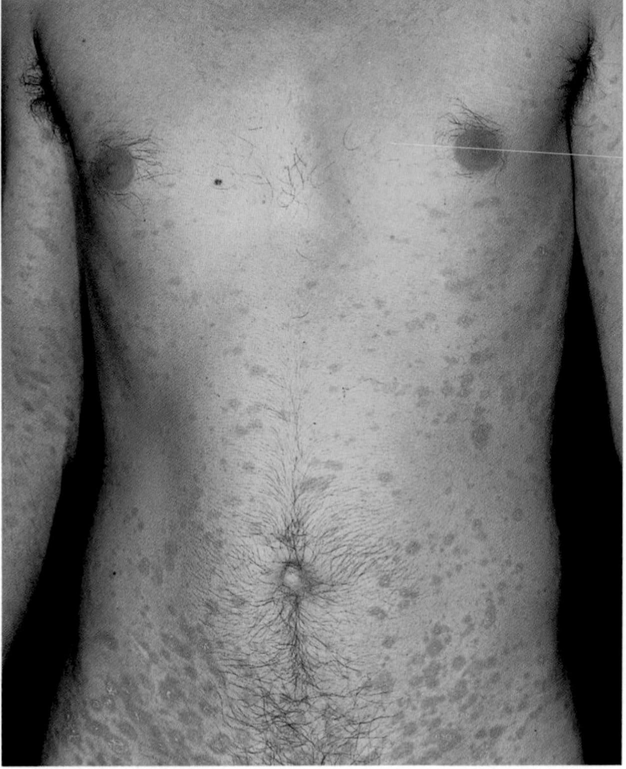

Figure 8-42 Pityriasis rosea. The fully evolved eruption 2 weeks after onset.

PITYRIASIS ROSEA

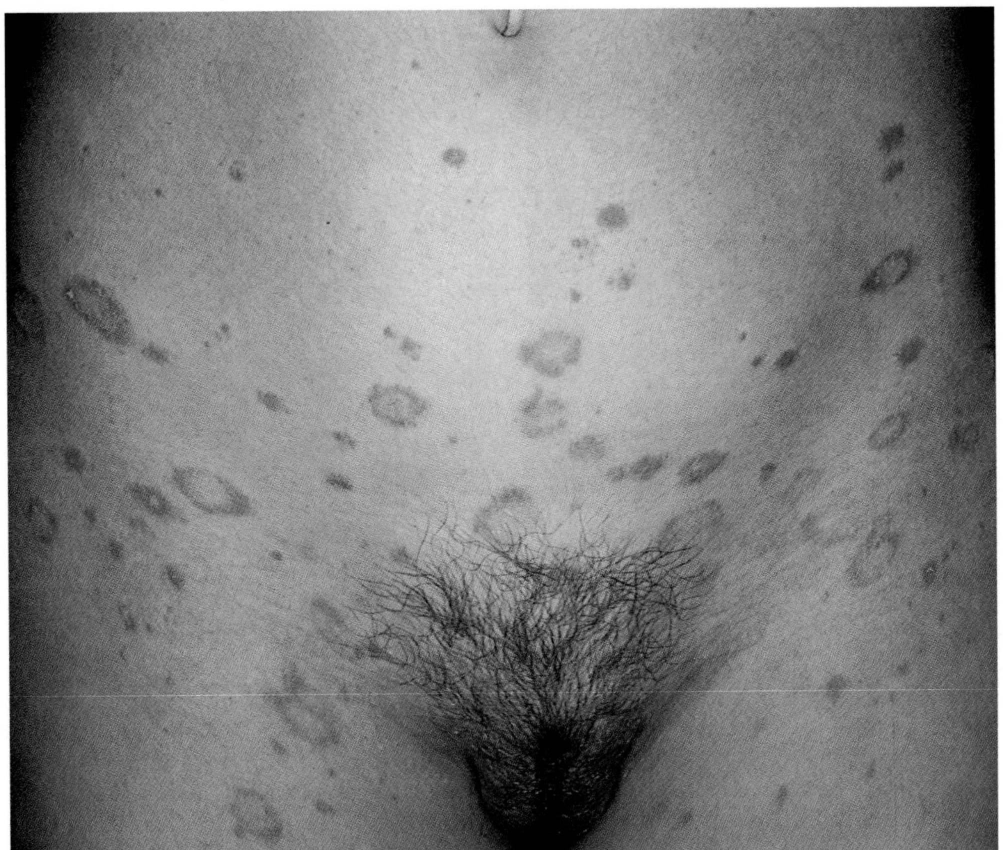

Figure 8-43 Lesions are typically concentrated in the lower abdominal area.

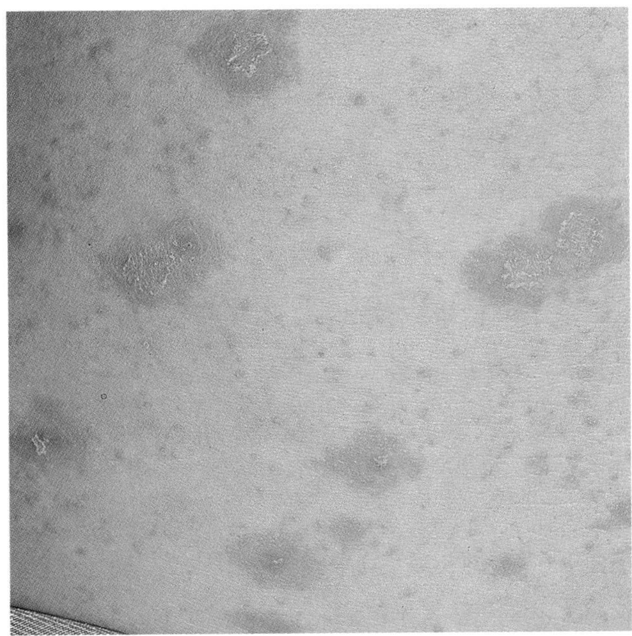

Figure 8-44 Both small, oval plaques and multiple, small papules are present. Occasionally the eruption consists only of small papules.

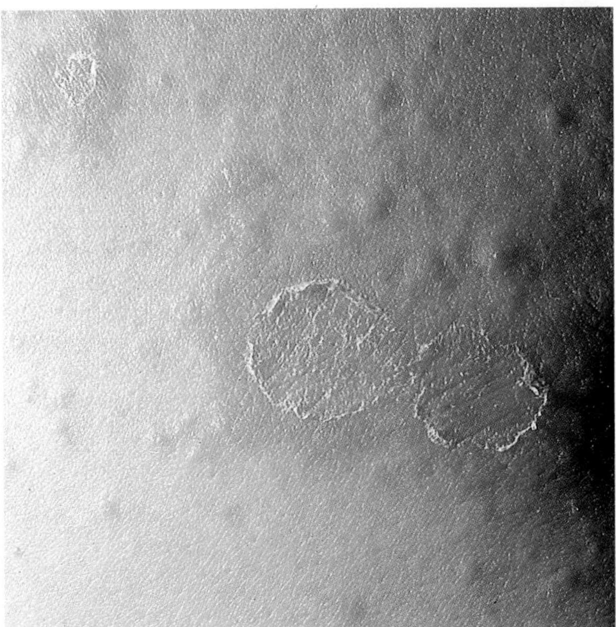

Figure 8-45 A ring of tissuelike scale (collarette scale) remains attached within the border of the plaque.

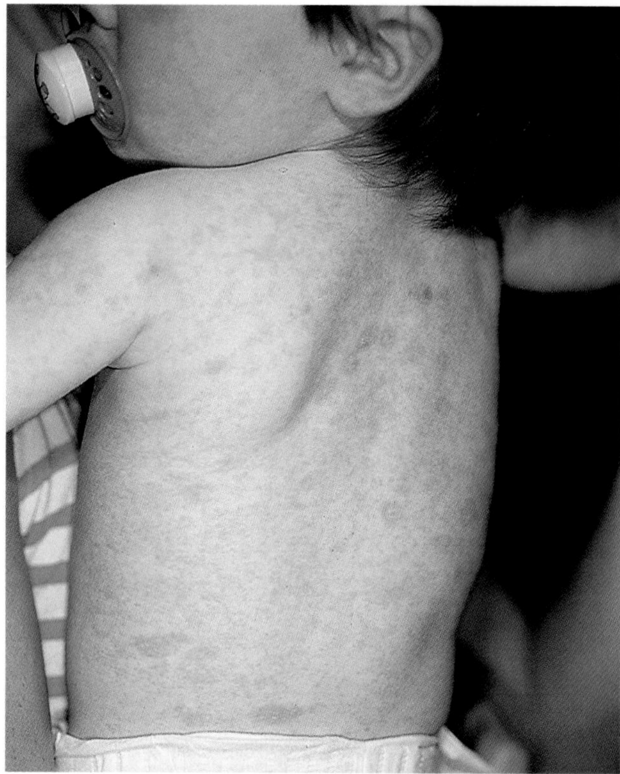

Figure 8-46 Pityriasis rosea. Papular lesions are seen in children, pregnant women, and blacks.

In some cases, other types of lesions predominate. The papular variety is more common in young children, pregnant women, and blacks (Figures 8-46 and 8-47). Vesicular and, rarely, purpuric lesions are seen in infants and children. Eczematized lesions were noted in 5.4% of cases. In rare instances the lesions seem to cover the entire skin surface (Figure 8-48). A variety of oral lesions have been reported.

Most lesions are asymptomatic, but many patients complain of mild transient itching. Severe itching may accompany extensive inflammatory eruptions. The disease clears spontaneously in 1 to 3 months. There may be postinflammatory hyperpigmentation, especially in blacks. Black American children have more frequent facial involvement (30%) and more scalp lesions (8%) than usually described in white populations. One third have papular lesions. The disease resolves in nearly one half of black patients within 2 weeks. Residual hyperpigmentation is seen in 48% of blacks. Hypopigmentation develops in 29% of blacks with purely papular or papulovesicular lesions. *PMID: 17485628*

DIAGNOSIS

The experienced observer can rely on a clinical impression to make the diagnosis. Tinea can be ruled out with a potassium hydroxide examination. Secondary syphilis may be indistinguishable from pityriasis rosea, especially if the herald patch is absent. A serologic test for syphilis should be ordered if a clinical diagnosis cannot be made. A biopsy is useful in atypical cases; it reveals extravasated erythrocytes within dermal papillae and dyskeratotic cells within the dermis. Pityriasis rosea may also be mimicked by psoriasis and nummular eczema.

Figure 8-47 Pityriasis rosea. Papular lesions may be the predominant lesion in children.

MANAGEMENT

Whether or not PR is contagious is unknown. The disease is benign and self-limited and does not appear to affect the fetus; therefore isolation is unnecessary. Oral erythromycin stearate daily (1 gm in four equally divided doses for 2 weeks in adults and 25 to 40 mg/kg in four divided doses in children) was used in a study to treat PR. In this study 33 patients achieved complete response in 2 weeks, four patients showed complete disappearance of lesions by the end of 6 weeks, and 8 patients did not respond. A more recent study reported that erythromycin was not effective. *PMID: 18246696* Group V topical steroids and oral antihistamines may be used as needed for itching. The rare extensive case with intense itching responds to a 1- to 2-week course of prednisone (20 mg twice a day). Direct sun exposure hastens the resolution of individual lesions, whereas those in protected areas, such as under bathing suits, remain (see Figure 8-36). Ultraviolet light B (UVB), administered in five consecutive daily erythemogenic exposures, results in decreased pruritus and hastens the involution of lesions. Therapy is most beneficial within the first week of the eruption. UVB phototherapy five times per week for 2 weeks resulted in decreased severity of disease during the treatment period. However, the itching and the course of the disease were unchanged. The possible association of human herpesvirus 6 (HHV-6) and HHV-7 with pityriasis rosea suggests that systemic drugs directed against HHV may hasten recovery of patients with pityriasis rosea. In one study patients were treated for 1 week with oral acyclovir (800 mg five times daily). The lesions cleared in 18.5 days in treated patients and in 37.9 days in the placebo group. Clearance was achieved in 17.2 days in patients treated in the first week from onset and in 19.7 days in the patients treated later. *PMID: 16384760*

PITYRIASIS ROSEA

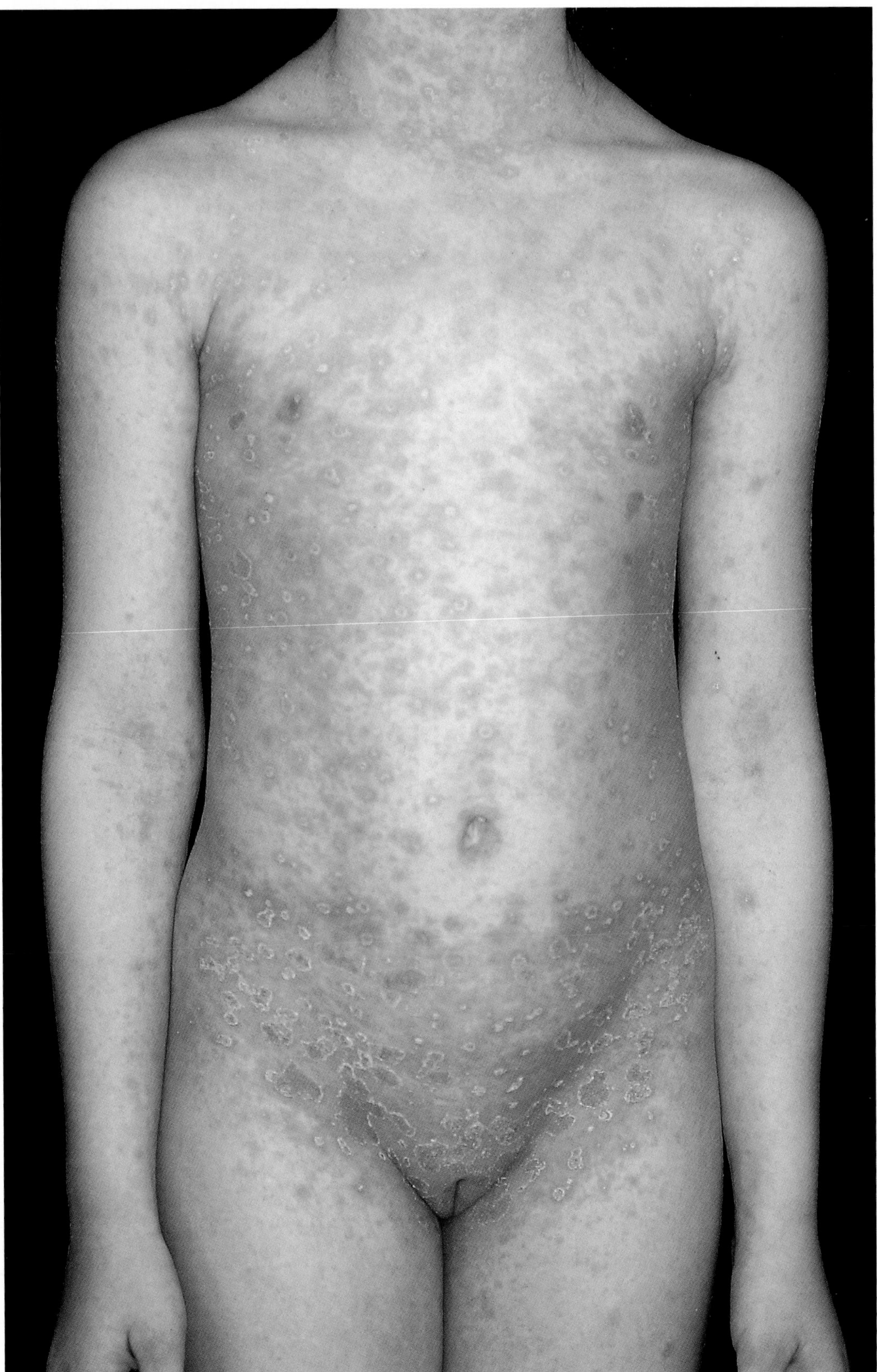

Figure 8-48 A rare extensive eruption. Eruption is concentrated in the commonly involved area (neck, trunk, and groin).

LICHEN PLANUS

Lichen planus (LP) is a unique inflammatory cutaneous and mucous membrane reaction pattern of unknown etiology. The mean age of onset is 40.3 years in males compared with 46.4 years in females. The main eruption clears within 1 year in 68% of patients, but 49% of eruptions recur. Although the disease may occur at any age, it is rare in children younger than 5 years. Approximately 10% of patients have a positive family history. This supports the hypothesis that genetic factors are of etiologic importance. Liver disease is a risk factor for LP although not a specific marker of it. Cutaneous and oral LP may be associated with hepatitis C virus (HCV)-related, chronic, active hepatitis. The virus may play a potential pathogenic role by replicating in cutaneous tissue and triggering lichen planus in genetically susceptible HCV-infected patients. No association between the hepatitis B surface antigen (HBsAg) carrier state and LP was found in one study. *PMID: 18693602* Another study shows that no clear association exists between oral lichen planus (OLP) and chronic HCV disease. *PMID: 17625433*

There are several clinical forms, and the number of lesions varies from a few chronic papules to acute generalized disease (Table 8-9).

Eruptions from drugs (e.g., gold, chloroquine, methyldopa, penicillamine), chemical exposure (film processing), bacterial infections (secondary syphilis), and post–bone marrow transplants (graft-versus-host reaction) that have a similar appearance are referred to as lichenoid.

Table 8-9 Various Patterns of Lichen Planus

Various patterns of lichen planus	Most common site
Actinic	Sun-exposed areas
Annular	Trunk, external genitalia
Atrophic	Any area
Erosioulcerative	Soles of feet, mouth
Follicular (lichen planopilaris)	Scalp
Guttate (numerous) small papules	Trunk
Hypertrophic	Lower limbs (especially ankles)
Linear	Zosteriform (leg), scratched area
Nail disease	Fingernails
Papular (localized)	Flexor surface (wrists and forearms)
Vesiculobullous	Lower limbs, mouth

PRIMARY LESIONS

The morphology and distribution of the lesions are characteristic (Figure 8-49). The clinical features of lichen planus can be remembered by learning the five Ps of lichen planus: *p*ruritic, *p*lanar (flat-topped), *p*olyangular, *p*urple *p*apules. The primary lesion is a 2- to 10-mm flat-topped papule with an irregular angulated border (polygonal papules). Close inspection of the surface shows a lacy, reticular pattern of crisscrossed, whitish lines (Wickham's striae) that can be accentuated by a drop of immersion oil (Figures 8-50 and 8-51). Histologically, Wickham's striae are areas of focal epidermal thickening.

Newly evolving lesions are pink-white, but over time they assume a distinctive violaceous, or purple, hue with a peculiar waxy luster. Lesions that persist for months may become thicker and dark red (hypertrophic lichen planus). Papules aggregate into different patterns. Patterns are usually haphazard clusters, but they may be annular, diffusely papular (guttate), or linear, appearing in response to a scratch (Koebner phenomenon). Rarely, a line of papules may extend the length of the extremity. Vesicles or bullae may appear on preexisting lesions or on normal skin. Many patients have persistent brown staining many years after the rash has cleared.

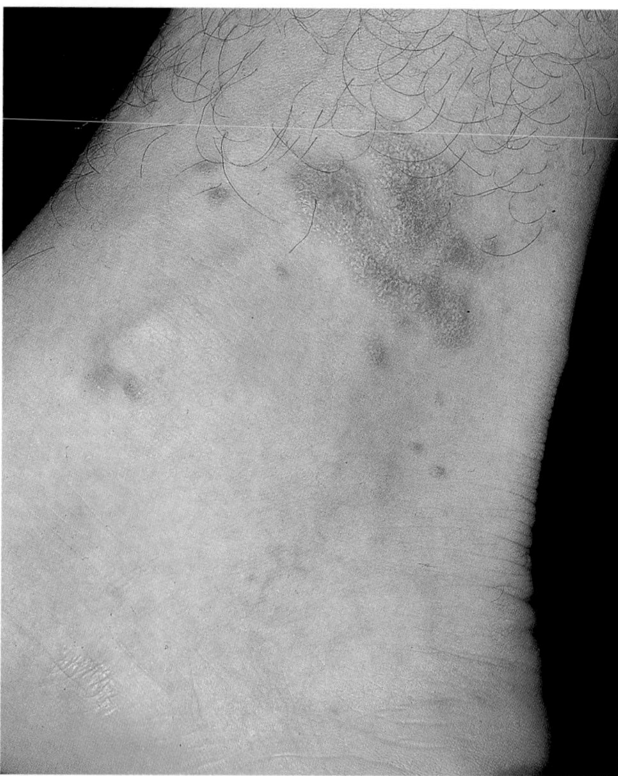

Figure 8-49 Lichen planus. A characteristic lesion of planar, polyangular, purple papules with lacy, reticular, crisscrossed whitish lines (Wickham's striae) on the surface.

LICHEN PLANUS

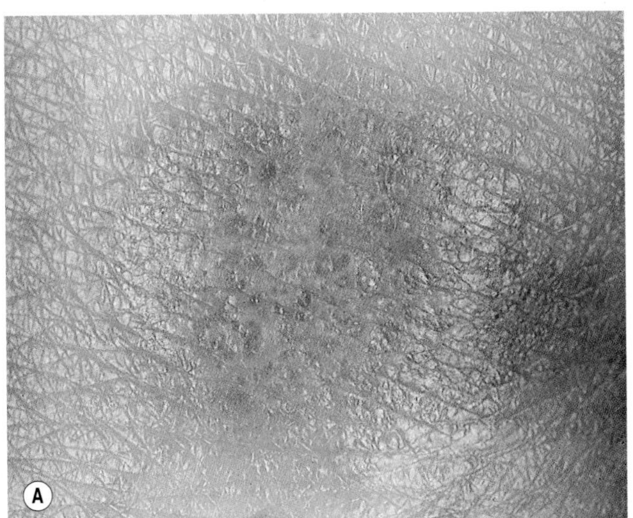

The primary lesion is a flat-topped papule with an irregular, angulated border (polygonal papules).

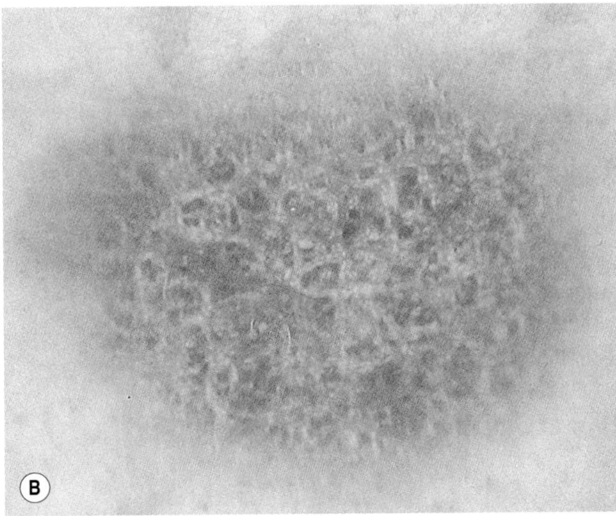

Close inspection of the surface shows a lacy, reticular pattern of crisscrossed whitish lines (Wickham's striae), accentuated here by a drop of immersion oil.

Figure 8-50 Primary lesions.

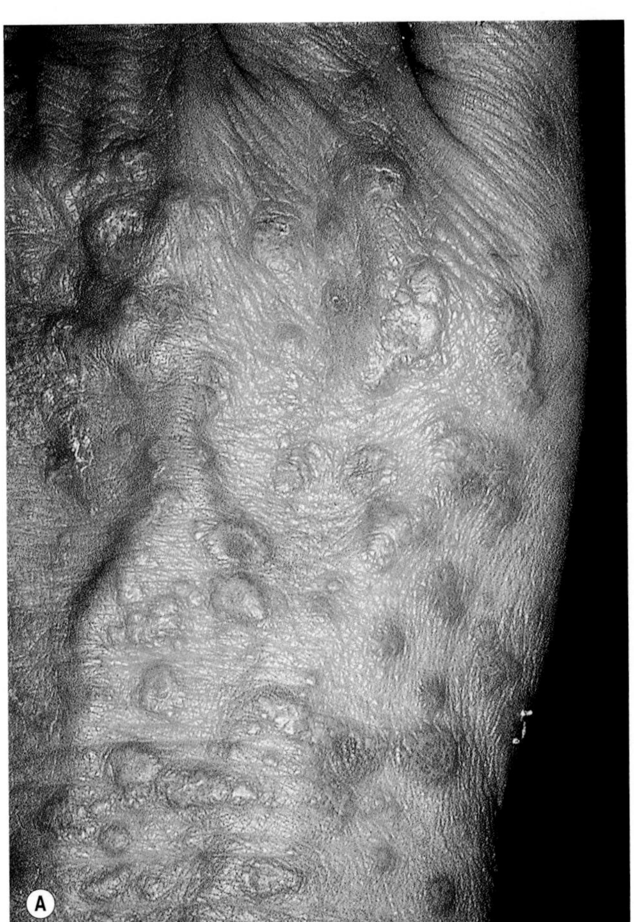

Large number of purple polycyclic lesions on the wrists.

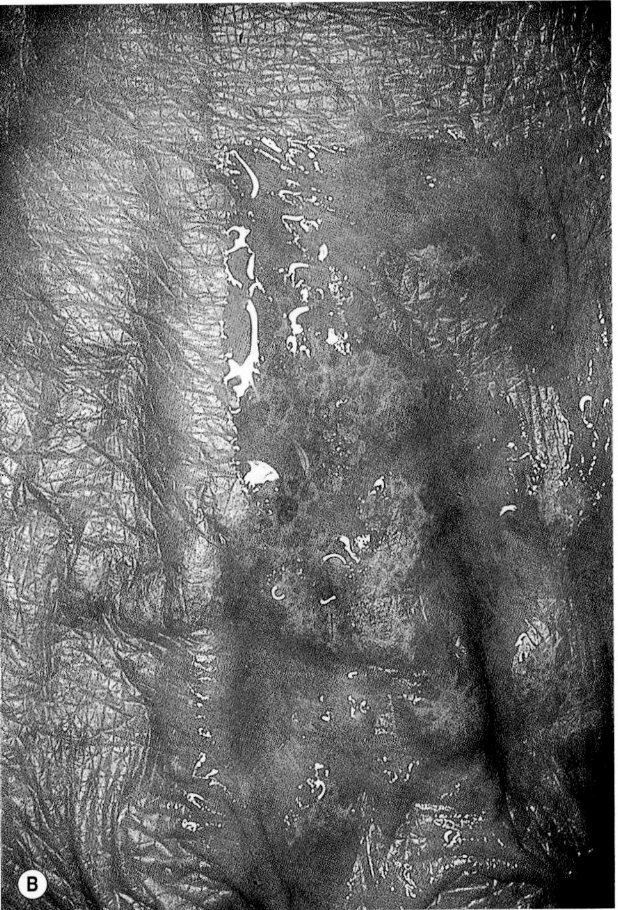

Oil accentuates the lacy, white Wickham's striae and helps confirm the clinical diagnosis.

Figure 8-51 Localized lesions.

Localized papules

Papules are most commonly located on the flexor surfaces of the wrists and forearms, the legs immediately above the ankles (Figures 8-52 and 8-53), and the lumbar region. Itching is variable; 20% of patients with lichen planus do not itch. Some patients with generalized involvement have minimal symptoms, whereas others display intolerable pruritus. The course is unpredictable. Some patients experience spontaneous remission in a few months, but the most common localized papular form tends to be chronic and endures for an average of approximately 4 years. Many patients have persistent brown staining many years after the rash has cleared.

Hypertrophic lichen planus

This second most common cutaneous pattern may occur on any body region, but it is typically found on the pretibial areas and ankles (Figures 8-54 and 8-56). After a long time, papules lose their characteristic features and become confluent as reddish brown or purplish, thickened, round-to-elongated (bandlike) plaques with a rough or verrucose surface; itching may be severe. Lesions continue for months or years, averaging approximately 8 years, and may be perpetuated by scratching. After the lesions clear, a dark brown pigmentation remains.

Generalized lichen planus and lichenoid drug eruptions

Lichen planus may occur abruptly as a generalized, intensely pruritic eruption (Figure 8-55). Initially, the papules are pinpoint, numerous, and isolated. The papules may remain discrete or become confluent as large, red, eczematous-like, thin plaques. A highly characteristic, diffuse, dark brown, postinflammatory pigmentation remains as the disease clears. Before resolving spontaneously, untreated generalized lichen planus continues for approximately 8 months. Lichenoid drug eruptions are frequently of this diffuse type. Low-grade fever may be present in the first few days, and lesions appear on the trunk, extremities, and lower back. The disease is seldom seen on the face or scalp and is rare on the palms and soles. Widespread inflammation can occur after sun exposure.

Lichen planus of the palms and soles

Lichen planus of the palms and soles generally occurs as an isolated phenomenon, but may appear simultaneously with disease in other areas. The lesions differ from classic lesions of lichen planus in that the papules are larger and aggregate into semitranslucent plaques with a globular waxy surface (Figure 8-57). Itching may be intolerable. Ulceration may occur and lesions of the feet may be so resistant to treatment that surgical excision and grafting are required. The disease may last indefinitely.

Follicular lichen planus

Follicular lichen planus is also known as lichen planopilaris. Lesions localized to the hair follicles may occur alone or with papular lichen planus. Follicular lichen planus, manifested as pinpoint, hyperkeratotic, follicular projections, is the most common form of lichen planus found in the scalp, where papular lesions are rarely observed. Hair loss occurs and may be permanent if the disease is sufficiently active to cause scarring. Lichen planus of the scalp is a cause of scarring alopecia. Patients with scarring alopecia should be evaluated histologically and with direct immunofluorescence. The immunofluorescence abnormalities differ from those associated with lichen planus, suggesting that lichen planopilaris and lichen planus are two different diseases.

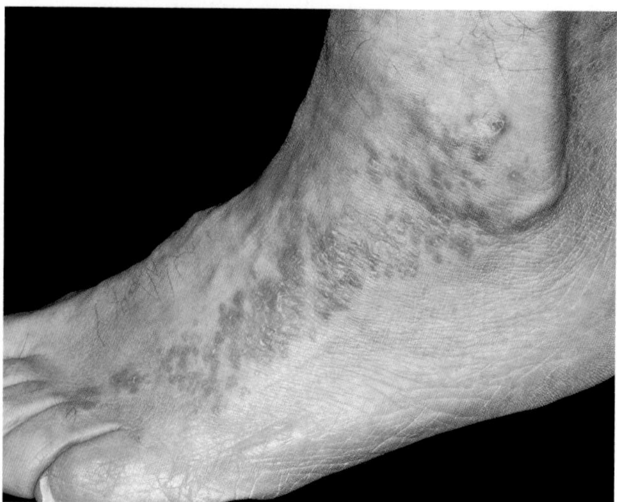

Figure 8-52 Localized lichen planus. Papules become thicker and confluent with time.

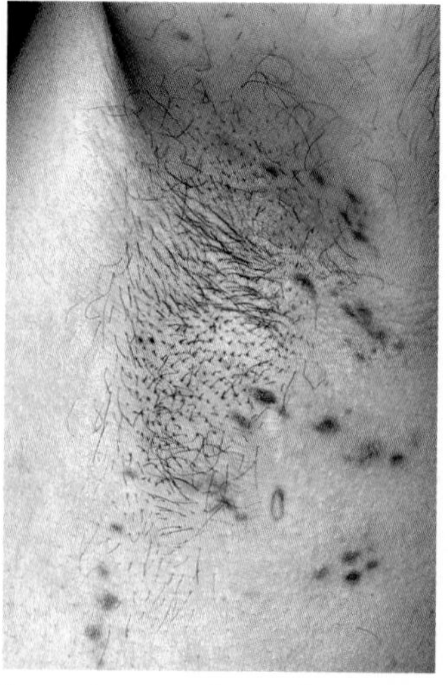

Figure 8-53 Hyperpigmented macules may occur after the active disease has cleared. This staining is often permanent.

LICHEN PLANUS

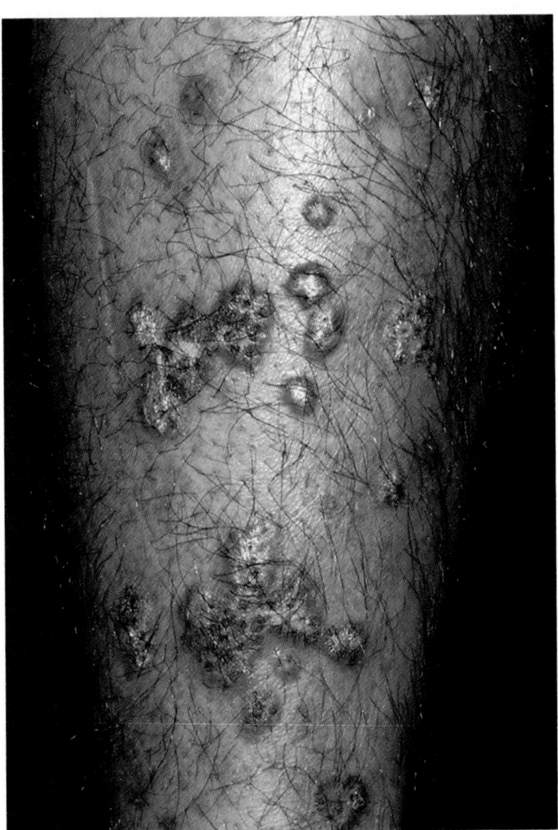

Figure 8-54 Hypertrophic lichen planus. Thick, reddish brown plaques are most often present on the lower legs.

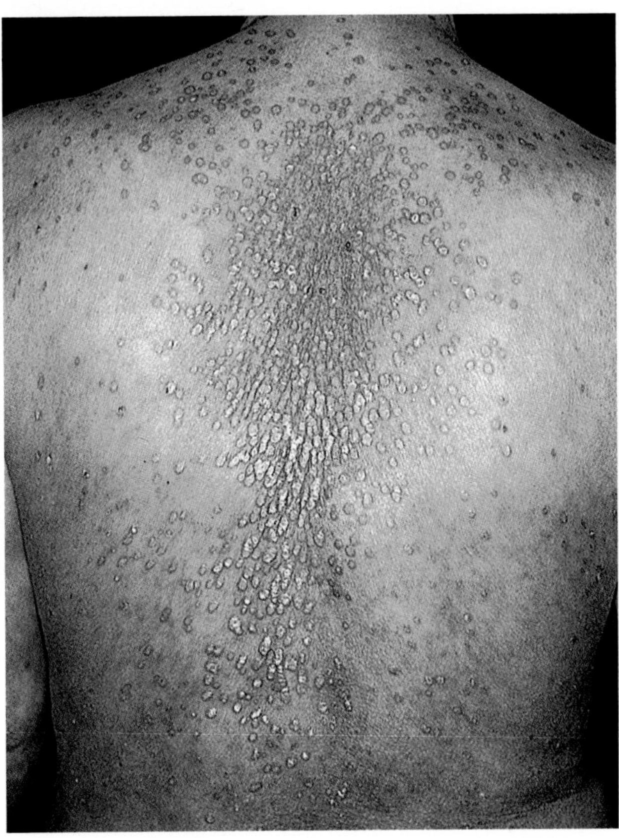

Figure 8-55 Generalized lichen planus. These discrete (guttate) lesions range from 1 mm to 1 cm in size. This generalized eruption occurred after starting antimalarial drugs.

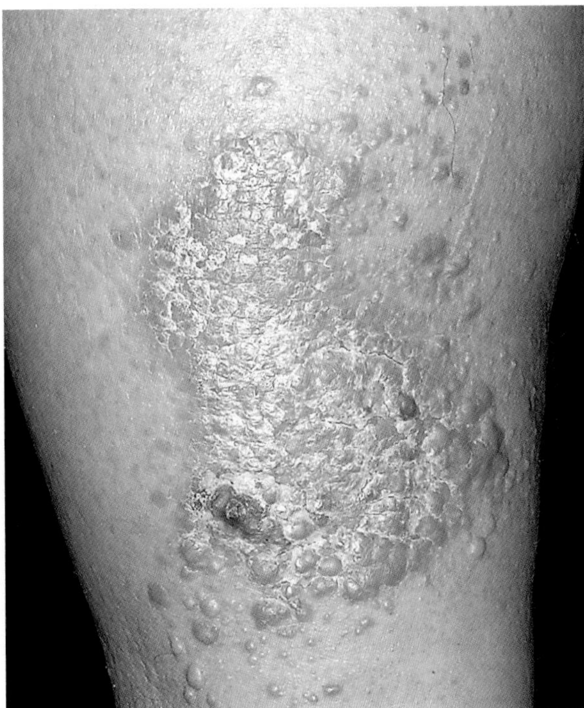

Figure 8-56 Confluent hypertrophic lichen planus. Lesions are extremely pruritic.

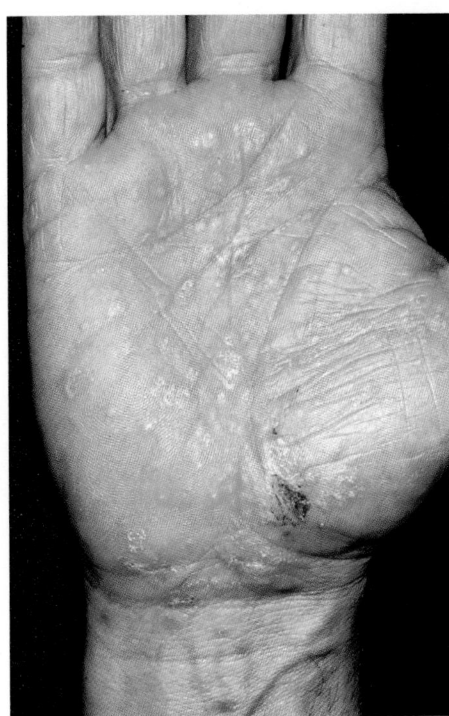

Figure 8-57 Lichen planus of the palms. Papules are large and become aggregated.

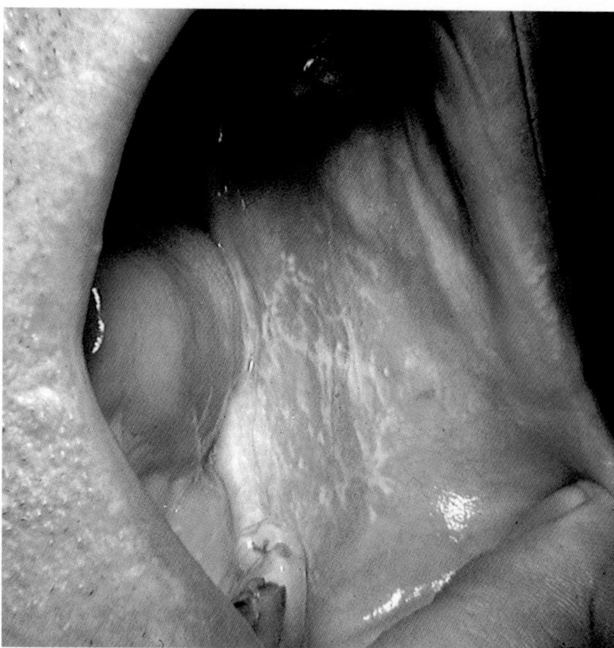

Figure 8-58 Mucous membrane lichen planus. A lacy, white pattern is present on the buccal mucosa. (Courtesy Gerald Shklar, BSc, DDS, MS, Harvard School of Dental Medicine.)

Oral and genital lichen planus

Oral lichen planus (OLP) can occur without cutaneous disease. Onset before middle age is rare; the mean age of onset is in the sixth decade. Women outnumber men by more than 2:1. Mucous membrane involvement is observed in more than 50% of patients with cutaneous lichen planus (Figures 8-58, 8-59, and 8-60). The most common location of OLP is the buccal mucosa (80% to 90%) followed by the tongue (30% to 50%) (see Figure 8-58). There are two stages of severity. The most common form is the nonerosive, generally asymptomatic, dendritic branching or lacy, white network pattern seen on the buccal mucosa; papules and plaques may appear with time. The oral cavity should always be examined if the diagnosis of cutaneous lichen planus is suspected. The presence of this dendritic pattern is solid supporting evidence for the diagnosis of cutaneous lichen planus.

A more difficult form is erosive mucosal lichen planus (see Figure 8-59). Localized or extensive ulcerations may involve any area of the oral cavity. Candidal infection was found in 17% to 25% of ulcerated and nonulcerated cases of lichen planus. Oral squamous cell carcinoma developed in 0.8% of patients at sites previously diagnosed by clinical examination as erosive or erythematous lichen planus.

Superficial and erosive lesions are less commonly found on the glans penis (Figure 8-61), vulvovaginal region (Figure 8-62), and anus.

One study shows that no clear association exists between OLP and chronic hepatitis C virus disease. *PMID: 17625433*

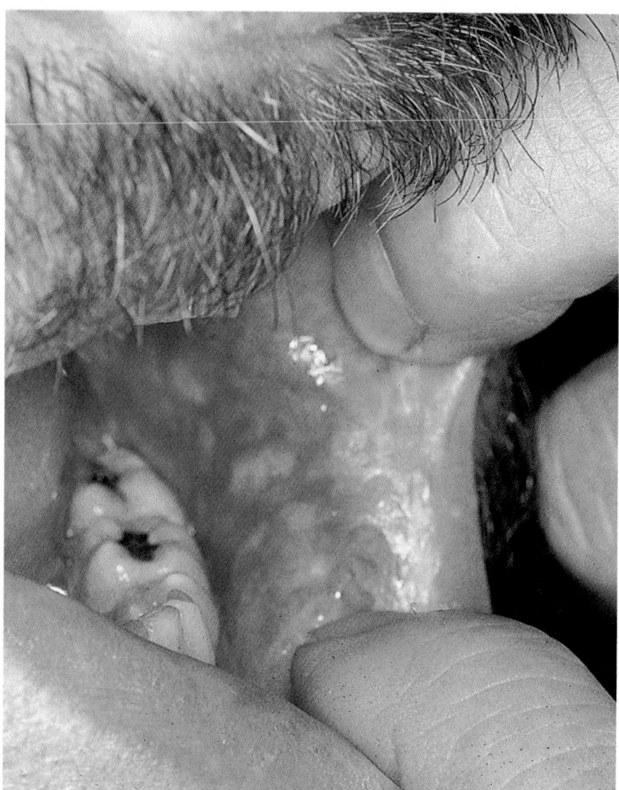

Figure 8-59 Erosive oral lichen planus. Localized or extensive ulcerations may involve any area of the oral cavity.

Erosive vaginal lichen planus

Lichen planus usually involves skin and oral cavity lesions, but erosive vaginal disease may be the first sign. Lichen planus may be the most common cause of desquamative vaginitis. There are flares and partial remissions but no tendency for complete remission. There is marked vaginal

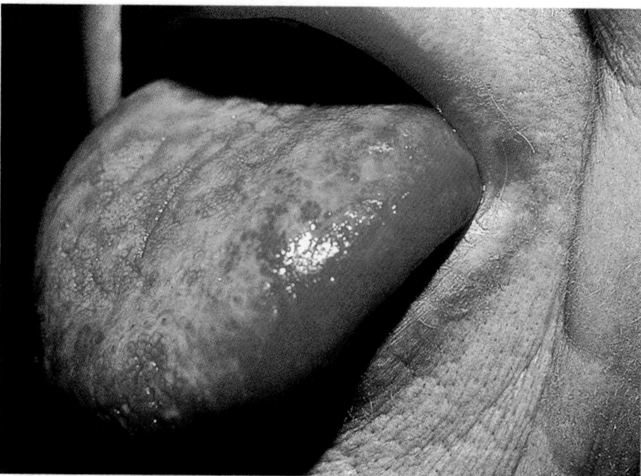

Figure 8-60 Lichen planus tongue. The surface is red and smooth with loss of papillae. White striae are an almost constant feature. *Candida* has a similar appearance.

mucosal fragility and erythema (see Figure 8-62). Agglutination of the labia minora may occur, and vaginal adhesions may render a patient unable to engage in sexual intercourse. Vaginal histology may be nonspecific, showing only a loss of epithelium. A biopsy taken from a white hyperkeratotic area on the labial skin may provide a specific histologic picture. Vaginal desquamation is not associated with lichen sclerosus. Topical and oral steroids are the most effective treatment. Topical tacrolimus (Protopic ointment) or pimecrolimus (Elidel cream) may be effective. Some patients respond to dapsone. Many other systemic agents have been used. Aloe vera gel is a safe and effective treatment for patients with vulval lichen planus. *PMID: 18940117*

The vulvovaginal-gingival syndrome is a variant of mucosal lichen planus characterized by erosions and desquamation of the vulva, vagina, and gingiva. Gingival lichen planus is present in all patients and is characterized by erosions, erythema, and white, reticulated lesions. Vulvovaginal lichen planus also displayed erosions in most patients. Concomitant use of several drugs is usually required to achieve beneficial results. Estrogens are not effective.

Nails

Nail changes frequently accompany generalized lichen planus but may occur as the only manifestation of disease. Approximately 25% of patients with nail LP have LP in other sites before or after the onset of nail lesions. Nail LP usually appears during the fifth or sixth decade of life. The changes include proximal to distal linear depressions or grooves and partial or complete destruction of the nail plate. The development of severe and early destruction of the nail matrix characterizes a small subset of patients with nail LP. Long-term observation indicates that permanent damage to the nail is rare even in patients with diffuse involvement of the matrix (see Figure 25-10). A case of treatment with combined topical therapy of tazarotene gel and clobetasol gel was reported. *PMID: 17373179*

Diagnosis

The diagnosis can be made clinically, but a skin biopsy eliminates any doubt. Direct immunofluorescence may help to establish the diagnosis. The skin shows ovoid globular deposits of IgG, IgM, IgA, and complement. Basement membrane zone deposits of fibrin and fibrinogen are present in a linear pattern in both cutaneous and oral lesions in almost all patients. Circulating antibodies have not been found; therefore indirect immunofluorescence is negative.

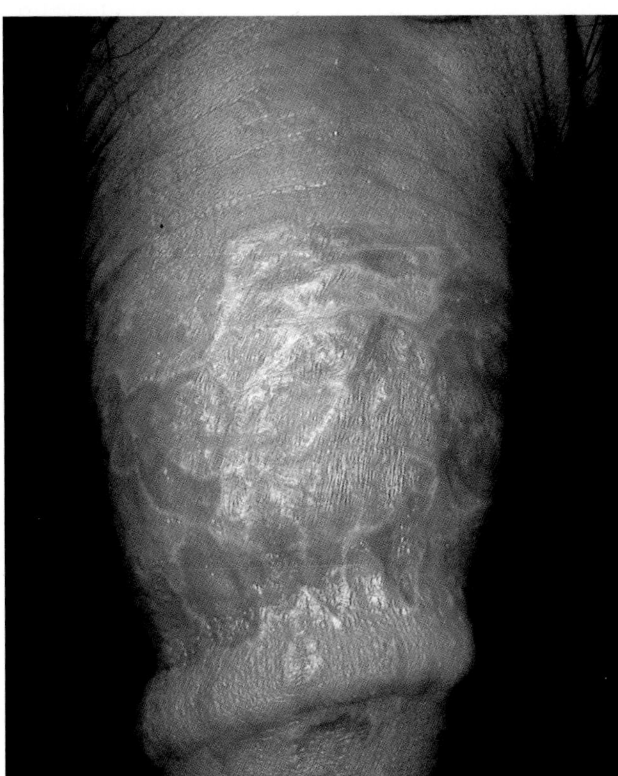

Figure 8-61 Lichen planus on the penis. A lacy, white pattern identical to that seen on the buccal mucosa.

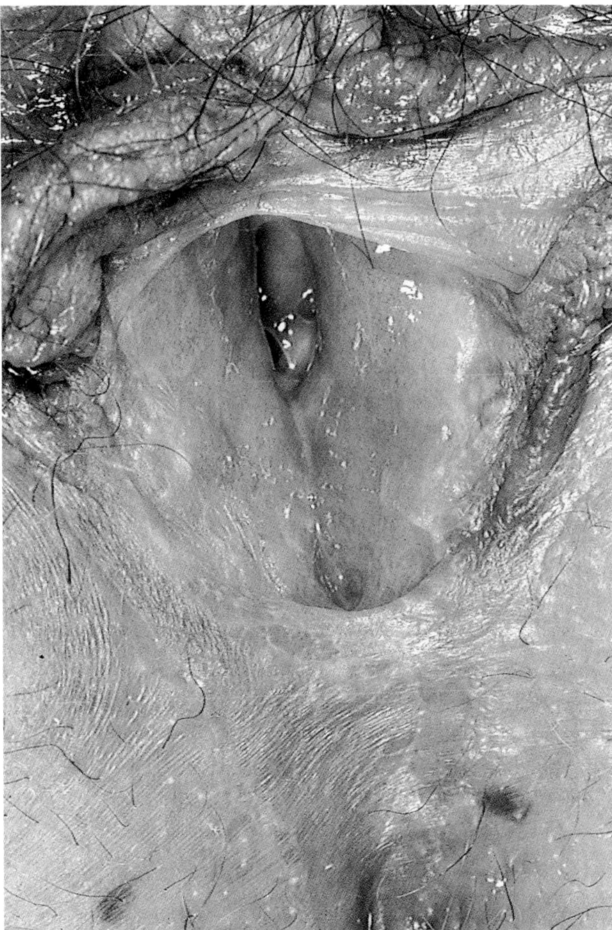

Figure 8-62 Erosive vaginal lichen planus. The entire vaginal tract is involved in this severe case.

Treatment

THERAPY FOR CUTANEOUS LICHEN PLANUS

Topical steroids. Group I or II topical steroids (in a cream or ointment base applied two times daily) are used as initial treatment for localized disease. They relieve itching, but the lesions are slow to clear. Plastic occlusion enhances the effectiveness of topical steroids.

Intralesional steroids. Triamcinolone acetonide (Kenalog 5 to 10 mg/ml) may reduce the hypertrophic lesions located on the wrists and lower legs. Injections may be repeated every 3 or 4 weeks.

Systemic steroids. Generalized, severely pruritic lichen planus responds to oral corticosteroids. For adults, a 2- to 4-week course of prednisone, 20 mg twice daily, is usually sufficient to clear the disease. To help prevent recurrence, gradually decrease the dosage over a 3-week period.

Acitretin. One large study showed that acitretin is an effective and acceptable therapy for severe cases of lichen planus. A significantly higher number of patients treated with 30 mg/day acitretin (64%) showed remission or marked improvement compared with placebo (13%). *PMID: 1829465* Furthermore, during the subsequent 8-week open phase, 83% of previously placebo-treated patients responded favorably to acitretin therapy.

Azathioprine. Azathioprine can be an effective steroid-sparing treatment for generalized lichen planus. Azathioprine alone is an alternative therapy, especially when there are risk factors against corticosteroid use.

Cyclosporine. Patients with severe, chronic lichen planus were successfully treated with oral cyclosporine (6 mg/kg/day). A response was noted within 4 weeks, and complete clearing was achieved after 8 weeks of treatment. No significant adverse effect was noted. The patients remained in remission up to 10 months after therapy.

Antihistamines. Antihistamines such as hydroxyzine, 10 to 25 mg every 4 hours, may provide relief from itching.

Light therapy. PUVA (psoralen + UVA light) and broadband and narrow-band UVB therapy are effective therapy for generalized, symptomatic lichen planus. Maintenance therapy might not be required once complete clearance is attained.

Tacrolimus ointment. Ulcerative lichen planus of the sole may respond to topical tacrolimus 0.1% ointment. *PMID: 18477162*

THERAPY OF MUCOUS MEMBRANE LICHEN PLANUS

The course of oral and vaginal lichen planus can extend for years. Treatment is challenging. Most treatment failures are due to improper diagnosis. Consider a biopsy to establish the diagnosis. Most patients are asymptomatic and do not need treatment. Most symptomatic forms of the disease are the erosive and atrophic types, which may need systemic therapy. The most effective treatment is short courses of systemic steroids (prednisone) and topical high-potency corticosteroids.

Tacrolimus and pimecrolimus. Topical tacrolimus (Protopic ointment 0.1%, 0.03%) and pimecrolimus (Elidel cream), immunomodulators approved for atopic dermatitis, have also been reported to be effective for erosive lichen planus. Long-term treatment may be required. Elevated blood levels of pimecrolimus have been documented. *PMID: 17438179* In view of the risk of malignant transformation of oral LP and the inherent immunosuppressive nature of calcineurin inhibitors, patients should be monitored closely. The medication can also be compounded by mixing tacrolimus powder in Orabase 0.1%.

Corticosteroids. These medicines are often the initial treatment for oral lichen planus. Topical application of corticosteroids (clobetasol propionate, fluocinonide, fluocinolone acetonide, triamcinolone acetonide [Kenalog]) in an adhesive base (Orabase) is safe and effective. Fluocinolone acetonide gel 0.1% is a safe and effective alternative therapy to fluocinolone acetonide in an oral base 0.1%. Clobetasol propionate in Orabase was more effective than fluocinonide ointment in Orabase for oral vesiculoerosive diseases. Do not rub in the Orabase formulations; simply place them on the lesions. Massaging the special cream base results in the loss of adhesiveness. Topical application of fluocinonide gel to the gingiva and buccal mucosa over a 3-week period in patients with erosive lichen planus produces no adrenal suppression. Acute candidiasis may occur during treatment but responds to topical antifungal therapy (e.g., Mycelex troches).

Intralesional steroids in a single submucosal injection, 0.5 to 1.0 ml of methylprednisolone acetate (Depo-Medrol 40 mg/ml), may be sufficient to heal erosive oral lichen planus within 1 week. Prednisone rapidly and effectively controls the disease, but recurrences may occur when the dosage is tapered.

Aloe vera gel. Aloe vera gel induces clinical and symptomatological improvement of OLP. *PMID: 18093246*

Dapsone (50 to 150 mg/day) may be tried if conservative medical treatment fails.

Hydroxychloroquine sulfate (Plaquenil), 200 to 400 mg daily, is useful for oral LP. Pain relief and reduced erythema occur after 1 to 2 months; erosions required 3 to 6 months of treatment before they resolved.

Azathioprine. Azathioprine is very effective for controlling oral lichen planus and may be considered for resistant, debilitating cases (see p. 302).

Mycophenolate mofetil. Mycophenolate mofetil in doses of 100 mg to 2000 mg/day is reported effective in a case of oral erosive lichen planus (see p. 298). *PMID: 17243970*

LICHEN SCLEROSUS ET ATROPHICUS

Lichen sclerosus et atrophicus (LSA) is an uncommon but distinctive chronic cutaneous disease of unknown origin.

There is some evidence that *Borrelia burgdorferi* or other similar strains are involved in the development, or as a trigger, of this disease. *PMID: 18490585* Cases in females outnumber those in males by 10:1. Although the trunk and extremities may be affected, the disease has a predilection for the vulva, perianal area, and groin. Most lesions appear spontaneously, but some may be induced by trauma or radiation (Koebner phenomenon).

At a glance, LSA may be confused with guttate morphea, lichen planus, or discoid lupus erythematosus. The difference becomes evident upon closer inspection of the surface features. Early lesions are small, smooth, pink or ivory, flat-topped, slightly raised papules. White-to-brown, horny follicular plugs appear on the surface; this feature is referred to as delling (Figures 8-63 and 8-64). Delling is not observed in lichen planus or morphea. In time, clusters of papules may coalesce to form small oval plaques with a dull or glistening, smooth, white, atrophic, wrinkled surface (Figure 8-58). Histologically, it appears that the interface area between the dermis and epidermis has dissolved. The overlying, unsupported, thin, atrophic epidermis contracts, giving the appearance of wrinkled tissue paper (Figure 8-65).

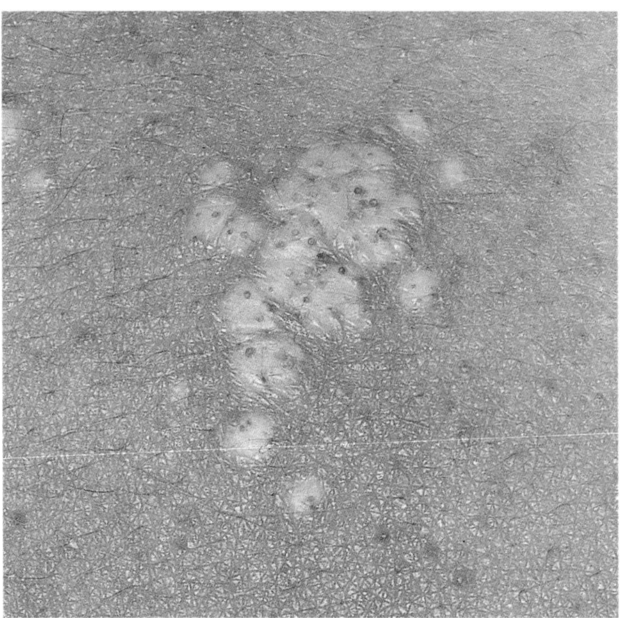

Figure 8-63 Lichen sclerosus et atrophicus. Early lesions are ivory-colored, flat-topped, slightly raised papules with follicular plugs.

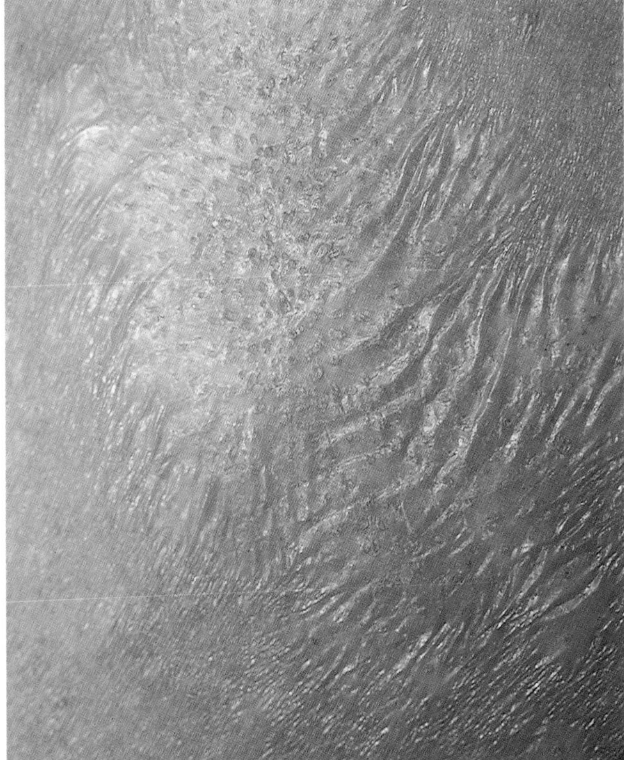

Figure 8-64 Papular lesions as illustrated in Figure 8-63 coalesce to form atrophic plaques with a wrinkled surface. White-to-brown, horny follicular plugs appear on the surface, a feature referred to as delling.

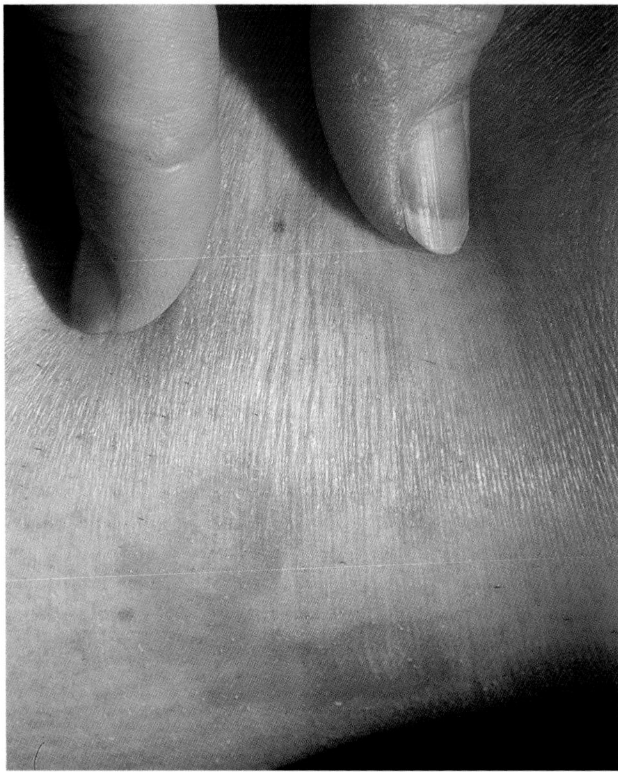

Figure 8-65 Lichen sclerosus et atrophicus. The epidermis is thin and atrophic and gives the appearance of wrinkled tissue paper when compressed.

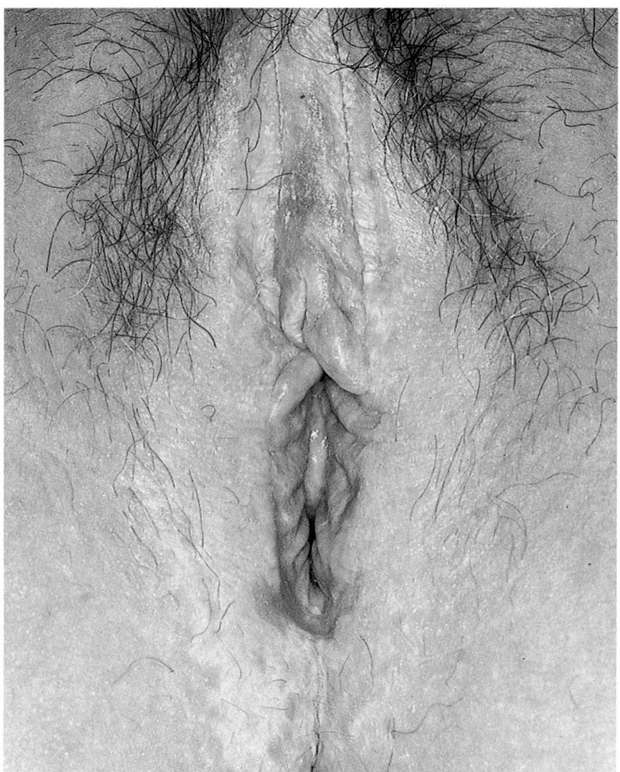

Figure 8-66 Lichen sclerosus et atrophicus. A white, atrophic plaque encircles the vagina and rectum (inverted keyhole pattern).

ANOGENITAL LESIONS IN FEMALES

In most cases, anogenital lesions are distinctive. All of the following patterns may be present in the same individual. The first is a white atrophic plaque in the shape of an hourglass or inverted keyhole encircling the vagina and rectum (Figures 8-66 and 8-67). This distinctive pattern is seen in prepubertal females (Figure 8-68) and adults. The lesions can extend to the entire vulva, giving it a pearly white appearance, or remain localized and require biopsy to confirm the diagnosis. Vulvar pruritus and dyspareunia are the most common symptoms. Dysuria and pain on defecation are common.

PREPUBERTAL LICHEN SCLEROSUS ET ATROPHICUS

Prepubertal LSA may occur in infants and resolves without sequelae in about two thirds of cases at or just before menarche, leaving a brown hyperpigmented area on skin that had been white and atrophic. Purpura of the vulva is an occasional manifestation of pediatric LSA. It mimics sexual abuse and has led to false accusations and investigations. The disease persists in approximately one third of patients.

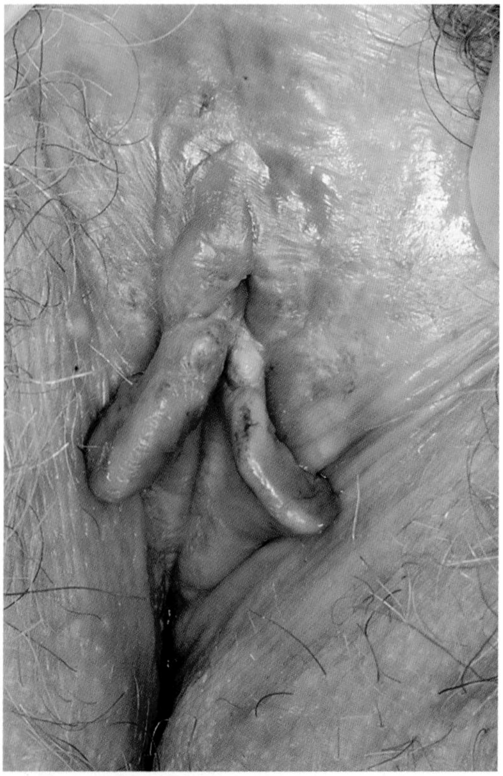

Figure 8-67 Lichen sclerosus et atrophicus of the vulva (kraurosis vulvae). The crease areas are atrophic and wrinkled, the labia is hyperpigmented, and the introitus is contracted and ulcerated.

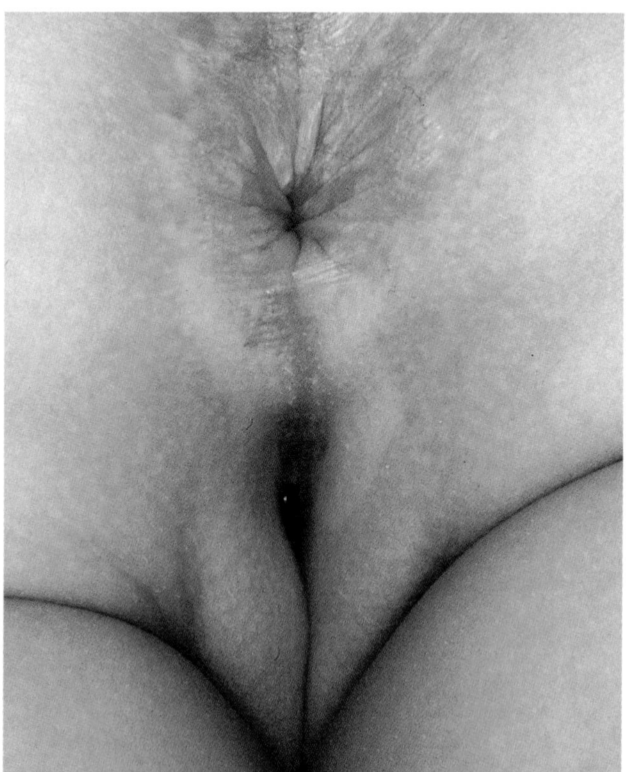

Figure 8-68 Lichen sclerosus et atrophicus. Prepubertal LSA typically involves the vulval and rectal areas. Spontaneous remission occurs in over two thirds of patients.

Intertriginous (skin crease) lesions involve the groin and anal area and are subject to friction and maceration. The delicate, thin, white, wrinkled, compromised skin breaks down to become hemorrhagic and eroded, simulating irritant or candidal intertrigo. Bullae may precede erosions.

ADULT LICHEN SCLEROSUS ET ATROPHICUS

LSA of the vulva is a distressing problem. Typically, the adult form appears after menopause and has a lengthy duration. Lesions itch and may show evidence of excoriation. The disease is chronic and painful, and interferes with sexual activity. Fragile, atrophic, thin, parchment-like tissue erodes, becomes macerated, and heals slowly. Repeated cycles of erosion and healing induce contraction and stenosis of the vaginal introitus and atrophy, and shrinkage of the clitoris and labia minora (see Figure 8-67). A watery discharge may be present. Squamous cell carcinoma, particularly of the clitoris or labia minora, has been reported in approximately 3% of patients with chronic LSA. Therefore biopsy should be considered in lesions that are white and raised (leukoplakia), fissured or ulcerated, and unresponsive to medical therapy.

LICHEN SCLEROSUS ET ATROPHICUS OF THE PENIS

ADULTS. LSA of the penis in the adult (balanitis xerotica obliterans) may present as recurrent balanitis, which may be intensified by intercourse; the shaft is rarely involved. The white atrophic plaques occur on the glans and prepuce and erode and heal with contraction (Figures 8-69, 8-70, and 8-71). Most patients are uncircumcised. LSA may be caused by chronic occlusion. Encroachment into the urinary meatus may lead to stricture. The incidence of neoplastic changes among patients with LS ranges from 2.3% to 8.4%. *PMID: 18374473* There appears to be an association between squamous cell carcinoma (SCC) of the penis and the presence of LSA. Fifty percent of SCC patients studied had a clinical history and/or histologic evidence of LSA. Clinical presentation of LSA or the need for circumcision may precede the SCC by many years.

BOYS. LSA in boys was thought to be rare, but recent reports suggest that it has been overlooked in the past. Most boys are between 4 and 12 years of age at onset. Nearly all affected boys had severe phimosis in a previously retractable penis, with obvious scarring or sclerosis near the tip of the prepuce. Purpura is an occasional manifestation of pediatric LSA. Genital purpura is also a sign of sexual abuse.

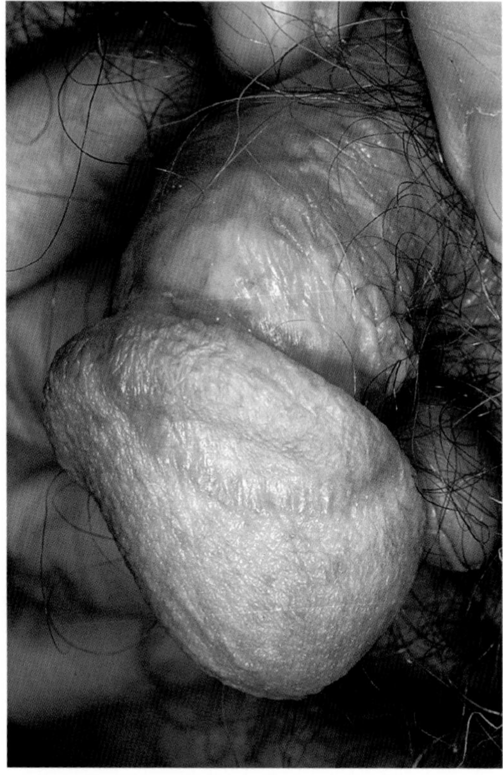

Figure 8-69 Penile shaft involvement is less common. Here an expanding sclerotic ring involves the shaft and glans.

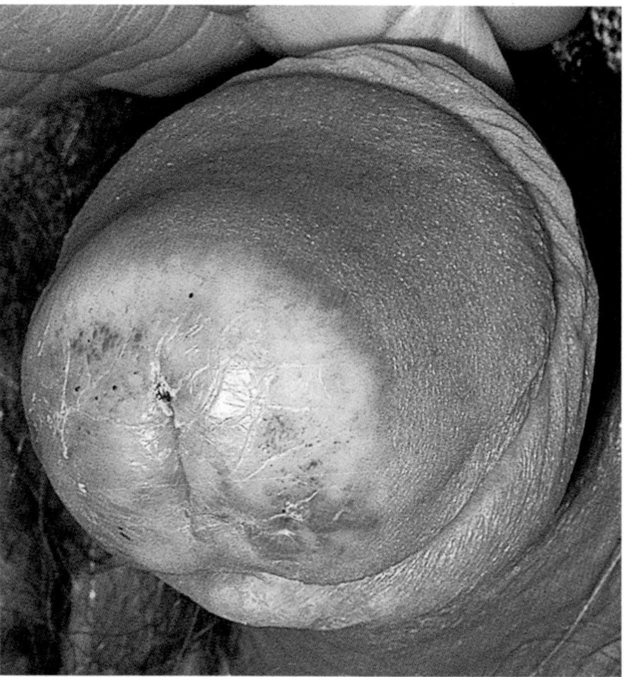

Figure 8-70 Lichen sclerosus et atrophicus of the penis (balanitis xerotica obliterans). The glans is smooth, white, and atrophic. Erosions are present on the prepuce.

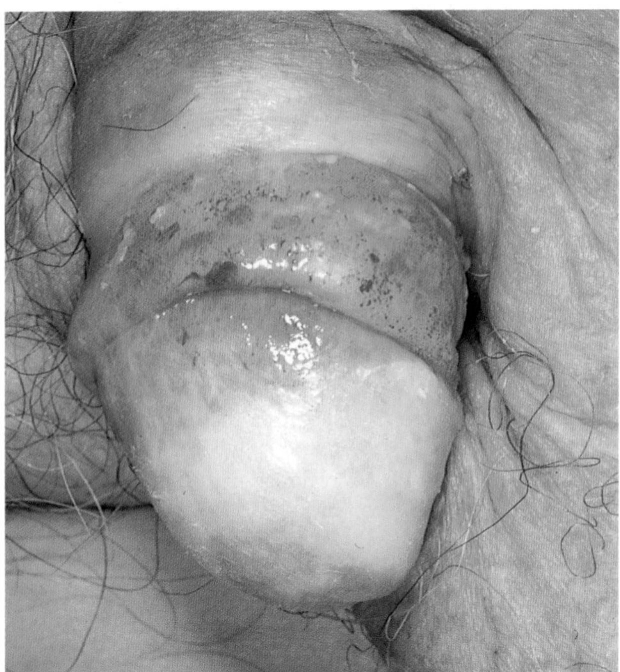

Figure 8-71 Lesions are usually confined to the glans and prepuce.

MANAGEMENT

In general, the diagnosis of LSA of the skin and vulva can be made by clinical observation, but a biopsy may be necessary for confirmation. Chronically fissured, ulcerated, or hyperplastic lesions should be biopsied to rule out SCC.

TOPICAL STEROIDS. Topical steroid creams should be the initial treatment for uncomplicated vulvar and penile lesions in adults and children. Vaginal and vulvar candidiasis may occur. Atrophy of the vulva may result from continual unsupervised application of topical steroids. Use should be discontinued when a favorable response is obtained, and bland lubricants can be used daily to soothe dry tissues.

CLOBETASOL. Clobetasol ointment 0.05% induces a remarkable relief of symptoms (itching, burning, pain, dyspareunia). The clinical signs of atrophy, hyperkeratosis, and sclerosis are improved and histologic alterations (atrophy of the epithelium, edema, inflammatory infiltrate, fibrosis) are reversed. Treatment with topical testosterone propionate 2% is less effective.

Calcineurin inhibitors. Case studies and small series report that extragenital and genital lichen sclerosus showed clinical and subjective improvement with tacrolimus ointment 0.1% and pimecrolimus cream 1%. The regimen used in one study was tacrolimus ointment 0.1% applied twice daily for 6 weeks, and then tapered over a further 6 weeks. *PMID: 17225019* These agents may reduce the incidence of flare ups, improve long-term disease control, and enhance the patient's quality of life, especially in postmenopausal women. Concern about the use of topical calcineurin inhibitors in this dermatosis where there is a risk of squamous carcinoma have been expressed. They may be considered in patients unresponsive to potent topical steroids.

Methotrexate and cyclosporine. Methotrexate may be considered for widespread cutaneous LS. *PMID: 1850766* Patients with refractory vulvar LS responded to oral cyclosporine (3 to 4 mg/kg/day) for 3 months. *PMID: 17442452*

Light therapy. Narrow-band (NB) UVB phototherapy and psoralen-UVA are reported effective in widespread extragenital lichen sclerosus (LS). Patients are advised that their skin disease might appear "deteriorated" during phototherapy because the healthy surrounding skin tans more strongly than LS lesions. Photodynamic therapy (PDT) with 20% 5-aminolevulinic acid and illumination with a red light may be considered for unresponsive cases. *PMID: 17637374*

Antibiotics. Some evidence suggests an infectious etiology of LS from *Borrelia*. Patients who failed potent topical steroids were treated for 3 to 21 months with intramuscular penicillin G benzathine suspension and/or oral penicillin V potassium, amoxicillin, or amoxicillin/clavulanate potassium, or with intramuscular ceftriaxone sodium or oral cefadroxil monohydrate. All patients showed a significant response, evident within a few weeks. *PMID: 16961523*

Vulvar lichen sclerosus et atrophicus in adults. The group I topical steroid ointment clobetasol propionate is reported effective for all age groups. The following regimen was reported for adults. Apply the ointment twice daily for 1 month and then once daily for 1 month; then taper down within the next month to two applications per week and remain on that regimen until a follow-up examination at 3 months after the initial visit. Treatment is then on an "as needed" basis. Follow-up examinations are important when using superpotent topical steroids. Long-term maintenance therapy of vulvar LS with a moisturizing cream can maintain the symptom relief induced by topical corticosteroids. This treatment may also be associated with a reduction in topical corticosteroid use. *PMID: 17603391*

Vulvar lichen sclerosus et atrophicus in children. Premenarchal LSA patients (averaging 5.7 years) responded to clobetasol ointment 0.05% for 2 to 4 weeks. Clobetasol is then stopped and tapered to a less potent steroid. Recurrences were common and required additional steroid treatment. Complications were infrequent, minor, and easily treatable. Betamethasone dipropionate 0.05% ointment applied three times each day for 3 weeks and then twice daily until the vulva appeared normal was effective. This required 1 to 6 months of treatment (average, 3 months). After this treatment course, patients received hydrocortisone 1% daily for 3 months, and then nothing. Recurrences were treated again with shorter courses. The appearance of the vulva returned to normal in most patients, leaving pigmentary changes in a few. Symptoms subsided within 6 weeks in all patients. No side effects were seen, except mild telangiectasia in three subjects. Recurrence manifested as a recurrence of symptoms.

Labial fusion is a common condition seen most frequently in infants and young children. Most cases are "physiological," but it can be the presenting feature of genital lichen sclerosus. Pain and scarring develop in young women with recurrent labial and periclitoral adhesions.

Vaginal and vulvar candidiasis may occur. Atrophy of the vulva may result from continual application of topical steroids. Use should be discontinued when a favorable response is obtained, and bland lubricants can be used daily to soothe dry tissues.

Penile lichen sclerosus et atrophicus in men. Topical treatment with clobetasol propionate 0.05% is safe and effective with little risk of epidermal atrophy. Treatment significantly improves itching, burning, pain, dyspareunia, phimosis, and dysuria after one to two daily applications, for a mean of 7.1 weeks. Histologic changes are significantly reduced after treatment. There is some potential for triggering latent infections, most importantly human papillomavirus.

Intralesional steroids such as triamcinolone acetonide (Kenalog 2.5 to 5.0 mg/ml) may be useful for areas that do not respond to topical therapy. Fissures and erosions are effectively treated with scarlet red gauze.

SURGERY

The high recurrence rate of all surgical modalities makes surgical treatment suitable only for patients who failed to respond to medical treatment. Surgical options in male patients with genital lichen sclerosus involving the anterior urethra and the foreskin include circumcision, meatotomy, circumcision and meatotomy, and one-stage penile oral mucosal graft urethroplasty. In patients with penile urethral strictures or panurethral strictures, the use of one-stage oral graft urethroplasty showed greater success than the staged procedures. *PMID: 18691809* Tacrolimus 0.1% ointment applied immediately after surgery for LS may lead to disease control for an extended period. *PMID: 18374471*

Surgical therapy of LSA of the vulva consists of vulvectomy (with or without a skin graft), cryosurgery, and laser ablation. It is indicated when malignant transformation is present or is likely to occur. Patients who fail medical treatment and still present with chronic debilitating pain may also be considered for surgical excision and reconstruction. Skinning and simple vulvectomies are associated with recurrence rates as high as 50%. However, better sexual function and cosmetic results have been reported in the former, especially with concomitant split skin grafting. Cryosurgery has high recurrence rates, although short-term results are favorable. Laser therapy may produce better long-term results than other treatments. Carbon dioxide laser ablation to a depth of 1 to 2 mm is acceptable treatment for patients who have LSA of the penis or vulva that is refractory to other measures. The procedure may be performed using a general anesthetic. Healing is complete 6 weeks postoperatively, and patients were free of symptoms for up to 3 years.

Young women with recurrent labial and periclitoral adhesions respond to sharp dissection of the clitoral hood and separation of the adherent labia. Surgicel, oxidized regenerated cellulose gauze (Johnson & Johnson, Arlington, Tex), is sutured to the exposed clitoral hood and labial surfaces with Vicryl suture. Complete dissolution of the Surgicel occurs between postoperative days 4 and 6 and without recurrence of adhesions. This technique has prevented the recurrence during the interval when these surfaces are at highest risk of reagglutination.

ACITRETIN. Acitretin (20 to 30 mg/day for 16 weeks) is effective in treating women with severe LSA of the vulva.

PITYRIASIS LICHENOIDES

Pityriasis lichenoides (PL) is a rare disease with two variants: acute (pityriasis lichenoides et varioliformis acuta [PLEVA] or Mucha-Habermann disease) and chronic (pityriasis lichenoides chronica [PLC]) (Table 8-10). The terms acute and chronic refer to the characteristics of the individual lesions and not to the course of the disease. A history of infection or drug intake preceded the skin manifestations in 30% and 11.2% of patients with PLC and PLEVA, respectively. The disease begins most commonly during winter (35%) or fall (30%). PLC and PLEVA are interrelated processes within the larger group of T-cell lymphoproliferative disorders. Most cases occur during the first 3 decades of the patient's life. The diseases are more common in males. Evidence suggests that PLEVA is a hypersensitivity reaction to an infectious agent. The prognosis for both forms is good. Pityriasis lichenoides chronica, PLEVA, and lymphomatoid papulosis share several clinical and immunohistologic features, suggesting that these disorders are interrelated and part of a spectrum of clonal-T-cell cutaneous lymphoproliferative disorders. An abnormal immune response to an antigenic trigger may be the inciting event. The histology of these entities is distinctive. PL in children is more likely to run an unremitting course, with greater lesional distribution, more dyspigmentation, and a poorer response to conventional treatment modalities. *PMID: 17854375*

PLEVA

Mucha-Habermann disease, or PLEVA, is usually a benign, self-limited papulosquamous disorder. PLEVA is a clonal T-cell-mediated lymphoproliferative disorder. PLEVA has been documented in all age groups, with most cases occurring in the second and third decades. PLEVA begins insidiously, with few symptoms other than mild itching or a low-grade fever. Crops of round or oval, reddish brown papules, usually 2 to 10 mm in diameter, appear either singly or in clusters. They can occur anywhere, but they typically appear on the trunk, thighs, and upper arms (Figure 8-72). The face, scalp, palms, and soles are involved in approximately 10% of cases.

The papules may develop a violaceous center and a surrounding rim of erythema. There may be micaceous scale. Lesions can become vesicular or pustular and then undergo hemorrhagic necrosis, usually within 2 to 5 weeks,

Table 8-10 Clinical Features and Management of Pityriasis Lichenoides Variants

Variant and % of cases	Clinical presentation	Median age of onset	Duration	Histopathology	Treatment	Comments
PLEVA 57.3%	Acute-to-subacute eruption of multiple, small, red papules that rapidly develop into polymorphic lesions (vesicles, pustules, ulcers) with periods of varying remission	60 months Peaks at 2-3 years (24.8%) and 5-7 years (32%)	Median duration: 18 months (range: 4-108 months)	Dermal-dense, wedge-shaped, mostly CD8+ T-cell infiltrate, with epidermal spongiosis, parakeratosis, necrosis, and ulceration	Erythromycin, azithromycin, phototherapy, topical or systemic corticosteroids, methotrexate, dapsone, cyclosporine, acitretin	Sequelae of hyper/hypopigmented and poxlike scars; rule out diagnosis of lymphomatoid papulosis; generally has good prognosis
PLC 37%	Gradually developing, very small, red-to-brown, flattened macules and papules with centrally adherent, micalike, shiny scales	72 months Peaks at 2-3 years (24.8%) and 5-7 years (32%)	Median duration: 20 months (range: 3-132 months)	Superficial, dermal, mostly CD4+ T-cell, bandlike infiltrate, and slight epidermal parakeratotic scale	Phototherapy, erythromycin, azithromycin, topical corticosteroids, antihistamines, methotrexate, acitretin, cyclosporine, calciferol, bromelain	May waver for years with a relapsing course; can progress to PLEVA
FUMHD Very rare	Sudden, dramatic, widespread eruption of purpuric-black ulceronecrotic plaques with systemic signs and symptoms	No data	No data	Intense inflammatory infiltrate and marked ulceration and eukocytoclastic vasculitis	Systemic corticosteroids, methotrexate, IVIg, oral antimicrobials, PUVA, DDS, consider biologics	Carries a potential lethality of up to 25%; dermatologic emergency

DDS, 4-diaminodiphenylsulfone (dapsone); *FUMHD,* febrile ulceronecrotic Mucha-Habermann disease; *IVIg,* intravenous immunoglobulin; *PLC,* pityriasis lichenoides chronica; *PLEVA,* pityriasis lichenoides et varioliformis acuta; *PUVA,* psoralen plus UVA.
Adapted from Pityriasis lichenoides: pathophysiology, classification, and treatment, *Am J Clin Dermatol* 8(1):29-36, 2007 (review). *PMID: 17298104*; and Pityriasis lichenoides in childhood: a retrospective review of 124 patients, *J Am Acad Dermatol* 56(2):205-210, 2007 (Epub 10/13/2006). *PMID: 17097385.*

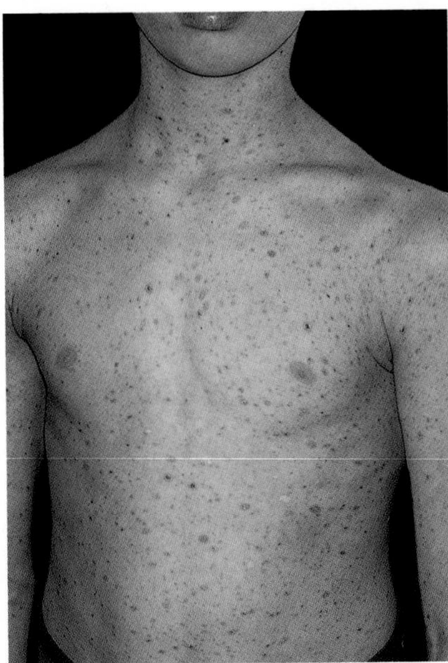

Figure 8-72 Pityriasis lichenoides et varioliformis acuta (PLEVA). A florid generalized eruption.

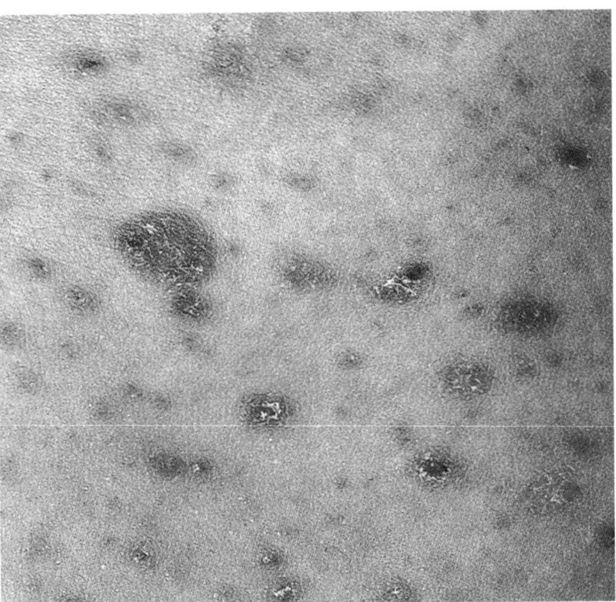

Figure 8-73 PLEVA. Scattered, discrete polymorphic red-brown papules, pustules, and erosions.

often leaving a postinflammatory hyperpigmentation and sometimes scars (Figure 8-73). Acute exacerbations are common and the disease may wax and wane for months or years. High fever is a rare complication, but it may be associated with an ulceronecrotic type of lesion. Complications include a self-limited arthritis and superinfection of the skin lesions. The mean duration of disease varies from 1.6 to 18 months. A rare, serious variant in children is an ulceronecrotic form (febrile ulceronecrotic Mucha-Habermann disease), which presents with large, coalescing, ulceronecrotic nodules and plaques with associated fever and other constitutional symptoms. The differential diagnosis includes varicella, arthropod bites, impetigo, pityriasis rosea, scabies, lymphomatoid papulosis, and other viral exanthems.

PITYRIASIS LICHENOIDES CHRONICA

Pityriasis lichenoides chronica (Juliusberg type) is a generalized eruption consisting of brownish papules with fine, micalike, adherent scale that becomes more evident when scratched. They can start de novo or can evolve from PLEVA lesions. PLEVA and PLC lesions can coexist. Lesions of PLC flatten with time and resolve with hypo- or hyperpigmentation without scarring. Each lesion can last weeks to months before resolving.

In a pediatric case series, the mean duration of disease ranges from 7.5 to 20 months. The disease may persist for years. Systemic symptoms are rare. The scale is less conspicuous than in psoriasis. Lesions clear without scarring and show only transient skin discoloration. The distribution is similar to that seen in PLEVA. The differential diagnosis includes guttate psoriasis, pityriasis rosea, postinflammatory hypopigmentation, secondary syphilis, and tinea corporis.

HISTOLOGY

PLEVA shows a perivascular and diffuse lymphocytic and histocytic infiltration at the dermo-epidermal junction. There is erythrocyte extravasation, epidermal necrosis, edema, and basal vacuolar degeneration. Similar changes are seen in PLC, but to a lesser extent.

TREATMENT

Erythromycin produced a remission in 73% of the cases. *PMID: 3722512* It frequently took as long as 2 months before a significant therapeutic effect was noted. Clearing with oral erythromycin was reported in most cases at dosages of 30 to 50 mg/kg/day. Erythromycin was tapered over several months, depending on the response. The disease usually recurred if erythromycin was tapered too rapidly. A case report demonstrated that azithromycin 500 mg on day 1 and 250 mg on days 2 through 5, taken on the first and third weeks of the month, was effective for an adult. After 3 weeks and two courses of azithromycin, the patient was clear of all lesions and remained clear for 6 months. A 5-year-old child was treated with the same dosage and cleared in 2 months after four courses of azithromycin. *PMID: 18280363* Psoralen ultraviolet light A (PUVA), ultraviolet light B (UVB) phototherapy, narrow-band UVB, tetracycline, gold, methotrexate, oral corticosteroids, and dapsone have all been used with some success. Bromelain, a crude aqueous extract of the stems and immature fruit of pineapple, was used to treat pityriasis lichenoides chronica. The following dose was prescribed: 40 mg 3 times a day for 1 month, 40 mg twice a day for 1 month, and 40 mg/day for 1 month. All patients showed complete recovery. Two patients experienced relapse 5 to 6 months after suspension of therapy but responded to another brief cycle of therapy. *PMID: 17671882*

GROVER'S DISEASE

Grover's disease (GD), also known as transient acantholytic dermatosis, is most common in men over 60 years of age. There is a significant association with atopy and dry skin, with peak incidence in winter. (Figure 8-74 and 8-75)

CLINICAL MANIFESTATIONS. There are pruritic papules and vesicles on the chest, back, and thighs. Itching may be transient and minimal. Persistent truncal, asymptomatic papules often localized to the submammary area, in men simulating folliculitis is a very common presentation. Lesions last days to weeks, and sometimes several years. Lesions are initiated or exacerbated by sunlight. The diagnosis is confirmed by finding focal acantholysis on skin biopsy.

TREATMENT. The disease is often transient and resolves without treatment. Avoid strenuous exercise and excessive exposure to sunlight. Group II-V topical steroids may be effective in controlling itch but may not clear the eruption. Soothing baths with emollient bath oils or colloidal oatmeal decrease itching and hydrate the skin. Phototherapy with ultraviolet B radiation may help. A one-month course of isotretinoin or acitretin may be effective.

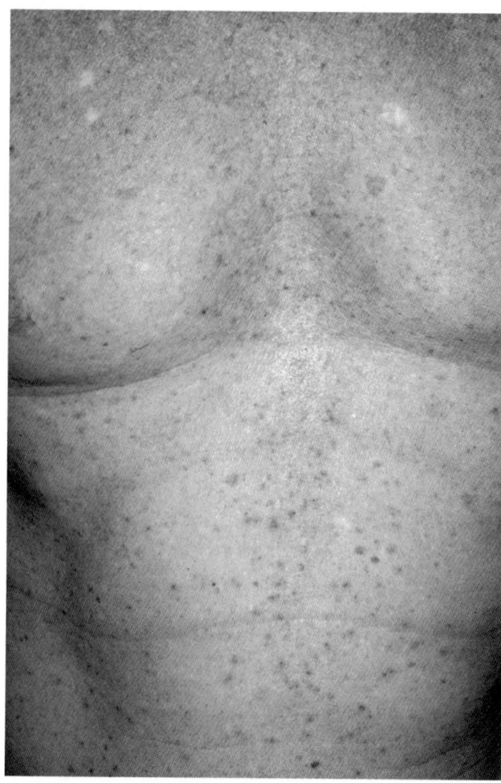

Figure 8-74 Grover's disease. Lesions may spread to involve the neck, shoulders, arms, legs, the upper part of the back, and the lower part of the rib cage.

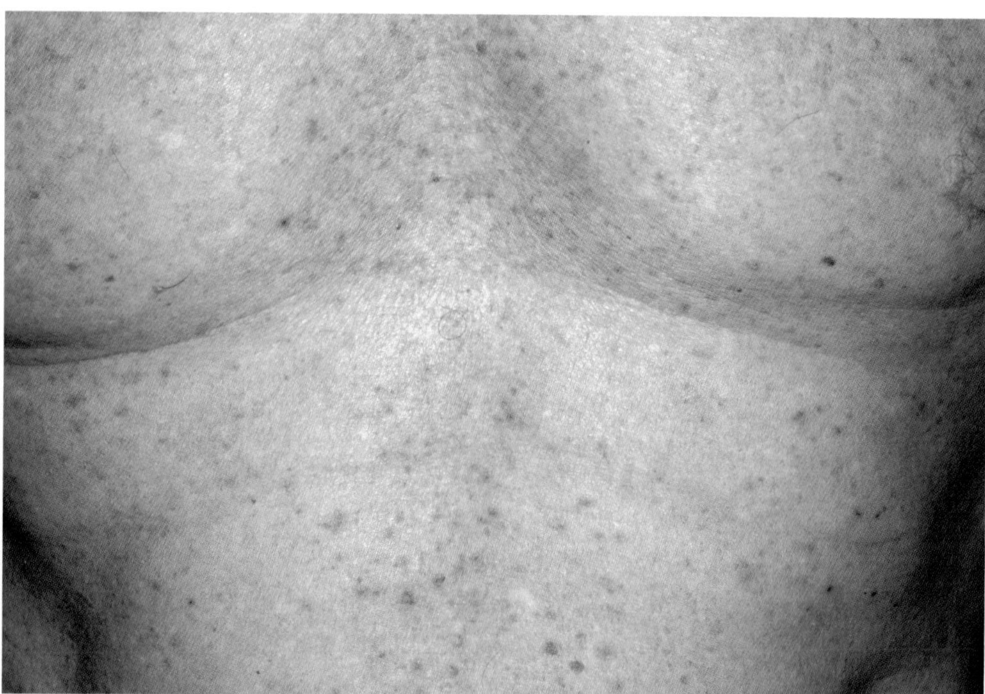

Figure 8-75 Grover's disease. Eruption begins on the anterior part of the chest as red to reddish-brown keratotic papules that remain discrete.

Chapter | 9 |

Bacterial Infections

CHAPTER CONTENTS

SKIN INFECTIONS

The two gram-positive cocci *Staphylococcus aureus* and group A beta-hemolytic streptococci account for the majority of skin and soft tissue infections. *S. aureus* invades skin and causes impetigo, folliculitis, cellulitis, and furuncles. Elaboration of toxins by *S. aureus* causes the lesions of bullous impetigo and staphylococcal scalded skin syndrome. The streptococci are secondary invaders of traumatic skin lesions and cause impetigo, erysipelas, cellulitis, and lymphangitis.

Impetigo

Impetigo is a common, contagious, superficial skin infection that is produced by streptococci, staphylococci, or a combination of both bacteria. There are two different clinical presentations: bullous impetigo and nonbullous impetigo. Both begin as vesicles with a very thin, fragile roof consisting only of stratum corneum. Bullous impetigo is primarily a staphylococcal disease. Nonbullous impetigo was once thought to be primarily a streptococcal disease, but staphylococci are isolated from the majority of lesions in both bullous and nonbullous impetigo. *S. aureus* is now known to be the primary pathogen in both bullous and nonbullous impetigo.

Children in close physical contact with each other have a higher rate of infection than do adults. Symptoms of itching and soreness are mild; systemic symptoms are infrequent. Impetigo may occur after a minor skin injury such as an insect bite, but it most frequently develops on apparently unimpaired skin. The disease is self-limiting, but when untreated it may last for weeks or months. Poststreptococcal glomerulonephritis may follow impetigo. Rheumatic fever has not been reported as a complication of impetigo.

BULLOUS IMPETIGO

Bullous impetigo (staphylococcal impetigo) is caused by an epidermolytic toxin produced at the site of infection and usually is not secondarily contaminated by streptococci. The toxin causes intraepidermal cleavage below or within the stratum granulosum.

CLINICAL MANIFESTATIONS. Bullous impetigo is most common in infants and children but may occur in adults. It typically occurs on the face, but it may infect any body surface. There may be a few lesions localized in one area, or the lesions may be so numerous and widely scattered that they resemble poison ivy. One or more vesicles enlarge rapidly to form bullae in which the contents turn from clear to cloudy. The center of the thin-roofed bulla collapses, but the peripheral area may retain fluid for many days in an inner tube–shaped rim. A thin, flat, honey-colored, "varnishlike" crust may appear in the center and, if removed, discloses a bright red, inflamed, moist base that oozes serum. The center may dry without forming a crust, leaving a red base with a rim of scale. In most cases, a tinea-like scaling border replaces the fluid-filled rim as the round lesions enlarge and become contiguous with the others (Figures 9-1 to 9-5). The border dries and forms a crust. The lesions have little or no surrounding erythema. In some untreated cases, lesions may extend radially and retain a narrow, bullous, inner tube rim. These individual lesions reach 2 to 8 cm and then cease to enlarge, but they may remain for months (Figure 9-5). Thick crust accumulates in these longer lasting lesions. Lesions heal with hyperpigmentation in black patients. Regional lymphadenitis is uncommon with pure staphylococcal impetigo. There is some evidence that the responsible staphylococci colonize in the nose and then spread to normal skin before infection.

Serious secondary infections (e.g., osteomyelitis, septic arthritis, and pneumonia) may follow seemingly innocuous superficial infections in infants.

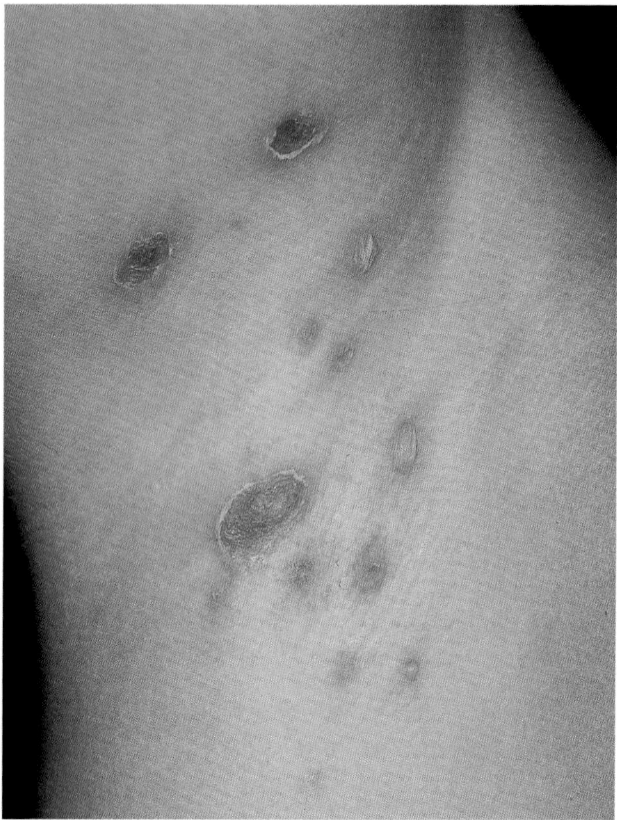

Figure 9-1 Lesions are present in all stages of development. Bullae rupture, exposing a lesion with an eroded surface and a peripheral scale.

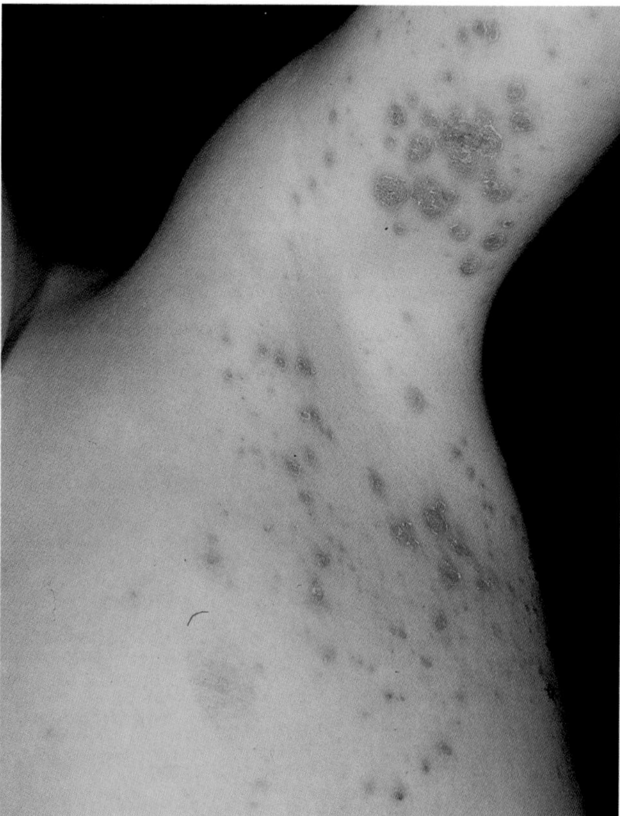

Figure 9-2 The lesions initially were present on the arm and autoinoculated the chest.

BULLOUS IMPETIGO

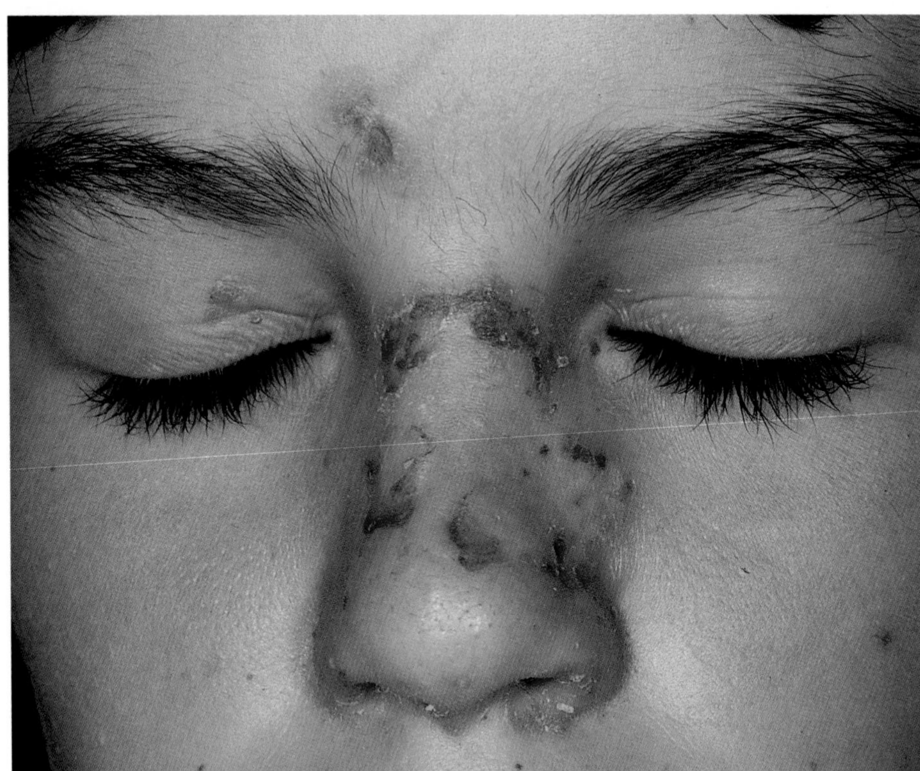

Figure 9-3 Bullae have collapsed and disappeared. The lesion is in the process of peripheral extension. Note involvement of both nares.

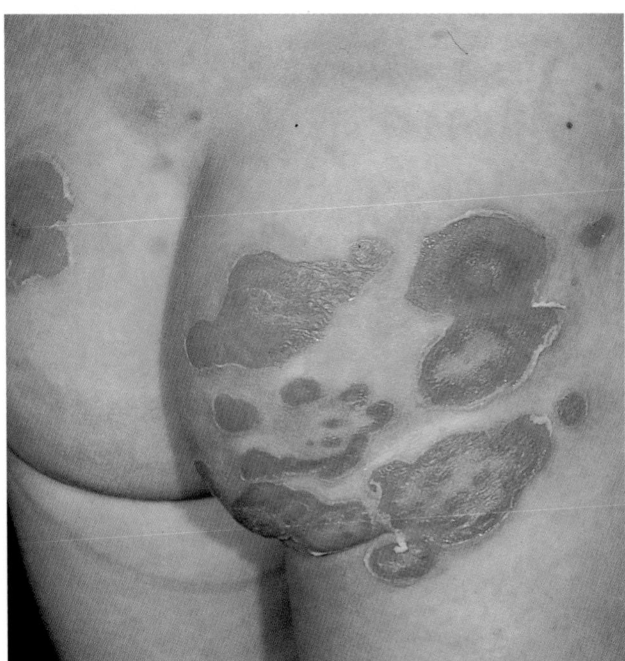

Figure 9-4 Huge lesions with a glistening, eroded base and a collarette of moist scale.

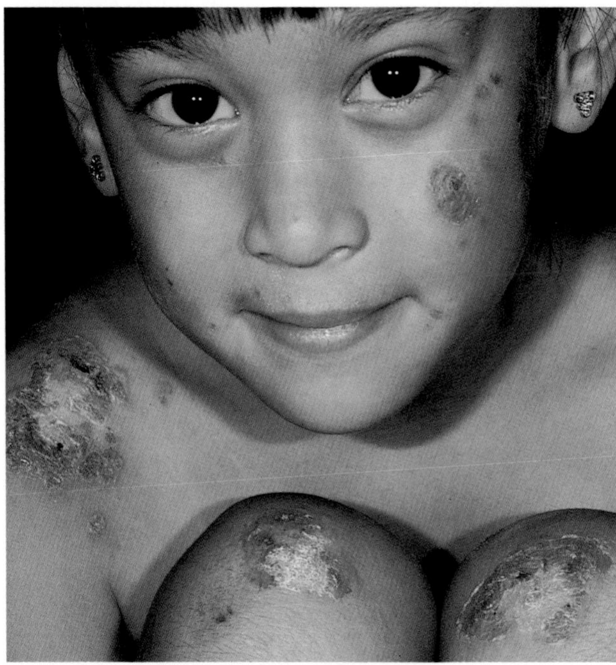

Figure 9-5 A bullous rim extended slowly for weeks. No topical or oral treatment had been attempted.

NONBULLOUS IMPETIGO

Nonbullous impetigo originates as a small vesicle or pustule that ruptures to expose a red, moist base. A honey-yellow to white-brown, firmly adherent crust accumulates as the lesion extends radially (Figures 9-6 to 9-10). There is little surrounding erythema. Satellite lesions appear beyond the periphery. The lesions are generally asymptomatic. The skin around the nose and mouth and the limbs are the sites most commonly affected. The palms and soles are not affected. Untreated cases last for weeks and may extend in a continuous manner to involve a wide area (see Figure 9-7). Most lesions heal without scarring. The sequence of events leading to nonbullous impetigo is exposure to the infectious agent, carriage on exposed normal skin, and finally skin infection after a minor trauma that is aggravated by scratching. The infecting strain has been found on normal skin surfaces 2 or more weeks before the appearance of lesions.

Intact skin is resistant to colonization or infection with group A beta-hemolytic streptococci, but skin injury by insect bites, abrasions, lacerations, and burns allows the streptococci to invade. A pure culture of group A beta-hemolytic streptococci may sometimes be isolated from early lesions, but most lesions promptly become contaminated with staphylococci. Regional lymphadenopathy is common. The reservoirs for streptococcus infection include the unimpaired normal skin or the lesions of other individuals rather than the respiratory tract. Children ages 2 to 5 years commonly have streptococcal impetigo. Warm, moist climates and poor hygiene are predisposing factors. The antistreptolysin O (ASO) titer does not increase to a significant level following impetigo. Antideoxyribonuclease B (anti-DNase B) increases to high levels and is a much more sensitive indicator of streptococcal impetigo.

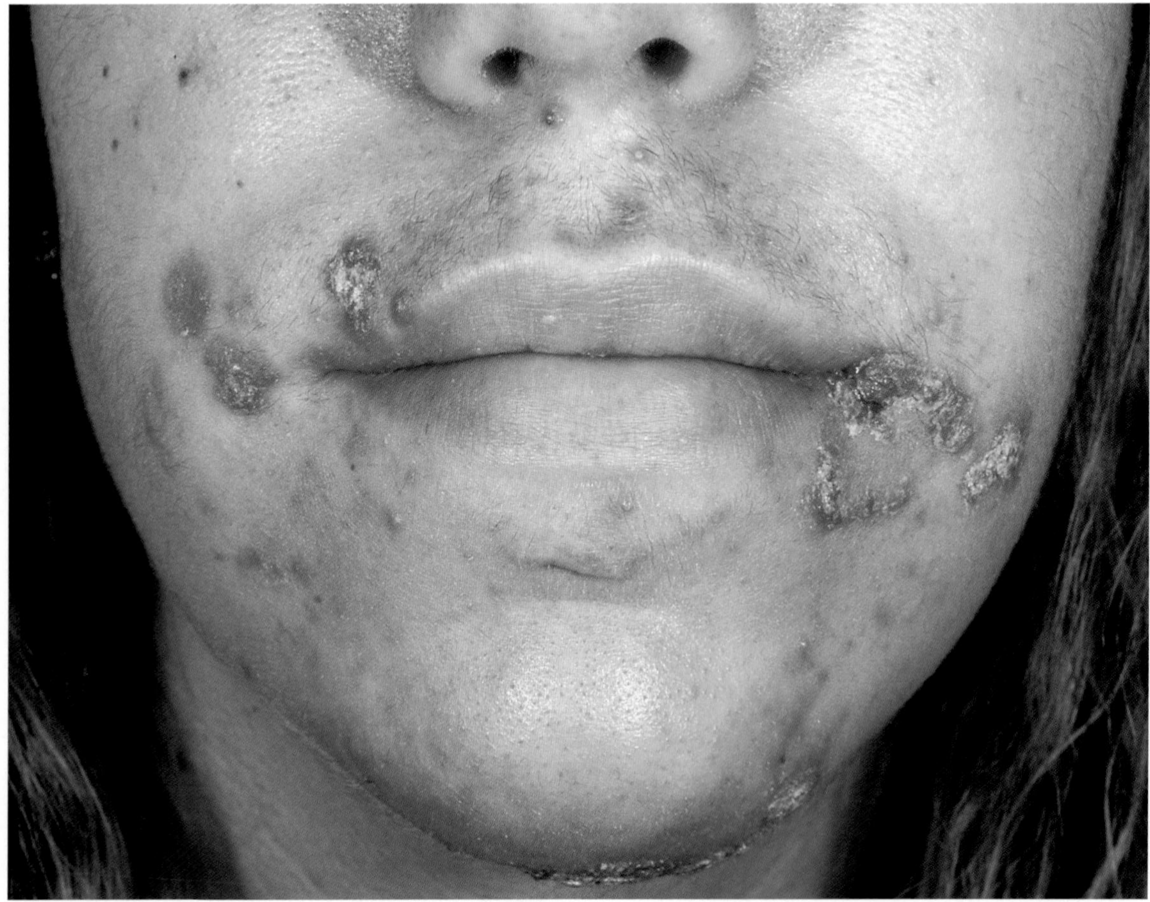

Figure 9-6 Nonbullous impetigo. Lesions begin as vesicles and then rupture, releasing serum, which dries and forms a honey-colored crust. Multiple lesions occur at the same site.

NONBULLOUS IMPETIGO

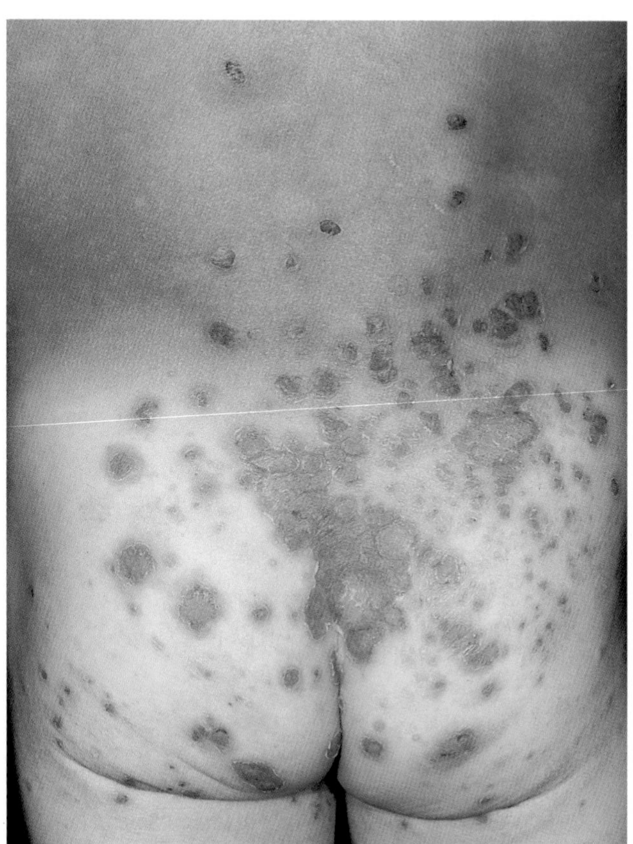

Figure 9-7 Widespread dissemination followed 3 weeks of treatment with a group IV topical steroid.

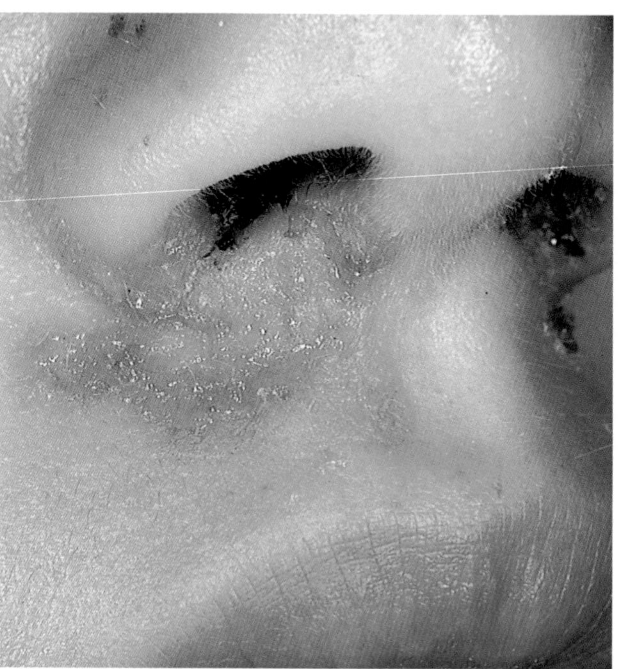

Figure 9-8 Serum and crust about the nostrils is a common presentation for impetigo.

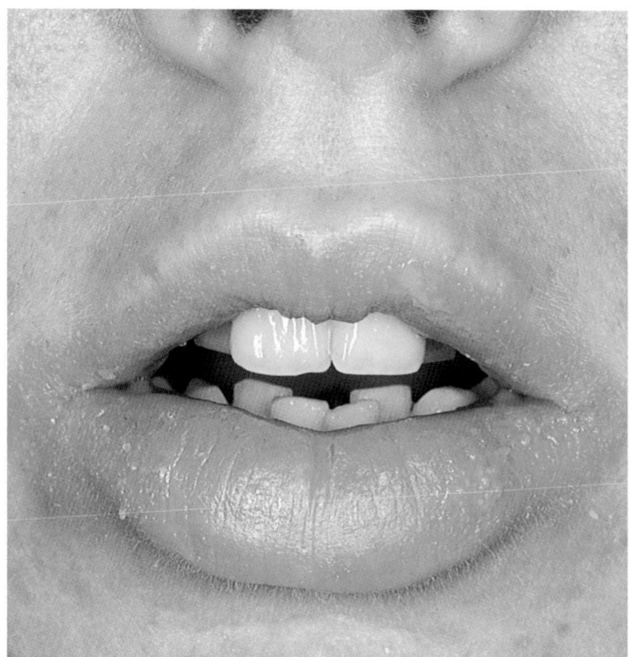

Figure 9-9 Serum and crust at the angle of the mouth is a common presentation for impetigo.

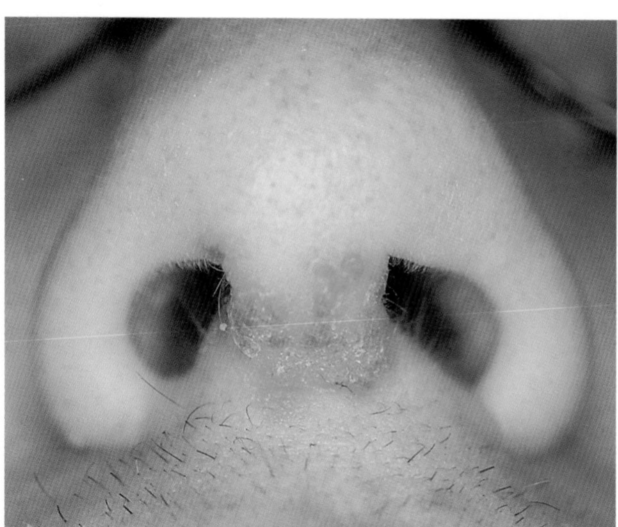

Figure 9-10 This crusted lesion was misinterpreted as recurrent herpes.

ACUTE NEPHRITIS

Acute nephritis tends to occur when many individuals in a family have impetigo.

Poststreptococcal glomerulonephritis (PSGN) usually develops 1 to 3 weeks following acute infection with specific nephritogenic strains of group A beta-hemolytic streptococcus. The overall incidence of acute nephritis with impetigo varies between 2% and 5%, but in the presence of a nephritogenic strain of streptococcus the rate varies between 10% and 25%.

PSGN occurs at any age but usually develops in children. Outbreaks in children aged 6 to 10 years are common. Children younger than 1½ years of age are rarely affected by nephritis following impetigo. Asymptomatic episodes of PSGN exceed symptomatic episodes by a ratio of 4:1.

LABORATORY FINDINGS. Diagnosis is based on history and clinical appearance. Culture is not routinely performed. Gram-stained smears of vesicles show gram-positive cocci. Culture of exudate beneath an unroofed crust reveals group A streptococci, *S. aureus,* or a mixture of streptococci and *S. aureus*. Evidence of previous streptococcal skin infection in patients with acute glomerulonephritis is accomplished by obtaining antideoxyribonuclease B (anti-DNase B) and antihyaluronidase (AH) titers. More than 90% of patients with impetigo-associated acute post-streptococcal glomerulonephritis have increased anti-DNase B titers.

The antistreptolysin O titer after streptococcal impetigo is low or absent. Total serum complement activity is low during the initial stages of acute nephritis. The C3 level parallels the total serum complement level. The sedimentation rate parallels the activity of the disease. The level of C-reactive protein is usually normal. Cultures of the pharynx and any skin lesion should be made, and the serotype of the group A streptococcus that is responsible should be determined by typing with M-group and T-type antisera. M-T serotypes associated with acute nephritis are 49, 55, 57, and 60.

Acute nephritis heals without therapeutic intervention. Symptoms and signs such as hypertension should be managed as they occur.

PREVENTION OF IMPETIGO

Mupirocin (Bactroban) or triple antibiotic ointment, containing bacitracin, Polysporin, and neomycin, applied three times daily to sites of minor skin trauma (e.g., mosquito bites and abrasions) can be efficacious as a preventative treatment.

Table 9-1 Antimicrobial Therapy for Impetigo and for Skin and Soft Tissue Infections

	DOSAGE		
Antibiotic therapy, by disease	**Adults**	**Children***	**Comment**
Impetigo†			
Dicloxacillin	250 mg 4 times per day PO	12 mg/kg/day in 4 divided doses PO	—
Cephalexin	250 mg 4 times per day PO	25 mg/kg/day in 4 divided doses PO	—
Erythromycin	250 mg 4 times per day PO‡	40 mg/kg/day in 4 divided doses PO	Some strains of *S. aureus* and *S. pyogenes* may be resistant
Clindamycin	300-400 mg 3 times per day PO	10-20 mg/kg/day in 3 divided doses PO	—
Amoxicillin/ clavulanate	875/125 mg 2 times per day PO	25 mg/kg/day of amoxicillin component in 2 divided doses PO	—
Mupirocin ointment	Apply to lesions 3 times per day	Apply to lesions 3 times per day	For patients with limited number of lesions
Retapamulin ointment	Apply to lesions 2 times per day for 5 days	Apply to lesions 2 times per day for 5 days	For patients with limited number of lesions For up to 2% total body surface area in pediatric patients aged 9 months or older

Adapted from Practice guidelines for the diagnosis and management of skin and soft-tissue infections, *Clin Infect Dis* 41:1373-1406, 2005. *PMID: 16231249*

*Larger doses listed are not appropriate for neonates.

†Infection caused by *Staphylococcus* and *Streptococcus* species. Duration of therapy is 7 days, depending on the clinical response.

‡Adult dosage of erythromycin ethylsuccinate is 400 mg four times per day PO.

IV, Intravenously; *MRSA,* methicillin-resistant *S. aureus; PO,* orally; *TMP-SMZ,* trimethoprim-sulfamethoxazole.

RECURRENT IMPETIGO

Patients with recurrent impetigo should be evaluated for carriage of *S. aureus*. The nares are the most common sites of carriage, but the perineum, axillae, and toe webs may also be colonized. Mupirocin ointment or cream (Bactroban) applied to the nares twice each day for 5 days significantly reduces *S. aureus* carriage in the nose and hands at 3 days and in the nasal carriage for as long as 1 year.

TREATMENT OF IMPETIGO

Impetigo may resolve spontaneously or become chronic and widespread. Studies show that 2% mupirocin ointment is as safe and effective as oral erythromycin in the treatment of patients with impetigo. Retapamulin ointment is also approved for treating impetigo. Local treatment does not treat lesions that evolve in other areas. Infected children should be briefly isolated until treatment has begun. Recommended treatment is found in Table 9-1.

Table 9-1 Antimicrobial Therapy for Impetigo and for Skin and Soft Tissue Infections—cont'd

Antibiotic therapy, by disease	DOSAGE Adults	Children*	Comment
Skin and soft tissue infection: Abscesses, cellulitis, erysipelas, furuncles, carbuncles (methicillin-susceptible *S. aureus*)			
Nafcillin or oxacillin	1-2 gm every 4 hr IV	100-150 mg/kg/day in 4 divided doses PO	Parental drug of choice; inactive against MRSA
Cefazolin	1 gm every 8 hr IV	50 mg/kg/day in 3 divided doses PO	For penicillin-allergic patients, except those with immediate hypersensitivity reactions
Clindamycin	600 mg/kg every 8 hr IV or 300-450 mg 3 times per day PO	25-40 mg/kg/day in 3 divided doses IV or 10-20 mg/kg/day in 3 divided doses PO	Bacteriostatic; potential of cross-resistance and emergence of resistance in erythromycin-resistant strains; inducible resistance in MRSA
Dicloxacillin	500 mg 4 times per day PO	25 mg/kg/day in 4 divided doses PO	Oral agent of choice for methicillin-susceptible strains
Cephalexin	500 mg 4 times per day PO	25 mg/kg/day in 4 divided doses PO	For penicillin-allergic patients, except those with immediate hypersensitivity reactions
Doxycycline, minocycline	100 mg 2 times per day PO	Not recommended for persons aged <8 years	Bacteriostatic; limited recent clinical experience
TMP-SMZ	1 or 2 double-strength tablets 2 times per day PO	8-12 mg/kg (based on trimethoprim component) in either 4 divided doses IV or 2 divided doses PO	Bactericidal; efficacy poorly documented
Skin and soft tissue infection: Abscesses, cellulitis, erysipelas, furuncles, carbuncles (methicillin-resistant *S. aureus*)			
Vancomycin	30 mg/kg/day in 2 divided doses IV	40 mg/kg/day in 4 divided doses IV	For penicillin-allergic patients; parenteral drug of choice for treatment of infections caused by MRSA
Linezolid	600 mg every 12 hr IV or 600 mg 2 times per day PO	10 mg/kg every 12 hr IV or PO	Bacteriostatic; limited clinical experience; no cross-resistance with other antibiotic classes; expensive; may eventually replace other second-line agents as a preferred agent for oral therapy of MRSA infections
Clindamycin	600 mg/kg every 8 hr IV or 300-450 mg 3 times per day PO	25-40 mg/kg/day in 3 divided doses IV or 10-20 mg/kg/day in 3 divided doses PO	Bacteriostatic; potential of cross-resistance and emergence of resistance in erythromycin-resistant strains; inducible resistance in MRSA
Daptomycin	4 mg/kg every 24 hr IV	Not applicable	Bactericidal; possible myopathy
Doxycycline, minocycline	100 mg 2 times per day PO	Not recommended for persons aged <8 years	Bacteriostatic, limited recent clinical experience
TMP-SMZ	1 or 2 double-strength tablets 2 times per day PO	8-12 mg/kg/day (based on trimethoprim component) in either 4 divided doses IV or 2 divided doses PO	Bactericidal; limited published efficacy data

ORAL ANTIBIOTICS. Some cases of impetigo have a mixed infection of staphylococci and streptococci. Oral antibiotics should be considered for patients with impetigo who have extensive disease or systemic symptoms. A 5- to 10-day course of oral antibiotics such as dicloxacillin, amoxicillin/clavulanate, cephalosporins, (e.g., cephalexin, cefadroxil) induces rapid healing and is effective for the treatment of impetigo; erythromycin is less effective (see Table 9-1). Oral penicillin V, amoxicillin, topical bacitracin, and neomycin are not recommended for the treatment of impetigo. Topical disinfectants such as hydrogen peroxide should not be used.

MUPIROCIN (BACTROBAN). Mupirocin ointment or cream was the first topical antibiotic approved for the treatment of impetigo. It is active against staphylococci (including methicillin-resistant strains) and streptococci. The drug is not active against Enterobacteriaceae, *Pseudomonas aeruginosa*, or fungi. It is as effective as oral antibiotics and is associated with fewer adverse effects. In superficial skin infections that are not widespread, mupirocin ointment offers several advantages. It is highly active against the most frequent skin pathogens, even those resistant to other antibiotics, and the topical route of administration allows delivery of high drug concentrations to the site of infection. Mupirocin is applied three times a day until all lesions have cleared. If topical treatment is elected, then it might be worthwhile to wash the involved areas once or twice a day with an antibacterial soap such as Hibiclens or Betadine. Washing the entire body with these soaps may prevent recurrence at distant sites. Crusts should be removed because they block the penetration of antibacterial creams. To facilitate removal, soften crusts by soaking with a wet cloth compress.

RETAPAMULIN (ALTABAX). Topical retapamulin (Altabax) is the first pleuromutilin antibacterial approved for the treatment of uncomplicated superficial skin infections caused by *S. aureus* (excluding methicillin-resistant *S. aureus* [MRSA]) and *Streptococcus pyogenes* in patients older than age 9 months. Retapamulin 1% ointment twice daily for 5 days is effective for impetigo but the efficacy is reduced in patients with MRSA infections or superficial abscesses.

Cellulitis and erysipelas

Cellulitis and erysipelas are skin infections characterized by erythema, edema, and pain. In most instances there is fever and leukocytosis. Both may be accompanied by lymphangitis and lymphadenitis. Pathogens enter at sites of local trauma or abrasions and at psoriatic, eczematous, or tinea lesions. Erysipelas involves the superficial layers of the skin and cutaneous lymphatics; cellulitis extends into the subcutaneous tissues.

Cellulitis is an infection of the dermis and subcutaneous tissue that is usually caused by a group A streptococcus, *S. aureus* in adults and *Haemophilus influenzae* type B in children younger than 3 years of age. Cellulitis is sometimes caused by other organisms. Cellulitis typically occurs near surgical wounds or a cutaneous ulcer or, like erysipelas, may develop in apparently normal skin. There are many anatomic variants of cellulitis (Table 9-2). There is no clear distinction between infected and uninfected skin. Recurrent episodes of cellulitis occur with local anatomic abnormalities that compromise the venous or lymphatic circulation. The lymphatic system can be compromised by a previous episode of cellulitis, surgery with lymph node resection, and radiation therapy.

Erysipelas is an acute, inflammatory form of cellulitis that differs from other types of cellulitis in that lymphatic involvement ("streaking") is prominent. The area of inflammation is raised above the surrounding skin, and there is a distinct demarcation between involved and normal skin. The lower legs, face, and ears are most frequently involved. The differential diagnosis of cellulitis is shown in Table 9-3.

DIAGNOSIS OF CELLULITIS

Recognizing the distinctive clinical features (erythema, warmth, edema, and pain) is the most reliable way of making an early diagnosis. Isolation of the etiologic agent is difficult and is usually not attempted. Fever, mild leukocytosis with a left shift, and a mildly increased sedimentation rate may be present. Patients with cellulitis of the leg often have a preexisting lesion, such as an ulcer or erosion that acts as a portal of entry for the infecting organism.

CELLULITIS VS. DEEP VEIN THROMBOSIS. Differentiating cellulitis from deep vein thrombosis (DVT) is a common clinical dilemma. Patients with cellulitis are more likely to have constitutional symptoms, rigors, and a history of diabetes and/or distinct margins of erythema. Diabetic patients are at increased risk for skin infections. Diabetes is not a known risk factor for DVT. Patients with DVT are more likely to have had recent surgery and a history of varicose veins and/or peripheral vascular disease. Patients with a diagnosis of DVT are more likely to have an elevated white blood cell (WBC) count. Aspiration and culture of fluid from the leading edge of the affected specimen is of limited value. Cellulitis is usually diagnosed clinically. Contrast venography is the accepted "gold standard" for the objective diagnosis of DVT. Venous duplex

Table 9-2 Specific Anatomic Variants of Cellulitis and Causes of Predisposition to the Condition

Anatomic variant or cause of predisposition	Location	Likely bacterial causes
Periorbital cellulitis	Periorbital	*Staphylococcus aureus,* pneumococcus, group A streptococcus
Buccal cellulitis	Cheek	*Haemophilus influenzae*
Cellulitis complicating body piercing	Ear, nose, umbilicus	*S. aureus,* group A streptococcus
Mastectomy (with axillary-node dissection) for breast cancer	Ipsilateral arm	Non–group A hemolytic streptococcus
Lumpectomy (with limited axillary-node dissection, breast radiotherapy)	Ipsilateral breast	Non–group A hemolytic streptococcus
Harvest of saphenous vein for coronary-artery bypass	Ipsilateral leg	Group A or non–group A hemolytic streptococcus
Liposuction	Thigh, abdominal wall	Group A streptococcus, peptostreptococcus
Postoperative (very early) wound infection	Abdomen, chest, hip	Group A streptococcus
Injection drug use ("skin popping")	Extremities, neck	*S. aureus;* streptococci (groups A, C, F, G)*
Perianal cellulitis	Perineum	Group A streptococcus
Crepitant cellulitis	Trunk, extremities	
Gangrenous cellulitis	Trunk, extremities	
Erythema migrans (bright red, circular lesion at initial sites; secondary annular lesions may develop elsewhere several days later because of hematogenous spread)	Extremities, trunk	*Borrelia burgdorferi* (agent of Lyme disease)

From *New Engl J Med* 350(9):904-912, 2004. *PMID: 14985488*

*Other bacteria to consider on the basis of isolation from skin or abscesses in this setting include *Enterococcus faecalis, viridans*-group streptococci, coagulase-negative staphylococci, anaerobes (including *Bacteroides* and *Clostridium* species), and *Enterobacteriaceae.*

ultrasonography is now the first-line diagnostic test for DVT because it does not use contrast media. *PMID: 18159459*

CULTURES. In adults with no underlying disease, yields of cultures of aspirate specimens, biopsy specimens, and blood are low. In adults with underlying diseases (e.g., diabetes mellitus, hematologic malignancies, intravenous drug abuse, human immunodeficiency virus infection, chemotherapy) results of culture are more productive. Cellulitis in these patients is often caused by organisms other than *S. aureus* or group A streptococcus, such as *Acinetobacter, Clostridium septicum, Enterobacter, Escherichia coli, H. influenzae, Pasteurella multocida, Proteus mirabilis, P. aeruginosa,* and group B streptococci. Cultures of entry sites, aspirate specimens, biopsy specimens, and blood facilitate the selection of the appropriate antibiotic for these patients.

Optimal methods for etiologic diagnosis in adults have not been delineated. Culture of the lesion is a more predictable source of information than more invasive procedures. Leading-edge and midpoint aspirates after saline injection and blood cultures are of little value in normal hosts. A higher concentration of bacteria may be found at the point of maximal inflammation. Needle aspiration from the point of maximal inflammation yielded a 45% positive culture rate, compared with a 5% rate from leading-edge cultures. Needle aspiration is performed by piercing the skin with a 20-gauge needle mounted on a tuberculin syringe. A 22-gauge needle is used for facial lesions. The needle is introduced into subcutaneous tissue. Suction is applied as the needle is withdrawn. Most clinicians do not culture, and proceed to treat with oral antibiotics.

Table 9-3 Cellulitis: Differential Diagnosis

Disease	Description
Anthrax (cutaneous)	Edema surrounding crusted lesion. Painless or itching. Animal contact.
Calciphylaxis (calcific uremic arteriolopathy)	Affects diabetic patients with end-stage renal disease and hyperparathyroidism who are receiving renal replacement therapy. Metastatic calcification leads to small vessel vasculopathy. Early stage: presents with nonulcerating plaques in the calves. Lesions eventually become necrotic and painful ulcers develop.
Carcinoma erysipelatoides	A form of metastatic carcinoma with lymphatic involvement. Seen on anterior chest wall in breast cancer and sites of distant metastasis. No fever, slow progression. If a suspected breast infection does not resolve with antibiotics, mammography and tissue biopsy are indicated.
Contact dermatitis (acute)	Lesion sharply demarcated and constricted to the area of exposure. Pruritus present, not in cellulitis. Topical steroids effective. Systemic corticosteroids are indicated for severe cases. Secondary infection may complicate dermatitis.
Deep venous thrombophlebitis	Unilateral leg edema, warmth, or erythema. Tenderness along involved veins. Can have low-grade fever, leukocytosis. Duplex ultrasonography diagnostic.
Eosinophilic cellulitis (Wells' syndrome)	Acute pruritic dermatitis. Hivelike lesions with central clearing. Lesions evolve over 2-3 days and resolve without scarring in 2-8 weeks. Disease recurs. Peripheral eosinophilia, during acute phase. Biopsy: eosinophils. Idiopathic or associated with myeloproliferative, immunologic, and infectious disorders and with medications. Responds to oral corticosteroids.
Erysipeloid (*Erysipelothrix rhusiopathiae*)	Acute bacterial infection (*Erysipelothrix rhusiopathiae*) of traumatized skin. Contact with infected meat or contact with infected animals or fish. Lesions affect hands; well-demarcated, bright red to purple plaques with a smooth, shiny surface.
Erythema migrans	Lyme disease rash that typically expands but clears in center. Often a single or multiple lesions occur that are round and red and expand to many centimeters but do not show central clearing.
Erythema nodosum	Most common panniculitis. Raised, painful, bilateral, tender lesions located over both shins. Lesions may coalesce and resemble cellulitis.
Factitial	Mechanical or chemical manipulation of skin can produce an area of erythema that resembles cellulitis.
Familial Hibernian fever	Irish ancestry; rare. Erysipelas-like lesion may occur anywhere on body; most common site is on a limb. Begins proximally and migrates distally during an attack. Lesion (about 15 cm in diameter) is well-demarcated, red, warm, and painful. Corticosteroids effective.
Familial Mediterranean fever	Autosomal recessive. Jews and Arabs from Mediterranean basin. Acute self-limited episodes of fever accompanied by peritonitis, pleuritis, pericarditis, or synovitis. Initial attack: childhood or early adolescence. Erysipelas-like erythema. Tender, red, well-demarcated, warm, swollen areas with a diameter of 10-15 cm. Occur below knee, on anterior leg or dorsum of foot (unilaterally or symmetrically). Erythema subsides in 24-48 hours as acute attack resolves. Recurs. Responds to colchicine.
Fixed drug eruption	A well-demarcated plaque that recurs at same site each time offending drug is taken. Itching or burning not seen in cellulitis. Most commonly affected areas are lips and genitalia.
Foreign-body granulomatous reactions (silicone injections, paraffin oils)	Material injected into skin can stimulate an overlying erythema.
Glucagonoma	Pancreatic tumor that is almost always malignant; presents with diabetes mellitus, diarrhea, and weight loss. Necrolytic migratory erythema is a rash that begins as an erythematous area and gradually spreads; after central crusting occurs, the lesions heal. Affects intertriginous, perioral, and perigenital areas.
Gouty arthritis (acute)	Joint inflamed with overlying erythema and warmth. May lead to tendonitis and bursitis. Chills, low-grade fever, elevated leukocyte count. Typically monoarticular, lower extremity, usually first metatarsophalangeal joint or knee.
Insect stings or bites and other envenomations	Swelling that can extend over a large area; peaks within 48 hours and lasts up to 7 days. No lymphangitis. Pruritus distinguishes this lesion from infectious cellulitis. Envenomations by marine animals cause a similar picture.
Leukemia/lymphoma	Lymphoma diagnosed after failure of antimicrobial therapy. Persisting fever or generalized lymphadenopathy may suggest the diagnosis.
Necrotizing fasciitis	A rapidly advancing erythema. Begins with fever and chills. Vesicles and bullae may form and drain fluid. Painless ulcers appear as the process spreads.

Table 9-3 Cellulitis: Differential Diagnosis—cont'd

Disease	Description
Panniculitis	Pancreatic disease, either inflammatory or neoplastic, may lead to panniculitis presenting as tender, red nodules located on pretibial regions, thighs, or buttocks. Lupus panniculitis occurs on face and upper extremities. α_1-Antitrypsin deficiency may present as cellulitis on trunk and proximal extremities, often precipitated by trauma. Panacinar emphysema, noninfectious hepatitis, and cirrhosis should suggest the diagnosis. Protein electrophoresis reveals low levels of α_1-antitrypsin. Some patients respond to dapsone or α_1-protease inhibitor concentrate. Other forms of panniculitis are Weber-Christian disease, cytophagic histiocytic panniculitis, post-steroid panniculitis, and nodular panniculitis. Deep excisional biopsies rather than punch biopsy are required to diagnose panniculitis.
Lipodermatosclerosis (chronic indurated cellulitis)	A form of panniculitis; affects middle-aged women, associated with venous insufficiency. Acute form resembles cellulitis. Painful, red, indurated, edematous area in medial aspect of leg. Lasts a few months. Superimposed cellulitis may occur. Compression therapy reduces venous hypertension and fluid extravasation.
Lymphedema	Nonpitting edema, erythema, induration of an extremity. No fever, no response to antibiotics. May be complicated by infection, recurrently. Lymphangioscintigraphy confirms diagnosis.
Pyoderma gangrenosum	An ulcerative cutaneous disease. Ulcers may follow trauma. An atypical form occurs on the hand. A red ulcer border may be misinterpreted as infection.
Relapsing polychondritis	Affects cartilaginous structures. Auricular chondritis is most common manifestation, usually both ears; cellulitis is usually unilateral with regional lymphadenopathy. Relapsing polychondritis spares earlobe because this structure is not cartilaginous. Recurrent inflammation causes auricular or saddle-nose deformity. Associated features include peripheral, nonerosive polyarthritis; episcleritis; keratitis or uveitis; and aortic valve insufficiency.
Polyarteritis nodosa	Subcutaneous, inflammatory, red to bluish nodules (2 cm in diameter) that follow the course of involved arteries; lower extremities, often bilateral; becomes confluent to form painful subcutaneous plaques that may resemble cellulitis. Ulcers may occur.
Sarcoidosis	Atypical lesions manifest as indurated red plaques with edema and pain.
Superficial thrombophlebitis	Gradual onset of localized tenderness, followed by erythema along the path of a superficial vein. Varicose veins, prolonged travel, or enforced stasis may be the cause.
Sweet's syndrome (acute febrile neutrophilic dermatosis)	Papules that coalesce to form inflammatory plaques (red and tender); upper extremities, face, and neck. Fever, arthralgia or arthritis. Moderate neutrophilia. Biopsy: dermal polymorphonuclear leukocytes. 10% have an associated malignant condition (e.g., acute myelogenous leukemia). Corticosteroids effective.

TREATMENT OF CELLULITIS

ADULTS. Therapy for erysipelas or cellulitis is an antibiotic active against streptococci. Either β-lactam or non-β-lactam antibiotics can be used to treat uncomplicated cellulitis (see Table 9-1 and Box 9-1). *PMID: 18456038* The use of empirical β-lactam antibiotics provided several minor advantages. The safety of cephalosporins and the propensity for adverse effects with trimethoprim-sulfamethoxazole, clindamycin, and the fluoroquinolones are known. Patients with uncomplicated cellulitis are those without ulceration or abscesses, significant immunosuppression, drainage or debridement, or intravenous therapy. These patients can receive oral medications from the start. Macrolide resistance among group A streptococci has increased regionally in the United States. Parenteral therapy is indicated for severely ill patients or for those unable to tolerate oral medications. A 5-day course of antibiotics is as effective as a 10-day course for uncomplicated cellulitis. Some patients are slow to respond. They may have a deeper infection, diabetes, chronic venous insufficiency, or lymphedema. Cutaneous inflammation sometimes worsens after

Box 9-1 **Antibiotic Utilization of Subjects Treated for Uncomplicated Cellulitis**

β-Lactam therapy

- Cephalexin
- Other β-lactam therapy
- Dicloxacillin
- Amoxicillin/clavulanate
- Other (cefuroxime, cefpodoxime, penicillin, amoxicillin)

Non-β-lactam therapy

- Clindamycin
- Trimethoprim-sulfamethoxazole
- Fluoroquinolone (gatifloxacin, ciprofloxacin)
- Macrolides (erythromycin, azithromycin, clarithromycin)
- Tetracyclines (tetracycline, doxycycline, minocycline)
- Combination therapy (two non-β-lactams)

Adapted from *Am J Med* 121(5):419-425, 2008. *PMID: 18456038*

starting antibiotics. This response can be attenuated with an 8-day tapering oral course of corticosteroid therapy beginning with 30 mg of prednisolone.

Elevation of the affected area promotes drainage of the edema and hastens recovery for lower leg infections. Pain can be relieved with cool compresses. Treat underlying conditions that may predispose to the infection, such as tinea pedis, stasis dermatitis, or trauma.

PREVENTING RECURRENT CELLULITIS

Each attack of cellulitis causes lymphatic inflammation and possibly some permanent damage. Severe or repeated episodes of cellulitis may lead to lymphedema, sometimes substantial enough to cause elephantiasis. Measures to reduce recurrences of cellulitis include treating interdigital maceration, keeping the skin well hydrated with emollients to avoid dryness and cracking, and reducing any underlying edema by such methods as elevation of the extremity, use of compressive stockings or pneumatic pressure pumps, and, if appropriate, diuretic therapy.

PROPHYLACTIC ANTIBIOTICS TO PREVENT RECURRENCE. Prolonged antimicrobial prophylaxis is effective and safe in preventing recurrent episodes of soft tissue infections and may be continued for months or years. Streptococci cause most recurrent cellulitis. Treatment options include monthly intramuscular benzathine penicillin injections of 1.2 milliunits in adults or oral therapy with twice-daily doses of either 250 mg of erythromycin or 1 gm of penicillin V. An alternative is to provide oral antibiotics to initiate therapy as soon as symptoms of infection begin. Low-dose oral clindamycin has been advocated for the prevention of recurrent staphylococcal skin infections and might also be useful for the prevention of recurrent cellulitis.

CHILDREN. *H. influenzae* cellulitis is now rare since the introduction of *Haemophilus influenzae* type b (Hib) vaccine. The vaccine is now used in the routine immunization schedule of more than 100 countries.

Cellulitis of specific areas

CELLULITIS AND ERYSIPELAS OF THE EXTREMITIES

Cellulitis of the extremities is most often caused by group A beta-hemolytic streptococci and is characterized by an expanding, red, swollen, tender-to-painful plaque with an indefinite border that may cover a small or wide area (Figures 9-11 and 9-12). Chills and fever occur as the red plaque spreads rapidly, becomes edematous, and sometimes develops bullae or suppurates. Less acute forms detected around a stasis leg ulcer spread slowly and may appear as an area of erythema with no swelling or fever. Erysipelas of the lower extremity is now more common than facial erysipelas. Group G streptococci may be a common pathogen, especially in patients older than 50 years. Red, sometimes painful, streaks of lymphangitis may ex-

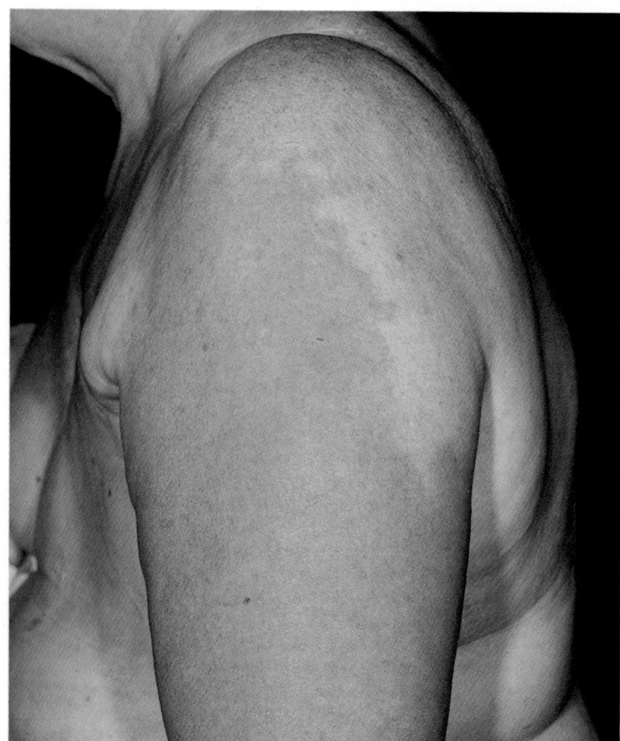

Figure 9-11 Cellulitis. Infected area is tender, deep red, and swollen.

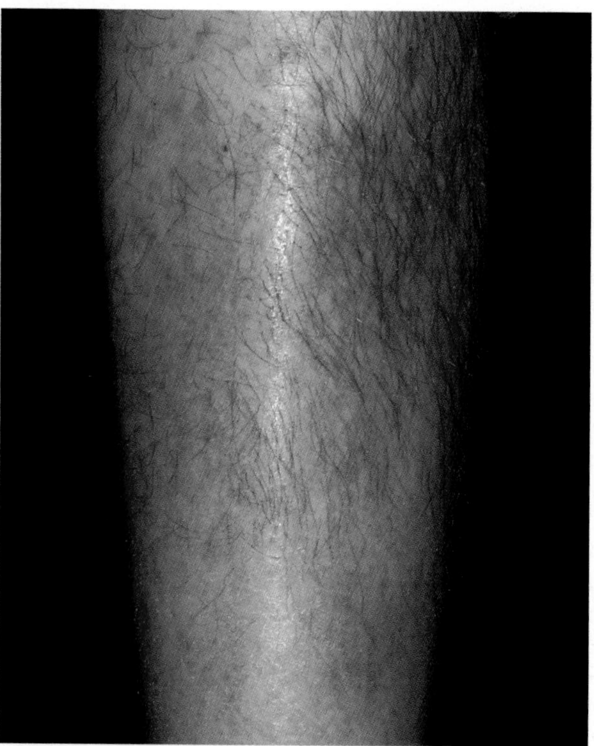

Figure 9-12 Cellulitis. There is erythema, edema, and tenderness.

tend toward regional lymph nodes. Repeated attacks can cause impairment of lymphatic drainage, which predisposes the patient to more infection and permanent swelling. This series of events takes place most commonly in the lower legs of patients with venous stasis and ulceration. The end stage, which includes dermal fibrosis, lymphedema, and epidermal thickening on the lower leg, is called elephantiasis nostras.

TREATMENT. Treatment with oral or intravenous antibiotics should be started immediately and, if appropriate, altered according to laboratory results (see Table 9-1). The mean time for healing after treatment is initiated is 12 days, with a range of 5 to 25 days. See the section Treatment of Cellulitis for more details.

FACIAL ERYSIPELAS AND CELLULITIS IN ADULTS

ERYSIPELAS. The archaic term St. Anthony's Fire accurately describes the intensity of this eruption. Erysipelas is a superficial cellulitis with lymphatic involvement. Isolated cases are the rule; epidemic forms are rare. Facial sites have become rare but erysipelas of the legs is common. It may originate in a traumatic or surgical wound, but no portal of entry can be found in most cases. In the preantibiotic era, erysipelas was a feared disease with a significant mortality rate, particularly in infants. Most contemporary cases are of moderate intensity and have a benign course. In the majority of cases, group A streptococci are the responsible organisms. The second most frequent causative organism is group G streptococci.

After prodromal symptoms that last from 4 to 48 hours and consist of malaise, chills, fever (101° to 104° F), and occasionally anorexia and vomiting, one or more red, tender, firm spots appear at the site of infection. These spots rapidly increase in size, forming a tense, red, hot, uniformly elevated, shining patch with an irregular outline and a sharply defined, raised border (Figure 9-13). As the process develops, the color becomes a dark, fiery red and vesicles appear at the advancing border and over the surface. Symptoms of itching, burning, tenderness, and pain may be moderate to severe. Without treatment, the rash reaches its height in approximately 1 week and subsides slowly over the next 1 or 2 weeks.

RECURRENCE. Recurrence after antibiotic treatment occurs in 18% to 30% of cases. In particularly susceptible people, erysipelas may recur frequently for a long period and, by obstruction of the lymphatics, cause permanent thickening of the skin (lymphedema). Subsequent attacks may be initiated by the slightest trauma or may occur spontaneously to cause further irreversible skin thickening. The pinna and lower legs are particularly susceptible to this recurrent pattern (Figure 9-14).

TREATMENT. Treatment is the same as that for streptococcal cellulitis (see Table 9-1). Recurrent cases may require long-term prophylactic treatment with low-dose penicillin or erythromycin. If other organisms are found on culture, a different agent is needed. See the section Treatment of Cellulitis for more details.

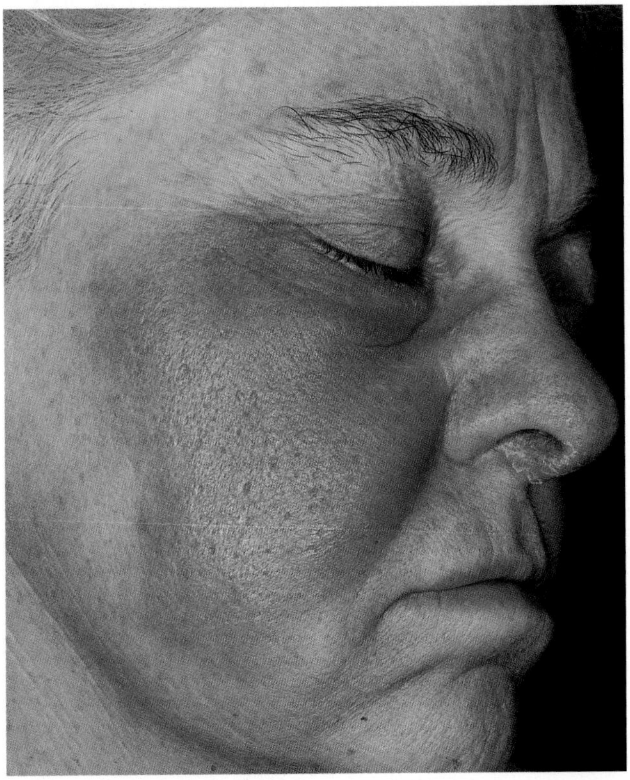

Figure 9-13 Erysipelas. Streptococcal cellulitis. The acute phase with intense erythema.

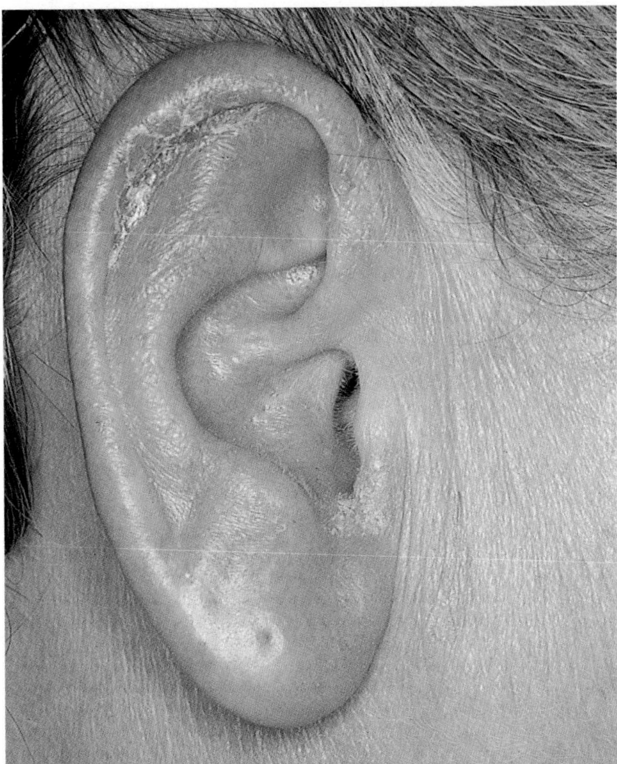

Figure 9-14 Erysipelas. Recurrent episodes of infection have resulted in lymphatic obstruction and caused permanent thickening of the skin.

PERIANAL CELLULITIS

Cellulitis (group A beta-hemolytic streptococcus) around the anal orifice is often misdiagnosed as candidiasis. It occurs more frequently in children than adults. Bright, perianal erythema extends from the anal verge approximately 2 to 3 cm onto the surrounding perianal skin (Figures 9-15 and 9-16). Boys are affected more than girls. Symptoms include painful defecation (52%), tenderness, soilage from oozing, and, sometimes, blood-streaked stool and perianal itching (78%). These children are not systemically ill. Pharyngitis may precede the infection. The differential diagnosis includes *Candida* intertrigo, psoriasis, pinworm infection, inflammatory bowel disease, a behavioral problem, and child abuse. Culture results confirm the diagnosis.

Initial treatment consists of a 10- to 14-day course of penicillin, amoxicillin-clavulanic acid, erythromycin, or other macrolides. Relapses occurred in 39% of the patients. After treatment, a new culture specimen should be taken to check for recurrence. The topical antibiotic mupirocin (Bactroban) may also provide rapid relief of symptoms, but systemic therapy is also required because it will treat any persistent oropharyngeal focus of streptococcal infection.

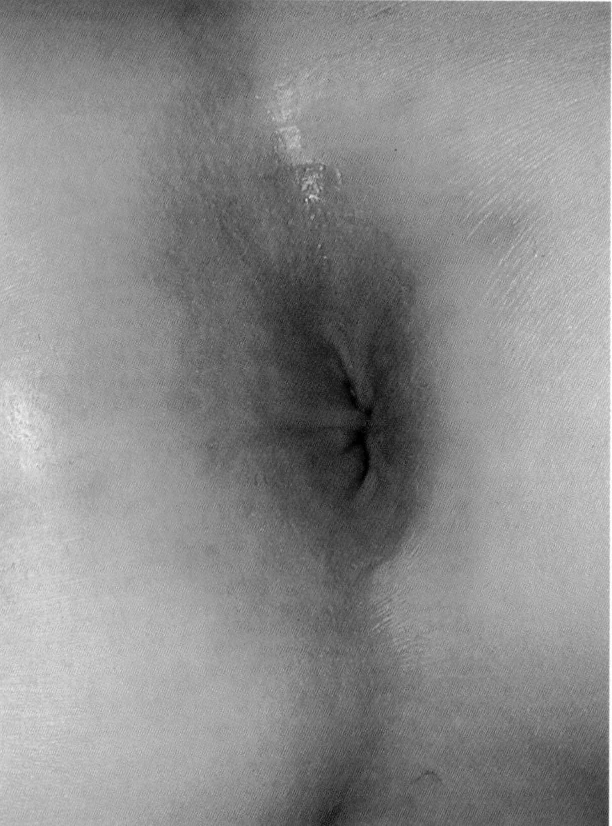

Figure 9-15 Perianal cellulitis (group A beta-hemolytic streptococcus). Bright perianal erythema extends from the anal verge approximately 2 to 3 cm onto the surrounding perianal skin. Candidiasis is usually accompanied by satellite pustules extending onto normal skin outside of the active border.

Necrotizing skin and soft tissue infections

Necrotizing skin and soft tissue infections are often deep and devastating. They may involve the fascial and/or muscle compartments and can cause destruction of tissue and be fatal. They are often secondary infections that develop from a break in the skin from trauma or surgery. They are usually caused by streptococci or a mixed bacterial flora. Features that suggest that deeper tissues are involved are shown in Box 9-2.

Necrotizing fasciitis

Necrotizing fasciitis (NF) is an infection of the subcutaneous tissue that results in the destruction of fascia and fat. The infection is most frequently polymicrobial. Ten per-

Box 9-2 Features That Suggest a Necrotizing Infection*

1. Severe, constant pain
2. Bullae related to occlusion of deep blood vessels
3. Skin necrosis or ecchymosis that precedes skin necrosis
4. Gas in the soft tissues, detected by palpation or imaging
5. Edema that extends beyond the margin of erythema
6. Cutaneous anesthesia
7. Hard, wooden feel of the subcutaneous tissue, extending beyond the area of apparent skin involvement
8. Rapid spread, especially during antibiotic therapy
9. Systemic toxicity—fever, leukocytosis, delirium, renal failure
10. CT scan or MRI may show edema extending along the fascial plane

Adapted from Practice guidelines for the diagnosis and management of skin and soft-tissue infections, *Clin Infect Dis* 41:1373-1406, 2005. *PMID: 16231249*
*Features that suggest that deeper tissues are involved.

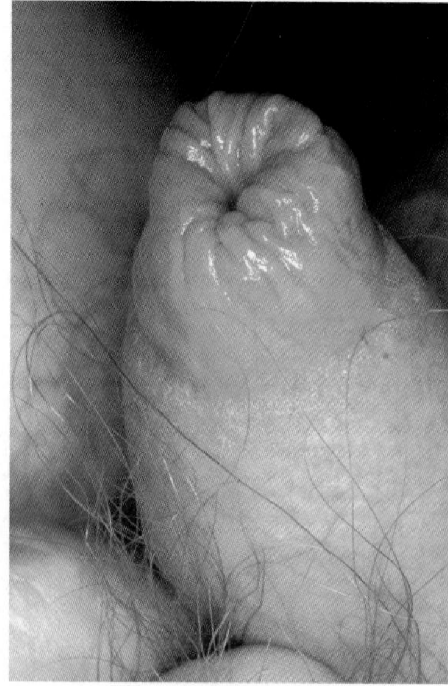

Figure 9-16 Streptococcal cellulitis occurred under the foreskin simultaneously with anal cellulitis in this adult.

cent of infections are caused by group A streptococcus and can lead to toxic shock. NF most frequently occurs in the extremities, with a predilection for the lower leg. NF may mimic deep vein thrombosis. Predisposing factors include trauma (often trivial), burns, splinters, surgery, childbirth, diabetes mellitus, varicella, immunosuppression, renal failure, arteriosclerosis, odontogenic infection, malignancy, and alcoholism. Nonsteroidal antiinflammatory agents may alter the immune response, causing a minor infection to become fulminant.

CLINICAL MANIFESTATIONS

Extension from a skin lesion occurs in 80% of cases. The initial lesion is often trivial, such as a minor abrasion, insect bite, injection site (drug addicts) or boil; 20% of patients have no visible skin lesion. Initially there is pain, erythema, edema, cellulitis, and high fever. The patient may be disoriented and lethargic. The local site shows cellulitis (90% of cases), edema (80%), skin discoloration or gangrene (70%), and anesthesia of involved skin. A wooden-hard feel of the subcutaneous tissues is characteristic.

Many patients are diagnosed with cellulitis and sent home; they return when the condition worsens. The most consistent clinical clue is unrelenting pain out of proportion to the physical findings even if there is only mild or no fever or erythema. Typically there is diffuse swelling of an arm or leg and intense pain on palpation. About 1 or 2 days after symptom onset, the patient has high fever, leukocytosis, edema with central patches of dusky blue discoloration, weeping blisters, and borders with cellulitis. Bullae with clear fluid rapidly turn violaceous. Septicemia may develop secondarily and should be strongly suspected in the presence of fever, anorexia, nausea, diarrhea, confusion, and hypotension. Progression to gangrene, sometimes with myonecrosis, and an extension of the inflammatory process along fascial planes are possible. Twenty-five percent will die of septic shock and organ failure.

BACTERIA

MONOMICROBIAL FORM. *S. pyogenes, S. aureus, V. vulnificus, A. hydrophila,* and anaerobic streptococci (e.g., *Peptostreptococcus* species) are most often isolated. Staphylococci and hemolytic streptococci can occur simultaneously. *S. pyogenes* are most often seen after varicella or minor scratches and insect bites. Mortality in this group approaches 50% to 70% in patients with hypotension and organ failure.

POLYMICROBIAL FORM. Most organisms originate from the bowel flora (e.g., coliforms and anaerobic bacteria). The polymicrobial necrotizing infection is associated with (1) surgical procedures involving the bowel or penetrating abdominal trauma, (2) decubitus ulcers or perianal abscesses, (3) sites of injection in injection drug users, and (4) extension from a Bartholin abscess or a minor vulvovaginal infection.

DIAGNOSIS. Computed tomography (CT) scan or magnetic resonance imaging (MRI) may show edema along the fascial plane. Gas may be present in clostridial and mixed aerobic/anaerobic infections but it is never present in group A streptococcal infections. Plain radiographs, CT, and ultrasound are useful in demonstrating the air bubbles in the soft tissues. Direct inspection at surgery shows the fascia is swollen and dull gray in appearance, with stringy areas of necrosis. A thin, brownish exudate emerges from the wound. There is no pus. Tissue planes can be dissected with a gloved finger or a blunt instrument. A Gram stain of the exudate demonstrates the presence of the pathogens. Gram-positive cocci in chains suggest *Streptococcus* organisms (either group A or anaerobic). Large gram-positive cocci in clumps suggest *S. aureus,* but this is an unusual primary organism in these spreading infections. Obtain samples for culture from the deep tissues and obtain blood cultures.

TREATMENT

NF requires surgical debridement of necrotic tissue, use of antimicrobial agents, and wound and supportive care. Patients in whom the etiologic agents cannot be definitively identified should be treated with broad-spectrum antimicrobial regimens. Surgical exploration is indicated when the diagnosis of infection is in doubt and the patient is very ill. Surgery can establish a diagnosis by providing material for culture, Gram staining, and histopathologic examination. A diagnosis can be made at surgery with a "finger test." When the site is incised and the finger is inserted, the skin peels off easily at the subcutaneous fascia. Simple drainage, radical debridement, or amputation are the options for treatment. Intravenous immunoglobulin may be a useful adjunct in the treatment of streptococcal toxic shock syndrome associated with necrotizing fasciitis. Early aggressive antimicrobial treatment may help avoid surgical intervention. Indications for surgery are shown in Box 9-3. Most patients return to the operating room 24 to 36 hours after the first debridement and daily thereafter until there is no further need for debridement. Wounds can discharge copious amounts of tissue fluid and administration of fluid is often necessary (Table 9-4).

Box 9-3 **Indications for Surgery in Necrotizing Fasciitis***

1. There is no response to antibiotics, no reduction in fever or toxicity, or no lack of advancement.
2. Profound toxicity, fever, hypotension, or advancement of the skin and soft tissue infection during antibiotic therapy occurs.
3. When the local wound shows any skin necrosis with easy dissection along the fascia by a blunt instrument, more complete incision and drainage are required.
4. Any soft tissue infection accompanied by gas in the affected tissue suggests necrotic tissue and requires operative drainage and/or debridement.

*Antimicrobial therapy (Table 9-4) is continued until operative procedures are no longer needed and fever has been absent for 48 to 72 hours.

Table 9-4 Treatment of Necrotizing Infections of the Skin, Fascia, and Muscle

First-line antimicrobial agent, by infection type	Adult dosage	Antimicrobial agent(s) for patients with severe penicillin hypersensitivity
Mixed infection		
Ampicillin-sulbactam **or** Piperacillin-tazobactam **plus** Clindamycin **plus** Ciprofloxacin	1.5-3.0 gm every 6-8 hr IV 3.37 gm every 6-8 hr IV 600-900 mg/kg every 8 hr IV 400 mg every 12 hr IV	Clindamycin or metronidazole* with an aminoglycoside or fluoroquinolone
Imipenem/cilastatin	1 gm every 6-8 hr IV	—
Meropenem	1 gm every 8 hr IV	—
Ertapenem	1 gm every day IV	—
Cefotaxime **plus** Metronidazole **or** Clindamycin	2 gm every 6 hr IV 500 mg every 6 hr IV 600-900 mg/kg every 8 hr IV	—
***Streptococcus* infection**		
Penicillin **plus** Clindamycin	2-4 milliunits every 4-6 hr IV (adults) 600-900 mg/kg every 8 hr IV	Vancomycin, linezolid, quinupristin/dalfopristin, or daptomycin
***S. aureus* infection**		
Nafcillin	1-2 gm every 4 hr IV	Vancomycin, linezolid, quinupristin/dalfopristin, daptomycin
Oxacillin	1-2 gm every 4 hr IV	—
Cefazolin	1 gm every 8 hr IV	—
Vancomycin (for resistant strains)	30 mg/kg/day in two divided doses IV	—
Clindamycin	600-900 mg/kg every 8 hr IV	Bacteriostatic; potential of cross-resistance and emergence of resistance in erythromycin-resistant strains; inducible resistance in methicillin-resistant *S. aureus*
Clostridium infection		
Clindamycin	600-900 mg/kg every 8 hr IV	—
Penicillin	2-4 milliunits every 4-6 hr IV	—

Adapted from Practice guidelines for the diagnosis and management of skin and soft-tissue infections, *Clin Infect Dis* 41:1373-1406, 2005. *PMID: 16231249*
IV, Intravenously.
*If *Staphylococcus* infection is present or suspected, add an appropriate agent.

FOLLICULITIS

Folliculitis is inflammation of the hair follicle caused by infection, chemical irritation, or physical injury. Inflammation may be superficial or deep in the hair follicle. Folliculitis is very common and is seen as a component of a variety of inflammatory skin diseases, which are listed in Table 9-5.

In superficial folliculitis, the inflammation is confined to the upper part of the hair follicle. Clinically, it is manifested as a painless or tender pustule that eventually heals without scarring. In many instances, the hair shaft in the center of the pustule cannot be seen. Inflammation of the entire follicle or the deeper portion of the hair follicle initially appears as a swollen, red mass, which eventually may point toward the surface, becoming a somewhat larger pustule than that seen in superficial folliculitis. Deeper lesions are painful and may heal with scarring.

Table 9-5 Diseases Initially Manifesting in Folliculitis

Superficial folliculitis	Deep folliculitis
Staphylococcal folliculitis	Furuncle and carbuncle
Pseudofolliculitis barbae (from shaving)	Sycosis (inflammation of entire depth of follicle)
Superficial fungal infections (dermatophytes)	Sycosis (beard area): sycosis barbae, bacterial or fungal
Cutaneous candidiasis (pustules also occur outside the hair follicle)	Sycosis (scalp): bacterial
Acne vulgaris	Acne vulgaris, cystic
Acne, mechanically or chemically induced	Gram-negative acne
Steroid acne after withdrawal of topical steroids	*Pseudomonas* folliculitis
Keratosis pilaris	Dermatophyte fungal infections

Staphylococcal folliculitis

Staphylococcal folliculitis is the most common form of infectious folliculitis. One pustule or a group of pustules may appear, usually without fever or other systemic symptoms, on any body surface (Figure 9-17). Staphylococcal folliculitis may occur because of injury, abrasion, or nearby surgical wounds or draining abscesses. It may also be a complication of occlusive topical steroid therapy (Figure 9-18, *A-B*), particularly if moist lesions are occluded for many hours. Follicular pustules are cultured, not by touching the pustule with a cotton swab, but by scraping off the entire pustule with a no. 15 blade and depositing the material onto the cotton swab of a transport medium kit. Some cases can be treated with a tepid, wet Burow's compress, but oral antibiotics are used in most cases.

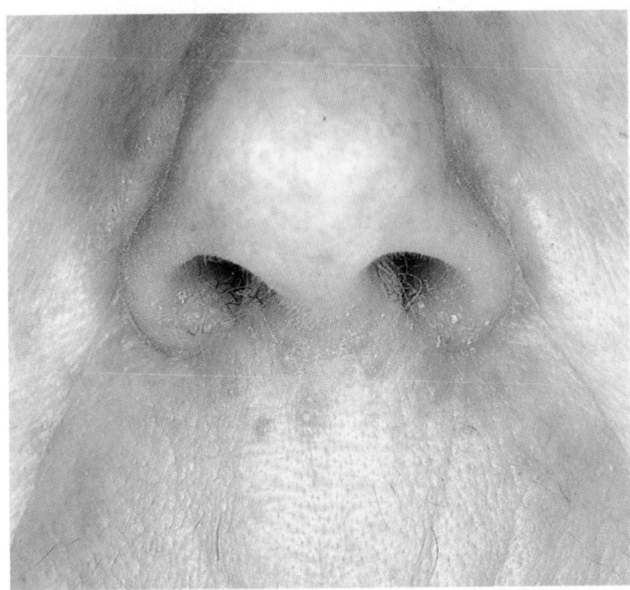

Figure 9-17 Staphylococcal folliculitis. The nares are a reservoir for *S. aureus*. Folliculitis may appear on the skin around the nose.

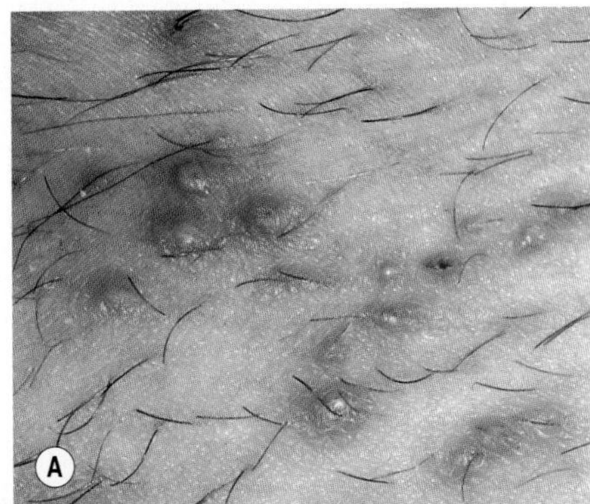

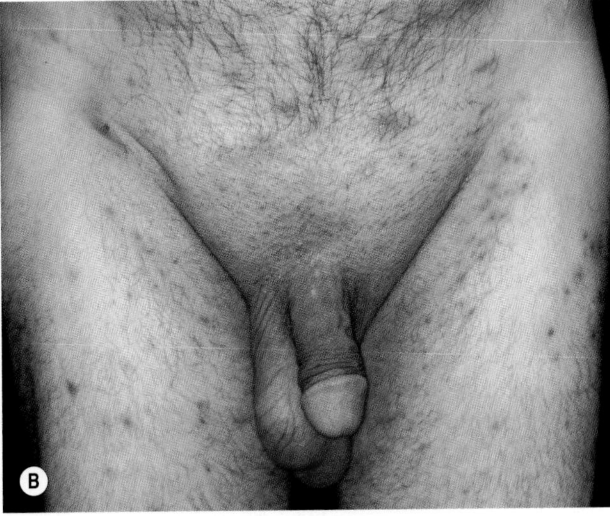

Figure 9-18 Methicillin-resistant *Staphylococcus aureus* (MRSA). **A,** Pustules are localized to the hair follicles (folliculitis). **B,** MRSA infections often begin as folliculitis, boils, abscess, and/or cellulitis. The face and groin are common sites.

Pseudofolliculitis barbae (razor bumps)

Pseudofolliculitis barbae (PFB) is a foreign body reaction to hair. Clinically, there is less inflammation than with staphylococcal folliculitis. The condition occurs on the cheeks and neck in individuals who are genetically inclined to have tightly curled, spiral hair, which can become ingrown (Figure 9-19). This condition is found in 50% to 75% of blacks and 3% to 5% of whites who shave. If cut below the surface by shaving, the sharp-tipped whisker may curve into the follicular wall or emerge and curve back to penetrate the skin. A tender, red papule or pustule occurs at the point of entry and remains until the hair is removed. Generally, the problem is more severe in the neck area where hair follicles are more likely to be oriented at low angles to the skin surface, making repenetration of the skin more likely. Pseudofolliculitis can occur also in the axillae, pubic area, and legs. Normal bacterial flora may eventually be replaced by pathogenic organisms if the process becomes chronic. Pseudofolliculitis of the beard is a significant problem in the armed services (see Figure 9-19) and in professions in which individuals are required to shave.

PREVENTION AND TREATMENT

Programs for treatment and prevention are outlined in Boxes 9-4 and 9-5. Wax depilation and tweezing may lead to transfollicular repenetration. Electrolysis tends to be expensive, painful, and often unsuccessful. The only definitive cure is permanent removal of the hair follicle with laser-assisted hair removal.

SHAVING TECHNIQUES. Use techniques that avoid close shaves and the production of sharply angled hair tips. Hydrating the beard before shaving by washing with soap and warm water softens the whiskers. The softened hairs are cut off directly, leaving a blunt hair and making ingrown hairs less likely. Use a highly lubricating shaving gel (e.g., Edge Gel). PFB Bump fighter razor is a special razor that does not shave close. Shaving closely with multiple razor strokes and shaving against the grain should be avoided. Electric clippers that cut hair as stubble can be an alternative to wet shaving. Depilatories with barium sulfide (Magic Shave and Royal Crown Powders) or calcium thioglycolate (Nair lotion, Magic Shave Gold Powder, Surgex cream) are available in all pharmacies. They are an effective

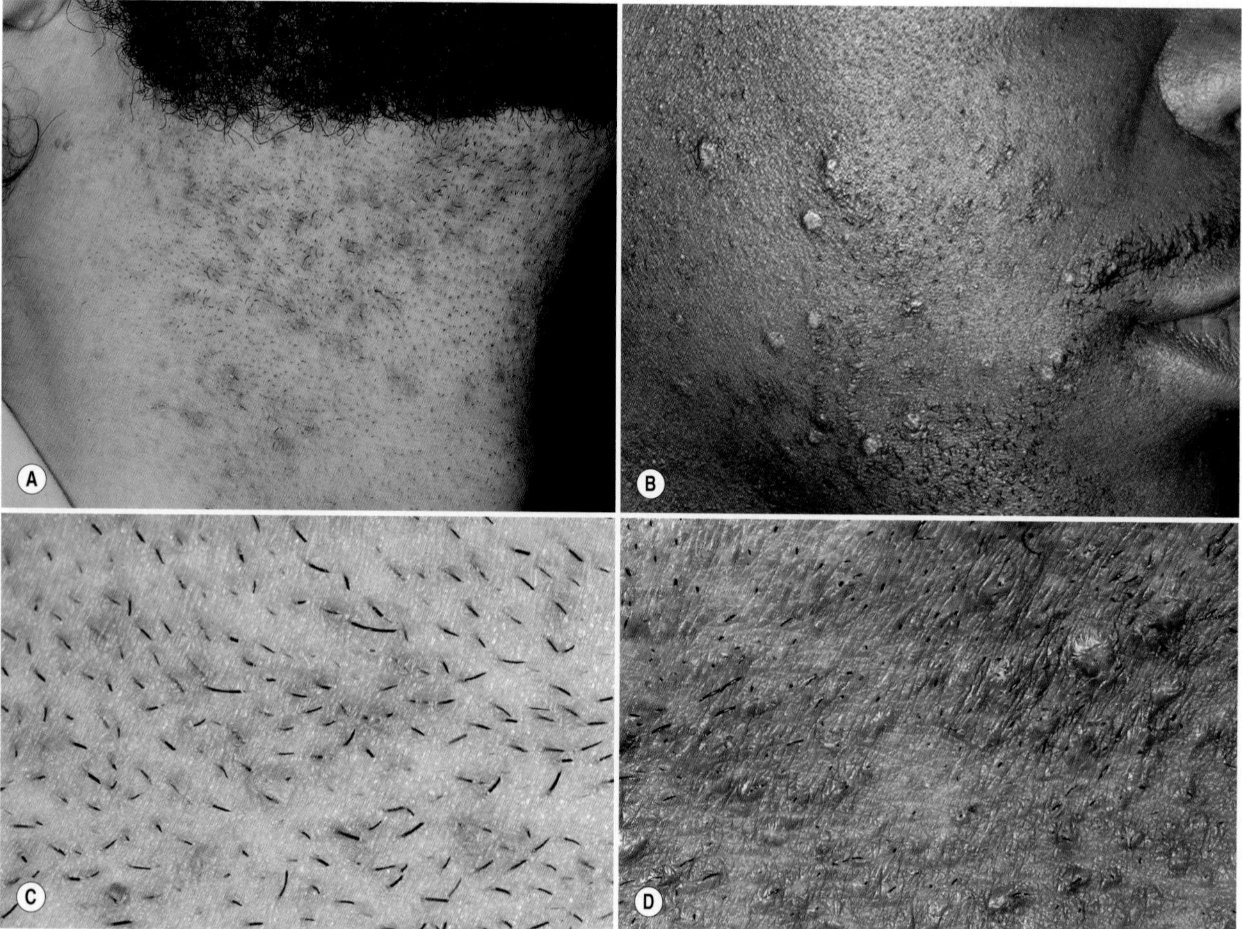

Figure 9-19 Pseudofolliculitis barbae. **A,** Papules and pustules persist after shaving. **B,** PFB is found mostly in black males. Scarring and keloids may occur in chronic cases. **C,** Red papules occur with a hair shaft imbedded in its center. **D,** Papules of different sizes may last indefinitely.

Box 9-4 Program for Treating Pseudofolliculitis Barbae

1. Stop shaving, electrolysis, tweezing, depilatory use, and waxing. (PFB may worsen during the first week because of regrowth.)
2. Use a hair-releasing technique. Wash the beard for several minutes in a circular motion with a washcloth or toothbrush to dislodge ingrown hairs.
3. Dislodge imbedded hair shafts by inserting a firm, pointed instrument such as syringe needle under the hair loop and firmly elevating it.
4. A short course of antibiotics (e.g., tetracyclines, cephalosporins) may hasten resolution.
5. Corticosteroids (prednisone at 40 to 60 mg/day for 5 to 10 days) may be used in moderate to severe cases to reduce inflammation around the hair follicles until the hair grows and is no longer an aggravating factor.
6. Intralesional triamcinolone acetonide (2.5 to 10 mg/ml) is useful for red papules that linger.
7. For a long-term solution to pseudofolliculitis barbae, laser hair removal may be the best option.

Box 9-5 Program for Preventing Pseudofolliculitis Barbae

1. Wet beard with warm water. This hydrates the hair so that it cuts more easily and leaves a tip that is not sharp.
2. Use a soft-bristled toothbrush, in a circular motion, to dislodge hair tips that are piercing the skin. Do this before shaving and at bedtime. Use a sterile needle to dislodge stubborn tips of hair.
3. Reduce the closeness of the shave. Avoid close shaves with twin- and triple-blade razors.
4. Shave hair with electric clippers (e.g., Norelco, Braun, Remington) to a minimum length of 1 mm. Purchase at beauty supply stores or at www.electricshaver.com.
5. Shave with The Bump Fighter® razor (American Safety Razor Co., Staunton, Va) (www.asrco.com), a single-edge blade with polymer coating and foil guard. This special razor cuts the hair at the correct length and prevents hair tip reentry into the skin. Lather with a thick gel (e.g., Aveeno, Edge Gel, or Bump Fighter Shaving Gel). Avoid taut skin by not pulling it while shaving. Shave with the grain (i.e., in the direction of hair growth). Rinse blade after each shaving stroke to prevent the traction that occurs with buildup of hair between the blade and guard. Apply cool compresses after shaving.
6. Alternatively, use an electric razor, avoiding the "closest" shave setting. Razors can be ordered from Delasco: 608 13th Avenue, Council Bluffs, Iowa 51501-6401. Telephone: 1-800-831-6273.
7. Apply a glycolic acid lotion (e.g., Nutraplus lotion) to reduce hyperkeratosis.
8. Consider use of chemical depilatories to remove hair.

Adapted from Crutchfield CE: *Cutis* 61:351, 1998; and Perry PK: *J Am Acad Dermatol* 46:S113, 2002. *PMID: 11807473*

way of removing hair and preventing pseudofolliculitis. They are applied to the skin for 3 to 10 minutes and wiped off. The chemical reduces sulfide bonds in the cortex of the medulla of the hair shaft. The weakened hair fibers shear when the material is wiped off, leaving a soft, fluffy hair tip that is less likely to become ingrown. These products are irritating and can only be tolerated once or twice each week. If these measures fail, shaving must be discontinued indefinitely.

LASER. Several different lasers are available for the permanent removal of the beard hair.

Keratosis pilaris

Keratosis pilaris is a common finding on the posterolateral aspects of the upper arms and anterior thighs. The eruption is probably more common in atopics (see p. 168). Clinically, a group of small, pinpoint, follicular pustules remains in the same area for years. Histologic studies show that the inflammation actually occurs outside of the hair follicle. Scratching, wearing tight-fitting clothing, or undergoing treatment with abrasives may infect these sterile pustules and cause a diffuse eruption (Figure 9-20). It is important to recognize this entity to avoid unnecessary and detrimental treatment. Many patients object to these small, sometimes unsightly bumps. Keratosis pilaris resists all types of treatment. Oral antibiotics active against *S. aureus* are used if folliculitis develops. Group V topical steroids provide temporary relief when the area becomes dry and inflamed. Urea creams (e.g., Vanamide) and lactic acid moisturizers (Lac-Hydrin, AmLactin) soften the skin.

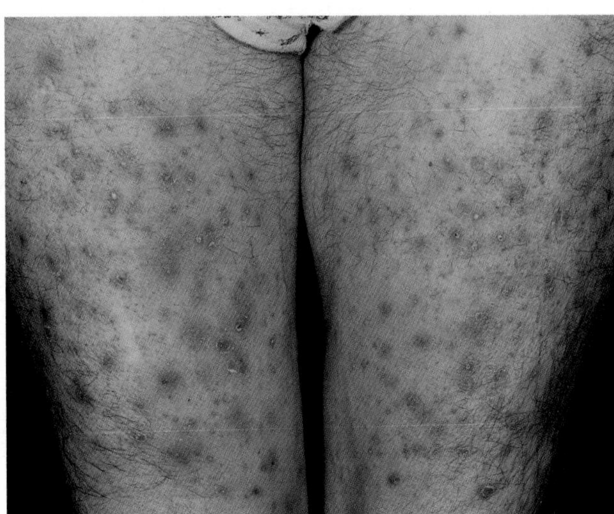

Figure 9-20 Keratosis pilaris and folliculitis. Keratosis pilaris is a common finding on the anterior thighs. A group of small, pinpoint, follicular pustules remains in the same areas for years. Scratching, wearing tight-fitting clothing, or treating with abrasives may infect these sterile pustules and cause a diffuse eruption.

Sycosis barbae

Sycosis implies follicular inflammation of the entire depth of the hair follicle and may be caused by infection with *S. aureus* or dermatophyte fungi. (See Chapter 13 on fungal infections for a discussion of fungal sycosis.) The disease occurs only in men who have commenced shaving. It begins with the appearance of small follicular papules or pustules and rapidly becomes more diffuse as shaving continues (Figures 9-21, 9-22, and 9-23). Reaction to the disease varies greatly among individuals. Infiltration about the follicle may be slight or extensive. The more infiltrated cases heal with scarring. In chronic cases, the pustules may remain confined to one area, such as the upper lip or neck. The hairs are epilated with difficulty in staphylococcal sycosis and with relative ease in fungal sycosis. Hairs should be removed and examined for fungi and the purulent material should be cultured. Fungal infections tend to be more severe, producing deeper and wider areas of inflammation; bacterial follicular infections usually present with discrete pustules. Pseudofolliculitis (see previous section) has a similar appearance.

Localized inflammation is treated topically with mupirocin (Bactroban ointment). Extensive disease is treated with oral antibiotics (e.g., dicloxacillin, cephalexin) for at least 2 weeks or until all signs of inflammation have cleared. Recurrences are not uncommon and require an additional course of oral antibiotics. Shaving should be performed with a clean razor.

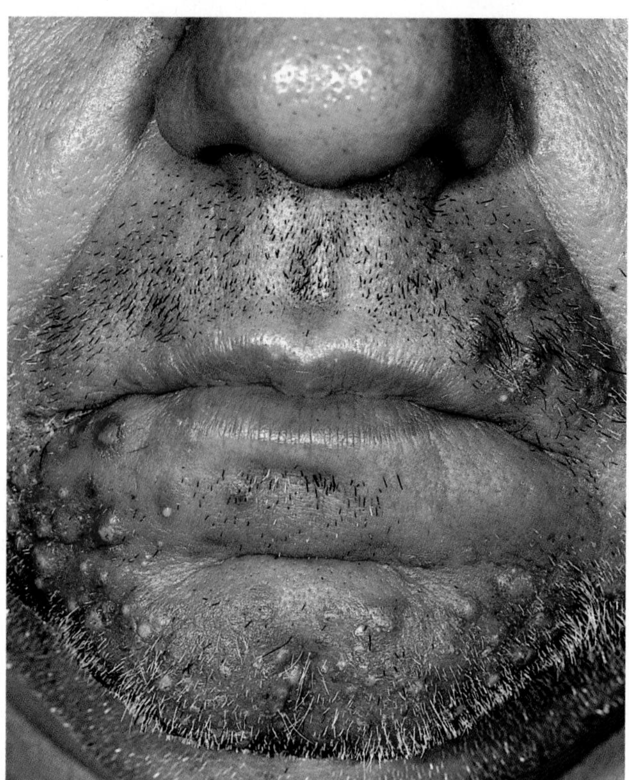

Figure 9-21 Sycosis barbae. Deep follicular pustules are concentrated in unshaved areas in this patient.

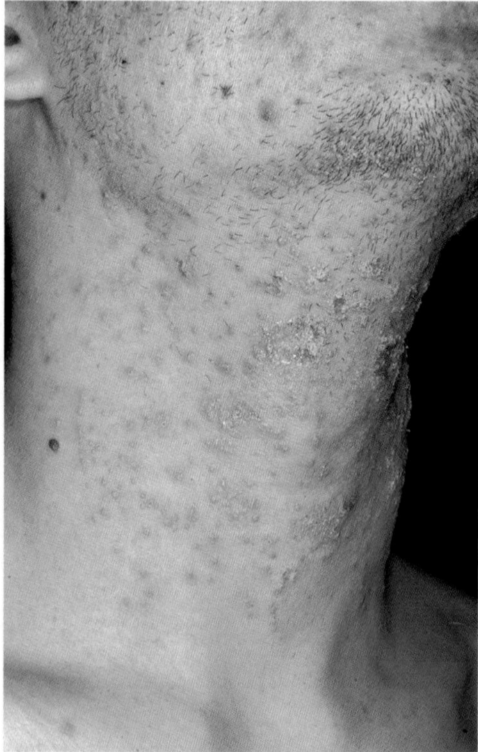

Figure 9-22 Sycosis barbae. An unusually extensive case involving the neck and face.

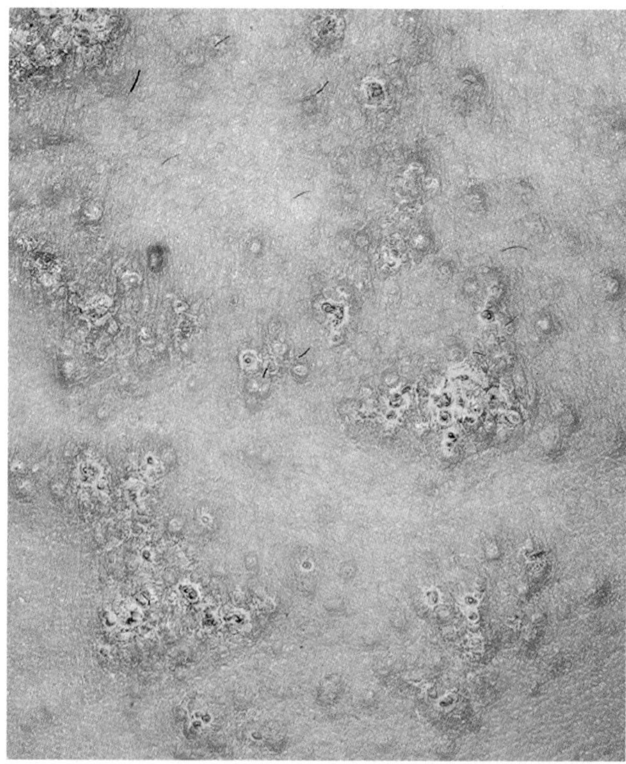

Figure 9-23 Sycosis barbae. Numerous pustules cleared rapidly with cephalexin 500 mg four times a day.

Acne keloidalis

Acne keloidalis (see Chapter 24) is a primary form of scarring alopecia. The word acne is a misnomer. It is a chronic scarring folliculitis of unknown etiology located on the posterior neck that eventually results in the formation of a group of keloidal papules. It occurs only in men and is more common in blacks. It may be initiated or aggravated by protective head devices. Follicular papules or pustules (Figure 9-24) develop on the back of the neck. They coalesce into firm plaques and nodules. Histologically there is inflammation, fibroplasia, and disappearance of sebaceous glands. The inflammatory stage may be asymptomatic. Extensive subclinical disease may be present and can account for some of the permanent hair loss. The patient eventually discovers a group of hard papules (Figure 9-25). The inflammatory stage lasts for months or years. The degree of inflammation varies from a group of discrete pustules to abscess formation on the entire back of the neck and scalp. Several hairs may protrude from a single follicle and look like tufted hair folliculitis.

Tufted hair folliculitis may not be a specific disease but secondary to progressive folliculitis like folliculitis decalvans, dissecting cellulitis, or acne keloidalis (see p. 942). Overgrowth of microorganisms does not appear to play an important role in the pathogenesis.

TREATMENT

A bacterial etiology has never been proven but acne keloidalis usually responds to short- or long-term courses of oral antibiotics. Different classes of antibiotics may have to be tried before control is achieved. Cephalosporins, trimethoprim-sulfamethoxazole (Bactrim, Septra), dicloxacillin, and amoxicillin-clavulanate potassium (Augmentin) have been successful in individual cases. Control with one antibiotic may diminish with time and the patient may have to be treated with a different antibiotic for continued long-term suppression. Topical steroid foams (Olux) applied twice daily in short courses may control inflammation and reduce the keloids. An intralesional injection of triamcinolone reduces the keloids, but this treatment should be delayed until infection has been controlled. Surgical excision may be necessary if persistent sinus tracts form. Successful surgical therapy of advanced cases can be carried out using a number of methods as long as subfollicular destruction of the process is achieved. Excision with primary closure is an excellent surgical treatment for extensive and refractory cases. Extremely large lesions should be excised in multiple stages.

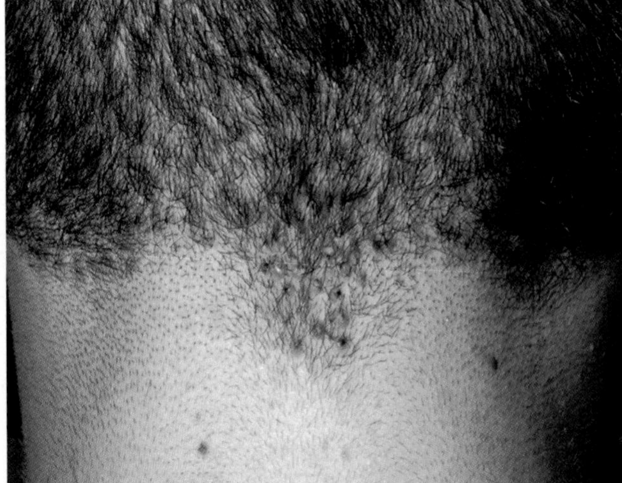

Figure 9-24 Deep folliculitis. Follicular pustules are surrounded by erythema and swelling. The entire follicular structure is inflamed. Staphylococci were isolated by culture.

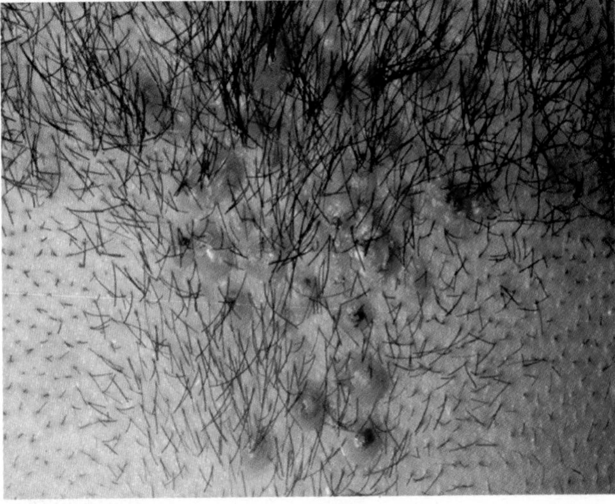

Figure 9-25 Acne keloidalis. Keloidal papules may eventually form on the back of the neck after chronic inflammation of the hair follicles.

FURUNCLES AND CARBUNCLES

A furuncle (abscess or boil) is a walled-off collection of pus that is a painful, firm, or fluctuant mass. Cellulitis may precede or occur in conjunction with it. An abscess is a cavity formed by fingerlike loculations of granulation tissue and pus that extends outward along planes of least resistance. Furuncles are uncommon in children, but increase in frequency after puberty. Furunculosis occurs as a self-limited infection in which one or several lesions are present or as a chronic, recurrent disease that lasts for months or years, affecting one or several family members. Most patients with sporadic or recurrent furunculosis appear to be otherwise normal and have an intact immune system.

Location

Lesions may occur at any site but favor areas prone to friction or minor trauma, such as underneath a belt, the anterior thighs, buttocks, groin, axillae, and waist.

Bacteria

S. aureus is the most common pathogen. The infecting strain may be found during quiescent periods in the nares and perineum. There is evidence that the anterior nares are the primary site from which the staphylococcus is disseminated to the skin. Other organisms, either aerobic (*E. coli, P. aeruginosa, S. faecalis*) or anaerobic (*Bacteroides, Lactobacillus, Peptococcus, Peptostreptococcus*) may cause furuncles. In general, the microbiology of abscesses reflects the microflora of the anatomic part of the body involved. Anaerobes are found in perineal and in some head and neck abscesses. Perirectal and perianal region abscesses often are reflective of fecal flora. Approximately 5% of abscesses are sterile. Bacteria colonize the skin in patients with atopic dermatitis, eczema, and scabies.

Predisposing conditions

Occlusion of the groin and buttocks by clothing, especially in patients with hyperhidrosis, encourages bacterial colonization. Follicular abnormalities, evident by the presence of comedones and acneiform papules and pustules, are often found on the buttocks and axillae of patients with recurrent furunculosis of those areas; these findings suggest the diagnosis of hidradenitis suppurativa (see p. 260).

CLINICAL MANIFESTATIONS

The lesion begins as a deep, tender, firm, red papule that enlarges rapidly into a tender, deep-seated nodule that remains stable and painful for days and then becomes fluctuant (Figures 9-26 to 9-28). The temperature is normal and there are no systemic symptoms. Pain becomes moderate to severe as purulent material accumulates. Pain is most intense in areas where expansion is restricted, such as the neck and external auditory canal. The abscess either remains deep and reabsorbs or points and ruptures through

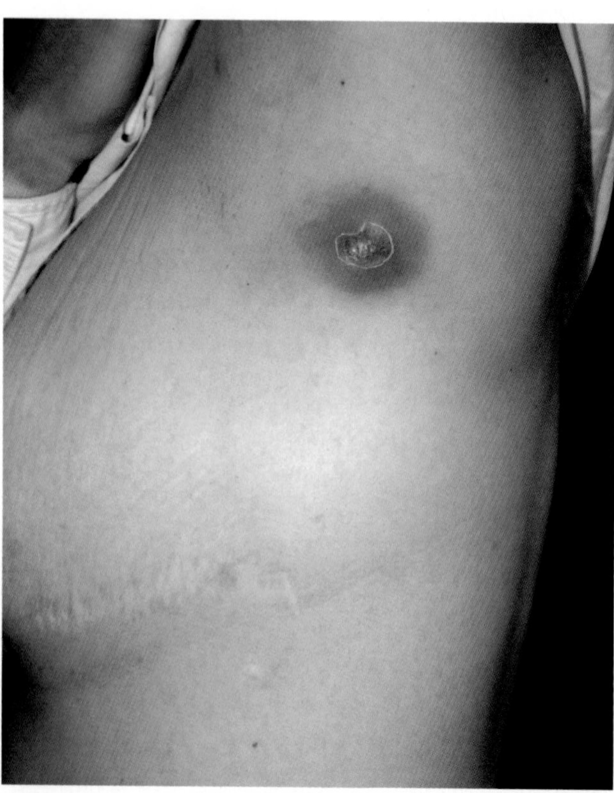

Figure 9-26 A furuncle is an abscess that exudes purulent material from a single opening. This picture shows a lesion of average size.

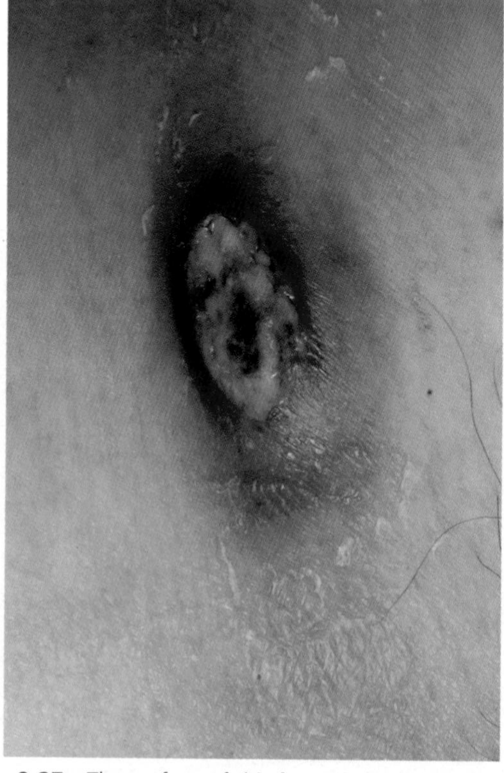

Figure 9-27 The surface of this furuncle has eroded and is exuding purulent material.

the surface. The abscess cavity contains a surprisingly large quantity of pus and white chunks of necrotic tissue. The point of rupture heals with scarring.

Carbuncles are aggregates of infected follicles. The infection originates deep in the dermis and the subcutaneous tissue, forming a broad, red, swollen, slowly evolving, deep, painful mass that points and drains through multiple openings. Malaise, chills, and fever precede or occur during the active phase. Deep extension into the subcutaneous tissue may be followed by sloughing and extensive scarring. Areas with thick dermis (i.e., the back of the neck, the back of the trunk, and the lateral aspects of the thighs) are the preferred sites. In the preantibiotic era, there were some fatalities.

DIFFERENTIAL DIAGNOSIS

Several diseases can be manifested as a furuncle (Table 9-6). The most common structure that is misinterpreted as a furuncle is a pilar cyst of the scalp or a ruptured epidermal cyst. The cyst wall ruptures spontaneously, leaking the white amorphous material into the dermis (Figure 9-29). An intense, foreign-body, inflammatory reaction occurs in hours, forming a sterile abscess. Treatment of a ruptured cyst consists of making a linear incision over the surface and evacuating the white material with manual pressure and a curette. Sometimes the cyst wall can be forced through the incision and cut out. In many cases the wall cannot be removed because it is fused to the dermis during the inflammatory process. Antibiotics are unnecessary.

Table 9-6 Diseases Initially Manifesting as Furunculosis ("Boils")

Disease	Location
Bacterial furunculosis	Any body surface
Recurrent furunculosis in scarred tissue	Buttock or any location
Ruptured epidermal cyst	Preauricular and postauricular areas, face, chest, back
Hidradenitis suppurativa	Axilla, groin, buttocks, under breasts
Cystic acne	Face, chest, back
Primary immunodeficiency diseases*	Any body surface
Secondary immunodeficiency†	Any body surface
Others: diabetes, alcoholism, malnutrition, severe anemia, debilitation	Any body surface

*Syndrome of hyperimmunoglobulinemia E associated with staphylococcal abscesses (Job's syndrome), chronic granulomatous disease, Chédiak-Higashi syndrome, C3 deficiency, C3 hypercatabolism, transient hypogammaglobulinemia of infancy, immunodeficiency with thymoma, Wiskott-Aldrich syndrome.

†Leukemia, leukopenia, neutropenia, therapeutic immunosuppression.

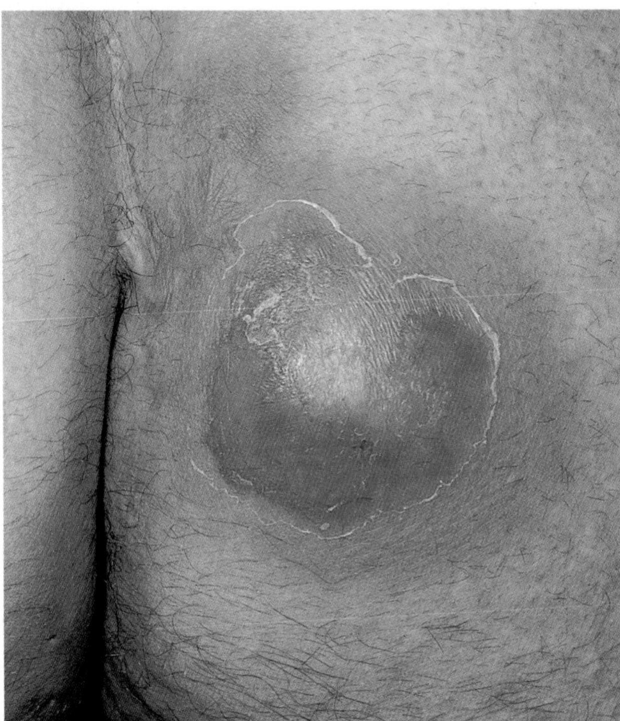

Figure 9-28 Furuncle (boil). Enlarged swollen mass with purulent material beginning to exude from several points on the surface.

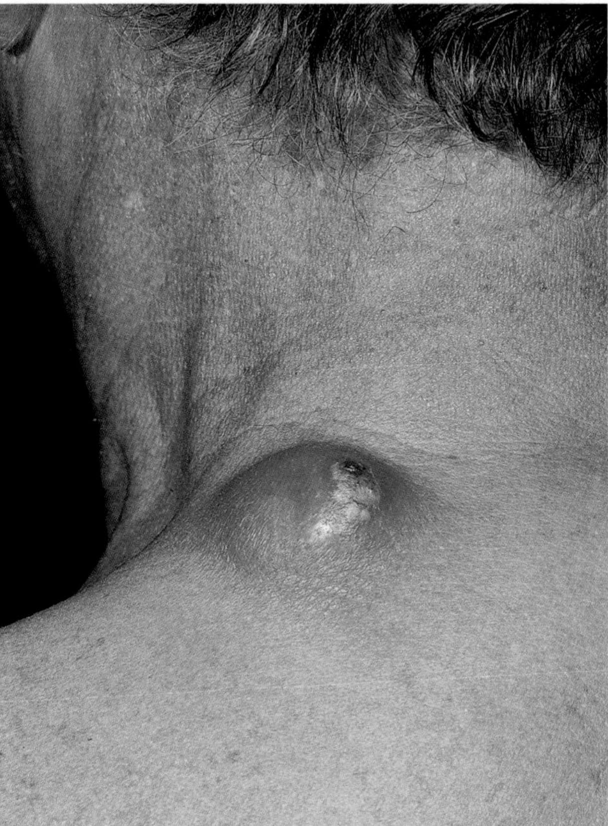

Figure 9-29 Ruptured epidermal cyst. This is commonly misinterpreted as a furuncle. A large mass of white, amorphous material and pus exudes after a linear incision is made over the surface.

TREATMENT OF FURUNCLES

WARM COMPRESSES. Many furuncles are self-limited and respond well to frequent applications of a moist, warm compress, which provide comfort and probably encourage localization and pointing of the abscess.

INCISION, DRAINAGE, AND PACKING. The primary management of cutaneous abscesses should be incision and drainage. In general, routine culture and antibiotic therapy are not indicated for localized abscesses in patients with presumably normal host defenses. The abscess is not ready for drainage until the skin has thinned and the underlying mass becomes soft and fluctuant. The skin around the central area is anesthetized with 1% lidocaine. A pointed, lance-shaped no. 11 surgical blade is inserted and drawn parallel to skin lines through the thin, effaced skin, creating an opening from which pus may be expressed easily with light pressure. Care must be taken to avoid extending the incision into firm, noneffaced skin. A curette is inserted through the opening and carefully drawn back and forth to break adhesions and dislodge fragments of necrotic tissue. Continuous drainage may be promoted in very large abscesses by packing the cavity with a long ribbon of iodoform gauze. The end of the ribbon is inserted through a curette loop. The curette is then turned to secure the gauze, inserted deep into the cavity, and twisted in the reverse direction and removed concurrently, while the gauze is held in place with a thin-tipped forceps. Next, the gauze is worked into the cavity with the forceps until resistance is met. The gauze quickly becomes saturated and should be removed hours later and replaced with a fresh packing.

CULTURE AND GRAM STAIN. These studies are indicated when there are recurrent abscesses, a failure to respond to conventional therapy, systemic toxicity, involvement of the central face, abscesses that contain gas or involve muscle or fascia, or when the patient is immunocompromised. Material for culture and Gram stain is collected in a sterile syringe by inserting the needle through the unbroken, effaced skin over the abscess. If anaerobic organisms are suspected, the material should be rapidly transported to the laboratory in the syringe or immediately inoculated into an anaerobic tube. Culturing of an abscess usually takes 48 hours or more to determine which bacteria are present. The Gram stain provides a rapid means of diagnosis.

ANTIBIOTICS. Patients with recurrent furunculosis learn that they can sometimes stop the progression of an abscess by starting antistaphylococcal antibiotics at the first sign of the typical localized swelling and erythema (see Table 9-1). They continue to use antibiotics for 5 to 10 days. Antibiotics should be started immediately to attenuate the evolving abscess. Antibiotics have little effect once the abscess has become fluctuant.

Recurrent furunculosis

Diseases manifesting as recurrent furunculosis are listed in Table 9-6.

MANAGEMENT

Although recurrent infection often ceases spontaneously after 2 years, a few patients have repeated episodes of furuncles that last for years. Several members of a family may be affected. Most of these patients are normal with an intact immune system. Most people do not carry *S. aureus* in the nose, but patients with recurrent furunculosis frequently carry the pathogenic strain of *S. aureus* in their nares and perineum. Therapy goals are to decrease or eliminate the pathogenic strain. The treatment program for recurrent furunculosis is described in Box 9-6.

Box 9-6 Treatment Program for Recurrent Furunculosis

ERADICATION OF *S. AUREUS* NASAL CARRIAGE

Program of first choice:

1. The major method of controlling recurrent furunculosis is the application of mupirocin ointment twice daily in the anterior nares for the first 5 days each month. This regimen reduces recurrences by 50%. *PMID: 8638999*
2. Culture the anterior nares every 3 months to check for the effectiveness of the above measure. Repeat with mupirocin or consider oral antibiotics for treatment failures.

Program for topical treatment failures:

1. Prescribe amoxicillin/clavulanate 375 or 625 mg three times a day for 7 to 10 days or a similar semisynthetic penicillin followed by 450 to 600 mg of rifampin once a day for 7 to 10 days. *PMID: 16787615* When culture of the anterior nares yields *S. aureus*, rifampin alone (given at 3-month intervals) significantly reduces the incidence of infection. Initial treatment with antibiotic for 2 months offers no benefit in preventing recurrences.
2. Another approach is to treat with oral clindamycin (150 mg daily) for 3 months. *PMID: 3184334* Treatment with systemic antibiotics eradicates the pathogenic organisms from the nares, perineum, and furuncles.)

OTHER MEASURES TO ERADICATE *S. AUREUS*

Instruct the patient to:

1. Wash the entire body and the fingernails with a nail brush each day for 1 to 3 weeks with Betadine, Hibiclens, or pHisoHex soap. The frequency of washing should be decreased if the skin becomes dry.
2. Change towels, washcloths, and sheets daily.
3. Change wound dressing frequently.
4. Clean shaving instruments thoroughly each day.
5. Avoid nose picking.

ERYSIPELOID

Erysipeloid is an acute skin infection caused by the gram-positive, rod-shaped, nonsporulating bacillus *Erysipelothrix rhusiopathiae* (or *E. insidiosa*). It has been found to cause infection in several dozen species of mammals and other animals and fish. Humans become infected through exposure to infected or contaminated animals or animal products. The disease is an occupational hazard for people who handle unprocessed meat and animal products, such as fishermen (fish poisoning, crab poisoning, seal finger, whale finger), meat handlers (swine erysipelas), butchers, farmers, and veterinarians. Patients who have repeated infections know that it responds to penicillin and treat themselves.

CLINICAL MANIFESTATIONS

The most common presentation is a localized, self-limited cutaneous lesion, erysipeloid. Diffuse cutaneous and systemic infections occur rarely. Approximately 1 to 7 days (an average of 3 days) after animal contact, a dull, red erythema appears at the inoculation site and extends centrifugally for 3 to 4 days to reach a fixed size of approximately 10 cm in diameter (Figure 9-30). Central clearing often occurs. Streptococcal cellulitis (erysipelas) is bright red and painful and spreads rapidly. Infection also occurs on the face, neck, and sole of the foot. There is burning, itching, and discomfort; lymphangitis or constitutional symptoms develop in a few patients. Arthropathy, sometimes longstanding, may develop. The disease is self-limited and may subside spontaneously. Relapse may occur from 4 days to 2 weeks after the lesions are completely resolved. Diffuse and systemic forms with extensive, red, diamond-shaped plaques, septic arthritis, and endocarditis are rare.

DIAGNOSIS

The organism may be isolated from biopsy or blood specimens on standard culture media.

TREATMENT

Although there are many instances of cutaneous forms of the disease running a self-limited course, all patients should receive antibiotics to prevent progression to systemic disease and the development of endocarditis. The disease responds to penicillin G, cephalosporins, erythromycin, and fluoroquinolones.

BLISTERING DISTAL DACTYLITIS

Blistering distal dactylitis (BDD) is a superficial infection of the anterior fat pad of the fingertips. The age range of most of the reported patients is 2 to 16 years but adult cases are also reported. Blistering distal dactylitis presents as oval bullae 10 to 30 mm in diameter. It is most commonly caused by group A beta-hemolytic streptococci (Figure 9-31). *S. aureus* is the cause in a few reported patients. A large blister filled with a watery, purulent fluid forms on the volar surface of the distal portion of the fingers. A firm diagnosis can be made with a Gram stain and culture of the blister fluid. Treatment consists of incision, drainage, and a 10-day course of antistreptococcal systemic antibiotics. BDD can occur on the proximal phalangeal and palmar areas of the hands and can manifest as multiple bullae.

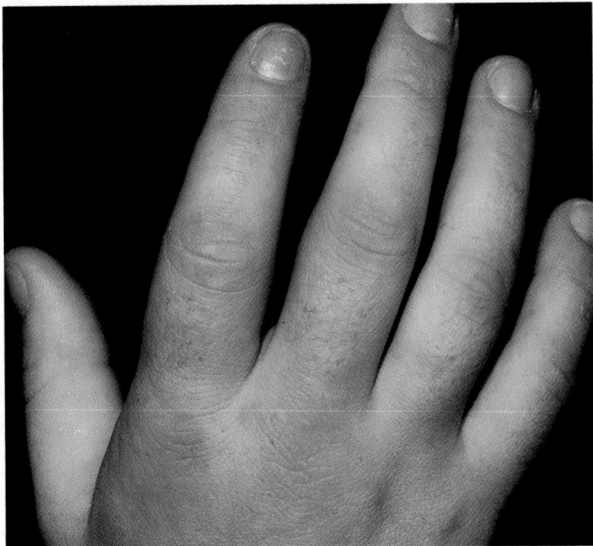

Figure 9-30 Erysipeloid. Approximately 3 days after animal or fish contact, a dull red erythema appears at the inoculation site and extends centrifugally.

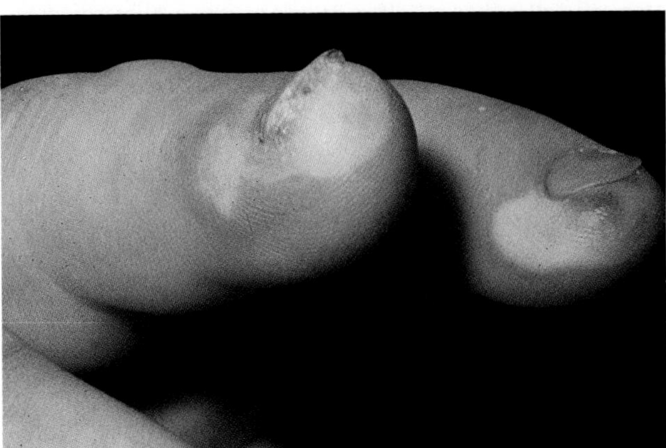

Figure 9-31 Blistering distal dactylitis. This superficial infection of the anterior fat pad of the distal portion of the fingers is caused most commonly by group A beta-hemolytic streptococci. (Courtesy Lucia Martin-Moreno, MD.)

STAPHYLOCOCCAL SCALDED SKIN SYNDROME

Staphylococcal scalded skin syndrome (SSSS) is a blistering disease caused by *Staphylococcus aureus* exfoliative toxins (ETs). These toxins cause intraepidermal splitting through the granular layer by cleavage of desmoglein 1, a desmosomal cadherin protein that mediates cell-cell adhesion of keratinocytes in the granular layer. Bullous impetigo is the localized form of SSSS. It begins with a skin infection with a *S. aureus* strain producing ETs that can be recovered from the bullae. The generalized form of SSSS affects newborns (Ritter's disease), infants, and children, but rarely adults. Fluid from bullae is sterile but the *S. aureus* can be isolated from distant sites, such as the nose. SSSS may then develop from systemic absorption of ETs from the colonized site that are then spread through the bloodstream to the skin. It is explained by a lack of immunity to the toxins and by renal immaturity in children that leads to poor clearance of toxins. There are three serological forms of staphylococcal ETs (ETA, ETB, and ETD). ETA and ETB cause SSSS. ETB is more frequently isolated than ETA in children with generalized SSSS.

Epidermolytic toxin

Blisters in bullous impetigo and the scalded skin syndrome (SSSS) are caused by exfoliative toxin released by staphylococcus. In patients with bullous impetigo, the toxin produces blisters locally at the site of infection. In cases of scalded skin syndrome, the toxin circulates throughout the body, causing blisters at sites distant from the infection. The toxin is antigenic and when elaborated elicits an antibody response. Two antigenically distinct forms—toxin A and toxin B—have been identified. Epidermolytic toxin antibody is present in 75% of normal people older than 10 years of age, a fact that explains the rarity of SSSS in adults. It is speculated that the toxins act on desmoglein 1, a component of desmosomes in epithelial cells that mediates cell-cell adhesion. This attack causes a blister just below the stratum corneum similar to that seen in pemphigus foliaceus.

Incidence

The childhood form of SSSS is most often seen in otherwise healthy children. About 62% of children are younger than 2 years old; 98% are 6 years or younger. The rare, adult type of generalized SSSS is associated with underlying diseases related to immunosuppression, abnormal immunity, and renal insufficiency. The risk of death from SSSS is less than 5% among children, but among adults the syndrome usually occurs in those who are immunosuppressed, and the risk of death can be as high as 60%.

CLINICAL MANIFESTATIONS

SSSS begins with a localized, often inapparent, *S. aureus* infection of the conjunctivae, throat, nares, or umbilicus. A diffuse, tender erythema appears; the skin has a sandpaper-like texture similar to that seen in scarlet fever. The erythema is often accentuated in flexural and periorificial areas. However, the rash of scarlet fever is not tender. The temperature rises and within 1 or 2 days the skin wrinkles, forms transient bullae, and peels off in large sheets, leaving a moist, red, glistening surface (Figures 9-32 through 9-36). Minor pressure induces skin separation (Nikolsky's sign). The area of involvement may be localized, but it is often generalized. Evaporative fluid loss from large areas is associated with increased fluid loss and dehydration. A yellow crust forms, and the denuded surface dries and cracks. Healing occurs in 7 to 10 days, accompanied by desquamation similar to that seen in scarlet fever. Reepithelialization is rapid because of the high level of the split in the epidermis. Distinguishing between the localized form of SSSS and bullous impetigo can be difficult. The criteria in favor of localized SSSS are (1) the absence of inflammatory cells in the dermis on biopsy, (2) erythematous skin with tenderness, (3) Nikolsky's phenomenon around lesions, and (4) a negative culture result from intact bullae. Staphylococcal scarlatiniform eruption is similar to SSSS, except that the skin does not blister or peel.

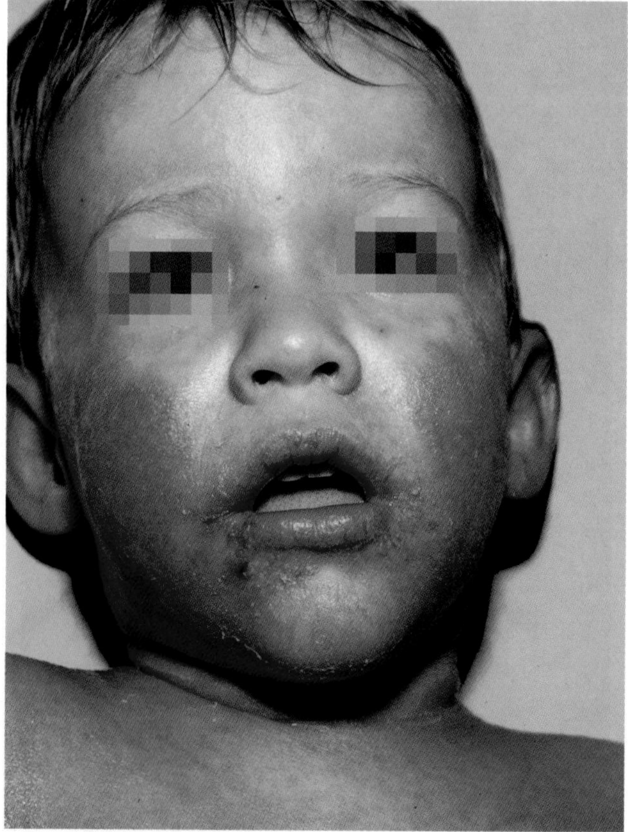

Figure 9-32 Staphylococcus scalded skin syndrome. The face is frequently involved. The skin becomes red followed by the formation of blisters. Blisters rupture leaving an eroded base that looks like a burn.

STAPHYLOCOCCAL SCALDED SKIN SYNDROME

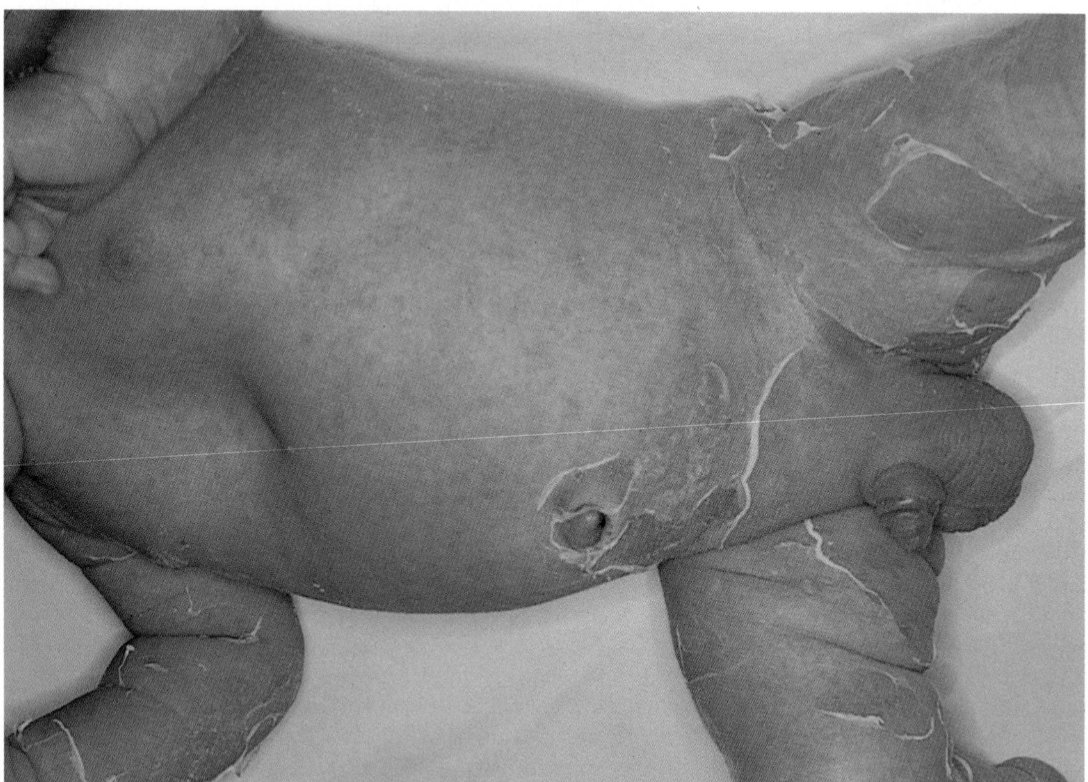

Figure 9-33 Staphylococcal scalded skin syndrome. A scarlatiniform eruption appears followed by a tissue paper–like wrinkling of the epidermis. Bullae then appear around body orifices and in the axillae and groin. Sheets of epidermis then shed and reveal a moist erythematous base. Healing occurs in 5 to 7 days.

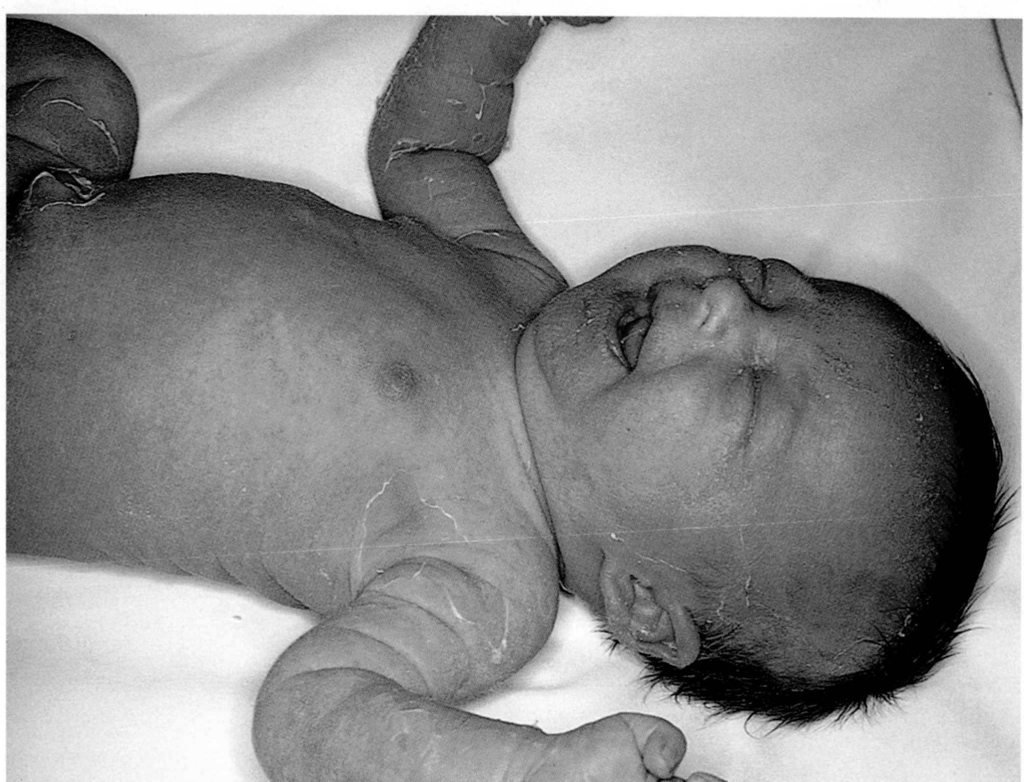

Figure 9-34 Staphylococcal scalded skin syndrome. Exfoliative phase, during which the upper epidermis is shed.

PATHOPHYSIOLOGY

The epidermolytic toxin is filtered through the glomeruli and partially reabsorbed in the proximal tubule where it undergoes catabolism by the proximal tubule cells. The glomerular filtration rate of infants is less than 50% of the normal adult rate, which is reached in the second year of life. This may explain why infants, patients with chronic renal failure, and those on hemodialysis may be predisposed to SSSS.

DIAGNOSIS

With SSSS, a biopsy shows splitting of the epidermis in the stratum granulosum near the skin surface; there is scant inflammation. Thin-roofed bullae are flaccid and rupture easily. Culture specimens should be taken from the eye, nose, throat, bullae, and any obviously infected area. Skin and blood culture results are often negative in children and positive in adults. SSSS must be differentiated from toxic epidermal necrolysis, a rare, life-threatening disease in which full-thickness epidermal necrosis occurs. Histologically, toxic epidermal necrolysis shows dermal-epidermal separation, rather than the granular layer split in the epidermis seen in SSSS and an intense inflammatory infiltrate. A frozen section of peeled skin is a reliable way of rapidly establishing the diagnosis. Many of the reported adult cases had positive blood culture results; children younger than 5 years infrequently have sepsis. Cultures from bullae have also been reported to be positive, but this may have been the result of contamination. Several reported adult patients were receiving systemic steroids.

TREATMENT

Corticosteroids are contraindicated because they interfere with host defense mechanisms. Hospitalization and intravenous antibiotic therapy are desirable for extensive cases. Most of the toxin-producing *S. aureus* bacteria produce penicillinase. First-line systemic therapy is oral or intravenous flucloxacillin or a similar drug active against beta-lactamase-producing *Staphylococcus aureus*. Patients with limited disease may be managed at home with oral antibiotics such as dicloxacillin 25 mg/kg per day, or a cephalosporin is prescribed for a minimum of 1 week. Topical antibiotics are not necessary. The patient's skin should be lubricated with bland, light lotions and washed infrequently. Wet dressings may cause further drying and cracking and should be avoided. Nasal swabs from the patient and relatives should be performed to identify asymptomatic nasal carriers of *Staphylococcus aureus*. Outbreaks on wards and in nurseries may develop from health care professionals, who should also be swabbed.

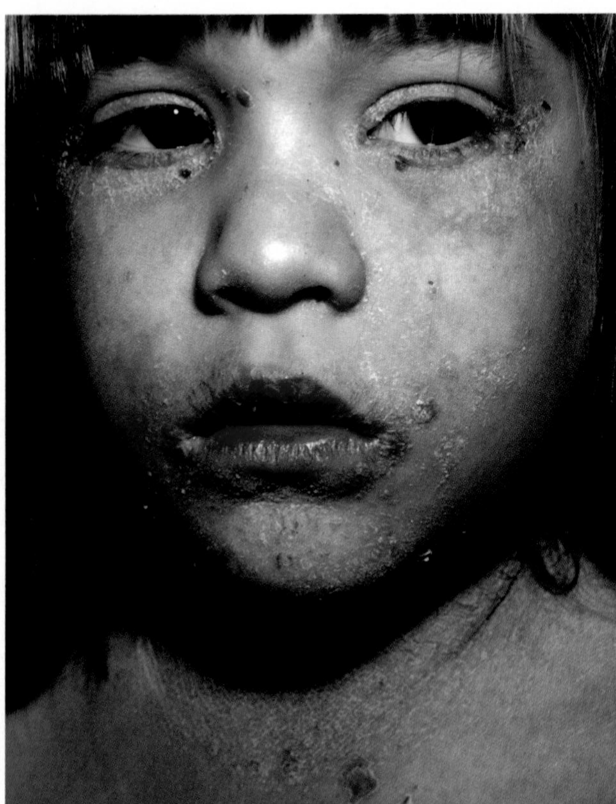

Figure 9-35 Staphyloccocal scalded skin syndrome. The infection often begins during the first few days of life in the diaper area; in older children, the face is the typical site. Toxin produced in these areas enters the circulation and affects the entire skin.

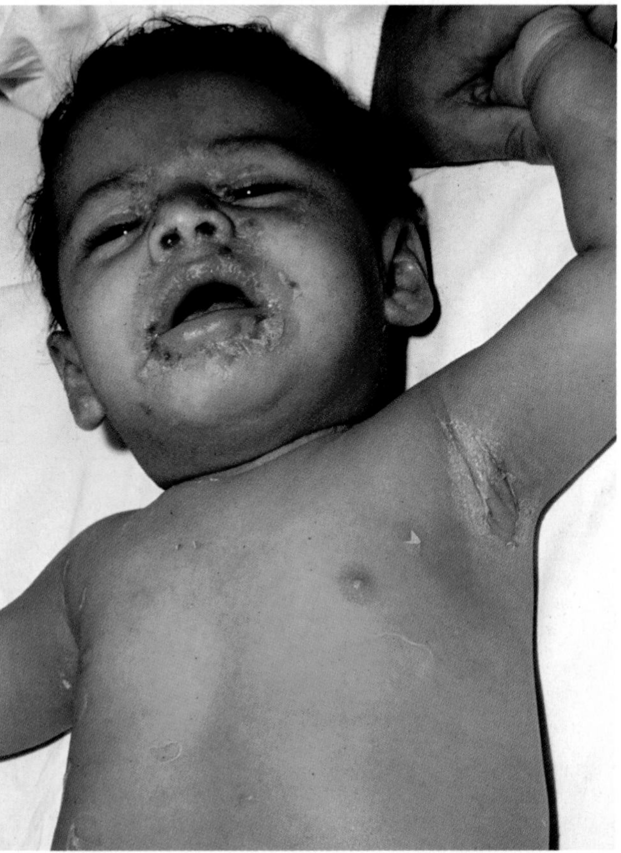

Figure 9-36 Staphyloccocal scalded skin syndrome. The rash spreads to the axillae, legs, and trunk. The diaper area is involved in newborns.

PSEUDOMONAS AERUGINOSA INFECTION

P. aeruginosa is a saprophytic intestinal gram-negative aerobic rod with a predilection for humid environments. In normal human skin, *Pseudomonas* species are part of the transitory skin flora and are found principally in the anogenital area, axillae, and external ear canal. Gram-positive cocci exert an inhibitory effect on the growth of *Pseudomonas* species. In immunocompromised hosts, skin fissures and erosions, venipuncture sites, nasogastric and endotracheal tubes, and urinary catheters are the usual portals of entry. The bacteria may colonize in warm, moist areas such as skin folds (toe webs), ear canals, burns, ulcers, and areas beneath nails. They are also found in the moist areas of sinks and drains and in poorly preserved topical creams and ointments. *P. aeruginosa* bacteria produce diffusible fluorescent pigments including pyoverdin and a soluble phenazine pigment called pyocyanin. Pyocyanin appears blue or green at neutral or alkaline pH and is the source of the name aeruginosa. An organic metabolite may impart a fruity odor to some cutaneous lesions. That same odor in culture is a specific quality of *P. aeruginosa*. *Pseudomonas* survives poorly in an acid environment. There are many serotypes.

Pseudomonas infects warm, moist areas in healthy people. Hot tub folliculitis and toe-web intertrigo occur because of a temporary change in the skin moisture content and temperature that allows pseudomonal overgrowth. Correction of the altered environment results in resolution of the infection. Severe, life-threatening infections occur in patients with impaired immunity, such as those with serious burns or acute leukemia or those receiving immunosuppressive therapy.

Oral treatment of *Pseudomonas* infections is possible with fluoroquinolones such as ciprofloxacin hydrochloride (Cipro).

Pseudomonas folliculitis

From 8 hours to 5 days or longer (mean incubation period is 48 hours) after using a contaminated whirlpool, home hot tub, waterslide, physiotherapy pool, or contaminated loofah sponge, *Pseudomonas* folliculitis develops in 7% to 100% of exposed patients. The attack rate is significantly higher in children than in adults, possibly because they tend to spend more time in the water. Showering after using the contaminated facility offers no protection.

CLINICAL MANIFESTATIONS

The typical patient has a few to more than 50 0.5- to 3-cm, pruritic, round, urticarial plaques with a central papule or pustule located on all skin surfaces except the head (Figure 9-37). The rash may be follicular, maculopapular, vesicular, pustular, or a polymorphous eruption that includes all these types of lesions. Women who wear one-piece bathing suits are at an increased risk (Figures 9-37 through 9-42). The eruption, in most cases, clears in 7 to 10 days, leaving round spots of red-brown, postinflammatory hyperpigmentation, but patients have been reported to have recurrent crops of lesions for as long as 3 months. The spread of infection from person to person is not likely. Malaise and fatigue may occur during the initial few days of the eruption. Fever is uncommon and low grade when it appears.

PATHOPHYSIOLOGY

Under normal conditions, *P. aeruginosa* infection cannot be induced by inoculation of the microorganism onto the intact skin surface of immune-competent persons. Occlusion and superhydration of the stratum corneum favor colonization of the skin with *P. aeruginosa*. This may explain why the rash is most severe in areas occluded by a snug bathing suit. *P. aeruginosa* serotypes 0:9 and 0:11 are most commonly isolated from skin lesions, but other serotypes have been reported. Three conditions are associated with folliculitis: prolonged exposure to the water, an excessive number of bathers, and inadequate pool care. The organism gains entry via the hair follicles or breaks in the skin. The increased water temperature promotes sweating, which enhances penetration of the skin by the bacteria. Also, with heavy use, there are desquamated skin cells in the water, providing a rich, organic nutrient source for the bacteria. The ubiquitous *P. aeruginosa* rapidly multiply in water at increased temperatures.

MANAGEMENT

The infection is self-limited, but a 5% acetic acid (white vinegar) wet compress applied for 20 minutes two to four times a day and/or silver sulfadiazine cream (Silvadene) might be of some help. Cases resistant to topical therapy can be treated orally with ciprofloxacin (Cipro) 500 or 750 mg twice each day.

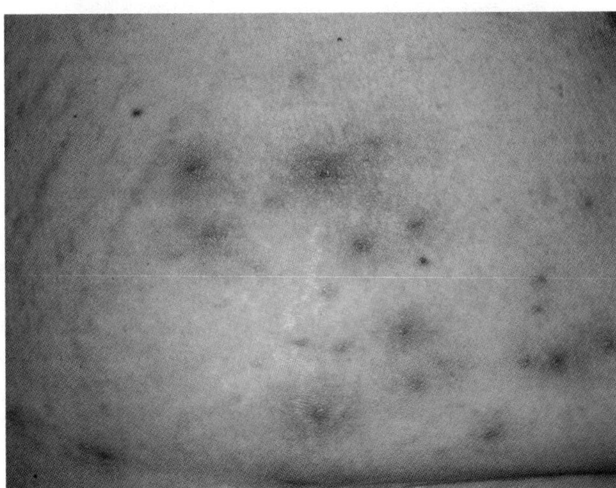

Figure 9-37 *Pseudomonas* folliculitis. Follicular papules, vesicles, and pustules progress to red papulopustules that have a central pustule.

PSEUDOMONAS FOLLICULITIS

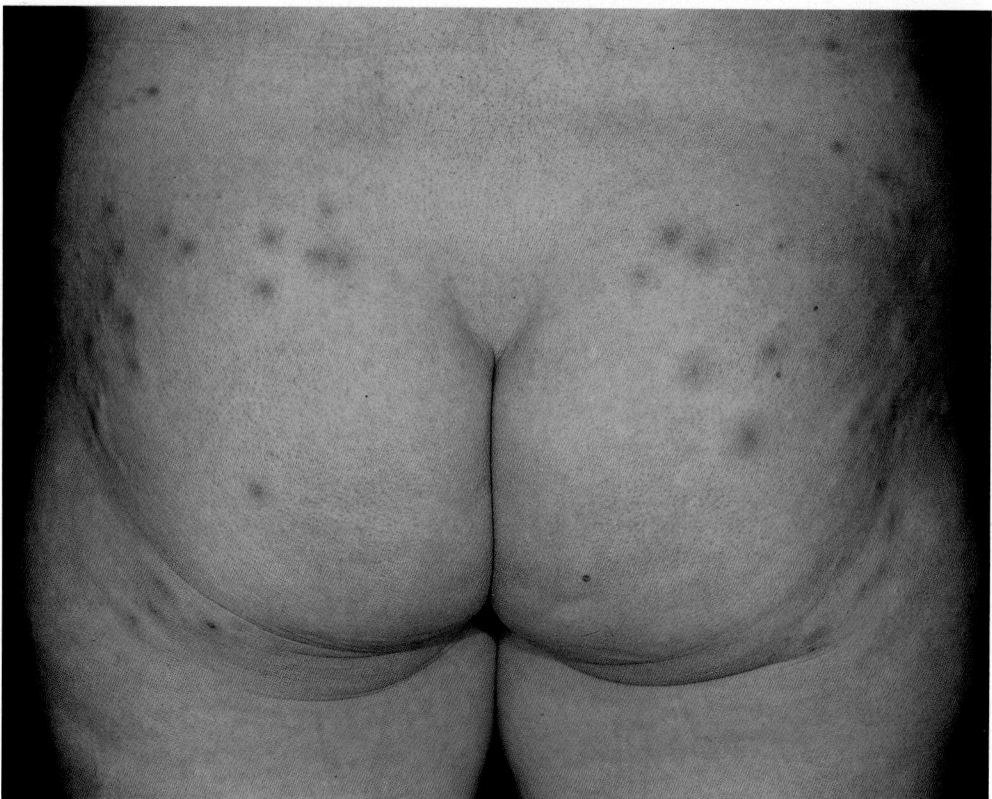

Figure 9-38 Urticarial plaques surmounted by pustules located primarily in the areas covered by the bathing suit.

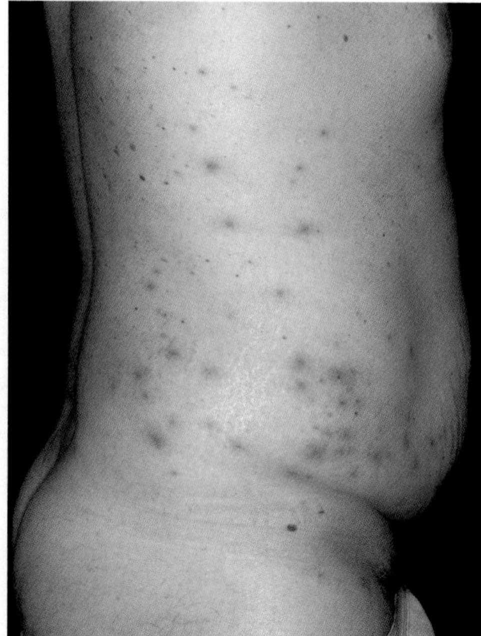

Figure 9-39 Lesions may begin as itchy red macules that progress to papules and pustules. Lesions are prevalent in intertriginous areas or under bathing suits.

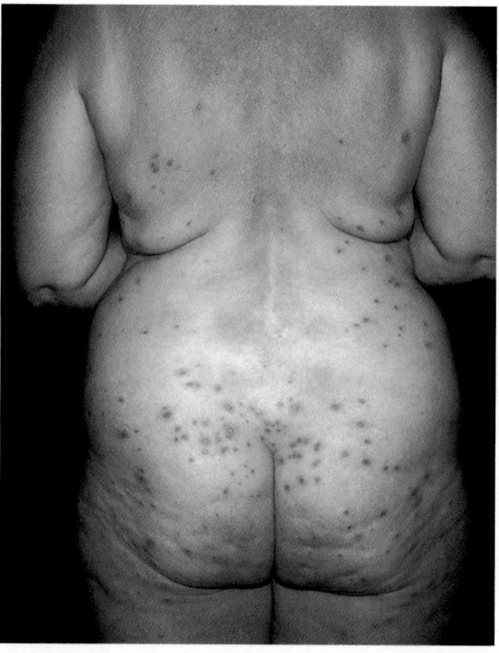

Figure 9-40 The rash usually clears in 7-14 days and heals without scarring.

Preventative measures include continuous water filtration to eliminate desquamated skin, frequent monitoring of the disinfectant levels, and frequent changing of the water, especially during heavy use. Public hot tubs and whirlpools with heavy use should be drained completely on a daily basis and the interior should be cleaned daily with an acidic solution. A heavy bather load, turbulent water, and aeration make it difficult to maintain satisfactory levels of chlorine. The Centers for Disease Control and Prevention recommends a free chlorine or bromine concentration of 3 to 6 ppm as health and safety guidelines for public spas and hot tubs. The recommended pH of a pool is between 7.6 and 7.8, because a higher water pH shifts the dissociation of chlorine or bromine, making them much less effective. In addition, more chlorine is often necessary to maintain the same chlorine levels at a higher temperature as in hot tub use. Infection may also be further prevented by reducing the abrasiveness of the floors of pools or hot tubs, given that most cases of *Pseudomonas* folliculitis hot-hand or hot-foot syndrome affect children with a thin stratum corneum layer of the epidermis on their palms and soles.

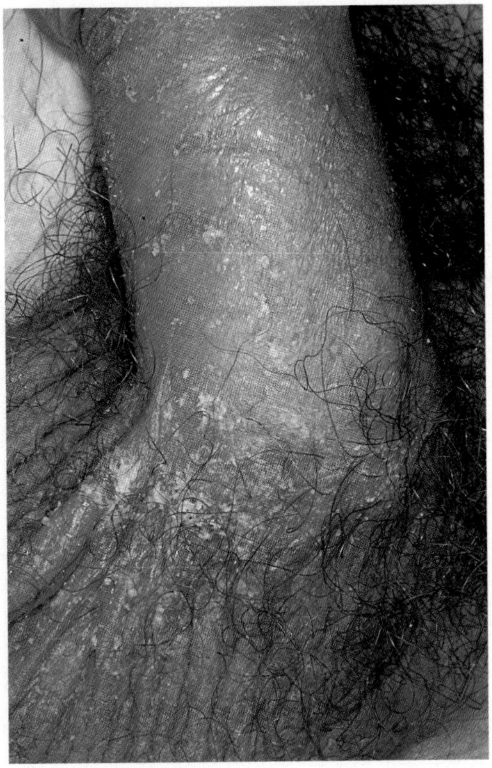

Figure 9-41 *Pseudomonas* cellulitis. Maceration occurred in the intertriginous area between the penis and scrotum. A painful cellulitis occurred. Culture showed pseudomonas.

Pseudomonas cellulitis

Pseudomonas cellulitis may be localized or may occur during *Pseudomonas* septicemia. The localized form occurs as a secondary infection of tinea of the toe webs or groin (Figure 9-42), bed sores, stasis ulcers, burns, grafted areas, under the foreskin of the penis, and following an injury. Maceration or occlusion of these cutaneous lesions encourages secondary infection with *Pseudomonas*. Suppression of normal bacterial flora by broad-spectrum antibiotics encourages secondary infection. *Pseudomonas* infection is often unsuspected and appropriate therapy is therefore delayed. Deep erosions and tissue necrosis may occur before the correct diagnosis is made. Severe pain is highly characteristic of an evolving infection. The skin turns a dusky red (see Figure 9-42). Bluish green, purulent material with a fruity or "mousey" odor accumulates as the red, indurated area becomes macerated and then eroded. Vesicles and pustules may occur as satellite lesions. The eruption may spread to cover wide areas and be accompanied by systemic symptoms. *Pseudomonas* septicemia may produce a deep, indurated, necrotic cellulitis that resembles other forms of infectious cellulitis.

TREATMENT

Treatment consists of 5% acetic acid (white vinegar) wet compresses applied 20 minutes four times a day. Localized infections respond to oral treatment with ciprofloxacin (Cipro) 500 or 750 mg twice each day. Severe infections may respond to clinafloxacin administered intravenously.

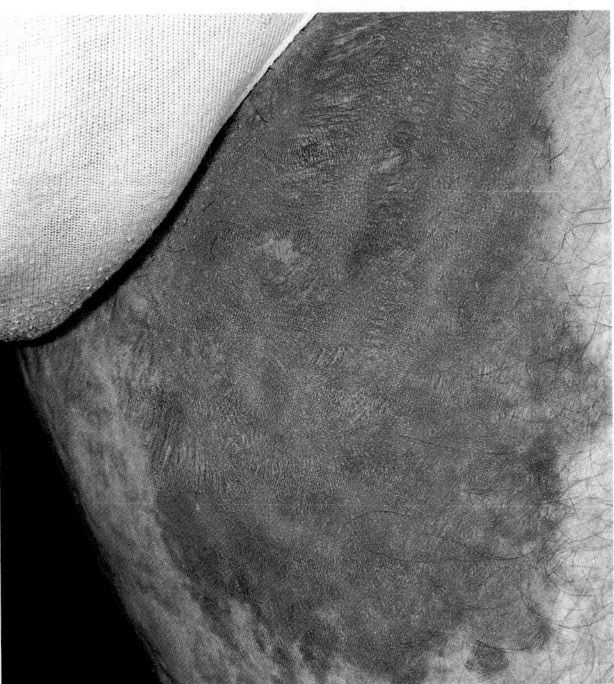

Figure 9-42 Inflamed area has a "mousey" or grape juice–like odor.

External otitis

Excessive moisture and trauma impairing the canal's natural defenses are the most common precipitants of otitis externa. Inflammation of the external auditory canal can be localized or diffuse and acute or chronic. Predisposing conditions include external trauma, loss of the canal's protective coating, maceration of the skin from water or humidity, and glandular obstruction. Acute otitis externa is generally caused by *P. aeruginosa* or *S. aureus*.

External otitis is an inflammation of the external auditory canal. It occurs in a mild, self-limited form (swimmer's ear) or as an acute and chronic, recurrent, debilitating disease. The normally acidic cerumen inhibits gram-negative bacterial growth and forms a protective layer that discourages maceration. Swimming or excessive manipulation while cleaning the canal may disrupt this natural barrier. Inflammatory diseases such as psoriasis, seborrheic dermatitis, and eczematous dermatitis disrupt the normal barrier and encourage infection. *Pseudomonas* is the most common bacteria isolated from both mild and severe external otitis. Most cases, however, represent a mixed infection with other gram-negative (*Proteus mirabilis, Klebsiella pneumoniae*) and gram-positive (*S. epidermidis,* beta-hemolytic streptococci) bacteria. Fungal infection with *Candida* or *Aspergillus niger* sometimes occurs, and these organisms may be the primary pathogens.

CLINICAL MANIFESTATIONS. Discomfort, erythema, and swelling of the canal with variable discharge are the common signs and symptoms. The early stages are characterized by erythema, edema, and an accumulation of moist, cellular debris in the canal. Traction on the pinna or tragus may elicit pain. If the disease progresses, erythema radiates into the pinna and purulent material partly obstructs and exudes from the canal. Pain becomes constant and more intense. Cellulitis of the pinna and skin surrounding the ear accompanied by a dense mucopurulent exudate discharging from the canal may result from infection with *Pseudomonas* (Figures 9-43, 9-44, and 9-45). However, in most cases, this indicates a secondary infection with staphylococci and streptococci.

The lymphatics of the external ear may be permanently damaged during an attack of cellulitis, predisposing the patient to recurrent episodes of streptococcal erysipelas of the pinna. Recurrent attacks are triggered by manipulation or even the slightest trauma. Eczematous inflammation and infection of the external ear and surrounding skin may occur for a variety of reasons, such as irritation from purulent exudate, scratching and manipulation, or allergy to topical medications. Habitual manipulation may cause this disease to persist for years.

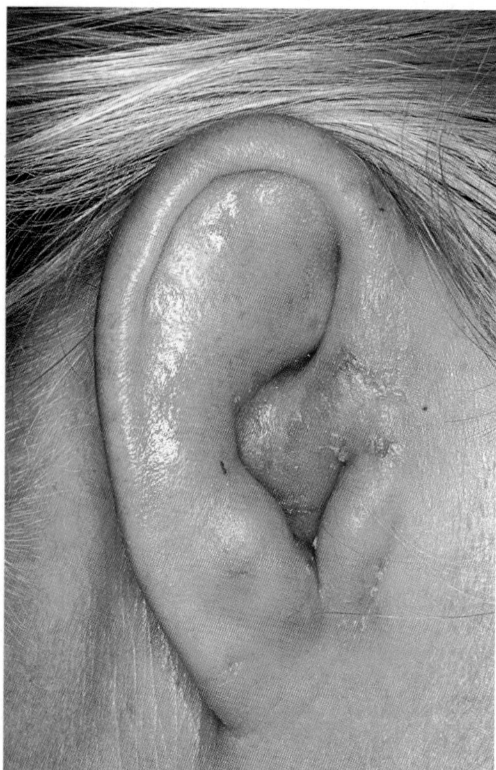

Figure 9-43 *Pseudomonas* cellulitis. The entire pinna and surrounding skin have become inflamed after an episode of external otitis.

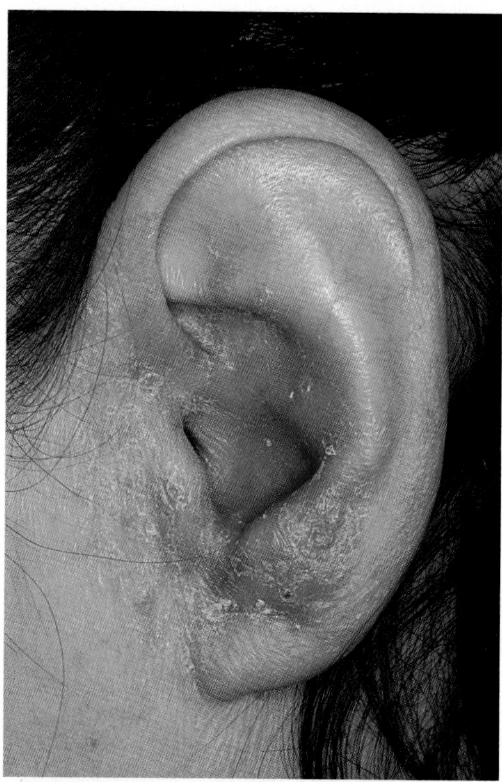

Figure 9-44 External otitis. Chronic inflammation of the canal progressed to involve the pinna. Erythema and scale (eczema) followed chronic manipulation of the pinna. Group V topical steroids were required for control

ECZEMATOUS EXTERNAL OTITIS

Eczema of the ear canal tends to be chronic or recurrent. Patients present with erythema and scaling. Allergy to topical preparations (such as neomycin sulfate and potassium dichromate) is a common cause. Patients suffering from eczematous external otitis who fail to respond to topical steroids should be patch tested for allergens.

TREATMENT. Treatment of patients with otitis externa includes debridement, topical therapy with acidifying and antimicrobial agents, and systemic antimicrobial therapy when indicated. The treatment of patients with chronic otitis externa includes cleansing and debridement accompanied by topical acidifying and drying agents.

CLEANSING AND DEBRIDEMENT. Cleansing is essential for treatment; flushing should be avoided. Squamous debris, cerumen, and pus are removed by suction or irrigation with an ear syringe.

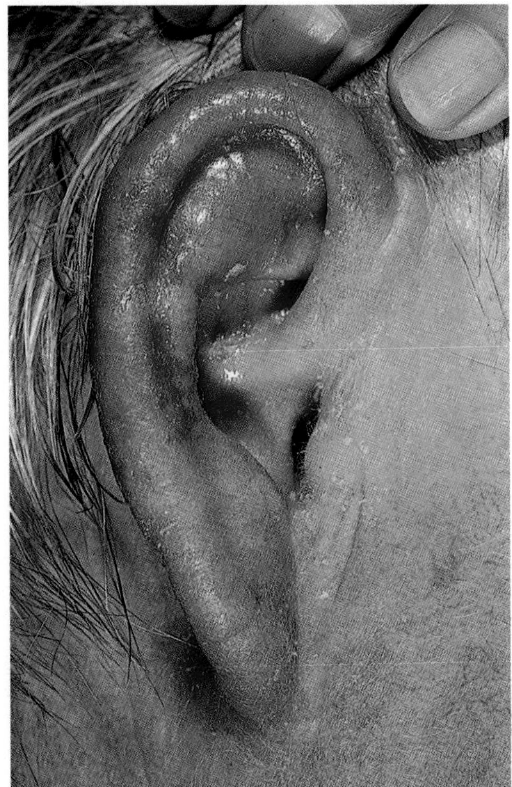

Figure 9-45 External otitis. Eczema of the pinna has become infected and painful. Culture showed staphylococcal infection and not *Pseudomonas*. Dicloxacillin 500 mg four times a day controlled the infection. Group V topical steroids were then used to treat the eczema.

TOPICAL THERAPY

TOPICAL STEROIDS. Ear drops containing 0.05% solution of betamethasone dipropionate (a group III steroid solution) applied twice daily cure external otitis whether or not there is infection. *PMID: 15949095* Fluocinolone acetonide in peanut oil 0.01% ear drops (DermOtic) are available for the treatment of chronic eczematous external otitis. With the supplied ear-dropper, apply 5 drops of oil into the affected ear.

TOPICAL ANTIBIOTICS. Topical antibiotics should be considered for infection localized to the canal. Ofloxacin given twice daily is as safe and effective as Cortisporin given four times daily for otitis externa. A culture specimen of canal drainage is obtained.

TACROLIMUS. The application of 0.1% tacrolimus ointment in the outer ear canal is an effective option in corticosteroid-free treatment of chronic therapy-resistant external otitis. An ear wick containing 0.1% tacrolimus ointment (Protopic) is inserted into the external auditory canal every second to third day. *PMID: 17440424*

ACIDIFICATION. Acidification is accomplished with a topical solution of 2% acetic acid (Domeboro otic). Some solutions add hydrocortisone for inflammation (VöSol HC otic). Acidification creates an environment that is inhospitable to gram-negative bacteria and fungi. These are effective treatments in most cases and, when used after exposure to moisture, are an excellent prophylactic.

WICKS. Ear wicks are made of strands of cotton or fine cloth and are inserted into the canal to act as a conduit for application of otic solutions. If properly saturated, they will keep medication in contact with all surfaces of the canal. Solution must be added almost hourly to maintain saturation. New wicks are inserted daily. The use of a wick is usually unnecessary for mild inflammation but may be considered when the canal is partially obstructed by swelling and edema. The wick must be introduced before the canal swells, which makes insertion painful or impossible.

SYSTEMIC ANTIMICROBIAL THERAPY. Infections that progress beyond the canal to the pinna and surrounding tissues are treated orally with ciprofloxacin (Cipro) 500 or 750 mg twice each day.

PREVENTION

Prevention of recurrent external otitis is aimed at minimizing ear canal trauma and the avoidance of exposure to water. Drying the ears with a hair dryer and avoiding manipulation of the external auditory canal may help prevent recurrence.

TREATING ECZEMA

Group III to IV topical steroids, wet compresses, and oral antibiotics are used when eczematous inflammation and infection occur on the external ear and surrounding skin. These can be instilled deep in the canal by connecting a syringe filled with medication to a Zollinger or disposable metal sucker tip, and then the ear canal can be filled under direct microscopic vision. (See the section on the treatment of eczematous inflammation in Chapter 3.)

Local injection of triamcinolone acetonide in the external auditory canal is effective in the management of chronic external otitis that may be accompanied by thickening of the skin in the external auditory canal.

Malignant external otitis

Malignant otitis externa is a life-threatening infection arising from the external auditory canal. The infection spreads to involve the temporal and adjacent bones. It is often initiated by self-inflicted or iatrogenic trauma to the external auditory canal. Patients with malignant external otitis present with a history of nonresolving otitis externa of many weeks' or months' duration (Figure 9-46). Most patients have diabetes mellitus. *Pseudomonas* infection penetrates the epithelium and invades underlying soft tissues. There is severe ear pain, which is worse at night, and purulent discharge. The external canal is edematous. Granulation tissue may be present, arising from the osseous cartilaginous junction at the floor of the canal or anteriorly. The infection then penetrates the floor of the canal at the bony cartilaginous junction and spreads to the base of the skull. Malignant external otitis is an osteomyelitis of the skull base. More advanced cases demonstrate cranial nerve palsies, most frequently involving cranial nerve VII. Diagnosis requires culture of ear secretions and pathologic examination of granulation tissue.

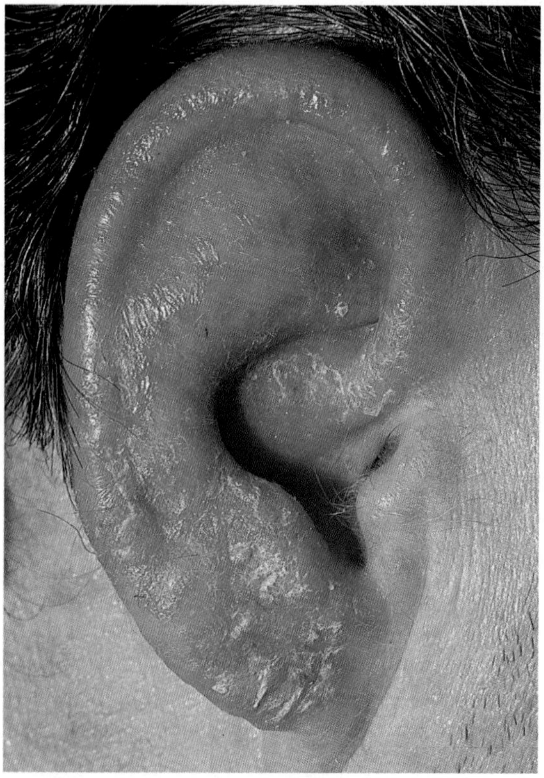

Figure 9-46 Malignant external otitis. Severe infection of the ear has occurred after months of chronic inflammation of the pinna.

IMAGING STUDIES

Imaging studies may include computed tomographic (CT) scanning, technetium (Tc) 99m medronate bone scanning, and gallium citrate (Ga) 67 scintigraphy. The diagnosis is confirmed by nuclear scanning studies and CT scanning of the temporal bone and skull base. CT scans show evidence of involvement of disease outside the external auditory canal; 70% of patients show bone erosion, and 25% show involvement of the petrous apex. Patients with petrous apical involvement present with cranial nerve palsies. CT findings of temporal bone involvement in itself are not closely correlated to the clinical outcomes of the patients. *PMID: 17680261* The criteria for diagnosis are listed in Box 9-7.

MANAGEMENT

The treatment of malignant external otitis has evolved from primarily surgical to one in which prolonged medical therapy of the underlying osteomyelitis with limited surgical debridement leads to a cure (see algorithm Manage-

Box 9-7 **Diagnostic Criteria of Malignant External Otitis**

Obligatory criteria:*

- Severe prolonged pain
- Edema
- Purulent exudate
- Granulation tissue
- Microabscess (when operated)
- Positive Tc99 bone scan of temporal bone (importance in detecting osteomyelitis)
- Failure of local treatment often more than 1 week
- Recovery of *Pseudomonas* in culture
- Soft tissue involvement and bone destruction (nasopharyngeal involvement) on CT scan

Occasional criteria:

- Diabetes
- Cranial nerve involvement (from subtemporal extension of the infection)
- Positive radiograph
- Debilitating condition
- Old age

*All obligatory criteria must be present to make the diagnosis.
Adapted from Cohen D, Friedman P: The diagnostic criteria of malignant external otitis, *J Laryngol Otol* 101(3):216-221, 1987. *PMID: 3106547*

MANAGEMENT OF MALIGNANT EXTERNAL OTITIS

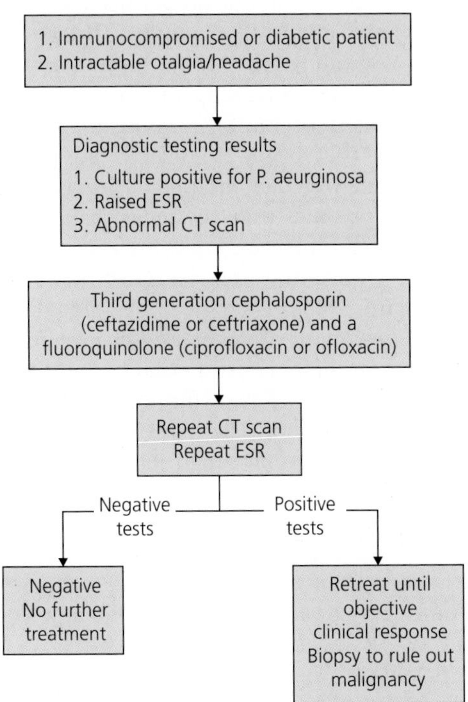

Figure 9-47 (With permission from Meningitis Research Foundation, 2008; accessed at www.meningitis.org.)

ment of malignant external otitis [Figure 9-47]). Therapy consists of using a third-generation cephalosporin (ceftazidime or ceftriaxone) and a fluoroquinolone (ciprofloxacin or ofloxacin). The association of ciprofloxacin and ceftazidime is efficient in countering the increasing resistance of *P. aeruginosa* to quinolones. Surgery is not indicated.

Toe web infection

Pseudomonas toe web infection is a distinctive clinical entity that is often misdiagnosed as tinea pedis. A thick, white, macerated scale with a green discoloration may appear in the toe webs of people who wear heavy, wet boots (Figure 9-48). The most constant clinical feature is soggy wetness of the toe webs and immediately adjacent skin. In its mildest form, the affected tissue is damp, softened, boggy, and white. The second, third, and fourth toe webs are the most common sites of initial involvement. More severe forms may progress to denudation of affected skin and profuse, serous, or purulent discharge. In most cases, this sopping-wet denudation involves all toe webs and extends onto the plantar surface and the dorsal and plantar surfaces of the toes, and an area approximately 1 cm wide beyond the base of the toes on the plantar surface of the foot. All patients are males with broad feet, square toes, and tight interdigital spaces. Close skin-to-skin contact and friction between the toes is a constant feature. Wood's light examination may show a green-white fluorescence resulting from elaboration of pyoverdin, and a green stain may be found on socks, bandages, toenails, and dried exudate. The green stain is due to elaboration of bacterial pyocyanin. *Pseudomonas* or a mixed flora of *Pseudomonas* organisms and fungi may be isolated from the soggy scale.

TREATMENT

First, the thickened, edematous, and devitalized layers of the epidermis are debrided. Repeated applications of silver nitrate (0.5%) soaks or 5% acetic acid (white vinegar) to the toe webs and the dorsal and plantar surfaces promote dryness and suppress bacteria. Gentamicin cream, silver sulfadiazine cream (Silvadene), or Castellani's paint (Derma-Cas gel) are then applied until the infection has resolved. Infections that do not respond to topical therapy are treated with ciprofloxacin (Cipro) 500 or 750 mg twice each day. Some *Pseudomonas* strains have developed resistance to Cipro.

Measures to prevent reinfection include the use of gauze pledgets between toes to prevent occlusion, the use of sandals or open-weave shoes to enhance evaporation of sweat, and the use of astringents such as 20% aluminum chloride (Drysol) to promote dryness.

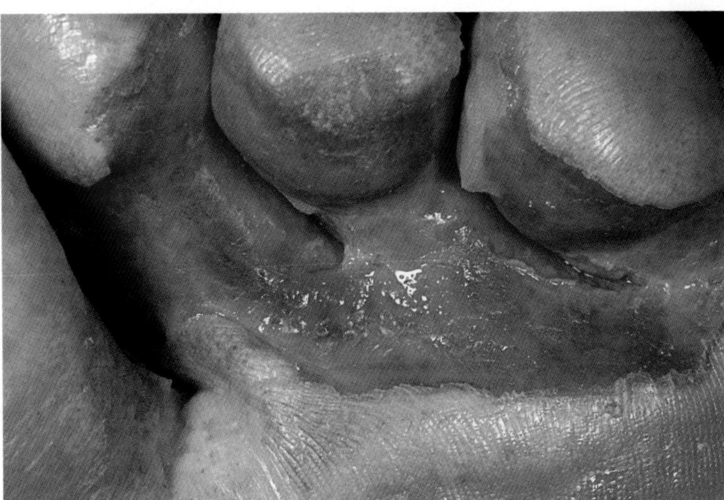

Figure 9-48 *Pseudomonas* cellulitis. A broad, eroded, ulcerated lesion started from macerated toe-web scale. The skin around the erosions was stained green.

Ecthyma gangrenosum

Ecthyma gangrenosum (EG) is the cutaneous manifestation of *P. aeruginosa* septicemia, typically affecting immunosuppressed patients, particularly those with neutropenia. Systemic *P. aeruginosa* usually complicates debilitating conditions, such as leukemia, burns, and cystic fibrosis. Many other pathogens can produce clinically indistinguishable lesions. It is not to be confused with pyoderma gangrenosum or streptococcal ecthyma. It is a rare but highly characteristic entity that is pathognomonic of *Pseudomonas* infection. The lesions represent either a bloodborne, metastatic seeding of *P. aeruginosa* to the skin or a primary lesion with no bacteremia. The mortality rate is high for the septicemic form and approximately 15% without bacteremia. The disease is rare, occurring in only 1.3% to 6.0% of patients with *Pseudomonas* sepsis. There are usually less than 10 lesions.

All patients have predisposing factors that increase their risk for infection. EG occurs in immunocompromised patients (neoplasia, leukemia, immunosuppressive treatment, graft recipients, malnutrition, diabetes), in burn patients, and in patients who have been treated with penicillin. Many patients have a disorder that leads to severe neutropenia or pancytopenia. Most cases arise during *P. aeruginosa* septicemia, but nonsepticemic forms are described in both infants and adults. The nonsepticemic cases occur without overt immunosuppression or neutropenia and may occur following antibiotic therapy.

Lesions consist of multiple noncontiguous ulcers or solitary ulcers. They begin as isolated, red, purpuric macules that become vesicular, indurated, and, later, bullous or pustular. The pustules may be hemorrhagic. The lesions remain localized or, more typically, extend over several centimeters. The central area becomes hemorrhagic and necrotic (Figure 9-49). The lesion then sloughs to form a gangrenous ulcer with a gray-black eschar and a surrounding erythematous halo. Lesions occur mainly in the gluteal and perineal regions (57%), the extremities (30%), the trunk (6%), and the face (6%) but may occur anywhere.

Septicemic patients have high temperatures, chills, hypotension, and tachycardia or tachypnea, or both. Neutropenia is a constant finding, and the absolute neutrophil count correlates closely with the clinical outcome. Most patients died when neutrophil counts were lower than $500/mm^3$ during or after appropriate therapy. The skin lesions are slow to heal (an average of 4 weeks).

The postulated mechanisms are a vasculitis caused by bacilli in the vessel wall, by circulating immune complexes, and/or by the effect of bacterial exotoxins or endotoxins.

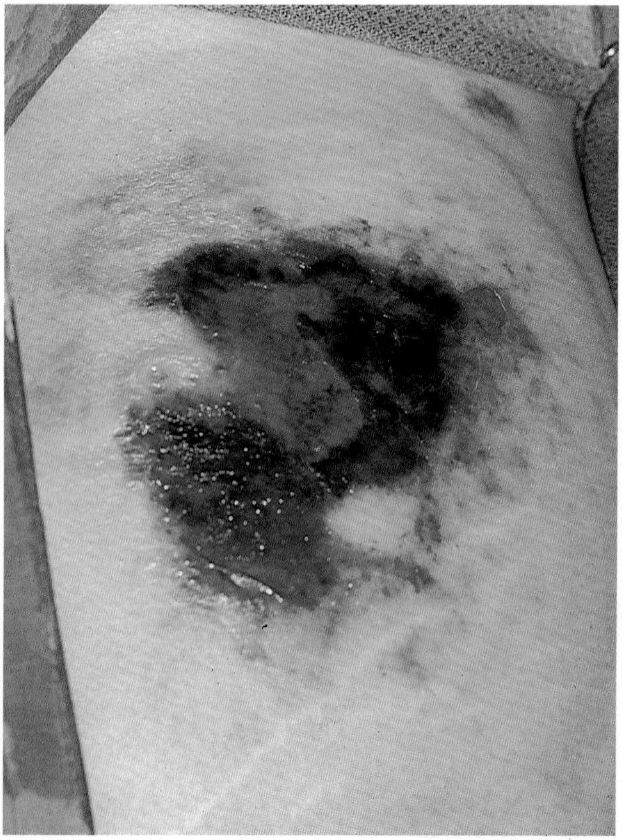

Figure 9-49 Ecthyma gangrenosum. A cutaneous manifestation of *Pseudomonas* septicemia. A large, vesicular, bullous, hemorrhagic mass is located on the thigh.

MANAGEMENT (SEPTICEMIC FORM)

1. Take a deep skin biopsy (4 or 5 mm) for histopathologic studies with special stains to identify bacteria in tissue.
2. Take a skin biopsy specimen for culture.
3. Perform needle aspiration of lesions to perform Gram stain for rapid diagnosis.
4. Take blood culture specimens, especially during fever spikes.
5. Start appropriate systemic antibiotics after cultures have been taken. Localized nonsepticemic disease may only require topical therapy such as silver nitrate (0.5%) or 5% acetic acid (white vinegar) wet compresses or silver sulfadiazine cream.

MENINGOCOCCEMIA

Meningococcemia is caused by the bacteria *Neisseria meningitidis*. It is transmitted by respiratory secretions. Meningitis is the most common presentation. Acute septicemia (meningococcemia) kills faster than any other infectious disease. Shock and death can occur in hours. Chronic meningococcemia is rare and resembles the arthritis-dermatitis syndrome of gonococcemia.

Transmission

Most cases are sporadic, but localized outbreaks occur.

Asymptomatic carriers are thought to be the major source of transmission. Meningococci are present in the nasopharynx of approximately 10% to 20% of healthy persons. Most cases begin with acquisition of a new organism by nasopharyngeal colonization, followed by systemic invasion and development of bacteremia. CNS invasion then occurs. Viral infection, household crowding, chronic illness, and persons who have deficiencies in the terminal common complement pathway (C3, C5-9) are at increased risk. Late complement components are required for bacteriolysis.

Incidence

Each year 2400 cases of meningococcal disease occur in the United States. Incidence is highest in infants; 32% of cases occur in persons 30 years of age or older. Serogroup C caused 35% of cases; serogroup B, 32%; and serogroup Y, 26%. More than half of cases among infants younger than 1 year of age are caused by serogroup B, for which no vaccine exists.

Pathophysiology

A viral infection may facilitate the invasion of *N. meningitidis* into the bloodstream. *N. meningitidis* invades small blood vessel endothelial cells and releases bacterial endotoxins. Endotoxin causes endothelial cells, monocytes, and macrophages to release cytokines. These cause severe hypotension, lowered cardiac output, and endothelial permeability. Organ anoxia and massive disseminated intravascular coagulation can result in organ failure, shock, and death.

Decreased permeability and thrombosis lead to infarction, producing small areas of purpura with an irregular pattern.

CLINICAL MANIFESTATIONS

See the chart titled Meningitis disease pathway. The incubation period varies from 2 to 10 days, but the disease typically begins 3 to 4 days after exposure. Clinical manifestations range from fever alone to fulminant septic shock with purpura fulminans. There is a sudden onset of fever, an intense headache, nausea, vomiting, a stiff neck, and a rash in more than 70% of cases. Purpuric lesions (60%), erythematous papules (32%) (Figures 9-50 through 9-53), faint pink macules (28%), and conjunctival petechiae

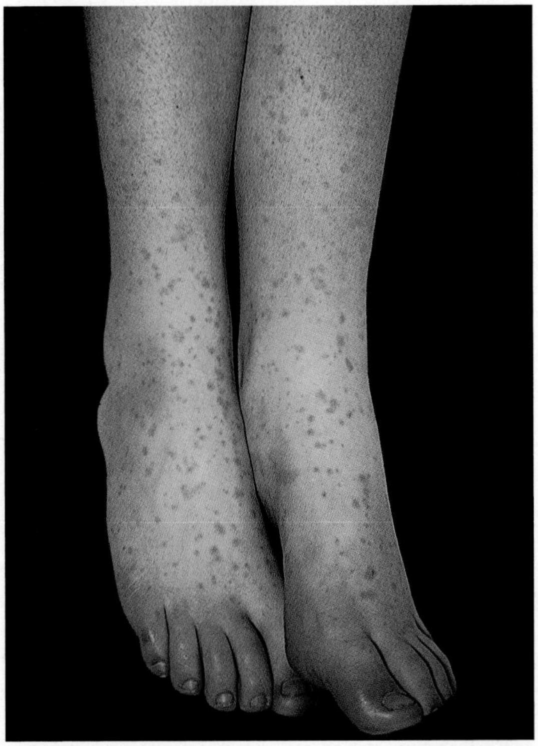

Figure 9-50 Meningococcemia. A papular nonhemorrhagic rash involves the axillae, trunk, wrists, and ankles. The rash subsequently became petechial.

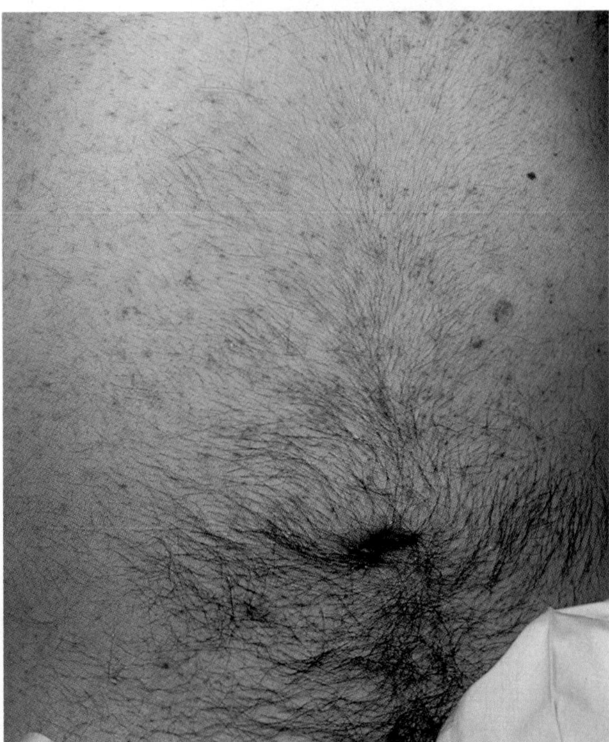

Figure 9-51 Meningococcemia. A maculopapular rash may develop and last for up to 48 hours. A petechial rash then begins on the trunk and legs in areas where pressure is applied.

MENINGOCOCCEMIA

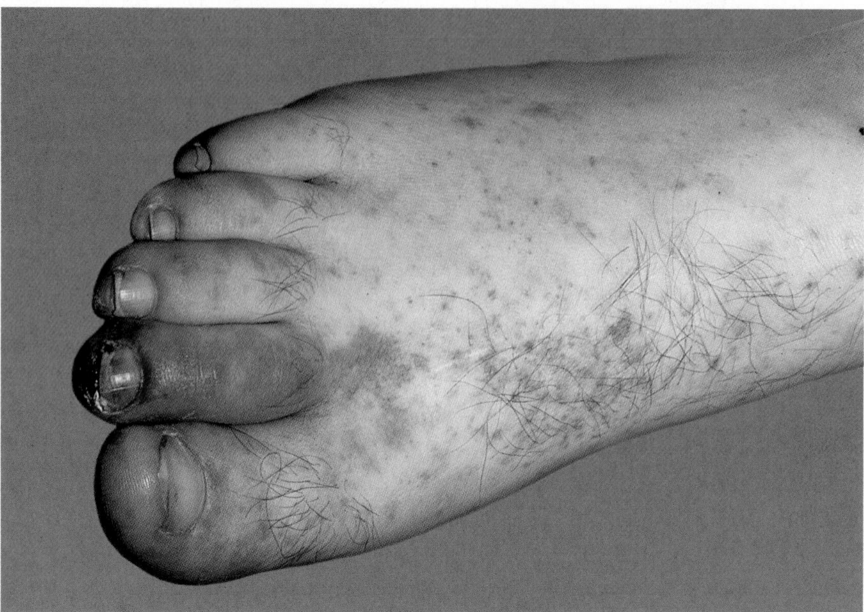

Figure 9-52 Meningococcemia. Lesions become confluent and form hemorrhagic patches, often with central necrosis as seen here on the toe.

Figure 9-53 Petechiae may be located in the center of lighter-colored macules. Confluence of lesions may then result in hemorrhagic patches, often with central necrosis.

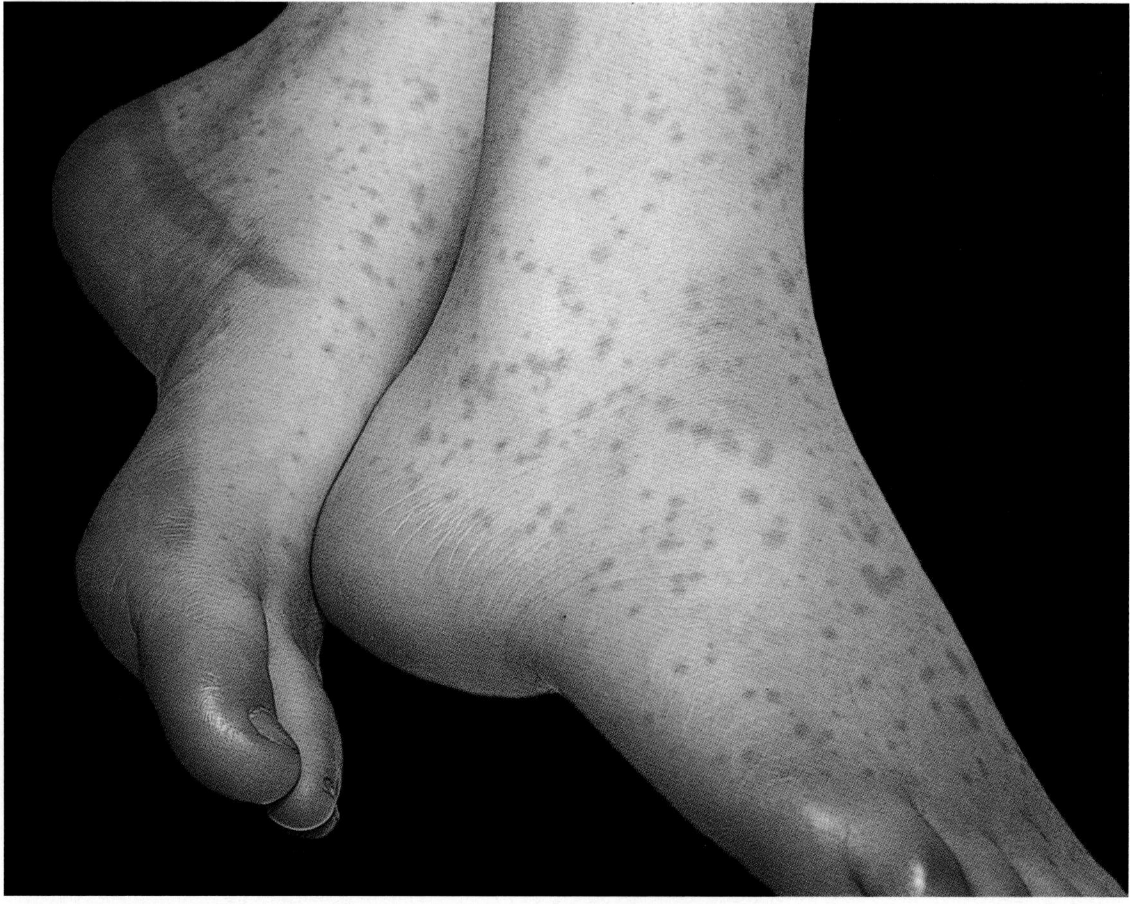

(10%) are the reported cutaneous signs. Petechiae of meningococcemia are usually larger and bluer than pinpoint petechiae caused by thrombocytopenia or leukocytoclastic vasculitis. Ecchymoses (diameter >10 mm) are mainly noted in patients with severe disseminated intravascular coagulation. Delirium and coma often appear. The fatality rate is 7%. The highest rate occurs among infants younger than 1 year of age. Meningococcal disease causes substantial morbidity: 9% to 11% have sequelae (e.g., neurologic disability, limb loss, and hearing loss).

Fulminant disease and purpura fulminans

Fulminant meningococcal septicemia is characterized by a rapid proliferation of meningococci in the circulation, resulting in very high concentrations of bacteria and meningococcal endotoxin. Large bacterial loads stimulate an intense intravascular inflammatory response, leading to progressive circulatory collapse and severe coagulopathy. Patients develop impaired renal, adrenal, and pulmonary function and disseminated intravascular coagulation with thrombotic lesions in the skin, limbs, kidneys, adrenals, choroid plexus, and occasionally the lungs. Vascular complications may lead to gangrene (Figure 9-54) and autoamputation of distal extremities. It is particularly likely to complicate meningococcemia in children younger than 2 years of age. The rapidly fatal Waterhouse-Friderichsen syndrome or fulminating septicemia results in massive bleeding into the skin and hemorrhagic destruction in both adrenal glands. Acquired deficiencies of proteins C and S may contribute to the pathogenesis of purpura fulminans. The immaturity of the protein C system in young children may explain the increased risk.

DIAGNOSIS

Meningococci (*N. meningitidis*) are encapsulated gram-negative diplococci. They are separated into 13 groups on the basis of seroagglutination of capsular polysaccharides. Serogroups A, B, C, Y, and W-135 are identified in most recent cases. Serogroups B and C are responsible for most cases throughout the world. A diagnosis of meningococcal meningitis is suspected in patients with fever, nonblanching rash, meningeal signs, and altered mental status, and is confirmed by pleocytosis and Gram stain with or without culture of cerebrospinal fluid (CSF) or blood or skin lesions. Early meningococcemia may present with no rash or meningeal signs. Petechiae are the clinical sign that best discriminates patients admitted with suspected meningococcal disease. Ecchymoses are specific for meningococcal disease. Reduced general condition and reduced consciousness are other valuable diagnostic signs. Evaluation of the CSF remains the gold standard for the diagnosis of bacterial meningitis. There is a polymorphonuclear leukocytosis in the CSF. Gram-negative diplococci are identified by Gram stain of the CSF, buffy coat, and smears taken from petechiae. A rapid diagnosis can be made with a biopsy of skin lesions. Bacteria are detected in specimens from hemorrhagic skin lesions by culture, Gram staining, or both in 63% of patients. Polymerase chain reaction (PCR) is increasingly used for diagnosis of meningococcal meningitis, including serogrouping and multilocus sequence typing. In meningococcal sepsis, a Gram-stained skin lesion is significantly more sensitive (72%) than Gram-stained CSF (22%). The results for punch biopsy specimens are not affected by antibiotics because Gram staining gives positive results up to 45 hours after the start of treatment and culture gives positive results up to 13 hours. Organisms are isolated by blood culture in almost 100% of cases, but the results are not available for 12 to 24 hours. Rule out complement deficiencies in complicated and recurrent or familial disease.

Text continued on p. 378.

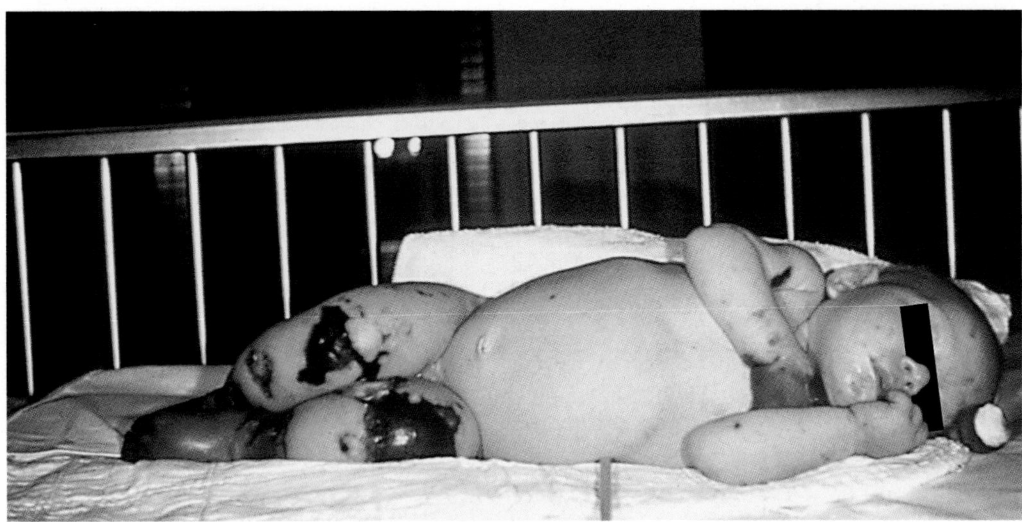

Figure 9-54 Purpura fulminans. Bacterial septicemia results in necrosis, small vessel thrombosis and disseminated intravascular coagulation and is often associated with multi-organ failure. Several amputations may be required.

Meningitis Disease Pathway

Meningococcal disease has two main clinical presentations: meningitis and septicaemia, which often occur together. Septicaemia is more common and more dangerous. It is most likely to be fatal when it occurs without meningitis[9].

A patient with septicaemia presents with very different symptoms from someone with meningitis.

This diagram illustrates the development of symptoms and signs at the far ends of the spectrum of meningococcal disease. It is important that the signs of underlying meningitis or septicaemia are looked for in all febrile patients without an obvious cause for fever, and patients who are currently afebrile who have a history of fever. Advanced meningococcal disease can be missed if the following signs are not looked for. The perceptions and concerns of parents and patients should be taken seriously[1].

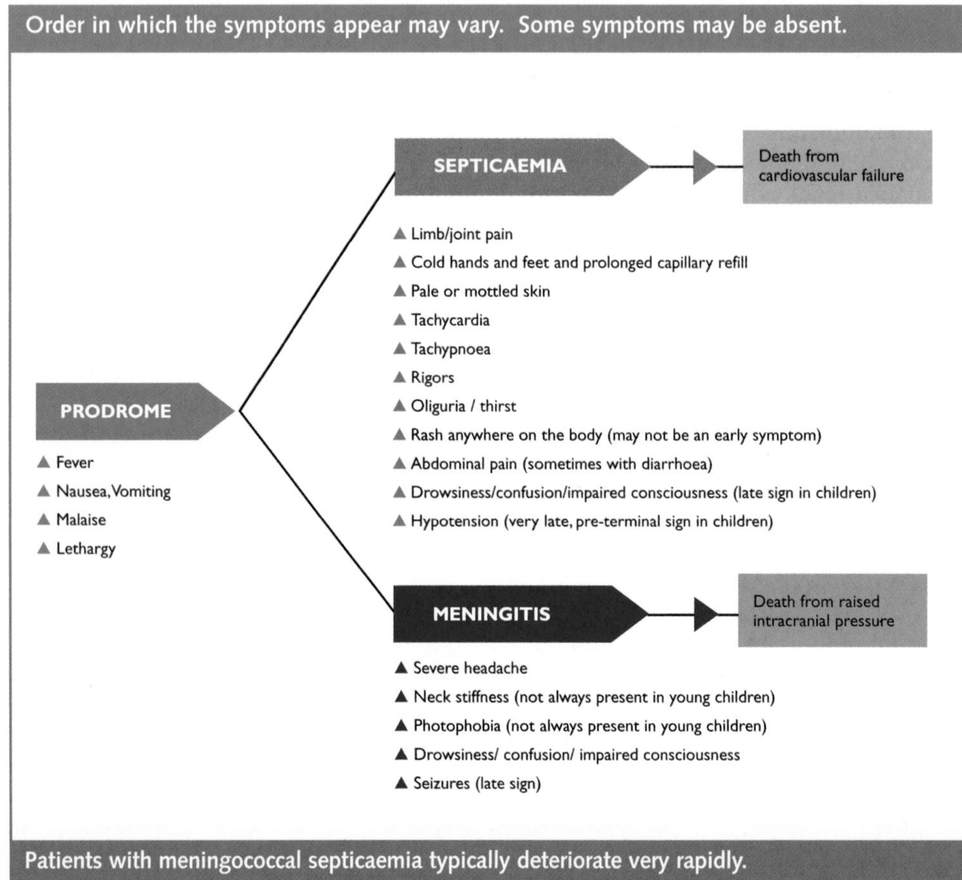

BABIES MAY ALSO SHOW THE FOLLOWING SYMPTOMS:

● Poor feeding ● Irritable particularly when handled, with a high pitched or moaning cry
● Abnormal tone, either increased or decreased, or abnormal posturing
● Vacant staring, poorly responsive or lethargic ● Tense fontanelle ● Cyanosis.

Meningitis disease pathway. (With permission from Meningitis Research Foundation, 2008; accessed at www.meningitis.org. See the website for references and footnotes.)

PHYSICAL SIGNS IN CHILDREN WITH MENINGOCOCCAL DISEASE

ORGAN SYSTEM	SEPTICAEMIA	MENINGITIS
Respiratory	▲ Increased respiratory rate and work of breathing occur early, secondary to acidosis and hypoxia as circulatory failure develops	▲ No changes early in disease ▲ Abnormal breathing patterns seen late with critically raised intracranial pressure. (Vary from hyperventilation to Cheyne-Stokes breathing or apnoea)
Cardiovascular	**Careful examination of this system is the key to recognition of septicaemia. Clinical features of circulatory failure (shock) develop:** ▲ Tachycardia is an early and important sign ▲ Peripheral vasoconstriction results in pallor, cold hands and feet, and mottling ▲ Capillary refill time ≥ 3 seconds on forehead or sternum is abnormal, ≥ 4 seconds on peripheries in conjunction with other signs suggests shock ▲ BP is normal until late in septicaemia. Hypotension is a pre-terminal sign	▲ No changes early in disease ▲ Later, raised intracranial pressure leads to bradycardia and hypertension
CNS	▲ Children have a normal conscious level until late in the illness and they may appear alert and responsive ▲ Hypoxia and hypoperfusion eventually lead to a decreased conscious level: this is a late and a pre-terminal sign in shock ▲ NO neck stiffness or photophobia occurs in septicaemia	**CNS function most likely to be abnormal** ▲ Irritability, drowsiness, confusion and decreased conscious level as intracranial pressure rises. **Babies** may have a vacant expression/full fontanelle. **Teenagers** can become confused and combative ▲ Neck stiffness and photophobia are uncommon signs in early meningitis in young children.
Renal	▲ Decreased urine output occurs early in shock	▲ No change in meningitis
Death	Results from **cardiovascular failure (shock)**	Results from **raised intracranial pressure**

Registered Office: Midland Way Thornbury Bristol BS35 2BS Tel 01454 281811 Fax 01454 281094 133 Gilmore Place Edinburgh EH3 9PP Tel 0131 228 3322 Fax 0131 221 0300
71 Botanic Avenue Belfast BT7 1JL Tel 028 9032 1283 Fax 028 9032 1284 Office also in the Republic of Ireland
Offices: Belfast, Bristol, Dublin, Edinburgh. A charity registered in England and Wales no 1091105, in Scotland no SC037586 & in Ireland CHY 12030.

Normal Values of Vital Signs
From Advanced Paediatric Life Support Manual

Age (years)	Heart Rate per minute	Respiratory Rate per minute	Systolic Blood Pressure
<1	110-160	30-40	70-90
1-2	100-150	25-35	80-95
2-5	95-140	25-30	80-100
5-12	80-120	20-25	90-110
over 12	60-100	15-20	100-120

RASH: The rash of meningococcal disease can start as a blanching rash in up to a third of patients: remember to check for underlying signs of meningitis and septicaemia in children who present with a maculopapular rash.

Patients with meningitis tend to have a more scanty (or absent) rash than those with septicaemia. Ideally, the whole skin surface of a febrile patient without an obvious cause for fever should be checked.

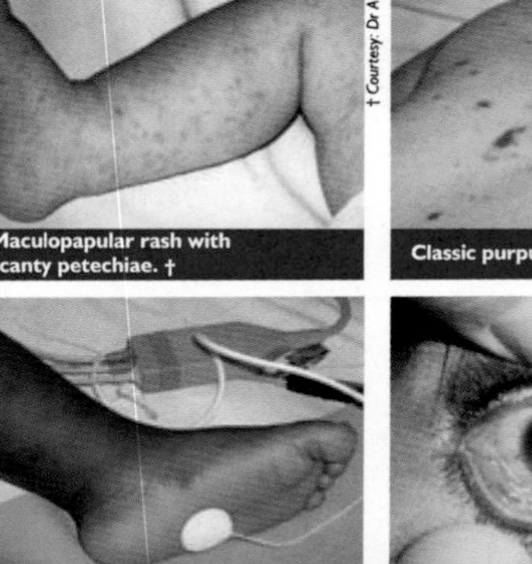

Maculopapular rash with scanty petechiae. †

† Courtesy: Dr A Riordan

Classic purpuric rash.

Purpuric rash on dark skin.

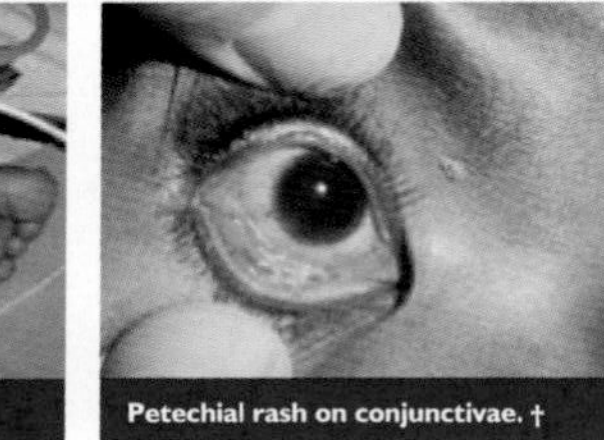

Petechial rash on conjunctivae. †

† Courtesy: D A Warrell

Benzylpenicillin dosage (BNF)

(except in severe penicillin allergy)

Adult and child aged 10 or older: **1200 mg**

Child 1-9 years: **600 mg**

Infant: **300 mg**

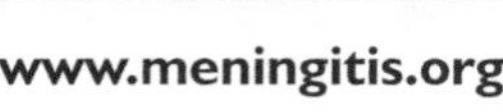

www.meningitis.org

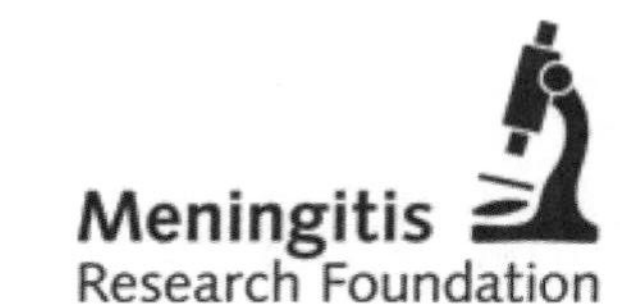

(With permission from Meningitis Research Foundation, 2008; accessed at www.meningitis.org.)

Early Management of Suspected Bacterial Meningitis and Meningococcal Septicaemia in Immunocompetent Adults*

Early Recognition

- Petechial/purpuric non-blanching rash or signs of meningitis
- A rash may be absent or atypical at presentation
- Neck stiffness may be absent in up to 30% of cases of meningitis
- Prior antibiotics may mask the severity of the illness

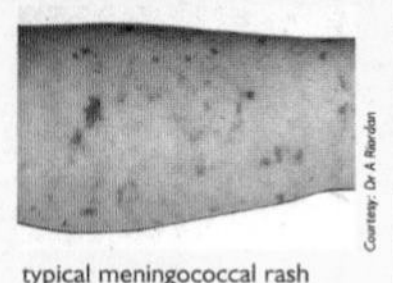

typical meningococcal rash

Assess Severity & Immediate Intervention[a]

- Airway
- Breathing - Respiratory Rate & O_2 Saturation
- Circulation - Pulse; Capillary Refill Time (hypotension late); Urine output
- Mental status (deterioration may be a sign of shock or meningitis)
- Neurology – Focal neurological signs; Persistent seizures; Papilloedema

Secure Airway
High Flow O_2
Large bore IV Cannula ± fluid resuscitation

Priority Investigations:

- FBC; U+Es; Blood sugar, LFTs; CRP
- Clotting profile
- Blood gases

Microbiology:

- Blood culture
- Throat swab
- Clotted blood
- EDTA blood for PCR

Predominantly Meningococcal Septicaemia

- Do not attempt LP
- IV 2g Cefotaxime or Ceftriaxone
- Call critical care team for review

Signs of Shock[a]: YES → Priorities; NO → Careful Monitoring / Repeated Review

Priorities

- Secure airway + High flow O_2
- Volume resuscitation
- Senior review
- Management in critical care unit

Poor response → Further interventions; Good response → Careful Monitoring / Repeated Review

Further interventions

- Pre-emptive Intubation + Ventilation
- Volume support
- Inotropic/ Vasopressor Support
- Consider activated protein C[12]
- Good glycaemic control[13]
- In refractory circulatory failure, physiological replacement corticosteroid therapy may be beneficial[14]

Predominantly Meningitis[b,c,d]

- Assess patient carefully before performing LP
- Call critical care team if any features of raised intracranial pressure, shock or respiratory failure
- If uncertain ask for senior review
- Monitor and stabilise circulation

No Raised ICP / No Shock / No Respiratory Failure[a,b] → Lumbar puncture

Signs of Raised ICP[a,b] → Priorities

Lumbar puncture[a,b]

- IV 2g Cefotaxime/ Ceftriaxone immediately after LP
- Consider corticosteroids[d]
- if LP will be delayed for more than 30 minutes give IV antibiotics first

Priorities

- Secure airway + High flow O_2
- Defer lumbar puncture
- IV 2g Cefotaxime/Ceftriaxone
- Consider corticosteroids[d]
- Careful volume resuscitation
- 30° head elevation
- Management in critical care unit
- Low threshold for elective Intubation + Ventilation (cerebral protection)

Careful Monitoring[a]
Repeated Review

Public Health/Infection Control

- Notify CCDC†
- If probable or confirmed meningococcal disease, contact CCDC† urgently regarding prophylaxis to contacts
- Notify microbiology
- Isolate patient for first 24 hours

Additional Information

[a] Warning Signs (see refs)

The following warn of impending/ worsening shock, respiratory failure or raised intracranial pressure and require urgent senior review and intervention (see algorithm):

- Rapidly progressive rash
- Poor peripheral perfusion, CRT > 4 secs, oliguria and systolic BP < 90 (hypotension often a late sign)
- RR < 8 or > 30
- Pulse rate < 40 or > 140
- Acidosis pH < 7.3 or BE worse than - 5
- WBC < 4

- Marked depressed conscious level (GCS < 12) or a fluctuating conscious level (fall in GCS > 2)
- Focal neurology
- Persistent seizures
- Bradycardia and hypertension
- Papilloedema

[b] CT scan and meningitis (see refs)

This investigation should only be used when appropriate:

- A normal CT scan does not exclude raised intracranial pressure
- If there are no clinical contraindications to LP, a CT scan is not necessary beforehand
- Subsequently a CT scan may be useful in identifying dural defects predisposing to meningitis

[c] Appropriate antibiotics for bacterial meningitis (see refs)

Review with microbiology:

- Ampicillin IV 2g qds should be added for individuals >55 years to cover Listeria
- Vancomycin ± rifampicin if pneumococcal penicillin resistance suspected
- Amend antibiotics on the basis of microbiology results

[d] Corticosteroids in adult meningitis (see refs)

- Dexamethasone 0.15mg/kg qds for 4 days started with or just before the first dose of antibiotics, particularly where pneumococcal meningitis is suspected
- Do not give unless you are confident you are using the correct antimicrobials
- Stop the dexamethasone if a non-bacterial cause is identified

See References Overleaf

www.britishinfectionsociety.org
Journal of Infection February 2003; Vol 46(2)

* *Community acquired meningitis in the immunocompetent host. In the immunocompromised seek additional expert advice*

†*CPHM in Scotland*

www.meningitis.org
For further copies contact
Meningitis Research Foundation 01454 281811

(With permission from Meningitis Research Foundation, 2008; see www.meningitis.org for references and footnotes.)

MENINGOCOCCEMIA: ANTIBIOTICS AND PREVENTING SHOCK

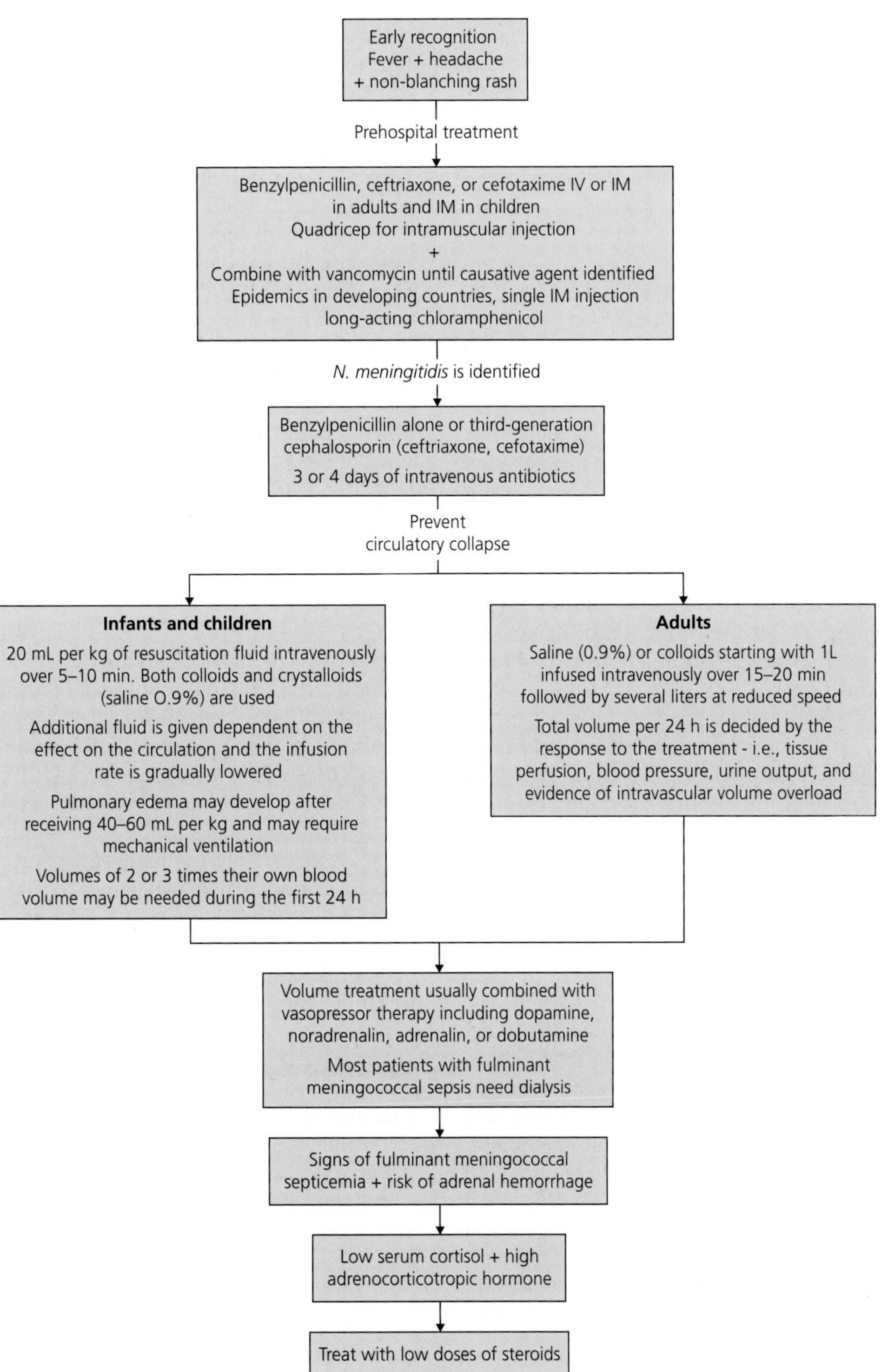

Figure 9-55

DIFFERENTIAL DIAGNOSIS

The differential diagnosis of acute petechial eruptions includes Rocky Mountain spotted fever, echovirus and coxsackievirus infections, and toxic shock syndrome. Gonococcemia and allergic vasculitis (Henoch-Schönlein purpura, leukocytoclastic vasculitis) produce petechial and purpuric lesions that are usually elevated and palpable.

Treatment

The key to successful treatment is speed. Patients with fever, headache, and a nonblanching rash may be candidates for prehospital antibiotic treatment to prevent fulminant meningococcal septicemia with rapidly increasing concentrations of meningococci and endotoxins in the circulation (Figure 9-55) and the British Infection Society algorithm: Early management of suspected bacterial meningitis and meningococcal septicaemia in immunocompetent adults [p. 376]). They are then rapidly transported to the hospital, and stabilized in an intensive care unit. Aggressive management of raised intracranial pressure reduces mortality. Management of shock through the use of volume expansion, inotropic support, and the correction of hemostatic metabolic abnormalities can substantially reduce rates of meningococcal sepsis.

ANTIBIOTICS. Early antibiotic treatment is the primary goal. All meningococci in cerebrospinal fluid are killed within 3 to 4 hours after intravenous treatment. Concentrations of endotoxin in plasma fall by 50% within 2 hours. Prehospital antibiotic treatment is used. The estimated doubling time of bacteria is 30 to 45 minutes and the concentrations of endotoxin rise rapidly.

Benzylpenicillin, cefotaxime, ceftriaxone, and chloramphenicol are effective and are injected intravenously or intramuscularly in adults and intramuscularly in children. The quadriceps muscle is the best site. During epidemics in developing countries, a single injection of long-acting chloramphenicol injected intramuscularly can cure the disease. A single injection of ceftriaxone is equally effective and may become the preferred treatment for epidemic meningitis. Patients in industrialized countries with suspected bacterial meningitis are usually given cefotaxime or ceftriaxone, often combined with vancomycin until the causative agent has been identified. When *N. meningitidis* is identified, antibiotic treatment should be continued with benzylpenicillin alone or a third-generation cephalosporin. Three or four days of intravenous treatment is effective.

MANAGEMENT OF SHOCK. Circulatory collapse is the primary cause of death. An altered endothelial barrier leads to capillary leak syndrome, vasodilation, and a reduction in myocardial function. There is increased flux of albumin and water across the altered capillary wall to the extravascular space. Large amounts of fluid accumulate in the extravascular tissue. Plasma albumin level falls and rises only temporarily after intravenous infusion of albumin. The concentration of albumin in the urine equals the concentration seen in patients with nephrotic syndrome. The primary goal is to increase the circulating blood volume by aggressive fluid treatment. The volume infused is more important than the type of fluid. Additional fluid is given dependent on the effect on the circulation, and the infusion rate is gradually lowered. The volume treatment is usually combined with vasopressor therapy including dopamine, noradrenaline, adrenaline, or dobutamine. Most patients with fulminant meningococcal sepsis need dialysis.

Patients with meningitis or mild meningococcemia are given the normal daily requirement of fluid intravenously supplemented with the volume lost before admission. Excessive volume treatment can induce fatal brain edema and herniation. Patients may need dialysis to compensate for the failing kidney's inability to reduce edema. The development of fulminant meningococcal septicemia can lead to adrenal hemorrhage. Adults with septic shock and indications of inadequate adrenal function are given low doses of steroids. Low doses of corticosteroids may be considered for children with shock caused by *N. meningitidis*.

Vaccines

At least 75% of cases of invasive meningococcal disease (IMD) in 11- to 18-year-olds are caused by serogroups A, C, Y, and W-135; thus IMD potentially is preventable by immunization with quadrivalent meningococcal vaccines. Meningococcal A, C, Y, W-135 conjugate vaccine (MCV4) was licensed in 2005 for use in people 11 to 55 years of age. The American Academy of Pediatrics recommends administration of MCV4 to young adolescents (11- to 12-year olds), students entering high school or 15-year-olds, and college freshmen who will be living in dormitories. For pediatric patients 11 years and older who are at increased risk of meningococcal disease, MCV4 also is recommended. See the American Academy of Pediatrics website (http://aappolicy.aappublications.org/) for full details.

Chemoprophylaxis

Chemoprophylaxis to prevent meningococcal infection is recommended for close contacts of patients with invasive meningococcal disease, including the following:

- Household members
- Childcare center contacts
- Anyone directly exposed to the patient's oral secretions (e.g., through kissing, mouth-to-mouth resuscitation, endotracheal intubation, or endotracheal tube management)

Chemoprophylaxis should be administered as soon as possible, ideally <24 hours after identification of the index patient. Administration of chemoprophylaxis >14 days after onset of illness in the index patient is probably of limited or no value. The recommended agents for chemoprophylaxis include rifampin, ciprofloxacin and ceftriaxone (Table 9-7).

Chemoprophylaxis is not recommended in the case of noninvasive meningococcal disease.

Table 9-7 Schedule for Administering Chemoprophylaxis Against Meningococcal Disease

Drug	Age group	Dosage	Duration and route of administration
Rifampin* (Rimactane)	<1 month	5 mg/kg every 12 hr	2 days, oral
Rifampin (Rimactane)	>1 month	10 mg/kg every 12 hr	2 days, oral
Rifampin (Rimactane)	Adult	600 mg every 12 hr	2 days, oral
Ciprofloxacin† (Cipro)	Adult	750 mg	Single dose, oral
Ceftriaxone	<15 yr	125 mg	Single dose, IM
Ceftriaxone	Adult	250 mg	Single dose, IM
Azithromycin (Zithromax)	Adult	500 mg	Single dose, oral

Adapted from Rosenstein NE et al: *New Engl J Med* 344:1378, 2001. *PMID: 11333996*
*Rifampin should not be used in pregnant women. Reliability of oral contraceptives may be affected by rifampin.
†Ciprofloxacin can be used for persons <18 years of age if no acceptable alternative therapy is available.

NONTUBERCULOUS MYCOBACTERIA

Mycobacteria are rods with a waxy coating that makes them resistant to stains and to many antibiotics. Once stained, they are not easily decolored and remain "acid-fast." The most common and important mycobacteria are *M. tuberculosis* and *M. leprae*. Nontuberculous mycobacteria (previously referred to as atypical mycobacteria) usually cause systemic disease, but they may just infect the skin (Table 9-8). They are widespread in nature and are found in soil, animal and human feces, and water in swimming pools and fish tanks. They differ in culture requirements, pigment production, disease manifestation, and drug susceptibility. The Runyon classification, which depends on colony pigment and growth rate characteristics, is no longer used. The bacteria are simply referred to by genus and species. Most cutaneous disease is caused by *M. marinum* (*Mycobacterium balnei*).

M. marinum

M. marinum is often called swimming pool granuloma and occurs in tropical fish enthusiasts, and fisherman as a chronic granulomatous infection, often manifesting as nodular lymphangitis. Because the organism requires a temperature of 30° to 32° C for optimal growth, infections are usually limited to the skin. The disease occurs at sites of minor trauma such as the fingers and hands; the elbows and knees follow. The incubation period is 2 to 6 weeks. A papule or nodule appears and may ulcerate and discharge a serosanguineous fluid or develop a verrucous surface. Lesions are usually solitary (Figure 9-56), but a sporotrichoid distribution, in which nodular or ulcerating lesions extend proximally along sites of lymphatic drainage, may occur (Figure 9-57). Tenosynovitis is commonly present in lesions of the fingers or hand. Localized adenopathy is rare. A positive tuberculin test result is present in 50% to 80% of patients. Minocycline is the treatment of choice.

M. ulcerans, M. fortuitum, M. chelonae, and *M. avium-intracellulare*

Mycobacterium-avium complex causes disseminated disease in as many as 15% to 40% of patients with human immunodeficiency virus infection in the United States, causing fever, night sweats, weight loss, and anemia. The bacteria are of low pathogenicity, and transmission between persons is rare. Predisposing conditions for infection are trauma, immunosuppression, human immunodeficiency virus infection, and chronic disease. Consider a nontuberculous mycobacterial infection when a lesion develops at the site of trauma and follows a chronic course.

Mycobacteria require different temperatures for culture. Instruct the laboratory to incubate the cultures at both 30° C and 37° C. Isolation of these opportunistic, widespread organisms in culture does not prove that they cause the disease. DNA probes are now available to identify the species of mycobacteria; time for identification is within 3 to 4 weeks.

Table 9-8 Nontuberculous Mycobacteria Infection

Characteristic	*M. marinum*	*M. ulcerans*	*M. fortuitum* and *M. chelonae*	*M. avium-intracellulare*	*M. kansasii*
Source of infection	Fresh water and salt-water (swimming pool, wells, contaminated fish, fish tanks); immunosuppressed patients	Water; swamp areas of Australia, Uganda, and Zaire	Ocean and fresh water, dirt, dust, animal feed, sporadic postoperative infections; trauma; dialysis equipment; postinjection abscesses	Gulf coast; Pacific coast; north central U.S.; soil, house dust, water; dried plants	Unclear; has been isolated from tap water; opportunistic infection
Symptoms	Asymptomatic to painful swelling of skin	Asymptomatic to painful swelling of skin; decreased mobility of joint	Often develops in patients with preexisting lung disease Disseminated disease associated with AIDS	Asymptomatic fever, weight loss, bone pain	Pruritus, fever, plaques, swelling Most common disease is a pulmonary infection in elderly men with chronic underlying pulmonary disease
Skin lesion	Lesions occur at inoculation site Papules; nodules; verrucous plaques; ulcers/abscesses, sporotrichoid; disseminated	Large, solitary, deep, painless ulcer on lower extremities Secondary necrosis occurs Primarily affects children and young adults	Granulomatous nodules; draining abscesses; ulcers; sporotrichoid lesions; cellulitis; disseminated disease	Granulomatous synovitis; deep hand infection; panniculitis; subcutaneous nodule	Verrucous papules, sporotrichoid eruption, cellulitis, granulomatous plaques, ulcers, and necrotic papulopustules
Treatment	Minocycline or doxycycline 100 mg twice daily; trimethoprim-sulfamethoxazole 160-800 mg twice daily; clarithromycin, rifampin 600 mg daily and ethambutol 800 mg daily for resistant strains, sporotrichoid lesions, and disseminated infections Treat for 1 mo to 1 yr	Wide excision with or without skin grafting is treatment of choice Trimethoprim-sulfamethoxazole 80/400 mg twice daily followed by rifampin 600 mg daily and minocycline 100 mg daily, or a combination of streptomycin, dapsone, and ethambutol Heat area with occlusive wraps because *M. ulcerans* is heat sensitive	Severe disease: surgical debridement; amikacin (15 mg/kg/day) plus cefoxitin (200 mg/kg/day) combined with oral administration of probenecid, followed by sulfonamide, erythromycin, or minocycline Less severe disease: sulfonamide with erythromycin Continue therapy for 4-6 weeks after wound healing	Aggressive therapy with multiple drugs including INH, clofazimine, rifampin, streptomycin, ethambutol, ethionamide, cycloserine, capreomycin, or clarithromycin	Rifampin in addition to ethambutol or isoniazid Drug resistance has been reported with isoniazid Treatment with higher dosages of isoniazid (900 mg) has been tried Sulfonamides and amikacin have been added when rifampin-resistant strains occur
Culture incubation temperature	30° to 33° C	30° to 33° C	Between 25° and 40° C	37° C	37° C

Adapted from Street ML et al: *J Am Acad Dermatol* 24:208, 1991. *PMID: 2007665*

MYCOBACTERIUM MARINUM

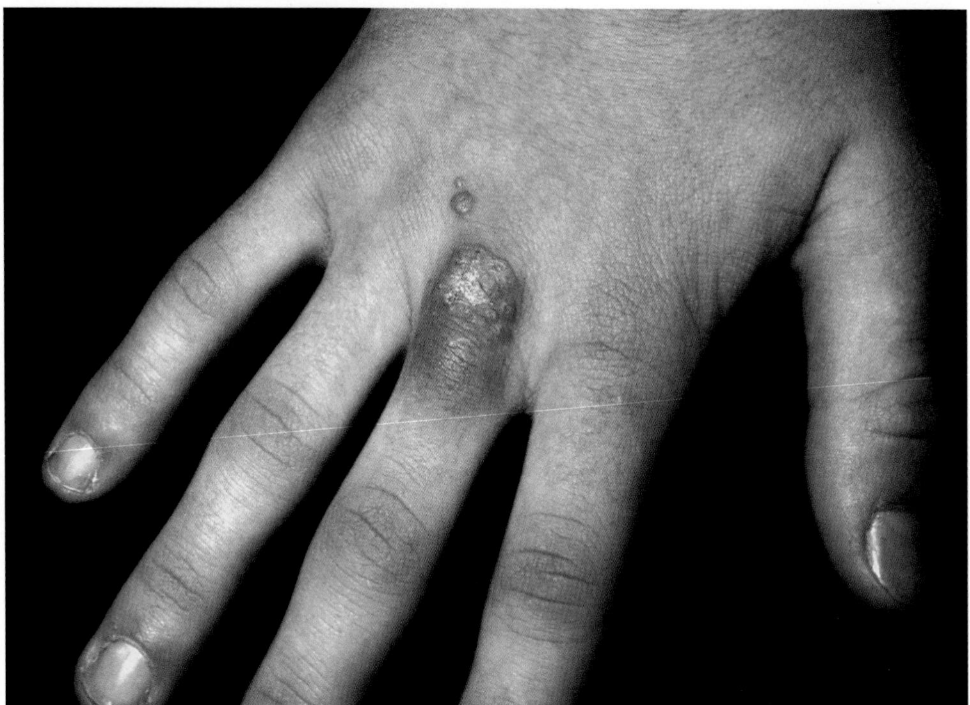

Figure 9-56 Patients may report that the painful nodules ulcerate.

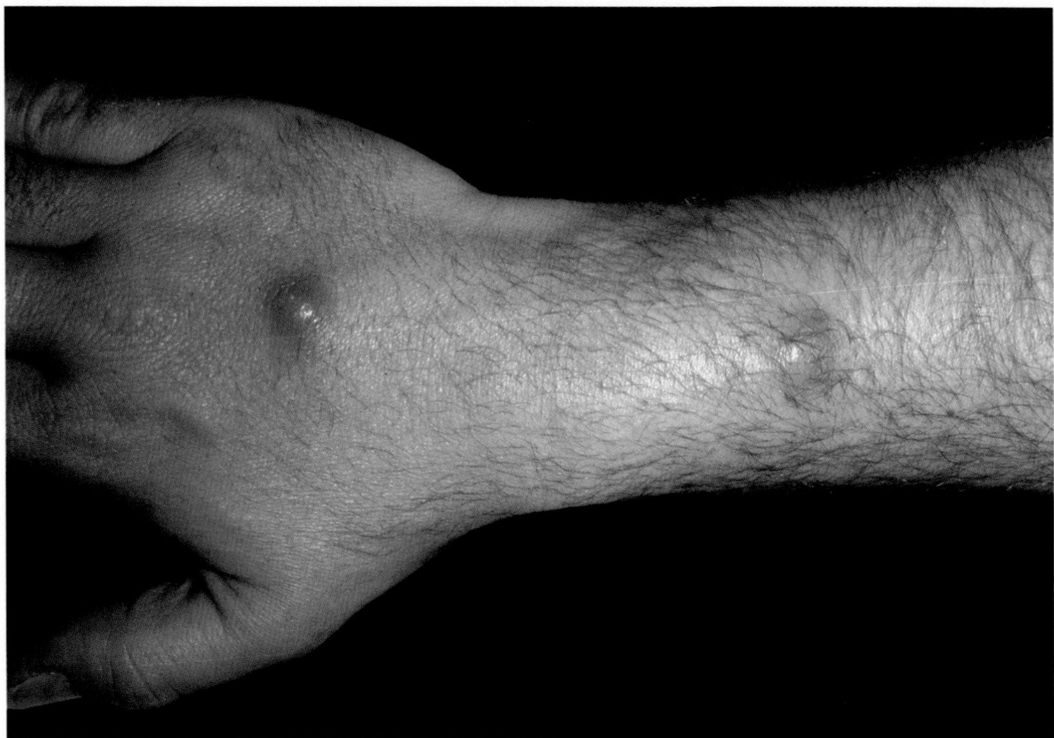

Figure 9-57 Patients who are exposed to home aquariums are at risk. A papule evolves into a nodule at the site of trauma 2-3 weeks earlier. New lesions then may progress up the arm as is seen in sporotrichosis.

Chapter 10

Sexually Transmitted Bacterial Infections

CHAPTER CONTENTS

SEXUALLY TRANSMITTED DISEASE PRESENTATIONS

Sexually transmitted diseases can present as follows:

- Genital ulcers or sores
- Urethral discharge
- Vaginal discharge
- Cervical infection
- Lower abdominal pain
- Inguinal bubo
- Scrotal swelling
- Rectal or pharyngeal inflammation
- Papules

The Centers for Disease Control criteria for the treatment of all sexually transmitted diseases (STDs) is presented in Box 10-1 (pp. 383-385). An overview of these diseases and their World Health Organization (WHO) syndromic diagnosis and management criteria is presented on pp. 388-395. An overview of these diseases and their syndromic diagnosis and management is presented in Figures 10-1 to 10-5.

Box 10-1 **Centers for Disease Control Sexually Transmitted Diseases**

Chancroid

*Recommended Regimens**

- Azithromycin 1 gm orally in a single dose
  OR
- Ceftriaxone 250 mg intramuscularly (IM) in a single dose
  OR
- Ciprofloxacin 500 mg orally twice a day for 3 days
  OR
- Erythromycin base 500 mg orally three times a day for 7 days
- Ciprofloxacin is contraindicated for pregnant and lactating women. Azithromycin and ceftriaxone offer the advantage of single-dose therapy. Worldwide, several isolates with intermediate resistance to either ciprofloxacin or erythromycin have been reported.

Herpes simplex viral infections

First clinical episode of genital herpes

*Recommended regimens**

- Acyclovir 400 mg orally three times a day for 7-10 days
  OR
- Acyclovir 200 mg orally five times a day for 7-10 days
  OR
- Famciclovir 250 mg orally three times a day for 7-10 days
  OR
- Valacyclovir 1 gm orally twice a day for 7-10 days

Suppressive therapy for recurrent genital herpes

Recommended regimens

- Acyclovir 400 mg orally twice a day
  OR
- Famciclovir 250 mg orally twice a day
  OR
- Valacyclovir 500 mg orally once a day
  OR
- Valacyclovir 1.0 gm orally once a day
  In patients who have very frequent recurrences (i.e., ≥10 episodes per year)

Episodic therapy for recurrent genital herpes

Recommended regimens

- Acyclovir 400 mg orally three times a day for 5 days
  OR
- Acyclovir 800 mg orally twice a day for 5 days
  OR
- Acyclovir 800 mg orally three times a day for 2 days
  OR
- Famciclovir 125 mg orally twice daily for 5 days
  OR
- Famciclovir 1000 mg orally twice daily for 1 day
  OR
- Valacyclovir 500 mg orally twice a day for 3 days
  OR
- Valacyclovir 1.0 gm orally once a day for 5 days

Daily suppressive therapy in persons infected with HIV

- Acyclovir 400-800 mg orally two to three times a day
  OR
- Famciclovir 500 mg orally twice a day
  OR
- Valacyclovir 500 mg orally twice a day

Episodic infection in persons infected with HIV

- Acyclovir 400 mg orally three times a day for 5-10 days
  OR
- Famciclovir 500 mg orally twice a day for 5-10 days
  OR
- Valacyclovir 1.0 gm orally twice a day for 5-10 days

Granuloma inguinale (donovanosis)

Recommended regimen

- Doxycycline 100 mg orally twice a day for at least 3 weeks and until all lesions have completely healed

Alternative regimens

- Azithromycin 1 gm orally once per week for at least 3 weeks and until all lesions have completely healed
  OR
- Ciprofloxacin 750 mg orally twice a day for at least 3 weeks and until all lesions have completely healed
  OR
- Erythromycin base 500 mg orally four times a day for at least 3 weeks and until all lesions have completely healed
  OR
- Trimethoprim-sulfamethoxazole 1 double-strength (160 mg/800 mg) tablet orally twice a day for at least 3 weeks and until all lesions have completely healed
- Some specialists recommend the addition of an aminoglycoside (e.g., gentamicin 1 mg/kg IV every 8 hours) to these regimens if improvement is not evident within the first few days of therapy.

Lymphogranuloma venereum

Recommended regimen

- Doxycycline 100 mg orally twice a day for 21 days

Alternative regimen

- Erythromycin base 500 mg orally four times a day for 21 days
- Some STD specialists believe that azithromycin 1.0 gm orally once weekly for 3 weeks is probably effective, although clinical data are lacking.

Primary and secondary syphilis

Adults

- Benzathine penicillin G 2.4 million units IM in a single dose
- Lidocaine as diluent for benzathine penicillin G (Bicillin) reduces injection pain without affecting penicillin concentration.

Alternatives (if penicillin-allergic and not pregnant)

- Doxycycline 100 mg PO twice daily or tetracycline 500 mg PO four times daily or minocycline 100 mg PO twice daily for 14 days
- Erythromycin 500 mg PO four times daily for 2 weeks but close follow-up needed since resistance reported
- Ceftriaxone 250 mg IM once daily for 10 days can be curative but close follow-up needed since resistance reported
- Azithromycin 2 gm PO once *PMID: 16177249* Treatment failures have been reported.

From www.cdc.gov/Treatment guidelines 2006 including 2007 revisions (modified)

Continued

*Treatment might be extended if healing is incomplete after 10 days of therapy.

†Consider concurrent treatment for gonococcal infection if prevalence of gonorrhea is high in the patient population under assessment.

‡The tablet formulation of cefixime is currently not available in the United States.

§Spectinomycin is currently not available in the United States.

Box 10-1 **Centers for Disease Control Sexually Transmitted Diseases—cont'd**

Children

- Benzathine penicillin G 50,000 units/kg IM, up to the adult dose of 2.4 million units in a single dose
- Lidocaine as diluent for benzathine penicillin G (Bicillin) reduces injection pain without affecting penicillin concentration.

Primary and secondary syphilis among HIV-infected persons

- Treatment with benzathine penicillin G 2.4 million units IM in a single dose is recommended. Some specialists recommend additional treatments (e.g., benzathine penicillin G administered at 1-week intervals for 3 weeks, as recommended for late syphilis) in addition to benzathine penicillin G 2.4 million units IM.

Early latent syphilis—adults

- Benzathine penicillin G 2.4 million units IM in a single dose

Late latent syphilis or latent syphilis of unknown duration—adults

- Benzathine penicillin G 7.2 million units total, administered as 3 doses of 2.4 million units IM each at 1-week intervals

Early latent syphilis—children

- Benzathine penicillin G 50,000 units/kg IM, up to the adult dose of 2.4 million units in a single dose

Late latent syphilis or latent syphilis of unknown duration—children

- Benzathine penicillin G 50,000 units/kg IM, up to the adult dose of 2.4 million units, administered as 3 doses at 1-week intervals (total 150,000 units/kg up to the adult total dose of 7.2 million units)
- See full CDC guidelines for management of latent syphilis among HIV-infected persons.

Tertiary syphilis

- Benzathine penicillin G 7.2 million units total, administered as 3 doses of 2.4 million units IM each at 1-week intervals

Nongonococcal urethritis

- Azithromycin 1 gm orally in a single dose
  OR
- Doxycycline 100 mg orally twice a day for 7 days

Alternative regimens

- Erythromycin base 500 mg orally four times a day for 7 days
  OR
- Erythromycin ethylsuccinate 800 mg orally four times a day for 7 days
  OR
- Ofloxacin 300 mg orally twice a day for 7 days
  OR
- Levofloxacin 500 mg orally once daily for 7 days

Recurrent and persistent urethritis

- Metronidazole 2 gm orally in a single dose
  OR
- Tinidazole 2 gm orally in a single dose
  PLUS
- Azithromycin 1 gm orally in a single dose (if not used for initial episode)

Cervicitis

Recommended regimen for presumptive treatment[†]

- Azithromycin 1 gm orally in a single dose
  OR
- Doxycycline 100 mg orally twice a day for 7 days

Chlamydial infections

- Azithromycin 1 gm orally in a single dose
  OR
- Doxycycline 100 mg orally twice a day for 7 days

Alternative regimens

- Erythromycin base 500 mg orally four times a day for 7 days
  OR
- Erythromycin ethylsuccinate 800 mg orally four times a day for 7 days
  OR
- Ofloxacin 300 mg orally twice a day for 7 days
  OR
- Levofloxacin 500 mg orally once daily for 7 days

Uncomplicated gonococcal infections of the cervix, urethra, and rectum

- Ceftriaxone 125 mg IM in a single dose
  OR
- Cefixime‡ 400 mg orally in a single dose or 400 mg by suspension (200 mg/5 ml)
  PLUS
- Treatment for chlamydia if chlamydial infection is not ruled out

Alternative regimens

- Spectinomycin[§] 2 gm in a single intramuscular (IM) dose
  OR
- Single-dose cephalosporin regimens
- Other single-dose cephalosporin therapies that are considered alternative treatment regimens for uncomplicated urogenital and anorectal gonococcal infections include ceftizoxime 500 mg IM; or cefoxitin 2 gm IM, administered with probenecid 1 gm orally; or cefotaxime 500 mg IM. Some evidence indicates that cefpodoxime 400 mg and cefuroxime axetil 1 gm might be oral alternatives.

Uncomplicated gonococcal infections of the pharynx

Recommended regimens

- Ceftriaxone 125 mg IM in a single dose
  PLUS
- Treatment for chlamydia if chlamydial infection is not ruled out

Disseminated gonococcal infection (DGI)

- Ceftriaxone 1 gm IM or IV every 24 hours

Alternative regimens

- Cefotaxime 1 gm IV every 8 hours
  OR
- Ceftizoxime 1 gm IV every 8 hours
  OR
- Spectinomycin[§] 2 gm IM every 12 hours
- A cephalosporin-based intravenous regimen is recommended for the initial treatment of DGI.
- Treatment should be continued for 24-48 hours after clinical improvement, at which time therapy may be switched to one of the following regimens to complete at least 1 week of antimicrobial therapy:
- Cefixime[†] 400 mg orally twice daily
  OR
- Cefixime 400 mg by suspension (200 mg/5 ml) twice daily
  OR

Box 10-1 Centers for Disease Control Sexually Transmitted Diseases—cont'd

- Cefpodoxime 400 mg orally twice daily
- Fluoroquinolones may be an alternative treatment option if antimicrobial susceptibility can be documented by culture.

Pelvic inflamatory disease (PID)

Parenteral regimen A

- Cefotetan 2 gm IV every 12 hours
  OR
- Cefoxitin 2 gm IV every 6 hours
  PLUS
- Doxycycline 100 mg orally or IV every 12 hours

Parenteral regimen B

- Clindamycin 900 mg IV every 8 hours
  PLUS
- Gentamicin loading dose IV or IM (2 mg/kg of body weight), followed by a maintenance dose (1.5 mg/kg) every 8 hours. Single daily dosing may be substituted.

Alternative parenteral regimens

- Ampicillin/sulbactam 3 gm IV every 6 hours
  PLUS
- Doxycycline 100 mg orally or IV every 12 hours

Oral treatment

Oral regimen

- Ceftriaxone 250 mg IM in a single dose
  PLUS
- Doxycycline 100 mg orally twice a day for 14 days
  WITH OR WITHOUT
- Metronidazole 500 mg orally twice a day for 14 days
  OR
- Cefoxitin 2 gm IM in a single dose and probenecid 1 gm orally administered concurrently in a single dose
  PLUS
- Doxycycline 100 mg orally twice a day for 14 days
  WITH OR WITHOUT
- Metronidazole 500 mg orally twice a day for 14 days
  OR
- Other parenteral third-generation cephalosporins (e.g., ceftizoxime or cefotaxime)
  PLUS
- Doxycycline 100 mg orally twice a day for 14 days
  WITH OR WITHOUT
- Metronidazole 500 mg orally twice a day for 14 days

Alternative oral regimens

- If parenteral cephalosporin therapy is not feasible, use of fluoroquinolones (levofloxacin 500 mg orally once daily or ofloxacin 400 mg twice daily for 14 days) with or without metronidazole (500 mg orally twice daily for 14 days) may be considered if the community prevalence and individual risk of gonorrhea are low. Tests for gonorrhea must be performed before instituting therapy.

Epididymitis

- Ceftriaxone 250 mg IM in a single dose
  PLUS
- Doxycycline 100 mg orally twice a day for 10 days
- For acute epididymitis most likely caused by enteric organisms or with negative gonococcal culture or nucleic acid amplification test:
  - Ofloxacin 300 mg orally twice a day for 10 days
    OR
  - Levofloxacin 500 mg orally once daily for 10 days

GENITAL ULCERS

Developed Countries

In developed countries, most patients who have genital ulcers have either herpes simplex virus (HSV), syphilis, or chancroid. The differential diagnosis of genital ulcers is presented in Table 10-1. The frequency of each differs by geographic area and patient population. Herpes is the most prevalent. A patient may have more than one of these diseases. Not all genital ulcers are caused by sexually transmitted infections. Each disease is associated with an increased risk for human immunodeficiency virus (HIV) infection. A diagnosis-based history and physical examination is often inaccurate. All patients who have genital ulcers should have a serologic test for syphilis and diagnostic tests for herpes. Tests include the following:

- Rapid plasma reagin (RPR) or Venereal Disease Research Laboratories (VDRL)
- Dark-field examination for *Treponema pallidum*
- Culture, polymerase chain reaction (PCR), and/or antigen test for HSV
- Culture for *Haemophilus ducreyi*
- Biopsy if treatment fails
- HIV testing if ulcers are caused by *T. pallidum* or *H. ducreyi*
- Consider HIV testing for patients with HSV

HIV testing should be performed in patients who have genital ulcers caused by *T. pallidum* or *H. ducreyi* and considered for those who have ulcers caused by HSV.

Treatment of genital ulcers is often desirable before test results are available. Treat for the most likely diagnosis. If the diagnosis is unclear, treat for syphilis or for both syphilis and chancroid if the patient lives in an area where *H. ducreyi* is a significant cause of genital ulcers. Even after complete diagnostic evaluation, at least 25% of patients who have genital ulcers have no laboratory-confirmed diagnosis (Tables 10-1 and 10-2).

Table 10-1 Differential Diagnosis of Genital Ulcerations*

	Chancroid	Granuloma inguinale	Lymphogranuloma venereum (LGV)	Primary syphilis	Herpes simplex
Etiology	*Haemophilus ducreyi*	*Calymmatobacterium (Donovania) granulomatis*	*Chlamydia*	*Treponema pallidum*	*Herpes virus hominis*
Incubation period	12 hr to 3 days	3-6 weeks	3 days to several weeks	3 weeks	3-10 days
Initial lesion	Single or multiple, round to oval, deep ulcers with outlines, ragged and undermined borders, and a purulent base; lesions are tender	Soft, nontender papule(s) that form(s) irregular ulcer with beefy-red, friable base, and raised, "rolled" border	Evanescent ulcer (rarely seen)	Nontender, eroded papule with clean base and raised, firm, indurated borders; multiple lesions occasionally seen	Primary lesions are multiple, edematous, painful erosions with yellow-white membranous coating; recurrent episodes may have grouped vesicles on an erythematous base
Duration	Undetermined (months)	Undetermined (years)	2-6 days	3-6 weeks	Primary 2-6 weeks; recurrent 7-10 days
Site	Genital or perianal	Genital, perianal, or inguinal	Genital, perianal, or rectal	Genital, perianal, or rectal	Genital or perianal
Regional adenopathy	Unilateral or bilateral tender, matted, fixed adenopathy that may become soft and fluctuant	Subcutaneous perilymphatic granulomatous lesions that produce inguinal swellings and are not lymphadenitis (pseudo buboes)	Unilateral or bilateral firm, painful inguinal adenopathy with overlying "dusky skin"; may become fluctuant and develop "grooves in the groin"	Unilateral or bilateral firm, movable, nonsupportive, painless inguinal adenopathy	Bilateral, tender inguinal adenopathy, usually present with primary vulvovaginitis and may or may not be present with recurrent genital lesions
Diagnostic tests	Smear, culture, or biopsy of lesion; smear from aspirated unruptured lymph node	Biopsy; touch preparation from biopsy stained with Giemsa	LGV complement fixation test, culture	Dark-field examination, VDRL, FTA-ABS	Tzanck smear; culture

*Modified from Margolis RJ, Hood AF: *J Am Acad Dermatol* 6:496, 1982.

GENITAL ULCERS

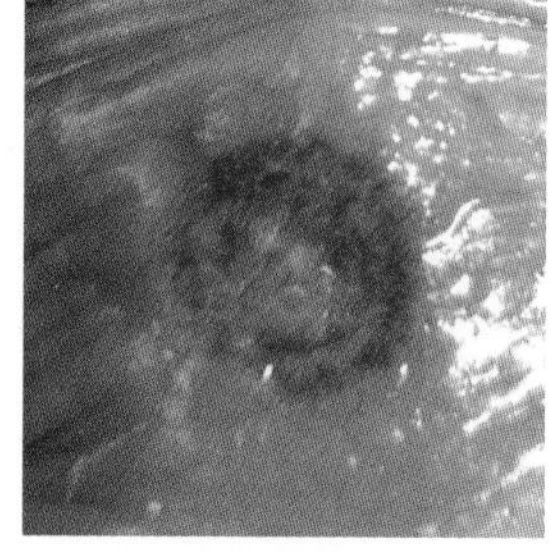

Syphilis

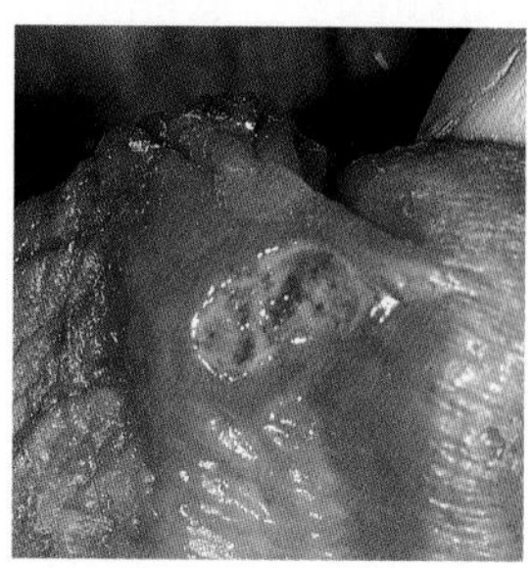

Chancroid

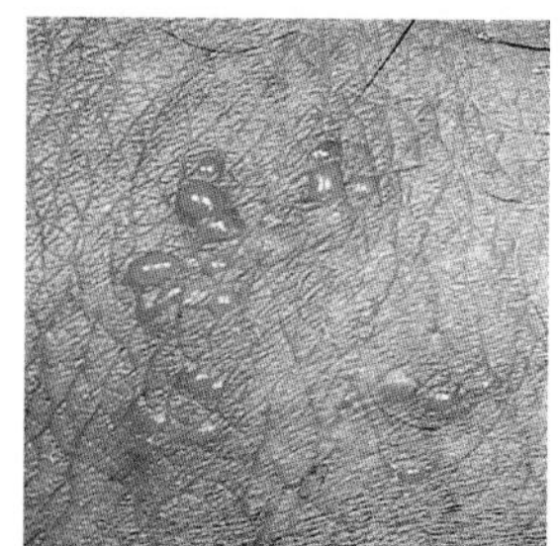

Herpes vesicles

SYNDROMIC MANAGEMENT OF SEXUALLY TRANSMITTED DISEASES

WORLD HEALTH ORGANIZATION (WHO). Many health care facilities in developing countries lack the equipment and trained personnel required for etiologic diagnosis of STDs. To overcome this problem, a syndrome-based approach rather than a conventional approach based on laboratory tests has been developed in a large number of countries. The syndromic management approach is based on the identification of consistent groups of symptoms and easily recognized signs (syndromes), and the provision of treatment that will handle the majority of, or the most serious, organisms responsible for producing a syndrome.

A more definite or etiologic diagnosis may be possible with sophisticated laboratory facilities, but this is often not possible. Laboratory tests require resources, add cost, may require extra visits, and may delay treatment. For these reasons, syndromic management guidelines are widely used for syndromes even in developed countries with advanced laboratory facilities.

WHO has developed a flow chart to guide health workers in the implementation of syndromic management of STDs. These charts in a modified form appear on the following pages.

The syndromes that cause sexually transmitted infections (STIs) are presented in Tables 10-2 through 10-10.

Text continued on p. 396

Table 10-2 Signs, Symptoms, and Causes for STI Syndromes (World Health Organization Terms and Definitions)

Syndrome	Symptoms	Signs	Most common causes
Genital ulcer	Genital sore	Genital ulcer	Syphilis Chancroid Genital herpes
Urethral discharge	Urethral discharge Dysuria Frequent urination	Urethral discharge (if necessary ask patient to milk urethra)	Gonorrhea Chlamydia
Vaginal discharge Cervical infection	Unusual vaginal discharge Vaginal itching Dysuria (pain on urination) Dyspareunia (pain during sexual intercourse)	Abnormal vaginal discharge	Vaginitis: Trichomoniasis Candidiasis Cervicitis: Gonorrhea Chlamydia
Lower abdominal pain	Lower abdominal pain Dyspareunia	Vaginal discharge Lower abdominal tenderness on palpation Temperature >38° C	Gonorrhea Chlamydia
Inguinal bubo	Painful enlarged inguinal lymph nodes	Enlarged inguinal lymph nodes Fluctuation Abscesses or fistulae	Lymphogranuloma venereum Chancroid

SYNDROMIC MANAGEMENT (WORLD HEALTH ORGANIZATION)

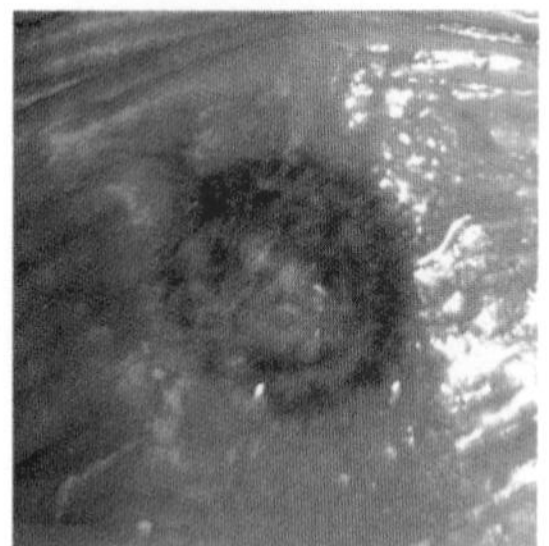
Syphilis

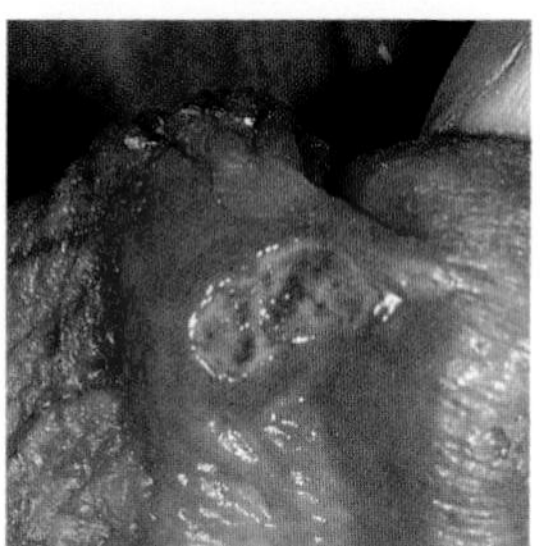
Chancroid

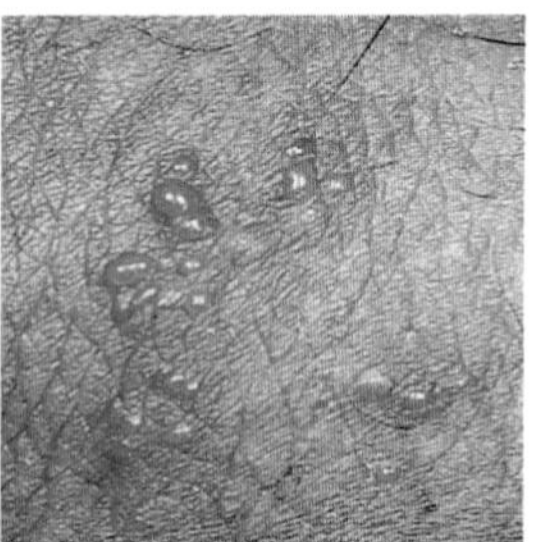
Herpes vesicles

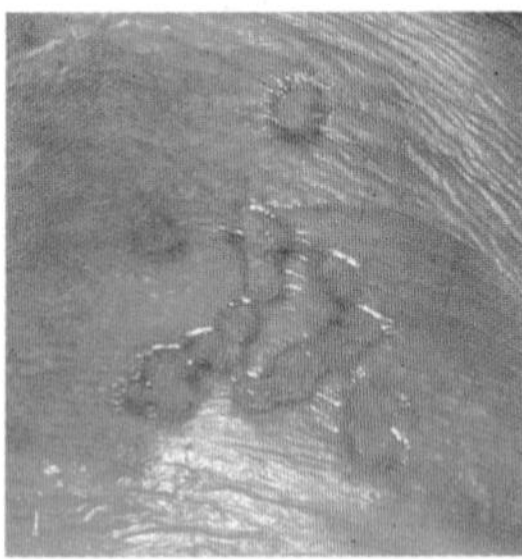
Herpes ulcers

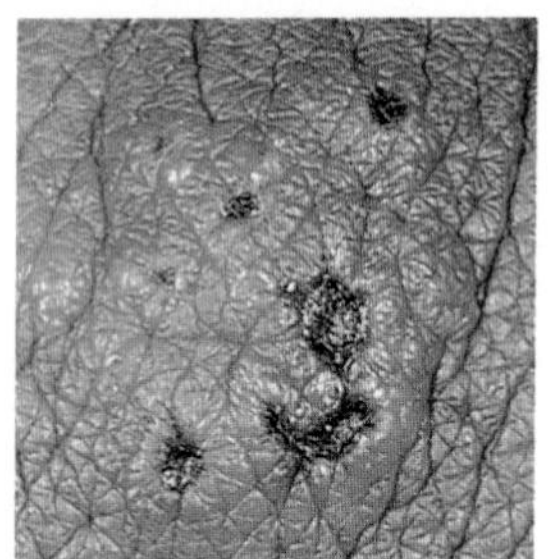
Herpes crust

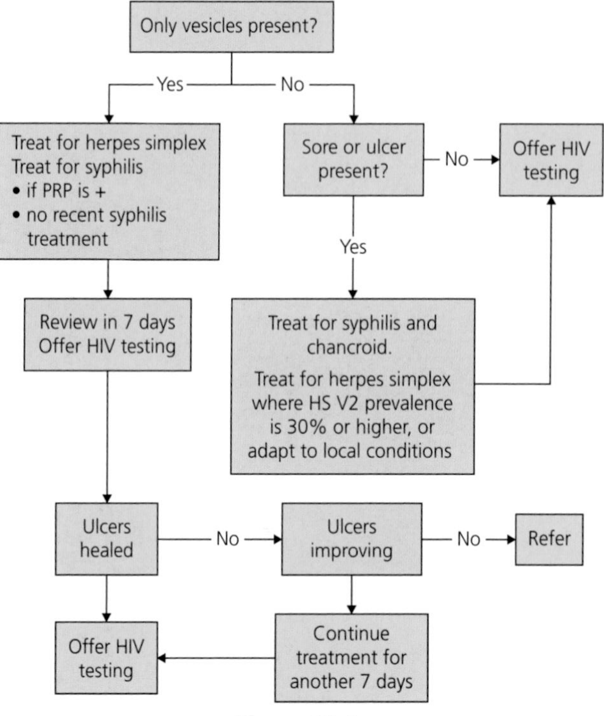

Figure 10-1

Table 10-3 Recommended Treatment for Genital Ulcers*

Coverage	***First choice*** **Choose 1 from each box (total of 2 drugs)**	**Effective substitutes**	***If patient is pregnant, breast-feeding, or <16 years old*** **Choose 1 from each box (total of 2 drugs)**
Syphilis	Benzathine penicillin 2.4 million units by single intramuscular injection NOTE: for patients with a positive syphilis test and no ulcer, administer same dose at weekly intervals for total of 3 doses	Doxycycline§ 100 mg twice a day for 13 days, or Tetracycline§ 500 mg orally 4 times a day for 14 days	Benzathine penicillin 2.4 million units by single intramuscular injection, or Erythromycin‡ 500 mg orally 4 times a day for 15 days
Chancroid	Ciprofloxacin† 500 mg orally twice a day for 3 days, or Azithromycin 1 gm orally as a single dose, or Erythromycin‡ 500 mg orally 4 times a day for 7 days	Ceftriaxone 250 mg as a single intramuscular injection	Erythromycin‡ 500 mg orally 4 times a day for 7 days, or Azithromycin 1 gm orally as a single dose, or Ceftriaxone 250 mg as a single intramuscular injection
Additional therapy for HSV-2 where HSV-2 is common			
Genital herpes	*Primary infection* Acyclovir§ 200 mg orally 5 times a day for 7 days, or Acyclovir§ 400 mg orally 3 times a day for 7 days	*Primary infection* Famciclovir§ 250 mg orally 3 times a day for 7 days, or Valacyclovir§ 1 gm twice a day for 7 days	Use acyclovir only when benefit outweighs risk
	Recurrent infection Acyclovir§ 200 mg orally 5 times a day for 5 days, or Acyclovir§ 400 mg orally 3 times a day for 5 days	*Recurrent infection* Famciclovir§ 125 mg orally 3 times a day for 5 days, or Valacyclovir§ 500 mg orally twice a day for 5 days	Dosage is the same as for primary infection

Adapted from *Sexually transmitted and other reproductive tract infections: A guide to essential practice,* World Health Organization, 2005.
*Recommended treatment for genital ulcers: (1) single-dose therapy for syphilis plus (2) single-dose or multidose therapy for chancroid. See Table 10-4 for additional GUD treatment that may be needed for some regions.
†The use of quinolones should take into consideration the patterns of *Neisseria gonorrhoeae* resistance, such as in the WHO South-East Asia and Western Pacific regions.
‡Erythromycin estolate is contraindicated in pregnancy because of drug-related hepatotoxicity; only erythromycin base or erythromycin ethylsuccinate should be used.
§These drugs are contraindicated for pregnant or breast-feeding women.

Table 10-4 Recommended Additional Treatment for Genital Ulcers (in areas where granuloma inguinale and lymlphogranuloma venereum are important causes of genital ulcers)

Coverage	**First choice**	**Effective substitutes**	**If patient is pregnant, breast-feeding, or <16 years old**
Granuloma inguinale (donovanosis): Treatment should be continued until all lesions have completely epithelialized.	Azithromycin 1 gm orally as a single dose followed by 500 mg once a day, or Doxycycline* 100 mg orally twice a day	Erythromycin† 500 mg orally 4 times a day, or Tetracycline† 500 mg orally 4 times a day, or Trimethroprim (80 mg)/ sulfamethoxazole (400 mg), 2 tablets orally twice a day	Azithromycin 1 gm orally as a single dose, or Erythromycin† 500 mg orally 4 times a day
Lymphogranuloma venereum	Doxycycline* 100 mg orally twice a day for 14 days, or Erythromycin† 500 mg orally 4 times a day for 14 days	Tetracycline† 500 mg orally 4 times a day for 14 days	Erythromycin† 500 mg orally 4 times a day for 14 days

From *Sexually transmitted and other reproductive tract infections: A guide to essential practice,* World Health Organization, 2005.
*These drugs are contraindicated for pregnant or breast-feeding women.
†Erythromycin estolate is contraindicated in pregnancy because of drug-related hepatotoxicity; only erythromycin base or erythromycin ethylsuccinate should be used.

SYNDROMIC MANAGEMENT (WORLD HEALTH ORGANIZATION)

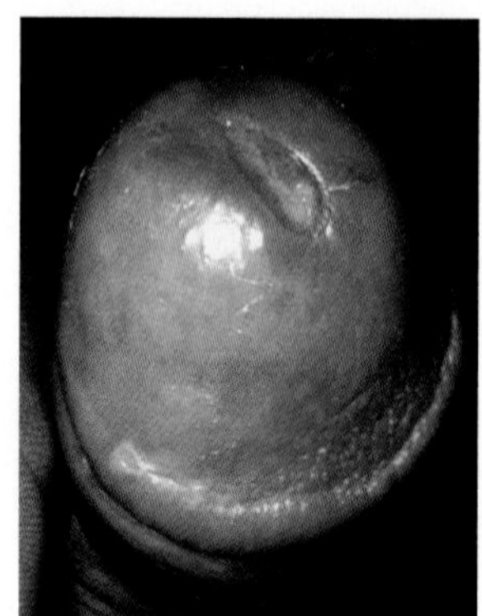

Gonorrhea

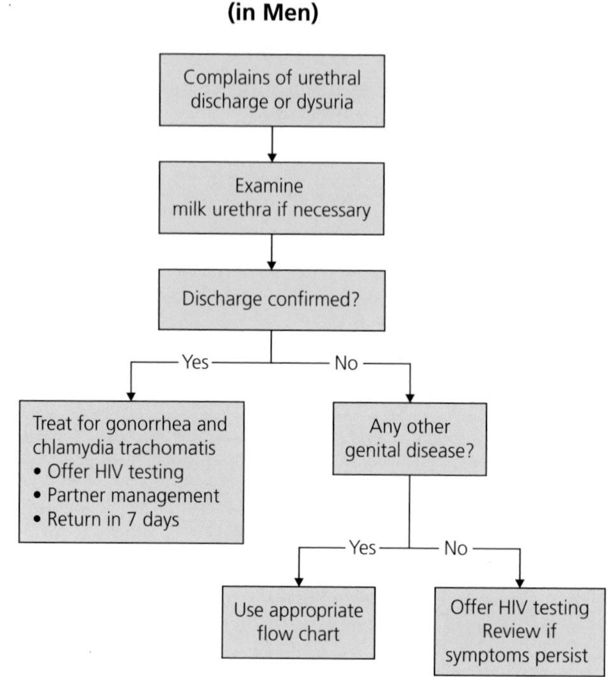

Figure 10-2

Table 10-5 Recommended Treatment for Urethral Discharge (Males Only) (Therapy for uncomplicated gonorrhoea plus therapy for chlamydia)

Coverage	***First choice*** **Choose 1 from each box (total of 2 drugs)**	**Effective substitutes**
Gonorrhoea	Cefixime 400 mg orally as a single dose, or	Ciprofloxacin* 500 mg orally as a single dose, or
	Ceftriaxone 125 mg by intramuscular injection	Spectinomycin 2 gm by intramuscular injection
Chlamydia	Azithromycin 1 gm orally as single dose, or	Ofloxacin*† 300 mg orally twice a day for 7 days, or
	Doxycycline 100 mg orally twice a day for 7 days	Tetracycline 500 mg orally 4 times a day for 7 days, or
		Erythromycin 500 mg orally 4 times a day for 7 days

From *Sexually transmitted and other reproductive tract infections: A guide to essential practice,* World Health Organization, 2005.
*The use of quinolones should take into consideration the patterns of *Neisseria gonorrhoeae* resistance, such as in the WHO South-East Asia and Western Pacific regions.
†Ofloxacin, when used as indicated for chlamydial infection, also provides coverage for gonorrhoea.

SYNDROMIC MANAGEMENT (WORLD HEALTH ORGANIZATION)

VAGINAL DISCHARGE IN NON-PREGNANT WOMEN

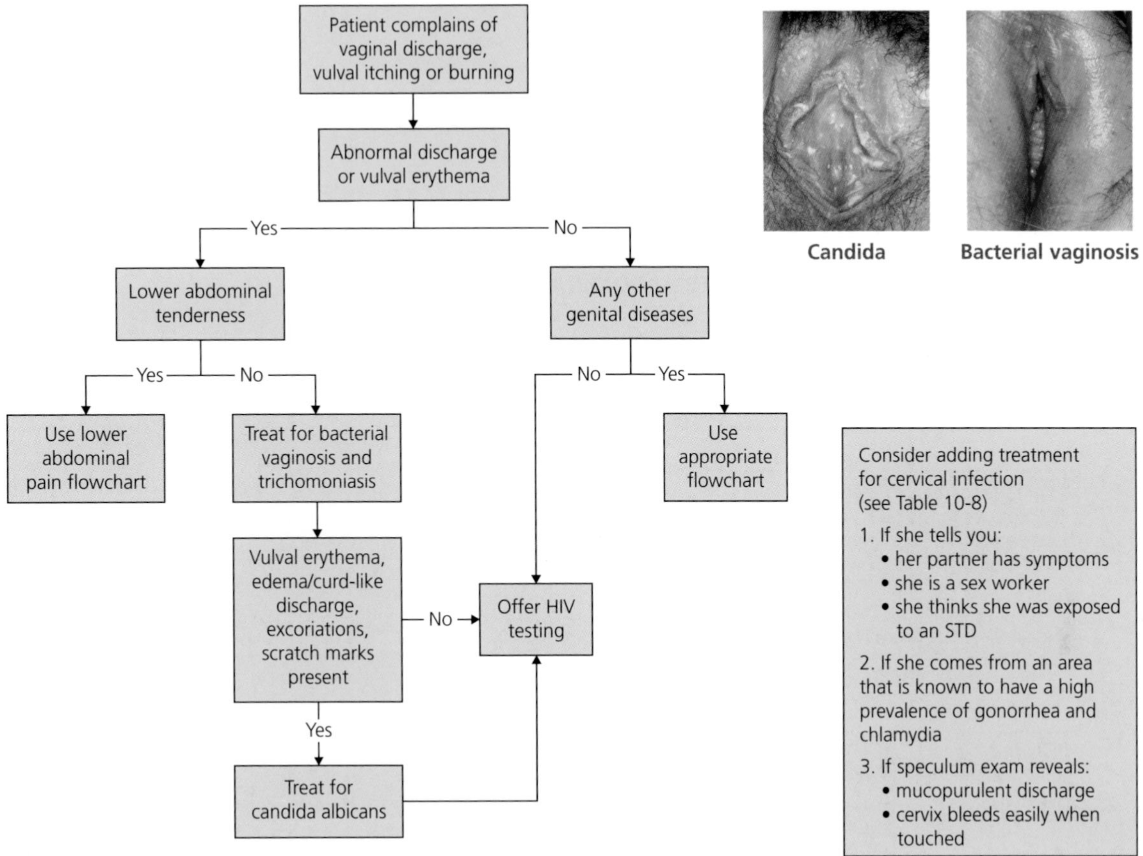

Figure 10-3

Table 10-6 Recommended Treatment for Vaginal Infection*

Coverage	***First choice*** **Choose 1 from BV/TV box, or 1 from each box if yeast infection is suspected**	**Effective substitutes**	***If patient is pregnant, breast-feeding*** **Choose 1 from BV/TV box below, or 1 from each box if yeast infection is suspected**
Bacterial vaginosis (BV)	Metronidazole† 2 gm orally in a single dose, or Metronidazole† 400 or 500 mg orally twice a day for 7 days	Clindamycin cream 2%, one full applicator (5 gm) intravaginally at bedtime for 7 days, or Clindamycin 300 mg orally twice a day for 7 days	*Preferably after first trimester* Metronidazole† 200 or 250 mg orally 3 times a day for 7 days, or Metronidazole† gel 0.75%, one full applicator (5 gm) intravaginally twice a day for 5 days, or Clindamycin 300 mg orally twice a day for 7 days
Trichomoniasis vaginalis (TV)		Tinidazole† 2 gm orally in a single dose, or Tinidazole† 500 mg orally twice a day for 5 days	
Candida albicans (CA) (yeast)	Miconazole 200-mg vaginal suppository, one a day for 3 days, or Clotrimazole‡ 100-mg vaginal tablet, 2 tablets a day for 3 days, or Fluconazole 150-mg oral tablet, in a single dose	Nystatin 100,000-unit vaginal tablet, one a day for 14 days	Miconazole 200-mg vaginal suppository, one a day for 3 days, or Clotrimazole‡ 100-mg vaginal tablet, 2 tablets a day for 3 days, or Nystatin 100,000-unit vaginal tablet, one a day for 14 days

From *Sexually transmitted and other reproductive tract infections: A guide to essential practice:* World Health Organization, 2005.

*Therapy for bacterial vaginosis and trichomoniasis plus therapy for yeast infection if curdlike white discharge, vulvovaginal redness, and itching are present.

†Patients taking metronidazole or tinidazole should be cautioned to avoid alcohol. Use of metronidazole is not recommended in the first trimester of pregnancy.

‡Single-dose clotrimazole (500 mg) available in some places is also effective for yeast infection (CA).

SYNDROMIC MANAGEMENT (WORLD HEALTH ORGANIZATION)

LOWER ABDOMINAL PAIN (in Women)

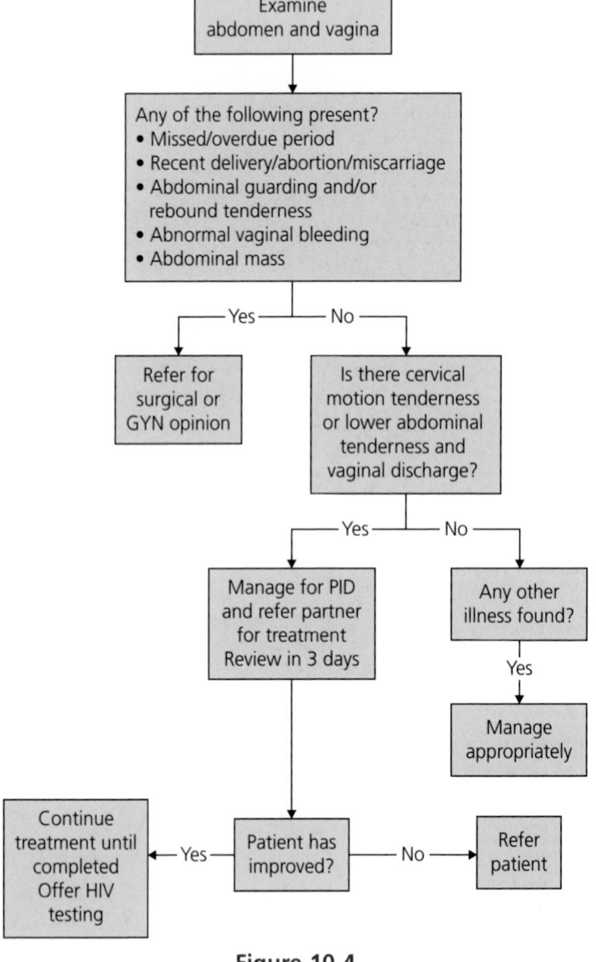

Figure 10-4

Table 10-7 Recommended Outpatient Treatment for PID (Single-dose therapy for gonorrhoea plus single-dose or multidose therapy for chlamydia plus therapy for anaerobic infections)

Coverage	Choose 1 from each box (total of 3 drugs)
Gonorrhoea	Ceftriaxone 250 mg by intramuscular injection, or Cefixime 400 mg orally as a single dose, or Ciprofloxacin* 500 mg orally as a single dose, or Spectinomycin 2 gm by intramuscular injection
Chlamydia	Doxycycline† 100 mg orally twice a day for 14 days, or Tetracycline† 500 mg orally 4 times a day for 14 days
Anaerobes	Metronidazole‡ 400-500 mg orally, twice a day for 14 days

From *Sexually transmitted and other reproductive tract infections: A guide to essential practice,* World Health Organization, 2005.
*The use of quinolones should take into consideration the patterns of *Neisseria gonorrhoeae* resistance, such as in the WHO South-East Asia and Western Pacific regions.
†These drugs are contraindicated for pregnant or breast-feeding women. PID is uncommon in pregnancy.
‡Patients taking metronidazole should be cautioned to avoid alcohol. Metronidazole should also be avoided during the first trimester of pregnancy.

Note: Hospitalization of patients with acute pelvic inflammatory disease should be seriously considered when: (a) a surgical emergency, such as appendicitis or ectopic pregnancy, cannot be excluded; (b) a pelvic abscess is suspected; (c) severe illness precludes management on an outpatient basis; (d) the patient is pregnant; (e) the patient is an adolescent; (f) the patient is unable to follow or tolerate an outpatient regimen; or (g) the patient has failed to respond to outpatient therapy (see Table 10-9).

Table 10-8 Recommended Treatment for Cervical Infection (Therapy for uncomplicated gonorrhoea plus therapy for chlamydia)

Coverage	***First choice*** Choose 1 from each box (total of 2 drugs)	Effective substitutes	***If patient is pregnant, breast-feeding or <16 years old*** Choose 1 from each box
Gonorrhoea	Cefixime 400 mg orally as a single dose, or Ceftriaxone 125 mg by intramuscular injection	Ciprofloxacin*† 500 mg orally as a single dose, or Spectinomycin 2 gm by intra-muscular injection	Cefixime 400 mg orally as a single dose, or Ceftriaxone 125 mg by intramuscular injection
Chlamydia	Azithromycin 1 gm orally as a single dose, or Doxycycline* 100 mg orally twice a day for 7 days	Ofloxacin*†‡ 300 mg orally twice a day for 7 days, or Tetracycline* 500 mg orally 4 times a day for 7 days, or Erythromycin 500 mg orally 4 times a day for 7 days	Erythromycin§ 500 mg orally 4 times a day for 7 days, or Azithromycin 1 gm orally as a single dose, or Amoxicillin 500 mg orally 3 times a day for 7 days

From *Sexually transmitted and other reproductive tract infections: A guide to essential practice,* World Health Organization, 2005.
*Doxycycline, tetracycline, ciprofloxacin, norfloxacin, and ofloxacin should be avoided in pregnancy and when breast-feeding.
†The use of quinolones should take into consideration the patterns of *Neisseria gonorrhoeae* resistance, such as in the WHO South-East Asia and Western Pacific regions.
‡Ofloxacin, when used as indicated for chlamydial infection, also provides coverage for gonorrhoea.
§Erythromycin estolate is contraindicated in pregnancy because of drug-related hepatotoxicity; only erythromycin base or erythromycin ethyl-succinate should be used.

Table 10-9 Recommended Inpatient Treatment for PID (Therapy for gonorrhoea plus therapy for chlamydia plus therapy for anaerobic infections)*

Coverage	***Option 1*** Choose 1 from each box (total of 3 drugs), and follow with oral outpatient therapy below	***Option 2*** Give both drugs and follow with oral outpatient therapy below	***Option 3*** Commonly available; give all 3 drugs plus oral outpatient therapy below
Gonorrhoea	Ceftriaxone 250 mg by intramuscular injection, once a day, or Ciprofloxacin† 500 mg orally as a single dose, or Spectinomycin 2 gm by intramuscular injection	Gentamicin 1.5 mg/kg of body weight by intravenous injection every 8 hr PLUS Clindamycin 900 mg by intravenous injection every 8 hr	Ampicillin 2 gm by intravenous or intramuscular injection, then 1 gm every 6 hr, PLUS Gentamicin 80 mg by intramuscular injection every 8 hr, PLUS Metronidazole 500 mg or 100 ml by intravenous infusion every 8 hr
Chlamydia	Doxycycline‡§ 100 mg orally or by intravenous injection, twice a day, or Tetracycline§ 500 mg orally 4 times a day		
Anaerobes	Metronidazole 400-500 mg orally or by intravenous injection, twice a day, or Chloramphenicol§ 500 mg orally or by intravenous injection, 4 times a day		

From *Sexually transmitted and other reproductive tract infections: A guide to essential practice,* World Health Organization, 2005.
*For all three options, therapy should be continued until at least 2 days after the patient has improved and should then be followed by one of the following oral treatments for a total of 14 days: doxycycline§ 100 mg orally twice a day, or tetracycline§ 500 mg orally 4 times a day.
†The use of quinolones should take into consideration the patterns of *Neisseria gonorrhoeae* resistance, such as in the WHO South-East Asia and Western Pacific regions.
‡Intravenous doxycycline is painful and has no advantage over the oral route if the patient is able to take medicine by mouth.
§Contraindicated for pregnant or breast-feeding women. PID is uncommon in pregnancy.

SYNDROMIC MANAGEMENT (WORLD HEALTH ORGANIZATION)

INGUINAL BUBO
(in Men and Women)

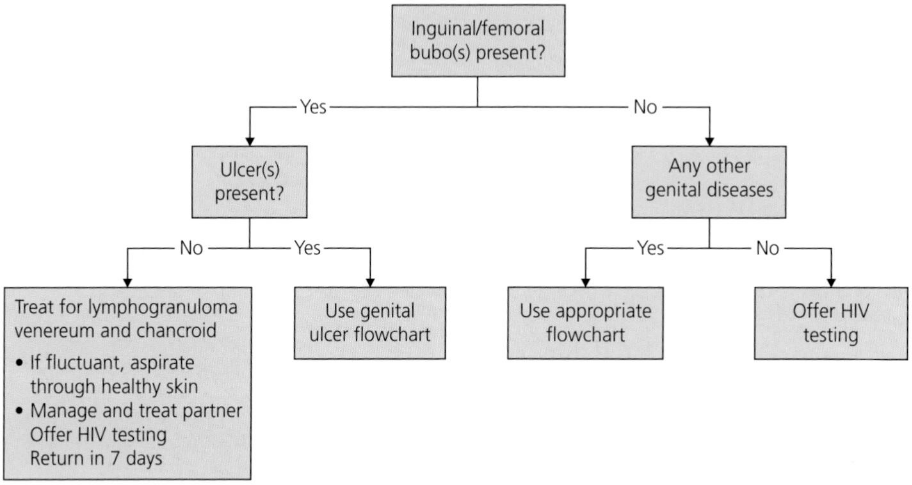

Inguinal/femoral bubo(s) present?

Yes → Ulcer(s) present?
- No → Treat for lymphogranuloma venereum and chancroid
  - If fluctuant, aspirate through healthy skin
  - Manage and treat partner

  Offer HIV testing
  Return in 7 days
- Yes → Use genital ulcer flowchart

No → Any other genital diseases
- Yes → Use appropriate flowchart
- No → Offer HIV testing

Figure 10-5

Table 10-10 Recommended Treatment for Inguinal Bubo (Single-dose or multidose therapies for chancroid plus multidose therapies for lymphogranuloma venereum [LGV])*

Coverage	***First choice*** **Choose 1 from each box (total of 2 drugs)**	**Effective substitutes**	**If patient is pregnant, breast-feeding, or <16 years old**
Chancroid	Ciprofloxacin*† 500 mg orally twice a day for 3 days, or Erythromycin‡ 500 mg orally 4 times a day for 7 days	Azithromycin 1 gm orally as a single dose, or Ceftriaxone 250 mg as a single intramuscular injection	Erythromycin‡ 500 mg orally 4 times a day for 14 days (covers both chancroid and LGV)
LGV	Doxycycline* 100 mg orally twice a day for 14 days	Tetracycline† 500 mg orally 4 times a day for 14 days	

From *Sexually transmitted and other reproductive tract infections. A guide to essential practice,* World Health Organization, 2005.

Note: Some cases may require longer treatment than the 14 days recommended. Fluctuant lymph nodes should be aspirated through healthy skin. Incision and drainage or excision of nodes may delay healing and should not be attempted.

*These drugs are contraindicated for pregnant or breast-feeding women.

†The use of quinolones should take into consideration the patterns of *Neisseria gonorrhoeae* resistance, such as in the WHO South-East Asia and Western Pacific regions.

‡Erythromycin estolate is contraindicated in pregnancy because of drug-related hepatotoxicity; only erythromycin base or erythromycin ethylsuccinate should be used.

WHO RECOMMENDED REGIMEN FOR WARTS

VENEREAL WARTS

Recommended regimen

Chemical (Self-applied by patient)

- Podophyllotoxin 0.5% solution or gel, twice daily for 3 days, followed by 4 days of no treatment; the cycle can be repeated up to 4 times (total volume of podophyllotoxin should not exceed 0.5 ml per day). **OR**
- Imiquimod 5% cream applied with a finger at bedtime, left on overnight, 3 times a week for as long as 16 weeks. The treatment area should be washed with soap and water 6 to 10 hours after application. Hands must be washed with soap and water immediately after application.
- The safety of both podophyllotoxin and imiquimod during pregnancy has not been established.

Chemical (Provider administered)

- Podophyllin, 10% to 25% in compound tincture of benzoin, is applied carefully to the warts, avoiding normal tissue. External genital and perianal warts should be washed thoroughly 1 to 4 hours after the application of podophyllin. Podophyllin applied to warts on vaginal or anal epithelial surfaces should be allowed to dry before the speculum or anoscope is removed. Treatment should be repeated at weekly intervals.
- Where available, podophyllotoxin 0.5%, one of the active constituents of podophyllin resin, is recommended. Its efficacy is equal to that of podophyllin, but it is less toxic and appears to cause less erosion.
- Some experts advise against the use of podophyllin for anal warts. Large amounts of podophyllin should not be used because it is toxic and easily absorbed. Its use during pregnancy and lactation is contraindicated. **OR**
- Trichloroacetic acid (TCA) 80% to 90%, applied carefully to the warts, avoiding normal tissue, followed by powdering of the treated area with talc or sodium bicarbonate (baking soda) to remove unreacted acid. Repeat application at weekly intervals.

Physical

- Cryotherapy with liquid nitrogen, solid carbon dioxide, or a cryoprobe. Repeat applications every 1 to 2 weeks. **OR**
- Electrosurgery **OR**
- Surgical removal

VAGINAL WARTS

- Cryotherapy with liquid nitrogen **OR**
- Podophyllin 10% to 25%. Allow to dry before removing speculum. **OR**
- TCA 80% to 90%

CERVICAL WARTS

Treatment of cervical warts should not be started until the results from a cervical smear test are known. Most experts advise against the use of podophyllin or TCA for cervical warts.

- Management should include consultation with an expert.
- Pap smear
- No TCA or podophyllin

MEATAL AND URETHRAL WARTS

Accessible meatal warts may be treated with podophyllin 10% to 25%, in compound tincture of benzoin, or podophyllotoxin 0.5%, where available. Great care should be taken to ensure that the treated area is dry before contact with normal, opposing epithelial surfaces is allowed. Low success rates with podophyllin are reported. Urethroscopy is necessary to diagnose intraurethral warts, but they should be suspected in men with recurrent meatal warts. Some experts prefer electrosurgical removal. Intraurethral instillation of a 5% cream of fluorouracil or thiotepa may be effective, but neither has been adequately evaluated. Podophyllin should not be used. Recommended treatments:

- Cryotherapy **OR**
- Podophyllin 10% to 25%

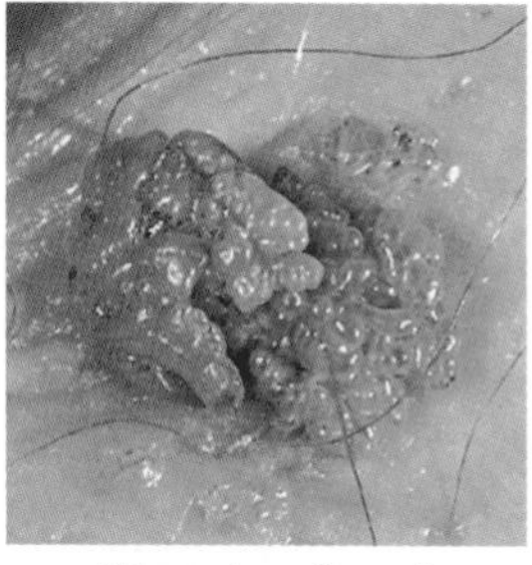

Warts (confluent)

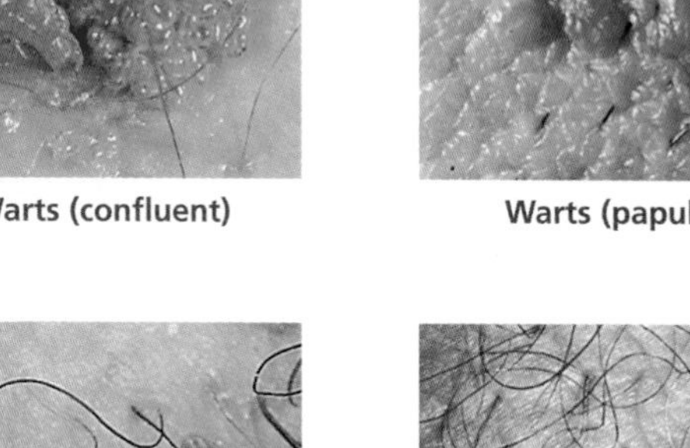

Warts (papules)

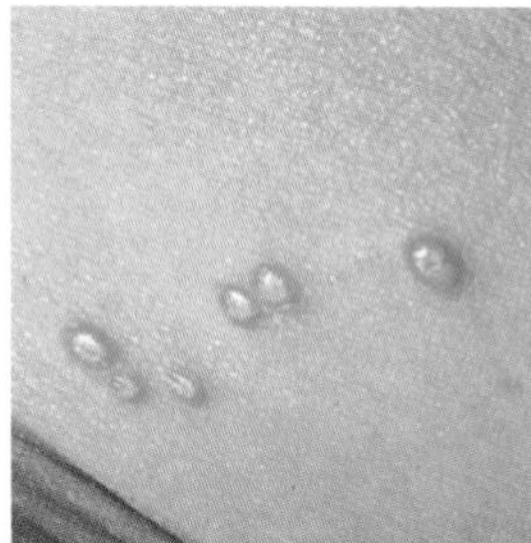

Molluscum contagiosum

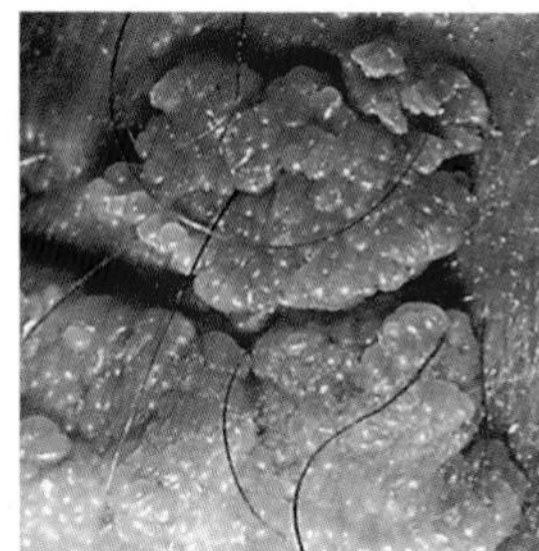

Warts (confluent)

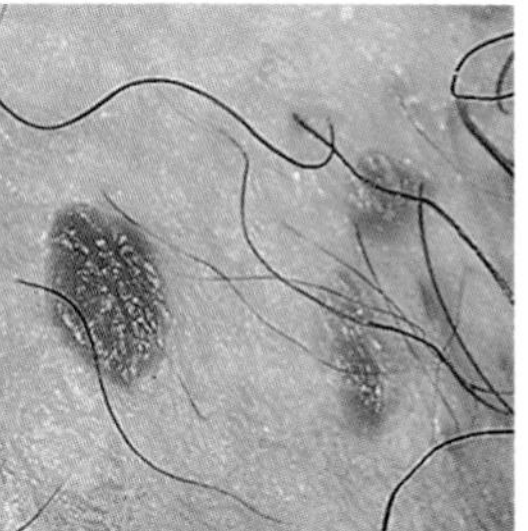

Bowenoid papulosis

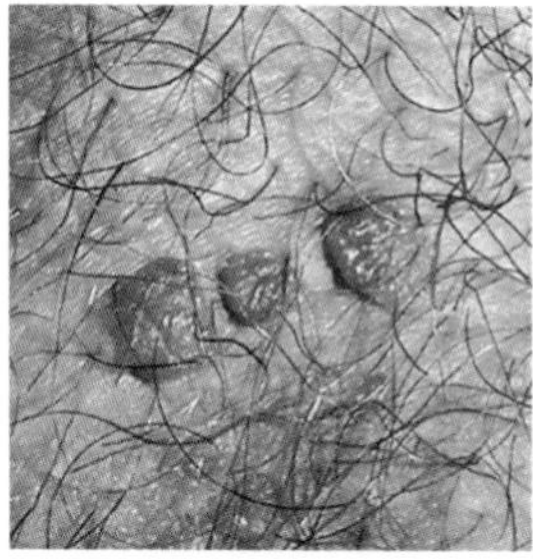

Warts (papules)

SYPHILIS

Syphilis is a human infectious disease caused by the bacterium *Treponema pallidum*. The disease is transmitted by direct contact with a lesion during the primary or secondary stage, in utero by the transplacental route, or during delivery as the baby passes through an infected canal. Like the gonococcus, this bacterium is fragile and dies when removed from the human environment. Unlike the gonococcus, *T. pallidum* may infect any organ, causing an infinite number of clinical presentations; thus the old adage, "he who knows syphilis knows medicine."

Incidence

The incidence of primary and secondary syphilis in the United States was 3.3 cases per 100,000 people in 2006 (9756 total cases). Blacks have a higher rate of syphilis than whites in the United States, based on 6862 cases reported in 2002; the incidence per 100,000 population was 9.4 in blacks and 1.1 in whites. Syphilis is found in the southern states, especially in blacks (Figure 10-6). Crack cocaine and the exchange of sex for drugs are contributing factors.

Stages

Untreated syphilis may pass through three stages. Syphilis begins with the infectious cutaneous primary and secondary stages that may terminate without further sequelae or may evolve into a latent stage that lasts for months or years before the now-rare tertiary stage, marked by the appearance of cardiovascular, neurologic, and deep cutaneous complications (Figure 10-7).

The Centers for Disease Control and Prevention defines the stages of syphilis as follows:

1. Infectious syphilis includes the stages of primary, secondary, and early latent syphilis of less than 1-year's duration.
2. Latent infections (i.e., those lacking clinical manifestations) are detected by serologic testing. Latent syphilis is divided into early latent disease of less than 1-year's duration and early latent disease of greater than 1-year's duration.
3. Late latent disease has a duration of 4 years or longer.

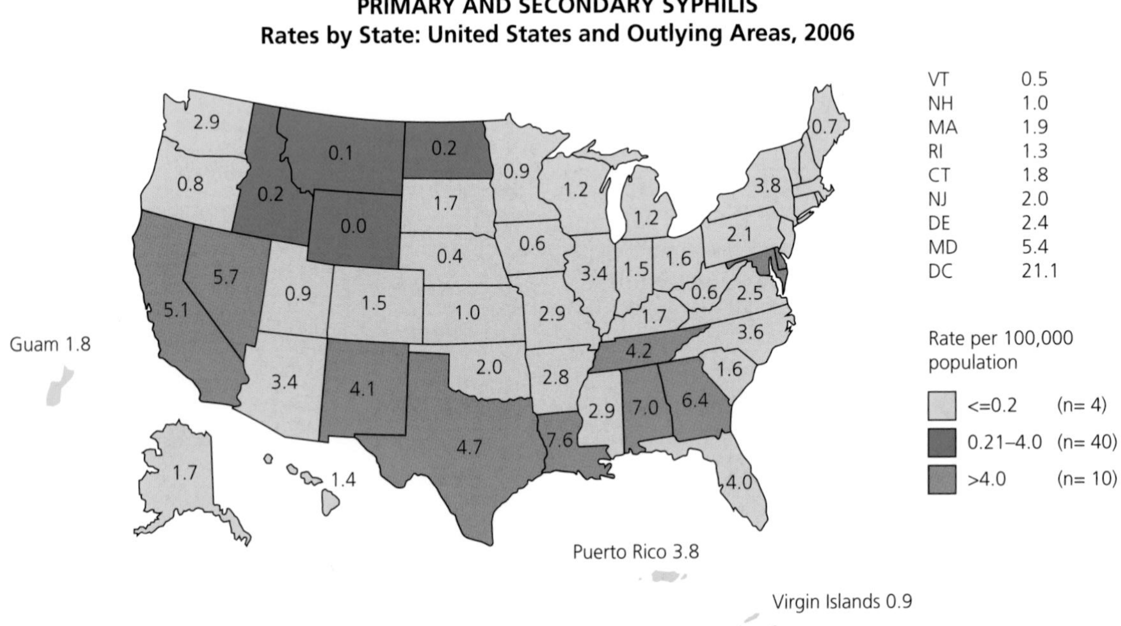

Figure 10-6

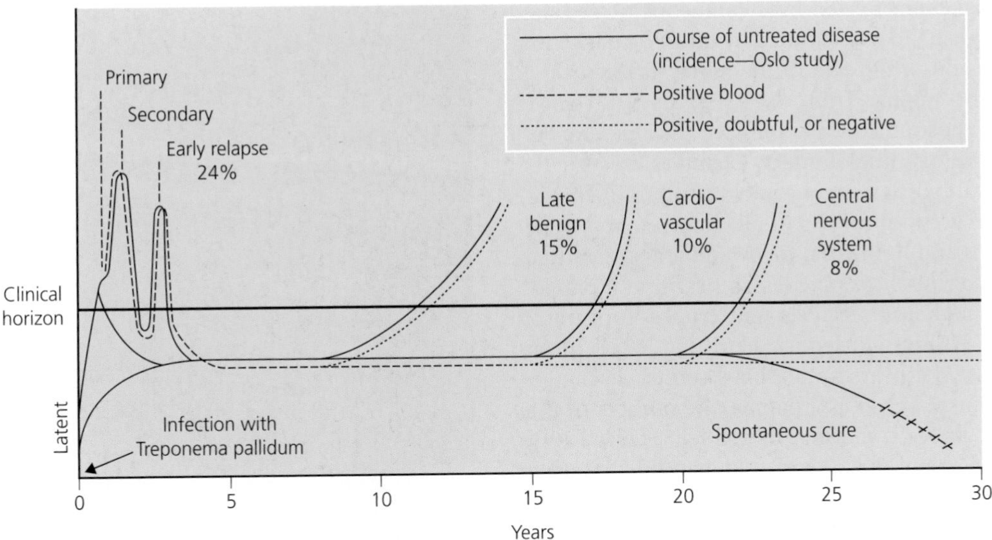

Figure 10-7 Natural history of untreated acquired syphilis. (From Morgan HJ: *South Med J* 26:18, 1933; incidence from Clark EG, Danbolt N: *J Chronic Dis* 2:311, 1955.)

Risk of transmission

The greatest risk of transmission occurs during the primary, secondary, and early latent stages of disease. The patient is most infectious during the first 1 to 2 years of infection. Patients with secondary syphilis are the most contagious because of the large number of lesions. The risk of acquiring syphilis from an infected partner is 10% to 60%. One third of persons with a single exposure to early syphilis will become infected.

T. pallidum

T. pallidum, the organism responsible for syphilis, is a very small, spiral bacterium (spirochete) whose form and corkscrew rotation motility can be observed only by dark-field microscopy (Figure 10-8). The reproductive time is estimated to be 30 to 33 hours, in contrast to most bacteria, which replicate every 30 minutes. Serum levels of antibiotics must therefore persist for at least 7 to 10 days to kill all replicating organisms. The Gram stain cannot be used, and growing the bacteria is difficult.

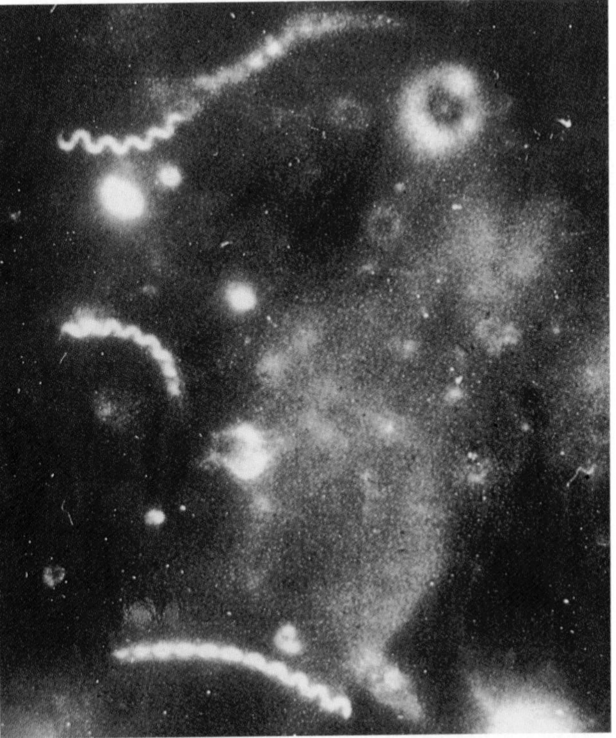

Figure 10-8 *Treponema pallidum*. Organism responsible for syphilis is seen here photographed through a dark-field microscope.

Primary syphilis

Primary syphilis, characterized by a cutaneous ulcer (Figures 10-9 through 10-13), is acquired by direct contact with an infectious lesion of the skin or the moist surface of the mouth, anus, or vagina. From 10 to 90 days (average, 21 days) after exposure, a primary lesion, the chancre, develops at the site of initial contact. Chancres are usually solitary, but multiple lesions are not uncommon. Extragenital chancres account for 6% of all chancres, and most occur on the lips and in the oral cavity and are transmitted by kissing or orogenital sex. The lesion begins as a papule that undergoes ischemic necrosis and erodes, forming a 0.3- to 2.0-cm, painless to tender, hard, indurated ulcer; the base is clean, with a scant, yellow, serous discharge. Because the chancre began as a papule, the borders of the ulcer are raised, smooth, and sharply defined (Figure 10-9). The chancre of chancroid is soft and painful. Painless, hard, discrete regional lymphadenopathy occurs in 1 to 2 weeks; the lesions never coalesce or suppurate unless there is a mixed infection. Without treatment, the chancre heals with scarring in 3 to 6 weeks. Painless vaginal (Figure 10-10) and anal lesions may never be detected. The differential diagnosis includes ulcerative genital lesions such as chancroid, herpes progenitalis, aphthae (Behçet's syndrome), and traumatic ulcers such as occur with biting. If untreated, approximately 25% of the infections progress directly to the second stage; the other 75% enter latency.

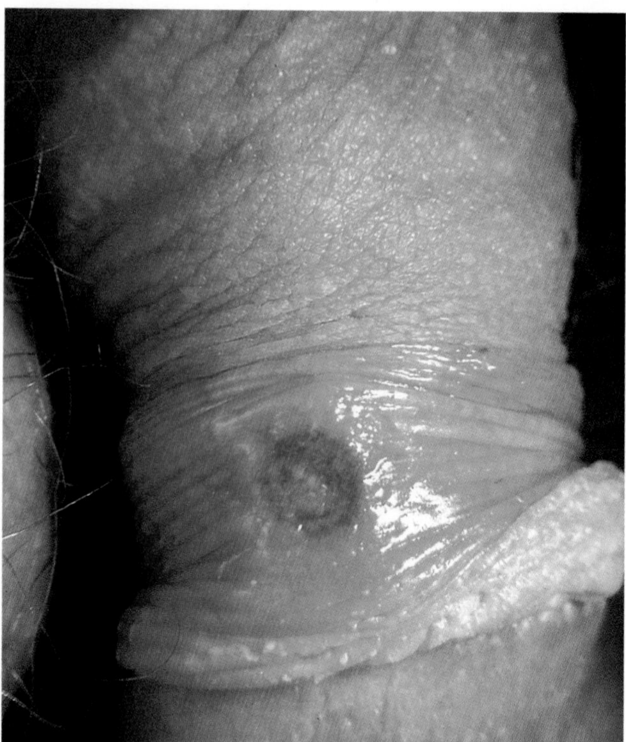

Figure 10-9 Primary syphilis. Syphilitic chancre is an ulcer with a clean, nonpurulent base and smooth, regular, sharply defined border.

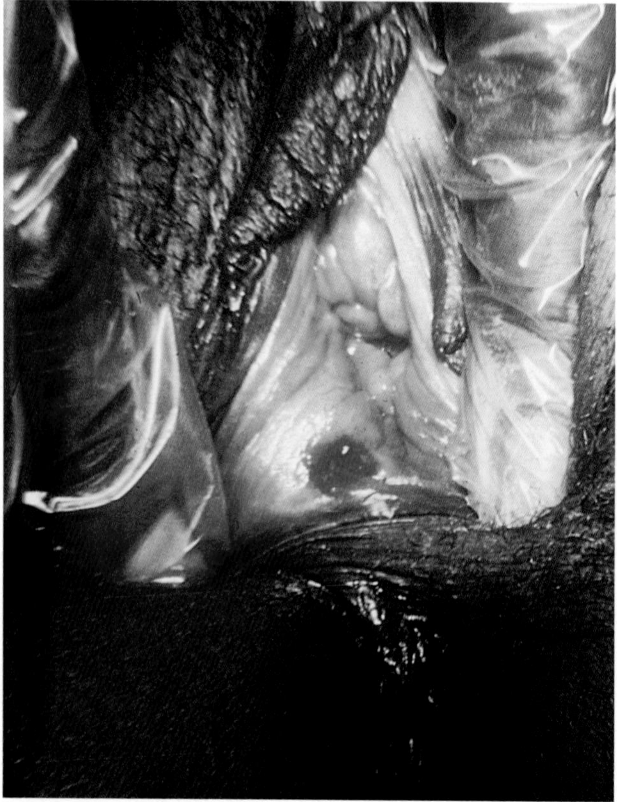

Figure 10-10 Primary syphilis. Chancre in vagina. Lesions are painless and may never be detected.

PRIMARY SYPHILIS

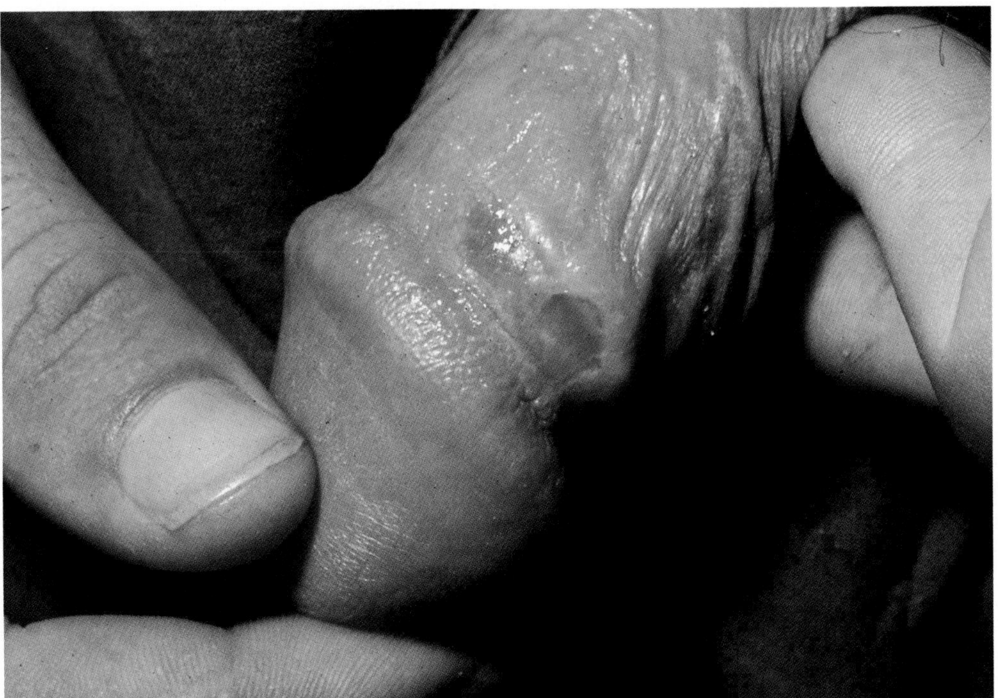

Figure 10-11 Two chancres located in close proximity. The base is well defined and clean.

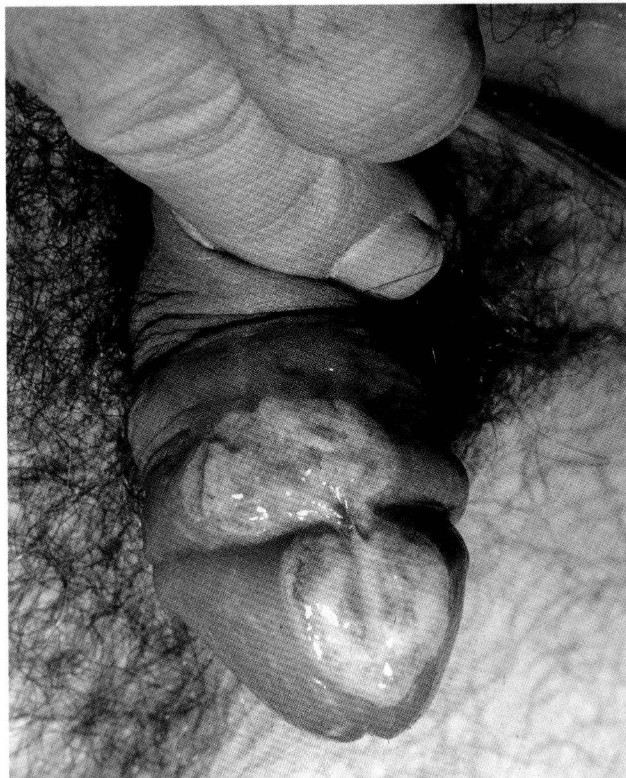

Figure 10-12 Two large ulcers with a purulent base look like chancroids. Lesions are "kissing" and were created by autoinoculation.

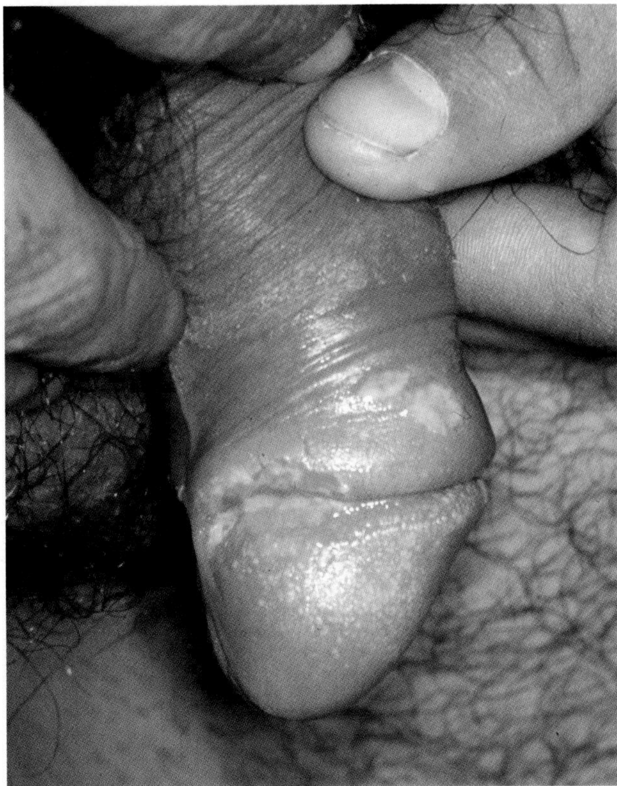

Figure 10-13 Three chancres with a purulent base. Chancres covered by a foreskin tend to develop a purulent exudate.

Secondary syphilis

Secondary syphilis is characterized by mucocutaneous lesions, a flulike syndrome, and generalized adenopathy. Asymptomatic dissemination of *T. pallidum* to all organs occurs as the chancre heals, and the disease then resolves in approximately 75% of cases (see Figure 10-2). In the remaining 25%, the clinical signs of the secondary stage begin approximately 6 weeks (range, 2 weeks to 6 months) after the chancre appears and last for 2 to 10 weeks. Cutaneous lesions are preceded by a flulike syndrome (sore throat, headache, muscle aches, meningismus, and loss of appetite) and generalized, painless lymphadenopathy. Hepatosplenomegaly may be present. In some cases lesions of secondary syphilis appear before the chancre heals. The distribution and morphologic characteristics of the skin and mucosal lesions are varied and may be confused with numerous other skin diseases. As with most other systemic cutaneous diseases, the rash is usually bilaterally symmetric (Figures 10-14 to 10-19).

LESIONS

The lesions of secondary syphilis have certain characteristics that differentiate them from other cutaneous diseases. There is little or no fever at the onset. Lesions are noninflammatory, develop slowly, and may persist for weeks or months. Pain or itching is minimal or absent. There is a marked tendency to polymorphism, with various types of lesions presenting simultaneously, unlike other eruptive skin diseases in which the morphologic appearance of the lesions is uniform. The color is characteristic, resembling a "clean-cut ham" or having a coppery tint. Lesions may assume a variety of shapes, including round, elliptic, or annular. Eruptions may be limited and discrete, profuse, generalized, or more or less confluent and may vary in intensity.

The types of lesions in approximate order of frequency are maculopapular, papular, macular, annular, papulopustular, psoriasiform, and follicular. The lesions in black individuals are marked by the absence of dull-red color. Lesions occur on the palms or soles in most patients with secondary syphilis (see Figure 10-15). Unlike the pigmented melanotic macules frequently seen on the palms and soles of older blacks, lesions of secondary syphilis of the palms and soles are isolated, oval, slightly raised, erythematous, and scaly. Temporary irregular ("moth eaten") alopecia of the beard, scalp, or eyelashes may occur (Figure 10-14). Moist, anal, wartlike papules (condylomata lata) are highly infectious (Figure 10-16). Lesions may appear on any mucous membrane. All cutaneous lesions of secondary syphilis are infectious; therefore, if you do not know what it is, do not touch it. The differential diagnosis is vast. The commonly observed diseases that may be confused with secondary syphilis are pityriasis rosea (especially if the herald patch is absent), guttate psoriasis (psoriasis that appears suddenly with numerous small papules and plaques), lichen planus, tinea versicolor, and exanthematous drug and viral eruptions.

The diagnosis is based primarily on clinical and serologic grounds. Histologic studies, in the majority of cases, may confirm the disease.

Cellular immune processes are responsible for the cutaneous manifestations of secondary syphilis. Coinfection with HIV-1 has little effect on the cutaneous response to *T. pallidum*.

Approximately 25% of untreated patients with secondary syphilis may experience relapse, most of them (approximately 90%) during the first year, a small percentage in the second year, and none after the fourth year.

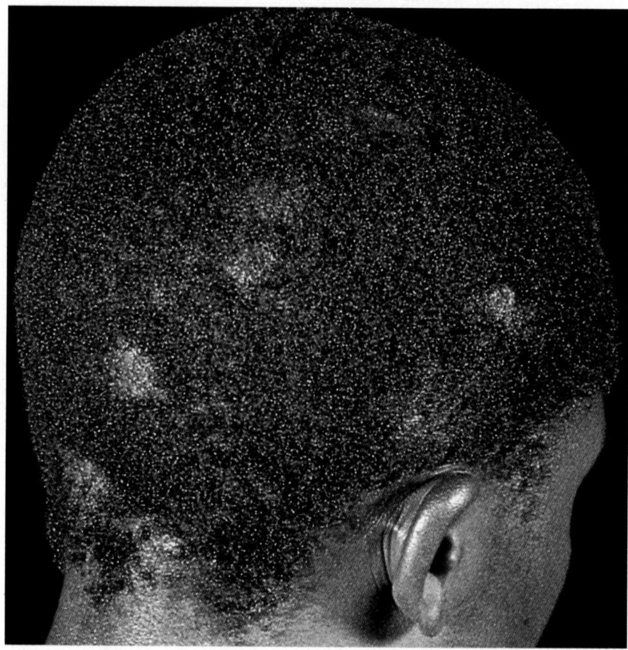

Figure 10-14 Secondary syphilis. Temporary, irregular ("moth eaten") alopecia of the scalp. (Courtesy Subhash K. Hira, MD.)

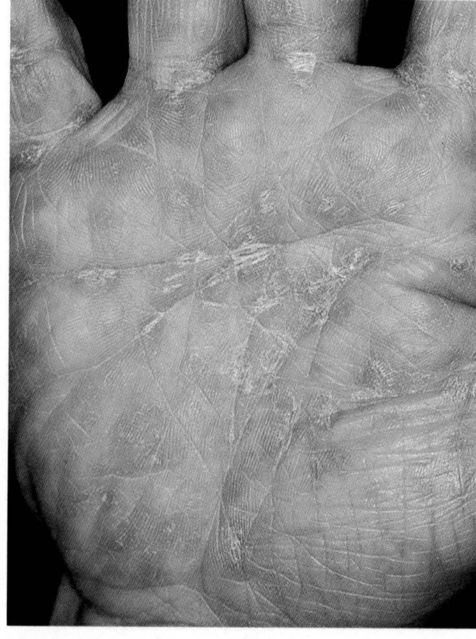

Figure 10-15 Secondary syphilis. A classic presentation for secondary syphilis with copper-colored scaly plaques on the palms and soles.

SECONDARY SYPHILIS

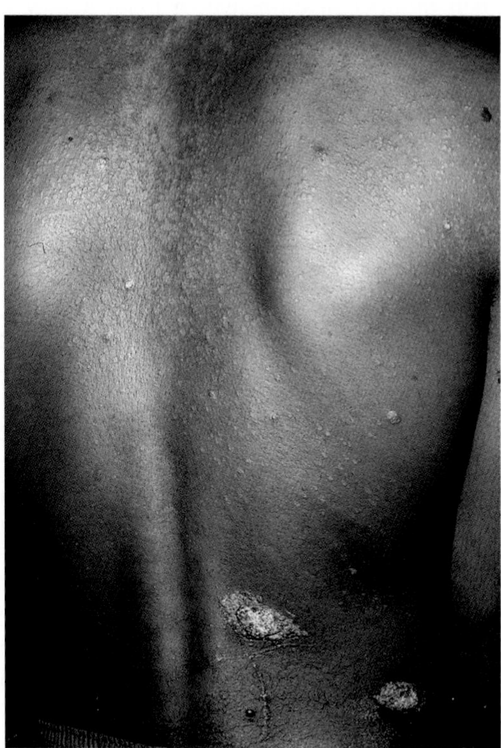

Figure 10-16 A diffuse eruption consisting of macules, papules, and pustules. Typical early lesions are usually less than 20, round, discrete, nonpruritic, and symmetric macules distributed on the trunk and proximal extremities. Red papular lesions also may appear on the palms, soles, face, and scalp and may become necrotic. Patchy and nonpatchy alopecia may occur. In intertriginous areas, papules may coalesce to form highly infectious lesions called condylomata lata. Lesions usually progress from red, painful, and vesicular to "gun-metal grey" as the rash resolves.

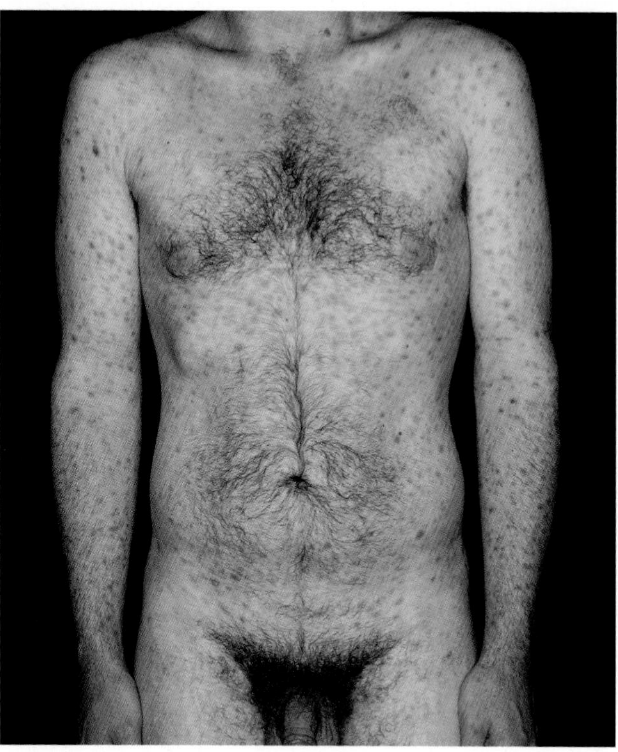

Figure 10-17 Numerous lesions are present on all body surfaces. This is a common presentation with maculopapular and psoriasiform lesions.

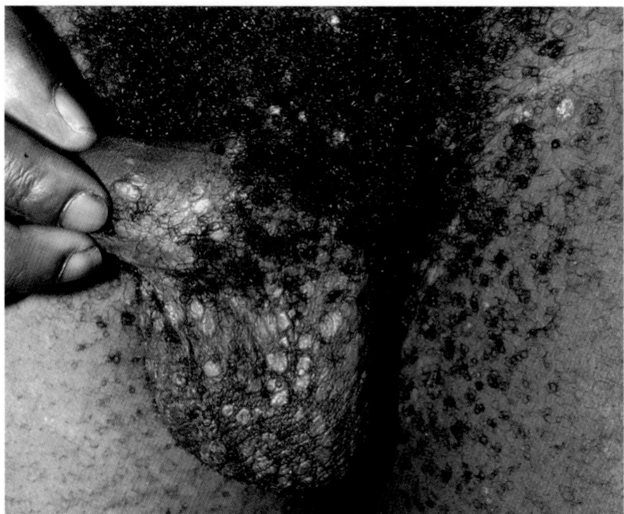

Figure 10-18 A cluster of red papules are located on the scrotum.

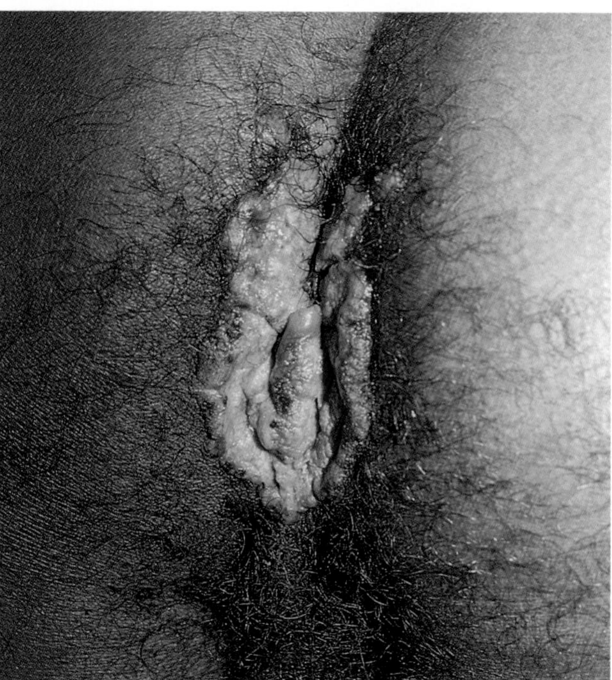

Figure 10-19 Moist, anal, wartlike papules (condylomata lata) are highly infectious.

Latent syphilis

Latent syphilis is defined as syphilis characterized by seroreactivity without other evidence of disease. Patients who have latent syphilis and who acquired syphilis within the preceding year are classified as having early latent syphilis. In latent syphilis, one depends on the accuracy of the patient's history that there were characteristic signs and symptoms or that the blood test, the result of which has been discovered to be positive, was nonreactive at a specific time.

Early latent syphilis can be diagnosed if, within the year preceding the evaluation, the patient reports the following:

1. There was a documented seroconversion (i.e., RPR, VDRL not a false-positive test result) without evidence of active disease. Often the physician is unable to confirm the specific time interval of conversion.
2. Unequivocal symptoms of primary or secondary syphilis were present.
3. A sex partner was documented to have primary, secondary, or early latent syphilis.

By convention, early latent syphilis is of 1-year or less duration and late latent syphilis is of more than 4-years' duration. The periods of 1 and 4 years were established to help predict a patient's chance of experiencing relapse with signs of secondary infectious syphilis. Approximately 25% of untreated patients in the secondary stage may experience a relapse, most of them (approximately 90%) during the first year, a small percentage in the second year, and none after the fourth year. The patient who experiences a relapse with secondary syphilis is infectious.

Patients who have latent syphilis of unknown duration should be treated as if they have late latent syphilis. Nontreponemal serologic titers (i.e., RPR, VDRL) usually are higher during early latent syphilis than late latent syphilis. However, early latent syphilis cannot be reliably distinguished from late latent syphilis solely on the basis of nontreponemal titers. All patients with latent syphilis should undergo careful examination of all accessible mucosal surfaces (i.e., the oral cavity, the perineum in women, and underneath the foreskin in uncircumcised men) to evaluate for internal mucosal lesions. All patients who have syphilis should be tested for HIV infection.

Tertiary syphilis

In a small number of untreated or inadequately treated patients, systemic disease develops, including cardiovascular disease, central nervous system (CNS) lesions, and systemic granulomas (gummas) (Figure 10-20).

Syphilis and human immunodeficiency virus

Syphilis (a genital ulcer disease) facilitates and is a cofactor for HIV transmission. Syphilis is associated with an increased risk of acquiring and transmitting HIV. The natural history of syphilis is altered by the human immunodeficiency virus. Reports describe an accelerated progression through the syphilitic stages in HIV patients.

Treatment of patients coinfected with syphilis and HIV is controversial; progression and relapse of neurosyphilis have been reported. Syphilis can increase the likelihood of HIV transmission and acquisition. HIV seroprevalence is high among patients with syphilis in the United States. The standard recommended doses of penicillin may not be effective for HIV-infected patients with syphilis. For most patients with coinfections of HIV and syphilis, laboratory tests for diagnosis and posttreatment follow-up can be interpreted as they would in an immunocompetent person.

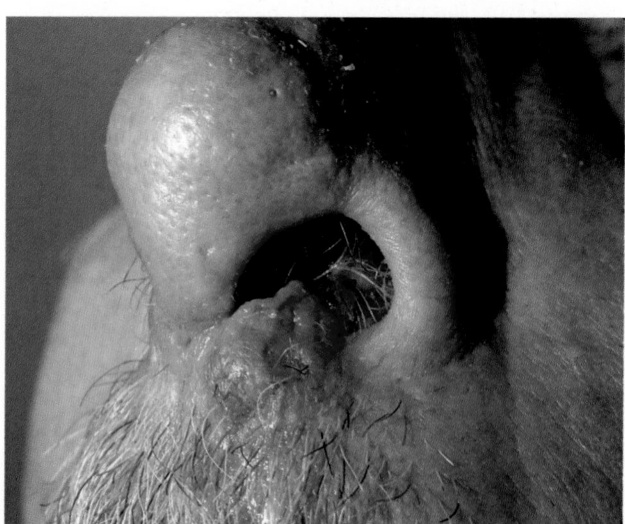

Figure 10-20 Tertiary syphilis. Gummatous syphilis with destructive lesions on the nose.

Congenital syphilis

Congenital syphilis is a problem in parts of the world where women do not receive prenatal care. *T. pallidum* can be transmitted by an infected mother to the fetus in utero. In untreated cases stillbirth occurs in 19% to 35% of reported cases, 25% of infants die shortly after birth, 12% are without symptoms at birth, and 40% will have late symptomatic congenital syphilis. The treponema can cross the placenta at any time during pregnancy. Adequate therapy of the infected mother before the sixteenth week of gestation usually prevents infection of the fetus. Treatment after 18 weeks may cure the disease but not prevent irreversible neural deafness, interstitial keratitis, and bone and joint changes in the newborn. The fetus is at greatest risk when maternal syphilis is of less than 2-years' duration. The ability of the mother to infect the fetus diminishes but never disappears in late latent stages. Condylomata lata and furuncles of Barlow can be seen toward the end of the first year of life. The clinical manifestations occur in an early and late form.

EARLY CONGENITAL SYPHILIS

Early congenital syphilis is defined as syphilis acquired in utero that becomes symptomatic during the first 2 years of life. It usually appears in the first week of life. The findings can be viewed as an exaggeration of those of acquired secondary syphilis. The fetal stigmata seen before the age of 2 years include eruptions characteristic of secondary syphilis. There are influenza-like respiratory symptoms in 20% to 50%, hepatosplenomegaly or lymphadenopathy in 50% to 75%, and mucocutaneous changes in 40% to 50%. Maculopapular rash and desquamating erythema of the palms and soles are common. Deep fissures at the angle of the mouth ("split papules") may be seen. A highly infectious hemorrhagic nasal discharge, "snuffles," is a characteristic early sign. Bone and joint symptoms are common.

A vesiculobullous variant, "pemphigus syphiliticus," may occur with vesicles, bullae, and erosions. Osteochondritis with the "sawtooth" metaphysis seen on radiographs and periostitis appear with tender limbs and joints. Nontender generalized adenopathy, alopecia, iritis, and failure to thrive occur less frequently.

LATE CONGENITAL SYPHILIS

Symptoms and signs of late congenital syphilis become evident after age 5 years. The average age at first diagnosis is 30 years. It may be difficult to distinguish from acquired syphilis. The most important signs are frontal bosses (bony prominences of the forehead) (87%), saddle nose (74%), short maxilla (83%), high arched palate (76%), mulberry molars (more than four small cusps on a narrow first lower molar of the second dentition), Hutchinson's teeth (peg-shaped upper central incisors of the permanent dentition that appear after age 6 years) (63%) (Figure 10-21), Higouménaki's sign (unilateral enlargement of the sternoclavicular portion of the clavicle as an end result of periostitis) (39%), and rhagades (linear scars radiating from the angle of the eyes, nose, mouth, and anus) (8%). Hutchinson's triad (Hutchinson's teeth, interstitial keratitis, and cranial nerve VIII deafness) is considered pathognomonic of late congenital syphilis.

Syphilis serology

Culture of *T. pallidum* is not available. The diagnosis of syphilis is based on serologic findings and/or dark-field microscopic examination of the organism or direct immunofluorescent microscopy. The latter two procedures require special equipment and an experienced technician.

The interpretation of reactive serologic tests for syphilis is shown in Figure 10-22. Two classes of immunoglobulin M (IgM) and IgG antibodies are produced in response to infection with *T. pallidum;* these are nonspecific antibodies measured by the VDRL and RPR tests and specific antibodies measured by the fluorescent treponemal antibody absorption (FTA-ABS) test (Table 10-11). The IgM antibodies

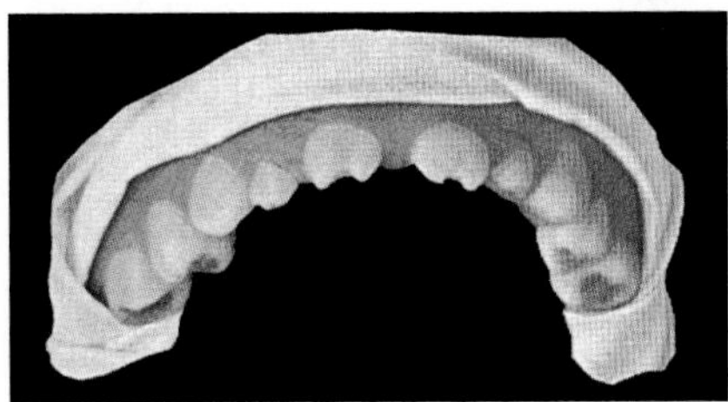

Figure 10-21 Late congenital syphilis. Hutchinson's teeth (peg-shaped upper central incisors of permanent dentition).

Table 10-11 Sensitivity of Serologic Tests in the Stages of Syphilis (Percent Positive)

Test	Primary	Secondary	Latent	Tertiary	Screening
VDRL*	72	100	73	77	86
FTA-ABS†	91	100	97	100	99

From Griner PF et al: *Ann Intern Med* 94:585, 1981.

FTA-ABS, Fluorescent treponemal antibody absorption; *VDRL,* Venereal Disease Research Laboratories.

*Specificity variable by stage and proportion of population tested with chronic and autoimmune diseases. Specificity in screening general population approximately 97%.

†Specificity for all stages probably 98% to 99%, including those with biologic false-positive results on nontreponemal test.

INTERPRETATION OF REACTIVE SEROLOGIC TESTS FOR SYPHILIS

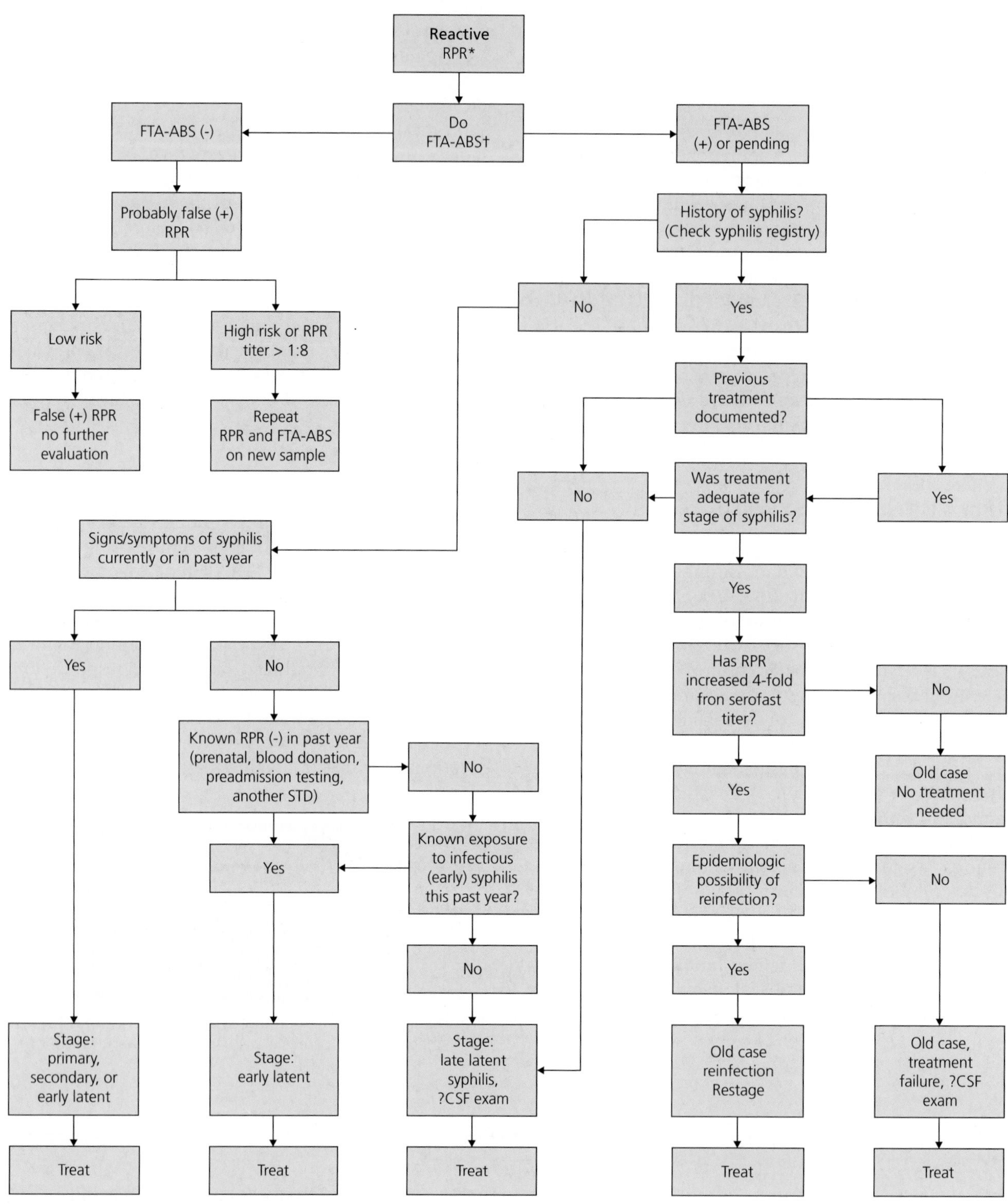

*Or other nontreponemal serologic test (e.g., VDRL or ART).
†Or other treponemal serologic test (e.g., MHA-TP).

Figure 10-22

are present in the second week of infection, and they disappear 3 months after treatment for early syphilis and 12 months afterward for late syphilis. They do not pass through the placenta or blood-brain barrier. IgG antibodies reach high levels in 4 to 5 weeks and may persist for life.

VENEREAL DISEASE RESEARCH LABORATORY AND RAPID PLASMA REAGIN TESTS

These tests are used for screening purposes and have a high degree of sensitivity (positive results in most patients with syphilis) but relatively low specificity (positive results in patients without syphilis). The primary chancre may be present for up to 2 weeks before serologic tests become reactive but the VDRL and RPR tests are usually reactive within 4 to 7 days of chancre development. When their results are positive, verification is by the more specific FTA-ABS test.

QUANTITATIVE TESTING. The tests give quantitative, as well as qualitative, results and can be used to monitor response to therapy. All reactive samples are titered to determine the highest reactive dilution. A rising titer indicates active disease; the titer falls in response to treatment. A fourfold change in titer, equivalent to a change of two dilutions (e.g., from 1:16 to 1:4 or from 1:8 to 1:32), is considered necessary to demonstrate a clinically significant difference between two nontreponemal test results that were obtained using the same serologic test. Nontreponemal tests usually become nonreactive with time after treatment; however, in some patients, nontreponemal antibodies can persist at a low titer for a long time, sometimes for the life of the patient. This response is referred to as the "serofast reaction."

FALSE-POSITIVE REACTIONS. Biologic false-positive reactions to nontreponemal tests (range, 3% to 20%) are defined as a positive nontreponemal antibody test result in patients for whom the FTA-ABS test result is negative (Table 10-12). False-positive test results may occur with collagen vascular disease, advancing age, narcotic drug use, chronic liver disease, several chronic infections such as HIV or tuberculosis, and several acute infections such as herpes. False-negative test results may occur if the patient has been applying topical antibiotics or ingesting systemic antibiotics. The VDRL test result is uniformly nonreactive in Lyme disease.

PROZONE PHENOMENON. Undiluted serum containing a high titer of nonspecific antibody, as occurs in secondary syphilis, may result in a negative result on the flocculation test. This is called the prozone phenomenon and occurs because the large quantity of antibody occupies all antigen sites and prevents flocculation. The laboratory may perform flocculation tests on diluted serum in anticipation of this problem.

Table 10-12 Diseases That Result in Positive Reactions to Tests Although Patients Do Not Have Syphilis (False-Positive Reactions)

NONTREPONEMAL TESTS		
Acute reactor (<6 months)	**Chronic reactor (>6 months)**	**FTA-ABS**
Pregnancy	Collagen vascular disease	Pregnancy
Drug-induced systemic lupus erythematosus	Senescence	Drug addiction
Acute infection	Leprosy	Herpes genitalis
Infectious mononucleosis	Metastasis to or cirrhosis of liver	Lupus erythematosus, scleroderma, rheumatoid arthritis (atypical beaded fluorescence pattern)
Malaria	Hashimoto's thyroiditis	Mixed connective tissue disease
Rubeola	Sjögren's syndrome	Alcoholic cirrhosis
Chickenpox	Sarcoidosis	
Atypical pneumonia	Lymphoma	
Smallpox vaccine	Myeloma	
Narcotic addiction	Narcotic addiction	
	Familial false-positive findings	

FLUORESCENT TREPONEMAL ANTIBODY ABSORPTION AND *T. PALLIDUM* PARTICLE AGGLUTINATION TESTS

Because of the decreased specificity of the nontreponemal tests, positive RPR and VDRL test results are confirmed with the more precise fluorescent treponemal antibody absorption test (FTA-ABS) or *T. pallidum* particle agglutination (TP-PA). The FTA-ABS test is also performed in patients with clinical evidence of syphilis for whom the nontreponemal test result is negative. Its main use is to rule out biologic false-positive reagin test reactions and to detect late syphilis in which the reagin test result may be nonreactive. FTA-ABS measures antibody directed against *T. pallidum* rather than from tissue (reagin), as with the RPR and VDRL tests. False-positive FTA-ABS test results occur most frequently in patients with autoantibodies. A patient who has a reactive treponemal test usually will have a reactive test for a lifetime, regardless of treatment or disease activity (15% to 25% of patients treated during the primary stage may revert to being serologically nonreactive after 2 to 3 years). Treponemal test antibody titers correlate poorly with disease activity and should not be used to assess response to treatment.

TESTS FOR NEUROSYPHILIS

Neurosyphilis is characterized by a cerebral spinal fluid (CSF) white blood cell (WBC) count >20/mm^3 or reactive CSF-VDRL. Consider testing for neurosyphilis if the serum RPR titer is 1:32 or higher. Risk factors for neurosyphilis are serum RPR titer 1:32 or higher, HIV infection, CD4 cell count 350/mm^3 or less, and (among HIV patients) ocular disease. *PMID: 14745693*

PATIENTS WITH HUMAN IMMUNODEFICIENCY VIRUS

Some HIV-infected patients can have atypical serologic test results (i.e., unusually high, unusually low, or fluctuating titers). For such patients, when serologic tests and clinical syndromes suggestive of early syphilis do not correspond with one another, use of other tests (e.g., biopsy and direct microscopy) should be considered. However, for most HIV-infected patients, serologic tests are accurate and reliable for the diagnosis of syphilis and for following the response to treatment.

Treatment of syphilis

Patients to be treated for syphilis should have a baseline serum RPR determination. The best indication of successful therapy is a decreasing RPR titer.

The drug of choice in the treatment of syphilis is benzathine penicillin G (see Box 10-1 and Table 10-3). The latest recommendations for treatment can be found at www.cdc.gov. Use this website to conduct a search for Sexually Transmitted Diseases Treatment Guidelines.

JARISCH-HERXHEIMER REACTION

A complex allergic response to antigens released from dead microorganisms can complicate the treatment of syphilis. A transient acute febrile reaction with headache and myalgia may develop within 24 hours of therapy. It is more prevalent with treatment of early syphilis.

MANAGEMENT OF THE PATIENT WITH A HISTORY OF PENICILLIN ALLERGY

No proven alternatives to penicillin are available for treating neurosyphilis, congenital syphilis, or syphilis in pregnant women. Penicillin is also recommended for use, whenever possible, in the treatment of HIV-infected patients. Only approximately 10% of persons who report a history of severe allergic reactions to penicillin are still allergic. Skin testing with the major and minor determinants can reliably identify persons at high risk for penicillin reactions. Those with positive test results should be desensitized. The protocol for desensitization can be found at www.cdc.gov. Use this website to conduct a search for Sexually Transmitted Diseases Treatment Guidelines.

Posttreatment evaluation of syphilis

SEROLOGIC RESPONSE TO TREATMENT

The lower the serologic titer before treatment, the quicker the blood test result will revert to normal. Patients with their first attack of primary syphilis will have a nonreactive RPR result within 1 year. Patients with secondary syphilis will have a nonreactive RPR test result within 2 years (Figures 10-23 and 10-24). Patients with early latent syphilis of less than 1-year's duration will have negative serologic findings within 4 years.

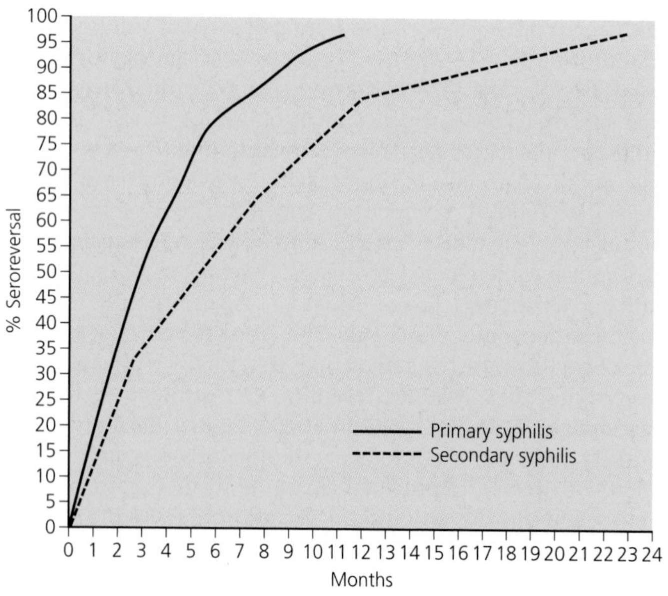

Figure 10-23 Speed of seroreversal of 500 patients with primary syphilis and 522 patients with secondary syphilis: 1977-1981.

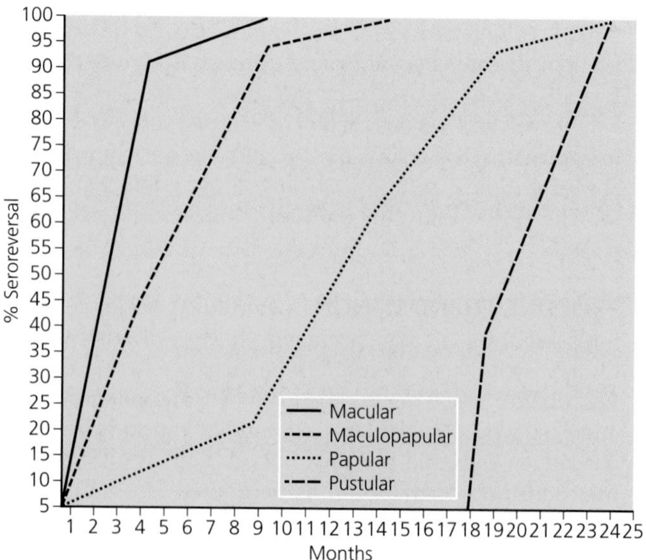

Figure 10-24 Speed of seroreversal of 522 patients with secondary syphilis by type of lesion: 1977-1981.

Table 10-13 Use of Nontreponemal Serologic Tests in Follow-Up After Treatment of Syphilis

Stage	Follow-up interval
Early syphilis (<1 year)	3, 6, 12 months after treatment
Late syphilis (>1 year)	2 years after treatment
Neurosyphilis	Blood and CSF levels every 6 months for 3 years after treatment
Retreatment	CSF level

Patients with a first attack of early latent syphilis of 1- to 4-years' duration treated with the schedules in Box 10-1 will have a nonreactive RPR finding in 5 years. Of patients with late latent syphilis, 45% will have negative serologic test results in 5 years, and the remainder will have reagin fast reactions. CSF examination is not performed unless the patient has neurologic or psychiatric signs and symptoms.

Persistent low-titer RPR reactivity may occur in 5% of successfully treated patients. The FTA-ABS test indicates past or present exposure and is not related to activity of the disease.

LATE LATENT SYPHILIS

In one study, 44% of patients with late latent syphilis had negative serologic findings within 5 years, and 56% had persistently positive reagin test results. The criteria of effectiveness in the treatment of patients with late latent syphilis are reversion of the reagin blood test for syphilis from reactive to nonreactive, a fourfold or greater decrease in the reagin titer, or a fixed titer with no significant change during the period of observation.

FREQUENCY OF FOLLOW-UP SEROLOGIC TESTS

All patients treated for syphilis must be followed to assess the effectiveness of initial treatment. Quantitative nontreponemal tests (VDRL or RPR) are obtained at 3, 6, and 12 months. If antibody titers do not decrease fourfold within 6 months for patients with primary or secondary syphilis, treatment failure or reinfection should be considered, and evaluation for possible HIV infection should be initiated. Patients with secondary syphilis should be observed for possible relapse or reinfection, with monthly follow-up for the first year and quarterly visits for the second year (Table 10-13). Repeat treatment should be considered for any patient who has a sustained fourfold increase in titer or when an initially high titer does not show a fourfold decrease within 1 year.

REINFECTION IN PRIMARY, SECONDARY, AND LATENT SYPHILIS

The titers of reagin antibody are higher than those during the first infection, and the serologic responses to treatment are slower, taking about twice the time to become nonreactive compared with the time expected after treatment of a first episode of syphilis (Figure 10-25).

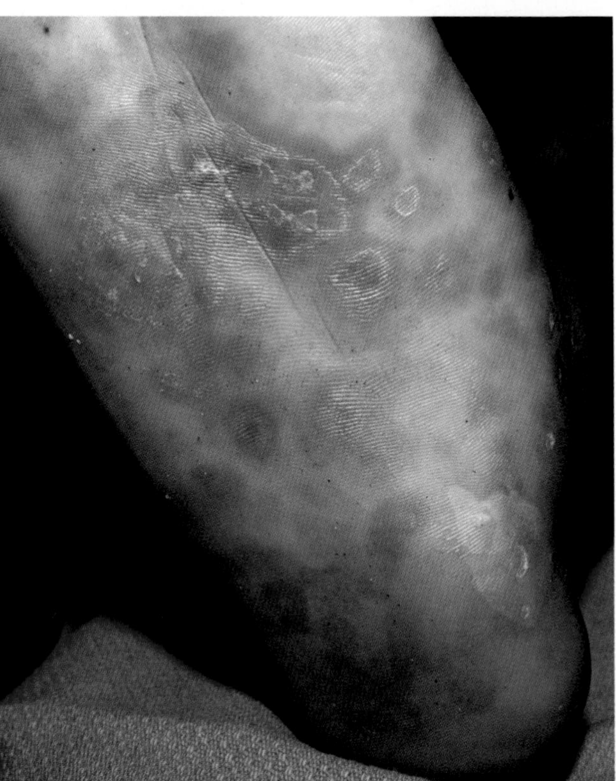

Figure 10-25 Secondary syphilis with classic papulosquamous lesion on the soles that may be mistaken for psoriasis.

RARE SEXUALLY TRANSMITTED DISEASES

Lymphogranuloma venereum

Lymphogranuloma venereum (LGV) is mainly a disease of lymphatic tissue that spreads to tissue surrounding lymphatics. LGV is endemic in Africa, India, Southeast Asia, and parts of Central and South America. It occurs sporadically in North America, Europe, and Australia. Cases have recently appeared in men who have sex with men, in the Netherlands, other cities in Western Europe, and the United States. These cases have presented with severe proctitis without inguinal lymphadenopathy, and predominance of the L2 serotype. *PMID: 15472852* It is more common in men (15 to 40 years). Asymptomatic female carriers are probably the primary source of infection. Men present with ulcers or tender inguinal and/or femoral lymphadenopathy that is usually unilateral. Women and male homosexuals might have proctocolitis or inflammatory involvement of perirectal or perianal lymphatic tissues that can result in fistulas and strictures. LGV is caused by the obligate intracellular bacteria *Chlamydia trachomatis* (serotypes L1, L2, and L3). These subtypes infect macrophages. The *C. trachomatis* serotypes that cause urethritis and cervicitis infect the squamocolumnar cells and infection is limited to mucous membranes. The diagnosis is usually made serologically and by exclusion of other causes of inguinal lymphadenopathy or genital ulcers.

PRIMARY LESIONS

After an incubation period of 5 to 21 days, a small, painless papule or viral (herpetiform) vesicle occurs on the penis, fourchette, posterior vaginal wall, or cervix (Figure 10-26). The lesion evolves rapidly to a small, painless erosion that heals without scarring within a week. The lesion in most cases is innocuous and most patients will not remember it. The primary lesion is rarely seen in women. A mucopurulent discharge affecting the urethra in men and the cervix in women may be present.

INGUINAL STAGE

The infected macrophages drain to the regional lymph nodes. Unilateral or sometimes bilateral inguinal lymphadenopathy accompanied by headache, fever, and migratory polymyalgia and arthralgia appears from 1 to 6 weeks after the primary lesion heals (Figure 10-27). In women, the deep pelvic nodes may also be involved. In a short time the lymph nodes become tender and fluctuant and are referred to as buboes when they ulcerate and discharge purulent material. Draining buboes may persist for months. Inflammation spreads to adjoining nodes and leads to matting. Abscesses rupture and sinus tracts eventually heal with scarring. Buboes are common in males but occur in only one third of infected females. Enlargement of inguinal nodes above and femoral nodes below Poupart's ligament creates the "groove sign" in approximately one fifth

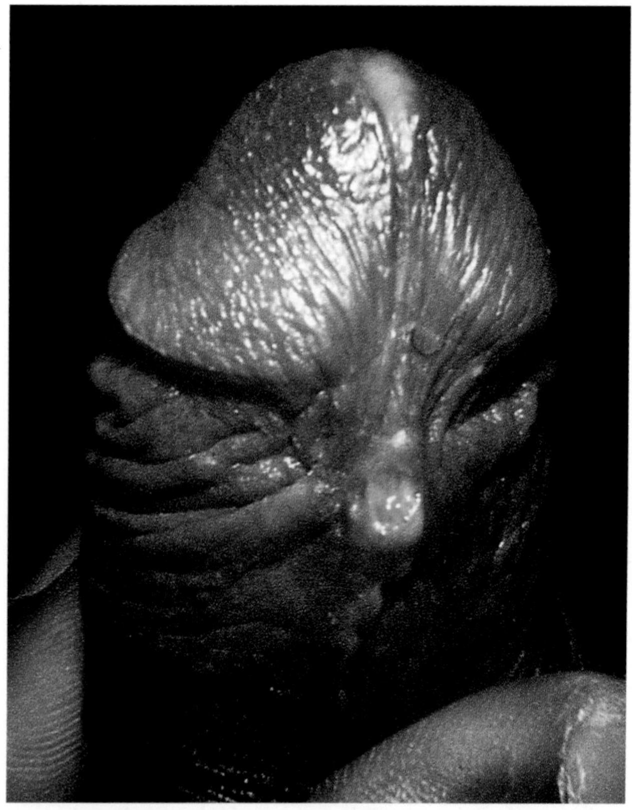

Figure 10-26 Lymphogranuloma venereum. Primary lesion consists of small, painless erosion that heals in a short time without scarring.

of patients, which is considered pathognomonic for LGV (see Figure 10-27). Inguinal lymphadenopathy occurs in only 20% to 30% of women. They have primary involvement of the rectum, vagina, cervix, or posterior urethra, which drain to the deep iliac or perirectal nodes. This produces lower abdominal or back pain.

Proctitis is the most common manifestation when the rectum is the site of primary inoculation, in both men and women. Fever and malaise are common. The most common infectious causes of proctitis in men who have sex with men are gonorrhea, herpes simplex, chlamydia, and syphilis. *PMID: 14699467* Patients may present with hemorrhagic proctitis and can be erroneously diagnosed with inflammatory bowel disease.

GENITOANORECTAL SYNDROME

This late stage occurs more often in women who were previously asymptomatic. Proctocolitis or inflammatory involvement of perirectal or perianal lymphatic tissues may lead to perirectal abscesses, fistulas, strictures, and stenosis of the rectum and ulceration of the labia, rectal mucosa, and vagina. Chronic edema (elephantiasis) of the female external genitals is a late manifestation of lymphatic obstruction. The enlargement, thickening, and fibrosis of the labia is termed esthiomene. Penile and/or scrotal edema and gross distortion of the penis is called "saxophone penis."

DIAGNOSIS

The organism is difficult to culture. The diagnosis depends mainly on serologic tests and nucleic acid amplification tests.

***CHLAMYDIA* TESTS.** A micro-immunofluorescent antibody (MIF) assay may be performed using acute and convalescent serum. Specimens are obtained in a red-top tube or a serum gel tube and refrigerated. Convalescent specimens should be drawn 2 to 3 weeks after onset. Nucleic acid testing is sensitive and convenient. Culture is expensive, and the sensitivity is low. Organisms are recovered approximately 30% of the time in the secondary phase of illness, probably because the inflammatory response reduces the organism load.

MANAGEMENT

In the absence of specific LGV diagnostic testing, patients with a clinical syndrome consistent with LGV, including proctocolitis or genital ulcer disease with lymphadenopathy, should be treated for LGV as described here.

DRUG REGIMEN. The drug regimen of choice is doxycycline 100 mg orally two times a day for 21 days. See Box 10-1 and Table 10-4 for complete prescribing information. Persons who have had sexual contact with a patient who has LGV within 60 days before the onset of the patient's symptoms should be examined, tested for urethral or cervical chlamydial infection, and treated with a standard chlamydia regimen (azithromycin 1 gm orally daily or doxycycline 100 mg orally twice a day for 7 days).

LESION MANAGEMENT. Fluctuant lymph nodes should be aspirated as needed through healthy, adjacent, normal skin. Incision and drainage or excision of nodes delays healing and is contraindicated. Late sequelae such as stricture or fistula may require surgical intervention.

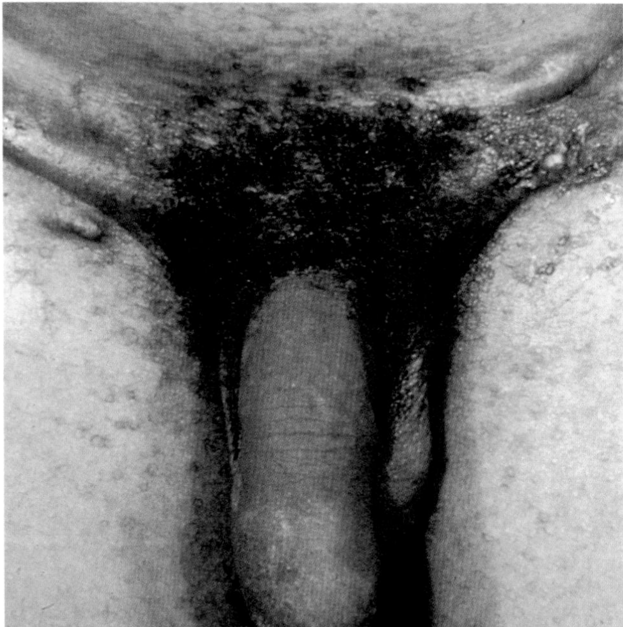

Figure 10-27 Lymphogranuloma venereum. Bilateral inguinal lymphadenopathy that discharges purulent material (buboes). Enlargement of inguinal nodes above and femoral nodes below Poupart's ligament creates the "groove sign."

Chancroid

Chancroid (soft chancre) is common and endemic in many parts of the world. It occurs in discrete outbreaks in some areas of the United States (New York, California, Texas, and South Carolina). It is common in Africa, the Caribbean basin, and Southwest Asia. The overall global incidence may surpass that of syphilis. In Kenya, Gambia, and Zimbabwe, chancroid is considered to be the most common cause of genital ulceration. Chancroid is a cofactor for HIV transmission. Ten percent of persons who have chancroid that was acquired in the United States are coinfected with *T. pallidum* or herpes simplex virus. This percentage is higher in persons who have acquired chancroid outside the United States.

BACTERIA

Chancroid is caused by the short gram-negative rod *H. ducreyi*. The male/female ratio is approximately 10:1. Chancroid predominantly affects heterosexual men, and many cases originate from prostitutes, who are often carriers with no symptoms.

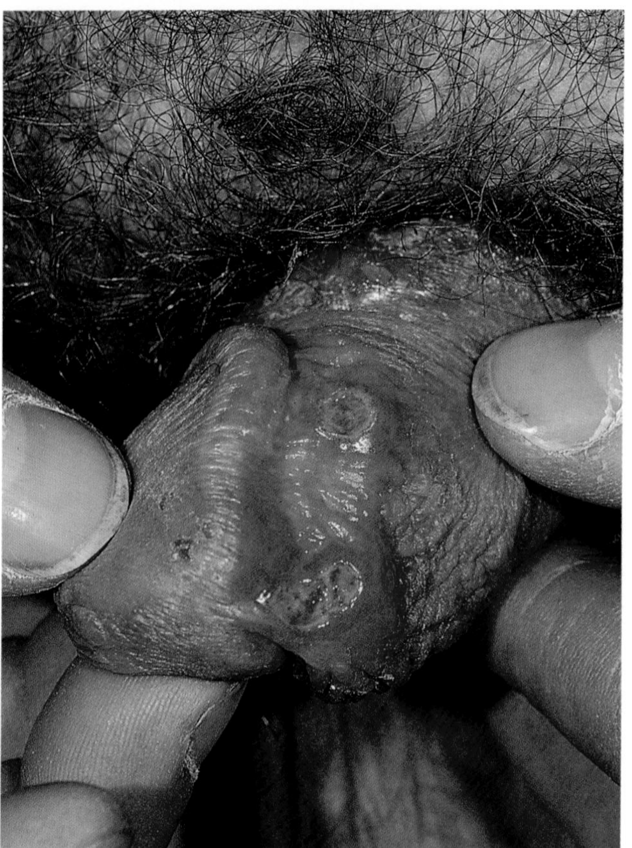

Figure 10-28 Chancroid. Several small, painful ulcers are usually present. Base is purulent, in contrast to the chancre of syphilis.

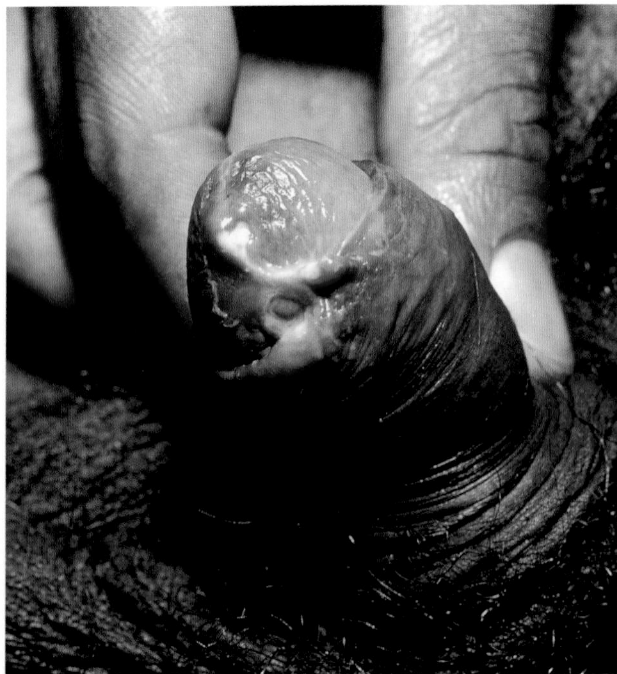

Figure 10-29 The soft chancre of chancroid with irregular borders.

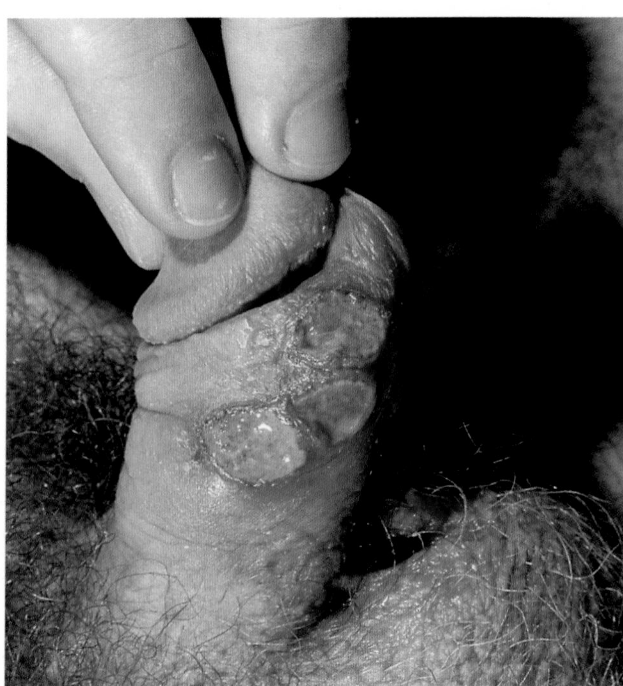

Figure 10-30 Chancroid. Large painful ulcers with a purulent "dirty" base.

PRIMARY STATE

After an incubation period of 3 to 5 days, a painful, red papule appears at the site of contact and rapidly becomes pustular and ruptures to form an irregular-shaped, ragged ulcer with a red halo (Figures 10-28, 10-29, and 10-30). The ulcer is deep, not shallow as in herpes; bleeds easily; and spreads laterally, burrowing under the skin and giving the lesion an undermined edge and a base covered by yellow-gray exudate. The ulcers are highly infectious, and multiple lesions appear on the genitals from autoinoculation. Unlike syphilis, the ulcers may be very painful. Untreated cases may resolve spontaneously or, more often, progress to cause deep ulceration, severe phimosis, and scarring. Systemic symptoms, including anorexia, malaise, and low-grade fever, are occasionally present. Females may have multiple, painful ulcers on the labia and fourchette and, less often, on the vaginal walls and cervix. Autoinoculation results in lesions on the thighs, buttocks, and anal areas. Female carriers may have no detectable lesions and may be without symptoms.

LYMPHADENOPATHY

Unilateral or bilateral inguinal lymphadenopathy develops in approximately 50% of untreated patients, beginning approximately 1 week after the onset of the initial lesion. The nodes then resolve spontaneously or they suppurate and break down.

DIAGNOSIS

The combination of a painful ulcer (syphilis is not painful) with tender inguinal adenopathy is suggestive of chancroid and, when accompanied by suppurative inguinal adenopathy, is almost pathognomonic.

A probable diagnosis is made when all the following criteria are met:

- One or more painful genital ulcers are present.
- There is no evidence of *T. pallidum* infection by dark-field examination of ulcer exudate or by a serologic test for syphilis performed at least 7 days after the onset of ulcers.
- The clinical presentation, appearance of genital ulcers, and, if present, regional lymphadenopathy are typical for chancroid.
- A test result for herpes simplex virus performed on the ulcer exudate is negative. Patients should be tested for HIV infection and tested 3 months later for syphilis and HIV if initial results are negative.

CULTURE

H. ducreyi is a difficult organism to culture, and it often takes several days for results to become available. Special media must be used and may not be immediately available. Therefore clinicians usually have to treat empirically at the first visit even if culture facilities are available.

A sterile swab or plastic loop is used to sample the base of the ulcers. Increased survival of *H. ducreyi* from less than 24 hours to up to 4 days was seen when specimens were held at 4° C with Stuart's, Amies', and thioglycolate hemin-based transport media.

GRAM STAIN

H. ducreyi possesses agglutination properties that account for the clumping of organisms when colonies are dispersed in saline. Agglutination may be responsible for the "school of fish" pattern seen on Gram staining. Gram-stained ulcer material should not be examined as a means to diagnose chancroid because of the poor sensitivity and specificity of this test. Smears taken from the surface areas are of little use. Material is obtained by drawing the flat surface of a toothpick under the undermined border of the ulcer. The cellular debris is then smeared on a glass slide. Exudate is obtained from the base of a new ulcer with a cotton swab. The swab is rolled in one direction over the slide to preserve the characteristic arrangement of the organisms. The slide is gently fixed with heat and stained with Gram stain. Gram-negative coccobacilli occur in parallel arrays (school-of-fish arrangement). This feature is infrequently seen and other gram-negative bacilli in the smear may result in a false-positive diagnosis. Bacteria may be intracellular. *H. ducreyi* may also be demonstrated with Wright's, Giemsa, or Unna-Pappenheim stains.

Herpes simplex genital ulcers can mimic chancroid. A herpes culture and Tzanck smear to look for virus-induced multinucleated giant cells help to establish the diagnosis. The histologic nature of chancroid is specific, but the biopsy procedure is so painful that other means of confirming the diagnosis should be used first.

TREATMENT

Patients who are not HIV-infected are treated with one dose of either azithromycin (1 gm orally) or ceftriaxone (250 mg IM). Ciprofloxacin (500 mg orally twice daily for 3 days) is an alternative. Erythromycin (500 mg four times daily for 7 days) is used when cost is an issue. HIV-infected patients and uncircumcised individuals are at higher risk for treatment failure and must be followed. Multiple dose regimens with azithromycin or ciprofloxacin have been successful. See Box 10-1 and Table 10-3 for complete prescribing information.

Asymptomatic carriage of *H. ducreyi* in males and females has been described; therefore aggressive tracing and treatment of sex partners, whether or not they have symptoms, is essential for control. Test patients for HIV infection and syphilis. HIV infection slows the healing rates of chancroid ulcers despite appropriate antibiotic therapy.

Fluctuant buboes should be aspirated for symptomatic relief and to avoid spontaneous rupture. Incision and drainage of fluctuant buboes, with subsequent packing of the wound, avoids the need for frequent bubo reaspirations. Suppurative lymphadenopathy may respond to appropriate antibiotic regimens. Surgical intervention for buboes may in some cases be delayed and used only for those recalcitrant to antibiotic therapy.

Granuloma inguinale (donovanosis)

Granuloma inguinale is a predominantly tropical cause of genital ulcer occurring chiefly in small endemic foci in all continents except Europe. It is endemic in Papua, New Guinea, South-East India, the Caribbean, and adjacent areas of South America, Durban South Africa, and among aborigines in Australia. It is a chronic, superficial, ulcerating disease of the genital, inguinal, and perianal areas. Granuloma inguinale is mildly contagious. The rate of infection between conjugal partners varies from 0.4% to 52%. It is caused by *Calymmatobacterium granulomatis,* a gram-negative, facultative, obligate-intracellular, encapsulated bacillus.

CLINICAL PRESENTATION

The incubation period is unknown, but 14 to 50 days is suspected. The disease begins as a single or multiple papules, nodules, or ulcers on the genitals and then evolves into a painless, broad, superficial ulcer with a distinct, raised, rolled margin and a friable, beefy-red, granulation tissue–like base raised above the skin surface (Figure 10-31). The ulceration spreads contiguously, causing progressive mutilation and destruction of local tissue. Autoinoculation produces lesions on adjacent skin, termed "kissing" lesions. The disease progresses to the genitocrural and inguinal folds in males and the perineal and perianal areas in females. It remains confined to areas of moist, stratified epithelium, sparing the columnar epithelium of the rectal area. Ulcers bleed to the touch and are not usually associated with inguinal lymphadenopathy as with LGV and chancroid. Women present with genital ulceration (88.5%) and genital tract bleeding (19.7%). The vulva is the most frequent anatomic site involved in women. Granuloma inguinale of the cervix presents as a proliferative growth and may mimic carcinoma. Systemic dissemination can occur. Most regular sexual partners of infected patients have no evidence of coexistent infection with donovanosis.

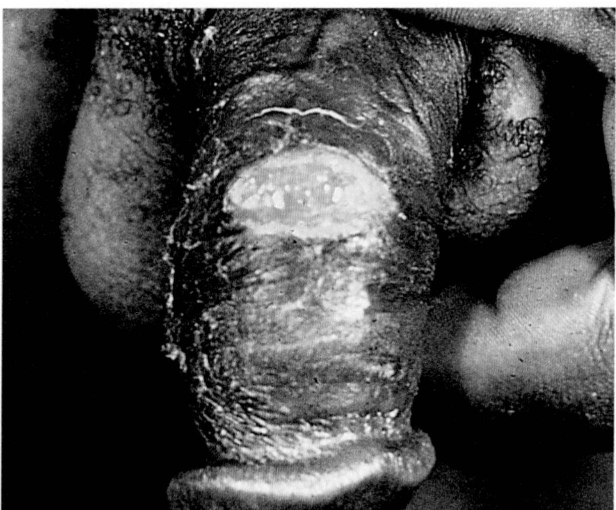

Figure 10-31 Granuloma inguinale. Painless, broad, superficial ulcer with beefy-red texture is raised above the skin surface.

Delay in treatment results in significant local destruction and morbidity. Extensive and multiple perianal fistulas and abscesses may form. Granuloma inguinale does not produce constitutional symptoms. Systemic symptoms suggest hematogenous dissemination, which may cause disease at distant sites and death. Extragenital sites become infected by autoinoculation (particularly the oral cavity) or extension into underlying organs, such as bone, bowel, or bladder.

Lymphatic obstruction causes genital edema. Scarring and mutilation of the anogenital region may require surgical correction.

DIAGNOSIS

Culture is very difficult on artificial culture media. The most reliable method of diagnosis involves direct visualization of the bipolar-staining intracytoplasmic inclusion bodies, called Donovan bodies. These "closed-safety-pin" appearing bodies can be seen within histiocytes of granulation tissue smears or biopsy specimens. Diagnosis can be confirmed in 1 hour with the following technique: The lesion is washed with saline. EMLA ointment is applied, removed in 10 minutes, reapplied, and again removed 10 minutes later. Two scoops are taken as deeply as possible from the lesion from the advancing edge of the ulceration with a curette or chalazion spoon. The first is submitted in formalin for histopathologic study. The second is rubbed together between two glass slides to ensure a uniform spread of cells from the material. Make tissue preparations immediately while the tissue is moist. Desiccation results in rupture of the involved histiocytes. Donovan bodies are more easily recognized in smears than in tissue biopsy sections. The slides are taken to the laboratory, immediately air-dried, and fixed in methyl alcohol for 5 minutes, followed by staining with 20% Giemsa for 10 minutes. Excess stain is washed off with water. Wright's or Leishman's stain is also suitable. Once dry, 100× oil-immersion, objective lens microscopic examination reveals bipolar-staining bacilli in vacuoles in the cytoplasm of large histiocytes. The intracellular organisms are called Donovan bodies and have a prominent clear capsule when mature. If slides cannot be immediately taken to the laboratory, they must be air-dried and fixed with an aerosol fixative, such as that used for Papanicolaou smear tests. The RapiDiff technique is suitable for use in the diagnosis of granuloma inguinale (donovanosis) in busy clinics that treat sexually transmitted diseases.

For histopathologic study, Warthin-Starry silver stains demonstrate the encapsulated bacilli within histiocytes.

TREATMENT

The recommended regimen is doxycycline 100 mg orally twice a day for at least 3 weeks and until all lesions have completely healed.

See Box 10-1 and Table 10-4 for complete prescribing information. Therapy should be continued at least 3 weeks and until all lesions have completely healed.

DISEASES CHARACTERIZED BY URETHRITIS AND CERVICITIS

Urethritis is characterized by urethral discharge of mucopurulent or purulent material and sometimes by dysuria or urethral pruritus (Box 10-2). Asymptomatic infections are common. *N. gonorrhoeae* and *C. trachomatis* are the principal pathogens. Gram stain can provide an immediate diagnosis of gonorrhea. Nucleic acid amplification tests enable detection of *N. gonorrhoeae* and *C. trachomatis* on all specimens. These tests are more sensitive than culture for *C. trachomatis* and are the preferred method for the detection of these organisms.

The presence of nongonococcal urethritis is demonstrated by the absence of gram-negative intracellular diplococci, a negative gonococcal culture result, and the detection of inflammatory cells (at least five polymorphonuclear leukocytes) in the urethral smear or in the urine sediment for each patient with clinical symptoms of urethral inflammation.

Box 10-2 **Signs of Urethritis**

1. Mucopurulent or purulent discharge.
2. Gram stain of urethral secretions demonstrating >5 WBCs per oil-immersion field. The Gram stain is the preferred rapid diagnostic test for evaluating urethritis.
3. Positive leukocyte esterase test on first-void urine or microscopic examination of first-void urine demonstrating >10 WBCs per high-power field.

Gonorrhea

Gonorrhea is the second most common notifiable infectious disease in the United States (the most common is chlamydia). A total of 358,366 cases of gonorrhea in the United States were reported to CDC in 2006 an incidence of 120.9 cases per 100,000. Blacks and adolescents account for the majority of cases. *N. gonorrhoeae* can survive only in a moist environment approximating body temperature. It is transmitted only by sexual contact (genital, genital-oral, or genital-rectal) with an infected person. It is not transmitted through toilet seats or the like. It most commonly infects superficial mucous membranes and initially produces discharge and dysuria. Purulent burning urethritis in males and asymptomatic endocervicitis in females are the most common forms of the disease, but gonorrhea is also found at other sites.

Gonorrhea may gain entry into the bloodstream from the primary source of infection and cause a disseminated gonococcal infection (arthritis-dermatitis syndrome) that consists of fever and chills, skin lesions, and articular involvement.

From an epidemiologic point of view the disease is becoming more difficult to control because of the increasing number of asymptomatic male carriers. "Core transmitters," or persons with repeated infections, are believed to be responsible for transmitting the majority of infections in urban areas. All forms of the disease previously responded to penicillin, but resistant strains have emerged.

Neisseria gonorrhoeae

N. gonorrhoeae is a gram-negative coccus that infects columnar or cuboidal epithelium. The neutrophilic response creates a purulent discharge, and stained smears show large numbers of phagocytosed gonococci in pairs (diplococci) within polymorphonuclear leukocytes. Nucleic acid amplification tests provide rapid and accurate diagnosis.

N. gonorrhoeae is a fragile organism that survives only in humans and quickly dies if all of its environmental requirements are not met. The organism can survive only in blood and on mucosal surfaces including the urethra, endocervix, rectum, pharynx, conjunctiva, and prepubertal vaginal tract. It does not survive on the stratified epithelium of the skin and postpubertal vaginal tract. The bacteria must be kept moist with isotonic body fluids and will die if not maintained at body temperature. A slightly alkaline medium is required, such as that found in the endocervix and in the vagina during the immediate premenstrual and menstrual phases. The antibodies produced during the disease offer little protection from future attacks. A fluorescent antibody test identifies the organism in tissue specimens such as in the skin in disseminated gonococcal infection (bacteremia-arthritis syndrome).

GENITAL INFECTION IN MALES

The risk of infection for a man after a single exposure to an infected woman is estimated to be 20% to 35%.

URETHRITIS. After a 3- to 5-day incubation period, most infected men have a sudden onset of burning, frequent urination, and a yellow, thick, purulent urethral discharge. In some men symptoms do not develop for 5 to 14 days. They then complain only of mild dysuria with a mucoid urethral discharge as observed in nongonococcal urethritis. Five percent to 50% of men who are infected never have symptoms and become chronic carriers for months, acting, as do women without symptoms, as major contributors to the ongoing gonorrhea epidemic. Infection may spread to the prostate gland, seminal vesicles, and epididymis, but presently these complications are uncommon because most men with symptoms are treated.

DIAGNOSIS. The diagnosis can be confirmed without culture in men with a typical history of acute urethritis by finding in urethral exudate containing gram-negative intracellular diplococci within polymorphonuclear leukocytes. Nucleic acid amplification tests (Gen-Probe, LCx Uriprobe) have high sensitivity and specificity, and they also test for *C. trachomatis*. Special transport kits provided by the laboratory are used to sample the urethra and endocervix. These tests are also performed on urine. Culture may be used for diagnostic problems.

GENITAL INFECTION IN FEMALES

Most cases occur in 15 to 19 year olds. The risk of infection for a woman after a single exposure to an infected man is estimated to be 50% to 90%. Female genital gonorrhea has traditionally been described as an asymptomatic disease, but symptoms of urethritis and endocervicitis may be elicited from 40% to 60% of the women. While the urethra and rectum are often involved, the locus of infection is typically the endocervix.

CERVICITIS. Endocervical infection may appear as a nonspecific, pale-yellow vaginal discharge, but in many cases this is not detected or is accepted as being a normal variation. The cervix may appear normal, or it may show marked inflammatory changes with cervical erosions and pus exuding from the os. Skene's glands, which lie on either side of the urinary meatus, exude pus if infected.

URETHRITIS. Urethritis begins with frequency and dysuria after a 3- to 5-day incubation period. These symptoms are of variable intensity. Pus may be seen exuding from the red external urinary meatus or after the urethra is "milked" with a finger in the vagina.

BARTHOLIN DUCTS. The Bartholin ducts, which open on the inner surfaces of the labia minora at the junction of their middle and posterior thirds near the vaginal opening, may, if infected, show a drop of pus at the gland orifice. After occlusion of the infected duct, the patient complains of swelling and discomfort while walking or sitting. A swollen, painful Bartholin gland may be palpated as a swollen mass deep in the posterior half of the labia majora.

DIAGNOSIS. The diagnosis of acute urethritis can be made with a high degree of certainty if gram-negative intracellular diplococci are found in the purulent exudate from the urethra (Figure 10-32). *Neisseria* species (e.g., *N. catarrhalis* and *N. sicca*) inhabit the female genital tract; thus the diagnosis is considered only if gram-negative diplococci are present inside polymorphonuclear leukocytes.

Nucleic acid amplification tests (Gen-Probe, LCx Uriprobe) are used on urethra and endocervix samples. These tests are also performed on urine. Culture may be used for diagnostic problems. A culture of the anal canal need be performed only if there are anal symptoms, a history of rectal sexual exposure, or follow-up of treated gonorrhea in women.

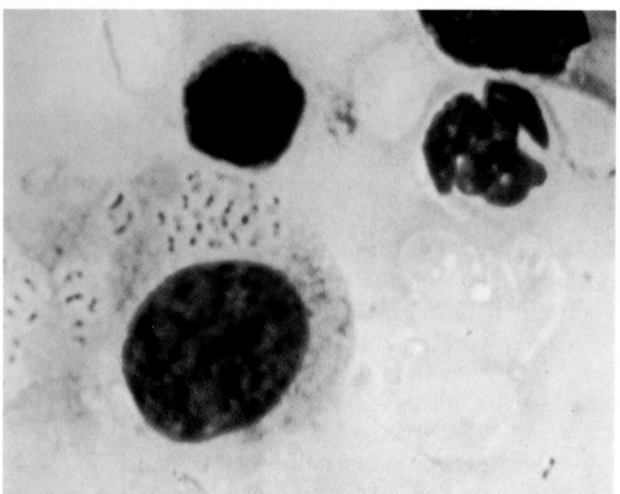

Figure 10-32 Gonorrhea. A gram stain shows gram negative diplococci in inflammatory cells.

Box 10-3 **Criteria for Diagnosis of Pelvic Inflammatory Disease (Centers for Disease Control and Prevention)**

Minimal (all present with no other cause)

- Lower abdominal tenderness
- Adnexal tenderness
- Cervical motion tenderness

Additional criteria that support a diagnosis of PID include

- Oral temperature >101° F (38.3° C)
- Abnormal cervical or vaginal discharge
- Elevated erythrocyte sedimentation rate
- Elevated level of C-reactive protein
- Laboratory documentation of cervical infection with *N. gonorrhoeae* or *C. trachomatis*

Definitive criteria for diagnosing PID

- Histopathologic evidence of endometritis on endometrial biopsy
- Laparoscopic abnormalities consistent with pelvic inflammatory disease
- Transvaginal sonography or other imaging techniques showing thickened fluid-filled tubes, with or without free pelvic fluid or tubo-ovarian complex
- Laparoscopic abnormalities consistent with PID

PELVIC INFLAMMATORY DISEASE

Pelvic inflammatory disease (PID), or salpingitis, is infection of the uterus, fallopian tubes, and adjacent pelvic structures. Organisms spread to these structures from the cervix and vagina. It is present in 10% to 20% of gonococcal infections in women. Most cases are caused by *C. trachomatis* and/or *N. gonorrhoeae*. Microorganisms that can be part of the normal vaginal flora (e.g., anaerobes, *G. vaginalis, H. influenzae,* enteric gram-negative rods, *Streptococcus agalactiae*) also can cause PID. In addition, *Mycoplasma hominis* and *Ureaplasma urealyticum* have been found in PID. Risk factors for ascending infection are age under 20 years, previous PID, vaginal douching, and bacterial vaginosis. Diagnostic criteria are listed in Box 10-3.

CLINICAL PRESENTATION. Symptoms range from minimal (e.g., lower abdominal tenderness) to severe pain accompanied by peritoneal signs. Pelvic inflammatory disease is an important cause of infertility. The most common presenting symptom is lower abdominal pain, usually bilateral. Gonococcal PID has an abrupt onset with fever and peritoneal irritation. The symptoms of nongonococcal disease are less dramatic. Any of these infections may be asymptomatic. Symptoms are more likely to begin during the first half of the menstrual cycle.

DIAGNOSIS. The diagnosis is usually made clinically. Lower abdominal tenderness and pain, adnexal tenderness, and pain on manipulation of the cervix are noted in most cases. Fever, leukocytosis, an increased erythrocyte sedimentation rate, elevated levels of C-reactive protein, and vaginal discharge may also occur.

Most women have either mucopurulent cervical discharge or evidence of WBCs on a microscopic evaluation of a saline preparation of vaginal fluid. If the cervical discharge appears normal and no white blood cells are found on the wet prep, the diagnosis of PID is unlikely, and alternative causes of pain should be investigated.

Endocervical specimens should be examined for *N. gonorrhoeae* and *C. trachomatis*. Direct visualization with the laparoscope of inflamed fallopian tubes and other pelvic structures is the most accurate method of diagnosis, but this procedure is usually not practical. A comprehensive microbiologic evaluation should be performed on specimens obtained through the laparoscope. The differential diagnosis includes acute appendicitis, pelvic endometriosis, hematoma of the corpus luteum, or ectopic pregnancy. Long-term complications (recurrent disease, chronic pain, ectopic pregnancy, infertility) occur from tubal damage and scarring.

MANAGEMENT. Empiric treatment of PID should be initiated in sexually active young women and others at risk for sexually transmitted diseases if all the minimum criteria in Box 10-3 are present and no other causes(s) of the illness can be identified. The recommended regimens are found in Box 10-1. Evaluate male sexual partners. Chlamydial and gonococcal infections in these men are often asymptomatic.

RECTAL GONORRHEA

Rectal gonorrhea is acquired by anal intercourse. Women with genital gonorrhea may also acquire rectal gonorrhea from contamination of the anorectal mucosa by infectious vaginal discharge. A history of anal intercourse is the most important clue to the diagnosis because the symptoms and signs of rectal gonorrhea are in most cases nonspecific.

Anoscopic examination of homosexual men reveals generalized exudate in 54% of culture-positive patients and 37% of culture-negative patients. Many infected patients have normal-appearing rectal mucosa. These figures emphasize what is generally observed—that the specificity of the most common signs and symptoms of rectal gonorrhea is low. Some patients report pain on defecation, blood in the stools, pus on undergarments, or intense discomfort while walking.

DIAGNOSIS. Anal culture should be considered for male homosexuals with symptoms and females with symptoms who have engaged in rectal intercourse. Gonococcal proctitis does not involve segments of bowel beyond the rectum. The area of infection is approximately 2.5 cm inside the anal canal in the pectinate lining of the crypts of Morgagni. An anoscope is unnecessary to obtain culture material. A sterile cotton-tipped swab is inserted approximately 2.5 cm into the anal canal. (If the swab is inadvertently pushed into feces, another swab must be used to obtain a specimen.) The swab is moved from side to side in the anal canal to sample crypts; 10 to 30 seconds are allowed for absorption of organisms onto the swab.

Gen-Probe assays are sensitive and specific for the detection of rectal and pharyngeal gonorrhea. If noncultural methods are used to screen for gonococcal infection, cultures should be obtained from patients with positive results so the antibiotic susceptibility and molecular epidemiology of the gonococcal population can be monitored.

Gram stain is unreliable because of the presence of numerous other bacteria.

GONOCOCCAL PHARYNGITIS

Gonococcal pharyngitis is acquired by penile-oral exposure and rarely by cunnilingus or kissing. The possibility of infection is increased when the penis is inserted deep into the posterior pharynx as practiced by most homosexuals. Most cases are asymptomatic, and the gonococcus can be carried for months in the pharynx without being detected. In those with symptoms, complaints range from mild sore throat to severe pharyngitis with diffuse erythema and exudates.

DIAGNOSIS. Culture is most productive if exudates are present. *N. meningitidis* is a normal inhabitant of the pharynx; consequently, sugar utilization tests are necessary on *Neisseria* species isolated from the pharynx to determine accurately if infectious organisms are present.

Gram stain is useful only if exudate is present and must therefore be interpreted with caution to avoid confusion with other *Neisseria* species. Gen-Probe assays are sensitive and specific for pharyngeal gonorrhea.

DISSEMINATED GONOCOCCAL INFECTION (ARTHRITIS-DERMATITIS SYNDROME)

Disseminated gonococcal infection (DGI) is the most common cause of acute septic arthritis in young sexually active adults. The classic clinical triad is dermatitis, tenosynovitis, and migratory polyarthritis. It follows a genitourinary, rectal, or pharyngeal mucosal infection, which is asymptomatic in most patients. The diagnosis should be considered in any young adult or adolescent who presents with a skin rash, joint swelling, and pain.

INCIDENCE. DGI develops in approximately 1% to 3% of patients with mucosal infections and is more common in young adults. It is the most common form of infectious arthritis. The male-to-female ratio is 1:4.

DISSEMINATION. Dissemination usually develops within 2 to 3 weeks of the primary infection. Hematogenous dissemination is more likely to occur within 1 week of the onset of the menstrual period. Women are more commonly affected with dissemination presumably because women more frequently have asymptomatic infection and remain untreated. Menses expose the submucosal blood vessels and increase the risk of dissemination. The risk of systemic infection increases during the second and third trimesters of pregnancy.

INITIAL PRESENTATION. Migratory polyarthralgias are the most common presenting symptoms, occurring in up to 80% of patients. Initial signs are tenosynovitis (67%), dermatitis (67%), and fever (63%). Less than 30% have symptoms or signs of localized gonorrhea, such as urethritis or pharyngitis; however, cervical culture results in women with DGI are positive in 80% to 90% of cases and men's urethral culture results are positive in 50% to 75% of cases.

JOINT DISEASE. Most patients have involvement of less than three joints. The upper extremity joints are more commonly involved, especially the wrist. The knee is the most commonly affected lower extremity joint. Tenosynovitis is present in two thirds of the patients, occurring in the hands and fingers, although the tendons around the small and large joints of the lower limbs also can be affected.

TWO PRESENTATIONS. Following a genitourinary, rectal, or pharyngeal mucosal infection, which is asymptomatic in most patients, the disseminated disease can present two clinical pictures. The initial bacteremic stage, associated with fever (rarely reaching 39° C), skin rash, and tenosynovitis, is followed by localization of the infection within the joints. Approximately 60% of patients present with the bacteremic picture, and 40% present with suppurative arthritis. The features of disseminated gonococcal infection are compared with those of nongonococcal bacterial arthritis in Table 10-14.

Table 10-14 Differential Features of Disseminated Gonococcal Infection and Nongonococcal Bacterial Arthritis

Disseminated gonococcal infection	Nongonococcal bacterial arthritis
Generally in young, healthy adults	Often in very young, elderly, or immunocompromised persons
Initial migratory polyarthralgia (common)	Polyarthralgia rare
Tenosynovitis in majority	Tenosynovitis rare
Dermatitis in majority	Dermatitis rare
>50% polyarthritis	>85% monoarthritis
Positive blood culture result in <10%	Positive blood culture result in 50%
Positive joint fluid culture result in 25%	Positive joint fluid culture result in 85% to 95%

From Goldenberg DL, Reed JI: *New Engl J Med* 312:767, 1985. Reprinted by permission of the *New England Journal of Medicine*.

ARTHRITIS-DERMATITIS SYNDROME. Chills (25%) and fever (more than 50%) are accompanied by pain, red-

GONOCOCCAL SEPTICEMIA

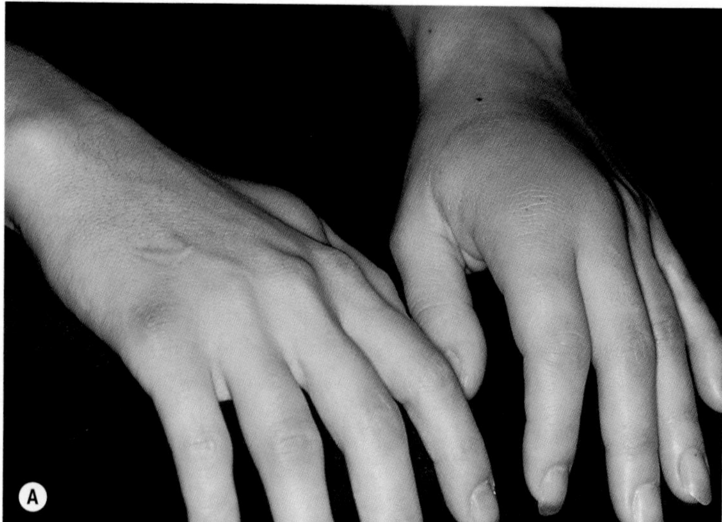

There is erythema and swelling of joints on the left hand. A single vesicle is present on the right hand.

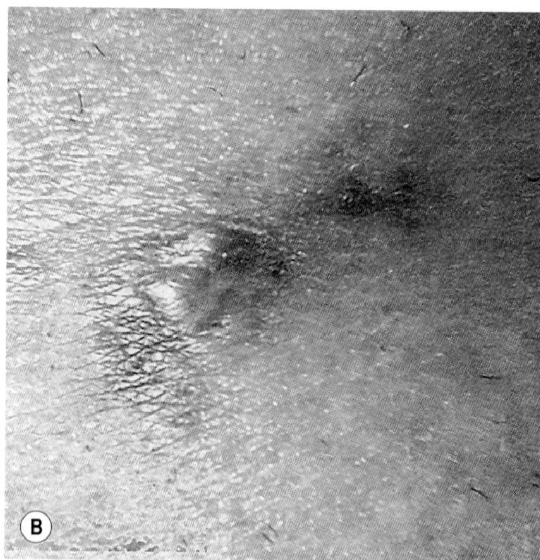

More advanced lesion than that shown in *A*. Base has become hemorrhagic and necrotic.

Figure 10-33

ness, and swelling of three to six small joints without effusion. This polyarthritis and tenosynovitis occur in the hands and wrists, with pain in the tendons of the wrist and fingers. Toes and ankles may also be affected. These patients are more likely to have positive results on blood culture and negative results on joint culture.

SKIN LESIONS. Dermatitis is seen in two thirds of cases. Chills and fever terminate as the rash appears on the extensor surfaces of the hands and dorsal surfaces of the ankles and toes. Lesions may develop on the trunk. The skin lesions are thought to be due to embolization of organisms to the skin with the development of microabscesses. The total number of lesions is usually less than ten. Lesions are seen in various stages of development. Many cases have only one or two lesions. The skin lesions begin as painless, nonpruritic, tiny, red papules or petechiae that either disappear or evolve through vesicular (Figure 10-33, *A*) and pustular stages, developing a grey necrotic and then hemorrhagic center (Figure 10-33, *B*). The central hemorrhagic area is the embolic focus of the gonococcus. These lesions heal in a few weeks. New lesions may appear even after antibiotic therapy has begun.

LOCALIZED SEPTIC ARTHRITIS. Usually one or two large joints are affected, most frequently the knee followed by the ankle, wrist, and elbow. The affected joint is hot, painful, and swollen, and movement is restricted. Permanent joint changes may occur. The mean leukocyte count in synovial fluid is often greater than 50,000 cells/mm^3. The joints are often sterile, possibly as a result of immunologic mechanisms. Dermatitis is usually absent.

Other less common complications of dissemination include endocarditis, myocarditis, and meningitis.

DIAGNOSIS. Diagnosis is based on the clinical picture and confirmed by isolation of gonococci from the primary infected mucosal site, such as the urethra, cervix, oropharynx, and rectum. Cultures of the joints, skin lesions, and blood are less apt to isolate the bacteria. Nucleic acid amplification tests allow identification of bacteria in synovial fluid even when the culture result is negative.

The most frequent laboratory findings are mild leukocytosis (10,500 to 12,500 cells/mm^3) and increased erythrocyte sedimentation rate (ESR). A positive culture result confirms the diagnosis and allows determination of drug susceptibility.

Culture. Obtain culture specimens of blood, synovial fluid, skin lesions, endocervix, urethra, rectum, and pharynx. *N. gonorrhoeae* is cultured from synovial fluid in approximately 50% of purulent joints and from 25% to 30% of all patients with DGI. More than 80% of culture specimens obtained from primary mucosal sites or from a sexual partner show positive results. Blood culture results are positive in 20% to 30% of DGI patients, and culture specimens from skin detect infection in less than 5% of cases. Blood culture results are usually positive only during the first few days.

Gram stain. Gram stain of the skin lesions is performed on the pus obtained by unroofing the pustule. Gram-stained smears on concentrated sediment of centrifuged synovial fluid show positive results in less than 25% of cases.

TREATMENT OF GONOCOCCAL INFECTION

Treatment recommendations for gonorrhea are found in Box 10-1, pp. 383-385.

Nongonococcal urethritis

Nongonococcal urethritis (NGU) and cervicitis are the most common sexually transmitted diseases in the United States. The diagnosis, as the name implies, used to be one of exclusion; however, routine diagnostic tests for identifying the various infecting organisms are now available. Epidemiologic control is difficult because many of those infected have no symptoms. Most women with cervical chlamydial infection, most homosexual men with rectal chlamydial infection, and as many as 30% of heterosexual men with chlamydial urethritis have few or no symptoms.

ORGANISMS

Genital chlamydial infection is responsible for about half of NGU cases. *Ureaplasma urealyticum* and *Mycoplasma genitalium* may cause 10% to 30% of NGU cases. Herpesviruses, *T. vaginalis, Haemophilus* species, and anaerobic bacteria account for less than 10% of NGU cases. In approximately one third of cases, no infectious cause can be found.

NONGONOCOCCAL URETHRITIS IN MALES

In males urethritis begins with dysuria and urethral discharge. Gonococcal urethritis begins 3 to 5 days after sexual contact and produces a burning, yellow, thick to mucopurulent urethral discharge (Figure 10-34). NGU begins 7 to 28 days after sexual contact with a smarting sensation while urinating and a mucoid discharge. Table 10-15 com-

Table 10-15 Comparison of Nongonococcal and Gonococcal Urethritis

	Nongonococcal urethritis	Gonococcal urethritis
Incubation period	7-28 days	3-5 days
Onset	Gradual	Abrupt
Dysuria	Smarting feeling	Burning
Discharge	Mucoid or purulent	Purulent
Gram stain of discharge	Polymorphonuclear leukocytes	Gram-negative intracellular diplococci

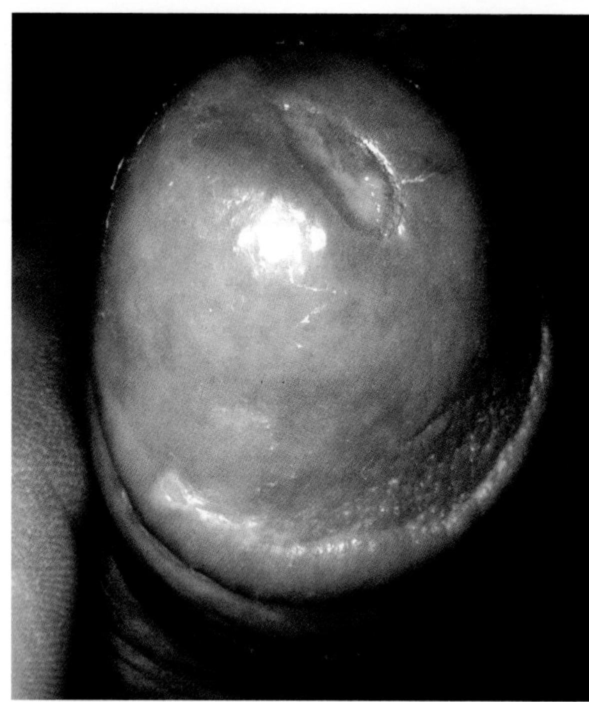

Figure 10-34 Gonorrhea. Dysuria and discharge are the most common symptoms in men.

pares the two forms of urethritis. *C. trachomatis* causes at least two thirds of the acute "idiopathic" epididymitis in sexually active men younger than 35 years.

NONGONOCOCCAL URETHRITIS IN FEMALES

The signs and symptoms in females are even more nonspecific. Nongonococcal cervicitis is asymptomatic or begins with a mucopurulent endocervical exudate or a mucoid vaginal discharge.

DIAGNOSIS

The diagnosis is made by confirming the presence of urethritis, demonstrating the presence of *C. trachomatis,* and excluding gonococcal infection.

MOLECULAR BIOLOGIC TESTS. Molecular biologic diagnostic methods have replaced culture and antigen tests. Amplifying assays (Gen-Probe, LCx Uriprobe) are highly effective in identifying genital chlamydial and gonococcal infections by testing urethral samples and first-voided urine. The results can be available in hours.

GRAM STAIN. A Gram stain is made of the urethral discharge. The presence of polymorphonuclear leukocytes confirms the diagnosis of urethritis, and the absence of gram-negative intracellular diplococci suggests urethritis is nongonococcal. Material for Gram stain is most effectively obtained at least 4 hours after urination. For those patients with urethral symptoms but without discharge, polymorphonuclear leukocytes may be seen in material obtained by a Calgiswab inserted approximately 2 cm beyond the urethral meatus.

CULTURE. Urethral discharge may be cultured for *N. gonorrhoeae.* These organisms are labile in vitro, and it is difficult to maintain viability during transport. If possible, culture specimens should be obtained from sexual partners of men with NGU and in pregnant women who may be transmitting the organism to the fetus during birth, causing neonatal conjunctivitis.

SPECIMEN COLLECTION. The proper collection and handling of specimens are important in all the methods used to identify *Chlamydia.* Because *Chlamydiae* are obligate intracellular organisms that infect the columnar epithelium, the objective of specimen collection procedures is to obtain columnar epithelial cells from the urethra.

- Delay obtaining specimens until 2 hours after the patient has voided.
- Obtain specimens for *Chlamydia* tests after obtaining specimens for Gram-stain smear or *N. gonorrhoeae* culture.
- For nonculture *Chlamydia* tests, use the swab supplied or specified by the manufacturer.
- Gently insert the urogenital swab into the urethra (females: 1 to 2 cm, males: 2 to 4 cm). Rotate the swab in one direction for at least one revolution for 5 seconds. Withdraw the swab and place it in the appropriate transport medium or use the swab to prepare a slide for direct fluorescent antibody (DFA) testing.

C. TRACHOMATIS–NEGATIVE NONGONOCOCCAL URETHRITIS

The most common cause of *C. trachomatis*–negative NGU is mycoplasmas, such as *U. urealyticum* and *M. genitalium. T. vaginalis,* yeasts, and anaerobic and aerobic bacteria are other possible sources of infection. Diagnosis requires cultures on specific media or detection by molecular biologic methods.

TREATMENT

Doxycycline and azithromycin are the drugs of choice (see Box 10-1).

Chapter 11

Sexually Transmitted Viral Infections

CHAPTER CONTENTS

GENITAL WARTS

Human papillomavirus

Human papillomavirus (HPV) causes warts. HPV can reside in epithelial basal cells and lead to subclinical or latent infection. More than 80 genotypes have been identified; HPV-6, HPV-11, and HPV-16 are most commonly associated with genital warts. HPV-6 and HPV-11 are rarely associated with cervical cancer. HPV-16 and HPV-18 are more likely to be present in subclinical infection and are the types most commonly associated with genital cancer. Bowenoid papulosis is most commonly caused by HPV-16. The rare verrucous carcinoma (Buschke-Löwenstein tumor) that resembles a large wart is locally aggressive but rarely metastatic. It is associated with HPV-6 and HPV-11.

Incidence

The incidence of genital warts is increasing rapidly and exceeds the incidence of genital herpes. It is the most common viral sexually transmitted disease. It is estimated that 30% to 50% of sexually active adults are infected with HPV. Only 1% to 2% of that group have clinically apparent anogenital warts. Most cervical dysplasias and cancers are related to oncogenic HPV.

Transmission

Risk factors for acquisition of condyloma in women have been identified as the number of sexual partners, frequency of sexual intercourse, and presence of warts on the sexual partner. Men have been found to be at increased risk if they fail to wear a condom. Condoms reduce the transmission of HPV but they do not eliminate it. Transmission of HPV during infant delivery may rarely occur.

Clinical presentation

Genital warts (condylomata acuminata or venereal warts) are pale pink with numerous, discrete, narrow-to-wide projections on a broad base. The surface is smooth or velvety and moist, and lacks the hyperkeratosis of warts found elsewhere (Figures 11-1 to 11-5). The warts may coalesce in the rectal or perineal area to form a large, cauliflower-like mass (Figures 11-6 and 11-7). Perianal warts may be present in persons who do not practice anal sex.

Another type is seen most often in young, sexually active patients. Multifocal, often bilateral, red- or brown-pigmented, slightly raised, smooth papules have the same virus types seen in exophytic condyloma, but in some instances these papules have histologic features of Bowen's disease. (See discussion of bowenoid papulosis later in this chapter.)

Warts spread rapidly over moist areas and may therefore be symmetric on opposing surfaces of the labia or rectum (Figure 11-7). Common warts can possibly be the source of genital warts, although they are usually caused by different antigenic types of virus. Warts may extend into the vaginal tract, urethra, and anal canal or the bladder, in which case a speculum or sigmoidoscope is required for visualization and treatment. Condyloma may spontaneously regress, enlarge, or remain unchanged. Genital warts frequently recur after treatment. There are two possible reasons. Latent virus exists beyond the treatment areas in clinically normal skin. Warts that are flat and inconspicuous, especially on the penile shaft and urethral meatus, escape treatment.

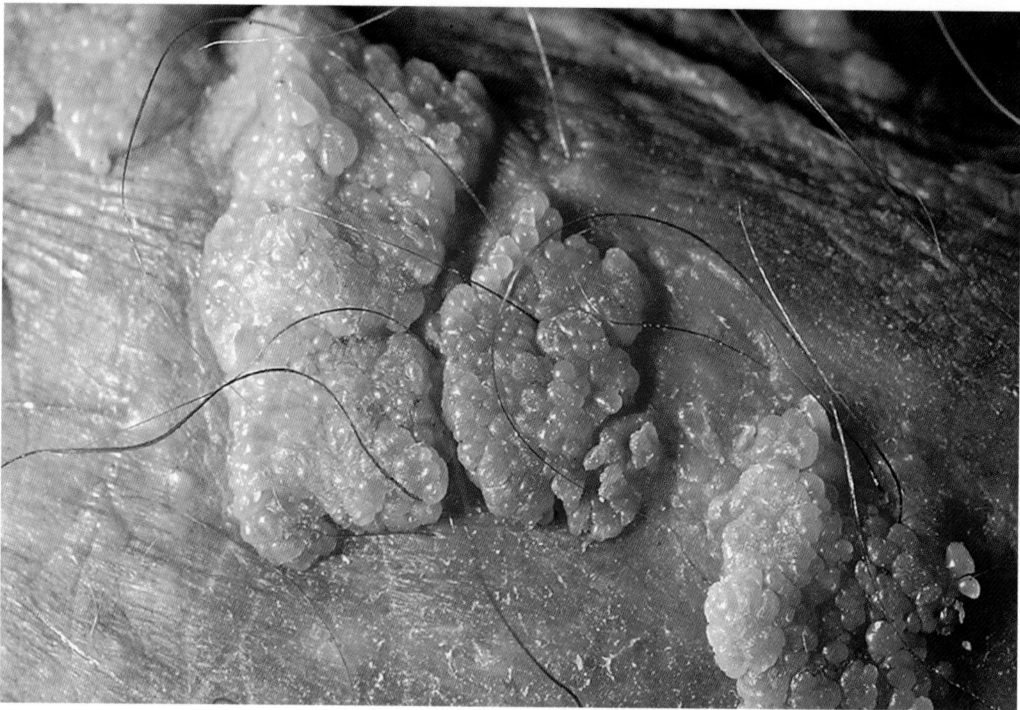

Figure 11-1 Warts on the shaft may have a papillomatous surface and a very broad base.

GENITAL WARTS

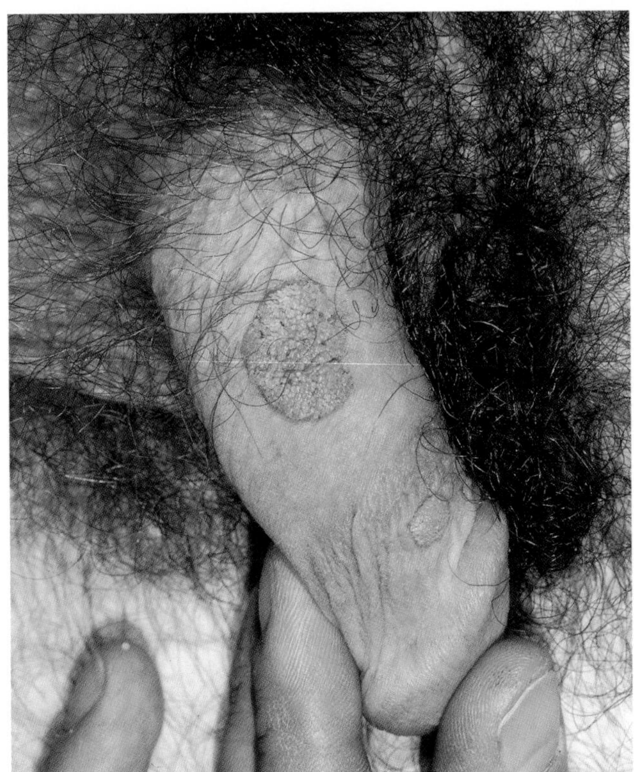

Figure 11-2 Broad-based wart on the shaft of a penis. There are numerous projections on the surface.

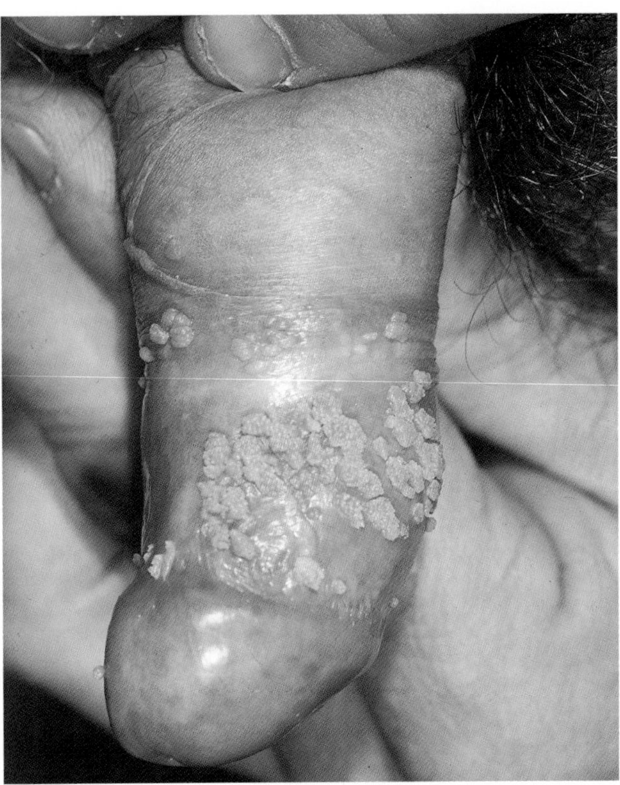

Figure 11-3 Multiple small warts under the foreskin. Multiple inoculations occur on a moist surface. Each wart is made up of many discrete, narrow projections.

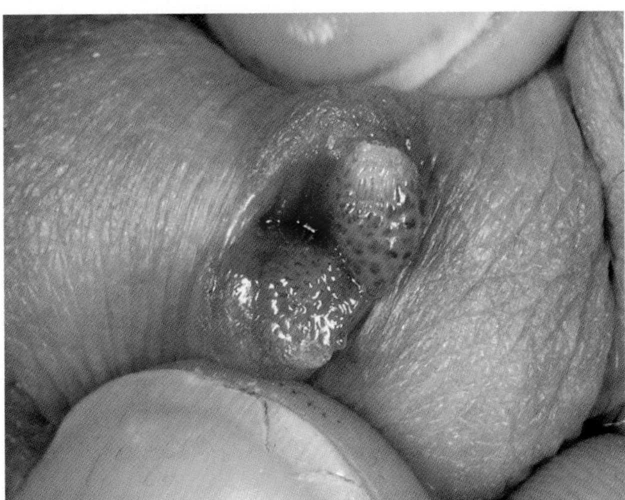

Figure 11-4 Wart at the urethral meatus.

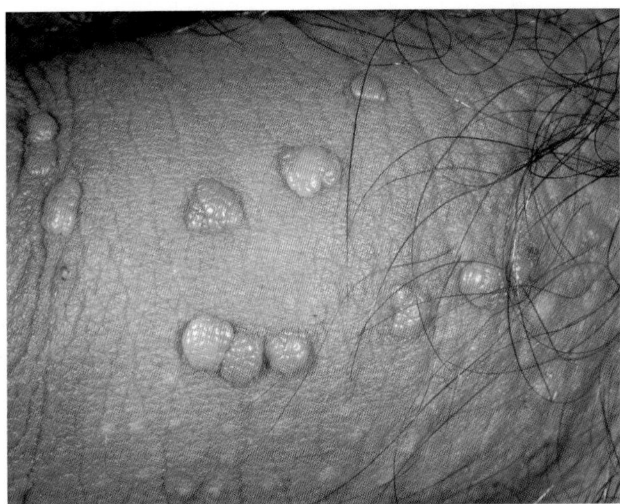

Figure 11-5 Small papular warts on the shaft of the penis. These smooth dome-shaped structures do not respond as well as broad-based papillomatous warts to topical medications. They are effectively treated with light electrodesiccation, cryosurgery, or scissor excision.

GENITAL WARTS

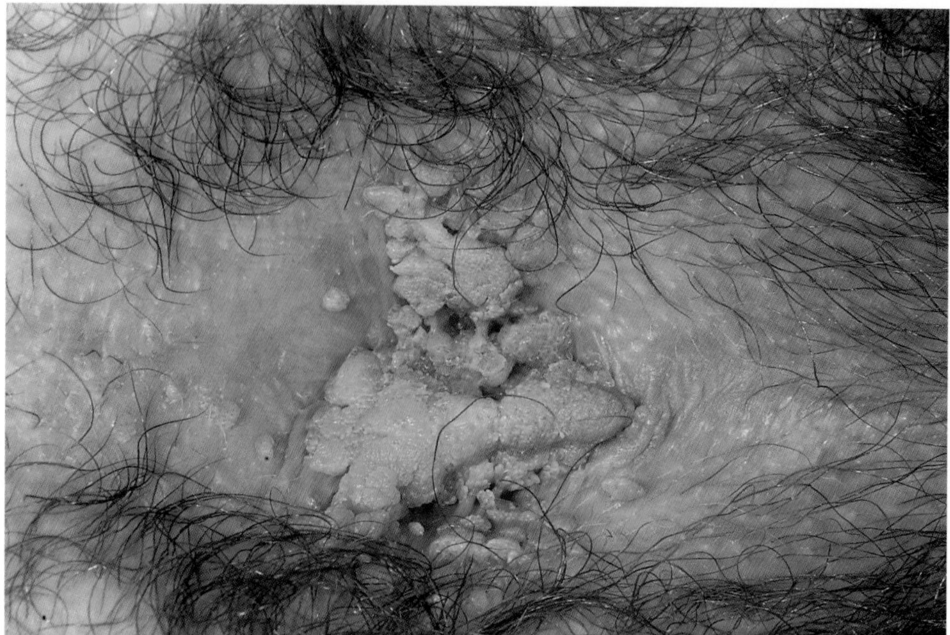

Figure 11-6 Mass of warts on opposing surfaces of the anus.

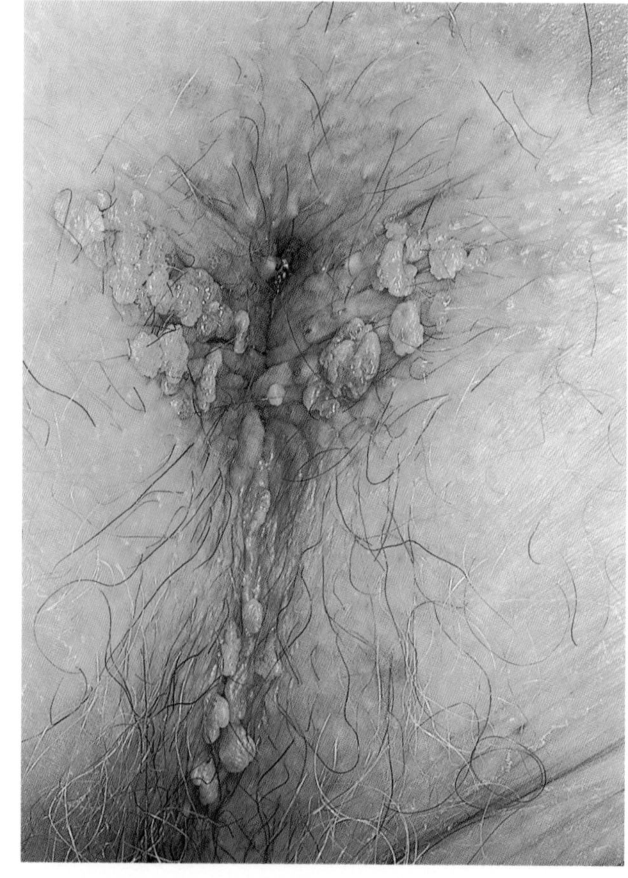

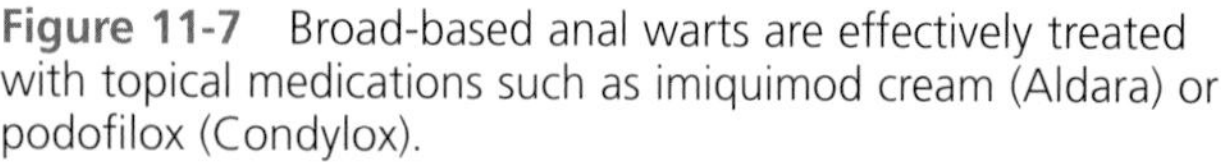

Figure 11-7 Broad-based anal warts are effectively treated with topical medications such as imiquimod cream (Aldara) or podofilox (Condylox).

ORAL CONDYLOMA IN PATIENTS WITH GENITAL HUMAN PAPILLOMAVIRUS INFECTION

One study showed that 50% of patients with multiple and widespread genital HPV infection who practiced orogenital sex have oral condyloma. All lesions were asymptomatic. Magnification was necessary to detect oral lesions. The diagnosis was confirmed by biopsy. The tongue was the site most frequently affected. Oral condyloma appeared as multiple, small, white or pink papules, sessile or pedunculate, and as papillary growths with filiform characteristics (Figure 11-8). The size of oral lesions was greater than 2 mm in more than 50% of lesions, and in 61% of cases more than five lesions were present. HPV-16, HPV-18, HPV-6, and HPV-11 were found. *PMID 1323211*

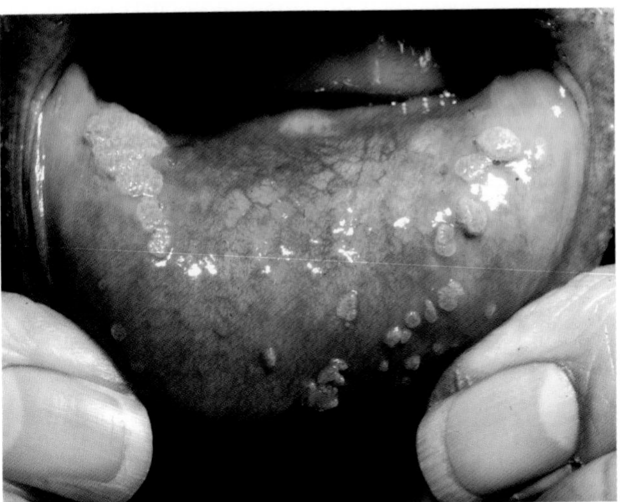

Figure 11-8 Oral condyloma that can be visualized without magnification are surprisingly uncommon.

PEARLY PENILE PAPULES

Dome-shaped or hairlike projections, called pearly penile papules, appear on the corona of the penis and sometimes on the shaft just proximal to the corona in up to 10% of male patients. These small angiofibromas are normal variants but are sometimes mistaken for warts. No treatment is required (Figure 11-9, *A* and *B*).

PEARLY PENILE PAPULES

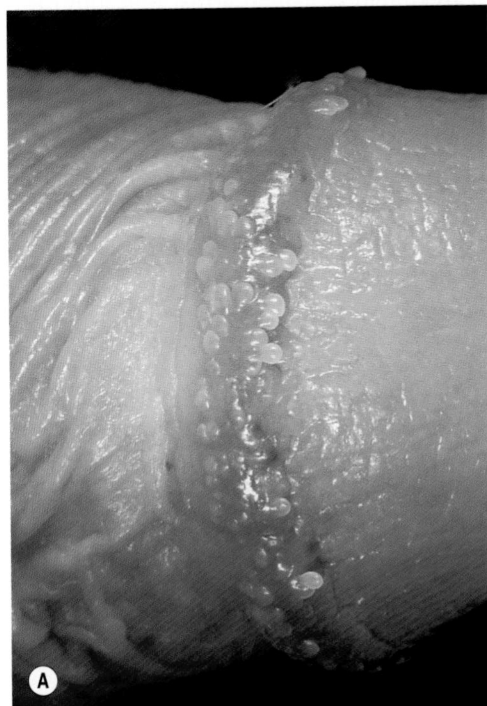

An anatomic variant of normal papules most commonly found on the corona of the penis. They are sometimes mistaken for warts. No treatment is required.

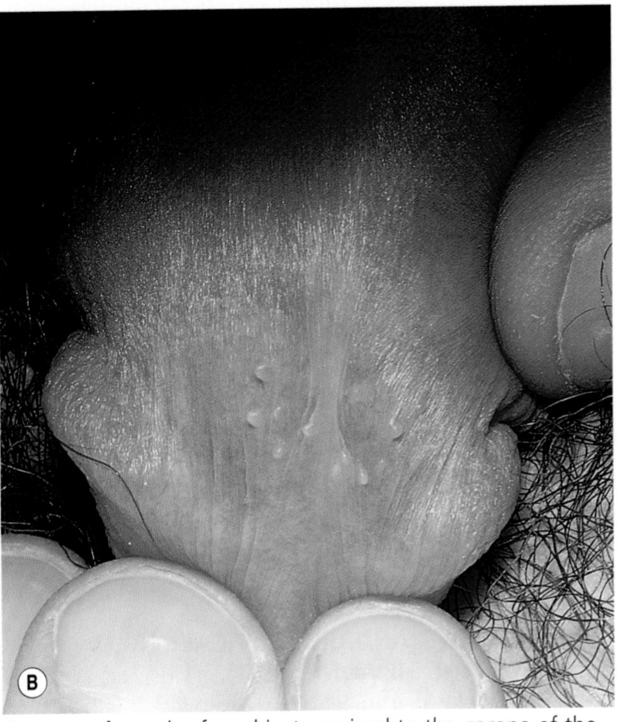

A group of papules found just proximal to the corona of the penis is sometimes mistaken for warts.

Figure 11-9

GENITAL WARTS IN CHILDREN

It has been estimated that at least 50% of the cases of condylomata acuminata in children are the result of sexual abuse. In all states there are laws that in effect declare, "If child abuse is recognized or suspected, it has to be reported to the authorities."

Warts in the genital area can be acquired without sexual abuse. A child with warts on the hands can transfer the warts to the mouth, genitals, and anal area. A mother with hand warts can transfer warts to the child. Sexual play among children is another possible mode of transmission. It is not known whether children can acquire condylomata acuminata from adults with anogenital warts through modes of transmission other than skin-to-skin contact. The incubation period for warts is often many months; this makes it difficult to associate past events.

GENITAL WARTS AND CANCER

There is strong evidence that several HPV types are associated with genital cancers. Genitoanal warts are predominantly induced by HPV-6, HPV-11, HPV-16, and HPV-18. A strong association has been established between infection by HPV-16 and HPV-18 and the subsequent development of cancer in the uterine cervix. When virus typing becomes generally available, it will be useful to identify patients harboring the high-risk HPV types. HPV-16 was demonstrated in 84% and HPV-18 in 8% of genital tumors.

Seventy-three percent of the nonmalignant, clinically and histologically normal tissue 2 to 5 cm from the tumors contained HPV-16. This implies that HPV can persist latently in tissue that appears normal. Cervical carcinomas and precancerous lesions in women may be associated with genital papillomavirus infection in their male sexual partners. Forty-three percent of male sexual partners of women with genital warts had lesions that could be detected only after application of acetic acid. Homosexual behavior in men is a risk factor for anal cancer. Squamous cell anal cancer is associated with a history of genital warts, which suggests that papillomavirus infection is a cause of anal cancer. Male circumcision is associated with a reduced risk of penile HPV infection and, in the case of men with a history of multiple sexual partners, a reduced risk of cervical cancer in their current female partners.

Diagnosis

A clinical diagnosis can be made in most cases. The differential diagnosis includes seborrheic keratoses, nevi, molluscum contagiosum, and pearly penile papules. Biopsy suspicious lesions.

VIRAL TYPING USING STANDARD CERVICAL SCREENING SPECIMENS (THE HPV-DNA TEST). This test is used to distinguish between infections with low-risk HPV types and infections with intermediate- to high-risk HPV types and uses nucleic acid hybridization. The test serves as an adjunct to the Pap smear in the identification of women who may be at increased risk for cervical intraepithelial neoplasia (CIN). The test is commonly performed. Cervical swab and cervical biopsies may be used. A special cervical swab must be used (e.g., Digene HPV specimen collection kit [for nonpregnant women only]). Then 3-mm cervical biopsy specimens are submitted into Digene specimen transport medium. This assay distinguishes between two groups of HPV: HPV types 6, 11, 42, 43, and 44 versus HPV types 16, 18, 31, 33, 35, 39, 45, 51, 52, 56, 58, 59, and 68. It does not identify specific viral types within these groups. HPV-DNA testing is likely to become the primary cervical cancer screening tool as vaccine use expands.

VIRAL TYPING USING PARAFFIN-EMBEDDED BIOPSIES. Human papillomavirus (HPV) typing in situ DNA hybridization testing detects the presence of nucleic acid in cells or tissues. Paraffin-embedded biopsies are used. The test is capable of detecting two distinct groups of the virus: HPV types 6/11 and HPV types 16/18/31/33/35/39/45/51/52/56/58/66. Other HPV types may appear in anogenital lesions but are not detectable with this assay. HPV types 6 and 11 are the predominant viruses associated with condylomata acuminata (genital warts). The condition usually remains benign. HPV types 16/18/31/33/35/39/45/51/52/56/58/66 frequently are found in CIN III (severe dysplasias and carcinoma in situ) and cervical cancer. This test is very expensive and is not routinely used.

VACCINATION. Gardasil is a vaccine indicated in girls and women 9 to 26 years of age for the prevention of cervical cancer, precancerous or dysplastic lesions, and genital warts caused by HPV types 6, 11, 16, and 18. It is used for treatment of genital warts. It is administered intramuscularly in a three-dose regimen, with the initial injection followed by subsequent doses at months 2 and 6. Studies on men are in progress. Other vaccines are being studied.

Treatment

A detailed overview of treatment is provided by the World Health Organization in Chapter 10.

HPV cannot be completely eliminated because of the surrounding subclinical HPV infection. Removal of visible lesions decreases viral transmission. All treatment methods are associated with a high rate of recurrence that is likely related to surrounding subclinical infection. Therapies with antiviral/immunomodulatory activity (e.g., imiquimod cream) may be associated with lower recurrence rates.

MANAGEMENT OF SEXUAL PARTNERS

Examination of sexual partners is not necessary for the management of genital warts because the role of reinfection is probably minimal. Many sexual partners have obvious warts and may desire treatment. The majority of partners are probably already subclinically infected with HPV, even if they do not have visible warts. The use of condoms may reduce transmission to partners likely to be uninfected, such as new partners. HPV infection may persist throughout a patient's lifetime in a dormant state and become infectious intermittently. Whether patients with subclinical HPV infection are as contagious as patients with exophytic warts is unknown. One study showed that the failure rate of treating women with condylomata acuminata did not decrease if their male sexual partners were also treated.

PREGNANCY

The use of podophyllin and podofilox is contraindicated during pregnancy. Genital papillary lesions have a tendency to proliferate and to become friable during pregnancy. Many experts advocate the removal of visible warts during pregnancy. HPV-6 and HPV-11 can cause laryngeal papillomatosis in infants. The route of transmission is unknown, and laryngeal papillomatosis has occurred in infants delivered by cesarean section. Cesarean delivery should not be performed solely to prevent transmission of HPV infection to the newborn. In rare instances, cesarean delivery may be indicated for women with genital warts if the pelvic outlet is obstructed or if vaginal delivery would result in excessive bleeding.

CHILDREN

Spontaneous resolution of pediatric condyloma occurs in more than half of cases in 5 years. Nonintervention is a reasonable initial approach to managing venereal warts in children.

PATIENT-APPLIED THERAPIES

IMIQUIMOD. Improved efficacy and lower recurrence rates occur with imiquimod (Aldara) by inducing the body's own immunologic defenses. Imiquimod has an immunomodulatory effect and does not rely on physical destruction of the lesion. It has antiviral properties by induction of cytokines, including interferon, tumor necrosis factor, and interleukin (IL)-6, IL-8, and IL-12. Imiquimod enhances cell-mediated cytolytic activity against HPV. The cream is applied at bedtime every other day, for a maximum of 16 weeks. On the morning after application, the treated area should be cleansed. Local mild-to-moderate irritation may occur. Systemic reactions have not been reported. Imiquimod has not been studied for use during pregnancy.

PODOFILOX. Podofilox, also known as podophyllotoxin, is the main cytotoxic ingredient of podophyllin. Podofilox gel (Condylox) is available for self-application and is useful for responsible, compliant patients. Patients are instructed to apply the 0.5% gel to their external genital warts twice each day for 3 consecutive days, followed by 4 days without treatment. It is recommended that no more than 10 cm^2 of wart tissue should be treated in a day. This cycle is repeated at weekly intervals for a maximum of 4 to 6 weeks. Approximately 15% of patients report severe local reactions to the treatment area after the first treatment cycle; this is reduced to 5% by the last treatment cycle. Local adverse effects of the drug, such as pain, burning, inflammation, and erosions, have occurred in more than 50% of patients. Podofilox is not recommended for perianal, vaginal, or urethral warts and is contraindicated in pregnancy.

PROVIDER-ADMINISTERED THERAPIES

CRYOSURGERY. Liquid nitrogen delivered with a probe, as a spray, or with a cotton applicator is very effective for treating smaller, flatter genital warts. It is too painful for patients with extensive disease. Exophytic lesions are best treated with excision, imiquimod, or podofilox. Warts on the shaft of the penis and vulva respond very well, with little or no scarring. Cryosurgery of the rectal area is painful. A conservative technique is best. Freeze the lesion until the white border extends approximately 1 mm beyond the wart. Overaggressive therapy causes pain, massive swelling, and scarring.

A blister appears and erodes to form an ulcer in 1 to 3 days, and the lesion heals in 1 to 2 weeks. Repeat treatment every 2 to 4 weeks as necessary. Two to three sessions may be required.

Use EMLA cream and/or 1% lidocaine injection for patients who do not tolerate the pain of cryotherapy.

Cryotherapy is effective and safe for both mother and fetus when applied in the second and third trimesters of pregnancy. An intermittent spray technique, using a small spray tip, is used to achieve a small region of cryonecrosis, limiting the runoff and scattering of liquid nitrogen. Cervical involvement that requires cervical cryotherapy does not increase the risk to mother or fetus.

SURGICAL REMOVAL AND ELECTROSURGERY. Excision with scissors, curettage, or electrosurgery produces immediate results. These methods are useful for both extensive condylomata or a limited number of warts. Small isolated warts on the shaft of the penis are best treated with conservative electrosurgery or scissor excision rather than subjecting the patient to repeated sessions with podophyllum. Large, unresponsive masses of warts around the rectum or vulva may be treated by scissor excision of the bulk of the mass, followed by electrocautery of the remaining tissue down to the skin surface. Removal of a very large mass of warts is a painful procedure and is best performed with the patient receiving a general or spinal anesthetic in the operating room.

TRICHLOROACETIC ACID. Application of trichloroacetic acid (TCA) and bichloroacetic acid (BCA) 80% to 90% is effective and less destructive than laser surgery, electrocautery, or liquid nitrogen application. It is most effective on small, moist warts.

This is an ideal treatment for isolated lesions in pregnant women. A very small amount is applied to the wart, which whitens immediately. The acid is then neutralized with water or bicarbonate of soda. The tissue slough heals in 7 to 10 days. Repeat each week or every other week as needed. Excessive application causes scars. Take great care not to treat normal surrounding skin.

PODOPHYLLUM RESIN. Podophyllin is a plant compound that causes cells to arrest in mitosis, leading to tissue necrosis. Podophyllum resin 10% to 25% in compound tincture of benzoin used to be the standard provider-administered therapy. Patient-applied medications are now commonly used. The medication can be very effective, especially for moist warts with a large surface area and lesions with many surface projections. Podophyllum is relatively ineffective in dry areas, such as the scrotum, penile shaft, and labia majora. It is not recommended for cervical, vaginal, or intraurethral warts. The compound is applied with a cotton-tipped applicator (Figure 11-10). The entire surface of the wart is covered with the solution, and the patient remains still until the solution dries in approximately 2 minutes. When lesions covered by the prepuce are treated, the applied solution must be allowed to dry for several minutes before the prepuce is returned to its usual position. Powdering the warts after treatment or applying petrolatum to the surrounding skin may help to avoid contamination of normal skin with the irritating resin. The medicine is removed by washing 1 hour later. The patient is treated again in 1 week. The podophyllum may then remain on the wart for 8 to 12 hours if there was little or no inflammation after the first treatment.

Overenthusiastic initial treatment can result in intense inflammation and discomfort that lasts for days. The procedure is simple and it is tempting to allow home treatment, but in most cases this should be avoided. Very frequently patients overtreat and cause excessive inflammation by applying podophyllum on normal skin. To avoid extreme discomfort, treat only part of a large warty mass in the perineal and rectal area. Warts on the shaft of the penis do not respond as successfully to podophyllum as do warts on the glans or under the foreskin; consequently, electrosurgery or cryosurgery should be used if two or three treatment sessions with podophyllum fail. Many warts disappear after a single treatment. Alternate forms of therapy should be attempted if there is no improvement after five treatment sessions.

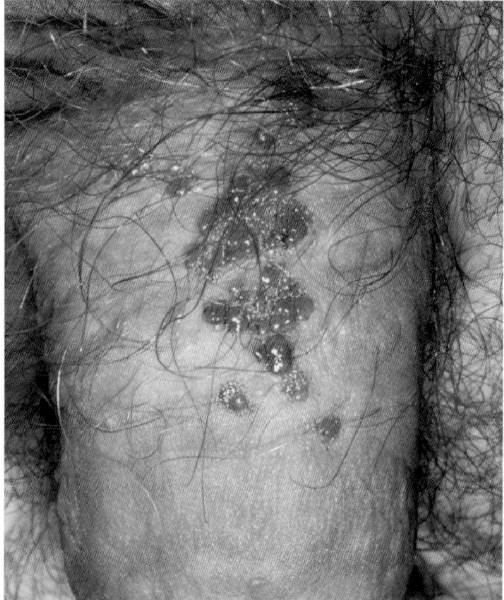

Figure 11-10 Podophyllin has just been applied to these papular warts. The medication is washed off several hours later.

Warning. Systemic toxicity occurs from absorption of podophyllum. Paresthesia, polyneuritis, paralytic ileus, leukopenia, thrombocytopenia, coma, and death have occurred when large quantities of podophyllum were applied to wide areas or allowed to remain in contact with the skin for an extended period. Only limited areas should be treated during each session. Very small quantities should be used in the mouth, vaginal tract, or rectosigmoid. Do not use podophyllum on pregnant women.

Alteration of histopathology. Podophyllum can produce bizarre forms of squamous cells, which can be mistaken for squamous cell carcinoma. The pathologist must be informed of the patient's exposure to podophyllum when a biopsy of a previously treated wart is submitted.

5-FLUOROURACIL CREAM. Application of a 5-fluorouracil cream (Carac, Efudex) may be considered in cases of genital warts that are resistant to all other treatments. A thin layer of cream is applied one to three times per week and washed off after 3 to 10 hours, depending on the sensitivity of the location. Treat for several weeks, as necessary. Irritation makes it intolerable for some patients.

Vaginal warts are treated by inserting an applicator (such as the one supplied by Ortho Pharmaceutical Corp. for the treatment of vaginal *Candida*) one-third full of 5% 5-fluorouracil cream (approximately 3 ml) deeply into the vagina at bedtime, once each week for up to 10 consecutive weeks. The vulva and urethra are protected with petrolatum. A tampon should be inserted just inside the introitus. In one study, there was no evidence of disease in 85% of patients 3 months after treatment. Resistant cases were treated twice each week. Mild irritation and vaginal discharge may develop. The vulva should be protected with zinc oxide or hydrocortisone ointments if the twice-each-week regimen is used. Application to the keratinized epithelium (vulva, anus, and penis) twice weekly on 2 consecutive days is well tolerated but less effective; such treatment should not be used for pregnant women. Patients should be warned to avoid thick coverage because the excess cream causes inflammation or ulceration in the labiocrural or anal folds. Protective gloves are not necessary, provided that the hands are carefully washed after applying the 5-fluorouracil cream. A single intravaginal dose of 1.5-gm, 5% 5-fluorouracil cream contains only 75 mg of 5-fluorouracil. This is less than 10% of the usual systemic dose and far lower than the toxicity level of the drug even if rapid and complete absorption occurs. 5-Fluorouracil (1%) in a vaginal hydrophilic gel was used in another study. A disposable applicator was used to insert

4 gm of medication deep into the vagina once at bedtime on every other day (e.g., days 1, 3, and 5) per week. A maximum of 12 applications were to be used in 4 weeks. A high rate of cure was reported. *PMID: 10872909*

CARBON DIOXIDE LASER. The CO_2 laser is an ideal method for treating both primary and recurrent condylomata acuminata in men and women because of its precision and the wound's rapid healing without scarring. The laser can be used with an operating microscope to find and destroy the smallest warts. For pregnant women, this is the treatment of choice for large or extensive lesions and for cases that do not respond to repeated applications of trichloroacetic acid.

INTERFERON ALFA-2B RECOMBINANT (INTRON A). Warts that do not respond to any form of conventional treatment and patients whose disease is severe enough to impose significant social or physical limitations on their activities may be candidates for treatment with interferon. Interferon-alfa is approved by the U.S. Food and Drug Administration for the treatment of condylomata acuminata in patients 18 years of age or older. There are two commercially available preparations for intralesional injection into the base of the wart. Alferon N injection (interferon alfa-n3) is available in 1-ml vials; 0.05 ml per wart is administered twice weekly for up to 8 weeks. Intron A (interferon alfa-2b, recombinant) is available in several-sized vials, but the vial of 10 million units is the only package size specifically designed for use in treatment of condylomata acuminata. Intron A (0.1 ml of reconstituted Intron A) is injected into each lesion three times per week on alternate days for 3 weeks. Influenza-like symptoms usually clear within 24 hours of treatment. Total clearing occurs in approximately 40% of treated warts. The medication is very expensive.

BOWENOID PAPULOSIS

Bowenoid papulosis is an uncommon condition seen in young, sexually active adults. It occurs on the genitals (vulva and circumcised penis) and histologically resembles Bowen's disease. The mean age is 30 years for male patients and 32 years for female patients. Patients' age range is from 3 to 80 years. The duration of disease has been from 2 weeks to 11 years. The natural history of the disease is unknown, but the lesions usually follow a benign clinical course and spontaneous regression is observed. Evolution of the lesions to invasive carcinoma is rare.

The papules are asymptomatic discrete, small (averaging 4 mm in diameter), flat, reddish violaceous or brown, often coalescent, and usually have a smooth, velvety surface. They may resemble flat warts, psoriasis, or lichen planus (Figure 11-11). In women the lesions are often darkly pigmented and are not as easily confused with other entities. They are located in men on the glans, the shaft, and the foreskin of the penis and in women on the labia majora and minora, on the clitoris, in the inguinal folds, and around the anus. The lesions in women are often bilateral, hyperpigmented, and confluent. Autoinoculation probably explains the bilateral, symmetric distribution in moist areas. Many patients have a history of genital infection with viral warts or herpes simplex. Genital warts are primarily caused by HPV types 6 and 11. HPV-16 has been found in a high percentage of women with bowenoid papulosis and in cervical and other genital neoplasias. Therefore the cervix of female patients with bowenoid papulosis and other genitoanal HPV infections should be examined routinely, with careful follow-up. Female partners of patients with bowenoid papulosis should also be observed closely.

Treatment should be conservative. Individual lesions can be adequately treated by electrosurgery, carbon dioxide laser, cryosurgery, or scissor excision, much as ordinary verrucae, without the need for wide surgical margins. Alternatively, lesions may be treated for 3 to 5 weeks with 5% 5-fluorouracil cream or imiquimod cream every other day until they become inflamed.

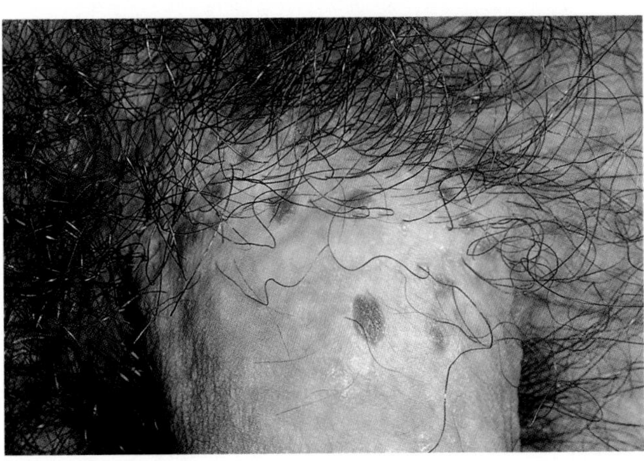

Figure 11-11 Bowenoid papulosis. Multiple brown verrucous papules on the shaft of the penis. This patient responded to imiquimod cream (Aldara) applied every other day. This is the same treatment regimen used to treat penile warts.

MOLLUSCUM CONTAGIOSUM

Molluscum contagiosum is a large double-stranded DNA virus that replicates entirely within the cytoplasm of keratinocytes. It is a member of the family Poxviridae and does not develop latency like the herpesvirus. The virion colony is encased in a protective sac that prevents triggering of the host immune response.

Clinical manifestations

Molluscum contagiosum papules are discrete, 2 to 5 mm in diameter, slightly umbilicated, flesh colored, and dome shaped. They spread by touching, by autoinoculation (particularly in atopic patients), and by scratching or secondary to shaving, and may result in a linear distribution of lesions. Transmission also occurs in wrestlers, masseurs, and steam and sauna bathers. The pubic and genital areas (Figures 11-12 through 11-15) are most commonly involved in adults. Molluscum lesions in other areas are described in Chapter 12. They are frequently grouped. There may be few or many covering a wide area. Erythema and scaling at the periphery of a single or several lesions may occur (Figure 11-16). This may be the result of inflammation from scratching, or it may be a hypersensitivity reaction.

Individual lesions last 6 to 8 weeks. Autoinoculation causes new lesions and the duration of infection can be up to 8 months.

The differential diagnosis includes warts and herpes simplex. Molluscum papules are dome shaped, slightly umbilicated, firm, and white. Warts have an irregular, often velvety surface. The vesicles of herpes simplex rapidly become umbilicated.

Genital molluscum contagiosum in children may be a manifestation of sexual abuse (see Figure 11-16).

Molluscum contagiosum is a common and at times severely disfiguring eruption in patients with HIV infection. It is often a marker of late-stage disease.

Diagnosis

The patient must be carefully examined because these discrete white-pink umbilicated papules are often camouflaged by pubic hair. Most patients have just a few lesions that can be easily overlooked. The focus of examination is the pubic hair, the genitals, anal area, thighs, and trunk. Lesions may appear anywhere except the palms and soles. If necessary, the diagnosis can be easily established by laboratory methods (see Chapter 12). Microscopic examination of a potassium hydroxide preparation of the soft material obtained from the umbilicated part of the lesion shows inclusion bodies (molluscum bodies) within the keratinocytes.

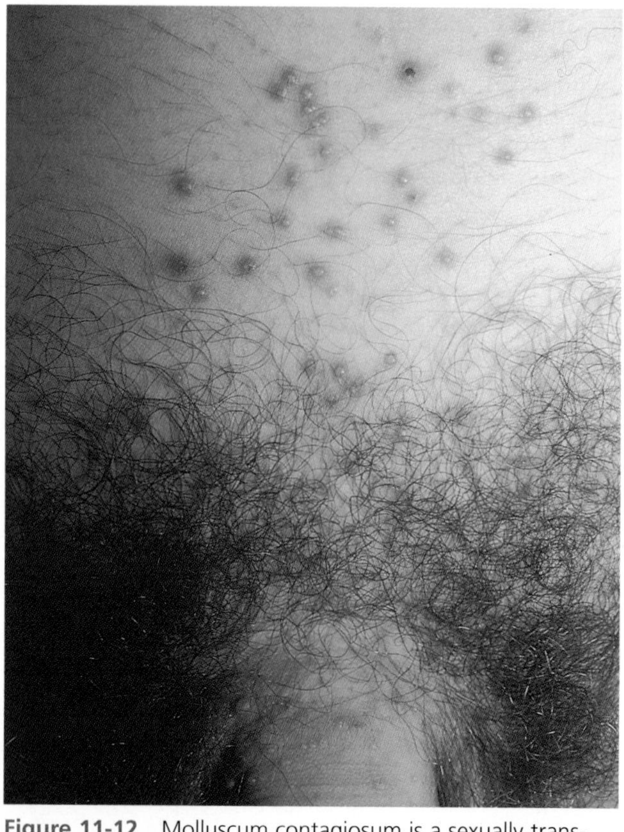

Figure 11-12 Molluscum contagiosum is a sexually transmitted disease in adults. Close observation of individual lesions is necessary to confirm the diagnosis. Lesions are often misdiagnosed as warts or herpes simplex.

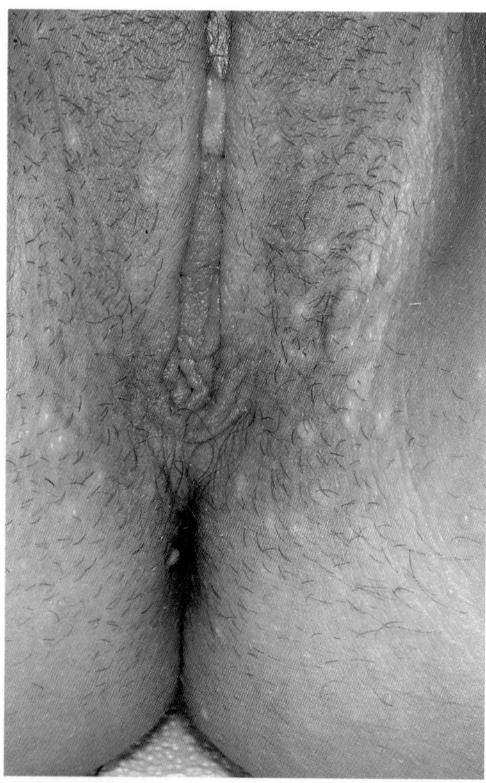

Figure 11-13 Molluscum contagiosum are easily misdiagnosed as genital warts. Lesions are never confluent or appear as a large mass as do warts.

MOLLUSCUM CONTAGIOSUM

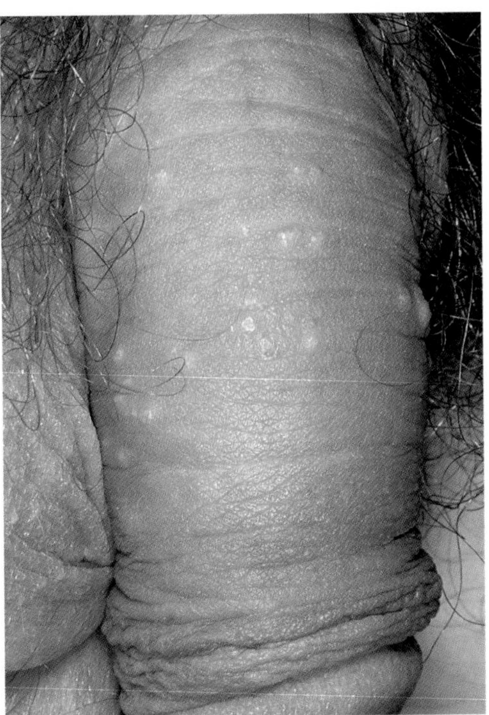

Figure 11-14 Molluscum contagiosum must be examined closely to differentiate them from warts, especially in the groin area.

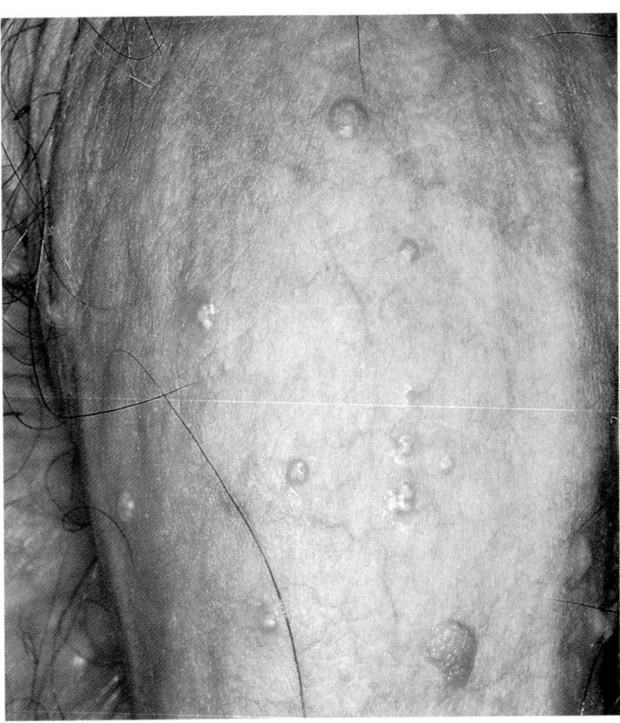

Figure 11-15 Molluscum contagiosum. Lesions are usually discrete, white, and dome shaped. They lack the many small projections found on the surface of genital warts.

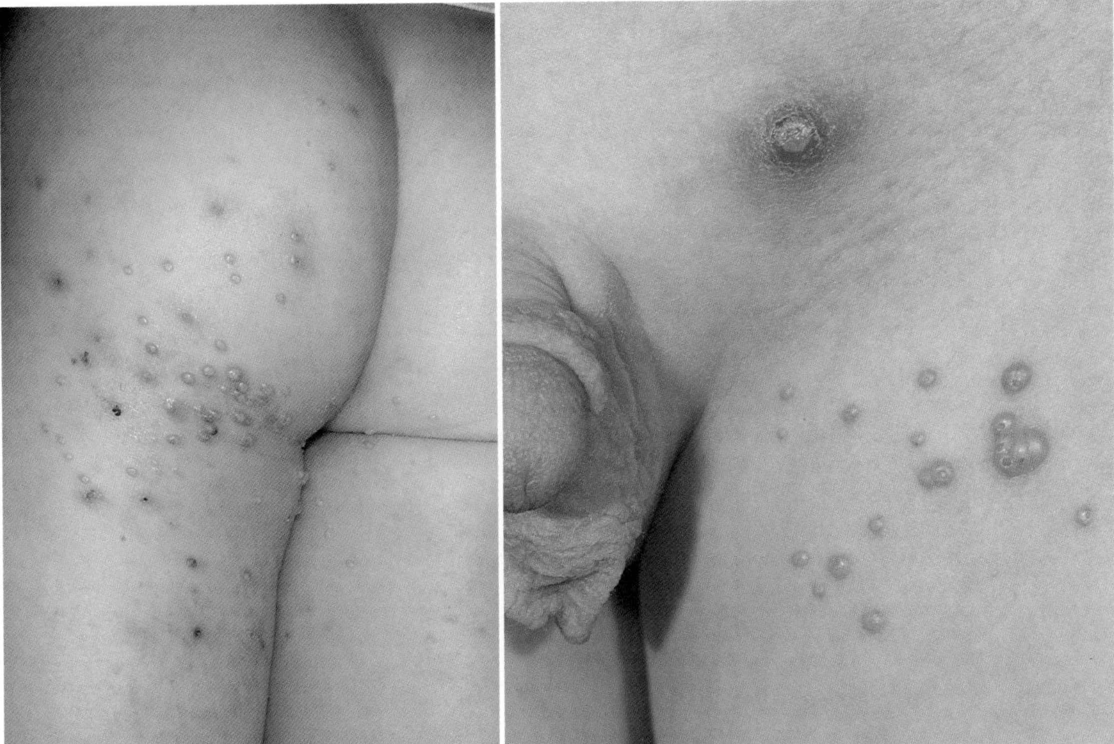

Figure 11-16 Molluscum contagiosum. A single lesion (or multiple lesions) may become inflamed and then disappear.

Treatment

Genital lesions should be definitively treated to prevent spread through sexual contact. New lesions that were too small to be detected at the first examination may appear after treatment and require attention at a subsequent visit.

OVER-THE-COUNTER TREATMENTS

There are several nonprescription "naturopathic" treatments that may be obtained on the Internet. Examples are MolluscumRx and ZymaDerm. Many patients report that these treatments are not effective.

CURETTAGE

Small papules can be quickly removed with a curette, with or without local anesthesia. Bleeding is controlled with gauze pressure or Monsel's solution. Warn the patient that Monsel's solution is painful. Curettage is useful when there are a few lesions because it provides the quickest, most reliable treatment. A small scar may form; therefore this technique should be avoided in cosmetically important areas.

Lidocaine/prilocaine (EMLA) cream applied 30 to 60 minutes before treatment helps prevent the pain of curettage for children.

CRYOSURGERY

Cryosurgery is the treatment of choice for patients who do not object to the pain. The papule is sprayed or touched lightly with a nitrogen-bathed cotton swab until the advancing, white, frozen border has progressed down the side of the papule to form a 1-mm halo on the normal skin surrounding the lesion. This should take approximately 5 seconds. A conservative approach is necessary because excessive freezing produces hypopigmentation or hyperpigmentation.

ANTIVIRAL AND IMMUNOMODULATORY THERAPIES

Males between 9 and 27 years of age with molluscum contagiosum self-administered an analog of imiquimod 5% cream (Aldara) three times daily for 5 consecutive days per week for 4 weeks. The cure rate was over 80%. Children may respond with less irritation if treated once each day or every other day. Children (mean age 7 years) were treated every night for 4 weeks. Adverse reactions were limited to application site reactions. There was no systemic toxicity. Imiquimod is most efficacious in patients with HIV-1 disease and in the genital area in immune-competent adults.

CANTHARIDIN

Cantharidin is a safe and effective therapy. A small drop of Cantharone (cantharidin 0.7%) is applied over the surface of the lesion, while contamination of normal skin is avoided. Temporary burning, pain, erythema, or pruritus may occur. Secondary bacterial infection does not occur. Lesions blister and may clear without scarring. New lesions occasionally appear at the site of the blister created by cantharidin. An alternate method is to apply a tiny amount of cantharidin or the more potent Verrusol (1% cantharidin, 30% salicylic acid, 5% podophyllin) and cover the area with tape for 1 day. The resulting small blister is treated with Polysporin until the reaction subsides.

POTASSIUM HYDROXIDE

Potassium hydroxide (KOH) 10% aqueous solution was applied twice daily, on each lesion. The therapy was continued until all lesions underwent inflammation and superficial ulceration. Of the 35 children tested, 32 achieved complete clinical cure after a mean treatment period of 30 days. Hypertrophic scarring occurred in one patient; pigmentary changes occurred in nine others.

ORAL CIMETIDINE

Pediatric patients were treated with a 2-month course of oral cimetidine 40 mg/kg/day. All but three children who completed treatment experienced clearance of all lesions. No adverse effects were observed. Response to cimetidine may be better in atopic compared to nonatopic children.

LASER THERAPY

The 585-nm pulsed dye laser is an effective, well-tolerated, and quick treatment for molluscum contagiosum.

TRICHLOROACETIC ACID PEEL

Peels performed with 25% to 50% trichloroacetic acid (average 35%) and repeated every 2 weeks as needed resulted in an average reduction in lesion counts of 40.5% (range 0% to 90%) in HIV patients with extensive molluscum contagiosum. No spread of molluscum lesions, scarring, or secondary infection developed at the 2-month follow-up examination.

GENITAL HERPES SIMPLEX

Genital herpes simplex virus (HSV) infection is primarily a disease of young adults. It is a recurrent, lifelong infection. There are two serotypes: HSV-1 and HSV-2. Most genital cases are caused by HSV-2. At least 50 million persons in the United States have genital HSV infection (Figure 11-17). Sexual encounters are often delayed or avoided for fear of acquiring or transmitting the disease. The psychologic implications are obvious. HSV-2 is not an etiologic factor in cervical cancer as was once suspected.

Most persons infected with HSV-2 have not been diagnosed. Many have mild or unrecognized infections but shed the virus intermittently in the genital tract. Most genital herpes infections are transmitted by persons unaware that they have the infection or who are asymptomatic when transmission occurs. The first-episode genital infection may be severe.

Herpes simplex infection of the penis and rectum (Figures 11-20, 11-21, and 11-22) is pathophysiologically identical to herpes infection in other areas.

Prevalence

From 1988 to 1994, the seroprevalence of HSV-2 in persons 12 years of age or older in the United States was 21.9%, corresponding to 50 million infected people. HSV-2 is now detectable in one of five persons 12 years of age or older nationwide.

Risk factors

Risk factors for genital herpes HSV-2 are strongly related to lifetime number of sexual partners (Figures 11-18 and 11-19), number of years of sexual activity, male homosexuality, black race, female gender, and a history of previous sexually transmitted diseases (STDs).

The seroprevalence is higher among women (25.6%) than men (17.8%) and higher among blacks (45.9%) than whites (17.6%). Less than 10% of all those who were seropositive reported a history of genital herpes infection.

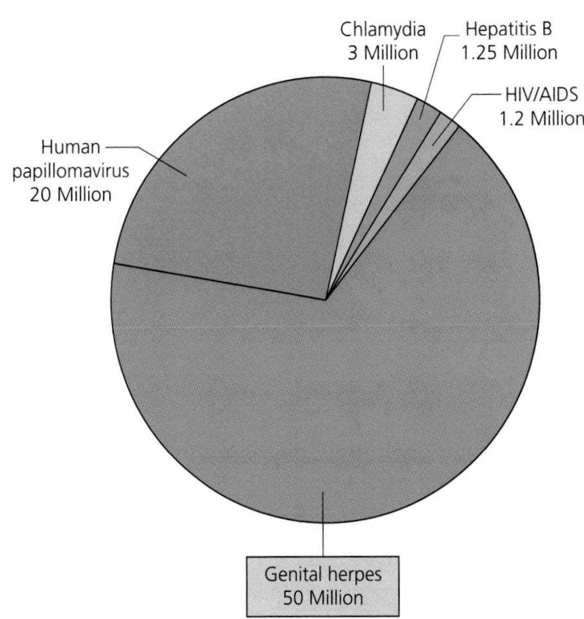

Figure 11-17 There are 1 million new genital herpes infections per year in the United States.

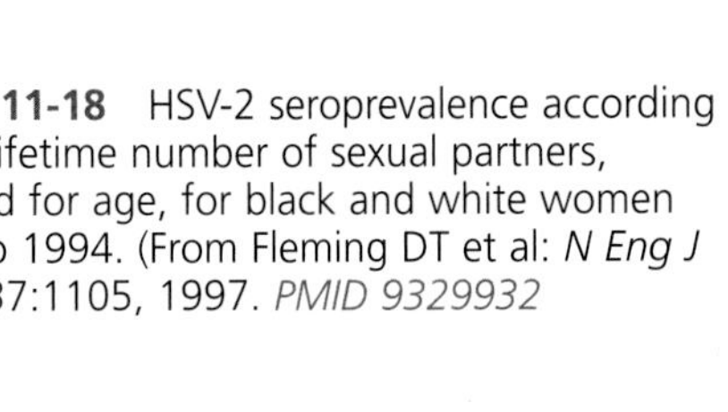

Figure 11-18 HSV-2 seroprevalence according to the lifetime number of sexual partners, adjusted for age, for black and white women 1998 to 1994. (From Fleming DT et al: *N Eng J Med* 337:1105, 1997. *PMID 9329932*

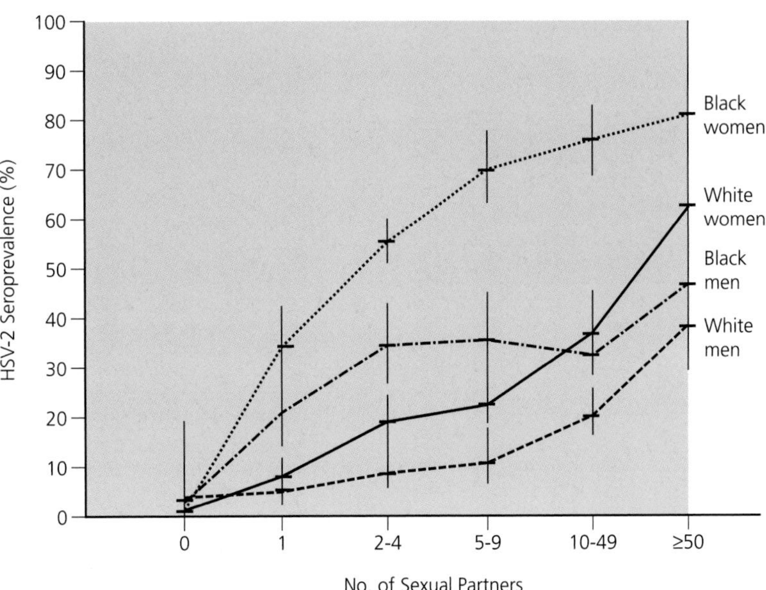

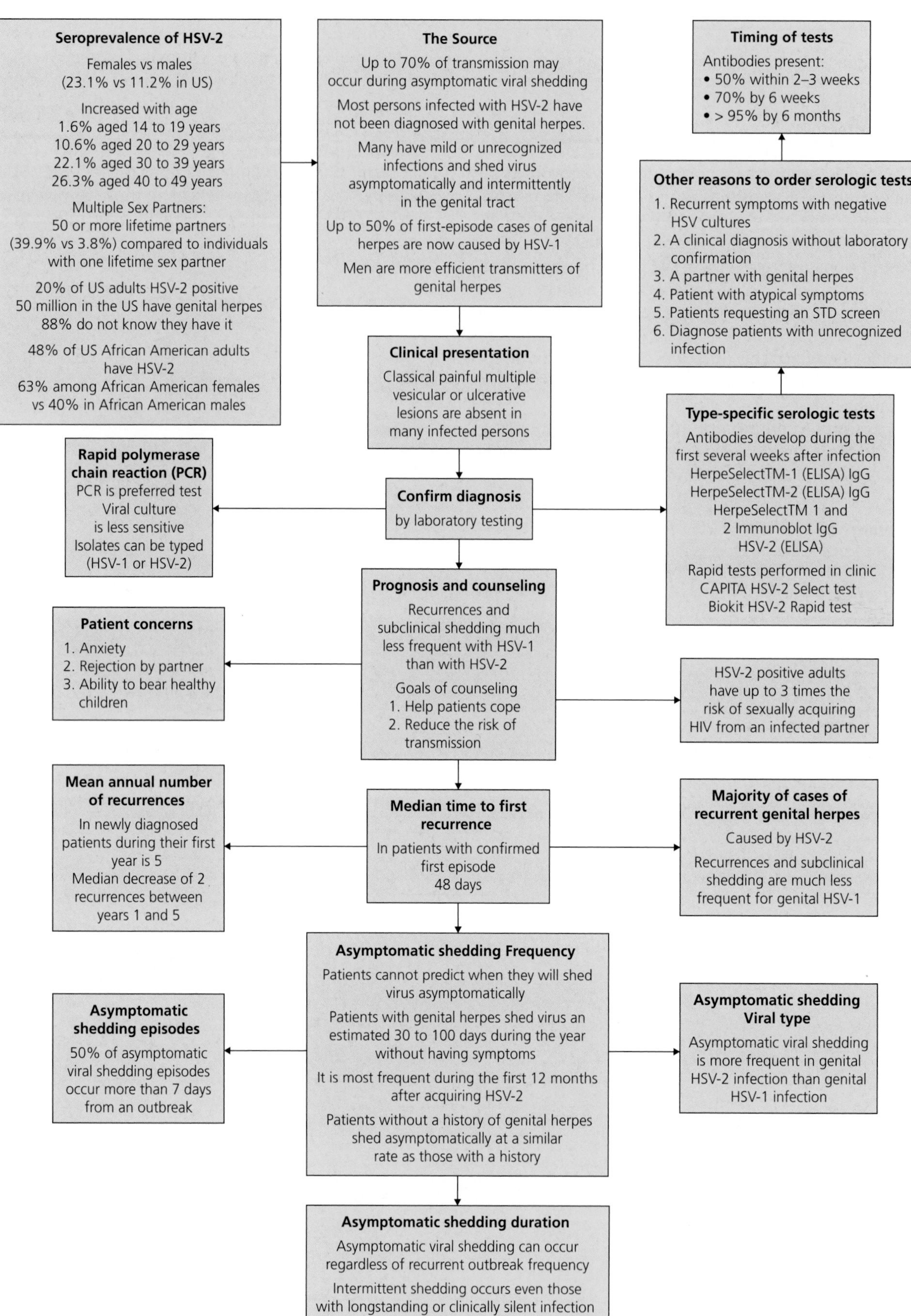
GENITAL HERPES
Seroprevalence of HSV-2
Females vs males
(23.1% vs 11.2% in US)
Increased with age
1.6% aged 14 to 19 years
10.6% aged 20 to 29 years
22.1% aged 30 to 39 years
26.3% aged 40 to 49 years
Multiple Sex Partners:
50 or more lifetime partners
(39.9% vs 3.8%) compared to individuals with one lifetime sex partner
20% of US adults HSV-2 positive
50 million in the US have genital herpes
88% do not know they have it
48% of US African American adults have HSV-2
63% among African American females vs 40% in African American males
The Source
Up to 70% of transmission may occur during asymptomatic viral shedding
Most persons infected with HSV-2 have not been diagnosed with genital herpes.
Many have mild or unrecognized infections and shed virus asymptomatically and intermittently in the genital tract
Up to 50% of first-episode cases of genital herpes are now caused by HSV-1
Men are more efficient transmitters of genital herpes
Timing of tests
Antibodies present:
• 50% within 2–3 weeks
• 70% by 6 weeks
• > 95% by 6 months
Other reasons to order serologic tests
1. Recurrent symptoms with negative HSV cultures
2. A clinical diagnosis without laboratory confirmation
3. A partner with genital herpes
4. Patient with atypical symptoms
5. Patients requesting an STD screen
6. Diagnose patients with unrecognized infection
Clinical presentation
Classical painful multiple vesicular or ulcerative lesions are absent in many infected persons
Type-specific serologic tests
Antibodies develop during the first several weeks after infection
HerpeSelectTM-1 (ELISA) IgG
HerpeSelectTM-2 (ELISA) IgG
HerpeSelectTM 1 and 2 Immunoblot IgG
HSV-2 (ELISA)
Rapid tests performed in clinic
CAPITA HSV-2 Select test
Biokit HSV-2 Rapid test
Rapid polymerase chain reaction (PCR)
PCR is preferred test
Viral culture is less sensitive
Isolates can be typed (HSV-1 or HSV-2)
Confirm diagnosis
by laboratory testing
Prognosis and counseling
Recurrences and subclinical shedding much less frequent with HSV-1 than with HSV-2
Goals of counseling
1. Help patients cope
2. Reduce the risk of transmission
Patient concerns
1. Anxiety
2. Rejection by partner
3. Ability to bear healthy children
HSV-2 positive adults have up to 3 times the risk of sexually acquiring HIV from an infected partner
Mean annual number of recurrences
In newly diagnosed patients during their first year is 5
Median decrease of 2 recurrences between years 1 and 5
Median time to first recurrence
In patients with confirmed first episode
48 days
Majority of cases of recurrent genital herpes
Caused by HSV-2
Recurrences and subclinical shedding are much less frequent for genital HSV-1
Asymptomatic shedding Frequency
Patients cannot predict when they will shed virus asymptomatically
Patients with genital herpes shed virus an estimated 30 to 100 days during the year without having symptoms
It is most frequent during the first 12 months after acquiring HSV-2
Patients without a history of genital herpes shed asymptomatically at a similar rate as those with a history
Asymptomatic shedding episodes
50% of asymptomatic viral shedding episodes occur more than 7 days from an outbreak
Asymptomatic shedding Viral type
Asymptomatic viral shedding is more frequent in genital HSV-2 infection than genital HSV-1 infection
Asymptomatic shedding duration
Asymptomatic viral shedding can occur regardless of recurrent outbreak frequency
Intermittent shedding occurs even those with longstanding or clinically silent infection

Figure 11-19

PRIMARY HERPES SIMPLEX

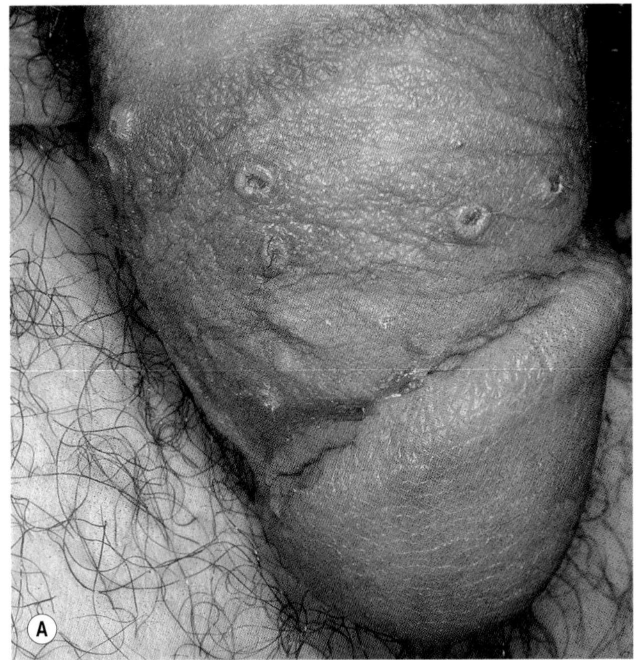

Vesicles are discrete and can be confused with warts and molluscum contagiosum. The primary lesion is a vesicle that rapidly becomes umbilicated.

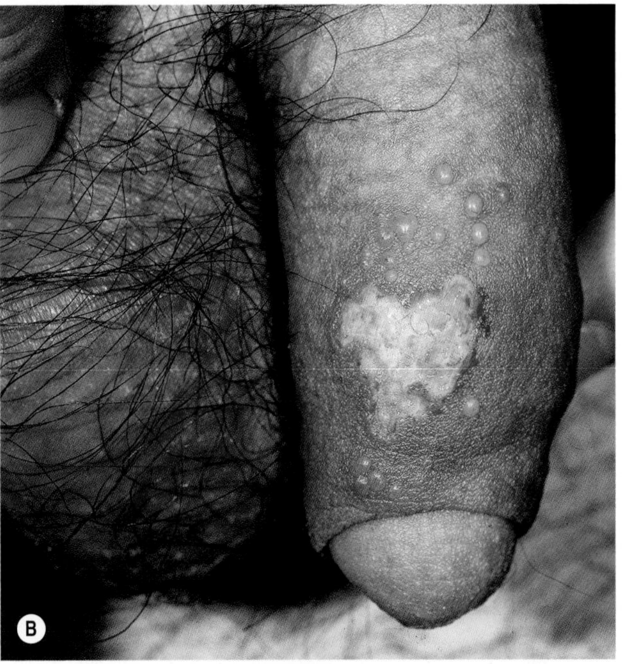

A group of vesicles has ruptured, leaving an erosion. Tense vesicles are at the periphery.

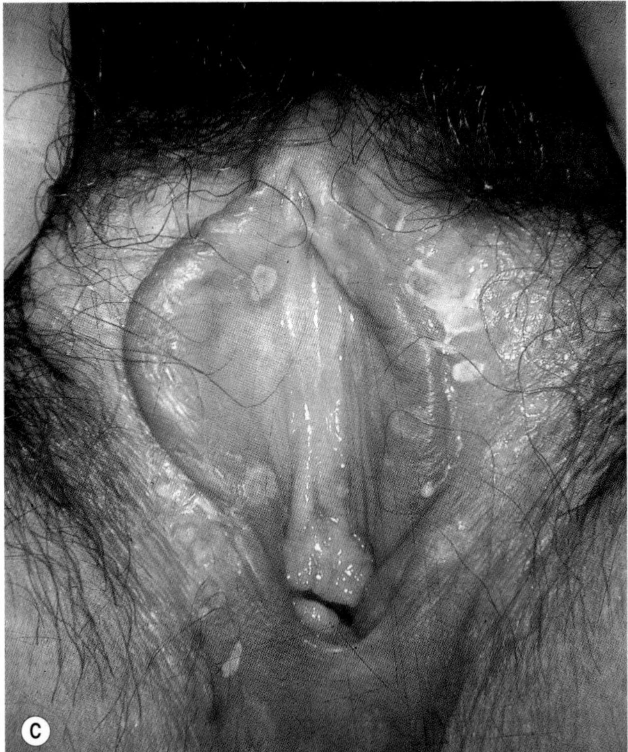

Scattered erosions covered with exudate.

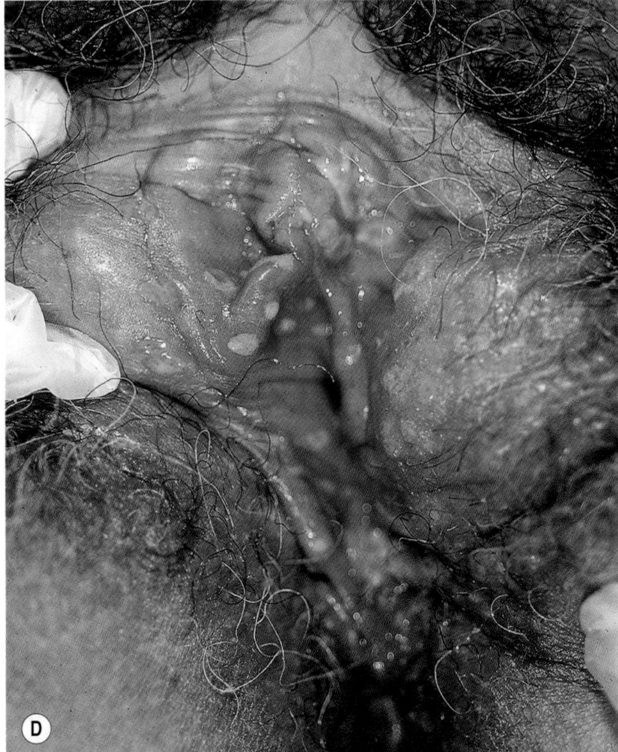

Numerous erosions appeared 6 days after contact with an asymptomatic carrier.

Figure 11-20

PRIMARY ANAL HERPES

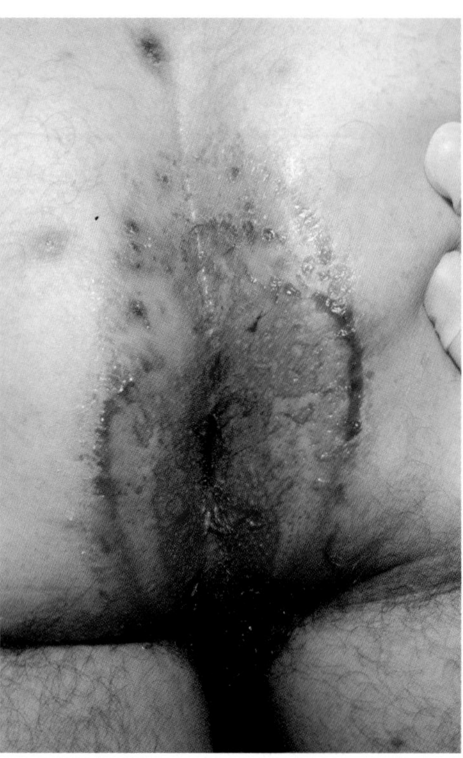

Figure 11-21 Lesions become numerous in this intertriginous area. Purulent material becomes trapped between apposing skin surfaces.

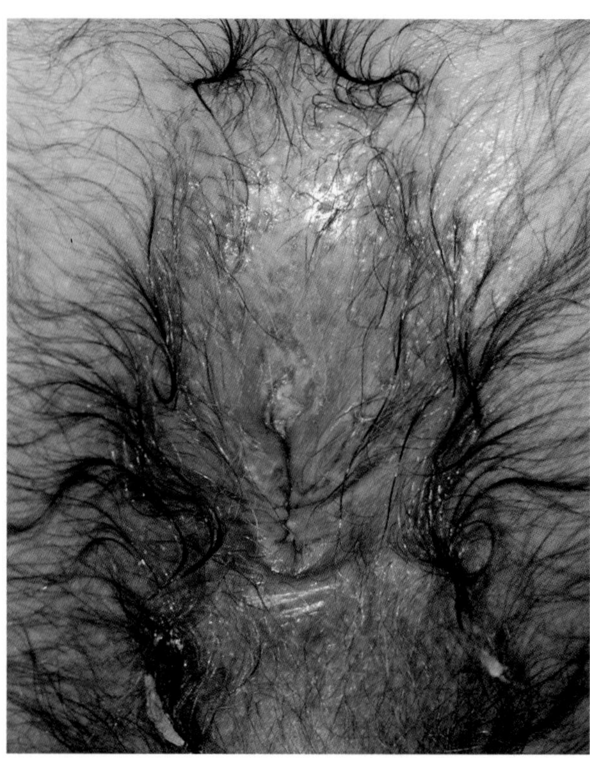

Figure 11-22 Numerous erosions are present in this intertriginous area. Crusts do not form on apposing skin surfaces.

RECURRENT GENITAL HERPES

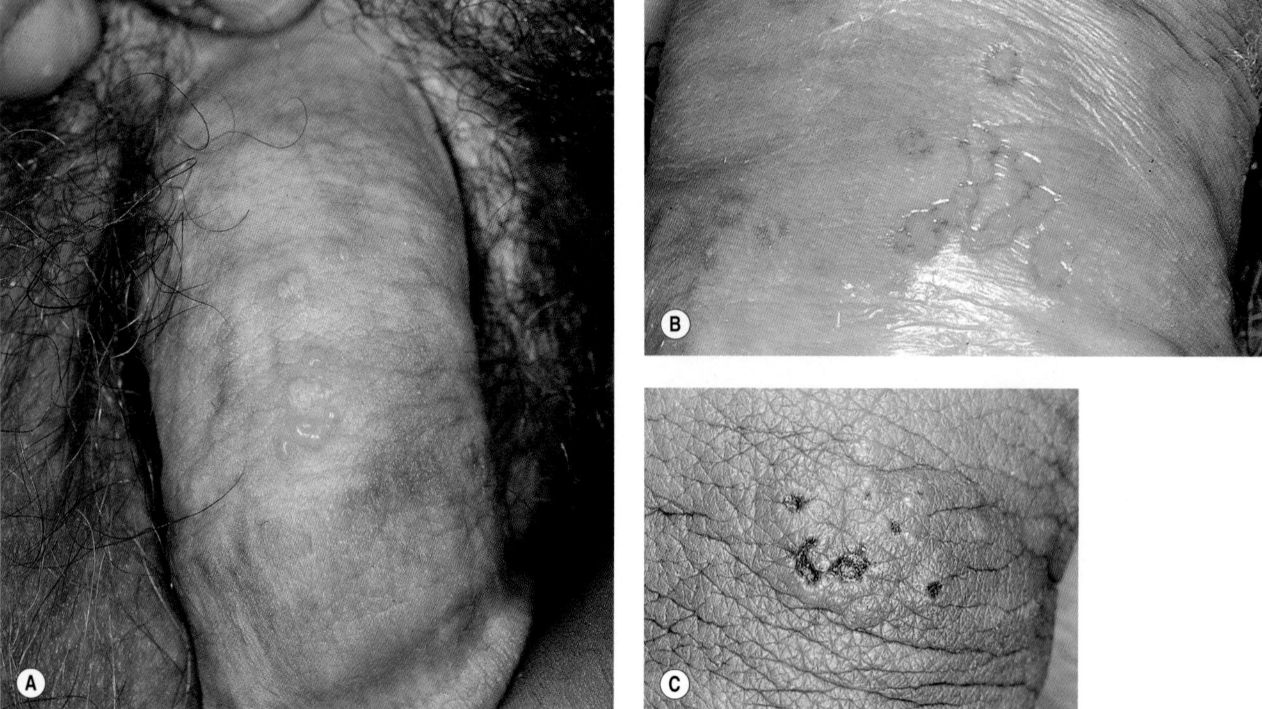

Figure 11-23 **A,** Grouped vesicles on a red base is the initial lesion. **B,** Vesicles do not appear under the foreskin. They are macerated to form punched-out erosions. **C,** Crusts form and then heal with or without scarring.

Rate of transmission

Transmission of HSV occurs through both symptomatic lesions and asymptomatic viral shedding. Symptomatic lesions are more efficient transmitters of the virus because they have higher viral titers. Herpes simplex is transmitted more efficiently from males to females than from females to males. This may be due to the increased rate of recurrence, and hence infectivity, in men. Seronegative female susceptible partners have the highest risk for acquiring genital herpes infection. The 32% annual risk in seronegative women was significantly higher than the 9% risk in HSV-1 seropositive women and than the 6% or less risk in susceptible male partners, regardless of previous HSV-1 infection. In a large study, women acquired HSV-2 at a rate of 8.9 per 10,000 episodes of sexual intercourse. Men acquired HSV-2 at a rate of 1.5 per 10,000 episodes of sexual intercourse.

PREVIOUS HERPES SIMPLEX VIRUS TYPE 1 INFECTION

Previous infection with HSV-1 reduces the rate of acquisition of genital HSV-2 infection, reduces the severity of initial HSV-2 infection, and may increase the proportion of persons acquiring HSV-2 asymptomatically or subclinically. The presence of HSV-1 antibody is associated with a decreased likelihood of detecting antibody to HSV-2 in women.

Genital infections with HSV-1 are associated with less asymptomatic shedding, lower rates of clinical recurrence, and lower rates of transmission.

HUMAN IMMUNODEFICIENCY VIRUS INFECTION

The rates of HSV infection are increasing; the highest prevalence is in patients with the human immunodeficiency virus (HIV). Genital ulcer disease is a risk factor in the transmission of human immunodeficiency virus-1 (HIV-1). HIV-1 virions can be detected in genital ulcers caused by HSV-2, which suggests that genital herpes infection likely increases the efficiency of the sexual transmission of HIV-1.

The treatment of genital herpes decreases the rates of HIV infection. Acyclovir resistance is more common in this group, but acyclovir use may prolong survival in some HIV-seropositive patients.

Primary and recurrent infections

FIRST-EPISODE INFECTIONS

First-episode infections include true primary infection and nonprimary first-episode infections. Patients with true primary infections have seronegative test results and have never been infected with any type of herpesvirus. Patients with nonprimary first-episode infections have been infected at another site with either type 1 or type 2 virus (e.g., the oral area) and have serum antibody and humoral immunity.

First-episode infections are more extensive and have more systemic symptoms. Viral shedding lasts longer (15 to 16 days) in primary first-episode infections. Virus infections spread easily over moist surfaces; 10% to 15% of patients with first-episode genital herpes have simultaneous infection in the pharynx, probably as a result of orogenital contact. They have extensive genital disease and exudative or ulcerative pharyngitis.

SIGNS AND SYMPTOMS. Vesicles appear approximately 6 days after sexual contact. Vesicles become depressed in the center (umbilicated) in 2 or 3 days, and then erode (Figure 11-20, *A*, *B*, *C*, and *D*). Crusts form and the lesion heals in the next week or two (Figure 11-23, *C*). Scars form if the inflammation has been intense. Discharge, dysuria, and inguinal lymphadenopathy are common. Systemic complaints, including fever, myalgias, lethargy, and photophobia, are present in approximately 70% of patients and are more common in women. The clinical diagnosis is insensitive and nonspecific. The typical painful multiple vesicular or ulcerative lesions are absent in many infected persons.

Women have more extensive disease than men and a higher incidence of constitutional symptoms probably because of the larger surface area involved. Wide areas of the female genitals may be covered with painful erosions (see Figure 11-20, *C-D*).

The cervix is involved in most cases, and erosive cervicitis is almost always associated with first-episode disease. The virus can be isolated from the cervix in only 10% to 15% of women with recurrent disease. Inflammation, edema, and pain may be so extreme that urination is difficult and catheterization is required. The patient may be immobilized and require bed rest at home or in the hospital.

A similar pattern of extensive involvement, with edema and possible urinary retention, develops in males, especially if uncircumcised. Crusts do not form under the foreskin (Figure 11-23, *B*). The eruption frequently extends onto the pubic area, and it is possibly spread from secretions during sexual contact. The anal area may be involved after anal intercourse (see Figures 11-21 and 11-22).

Nearly 40% of newly acquired HSV-2 infections and nearly two thirds of new HSV-1 infections are symptomatic. Among sexually active adults, new genital HSV-1 infections are as common as new oropharyngeal HSV-1 infections.

The virus ascends the peripheral sensory nerves after the primary infection and establishes latency in the nerve root ganglia. Intercourse, skin trauma, cold or heat, stress, concurrent infection, and menstruation can trigger reactivation.

RECURRENT INFECTION

CLINICAL SIGNS AND SYMPTOMS. Recurrent infection in females may be so minor or hidden from view in the vagina or cervix that it is unnoticed. This explains why some males with primary disease are not aware of the source. Recurrences cannot be predicted, but they often follow sexual intercourse. Itching or pain may precede the recurrent lesion. A small group of vesicles appears, umbilicates in 1 or 2 days, and then erodes and crusts. The lesion heals in 10 to 14 days. Vesicles are not seen under the foreskin or on the moist surfaces of the vulva or vagina (see Figures 11-20 and 11-23).

The virus can be cultured for approximately 5 days from active genital lesions, and the lesions are almost certainly infectious during this time. Males and females who have no symptoms can transmit the disease. Infection can develop in male patients from contact with female carriers who have no obvious disease. The infection may be acquired from an active cervical infection or from cervical secretions of a female who chronically carries the virus, from vulvar ulcers, from fissures, and from anorectal infection.

FREQUENCY OF RECURRENCE. A study documented the recurrence rates in patients with a symptomatic first-episode HSV-2 genital infection (Box 11-1).

Approximately 80% to 90% of persons with symptomatic first episodes of HSV-2 genital infection will have a recurrent episode within the following year, compared with 50% to 60% of patients with HSV-1 infection.

Box 11-1 **Genital Herpes Recurrence Rates during the First Year After Symptomatic First-Episode HSV-2 Infection**

89% have at least 1 recurrence
38% have >6 recurrences
20% have >10 recurrences

None or 1 recurrence

26% of women
8% of men

More than 10 recurrences

14% of women
26% of men
Patients who had severe primary infection had recurrences nearly twice as often and had a shorter time to first recurrence compared with those who had shorter first episodes.

From Benedetti J et al: *Ann Intern Med* 121:847, 1994.
PMID 7978697

Reactivation decreases in frequency over time in most patients. Ninety-five percent of patients with primary HSV-2 have recurrences, with a median time to the first recurrence of approximately 50 days. The recurrence rates in patients with a symptomatic first-episode HSV-2 genital infection are documented in Box 11-1. Fifty percent of patients with primary HSV-1 have recurrent outbreaks, and the median time to the first recurrence is 1 year.

Median recurrence rates in the first year are one (HSV-1) and five (HSV-2) per year in patients with newly acquired infection. Patients infected with HSV-2 who were observed for longer than 4 years had a median decrease of two recurrences between years 1 and 5. However, 25% of these patients had an increase of at least one recurrence in year 5. Decreases among patients who never received suppressive therapy were similar to decreases during untreated periods in patients who received suppressive therapy.

ANATOMIC SITE. The frequency of recurrence varies with the anatomic site and the virus type. The frequency of recurrences of genital HSV-2 herpes is higher than that of HSV-1 orolabial infection. HSV-1 oral infections recur more often than genital HSV-1 infections. HSV-2 genital infections occur six times more frequently than HSV-1 genital infections. The frequency of recurrence is lowest for orolabial HSV-2 infections.

ASYMPTOMATIC TRANSMISSION. Asymptomatic viral shedding is the primary mode of herpesvirus transmission. The infected partner is almost always unaware of the herpes infection. Therefore highly motivated couples who are aware of the signs and symptoms of genital herpes and attempt to avoid sexual contact with lesions remain at substantial risk for transmission of genital herpes to the uninfected partner. Acyclovir therapy substantially decreases but does not totally eliminate symptomatic or asymptomatic viral shedding or the potential for transmission.

ASYMPTOMATIC SHEDDING. Most persons who have serologic evidence of infection with HSV-2 are asymptomatic. The site of asymptomatic shedding is unknown. Virus has not been isolated from the semen or urethra after primary infection. Viral shedding can occur at any time. Asymptomatic shedding occurs most commonly in the first year after the primary episode (particularly the first 3 months), during the prodromal period, in the week after a symptomatic recurrence, and in HSV-2 infections versus HSV-1.

The rate of subclinical shedding of HSV in the subjects with no reported history of genital herpes was similar to that in the subjects with such a history (3.0% vs. 2.7%).

Among women with genital HSV-2 infection, subclinical shedding occurred on a mean of 2% of the days. The mean duration of viral shedding during subclinical episodes was 1.5 days, as compared with 1.8 days during symptomatic episodes. Women with frequent symptomatic recurrences also have frequent subclinical shedding and may be at high risk for transmitting HSV.

Prevention

Virus can be recovered from the eroded lesions for approximately 5 days after onset, but sexual contact should be avoided until reepithelialization is complete. Male (urethra) and female (cervix) carriers who have no symptoms can conceivably transmit the infection at any time. The use of spermicidal foams and condoms should be recommended to patients who have a history of recurrent genital herpes. For sexual partners who have both had genital herpes, protective measures are probably not necessary if both carry the same virus type (one partner infected the other) and active lesions are not present. Remember that having herpes in one area is not a guarantee from acquiring the infection in another location. Contact should be avoided when active lesions are present.

One study showed that condom use during more than 25% of sex acts was associated with protection against HSV-2 acquisition for women but not for men. Therefore identification of heterosexual couples in which the male partner has HSV-2 infection and the female is HSV-2 negative can reduce transmission of HSV-2 for women.

Laboratory diagnosis

The sensitivity of all laboratory methods depends on the stage of lesions (sensitivity is higher in vesicular than in ulcerative lesions), on whether the patient has a first or a recurrent episode of the disease (higher in first episodes), and on whether the sample is from an immunosuppressed or an immunocompetent patient (more antigen is found in immunosuppressed patients). It is crucial to document genital herpes simplex infection in pregnant women and cutaneous herpes in newborn infants. Consequently, in these instances, suspicious vesicular and eroded lesions should be tested or cultured. In all other forms the clinical presentation is usually so characteristic that an accurate diagnosis can be made by inspection. A number of laboratory procedures are available if confirmation is desired.

POLYMERASE CHAIN REACTION

Rapid polymerase chain reaction (PCR) is the new gold standard for detection of HSV in genital specimens. Several laboratories have discontinued using cell cultures. Collect a specimen of the cervix, rectum, urethra, vagina, or other genital sites using a culture transport swab. (Calcium alginate-tipped swab, wood swab, or transport swab containing gel is not acceptable for PCR testing.) Specimen volume is usually small with PCR assays (0.5 m). Specimens are refrigerated. Positive results are reported as herpes simplex type 1 DNA detected or herpes simplex type 2 DNA detected. The rapid test provides results the same day.

CULTURE

Some laboratories have stopped performing cultures now that rapid PCR is available. Viral culture can distinguish between HSV-1 and HSV-2. The culture specimen must be obtained from active lesions during viral shedding, which, on average, lasts 4 days. Fifty percent of culture results are negative in recurrent lesions. Vesicles and wet erosions give a higher yield than dry erosions or crusts. Vesicles are punctured and the fluid is absorbed into the swab, which is then rubbed vigorously onto the base of the lesion.

Cervical samples are taken from the endocervix with the swab. From the viewpoint of cost, the insertion of separate swabs from a number of anatomic sites (cervix, vaginal ulcers, vaginal fissures, anus) into one culture vial is the most efficient way to collect genital samples for viral culture.

Specimens are inoculated into tube cell cultures and monitored microscopically for characteristic morphologic changes (cytopathic effects for up to 5 to 7 days after inoculation for maximum sensitivity). Results may be available in 1 or 2 days.

HISTOPATHOLOGIC STUDIES

A biopsy specimen should be obtained from an intact vesicle. The histologic picture is characteristic but not unique for herpes simplex.

Serology

Approximately 50% to 90% of adults have antibody to HSV. More than 70% of the population have antibody levels ranging from 1:10 to 1:160; only 5% have titers greater than 1:160. Because of the high incidence of antibodies to herpes simplex in the population, assay of a single serum specimen is not of great value.

SUBTYPING

There are two serotypes of HSV. HSV-1 infections are primarily oropharyngeal; genital infections can also be caused by this serotype. HSV-2 infections are primarily genital, but are also detected in the mouth.

HERPES SIMPLEX VIRUS TYPE 1. HSV-1 seropositivity is usually associated with orolabial infection. Herpes simplex virus type 2 seropositivity is usually associated with genital infection. HSV-1 is now a significant cause of genital herpes and is implicated in 5% to 30% of all first-episode cases. The proportion of HSV-1 among initial genital herpes infections is higher among men who have sex with men (46.9%) than among women (21.4%) and is lowest among heterosexual men (14.6%). Receptive oral sex significantly increases the odds that initial infections are HSV-1 rather than HSV-2. Genital HSV-1 may often be acquired through contact with a partner's mouth.

TYPE-SPECIFIC SEROLOGIC TESTS

Type-specific and nonspecific antibodies develop during the first several weeks following infection and persist indefinitely. Almost all HSV-2 infections are sexually acquired. Therefore HSV-2 antibody indicates anogenital infection, but the presence of HSV-1 antibody does not distinguish anogenital from orolabial infection.

The assays include POCkit HSV-2; Meridian's Premier test; HerpeSelect-1 enzyme-linked immunosorbent assay (ELISA) IgG or HerpeSelect-2 ELISA IgG; and HerpeSelect 1 and 2 Immunoblot IgG.

The POCkit HSV-2 assay is a point-of-care (performed in the office) test that provides results for HSV-2 antibodies from capillary blood or serum during a clinic visit. The other assays are laboratory-based. The sensitivities of these tests for detection of HSV-2 antibody vary from 80% to 98%, and false-negative results may occur, especially at early stages of infection. The specificities of these assays are greater than 96%. False-positive results can occur, especially in patients with low likelihood of HSV infection. Therefore repeat testing or a confirmatory test (e.g., an immunoblot assay if the initial test was an ELISA) may be indicated in some settings.

The POCkit HSV-2 Rapid Test provides rapid (6 minutes) results. It determines HSV-2 seropositivity and cannot test for HSV-1 antibodies. With Meridian's Premier test, a blood sample is sent to the laboratory. The Meridian Premier tests can detect both HSV-1 and HSV-2 type-specific HSV antibodies. With the Premier tests, seroconversion to HSV-2 can take up to 4 months, so negative results should be confirmed with Western blot analysis or a later serum sample should be tested if seroconversion is suspected.

INDICATIONS TO TEST

Subclinical or unrecognized infections are best diagnosed with type-specific antibody tests.

PREGNANT WOMEN. Consider testing pregnant women who are at risk of acquiring herpes in the third trimester. These are women without a history of genital herpes whose partner is known to be infected or is seropositive. Infection of the neonate is most common when primary infection develops late in pregnancy. Transmission of herpes to the neonate during birth results in neonatal herpes, with devastating results.

A pregnant seronegative woman could be identified and counseled to avoid transmission during the third trimester. An HSV-2–seropositive woman can be informed that her risk of transmission to her fetus is low and that most patients can have a vaginal delivery. If a woman is entirely seronegative and her partner is HSV-1 positive, they should be instructed to avoid oral-genital and genital-genital contact in the last trimester because HSV-1 accounts for up to 30% of cases of neonatal herpes. Consider suppressive therapy for seropositive men unwilling to abstain or to use condoms.

MONOGAMOUS COUPLES. Test results can be used to counsel couples in monogamous relationships in which one partner has clinical or serologic evidence of herpes. Serologic testing can identify partners at risk. Many people are unaware of their infection. Explain the risks when one partner has antibodies and the other does not. Educate patients about the frequency of transmission, asymptomatic shedding, condoms, and suppressive therapy.

DIAGNOSIS OF RECURRENT GENITAL ERUPTIONS. Testing can be used to diagnosis or exclude the diagnosis of genital herpes as a cause of recurrent genital eruption when the diagnosis cannot be made by other means. Patients with recurrent genital eruptions frequently present after the virus can no longer be cultured. The presence of HSV-2 antibodies provides evidence of infection. The absence of seropositivity excludes genital herpes. Some patients with a clinical history of what was diagnosed as genital herpes are surprised to find that they have no serologic evidence of infection. A seropositive HSV-1 or HSV-2 result does not determine whether the infection is orolabial or genital. Viral cultures are required to confirm the diagnosis. HSV-1 recurs less frequently than HSV-2; therefore typing helps determine prognosis.

IDENTIFYING HERPES SIMPLEX VIRUS AS A RISK FACTOR FOR HUMAN IMMUNODEFICIENCY VIRUS TRANSMISSION. Testing can be used to identify HSV-2 infection in patients at high risk for HIV acquisition. Genital HSV ulcers facilitate the transmission of HIV through mucosal disruption. CD4+ lymphocytes in herpetic lesions are targets for HIV attachment and entry. Consider suppressive therapy for seropositive people at risk of HIV acquisition.

Psychosocial implications

Herpes is a benign disorder that has a tremendous psychosocial impact. The sensitive physician is aware of the spectrum of symptoms that can evolve and provides emotional support, especially at initial diagnosis. The victim's response usually begins with initial shock and emotional numbing, and then a frantic search for a cure. A sense of loneliness and isolation occurs after the patient becomes aware that the disease is chronic and incurable. The anxiety then generalizes to concerns about establishing relationships and that sexual gratification, marriage, and normal reproduction might not be possible. There is diminished self-esteem, social isolation, anxiety, and reluctance to initiate close relationships. Sexual drive persists, but there is a fear of initiating sexual relationships and an inhibition of sexual expression. These emotional problems appear to be worse in women than in men. A minority of patients experience deepening of depression with each recurrence, and all aspects of their lives are affected, including job performance. Recurrent disease can now be controlled by daily oral dosing with antiviral drugs such as acyclovir. This drug has significantly improved the quality of life for many herpes victims.

Treatment of genital herpes (CDC guidelines)

Antiviral oral medication and counseling are the mainstays of management. Systemic antiviral drugs partially control symptoms and signs. They do not eradicate latent virus or affect the risk, frequency, or severity of recurrences after the drug is stopped. Topical antiviral drugs offer minimal benefit.

Figure 11-24 summarizes the indications and effects of treatment.

DRUGS

Three antiviral medications are effective: acyclovir, valacyclovir, and famciclovir. Valacyclovir is a valine ester of acyclovir with enhanced absorption after oral administration. Famciclovir, a prodrug of penciclovir, also has high oral bioavailability. Topical therapy with acyclovir is less effec-

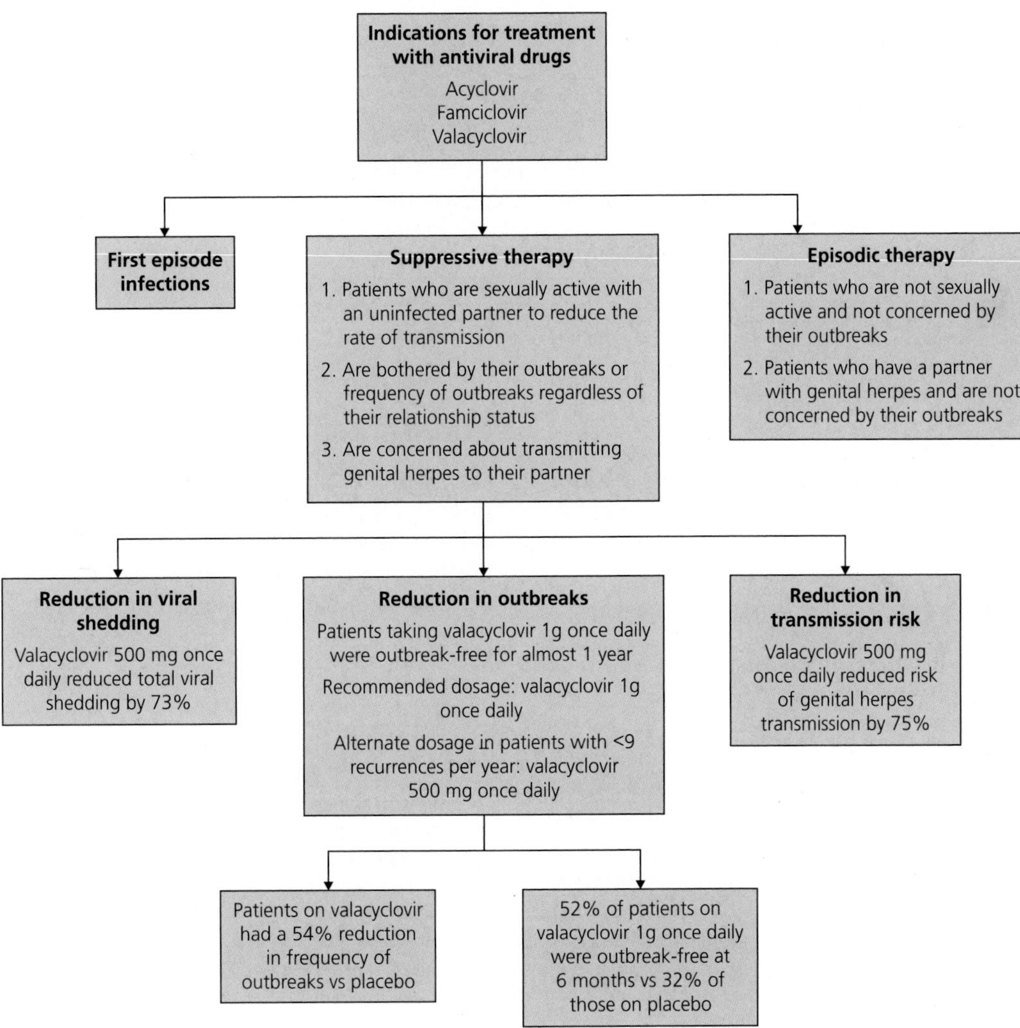

2006 CDC Guidelines recommendations for counseling:

1. Educate on the potential for recurrent episodes, asymptomatic viral shedding and the risk of sexual transmission.
2. Persons with a first episode of GH should be advised that suppressive daily therapy is available and effective and that episodic therapy is sometimes useful in shortening the duration of recurrent episodes.
3. Sexual transmission of HSV can occur during asymptomatic periods. The risk of HSV-2 sexual transmission can be decreased by the daily use of valacyclovir by the infected person.
4. All persons with genital herpes should avoid sexual contact when lesions and/or symptoms are present.

Figure 11-24

Table 11-1 Treatment of Genital Herpes (Oral)

Condition	Immunocompetent	Immunocompromised (HIV-infected persons)
Primary genital herpes	Acyclovir 200 mg five times/day for 7-10 days Acyclovir 400 mg three times/day for 7-10 days Valacyclovir 1 gm two times/day for 7-10 days Famciclovir 250 mg three times/day for 7-10 days	
Recurrent genital herpes (episodic therapy)	Acyclovir 400 mg three times/day for 5 days Acyclovir 800 mg two times/day for 5 days Acyclovir 800 mg three times/day for 2 days Valacyclovir 500 mg two times/day for 3 days Valacyclovir 1 gm once daily for 5 days Famciclovir 125 mg two times/day for 5 days Famciclovir 1000 mg two times/day for 1 day	Acyclovir 400 mg three times/day for 5-10 days Valacyclovir 1 gm two times/day for 5-10 days Famciclovir 500 mg two times/day for 5-10 days
Recurrent genital herpes (long-term suppressive therapy)	Acyclovir 400 mg two times/day Valacyclovir 500 mg once daily for <9 episodes/year Valacyclovir 1 gm once daily for >10 episodes/year Famciclovir 250 mg two times/day	Acyclovir 400-800 mg two or three times/day Valacyclovir 500 mg two times/day Famciclovir 500 mg two times/day
Severe disease	Acyclovir 5-10 mg/kg/body weight IV every 8 hr	

Centers for Disease Control and Prevention Guidelines, 2006.

tive than the systemic drug, and its use is discouraged. Acyclovir, valacyclovir, and famciclovir reduce the duration of viral shedding, the time to healing, and the development of new lesions. Dosages are listed in Table 11-1.

FIRST CLINICAL EPISODE OF GENITAL HERPES

Many patients with first-episode herpes present with mild clinical manifestations but severe or prolonged symptoms develop later. Therefore most patients with initial genital herpes should receive antiviral therapy. Counseling regarding the natural history of genital herpes, sexual and perinatal transmission, and methods to reduce such transmission is essential. About 5% to 30% of first-episode cases of genital herpes are caused by HSV-1, but clinical recurrences are much less frequent for HSV-1 than HSV-2 genital infections. Therefore identification of the type of the infecting strain has prognostic importance and may be useful for counseling purposes. Recommended treatment regimens are shown in Table 11-1.

COOL COMPRESSES

Extensive erosions on the vulva and penis may be treated with cool water, silver nitrate 0.5%, or Burow's compresses applied for 20 minutes several times daily. This effective local therapy reduces edema and inflammation, macerates and debrides crust and purulent material, and relieves pain. The legs may be supported with pillows under the knees to expose the inflamed tissues and promote drying.

COUNSELING

Counseling is an important aspect of management. Although initial counseling can be provided at the first visit, patients benefit from learning about the chronic aspects of the disease after the acute illness subsides. Provide patients with the information presented in Box 11-2.

Box 11-2 **Counseling Patients with Genital Herpes**

- Explain the natural history of the disease, with emphasis on the potential for recurrent episodes, asymptomatic viral shedding, and sexual transmission.
- Abstain from sexual activity when lesions or prodromal symptoms are present and inform their sex partners that they have genital herpes. The use of condoms during all sexual exposures with new or uninfected sex partners should be encouraged.
- Sexual transmission of HSV can occur during asymptomatic periods. Asymptomatic viral shedding occurs more frequently in patients who have genital HSV-2 infection than HSV-1 infection and in patients who have had genital herpes for <12 months.
- Childbearing-aged women who have genital herpes should inform health care providers who care for them during pregnancy about the HSV infection.
- Episodic antiviral therapy during recurrent episodes might shorten the duration of lesions.
- Suppressive antiviral therapy can ameliorate or prevent recurrent outbreaks and prevent asymptomatic transmission.

RECURRENT EPISODES OF HERPES SIMPLEX VIRUS DISEASE

Most patients with first-episode genital HSV-2 infection will have recurrent episodes. Episodic or suppressive antiviral therapy might shorten the duration of lesions or ameliorate recurrences. Treatment is most effective when started during the prodrome or within 1 day after onset of lesions. Patient-initiated episodic treatment is more effective than provider-initiated therapy in decreasing the healing time in recurrent genital HSV infections. If episodic treatment of recurrences is chosen, the patient should be provided with antiviral therapy or a prescription for the medication, so that treatment can be initiated at the first sign of prodrome or genital lesions.

DAILY SUPPRESSIVE THERAPY

The decision to initiate continuous suppressive therapy is subjective and is based on the frequency and severity of recurrences and psychosocial factors. Continuous daily suppressive therapy significantly reduces, but does not completely suppress, the amount of asymptomatic shedding and clinical outbreaks. Therefore the extent to which suppressive therapy may prevent HSV transmission is unknown. Daily suppressive therapy reduces the frequency of genital herpes recurrences by 75% among patients who have frequent recurrences (i.e., six or more recurrences per year). Safety and efficacy have been documented among patients receiving daily therapy with acyclovir for as long as 6 years, and with valacyclovir and famciclovir for 1 year.

Suppressive therapy has not been associated with emergence of clinically significant acyclovir resistance among immunocompetent patients. After 1 year of continuous suppressive therapy, discontinuation of therapy should be discussed with the patient to assess the patient's psychologic adjustment to genital herpes and rate of recurrent episodes, since the frequency of recurrences decreases over time in many patients. Patients with a history of less than 10 recurrences per year are effectively managed with 500 mg of valacyclovir once daily. One gram of valacyclovir once daily or 400 mg of acyclovir twice daily is more effective in patients with greater than 10 recurrences per year. Once-daily regimens offer a useful option for patients who require suppressive therapy for management of genital herpes.

LUBRICATION

Occlusive ointments such as petroleum jelly should not be applied to eroded lesions. Light lubricating body lotions are soothing when inflammation subsides and tissues become dry.

Women with multiple eroded lesions on the labia experience great discomfort while urinating. Pain can be avoided by sitting in a bathtub of water and urinating while holding the labia apart.

Genital herpes simplex during pregnancy

Most mothers of infants who acquire neonatal herpes lack histories of clinically evident genital herpes. Many neonatal infections result from asymptomatic cervical shedding of the virus after a primary episode of genital HSV in the third trimester. The risk for transmission to the neonate from an infected mother is high (30% to 50%) among women who acquire genital herpes near the time of delivery and is low (<1%) among women with histories of recurrent herpes at term or who acquire genital HSV during the first half of pregnancy. However, because recurrent genital herpes is much more common than initial HSV infection during pregnancy, the proportion of neonatal HSV infections acquired from mothers with recurrent herpes remains high. Prevention of neonatal herpes depends both on preventing acquisition of genital HSV infection during late pregnancy and on avoiding exposure of the infant to herpetic lesions during delivery.

PREGNANCY COMPLICATIONS

The acquisition of genital herpes during pregnancy has been associated with spontaneous abortion, prematurity, and congenital and neonatal herpes. Two percent or more of susceptible women acquire HSV infection during pregnancy. Acquisition of infection with seroconversion completed before labor was not associated with an increase in neonatal morbidity or with any cases of congenital herpes infection, but infection acquired shortly before labor is associated with neonatal herpes and perinatal morbidity.

PRENATAL SCREENING AND MANAGEMENT

Most newborns acquire their infection by contact with infected genital secretions during delivery from an asymptomatic mother who acquired a first episode of genital herpes near the time of labor. The majority of cases of first-episode genital herpes during pregnancy are unrecognized. Some experts recommend HSV serologic testing for HSV-1 and HSV-2 at the first prenatal visit. This would identify patients already infected and those at risk for acquiring genital herpes. Pregnant women who are not infected with HSV-2 are advised to avoid intercourse during the third trimester with men who have genital herpes. Pregnant women who are not infected with HSV-1 should be counseled to avoid genital exposure to HSV-1 during the third trimester (e.g., cunnilingus with a partner with oral herpes and vaginal intercourse with a partner with genital HSV-1 infection). Antiviral prophylaxis with acyclovir may be considered in late pregnancy for women with a known history of genital herpes.

PREVENTION

Prevention of neonatal herpes should emphasize prevention of acquisition of genital HSV infection during late pregnancy. Susceptible women whose partners have oral or genital HSV infection, or those whose sex partners' infection status is unknown, should be counseled to avoid unprotected genital and oral sexual contact during late pregnancy or to take suppressive therapy with an oral antiviral (see Box 11-2).

ANTIVIRAL THERAPY

The safety of systemic acyclovir and valacyclovir therapy in pregnant women has not been established. Current findings do not indicate an increased risk for major birth defects after acyclovir treatment. The first clinical episode of genital herpes during pregnancy may be treated with oral acyclovir. Acyclovir treatment near term decreases the incidence of active lesions, thus reducing the rate of abdominal deliveries among women who have frequently recurring or newly acquired genital herpes. Routine administration of acyclovir to pregnant women who have a history of recurrent genital herpes is not recommended by most clinicians.

VIRAL CULTURES

The results of viral cultures during pregnancy do not predict viral shedding at the time of delivery, and such cultures are not indicated routinely.

MANAGEMENT AT LABOR

At the onset of labor, all women should be examined and carefully questioned regarding whether they have symptoms of genital herpes. Infants of women who do not have symptoms or signs of genital herpes infection or its prodrome may be delivered vaginally. A study does not support the policy of cesarean section in case of maternal recurrent herpes simplex infection at delivery. If a woman experiences her first attack of genital HSV infection around the time of delivery, the risk that her neonate will acquire an HSV infection is high. In this circumstance a cesarean delivery is probably prudent. Cesarean section, where the amniotic membranes are intact or have been ruptured for less than 4 hours, is recommended for those women who have clinical evidence of active herpes lesions on the cervix or vulva at the time of labor.

Abdominal delivery does not completely eliminate the risk for HSV infection in the neonate. Infants exposed to HSV during birth, as proven by virus isolation or presumed by observation of lesions, should be observed carefully. Some authorities recommend that such infants undergo surveillance cultures of mucosal surfaces to detect HSV infection before development of clinical signs. Available data do not support the routine use of acyclovir for asymptomatic infants exposed during birth through an infected birth canal, because the risk for infection in most infants is low. However, infants born to women who acquired genital herpes near term are at high risk for neonatal herpes, and some experts recommend acyclovir therapy for these infants. Such pregnancies and newborns should be managed in consultation with an expert. All infants who have evidence of neonatal herpes should be promptly evaluated and treated with systemic acyclovir.

Neonatal herpes simplex virus infection

Neonatal infection is serious but rare. Approximately half the infected babies are born prematurely, which raises the question of whether reactivation can trigger early onset of labor. The mortality rate is approximately 50% in the absence of therapy, and many survivors have ocular or neurologic complications. Most infected neonates are exposed to the virus during vaginal delivery, but infection may occur in utero, by transplacental or ascending infection, or postnatally from relatives or attendants. Many of the infections result from asymptomatic cervical shedding of virus after a primary episode of genital HSV in the third trimester. HSV-positive papules may be present on the skin at birth. Infants born to women who have an active primary HSV infection have a risk of approximately 50% of acquiring an infection. HSV transmission to neonates may occur through contact with infected health care workers or family members in the postpartum period. Nearly 10% of infections are attributed to postnatal HSV exposure.

HSV-2 accounts for nearly 70% of cases of neonatal herpes, a majority of which are due to intrapartum asymptomatic viral shedding in mothers without any signs or symptoms of genital herpes.

CLINICAL SIGNS

The diagnosis of neonatal HSV should be suspected in any newborn with irritability, lethargy, fever, or poor feeding at 1 week of age. Clinical signs of infection in the neonate are usually present between 1 and 7 days of life. Neonatal infections are clinically categorized according to the extent of the disease, as follows: (1) skin, eye, and mouth (SEM) infections (17%); (2) central nervous system (CNS) infection (encephalitis)—neonatal encephalitis can include SEM infections (32%); and (3) disseminated infection involving several organs, causing hepatitis, pneumonitis, intravascular coagulopathy, or encephalitis (39%). The CNS may also be involved in disseminated infections. A significant minority of patients do not have skin vesicles at presentation, and vesicles do not develop during the acute HSV disease.

Progression to systemic infection from isolated skin vesicles can occur in a matter of days. The mean age at diagnosis is 12.8 days, but at the time of diagnosis these infants have had symptoms for an average of 5 days. This delay in diagnosis puts the infant at great risk of internal disease, which is preventable with antiviral therapy if treatment is started when only skin disease is present. The infection can be limited to the skin, eyes, or mouth, or can affect the CNS or visceral organs.

DIAGNOSIS

Diagnosis is made by culturing the blood, cerebrospinal fluid, urine, and fluid from the eyes, nose, and mucous membranes. Herpes simplex virus was detected earlier and frequently in pharyngeal swabs (in one third on postnatal days 2 to 5).

PROGNOSIS

A large collaborative study showed no deaths among infants with localized HSV infection. The mortality rate was 57% in neonates with disseminated infection and 15% in neonates with encephalitis. Therefore the most important predictor of death is visceral involvement. The risk of death was increased in neonates who were in or near coma, had disseminated intravascular coagulopathy, or were premature. In babies with disseminated disease, HSV pneumonitis was associated with greater mortality. In the survivors, morbidity was most frequent in infants with encephalitis, disseminated infection, seizures, or infection with HSV type 2. With HSV infection limited to the skin, eyes, or mouth, the presence of three or more recurrences of vesicles was associated with an increased risk of neurologic impairment as compared with two or fewer recurrences. Death is unusual when disease is limited to the skin but occurs in 15% to 50% of cases of brain and disseminated disease, even with antiviral therapy. Despite antiviral therapy, there is evidence of impairment in approximately 10% of children and debility in more than 50% with CNS and visceral disease.

Babies with HSV-1 cutaneous, ocular, and oral disease fare better than those with HSV-2–associated cutaneous involvement. Infants with HSV-1–associated encephalitis suffer less neurologic morbidity compared with those with HSV-2 infection. HSV-1 disseminated disease leads to more significant sequelae than HSV-2.

Strategies to reduce the risk of neonatal transmission are listed in Box 11-3.

TREATMENT

Early institution of antiviral therapy is crucial to the outcome of the disease.

The early identification of skin lesions is critical for the outcome of infections that originate in the skin. Ninety percent of infants with initial herpetic skin lesions treated with acyclovir 30 mg/kg/day had no sequelae.

All infants who have evidence of neonatal herpes should be promptly treated with systemic acyclovir. The recommended regimen for infants treated for known or suspected neonatal herpes is acyclovir 20 mg/kg of body weight intravenously every 8 hours for 21 days for disseminated and CNS disease, or 14 days for disease limited to the skin and mucous membranes.

Box 11-3 **Strategies to Reduce the Risk of Neonatal Transmission**

1. Obtain history of HSV from pregnant women and partner.
2. An HSV-2-seropositive male and an HSV-2–seronegative female should consider sexual abstinence, protective condoms, or prophylactic antivirals.
3. Suppress HSV reactivation with antivirals; this treatment is recommended from 36 weeks of gestation in HSV-2–seropositive women at high risk for an active HSV outbreak at the time of labor.
4. Provide antiviral treatment for pregnant females with an active primary or recurrent genital outbreak near or at the time of delivery.
5. Abstain from oral sex between an HSV-1–seronegative female and an HSV-1–seropositive male or a male partner with active oral lesions during the last trimester.
6. Administer occlusive coverage to nongenital HSV lesions before vaginal delivery.
7. Cesarean deliveries are considered when a mother experiences primary genital herpes or symptomatic outbreaks near or at the time of delivery.
8. Cesarean delivery is probably not justified in the absence of active lesions of recurrent genital herpes and in the presence of protective, maternal transplacental antibodies.

Adapted from Fatahzadeh M, Schwartz RA: Human herpes simplex virus infections: epidemiology, pathogenesis, symptomatology, diagnosis, and management, *J Am Acad Dermatol* 57(5):737-763, 2007. *PMID: 17939933*

ACQUIRED IMMUNODEFICIENCY SYNDROME

Acquired immunodeficiency syndrome (AIDS) is the end stage of HIV infection. The infection causes a profound defect in cell-mediated immunity, which causes complicating opportunistic infections and neoplastic processes. The initial event is a symptomatic or an asymptomatic HIV infection. The infection may not be apparent for months or years. In an undetermined number of patients, symptoms emerge and the disease progresses to AIDS. Internal infections are the major cause of death. Infections can be controlled but are rarely curable. Most result from reactivation of previously acquired organisms. Concurrent or consecutive infections with a different organism are common. Infections are severe and commonly disseminated.

Human immunodeficiency virus pathogenesis

HIV is a retrovirus. Retroviruses carry a positive-stranded ribonucleic acid (RNA) and use a deoxyribonucleic acid (DNA) polymerase enzyme called reverse transcriptase to convert viral RNA to DNA. This reverses the usual process of transcription whereby DNA is converted to RNA, thus the term retrovirus. HIV attaches to a protein receptor site (CD4) on the surface of CD4+ lymphocytes, penetrates the cell, and exposes its RNA core; then reverse transcriptase converts viral RNA to DNA, which becomes part of the host genome. New viral particles are then produced during normal cellular division and CD4+ lymphocytes are destroyed. A repetitive cycle of immune activation, and partial clearing of the virus, and reinfection of immune cells by replicating virus occurs. Every component of the immune system attempts to stop the disease but fails. Components of the immune system wear down or are destroyed, leading to severe immunosuppression and progression of HIV disease to AIDS and death. The immune system produces cytokines that have an inflammatory effect that promotes spread of HIV infection and penetrance of HIV into several types of cells.

CD4+ T-LYMPHOCYTE DESTRUCTION LEADS TO INFECTION

HIV selectively attacks helper/inducer CD4+ T lymphocytes, decreases their number, and interferes with their function. CD4+ T lymphocytes are responsible for modulation of essentially the entire immune response. Lymphopenia occurs because of the reduced numbers of CD4+ T lymphocytes. Infections normally controlled by cellular immunity occur with markedly increased frequency.

THE INITIAL HUMAN IMMUNODEFICIENCY VIRUS INFECTION

The incubation period is unknown but has been estimated to be 3 to 6 weeks. An acute mononucleosis-like syndrome develops in 50% to 70% of patients approximately 3 to 6 weeks after initial infection. There is fever, myalgia-arthralgias, pharyngitis, and a diffuse red eruption consisting of macules 0.5 to 2.0 cm in diameter. The symptoms resolve spontaneously within 8 to 12 days. Seroconversion may take place within 1 week to 3 months, and then there is a dramatic decline in viremia. The CD4+ cells remain at a normal level of more than 500/mm^3, and the patient is without symptoms. After the initial infection viremia may persist for life.

THE EVOLUTION OF DISEASE

After primary infection, viral dissemination, and the appearance of HIV-specific immunity, most patients have a period of "clinical latency" that lasts for years (Figure 11-25). The clinical presentation of patients with HIV infections ranges from asymptomatic, through chronic generalized lymphadenopathy, to subclinical and clinical T-cell deficiency. There is strong association between the development of life-threatening opportunistic illnesses and the absolute number of CD4+ T lymphocytes. As the number of CD4+ T lymphocytes decreases, the risk and severity of opportunistic illnesses increase. The revised Centers for Disease Control and Prevention Classification System for HIV Infection categorizes persons on the basis of clinical conditions associated with HIV infection and CD4+ T-lymphocyte counts. Measures of CD4+ T lymphocytes are used to guide clinical and therapeutic management.

PROGRESSION TO ACQUIRED IMMUNODEFICIENCY SYNDROME

Patients have a number of symptoms during disease progression. They exhibit prolonged constitutional symptoms such as chronic fatigue, night sweats, fever, weight loss, and diarrhea. They frequently have clinical manifestations of T-cell dysfunction such as mucous membrane disease (oral candidiasis, hairy leukoplakia) and dermatologic diseases (herpes simplex/zoster, fungal infections).

AIDS is the end stage of HIV infection. It is characterized by a variety of unusual tumors and opportunistic infections. There appears to be a spectrum of disease, and long-term survival with new drug regimens may be possible.

AIDS—EVOLUTION OF THE DISEASE

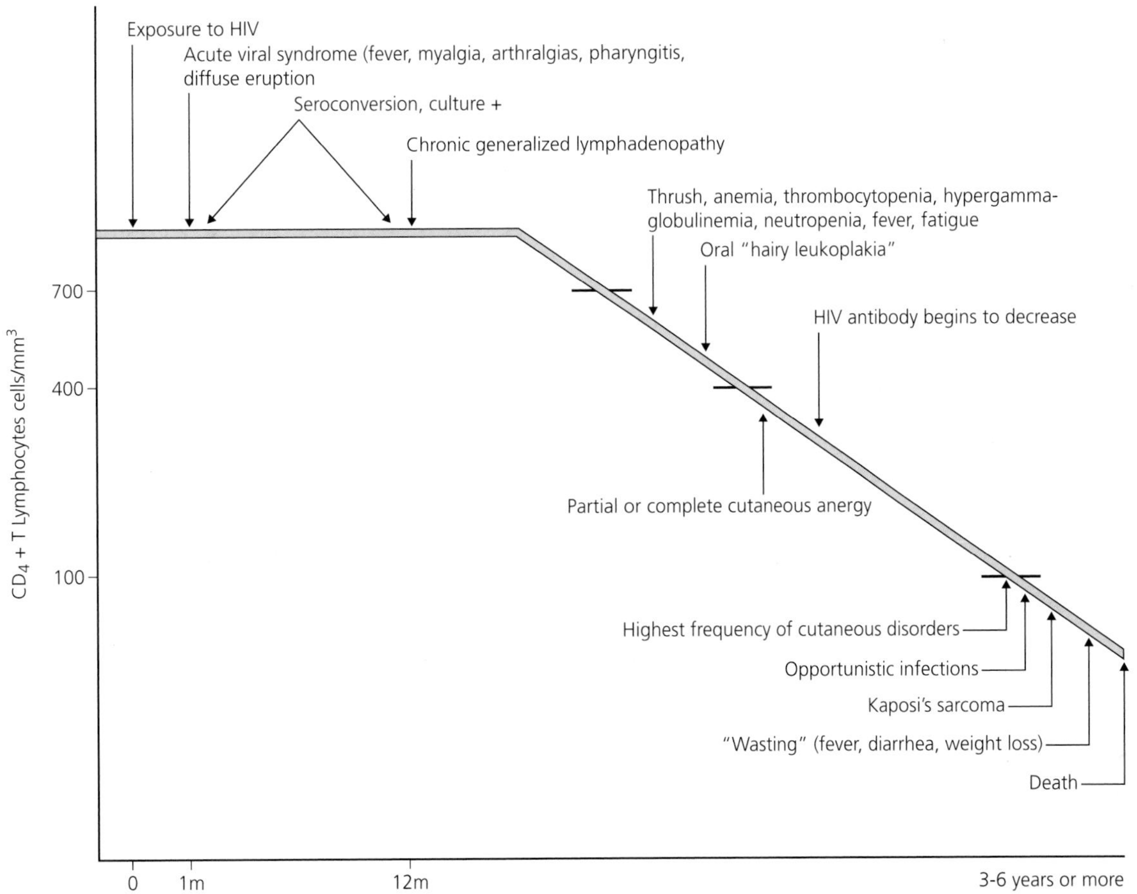

Note: The natural history of HIV infection is highly variable.
This chart shows approximate relationships of signs and symptoms.

Figure 11-25

Diagnosis

In adults, the diagnosis is made with serologic tests (ELISA) and is confirmed with the Western blot antibody test. These tests are then repeated to confirm the diagnosis.

Several rapid tests are available. They produce results in approximately 20 minutes. Rapid tests use blood from a vein or from a finger stick, or oral fluid. A reactive rapid HIV test result must be confirmed with a follow-up confirmatory test.

Viral burden

The onset of infection, the initial immune response, and the long-term prognosis of the disease can be monitored by determining the viral burden. This is measured with PCR tests for the level of HIV RNA. HIV-RNA level increases soon after infection in adults, declines within 3 weeks because of an immune response, and adjusts to a viral set point, which is predictive of outcome. Patients with a high viral set point experience early onset of AIDS and death; those with a low viral set point live longer with relatively asymptomatic disease.

Assessment of immune status (CD4+ T-cell determinations)

The pathogenesis of AIDS is attributable to the decrease in T lymphocytes that bear the CD4 receptor. The degree of immunosuppression is indicated by the T-helper (CD4+) lymphocyte count. Measures of CD4+ T lymphocytes (CD4+ T cells) are essential to the assessment of the immune system of HIV-infected persons. Progressive depletion of CD4+ T lymphocytes is associated with an increased likelihood of clinical complications. CD4+ T-cell levels are monitored every 3 to 6 months in all HIV-infected persons.

The measurement of CD4+ T-cell levels is used to establish decision points for initiating antiviral therapy, determining prophylaxis for opportunistic infections, and monitoring the efficacy of treatment.

Revised CDC classification and management

The revised Centers for Disease Control and Prevention Classification System (1993) for HIV-infected adolescents and adults is primarily intended for use in public health practice. It categorizes persons on the basis of clinical conditions associated with HIV infection and CD4+ T-lymphocyte counts. The system is based on three ranges of CD4+ T-lymphocyte counts and three clinical categories of conditions associated with HIV infection and is represented by a matrix of nine mutually exclusive categories. The three CD4+ T-lymphocyte categories are defined as follows:

- Category 1: greater than 500 cells/ml
- Category 2: 200 to 499 cells/ml
- Category 3: less than 200 cells/ml

Antimicrobial prophylaxis and antiretroviral therapies have been shown to be most effective within certain levels of immune dysfunction. Therefore CD4+ T-lymphocyte determinations are an integral part of medical management of HIV-infected persons.

INCIDENCE

The incidence, severity, and number of skin disorders increase as immune function deteriorates (Tables 11-2 and 11-3). The number of mucocutaneous diseases, like the CD4+ T-cell count, is an indicator of the status of the immune system and the prognosis. Cutaneous disorders found to correlate with CD4 cell counts are shown in Figure 11-26. Herpes zoster and drug reactions correlated with a higher CD4+ T-cell count (424/mm^3 and 301/mm^3, respectively), whereas the other seven disorders correlated with a more advanced degree of immunosuppression with CD4+ T-cell counts less than 75/mm^3. Therefore, in the majority of patients infected with HIV, cutaneous manifestations may reflect the underlying degree of immunosuppression.

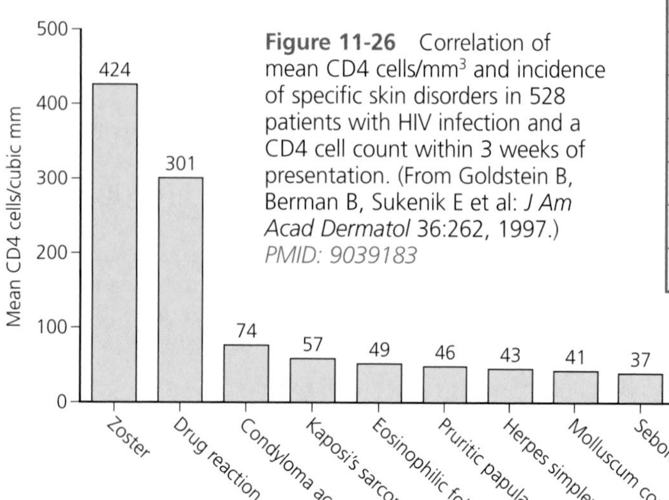

Figure 11-26 Correlation of mean CD4 cells/mm^3 and incidence of specific skin disorders in 528 patients with HIV infection and a CD4 cell count within 3 weeks of presentation. (From Goldstein B, Berman B, Sukenik E et al: *J Am Acad Dermatol* 36:262, 1997.) PMID: 9039183

Dermatologic diseases associated with human immunodeficiency virus infection

Disorders of the skin and mucous membranes occur throughout the course of HIV infection, affecting more than 90% of patients at some time. Cutaneous disease may be the initial or only problem for much of the course of the HIV infection and may be the most debilitating element of the patient's condition. Serious opportunistic infections may present for the first time in the skin. Skin disorders in patients with HIV may look unusual and may not be accurately diagnosed. Response to treatment may be poorer than expected.

Complete lists of diseases and treatments are found in Tables 11-2 and 11-3. Illustrations of these diseases are found in Figures 11-26 to 11-41. The most common skin disorders in HIV disease are caused by infections.

The frequency and percentage of patients presenting with specific skin disorders in a population of 528 patients infected with HIV are shown in Table 11-2.

Table 11-2 Frequency and Percentage of Patients Presenting with Specific Skin Disorders in a Population of 528 Patients Infected with HIV

Presenting diagnosis	No.	%
Pruritic papular eruption	60	11.4
Herpes simplex	57	10.8
Kaposi's sarcoma	45	8.5
Molluscum contagiosum	43	8.1
Condylomata acuminata	42	8.0
Seborrheic dermatitis	39	7.4
Drug eruption	33	6.3
Xerosis	28	5.3
Eosinophilic folliculitis	21	4.0
Tinea	19	3.6
Verruca vulgaris	18	3.4
Scabies	17	3.2
Bacterial cellulitis	15	2.8
Syphilis	12	2.3
Psoriasis	12	2.3
Herpes zoster	11	2.1
Nonmelanoma skin cancer	10	1.9

Adapted from Goldstein B, Berman B, Sukenik E et al: *J Am Acad Dermatol* 36:262, 1997. PMID: 9039183

Table 11-3 HIV Infection—Cutaneous Manifestations

Disease	Clinical manifestations	Diagnosis	Treatment
Viral infections			
Acute HIV exanthema (HIV primary infection)	Fever, myalgias, urticaria Truncal maculopapular eruption Mononucleosis-like syndrome Generalized lymphadenopathy follows later	Time to seroconversion unknown Antibodies found 3 wk to 6 mo after initial infection Low white blood cell count, thrombocytopenia, hypergammaglobulinemia	Antiretroviral drugs
Herpes simplex (common)	Persistent erosions and ulcerations Widely disseminated Resembles other infections Intractable perirectal ulcerations Regional lymphadenopathy	HSV culture Tzanck smear for multinucleated giant cells HSV-2 infection is risk factor for subsequent or concurrent HIV infection	Acyclovir, valacyclovir, or famciclovir Acyclovir or penciclovir (Denavir) ointment Foscarnet
Herpes zoster Shingles (common sign of AIDS)	Shingles may be severe, resulting in deep scarring Persistent disseminated lesions Intractable herpetic pain	Herpesvirus culture Tzanck smear for multinucleated giant cells	Acyclovir, valacyclovir, or famciclovir
Chickenpox (uncommon)	Chickenpox with numerous lesions and pneumonia		Same treatment as for herpes zoster
Molluscum contagiosum	Clusters of white, umbilicated papules Persistent on face, groin Cutaneous cryptococcus can mimic molluscum contagiosum	KOH preparations of soft material in center of lesion show large viral inclusions Biopsy—large viral inclusions	Cryosurgery, curettage Scissor excision with blunt-tipped scissors Trichloroacetic acid peels for extensive cases Imiquimod cream (Aldara)
Warts/condyloma (common) Human papillomavirus (HPV)	Common warts—extensive and persistent Condylomata—increased prevalence, number, size Cervical, anal squamous cell carcinoma (HPV types 16, 18)	Biopsy or clinical appearance Profound reduction in CD4+ T-cells	Cryosurgery, blunt dissection, excision, surgery Imiquimod cream (Aldara) Podophyllotoxin (Condylox)
Hairy leukoplakia (Epstein-Barr virus) (common)	Whitish, nonremovable verrucous hairy plaques on sides of tongue May resemble fungal tongue infections	Biopsy—acanthosis and parakeratosis with large pale-staining cells with pyknotic nuclei	Treating oral *Candida* improves appearance Podophyllin resin 25% in ethanol and acetone Gentian violet solution (OTC)
Fungal infections			
Candida albicans (very common)	White plaques on cheeks, tongue Sore throat, dysphagia Deep tongue erosions, thick plaques on back of throat Esophageal infection Intractable vaginal infection *Candida* nail infection	Culture Obtain specimen for KOH slide preparation with cotton swab	Nystatin oral suspension Clotrimazole (Mycelex Troche) 10 mg 5×/day PO Ketoconazole (200 mg PO daily) Fluconazole (100-200 mg PO daily) Amphotericin B (severe cases) 0.3 mg/kg IV daily

Continued

Table 11-3 HIV Infection—Cutaneous Manifestations—cont'd

Disease	Clinical manifestations	Diagnosis	Treatment
Tinea versicolor (common)	Common early and late in HIV infection Thick, scaly hypopigmented or light-brown plaques on trunk	KOH slide preparation shows numerous short hyphae and spores Wood's light accentuates lesions	Oral: fluconazole, itraconazole, ketoconazole (various dosages) Topical: many (see Chapter 13)
Dermatophytes Tinea corporis Tinea pedis Tinea cruris Onychomycoses (common)	Extensive involvement, especially groin and feet Thick keratoderma—blennorhagic-like lesions on feet Proximal subungual onychomycosis	KOH slide preparation shows branched, septated hyphae	Dosage schedules: see Table 13-2, page 519
Cryptococcus neoformans (rare)	White papules that resemble molluscum contagiosum	Assays for antigen in serum or cerebrospinal fluid, India ink or Wright's stain Culture Biopsy	Amphotericin B or add flucytosine followed by fluconazole 200-400 mg PO daily
Histoplasma capsulatum (rare)	Multiple papules, nodules, macules, and oral and skin ulcers on arms, face, trunk Travel history (South America)	Biopsy—PAS stain Crushed tissue preparation—rapid diagnosis Culture—several weeks required	Amphotericin B Itraconazole 200 mg PO 2×/day
Bacterial infections			
Staphylococcus aureus (common)	Bullous impetigo—axillae or groin Facial or truncal folliculitis (resembling acne) Impetigo of beard and body	Culture	Dicloxacillin Cefadroxil Many others
Syphilis (uncommon)	Generalized papulosquamous papules and plaques Can mimic almost any inflammatory cutaneous disorder Incubation period for neurosyphilis may be very brief (months)	VDRL titer may be very high or negative; obtain sequential tests or skin biopsy with special stains	Standard recommended treatment may not be sufficient to prevent central nervous system disease; see Chapter 10
Arthropod			
Scabies (uncommon)	Generalized crusted papules Norwegian scabies—generalized hyperkeratotic eruption	KOH or oil preparation shows mites	Lindane (Kwell) Permethrin (Elimite) Ivermectin (Stromectol) oral
Proliferative disorders			
Seborrheic dermatitis (common)	Red scaling plaques with yellowish, greasy scales and crust Distinct margins, hypopigmentation of scalp, face; sometimes groin, extremities Severity correlates with degree of clinical deterioration	Biopsy differs from ordinary seborrheic dermatitis Parakeratosis is widespread Necrotic keratinocytes Dermoepidermal obliteration by lymphocytes Sparse spongiosis Thick-walled vessels Do KOH to rule out tinea	Ketoconazole cream Ciclopirox gel

Table 11-3 HIV Infection—Cutaneous Manifestations—cont'd

Disease	Clinical manifestations	Diagnosis	Treatment
Psoriasis (uncommon)	Activation of previous disease or no history	Biopsy	Treatment-resistant cases may respond to acitretin or antiretroviral drugs
Xeroderma (common) Ichthyosis (uncommon)	Severe dry skin may be associated with erythroderma, seborrheic dermatitis, and dementia Ichthyosiform scaling of legs, keratoderma of palms and soles	Clinical presentation	Ammonium lactate emollients (Lac-Hydrin cream or lotion; AmLactin cream or lotion) Most topical lubricating lotions or creams
Pruritic papular eruption (common)	2-5 mm skin-colored papules on head, neck, upper trunk Pruritus and number of papules may wax and wane with time	Biopsy—lymphocytic perivascular infiltrate with numerous eosinophils Follicular damage	Ultraviolet B phototherapy Often resistant to topical steroids and oral antihistamines Antipruritic lotions (Sarna) Dapsone 100 mg PO daily possibly effective
Eosinophilic pustular folliculitis (rare)	Groups of small vesicles and pustules becoming confluent to form irregular pustular lakes and erosions Polycyclic plaques with central hyperpigmentation Severe, intractable pruritus Chronic and persistent Many nonfollicular lesions	Biopsy is diagnostic Eosinophils that invade sebaceous glands and outer root sheaths of hair follicles Moderate eosinophilia and leukocytosis (50%) CD4+ counts <250-300 cells/mm^3	Permethrin cream (Elimite) daily until lesions clear Ultraviolet B phototherapy Antihistamines Group I topical steroids: tacrolimus topically Itraconazole 100-400 mg/day Dapsone 100 mg PO daily possibly effective Metronidazole Acitretin Doxicyline
Vascular disorders			
Telangiectasias of anterior chest wall (uncommon)	Linear telangiectasia in broad, crescent distribution across chest Associated with erythema in same distribution	Biopsy shows dilated blood vessels with perivascular small cell infiltrate No endothelial proliferation	None
Bacillary (epithelioid) angiomatosis (rare)	Solitary or multiple dome-shaped friable, bright-red granulation tissue-like papules and subcutaneous nodules (1 mm-2 cm) of face, trunk, extremities Visceral angiomatosis Cat bite or scratch	Biopsy—proliferation of small blood vessels lined with plump endothelial cells projecting into lumen *Bartonella* bacilli seen with Warthin-Starry silver stain	Erythromycin, azithromycin, tetracycline, doxycycline, trimethoprim-sulfamethoxazole, rifampin
Thrombocytopenic purpura (common)	Petechia	Complete blood count	Treat HIV

Continued

Table 11-3 HIV Infection—Cutaneous Manifestations—cont'd

Disease	Clinical manifestations	Diagnosis	Treatment
Neoplastic disorders			
Kaposi's sarcoma	Pale to deep violaceous, thin, oval plaques Long axis of lesions aligned with skin tension lines Many unusual presentations Numbers vary from few to numerous lesions Any skin surface and mouth, usually palate Visceral lesions Lesions induced by trauma	Biopsy Proliferation of small vessels Proliferation of bundles of interweaving plump spindle cells Slitlike intercellular spaces with extravasated red blood cells	Radiation for individual lesions Intralesional vinblastine (0.1-0.5 mg/ml every 4 wk) Liquid nitrogen cryotherapy (keep blister covered to prevent exposure of others to HIV) Many others
Miscellaneous			
Cutaneous drug reactions	Morbilliform eruptions predominate Urticaria Much greater incidence than general population	Trimethoprim-sulfamethoxazole Dapsone Aminopenicillins	Stop drug if possible
Pruritus (uncommon)	Intractable pruritus without internal malignancy May be presenting symptom of AIDS	Numerous excoriations Rule out other causes of pruritus (e.g., renal, thyroid, hepatic dysfunction; drugs; malignancy; diabetes; iron deficiency anemia)	Emollients, topical steroids, and prednisone are not effective
Yellow nails	Yellow discoloration of nail plate Many associated with *Pneumocystis jiroveci* pneumonia	Differentiate from yellow nail syndrome: yellow nail plate + absent cuticles + diminished growth rate + transverse overcurvature of nail plate + subungual hyperkeratosis	Treat possible aggravating conditions (e.g., *P. jiroveci* pneumonia)
Dark-blue nails	Darkened bluish appearance at bases of fingernails (black patients > white patients)	Recent history of zidovudine treatment	None
Vitiligo (uncommon) Premature graying of hair (common)	Loss of pigmentation of hair and skin usually follows other AIDS signs and symptoms	Physical examination	None
Straightened hair	May be caused by denutrition	Physical examination	None

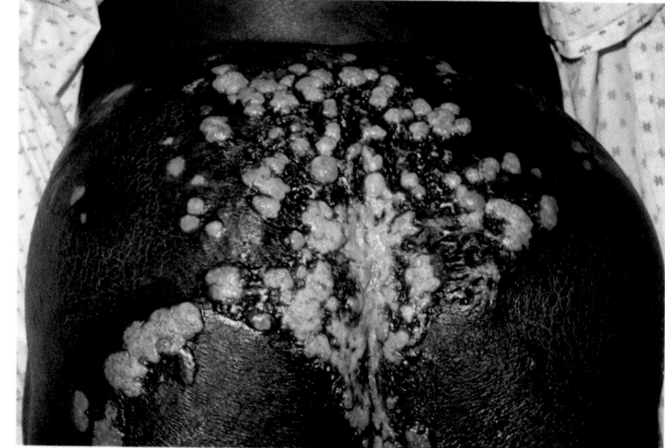

Figure 11-27 Chronic herpes simplex infection of the anal and buttocks area.

CUTANEOUS MANIFESTATIONS OF HIV

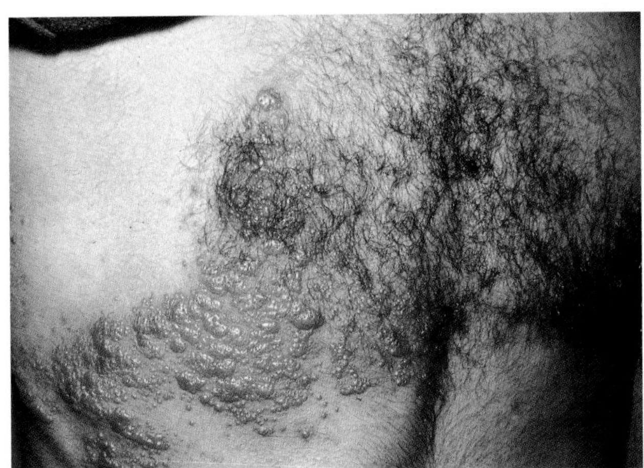

Figure 11-28 Herpes zoster. (Courtesy Benjamin K. Fisher, MD.)

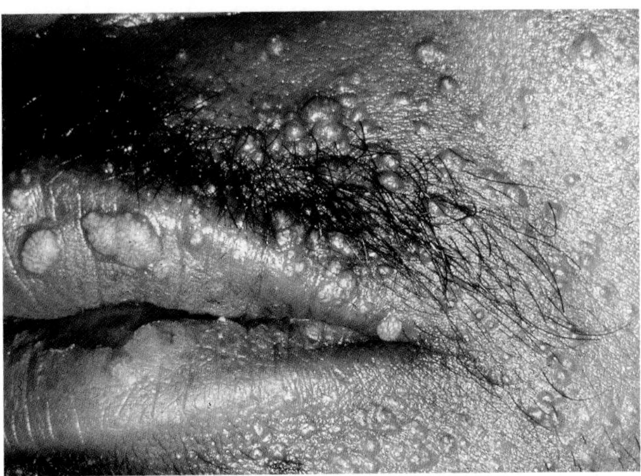

Figure 11-29 Molluscum contagiosum. (From Redfield RR, James WD, Wright DC: *J Am Acad Dermatol* 13:821, 1985.)

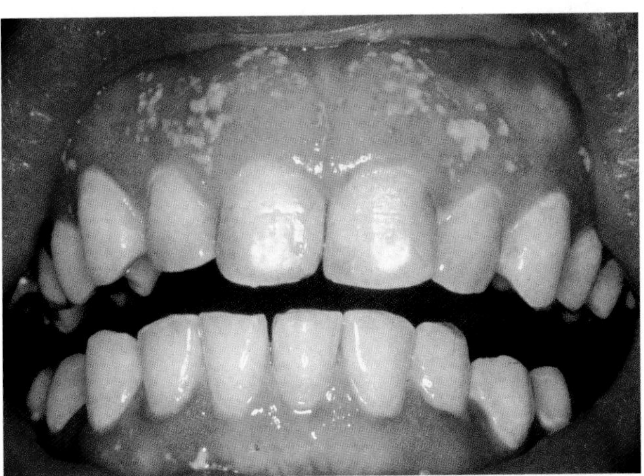

Figure 11-30 *Candida albicans*. (Courtesy William D. James, MD.)

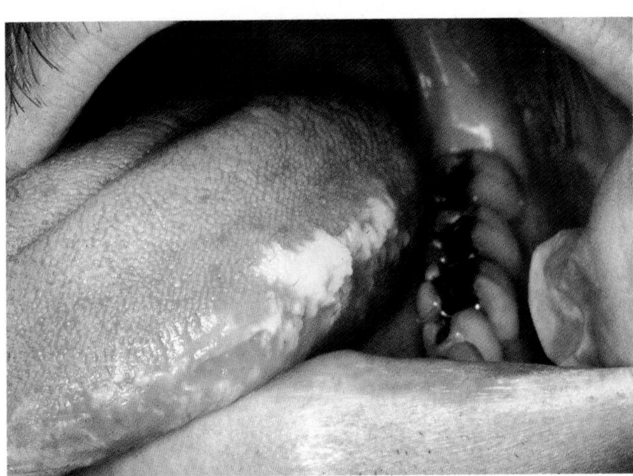

Figure 11-31 Hairy leukoplakia. (Courtesy Deborah S. Greenspan.)

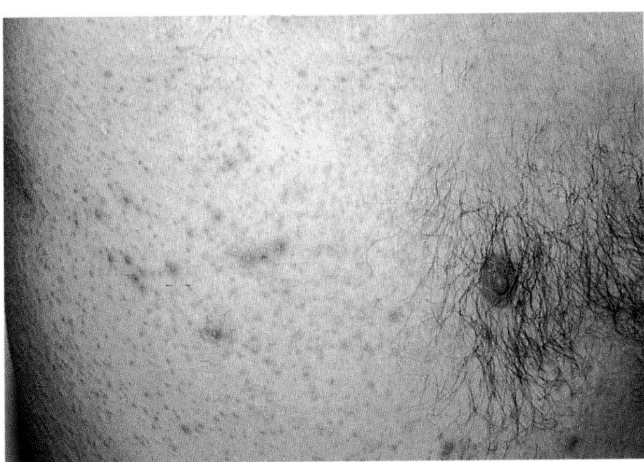

Figure 11-32 Papular eruption. (Courtesy David Goodman, MD.)

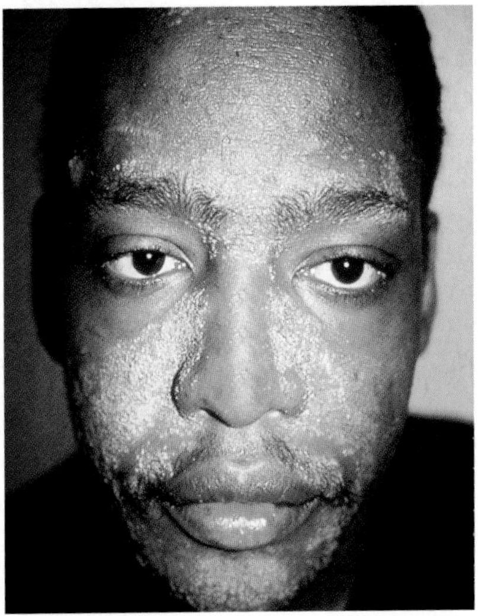

Figure 11-33 Seborrheic dermatitis. (Courtesy William D. James, MD.)

CUTANEOUS MANIFESTATIONS OF HIV

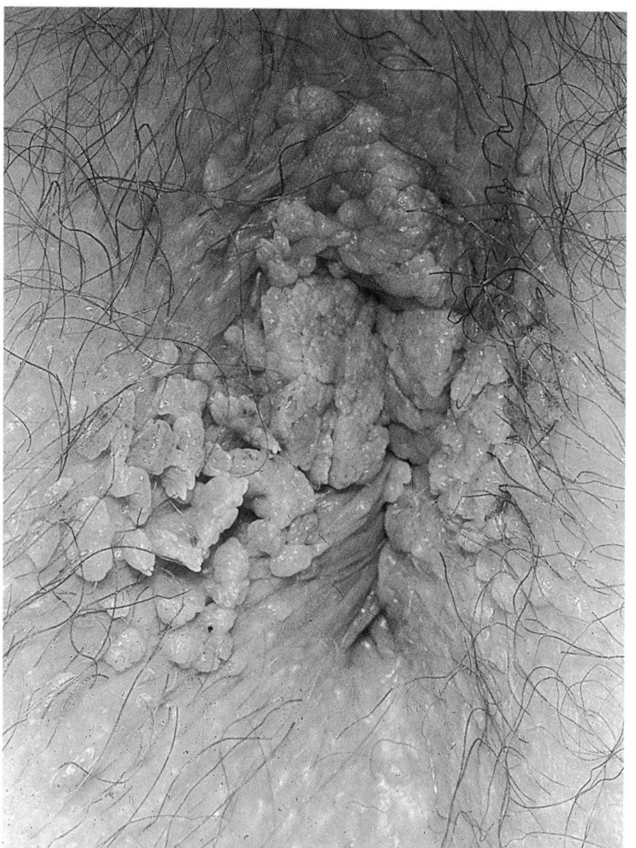

Figure 11-34 Anal warts.

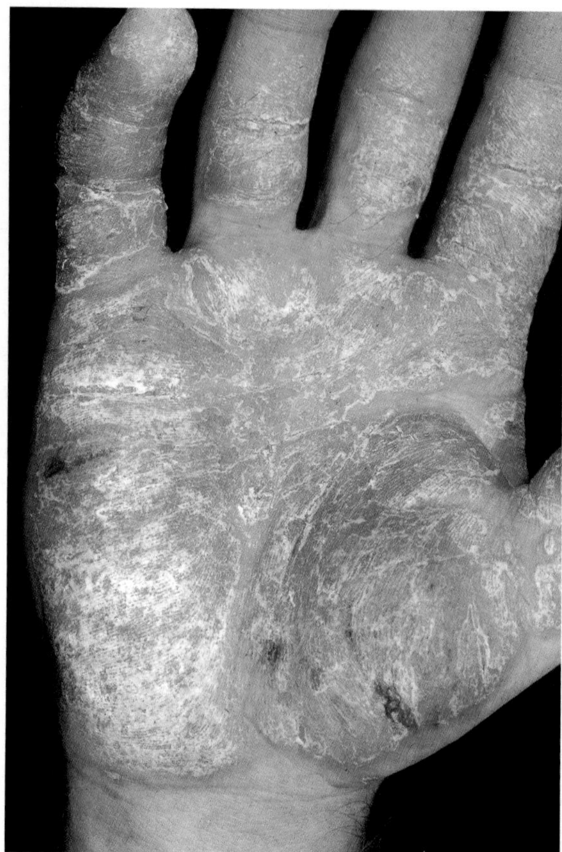

Figure 11-35 Psoriasis. (Courtesy William D. James, MD.)

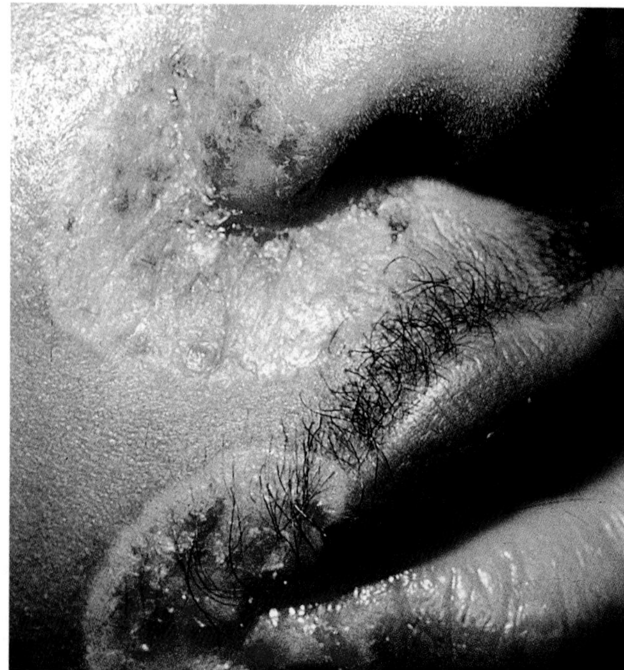

Figure 11-36 Herpes simplex. Erosive. (Courtesy Neal S. Penneys, MD, PhD.)

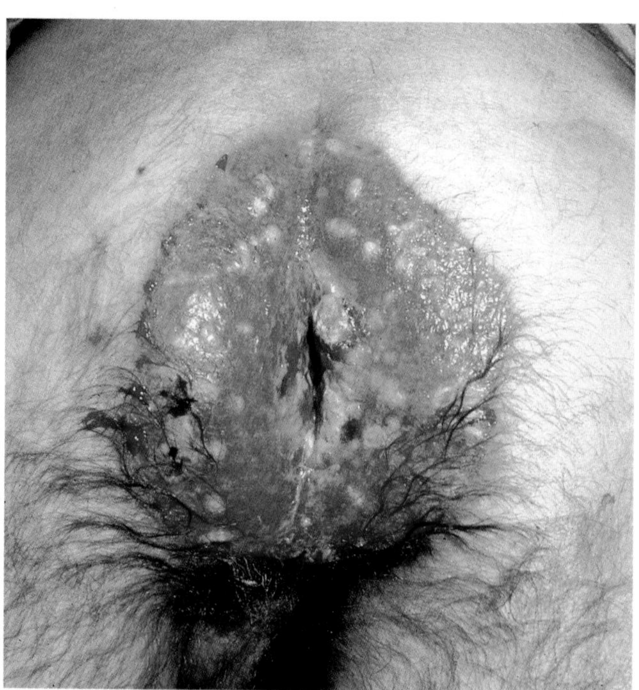

Figure 11-37 Herpes simplex. Erosive. (Courtesy Benjamin K. Fisher, MD.)

KAPOSI'S SARCOMA IN HIV PATIENTS

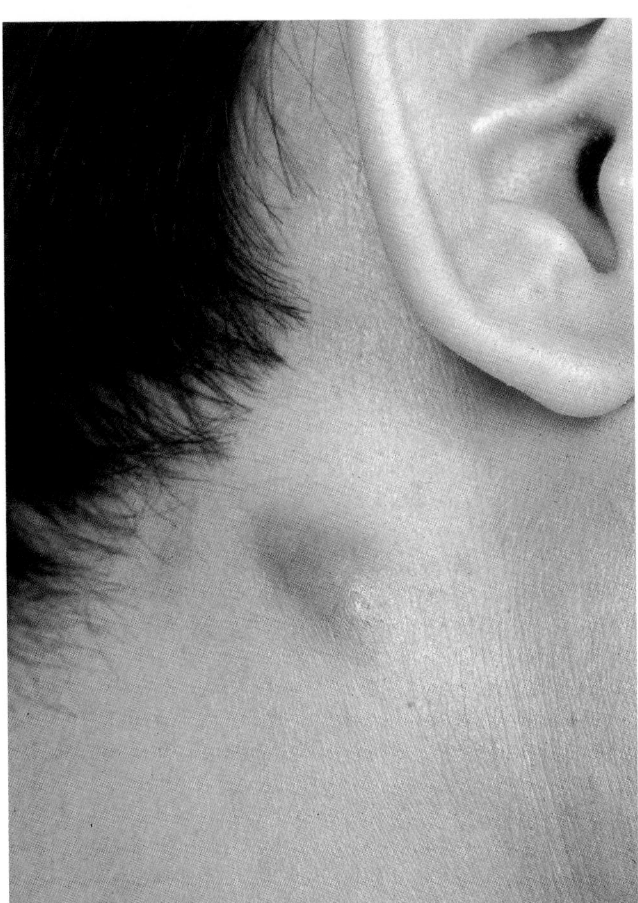

Figure 11-38 Kaposi's sarcoma. (Courtesy H.J. Hulsebosch, MD.)

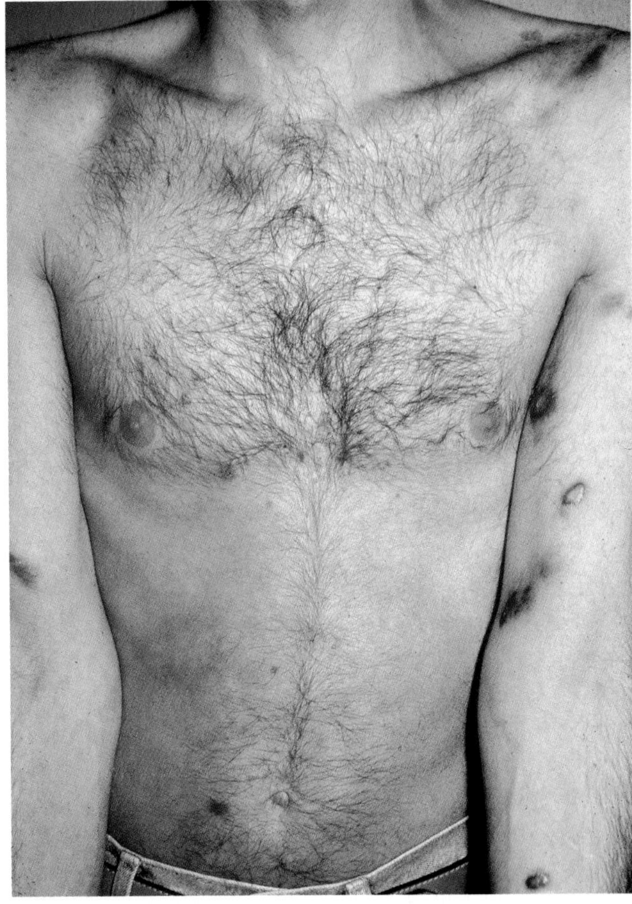

Figure 11-39 Kaposi's sarcoma. (Courtesy Benjamin K. Fisher, MD.)

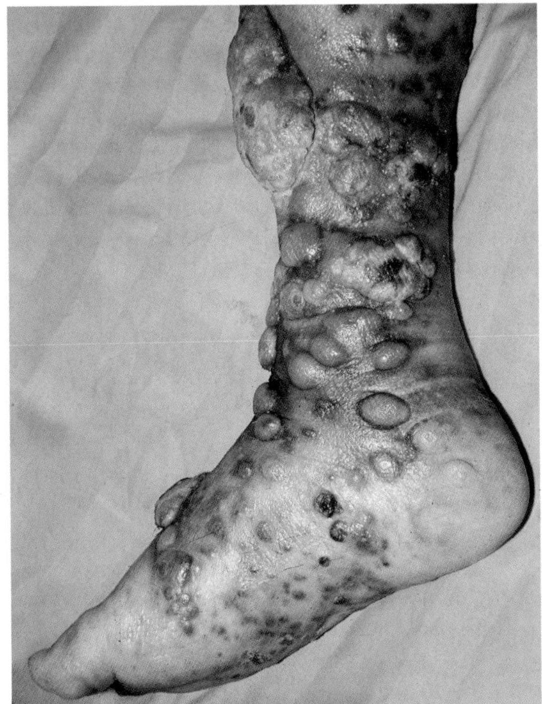

Figure 11-40 Kaposi's sarcoma. (Courtesy Benjamin K. Fisher, MD.)

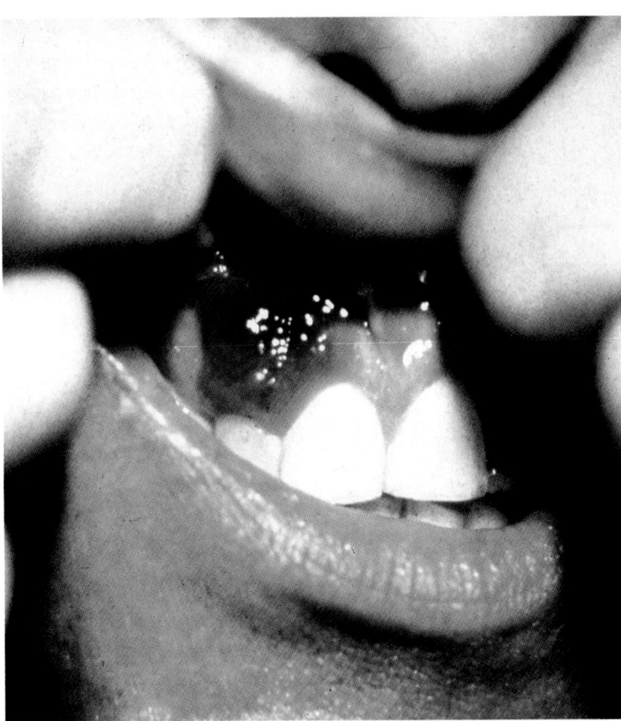

Figure 11-41 Kaposi's sarcoma. (Courtesy William D. James, MD.)

Chapter 12

Warts, Herpes Simplex, and Other Viral Infections

CHAPTER CONTENTS

WARTS

Warts are benign epidermal neoplasms that are caused by human papillomaviruses (HPVs), which are small DNA viruses. There are more than 100 different types of HPVs, and new types are discovered each year. HPVs infect epithelial cells of the skin, mouth, esophagus, larynx, trachea, and conjunctiva and cause both benign and malignant lesions. They induce a variety of infections (Table 12-1).

Clinical infection

Warts commonly occur in children and young adults, but they may appear at any age. Warts are transmitted simply by touch; it is not unusual to see warts on adjacent toes ("kissing lesions"). Warts commonly appear at sites of trauma, on the hands, in periungual regions as a result of nail biting, and on plantar surfaces. Plantar warts may be acquired from moist surfaces in communal swimming areas. Their course is highly variable; most resolve spontaneously in weeks or months, and others may last years or a lifetime. Infection with HPV can be latent, subclinical, or clinical. Latent infections are detected with molecular biologic techniques. Subclinical infections are found with a colposcope or microscope. HPVs induce hyperplasia and hyperkeratosis.

Table 12-1 Different Types of HPV and Their Clinical Manifestations

Clinical manifestation	HPV types
Plantar warts	1, 2, 3, 4, 27, 29, 57
Common warts	1, 2, 3, 4, 27, 57
Flat warts	3, 10, 28
Epidermodysplasia verruciformis	5, 8, 9, 12, 14, 15, 17, 19-25, 36, 47, 50
Genital warts, laryngeal papillomas	6, 11
Butcher's warts	7
Focal epithelial hyperplasia (Heck disease)	13, 32
Anogenital dysplasias and neoplasms (rarely laryngeal carcinomas)	16, 18, 31, 33, 35, 42, 43, 44, 45, 51, 52, 56, 58, 59, 68
Keratoacanthoma	37
Cutaneous squamous cell carcinoma	38, 41, 48
Oral papillomas, inverted nasal and papillomas	57
Buschke-Löwenstein tumors	6, 11
Bowenoid papulosis	16, 18, 33, 39
Cystic warts	60
Pigmented wart	65
Vulvar papilloma	70
Oral papillomas (in HIV-infected patients)	72, 73
Common wart in renal allograft recipient	75-77
Cutaneous wart	78

Immunologic response

The regression of virus-infected cells involves a multifactorial response that includes cell-mediated immunity and induction of interferons. Individual variations in cell-mediated immunity may account for differences in severity and duration. Warts develop on many immunosuppressed patients. Warts occur more frequently, last longer, and appear in greater numbers in patients with acquired immunodeficiency syndrome (AIDS) or lymphomas and in those taking immunosuppressive drugs. Patients with atopic eczema may not be at increased risk for viral warts, as was once suspected.

TREATMENT

Some types of warts respond quickly to routine therapy, whereas others are resistant. It should be explained to patients that warts often require several treatment sessions before a cure is realized. Because warts are confined to the epidermis, they can be removed with little, if any, scarring. To avoid scarring, treatment should be conservative. Treatment that results in a hand with many scars is not worthwhile for lesions that undergo spontaneous resolution (Figure 12-1).

Warts obscure normal skin lines; this is an important diagnostic feature. When skin lines are reestablished, the warts are gone. Warts vary in shape and location and are managed in several different ways.

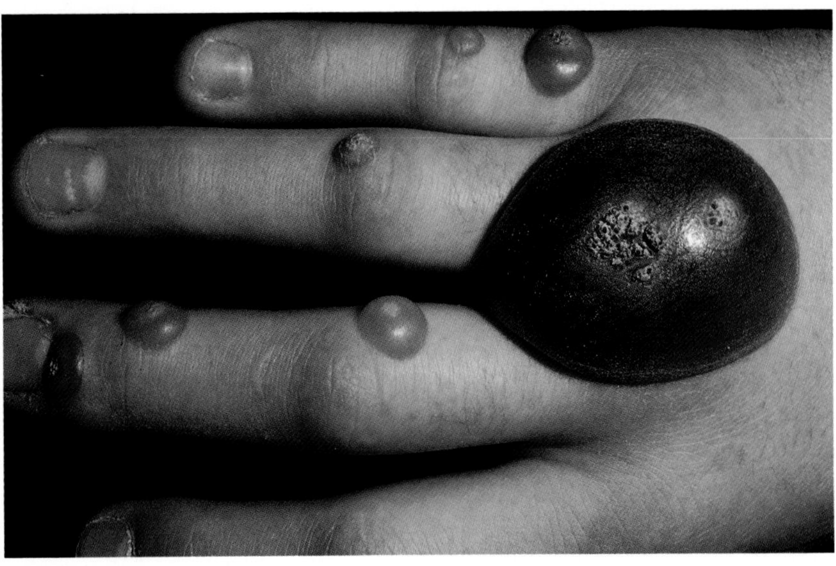

Figure 12-1 Cryosurgery for warts. Excessive, prolonged freezing with liquid nitrogen resulted in a huge blister that healed with scarring.

WARTS: THE PRIMARY LESION

Viral warts are tumors initiated by a viral infection of keratinocytes. The cells proliferate to form a mass but the mass remains confined to the epidermis. There are no "roots" that penetrate the dermis. Several types of warts form cylindrical projections. These projections are clearly seen in digitate warts that occur on the face (Figure 12-2). The projections become fused together in common warts on thicker skin (Figure 12-3); this produces a highly organized mosaic pattern on the surface. This pattern is unique to warts and is a useful diagnostic sign (Figure 12-4). Thrombosed black vessels become trapped in these projections and are seen as black dots on the surface of some warts (Figure 12-5). Although warts remain confined to the epidermis, the growing mass can protrude down and displace the dermis. Blunt dissection of a wart shows that the undersurface is smooth (Figure 12-6).

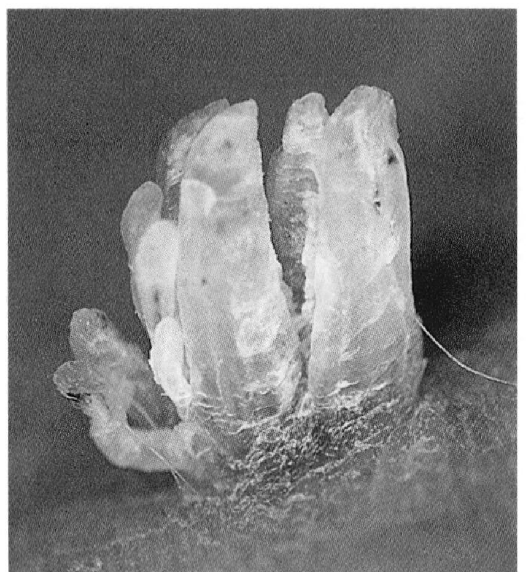

Figure 12-2 Warts form cylindrical projections. They diverge when the wart grows in thin skin.

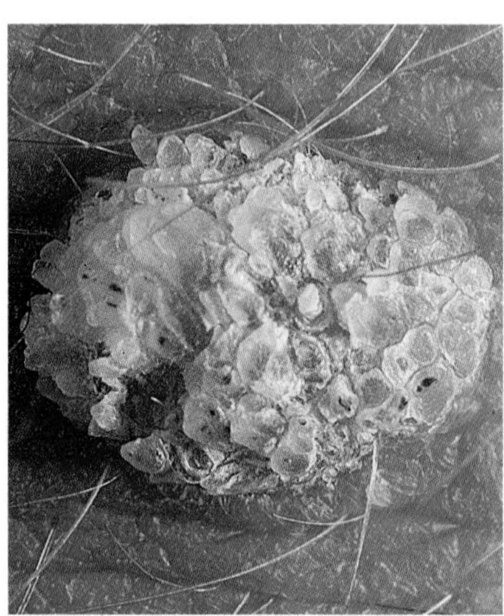

Figure 12-3 The cylindrical projections are partially fused in this larger wart.

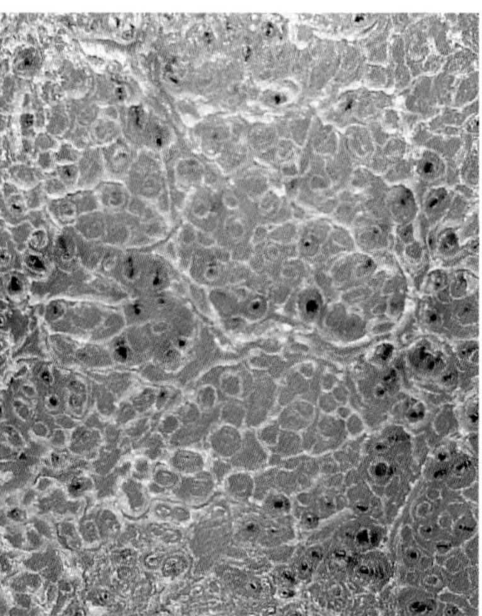

Figure 12-4 The cylindrical projections are tightly packed together, confined by the surrounding skin. This uniform mosaic surface pattern is unique to warts and is a useful diagnostic sign. The pattern can be easily seen with a hand lens.

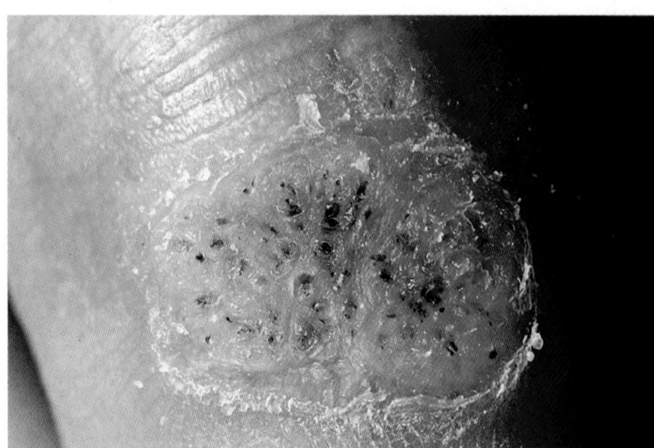

Figure 12-5 Thrombosed black vessels are trapped in the cylindrical projections. They appear as black dots when only the surface of the projections can be seen.

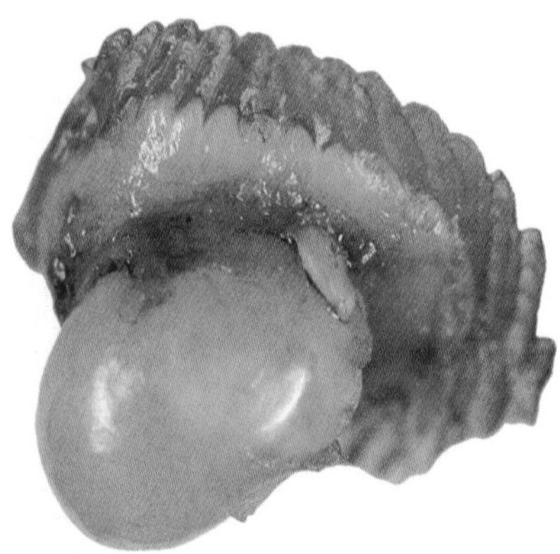

Figure 12-6 The undersurface of a wart. Contrary to popular belief, warts do not have roots. The undersurface is round and smooth. The wart is confined to the epidermis, but it expands and displaces the dermis, giving the impression that it extends into the dermis or subcutaneous tissue.

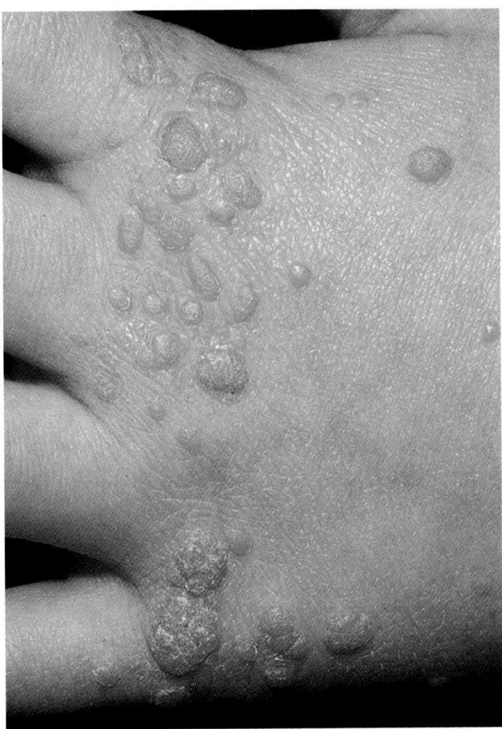

Figure 12-7 Common warts on the back of the hand.

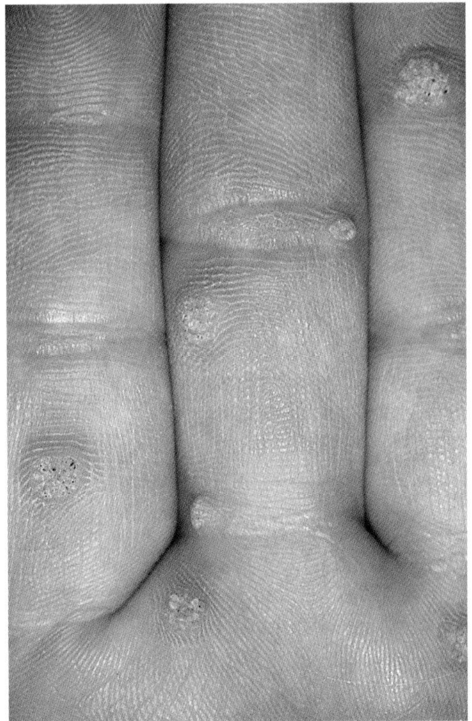

Figure 12-8 A common wart with black dots on the surface.

Common warts

Common warts (verruca vulgaris) begin as smooth, flesh-colored papules and evolve into dome-shaped, gray-brown, hyperkeratotic growths with black dots on the surface (Figures 12-7 and 12-8). The black dots, which are thrombosed capillaries, are a useful diagnostic sign and may be exposed by paring the hyperkeratotic surface with a #15 surgical blade. The hands are the most commonly involved areas, but warts may be found on any skin surface. In general, warts are few in number, but it is not unusual for common warts to become so numerous that they become confluent and obscure large areas of normal skin.

TREATMENT. Topical salicylic acid preparations, liquid nitrogen (Figures 12-9 and 12-10), and very light electrocautery are the best methods of initial therapy. Blunt dissection is used for resistant or very large lesions. The technique for the application of salicylic acid is described in the treatment section for plantar warts. Duct tape occlusion is not effective.

CRYOTHERAPY. The hyperkeratotic surface should be pared and liquid nitrogen applied with either a spray or a cotton-tipped applicator so that a 1- to 2-mm zone of frozen tissue is created and maintained around lesional skin for about 5 seconds. A small blister, sometimes hemorrhagic, is expected. Excessive freezing causes massive swelling, hemorrhagic blisters, hypopigmentation or hyperpigmentation, and scarring. Sharp pain lasts for minutes and sometimes hours; some children tolerate the pain. Freezing may be repeated in 2 to 4 weeks.

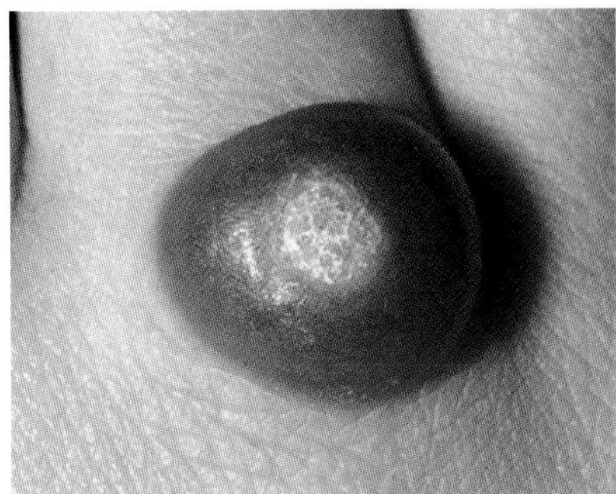

Figure 12-9 Cryosurgery produced the expected hemorrhagic blister.

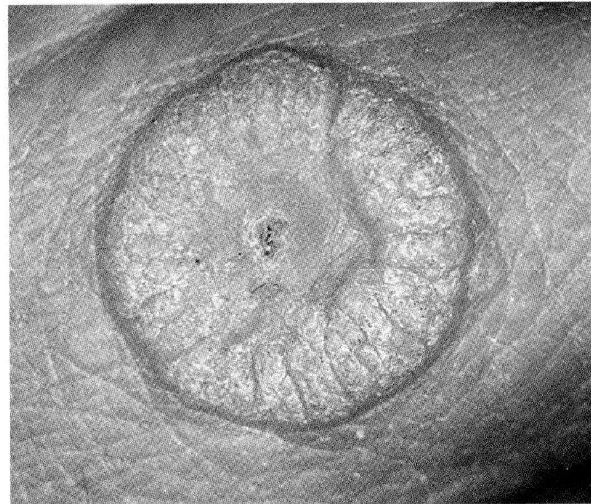

Figure 12-10 A side effect of cryosurgery. The wart spreads to the blister edge.

TREATMENT OF RECALCITRANT WARTS

IMIQUIMOD. Nightly application of the immunomodulatory drug imiquimod (Aldara cream) may be effective. The patient is instructed to soak the wart to soften the keratin surface. Removal of the keratin with an abrasive material, such as a pumice stone, and application of tape to cover the area facilitate penetration of the imiquimod cream.

APPLE CIDER VINEGAR. Many people claim success with this technique. Dip the wart in vinegar for 20 minutes. Apply Vaseline around the wart to protect the skin. Soak a small piece of cotton in vinegar and tape it to the wart overnight. Repeat each night until the wart is gone.

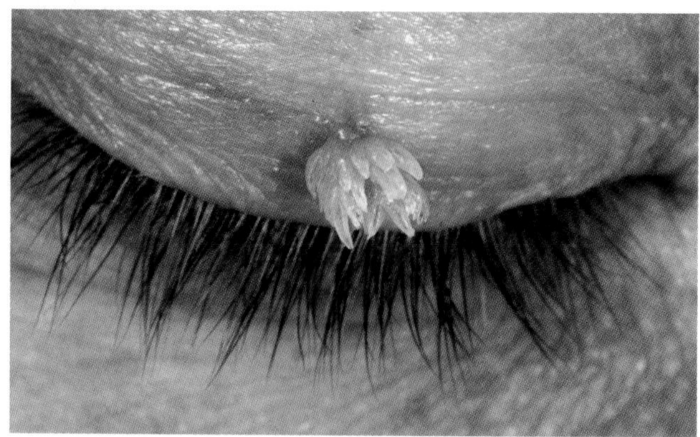

Figure 12-11 Filiform wart with fingerlike projections. These are most commonly observed on the face.

Filiform and digitate warts

These growths consist of a few or several fingerlike, flesh-colored projections emanating from a narrow or broad base. They are most commonly observed about the mouth, beard, eyes, and ala nasi (Figures 12-11 to 12-13).

TREATMENT. These are the easiest warts to treat. Those with a very narrow base do not require anesthesia. A firm base is created by retracting the skin on either side of the wart with the index finger and thumb. A curette is then firmly drawn across the base, removing the wart with one stroke. Bleeding is controlled with gauze pressure rather than by using Monsel's solution, which is painful. This technique is particularly useful for young children who refuse local anesthesia with a needle. Light electrocautery is an alternative.

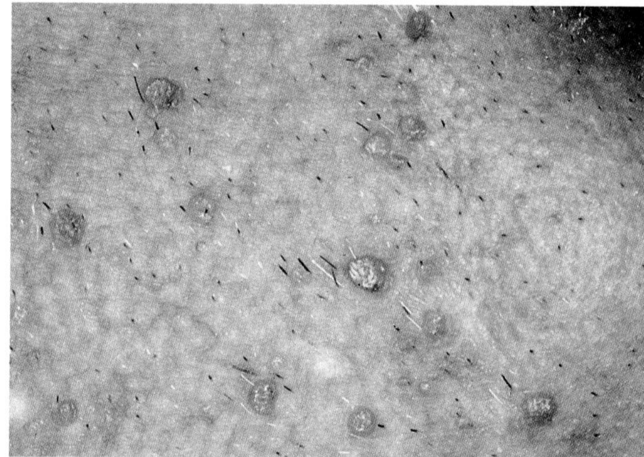

Figure 12-12 Small digitate and filiform warts in the beard area. Shaving spreads the virus over wide areas of the beard. Recurrences are common after cryotherapy or curettage. The infection may last for years.

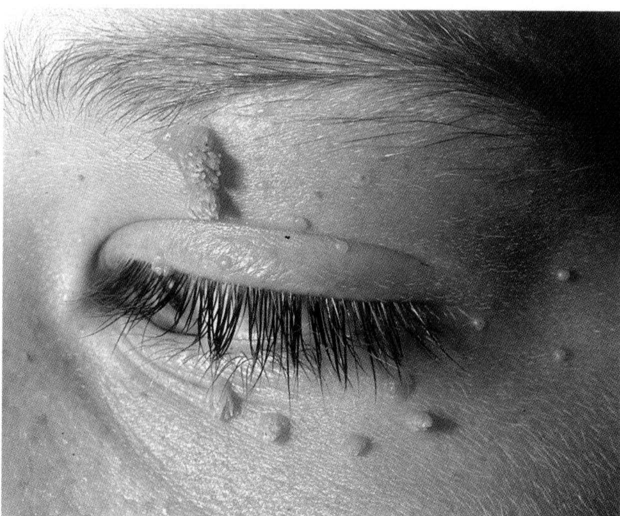

Figure 12-13 A group of digital warts. They may be misinterpreted as skin tags.

Flat warts

Flat warts (verruca plana) are pink, light brown, or light yellow and are slightly elevated, flat-topped papules that vary in size from 0.1 to 0.5 cm. There may be only a few, but in general they are numerous. Typical sites of involvement are the forehead (Figure 12-14, *A,*), around the mouth (Figure 12-15), the backs of the hands, and shaved areas such as the beard area in men and the lower legs in women. A line of flat warts may appear as a result of scratching these sites.

TREATMENT. Flat warts present a special therapeutic problem. Their duration may be lengthy, and they may be very resistant to treatment. In addition, they are usually located in cosmetically important areas where aggressive, scarring procedures are to be avoided. Imiquimod 5% cream (Aldara) applied every day or every other day may be effective. Freezing of individual lesions with liquid nitrogen or exercising a very light touch with the electrocautery needle may be performed for patients who are concerned with cosmetic appearance and desire quick results. Treatment with 5-fluorouracil cream (Carac) applied once or twice a day for 3 to 5 weeks may produce dramatic clearing of flat warts; it is worth the attempt if other measures fail. Persistent hyperpigmentation may occur following 5-fluorouracil use. This result may be minimized by applying the ointment to individual lesions with a cotton-tipped applicator. Warts may reappear in skin inflamed by 5-fluorouracil.

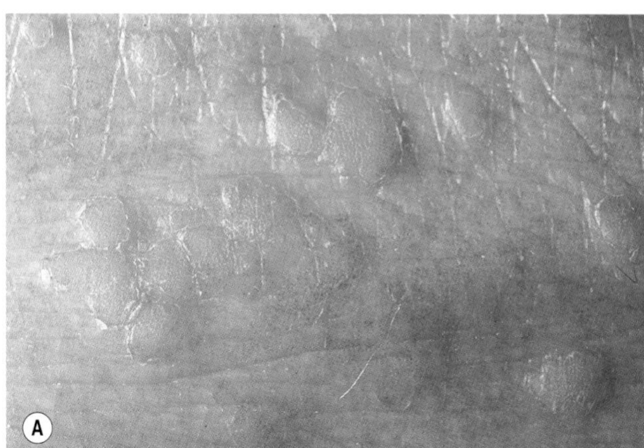

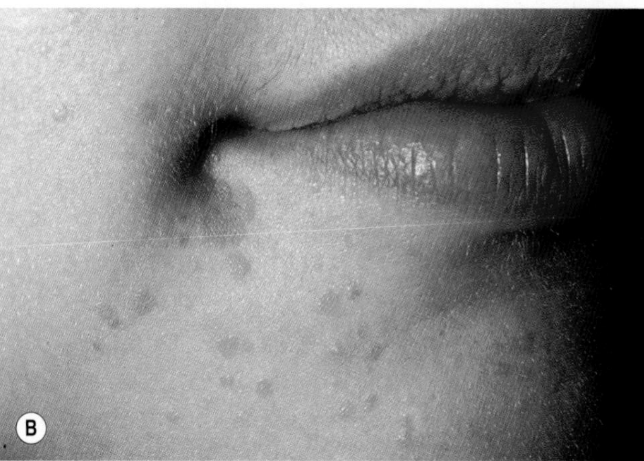

Figure 12-14 Flat warts. **A,** Lesions are slightly elevated, flesh-colored papules that often appear grouped. **B,** The face, back of the hands, and shins are the most common areas affected. Flatter lesions are brown.

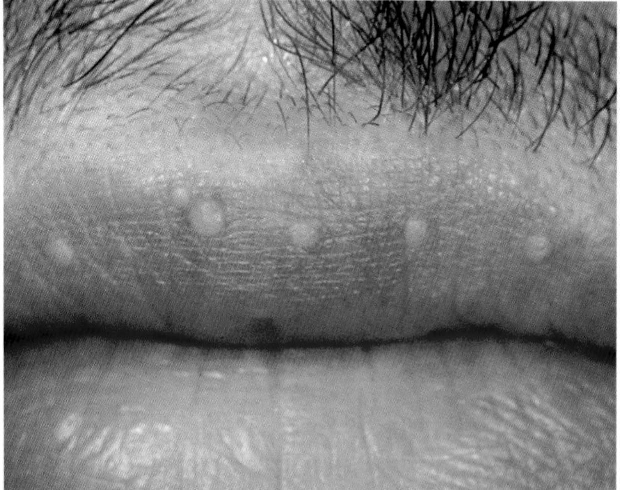

Figure 12-15 Flat warts on the vermillion surface of the lip.

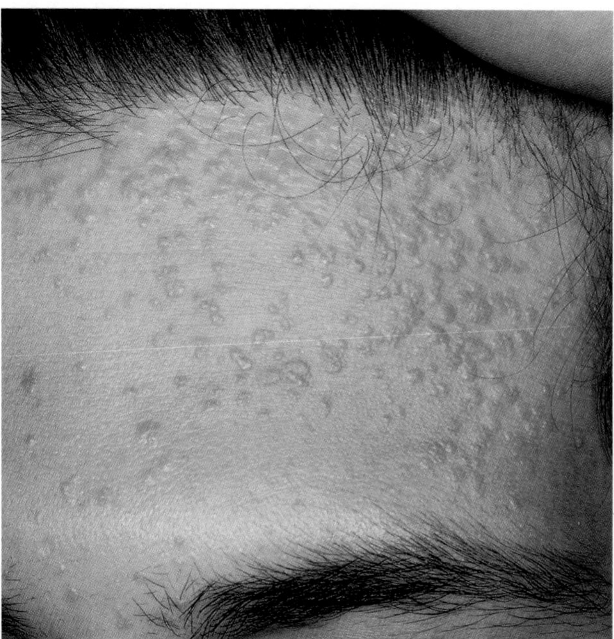

Figure 12-16 Lesions may be numerous and often appear in a linear distribution as a result of scratching.

Plantar warts

Warts of the soles are called plantar warts. Patients may, incorrectly, refer to warts on any surface as plantar warts. Plantar warts frequently occur at points of maximum pressure, such as over the heads of the metatarsal bones or on the heels (Figure 12-17). A thick, painful callus forms in response to pressure and the foot is repositioned while walking. This may result in distortion of posture and pain in other parts of the foot, leg, or back. A little wart can cause a lot of trouble.

Warts may appear anywhere on the plantar surface. A cluster of many warts that appears to fuse is referred to as a mosaic wart (Figure 12-18).

DIFFERENTIAL DIAGNOSIS

Corns. Corns are a mechanically induced lesion that forms over or under a weight-bearing surface or structure. Corns (clavi) over the metatarsal heads are frequently mistaken for warts. The two entities can be easily distinguished by paring the callus with a #15 surgical blade. Warts lack skin lines that cross their surface and have centrally located black dots that bleed with additional paring. Examination with a hand lens shows a highly organized mosaic pattern on the surface (see Figure 12-4). Clavi or corns also lack skin lines crossing the surface, but they have a hard, painful, well-demarcated, translucent central core (Figure 12-19, *A*). The core or kernel can be removed easily by inserting the point of a #15 surgical blade into the cleavage plane between normal skin and the core, holding the scalpel vertically, and smoothly drawing the blade circumferentially. The hard kernel is freed by drawing the blade horizontally through the base to reveal a deep depression. Pain is greatly relieved by this simple procedure. Lateral pressure on a wart causes pain, but pinching a plantar corn is painless.

The treatment of corns is targeted at reducing the friction or pressure at a specific location. This can be accomplished with orthotic therapy and/or surgical correction of the osseous deformity creating the mechanical pressure point. Podiatric or orthopedic surgeons familiar with biomechanics and reconstructive surgery perform these corrective procedures.

Black heel. Horizontally arranged clusters of blue-black dots (ruptured capillaries or petechiae) may appear on the upper edge of the heel or anywhere on the plantar surface following the shearing trauma of sports that involve sudden stops or position changes (Figure 12-20, *A*). It is caused by the shearing force of the epidermis sliding over the rete pegs of the papillary dermis. At first glance, this may be confused with a wart or acral-lentiginous melanoma, but closer examination reveals normal skin lines, and paring does not cause additional bleeding (Figure 12-20, *B*). The condition resolves spontaneously in a few weeks.

Black warts. Warts in the process of undergoing spontaneous resolution, particularly on the plantar surface, may turn black (Figure 12-21) and feel soft when pared with a blade. Cell-mediated immunity against virus-infected keratinocytes may take place in the process of regression of some warts.

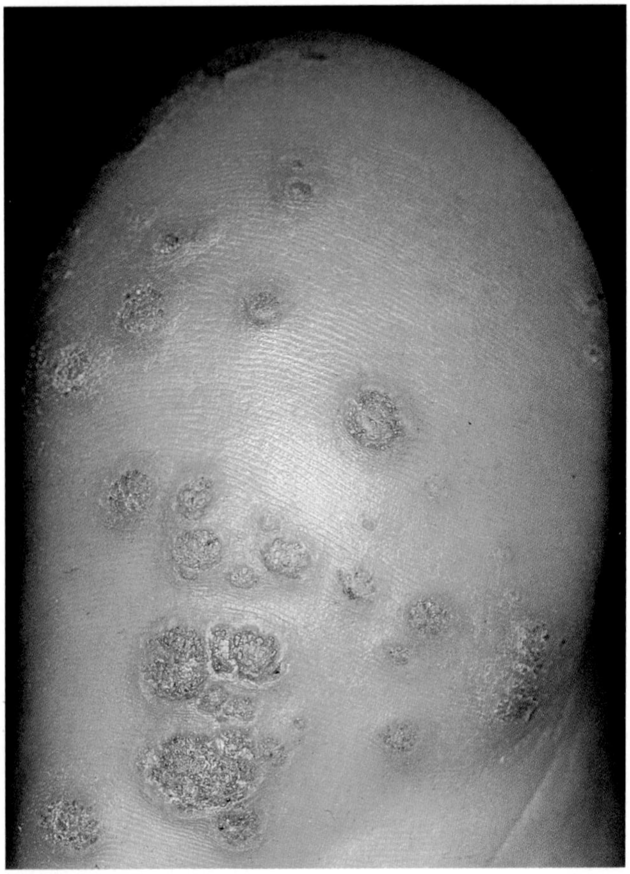

Figure 12-17 Plantar warts. Warts on weight-bearing surfaces accumulate callus and may become painful.

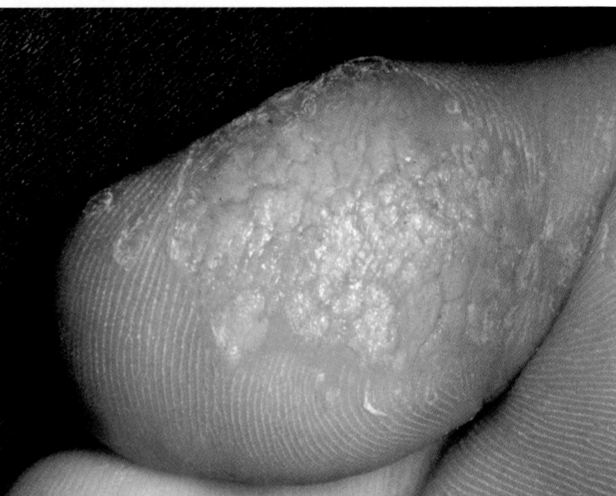

Figure 12-18 Plantar wart. Fusion of numerous small warts to form a mosaic wart. Examination with a hand lens shows a highly organized mosaic pattern on the surface.

DEBRIDEMENT OF CORNS

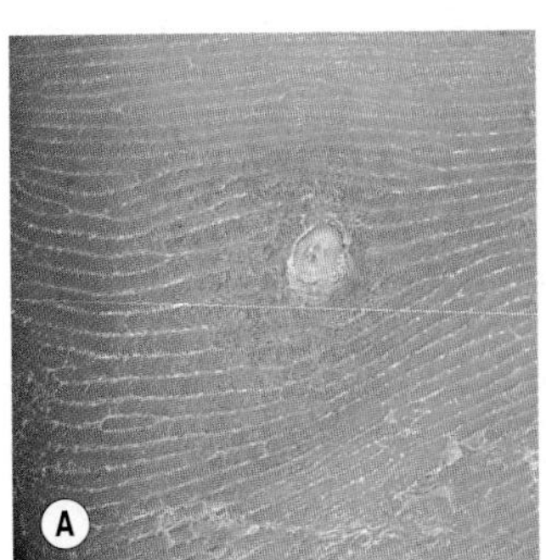

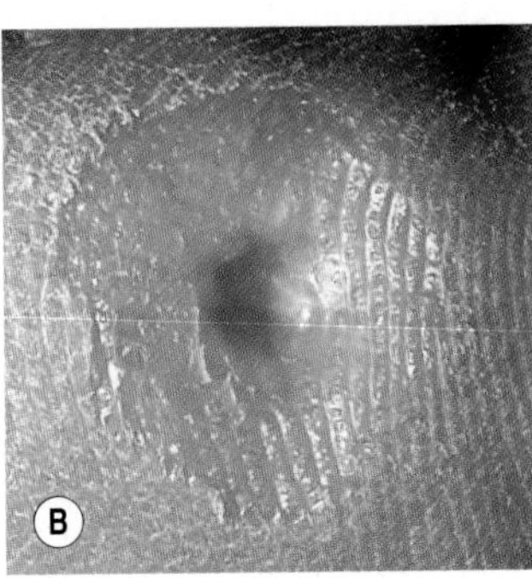

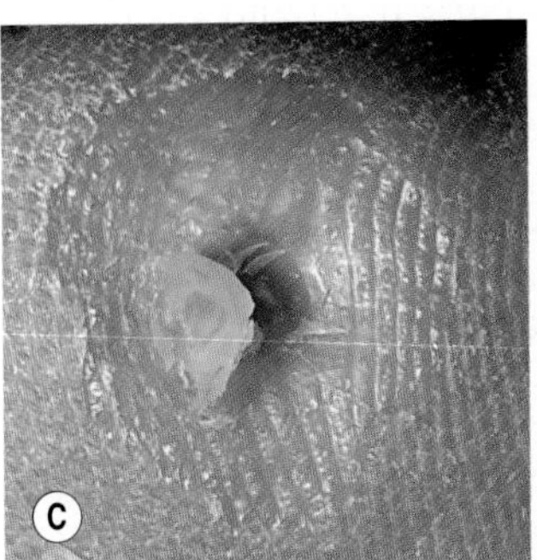

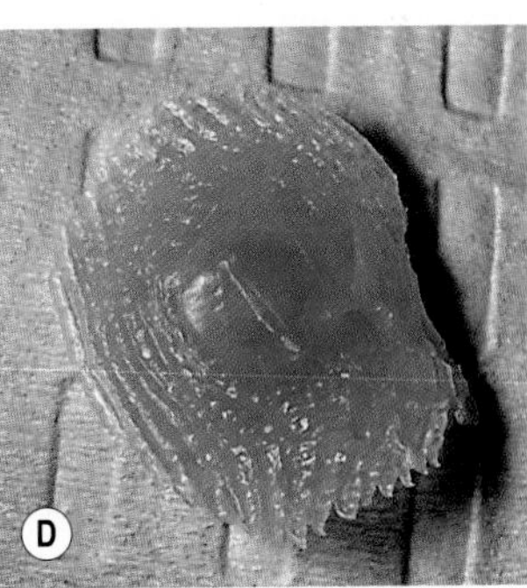

Figure 12-19 **A,** Corns (clavi) on the plantar surface are frequently mistaken for warts. **B,** Plantar surface depicted in **A** with soft and hard callus removed from the corn to reveal a deep depression. Examination with a hand lens shows no organized surface pattern as is seen in a plantar wart. **C** and **D** show the hard callus that was removed.

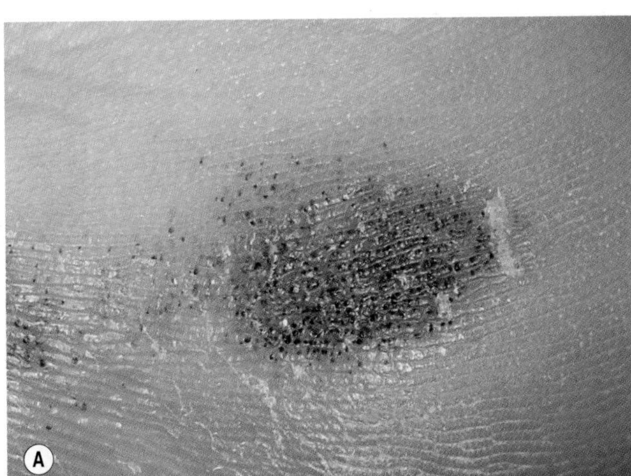

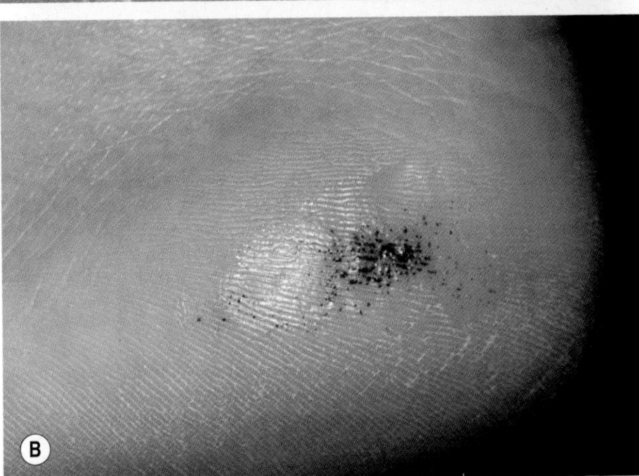

Figure 12-20 **A,** Black heel. Trauma causes capillaries to shear, resulting in a group of black dots; appearance may be confused with warts. **B,** Paring the skin over the black dots in **A** reveals normal skin lines, proving that a wart is not present.

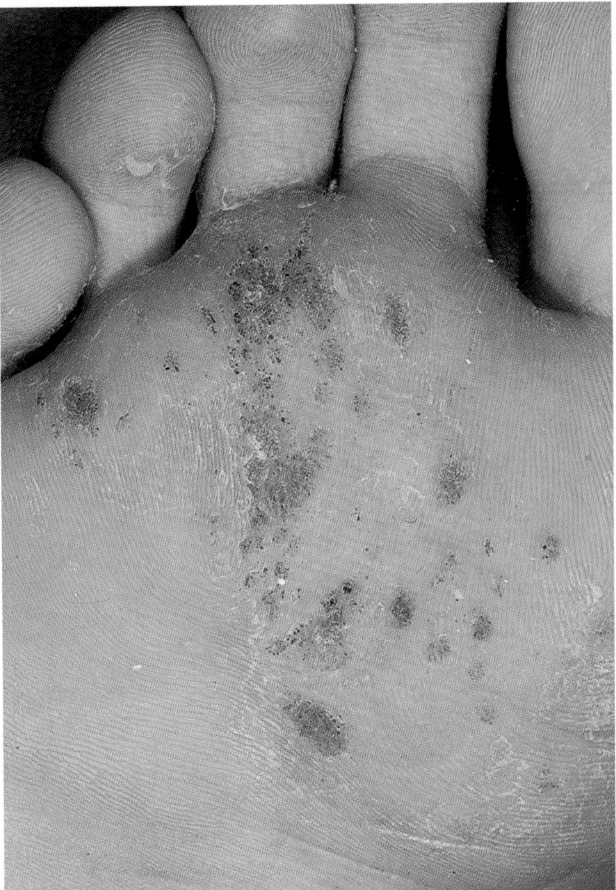

Figure 12-21 Spontaneous resolution. Warts in the process of resolving may be painful and turn black. They are easily removed without anesthesia by using a curette.

TREATMENT. Plantar warts do not require therapy as long as they are painless. Although their number may increase, it is sometimes best to explain the natural history of the virus infection and wait for resolution rather than subject the patient to a long treatment program. Minimal discomfort can be relieved by periodically removing the callus with a blade or pumice stone.

Painful warts must be treated (Figures 12-22 and 12-23). A technique that does not cause scarring should be used; scars on the soles of the feet may be painful for years.

DEBRIDEMENT. It is very important to debride the hyperkeratotic tissue over and around plantar warts to ensure that the medication can penetrate. This may require seeing the patient every 2 to 3 weeks.

COMBINATION THERAPY. Multiple simultaneous techniques are often required to successfully treat plantar warts and may include the following regimens.

Keratolytic therapy (salicylic acid liquid). Keratolytic therapy with salicylic acid (over-the-counter) is conservative initial therapy for plantar warts. The treatment is nonscarring and relatively effective but requires persistent application of medication once each day for many weeks.

The wart is pared with a blade, pumice stone, or sandpaper (emery board). The affected area is soaked in warm water to hydrate the keratin surface; this facilitates penetration of the medicine. A drop of solution is applied with the applicator and allowed to dry. Solution may be added as needed to cover the entire surface of the wart. Penetration of the acid mixture is enhanced if the treated wart is covered with a piece of adhesive tape. Inflammation and soreness may follow tape occlusion, necessitating periodic interruption of treatment; consequently, the patient may be satisfied with the longer, more comfortable process of simply applying the solution at bedtime. White, pliable keratin forms in a few days and should be pared with a blade or worn away with abrasives such as sandpaper or a pumice stone. Ideally, the white keratin should be removed to expose pink skin; to accomplish this, an occasional visit to the office may be necessary.

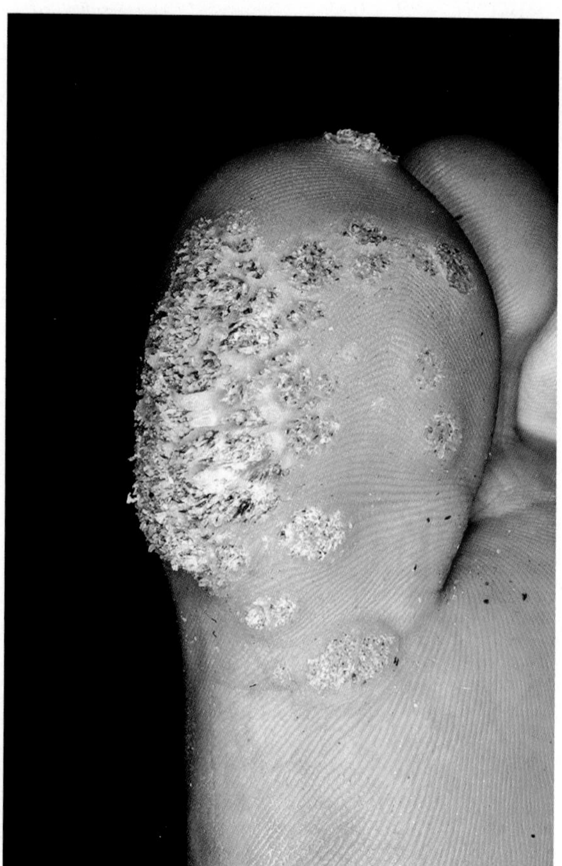

Figure 12-22 Plantar wart. This large mosaic wart is not on a pressure area. It has very long projections. Cryosurgery combined with other treatments would be appropriate.

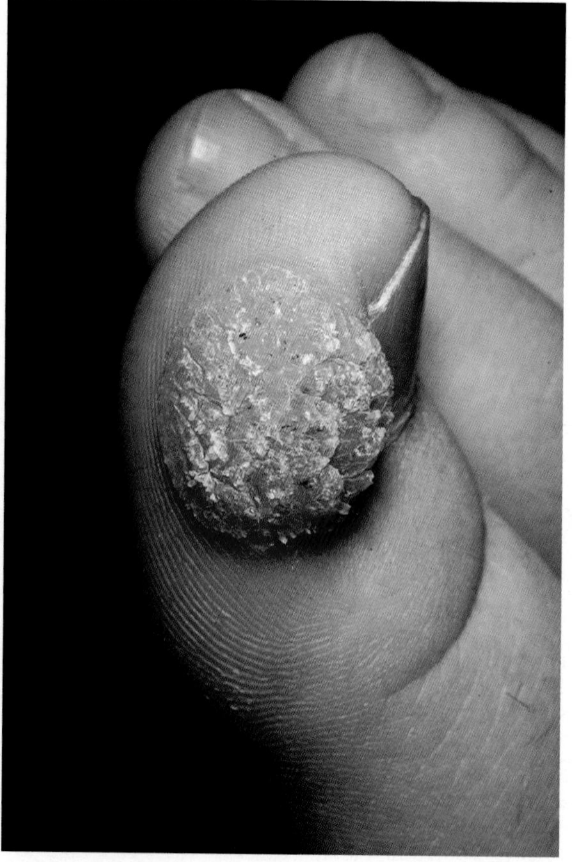

Figure 12-23 Plantar wart. Warts on the plantar surface are elevated and exophytic like common warts in other locations and could be treated with cryosurgery and other techniques.

Keratolytic therapy (40% salicylic acid plasters). This is a safe, nonscarring treatment similar to keratolytic therapy with salicylic acid liquid except the salicylic acid has been incorporated into a pad. Salicylic acid plasters are particularly useful in treating mosaic warts that cover a large area.

The plaster is cut to the size of the wart. The backing of the plaster is removed and the sticky surface is applied to the wart and secured with tape. The plaster is removed in 24 to 48 hours, the pliable white keratin is reduced in the manner previously described, and another plaster is applied. The treatment requires many weeks, but it is effective and less irritating than salicylic acid and lactic acid liquid. Pain is relieved because a large amount of keratin is removed during the first few days of treatment.

Apple cider vinegar. Many people claim success with this technique. Dip the wart in vinegar for 20 minutes. Apply Vaseline around the wart to protect the skin. Soak a small piece of cotton in vinegar and tape it to the wart overnight. Repeat each night until the wart is gone.

Blunt dissection. Blunt dissection is a surgical alternative that is fast, effective (90% cure rate), and usually nonscarring. It is superior to both electrodesiccation-curettage and excision because normal tissue is not disturbed. (See Chapter 27 for surgical techniques.)

Imiquimod. The immunomodulating drug imiquimod (Aldara cream) is more effective on thicker keratinized (nongenital) skin when occluded and used in combination with cryotherapy or a keratolytic agent. It is essential to debride the thick scale before applying imiquimod. The patient applies the cream daily and covers with tape (for ≥12 hours) to enhance penetration. Response to the use of imiquimod on the plantar surface is usually not preceded by an inflammatory reaction.

Suggestive therapy. Suggestive therapy generally works through the age of 10 years. A banana peel, potato eye, or a penny applied to the skin and covered with tape for a 1- to 2-week period has been effective in young children. Another technique is to draw the body part on a piece of paper and then draw a picture of the wart on the diagram. Crumble the pictures and throw them in the wastebasket.

Cantharidin. Cantharidin mixtures are very effective for plantar warts. Apply Canthacur PS (cantharone plus podophyllin 5% plus salicylic acid 30%) in the office and allow to dry. Avoid touching normal skin. Cover with occlusive tape (e.g., Blenderm) or moleskin and remove in 24 hours, or earlier if there is significant discomfort. A blister usually appears. Patients can relieve pain by breaking the blister. Patients may apply moleskin or felt padding around but not over the lesion to reduce pressure. In 2 to 3 days, remove the blister by excising with a scissors or using a curette after administering a local anesthestic. Repeat weekly if necessary.

Laser. Various lasers are available for treating resistant warts. The procedure is expensive and at times painful.

Chemotherapy. For years a variety of acids have been successfully used to treat plantar warts. This technique is occasionally used to treat warts that have recurred after treatment with other techniques and is occasionally used as initial therapy. Like keratolytic therapy, repeated application is required. Home application of acids is too dangerous; therefore weekly or biweekly visits to the office are required. A number of acids may be used (bichloroacetic acid is commercially available).

Treatment is as follows. The excess callus is pared. The surrounding area is protected with petrolatum. The entire lesion is coated with acid and the acid is worked into the wart with a sharp toothpick. This procedure is repeated every 7 to 10 days.

Formalin. This may be considered for resistant cases. Mosaic warts or other large involved areas may be treated with daily soaking for 30 minutes in 4% formalin solution. The firm, fixed tissue is pared before subsequent soaking. Lazerformaldehyde solution (10% formaldehyde) is commercially available for direct application to warts. There is a risk of inducing sensitization to formalin.

Cryosurgery. Cryosurgery on the sole may produce a deep, painful blister and interfere with mobility. Repeated light applications of liquid nitrogen are preferred to aggressive treatment. Cryotherapy is equally effective when applied with a cotton wool bud or by means of a spray. A surgical blade is used to debulk the wart before freezing. Liquid nitrogen is applied until ice-ball formation has spread from the center to include a margin of 2 mm around each wart. A double or triple freeze-thaw cycle may be more effective than a single freeze. Treatment is given every 2 to 4 weeks for up to 3 months.

Subungual and periungual warts

Subungual and periungual warts (Figures 12-24 and 12-25) are more resistant to both chemical and surgical methods of treatment than are warts located in other areas. A wart next to the nail may simply be the tip of the iceberg; much more of the wart may be submerged under the nail.

TREATMENT. The tips of the fingers and toes are a confined area. Therapeutic measures that cause inflammation and swelling, such as cryosurgery, may produce considerable pain.

Cryosurgery. Small periungual warts respond to conservative cryosurgery; warts that extend under the nail do not respond. The use of aggressive cryosurgery over superficial nerves on the volar or lateral aspects of the proximal phalanges of the fingers has caused neuropathy. Permanent nail changes may occur if the nail matrix is frozen.

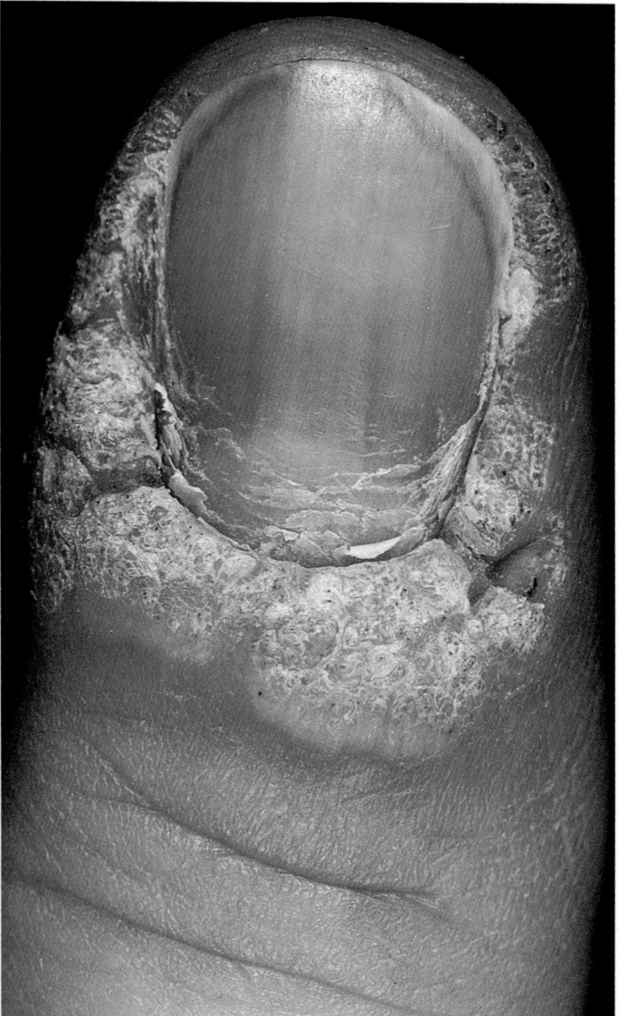

Figure 12-24 Periungual wart. Warts may extend under a nail. Cuticle biting may spread warts.

Cantharidin. Cantharidin (Cantharone) causes blister formation at the dermoepidermal junction but does not cause scarring. Adverse effects are postinflammatory hyperpigmentation, painful blistering, and dissemination of warts to the area of blistering.

In treatment, the solution is applied to the surface and allowed to dry. The patient is seen 1 week later for evaluation. Blisters are opened and the remaining wart is retreated. If blistering does not occur, then cantharidin is applied in one to three layers and covered with tape for 48 hours. Each layer should be dry before the next application of cantharidin. The treatment is very effective for some patients, but there are some warts that do not respond to repeated applications.

Keratolytic preparations. The same procedures described for treating plantar warts with salicylic acid and lactic acid paint and salicylic acid plasters are useful for periungual warts.

Blunt dissection. When conventional measures fail, blunt dissection offers an excellent surgical alternative (see Chapter 27). Local anesthesia is induced with 2% lidocaine without epinephrine around and under small warts. A digital block is required for larger warts. Hemostasis during the procedure is maintained by firm pressure over the digital arteries or with a rubber-band tourniquet. The nail should be removed only if the wart is very large and imbedded. The procedure is exactly the same as that described for blunt dissection of plantar warts.

Duct tape occlusion. Duct tape occlusion therapy may be more effective than cryotherapy for common warts. To completely cover the wart, the tip of the finger is wrapped with duct tape. The tape remains in place for 6 days, is removed at home, is then reapplied in a similar manner 12 hours later, and remains in place for an additional 6 days. This procedure is repeated for up to 2 months.

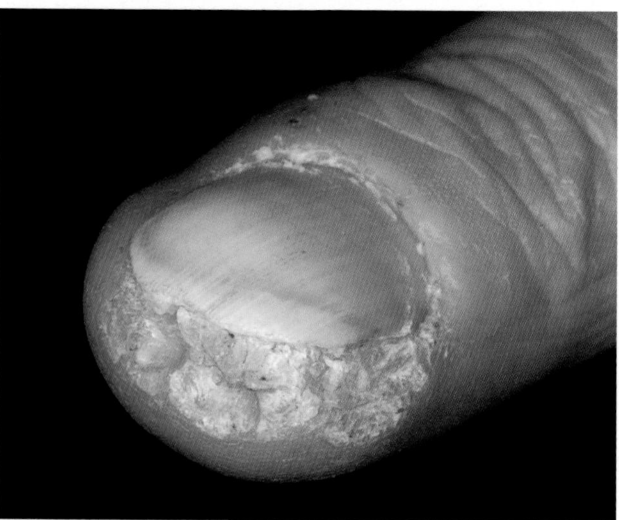

Figure 12-25 Periungual warts may extend deep under the nail.

MOLLUSCUM CONTAGIOSUM

CLINICAL MANIFESTATIONS. Molluscum contagiosum is a double-stranded DNA poxvirus infection of the skin characterized by discrete, 2- to 5-mm, slightly umbilicated, flesh-colored, dome-shaped papules (Figure 12-26). It spreads via autoinoculation, scratching, or touching a lesion and fomites. The areas most commonly involved are the face (Figure 12-27), trunk, axillae, extremities in children, and the pubic and genital areas in adults. Lesions are frequently grouped; there may be few or many covering a wide area. Unlike warts, the palms and soles are not involved. It is not uncommon to see erythema and scaling at the periphery of a single lesion or several lesions. This may be the result of inflammation from scratching or may be a hypersensitivity reaction. Lesions spread to inflamed skin, such as areas of atopic dermatitis (Figure 12-28). The individual lesion begins as a smooth, dome-shaped, white- to flesh-colored papule. With time, the center becomes soft and umbilicated. Most lesions are self-limiting and clear spontaneously in 6 to 9 months; however, they may last 2 to 4 years or longer. Genital molluscum contagiosum may be a manifestation of sexual abuse in children.

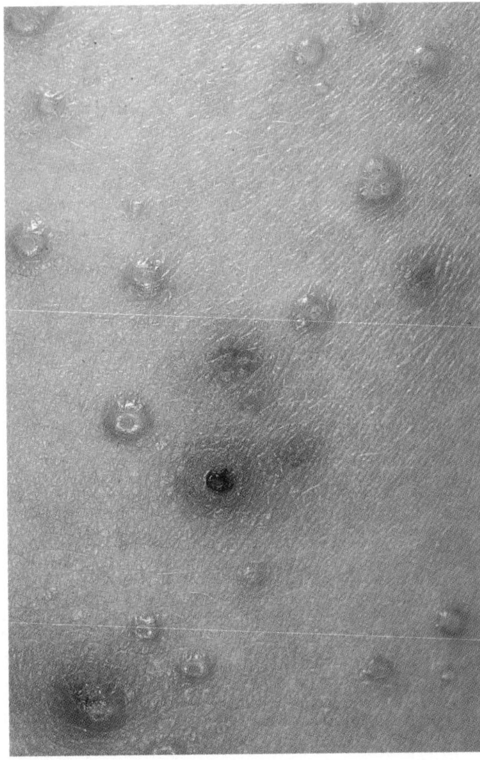

Figure 12-26 Molluscum contagiosum. Individual lesions are

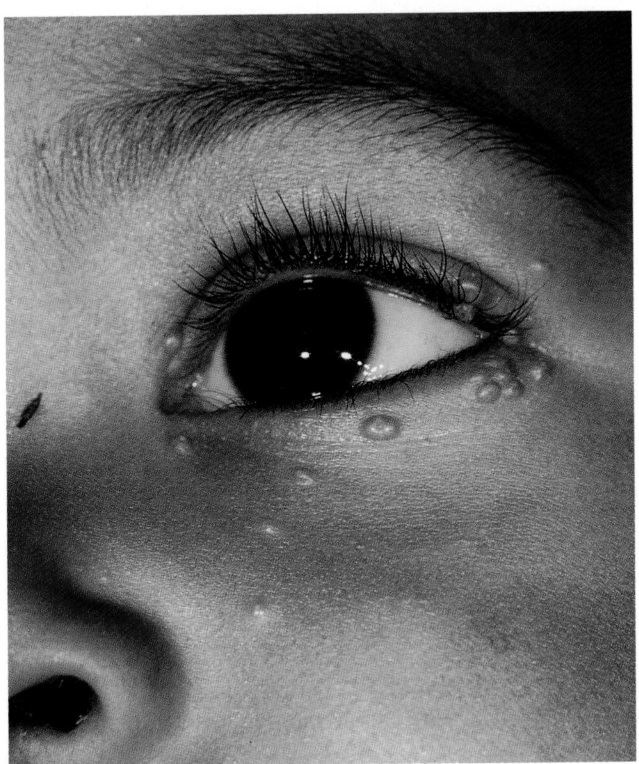

Figure 12-27 Molluscum contagiosum. Inoculation around

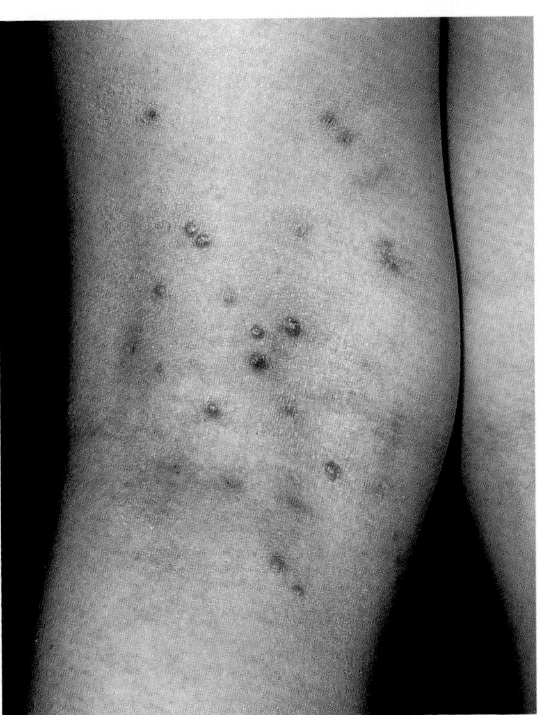

Figure 12-28 Molluscum contagiosum spreads rapidly in eczematous skin. This patient has atopic dermatitis of the popliteal fossa.

MOLLUSCUM CONTAGIOSUM IN HIV-INFECTED PATIENTS. Molluscum contagiosum is a common and at times severely disfiguring cutaneous viral infection in patients with HIV. Atypical facial lesions occur with either multiple small papules or giant nodular tumors. Cutaneous cryptococcosis may resemble molluscum contagiosum in AIDS patients. Cytologic examination of skin brushing reveals encapsulated budding yeasts. An inverse relation between CD4+ count and the number of molluscum contagiosum lesions is observed.

DIAGNOSIS. If necessary the diagnosis can be established easily with laboratory methods. The virus infects epithelial cells, creating very large intracytoplasmic inclusion bodies and disrupting cell bonds by which epithelial cells are generally held together. This lack of adhesion causes the central core of the lesion to be soft. Rapid confirmation can be made by removing a small lesion with a curette and placing it with a drop of potassium hydroxide between two microscope slides. The preparation is gently heated and then crushed with firm, twisting pressure. Larger umbilicated papules have a soft center, the contents of which can be obtained by scooping with a needle. This material contains only infected cells and can be examined directly in a heated potassium hydroxide preparation. The infected cells are dark and round and disperse easily with slight pressure, whereas normal epithelial cells are flat and rectangular and tend to remain stuck together in sheets. Virions streaming out of the amorphous mass can be seen if Sedi-Stain, a supravital stain used to stain urine sediments, is used. Toluidine blue gives the same results. Viral inclusions (large, eosinophilic, round, intracytoplasmic bodies) are easily seen in a fixed and stained biopsy specimen.

TREATMENT. Treatment must be individualized. Conservative nonscarring methods should be used for children who have many lesions. Genital lesions in adults should be definitively treated to prevent spread by sexual contact (see Chapter 11). New lesions that are too small to be detected may appear after treatment and may require additional attention. Topical corticosteroids are used to treat dermatitis near or involving the lesions.

Curettage. Small papules can be quickly removed with a curette and without local anesthesia in adults. Children might tolerate curettage after using a lidocaine/prilocaine cream (EMLA) for analgesia. The cream is applied 30 to 60 minutes before treatment. Bleeding is controlled with gauze pressure. Monsel's solution is painful to use in an unanesthetized area in children. Curettage is useful when there are a few lesions because it provides the quickest, most reliable treatment. A small scar may form; therefore this technique should be avoided in cosmetically important areas.

Cryosurgery. Cryosurgery is the treatment of choice for patients who do not object to the pain. Most children will not tolerate cryosurgery. The papule is touched lightly with a nitrogen-bathed cotton swab or spray until the advancing, white, frozen border has progressed to form a 1-mm halo on the normal skin surrounding the lesion. This should take approximately 5 seconds. This conservative method destroys most lesions in one to three treatment sessions at 1- or 2-week intervals and rarely produces a scar.

Cantharidin. Cantharidin, a chemovesicant extract from the blister beetle, is very effective, well tolerated, and safe in children. It penetrates the epidermis and induces vesiculation through acantholysis. Cantharidin is sparingly applied to each nonfacial lesion with the blunt wooden end of a cotton-tipped applicator. Contact with surrounding skin is avoided, and a maximum of 20 lesions are treated per visit. The treated areas are washed with soap and water after 4 to 6 hours, or sooner if burning, discomfort, or vesiculation occurs; therapy is repeated at 2- to 4-week intervals. Lesions blister and may clear without scarring. Occasionally, new lesions appear at the site of the blister created with cantharidin. Blistering and pain are mild to moderate. Pitted shallow depressions sometimes occur.

Imiquimod. Nightly application of the immunomodulatory drug imiquimod (Aldara cream) has been reported to be effective in both immunocompromised and immunocompetent children and adults. The cream is applied for several weeks.

Potassium hydroxide 5%. Parents are instructed to apply the pharmacist-prepared solution twice daily with a cotton swab. A brief stinging may occur shortly after the application. Most lesions clear in 4 weeks.

Podophyllotoxin 0.5%. The daily application of podophyllotoxin 0.5% (Condylox) may be tried for cases resistant to other therapies.

Hypoallergenic surgical adhesive tape. Tape is applied once each day after showering and is used each day until the lesion ruptures and the core is discharged. The average time to clearance is 16 weeks.

Salicylic acid. Salicylic acid (Occlusal) applied each day without tape occlusion may cause irritation and encourage resolution.

Laser therapy. Lesions on the genital area may be treated with the carbon dioxide laser.

Trichloroacetic acid peel in immunocompromised patients. Patients with HIV infection who have extensive facial molluscum contagiosum infection were treated with trichloroacetic acid peels. Peels were performed with 25% to 50% trichloroacetic acid (average, 35%) and were repeated every 2 weeks as needed. A total of 15 peels were performed with an average reduction in lesion counts of 40.5% (range, 0% to 90%).

HERPES SIMPLEX

Genital herpes simplex virus (HSV) infections are discussed in Chapter 11.

HSV infections are caused by two different virus types (HSV-1 and HSV-2), which can be distinguished by laboratory and office tests. HSV-1 is generally associated with oral infections, and HSV-2 is associated with genital infections. HSV-1 genital infections and HSV-2 oral infections are becoming more common, possibly as a result of oral-genital sexual contact. Both types seem to produce identical patterns of infection. Many infections are asymptomatic, and evidence of previous infection can be detected only by an elevated IgG antibody titer. HSV infections have two phases: the primary infection, after which the virus becomes established in a nerve ganglion; and the secondary phase, characterized by recurrent disease at the same site. The rate of recurrence varies with virus type and anatomic site. Genital recurrences are nearly 6 times more frequent than oral-labial recurrences; genital HSV-2 infections recur more often than genital HSV-1 infections; and oral-labial HSV-1 infections recur more often than oral HSV-2 infections. Infections can occur anywhere on the skin. Infection in one area does not protect the patient from subsequent infection at a different site. Lesions are intraepidermal and usually heal without scarring.

Primary infection

Many primary infections are asymptomatic and can be detected only by an elevated IgG antibody titer. Like most virus infections, the severity of disease increases with age. The virus may be spread via respiratory droplets, direct contact with an active lesion, or contact with virus-containing fluid such as saliva or cervical secretions in patients with no evidence of active disease. Symptoms occur from 3 to 7 or more days after contact. Tenderness, pain, mild paresthesias, or burning occurs before the onset of lesions at the site of inoculation. Localized pain, tender lymphadenopathy, headache, generalized aching, and fever are characteristic prodromal symptoms. Some patients have no prodromal symptoms.

LESIONS

Grouped vesicles on an erythematous base appear and subsequently umbilicate (Figure 12-29). The vesicles in primary herpes simplex (see Figures 12-32 and 12-33) are more numerous and scattered than those in the recurrent infection (see Figures 12-34 and 12-37). The vesicles of herpes simplex are uniform in size in contrast to the vesicles seen in herpes zoster, which vary in size. Mucous membrane lesions accumulate exudate, whereas skin lesions form a crust. Lesions last for 2 to 4 weeks unless secondarily infected and heal without scarring.

The virus replicates at the site of primary infection. Virons are then transported by neurons via retrograde axonal flow to the dorsal root ganglia, and latency is established in the ganglion.

HERPES SIMPLEX—EVOLUTION OF LESIONS

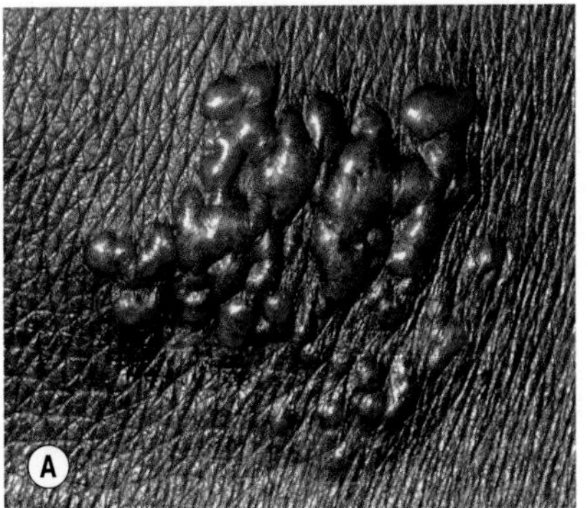

Vesicles on a red base are the primary lesions.

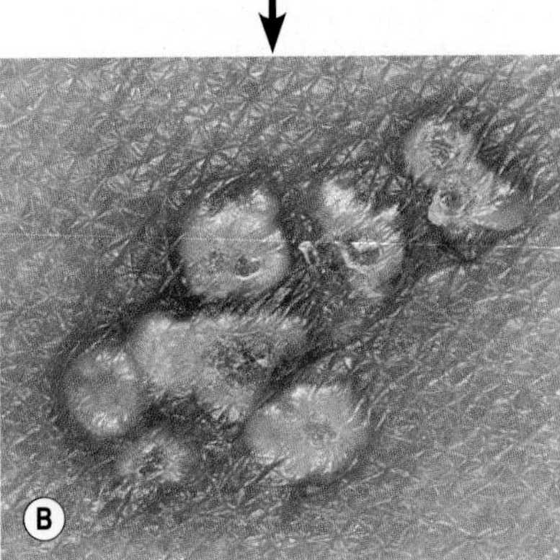

Vesicles evolve to pustules and become umbilicated.

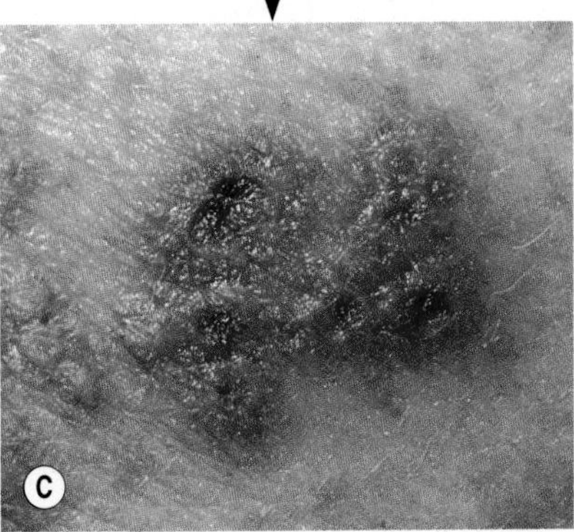

Umbilication becomes more pronounced.

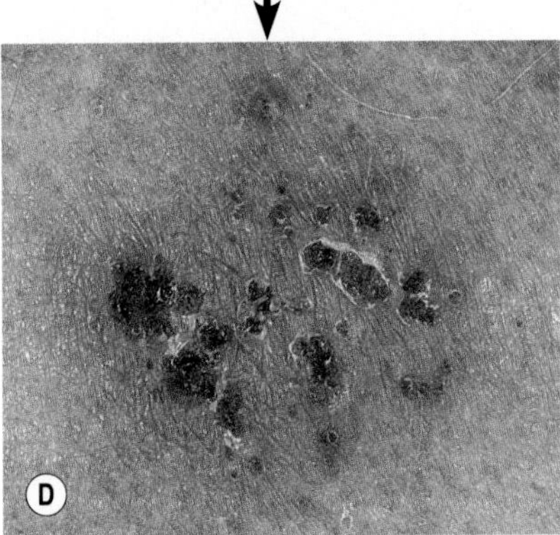

Lesions dry and form discrete crusts.

Figure 12-29

Recurrent infection

Local skin trauma (e.g., ultraviolet light exposure, chapping, abrasion) or systemic changes (e.g., menses, fatigue, fever) reactivate the virus, which then travels down the peripheral nerves to the site of initial infection and causes the characteristic focal, recurrent infection. Recurrent infection is not inevitable. Many individuals have a rise in antibody titer and never experience recurrence. The prodromal symptoms of itching or burning, lasting 2 to 24 hours, resemble those of the primary infection. Within 12 hours, a group of lesions evolves rapidly from an erythematous base to form papules and then vesicles (Figures 12-30 and 12-31). The dome-shaped, tense vesicles rapidly umbilicate. In 2 to 4 days, they rupture, forming aphthaelike erosions in the mouth and vaginal area or erosions covered by crusts on the lips and skin. Crusts are shed in approximately 8 days to reveal a pink, reepithelialized surface. In contrast to the primary infection, systemic symptoms and lymphadenopathy are rare unless there is secondary infection.

The frequency of recurrence varies with anatomic site and virus type. HSV-1 oral infections recur more often than genital HSV-1 infections; HSV-2 genital infections recur 6 times more frequently than HSV-1 genital infections; and the frequency of recurrence is lowest for oral-labial HSV-2 infections.

LABORATORY DIAGNOSIS. The laboratory diagnosis of herpes simplex is covered in Chapter 11, which discusses sexually transmitted viral infections. Herpes simplex virus detection by rapid polymerase chain reaction (PCR) is the most accurate and reliable method of detecting the virus. Culture and serology are also available.

TREATMENT. A number of measures can be taken to relieve discomfort and promote healing; these are described in the following sections. The appropriate use of topical, oral, and intravenous antiviral agents is outlined (Table 12-2 and Box 12-1). Oral drugs decrease the duration of viral excretion, new lesion formation, and vesicles and promote rapid healing. The subsequent recurrence rate is not influenced by acyclovir. Acyclovir-resistant HSV infections are becoming a problem in patients with AIDS. L-Lysine is not effective.

Table 12-2 Treatment of HSV-1 Oral-Labial Herpes Simplex

Condition	Immunocompetent	Immunocompromised (HIV-infected persons)
Primary herpes	Acyclovir 200 mg five times/day for 7-10 days	
	Acyclovir 400 mg three times/day for 7-10 days	
	Valacyclovir 1 gm twice a day for 7-10 days	
	Famciclovir 250 mg three times/day for 7-10 days	
Recurrent herpes (episodic therapy)	Acyclovir 400 mg three times/day for 5 days	Acyclovir 400 mg five times/day for 7-14 days
	Acyclovir 800 mg two times/day for 5 days	Valacyclovir 1 gm twice a day for 5-10 days
	Acyclovir 800 mg three times/day for 2 days	Famciclovir 500 mg twice a day for 7 days
	Valacyclovir 2 gm twice a day for 1 day	
	Valacyclovir 500 mg twice a day for 3 days	
	Valacyclovir 1 gm once a day for 5 days	
	Famciclovir 125 mg twice a day for 5 days	
	Famciclovir 1500 mg as a single dose	
	Penciclovir 1% cream applied every 2 hr (while awake) for 4 days	
	Acyclovir 5% ointment applied every 3 hr, six times/day for 7 days	
	n-Docosanol (OTC Abreva) applied five times/day until healed	
Recurrent herpes (long-term suppressive therapy)	Acyclovir 400 mg twice a day	Acyclovir 400-800 mg two or three times/day
	Valacyclovir 500 mg once a day for <9 episodes/year	Valacyclovir 500 mg twice a day
	Valacyclovir 1 gm once a day for >10 episodes/year	Famciclovir 500 mg twice a day
	Famciclovir 250 mg twice a day	
Severe disease	Acyclovir 5-10 mg/kg/body weight IV every 8 hr	

RECURRENT INFECTION

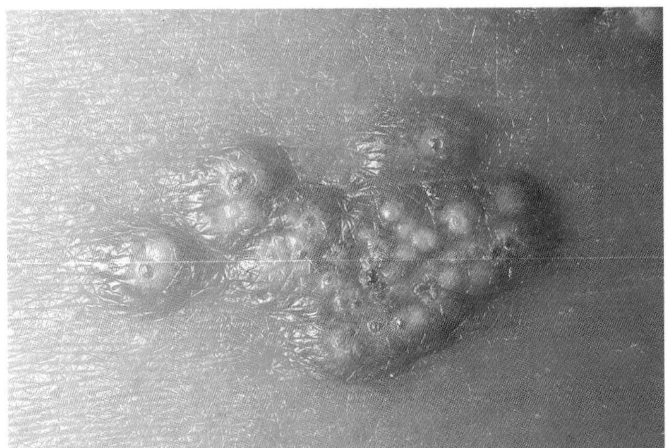

Figure 12-30 The recurrent lesion is a small group of vesicles that, like primary lesions, evolve to form umbilicated pustules and then crusts.

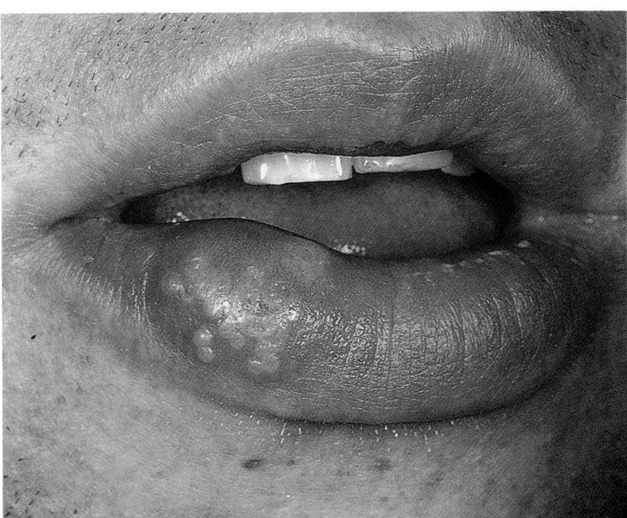

Figure 12-31 A small group of vesicles on an erythematous base are the initial lesion.

Box 12-1 **Recurrent Herpes Simplex Infection (Topical Medication)**
Apply the creams frequently (e.g., every 2 hours)
Acyclovir cream
Penciclovir cream (Denavir)
n-Docosanol cream (Abreva) over-the-counter
Topical corticosteroids plus oral antiviral drug
Famciclovir (500 mg three times a day × 5 days) + topical fluocinonide (0.05% three times a day × 5 days)

Oral-labial herpes simplex

PRIMARY INFECTION

Transmission is dependent on intimate, personal contact with someone excreting HSV. Gingivostomatitis and pharyngitis are the most frequent manifestations of first-episode HSV-1 infection. Infection occurs most commonly in children between ages 1 and 5 years. The incubation period is 3 to 12 days. Although most cases are mild, some are severe. Sore throat and fever may precede the onset of painful vesicles occurring anywhere in the oral cavity or on the face (see Figures 12-32 and 12-33). The vesicles rapidly coalesce and erode with a white, then yellow, superficial, purulent exudate. Children are unable to swallow liquids because of the edema, ulcerations, and pain. Tender cervical lymphadenopathy develops. Fever subsides in 3 to 5 days, and oral pain and erosions are usually gone in 2 weeks; in severe cases, they may last for 3 weeks.

RECURRENT INFECTION

Recurrences average two or three each year but may occur as often as 12 times a year. Oral HSV-1 infections recur more often than oral HSV-2 infections. Recurrent oral herpes simplex can appear as a localized cluster of small ulcers in the oral cavity, but the most common manifestation consists of eruptions on the vermilion border of the lip (recurrent herpes labialis) (Figures 12-34 to 12-37). Fever (fever blisters), upper respiratory tract infections (cold sores), and exposure to ultraviolet light, among other things, may precede the onset. The course of the disease in the oral-labial area is the same as it is in other areas. Immunosuppressed patients are at greater risk of developing lesions on the lips, in the oral cavity, and on surrounding skin. Lesions may also appear on the upper lip and chin. The recurrence rate and long-term natural history are not well-defined. Many people experience a decrease in the frequency of recurrences, but others experience an increase. A history of recurrent herpes labialis is present in 38% of college students. The prevalence of asymptomatic excretion of HSV following recurrence varies from 1% to 5% in adults.

TREATMENT. A number of treatment modalities have been used for herpes on the vermilion border. Oral acyclovir, famciclovir, and valacyclovir can be used to treat the primary infection and episodic recurrences and for suppression (see Table 12-2 and Box 12-1). Oral antiviral drugs have a modest clinical benefit only if initiated very early after recurrence. They may be of value in patients whose recurrences are associated with protracted clinical illness. Oral antiviral drugs can alter the severity of sun-induced reactivation. Short-term prophylactic treatment may help patients who anticipate high-risk activity (e.g., intense sunlight exposure). Intermittent administration does not alter the frequency of subsequent recurrences.

PRIMARY HERPES SIMPLEX LESIONS

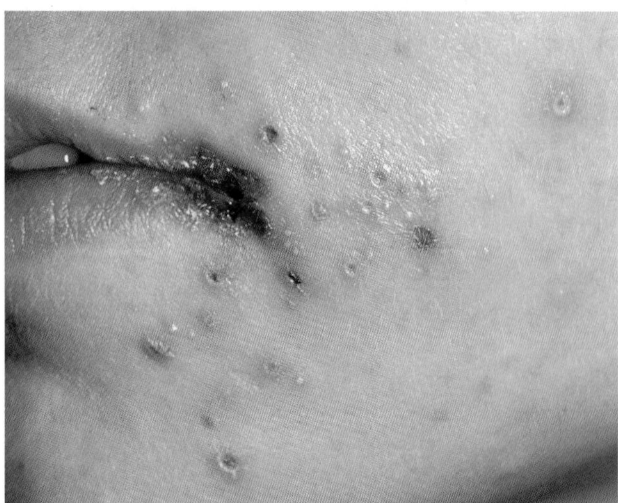

Figure 12-32 The mouth is inflamed. Umbilicated vesicles are widely scattered about the perioral area.

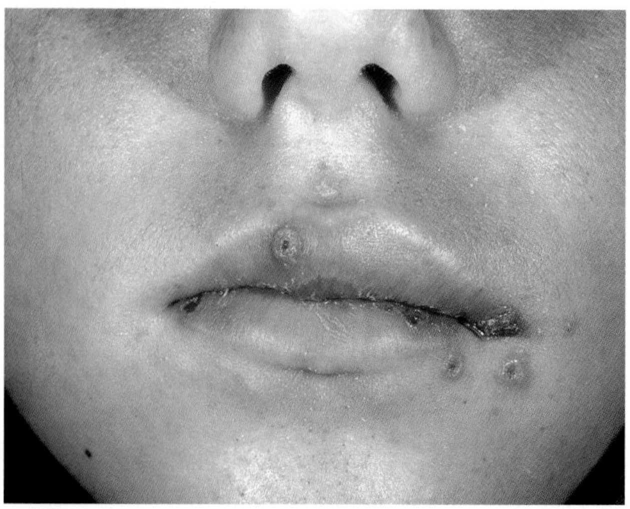

Figure 12-33 The patient is febrile. Lesions are not grouped as in recurrent herpes.

RECURRENT HERPES LESIONS

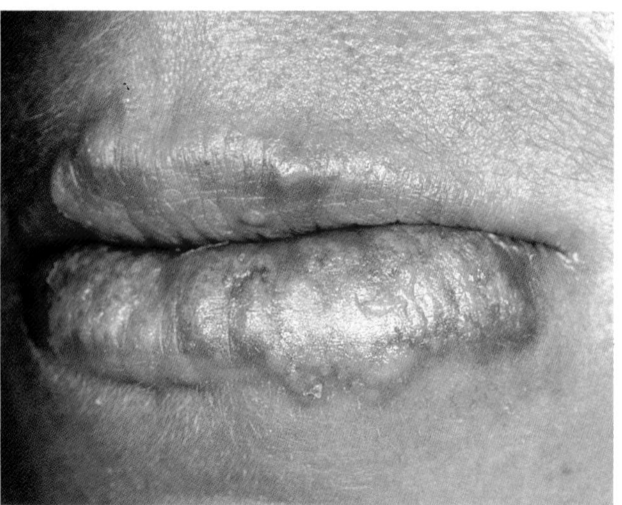

Figure 12-34 The entire surface of the lips is involved in this case stimulated by sun exposure.

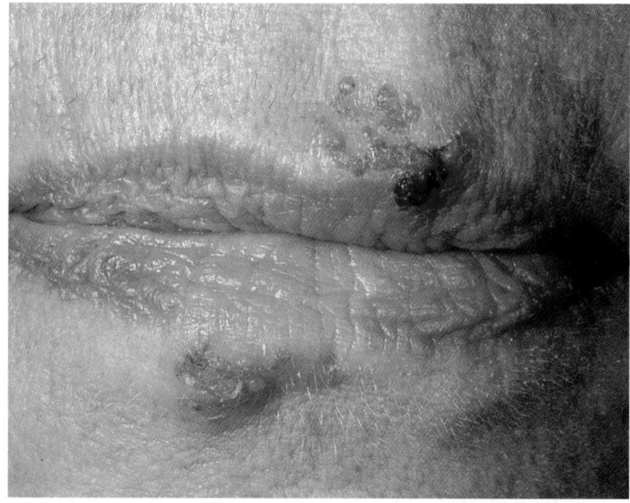

Figure 12-35 The recurrence involves two areas simultaneously.

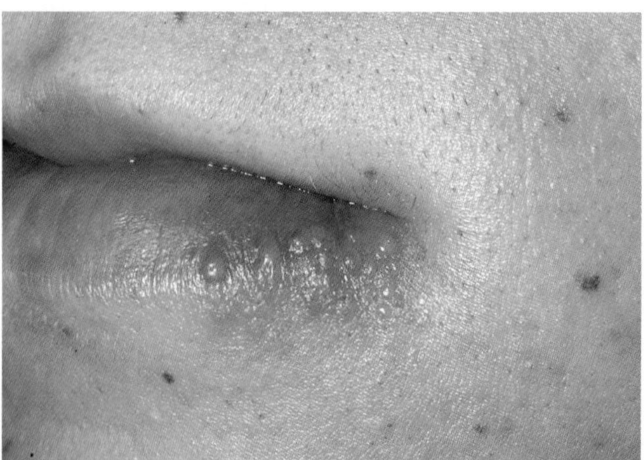

Figure 12-36 Recurrent herpes begins with a prodrome of itching or burning. A group of vesicles appears on an erythematous base. Previous episodes in the same area are typical.

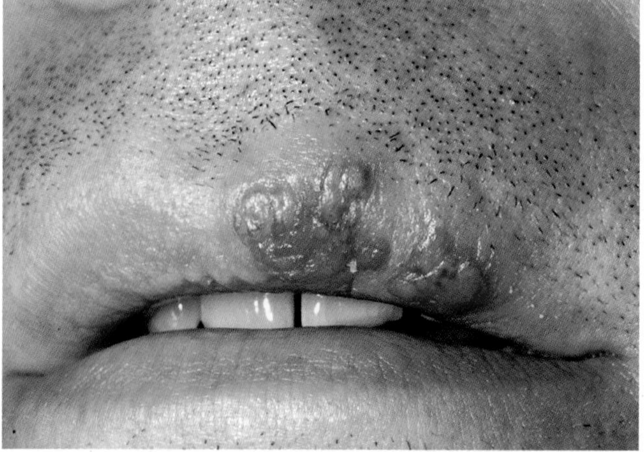

Figure 12-37 Vesicles of recurrent herpes evolve in a few days to form crusts. The diagnosis is suspected because crusts are small, round, and grouped. Previous episodes support the diagnosis.

COMBINATION TREATMENT. Corticosteroids in combination with an oral antiviral agent may be beneficial for episodic treatment of herpes labialis. Famciclovir (500 mg three times a day for 5 days) and topical fluocinonide (0.05% three times a day for 5 days) significantly reduced lesion size and pain.

TOPICAL TREATMENT. Topical treatments include penciclovir cream (Denavir), *n*-docosanol cream (Abreva), and acyclovir cream. Abreva is an over-the-counter drug. The cream is applied frequently (e.g., every 2 hours while awake) at the first sign of prodromal symptoms or erythema. These creams may shorten an episode of herpes labialis by a few hours or a day and may not be worth the high cost. Many patients believe that these creams are effective and prefer them to oral medication.

The lips should be protected from sun exposure with an opaque cream such as zinc oxide or with sun-blocking agents incorporated into a lip balm (e.g., ChapStick). A cool water or Burow's solution compress decreases erythema and debrides crusts to promote healing.

Lubricating creams may be applied if the lips become too dry.

Cutaneous herpes simplex

Herpes simplex may appear on any skin surface (Figures 12-38 and 12-39). It is important to identify all of the characteristic features when attempting to differentiate cutaneous herpes from other vesicular eruptions.

HERPES GLADIATORUM. Cutaneous herpes in athletes involved in contact sports is transmitted via direct skin-to-skin contact. This is a recognized health risk for wrestlers (wrestler's herpes) (Figure 12-40). Prompt identification and exclusion of wrestlers with skin lesions may reduce transmission. Outbreaks may lead to exclusion of athletes from sports events and necessitate prophylactic antiviral therapy throughout the sport season.

OCULAR HERPES. Ocular HSV infection is a cause of corneal blindness. Patients with ocular herpes often report a prior history of primary herpes in the oral cavity. Ocular HSV inoculation may lead to unilateral or bilateral keratoconjunctivitis, recurrent ocular ulcerations, and sight impairment that requires antiviral therapy.

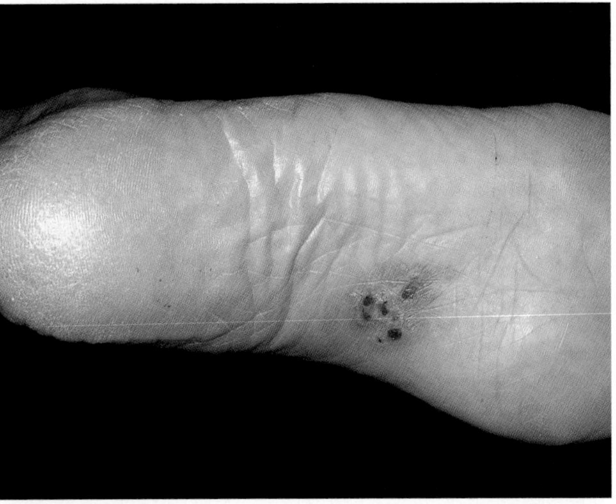

Figure 12-38 Herpes can infect any cutaneous surface. Here the initial diagnosis was a bacterial infection.

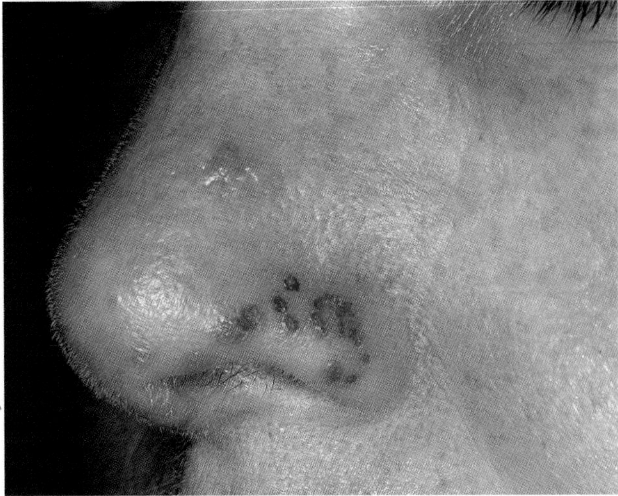

Figure 12-39 This is a typical picture of recurrence. The initial diagnosis was impetigo.

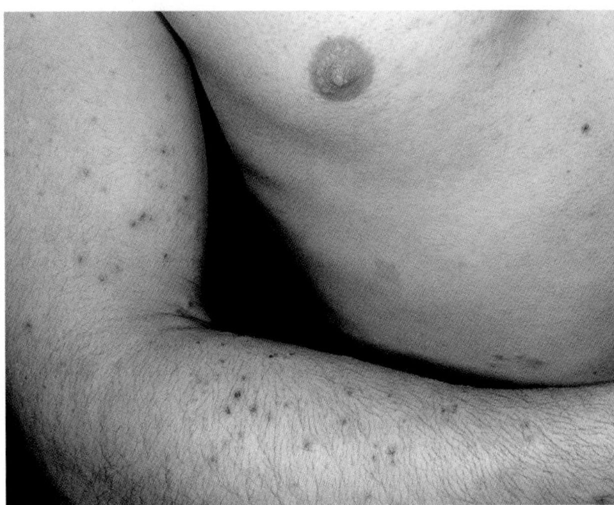

Figure 12-40 Herpes gladiatorum. Lesions may be numerous in wrestlers and involve a wide area of the skin surface.

CUTANEOUS HERPES SIMPLEX

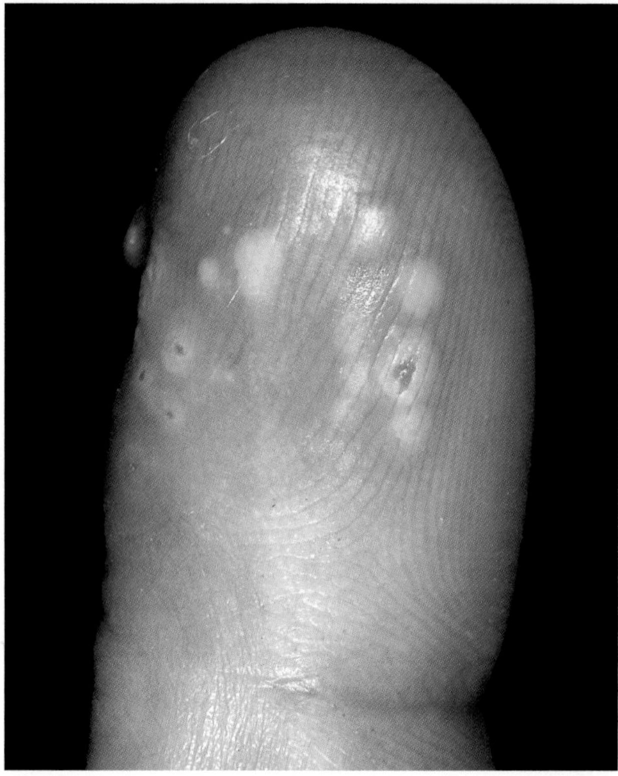

Figure 12-41 Herpetic whitlow. Grouped pustules may be diagnosed as a bacterial infection. Recurrence at the same location was the clue to the diagnosis.

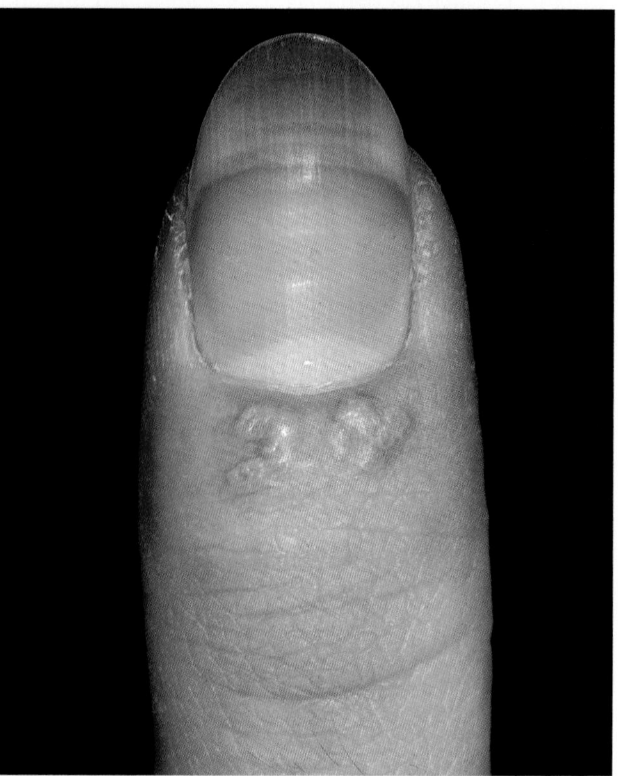

Figure 12-42 Herpetic whitlow. Inoculation followed examination of the patient's mouth.

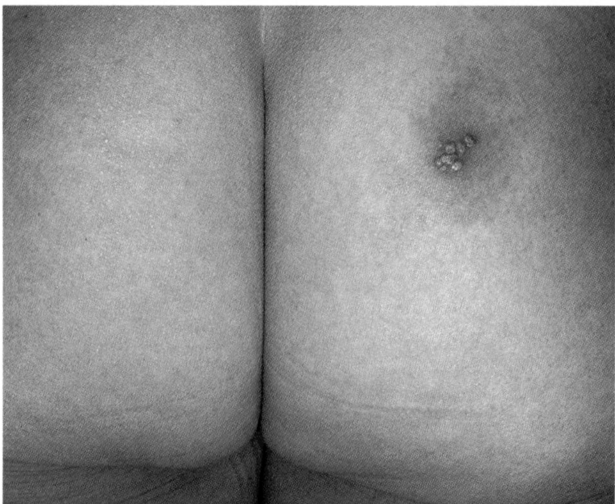

Figure 12-43 Herpes of the buttocks. The diagnosis is suspected because of the classic presenation of recurrent disease with highly characteristic grouped vesicles of uniform size on an erythematous base. This presentation is seen almost exclusively in women. Recurrences may be frequent and very annoying; suppressive therapy can greatly improve the quality of life.

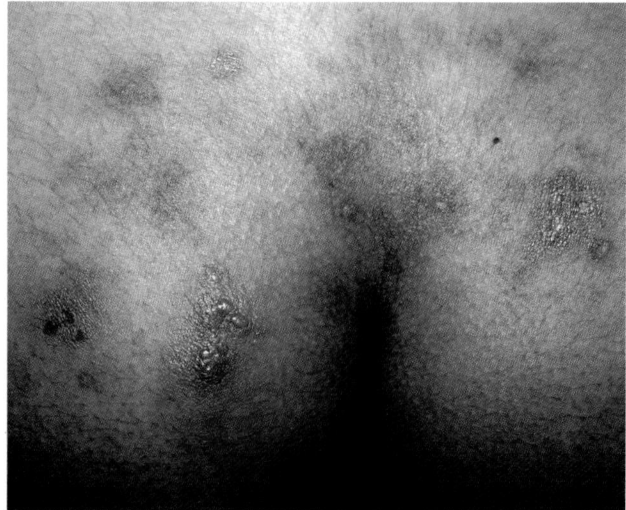

Figure 12-44 Recurrent herpes of the buttocks. Recurrent lesions in the same area that progress from vesicles to crusts make the clinical diagnosis. Patients with herpes of the buttocks may have recurrences in several different areas of the buttocks. Groups of small round scars may be the only evidence of past recurrences.

HERPETIC WHITLOW. Herpetic whitlow is the cutaneous herpetic infection of the pulp of the distal phalanx of the hand. It results from direct inoculation of the involved digit through the abraded skin by either HSV-1 or HSV-2. Herpes simplex of the fingertip (Figures 12-41 and 12-42) can resemble a group of warts or a bacterial infection. Health care professionals who had frequent contact with oral secretions used to be the most commonly affected group; the incidence has decreased, probably as a result of heightened awareness of the condition and stricter infection-control precautions. In young children, it is associated with HSV-1 inoculation through thumb sucking during primary herpetic gingivostomatitis. In adolescents and adults it is associated with digital-genital contact.

HERPES SIMPLEX OF THE BUTTOCK. Herpes simplex of the buttock area is much more common in women (Figures 12-43 and 12-44). The cause of infection in this area has not been identified.

HERPES SIMPLEX OF THE TRUNK. Herpes simplex of the lumbosacral region or trunk may be very difficult to differentiate from herpes zoster; the diagnosis becomes apparent only at the time of recurrence.

TREATMENT. Oral antiviral drugs are useful for suppressive therapy, particularly for recurrent fingertip and buttock infections.

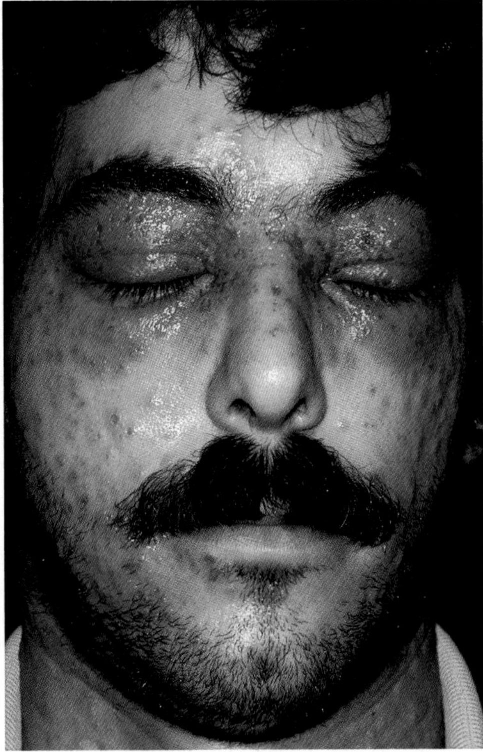

Figure 12-45 Eczema herpeticum. Numerous lesions spread over the face in this patient with active atopic dermatitis.

Eczema herpeticum

Eczema herpeticum (Kaposi's varicelliform eruption) is the association of two common conditions: atopic dermatitis and HSV infection. Certain atopic infants and adults may develop the rapid onset of diffuse cutaneous herpes simplex. The severity of infection ranges from mild and transient to fatal. The disease is most common in areas of active or recently healed atopic dermatitis, particularly the face, but normal skin can be involved. The disease in most cases is a primary HSV infection. In one third of the patients in a particular study, there was a history of herpes labialis in a parent in the previous week. Recurrences are uncommon and usually limited. Approximately 10 days after exposure, numerous vesicles develop, become pustular, and umbilicate markedly (Figures 12-45 and 12-46). Secondary staphylococcal infection commonly occurs. New crops of vesicles may appear during the following weeks. The most intense viral dissemination is located in the areas of dermatitis, but normal appearing skin may ultimately be involved. High fever and adenopathy occur 2 to 3 days after the onset of vesiculation. The fever subsides in 4 to 5 days in uncomplicated cases, and the lesions evolve in the typical manner. Viremia with infection of internal organs can be fatal. Recurrent disease is milder and usually without constitutional symptoms.

TREATMENT. Eczema herpeticum of the young infant is a medical emergency; early treatment with acyclovir can be life-saving. Eczema herpeticum is managed with cool, wet compresses, similar to the management of diffuse genital herpes simplex. Oral dosages of acyclovir 25 to 30 mg/kg/day have been effective. Infants were successfully treated with intravenous acyclovir, 1500 mg/m^2/day administered over a 1-hour period three times/day. Oral antistaphylococcal antibiotics are an important part of treatment. Minor relapses do not require a second course of acyclovir. Adults respond to the standard intravenous acyclovir dosage of 250 mg three times a day. Oral antiviral drugs (see Table 12-2) are expected to be equally effective.

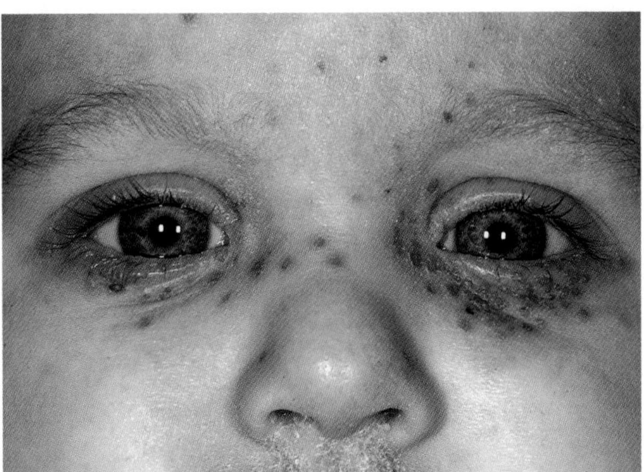

Figure 12-46 Eczema herpeticum. Lesions about the eyes are a common presentation in children.

CHICKENPOX—EVOLUTION OF LESIONS

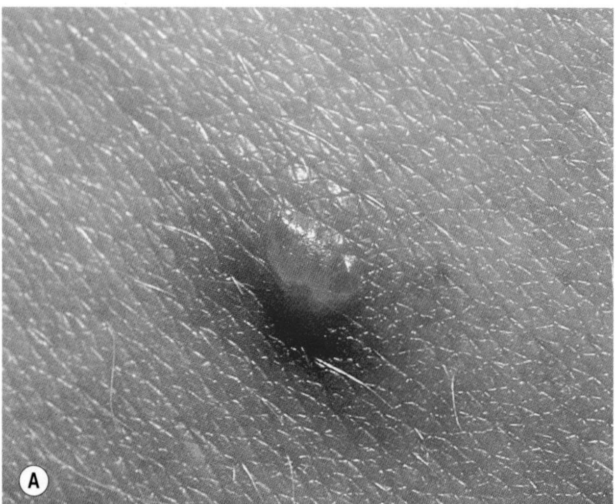

"Dewdrop on a rose petal"; a think-walled vesicle with clear fluid forms on a red base.

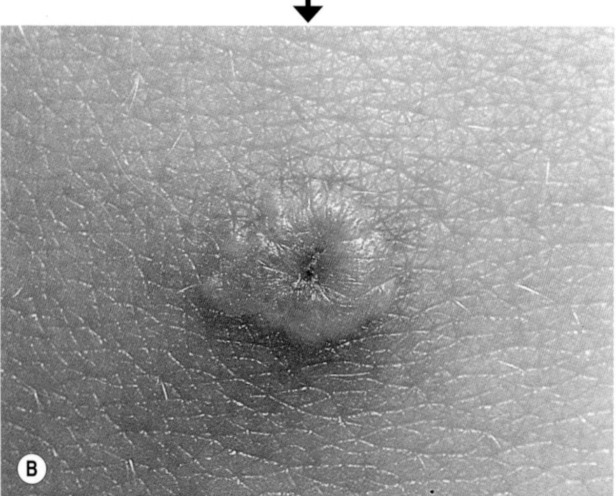

The vesicle becomes cloudy and depressed in the center (umbilicated), the border is irregular (scalloped).

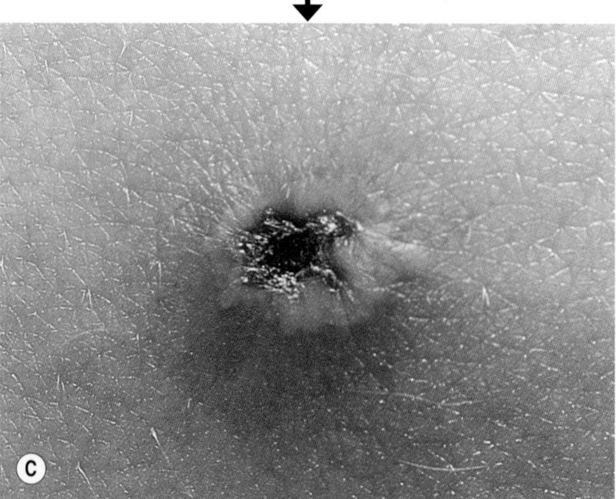

A crust forms in the center and eventually replaces the remaining portion of the vesicle at the periphery.

Figure 12-47

VARICELLA

Varicella, or chickenpox, is a highly contagious viral infection that, during epidemics, affects the majority of urban children before puberty. The incidence peaks sharply in March, April, and May in temperate climates. Transmission occurs via airborne droplets or vesicular fluid. Patients are contagious from 2 days before onset of the rash until all lesions have crusted. The systemic symptoms, extent of eruption, and complications are greater in adults than in children; thus some parents intentionally expose their young children. Patients with defective, cell-mediated immunity or those using immunosuppressive drugs, especially systemic corticosteroids, have a prolonged course with more extensive eruptions and a greater incidence of complications. An attack of chickenpox usually confers lifelong immunity. After it has produced chickenpox, varicella-zoster virus (VZV) becomes latent in ganglia along the entire neuraxis. Unlike HSV, however, VZV cannot be cultured from human ganglia. Varicella vaccine is effective and approved for use in children and adults.

CLINICAL COURSE. The incubation period averages 14 days, with a range of 9 to 21 days; in the immunosuppressed host, the incubation period can be shorter. The prodromal symptoms in children are absent or consist of low fever, headache, and malaise, which appear directly before or with the onset of the eruption. Symptoms are more severe in adults. Fever, chills, malaise, and backache occur 2 to 3 days before the eruption.

ERUPTIVE PHASE. Lesions of different stages are present at the same time in any given body area. New lesion formation ceases by day 4 and most crusting occurs by day 6; the process lasts longer in the immunosuppressed patient. The lesion starts as a 2- to 4-mm red papule that develops an irregular outline (rose petal) as a thin-walled clear vesicle appears on the surface (dewdrop) (Figure 12-47). This lesion, "dewdrop on a rose petal," is highly characteristic. The vesicle becomes umbilicated and cloudy and breaks in 8 to 12 hours to form a crust as the red base disappears. Fresh crops of additional lesions undergoing the same process occur in all areas at irregular intervals during the following 3 to 5 days, giving the characteristic picture of intermingled papules, vesicles, pustules, and crusts. Moderate to intense pruritus is usually present during the vesicular stage. The degree of temperature elevation parallels the extent and severity of the eruption and varies from 101° to 105° F. The temperature returns to normal when the vesicles have disappeared. Crusts fall off in 7 days (with a range of 5 to 20 days) and heal without scarring. Secondary infection or excoriation extends the process into the dermis, producing a craterlike, pockmark scar. Vesicles often form in the oral cavity and vagina and rupture quickly to form multiple, aphthaelike ulcers.

CHICKENPOX—PROGRESSION OF ERUPTION

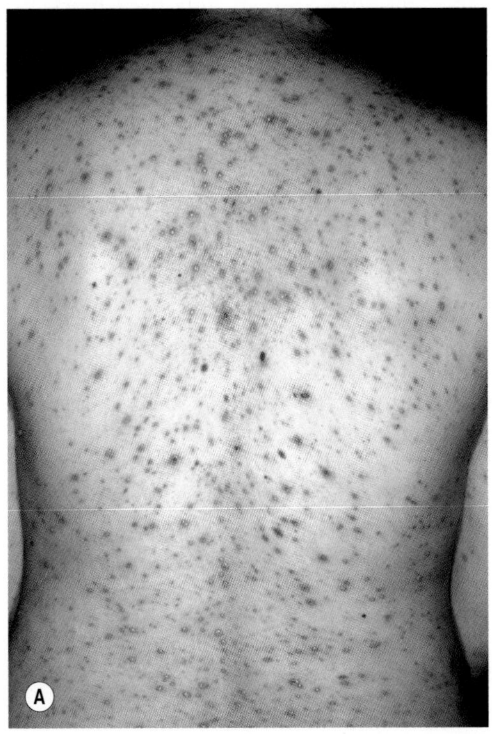

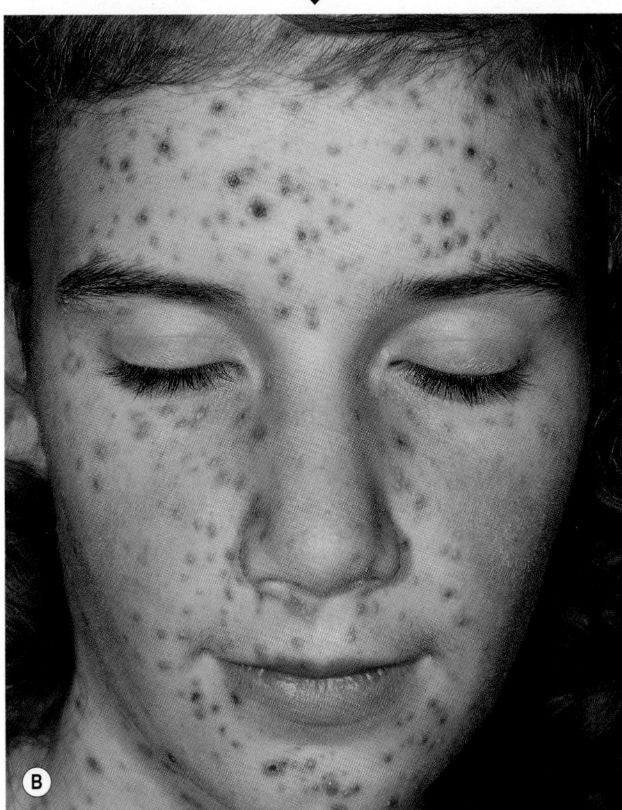

Figure 12-48 The disease starts with lesions on the trunk and then spreads to the face and extremities.

The rash begins on the trunk (centripetal distribution) (Figure 12-48, *A*) and spreads to the face (Figure 12-48, *B*) and extremities (centrifugal spread). The extent of involvement varies considerably. Some children have so few lesions that the disease goes unnoticed. Older children and adults have a more extensive eruption involving all areas, sometimes with lesions too numerous to count.

DIFFERENTIAL DIAGNOSIS. The differential diagnosis includes drug eruptions, smallpox, other viral exanthemas, scabies, erythema multiforme, and insect bites.

COMPLICATIONS

Skin infection. The most common complication in children is bacterial skin infection (Figure 12-49). Secondary infection should be suspected when the vesiculopustules develop large, moist, denuded areas, and particularly when the lesions become painful.

Neurologic complications. The most common extracutaneous complication is central nervous system involvement. Encephalitis and Reye's syndrome are complications of chickenpox. There are two forms of encephalitis. The cerebellar form seen in children is self-limited and complete recovery occurs. There is ataxia with nystagmus, headache, nausea, vomiting, and nuchal rigidity. Adult patients with encephalitis have altered sensorium, seizures, and focal neurologic signs with a mortality rate of up to 35%. Reye's syndrome is an acute, noninflammatory encephalopathy associated with hepatitis or fatty metamorphosis of the liver; 20% to 30% of Reye's syndrome cases are preceded by varicella. The fatality rate is 20%. Salicylates used during the varicella infection may increase the risk of the development of Reye's syndrome.

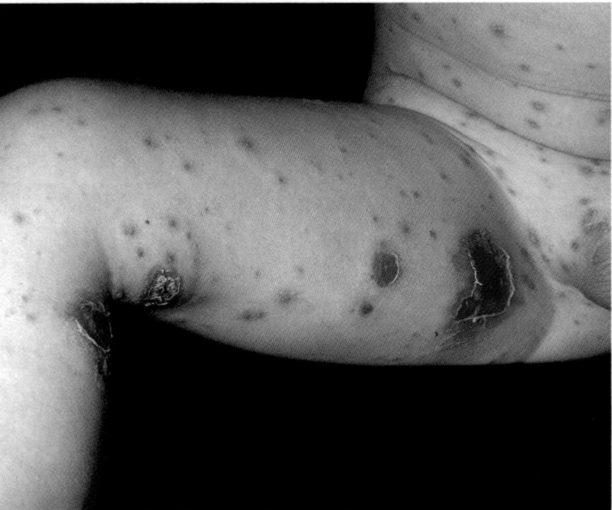

Figure 12-49 Secondary infection with impetigo is common in children. Excoriation may predispose to infection.

Pneumonia. Varicella pneumonia occurs in 1 of every 400 cases. Pneumonia is rare in normal children, but it is the most common serious complication in normal adults. Viral pneumonia develops 1 to 6 days after onset of the rash. In most cases it is asymptomatic and can be detected only with a chest x-ray examination. Cough, dyspnea, fever, and chest pain can occur. The mortality rate for adult varicella pneumonia is 10% of immunocompetent patients and 30% of immunocompromised patients.

Other. Hepatitis is the most common complication in immunosuppressed patients. Mild degrees of thrombocytopenia can accompany routine cases.

Chickenpox in the immunocompromised patient

Patients with cancer or patients who are taking immunosuppressive drugs, particularly systemic and intranasal corticosteroids, have extensive eruptions and more complications. The mortality rate for immunosuppressed children or children with leukemia is 7% to 14%. Adults with malignancy and varicella have a mortality rate as high as 50% (Figure 12-50). Hemorrhagic chickenpox, also called malignant chickenpox, is a serious complication in which the lesions are numerous and often bullous and bleeding occurs in the skin at the base of the lesion. The bullae turn dark brown and then black as blood accumulates in the blister fluid. Patients are usually toxic, have high fever and delirium, and may develop convulsions and coma. They frequently bleed from the gastrointestinal tract and mucous membranes. Pneumonia with hemoptysis commonly occurs. The mortality rate was 71% in one series.

Chickenpox and HIV infection

Many children with HIV infection who acquire varicella have an uncomplicated clinical course and have a significant antibody response to VZV. Some, however, have chronic, recurrent, or persistent varicella. Varicella in adult HIV-infected patients is a potentially severe infection, but these patients respond well to acyclovir therapy. Immune status to varicella does not correlate with the declining CD4+ counts and is well preserved, even in patients with fewer than 200 CD4+ cells/mm^3.

Figure 12-50 Hemorrhagic chickenpox. Numerous vesicular and bullous lesions with hemorrhage at the base.

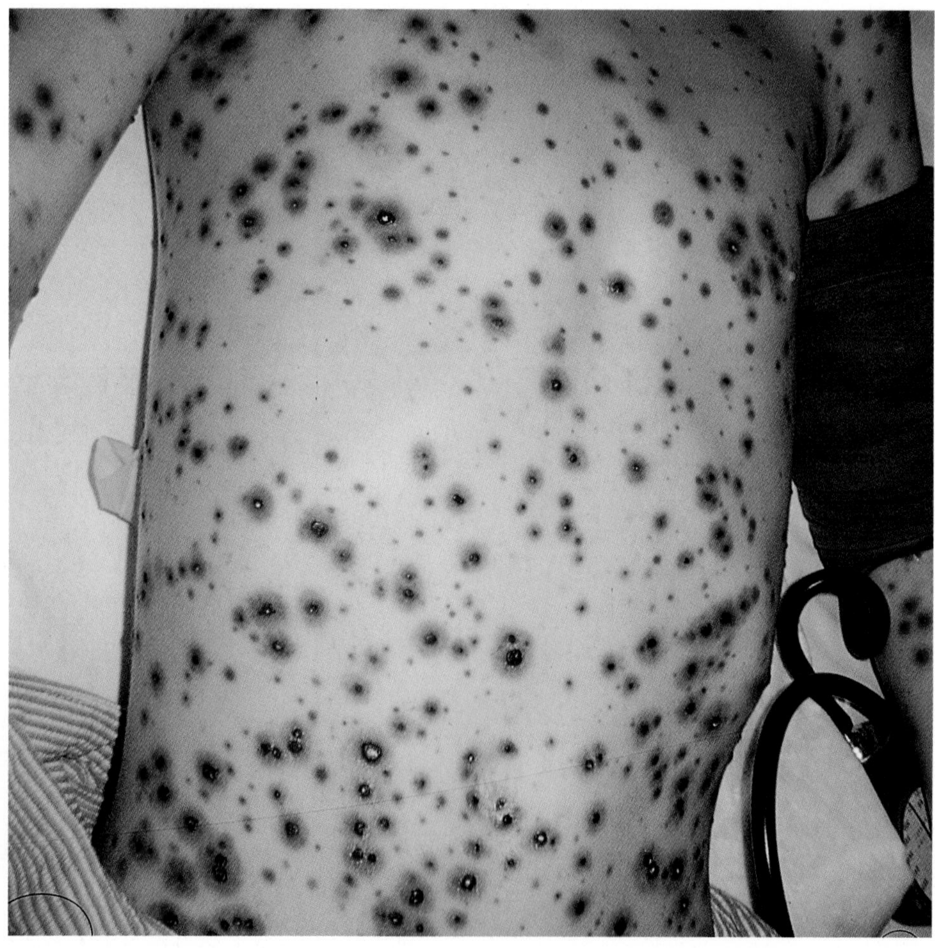

Chickenpox during pregnancy

Varicella during pregnancy poses a risk for both the mother and the unborn child. In a study of 43 pregnant women, 4 developed symptomatic pneumonia and 1 died of the infection. Smoking is a possible risk factor. Pregnant women with pneumonitis who received high-dose intravenous acyclovir, ranging from 10 to 18 mg/kg every 8 hours, showed rapid improvement. Lower dosages may not be effective.

Congenital and neonatal chickenpox

MATERNAL VARICELLA

FIRST TRIMESTER. Infection with the VZV during pregnancy can produce an embryopathy characterized by limb hypoplasia, chorioretinitis, cortical atrophy, and cutaneous scars (congenital varicella syndrome). The risk is greatest when infection occurs during the first 20 weeks of pregnancy. The absolute risk of embryopathy after maternal varicella infection in the first 20 weeks of pregnancy is approximately 2%.

SECOND TRIMESTER. Maternal varicella in the middle months of pregnancy may result in undetected fetal chickenpox. The newborn child who has already had chickenpox is at risk for developing herpes zoster (shingles). This may explain why some infants and children develop herpes zoster without the expected history of chickenpox.

NEAR BIRTH. The time of onset of maternal lesions correlates directly with the frequency and severity of neonatal disease (Figure 12-51). If the mother has varicella 2 to 3 weeks before delivery, the fetus may be infected in utero and be born with or develop lesions 1 to 4 days after birth. Transplacental maternal antibody protects the infant and the course is usually benign. The risk of infection and complications is greatest when the maternal onset of varicella is from 5 days before to 2 days after delivery. When maternal infection appears more than 5 days before delivery, maternal antibody can develop and transfer via the placenta. Maternal infection that develops more than 2 days after delivery is associated with onset of disease in a newborn approximately 2 weeks later, at which point the immune system is better able to respond to the infection.

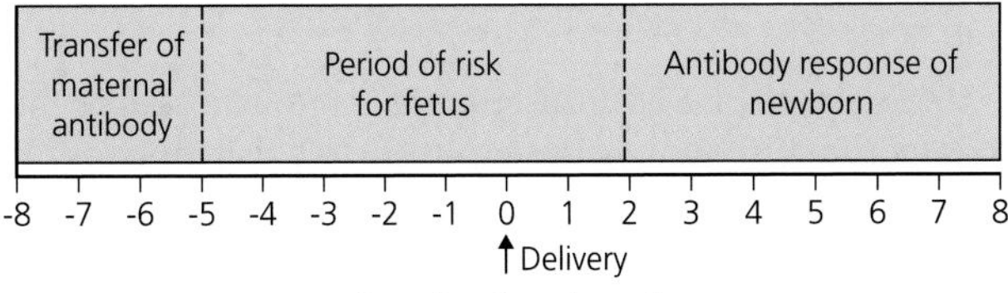

Figure 12-51 Varicella in newborns. For neonates, the risk of varicella infection and its associated complications is greatest when maternal onset of disease occurs in a 7-day period from 5 days before delivery to 2 days after delivery.

There is a high incidence of disseminated varicella in the infant when the mother's eruption appears 1 to 4 days before delivery or the child's eruption appears 5 to 10 days after birth. When the maternal rash appears within 5 days before delivery, approximately one third of infants become infected. After 5 days, transmission occurs in approximately 18%. When the rash appears in infants between 5 and 10 days old, the mortality rate may be as high as 20%. In this situation, the virus is either acquired transplacentally or from contact with maternal lesions during birth; there is insufficient time to receive adequate maternal antibody. The infant is immunologically incapable of controlling the infection and is at great risk of developing a disseminated disease. These infants should be given zoster immune globulin (ZIG), varicella-zoster immune globulin (VZIG), or gamma-globulin if ZIG or if VZIG is not available.

LABORATORY DIAGNOSIS

Rapid PCR. Rapid polymerase chain reaction (PCR) is the fastest and most accurate method of establishing the diagnosis. Collect lesion specimens using a culture transport swab. Use of a calcium alginate–tipped swab, wood swab, or transport swab containing gel is not acceptable for PCR testing. Send the specimen refrigerated.

Culture. In questionable cases, virus can be cultured from vesicular fluid. Culture is not easily obtained because VZV is a labile virus that is cultured much less readily than HSV.

Serology. The main value of serologic testing is the assessment of the immune status of immunocompromised patients, such as children with neoplastic diseases, who are at risk of developing severe disease with VZV infection. There are qualitative and quantitative tests that measure IgG and IgM antibodies. The presence of IgM antibodies or a fourfold or greater rise in paired sera IgG titer indicates recent infection. The presence of IgG indicates past exposure and immunity.

A chest x-ray examination should be obtained if respiratory symptoms develop. The white blood cell count is variably elevated, but it is necessary to obtain a count only if the disease progresses.

VARICELLA VACCINE

Varicella vaccine is made with live, attenuated varicella virus. It was licensed in the United States in 1995. It prevents chickenpox in 70% to 90% of people who get it, and it prevents severe chickenpox in more than 95%. It is expected to provide lifelong immunity. Two doses of varicella vaccine are recommended for children. The first dose is recommended at 12 to 15 months of age. It is usually given at the same time as the measles-mumps-rubella (MMR) vaccine. The second dose is recommended at 4 to 6 years, before entering kindergarten or first grade. It may be given sooner, as long as it is separated from the first dose by at least 3 months. People 13 years of age and older (who have never had chickenpox or received chickenpox vaccine) should get two doses at least 28 days apart.

People should not get the chickenpox vaccine if they have ever had a life-threatening allergic reaction to gelatin, the antibiotic neomycin, or a previous dose of chickenpox vaccine. Pregnant women should wait to get chickenpox vaccine until after they have given birth. Women should not get pregnant for 1 month after getting chickenpox vaccine. The live attenuated vaccine should not be given to patients with HIV infection or to other immunosuppressed patients.

Anyone who has had chickenpox does not need the vaccine. Each year, about 1% of people who have received the varicella vaccine develop chickenpox. Breakthrough infections are milder than normal chickenpox. Patients generally have fewer than 50 lesions, which do not form blisters. They also are afebrile and have no complications.

The incidence of zoster in children with leukemia is no greater than that in children who have had natural varicella infection.

TREATMENT

Bland antipruritic lotions (e.g., Sarna Anti-Itch [camphor and menthol over-the-counter]); cool, wet compresses; tepid baths; and antipyretics (excluding aspirin because of its association with Reye's syndrome) provide symptomatic relief. Antihistamines (e.g., hydroxyzine) may help control excoriation. Oral antibiotics active against *Streptococcus* and *Staphylococcus* are indicated for secondarily infected lesions.

ACYCLOVIR

Children and adolescents. Oral acyclovir therapy initiated within 24 hours of illness for otherwise healthy children with varicella typically results in a 1-day reduction in fever and an approximately 15% to 30% reduction in the severity of cutaneous and systemic signs and symptoms. Therapy has not been shown to reduce the rate of acute complications, pruritus, spread of infection, or duration of absence from school.

The American Academy of Pediatrics Committee on Infectious Diseases published recommendations for the use of oral acyclovir in otherwise healthy children with varicella. Recommendations are that (1) oral acyclovir therapy is not routinely recommended for the treatment of uncomplicated varicella in otherwise healthy children, and that (2) for certain groups at increased risk of severe varicella or its complications, oral acyclovir therapy for varicella should be considered if it can be initiated within the first 24 hours after the onset of rash. These groups include otherwise healthy, nonpregnant individuals 13 years of age or older; children older than 12 months with a chronic cutaneous or pulmonary disorder; and those receiving long-term salicylate therapy, although in the latter instance a reduced risk for Reye's syndrome has not been shown to result from oral acyclovir therapy or from milder illness with varicella.

Adults. Early therapy with oral acyclovir (800 mg 5 times per day for 7 days) decreases the time to cutaneous healing of adult varicella, decreases the duration of fever, and lessens symptoms. Initiation of therapy after the first day of illness is of no value in uncomplicated cases of adult varicella.

Immunocompromised patients. Studies show that immunosuppressed patients treated with acyclovir had decreased morbidity from visceral dissemination; there was a modest effect on the cutaneous disease (see Table 12-2). Acyclovir (500 mg/m^2 intravenous every 8 hours for 7 to 10 days) is the drug of choice for treatment of varicella in immunocompromised patients.

A continuous infusion of acyclovir may be beneficial for severe, life-threatening VZV infections that are resistant to treatment with the conventional regimen, and perhaps even acyclovir-resistant herpesvirus infections. A continuous infusion of acyclovir at a rate of 2 mg/kg body weight/hour (2250 mg/day) was effective in one report.

Acyclovir-resistant strains of VZV have been reported in AIDS patients. Foscarnet is a potentially effective with acyclovir-resistant VZV strains.

VZIG. Preventive treatment is available after exposure to chickenpox for susceptible persons who are not eligible to receive chickenpox vaccine. Varicella-zoster immune globulin (VZIG) can prevent or modify disease after exposure to someone with chickenpox. VZIG is only recommended for persons at high risk of developing severe disease who are not eligible to receive chickenpox vaccine.

The following individuals may be included in this group:

- Newborns whose mothers have chickenpox 5 days before to 2 days after delivery
- Premature babies exposed to varicella in the first month of life
- Children with leukemia or lymphoma who have not been vaccinated
- Persons with cellular immunodeficiencies or other immune system problems
- Persons receiving medications, such as high-dose systemic steroids, that suppress the immune system
- Women who are pregnant

VZIG is not known to be useful in treating clinical varicella or zoster or in preventing disseminated zoster. The duration of protection is estimated to be 3 weeks. Patients exposed again more than 3 weeks after a dose of VZIG should receive another full dose. VZIG is given intramuscularly.

VZIG should be administered as soon as possible, but no later than 96 hours, after exposure to chickenpox. VZIG production was discontinued in the United States in 2006. A similar product, VariZIG, is now available.

GAMMAGLOBULIN. Intravenous gammaglobulin may be an acceptable substitute if VZIG is not available.

HERPES ZOSTER

Herpes zoster, or shingles, a cutaneous viral infection generally involving the skin of a single dermatome (Figure 12-52), occurs during the lifetime of 10% to 20% of all persons. People of all ages are afflicted; it occurs regularly in young individuals, but the incidence increases with age as T-cell immunity to the virus wanes. Patients who have T-cell immunosuppression are at greater risk. There is an increased incidence of zoster in normal children who acquire chickenpox when younger than 2 months. Patients with zoster are not more likely to have an underlying malignancy. Zoster may be the earliest clinical sign of the development of AIDS in high-risk individuals.

Zoster results from reactivation of varicella virus that entered the cutaneous nerves during an earlier episode of chickenpox, traveled to the dorsal root ganglia, and remained in a latent form. Age, immunosuppressive drugs, lymphoma, fatigue, emotional upsets, and radiation therapy have been implicated in reactivating the virus, which subsequently travels back down the sensory nerve, infecting the skin. Some patients, particularly children with zoster, have no history of chickenpox. They may have acquired chickenpox via the transplacental route. Although reported, herpes zoster acquired through direct contact with a patient with active varicella or zoster is rare. After contact with such patients, infections are more inclined to result from reactivation of latent infection. Virus reactivation usually occurs once in a lifetime; the incidence of a second attack is less than 5%.

Varicella-zoster virus can be cultured from vesicles during an eruption. It may also cause chickenpox in those not previously infected.

The elderly are at greater risk to develop segmental pain, which can continue for months after the skin lesions have healed.

CLINICAL PRESENTATION. Preeruptive pain (preherpetic neuralgia), itching, or burning, generally localized to the dermatome, precedes the eruption by 4 to 5 days. An extended period of pain (7 to 100 days) has been reported. The pain may simulate pleurisy, myocardial infarction, abdominal disease, or migraine headache and may present a difficult diagnostic problem until the characteristic eruption provides the answer. Preeruptive tenderness or hyperesthesia throughout the dermatome is a useful predictive sign. Zoster sine herpete refers to segmental neuralgia without a cutaneous eruption and is rare. Constitutional symptoms of fever, headache, and malaise may precede the eruption by several days. Regional lymphadenopathy may be present. Segmental pain and constitutional symptoms

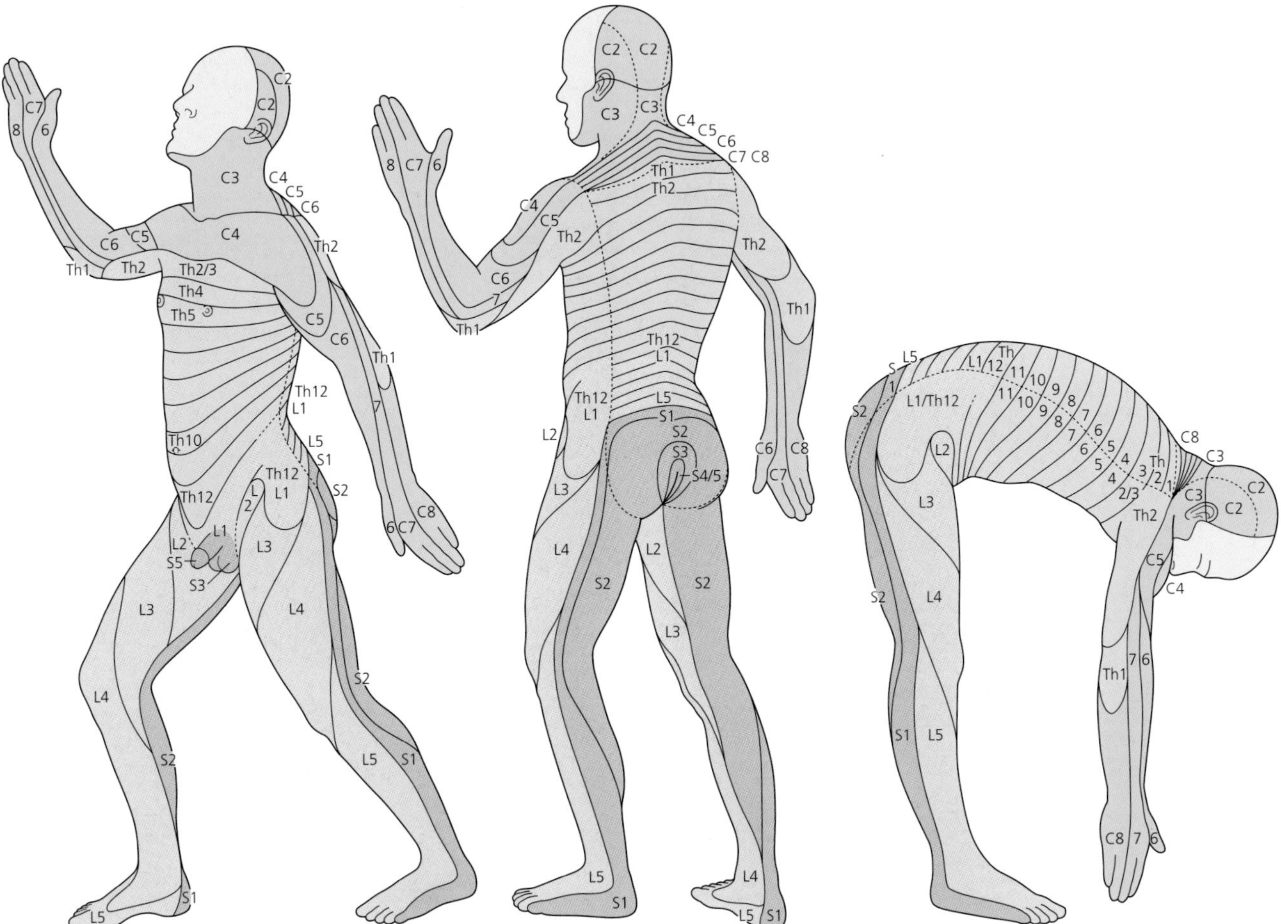

Figure 12-52 Dermatome areas.

HERPES ZOSTER—EVOLUTION OF LESIONS

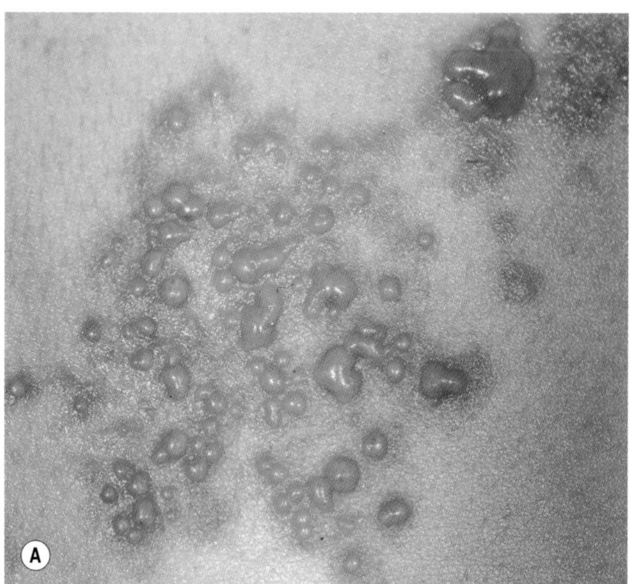

A group of vesicles that vary in size. Vesicles of herpes simplex are of uniform size.

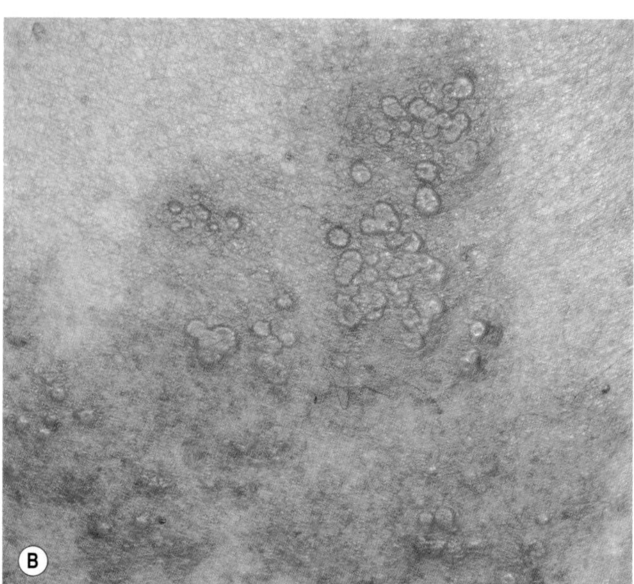

Vesicles become umbilicated and then form crusts.

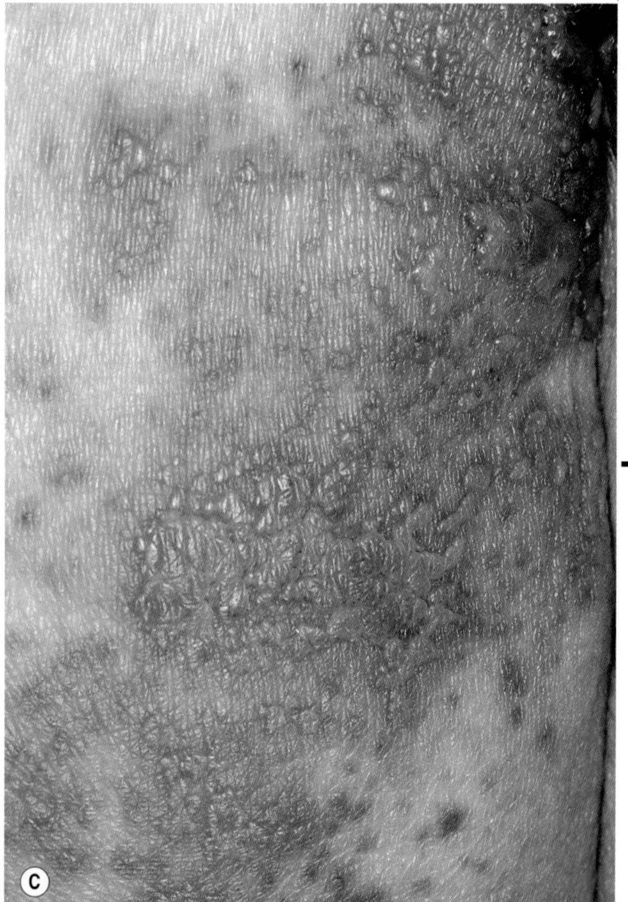

Confluent groups of vesicles in a highly inflamed case.

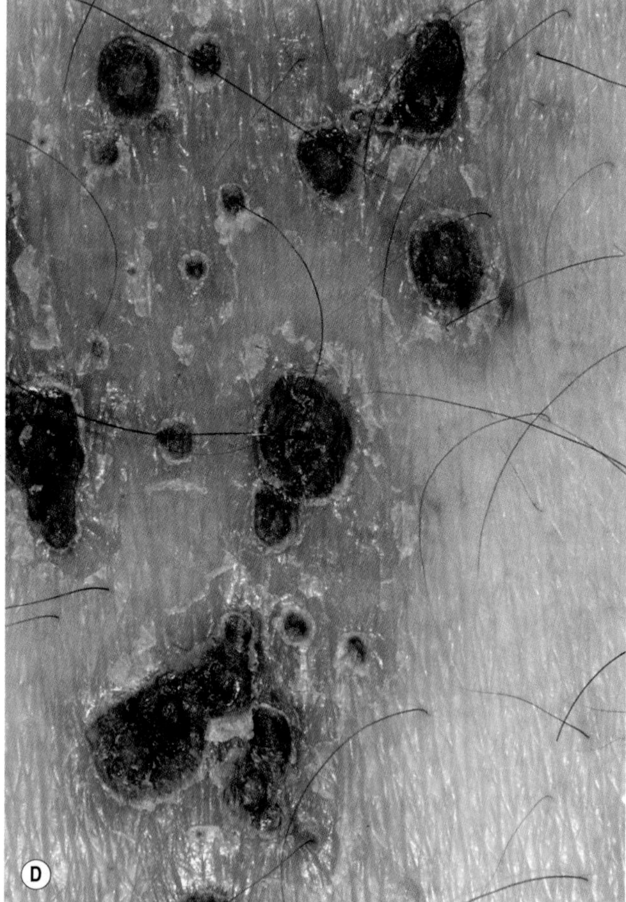

Vesicles evolve to crusts and may eventually scar if inflammation is intense.

Figure 12-53

gradually subside as the eruption appears and then evolves (Figure 12-53). Prodromal symptoms may be absent, particularly in children.

ERUPTIVE PHASE. The eruption begins with red, swollen plaques of varying sizes and spreads to involve part or all of a dermatome (Figures 12-54 through 12-61). The vesicles arise in clusters from the erythematous base and become cloudy with purulent fluid by day 3 or 4. In some cases vesicles do not form or are so small that they are difficult to see. The vesicles vary in size, in contrast to the cluster of uniformly sized vesicles noted in herpes simplex. Successive crops continue to appear for 7 days. Vesicles either umbilicate (Figure 12-53) or rupture before forming a crust, which falls off in 2 to 3 weeks. The elderly or debilitated patients may have a prolonged and difficult course. For them, the eruption is typically more extensive and inflammatory, occasionally resulting in hemorrhagic blisters, skin necrosis, secondary bacterial infection, or extensive scarring, which is sometimes hypertrophic or keloidal.

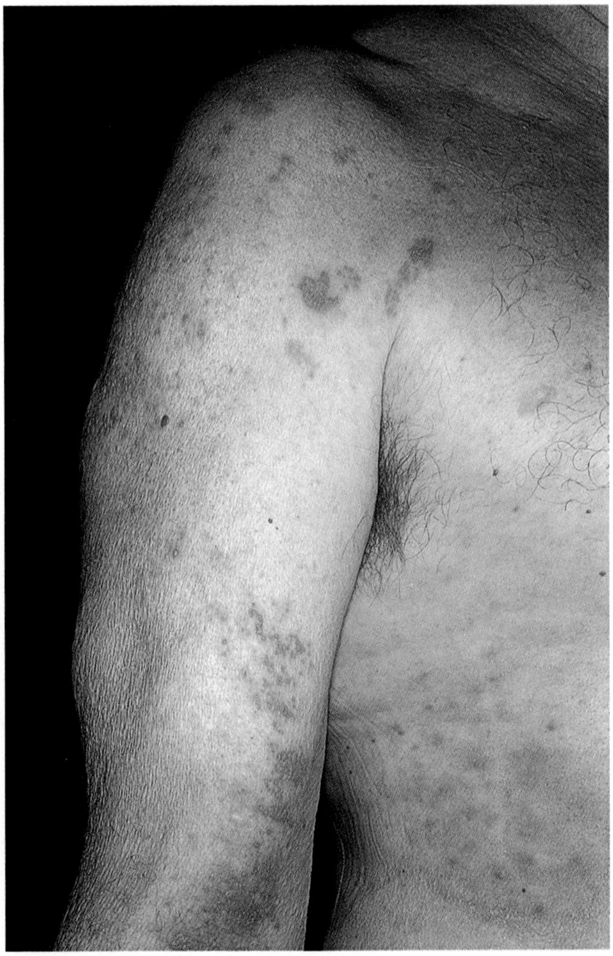

Figure 12-54 Herpes zoster may involve any dermatome. Patients are confused by this presentation. They think that "shingles" can appear only on the trunk.

Although generally limited to the skin of a single dermatome (Figure 12-54), the eruption may involve one or two adjacent dermatomes (Figure 12-55). Occasionally, a few vesicles appear across the midline. Eruption is rare in bilaterally symmetric or asymmetric dermatomes. Approximately 50% of patients with uncomplicated zoster have a viremia, with the appearance of 20 to 30 vesicles scattered over the skin surface outside the affected dermatome. Possibly because chickenpox is centripetal (located on the trunk), the thoracic region is affected in two thirds of herpes zoster cases. An attack of herpes zoster does not confer lasting immunity, and it is possible, although very unusual, to have two or three episodes in a lifetime.

PAIN. The pain associated with acute zoster and postherpetic neuralgia (PHN) is neuropathic and results from injury of the peripheral nerves and altered central nervous system signal processing. After the injury, peripheral neurons discharge spontaneously, have lower activation thresholds, and display exaggerated responses to stimuli. Axonal regrowth after the injury produces nerve sprouts that are also prone to unprovoked discharge. The excessive peripheral activity is thought to lead to hyperexcitability of the dorsal horn, resulting in exaggerated central nervous system responses to all input. These changes may be so complex that no single therapeutic approach will ameliorate all the abnormalities.

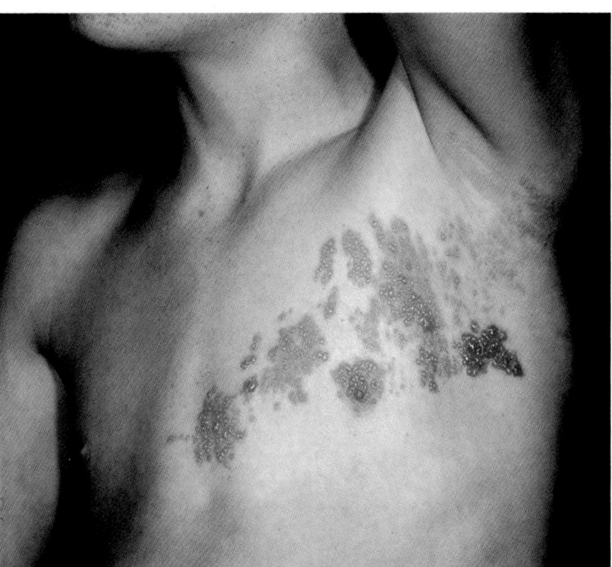

Figure 12-55 Herpes zoster may involve one, two, or three adjacent dermatomes.

HERPES ZOSTER

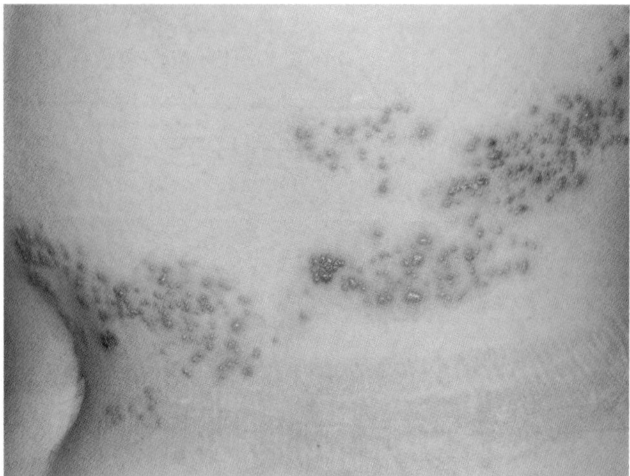

Figure 12-56 A common presentation with involvement of a single thoracic dermatome.

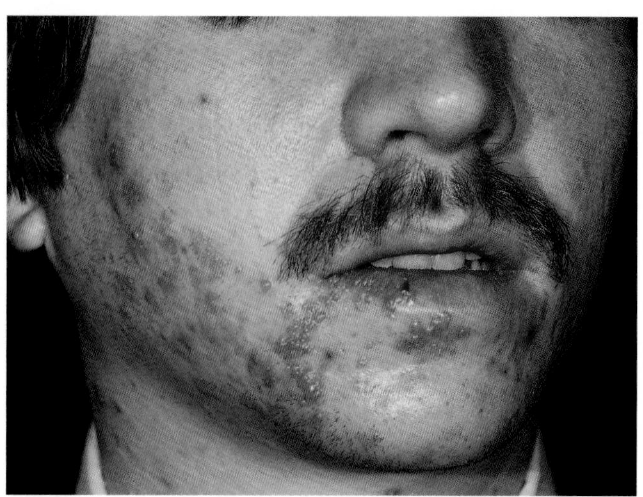

Figure 12-57 Unilateral single-dermatome distribution involving the mandibular branch of the fifth nerve.

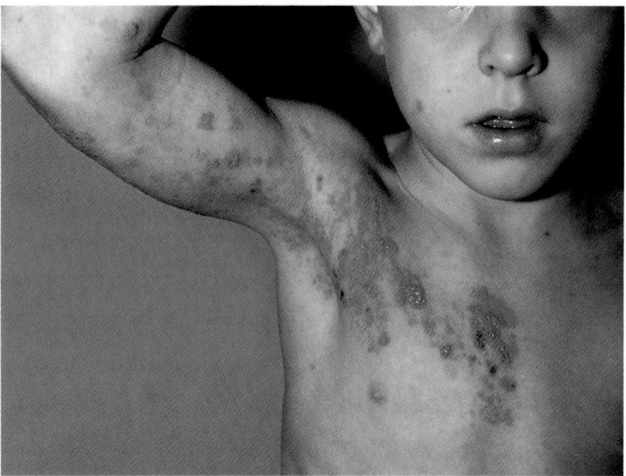

Figure 12-58 Almost the entire skin surface of a dermatome is involved. Zoster is seen in children.

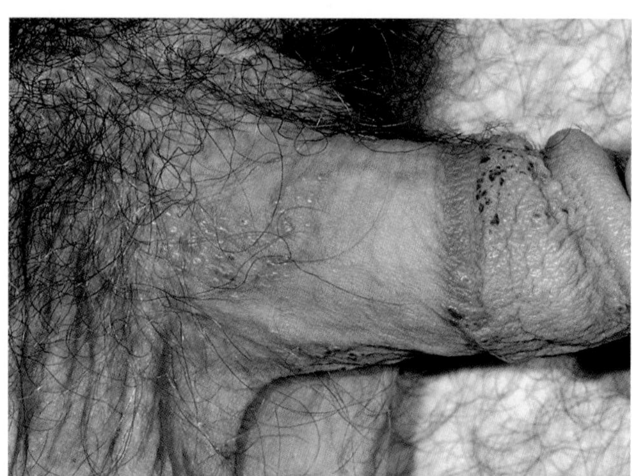

Figure 12-59 Zoster of the penis looks just like herpes simplex.

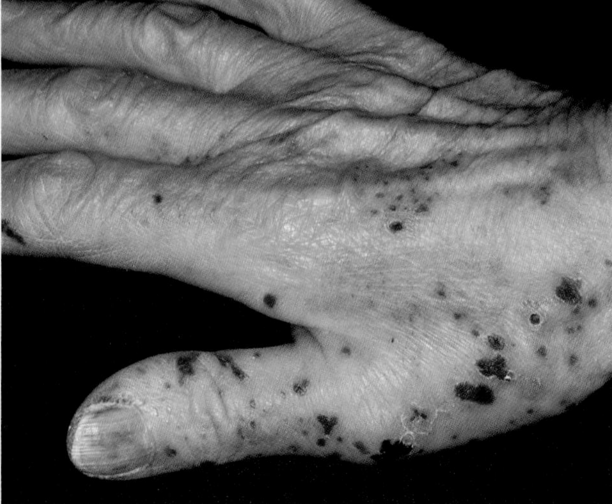

Figure 12-60 Zoster of the hand is a confusing presentation. Poison ivy was the initial diagnosis here.

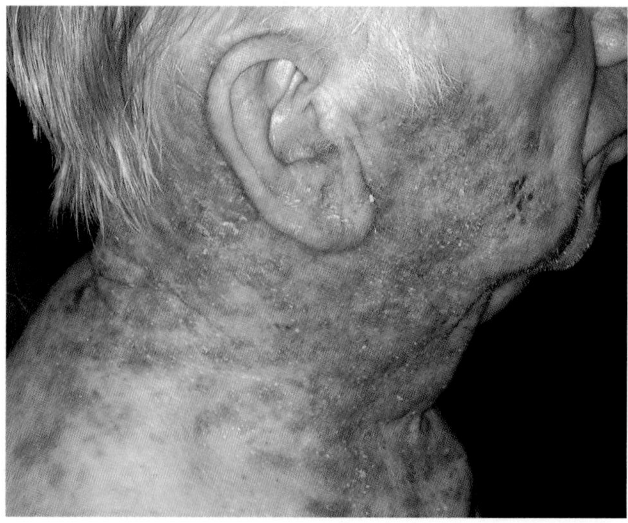

Figure 12-61 Zoster with infection of almost the entire skin surface of two or three dermatomes.

Herpes zoster after varicella immunization

Herpes zoster may be less common after immunization than after natural infection. The incidence of zoster in children with leukemia who receive the vaccine is lower than that in leukemic children who have natural varicella infection.

Herpes zoster and HIV infection

Zoster may be the earliest clinical sign of the development of AIDS in high-risk individuals. The incidence of herpes zoster is significantly higher among HIV-seropositive patients. The risk of herpes zoster is not associated with duration of HIV infection and is not predictive of faster progression to AIDS.

Herpes zoster during pregnancy

Herpes zoster during pregnancy, whether it occurs early or late in the pregnancy, appears to have no deleterious effects on either the mother or the infant.

Syndromes

OPHTHALMIC ZOSTER

Herpes zoster ophthalmicus presents with vesicular and erythematous involvement of the cranial nerve VI dermatome, ipsilateral forehead, and upper eyelid. The fifth cranial, or trigeminal, nerve has three divisions: the ophthalmic, maxillary, and mandibular. The ophthalmic division further divides into three main branches: the frontal, lacrimal, and nasociliary nerves. Involvement of any branch of the ophthalmic nerve is called herpes zoster ophthalmicus. It constitutes 10% to 15% of all zoster cases. Involvement of the ophthalmic branch of the fifth cranial nerve is five times as common as involvement of the maxillary or mandibular branches.

CLINICAL PRESENTATION. Headaches, nausea, and vomiting are prodromal symptoms. Ipsilateral preauricular and, sometimes, submaxillary nodal involvement is a common prodromal event. Reactive lymphadenopathy can occur later with secondary infection of vesicles. The ophthalmic branch of the fifth cranial nerve sends branches to the tentorium and to the third and sixth cranial nerves, which may explain the meningeal signs and, occasionally, the third and sixth cranial palsies associated with herpes zoster ophthalmicus. The rash extends from eye level to the vertex of the skull but does not cross the midline (Figures 12-62 and 12-63). Herpes zoster ophthalmicus may be confined

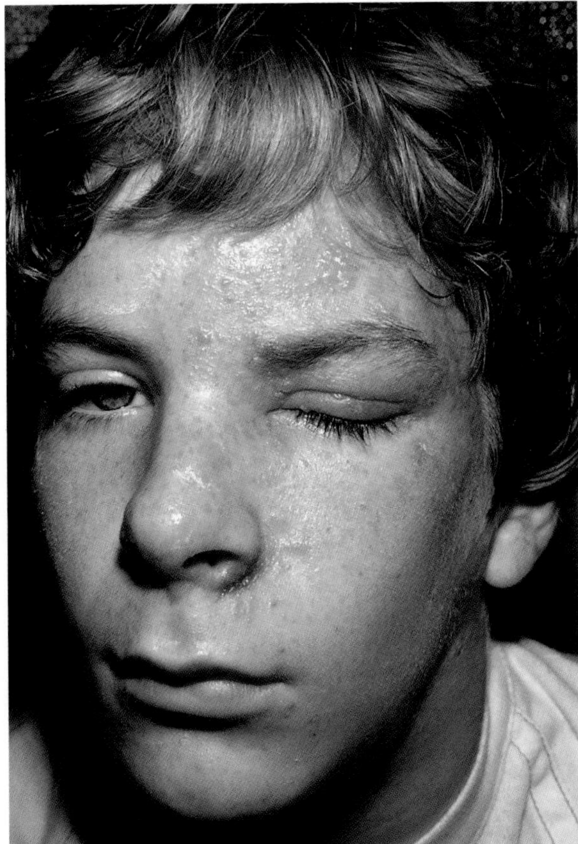

Figure 12-62 Herpes zoster (ophthalmic zoster). Involvement of the first branch of the fifth nerve. Vesicles on the side of the nose are associated with the most serious ocular complications.

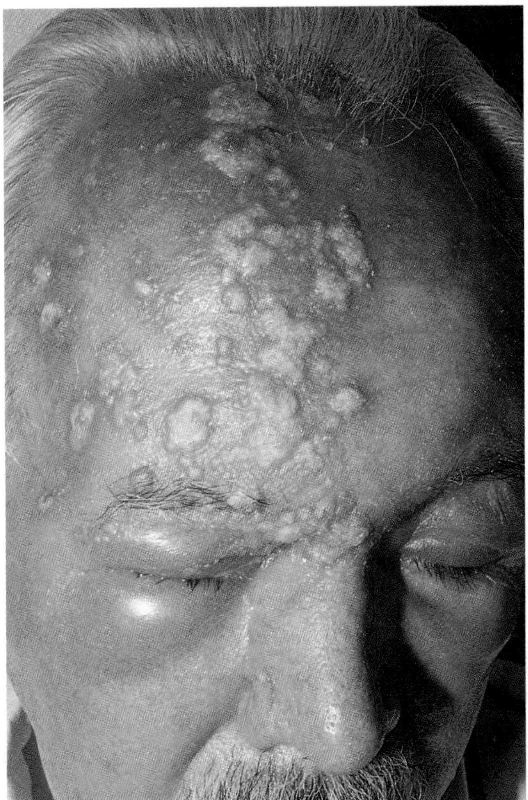

Figure 12-63 Herpes zoster (ophthalmic zoster). A virulent infection of the skin and eye.

to certain branches of the trigeminal nerve. The tip and side of the nose and eye are innervated by the nasociliary branch of the trigeminal nerve. Vesicles on the side or tip of the nose (Hutchinson's sign) that occur during an episode of zoster are associated with the most serious ocular complications, including conjunctival, corneal, scleral, and other ocular diseases, although this is not invariable. Involvement of the other sensory branches of the trigeminal nerve is most likely to yield periocular involvement but spare the eyeball. Acute pain occurs in 93% of patients and remains in 31% of patients at 6 months. Of patients aged 60 and older, pain persists in 30% for 6 months or longer, and this rises to 71% in those aged 80 and older.

Table 12-3 Ocular Complications in 86 Patients with Herpes Zoster Ophthalmicus*

Complication	No. of patients
Lid involvement	11
Corneal involvement	66
Scleral involvement	4
Canalicular scarring	2
Uveitis	37
Glaucoma (secondary)	10
Glaucoma (persistent)	2
Cataract	7
Neuroophthalmic involvement	7
Postherpetic neuralgia	15

*Some patients had more than one manifestation of involvement. Modified from Womack LW, Liesegang TJ: *Arch Ophthalmol* 101:44, 1983. By permission of Mayo Foundation. *PMID: 6600391*

Eye involvement. Between 20% and 72% develop ocular complications. Anterior uveitis and the various varieties of keratitis are most common, affecting 92% and 52% of patients with ocular involvement, respectively. Sight-threatening complications include neuropathic keratitis, perforation, secondary glaucoma, posterior scleritis/orbital apex syndrome, optic neuritis, and acute retinal necrosis (Table 12-3). Twenty-eight percent of initially involved eyes develop long-term ocular disease (6 months), with chronic uveitis, keratitis, and neuropathic ulceration being the most common.

Prompt treatment with oral antiviral drugs (Table 12-4) reduces the severity of the skin eruption, the incidence and the severity of late ocular manifestations, and the intensity of PHN. At 6 months, late ocular inflammatory complications are seen in 29.1% of acyclovir-treated patients versus 50% to 71% of untreated patients. Ophthalmic 3% acyclovir ointment may be used for established ocular complications.

Ramsay Hunt syndrome. The strict definition of the Ramsay Hunt syndrome (geniculate ganglion zoster) is peripheral facial nerve palsy accompanied by a vesicular rash on the ear (zoster oticus) or in the mouth. It is caused by zoster of the geniculate ganglion. Other frequent signs and symptoms include tinnitus, hearing loss, nausea, vomiting, vertigo, and nystagmus. These eighth cranial nerve features are caused by the close proximity of the geniculate ganglion to the vestibulocochlear nerve within the bony facial canal. Bell's palsy (facial paralysis without rash) is significantly associated with herpes simplex virus infection.

There is involvement of the sensory portion and motor portion of the seventh cranial nerve. There may be unilateral loss of taste on the anterior two thirds of the tongue as well as vesicles on the tympanic membrane, external auditory meatus, concha, and pinna. Involvement of the motor division of the seventh cranial nerve causes unilateral facial paralysis. Auditory nerve involvement occurs in 37.2% of

Table 12-4 Drugs for Varicella-Zoster Infections*

	Acyclovir (Zovirax) (200-, 400-, and 800-mg capsules)	Famciclovir (Famvir) (125-, 250-, and 500-mg tablets)	Valacyclovir (Valtrex) (500- and 1000-mg caplets)
Varicella-zoster	800 mg four times/day × 7 days	500 mg q8h × 7 days	1 gm three times a day × 7 days
Varicella chickenpox	20 mg/kg per dose (800 mg maximum) four times/day × 5 days		
Varicella or zoster in immuno-compromised patients	10 mg/kg IV q8h × 10 days (adult dose)		
Acyclovir-resistant infections: foscarnet (Foscavir) 40 mg/kg IV q8h × 10 days			

*Higher doses of medication may be needed in HIV-infected patients.

patients, resulting in hearing deficits and vertigo. Recovery from the motor paralysis is generally complete, but residual weakness is possible. Sweeney discusses and diagrams the complex neuroanatomy of this syndrome. PMID: 11459884

The syndrome also may result from zoster of the ninth or tenth cranial nerves since the external ear has complex innervation by branches of several cranial nerves.

Compared with Bell's palsy (facial paralysis without rash), patients with Ramsay Hunt syndrome often have more severe paralysis at onset and are less likely to recover completely. About 14% developed vesicles after the onset of facial weakness. Thus Ramsay Hunt syndrome may initially be indistinguishable from Bell's palsy.

Some patients develop peripheral facial paralysis without ear or mouth rash, associated with a fourfold rise in antibody to VZV. This indicates that a proportion of patients with "Bell's palsy" have Ramsay Hunt syndrome zoster sine herpete (zoster without the rash). Treatment of these patients with acyclovir and prednisone within 7 days of onset has been shown to improve the outcome of recovery from facial palsy.

Sacral zoster (S2, S3, or S4 dermatomes). A neurogenic bladder with urinary hesitancy or urinary retention has reportedly been associated with zoster of the sacral dermatome S2, S3, or S4 (Figures 12-64 and 12-65). Migration of virus to the adjacent autonomic nerves is responsible for these symptoms.

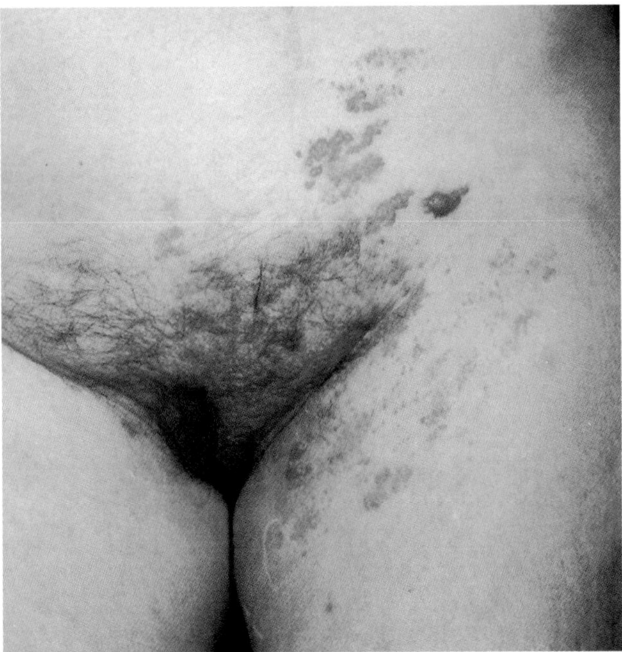

Figure 12-64 Ilioinguinal and sacral zoster. Zoster of T12, L1-L2, and S2-S4 dermatomes can occasionally cause a neurogenic bladder. Acute urinary retention and polyuria are the most common symptoms.

COMPLICATIONS

Pain and postherpetic neuralgia. Pain persisting after herpes zoster is called *postherpetic neuralgia*. It is the most common and most feared complication and the major cause of morbidity. The risk of PHN increases with age (especially in patients older than 50 years) and increases in patients who have severe pain or severe rash during the acute episode or who have a prodrome of dermatomal pain before the rash appears. The pain is often severe, intractable, and exhausting. The patient protects areas of hyperesthesia to avoid the slightest pressure, which activates another wave of pain. There is a yearning for a few hours of sleep, but sharp paroxysms of lancinating pain invade the mind and the patient is again awakened. "The pain is sometimes so severe as to make the patient weary of existence."PMID: 11087888 These words were written more than 100 years ago. Despair and sometimes suicide occur if hope and encouragement are not provided.

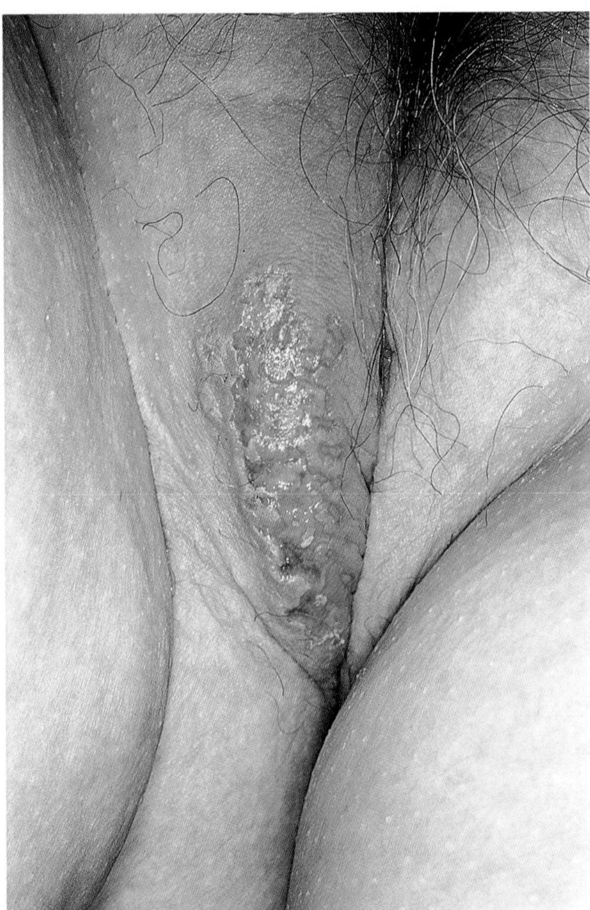

Figure 12-65 Herpes zoster may not be expected when lesions appear in unusual areas. The prodome of pain and sudden appearance of grouped vesicles, crusts, or erosions support the diagnosis. Vesicles are macerated to form erosions in intertriginous areas.

Duration of pain. Pain can persist in a dermatome for months or years after the lesions have disappeared. The probability of longstanding pain in patients not treated with antiviral drugs is low. One large study provided the following data. Regardless of age, the incidence of pain was 19.2% at 1 month, 7.2% at 3 months, and 3.4% at 1 year. Among patients younger than 60 years, the risk of PHN 3 months after the start of the zoster rash was 2% and pain was mild in all cases. After the age of 60, both the frequency and the severity of pain increased, although moderate pain was rare after 3 months and severe pain was uncommon at all times (Figure 12-66). The probability of having severe PHN after 3 months in this age group was less than 7%, and it was less than 3% at 12 months.

Once present, neuralgia can persist for years, but spontaneous remission may occur after several years.

Pathophysiology of pain. Postherpetic neuralgia is associated with scarring of the dorsal root ganglion and atrophy of the dorsal horn on the affected side. These changes are caused by the extensive inflammation that occurs during the active infection.

Dissemination. A few vesicles may be found remote from the affected dermatome in immunocompetent patients and is probably a result of hematogenous spread of the virus. Cutaneous dissemination is defined as more than 20 vesicles outside the primary and immediately adjacent dermatomes. Visceral dissemination (lungs, liver, brain) occurs in 10% of immunocompromised patients. In addition, patients with Hodgkin's disease are uniquely susceptible to herpes zoster. Furthermore, 15% to 50% of zoster patients with active Hodgkin's disease have disseminated disease involving the skin, lungs, and brain; 10% to 25% of those patients die. In patients with other types of cancer, death from zoster is unusual. HIV-infected patients with zoster have increased neurologic (e.g., aseptic meningitis, radiculitis, and myelitis) and ophthalmologic complications.

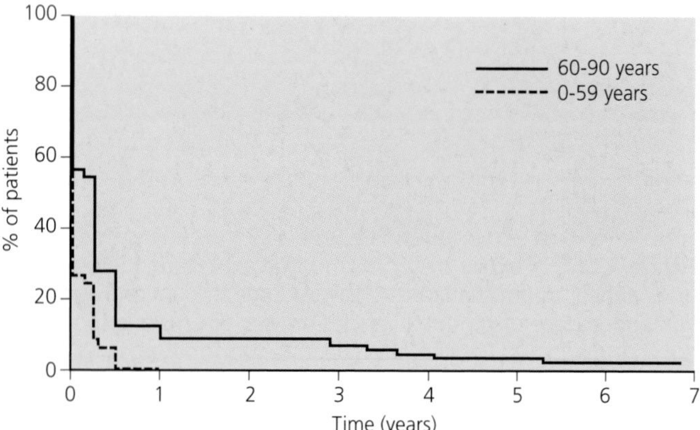

Figure 12-66 Plot of duration of any pain from start of herpes zoster among patients in two age groups.

Motor paresis. Muscle weakness in the muscle group associated with the infected dermatome may be observed before, during, or after an episode of herpes zoster. The paralysis usually occurs in the first 2 to 3 weeks after rash onset and can persist for several weeks. The weakness results from the spread of the virus from the dorsal root ganglia to the anterior root horn. Patients in the sixth to eighth decade of life are most commonly involved. Motor neuropathies are usually transient and approximately 75% of patients recover. They occur in approximately 5% of all cases of zoster but in up to 12% of patients with cephalic zoster. Ramsay Hunt syndrome accounts for more than half of the cephalic motor neuropathies.

Encephalitis. Neurologic symptoms characteristically appear within the first 2 weeks of onset of the skin lesions. It is possible that encephalitis is immune mediated rather than a result of viral invasion. Patients at greatest risk are those with trigeminal and disseminated zoster, as well as the immunosuppressed. The mortality rate is 10% to 20%; most survivors recover completely. The diagnosis is hampered by the fact that the virus is rarely isolated from the spinal fluid. Cell counts and protein concentration of the spinal fluid are elevated in encephalitis and in approximately 40% of typical zoster patients.

Necrosis, infection, and scarring. Elderly, malnourished, debilitated, or immunosuppressed patients tend to have a more virulent and extensive course of disease. The entire skin area of a dermatome may be lost after diffuse vesiculation. Large adherent crusts promote infection and increase the depth of involvement (Figure 12-67). Scarring, sometimes hypertrophic or keloidal, follows.

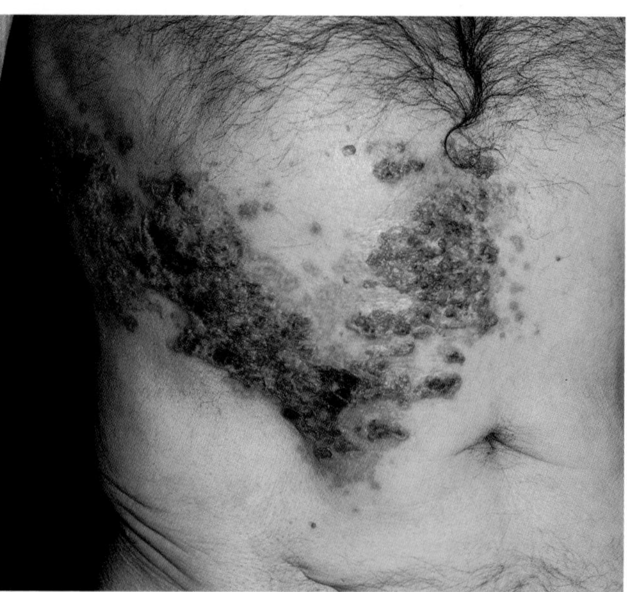

Figure 12-67 Herpes zoster. Massive involvement of a dermatome: numerous vesicles have been replaced by large crusts.

PREGNANCY

Herpes zoster during pregnancy is not associated with maternal or fetal morbidity.

DIFFERENTIAL DIAGNOSIS

Herpes simplex. The diagnosis of herpes zoster is usually obvious. Herpes simplex can be extensive, particularly on the trunk. It may be confined to a dermatome and possess many of the same features as zoster (zosteriform herpes simplex). The vesicles of zoster vary in size, whereas those of simplex are uniform within a cluster. A later recurrence proves the diagnosis.

Poison ivy. A group of vesicles on a red, inflamed base may be mistaken for poison ivy.

"Zoster sine herpete." Neuralgia within a dermatome without the typical rash can be confusing. A concurrent rise in varicella-zoster complement-fixation titers has been demonstrated in a number of such cases.

Cellulitis. The eruption of zoster may never evolve to the vesicular stage. The red, inflamed, edematous, or urticarial-like plaques may appear infected, but they usually have a fine, cobblestone surface indicative of a cluster of minute vesicles. A skin biopsy shows characteristic changes.

LABORATORY DIAGNOSIS

A clinical diagnosis is made in most cases; laboratory confirmation is usually unnecessary. The laboratory methods for identification are the same as those for herpes simplex. Tzanck smears, skin biopsy, antibody titers, vesicular fluid immunofluorescent antibody stains, electron microscopy, and culture of vesicle fluid are some of the studies to consider. The initial test of choice is a cytologic smear (Tzanck smear). The test does not differentiate herpes simplex from varicella. The base of an early lesion is scraped and stained with hematoxylin-eosin, Giemsa, Wright's, toluidine blue, or Papanicolaou's stain. Multinucleated giant cells and epithelial cells containing acidophilic intranuclear inclusions are seen. Zoster is seen about 7 times more frequently in HIV patients. An HIV test should be ordered if indicated.

VARICELLA–ZOSTER VACCINE. Immunization with a varicella vaccine boosts waning cell-mediated immunity in older adults. A large trial of a live attenuated Oka/Merck VZV vaccine (Zostavax) was conducted in individuals who were 60 years of age or older. The incidence of herpes zoster was 51% lower in the vaccinated group (5.4 cases per 1000 person-years vs. 11.1 cases per 1000 person-years, $P < 0.001$). The incidence of postherpetic neuralgia was 67% lower (0.5 case per 1000 person-years vs. 1.4 cases per 1000 person-years, $P < 0.001$). The median duration of pain among subjects in whom herpes zoster developed was shorter in the vaccine group than in the placebo group (21 days vs. 24 days, $P = 0.03$), and the degree of pain also was lower among the vaccine recipients ($P = 0.008$). The vaccine was more efficacious in preventing herpes zoster among persons who were 60 to 69 years of age than among those who were 70 years or older. However, it prevented postherpetic neuralgia to a greater extent among those who were 70 years or older than among those who were 60 to 69 years old. *PMID: 15930418*

A single dose of zoster vaccine is recommended for adults 60 years of age or older, whether or not they have had a previous episode of herpes zoster. Persons with chronic medical conditions may be vaccinated unless there is an applicable precaution or contraindication. Because virtually all adults 60 years of age or older will have had clinical or subclinical primary VZV infection (chickenpox), it is not necessary to determine whether there is a history of chickenpox for routine vaccination of people in this age group.

TREATMENT

The aim of treatment is the suppression of inflammation, pain, and infection.

TREATMENT STRATEGY. Treatment for acute zoster can accelerate healing, control pain, and reduce the risk of complications. Acute herpes zoster causes mixed somatic and neuropathic pain (pain from nerve injury) of varying intensity. Pain must be controlled. Antiviral therapy within the first 72 hours from the onset of rash or radicular pain and the use of analgesics, including opioids (if necessary), nerve blocks, and early antidepressant therapy, are treatment options. The dose and drug should be selected according to the needs of the individual patient. If less potent analgesic medications are ineffective, stronger agents should be prescribed until pain is relieved or dose-limiting side effects occur. It is possible that early, aggressive treatment may prevent PHN. Treatment with amitriptyline and related drugs, nerve blocks, and/or opioids soon after the development of acute pain may help prevent the sensitization of the central nervous system that may lead to persistence of the pain. Patients who develop postherpetic neuralgia are treated with gabapentin, pregabalin, opioids, tricyclic antidepressants, lidocaine patch 5%, and capsaicin. Treatment-refractory postherpetic neuralgia may respond to nonpharmacologic approaches by a pain-management specialist.

Topical therapy. Burow's solution or cool tap water can be used in a wet compress. The compresses, applied for 20 minutes several times a day, macerate the vesicles, remove serum and crust, and suppress bacterial growth. A whirlpool with Betadine (povidone-iodine) solution is particularly helpful in removing the crust and serum that occur with extensive eruptions in the elderly.

Antiviral drugs. Antiviral drugs reduce the severity, duration, and prevalence of PHN by as much as 50%, but 20% of patients over 50 years of age treated with famciclovir or valacyclovir report pain at 6 months (see Table 12-4).

Topical acyclovir. Topical acyclovir ointment applied 4 times a day for 10 days to immunocompromised patients significantly shortened complete-healing time.

Valacyclovir (Valtrex). Valacyclovir is available only as an oral formulation. After ingestion, the drug is converted to acyclovir in the gastrointestinal tract and liver. Its oral bioavailability is three to five times that of acyclovir. Studies demonstrate a significant advantage of Valtrex compared with Zovirax on decreasing the duration and incidence of pain, including both acute pain and PHN. Valacyclovir reduced the median duration of pain from 60 days after healing (with acyclovir) to 40 days. Six months after healing, only 19% of patients taking valacyclovir had pain compared with 26% of patients taking acyclovir. Patients who may have trouble complying with five-times-daily dosing of oral Zovirax and patients at highest risk for PHN (e.g., older patients and those with prodromal pain) may benefit from valacyclovir.

Famciclovir (Famvir). Famciclovir is an analog of penciclovir. It is well absorbed after oral administration and is rapidly metabolized to penciclovir in the gastrointestinal tract, blood, and liver. The intracellular half-life of the active drug, penciclovir triphosphate, is very long. Famciclovir is available for oral treatment of acute uncomplicated herpes zoster. The benefits appear to be similar to those of acyclovir. It was found to decrease the duration of PHN among elderly patients compared with placebo.

Oral and intravenous acyclovir. Acyclovir decreases acute pain, inflammation, vesicle formation, and viral shedding. The median duration of pain in acyclovir recipients is 20 days vs. 62 days for their placebo counterparts. Several studies show no effect on the subsequent development of PHN, even in patients who experience immediate pain relief. A study showed a possible reduction in the incidence of PHN if treatment began within 4 days of the onset of pain or within 48 hours of the onset of rash. Acyclovir appears to change the nature of PHN. Its use should be considered for immunosuppressed, debilitated patients who appear to be developing extensive cutaneous disease and for patients with ophthalmic zoster who are at increased risk of ocular complications. Treatment is most effective when started within the first 72 hours of infection. If lesions are not completely crusted and the patient is older than 50 years, immunocompromised, and/or has trigeminal zoster, treatment after 72 hours of the onset of vesicles should be considered. The recommended oral dosage is shown in Table 12-4. Proper hydration and urine flow must be maintained.

Acyclovir-resistant infection. Persons with AIDS who have CD4+ counts of less than 100 cells/mm^3 and transplant recipients, especially bone marrow allograft recipients, may experience infections with acyclovir-resistant VZV. Patients who have received prior repeated acyclovir treatment appear to be at the highest risk of harboring acyclovir-resistant strains. Treatment with foscarnet (40 mg/kg intravenously every 8 hours) should be initiated within 7 to 10 days in patients suspected to have acyclovir-resistant VZV infections. Foscarnet therapy should be continued for at least 10 days or until lesions are completely healed.

Disseminated herpes zoster in the immunocompromised host. Acyclovir (30 mg/kg/day at 8-hour intervals) and vidarabine (continuous 12-hour infusion at 10 mg/kg/day) for 7 days (longer if resolution of cutaneous or visceral disease is incomplete) are equally effective for the treatment of disseminated herpes zoster. The resultant mortality rate is low.

Oral steroids. Studies have shown that the addition of corticosteroids to antivirals offers no benefit in reducing time to complete cessation of pain and leads to no further reduction in the incidence of postherpetic neuralgia. Treatment with corticosteroids may initially reduce pain but it is associated with a risk of serious adverse effects.

Nerve blocks. Sympathetic blocks (stellate ganglion or epidural) with 0.25% bupivacaine terminate the pain of acute herpes zoster and possibly prevent or relieve PHN in patients treated within 2 months of onset of the acute phase of the disease. Three injections are made on alternate days. When thoracic dermatomes are involved, an epidural catheter is left in place for the 5 days of therapy to avoid having to replace the needle each time. Epidural injections are made at or just above the highest dermatome of the rash. There is prompt relief of pain and all symptoms are usually gone after the second injection. Sympathetic blockade applied within the first 2 months after the onset of acute herpes zoster terminates the acute phase of the disease, probably by restoring intraneural blood flow and thus preventing the death of the large fibers and avoiding the development of PHN. After 2 months, the damage to the large fibers is irreversible.

Treatment of postherpetic neuralgia

The nature of the pain. PHN has many characteristics. There is frequently a steady, burning pain; a paroxysmal pain like that of an electric shock; and exquisite sensitivity of the skin, often with allodynia (pain from an ordinarily nonpainful stimulus). Allodynic pain from light tactile stimulation, such as that from clothing, hair, or even a breeze, can be one of the most debilitating problems faced by patients with PHN. There may be deterioration in the quality of life; patients may become reclusive, unable to bear the lightest contact of clothing against the affected skin.

POSTHERPETIC NEURALGIA TREATMENT OPTIONS. First-line therapy for neuropathic pain may be an anticonvulsant or if that fails an older-generation antidepressant such as amitriptyline or nortriptyline. For refractory cases, chronic opioid therapy may be the only avenue of relief, and evidence is accumulating that this approach is safe if proper guidelines are observed. Some of the patients who develop postherpetic neuralgia will receive adequate pain relief from topical treatments such as lidocaine patch 5% and capsaicin cream, anticonvulsants, tricyclic antidepressants, or opioids. Others will have little or no relief. Adverse side effects of these drugs limit their use.

See Figure 12-68 for the treatment of herpes zoster and PHN.

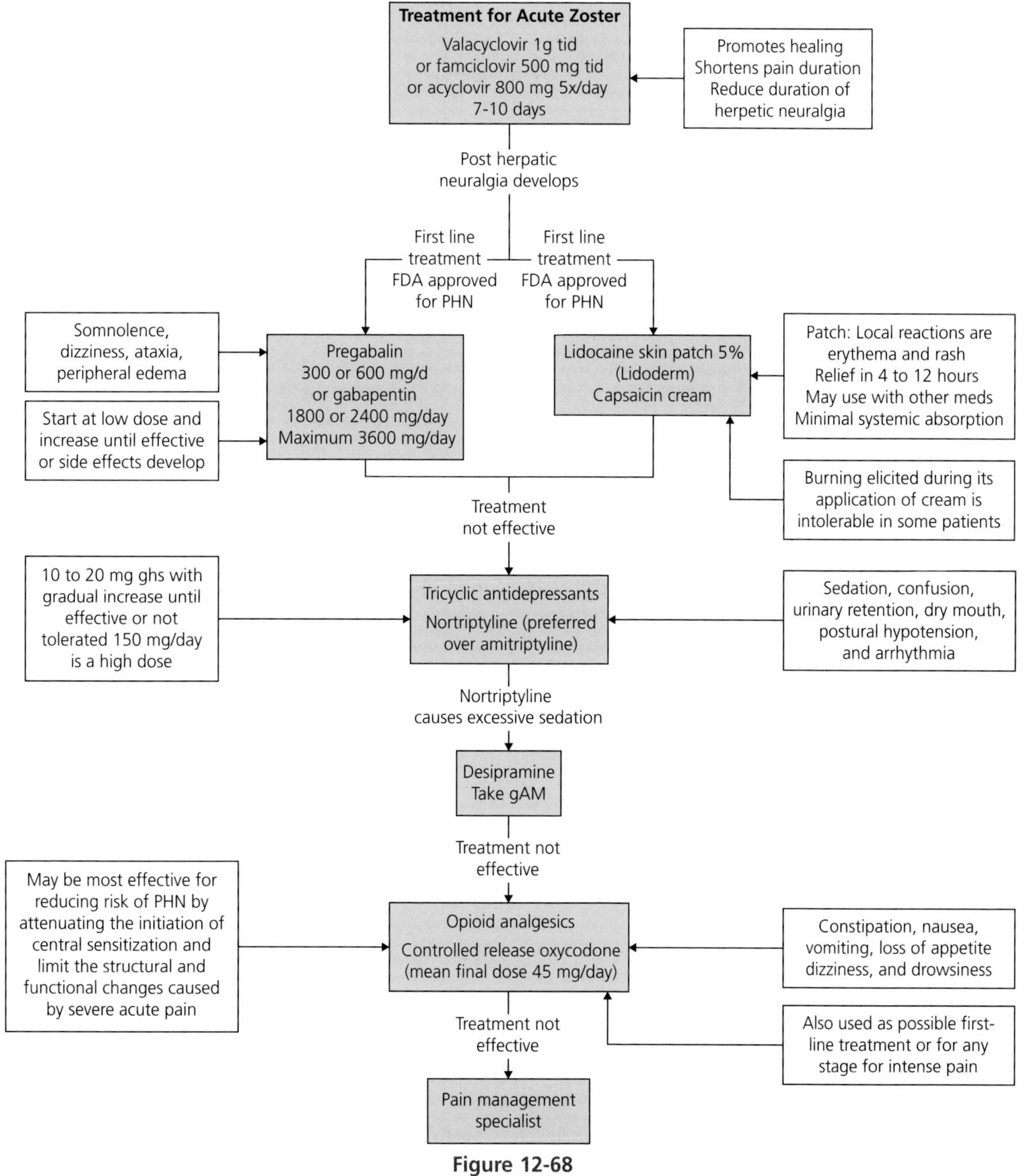

Figure 12-68

TREATMENT OF HERPES ZOSTER AND POSTHERPETIC NEURALGIA

Topical lidocaine patch (Lidoderm). The topical lidocaine patch is the first FDA-approved drug for PHN. It has no systemic side effects and is easy to use.

Analgesics. Oral analgesics (e.g., Tylenol [acetaminophen] with codeine, Percodan [oxycodone HCl], Percocet [oxycodone HCl and acetaminophen]) should be used as needed. Aspirin and other mild analgesic drugs are commonly used in patients with PHN, but their value is limited. Ibuprofen is ineffective.

Pregabalin and gabapentin. These anticonvulsant drugs are effective in the treatment of pain and sleep interference associated with PHN. They are FDA approved for the treatment of postherpetic neuralgia. Mood and quality of life also improve. Treatment with pregabalin or gabapentin results in a significant reduction in pain and improved sleep. Pregabalin is administered in two or three divided doses per day. Begin dosing at 150 mg/day; dosing may be increased to 300 mg/day within 1 week. Maximum dose is 600 mg/day.

Gabapentin is started as a single 300-mg dose on day #1, 600 mg/day on day 2 (two 300-mg doses), and 900 mg/day on day 3 (three 300-mg doses). The dose can subsequently be titrated up as needed for pain relief to a daily dose of 1800 mg (three 600-mg doses per day). In clinical studies, efficacy was demonstrated over a range of doses from 1800 mg/day to 3600 mg/day with comparable effects across the dose range. Additional benefit of using doses greater than 1800 mg/day was not demonstrated.

Tricyclic antidepressants. Tricyclic antidepressants provide moderate-to-excellent pain relief for treating postherpetic neuralgia. They are thought to act independently of their antidepressant actions (because relief of PHN occurs at less than antidepressant dosages). Crossover trials comparing nortriptyline with amitriptyline demonstrate that nortriptyline is the preferred tricyclic antidepressant; desipramine may be used in patients who experience excessive sedation with nortriptyline. Nortriptyline is a noradrenergic metabolite of amitriptyline. Pain relief occurs without an antidepressant effect with nortriptyline, and there are fewer side effects with nortriptyline. Therefore nortriptyline is the preferred antidepressant, although desipramine may be used if the patient experiences unacceptable sedation from nortriptyline. Desipramine has a low incidence of anticholinergic and sedative effects. As many as half the patients do not have a response to these drugs or have intolerable side effects. These drugs have only a moderate effect.

Side effects include confusion, urinary retention, postural hypotension, and arrhythmias. Dry mouth occurs in up to 40% of patients with amitriptyline and 25% with nortriptyline. Constipation, sweating, dizziness, disturbed vision, and drowsiness occur in up to 30% of patients with amitriptyline and 15% with nortriptyline. Use tricyclic antidepressants with caution in patients with cardiovascular disease, glaucoma, urinary retention, and autonomic neuropathy. Screen patients over age 40 for cardiac conduction abnormalities.

Oxycodone. Controlled-release oxycodone (10 mg every 12 hours) is an effective analgesic for the management of steady pain, paroxysmal spontaneous pain, and allodynia. The dose is increased weekly up to a maximum of 30 mg every 12 hours. Others have found narcotics ineffective for the long-term control of pain from PHN and to be associated with unacceptable side effects. The most common side effects are constipation, nausea, and sedation.

Capsaicin. Capsaicin is a chemical that depletes the pain impulse transmitter substance P and prevents its resynthesis within the neuron. Substantial relief of pain follows the application (three to five times daily) of this chemical in the form of a white cream (Zostrix and Zostrix-HP). Substantial pain relief occurs in 4 weeks in most patients. Maximum benefit occurs when capsaicin cream is applied for many weeks. The application of EMLA or topical lidocaine before capsaicin may prevent burning. Do not apply capsaicin to the unhealed skin lesions of acute zoster. Capsaicin is available without prescription. Some experts believe that this medication is not effective.

Emotional support. Patients with PHN can be miserable for several months. Emotional support is another important therapeutic measure.

Chapter 13

Superficial Fungal Infections

CHAPTER CONTENTS

- **Dermatophyte fungal infections**
  - Tinea
  - Pitted keratolysis
  - Treatment of fungal infections
- **Candidiasis (moniliasis)**
  - Candidiasis of normally moist areas
  - Candidiasis of large skin folds
  - Candidiasis of small skin folds
- **Tinea versicolor**
  - *Pityrosporum* folliculitis

DERMATOPHYTE FUNGAL INFECTIONS

These dermatophytes include a group of fungi (ringworm) that under most conditions have the ability to infect and survive only on dead keratin, that is, the top layer of the skin (stratum corneum or keratin layer), the hair, and the nails. They cannot survive on mucosal surfaces such as the mouth or vagina where the keratin layer does not form. Very rarely, dermatophytes undergo deep local invasion and multivisceral dissemination in the immunosuppressed host. Dermatophytes are responsible for the vast majority of skin, nail, and hair fungal infections. Lesions vary in presentation and closely resemble other diseases; therefore laboratory confirmation is often required. There is evidence that genetic susceptibility may predispose a patient to dermatophyte infection. Studies show that although several blood-related members of a family may share similar manifestations of disease, spouses, despite prolonged exposure, do not become infected. Patients with chronic dermatophytosis have a relatively specific defect in delayed hypersensitivity to *Trichophyton,* but their cell-mediated responses to other antigens are somewhat depressed. There also is a greater frequency of atopy in chronically infected patients.

CLASSIFICATION. Dermatophytes are classified in several ways. The ringworm fungi belong to three genera: *Microsporum, Trichophyton,* and *Epidermophyton*. There are several species of *Microsporum* and *Trichophyton* and one species of *Epidermophyton*.

Place of origin. The anthropophilic dermatophytes grow only on human skin, hair, or nails. The zoophilic varieties originate from animals but may infect humans. Geophilic dermatophytes live in soil but may infect humans.

Types of inflammation. The inflammatory response to dermatophytes varies. In general, zoophilic and geophilic dermatophytes elicit a brisk inflammatory response on skin and in hair follicles. The inflammatory response to anthropophilic fungi is usually mild.

Types of hair invasion. Some species are able to infect the hair shaft. Microscopic examination of infected hairs shows fungal spores and hyphae either inside the hair shaft or both inside and on the surface. The endothrix pattern consists of fungal hyphae inside the hair shaft, whereas the ectothrix pattern consists of fungal hyphae inside and on the surface of the hair shaft.

Spores of fungi are either large or small. The type of hair invasion is further classified as large- or small-spored ectothrix or large-spored endothrix.

CLINICAL CLASSIFICATION. *Tinea* means fungal infection. Clinically, dermatophyte infections are classified by body region. The dermatophytes, or ringworm fungi, produce a variety of disease patterns that vary with the location and species. Learning the numerous patterns of disease produced by each species is complicated and unnecessary because all dermatophytes respond to the same topical and oral agents. It is important to be familiar with the general patterns of inflammation in different body regions and to be able to interpret accurately a potassium hydroxide wet mount preparation of scale, hair, or nails. Species identification by culture is necessary only for scalp infections, inflammatory skin infections, and some nail infections.

The active border. One very characteristic pattern of inflammation is the active border of infection. The highest numbers of hyphae are located in the active border, and this is the best area to obtain a sample for a potassium hydroxide examination. Typically the active border is scaly, red, and slightly elevated (Figure 13-1). Vesicles appear at the active border when inflammation is intense (Figure 13-2). This pattern is present in all locations except the palms and soles.

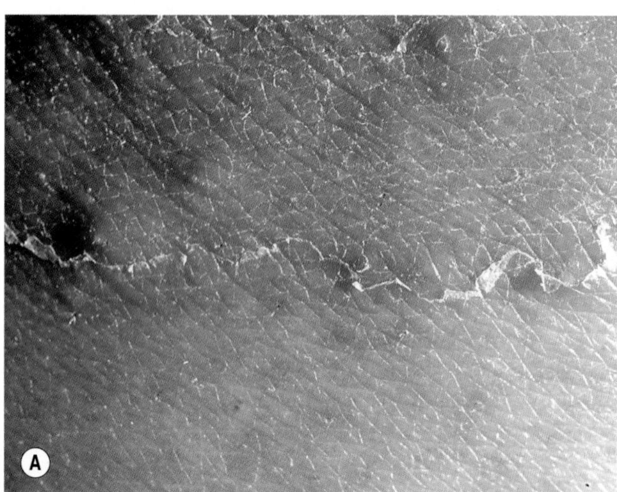

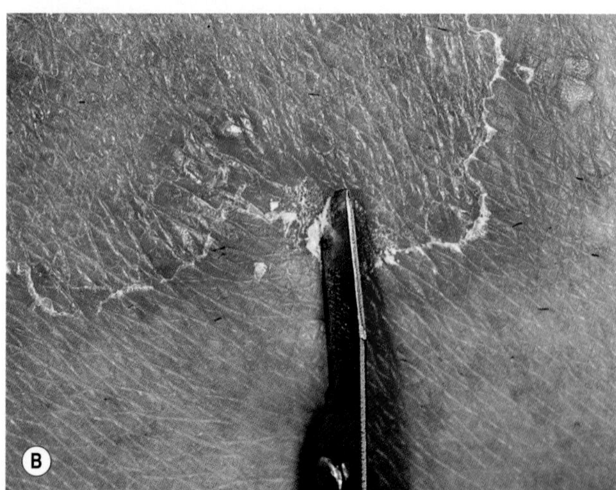

Figure 13-1 Tinea infection.
A, Active border (classic presentation). The border is red, scaly, and slightly raised. The central area is often lighter than the surrounding normal skin.
B, Sample this scale by scraping perpendicular to the border.

DIAGNOSIS

Potassium hydroxide wet mount preparation. The single most important test for the diagnosis of dermatophyte infection is direct visualization under the microscope of the branching hyphae in keratinized material.

Sampling scale. Scale is obtained by holding a #15 surgical blade perpendicular to the skin surface and smoothly but firmly drawing the blade with several short strokes against the scale. If an active border is present, the blade is drawn along the border at right angles to the fringe of the scale. If the blade is drawn from the center of the lesion out and parallel to the active border, some normal scale may also be included.

Wet mount preparation. The small fragments of scale are placed on a microscope slide and gently separated, and a coverslip is applied. Potassium hydroxide (10% or 20% solution) is applied with a toothpick or eye dropper to the edge of the coverslip and allowed to run under via capillary action. The preparation is gently heated under a low flame and then pressed to facilitate separation of the epithelial cells and fungal hyphae. Potassium hydroxide dissolves material that fuses cells but does not distort the epithelial cells or fungi. Lowering the condenser of the microscope and dimming the light enhance contrast, making hyphae easier to identify.

Nail plate keratin is thick and difficult to digest. The nail plate can be adequately softened by leaving the fragments along with several drops of potassium hydroxide in a watch glass covered with a Petri dish for 24 hours. Hair specimens require no special preparation or digestion and can be examined immediately.

Microscopy. The preparation is studied carefully by scanning the entire area under the coverslip at low power. The presence of hyphae should be confirmed by examination with the ×40 objective. Slight back-and-forth rotation of the focusing knob aids visualization of the entire segment

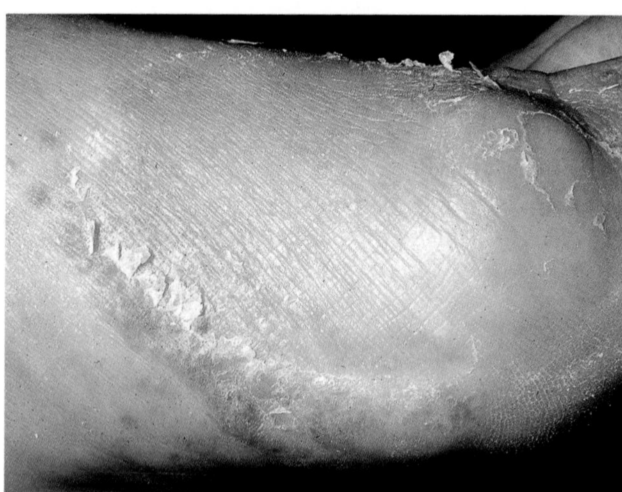

Figure 13-2 Tinea infection. Active border, which contains vesicles that indicate acute inflammation.

of the hyphae, which may be at different depths. It is not uncommon to find one small fragment of scale containing many hyphae and the rest of the preparation free of hyphae. The entire preparation should be studied carefully.

Interpretation. The interpretation of potassium hydroxide wet mounts takes experience. Dermatophytes appear as translucent, branching, rod-shaped filaments (hyphae) of uniform width, with lines of separation (septa) spanning the width and appearing at irregular intervals (Figures 13-3 and 13-4). The uniform width and characteristic bending and branching distinguish hyphae from hair and other debris. Hair tapers at the tip. Lines that intersect across cell walls at different planes of the scale are viewed using the fine adjustment knob of the microscope. Some hyphae contain a single-file line of bubbles in their cytoplasm. Hyphae may fragment into round or polygonal fragments that look like spores. Hyphae may be seen in combination with scale or floating free in the potassium hydroxide.

Artifact. Confusion may arise with the so-called mosaic artifact produced by lipid droplets appearing in a single-file line between cells, especially from specimens taken from the palms and soles (Figure 13-5). These lipid droplets disappear when the cells are separated further by additional heating and pressure. Although spores and branching hyphae as well as short, nonbranching hyphae are seen in superficial *Candida* infections and tinea versicolor, only branching hyphae are seen in dermatophyte infections. Longitudinal, rod-shaped potassium hydroxide crystals that simulate hyphae may appear if the wet mount is heated excessively.

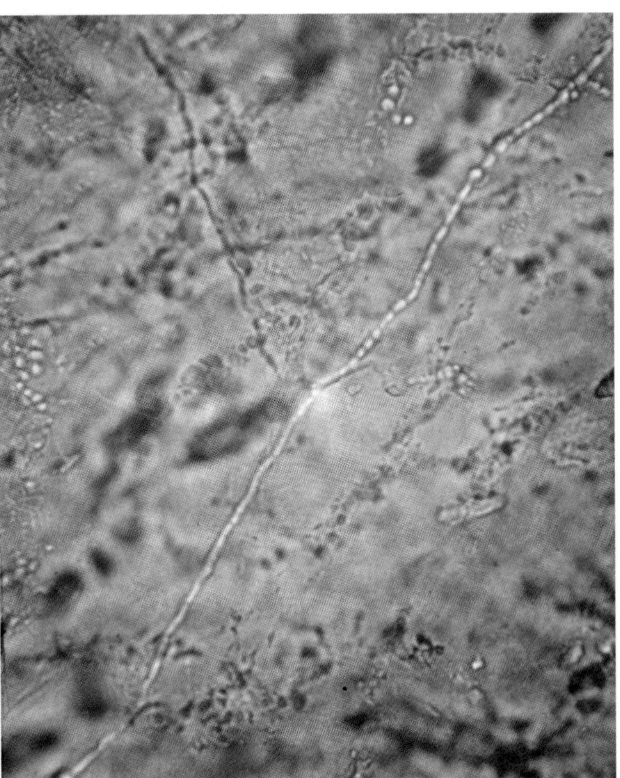

Figure 13-4 A drop of ink added to the potassium hydroxide wet mount accentuates hyphae. (Courtesy Dr. Leanor Haley, Centers for Disease Control and Prevention.)

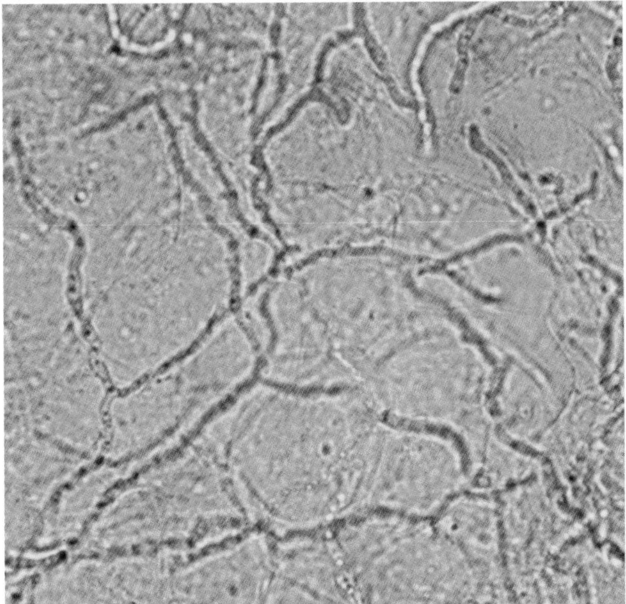

Figure 13-3 Fungal hyphae in a potassium hydroxide wet mount. The identifying characteristic is the branching, filamentous structure that is uniform in width.

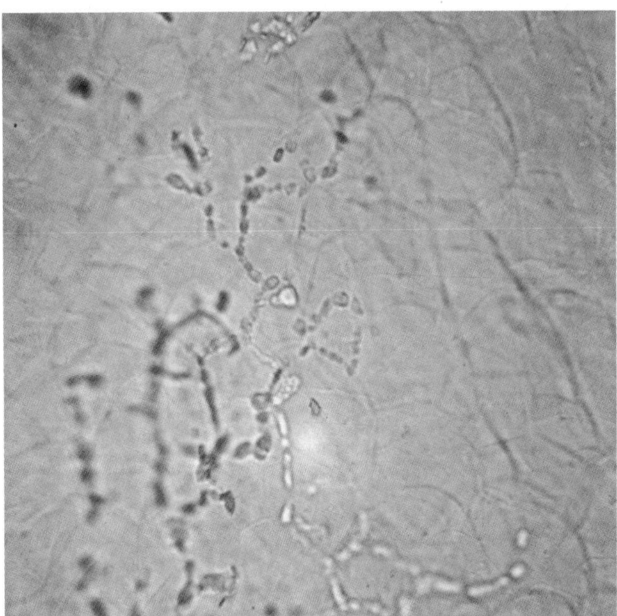

Figure 13-5 Mosaic artifact. Lipid droplets appearing in a single-file line between epithelial cells simulate fungal hyphae in potassium hydroxide wet mounts. Heat encourages cell separation and the artifact disappears. (Courtesy Dr. Leanor Haley, Centers for Disease Control and Prevention.)

Special stains. Hyphae may be difficult to find in a potassium hydroxide wet mount. Chlorazol fungal stain, Swartz Lamkins fungal stain, or Parker's blue ink clearly stains hyphae, rendering them visible under low power. The specialized stains are available from Dermatologic Lab and Supply, Inc. (www.delasco.com).

Culture. In most cases it is not necessary to know the species of dermatophyte infecting skin because the same oral and topical agents are active against all of them. Fungal culture is necessary for hair and nail fungal infections. Scalp hair infections in children may originate from an animal that carries a typical species of dermatophyte. The animal can then be traced and treated or destroyed to prevent further infection of other humans. Nail plate, especially of the toenails, may be infected with nondermatophytes, such as the saprophytic mold *Scopulariopsis,* which do not respond to treatment. Identification of the genus of fungus responsible for nail plate infection is therefore necessary before embarking on a long course of treatment.

Cotton swab technique for culture. A sterile cotton swab that is moistened with sterile water or agar from an agar plate and rubbed vigorously over the lesion produces results comparable to those obtained by scraping with a scalpel blade. A light sweep over the lesion does not collect sufficient material; therefore the swab must be rubbed vigorously over the active part of the lesion and then over the surface of the agar. The swab is useful in areas that are difficult to scrape, such as the scalp, eyelids, ears, nose, and between the toes. The sterile swab is less threatening than a blade, and it is safer in situations in which the sudden movement of a child could lead to a painful stab or cut.

Culture media for tinea. Dermatophytes are aerobic and grow on the surface of media. The three types of culture media used most often for isolation and identification are dermatophyte test medium (DTM), mycobiotic agar, and Sabouraud's dextrose agar. Many hospital laboratories lack the experience to interpret fungal cultures and instead send them to outside laboratories for analysis. Material to be cultured can be sent directly to a laboratory because, unlike many bacteria, fungi remain viable for days in scale and hair without being inoculated onto media. Alternatively, many hospitals and individual practitioners now rely on DTM for faster but slightly less accurate results.

DTM is a commercially available medium supplied in vials that are ready for direct inoculation. The yellow medium, which contains the indicator phenol red, turns pink in the presence of the alkaline metabolic products of dermatophytes in approximately 6 or 7 days but remains yellow in the presence of the acid metabolic products of nonpathogenic fungi. It must be discarded after 2 weeks because saprophytes can induce a similar color change after the 2-week period. Species identification is possible with DTM but is more accurately determined with mycobiotic agar and Sabouraud's agar because the dye in DTM may interfere with interpretation.

DTM and onychomycosis. DTM can be used to confirm dermatophyte infections in patients with presumed onychomycosis. Diagnosis of onychomycosis requires confirmation of dermatophyte infection only, not identification of genus and species. DTM fulfills this requirement and has a diagnostic yield comparable to central laboratory culture. This allows diagnosis in the office and should fulfill the requirement when insurers demand confirmation of toenail infection before approving the use of oral antifungals.

Mycobiotic agar is a modification of Sabouraud's medium that contains cycloheximide and chloramphenicol to prevent the growth of bacteria and saprophytic fungi; the dextrose content of Mycosel agar has been lowered and the pH has been raised to allow for better growth of dermatophytes.

Sabouraud's agar, which does not contain antibiotics, allows the growth of most fungi, including nondermatophytes. This may be useful for nail infections because the detection of nondermatophytes is desirable in nail infections; but the more selective mycobiotic agar is best for evaluation of hair tinea because only dermatophytes cause hair tinea. Cultures usually become positive in 1 to 2 weeks.

Culture media for yeast. Yeast may be isolated on plates obtained from the hospital laboratory. Acu-Nickerson is a commercially available medium in a slant for use in the isolation and identification of *Candida* species.

Wood's light examination. Light rays with a wavelength above 365 nm are produced when ultraviolet light is projected through a Wood's filter. Hair, but not the skin of the scalp, fluoresces with a blue-green color if infected with *Microsporum canis* or *Microsporum audouinii*. The rarer *Trichophyton schoenleinii* produces a paler green fluorescence of infected hair; no other dermatophytes that infect hair produce fluorescence. Fungal infections of the skin do not fluoresce, except for tinea versicolor, which produces a pale white-yellow fluorescence. Erythrasma—a noninflammatory, pale brown, scaly eruption of the toe webs, groin, and axillae caused by the bacteria *Corynebacterium minutissimum*—shows a brilliant coral-red fluorescence with the Wood's light. Wood's light examination should be performed in a dark room with a high-intensity instrument. The fluorescence of hair may be caused by tryptophan metabolites.

Tinea

Clinically, dermatophyte infections have traditionally been classified by body region. *Tinea* means fungus infection. The term *tinea capitis,* for example, indicates "dermatophyte infection of the scalp."

TINEA OF THE FOOT

The feet are the most common area infected by dermatophytes (*tinea pedis,* or "athlete's foot"). Shoes promote warmth and sweating, which encourage fungal growth. Fungal infections of the feet are common in men and uncommon in women; although uncommon, tinea pedis does occur in prepubertal children. Tinea should be considered in the differential diagnosis of children with foot dermatitis. The occurrence of tinea pedis seems to be inevitable in immunologically predisposed individuals regardless of elaborate precautions taken to avoid the infecting organism. Locker-room floors contain fungal elements, and the use of communal baths may create an ideal condition for repeated exposure to infected material. White socks do nothing to prevent tinea pedis. Once established, the individual becomes a carrier and is more susceptible to recurrences. There are many different clinical presentations of tinea pedis. The clinical diagnosis of tinea pedis can be misleading, since it features lesions that can also be present in some other skin diseases, and direct microscopy may be insufficient to confirm the diagnosis. Culture may be necessary for a definitive diagnosis.

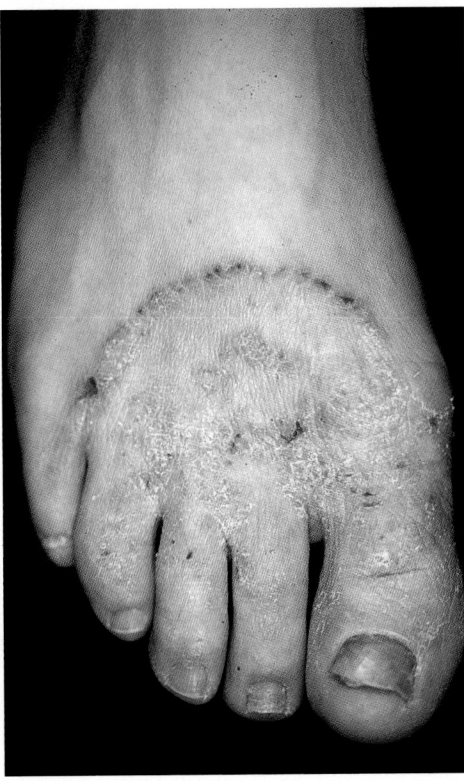

Figure 13-6 Tinea pedis. The classic "ringworm" pattern of tinea can appear on any body surface.

CLINICAL PRESENTATIONS. Tinea of the feet may present with the classic "ringworm" pattern (Figure 13-6), but most infections are found in the toe webs or on the soles.

Interdigital tinea pedis (toe web infection). Tight-fitting shoes compress the toes, creating a warm, moist environment in the toe webs; this environment is suited to fungal growth. The web between the fourth and fifth toes is most commonly involved, but all webs may be infected. The web can become dry, scaly, and fissured or white, macerated, and soggy (Figure 13-7). Itching is most intense when the shoes and socks are removed. The bacterial flora is unchanged when the tinea-infected webs demonstrate scale and peeling without maceration. Overgrowth of the resident bacterial population determines the severity of interdigital toe web infection. The macerated pattern of

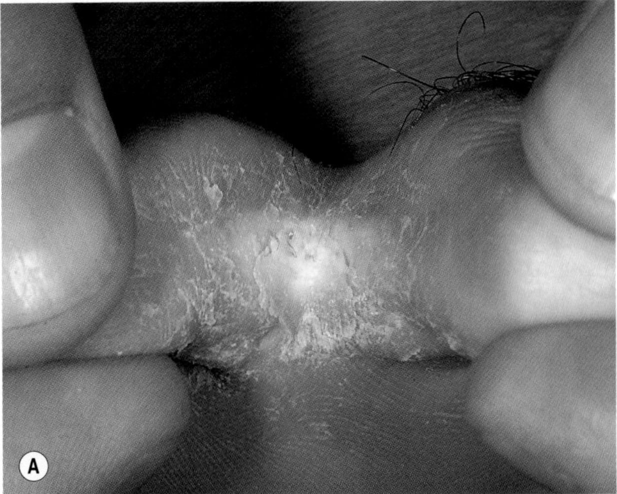

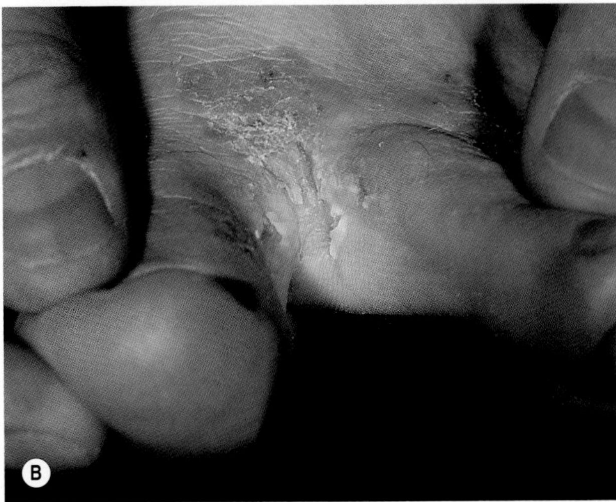

Figure 13-7 Tinea pedis (toe web infection).
A, Scale is either dry or **B,** the toe web space contains wet macerated scale. The fourth web is the most commonly involved web space.

infection occurs from an interaction of bacteria and fungus. Dermatophytes initiate the damage to the stratum corneum and, by the production of antibiotics, influence the selection of a more antibiotic-resistant bacterial population. The prevalence of *Staphylococcus aureus,* gram-negative bacteria, *Corynebacterium minutissimum, Staphylococcus epidermidis,* and *Micrococcus sedentarius* increases. Extension out of the web space onto the plantar surface or the dorsum of the foot is common and occurs with the typical, chronic, ringworm type of scaly, advancing border or with an acute, vesicular eruption (Figure 13-8). Identification of fungal hyphae in the macerated skin of the toe webs may be difficult.

TWO FEET-ONE HAND SYNDROME

The two feet-one hand syndrome involves dermatophyte infection of both feet, with tinea of the right or left palm (Figure 13-9). Nail infection of the hands and feet may also be present. Most cases occur in men. The same organism infects the feet, hand, and nails. *T. rubrum* is the causative organism in most cases. The development of tinea pedis/onychomycosis generally precedes the development of tinea of the hand. Tinea manuum usually develops in the hand used to excoriate the feet or pick toenails. Patients whose occupation involves a high intensity of use of the hands are more likely to develop the disease at an earlier age.

TREATMENT. The newest class of antifungal agents produces higher cure rates and more rapid responses in dermatophyte infections than do older agents such as clotrimazole. They produce a higher cure rate and lower relapse rate than the antifungal/corticosteroid combination (e.g., Lotrisone [clotrimazole/betamethasone]).

Terbinafine 1% cream (Lamisil over-the-counter) applied twice daily for 1 week results in a high cure rate in interdigital tinea pedis. In one series, terbinafine gave progressive mycologic improvement; at 5 weeks after treatment, 88% of the patients were clear of infection. Effective short-course therapy with potent fungicidal drugs such as terbinafine may avoid treatment failure caused by noncompliance with fungistatic agents, such as clotrimazole, that require 4 weeks of treatment. Butenafine (Mentax cream, Lotrimin Ultra over-the-counter) applied twice daily for 1 week is also highly effective in treating interdigital tinea pedis. Econazole nitrate (Spectazole) has activity against several bacterial species associated with severely macerated interdigital interspaces. Recurrence is prevented by wearing wider shoes and expanding the web space with a small strand of lamb's wool (Dr. Scholls' lamb's wool). Powders, not necessarily medicated, absorb moisture. The powders should be applied to the feet rather than to the shoes. Wet socks should be changed.

Hyperkeratotic, moccasin-type tinea of the plantar surface responds slowly to conventional therapy. Oral terbinafine 125 mg daily for 4 weeks produced sustained cure rates of 95%. *PMID: 18076589* Griseofulvin 250 to 500 mg twice a day for 6 weeks resulted in a 27% to 35% cure rate.

Acute vesicular tinea pedis responds to wet Burow's solution compresses applied for 30 minutes several times each day. Oral antifungal drugs control the acute infection. Secondary bacterial infection is treated with oral antibiotics. A vesicular id reaction sometimes occurs at distant sites during an inflammatory foot infection. Wet dressings, group V topical steroids, and, occasionally, prednisone 20 mg twice a day for 8 to 10 days are required for control of id reactions.

Tinea pedis has been effectively treated with pulse doses of fluconazole 150 mg orally once weekly, with 200 mg itraconazole daily for 2 weeks or 200 mg twice a day for 1 week, and with 250 mg terbinafine daily for 2 weeks.

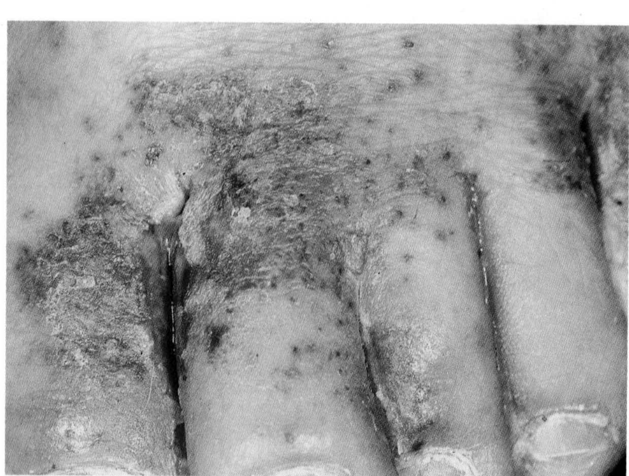

Figure 13-8 Tinea pedis. The infection has spread beyond the toe web.

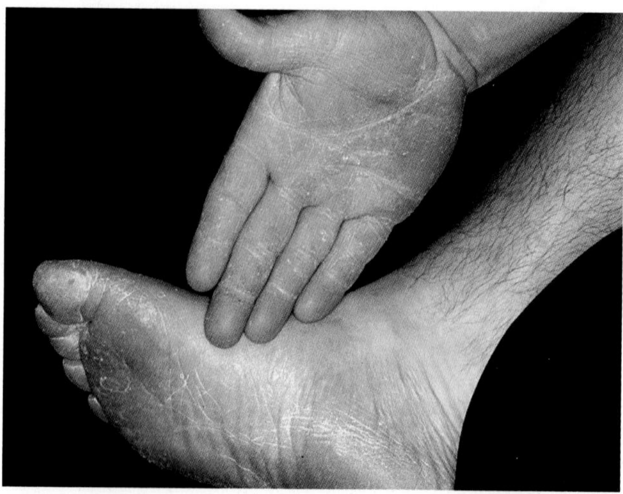

Figure 13-9 It is common to see infection of one hand and two feet or two hands and one foot but not infection of both hands and feet at the same time.

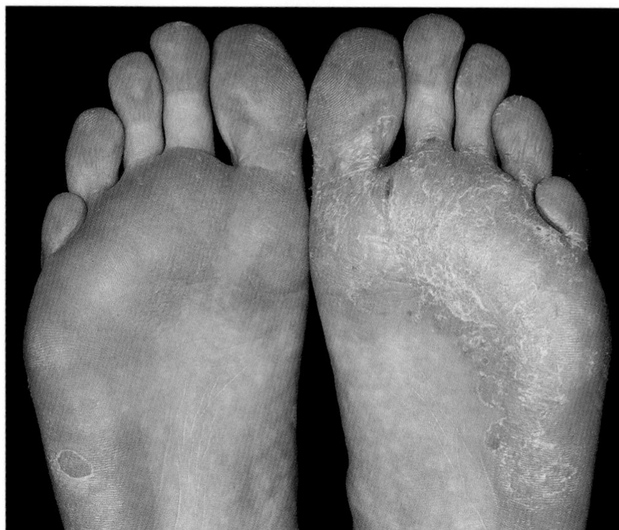

Figure 13-10 Tinea pedis. Web spaces and plantar surfaces of one foot have been inflamed for years; the other foot remains clear.

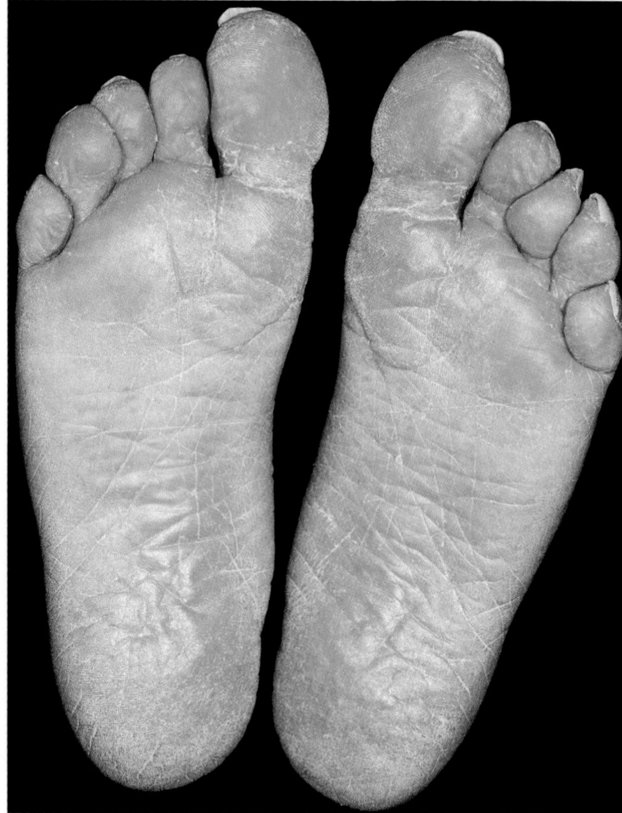

Figure 13-11 Tinea pedis. The entire plantar surface of both feet is thickened, tan colored, and covered with a fine, white scale.

Chronic scaly infection of the plantar surface. Plantar hyperkeratotic or moccasin-type tinea pedis is a particularly chronic form of tinea that is resistant to treatment. The entire sole is usually infected and covered with a fine, silvery white scale (Figures 13-10 to 13-12). The skin may be pink, tender, and/or pruritic. The hands may be similarly infected. It is rare to see both palms and soles infected simultaneously; rather, the pattern is infection of two feet and one hand or of two hands and one foot. *Trichophyton rubrum* is the usual pathogen. This pattern of infection is difficult to eradicate. *T. rubrum* produce substances that diminish the immune response and inhibit stratum corneum turnover.

Acute vesicular tinea pedis. A highly inflammatory fungal infection may occur, particularly in people who wear occlusive shoes. This acute form of infection often originates from a more chronic web infection. A few or many vesicles evolve rapidly on the sole or on the dorsum of the foot. The vesicles may fuse into bullae or remain as collections of fluid under the thick scale of the sole and never rupture through the surface. Secondary bacterial infection occurs commonly in eroded areas after bullae rupture. Fungal hyphae are difficult to identify in severely inflamed skin. Specimens for potassium hydroxide examination should be taken from the roof of the vesicle. A second wave of vesicles may follow shortly in the same areas or at distant sites such as the arms, chest, and along the sides of the fingers. These itchy sterile vesicles represent an allergic response to the fungus and are termed a *dermatophytid,* or *id, reaction*. They subside when the infection is controlled. At times the id reaction is the only clinical manifestation of a fungus infection. Careful examination of these patients may show an asymptomatic fissure or area of maceration in the toe webs.

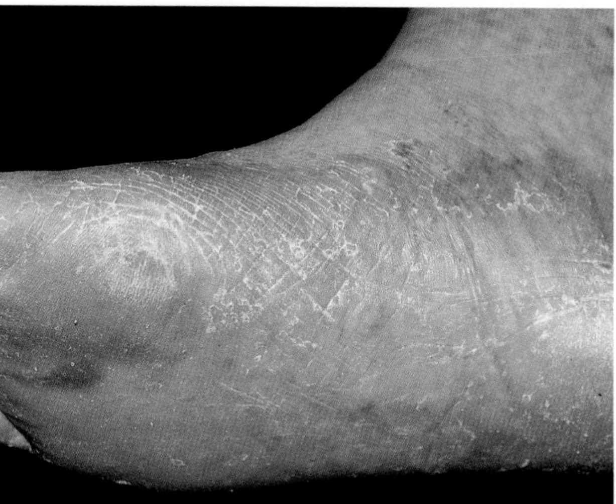

Figure 13-12 Tinea pedis. This patient has chronic inflammation of the soles that periodically flares on the dorsum and ankle.

Pitted keratolysis

Pitted keratolysis, a disease mimicking tinea pedis, is an eruption of the weight-bearing surfaces of the soles. The most common sites of onset are the pressure-bearing areas, such as the ventral aspect of the toe, the ball of the foot, and the heel. Lesions are rarely seen on the non–pressure-bearing locations. Hyperhidrosis is the most frequently observed symptom. Malodor and sliminess of the skin are also distinctive features.

The disease is bacterial in origin but is often misinterpreted as a fungal infection. It is characterized by many circular or longitudinal, punched-out depressions in the skin surface (Figures 13-13 and 13-14). Most cases are asymptomatic, but painful, plaquelike lesions may occur in both adults and children. The eruption is limited to the stratum corneum and causes little or no inflammation. Hyperhidrosis, moist socks, or immersion of the feet favors its development. There may be a few circular pits that remain unnoticed, or the entire weight-bearing surface may be covered with annular furrows. Several bacteria have been implicated, including *Dermatophilus congolensis* and *Micrococcus sedentarius*. These bacteria produce and excrete exoenzymes (keratinase) that are able to degrade keratin and produce pitting in the stratum corneum when the skin is hydrated and the pH rises above neutrality. These organisms are not easily cultured, but the filamentous and coccoid microorganisms can be demonstrated by hematoxylin and eosin staining of a formalin-fixed section of shaved stratum corneum prepared for histopathology. The clinical presentation is so characteristic that laboratory confirmation is usually not necessary.

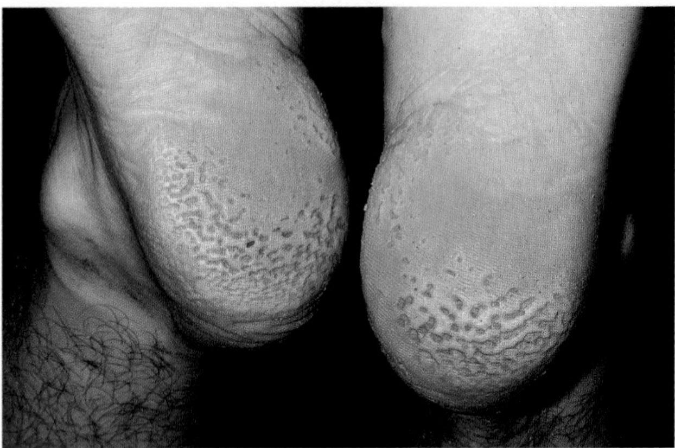

Figure 13-13 Pitted keratolysis. Deep longitudinal furrows are located primarily on weight-bearing surfaces.

TREATMENT. Wash feet daily with soap or antibacterial cleanser. Treatment consists of promoting dryness. Socks should be changed frequently. Rapid clearing occurs with application of 20% aluminum chloride (Drysol) twice a day. Lazerformalyde solution (10% formaldehyde), which is a potent antiperspirant, is useful. Treatment can then be applied periodically when necessary. Antibiotics are effective even without aluminum chloride or formaldehyde. The application twice a day of alcohol-based benzoyl peroxide may also be useful. Treatment with acne medications such as topical erythromycin solution or clindamycin solution is also curative. Mupirocin (Bactroban) ointment or cream and fusidic acid cream may also be effective. Oral erythromycin is an alternative.

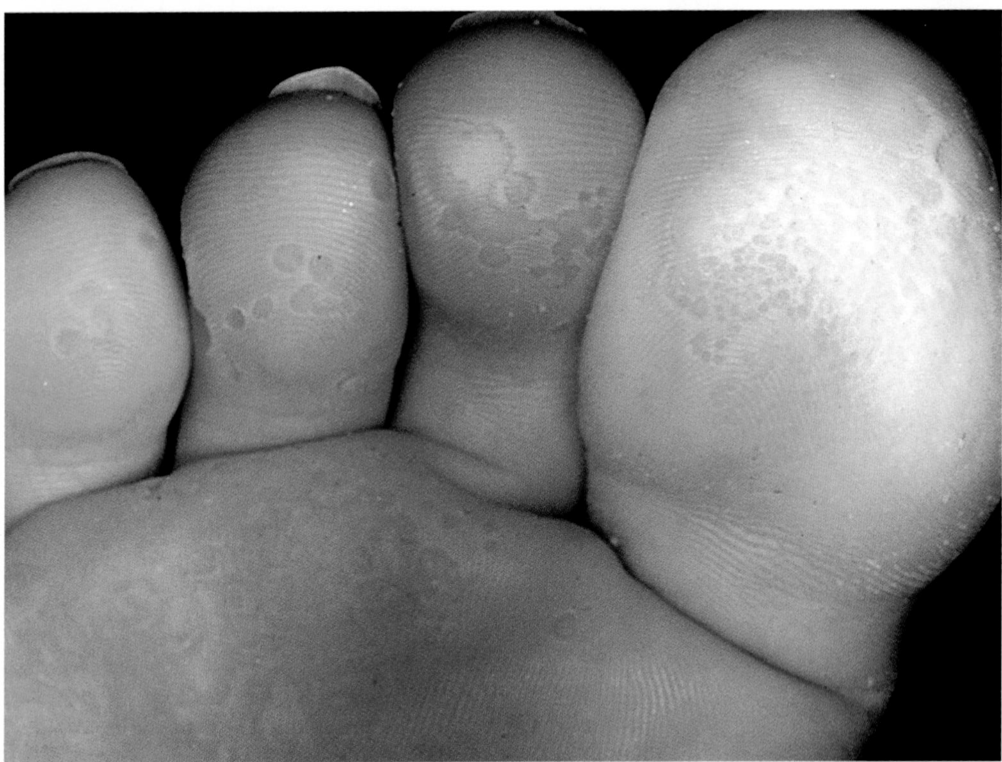

Figure 13-14 Pitted keratolysis. The skin around the deep pits is often wet and macerated.

TINEA OF THE GROIN

Tinea of the groin (*tinea cruris,* "jock itch") occurs often in the summer months after sweating or wearing wet clothing and in the winter months after wearing several layers of clothing. The predisposing factor, as with many other types of superficial infection, is the presence of a warm, moist environment. Men are affected much more frequently than are women; children rarely develop tinea of the groin. Itching becomes worse as moisture accumulates and macerates this intertriginous area.

The lesions are most often unilateral and begin in the crural fold. A half-moon–shaped plaque forms as a well-defined scaling, and sometimes a vesicular border advances out of the crural fold onto the thigh (Figure 13-15). The skin within the border turns red-brown, is less scaly, and may develop red papules. Acute inflammation may appear after a person has worn occlusive clothing for an extended period. The infection occasionally migrates to the buttock and gluteal cleft area. Involvement of the scrotum is unusual—unlike *Candida* reactions, in which it is common (Figure 13-16). Specimens for potassium hydroxide examination should be taken from the advancing scaling border.

Topical steroid creams are frequently prescribed for inflammatory skin disease of the groin, and they modify the typical clinical presentation of tinea. The eruption may be much more extensive, and the advancing, scaly border may not be present (see Figure 13-34). Red papules sometimes appear at the edges and center of the lesion. This modified form (tinea incognito) may not be immediately recognized as tinea; the only clue is the history of a typical, half-moon–shaped plaque treated with cortisone cream. Scale, if present, contains numerous hyphae.

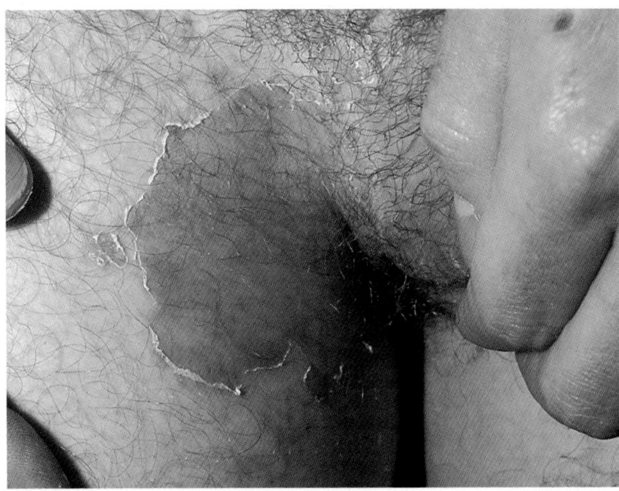

Figure 13-15 Tinea cruris. A half-moon–shaped plaque has a well-defined, scaling border.

Figure 13-16 *Candida* groin infection. Tinea cruris usually presents as a unilateral half-moon–shaped plaque that does not extend onto the scrotum. *Candida* groin infections are more extensive and often bilateral. They infect the scrotum and show the typical fringe of scale at the border and satellite pustules.

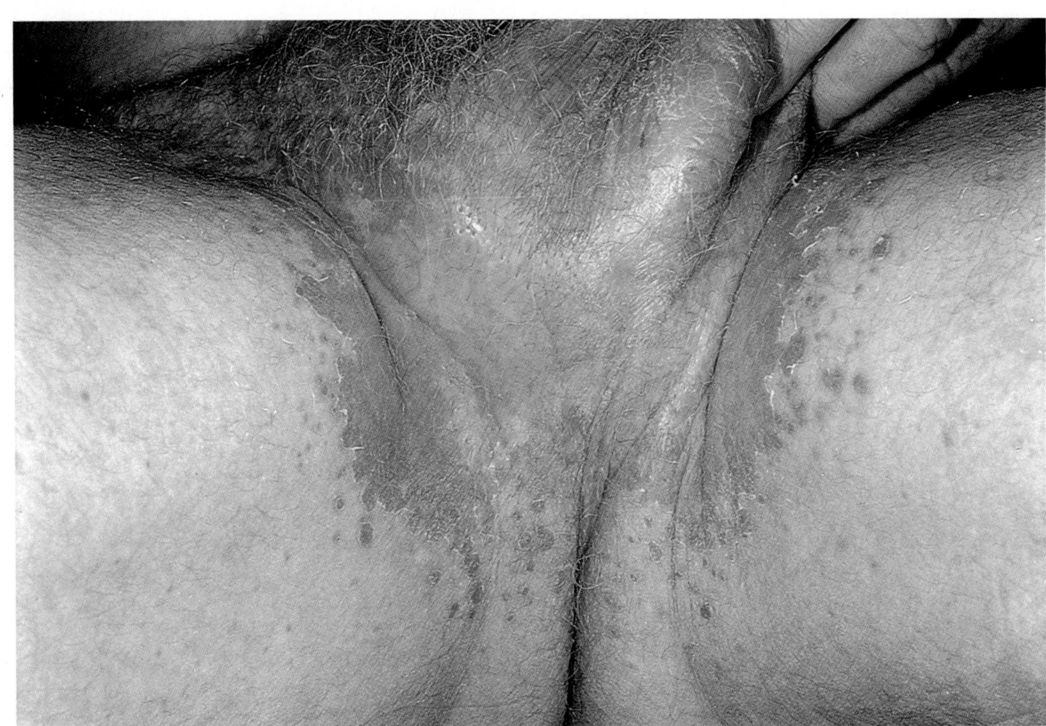

INTERTRIGO

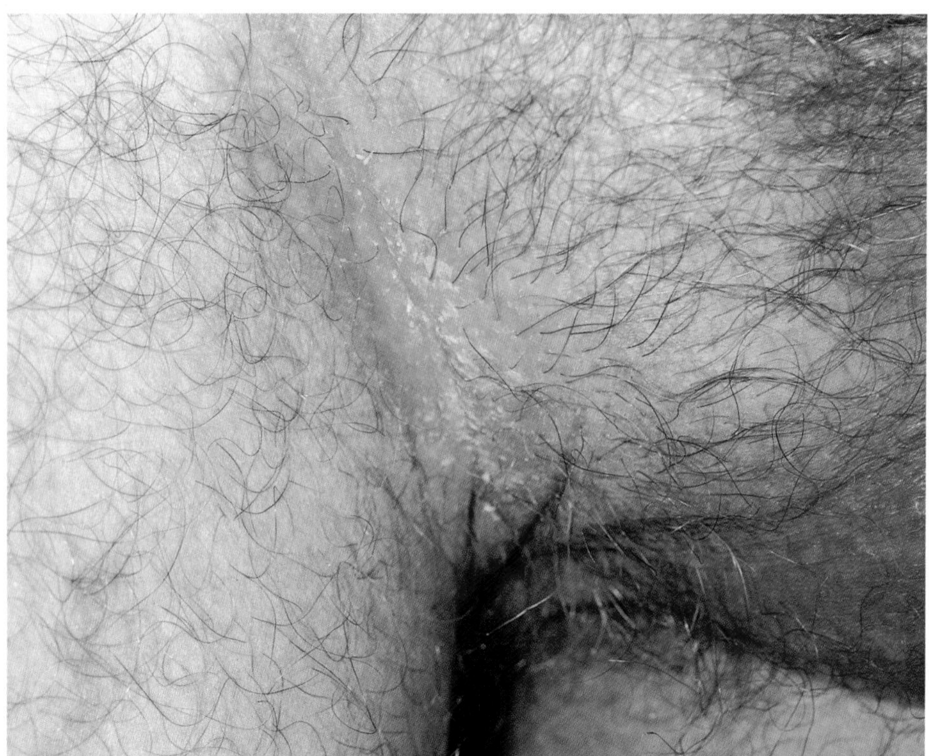

Figure 13-17 A tender, red plaque with a moist macerated surface extends to an equal extent onto the scrotum and thigh.

Figure 13-18 An advanced case with deep longitudinal fissuring in the crural fold.

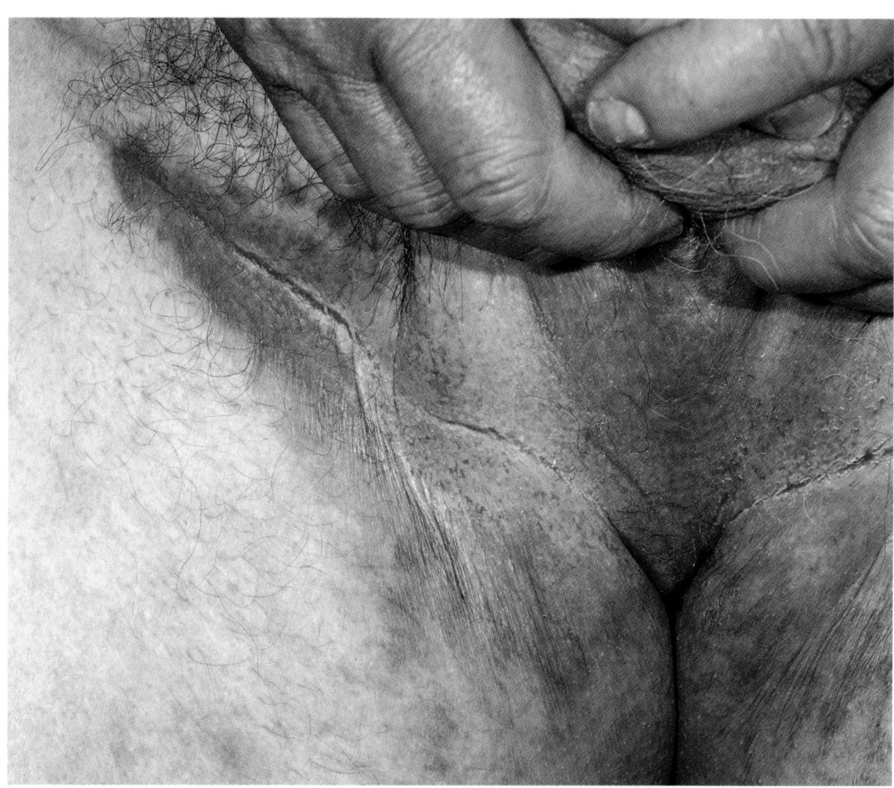

DIFFERENTIAL DIAGNOSIS

Intertrigo. A red, macerated, half-moon–shaped plaque, resembling tinea of the groin and extending to an equal extent onto the groin and down the thigh, forms after moisture accumulates in the crural fold (Figure 13-17). The sharp borders touch where the opposed surfaces of the skin folds of the groin and thigh meet. Obesity contributes to this inflammatory process, which may be infected with a mixed flora of bacteria, fungi, and yeast. Painful, longitudinal fissures occur in the crease of the crural fold (Figure 13-18). Groin intertrigo recurs after treatment unless weight and moisture are controlled. Psoriasis and seborrheic dermatitis of the groin may mimic intertrigo (see the section Candidiasis of Large Skin Folds).

Erythrasma. This bacterial infection (*C. minutissimum*) may be confused with tinea cruris because of the similar, half-moon–shaped plaque (Figure 13-19). Erythrasma differs in that it is noninflammatory, it is uniformly brown and scaly, and it has no advancing border. The organism produces porphyrins, which fluoresce coral-red with the Wood's light; tinea of the groin does not fluoresce. Erythrasma of the vulva may be misinterpreted as a candidal infection, especially if the Wood's light examination is negative. The most common site of erythrasma is in the fourth interdigital toe space, but infection is also seen in the inframammary fold and the axillae. Gram stain of the scale shows gram-positive, rodlike organisms in long filaments. However, the scale is difficult to fix to a slide for Gram stain. One technique is to strip the scale with clear tape and then carefully stain the taped-scale preparation. A biopsy demonstrates rods and filamentous organisms in the keratotic layer. Erythrasma responds to erythromycin (250 mg four times a day for 5 days) or clarithromycin (single 1-gm dose) or topically to miconazole, clotrimazole, and econazole creams (but not ketoconazole). Topical acne medication such as clindamycin (Cleocin-T lotion) or erythromycin applied two times a day for 2 weeks is effective. Some topical antibiotics contain alcohol and may be irritating when applied to the groin.

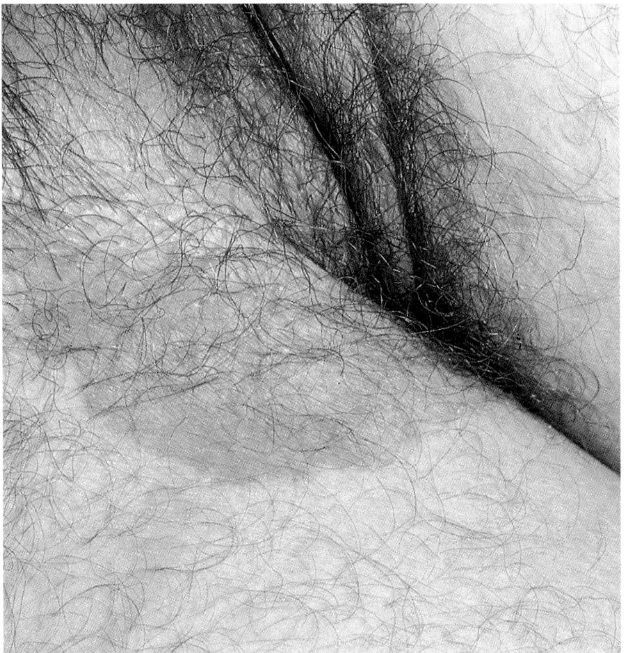

Figure 13-19 Erythrasma: a bacterial infection (*Corynebacterium minutissimum*). The diffuse brown, scaly plaque resembles tinea cruris.

TREATMENT FOR TINEA OF THE GROIN. Tinea of the groin responds to any of the topical antifungal creams listed in the Formulary. Lesions may appear to respond quickly, but creams should be applied twice a day for at least 10 days. The fungicidal allylamines (naftifine and terbinafine) and butenafine (allylamine derivative) allow for a shorter duration of treatment compared with fungistatic azoles (clotrimazole, econazole, ketoconazole, oxiconazole, miconazole, and sulconazole).

Moist intertriginous lesions may be contaminated with dermatophytes, other fungi, or bacteria. Antifungal creams with activity against *Candida* and dermatophytes (e.g., miconazole) are applied and covered with a cool, wet Burow's solution, water, or saline compress for 20 to 30 minutes two to six times daily until macerated, wet skin has been dried. The wet dressings are discontinued when the skin is dry, but the cream is continued for at least 14 days or until all evidence of the fungal infection has disappeared. Any residual inflammation from the intertrigo is treated with a group V through VII topical steroid twice a day for a specified length of time (e.g., 5 to 10 days). A limited amount of topical steroid cream is prescribed to discourage long-term use. Absorbent powders, not necessarily medicated (e.g., Z-Sorb), help to control moisture but should not be applied until the inflammation is gone. Resistant infections respond to any of the oral agents listed in Table 13-2, p. 519.

Lotrisone solution or cream (betamethasone dipropionate/clotrimazole) may be used for initial treatment if lesions are red, inflamed, and itchy. A pure antifungal cream should be used once symptoms are controlled. Prolonged use of this steroid antifungal preparation may not cure the infection and may cause striae in this intertriginous area.

Systemic therapy is sometimes necessary. Tinea cruris is effectively treated by 50 to 100 mg fluconazole daily or 150 mg once weekly for 2 to 3 weeks. Itraconazole 100 mg twice daily immediately after meals on days 1 and 8 or on days 1 and 2 may be effective. *PMID: 12950901* The standard treatments are itraconazole 100 mg daily for 2 weeks or 200 mg daily for 7 days, or 250 mg terbinafine daily for 1 to 2 weeks. Griseofulvin 500 mg daily for 4 to 6 weeks is also effective.

TINEA OF THE BODY AND FACE

Tinea of the face (excluding the beard area in men), trunk, and limbs is called *tinea corporis* ("ringworm of the body"). The disease can occur at any age and is more common in warm climates. There is a broad range of manifestations, with lesions varying in size, degree of inflammation, and depth of involvement. This variability is explained by differences in host immunity and the species of fungus. An epidemic of tinea corporis caused by *Trichophyton tonsurans* was reported in student wrestlers.

ROUND ANNULAR LESIONS. In classic ringworm, lesions begin as flat, scaly spots that then develop a raised border that expands at varying rates in all directions. The advancing, scaly border may have red, raised papules or vesicles. The central area becomes brown or hypopigmented and less scaly as the active border progresses outward (Figure 13-20). However, it is not uncommon to see several red papules in the central area (Figure 13-21). There may be just one ring that grows to a few centimeters in diameter and then resolves or several annular lesions that enlarge to cover large areas of the body surface (Figures 13-22, 13-23, and 13-24). These larger lesions tend to be mildly itchy or asymptomatic. They may reach a certain size and remain for years with no tendency to resolve. Clear, central areas of the larger lesions are yellow-brown and usually contain several red papules. The borders are serpiginous or annular and very irregular.

Pityriasis rosea and multiple small annular lesions of ringworm may appear to be similar. However, the scaly ring of pityriasis rosea does not reach the edge of the red border as it does in tinea. Other distinguishing features of pityriasis rosea include rapid onset of lesions and localization of the trunk. Tinea from cats may appear suddenly as multiple round-to-oval plaques on the trunk and extremities (Figure 13-25).

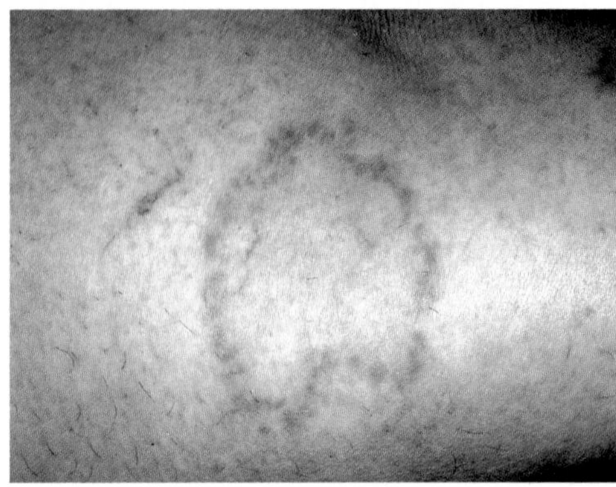

Figure 13-20 The classic ring worm pattern of infection of the body.

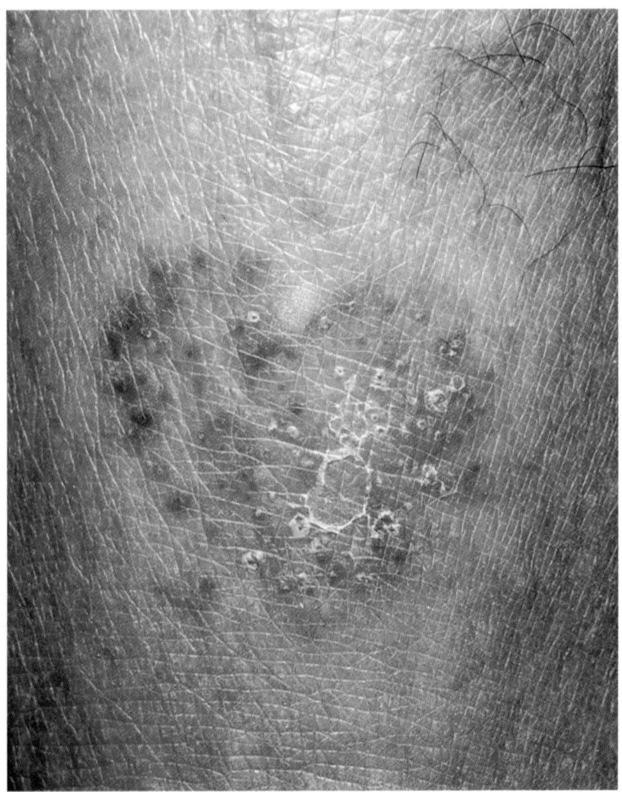

Figure 13-21 Papules and pustules may appear within the border and indicate deeper follicular infection.

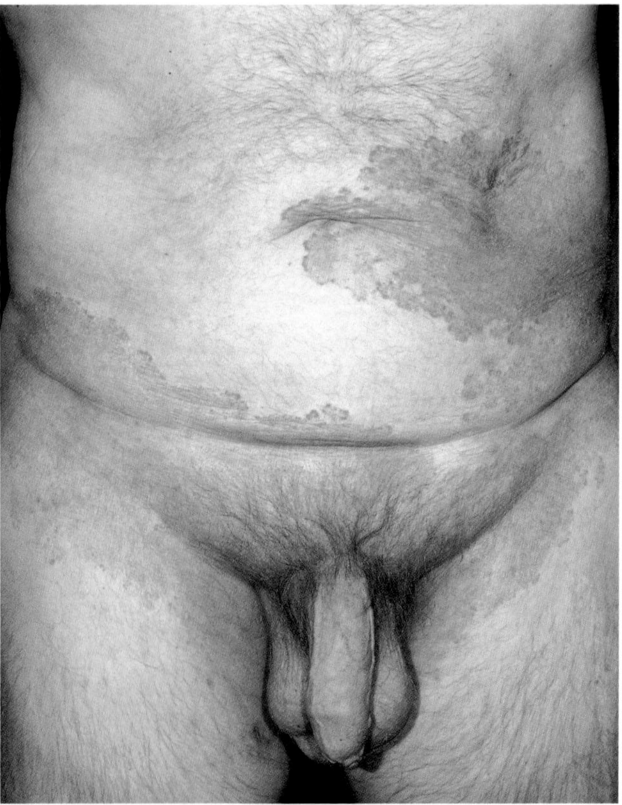

Figure 13-22 Tinea corporis. The border areas are fairly distinct and contain red papules. The central area is light brown and scaly.

TINEA OF THE BODY AND FACE

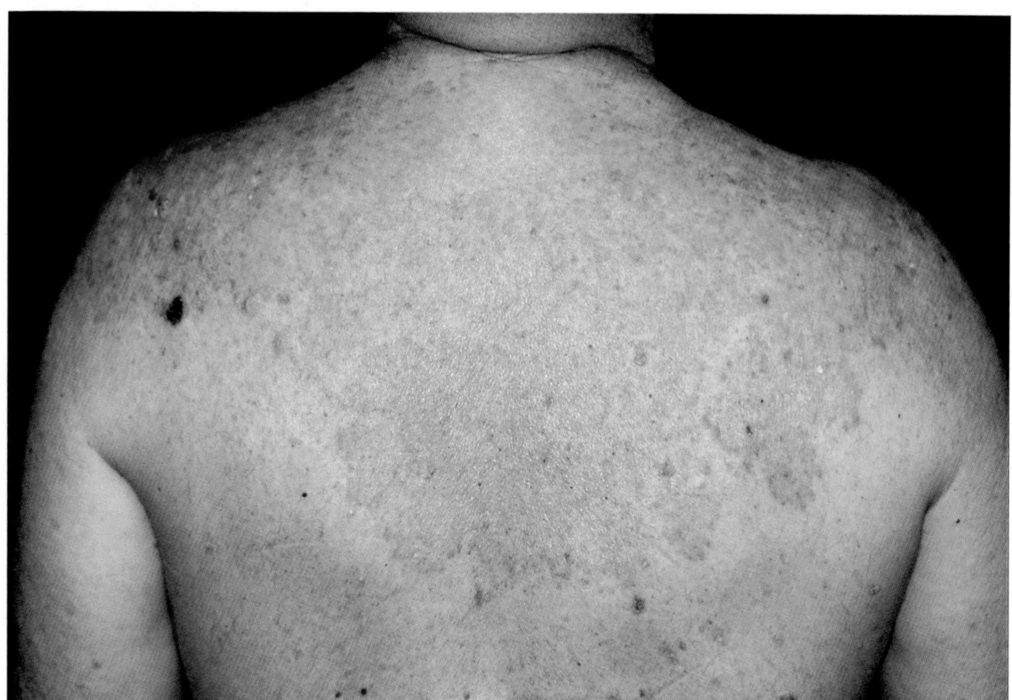

Figure 13-23 Tinea corporis can extend over huge areas and persist for years. There may be few or no symptoms.

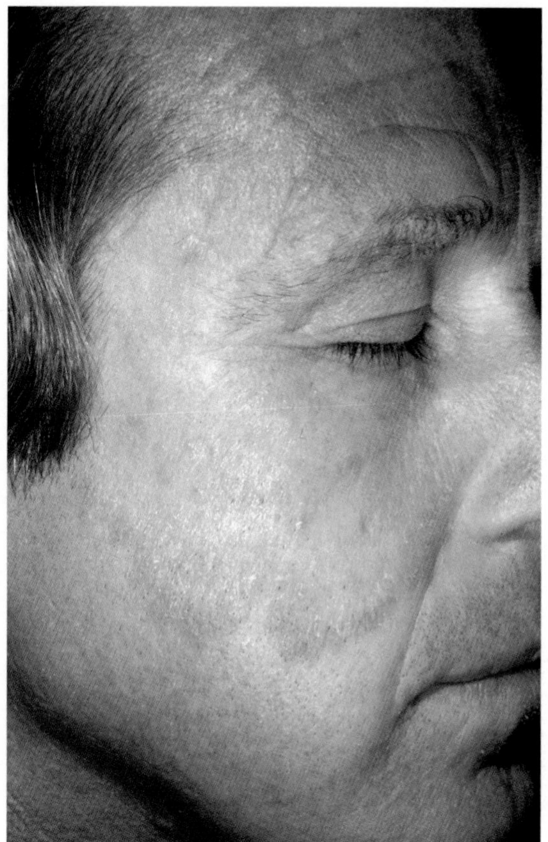

Figure 13-24 Tinea of the face. The active border is sharply defined. The initial diagnosis was eczema.

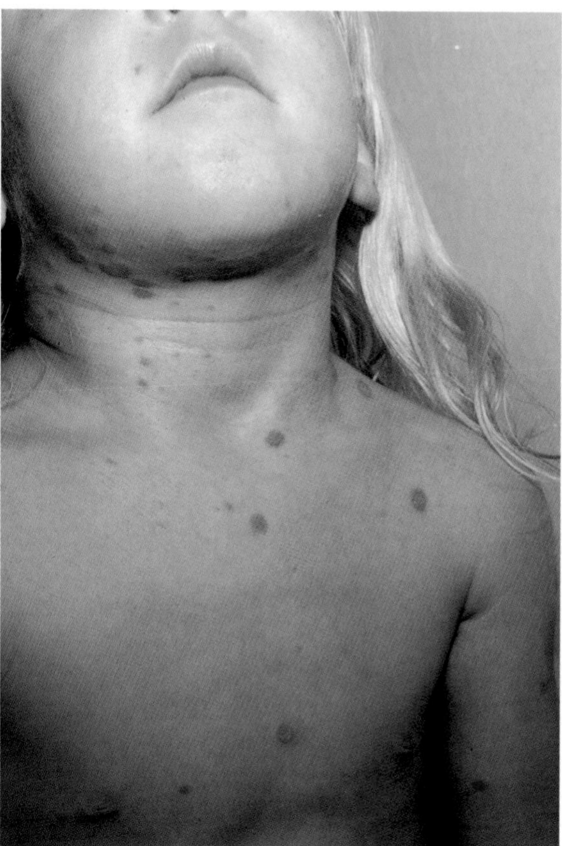

Figure 13-25 Tinea from cats may present with many small plaques on the trunk and extremities.

TINEA CORPORIS (TINEA GLADIATORUM)

Tinea corporis has become common in competitive wrestling. Most reported cases are caused by *T. tonsurans*. Person-to-person contact is probably the main source of transmission. The role of potential asymptomatic carriers of dermatophytes is unknown.

DEEP INFLAMMATORY LESIONS. Zoophilic fungi such as *T. verrucosum* from cattle may produce a very inflammatory skin infection (Figures 13-26, 13-27, and 13-28). The infection is more common in northern regions, where cattle are confined in close quarters during the winter. The round, intensely inflamed lesion has a uniformly elevated, red, boggy, pustular surface. The pustules are follicular and represent deep penetration of the fungus into the hair follicle (Figures 13-26 and 13-28). Secondary bacterial infection can occur. The process ends with brown hyperpigmentation and scarring (Figure 13-27). A fungal culture helps to identify the animal source of the infection.

A distinctive form of inflammatory tinea called *Majocchi's granuloma*, caused by *T. rubrum* and other species, was originally described as occurring on the lower legs of women who shave, but it is also seen at other sites on men and children. The primary lesion is a follicular papulopustule or inflammatory nodule. Intracutaneous and subcutaneous granulomatous nodules arise from these initial inflammatory tinea infections. Lesions have necrotic areas containing fungal elements; they are surrounded by epithelioid cells, giant cells, lymphocytes, and polymorphonuclear leukocytes, and they are believed to result from the rupturing of infected follicles into the dermis and subcutis: thus the term *granuloma*. There is marked variation from the usual hyphal forms. These include yeast forms, bizarre hyphae, and mucinous coatings. These variations may be a factor in allowing the dermatophytes to persist and grow in an abnormal manner. Lesions are single or multiple and discrete or confluent. The area involved covers a few to 10 cm and may be red and scaly, but it is not as intensely inflamed as the *T. verrucosum* infection described earlier. The border may not be well-defined. Skin biopsy with special stains for fungi is required for diagnosis if hyphae cannot be demonstrated in scale or hair.

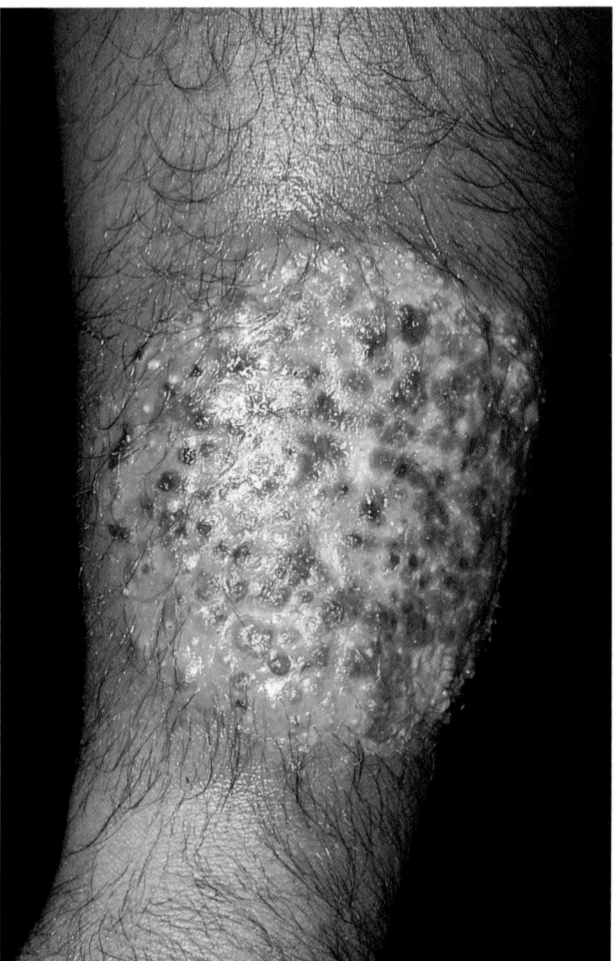

Figure 13-26 *Trichophyton verrucosum*, a zoophilic fungi from cattle that causes intense inflammation in humans.

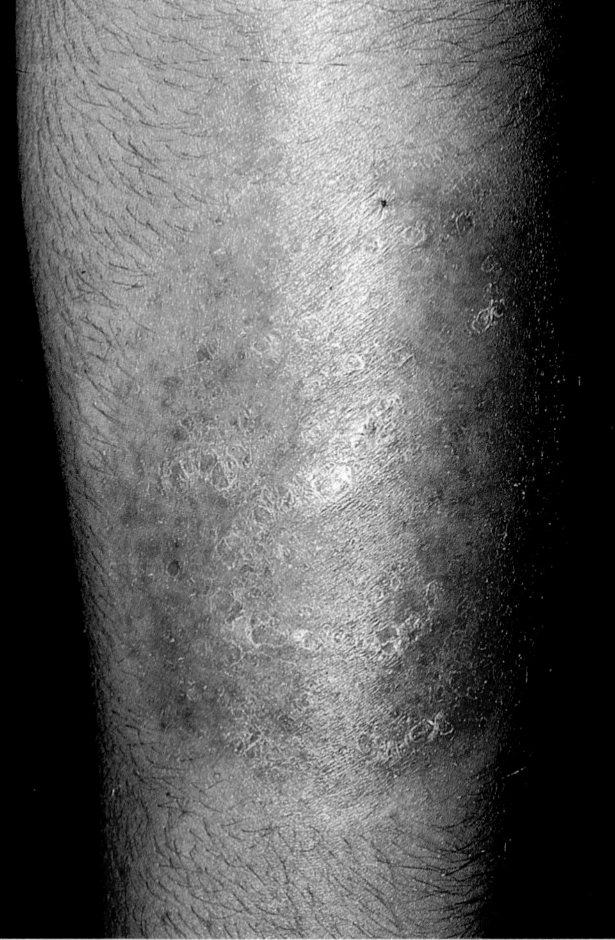

Figure 13-27 *Trichophyton verrucosum*. The deep inflammatory infection has caused brown hyperpigmentation and scarring. The hair follicles were destroyed.

TREATMENT. The superficial lesions of tinea corporis respond to the antifungal creams described in the Formulary. Lesions usually respond after 2 weeks of twice-a-day application, but treatment should be continued for at least 1 week after resolution of the infection. Extensive superficial lesions or those with red papules respond more predictably to oral therapy (see Table 13-2, p. 519). Tinea corporis is treated by 50 to 100 mg fluconazole daily or 150 mg once weekly for 2 to 4 weeks, or by 100 mg itraconazole daily for 2 weeks or 200 mg daily for 7 days. Itraconazole 100 mg twice daily immediately after meals on days 1 and 8 or on days 1 and 2 may also be effective. *PMID: 12950901* Terbinafine 250 mg daily for 1 to 2 weeks is also effective. The recurrence rate is high for those with extensive superficial infections. Deep inflammatory lesions require 1 to 3 or more months of oral therapy. Inflammation can be reduced with wet Burow's solution compresses, and bacterial infection is treated with the appropriate oral antibiotics. Some authors believe that oral or topical antifungal agents do not alter the course of highly inflammatory tinea (e.g., tinea verrucosum), because the intense inflammatory response destroys the organisms. However, oral antifungals are safe, and few physicians would withhold such therapy. As with tinea capitis kerion infections, a short course of prednisone may be considered for patients who have highly inflamed kerions, such as the patient depicted in Figure 13-26.

INVASIVE DERMATOPHYTE INFECTION. Dermatophytes are typically confined within the keratinized, epithelial layer of the skin. The pathogenic potential is dependent, however, on a variety of local and systemic factors affecting the natural host resistance to dermatophytic infection. Underlying systemic conditions that cause depressed cellular immunity, such as malignant lymphomas and Cushing's disease, as well as the administration of exogenous steroids or immunosuppressive agents, can lead to atypical, generalized, or invasive dermatophyte infection. Invasive dermatophyte infection should be included in the differential diagnosis of nodular, firm, or fluctuant masses (particularly on the extremities). Several dermatophyte species have caused a deep, generalized infection in which the organism invaded various visceral organs.

Figure 13-28 *Trichophyton verrucosum*. "Barn itch" occurred in this farmer who rested his head against the cow while milking. Fungal infections caught from animals are often intensely inflamed.

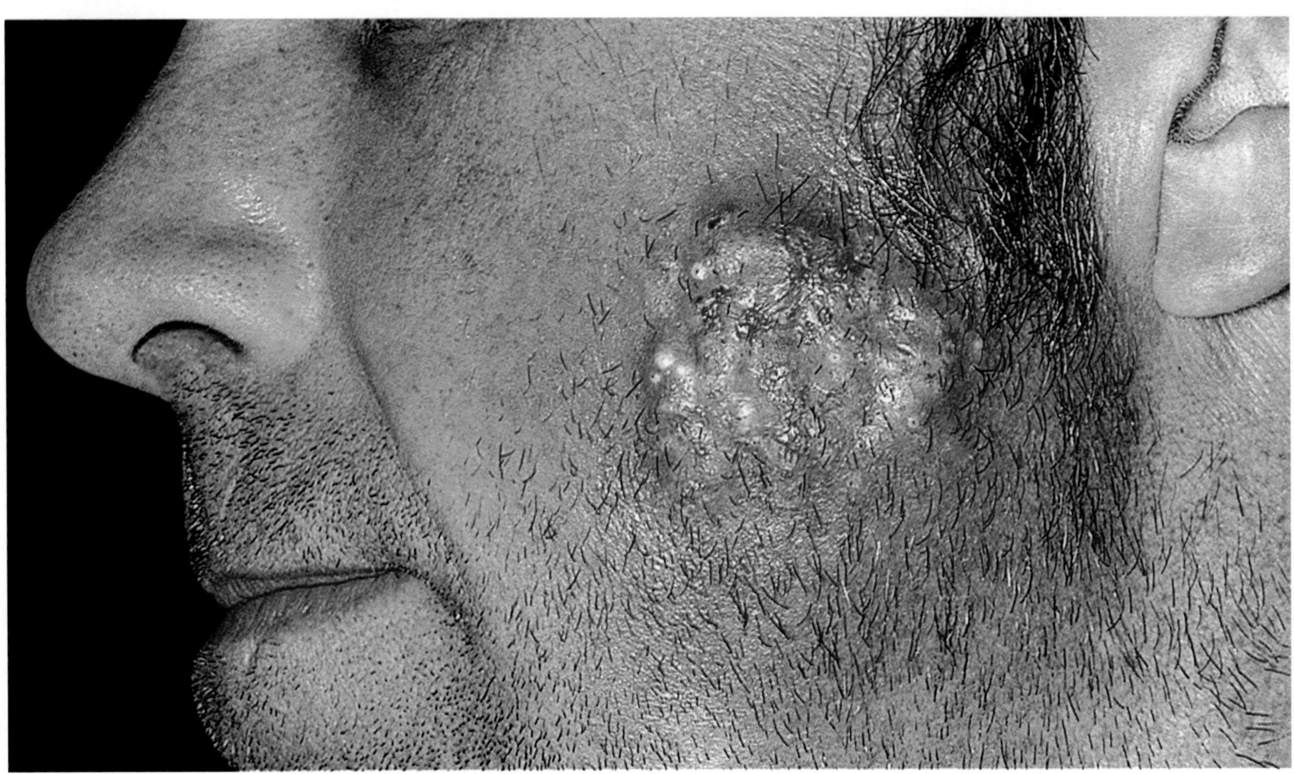

TINEA OF THE HAND

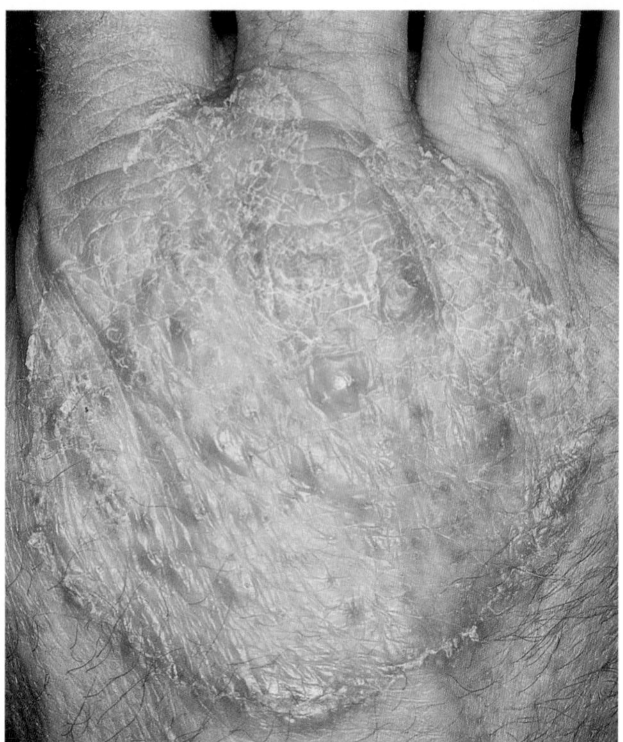

Figure 13-29 The classic "ringworm" pattern of infection with a prominent scaling border.

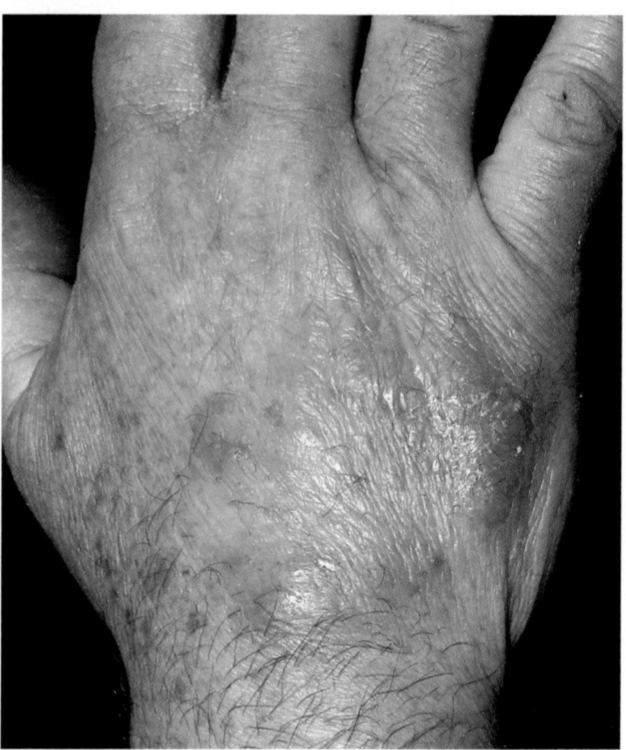

Figure 13-30 The infected areas are red with little or no scale.

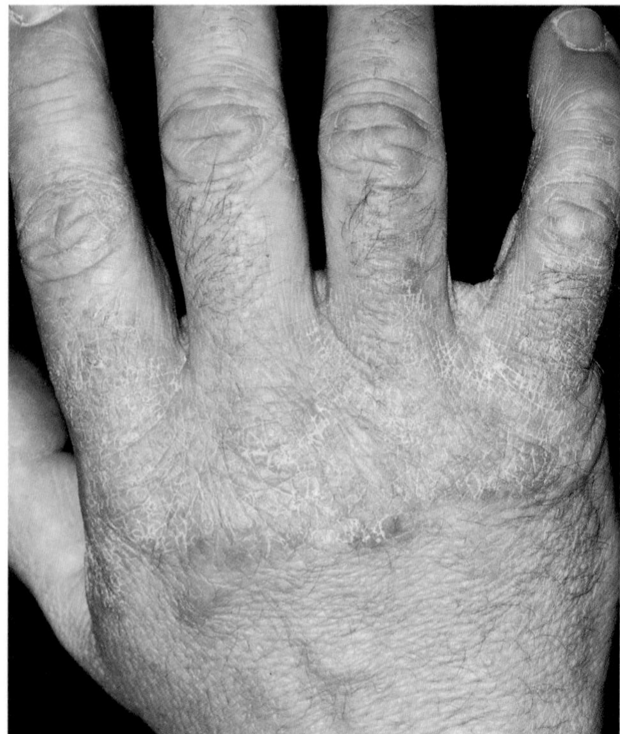

Figure 13-31 There is a well-defined red border. Scaling is present, in contrast to the case illustrated in Figure 13-30.

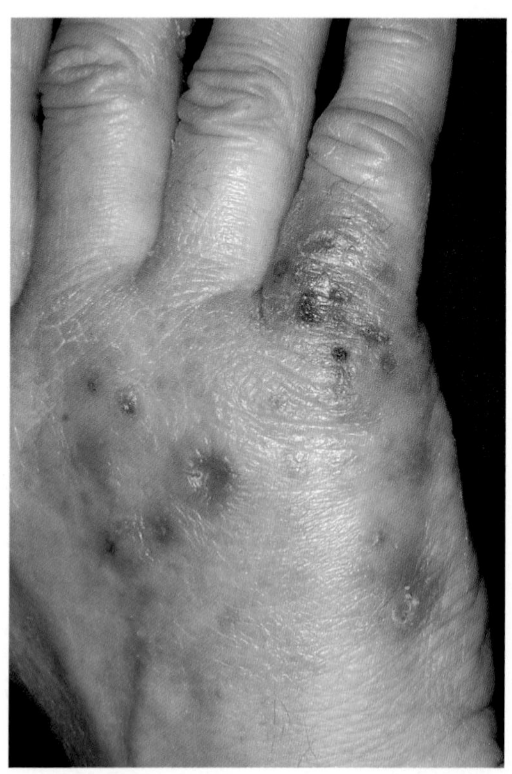

Figure 13-32 There is diffuse erythema and scaling, simulating contact dermatitis.

TINEA OF THE HAND

Tinea of the dorsal aspect of the hand (tinea manuum) (Figures 13-29 to 13-32) has all of the features of tinea corporis; tinea of the palm (Figure 13-33) has the same appearance as the dry, diffuse, keratotic form of tinea on the soles. The dry keratotic form may be asymptomatic and the patient may be unaware of the infection, attributing the dry, thick, scaly surface to hard physical labor. Tinea of the palms is frequently seen in association with tinea pedis. The usual pattern of infection is involvement of one foot and two hands or of two feet and one hand. Fingernail infection often accompanies infection of the dorsum of the hand or palm. Treatment is the same as that for tinea pedis and, as with the soles, a high recurrence rate can be expected for palm infection.

Figure 13-33 The involved palm is thickened, very dry, and scaly. The patient is often unaware of the infection and feels that these changes are secondary to dry skin or hard physical labor.

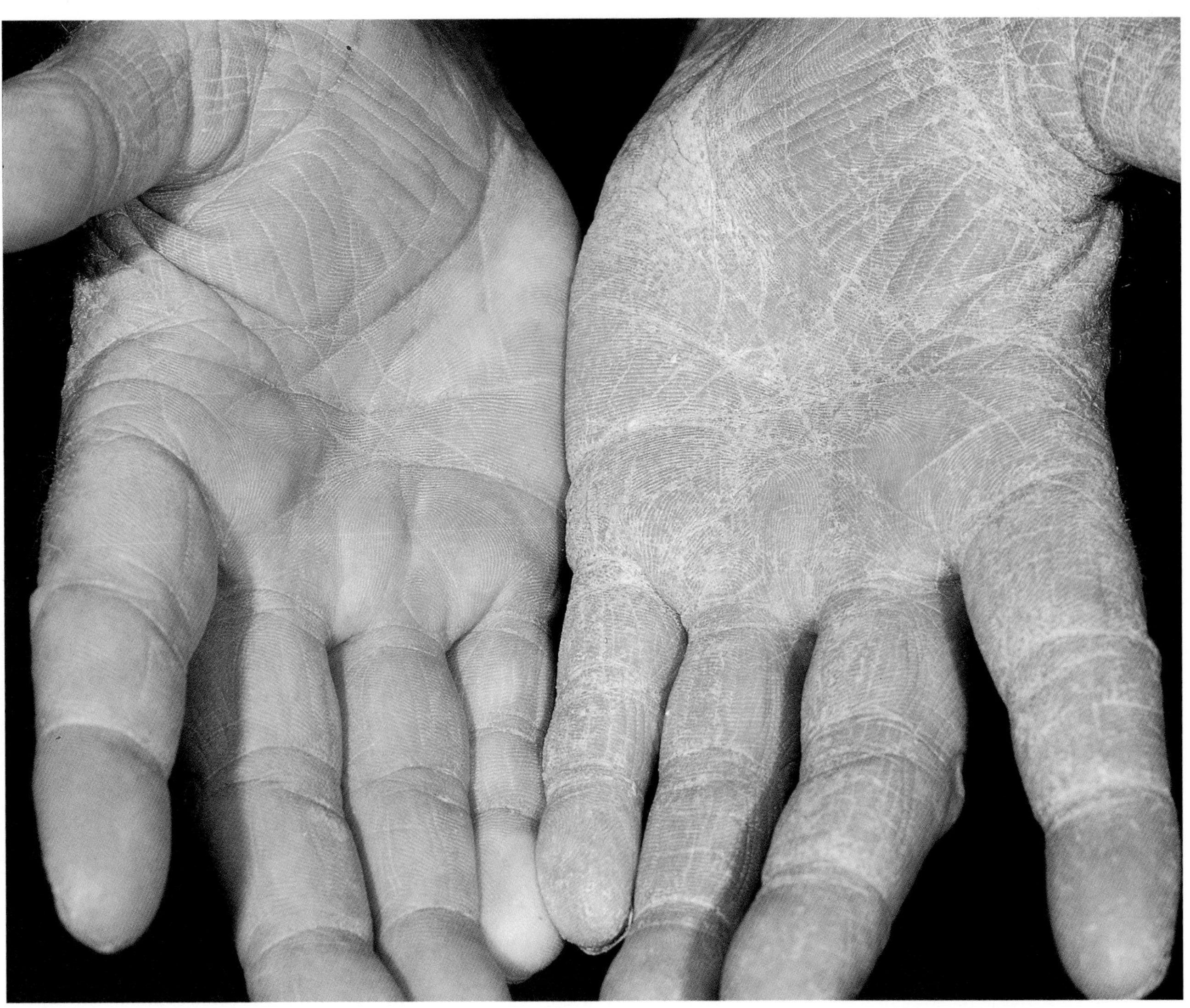

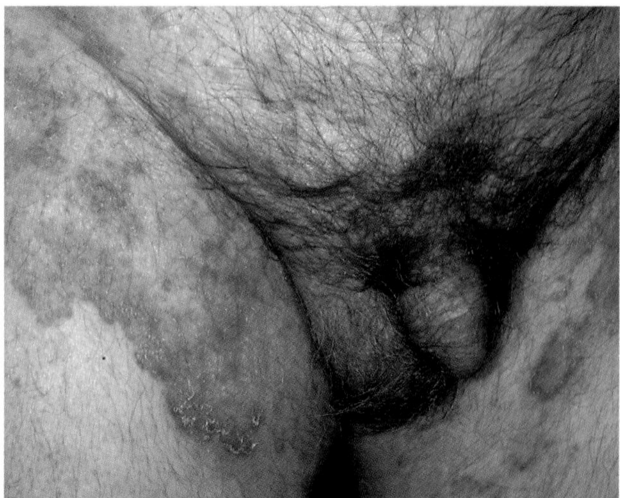

Figure 13-34 Tinea incognito. Inappropriate treatment of groin tinea with topical steroids has allowed the once localized infection to extend over a wide area.

TINEA INCOGNITO

Fungal infections treated with topical steroids often lose some of their characteristic features. Topical steroids decrease inflammation and give the false impression that the rash is improving while the fungus flourishes secondary to cortisone-induced immunologic changes. Treatment is stopped, the rash returns, and memory of the good initial response prompts reuse of the steroid cream, but by this time the rash has changed. Scaling at the margins may be absent. Diffuse erythema, diffuse scale, scattered pustules (Figures 13-34 and 13-35) or papules, and brown hyperpigmentation may all result. A well-defined border may not be present and a once-localized process may have expanded greatly. The intensity of itching is variable. Tinea incognito is most often seen on the groin, on the face, and on the dorsal aspect of the hand. Tinea infections of the hands are often misdiagnosed as eczema and treated with topical steroids. Hyphae are easily demonstrated, especially a few days after discontinuing use of the steroid cream when scaling reappears.

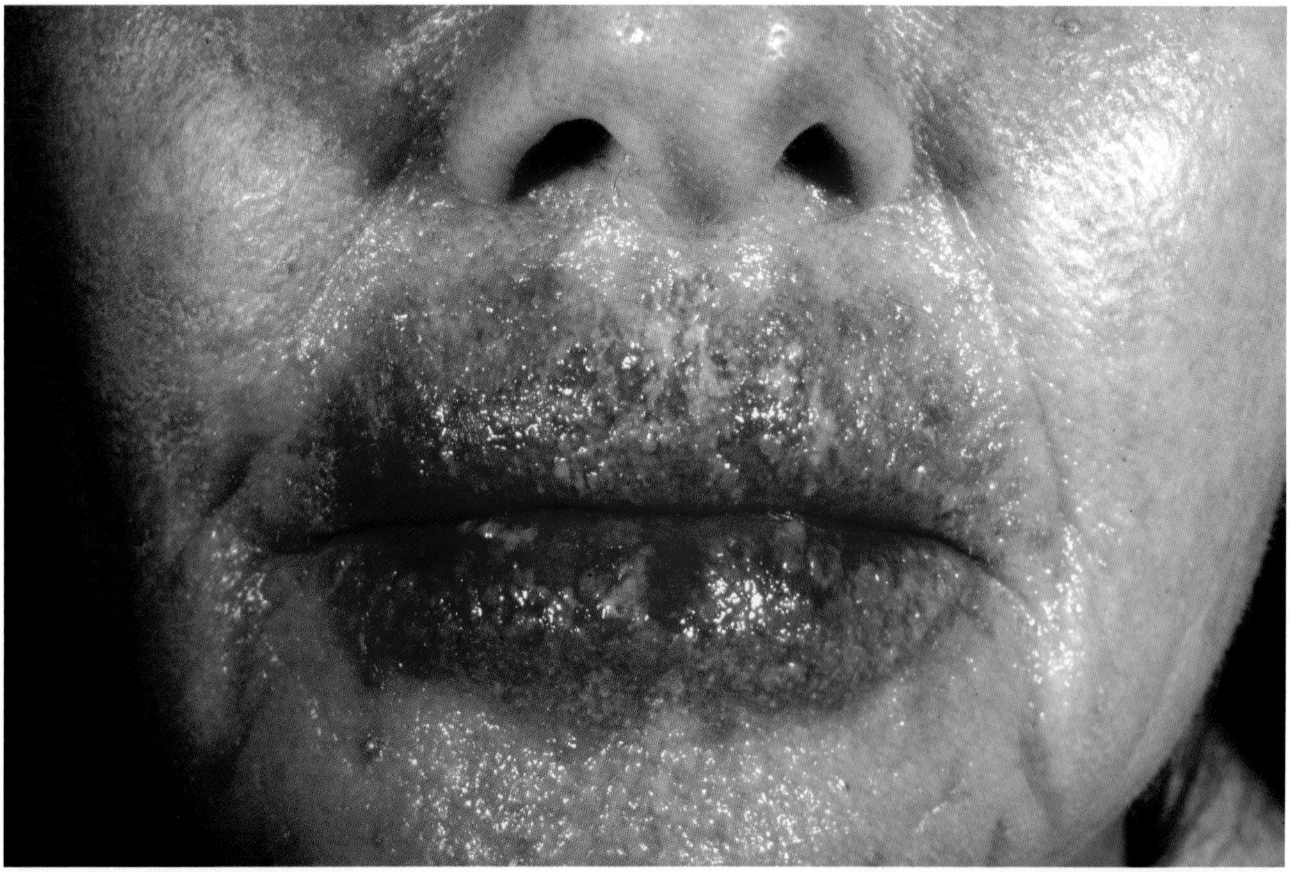

Figure 13-35 Tinea incognito. Initial treatment was oral antibiotics. This was followed by a trial of topical steroids and the infection became more intense. Another course of oral antibiotics failed. A potassium hydroxide examination revealed numerous fungal hyphae and the patient cleared with a 2-week course of oral terbinafine.

TINEA OF THE SCALP

Tinea of the scalp (tinea capitis) occurs most frequently in prepubertal children between 3 and 7 years of age. The infection has several different presentations. The species of dermatophyte likely to cause tinea capitis varies from country to country, but anthropophilic species (found in humans) predominate in most areas. Tinea capitis is most common in areas of poverty and crowded living conditions. The infection originates from contact with a pet or an infected person. Each animal is associated with a limited number of fungal species; therefore an attempt should be made to identify the fungus by culture to help locate and treat a possible animal source. Spores are shed in the air in the vicinity of the patient. Therefore direct contact is not necessary to spread infection. Unlike other fungal infections, tinea of the scalp may be contagious by direct contact or from contaminated clothing; this provides some justification for briefly isolating those with proven infection.

ORGANISM AND TRANSMISSION. Large family size, crowding, and low socioeconomic status increase the chance of infection. Infectious fungal particles that have fallen from the infected person may be viable for months. Tinea capitis can be transmitted by infected persons, fallen hairs, animals, fomites (clothing, bedding, hairbrushes, combs, hats), and furniture. Zoophilic dermatophytes are acquired from contact with pets or wild animals. *Microsporum canis* is the most common cause of tinea capitis in central Europe. Sources of *M. canis* infection are cats, dogs, and guinea pigs. The animals may harbor the pathogen in their fur (colonization) although clinical symptoms may not be visible. Of the 3775 cases of tinea capitis reported to the European Confederation of Medical Mycology, 37.9% were *M. canis,* 23.1% *T. tonsurans,* 10.8% *M. audouinii,* 10.4% *Trichophyton soudanense,* and 9.7% *Trichophyton violaceum*. The pathogen spectrum shows clear geographical differences. A dramatic rise in *T. tonsurans* infections has been reported in the United States, which has not been the case in Europe. Farmers acquire *T. verrucosum* from touching the hide of infected cattle. *Microsporum gypseum* infection comes from contaminated soil.

Asymptomatic scalp carriage of dermatophytes by classmates and adults is probably an important factor contributing to disease transmission and reinfection. The asymptomatic carriage persists for an indefinite period.

HAIR SHAFT INFECTION. Hair shaft infection is preceded by invasion of the stratum corneum of the scalp. (See Chapter 24.) The fungus grows down through this dead protein layer into the hair follicle and gains entry into the hair in the lower intrafollicular zone, just below the point where the cuticle of the hair shaft is formed. Because of the cuticle, the fungi cannot cross over from the perifollicular stratum corneum into the hair but must go deep into the hair follicle to circumvent the cuticle. This may explain why topical antifungal agents are ineffective for treating tinea capitis. The fungi then invade the keratinized, outer root sheath; enter the inner cortex; and digest the keratin contained inside the hair shaft. The growth of hyphae occurs within the hair above the zone of keratinization of the hair shaft and keeps pace with the growth of hair. Distal to this zone of active growth, arthrospores are formed within or on the surface of the hair, depending on the species of dermatophytes. Hyphae grow inside and fragment into short segments called *arthrospores*. The arthrospores remain inside the hair shaft in the endothrix pattern (Figure 13-36). In the ectothrix type, they dislodge (Figure 13-37), obscure and penetrate the surface cuticle on the hair shaft surface, and form a sheath of closely packed spheres. The arthrospores are either large (6 to 10 mm) or small (2 to 3 mm). Large spores can be seen as separate structures with the low-power microscope objective. Higher power is needed to see the small spores.

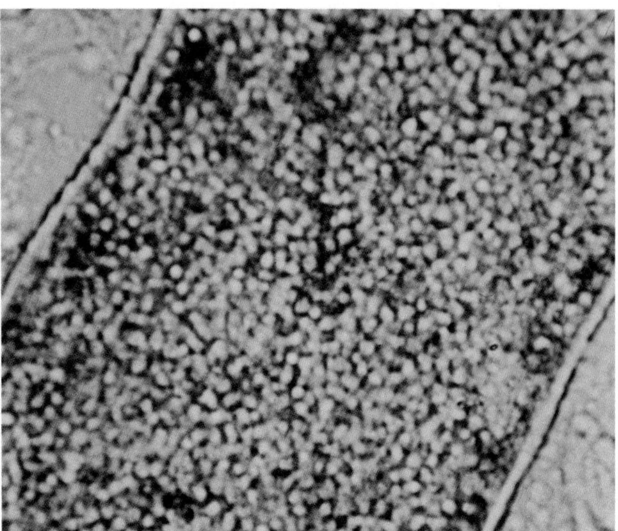

Figure 13-36 Large-spore endothrix pattern of hair invasion (*Trichophyton tonsurans,* "a sack of marbles").

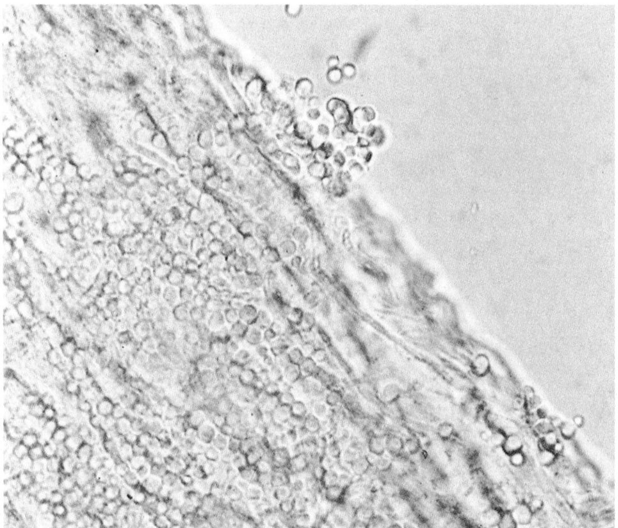

Figure 13-37 Large-spore ectothrix pattern of hair invasion (*Trichophyton verrucosum*).

ENDOTHRIX PATTERN OF INVASION. Endothrix hair invasion is produced predominantly by *T. tonsurans, T. soudanense,* and *T. violaceum*. The fungus grows completely within the hair shaft, and the cuticle surface of the hair remains intact. The hyphae within the hair are converted to arthroconidia (spores). The spores remain in the hair shaft. In "black dot" tinea capitis caused by *T. tonsurans* and *T. violaceum,* the hair cortex is almost completely replaced by spores and swells at the infundibular level, impeding further exit of the growing hair and causing the already weakened hair to coil inside the infundibulum, forming a black dot. Endothrix infections tend to progress, become chronic, and may last into adult life.

ECTOTHRIX PATTERN OF INVASION. Ectothrix hair invasion is associated with *M. audouinii, M. canis,* and *T. verrucosum*. Inflammatory tinea related to exposure to a kitten or puppy usually is a fluorescent small-spore ectothrix. Some of the hyphae destroy and break through the surface of the hair shaft (cuticle) and then invade the keratinized inner root sheath that grows around the exterior of the hair shaft. The hyphae are subsequently converted into infectious arthrospores (arthroconidia). The arthrospores are located both on the inside of the hair shaft and on the outer surface to produce the ectothrix pattern seen under the microscope. The arthroconidia that surround the hair have the appearance of a sheath.

MICROSCOPIC PATTERNS OF HAIR INVASION. There are three patterns of hair invasion: small-spored ectothrix, large-spored ectothrix, and large-spored endothrix. Infection originates inside the hair shaft in all patterns.

CLINICAL PATTERNS OF INFECTION. The clinical patterns of tinea capitis are summarized in Box 13-1. An approach for the clinical diagnosis, laboratory investigations, and management of tinea capitis is presented in Box 13-1 and Box 13-2. The inflammatory response to infection is variable. Noninflammatory tinea of the scalp is illustrated in Figure 13-38. A severe, inflammatory reaction with a boggy, indurated, tumorlike mass that exudes pus is called a kerion; it represents a hypersensitivity reaction to fungus and heals with scarring and some hair loss. The hair loss is less than would be expected from the degree and depth of inflammation. Cervical or occipital lymphadenopathy occurs in all types of tinea capitis. The diagnosis of tinea capitis should be questioned if lymphadenopathy is not present. A fungal infection is rarely the cause when neither adenopathy nor alopecia is present.

Box 13-1 **Systematic Approach to Investigation of Tinea Capitis**

Determine clinical presentation

- Most forms of tinea capitis begin with one or several round patches of scale or alopecia.
- Inflammatory lesions, even if untreated, tend to resolve spontaneously in a few months; the noninflammatory infections are more chronic.
- Presents as patchy alopecia plus fine, dry scale with no inflammation:
  - –Short stubs of broken hair ("gray patch ringworm"): *M. audouinii*
  - –Hairs broken off at surface ("black dot ringworm"): *T. tonsurans* (most common), *T. violaceum*
  - –Patchy alopecia plus swelling plus purulent discharge: *M. canis, T. mentagrophytes* (granular), *T. verrucosum*
- Kerion is a severe inflammatory reaction with boggy induration; caused by any fungus, but especially *M. canis, T. mentagrophytes* (granular), and *T. verrucosum.*

Wood's light examination

Blue-green fluorescence of hair—only *M. canis* and *M. audouinii* have this feature. Scale and skin do not fluoresce.

Potassium hydroxide wet mount of plucked hairs

- The pattern of hair invasion is characteristic for each species of fungus. Hairs that can be removed with little resistance are best for evaluation.
- Large-spored endothrix pattern: Appears as chains of large spores densely packed within the hair, "like a sack full of marbles." Causative organisms are *T. tonsurans* and *T. violaceum.*
- Large-spored ectothrix pattern: Appears as chains of large spores inside and on the surface of the hair shaft and visible with the low-power objective. Caused by *T. verrucosum* and *T. mentagrophytes.*
- Small-spored ectothrix pattern: Small spores are randomly arranged in masses inside and on the surface of the hair shaft; it is not visible with the low-power objective. Looks like a stick dipped in maple syrup and rolled in sand. Causative organisms are *M. canis* and *M. audouinii.*

Identification of source after species is verified by culture

- Anthropophilic (parasitic on humans): Infection from other humans: *M. audouinii, T. tonsurans, T. violaceum*
- Zoophilic (parasitic on animals): Infection from animals or other infected humans: *M. canis*—dog, cat, monkey; *T. mentagrophytes* (granular)—dog, rabbit, guinea pig, monkey; *T. verrucosum*—cattle

TRICHOPHYTON TONSURANS

Since the 1950s *T. tonsurans* (large-spored endothrix) has been responsible for more than 90% of the scalp ringworm in the United States, but *M. canis* (small-spored ectothrix) is still a major cause in some parts of the United States. The occurrence rate is equal in boys and girls, and most cases involve blacks or Hispanics in the crowded inner cities. Cases of tinea capitis before the 1950s were caused by *M. audouinii,* which spontaneously clears in adolescence and fluoresces green with the Wood's light. *T. tonsurans* does not fluoresce and infects people of all ages.

It can remain viable for long periods on inanimate objects such as combs, brushes, blankets, and telephones. *T. tonsurans* lesions may occur outside of the scalp in patients, their families, and their close friends. These lesions serve as a reservoir for reinfection; therefore all siblings or close contacts within the family should be examined. The peak incidence of infection occurs at ages 3 through

Box 13-2 **British Guidelines for the Management of Tinea Capitis (2000), Modified**

Definition

Tinea capitis is an infection caused by dermatophyte fungi (usually species in the genera *Microsporum* and *Trichophyton*) of scalp hair follicles and the surrounding skin.

Epidemiology

Tinea capitis is predominantly a disease of preadolescent children, adult cases being rare. The main pathogens are anthropophilic organisms, with *Trichophyton tonsurans* now accounting for >90% of cases in the U.K. and North America. These infections frequently spread among family members and classmates. In nonurban communities, sporadic infections acquired from puppies and kittens are due to *M. canis,* which accounts for less than 10% of cases in the U.K. Occasional infection from other animal hosts (e.g., *T verrucosum* from cattle) occurs in rural areas.

Pathogenesis

There are three patterns: endothrix, ectothrix, and favus. The latter, a pattern of hair loss caused by *T. schoenleinii,* is rarely seen in the U.K., being largely confined to eastern Europe and Asia; therefore it is not considered further here. Endothrix infections are characterized by arthroconidia (spores) within the hair shaft. The cuticle is not destroyed. Ectothrix infections are characterized by hyphal fragments and arthroconidia outside the hair shaft, which lead eventually to cuticle destruction.

Clinical diagnosis

A variety of clinical presentations are recognized as being either inflammatory or noninflammatory and are usually associated with patchy alopecia (see "Summarizing the clinical patterns of tinea capitis"). However, the infection is so widespread, and the clinical appearances can be so subtle, that in urban areas tinea capitis should be considered in the diagnosis of any child over the age of 3 months with a scaly scalp, until dismissed by negative mycology. Infection may also be associated with painful regional lymphadenopathy, particularly in the inflammatory variants. A generalized eruption of itchy papules particularly around the outer helix of the ear may occur as a reactive phenomenon (an "id" response). This may start with the introduction of systemic therapy and consequently be mistaken for a drug reaction.

Summarizing the clinical patterns of tinea capitis

Clinical patterns	Clinical description	Differential diagnosis
Diffuse scale	Generalized diffuse scaling of the scalp	Seborrheic and atopic dermatitis, psoriasis
Grey patch	Patchy, scaly alopecia	Seborrheic and atopic dermatitis, psoriasis
Black dot	Patches of alopecia studded with broken-off hair stubs	Alopecia areata, trichotillomania
Diffuse pustular	Scattered pustules associated with alopecia scaling ± associated lymphadenopathy	Bacterial folliculitis, dissecting folliculitis
Kerion	Boggy tumor studded with pustules ± associated lymphadenopathy	Abscess, neoplasia

Laboratory diagnosis

Specimens should be taken to confirm the diagnosis as systemic therapy will be required.

Taking specimens

Affected areas should be scraped with a blunt scalpel to harvest affected hairs, broken-off hair stubs, and scalp scale. This is preferable to plucking, which may remove uninvolved hairs. Scrapings should be transported in a folded square of paper preferably fastened with a paper clip, but commercial packs are also available. Alternatively, the area can be rubbed with a moistened gauze swab or brushed gently 10 times with a plastic, sterile, single-use toothbrush. The brush can then be sent in the container provided to the laboratory for culture.

Microscopy and culture

Potassium hydroxide wet mounts

Microscopy provides the most rapid means of diagnosis. Firmly rub tap water–moistened gauze or a toothbrush over the involved area. Each hair is lifted off the gauze with a needle or forceps and placed on a slide for potassium hydroxide preparation. Potassium hydroxide 10% to 20% solution is added, the slide is gently heated, and the slide is microscopically examined for fungal hyphae and spores. Early or inflammatory lesions may only contain very few hyphae. Overheating of the slide may burst the hair and make it difficult to differentiate the endothrix pattern from the ectothrix pattern. Positive microscopy (when the hairs or scales are seen to be invaded by spores or hyphae) confirms the diagnosis and allows treatment to commence at once.

Brush-culture method

The brush-culture method involves gently rubbing a previously sterilized toothbrush in a circular motion over areas where scale is present or over the margins of patches of alopecia. The brush fibers are then pressed into the culture media (e.g., Sabouraud's media) and the brush is discarded. A cotton swab produces similar results. Cultures turn positive faster when using these collection techniques. Culture allows accurate identification of the organism involved, and this may alter the treatment schedule. Culture is more sensitive than microscopy; results may be positive even when microscopy is negative. Cultures usually show signs of growth in 7 to 10 days, but may take up to 4 weeks.

Modified from Higgins EM, Fuller LC, Smith CH: Guidelines for the management of tinea capitis, *Brit J Dermatol* 143(1):53-58, 2000 (doi:10.1046/j.1365). *PMID: 10886135*

Continued

Box 13-2 **British Guidelines for the Management of Tinea Capitis (2000), Modified—cont'd**

Brush-culture method—cont'd

Conventional sampling of a kerion can be difficult. In these cases negative results are not uncommon and the diagnosis and decision to treat may need to be made clinically. A moistened standard bacteriologic swab taken from the pustular areas and inoculated onto the culture plate may yield a positive result.

Wood's light examination

Examination with Wood's ultraviolet light will show a yellow-green fluorescence with the ectothrix organisms *M. audouinii, M. canis*, and *T. tonsurans*. Endothrix-producing organisms do not fluorescence.

Most of the current infections in the U.K. are endothrix and therefore negative under Wood's light; it is of limited value to screen and monitor these infections.

Therapy of tinea capitis

The aim of treatment is to achieve a clinical and mycological cure as quickly as possible. Oral antifungal therapy is generally needed.

Topical

Topical treatment alone is not recommended for the management of tinea capitis. Local treatment with a topical antifungal with a fungicidal mechanism of action, such as ciclopiroxolamine or terbinafine cream, may reduce the risk of infecting other people and shortens the duration of systemic treatment. The entire hair of the scalp in all its length should be treated with the antifungal. Treatment should be administered once daily for approximately 1 week. The hair should be washed two times weekly using an antifungal shampoo (povidone-iodine, selenium disulfide).

Other supportive measures: Cutting the hair or shaving the head may significantly shorten the duration of treatment with a systemic antifungal. Shaving the affected areas of the scalp significantly reduces the infectious load. Shaving should be performed at the beginning of systemic treatment and again 3 to 4 weeks later. Shaving the hair once each week may significantly shorten treatment.

Oral

All systemic antifungals are more effective in the presence of endothrix infection (e.g., *Trichophyton* spp.) than in patients with ectothrix disease (e.g., *M. canis*). Current data suggest that *M. canis* infections might respond better to itraconazole.

Griseofulvin

Griseofulvin is the current drug of choice in children. It has a long track record of safety, has the least known drug interactions, and is well tolerated. It is fungistatic and antiinflammatory. Available in tablet or suspension form. The recommended dose, for those older than 1 month is, 10 mg/kg per day. Taking the drug with fatty food increases absorption and aids bioavailability. Dosage recommendations vary according to the formulation used, with higher doses being recommended by some authors for micronized griseofulvin as opposed to ultramicronized griseofulvin, but up to 25 mg/kg may be required. The duration of therapy depends on the organism (e.g., *T. tonsurans* infections may require prolonged treatment schedules) but varies between 8 and 10 weeks. Shorter courses may lead to higher relapse rates. Side effects include nausea and rashes in 8% to 15% of cases. The drug is contraindicated in pregnancy and the manufacturers caution against men fathering a child for 6 months after therapy.

Advantages: Licensed; inexpensive; syrup formulation is more palatable; suspension allows accurate dosage adjustments in children; and extensive experience.

Disadvantages: Prolonged treatment required. Contraindicated in lupus erythematosus, porphyria, and severe liver disease.

Drug interactions: Warfarin, cyclosporine, and the oral contraceptive pill.

Terbinafine

Fungicidal. It is effective against all dermatophytes. It is at least as effective as griseofulvin and is safe for the management of scalp ringworm caused by *Trichophyton* sp. in children. Its role in management of *Microsporum* sp. is debatable. Early evidence suggests that higher doses or longer therapy (>4 weeks) may be required in *Microsporum* infections. Dosage depends on the weight of the patient, but typical range is between 3 and 6 mg/kg per day. Side effects include gastrointestinal disturbances and rashes in 5% and 3% of cases, respectively. Gastrointestinal symptoms subside with continuing therapy.

Advantages: Fungicidal so shorter therapy required (cf. griseofulvin); therefore increased compliance more likely.

Disadvantages: No suspension formulation.

Drug interactions: Plasma concentrations are reduced by rifampicin and increased by cimetidine.

Itraconazole

Both fungistatic and fungicidal activity depending on the concentration of drug in the tissues. 100 mg/day for 4 weeks or 5 mg/kg per day in children is as effective as griseofulvin and terbinafine. Bioavailability is improved when it is taken with a fatty meal. Nausea and vomiting occur; abnormalities in liver functions occur in more than 1% of patients.

Advantages: Pulsed shorter treatment regimens are possible.

Disadvantages: Potential drug interactions.

Drug interactions: Enhanced toxicity of anticoagulants (warfarin), antihistamines (terfenadine and astemizole), antipsychotics (sertindole), anxiolytics (midazolam), digoxin, cisapride, cyclosporine, and simvastatin (increased risk of myopathy). Reduced efficacy of itraconazole with concomitant use of H_2-blockers, phenytoin, and rifampicin.

Box 13-2 British Guidelines for the Management of Tinea Capitis (2000), Modified—cont'd

Fluconazole

Use has mainly been limited by side effects. Dosages of 3-5 mg/kg per day for 4 weeks are effective in children with tinea capitis. The most common side effects are nausea and vomiting, but liver function test abnormalities are also found. Fluconazole is approved by the Food and Drug Administration for use in children older than 6 months. It is available in a pleasant-tasting liquid formula (10 and 40 mg/ml).

Ketoconazole

Use limited by side effects. Dosages between 3.3 and 6.6 mg/kg per day. Resolution is comparable with griseofulvin but the response may be slower. However, side effects are arguably sufficiently significant to lead to the recommendation by some authors that it should not be used in children. Studies have not shown it to be consistently superior to griseofulvin and its use in children is limited by hepatotoxicity.

Additional measures

Exclusion from school

Although there is a risk of transmission of infection from patients to unaffected classmates, for practical reasons children should be allowed to return to school once they have started receiving appropriate systemic and adjuvant topical therapy.

Familial screening

Index cases resulting from the anthropophilic *T. tonsurans* are highly infectious. Family members and other close contacts should be screened (both for tinea capitis and for tinea corporis) and appropriate mycological samples taken preferably using the brush technique, even in the absence of clinical signs.

Cleansing of fomites

T. tonsurans spores may remain viable on furniture, combs, and brushes. Scrupulous cleaning of all possibly contaminated objects helps to prevent reinfection. For all anthropophilic species these should be cleansed with disinfectant. Simple bleach or Milton can be used. All family members should be examined carefully for tinea capitis and tinea corporis. Soaking off crust from kerions or pustules may be soothing.

Steroids

The use of corticosteroids (both oral and topical) for inflammatory varieties (e.g., kerions and severe id reactions) is controversial, but may help to reduce itching and general discomfort. Although in the past steroids have been thought to minimize the risk of permanent alopecia secondary to scarring, current evidence does not suggest any reduction in clearance time compared with griseofulvin alone.

Treatment failures

Some individuals are not clear at follow-up. The following are reasons why this occurs:

1. Lack of compliance with the long courses of treatment
2. Suboptimal absorption of the drug
3. Relative insensitivity of the organism
4. Reinfection

T. tonsurans and *Microsporum* sp. are typical culprits in persistently positive cases. If fungi can still be isolated at the end of treatment, but the clinical signs have improved, the authors recommend continuing the original treatment for a further month.

If there has been no clinical response and signs persist at the end of the treatment period, then the options include the following:

1. Increase the dose or duration of the original drug: both griseofulvin (in dosages up to 25 mg/kg for 8-10 weeks) and terbinafine have been used successfully and safely at higher dosages or for longer courses to clear resistant infections.
2. Change to an alternative antifungal (e.g., switch from griseofulvin to terbinafine or itraconazole).

Carriers

The optimal management of symptom-free carriers (i.e., individuals without overt clinical infection, but who are culture-positive) is unclear. In those with a heavy growth/high spore count on brush culture, systemic antifungal therapy may be justified as these individuals are especially likely to develop an overt clinical infection, are a significant reservoir of infection, and are unlikely to respond to topical therapy alone. Alternatively, they may represent a missed overt clinical infection. For those with light growth/low spore counts on brush culture, use shampoos containing 1%-2.5% selenium sulfide, 1%-2% zinc pyrithione, povidone-iodine, or ketoconazole 2% to inhibit the growth of fungi. They may be useful as adjunctive therapy to control spore loads in infected children and asymptomatic carriers. These agents are lathered, massaged well, and left on the scalp for 5 minutes. They are used two to three times each week during the course of treatment or longer.

Follow-up

The definitive end-point for adequate treatment is not clinical response but mycological cure; therefore follow-up with repeat mycology sampling is recommended at the end of the standard treatment period and then monthly until mycological clearance is documented. Treatment should, therefore, be tailored for each individual patient according to response.

9 years. This fungal infection does not tend to resolve spontaneously at puberty, resulting in a large population of infected carriers.

FOUR PATTERNS OF INFECTION. *T. tonsurans* has four different clinical infection patterns. There may be multiple cases within a family, and each person may have a different infection pattern. The clinical presentation may be related to specific host T-lymphocyte response. This dermatophytosis is most frequently incurred from contact with an infected child, either directly or via a variety of fomites. Current studies indicate that an asymptomatic adult carrier state exists and may provide a source for continued reinfection in children.

Noninflammatory black dot pattern. In the black dot pattern, there are well-demarcated areas of hair loss, with hairs broken off at the follicular orifice, giving the characteristic appearance of black dots if the patient's hair is black. Red hairs will produce a "red dot" pattern. This is the most distinctive pattern. Large areas of alopecia are present without inflammation (Figures 13-38 and 13-39). There is a mild-to-moderate amount of scalp scale. Occipital adenopathy may be present. Lack of inflammation may be explained by the fact that cell-mediated immunity to *Trichophyton* antigen skin tests is negative in these patients. The infected hairs of *T. tonsurans* have arthrospores inside the hair shaft; the arthrospores weaken the hair and cause it to break off at or below the scalp surface, resulting in a black dot appearance of the scalp surface (see Figure 13-36). Broken hairs are typically less than 2 mm long. Hairs long enough to be pulled are generally not infected.

Inflammatory tinea capitis (kerion). Most patients with this infection pattern have a positive skin test to the *Trichophyton* antigen, suggesting that the patient's immune response may be responsible for intense inflammation. Approximately 35% of patients infected with *T. tonsurans* have this pattern. There are one or multiple inflamed, boggy, tender areas of alopecia with pustules on and/or in surrounding skin (Figures 13-40 and 13-41). Fever, occipital adenopathy, leukocytosis, and a diffuse, morbilliform rash may occur. Potassium hydroxide wet mounts and fungal cultures are often negative because of destruction of fungal structures by inflammation, and treatment may have to be initiated based on clinical appearance. Cultures are best obtained with a toothbrush (Figure 13-42). Scarring alopecia may occur.

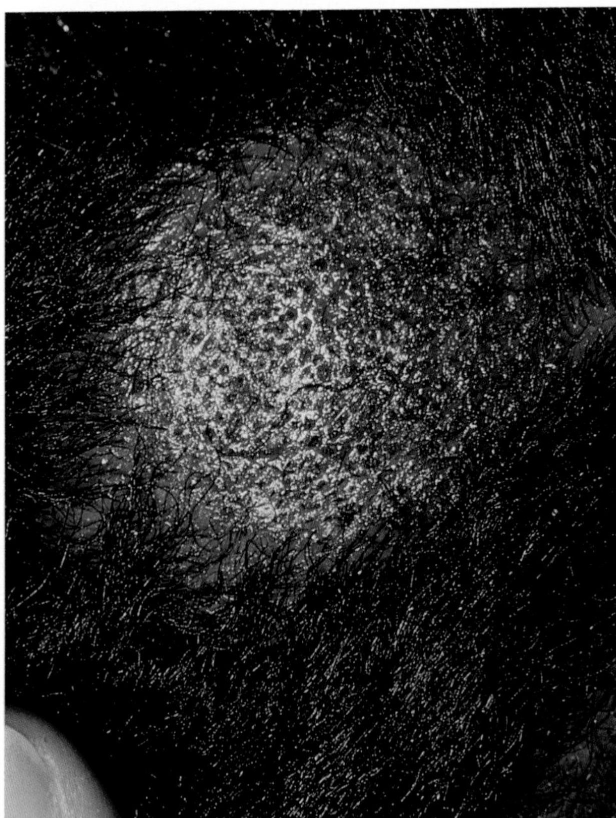

Figure 13-38 *Trichophyton tonsurans*. Black dot ringworm. There are areas of alopecia with scale but no inflammation. Arthrospores inside the shafts of infected hairs weaken the hair and cause it to break off at or below the scalp surface, resulting in the "black dot" appearance of the surface. (From Solomon LM et al: *Current Concepts* 2[3]:224, 1985; reproduced by permission of Blackwell Scientific Publications.)

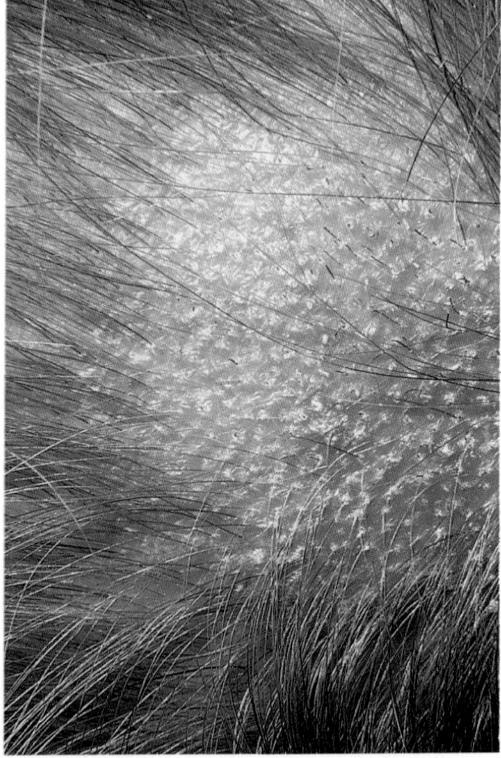

Figure 13-39 *Trichophyton tonsurans*. Noninflammatory black dot scaling pattern. Infection of the hair shaft causes the shaft to fracture, leaving infected hair stubs. The color of the hair determines the color of the dots. Black hair presents with black dots. Light hair presents with white dots.

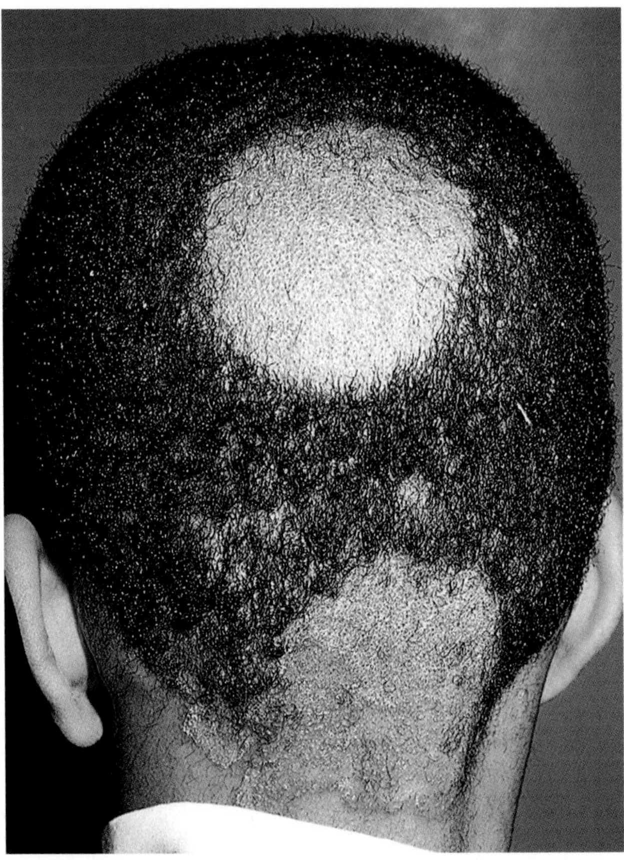

Figure 13-40 Inflammatory tinea capitis. A very extensive infection with extension onto the neck.

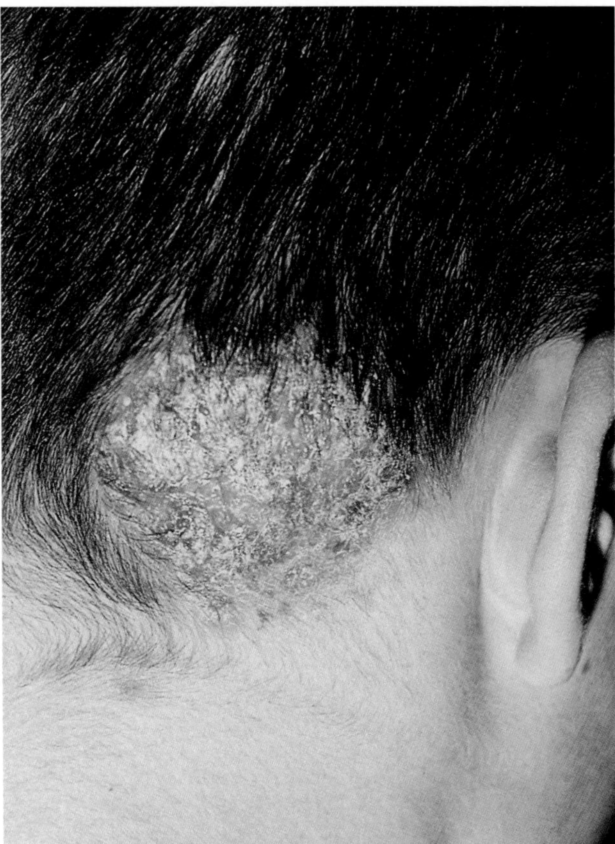

Figure 13-41 This severely inflamed deep lesion has accumulated serum and crust on the surface. Cervical lymphadenopathy was present.

Seborrheic dermatitis type. This type is common and the most difficult to diagnosis because it resembles dandruff. There is diffuse or patchy, fine, white, adherent scale on the scalp. Close examination shows tiny, perifollicular pustules and/or hair stubs that have broken off at the level of the scalp: the black dot pattern. Less commonly, there is patchy or diffuse hair loss. Adenopathy is often present. Culture is often necessary to make the diagnosis because only 29% of affected patients have a positive potassium hydroxide examination.

Pustular type. There are discrete pustules or scabbed areas without scaling or significant hair loss. Pustules suggest bacterial infection, and patients with pustules may receive several courses of antibiotics before the correct diagnosis is made. The pustules may be sparse or numerous. As with kerions, the cultures and potassium hydroxide wet mounts may be negative.

DIFFERENTIAL DIAGNOSIS. Seborrheic dermatitis and psoriasis may be confused with tinea of the scalp. Tinea amiantacea, a form of seborrheic dermatitis that occurs in children, is frequently misdiagnosed as tinea. Tinea amiantacea is a localized 2- to 8-cm patch of large, brown, polygonal-shaped scales that adheres to the scalp and mats the hair. The matted scale grows out, attached to the hair (see Figure 8-34). There is little or no inflammation.

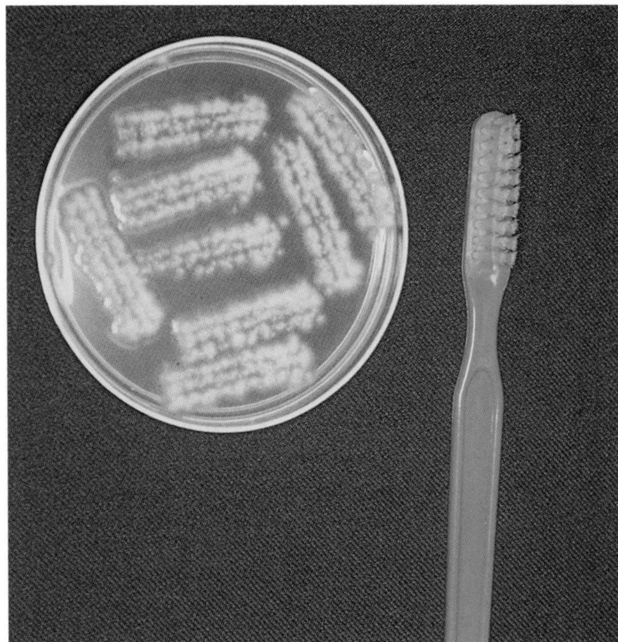

Figure 13-42 *Trichophyton tonsurans.* Culture technique for sampling dry scale in the scalp. (From Solomon LM et al: *Current Concepts* 2(3):224, 1985; reproduced by permission of Blackwell Scientific Publications.)

ID REACTION TO THERAPY. A dermatophytid (id) reaction may accompany oral antifungal therapy. The id reaction is not a widespread fungal infection but may be a cell-mediated immune response to the dermatophyte after therapy has been started. The id eruption is typically pruritic, papular or vesicular, and sometimes follicular. It usually begins on the face and spreads to the trunk. The palms and soles may be involved. A drug eruption is usually macular, papular, or urticarial and begins on the trunk. Topical steroids may be required to control symptoms. It is usually not necessary to stop the oral antifungal drug.

TREATMENT. The treatment of tinea capitis in children is summarized in Table 13-1. The British Guidelines for the diagnosis and management are summarized in Box 13-2.

Table 13-1 Tinea Capitis—Oral Drugs Used to Treat Children

Drug	Dosage	Suspension, capsule, tablet	Duration for *Trichophyton* (T), *Microsporum* (M) infections	Cochrane Database info for *Trichophyton* species + risks and benefits
Griseofulvin	10-25 mg/kg/day (microsize) or 15 mg/kg/day (ultramicrosize)	25 mg/ml 125-mg tablets 250-mg tablets 333-mg tablets 500-mg tablets Take with fatty food	(T) 6-8 weeks or longer until cultures are negative (M) 8-12 weeks or longer until fungal cultures are negative	Treatment of choice Long experience of safety No laboratory monitoring Terbinafine for 4 weeks and griseofulvin for 8 weeks showed similar efficacy
Terbinafine	<20 kg: 62.5 mg daily 21-40 kg: 125 mg daily >40 kg: 250 mg daily	250-mg tablet	(T) 4 weeks (M) Efficacy in pediatric *Microsporum* infections is disputed	Shortest duration of therapy Drug interactions Liver function tests baseline + if therapy is continued for >4 weeks
Itraconazole	5 mg/kg/day 3 mg/kg/day (oral suspension) Capsule: simplified dosing 10-20 kg: 100 mg every other day 21-30 kg: 100 mg daily 31-40 kg: 100 and 200 mg on alternate days 41-50 kg: 200 mg daily >50 kg: 200-300 mg daily	100-mg tablet or oral suspension NOTE: Oral solution is better absorbed Take with a main meal	(T) 4 weeks, fungal monitoring, another 2 weeks of treatment if test is positive (M) 6 weeks, fungal monitoring, another 2 weeks of treatment if test is positive	Cytochrome P-450/drug interactions Liver function tests baseline + if therapy is continued for >4 weeks Cure rates following treatment with itraconazole and griseofulvin for 6 weeks were similar No significant difference in cure between itraconazole for 2 weeks compared with griseofulvin for 6 weeks No difference between itraconazole and terbinafine for treatment periods lasting 2-3 weeks
Fluconazole	Dose range studies still ongoing, 6 mg/kg body weight daily; alternatively, 6-8 mg/kg body weight once weekly	50-, 100-, and 200-mg tablets or oral suspension	(T) 3-4 weeks daily regimen; 4-8 weeks weekly regimen (M) 6-8 weeks or longer	Cytochrome P-450/drug interactions Liver function tests baseline + if therapy is continued for >4 weeks Similar cure rates between 2-4 weeks of fluconazole with 6 weeks of griseofulvin

Adapted from Elewski BE: *J Am Acad Dermatol* 42:1-20, 2000 *PMID: 10607315*; Gupta AK et al: *Pediatr Dermatol* 16:171, 1999 *PMID: 10383772*; González U et al: Systemic antifungal therapy for tinea capitis in children, *Cochrane Database Syst Rev* Oct 17(4):CD004685, 2007 (review) *PMID: 17943825*; Seebacher C et al: (2007) Tinea capitis: ringworm of the scalp, *Mycoses* 50(3):218-226, 2007 (doi:10.1111/j.1439-0507.2006.01350.x). *PMID: 17472621*

TINEA OF THE BEARD

Tinea barbae is a dermatophytic infection that is limited to the coarse hair-bearing beard and mustache areas in men. Infection usually occurs after minor trauma such as from shaving.

Fungal infection of the beard area (tinea barbae) should be considered when inflammation occurs in this area. Bacterial folliculitis and inflammation secondary to ingrown hairs (pseudofolliculitis) are common. However, it is not unusual to see patients who have finally been diagnosed as having tinea after failing to respond to several courses of antibiotics. A positive culture for *Staphylococcus* does not rule out tinea, in which purulent lesions may be infected secondarily with bacteria. Like tinea capitis, the hairs are almost always infected and easily removed. The hairs in bacterial folliculitis resist removal. Cases may be associated with topical steroid therapy, pet contact, and contact with the hide of dairy cattle or horses.

Lesions are usually unilateral and are found on the chin, neck, and maxillary or submaxillary areas. Upper lip involvement is usually seen as scattered, discrete, follicular pustules; kerion formation rarely occurs.

SUPERFICIAL INFECTION. This pattern resembles the annular lesions of tinea corporis. The hair is usually infected (Figure 13-43).

DEEP FOLLICULAR INFECTION. This pattern clinically resembles bacterial folliculitis except that it is slower to evolve and is usually restricted to one area of the beard. Bacterial folliculitis spreads rapidly over wide areas after shaving. Tinea begins insidiously with a small group of follicular pustules. The process becomes confluent in time with the development of a boggy, erythematous, tumorlike abscess covered with dense, superficial crust similar to that of fungal kerions seen in tinea capitis (Figures 13-43 through 13-46). Hairs may be painlessly removed at almost any stage of the infection and examined for hyphae. Zoophilic *Trichophyton mentagrophytes* and *T. verrucosum* are the most common pathogens. *T. verrucosum* infection is acquired from the hide of dairy cattle and causes a severe pustular eruption on the face and neck. Many patients are dairy farmers (see Figure 13-28). Pustular tinea barbae in farmers may be mistaken for a *S. aureus* infection. Species identification by culture helps to identify the possible animal reservoir of infection.

TREATMENT. Treatment is the same as that for tinea capitis. Oral agents (Tables 13-2 and 13-3) are usually required because creams do not penetrate to the depths of the hair follicle.

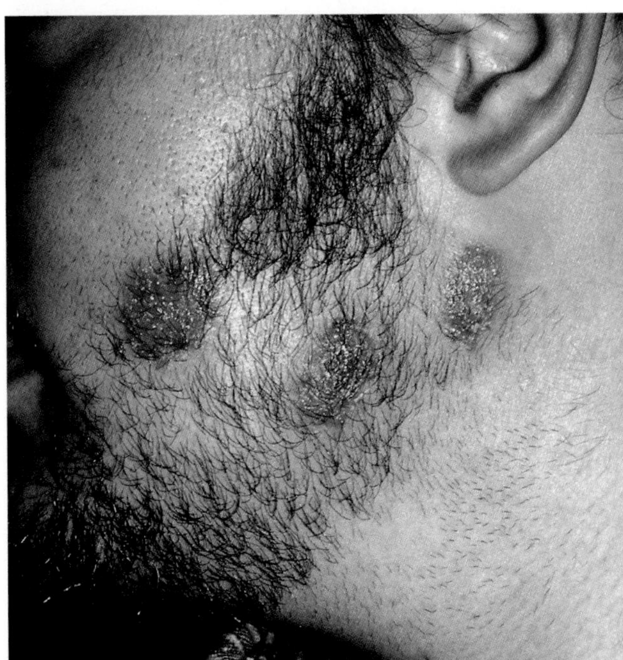

Figure 13-43 Classic ringworm pattern may be mistaken for impetigo.

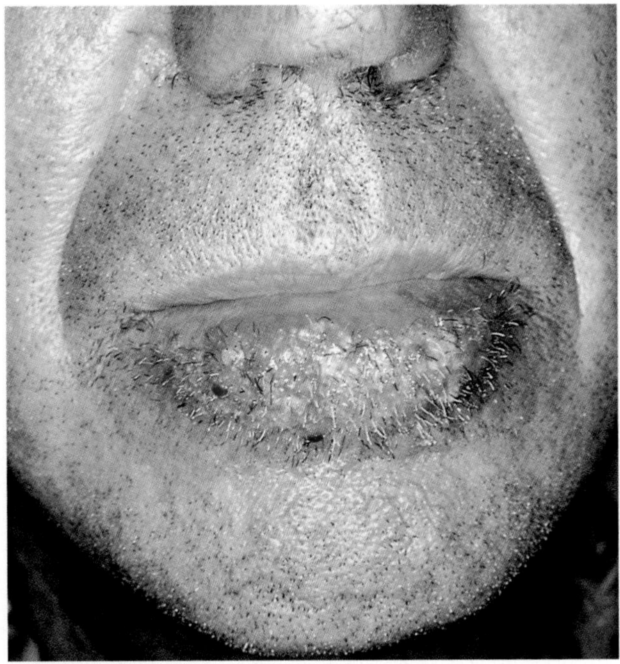

Figure 13-44 Tinea of the beard. A deep boggy infection of the follicles. The patient had been treated with several different oral antibiotics before the diagnosis of tinea was finally made. Oral antifungal agents are required to treat this deep infection.

TINEA BARBAE

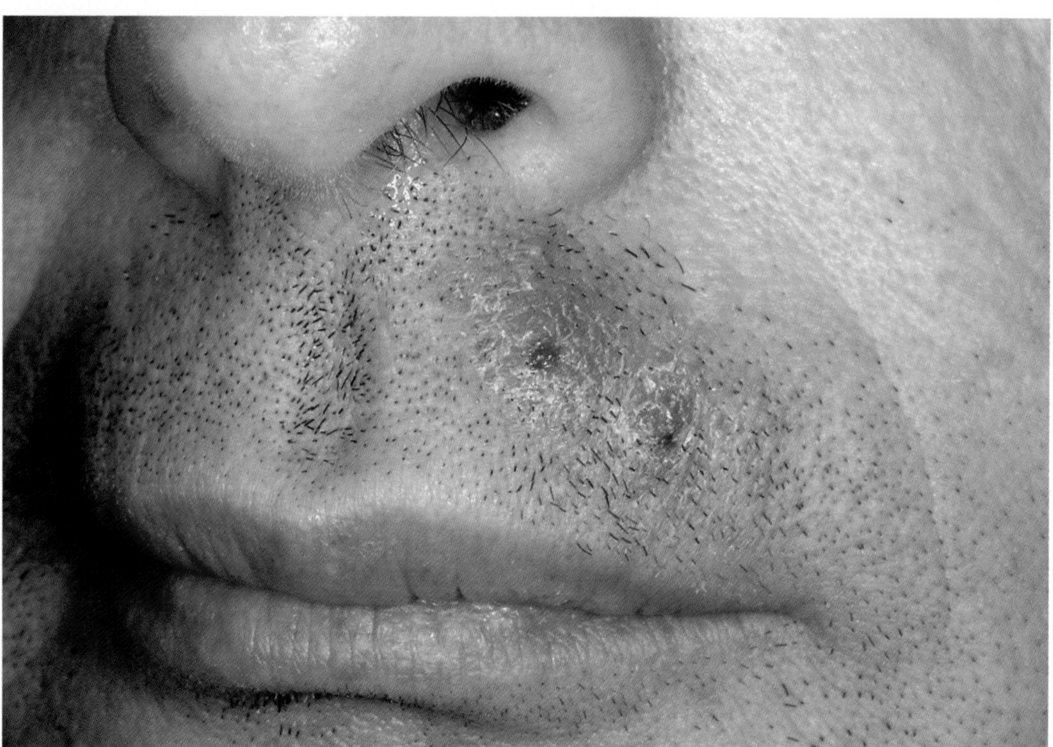

Figure 13-45 Tinea at an early stage can easily be misdiagnosed as staphylococcal folliculitis. This explains why many of these cases become more extensive after failing to respond to antibacterial antibiotics.

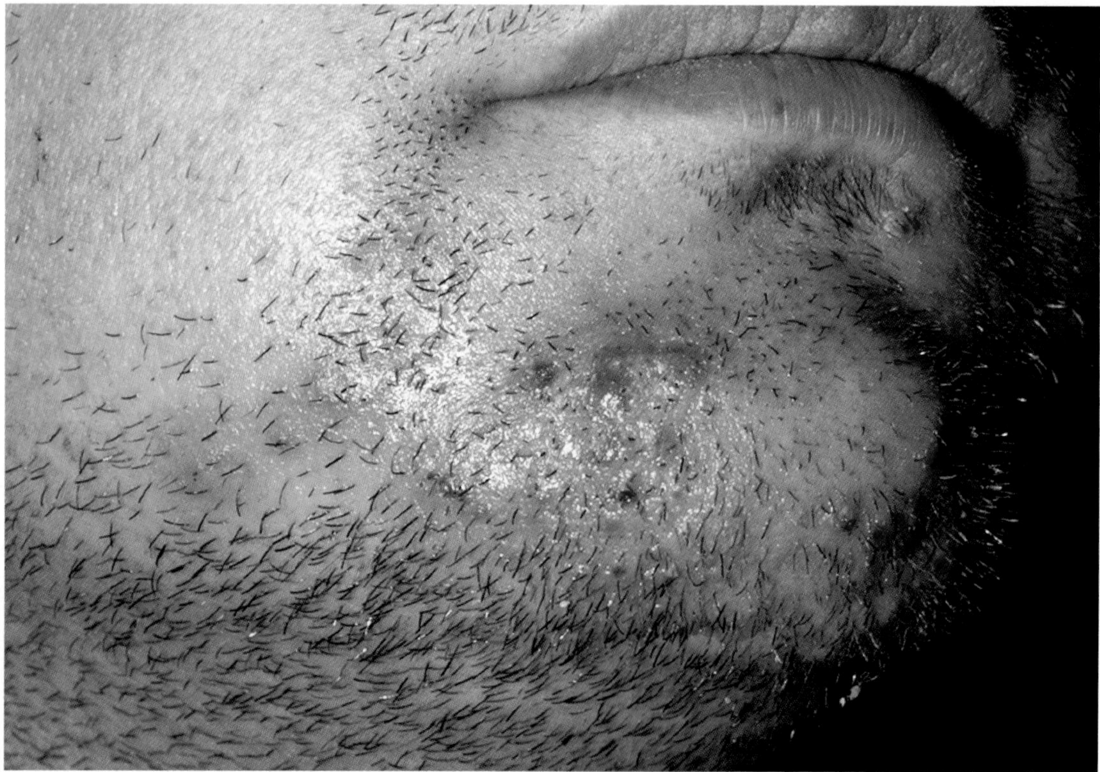

Figure 13-46 Inflamed areas are indurated and eroded on the surface. Hairs may be painlessly removed. Removal of beard hair in bacterial infections is usually painful.

Table 13-2 Oral Antifungal Drug Dosages

	Griseofulvin (ultramicrosize)	Ketoconazole (Nizoral)	Fluconazole (Diflucan)	Itraconazole (Sporanox)	Terbinafine (Lamisil)
Tinea corporis and cruris	Adult: 500 mg daily 2-4 wk Child: 5-7 mg/kg/day 2-6 wk	200-400 mg/day 2 wk	150 mg once a week for 2-4 wk	100 mg daily 1-2 wk 200 mg daily 1 wk	250 mg daily 1-2 wk
Tinea capitis	15-25 mg/kg/day (microsize) or 15 mg/kg/day (ultramicrosize) 6-8 wk	NR	5 mg/kg/day 4-6 wk 6 mg/kg/day 20 days 8 mg/kg once weekly 4-16 wk	5 mg/kg/day 4 to-6 wk 5 mg/kg/day for 1 week plus 1-3 pulses 3 weeks apart 3 mg/kg/day (oral suspension) for 1 week plus 1-3 pulses 3 weeks apart *Capsule-simplified dosing:* 10-20 kg: 100 mg every other day 21-30 kg: 100 mg daily 31-40 kg: 100 mg and 200 mg on alternate days 41-50 kg: 200 mg daily >50 kg: 200-300 mg daily	20-40 kg: 125 mg daily 2-4 wk >40 kg: 250 mg daily 2-4 wk
Onychomycosis	NR	NR	150 mg once a week for 9 months	200 mg daily Fingernails: 6 wk Toenails: 12 wk *Pulse dosing:* 200 mg bid 1 wk on, 3 wk off Toenails: 3-4 months Fingernails: 2-3 months	250 mg daily Fingernails: 6 wk Toenails: 12 wk
Tinea pedis	Adult: 500 mg daily 6-12 wk Child: 5-7 mg/kg/day 6-12 wk	NR	50 mg once a week for 3-4 wk	*Moccasin tinea pedis:* 200 mg bid 1 week	*Moccasin tinea pedis:* 250 mg daily 2 wk 200 mg daily 3 wk
Tinea versicolor	Not effective	400-mg single dose 200-mg daily 5 days Prophylaxis with 400 mg once monthly for recurrent disease	300- or 400-mg single dose; repeat in 2 wk if needed	200 mg daily for 1 wk *Prophylaxis:* 200 mg bid 1 day per month for 6 months for recurrent disease	Oral not effective Topical is effective
Vaginal candidiasis	Not effective	200-400 mg daily for 5 days	150-mg single dose 100 mg every 5-7 days	200 mg 3-5 days	Not effective

NR, not recommended.

Table 13-3 Oral Antifungal Drugs

	Griseofulvin (ultramicrosize)	Ketoconazole (Nizoral)
Dosage forms	125-, 250-, and 333-mg ultramicronized tablets 125 mg/5 ml	200-mg tablet
Gastrointestinal absorption	Fatty foods enhance absorption	Acid environment enhances absorption Take with breakfast with an acidic fruit juice Absorption reduced by antacids, histamine-2 blockers (cimetidine, ranitidine, famotidine, nizatidine), acid pump inhibitors (omeprazole, lansoprazole), and didanosine
Persistent in plasma	2 wk	2 days
Persistent in skin and nails	1-2 wk	Unknown
Laboratory monitoring*	Rx 6 wk CBC, LFT	Baseline CBC, LFT; repeat each month
Abnormal LFT elevations	Rare	Hepatotoxic drug; see package insert
Mechanism of adverse drug reactions	Potent inducer of microsomal cytochrome P-450 enzymes	Metabolized by and inhibits liver cytochrome P-450 enzyme
Adverse events	—	3%
Adverse drug interactions	Decreases levels of warfarin, estrogen, birth control pills Effect of alcohol is potentiated Barbiturates depress activity of griseofulvin	Raises serum levels of astemizole, cisapride, quinidine Quinidine: tinnitus, cardiac arrhythmias Anticoagulants: bleeding Sulfonylureas: hypoglycemia Cyclosporine, tacrolimus: renal toxicity Calcium channel blockers: edema Midazolam, triazolam: increased sedation Phenytoin: dizziness, ataxia Induce synthesis of cortisol-producing symptoms of hypoadrenalism (fatigue, malaise) Reduces synthesis of testosterone: impotence, gynecomastia
Adverse drug reactions	Nausea, vomiting, diarrhea, headache, dizziness, insomnia, cutaneous eruptions, photosensitivity (rare)	Gastrointestinal disturbances, disulfiram-like effect when alcohol is ingested, hepatitis (1:10,000)—stop drug if nausea, vomiting, fatigue, malaise, dark urine, pale stools, jaundice, or cutaneous eruptions occur

*Patient education regarding the symptoms of early hepatitis and advice to stop the drug at first sign of symptoms (nausea, malaise, fatigue) are essential to prevent progression to severe liver injury.
CBC, complete blood cell count; LFT, liver function test.

Fluconazole (Diflucan)	Itraconazole (Sporanox)	Terbinafine (Lamisil)
50-, 100-, and 200-mg tablets 150-mg tablet (for vaginal infections)	100-mg capsule	250 mg
Food does not affect absorption	Acid environment enhances absorption Take with breakfast with an acidic fruit juice Absorption reduced by antacids, histamine-2 blockers (cimetidine, ranitidine, famotidine, nizatidine), acid pump inhibitors (omeprazole, lansoprazole), and didanosine	Food enhances absorption by 20%
30-50 hr half-life	1 wk	4-6 wk
3 months	6-9 months lipophilic	4-6 wk lipophilic
For continuous therapy: baseline CBC, LFT; repeat every 4-6 wk	For continuous therapy: baseline CBC, LFT; repeat every 4-6 wk	Baseline CBC, LFT; repeat every 4-6 wk
Low incidence	2.0% pulse dosing 4.0% continuous dosing	3.3-7%
Metabolized by and inhibits liver cytochrome P-450 enzyme	Metabolized by liver and inhibits cytochrome P-450 enzymes	Metabolized by liver cytochrome P-450 enzymes; cytochrome P-450 enzymes CYP2D6 inhibited by terbinafine
26%	8.3%	10.5%
Possibly same type of drug interactions as ketoconazole but less likely when drug is given on an intermittent basis *Cautions:* Astemizole (Hismanal) Cisapride (Propulsid) Warfarin (Coumadin) Cyclosporine (Neoral) Phenytoin (Dilantin) Sulfonylureas	Drugs that induce cytochrome P-450 enzymes will increase catabolism and reduce plasma concentration of itraconazole (phenytoin, rifampin, rifabutin, isoniazid, carbamazepine) May be involved in same drug interactions as ketoconazole *Cautions:* Atorvastatin (Lipitor) Digoxin Quinidine Warfarin (Coumadin) Cyclosporine (Neoral) Calcium channel blockers *Contraindications:* Astemizole (Hismanal) Triazolam (Halcion) Cisapride (Propulsid) Lovastatin (Mevacor) Simvastatin (Zocor) Midazolam (Versed)	CYP2D6 involved in metabolism of tricyclic antidepressants and other psychotropic drugs Increases clearance and thus lowers levels of cyclosporine Decreases clearance of caffeine Terbinafine blood levels are increased by cimetidine, and decreased by rifampin and rifabutin Monitor theophylline levels
Gastrointestinal disturbances Hepatitis much less likely than with ketoconazole	Headache, gastrointestinal disturbances, cutaneous eruptions Hepatitis much less likely than with ketoconazole Peripheral edema especially if taken with calcium channel blockers	Gastrointestinal disturbances, alteration in taste (2.8%), cutaneous eruptions, neutropenia, agranulocytosis

Treatment of fungal infections

TOPICAL PREPARATIONS. A variety of preparations are commercially available. Studies have shown that undecylenic acid (e.g., Desenex) may be almost as effective for treating dermatophyte infections as the newer agents. Most of the medicines are available as creams or lotions; some are available as powders or aerosols. They are effective for all dermatophyte infections except for deep, inflammatory lesions of the body and scalp. They have no effect on tinea of the nail. Creams or lotions should be applied twice a day until the infection is clear. (See Box 13-3 and the Formulary for a list of the available topical agents.)

SYSTEMIC AGENTS (see Tables 13-1 to 13-3)

GRISEOFULVIN. Griseofulvin is active only against dermatophytes; yeast infections, including those caused by *Candida* organisms and *Pityrosporum* organisms (tinea versicolor), and deep fungi do not respond. The drug has been available for more than 40 years and has been proved to be safe. Griseofulvin has a fungistatic effect; therefore it works best on actively growing dermatophytes, in which it may inhibit fungal cell wall synthesis. Griseofulvin probably diffuses into the stratum corneum from the extracellular fluid and sweat. Increased sweating may increase the concentration in the stratum corneum, thereby enhancing the drug's effect. Griseofulvin produces a sustained blood level so that a daily or twice-a-day schedule is adequate. Absorption varies from person to person; individual patients attain consistently high or low levels of the drug. Taking the drug with fatty foods may enhance absorption. Two types of preparations are available: microsize and ultramicrosize. The newer, ultramicrosize forms are better absorbed and require approximately 50% to 70% of the dosage of the microsize form. Many brands are available in both forms. In microsize forms, the drug is supplied as 125-, 250-, and 500-mg tablets; in ultramicrosize forms, it is supplied as 125-, 250-, and 330-mg tablets. A liquid formulation is available. Reported treatment failures are probably the result of using too small a dosage rather than treating resistant organisms.

Box 13-3 Topical Antifungals and Spectrum of Coverage

Class	Drug	Dermatophytes	Yeasts	Bacteria
Allylamine/benzylamine	Butenafine	X		
	Naftifine	X		
	Terbinafine	X		
Imidazole	Clotrimazole	X	X	
	Econazole	X	X	X
	Ketoconazole	X	X	
	Miconazole	X	X	
	Oxiconazole	X	X	
	Sulconazole	X	X	
Pyridone	Ciclopirox-olamine	X	X	X
Polyene	Nystatin		X	

Adverse reactions. Griseofulvin is a safe drug. Headaches and gastrointestinal symptoms are the most common side effects. The dosage can be temporarily lowered to see if the symptoms clear, but sometimes the drug must be discontinued. Hepatotoxicity, leukopenia, and photosensitivity rarely occur; therefore routine blood studies are not necessary unless treatment is to last for many months or the dosage is exceptionally high. If a headache occurs, it usually does so during the first few days of treatment and may disappear as treatment is continued. A trial at a lower dosage level is warranted for those with headaches lasting longer than 48 hours. Patients with persistent headaches after a lower dosage trial need alternative treatment. Bone marrow suppression, once attributed to griseofulvin, probably never occurs, and routine complete blood cell counts are not necessary. Gastrointestinal upset, urticaria, photosensitivity, and morbilliform skin eruptions have been reported. Griseofulvin activates hepatic enzymes that cause degradation of warfarin and other drugs. Appropriate steps should be taken if combined treatment is used.

ALLYLAMINES. Allylamines, like the azoles, inhibit ergosterol synthesis, but they do so at an earlier point. The result, as with the azoles, is membrane disruption and cell death.

TERBINAFINE. Terbinafine belongs to the allylamine class of antifungal agents. It inhibits squalene epoxidase, a membrane-bound enzyme that is not part of the cytochrome P-450 superfamily and is fungicidal to dermatophytes. Terbinafine is well absorbed and highly lipophilic and keratophilic, and is distributed throughout adipose tissue, dermis, epidermis, and nails. The drug persists in plasma, dermis-epidermis, hair, and nails for weeks. Persistence of the drug in plasma is of concern when side effects are experienced. Terbinafine is delivered to the stratum corneum via the sebum and, to a lesser extent, through incorporation into the basal keratinocytes and diffusion through the dermis-epidermis. Terbinafine is not found in eccrine sweat. It remains in skin at concentrations above the mean inhibitory concentration (MIC) for most dermatophytes for 2 to 3 weeks after discontinuation of long-term oral therapy. After 6 and 12 weeks of oral therapy, terbinafine has been detected in the nail plate for 30 and 36 weeks, respectively, at a concentration well above the MIC for most dermatophytes. Terbinafine is metabolized in the liver. Dose adjustments may be needed for patients with liver dysfunction. In patients with renal disease, the elimination half-life can become prolonged. The dose of terbinafine should be halved when the serum creatinine level exceeds 300 μmol/L, or when the creatinine clearance rate is less than or equal to 50 ml/minute (0.83 ml/second).

Indications. Oral terbinafine is effective for onychomycosis and other dermatomycoses.

TRIAZOLES. Triazoles are similar to imidazoles in chemical structure and mechanism of action.

Itraconazole (Sporanox). Itraconazole, like the other antifungal azoles, inhibits fungal cytochrome P-450–dependent enzymes, blocking the synthesis of ergosterol, the principal sterol in the fungal cell membrane. Itraconazole is lipophilic and has a high affinity for keratinizing tissues. It adheres to the lipophilic cytoplasm of keratinocytes in the nail plate, allowing progressive buildup and persistence in the nail plate. The drug reaches high levels in the nails that persist for at least 6 months after discontinuation of 3 months of therapy and during pulsed cycles. The concentration in the stratum corneum remains detectable for 4 weeks after therapy. Itraconazole levels in sebum are five times higher than those in plasma and remain high for as long as 1 week after therapy. This suggests that secretion in sebum may account for the high concentrations found in skin. Itraconazole has an affinity for mammalian cytochrome P-450 enzymes, as well as for fungal P-450–dependent enzyme, and thus has the potential for clinically important interactions (e.g., astemizole, rifampin, oral contraceptives, H_2-receptor antagonists, warfarin, cyclosporine). Absorption of itraconazole is significantly increased by the presence of food; it should be taken with a full meal.

Fluconazole (Diflucan). Fluconazole is much more specific and effective at inhibiting cytochrome P-450 than are the imidazole agents. Fluconazole is highly water soluble and is transported to the skin through sweat and concentrated by evaporation. It achieves high concentrations in the epidermis and nails and persists for long periods of time.

Ketoconazole (Nizoral). The use of ketoconazole for the treatment of dermatophyte infections has greatly diminished with the introduction of itraconazole, fluconazole, and terbinafine. These newer drugs are more effective and less likely to cause hepatic toxicity.

CANDIDIASIS (MONILIASIS)

The yeastlike fungus *C. albicans* and a few other *Candida* species are capable of producing skin, mucous membrane, and internal infections. The organism lives within the normal flora of the mouth, vaginal tract, and gut, and it reproduces through the budding of oval yeast forms. Pregnancy, oral contraception, antibiotic therapy, diabetes, skin maceration, topical steroid therapy, certain endocrinopathies, and factors related to depression of cell-mediated immunity may allow the yeast to become pathogenic and produce budding spores and elongated cells (pseudohyphae) or true hyphae with septate walls. The pseudohyphae and hyphae are indistinguishable from dermatophytes in potassium hydroxide preparations (Figure 13-47). Culture results must be interpreted carefully because the yeast is part of the normal flora in many areas.

The yeast infects only the outer layers of the epithelium of mucous membranes and skin (the stratum corneum). The primary lesion is a pustule, the contents of which dissect horizontally under the stratum corneum and peel it away. Clinically, this process results in a red, denuded, glistening surface with a long, cigarette paper–like, scaling, advancing border. The infected mucous membranes of the mouth and vaginal tract accumulate scale and inflammatory cells that develop into characteristic white or white-yellow, curdy material.

Yeast grows best in a warm, moist environment; therefore infection is usually confined to the mucous membranes and intertriginous areas. The advancing infected border usually stops when it reaches dry skin.

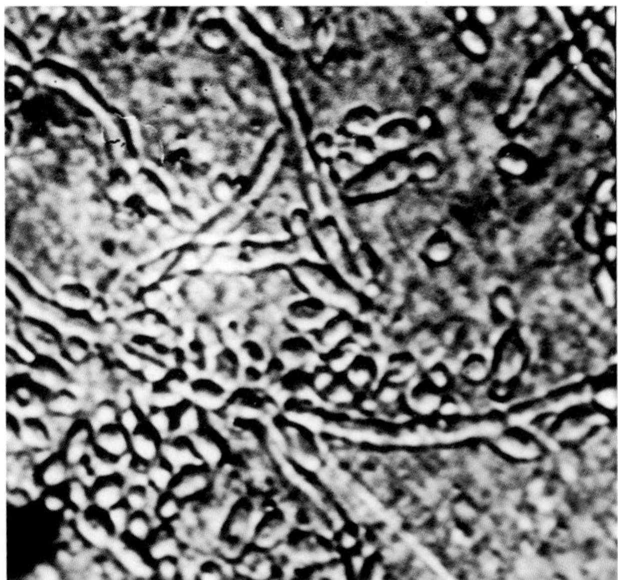

Figure 13-47 *Candida albicans.* A potassium hydroxide wet mount of skin scrapings showing both elongated pseudohyphae and budding spores.

Candidiasis of normally moist areas

Candidiasis affects normally moist areas such as the vagina, the mouth, and the uncircumcised penis. In the vagina, it causes vulvovaginitis; in the mouth, it causes thrush; and in the uncircumcised penis, it causes balanitis.

VULVOVAGINITIS

Vulvovaginitis has infectious (Box 13-4) and noninfectious causes. Infectious vaginitis is the most common cause of a vaginal discharge. Common infectious causes include several species of yeasts, *Trichomonas vaginalis,* and *Gardnerella vaginalis* and its associated proliferation of anaerobic bacteria. Other causes include infectious cervicitis, a physiologic discharge, and allergic or irritant contact vaginitis. Atrophic vaginitis is the most common noninfectious cause of vaginitis in the postmenopausal woman. *Neisseria gonorrhoeae,* group A β-hemolytic *Streptococcus (Streptococcus pyogenes),* other bacteria, pinworms, and foreign bodies in the vagina are also possible causes of vaginitis in prepubertal girls.

VAGINAL DISCHARGE

NON–SEXUALLY-ACQUIRED DISCHARGE. Bacterial vaginosis and candidiasis are possibly due to a disturbance of vaginal flora. They are not sexually transmitted, unlike most trichomoniasis (*Trichomonas vaginalis*) cases. Many patients are initially managed as having candidiasis even though bacterial vaginosis is more common. Group B *Streptococcus* is often reported on vaginal swabs, but this organism does not typically cause discharge and only needs treatment in pregnancy. Patients who present with symptoms suggestive of bacterial vaginosis and *vulvovaginal candidiasis* can be treated without sampling.

Box 13-4 **Causes of Vaginal Discharge**
Noninfective
Physiologic
Cervical ectopy
Foreign bodies, such as retained tampon
Vulval dermatitis
Non–sexually-transmitted infection
Bacterial vaginosis
Candida infections
Sexually transmitted infection
Chlamydia trachomatis
Neisseria gonorrhoeae
Trichomonas vaginalis

BACTERIAL VAGINOSIS. Bacterial vaginosis (e.g., *Gardnerella vaginalis,* among others) is the most common cause of infective vaginal discharge. The symptoms are fishy-smelling discharge without itch or soreness. Anaerobic bacteria occur and remit spontaneously. Asymptomatic bacterial vaginosis in nonpregnant women does not require treatment. The condition is associated with poor pregnancy outcomes, endometritis after miscarriage, and pelvic inflammatory disease.

SEXUALLY ACQUIRED DISCHARGE. Much less often, vaginal discharge may be the result of mucopurulent cervicitis caused by *Neisseria gonorrhoeae* or *Chlamydia trachomatis. Chlamydia trachomatis, Neisseria gonorrhoeae,* and p. 393*Trichomonas vaginalis* present with vaginal discharge or are asymptomatic (see). *Chlamydia trachomatis* and gonorrhea may be complicated by pelvic inflammatory disease.

Trichomonas vaginalis can cause an offensive, yellow, profuse, frothy discharge with vulvar itch, soreness, dysuria, and superficial dyspareunia. Detection of cervical infection in women with or without vaginal discharge requires laboratory confirmation.

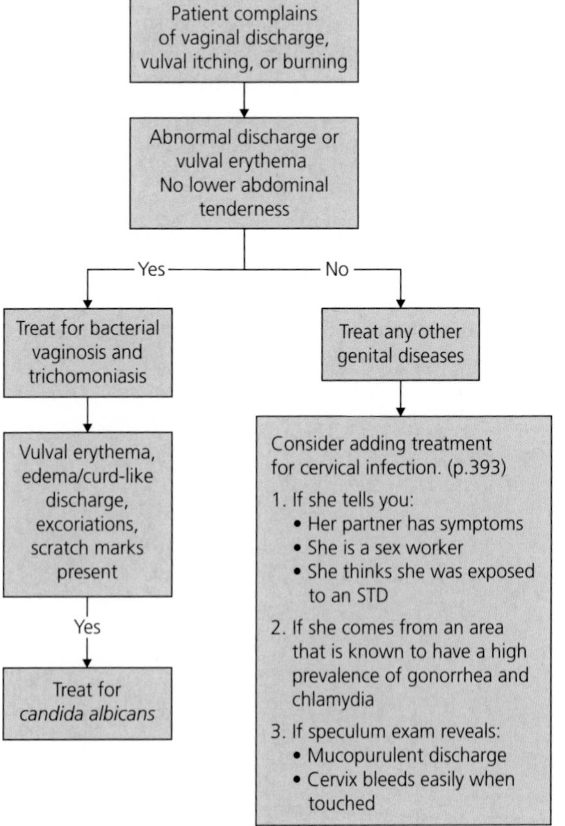

Figure 13-48

SYNDROMIC MANAGEMENT. Many diseases can be identified and treated on the basis of characteristic symptoms and signs, which can be grouped into syndromes. It is often difficult to know exactly what organism is causing the syndrome, however, and treatment may need to cover several possible infections. Syndromic management refers to the approach of treating symptoms and signs based on the organisms most commonly responsible for each syndrome. A more definite or etiologic diagnosis may be possible in some settings with laboratory facilities, but this is often difficult in clinic settings that lack laboratory facilities. Laboratory tests require resources, add to the cost of treatment, may require clients to make extra visits to the clinic, and almost always result in delays in treatment. For these reasons, syndromic management guidelines are widely used for syndromes such as urethral discharge, vaginal discharge, and genital ulcer even in developed countries with advanced laboratory facilities.

The World Health Organization (WHO) has developed flowcharts (algorithms) to guide health care providers in using the syndromic approach to manage several sexually transmitted infection syndromes. The WHO method for managing vaginal discharge is presented in Figure 13-48 and Table 13-4.

Optional tests. Testing provides a more accurate diagnosis (see Boxes 13-5 and 13-6).

MONILIAL VULVOVAGINITIS

Vaginal candidiasis is the most common cause of vaginal discharge. Greater than 50% of women older than 25 years develop vulvovaginal candidiasis at some time; fewer than 5% of these women experience recurrences. Infection is usually caused by *C. albicans*. The incidence of infections resulting from yeasts other than *C. albicans* has increased in the last few years. Of these non-*albicans* species, *Candida tropicalis* and *Candida glabrata* are the most important. Currently used drug therapies (e.g., imidazoles) do not adequately eradicate non-*albicans* species. A possible explanation for the recent increased selection of these species may be the shortened antifungal therapies (1- to 3-day regimens) that suppress *C. albicans* but create an imbalance of flora that facilitates an overgrowth of non-*albicans* species.

Candida is present in the normal flora of the vaginal tract and rectum in 10% of women. Candidal vaginitis develops in approximately one fourth of women in their child-bearing years. Heat and moisture are increased under large folds of fat and occlusive undergarments. Symptoms may worsen a few days before menstruation. One study showed that 30% of women treated with antibiotics developed candidal vaginitis.

Table 13-4 Recommended Treatment for Vaginal Infection*

<table>
<tr><th>Coverage</th><th>First choice
Choose 1 from BV/TV box, or 1 from each box if yeast infection is suspected</th><th>Effective substitutes</th><th>If patient is pregnant, breast-feeding
Choose 1 from BV/TV box below, or 1 from each box if yeast infection is suspected</th></tr>
<tr><td>Bacterial vaginosis (BV)</td><td rowspan="2">Metronidazole† 2 gm orally in a single dose, or
Metronidazole† 400 or 500 mg orally twice a day for 7 days</td><td>Clindamycin cream 2%, one full applicator (5 gm) intravaginally at bedtime for 7 days, or
Clindamycin 300 mg orally twice a day for 7 days</td><td rowspan="2">Preferably after first trimester
Metronidazole† 200 or 250 mg orally 3 times a day for 7 days, or
Metronidazole† gel 0.75%, one full applicator (5 gm) intravaginally twice a day for 5 days, or
Clindamycin 300 mg orally twice a day for 7 days</td></tr>
<tr><td>Trichomoniasis vaginalis (TV)</td><td>Tinidazole† 2 gm orally in a single dose, or
Tinidazole† 500 mg orally twice a day for 5 days</td></tr>
<tr><td>Candida albicans (CA) (yeast)</td><td>Miconazole 200-mg vaginal suppository, one a day for 3 days, or
Clotrimazole‡ 100-mg vaginal tablet, 2 tablets a day for 3 days, or
Fluconazole 150-mg oral tablet, in a single dose</td><td>Nystatin 100,000-unit vaginal tablet, one a day for 14 days</td><td>Miconazole 200-mg vaginal suppository, one a day for 3 days, or
Clotrimazole† 100-mg vaginal tablet, 2 tablets a day for 3 days, or
Nystatin 100,000-unit vaginal tablet, one a day for 14 days</td></tr>
</table>

From *Sexually transmitted and other reproductive tract infections: A guide to essential practice:* World Health Organization, 2005.

*Therapy for bacterial vaginosis and trichomoniasis plus therapy for yeast infection if curdlike white discharge, vulvovaginal redness, and itching are present.

†Patients taking metronidazole or tinidazole should be cautioned to avoid alcohol. Use of metronidazole is not recommended in the first trimester of pregnancy.

‡Single-dose clotrimazole (500 mg) available in some places is also effective for yeast infection (CA).

CLINICAL PRESENTATION. Vaginal candidiasis usually begins with vaginal itching and/or a white, thin-to-creamy discharge (Figure 13-49). Symptoms may resolve spontaneously after several days, or they may progress. The vaginal mucous membranes and external genitalia become red, swollen, and sometimes eroded and painful (Figure 13-50). They are covered with a thick, white, crumbly discharge, which becomes more copious during pregnancy. The infection may spread onto the thighs and anus, producing a tender, red skin surface with discrete pustules, called *satellite lesions,* that appear outside the edges of the advancing border. The diagnosis is confirmed by a potassium hydroxide preparation of the discharge.

MANAGEMENT. First-line therapy consists of antifungal creams or pills (Box 13-7). A Cochrane Database review in 2007 showed that no statistically significant differences were observed in clinical cure rates of antifungals administered by the oral and intravaginal routes for the treatment of uncomplicated vaginal candidiasis. No definitive conclusion can be made regarding the relative safety of oral and intravaginal antifungals for uncomplicated vaginal candidiasis. The decision to prescribe or recommend the purchase of an antifungal for oral or intravaginal administration should take into consideration safety, cost, and treatment preference. Decision-makers should consider whether the higher cost of some oral antifungals is worth the gain in convenience, if this is the patient's preference. *PMID: 17943774*

Topical antifungal agents. There are a large variety of topical medications in many forms, including tablets, creams, and tampons (see Box 13-7 and the Formulary). Clotrimazole and miconazole are the most widely used. The cure rate with polyenes (e.g., nystatin) is 70% to 80%; the cure rate with azole derivatives is 85% to 90%. Topical antimycotic therapy is free of systemic side effects. The initial application may cause local burning, especially if inflammation is severe. The burning is a local irritant reaction rather than an allergy. Treatment schedules are listed in Box 13-7 and the Formulary. The course should be repeated if symptoms have not subsided. Cream is useful if the external areas are also infected; the cream can be used to coat the vulva. Cream may also be applied directly from the tube. There is sufficient cream supplied for both external and internal application. Nystatin (Mycostatin) has been used for years. The applicator is used to insert one tablet high in the vaginal tract twice a day for 2 weeks. The duration of treatment is extended if signs or symptoms persist. Although nystatin must be used longer than the azoles, it is still an effective and safe medicine.

Box 13-5 **Optional Tests for Vaginal Discharge**

Swab testing

1. High vaginal swab to culture bacterial vaginosis, *Candida* infections, and *Trichomonas vaginalis*
2. Endocervical and/or vaginal swab in transport medium to culture gonorrhea (not a preferred test)
3. Endocervical swab for a chlamydial DNA amplification test to diagnose *Chlamydia trachomatis*

Vaginal pH testing

1. Bacterial vaginosis (pH >4.5)
2. Candidiasis (pH <4.5)

Nucleic acid amplification tests (polymerase chain reaction)

1. Highly sensitive and specific
2. For detecting *Chlamydia* and gonorrhea

Box 13-6 **Diagnosis of Vaginal Infections***

	Monilial (*Candida*)	Bacterial vaginosis (*G. vaginalis* and anaerobic bacteria)	Trichomoniasis
Vaginal discharge	White, clumpy	Gray, homogeneous	Profuse greenish, sometimes frothy
Symptoms	Itching	Malodorous discharge	Malodorous discharge, itching, dyspareunia, dysuria
Saline or potassium hydroxide wet mount	Budding yeast, pseudohyphae; 30% will be negative	Clue cells (epithelial cells) with adherent bacteria	Motile trichomonads, white blood cells (do not use potassium hydroxide)
pH	<4.5	>4.7	4.5
Amine whiff test (add 10% potassium hydroxide to discharge)	Not applicable	+ (fishy odor caused by release of amines)	+ (strong odor because of a proliferation of anaerobic organisms)
Culture	Standard transport media	Standard transport media	Diamond's media
Partner treatment	Treat sexual partners if partners are symptomatic	Treat sexual partners if recurrent	Treat sexual partner to prevent reinfection

*The laboratory personnel can perform all of these tests if provided with sufficient material. Discharge specimens should be taken to the laboratory immediately if trichomoniasis is suspected; motility of the organism may not be visible after 15 to 30 minutes.

Oral antifungal agents. Oral preparations include fluconazole and itraconazole. Fluconazole (Diflucan) is the preferred oral drug for *Candida vaginitis*. A single 150-mg oral tablet was shown to be as effective as other oral and intravaginal regimens, with minimal adverse effects.

ACUTE VAGINAL CANDIDIASIS. The imidazoles and triazoles are the first choice of treatment for vulvovaginal candidiasis. There is a lack of clear superiority of one azole agent or dosing regimen. Most patients are treated with a short course of intravaginal therapy (1 to 3 days) for acute, uncomplicated candidal vaginitis. The physician's judgment and the patient's preference determine the specific antifungal agent and route of administration; cost, distribution of inflammation, and medicine vehicle characteristics are factors in the decision. Many patients prefer oral treatment. Oral and vaginal medications are almost equally effective in treating acute disease. Fluconazole administered as a single 150-mg oral dose proved to be as safe and effective as 7 days of intravaginal clotrimazole therapy for *C. vaginitis*.

PATIENT PREFERENCE. Half of patients prefer oral medication; only 5% prefer intravaginal therapy, and the others have no clear preference. Before treating vaginal candidiasis, the physician should ask the patient about her preference.

PARTNER TREATMENT. Vaginal candidiasis is usually not a sexually transmitted disease and routine treatment of male partners is not necessary. One study showed that treatment of male partners with a brief course of ketoconazole was not of value in reducing the incidence of relapse in women with recurrent vaginal candidiasis. Partner treatment is indicated for men with balanoposthitis or for chronic recurrent cases.

Box 13-7 **Common Treatments for Acute Vulvovaginal Candidiasis**

Route	Drug	Dose
Topical	Miconazole 2% cream	Apply twice daily × 5 days
Vaginal	Nystatin	Insert daily × 1 wk
	Tioconazole 6.5%	1 day
	Miconazole nitrate 2%	1200 gm/1 day
	Miconazole nitrate 4%	3 days
	Clotrimazole 2%	3 days
	Miconazole nitrate 2%	7 days
	Clotrimazole 1%	7 days
Suppository	Clotrimazole	Insert daily × 1 wk
	Miconazole nitrate	3 days
Systemic	Fluconazole	150 mg × 1 dose, or 100 mg/day × 5-7 days
	Itraconazole	200 mg/day × 3-5 days

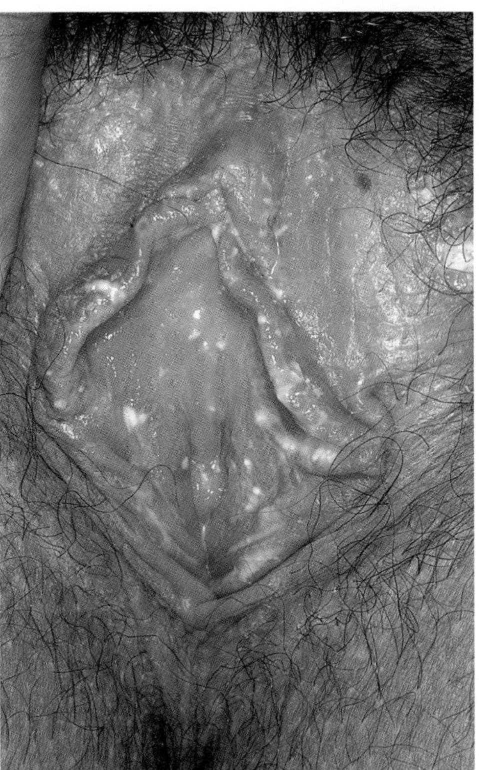

Figure 13-49 The most common presentation for acute vaginal candidiasis is a red inflamed vulva and vagina and a white, thick discharge.

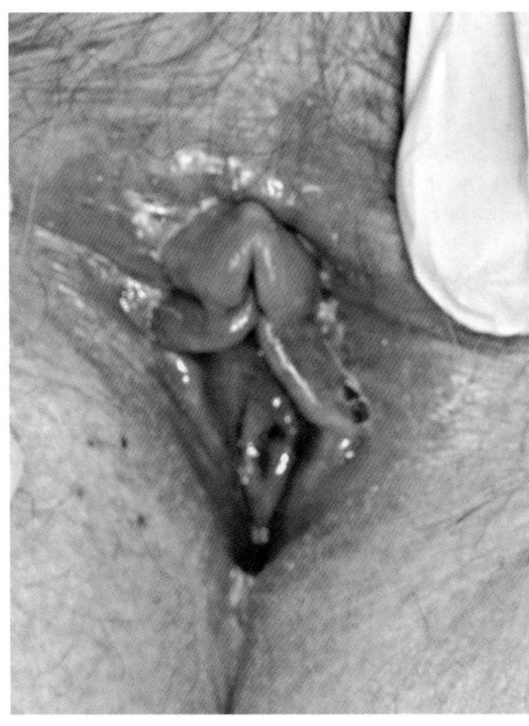

Figure 13-50 Vulvar and vaginal candidiasis with intense erythema and no white discharge. A culture proved the diagnosis.

SIDE EFFECTS. Side effects of treatment for vaginal candidiasis are rare.

PREGNANCY. Oral therapy should not be given to pregnant patients or to patients who are not using reliable contraceptive measures. Topical therapy during pregnancy may require a longer treatment regimen (6 to 14 days). Women who do not use reliable contraception should use oral treatment only during the first 10 days of the menstrual cycle.

Candida strains can be cultured from the vagina in 10% to 20% of pregnant women. The incidence of vaginal candidiasis in pregnancy is twice as high as in the nonpregnant state. The incidence is higher late in pregnancy. In 80% to 90% of the cases, candidiasis is caused by *C. albicans*. Treatment of vaginal candidiasis in pregnancy is indicated not only to make the woman symptom-free but also to protect the fetus from a life-threatening *Candida* sepsis. Itraconazole cannot be used for oral treatment of vaginal candidiasis in pregnant women because of possible teratogenic effects.

RECURRENT (RESISTANT) DISEASE

Vulvovaginal candidiasis is considered recurrent when at least four episodes occur in 1 year or at least three episodes unrelated to antibiotic therapy occur within 1 year. Patients with chronic and recurrent candidal vaginitis rarely have recognizable precipitating or causal factors. Appearance of non-*albicans* species is possible but unusual. Relapse is due to persistent yeast in the vagina rather than to frequent vaginal reinfection. Causes include treatment-resistant *Candida* species other than *C. albicans,* frequent antibiotic therapy, contraceptive use, compromise of the immune system, increasing frequency of sexual intercourse, and hyperglycemia. Women with recurrent candidal vaginitis are more likely to use solutions for vulvoperineal cleansing or vaginal douching. Frequent yeast infections could be an early sign of human immunodeficiency virus (HIV) infection.

LABORATORY TESTS. Potassium hydroxide preparations of vaginal secretions are not sufficiently sensitive to exclude fungal infection in recurrent disease. If microscopic examination is negative but clinical suspicion is high, fungal cultures should be obtained.

TREATING RESISTANT CASES. Some women have repeated or ongoing infection even after several courses of anti-yeast therapy. The pathogenesis is poorly understood and the majority of patients have no recognizable predisposing factors.

There is no definitive cure for recurrent disease, but long-term maintenance regimens with oral or topical medication are effective.

Weekly applications of terconazole 0.8% cream were effective in preventing recurrent episodes of candidal vaginitis and were well tolerated.

Patients with recurrent disease should be advised to lose excess weight and to wear loose-fitting, cotton undergarments. Daily ingestion of 8 ounces of yogurt containing *Lactobacillus acidophilus* decreased both candidal colonization and infection in one study. The efficacy of yeast-elimination diets is unknown.

Attempts to reduce the number of attacks by treating sexual partners and by suppressing a gastrointestinal tract focus with Mycostatin have failed. Many patients experience recurrences once prophylaxis is discontinued; therefore long-term therapy may be necessary. Patients are more likely to comply when antifungal therapy is administered orally.

Table 13-5 Treatment Options for Acute and Recurrent Vulvovaginal Candidiasis

Agent	Dosing regimen
Treatment of acute episode	
Clotrimazole (Gyne-Lotrimin)	100-mg tablets administered intravaginally for 7 days
Terconazole 0.8% cream (Terazol 3)	One full applicator (5 gm) administered intravaginally for 3 days
Fluconazole (Diflucan)	150 mg administered orally (one dose) 100 mg administered orally for 5 to 7 days
Ketoconazole (Nizoral)	200 mg administered orally once daily for 14 days 400 mg administered orally once daily for 14 days
Itraconazole	200 mg administered orally for 3 to 5 days
Boric acid	600-mg vaginal suppository administered twice daily for 14 days (must be compounded)
Prophylaxis (maintenance)	
Clotrimazole (Gyne-Lotrimin)	Two 100-mg tablets administered intravaginally twice weekly for 6 months
Terconazole 0.8% cream (Terazol 3)	One full applicator (5 gm) administered vaginally once a week
Fluconazole (Diflucan)	150 mg administered orally once a month 100 to 200 mg weekly
Itraconazole (Sporanox)	50 to 100 mg administered daily 200 mg bid administered orally once a month
Ketoconazole (Nizoral)	Two 200-mg tablets administered orally for 5 days after the menses for six months One half of a 200-mg tablet administered orally once daily for 6 months
Boric acid	600-mg vaginal suppository administered once daily during menstruation (5-day menses)

Adapted from Ringdahl EN: *Am Fam Physician* 61: 3306, 2000.
PMID: 10865926

Candida should be documented by culture for any patient who has recurrent or persistent disease and a negative potassium hydroxide slide.

Long-term maintenance therapy schedules are listed in Table 13-5.

Resistant organisms. Vaginal candidiasis resulting from *C. glabrata* may not respond to any of the azole drugs. Vaginal nystatin or local application of 1% gentian violet may eradicate this species. Recurrent infections after treatment may be caused by more common *Candida* species.

ORAL CANDIDIASIS

C. albicans may be transmitted to the infant's oral cavity during passage through the birth canal. It is part of the normal mouth flora in many adults.

Non-*albicans Candida* species are causing an increasing number of infections. Most of these occur in immunocompromised individuals, especially in those infected with HIV. Oral candidiasis is common in advanced cancer. In a study of patients with advanced cancer, the two most prevalent species were *C. albicans* and *C. glabrata,* with fewer numbers of *C. tropicalis, C. parapsilosis, C. guilliermondi,* and *C. inconspicua*. Non-*albicans Candida* yeasts are common in the mouths of patients with advanced-stage cancer, and these patients may have reduced sensitivity to fluconazole. *Candida dubliniensis* is a recently identified yeast, mostly isolated in HIV-positive individuals with oral candidiasis.

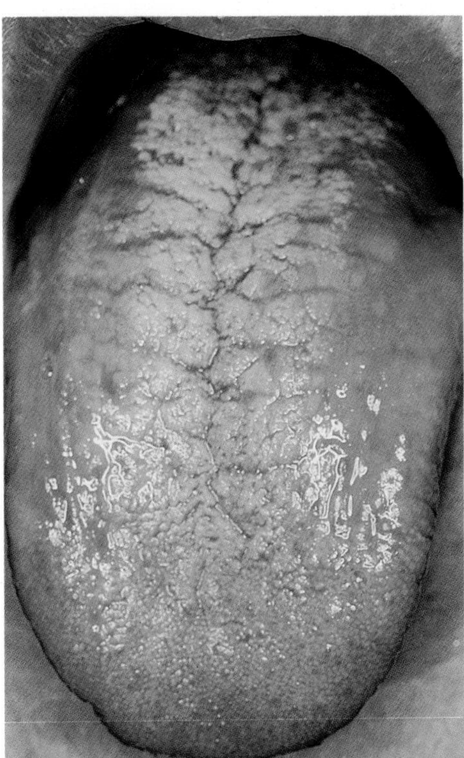

Figure 13-51 Oral candidiasis. A chronic infection with white debris covering the surface of the tongue.

HIV INFECTION. Oropharyngeal candidiasis may be the first manifestation of HIV infection, and more than 90% of patients with AIDS develop the disease. A concern in these patients is clinical relapse after treatment, which appears to be dependent on degree of immunosuppression and is more common with treatment regimens of clotrimazole and ketoconazole than with fluconazole or itraconazole.

Infants. Oral candidiasis in children is called thrush. Healthy, newborn infants, especially if premature, are susceptible. In older infants, thrush usually occurs in the presence of predisposing factors such as antibiotic treatment or debilitation. In the healthy newborn, thrush is a self-limited infection, but it should be treated to avoid interference with feeding. The infection appears as a white, creamy exudate or white, flaky, adherent plaques. The underlying mucosa is red and sore. The mother should be examined for vaginal candidiasis.

Adults. In the adult, oral candidiasis occurs for several reasons; clinically, it is found in a variety of acute and chronic forms. Extensive oral infection may occur in patients with diabetes or depressed cell-mediated immunity, the elderly, and patients with cancer, especially leukemia. Prolonged use of corticosteroids, immunosuppressive or broad-spectrum antibiotics, and inhalant steroids may also cause infection.

The acute process in adults is similar to the infection in infants. The tongue is almost always involved (Figure 13-51). Infection may spread into the trachea or esophagus and cause very painful erosions, appearing as dysphagia, or it may spread onto the skin at the angles of the mouth (perlèche). A specimen may be taken by gently scraping with a tongue blade. Pseudohyphae are easily demonstrated. In other cases, the oral cavity may be red, swollen, and sore, with little or no exudate (Figure 13-52). In this instance, pseudohyphae are often difficult to find and treatment may have to be started without laboratory verification.

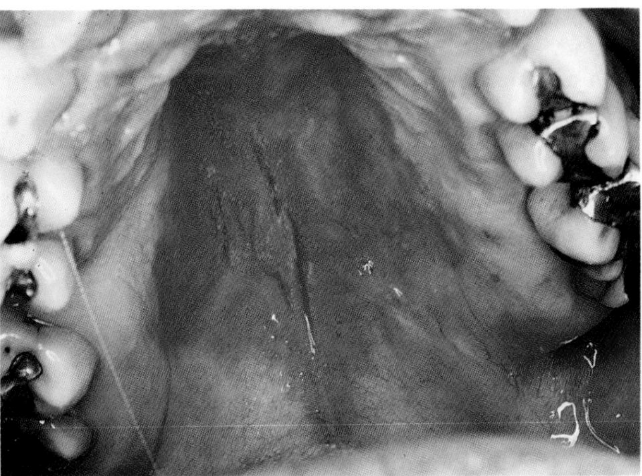

Figure 13-52 Oral candidiasis. The hard palate is red and swollen.

Box 13-8 **Topical and Systemic Treatment for Oral Candidiasis**

	Drug	Dose
Topical	Mycostatin pastilles 200,000 units/ml	1-2 pastilles orally 4-5 times/ day × 2 wk
	Clotrimazole troches 10 mg	1-2 tablets orally 4-5 times/ day × 2 wk
Systemic	Fluconazole	200 mg/day × 1 wk
	Itraconazole	200 mg/day × 1-3 wk
	Ketoconazole	200 mg/day × 2 wk

Chronic infection appears as localized, firmly adherent plaques with an irregular, velvety surface on the buccal mucosa. They may occur from the mechanical trauma of cheek biting, poor hygiene of dental prostheses, pipe smoking, or irritation from dentures. A biopsy is indicated to rule out leukoplakia and lichen planus if organisms cannot be demonstrated.

Localized erythema and erosions with minimal white exudate may be caused by candidal infection beneath dentures and is commonly called *denture sore mouth*. The border is usually sharply defined. Hyperplasia with thickening of the mucosa occurs if the process is long lasting. The gums and hard palate are most frequently involved. Organisms may be difficult to find. Adult treatment schedules are shown in Box 13-8.

TREATMENT

Fluconazole. Fluconazole (200 mg/day for adults) is the first-line management option for the treatment and prophylaxis of localized and systemic *C. albicans* infections. It is effective, well tolerated, and suitable for use in most patients with *C. albicans* infections, including children, the elderly, and those with impaired immunity. Prophylactic administration of fluconazole can help to prevent fungal infections in patients receiving cytotoxic cancer therapy. The increasing use of fluconazole for the long-term prophylaxis and treatment of recurrent oral candidiasis in AIDS patients has led to the emergence of *C. albicans* infections that are not responsive to conventional doses. Second-line therapy with a wider spectrum antifungal, such as itraconazole, should be sought if treatment with fluconazole is not successful. *Candida* spp. other than *C. albicans* may develop resistance to fluconazole in a patient who is repeatedly exposed to the drug.

Itraconazole. Itraconazole solution is as effective as fluconazole but is less well tolerated as first-line therapy. Itraconazole oral solution is a useful therapy in the treatment of HIV-infected patients with fluconazole-refractory oropharyngeal candidiasis. HIV-infected patients with oropharyngeal candidiasis for whom fluconazole therapy (200 mg/day) failed were treated with 100 mg of itraconazole oral solution administered twice daily (200 mg/day) for 14 days. Patients who demonstrated an incomplete response to treatment were treated for an additional 14 days (28 days total).

Clotrimazole (Mycelex) troche. Children and adults are effectively treated by slowly dissolving a clotrimazole (Mycelex) troche in the mouth five times a day for 14 days.

Ketoconazole (Nizoral). Ketoconazole (Nizoral 200-mg oral tablet) given once a day is a second-line drug for treatment of oropharyngeal candidiasis.

Nystatin (Mycostatin) oral suspension. For infants, the dosage is 2 ml of nystatin (Mycostatin) oral suspension four times a day, 1 ml in each side of the mouth. For adults, the dosage is 4 to 6 ml, with half of the dose in each side of the mouth retained as long as possible before swallowing. Treatment is continued for 48 hours after symptoms have disappeared; a 10-day course is typical. The oral suspension is useful for infants but less effective for adults, probably because the liquid may not come in contact with the entire surface of the oral cavity.

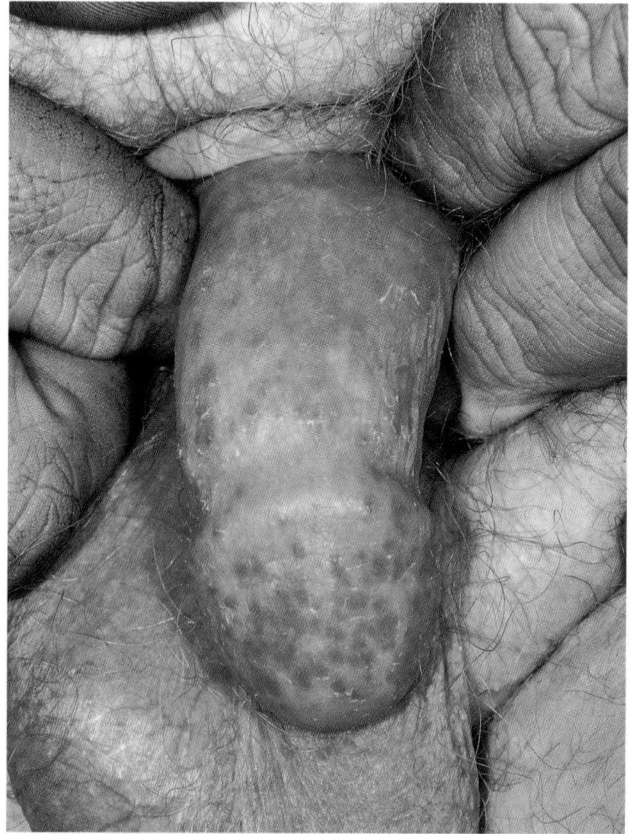

Figure 13-53 *Candida balanitis*. Multiple red, round erosions are present on the glans and shaft of the penis. There is a white exudate.

CANDIDA BALANITIS

The uncircumcised penis provides the warm, moist environment ideally suited for yeast infection, but the circumcised male is also at risk. *Candida balanitis* sometimes occurs after intercourse with an infected female and is more common in those who had vaginal intercourse than in those who had anal intercourse within the previous 3 months. Tender, pinpoint, red papules and pustules appear on the glans and shaft of the penis. The pustules rupture quickly under the foreskin and may not be noticed (Figure 13-53). Typically, 1- to 2-mm, white, doughnut-shaped, possibly confluent rings are seen after the pustules break. In some cases pustules never evolve, and the multiple red papules may be transient, resolving without treatment. The presence of pustules is highly suggestive of candidiasis. White exudate similar to that seen in *Candida* vaginal infections may be present (Figures 13-54 and 13-55). The infection may occur and persist without sexual exposure.

TREATMENT. The eruption responds quickly with twice-a-day application for 7 days of miconazole, clotrimazole, or several of the other medications listed in the Formulary. Relief is almost immediate, but treatment should be continued for 7 days. Preparations containing topical steroids give temporary relief by suppressing inflammation, but the eruption rebounds and worsens, sometimes even before the cortisone cream is discontinued. A single 150-mg dose of fluconazole was comparable in efficacy and safety to clotrimazole cream applied topically for 7 days when administered to patients with balanitis.

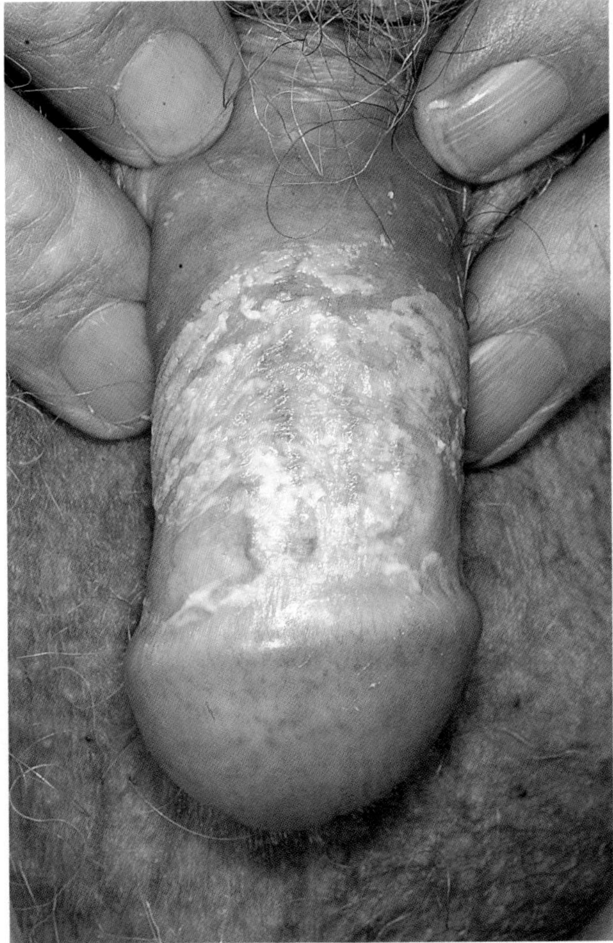

Figure 13-54 *Candida balanitis.* The moist space between the skin surfaces of the uncircumcised penis is an ideal environment for *Candida* infection. This thick white exudate is typical of a severe acute infection.

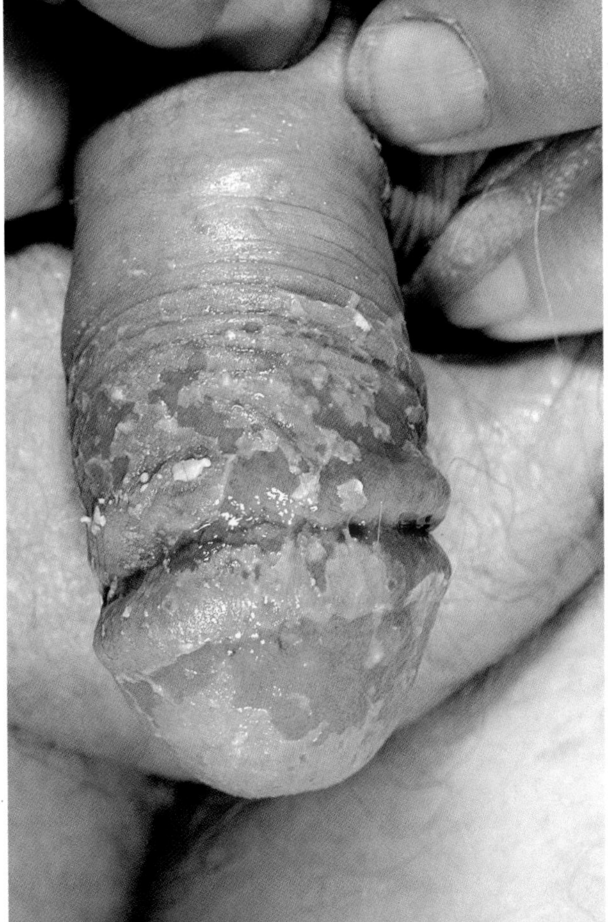

Figure 13-55 *Candida balanitis.* This persistent infection has resulted in erosions forming on the glans and under the foreskin.

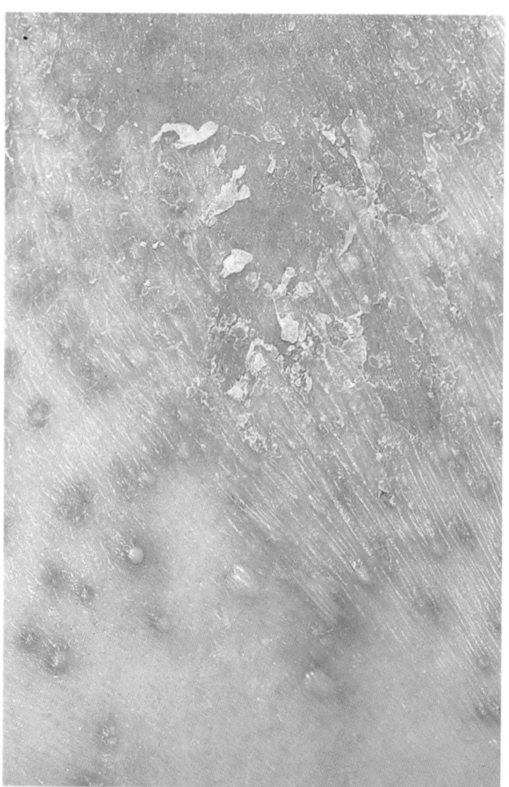

Figure 13-56 Candidiasis under the breast. There are several moist, red papules and pustules with a fringe of white scale.

Candidiasis of large skin folds

Candidiasis of large skin folds (*Candida* intertrigo) occurs under pendulous breasts, between overhanging abdominal folds, in the groin and rectal area, and in the axillae. *Skin folds* (intertriginous areas where skin touches skin) contain heat and moisture, providing the environment suited for yeast infection. Hot, humid weather; tight or abrasive underclothing; poor hygiene; and inflammatory diseases occurring in the skin folds, such as psoriasis, make a yeast infection more likely.

There are two presentations. In the first type, pustules form but become macerated under apposing skin surfaces and develop into red papules with a fringe of moist scale at the border. Intact pustules may be found outside the apposing skin surfaces (Figures 13-56 and 13-57). The second type consists of a red, moist, glistening plaque that extends to or just beyond the limits of the apposing skin folds (Figure 13-58). The advancing border is long and sharply defined and has an ocean wave–shaped fringe of macerated scale (see Figure 13-47). The characteristic pustule of candidiasis is not observed in intertriginous areas because it is macerated as soon as it forms. Pinpoint pustules do appear outside the advancing border and are an important diagnostic feature when present (Figures 13-56, 13-57, and 13-59). There is a tendency for painful fissuring in the skin creases.

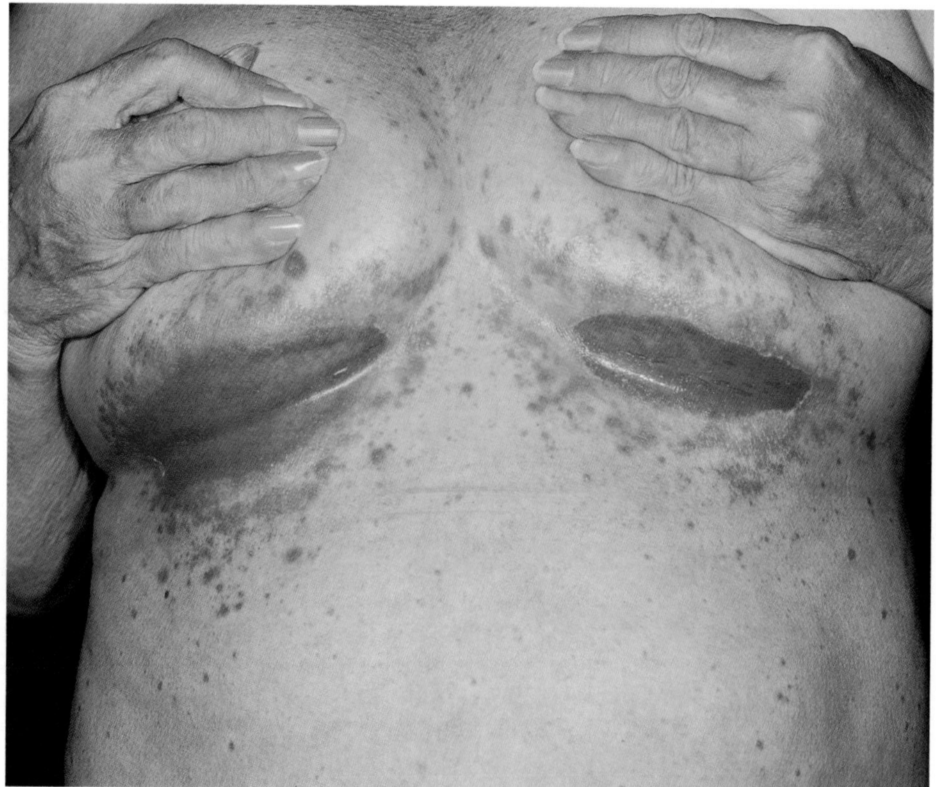

Figure 13-57 *Candida* intertrigo. An acute infection. The fringe of scale is present on the opposing borders. There are numerous satellite pustules beyond the intertriginous area.

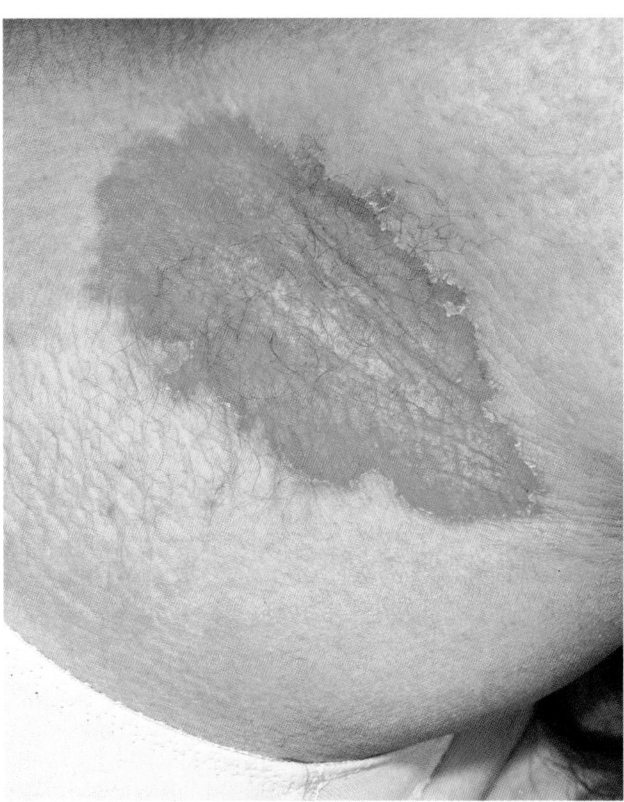

Figure 13-58 Candidiasis of the axillae. A prominent fringe of scale is present at the border.

TREATMENT. Eradication of the yeast infection must be accompanied by maintained dryness of the area. A cool, wet Burow's solution, water, or saline compress is applied for 20 to 30 minutes several times each day to promote dryness. Antifungal cream is applied in a thin layer twice a day until the rash clears. Some of these medicines are also available in lotion form, but the liquid base may cause stinging when applied to intertriginous areas. Miconazole nitrate is the least irritating. Application of compresses should be continued until the skin remains dry. An absorbent powder, not necessarily medicated, such as Z-Sorb, may be applied after the inflammation is gone. The powder absorbs a small amount of moisture and acts as a dry lubricant, allowing skin surfaces to slide freely, thus preventing moisture accumulation in a potentially stagnant area.

Figure 13-59 *Candida* intertrigo. The overhanging abdominal fold and groin area are infected in this obese patient.

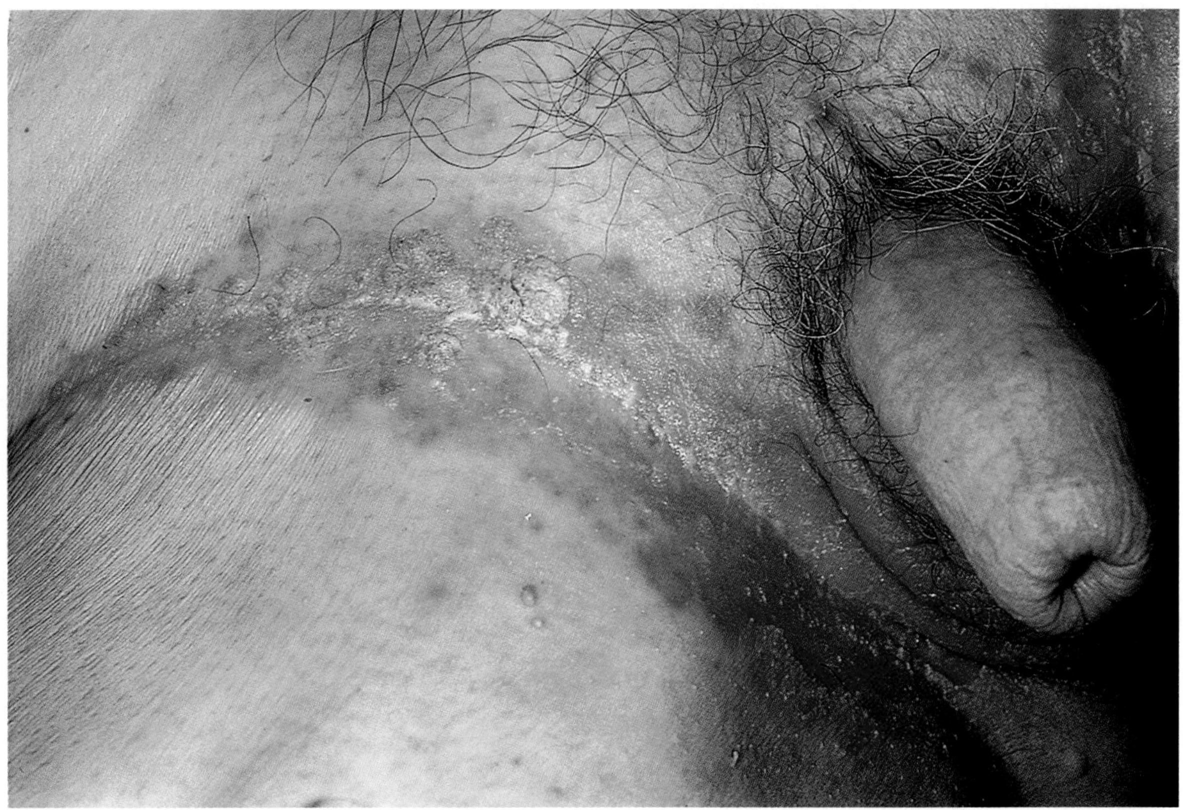

INTERTRIGO

Intertrigo is an inflammatory condition of skin folds of the axillae, breasts, abdomen, groin, or buttocks (see p. 500). Obese people are at greatest risk. Itching, burning, and stinging are the most common symptoms. Apposing skin folds retain moisture and become warm, macerated, and inflamed. *Candida* is the most common secondary infection but bacteria, fungi, or viruses may be a factor. Erosions are possible. Sweat, feces, urine, and vaginal discharge may aggravate intertrigo. The course can be recurrent and chronic.

TREATMENT. A 1- or 2-week course of group VI to VII topical steroids (desonide, hydrocortisone) may be all that is necessary. Long-term continuous use of topical steroids in skin fold areas may result in the formation of atrophy and striae; 0.1% tacrolimus may be used as an antiinflammatory agent instead of topical steroids for initial treatment or for cases requiring long-term intermittent treatment. Some patients respond to just 1% hydrocortisone cream or lotion. This is safe for intermittent long-term treatment and has a low potential for causing striae or atrophy. Add topical anti-yeast medications such as econazole cream if *Candida* infection is suspected. Alternate these creams with topical steroids. To separate and expose skin effectively in order to promote dryness, administer while the patient is in the supine position. Cool water compresses $^1/_2$ hour two or three times a day for just a few days are rapidly effective in controlling moisture and suppressing inflammation.

Castellani's paint (carbolfuchsin paint) is very effective but not readily available at all pharmacies.

"Greer's goo" is prepared by the pharmacist. It is composed of nystatin powder 4 million units, hydrocortisone powder 1.2 gm, and zinc oxide paste 4 oz and is applied daily or twice a day as another treatment. Thick barrier creams such as Desitin may prevent recurrences. Powders may be used after resolution to promote dryness. Oral fluconazole is usually not as effective in localized cutaneous *Candida* secondary infections as topical anti-yeast creams.

DIAPER CANDIDIASIS

An artificial intertriginous area is created under a wet diaper, predisposing the area to a yeast infection with the characteristic red base and satellite pustules as described earlier (Figure 13-60). Diaper dermatitis is often treated with steroid combination creams and lotions that contain antibiotics. Although these medications may contain the anti-yeast agent clotrimazole, its concentration may not be sufficient to control the yeast infection. The cortisone component may alter the clinical presentation and prolong the disease. A nodular, granulomatous form of candidiasis in the diaper area, appearing as dull, red, irregularly shaped nodules, sometimes on a red base, has been described and may represent an unusual reaction to *Candida* organisms or to a *Candida* organism infection modified by steroids. Although dermatophyte infections are unusual in the diaper area, they do occur. Every effort should be made to identify the organism and treat the infection appropriately.

TREATMENT. Dryness should be maintained by changing the diaper frequently or not using a diaper for short periods. Antifungal creams should be applied twice a day until the eruption is clear, in approximately 10 days. Some erythema from irritation may be present after 10 days; this can be treated by alternately applying 1% hydrocortisone cream followed in a few hours by creams active against yeasts (see the Formulary). Apply each agent twice a day. Baby powders may help prevent recurrence by absorbing moisture. Mupirocin ointment 2% (Bactroban) applied three or four times daily is effective for severe *Candida* and bacterial diaper dermatitis.

DIFFERENTIAL DIAGNOSIS. Any recalcitrant diaper dermatitis must be further investigated to uncover underlying disease. Inflammation in the diaper area can be caused by psoriasis, seborrheic dermatitis, Langerhans cell histiocytosis (Letterer-Siwe disease), acrodermatitis enteropathica (zinc deficiency), biotin deficiency, Kawasaki disease, and HIV infection.

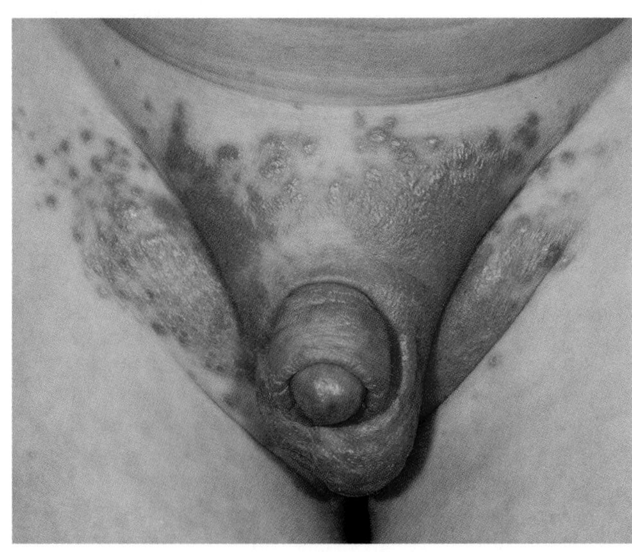

Figure 13-60 Diaper candidiasis, an advanced case. The skin folds are deeply erythematous. The urethral meatus is infected and numerous satellite pustules are on the lower abdominal area.

Candidiasis of small skin folds

FINGER AND TOE WEBS

Web spaces are like small intertriginous areas. Cooks, bartenders, dishwashers, dentists, and others who work in a moist environment are at risk. White, tender, macerated skin erodes, revealing a pink, moist base (Figures 13-61, 13-62, and 13-63). Candidiasis of the toe webs occurs most commonly in the narrow interspace between the fourth and fifth toes, where it may coexist with dermatophytes and gram-negative bacteria. Clinically and in potassium hydroxide preparations, infection by *Candida* and dermatophytes may appear to be identical. Macerated, white scale becomes thick and adherent. Diffuse candidiasis of the webs and feet is unusual. Both areas are treated with any of the antifungal creams or lotions listed in the Formulary. Strands of lamb's wool (Dr. Scholl's lamb's wool) can be placed between the toe webs to separate and promote dryness.

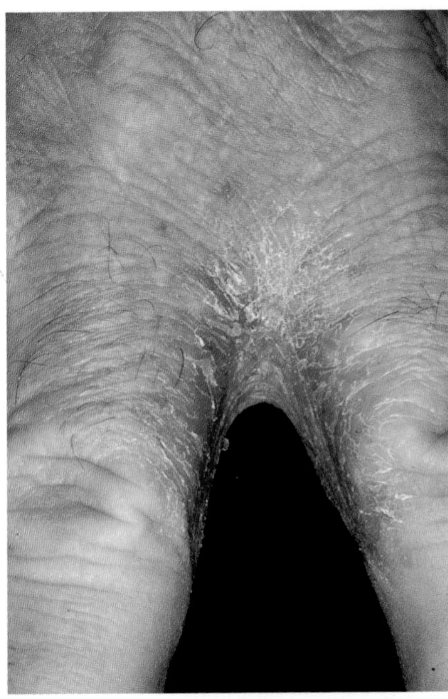

Figure 13-61 Intertrigo of the finger web. This lesion is not wet and macerated like that depicted in Figure 13-62. This eczematous process occurred in a bartender whose hands were constantly wet.

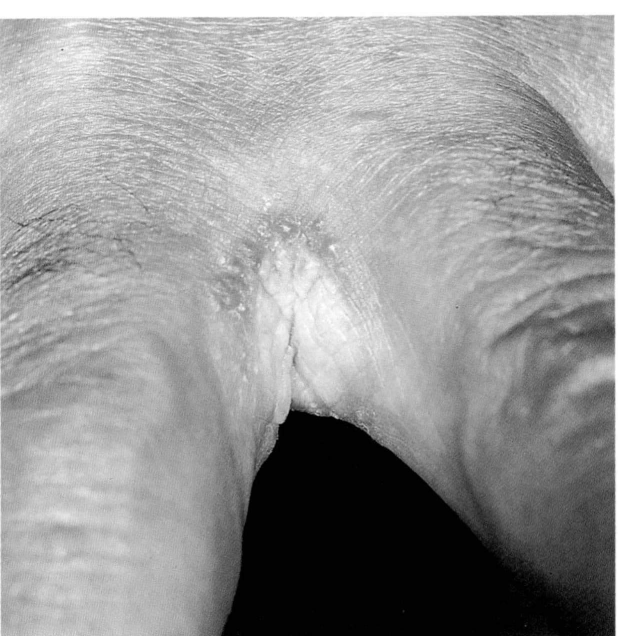

Figure 13-62 Candidiasis of the finger web. The acute phase with maceration of the web. Pustules are present at the border.

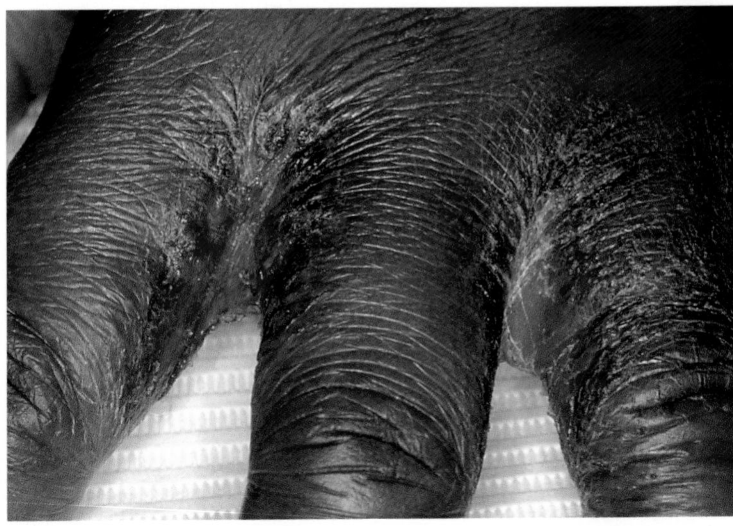

Figure 13-63 Candidiasis of the finger webs. All webs are infected except the wide space between the thumb and index finger.

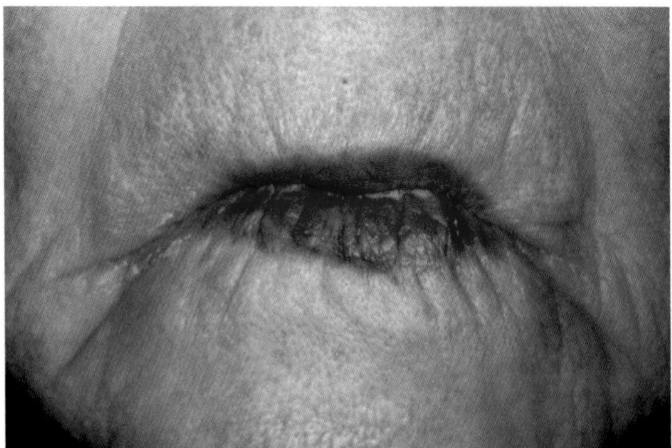

Figure 13-64 Angular cheilitis (perlèche). Skin folds at the angles of the mouth are red and eroded.

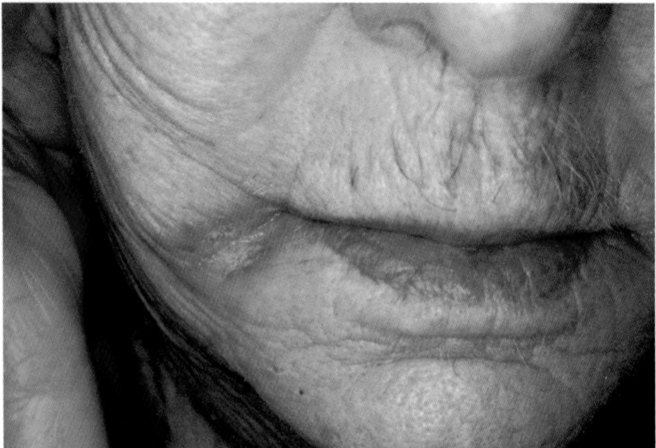

Figure 13-65 Angular cheilitis. Inflammation starts in the small intertriginous crease at the angle of the mouth and extends to the adjacent skin.

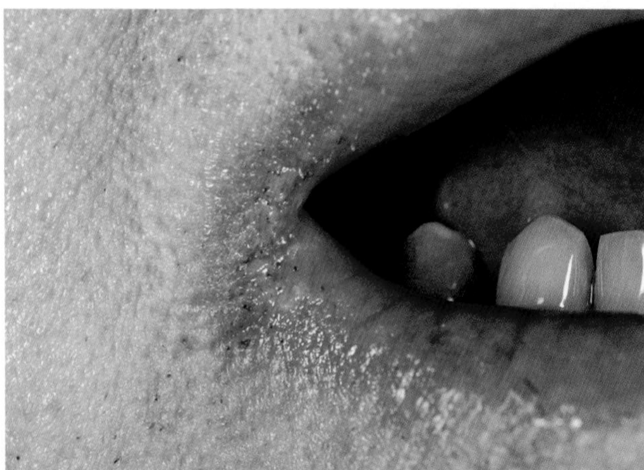

Figure 13-66 Angular cheilitis. Interigo of the mouth angle is a combination of eczema, *Candida,* and bacterial infection.

ANGLES OF THE MOUTH

Angular cheilitis or perlèche, an inflammation at the angles of the mouth, can occur at any age. Patients may have the misconception that they have a vitamin B deficiency; yeast and bacteria may be involved in the process. Lip licking, biting the corners of the mouth, or thumb sucking causes perlèche in the young. Continued irritation may lead to eczematous inflammation. The presence of saliva at the angles of the mouth is the most important factor. Excess saliva occurs as a result of mouth breathing secondary to nasal congestion and of malocclusion resulting from poorly fitting dentures and compulsive lip licking. Aggressive use of dental floss may cause mechanical trauma to mouth angles. A moist, intertriginous space forms in skin folds at the angles of the mouth as a result of advancing age, congenital excessive-angle skin folds, sagging that occurs with weight loss, or abnormal vertical shortening of the lower one third of the face from loss of teeth and resultant resorption of the alveolar bone. Capillary action draws fluid from the mouth into the fold, creating maceration, chapping, fissures, erythema, exudation, and secondary infection with *Candida* organisms and/or staphylococci.

The infection starts as a sore fissure in the depth of the skin fold (Figure 13-64). Erythema, scale, and crust form at the sides of the fold (Figures 13-65 and 13-66). Patients lick and moisten the area in an attempt to prevent further cracking. This attempt at relief only aggravates the problem and may lead to eczematous inflammation, staphylococcal infection, or hypertrophy of the skin fold.

Consider contact dermatitis, diabetes mellitus, and HIV infection in chronic treatment–resistant cases.

TREATMENT. Treatment consists of applying antifungal creams (see the Formulary), followed in a few hours by a group V steroid cream with a nongreasy base until the area is dry and free of inflammation. As an alternative, Lotrisone lotion may be applied twice a day until symptoms resolve. Patients should discontinue topical steroids when inflammation has resolved. Thereafter, a thick, protective lip balm (e.g., ChapStick) is applied frequently. Cosmetic fillers injected at the mouth angles can decrease the depth of the grooves and fill the depression that often occurs below the lateral lower lip, thereby correcting the anatomic defect causing the problem. Culture resistant cases for bacteria and yeast. Mupirocin ointment or cream 2% (Bactroban) applied three or four times daily may be effective for both yeast and bacteria.

TINEA VERSICOLOR

Tinea versicolor is a common fungal infection of the skin caused by the dimorphic lipophilic yeasts *Pityrosporum orbiculare* (round form) and *Pityrosporum ovale* (oval form). Some authors believe these are different forms of the same organism. (Both were previously called *Malassezia furfur*.) The organism is part of the normal skin flora and appears in highest numbers in areas with increased sebaceous activity. It resides within the stratum corneum and hair follicles, where it thrives on free fatty acids and triglycerides. Certain predisposing endogenous factors (adrenalectomy, Cushing's disease, pregnancy, malnutrition, burns, corticosteroid therapy, immunosuppression, depressed cellular immunity, oral contraceptives) or exogenous factors (excess heat, humidity) cause the yeast to convert from budding yeast form to its mycelial form, leading to the appearance of tinea versicolor. Whether the disease is contagious is unknown. The disease may occur at any age, but it is much more common during the years of higher sebaceous activity (i.e., adolescence and young adulthood). Some individuals, especially those with oily skin, may be more susceptible.

CLINICAL PRESENTATION. The individual lesions and their distribution are highly characteristic. Lesions begin as multiple small, circular macules of various colors (white, pink, or brown) that enlarge radially (Figures 13-67 to 13-71). Tinea versicolor infections produce a spectrum of clinical presentations and colors that include (1) red to fawn-colored macules, patches, or follicular papules that are predominantly caused by a hyperemic inflammatory response; (2) hypopigmented lesions; and (3) tan to dark brown macules and patches. Melanocyte damage appears to be the basis for hypopigmentation. Dicarboxylic acids produced by the *Pityrosporum* may have a cytotoxic effect on melanocytes and inhibit the dopa tyrosinase reaction. There is a reduction in number, size, and aggregation of melanosomes in melanocytes and in surrounding keratinocytes. The lesions may be hyperpigmented in blacks. The color is uniform in each individual. The lesions may be inconspicuous in fair-complexed individuals during the winter. White hypopigmentation becomes more obvious as unaffected skin tans. The upper trunk is most commonly affected, but it is not unusual for lesions to spread to the upper arms, neck, and abdomen. Involvement of the face, back of the hands, and legs can occur. Facial lesions are more common in children; the forehead is the site of facial involvement usually affected. The eruption may itch if it is inflammatory, but it is usually asymptomatic. The disease may vary in activity for years, but it diminishes or disappears with advancing age. The differential diagnosis includes vitiligo, pityriasis alba, seborrheic dermatitis, secondary syphilis, and pityriasis rosea.

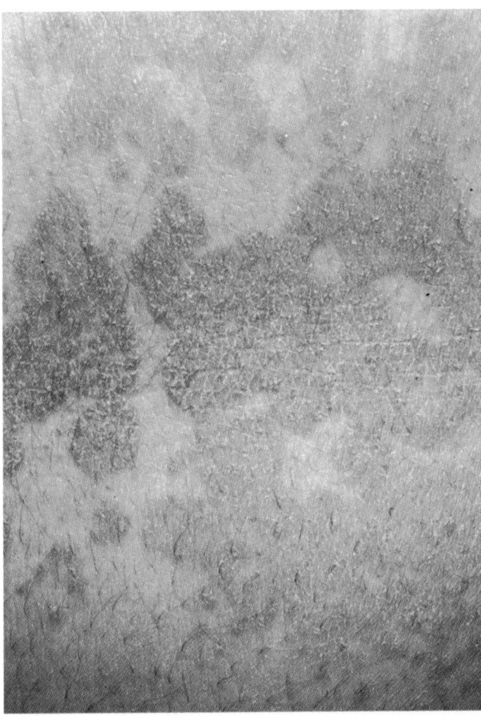

Figure 13-67 Tinea versicolor. Numerous circular, scaly lesions. The eruption is light brown or fawn colored in fair-complected, untanned skin.

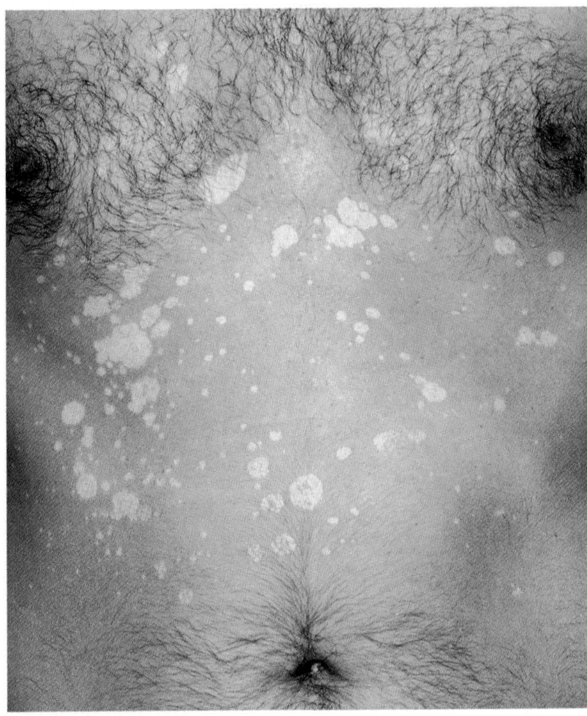

Figure 13-68 The classic presentation of tinea versicolor with white, oval, or circular patches on tan skin.

TINEA VERSICOLOR

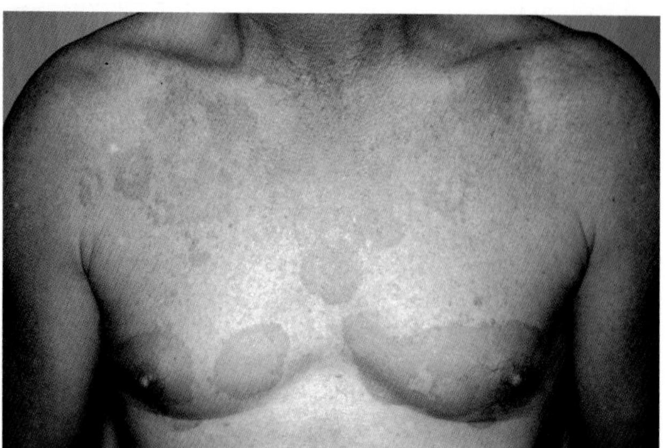

Figure 13-69 Broad, confluent, scaly patches in a fair-skinned individual.

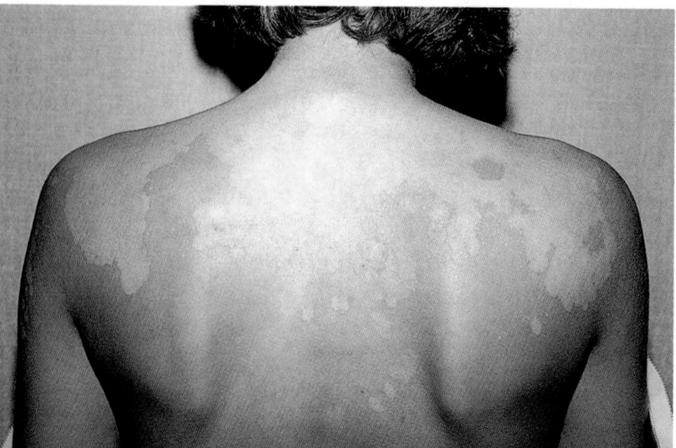

Figure 13-70 Scaling macules coalesce to form broad, irregularly shaped areas that can be either lighter or darker than the surrounding skin.

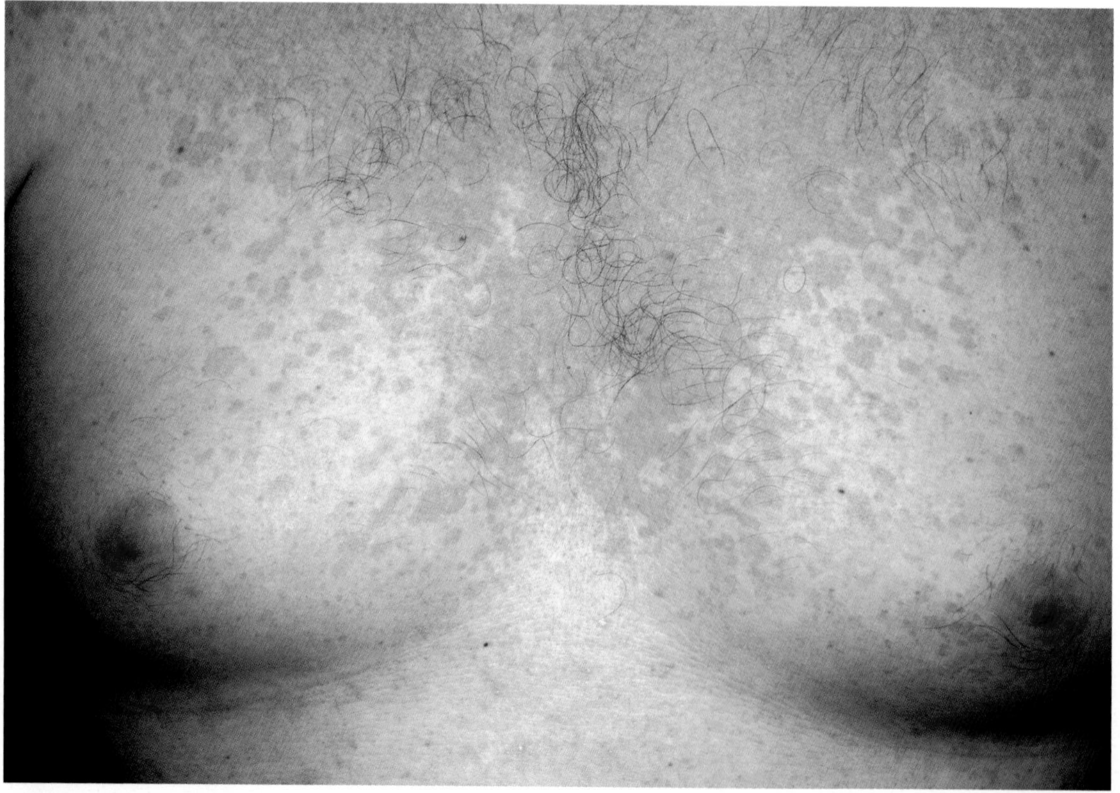

Figure 13-71 Tinea versicolor. The most common presentation with thin fawn-colored scaling papules on the upper chest.

DIAGNOSIS. A powdery scale that may not be obvious on inspection can easily be demonstrated by scraping lightly with a #15 surgical blade (Figure 13-72). Potassium hydroxide examination of the scale shows numerous hyphae that tend to break into short, rod-shaped fragments intermixed with round spores in grapelike clusters, giving the so-called spaghetti-and-meatballs pattern (Figure 13-73). Wood's light examination shows irregular, pale, yellow-to-white fluorescence that fades with improvement. Some lesions do not fluoresce. Culture is possible but rarely necessary.

TREATMENT. Griseofulvin is not active against tinea versicolor. A variety of medicines eliminate the fungus, but relief is usually temporary and recurrences are common (40% to 60%). Patients must understand that the hypopigmented areas will not disappear immediately after treatment. Sunlight accelerates repigmentation. The inability to produce powdery scale by scraping with a #15 surgical blade indicates the fungus has been eradicated. Fungal elements may be retained in frequently worn garments that are in contact with the skin; discarding or boiling such clothing might decrease the chance of recurrence. Patients without obvious involvement who have a history of multiple recurrences might consider repeating a treatment program just before the summer months to avoid uneven tanning.

TOPICAL TREATMENT. Topical treatment is indicated for limited disease. Recurrence rates are high.

Ketoconazole shampoo. Ketoconazole 2% shampoo, used as a single application or daily for 3 days, is highly effective and is the treatment of first choice. Apply the shampoo to the entire skin surface from the lower posterior scalp area down to the thighs. The shampoo is left in place for 5 minutes and then rinsed thoroughly. Wash the scalp with the shampoo at the same time.

Selenium sulfide suspension 2.5%. When applied for 10 minutes every day for 7 consecutive days, the suspension (available as Selsun or in generic forms) resulted in an 87% cure rate at a 2-week follow-up evaluation. Blood and urine samples showed that no significant absorption of selenium took place. The suspension is applied to the entire skin surface from the lower posterior scalp area down to the thighs. Another commonly recommended schedule is to apply the lotion and wash it off in 24 hours. This is repeated once each week for a total of 4 weeks. There are many suggested variations of this treatment schedule. Wash the scalp with the lotion at the same time.

Terbinafine solution (Lamisil solution 1% spray bottle). Application of the spray to the affected areas twice a day for 1 week is effective. Lamisil spray is available as an over-the-counter product.

Antifungal antibiotics. Miconazole, ketoconazole, clotrimazole, econazole, or ciclopiroxolamine is applied to the entire affected area one or two times a day for 2 to 4 weeks. The creams are odorless and nongreasy but expensive.

ORAL TREATMENT (See Box 13-9 and Table 13-2). Oral treatment may be used in patients with extensive disease and those who do not respond to conventional treatment or have frequent recurrences.

Itraconazole. Prophylactic treatment with itraconazole 200 mg twice a day 1 day per month for 6 consecutive months is effective to maintain control.

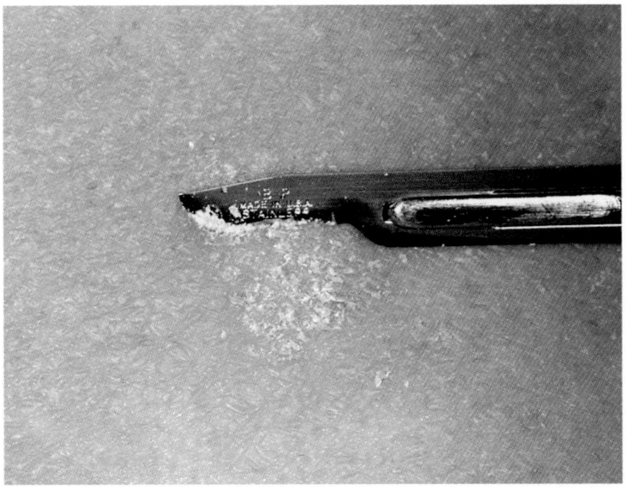

Figure 13-72 Tinea versicolor. The central area was scraped with a #15 surgical blade to demonstrate white, powdery scale.

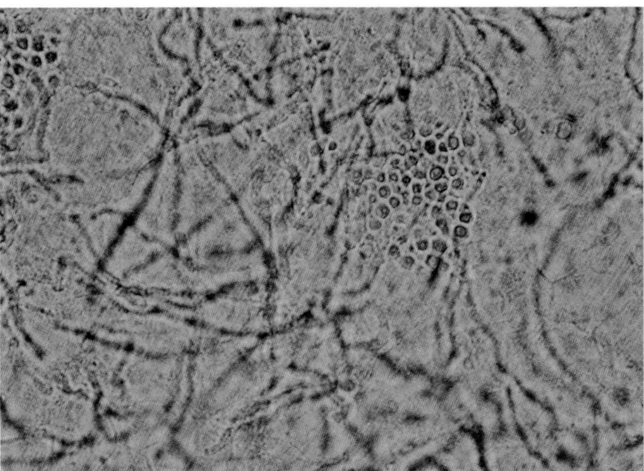

Figure 13-73 Tinea versicolor. A potassium hydroxide wet mount. A low-power view showing numerous short, broad hyphae and clusters of budding cells, which have been described as having the appearance of "spaghetti and meatballs."

Box 13-9 **Dosage Regimens of Oral Antifungal Agents for Tinea Versicolor**	
Ketoconazole	
200 mg/day	5 days
400 mg	Once a week for 2 weeks
400 mg	3 doses 12 hours apart
Itraconazole	
200 mg/day	5 or 7 days
Fluconazole	
150 mg	Once a week for 4 weeks
300 mg	Once a week for 2 doses
300 mg	Single dose repeated 2 weeks later

Adapted from: Gupta AK et al: *Clin Dermatol* 21(5):417-425, 2003. *PMID: 14678722*

Ketoconazole. Several dose regimens have been used (see Box 13-9). Prophylaxis with ketoconazole 400 mg once monthly resulted in no recurrence during follow-up of 4 to 15 months. Efficacy can be enhanced by refraining from antacids and taking the drug at breakfast with fruit juice. The patient should not bathe for at least 12 hours after treatment; this allows the medication to accumulate in the skin.

Terbinafine and griseofulvin. Terbinafine or griseofulvin taken orally is not effective.

PREVENTING RECURRENCES. Once-weekly application of ketoconazole 2% shampoo (Nizoral), applied as a lotion to the neck, trunk, and proximal extremities 5 to 10 minutes before showering, may help prevent recurrences.

Pityrosporum folliculitis

Pityrosporum folliculitis is an infection of the hair follicle caused by the yeast *Pityrosporum orbiculare,* the same organism that causes tinea versicolor. The typical patient is a young woman with asymptomatic or slightly itchy follicular papules and pustules localized to the upper back and chest, upper arms, and neck. Occlusion and greasy skin may be important predisposing factors. It is frequently diagnosed as acne (Figure 13-74). Diabetes mellitus and administration of broad-spectrum antibiotics or corticosteroids are predisposing factors. Follicular occlusion may be a primary event, with yeast overgrowth as a secondary occurrence. Hodgkin's disease may predispose to *Pityrosporum* folliculitis. These patients complain of severe generalized pruritus; the eruption may involve the trunk and extremities.

Pityrosporum is very common in the tropics, where it presents as a polymorphous eruption with the following characteristics. The primary lesion is a keratinous plug that underlies four clinical types of lesion: follicular papules (dome-shaped papules with a central depression), pustules, nodules, and cysts. The lesions evolve from follicular plugs colonized by *Pityrosporum*. The face is often affected—this is the most common site in female patients and the second most common site in male patients. The lesions are localized to the mandible, chin, and sides of the face. This is in contrast to the usually more central facial location of acne vulgaris. Lesions also are found on the nape of the neck, abdomen, buttocks, and thighs. Both young men and young women are equally affected. Their active sebaceous glands presumably provide the lipid-rich environment required by the yeast.

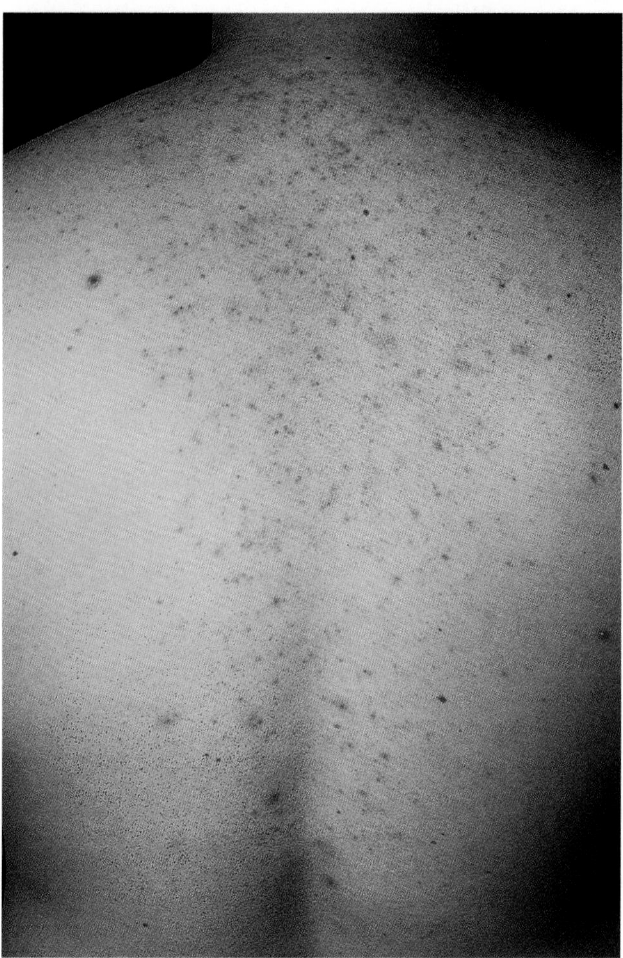

Figure 13-74 *Pityrosporum* folliculitis. Asymptomatic or slightly itchy follicular papules and pustules located on the upper back. It is frequently diagnosed as acne.

A potassium hydroxide examination reveals abundant round, budding yeast cells, and sometimes hyphae. Treatment is the same as that for tinea versicolor. Combined ketoconazole shampoo and systemic ketoconazole (200 mg daily for 4 weeks) produced clearance of the lesions in 100% of patients, whereas systemic therapy resulted in only a 75% clearance rate. Topical econazole and miconazole failed in 90% of patients. Salicylic acid wash (SalAc) is keratolytic and effective.

Chapter 14

Exanthems and Drug Eruptions

CHAPTER CONTENTS

- **Exanthems**
  - Measles
  - Hand-foot-and-mouth disease
  - Scarlet fever
  - Rubella
  - Erythema infectiosum
  - Roseola infantum
  - Enteroviruses: echovirus and coxsackievirus exanthems
  - Kawasaki disease
  - Superantigen toxin-mediated illnesses
  - Toxic shock syndrome
  - Cutaneous drug reactions
- **Drug eruptions: clinical patterns and most frequently causal drugs**
  - Exanthems (maculopapular)
  - Urticaria
  - Pruritus
- **Drug eruptions**
  - Acute generalized exanthematous pustulosis
  - Acneiform (pustular) eruptions
  - Eczema
  - Fixed drug eruptions
  - Blistering drug eruptions
  - Erythema multiforme and toxic epidermal necrolysis
  - Exfoliative erythroderma
  - Lichenoid (lichen planus–like drug eruptions)
  - Lupus erythematosus–like drug eruptions
  - Chemotherapy-induced acral erythema
  - Pigmentation
  - Photosensitivity
  - Vasculitis
  - Lymphomatoid drug eruptions
  - Skin eruptions associated with specific drugs

The word *exanthem* means a skin eruption that bursts forth or blooms. Exanthematous diseases are characterized by widespread, symmetric, erythematous, discrete, or confluent macules and papules that initially do not form scale. Exanthematous disease is one of the few diseases for which the term *maculopapular* is an appropriate descriptive term. Other lesions, such as pustules, vesicles, and petechiae, may form, but most of the exanthematous diseases begin with red macules or papules. Widespread red eruptions such as guttate psoriasis or pityriasis rosea may have a similar beginning and are often symmetric, but these conditions have typical patterns of scale and are therefore referred to as *papulosquamous eruptions*. Diseases that begin with exanthems may be caused by bacteria, viruses, or drugs. Most have a number of characteristic features such as a common primary lesion, distribution, duration, and systemic symptoms. Some are accompanied by oral lesions that are referred to as *enanthems*. Pediatric exanthems are summarized in Table 14-1.

Exanthems were previously consecutively numbered according to their historical appearance and description: first disease, measles; second disease, scarlet fever; third disease, rubella; fourth disease, "Dukes' disease" (probably coxsackievirus or echovirus); fifth disease, erythema infectiosum; and sixth disease, roseola infantum.

Table 14-1 Exanthems

Disease	Age group	Prodrome incubation	Morphology
Measles (rubeola)	Birth to 20 yr	Rhinitis, cough, fever, conjunctivitis, Koplik's spots 8-12 days	Erythematous macules and papules later become confluent; turns coppery-colored
German measles (rubella)	5 -25 yr	Mild URI symptoms 14-23 days	Generalized maculopapular becomes pinpoint
Roseola (exanthem subitum HHV-6)	Birth to 3 yr	High fever for 3-5 days; diarrhea, cough 5-15 days	Pale pink, almond-shaped macules and papules
Erythema infectiosum (fifth disease parvovirus B19)	4 yr (1-17 yr) Non-immune adults	Nonspecific fever and malaise 13-18 days	Macular erythema on face (1-4 days), erythematous macular eruption for first week followed by lacy erythema
Unilateral laterothoracic exanthem	12-63 mo	URI symptoms	Discrete, mild, pruritic, 1-mm erythematous papules and morbilliform, eczematous plaques Spontaneous resolution after 5 wk
Papular-purpuric gloves and socks syndrome (parvovirus B19)	Children, mean age 24 mo	Fever	Finely papular, purpuric, petechial edema and erythema; resolves spontaneously within 1-2 wk
Chickenpox (varicella)	1-14 yr	Fever, malaise, headache, anorexia, abdominal pain for 48 hr	Erythematous macules that evolve into vesicles containing serous fluid Different stages of lesions present simultaneously
Kawasaki disease (mucocutaneous syndrome, lymph node syndrome)	Usually <5 yr	High fever, irritability	Erythematous maculopapular Desquamation of tips of fingers (morbilliform or vesiculobullous form) and toes
Gianotti-Crosti syndrome (papular acrodermatitis of childhood)	Peak 1-6 yr; can occur in adults	URI; generalized adenopathy	Lichenoid, flesh-colored to red papules; may form plaques
Meningococcemia (*Neisseria meningitidis*)	<2 yr	Hepatosplenomegaly; fever, malaise, URI symptoms	Petechiae, purpura; bullous lesions seen
Rocky Mountain spotted fever (*Rickettsia rickettsii*)	Any age	Fever, malaise, headache	Pale red or rose-colored macules; evolves to petechiae and purpura

Distribution of rash	Associated findings	Laboratory findings
Begins in hairline on neck and face Moves down and covers entire body Becomes confluent as it fades and leaves a brownish hue with fine desquamation	Koplik's spots, exudative conjunctivitis, photophobia, and severe cough; pneumonia, swelling of hands and feet Otitis media, encephalitis 1:1000, subacute sclerosing panencephalitis (late)	WBC count and ESR are low Measles immunoglobulin M (IgM) titer
Begins on face Migrates to trunk	Tender retroauricular, posterior cervical, and occipital adenopathy Slight fever Transient polyarthralgia and polyarthritis in adolescents and adults, especially females	Nasal culture for virus Antibody titer
Trunk, neck, and proximal extremities	Rash appears as fever resolves Irritability, febrile seizures possible	Leukocytosis at onset of fever, but leukopenia as temperature increases
Face ("slapped cheek") followed by extremities; lacy rash over extensor surfaces Rash can recur	Spontaneous abortion (from severe fetal anemia and hydrops fetalis) Aplastic crises in sickle cell disease Women may develop arthralgia or arthritis	IgM antibodies CBC Evaluate immune status of exposed pregnant women (IgG)
Predominantly unilateral Begins close to axilla and spreads to become bilateral Retains a unilateral predominance on trunk or flexures and may become bilateral	Fever, upper respiratory tract infection, vomiting, diarrhea	Relative lymphocytosis 37%
Sharply demarcated gloves and socks distribution Groin, buttock, antecubital, and popliteal fossae Nose may be involved	Fever, lymphadenopathy, oral lesions Clears in 1-2 wk	Leukopenia
Begins on face, scalp, or trunk Spreads peripherally	Pruritus present Lesions seen on mucous membranes	Culture of vesicle Acute and convalescent serum samples for IgG
Most prominent on trunk and extremities Perineal accentuation typical of KD but fades abruptly without residual of measles Desquamation around perineum and fingertips after first week	Conjunctivitis; strawberry tongue, fissured lips, adenopathy; coronary artery aneurysms Swelling of hands and feet No hypotension or renal involvement	WBC count and ESR are high Thrombocytosis during second to third week Sterile pyuria in first week
Face, buttocks, extremities	Fever, malaise, diarrhea	Skin biopsy Some cases, surface antigenemia Elevation of serum transaminase and alkaline phosphatase without hyperbilirubinemia
Trunk, extremities, palms, and soles	Temperature >40° C Shock DIC	Culture blood and CSF Antigen detection in CSF
Begins on wrists, ankles; spreads centrally; seen on palms and soles	Hepatosplenomegaly, hyponatremia, myalgias, CNS involvement	Any of rickettsial group–specific serologic tests

Continued

Table 14-1 Exanthems—cont'd

Disease	Age group	Prodrome incubation	Morphology
Henoch-Schönlein (purpura)	6 mo to young child	Arthralgia or abdominal pain	Symmetric palpable purpura
Erythema multiforme	10-30 yr	Infection with HSV or mycoplasma may precede; drug exposure	Erythematous macules with darker center "target lesion"
Scarlet fever	1-10 yr	2-4 days	Pinpoint papules Desquamation of tips of fingers and toes
Toxic shock syndrome	Children with burns and tracheitis	Sudden onset	Macular erythroderma, desquamation of tips of finger and toes
Drug exanthem	Any age	7-10 days after drug is first taken	Maculopapular, urticarial, pruritus
Hand-foot-and-mouth disease (coxsackievirus A16 and others)	Children	4-6 days, 50% fever, malaise	Vesiculopustules
Staphylococcal scalded skin syndrome	<5 yr	Malaise, fever, irritability	Tender, generalized, macular erythema becomes vesicular and bullous

Adapted from Gable EK et al: *Prim Care* 27:353, 2000. *PMID: 10815048*
*Twenty-five percent of all children may be group A streptococcal carriers.

EXANTHEMS

Measles

TRANSMISSION AND RISK. Measles (rubeola or morbilli) is a highly contagious viral disease transmitted by contact with droplets from infected individuals. The virus is spread by coughing and sneezing, close personal contact, or direct contact with infected nasal or throat secretions. The virus remains active and contagious in the air or on infected surfaces for up to 2 hours. It can be transmitted by an infected individual from 4 days before the onset of the rash to 4 days after the onset. If one person has the disease, a high proportion of their susceptible close contacts will also become infected. Unimmunized young children are at highest risk for measles and its complications, including death. Measles can be particularly deadly in countries experiencing or recovering from war, civil strife, or a natural disaster. Infection rates soar because damage to health services interrupts routine immunization. Overcrowding in camps for refugees and internally displaced people greatly increases the risk of infection.

COMPLICATIONS. Most cases have a benign course.

Severe measles is likely in poorly nourished young children, especially if they do not receive sufficient vitamin A, or are immunocompromised by human immunodeficiency virus/acquired immunodeficiency syndrome (HIV/AIDS) or other diseases.

Children die from complications. Complications are more common in children under the age of 5 or adults over the age of 20. The most serious complications include blindness, encephalitis, severe diarrhea, and ear infections. Pneumonia is the most common cause of death associated with measles. Encephalitis occurs in 1 out of 1000 cases; otitis media is reported in 5% to 15% of cases and pneumonia in 5% to 10% of cases. Survivors of this encephalitis often have permanent brain damage and mental retardation. The case fatality rate in developing countries is 1% to 5%, but may be as high as 25% in populations where high levels of malnutrition and poor access to health care exist. People who recover from measles are immune for life. Measles occurring during pregnancy may affect the fetus. Most commonly, this involves premature labor, moderately increased rates of spontaneous abortion, and low-birth-weight infants. Measles infection in the first trimester of pregnancy may be associated with an increased rate of congenital malformation.

INCIDENCE. The World Health Organizations (WHO) estimated deaths as a result of measles during 2006 are listed in Table 14-2. Between 1990 to 2000, implementation of national vaccination and surveillance programs reduced measles incidence in the Americas by 99%. Haiti and Venezuela are the last countries in the Americas where measles is endemic. Measles can be imported to measles-free countries from countries where measles is endemic; therefore all countries in the Americas must maintain the highest possible population immunity (i.e., >95% among

Distribution of rash	Associated findings	Laboratory findings
Buttocks, extensor extremities	Gastrointestinal, musculoskeletal, renal involvement	Skin biopsy H&E Immunofluorescences
Extensor surfaces of extremities, palms, and soles can be involved	May progress to involve mucous membranes, Stevens-Johnson syndrome	Skin biopsy
Generalized; spares palms and soles	Exudative pharyngitis	Group A streptococcal positive throat culture* Elevated WBC count and ESR
Diffuse	Hypotension, renal involvement, a focus of infection	Elevations of serum creatinine phosphokinase level
Generalized, symmetric; often spares face; palms and soles may be involved	Periorbital edema, fever	ESR is low
Hands, feet, buttock Erosions on mouth	Submandibular and/or cervical lymphadenopathy Dysphagia 90%	Biopsy
Face, neck, axilla, and groin	Staphylococcal infection of nasopharynx or conjuctiva	Elevated WBC count and ESR

infants and children). Measles is the leading cause of vaccine-preventable death in Africa.

VACCINE. Lifelong immunity is established with a single injection of live measles virus vaccine given at approximately 15 months of age. From 1963 to 1967, both live and inactivated measles vaccines were in use; since 1968 only the live vaccine has been used. Susceptible persons include those who were vaccinated between 1963 and 1967 with inactivated vaccine, patients given live measles virus vaccine before their first birthdays, and those patients who have never had measles. Prior recipients of killed measles vaccine may develop atypical measles syndrome when exposed to natural measles and should be revaccinated with live measles virus.

Table 14-2 Measles—Estimated Number of Deaths by the World Health Organization (WHO), 2006

Region	Deaths
Africa	36,000
Americas	<1,000
Eastern Mediterranean	23,000
European	<1,000*
South-East Asia	178,000
Western Pacific	5,000
TOTAL	**242,000**

TYPICAL MEASLES

The incubation period of measles (rubeola) (Figure 14-1) averages 10 to 12 days from exposure to prodrome and 14 days from exposure to rash (range, 7 to 18 days). The disease is spread by respiratory droplets and can be communicated from slightly before the beginning of the prodromal period to 4 days after appearance of the rash; com-

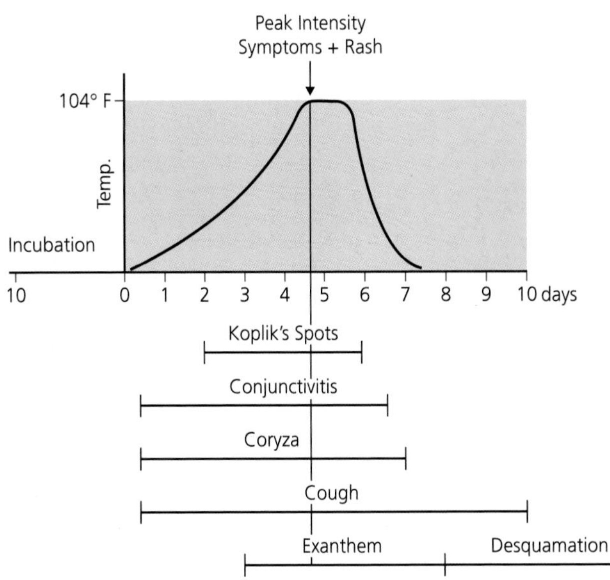

Figure 14-1 Measles. Evolution of the signs and symptoms.

MEASLES—PROGRESSION OF DISEASE

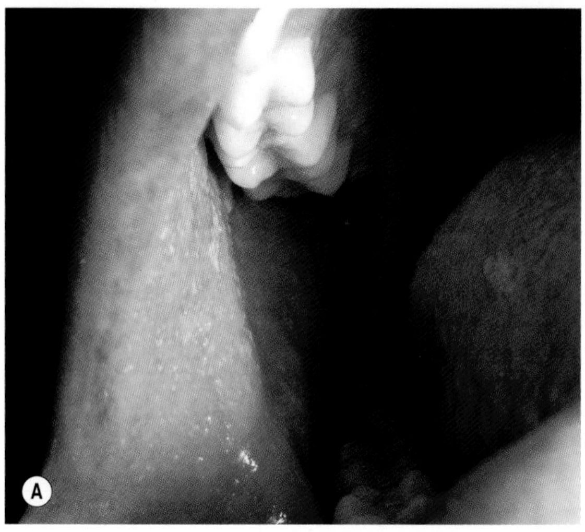

Koplik's spots appear as red spots with bluish-white centers "grains of sand." They may occur anywhere in the mouth.

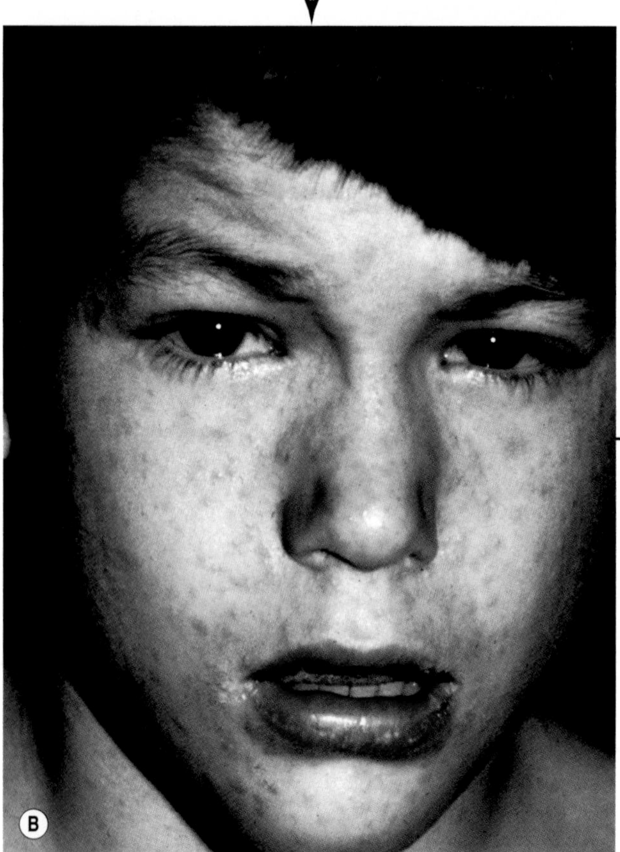

A maculopapular rash appears on the face and becomes confluent.

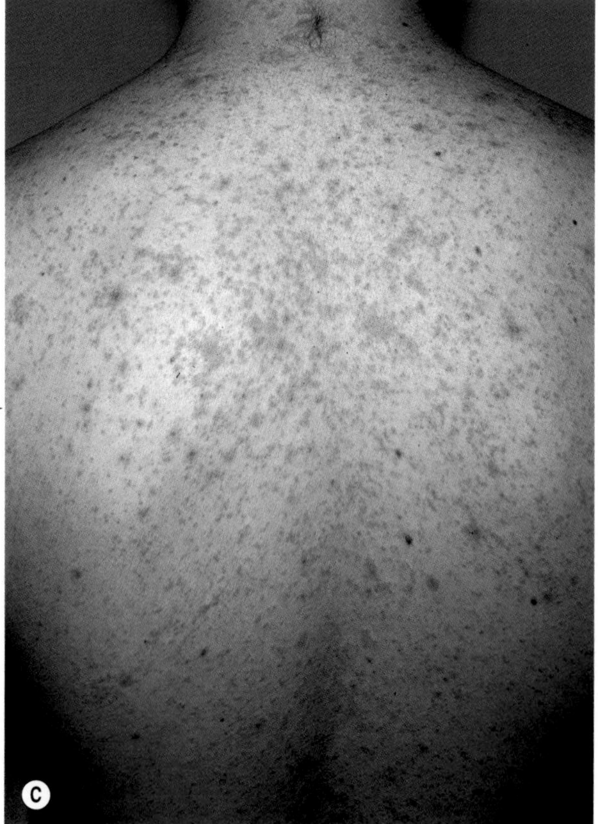

The rash then appears on the trunk.

Figure 14-2

municability is minimal after the second day of the rash. Prodromal symptoms of severe, brassy cough; nasal congestion; conjunctivitis; photophobia; and fever appear 3 to 4 days before the exanthem and increase daily in severity. The nose and eyes run continuously: the classic sign of measles. Koplik's spots (blue-white spots with a red halo) appear on the buccal mucous membrane opposite the premolar teeth 24 to 48 hours before the exanthem and remain for 2 to 4 days.

ERUPTIVE PHASE. The rash begins on the fourth or fifth day on the face and behind the ears, but in 24 to 36 hours it spreads to the trunk and extremities (Figure 14-2). It reaches maximum intensity simultaneously in all areas in approximately 3 days and fades after 5 to 10 days. The rash consists of slightly elevated maculopapules that vary in size from 0.1 to 1.0 cm and vary in color from dark red to a purplish hue. They are frequently confluent on both the face and the body, a feature that is such a distinct characteristic of measles that eruptions of similar appearance in other diseases are termed *morbilliform* (looks like measles). The early rash blanches on pressure; the fading rash is yellowish brown with a fine scale, and it does not blanch. Supportive treatment is the only necessity unless complications, such as bacterial infection or encephalitis, appear.

MANAGEMENT OF MEASLES

Nutritional support and prevention of dehydration with oral rehydration are necessary. Antibiotics treat eye and ear infections and pneumonia. Vitamin A deficiency impairs epithelial integrity and systemic immunity and increases the incidence and severity of infections during childhood. Vitamin A supplementation is effective in reducing total mortality and complications from measles infections; it is likely to be more effective in populations with nutritional deficiencies.

VITAMIN A TREATMENT. Vitamin A, retinol-binding protein (RBP), and albumin are significantly reduced early in the exanthem. Treatment with vitamin A reduces morbidity and mortality in measles, and all children with severe measles should be given vitamin A supplements regardless of whether they are thought to have a nutritional deficiency. This can help prevent eye damage and blindness. Vitamin A–treated children recover more rapidly from pneumonia and diarrhea, have less croup, and spend fewer days in the hospital. Treated patients have an increase in the total number of lymphocytes and measles IgG antibody. The risk of death or a major complication during a hospital stay is half that of untreated patients.

The following are appropriate dose regimens for safe administration of vitamin A in complicated measles: age younger than 6 months, 50,000 international units; age between 6 months and 2 years, 100,000 international units; age older than 2 years, 200,000 international units, administered via mouth on admission. A repeated dose can be administered on the next day.

Immunity. Persons are considered immune if they have documentation of adequate immunization with live measles vaccine on or after the first birthday, physician-diagnosed measles, or laboratory evidence of measles immunity. Most persons born before 1957 are likely to have been naturally infected and generally need not be considered susceptible. Routine serologic screening to determine measles immunity is not recommended.

Individuals exposed to disease. Live vaccine, if given within 72 hours of measles exposure, may provide protection and is preferable to the use of human immunoglobulin in persons at least 12 months of age if there is no contraindication.

Use of human immunoglobin. Human immunoglobulin (Ig) can be given to prevent or modify measles in a susceptible person within 6 days after exposure. The recommended dose of Ig is 0.25 ml/kg (0.11 ml/lb) of body weight (maximum dose, 15 ml).

Revaccination risks. There is no enhanced risk from administering live measles vaccine to persons who are already immune to measles.

Pregnancy. Live measles vaccine should not be given to women known to be pregnant or who are considering becoming pregnant within 3 months after vaccination. This precaution is based on the theoretical risk of fetal infection.

Hand-foot-and-mouth disease

Hand-foot-and-mouth disease (HFMD), which has no relation to hoof-and-mouth disease in cattle, is a contagious enteroviral infection occurring primarily in children and characterized by a vesicular palmoplantar eruption and erosive stomatitis. It is most often caused by coxsackievirus A16 and enterovirus 71 (EV71). Enteroviruses are believed to be spread via the fecal-oral and perhaps respiratory routes. This disease may occur as an isolated phenomenon, or it may occur in epidemic form. It is more common among children.

CLINICAL PRESENTATION. The incubation period is 4 to 6 days. There may be mild symptoms of low-grade fever, sore throat, and malaise for 1 or 2 days. Twenty percent of patients develop submandibular and/or cervical lymphadenopathy.

ERUPTIVE PHASE. Oral lesions, present in 90% of cases, are generally the initial sign. Aphthae-like erosions varying from a few to 10 or more appear anywhere in the oral cavity and are most frequently small and asymptomatic (Figure 14-3). The cutaneous lesions, which occur in approximately two thirds of patients, appear less than 24 hours after the enanthem. They begin as 3- to 7-mm, red macules that rapidly become pale, white, oval vesicles

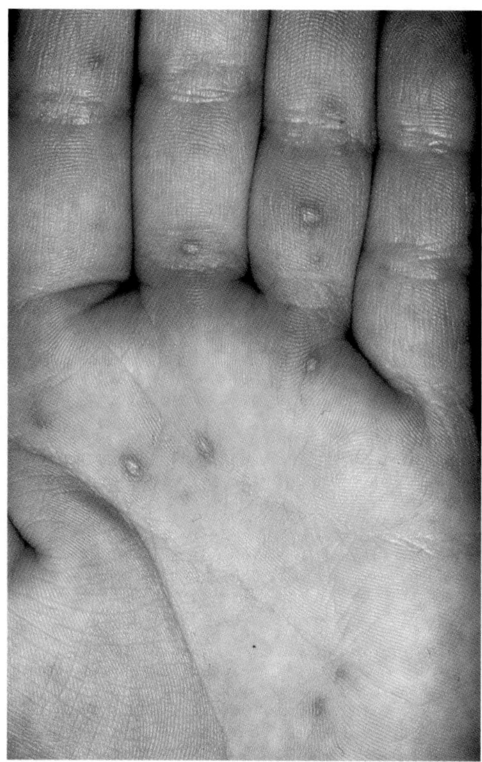

Figure 14-3 Cloudy vesicles with a red halo are highly characteristic of this disease.

with a red areola (Figure 14-4). There may be a few inconspicuous lesions, or there may be dozens. The vesicles occur on the palms, soles (Figure 14-5), dorsal aspects of the fingers and toes, and occasionally on the face, buttocks, and legs. They heal in approximately 7 days, usually without crusting or scarring. Nail matrix arrest was reported in a small group of children after HFMD. Beau's lines (transverse ridging) and/or onychomadesis (nail shedding) followed HFMD by 3 to 8 weeks.

SERIOUS AND FATAL CASES. EV71 can result in disability and death. Pulmonary edema/hemorrhage can kill a child within 1 day. In 2000 Human enterovirus 71 (HEV71) caused the largest HFMD epidemic recorded in Singapore, an epidemic that involved mainly young children <4 years of age. Five deaths occurred, and HEV71 was isolated from four case-patients. Autopsies showed encephalitis, interstitial pneumonitis, and myocarditis. HFMD caused by HEV71 produced a high number of cases of fatal encephalitis during an outbreak in Malaysia in 1997 and Taiwan in 1998. Thousands of people in Taiwan were infected. Most of those who died were young, and the majority died of pulmonary edema and pulmonary hemorrhage. Death attributable to HEV71 infection likely results from brainstem lesions that cause an increase in the sympathetic drive. Hyperglycemia is an important prognostic factor.

DIFFERENTIAL DIAGNOSIS. When cutaneous lesions are absent, the disease may be confused with aphthous stomatitis. The oral erosions of HFMD are usually smaller and more uniform. The vesicles of herpes appear in clusters, and those of varicella endure longer and always crust. Both varicella and herpes have multinucleated, giant cells in smears taken from the moist skin exposed when a vesicle is removed (Tzanck smear). Giant cells are not present in lesions of HFMD.

TREATMENT. Symptomatic relief and reassurance are all that are required.

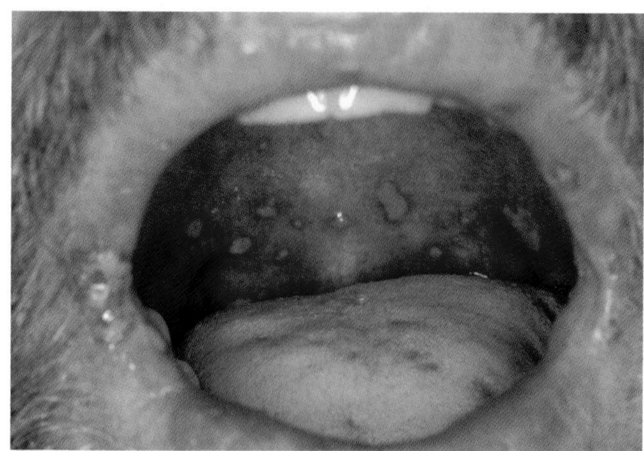

Figure 14-4 Hand-foot-and-mouth disease. Aphthae-like erosions may appear anywhere in the oral cavity.

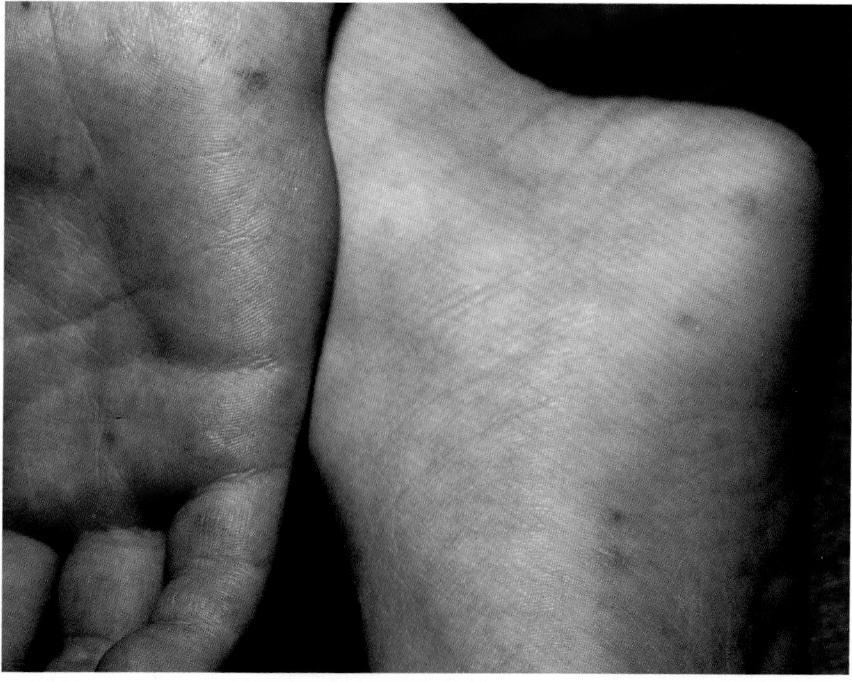

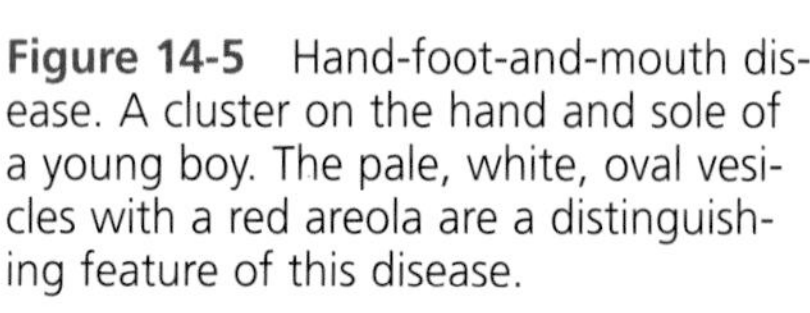

Figure 14-5 Hand-foot-and-mouth disease. A cluster on the hand and sole of a young boy. The pale, white, oval vesicles with a red areola are a distinguishing feature of this disease.

Scarlet fever

Scarlet fever (scarlatina) is an endemic, contagious disease produced by a streptococcal, erythrogenic toxin. The circulating toxin is responsible for the rash and systemic symptoms. The infection may originate in the pharynx or skin and is most common in children (ages 1 to 10 years) who lack immunity to the toxin. An outbreak of scarlet fever caused by group A streptococci in contaminated food was reported in China in 2006. *PMID: 17719644* Scarlet fever was a feared disease in the nineteenth and early twentieth centuries, when it was more virulent, but presently scarlet fever is usually benign. Virulent strains may appear in the future. New waves of scarlet fever are associated with an increase in frequency of *Streptococcus pyogenes* clones carrying variant gene alleles encoding streptococcal pyrogenic exotoxin A (scarlet fever toxin). Previous exposure to the toxin is required for expression of disease. Streptococcal pyrogenic exotoxin A causes disease by enhancing delayed-type hypersensitivity to streptococcal products.

INCUBATION PERIOD. The incubation period of scarlet fever (Figure 14-6) is 2 to 4 days.

PRODROMAL AND ERUPTIVE PHASE. The sudden onset of fever and pharyngitis is followed shortly by nausea, vomiting, headache, and abdominal pain. The entire oral cavity may be red, and the tongue is covered with a yellowish white coat through which red papillae protrude. Diffuse lymphadenopathy may appear just before the onset of the eruption. The systemic symptoms continue until the fever subsides. The rash begins about the neck and face and spreads in 48 hours to the trunk and extremities; the palms and soles are spared (Figure 14-7). The face is flushed except for circumoral pallor, whereas all other involved areas exhibit a vivid scarlet hue with innumerable pinpoint papules that give a sandpaper quality to the skin (Figure 14-8). The rash is more limited and less dramatic in milder cases. Linear petechiae (Pastia's sign) are characteristic; they are found in skin folds, particularly the antecubital fossa and inguinal area. The tongue sheds the white coat to reveal a red, raw, glazed surface with engorged papillae (Figure 14-9).

The fever and rash subside and desquamation appears, more pronounced than in any of the eruptive fevers. It begins on the face, where it is sparse and superficial; progresses to the trunk, often with a circular, punched-out appearance; and finally spreads to the hands (Figure 14-10) and feet (Figures 14-11 and 14-12), where the epidermis is the thickest. Clinically, the hands and feet appear normal during the initial stages of the disease. Large sheaths of epidermis may be shed from the palms and soles in a glovelike cast, exposing new and often tender epidermis beneath. A transverse groove may be produced in all of the nails (Beau's lines) (Figure 14-13). The pattern of desquamation of the palms and soles and grooving of the nails is such a distinct characteristic of scarlet fever that it is helpful in making a retrospective diagnosis in cases where the eruption is minimal. A rising antistreptolysin-O titer constitutes additional supporting evidence for a recent infection. Desquamation is generally complete in 4 weeks, but it may last for 8 weeks. Recurrence rates of scarlet fever as high as 18% have been reported.

TREATMENT. Treat with penicillin, cephalosporins, erythromycin, ofloxacin, rifampin, or the newer macrolides.

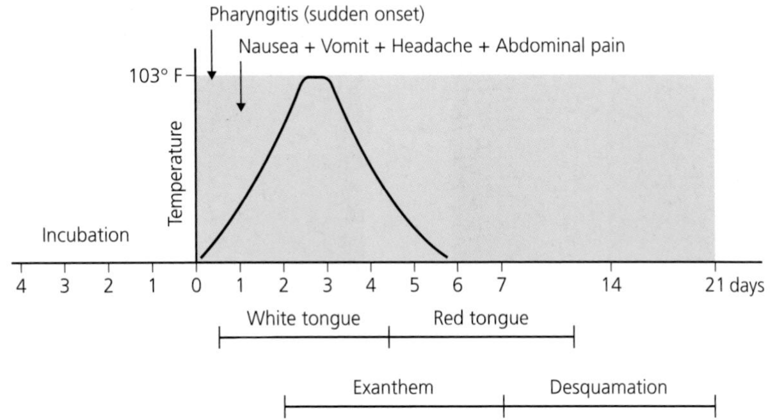

Figure 14-6 Scarlet fever. Evolution of signs and symptoms.

SCARLET FEVER

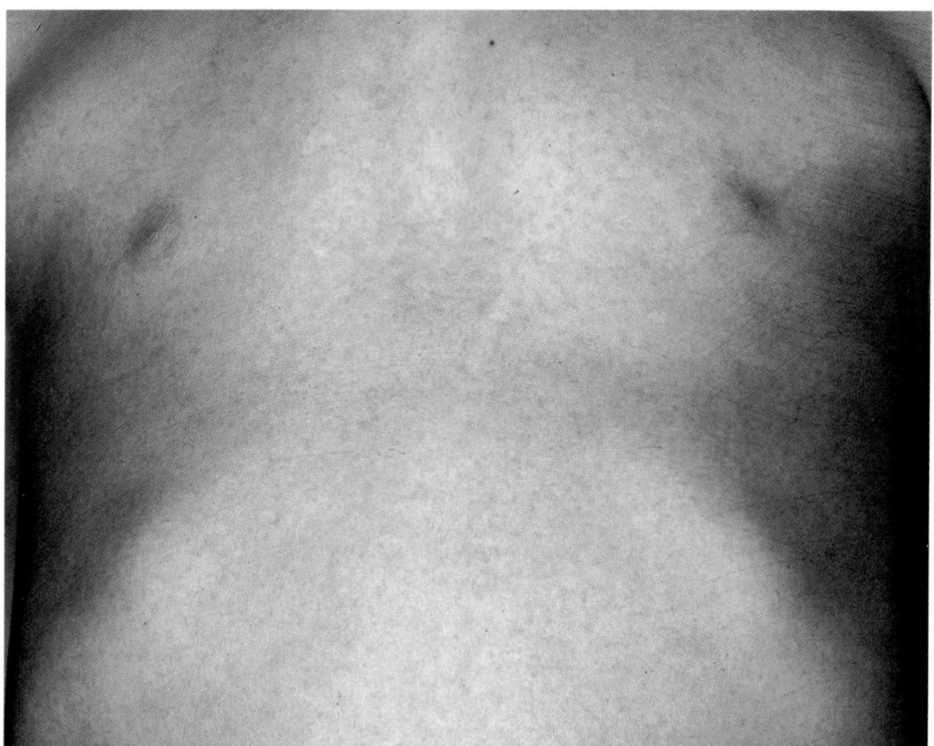

Figure 14-7 Early eruptive stage on the trunk showing numerous pinpoint red papules.

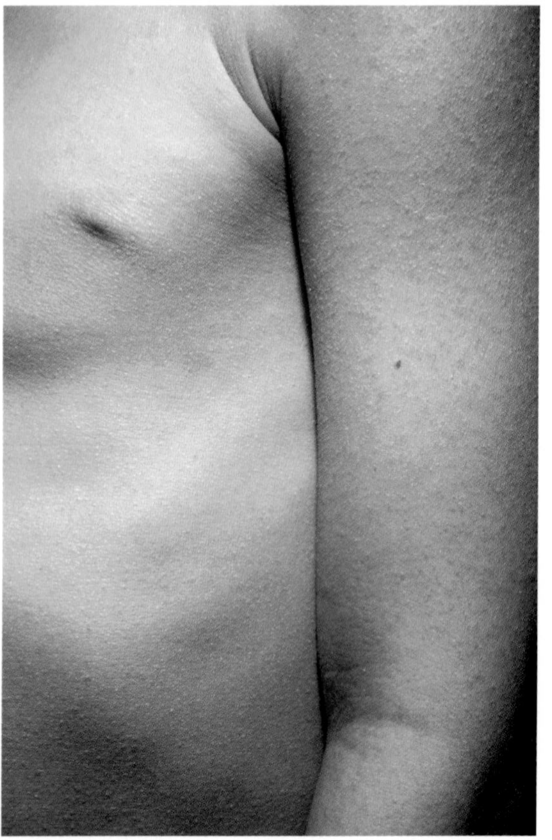

Figure 14-8 Fully evolved eruption. Numerous papules giving a sandpaper-like texture to the skin.

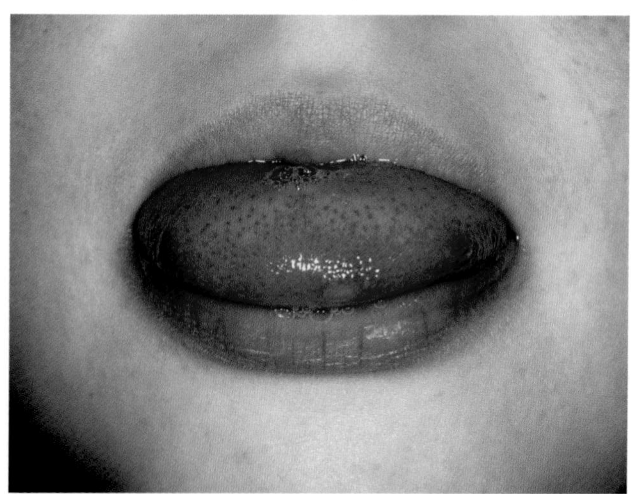

Figure 14-9 Portions of the white coat remain in the center, but the remainder of the tongue is red with engorged papillae ("strawberry tongue").

SCARLET FEVER

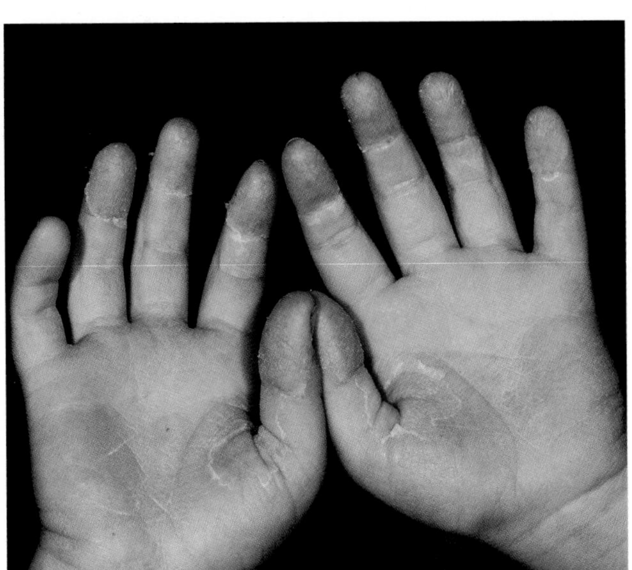

Figure 14-10 Desquamation of the hands begins 7-10 days after resolution of the rash. Peeling occurs in the axillae, groin, and on the tips of the fingers.

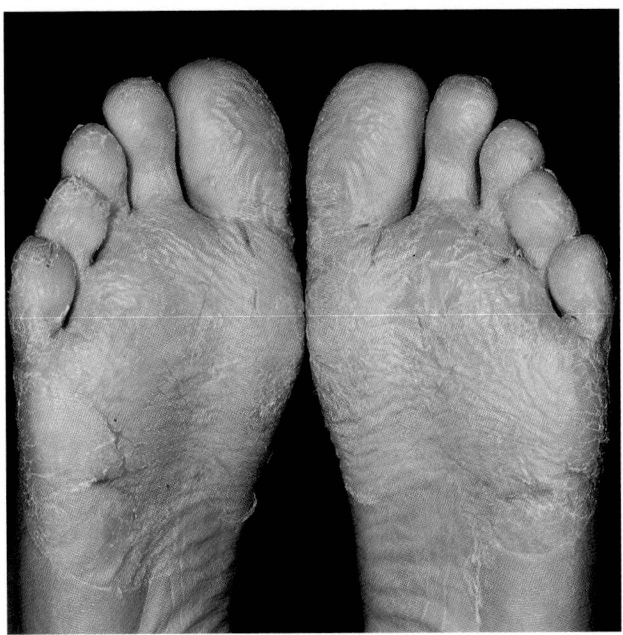

Figure 14-11 Desquamation of the feet.

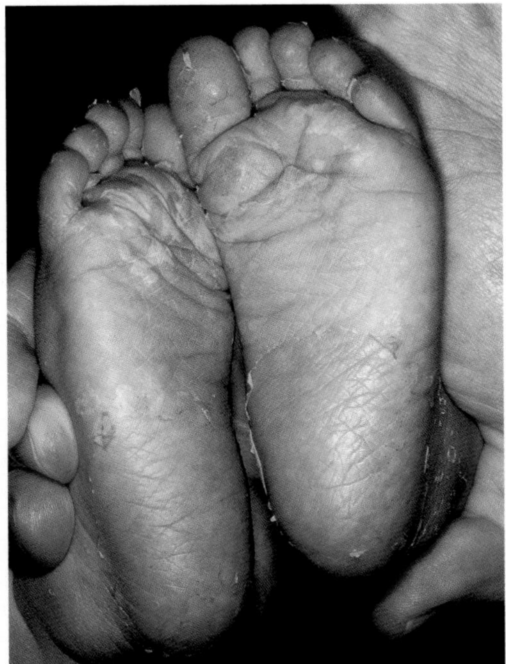

Figure 14-12 Desquamation of the feet.

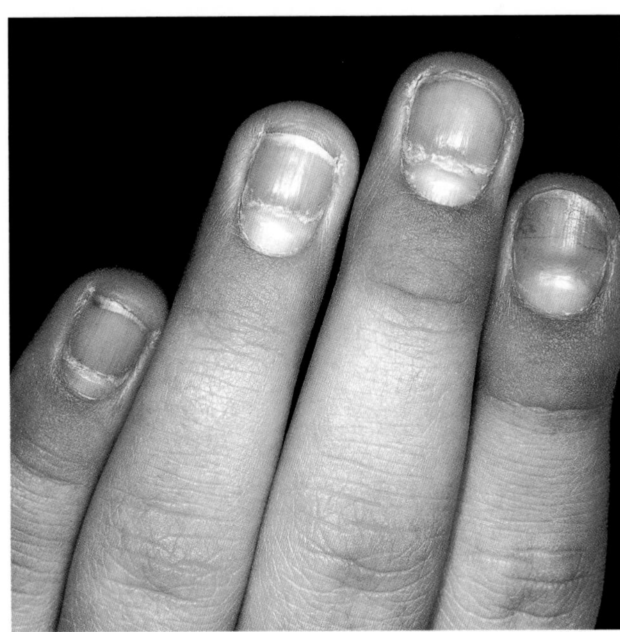

Figure 14-13 Beau's lines: transverse grooves on all nails several weeks after skin signs of scarlet fever have cleared.

Rubella

Rubella (German measles, 3-day measles) is a benign, contagious exanthematous viral infection characterized by nonspecific signs and symptoms including transient erythematous and sometimes pruritic rash, postauricular or suboccipital lymphadenopathy, arthralgia, and low-grade fever. Clinically similar exanthematous illnesses are caused by parvovirus, adenoviruses, and enteroviruses. Moreover, 25% to 50% of rubella infections are subclinical. The most important consequences of rubella are the miscarriages, stillbirths, fetal anomalies, and therapeutic abortions that result when rubella infection occurs during early pregnancy, especially during the first trimester.

CONGENITAL RUBELLA SYNDROME. Pregnant women who have rubella early in the first trimester may transmit the disease to the fetus, which may consequently develop a number of congenital defects (congenital rubella syndrome).

INCUBATION PERIOD. The incubation period of rubella (Figure 14-14) is 18 days, with a range of 14 to 21 days.

PRODROMAL PHASE. Mild symptoms of malaise, headache, and moderate temperature elevation may precede the eruption by a few hours or a day. Children are usually asymptomatic. Lymphadenopathy, characteristically postauricular, suboccipital, and cervical, may appear 4 to 7 days before the rash and be maximal at the onset of the exanthem. In 2% of cases, petechiae on the soft palate occur late in the prodromal phase or early in the eruptive phase.

ERUPTIVE PHASE. The eruption begins on the neck or face and spreads in hours to the trunk and extremities (Figure 14-15). The lesions are pinpoint to 1 cm, round or oval, pinkish or rosy red macules or maculopapules. The color is less vivid than that of scarlet fever and lacks the blue or violaceous tinge seen in measles. The lesions are usually discrete but may be grouped or coalesced on the face or trunk. The rash fades in 24 to 48 hours in the same order in which it appeared and may be followed by a fine desquamation.

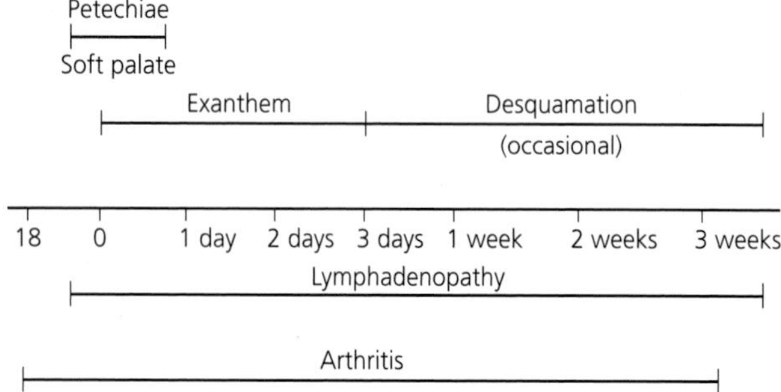

Figure 14-14 Rubella. Evolution of signs and symptoms.

Among adults infected with rubella, transient polyarthralgia or polyarthritis occurs frequently. These manifestations are particularly common among women.

Arthritis, affecting primarily the phalangeal joints of women, may occur in the prodromal period and may last for 2 to 3 weeks after the rash has disappeared. No treatment is required.

Central nervous system complications (e.g., encephalitis) occur at a ratio of 1:6000 cases and are more likely to affect adults. Thrombocytopenia occurs at a ratio of 1:3000 cases and is more likely to affect children.

Vaccine. The rubella vaccine is a live attenuated virus. Although it is available as a single preparation, it is recommended that in most cases rubella vaccine be given as part of the measles-mumps-rubella (MMR) vaccine. MMR is recommended at 12 to 15 months (not earlier) and a second dose when the child is 4 to 6 years old (before kindergarten or first grade). Rubella vaccination is important for nonimmune women who may become pregnant because of the risk for serious birth defects if they acquire the disease during pregnancy

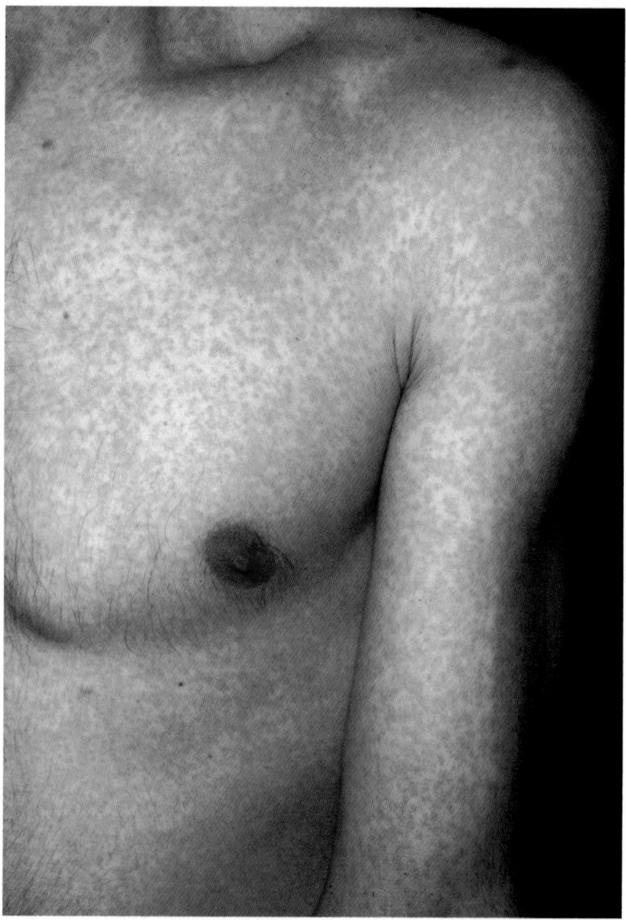

Figure 14-15 Rubella. The rash begins as macules on the face that spread to the trunk and the extremities. The macules may coalesce on the trunk.

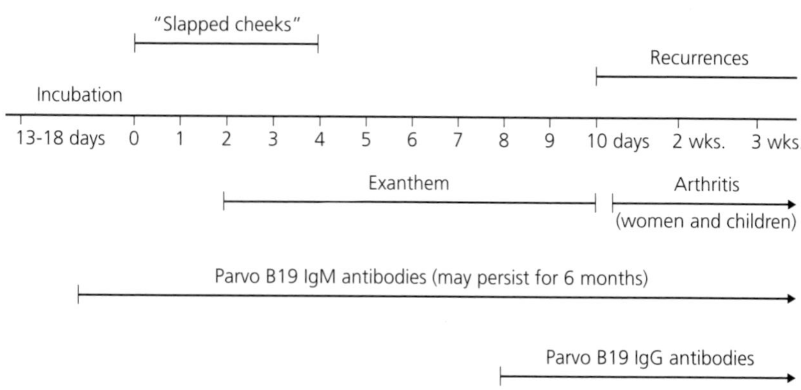

Figure 14-16 Erythema infectiosum. Evolution of signs and symptoms.

Erythema infectiosum (parvovirus B19 infection)

Parvovirus B19 is associated with many disease manifestations that vary with the immunologic and hematologic status of the patient. The main target of B19 infection is the red cell receptor globoside (blood group P antigen) of erythroid progenitor cells of the bone marrow. People who do not have the virus receptor (erythrocyte P antigen) are naturally resistant to infection with this virus.

ERYTHEMA INFECTIOSUM. Erythema infectiosum (fifth disease) is caused by the B19 parvovirus. It is relatively common and mildly contagious and appears sporadically or in epidemics. Peak attack rates occur in children between 5 and 14 years of age. Asymptomatic infection is common.

Infection causes erythema infectiosum in immunocompetent patients. It is the primary cause of transient aplastic crisis in patients with underlying hemolytic disorders. Persistent infection in immunosuppressed patients may present as red cell aplasia and chronic anemia. In utero infection may result in hydrops fetalis or congenital anemia. There is no evidence of reinfection in immunocompetent individuals.

Seroprevalence is 2% to 10% in children younger than 5 years, 40% to 60% in adults older than 20 years, and 85% or more in those older than 70 years. The average annual seroconversion rate of women of childbearing age is 1.5%.

The virus may be transmitted via the respiratory route and via the transfusion of infected blood and blood products. Nosocomial transmission has been well documented. Individuals are not viremic or infectious at the rash or arthropathy stage of disease.

INCUBATION PERIOD. The incubation period of erythema infectiosum (Figure 14-16) is 13 to 18 days. Viremia occurs after the incubation period and reticulocyte numbers fall, resulting in a temporary drop in hemoglobin concentration of 1 g/dl in a normal person.

There is a nonspecific prodromal illness, followed by a three-stage erythematous disease.

PRODROMAL SYMPTOMS. Symptoms are usually mild or absent. Pruritus, low-grade fever, malaise, and sore throat precede the eruption in approximately 10% of cases. Lymphadenopathy is absent. Older individuals may complain of joint pain.

ERUPTIVE PHASE. There are three distinct, overlapping stages.

Facial erythema ("slapped cheek"). Red papules on the cheeks rapidly coalesce in hours, forming fiery red, slightly edematous, warm, erysipelas-like plaques that are symmetric on both cheeks and spare the nasolabial fold and the circumoral region (Figure 14-17). The "slapped cheek" appearance fades in 4 days. The classic slapped cheek is much more common in children than in adults.

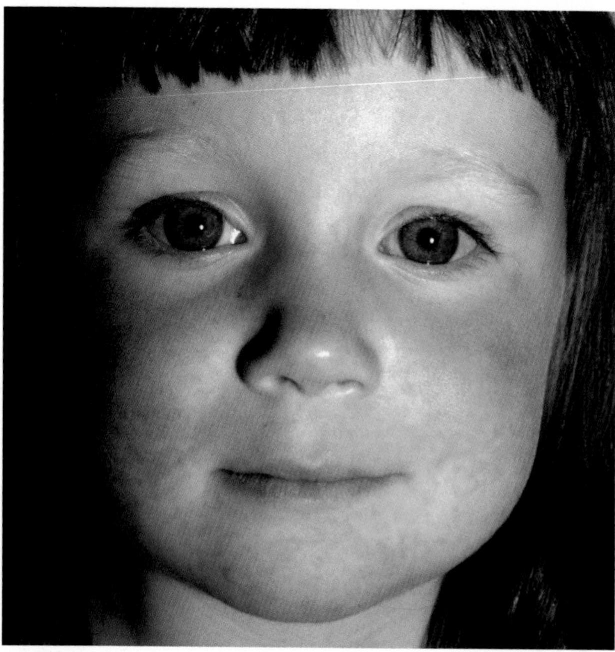

Figure 14-17 Erythema infectiosum. Facial erythema "slapped cheek." The red plaque covers the cheek and spares the nasolabial fold and the circumoral region.

Net pattern erythema. This unique characteristic eruption—erythema in a fishnet-like pattern—begins on the extremities approximately 2 days after the onset of facial erythema and extends to the trunk and buttocks, fading in 6 to 14 days (Figure 14-18). At times, the exanthem begins with erythema and does not become characteristic until irregular clearing takes place. This second-stage rash may vary from very faint erythema to a florid exanthem. Livedo reticularis has a similar netlike pattern, but it does not fade quickly.

Recurrent phase. The eruption may fade and then reappear in previously affected sites on the face and body during the next 2 to 3 weeks. Temperature changes, emotional upsets, and sunlight may stimulate recurrences. The rash fades without scaling or pigmentation. There may be a slight lymphocytosis or eosinophilia.

POLYARTHROPATHY SYNDROME AND PRURITUS

Adults. Women exposed to the parvovirus during outbreaks may develop itching and arthralgia or arthritis. Men are not affected. The itching varies from mild to intense and is localized or generalized. In most cases a nonspecific macular eruption occurs without the appearance of the typical netlike pattern before the arthritis.

Women develop moderately severe, symmetric polyarthritis that may evolve to a form that is often indistinguishable from rheumatoid arthritis. Most have involvement of the knees and other joints, as well as migratory arthritis.

B19 patients present with the sudden onset of symmetric peripheral polyarthropathy of moderate severity. B19 infection mimics rheumatoid arthritis in the acute stage, and the rheumatoid factor test can be positive.

The joints can be painful, with accompanying swelling and stiffness. Symptoms continue for 1 to 3 weeks. In some women, arthropathy or arthritis may persist or recur for months or years.

There are striking similarities between B19 infection and systemic lupus erythematosus: both may present with malar rash, fever, arthropathy, myalgia, cytopenia, hypocomplementemia, and anti-DNA and antinuclear antibodies (ANAs).

The differential diagnosis includes acute rheumatoid arthritis, seronegative arthritis, Lyme disease, and lupus. Parvovirus infection should be considered when an adult woman has acute polyarthropathy associated with pruritus, especially if she has been exposed to children with erythema infectiosum.

The demonstration of anti-parvovirus-B19 immunoglobulins (IgM) and anti-parvovirus-B19 IgG is a most important diagnostic finding. Measurement of IgM must be done within the first months, as it disappears later on. Immunosuppressive agents used to treat rheumatoid arthritis may prolong the persistence of the virus and disease in parvovirus B19–induced arthritis/arthropathy.

B19 infection is not associated with joint destruction seen in rheumatoid arthritis. Prolonged symptoms do not correlate with serologic studies, such as the duration of B19 immunoglobulin M (IgM) response, or persistent viremia.

Adult flulike symptoms and arthropathies begin coincidentally with IgG antibody production in 18 to 24 days after exposure and are probably immune-complex mediated.

Children. Both male and female children may develop joint symptoms. Most cases have acute arthritis of brief duration; a few have arthralgias. Two patterns are seen: polyarticular, affecting more than five joints; and pauciarticular, affecting four or fewer joints. Large joints are affected more often than small joints. The knee is the most common joint affected (82%). Laboratory findings are normal. The duration of joint symptoms is usually less than 4 months, but some have persistent arthritis for 2 to 13 months, which fulfills the criteria for the diagnosis of juvenile rheumatoid arthritis.

INFECTION IN THE PREGNANT WOMAN (INTRAUTERINE INFECTION AND SPONTANEOUS ABORTION).

In pregnant women, infection can, but usually does not, lead to fetal infection (Box 14-1). Fetal infection sometimes causes severe anemia, congestive heart failure, generalized edema (fetal hydrops), and death. Many fetuses dying because of this infection are not noticeably hydropic.

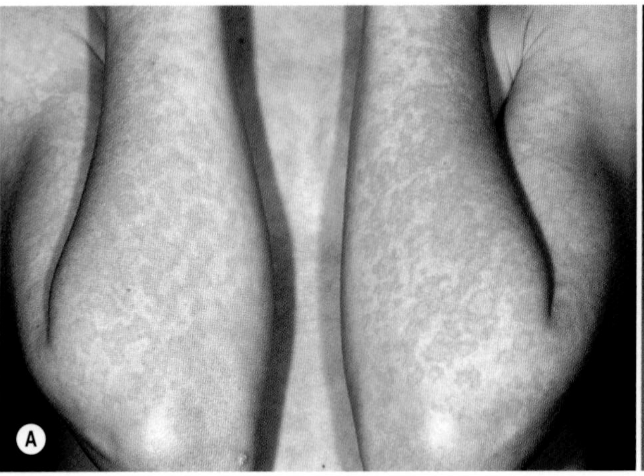

A macular eruption appears on the extensor extremities.

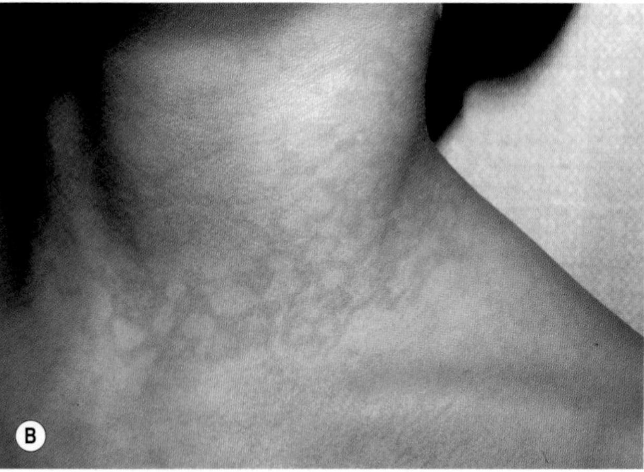

The eruption fades into a lacy net-like pattern.

Figure 14-18 Erythema infectiosum.

Box 14-1 Facts and Recommendations for Pregnant Women Exposed to B19 Parvovirus

Risk of maternal infection during an epidemic: 30% to 65%

Infected women may be asymptomatic.

Nurses and school teachers: High rate of infection if exposed

- People with fifth disease are contagious before they develop the rash; therefore exposure at the onset of an outbreak cannot be avoided.
- Pregnant personnel should remain at home until 2 to 3 weeks after the last identified case.

Laboratory tests

- IgM tests for symptomatic exposed women
- Fetal ultrasonography for confirmed or suspected cases
- Polymerase chain reaction testing of amniotic fluid and fetal serum—a sensitive and rapid method for diagnosis of intrauterine infection
- Monitor alpha-fetoprotein* levels in exposed and infected women
- Ultrasonography when alpha-fetoprotein levels are increased
- Abnormal ultrasound: fetal blood sampling as a guide for possible fetal transfusion
- Teratogenic effects not demonstrated
- Therapeutic abortion not indicated

Adapted from Levy M, Stanley ER: *Can Med Assoc J* 143:849, 1990. *PMID: 2171743*

*Maternal serum alpha-fetoprotein is a marker for fetal aplastic crisis during intrauterine human parvovirus infection.

Parvovirus B19 probably causes 10% to 15% of all cases of nonimmune hydrops. If the fetus survives fetal hydrops caused by B19, there usually are no long-term sequelae.

The fetus has a high rate of red cell production; its immature immune system may not be able to mount an adequate immune response. Parvovirus has been implicated as a cause of spontaneous abortion (from severe fetal anemia and hydrops fetalis).

Maternal infection in the first half of pregnancy is associated with 10% excess fetal loss and hydrops fetalis in 3% of cases (of which up to 60% resolve spontaneously or with appropriate management). B19-associated congenital abnormalities have not been reported among several hundred live-born infants of B19-infected mothers. The overall risk of serious adverse outcome from occupational exposure to parvovirus B19 infection during pregnancy is low (excess early fetal loss in 2 to 6 of 1000 pregnancies and fetal death from hydrops in 2 to 5 of 10,000 pregnancies). It is not recommended that susceptible pregnant women be excluded routinely from working with children during epidemics.

The polymerase chain reaction is a sensitive and rapid method for the diagnosis of intrauterine infection.

ANEMIA. The virus has the propensity to infect and lyse erythroid precursor cells and interrupt normal red cell production. In a person with normal hematopoiesis, B19 infection produces a self-limited red cell aplasia that is clinically inapparent. In patients who have increased rates of red cell destruction or loss and who depend on compensatory increases in red cell production to maintain stable red cell indices, B19 infection may lead to transient aplastic crisis. Patients at risk for transient aplastic crisis include those with hemoglobinopathies (sickle cell disease, thalassemia, hereditary spherocytosis, and pyruvate kinase deficiency) and those with anemias associated with acute or chronic blood loss. B19 infection accounts for most, if not all, aplastic crises in sickle cell disease, but at least 20% of infections do not result in aplasia. Up to 30% of hospital staff members may be infected when exposed to infected sickle cell patients. In immunodeficient persons and those with AIDS, B19 may persist, causing chronic red cell aplasia, which results in chronic anemia. Some of these patients may be cured with immune globulin therapy.

LABORATORY EVALUATION. Most acute infections with B19 are diagnosed in the laboratory by serologically detecting IgG and IgM class antibodies with enzyme immunoassay. IgM antibodies are the most sensitive indicator of acute B19 infection in immunologically normal persons. Measuring IgM is useful for diagnosing recent parvovirus infection. Both IgG and IgM may be present at or soon after onset of illness and reach peak titers within 30 days. Because IgG antibody may persist for years, diagnosis of acute infection is made by the detection of IgM antibodies. The prevalence of parvovirus B19 IgG antibodies increases with age. The age-specific prevalence of antibodies to parvovirus is 2% to 9% of children under 5 years, 15% to 35% in children 5 to 18 years of age, and 30% to 60% in adults (19 years or older). IgM is detectable for as long as 3 months after exposure. Parvovirus B19 can be detected in blood, amniotic fluid, and synovial fluid by rapid polymerase chain reaction (PCR).

MANAGEMENT. Parents need only to be assured that this unusual eruption will fade and does not require treatment. Most health departments do not recommend exclusion from school for children with fifth disease. Many infections are inapparent, and exposure may occur in the community, as well as in school.

Evaluate the immune status of exposed pregnant women. The risks are nil if the women is IgG positive. If she is not immune (although the risk of the fetus being affected is very low), fetal surveillance by repeated ultrasonographic examination and immune status reevaluation is recommended.

Because the major immune response appears to be humoral, patients with chronic infection have been treated with immune globulin. These patients often respond with a marked reduction in the level of B19 viremia and with reticulocytosis, followed within a few weeks by resolution of the anemia. Patients with persistent infection should be monitored for evidence of relapse by observation of the reticulocyte counts and by assays for B19 viremia when indicated.

Roseola infantum (human herpesvirus 6 and 7 infection)

Roseola infantum (exanthem subitum, "sudden rash," sixth disease, rose rash of infants, 3-day fever) is caused primarily by human herpesvirus 6 (HHV-6), which is epidemiologically and biologically similar to cytomegalovirus. As with other herpesviruses, HHV-6 shows persistent and intermittent or chronic shedding in the normal population, making the unusually early infection of children (seroconversion in the first year of life in up to 80% of all children) understandable. The virus remains latent in monocytes and macrophages and probably in the salivary glands. Virus may infect infants through the saliva mainly from mother to child. A severe, infectious, mononucleosis-like syndrome in adults may be caused by a primary infection with HHV-6. HHV-6 has also been implicated in idiopathic pneumonitis in immunocompromised hosts.

Most cases are asymptomatic or present with fever of unknown origin and occur without a rash. The disease is sporadic, and the majority of cases occur between the ages of 6 months and 4 years. Primary HHV-7 infection occurs later in childhood (at approximately 3 years of age) and also causes exanthema subitum, although less often than HHV-6. HHV-6 antibody is present in 90% to 100% of the population over age 2. The development of high fever, as is seen in roseola, is worrisome, but the onset of the characteristic rash is reassuring.

One study showed that HHV-6 was responsible for 10% of hospital visits for acute illness in infants younger than 25 months of age and 33% of the febrile seizures occurring in children younger than 2 years.

In infants and young children HHV-6 is a major cause of visits to the emergency department, febrile seizures, and hospitalizations.

INCUBATION PERIOD. The incubation period of roseola infantum (Figure 14-19) is 12 days, with a range of 5 to 15 days.

PRODROMAL SYMPTOMS. There is a sudden onset of high fever of 103° to 106° F, with few or minor symptoms. Most children appear inappropriately well for the degree of temperature elevation, but they may experience slight anorexia or one or two episodes of vomiting, running nose, cough, and hepatomegaly. Seizures (but more frequently general cerebral irritability) may occur before the eruptive phase. Most recover without sequelae. Cases of encephalitis/encephalopathy with abnormal electroencephalograms and cerebral computed tomograms have been reported; epilepsy developed in one case and in another case the patient died. HHV-6 DNA has been detected in the cerebrospinal fluid (CSF); this suggests that HHV-6 may invade the brain during the acute phase. HHV-6 infection should be suspected in infants with febrile convulsions, even those without the exanthem. Mild-to-moderate lymphadenopathy, usually in the occipital regions, begins at the onset of the febrile period and persists until after the eruption has subsided.

ERUPTIVE PHASE. The rash begins as the fever subsides. The term exanthem subitum indicates the sudden "surprise" of the blossoming rash after the fall of the fever. Numerous pale pink, almond-shaped macules appear on the trunk and neck, become confluent, and then fade in a few hours to 2 days without scaling or pigmentation (Figures 14-20 and 14-21). The exanthem may resemble rubella or measles, but the pattern of development, distribution, and associated symptoms of these other exanthematous diseases are different.

LABORATORY EVALUATION. Leukocytosis develops at the onset of fever, but leukopenia with a granulocytopenia and relative lymphocytosis appears as the temperature increases and persists until the eruption fades. Seroconversion during the convalescent phase can be detected with immunofluorescence or enzyme immunoassays. HHV-6 can be detected by rapid PCR.

TREATMENT. Control temperature with aspirin and provide reassurance. HHV-6 is inhibited by several antiviral drugs in the laboratory, including ganciclovir and foscarnet. Treatment may be considered for patients with serious HHV-6-associated disease confirmed with virologic tests.

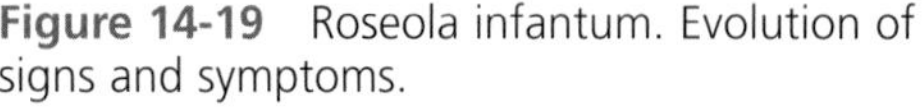

Figure 14-19 Roseola infantum. Evolution of signs and symptoms.

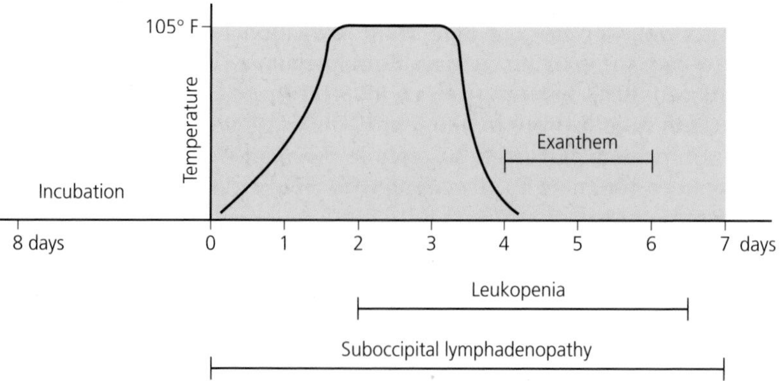

ROSEOLA

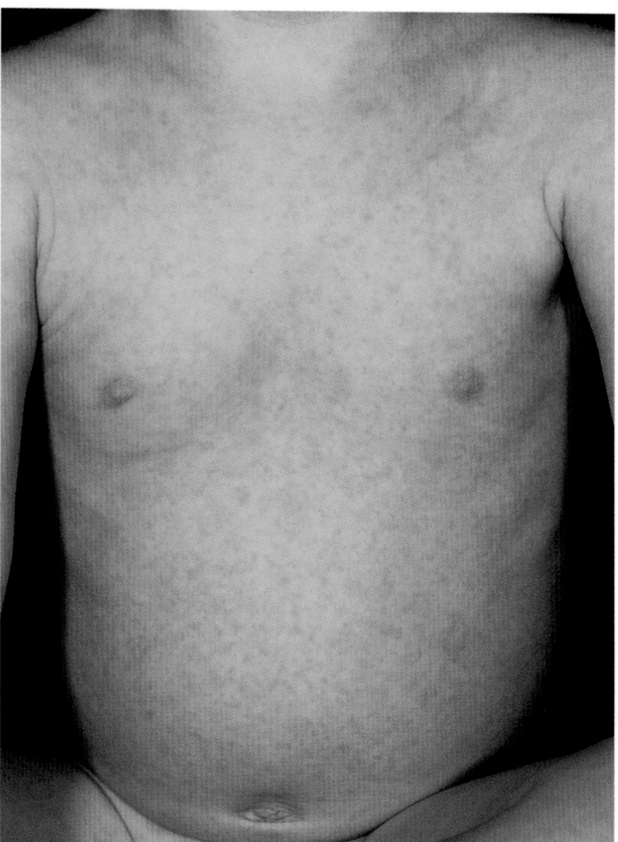

Figure 14-20 Numerous pale pink, almond-shaped macules.

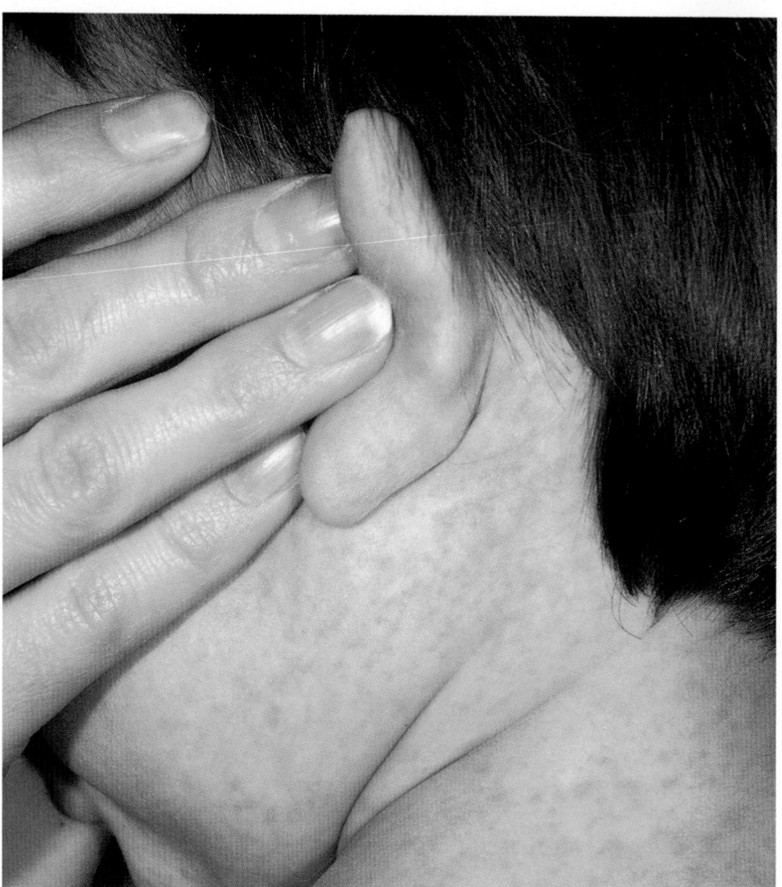

Figure 14-21 Pale pink macules may appear first on the neck.

Enteroviruses: echovirus and coxsackievirus exanthems

The previously described diseases characteristically display a predictable set of signs and symptoms. Roseola and erythema infectiosum are relatively common. Many physicians never see cases of measles, German measles, or scarlet fever. The most common exanthematous eruptions are caused by the enteroviruses echovirus and coxsackievirus. A large number of these viruses may begin with a skin eruption. Some of these eruptions are characteristic of the virus type, but in most cases one must be satisfied with the diagnosis of "viral rash." In many cases, drug eruptions cannot be distinguished from the nonspecific exanthems of these enteroviruses.

SYSTEMIC SYMPTOMS. Many are possible, such as fever, nausea, vomiting, and diarrhea, along with typical viral symptoms of photophobia, lymphadenopathy, sore throat, and possibly encephalitis.

EXANTHEM. The rash may appear at any time during the course of the illness, and it is usually generalized. Lesions are erythematous maculopapules with areas of confluence, but they may be urticarial, vesicular, or sometimes petechial (Figures 14-22 to 14-26). The palms and soles may be involved. The eruptions are more common in children than in adults. In most cases, the rash fades without pigmentation or scaling.

TREATMENT. Treatment consists of relieving symptoms.

Figure 14-22 Viral exanthem. Symmetric erythematous maculopapular eruption.

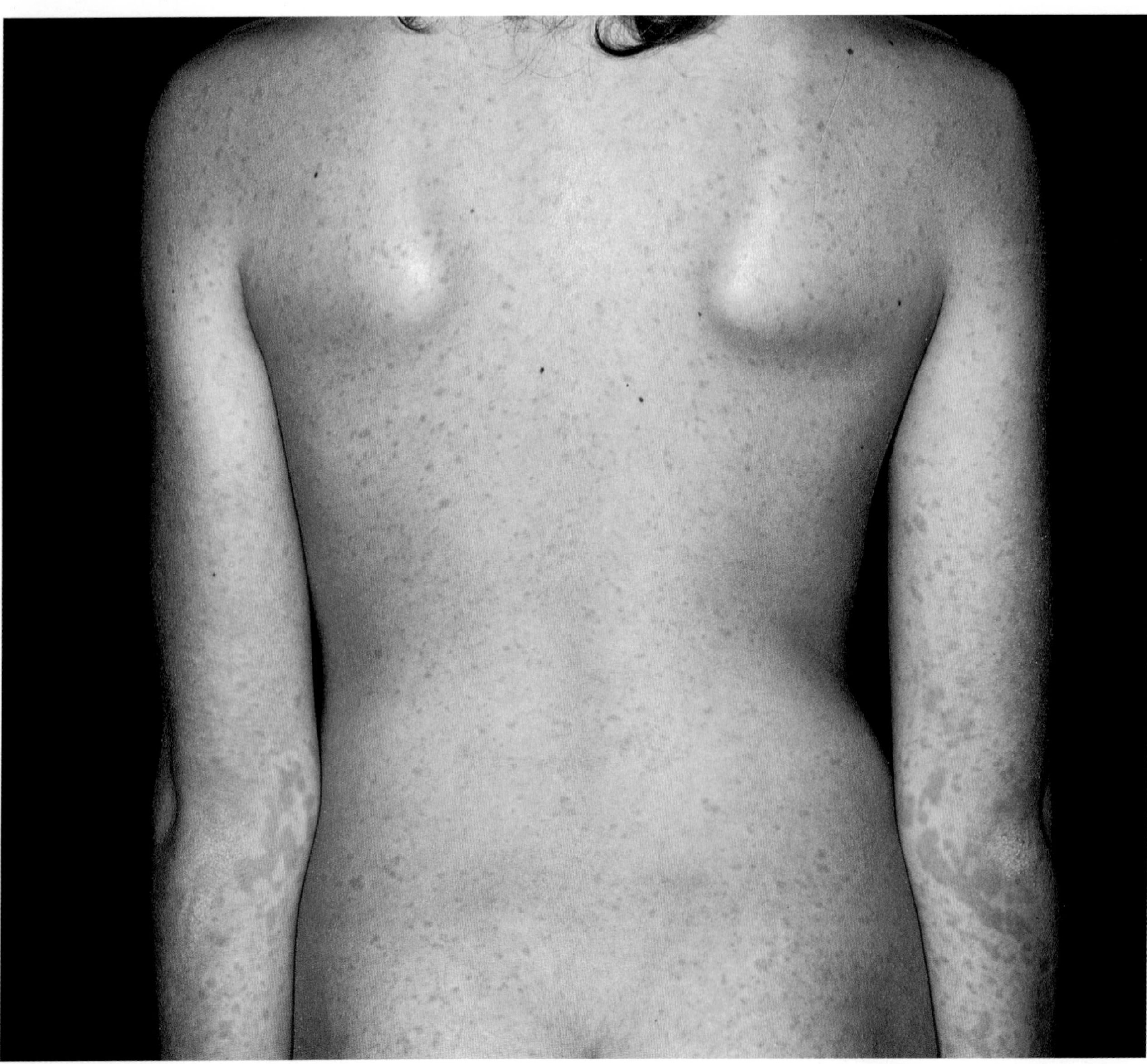

VIRAL EXANTHEM

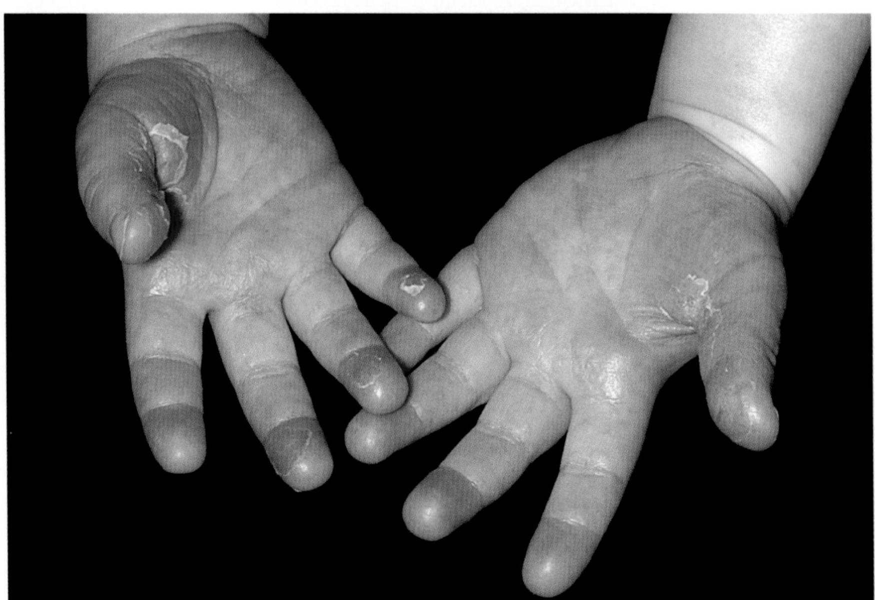

Figure 14-23 Viral exanthems can present with a variety of patterns on the palms. Papules, vesicles or diffuse erythema are seen.

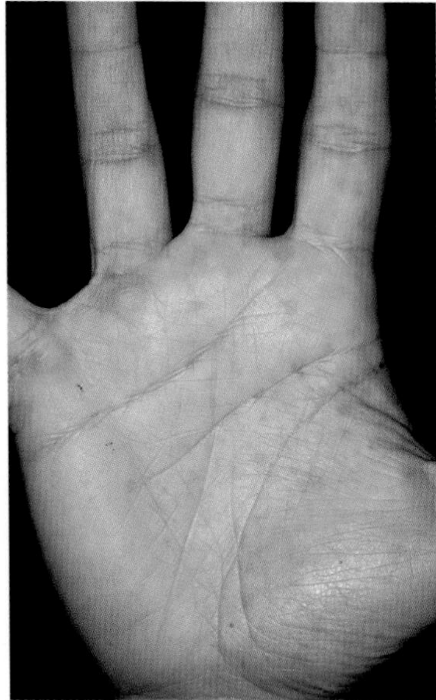

Figure 14-24 Viral exanthem with a maculopapular and vesicular pattern on the palm.

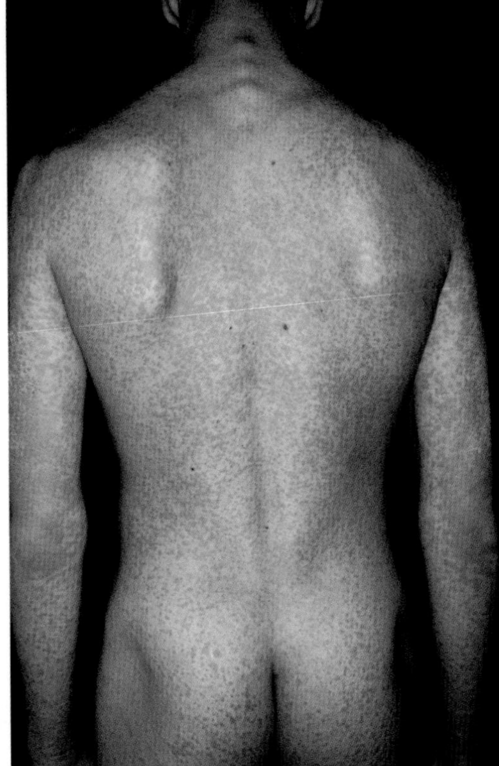

Figure 14-25 Viral exanthems may have several patterns. A diffuse maculopapular, blanching rash is a common pattern. Vesicular, urticarial, and petechial lesions may predominate.

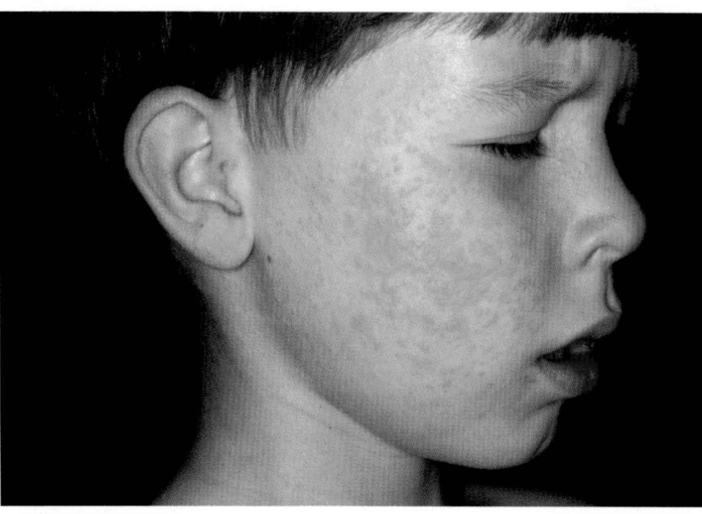

Figure 14-26 Viral exanthem with a papular urticarial pattern on the face.

Kawasaki disease

Kawasaki disease (KD), or mucocutaneous lymph node syndrome, was first described in Japan in 1967 but now is reported in both endemic and epidemic forms worldwide (Figure 14-27). Patients' ages range from 7 weeks to 12 years (mean, 2.6 years); rare adult cases are reported. Kawasaki disease is an acute multisystem vasculitis of unknown etiology that is associated with marked activation of T cells and monocytes/macrophages. An infectious agent is strongly suggested by its occurrence primarily in young children (who apparently lack immunity) and by the existence of outbreaks. Recurrences are rare. The major causes of short- and long-term morbidity are the cardiovascular manifestations. The histopathologic features of vasculitis involving arterioles, capillaries, and venules appear in the earliest phase of the disease.

THREE CLINICAL PHASES

Acute. The acute febrile phase lasts 7 to 14 days and ends with the resolution of fever. There is conjunctival infection, mouth and lip changes, swelling and erythema of the hands and feet, rash, and cervical lymphadenopathy.

Subacute. The subacute phase covers the period from the end of the fever to about day 25. Symptoms include desquamation of the fingers and toes, arthritis and arthralgia, and thrombocytosis.

Convalescent. The convalescent phase begins when clinical signs disappear and continues until the erythrocyte sedimentation rate (ESR) becomes normal, usually 6 to 8 weeks after the onset of illness.

CLINICAL MANIFESTATIONS. There is no single clinical finding or laboratory test that is diagnostic, but the diagnosis should be considered in children with rash and fever of unknown origin. The Centers for Disease Control and Prevention (CDC) definition is shown in Table 14-3. The evolution of signs and symptoms is shown in Figure 14-28. Children have high fever for 1 to 2 weeks, rash, and edema of the extremities that is painful and interferes with walking, and they are extremely irritable.

MAJOR DIAGNOSTIC FEATURES

Fever. The fever, without chills or sweats, is a constant feature (range, 5 to 30 days; mean, 8.5 days) in untreated patients. It begins abruptly, spikes from 101° to 104° F (usually 39° C), and does not respond to antibiotics or antipyretics. KD should be in the differential diagnosis of prolonged fever in infants; occasionally, prolonged fever is the only manifestation of KD. In patients treated with aspirin at 80 to 100 mg/kg/day and a single 2 gm/kg dose of intravenous gamma-globulin (IVGG), fever usually resolves in 1 or 2 days.

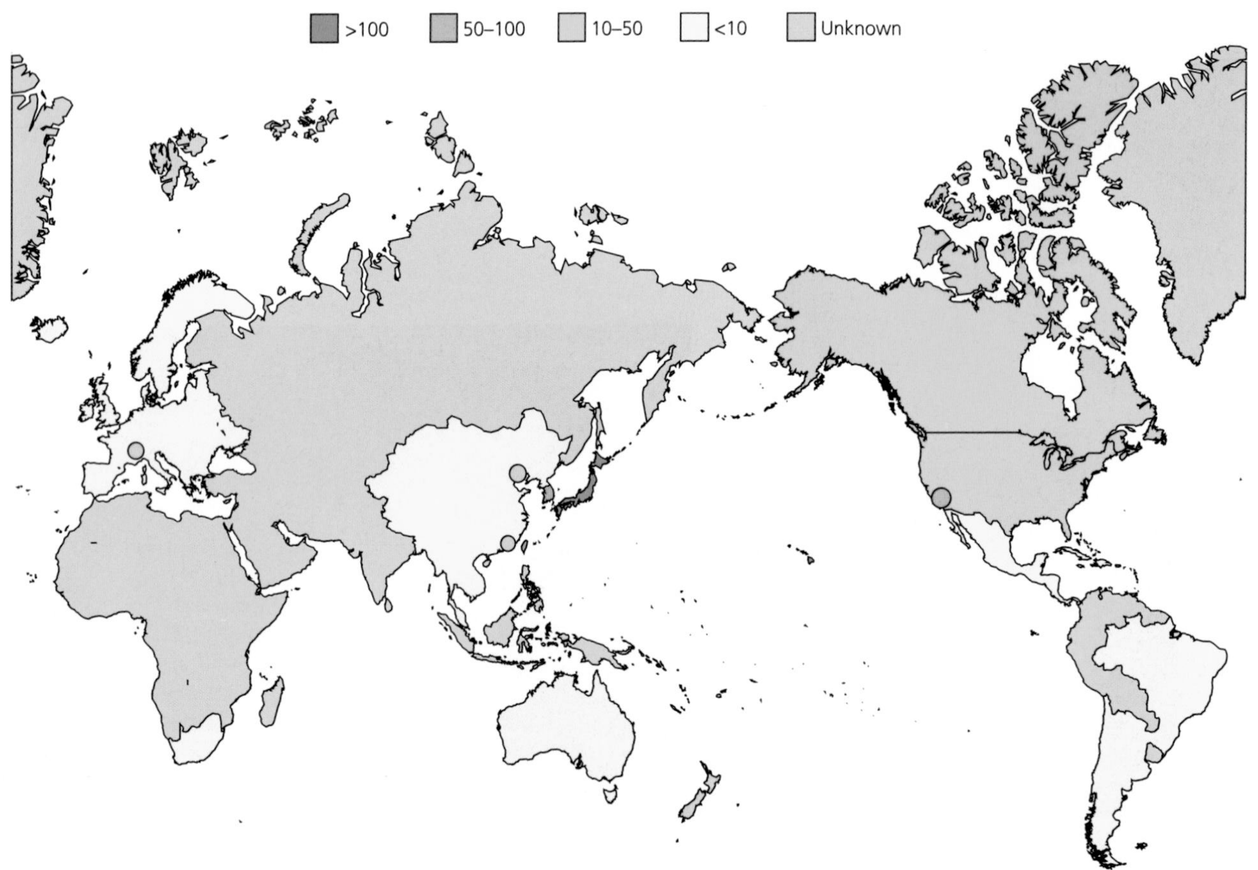

Figure 14-27 Cases of Kawasaki disease per 100,000 children younger than 5 years. (From *Lancet* 364(9433): 533-544, 2004. PMID: 15302199)

Table 14-3 Clinical and Laboratory Features of Kawasaki Disease

Epidemiological case definition (classic clinical criteria)—CDC*

Fever persisting at least 5 days + presence of at least 4 of the following:

1. Bilateral bulbar conjunctival injection without exudate
2. Changes in lips and oral cavity: Erythema, lips cracking, strawberry tongue, diffuse injection of oral and pharyngeal mucosae
3. Changes in extremities: Acute: Erythema of palms, soles; edema of hands, feet
   Subacute: Periungual peeling of fingers, toes in weeks 2 and 3
4. Polymorphous exanthem
5. Cervical lymphadenopathy (>1.5-cm diameter), usually unilateral

In the presence of 4 principal criteria, Kawasaki disease diagnosis can be made on day 4 of illness. Experienced clinicians who have treated many Kawasaki disease patients may establish diagnosis before day 4.

Other clinical and laboratory findings

Cardiovascular findings	
Congestive heart failure, myocarditis, pericarditis, valvular regurgitation Coronary artery abnormalities	Aneurysms of medium-size noncoronary arteries Raynaud's phenomenon Peripheral gangrene
Musculoskeletal system	
Arthritis, arthralgia	
Gastrointestinal tract	
Diarrhea, vomiting, abdominal pain Hepatic dysfunction	Hydrops of gallbladder
Central nervous system	
Extreme irritability Aseptic meningitis	Sensorineural hearing loss
Genitourinary system	
Urethritis/meatitis	
Other findings	
Erythema, induration at bacille Calmette-Guérin (BCG) inoculation site Anterior uveitis (mild)	Desquamating rash in groin

Laboratory findings in acute Kawasaki disease

Leukocytosis with neutrophilia and immature forms Elevated ESR Elevated CRP Anemia Abnormal plasma lipids Hypoalbuminemia	Hyponatremia Thrombocytosis after week 1 Sterile pyuria Elevated serum transaminases Elevated serum γ-glutamyl transpeptidase	Pleocytosis of cerebrospinal fluid Leukocytosis in synovial fluid Some infants present with thrombocytopenia and disseminated intravascular coagulation.

Exclusion of other diseases with similar findings

Differential diagnosis of Kawasaki disease: Diseases and disorders with similar clinical findings

Viral infections (e.g., measles, adenovirus, enterovirus, Epstein-Barr virus) Scarlet fever Staphylococcal scalded skin syndrome	Toxic shock syndrome Bacterial cervical lymphadenitis Drug hypersensitivity reactions Stevens-Johnson syndrome	Juvenile rheumatoid arthritis Rocky Mountain spotted fever Leptospirosis Mercury hypersensitivity reaction (acrodynia)

*Patients with fever at least 5 days and <4 principal criteria can be diagnosed with Kawasaki disease when coronary artery abnormalities are detected by two-dimensional (2DE) echocardiographic examinations or angiography.

Adapted from *Pediatrics* 114(6):1708-1733, 2004. *PMID: 15574639*

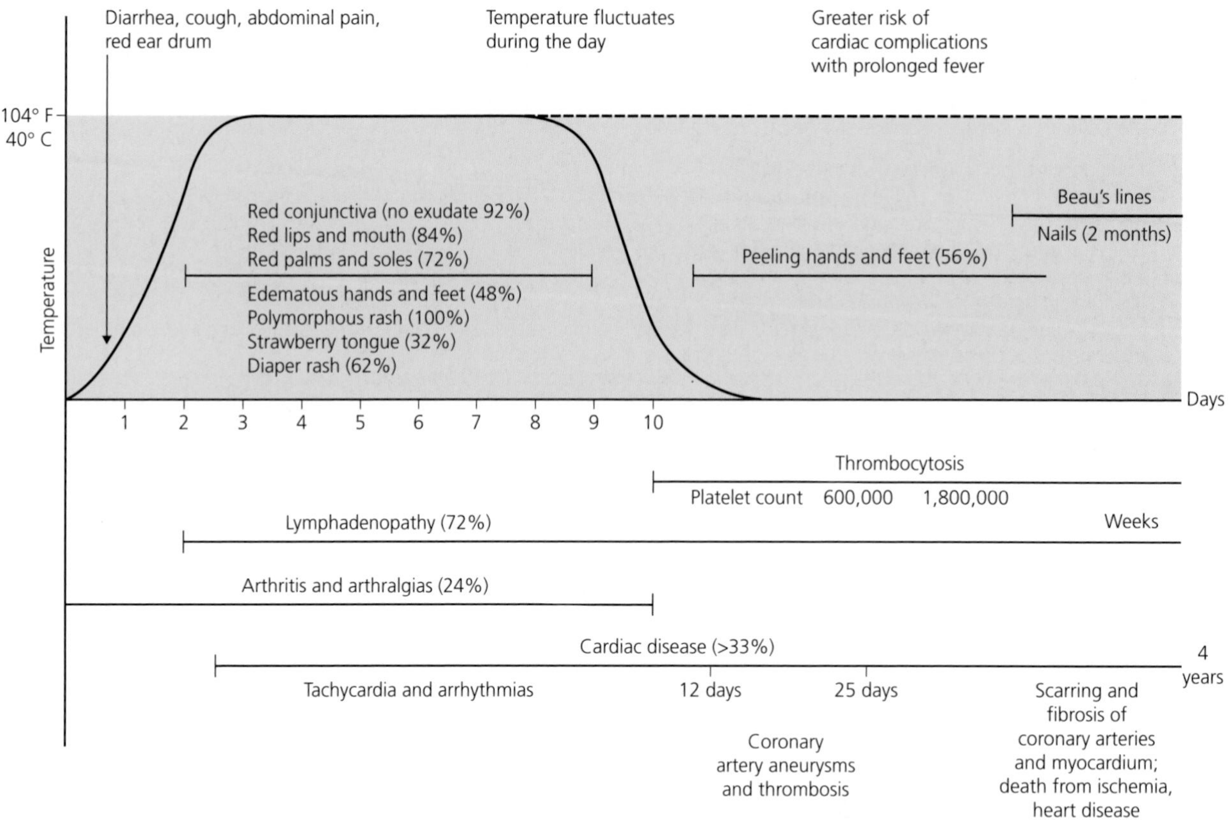

Figure 14-28 Kawasaki syndrome—distribution, signs and symptoms, and incidence.

Conjunctival injection. Self-limited, bilateral congestion of the bulbar and sometimes the palpebral conjunctivae is an almost constant feature. Typically, the inflammation spares the area of the conjunctiva around the limbus. Uveitis occurs in 70% of cases. There is no discharge or ulceration, as seen in Stevens-Johnson syndrome.

Oral mucous membrane changes. The lips and oral pharynx become red 1 to 3 days after the onset of the fever. The lips become dry, fissured, cracked, and crusted (Figures 14-29, *A-B*). Secondary infection of the lips can occur. Hypertrophic tongue papillae result in the "strawberry tongue" typically seen in scarlet fever. There is no sore throat, but small ulcerations may form. Cough occurs in 25% of patients.

Extremity changes. Within 3 days of the onset of fever, the palms and soles become red, and the hands and feet become edematous (Figures 14-29, *C-D*). The edema is nonpitting. The tenderness can be severe enough to limit walking and use of the hands. The edema lasts for approximately 1 week. Peeling of the hands and feet occurs 10 to 14 days after the onset of fever (see Figure 14-29, *D*). The peeling is similar to that seen in scarlet fever. Generalized desquamation of the skin is uncommon. The skin peels off in sheets, beginning around the nails and fingertips and progressing down to the palms and soles. The skin of children with diaper area inflammation peels at the margins of the rash and on the labia and scrotum. About 1 to 2 months after the onset of KD, transverse grooves across the nails may develop (Beau's lines).

Rash. A rash appears soon after the onset of fever. Several symptoms have been described. The most common forms are urticarial and a diffuse, deep red, maculopapular eruption (Figure 14-30, *A*). Less often the rash resembles erythema multiforme, scarlet fever, or the erythema marginatum seen in rheumatic fever. Dermatitis in the diaper area is common. The perineal rash usually occurs in the first week of the onset of symptoms. Red macules and papules become confluent (Figure 14-30, *B*). Desquamation occurs within 5 to 7 days. Perineal desquamation occurs 2 to 6 days before desquamation of the fingertips and toes (Figure 14-30, *C*). Vesiculopustules may develop over the elbows and knees.

Cervical lymphadenopathy. Firm, nontender, nonsuppurative lymphadenopathy is often limited to a single node and occurs in only 50% to 75% of patients. Children with acute cervical adenitis unresponsive to antibiotic therapy may have KD.

KAWASAKI DISEASE

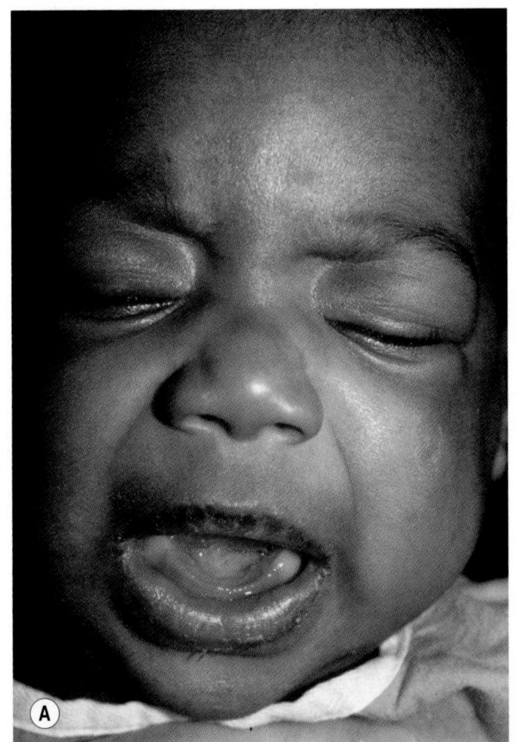

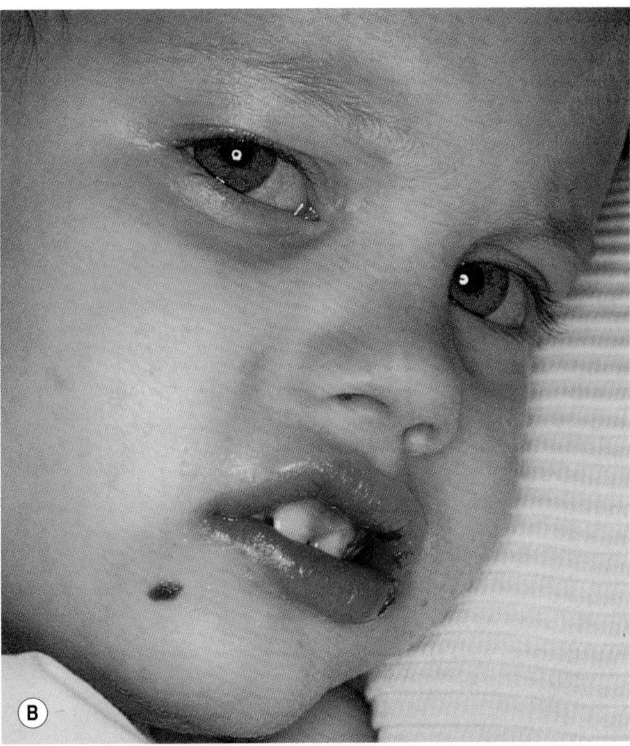

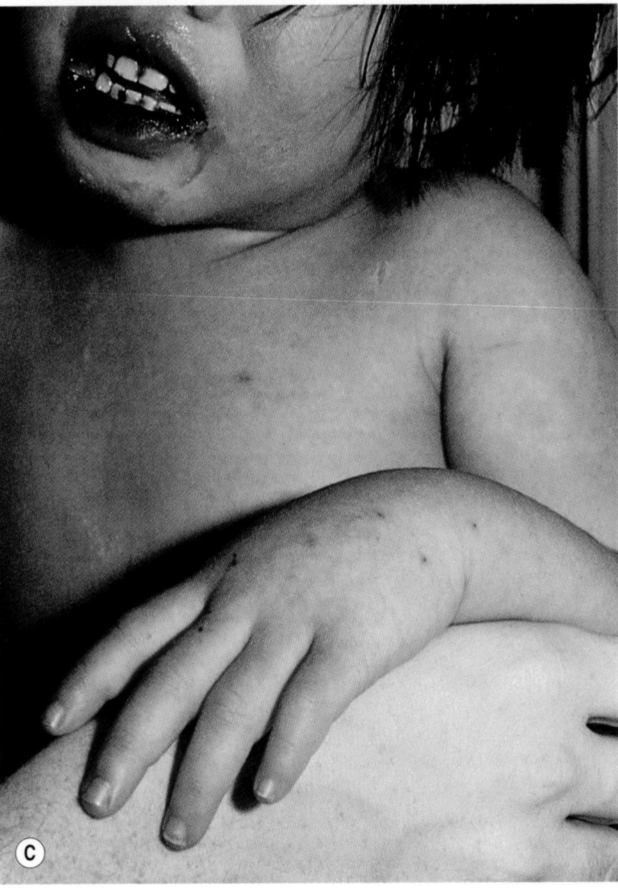

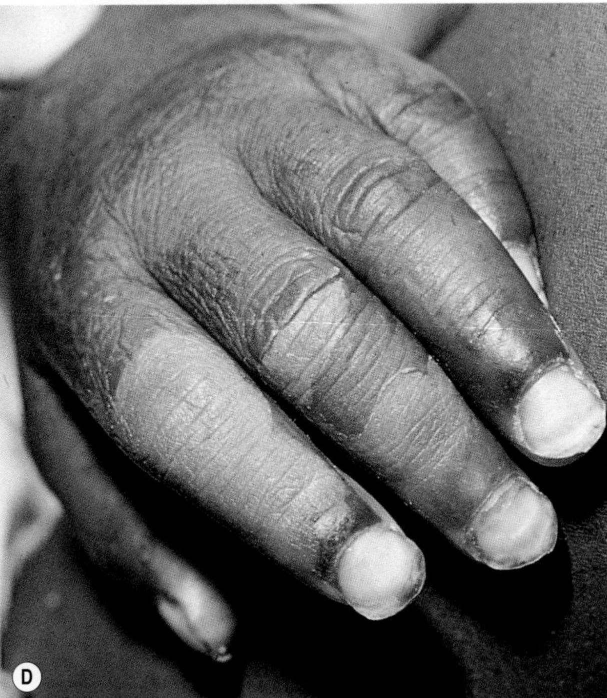

Figure 14-29 **A-B,** Nonpurulent conjunctival injection and "cherry red" lips with fissuring and crusting are early signs of the disease. (Courtesy Anne W. Lucky, M.D.)
C-D, The hands become red and swollen; they peel approximately 2 weeks after the onset of fever. (Courtesy Nancy B. Esterly, M.D.)

OTHER CLINICAL FEATURES

Abdominal symptoms. Acute distention of the gallbladder (hydrops) is common and presents with a right upper quadrant mass, jaundice, and pain or guarding in the first or second week of the illness; ultrasound is useful. The distention resolves in a few days without surgery.

Urethritis. Inflammation of the mucosa of the urethra causes sterile pyuria and is seen in more than 75% of patients.

Arthritis and arthralgias. A polyarticular arthritis or arthralgia of the feet and hands often develops in the first 10 days. This process may evolve to a pauciarticular arthritis that involves the larger joints such as the knees and hips. Early-onset arthritis is associated with synovial fluid white blood cell (WBC) counts of 100,000 to 300,000/μL with a polymorphonuclear (PMN) predominance; late-onset arthritis has a lower synovial WBC count of approximately 50,000/μL with 50% mononuclear cells.

Aseptic meningitis. Approximately 25% of patients have irritability or severe lethargy and stiff neck. Lumbar puncture reveals 25 to 100 WBCs/μL, predominantly lymphocytes, and normal glucose and normal to mildly elevated protein levels.

CARDIAC AND OTHER ORGAN VESSEL INVOLVEMENT. Kawasaki disease is the major cause of acquired heart disease in children in the United States. Cardiovascular manifestations are the leading cause of morbidity and mortality. Coronary artery aneurysms occur as a sequela of the vasculitis in 20% to 25% of untreated children. Echo-

KAWASAKI DISEASE

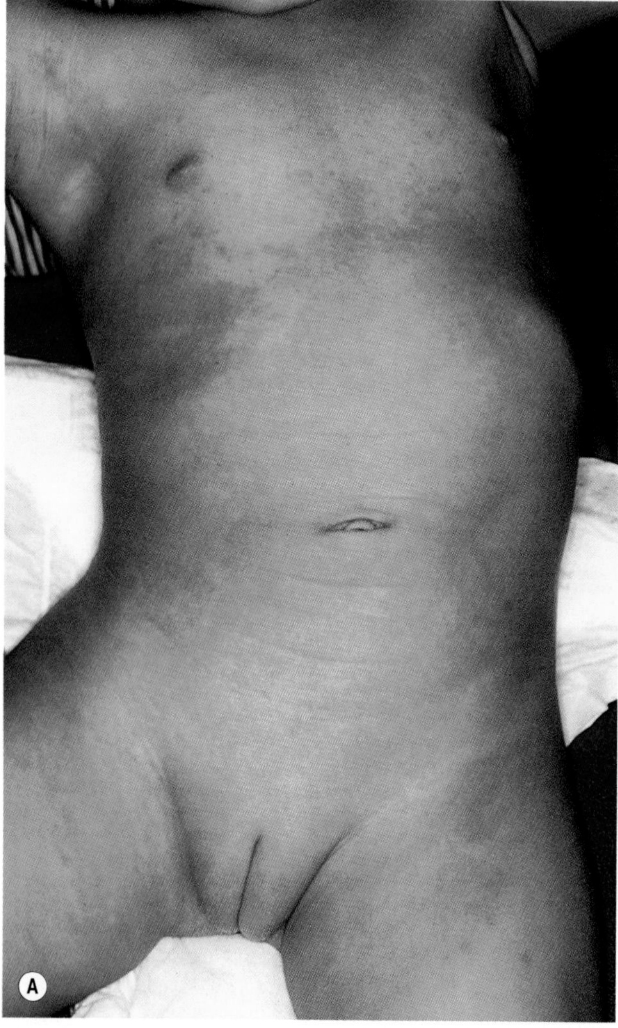

Diffuse, blanching, erythematous, macular exanthem.
The eruption is frequently concentrated in the perineal area.

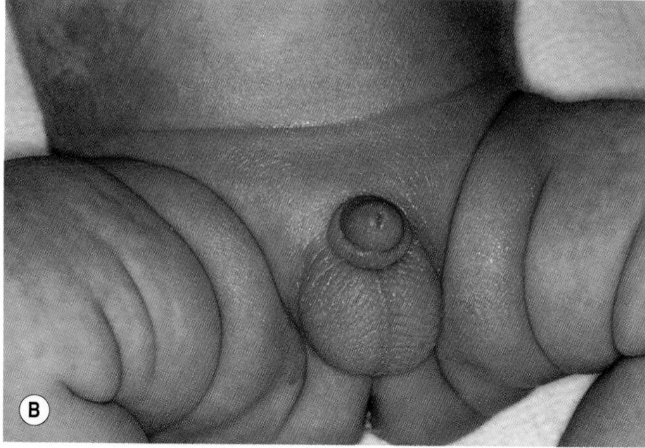

Red macules and papules appear in the perineal area 3 to 4 days after the onset of the illness. The rash becomes confluent and desquamates within 5 to 7 days. Desquamation of the fingertips and toes occurs 2 to 6 days later.

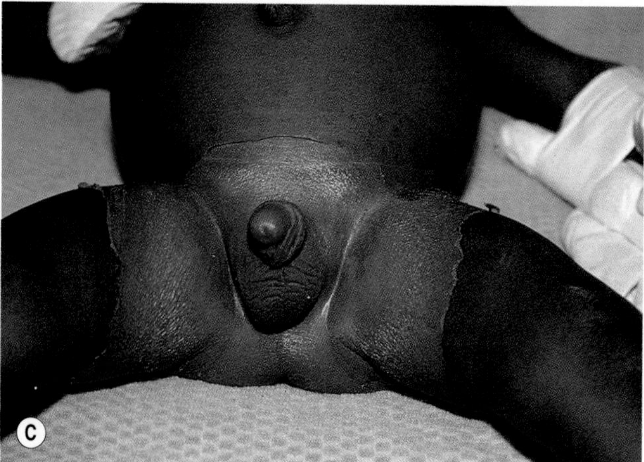

The skin of children with diaper-area inflammation peels at the margin of the rash. (Courtesy Anne W. Lucky, MD.)

Figure 14-30

cardiography is a reliable method to detect coronary artery aneurysms in the acute and subacute stages of the disease. Patients with no coronary artery aneurysms detected by echocardiography during the acute and subacute phases are clinically asymptomatic at least 10 years later. About 20% of patients who develop coronary artery aneurysms during the acute disease will develop coronary artery stenosis and might subsequently need treatment. Predictors of coronary artery aneurysms include persistent fever after IVIG therapy, low hemoglobin concentrations, low albumin concentrations, high white blood cell count, high band count, high C-reactive protein concentrations, male gender, and age under 1 year. Therefore laboratory evidence of increased inflammation combined with male gender, age under 6 months or over 8 years, and incomplete response to IVIG therapy create a profile of a high-risk patient with Kawasaki disease.

LABORATORY EVALUATION. The lack of a specific diagnostic test is a problem. Physicians use laboratory markers of inflammation (e.g., high levels of white blood cell count, C-reactive protein, and erythrocyte sedimentation rate) to support the diagnosis of Kawasaki disease in patients with rash/fever syndromes (Figure 14-31). The acute phase is characterized by marked inflammation and immune activation. Leukocytosis (20,000 to 30,000/μL) with a shift to the left (80%), thrombocytosis, anemia, and T-cell and monocyte-macrophage activation occur. Acute-phase reactants, such as ESR (90%), C-reactive protein, and serum alpha$_1$-antitrypsin, are elevated with the onset of fever and persist for up to 10 weeks after onset of illness. Other findings include mild transaminase elevations, abnormal urinalysis consisting of sterile pyuria (68%), and CSF pleocytosis (25%). Thrombocytosis is a distinctive sign of this disease. The platelet count begins to rise on the tenth day of the illness, peaks at 600,000 to 1.6 million/mm^3, and returns to normal by the thirtieth day of the illness. Echocardiography is obtained as soon as the diagnosis is suspected.

TREATMENT

IVIG. A single dose of 2 gm/kg IVIG infused over 10 to 12 hours is standard therapy. This therapy should be instituted within the first 10 days of illness and, if possible, within 7 days of illness. Treatment of Kawasaki disease before day 5 of illness appears no more likely to prevent cardiac sequelae than does treatment on days 5 to 7, but it may be associated with an increased need for IVIG retreatment. IVIG also should be administered to children presenting after the tenth day of illness (i.e., children in whom the diagnosis was missed earlier) if they have either persistent fever without other explanation or aneurysms and ongoing systemic inflammation, as manifested by elevated ESR or C-reactive protein (CRP) .

Aspirin. Aspirin is used to reduce inflammation and to inhibit platelet aggregation but has no effect on the development of coronary artery aneurysms. High doses of aspirin (80 to 100 mg/kg daily divided into four doses) are used in the acute inflammatory stage of the disease. Once the patient has been afebrile for 3 to 7 days, the dose of aspirin is decreased to a single daily dose of 3 to 5 mg/kg. This antiplatelet dose is continued for 4 to 6 weeks, until the concentrations of all inflammatory markers have returned to normal and no coronary artery damage has been noted by echocardiography. Because antipyretic doses of aspirin (40 mg/kg daily) in conjunction with influenza and varicella viruses have been epidemiologically linked to Reye's syndrome, immunization against influenza may be prudent in patients who need long-term aspirin therapy.

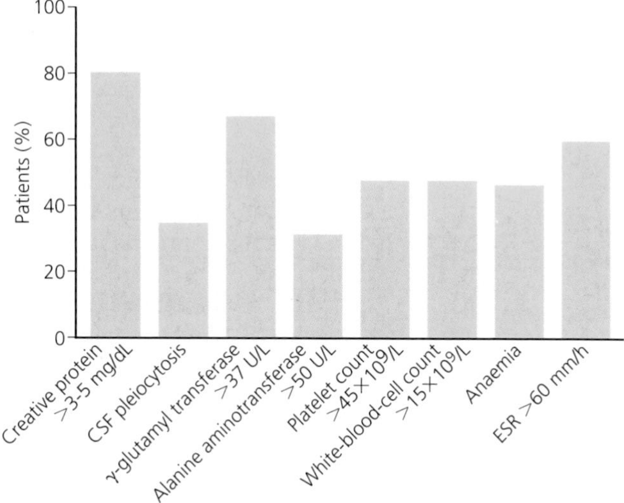

Laboratory findings in acute Kawasaki syndrome. Proportion of patients with laboratory abnormalities when investigated within 10 days of fever onset. Anaemia is defined as haemoglobulin concentration <2 SD below the mean for age. Cerebrospinal-fluid (CSF) pleiocytosis is defined as >10 white blood cells per high-power field. ESR=erythrocyte sedimentation rate.

Figure 14-31 Laboratory markers of inflammation in Kawasaki disease. (From *Lancet* 364(9433):533-544, 2004. *PMID: 15302199*)

Superantigen toxin-mediated illnesses

Streptococcus and *Staphylococcus* can produce circulating toxins that cause clinical disease. Many of these toxins function as superantigens.

Pyrogenic toxin superantigens comprise a large family of exotoxins made by *Staphylococcus aureus* and group A streptococci. These toxins include toxic shock syndrome toxin-1, the staphylococcal enterotoxins, and the streptococcal pyrogenic exotoxins (synonyms: scarlet fever toxins and erythrogenic toxins), all of which have the ability to cause toxic shock syndromes and related illnesses (Box 14-2).

SUPERANTIGENS. Normally antigens are processed inside antigen-presenting cells. A protein fragment of the antigen is then expressed on the cell surface in the groove of the major histocompatibility type II complex (MHCII). The antigen-MHCII complex then interacts with a receptor on a T cell, which results in cytokine production.

Superantigens are proteins with a special chemical structure and they are manufactured by bacteria and viruses that are not processed by antigen-presenting cells. They bind directly to the MHCII complex outside of the groove and cause a nonspecific stimulation of T cells.

Conventional antigens activate 0.01% or more of the body's T cells. A superantigen/T-cell interaction activates 5% to 30% of the entire T-cell population. This leads to massive cytokine production, especially of tumor necrosis factor-α (TNF-α), interleukin-1 (IL-1), and interleukin-6 (IL-6). Fever, emesis, hypotension, shock, tissue injury, and cutaneous signs including strawberry tongue, acral erythema with desquamation, and erythematous eruption with perineal accentuation are the result of massive cytokine production.

The best-characterized superantigens are staphylococcal enterotoxins A through E, toxic shock syndrome toxin-1, and exfoliating toxin; these are all toxins released from *S. aureus*. Other bacterial proteins known to have superantigen properties are streptococcal pyrogenic exotoxins A through C and streptococcal M protein.

Box 14-2 Toxin-Mediated Streptococcal and Staphylococcal Diseases

- Necrotizing fasciitis
- Recalcitrant erythematous desquamating disorder
- Scarlet fever
- Staphylococcal scalded skin syndrome
- Streptococcal toxic shock syndrome (STSS)
- Toxic shock syndrome
- Atopic dermatitis*
- Guttate psoriasis*
- Kawasaki disease*

*Possibly toxin mediated.

Toxic shock syndrome

Toxic shock syndrome (TSS), originally described in 1978, is a rare, potentially fatal, multisystem illness associated with *S. aureus* infection and production of superantigen toxins. Early cases were associated with tampon use. Most cases now occur in the postoperative setting, but TSS has been described in association with influenza, sinusitis, tracheitis, postpartum state, intravenous drug use, HIV infection, cellulitis, burn wounds, and allergic contact dermatitis.

Infected burn wounds in hospitalized children and bacterial tracheitis are relatively high-risk settings for pediatric TSS.

SUPERANTIGEN PRODUCTION. Five enterotoxins are elaborated by staphylococci (SE A to E) plus TSS toxin-1 (TSST-1). Many cases of TSS are mediated by TSST-1 and enterotoxin B and C production, which is associated with massive release of cytokines (TNF-α and IL-1). These cytokines produce fever, rash, hypotension, tissue injury, and shock. Absence of antibody to TSST-1 is a major risk factor for acquisition of TSS.

Erythrogenic toxins (pyrogenic exotoxins) A, B, and C produced by group A beta-hemolytic streptococci (*S. pyogenes*) may cause a disease with all the defining criteria for TSS. Streptococci toxic shock syndrome (STSS) differs from that caused by *S. aureus* in two ways: (1) a focus of infection in soft tissue and skin is usually present in STSS, and (2) many STSS patients have bacteremia.

CLINICAL MANIFESTATIONS. The evolution of signs and symptoms is illustrated in Figure 14-32. The CDC definition of TSS requires a temperature greater than 38.9° C, hypotension with a systolic blood pressure less than 90 mm Hg (or postural dizziness), rash, desquamation, evidence of multiple organ system involvement, and exclusion of other reasonable pathogens. Recurrences occur in as many as 30% to 40% of cases.

DERMATOLOGIC MANIFESTATIONS. The disease has several features in common with KD and scarlet fever. A diffuse scarlatiniform erythroderma, bulbar conjunctiva hyperemia, and palmar edema are highly characteristic early signs. Desquamation of the tips of the fingers and toes occurs 1 to 2 weeks after the onset in exactly the same manner as is seen in scarlet fever and KD.

DIFFERENTIAL DIAGNOSIS. TSS can mimic many diseases. The differential diagnosis of TSS is drug eruptions, KD, scarlet fever, staphylococcal scalded skin syndrome, toxic epidermal necrolysis, and viral exanthems.

DIAGNOSIS. A biopsy may be helpful in the early stages. Assays for toxin and antibody can be performed.

TREATMENT. Treatment of TSS includes hydration, administration of vasopressors, removal of tampons, and incision and drainage of abscesses.

TOXIC SHOCK SYNDROME

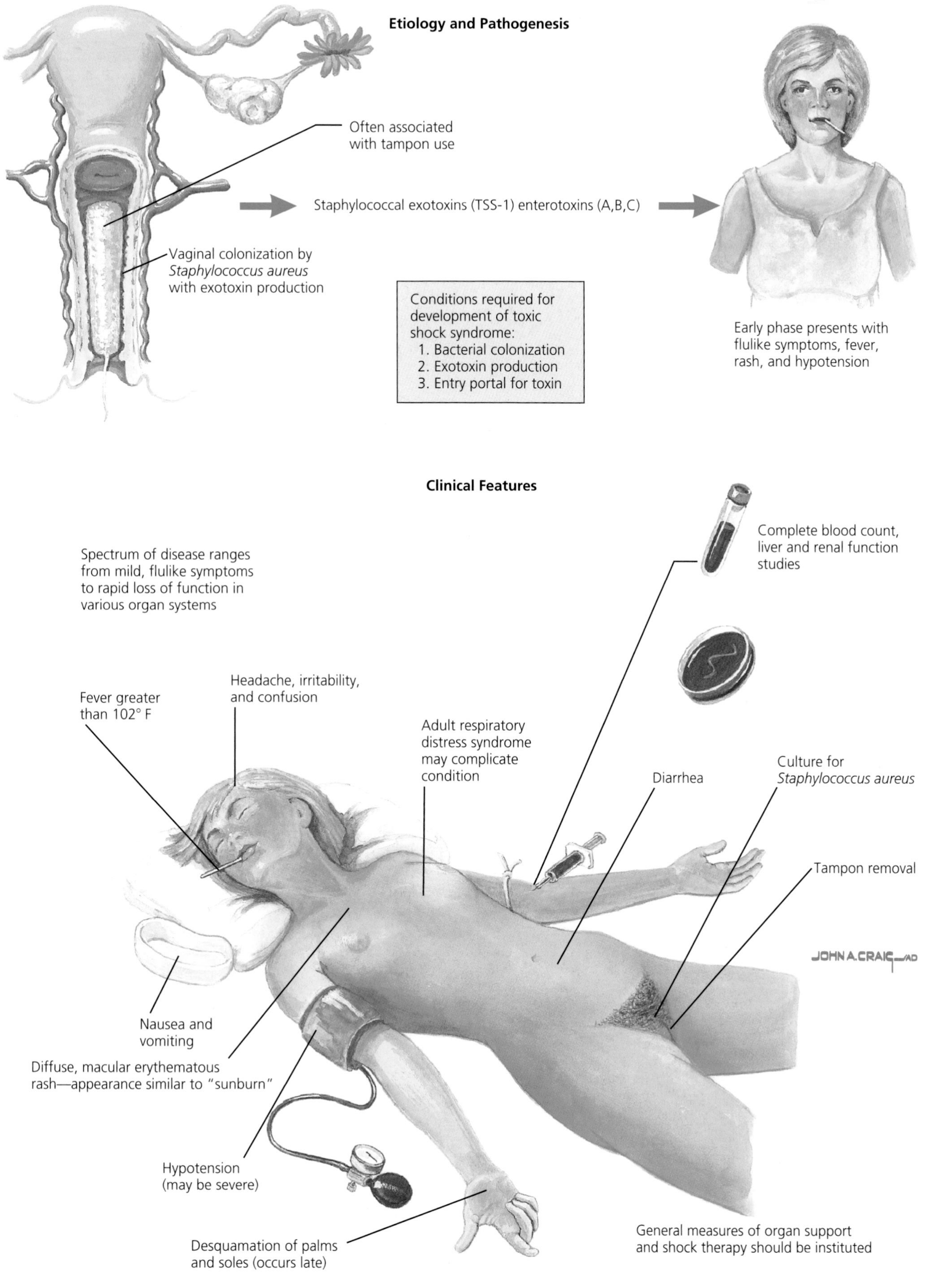

Etiology and Pathogenesis
Often associated with tampon use
Staphylococcal exotoxins (TSS-1) enterotoxins (A,B,C)
Vaginal colonization by *Staphylococcus aureus* with exotoxin production
Conditions required for development of toxic shock syndrome:
1. Bacterial colonization
2. Exotoxin production
3. Entry portal for toxin
Early phase presents with flulike symptoms, fever, rash, and hypotension
Clinical Features
Spectrum of disease ranges from mild, flulike symptoms to rapid loss of function in various organ systems
Complete blood count, liver and renal function studies
Fever greater than 102° F
Headache, irritability, and confusion
Adult respiratory distress syndrome may complicate condition
Diarrhea
Culture for *Staphylococcus aureus*
Tampon removal
JOHN A.CRAIG—AD
Nausea and vomiting
Diffuse, macular erythematous rash—appearance similar to "sunburn"
Hypotension (may be severe)
Desquamation of palms and soles (occurs late)
General measures of organ support and shock therapy should be instituted

Figure 14-32

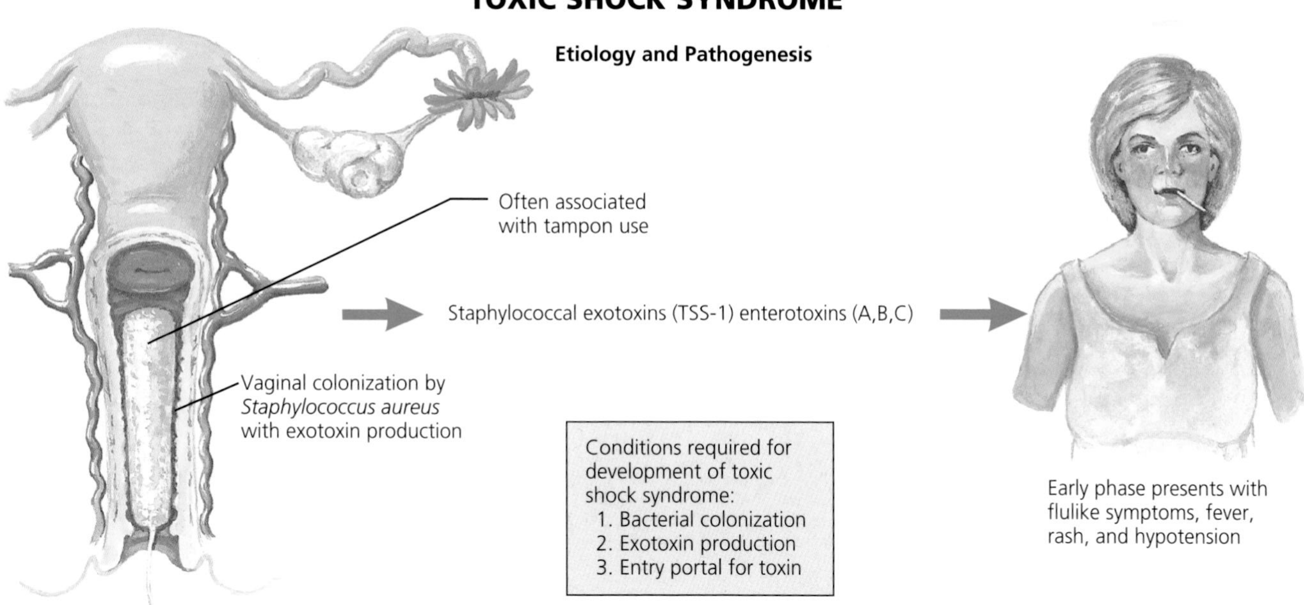

Cutaneous drug reactions

INCIDENCE. Rashes are among the most common adverse reactions to drugs. They occur in many forms and mimic many dermatoses. They occur in 2% to 3% of hospitalized patients (Table 14-4); in those patients there is no correlation between the development of an adverse reaction and the patient's age, diagnosis, or survival. The last Boston Collaborative Drug Surveillance Project estimated that approximately 30% of hospitalized patients experience adverse events attributable to drugs and that 3% to 28% of all hospital admissions are related to adverse drug eruptions.

Any dermatologic condition that appears within 2 weeks of starting a medication should include "drug-induced" in the differential.

Online and other resources: The websites pdr.net and MEDLINE provide current information on drug interactions. *The Drug Eruption Reference Manual* by Jerome Litt is available in paperback and online (www.drugeruptiondata.com). Drug interaction information is found at www.druginteractions.com and www.epocrates.com.

When drug-specific IgE antibodies bind to corresponding mast cell or basophil surface receptors, vasoactive mediators are released within minutes, causing an immediate-type reaction, clinically noted as pruritus, erythema, urticaria, angioedema, or anaphylaxis.

Table 14-4 Rates of Allergic Skin Reactions to Specific Drugs (Urticaria, Generalized Maculopapular Eruption, Generalized Pruritus)

Drug or substance	Reactions (%)
Platelet	45
Amoxicillin	5
Trimethoprim-sulfamethoxazole	3
Ampicillin	3
Ipodate	3
Blood	2
Penicillin	2
Cephalosporins	2
Erythromycin	2
Dihydralazine hydrochloride	2
Cyanocobalamin	2
Quinidine	1
Hyoscine butylbromide	1
Cimetidine	1
Phenylbutazone	1

Data from Bigby M et al: *JAMA* 256:3358, 1986.
PMID: 2946876

The drugs that commonly trigger this IgE mechanism are the beta-lactam antibiotics (especially the penicillins and first-generation cephalosporins) or autologous sera. These reactions are not dose dependent and require that the patient be sensitized before the "allergic" episode. On discontinuance or dissipation of the triggering agent, the cutaneous reaction usually resolves spontaneously within 48 hours.

MECHANISM. Two groups of mechanisms are involved in the pathogenesis of drug reactions: immunologic, with all four types of hypersensitivity reactions described; and nonimmunologic, accounting for at least 75% of all drug reactions.

Toxic epidermal necrolysis and other severe cutaneous adverse drug reactions may be linked to an inherited defect in the detoxification of drug metabolites. In a few predisposed patients a drug metabolite may bind to proteins in the epidermis and trigger an immune response leading to immunoallergic cutaneous adverse drug reactions. The drugs most often responsible for the eruptions are antimicrobial agents and antipyretic/antiinflammatory analgesics.

CLINICAL CHARACTERISTICS. The most common types of reactions are maculopapular (exanthematous eruptions), urticarial, and fixed drug eruptions (Box 14-3). Toxic epidermal necrolysis, erythema multiforme, and fixed drug eruptions share similar pathologic features and are caused by many of the same drugs. Photoallergic drug reactions require the interaction of drugs, UV irradiation, and the immune system. Eruptions seen in serum sickness include exanthem, urticaria, vasculitis, urticarial vasculitis, and erythema multiforme.

The typical patient seen by the dermatologist is a hospitalized patient who is receiving several medications. A fever occurs and hours later a diffuse maculopapular rash, hives, and/or generalized pruritus develop; the attending physician stops all medications and consults the dermatologist. Although maculopapular and urticarial eruptions are the most common examples of a drug eruption, several other patterns occur.

Box 14-3 **Cutaneous Patterns of Drug Eruptions**

Acneiform	Photosensitivity
Alopecia	Pigmentation
Eczema	Pityriasis rosea–like
Erythema multiforme	Purpura
Erythema nodosum	Seborrheic dermatitis–like
Exanthems (maculopapular, morbilliform)	Toxic epidermal necrolysis
Exfoliative erythroderma	Urticarial vasculitis
Fixed eruption	Vesiculobullous (pemphigus-like)
Lichenoid (lichen planus–like)	Lupus erythematosus–like

Knowledge of these patterns and the drugs that commonly cause them helps to solve what is often a difficult problem when patients take many drugs simultaneously (Box 14-3).

CLINICAL DIAGNOSIS. Examine the patient and determine the primary lesion and distribution. Then ask the following questions: "When did it start? Does it itch?" Drugs can cause skin symptoms without a rash (itching, burning, pain). Maculopapular and urticarial eruptions are the most frequent patterns. Maculopapular eruptions occur suddenly, often with fever, 7 to 10 days after the drug is first taken. They are generalized, symmetric, and often pruritic. Drug eruptions are always suspected when hives are present. One must be familiar with the many other patterns of skin eruptions and the types of eruptions caused by specific drugs in order to diagnose drug-related disease (see Box 14-3). Knowledge of the frequency with which certain drugs cause allergic drug reactions also helps to identify offending agents. The clinical characteristics of each type of reaction are described here.

DIAGNOSTIC TESTS. Box 14-4 lists tests to consider.

Serum tryptase. Serum tryptase is a biochemical marker of the release of mast cell granules that occurs during an allergic reaction.

Mast cells release histamine and tryptase. Tryptase is secreted exclusively by mast cells. It is not detectable in the serum of healthy or allergic individuals. Tryptase levels greatly increase after an anaphylactic reaction caused by drugs, insect venom, and food. Increased serum tryptase levels have been associated with acute anaphylaxis with or without itching, flushing, or urticaria, especially in severe reactions with cardiovascular involvement. For less severe acute reactions, a negative serum tryptase level does not rule out drug-induced anaphylaxis.

Tryptase may be used to verify an anaphylactic event attributable to allergen or drug exposure. Patients with allergic urticaria and those with idiosyncratic responses to acetylsalicylic acid (ASA) exhibited a small increase in serum tryptase level. Increased levels of tryptase can be detected up to 3 to 6 hours after the anaphylactic reaction. Tryptase is stable and may even be determined on postmortem serum (up to 24 hours) if anaphylaxis is suspected as the cause of death. Serial measurements may be needed to confirm mast cell participation in milder reactions. Levels return to normal within 12 to 14 hours after release.

MANAGEMENT. The management of patients suspected of having a drug eruption is listed in Box 14-5.

Box 14-4 **Diagnostic Tests to Consider in the Evaluation of a Possible Drug Eruption**

- Skin biopsy to categorize an eruption (i.e., urticaria, perivascular dermatitis, leukocytoclastic vasculitis) or to differentiate it from psoriasis, lichen planus, or cutaneous T-cell lymphoma.
- Drug levels for overdose or in a comatose or noncommunicative patient
- Patch test for allergic contact dermatitis
- Prick, radioallergosorbent test (RAST), or intradermal testing indicated only for IgE-induced, immediate-type (urticarial) reactions (e.g., penicillin, insulin, papain, protamine, streptokinase, heterologous antisera, tetanus toxoid, cephalosporins). These require expertise for antigen selection.
- Serum tryptase levels are associated with acute anaphylaxis with or without itching, flushing, or urticaria, especially in severe reactions with cardiovascular involvement. For less severe acute reactions, negative serum tryptase level does not rule out drug-induced anaphylaxis.
- Immunoassays for drug-specific antibody isotypes other than IgE high titers of drug-specific IgG antibodies have been associated with drug-induced immune complex syndromes (e.g., serum sickness).

Box 14-5 **Management of Patients with a Suspected Dermatologic Drug Reaction**

- Make a flow sheet documenting time of onset of eruption, drugs, dosages, duration, and interruptions in the use of drugs.
- Determine the frequency of adverse reactions to the drug in the general population.
- Is the drug likely to be responsible for the cutaneous reaction, or is the eruption an unrelated dermatologic disease?
- Determine time of onset. Most cutaneous drug reactions occur 1 to 2 weeks after starting the drug.
- Consider ordering drug levels. Some cutaneous reactions may be dependent on dose or cumulative toxicity.
- Discontinue suspected offending drugs. Most adverse dermatologic reactions to drugs will improve when the drug is stopped.
- Rechallenge is the most accurate way to identify the offending drug. The decision to rechallenge a patient is made on an individual basis. Rechallenge in patients who have had urticarial-like, bullous-like, or erythema multiforme–like eruptions can be very dangerous. A reaction that fails to recur on rechallenge with a drug is unlikely to be caused by that agent.
- Symptomatic relief is provided with antihistamines and group V topical steroids.

DRUG ERUPTIONS: CLINICAL PATTERNS AND MOST FREQUENTLY CAUSAL DRUGS (Box 14-6)

Exanthems (maculopapular)

Maculopapular eruptions, the most frequent of all cutaneous drug reactions, are often indistinguishable from viral exanthems. They are the classic ampicillin and amoxicillin drug rashes, but practically any drug can trigger a maculopapular eruption (see Box 14-6). Red macules and papules become confluent in a symmetric, generalized distribution that often spares the face (Figures 14-33 through 14-36). Itching is common. Mucous membranes, palms, and soles may be involved. Fever may be present from the onset. These eruptions are identical in appearance to a viral exanthem and routine laboratory tests usually fail to differentiate the two diseases. Onset is 7 to 10 days after starting the drug but may not occur until after the drug is stopped. The rash lasts for 1 to 2 weeks and fades in some cases even if the drug is continued. Lesions clear rapidly following withdrawal of the implicated agent and may progress to a generalized exfoliative dermatitis if use of the drug is not discontinued. The pathogenesis is unknown.

AMPICILLIN RASHES. Two types of skin reactions occur: a urticarial reaction mediated by skin-sensitizing antibody and a much more common exanthematous maculopapular reaction for which no allergic basis can be established (see Figure 14-34). Ampicillin and other penicillins should not be given to patients who have had previous urticarial reactions while taking ampicillin. Ampicillin may safely be given to patients who have previously had a maculopapular ampicillin rash. The exanthematous reaction occurs in 50% to 80% of patients with infectious mononucleosis who take ampicillin. One study reported a high rate of drug exanthems in patients taking ampicillin in combination with allopurinol, but another study found no increased rate.

CLINICAL PRESENTATION. The rash begins 5 to 10 days (range, 1 day to 4 weeks) after starting the drug and may occur after the drug is terminated.

Latent periods of 2 to 3 weeks are seen with allopurinol, nitrofurantoin, and phenytoin. Eruptions may subside with continued use of the drug and may not recur on repeat exposure.

The rash starts on the trunk as a mildly pruritic, red, maculopapular, sometimes confluent eruption and spreads in hours in a symmetric fashion to the face and extremities. The palms, soles, and mucous membranes are spared. Lesions appear confluent in intertriginous areas (axilla, groin, and inframammary skin). Pruritus occurs frequently, and the intensity varies. A transient mild-to-moderate fever is common. Previously sensitized patients develop fever within hours of drug administration. Transient lymphadenopathy can accompany severe cases. Sometimes the eruption progresses to generalized erythroderma or exfoliative dermatitis. The rash begins to fade in 3 days and is gone in 6 days, even if the drug is continued.

DIFFERENTIAL DIAGNOSIS. Viral eruptions look and feel like drug-induced maculopapular eruptions. Drug maculopapular eruptions can be scarlatiniform, rubelliform (lentil-sized macules and faint papules), or morbilliform (resembles measles). Drug eruptions usually develop within 1 week of starting treatment and last 1 to 2 weeks. Features that support a viral exanthem are hemorrhage and the absence of tissue eosinophilia.

Drug-induced morbilliform eruptions are common with ampicillin, amoxicillin, allopurinol, and trimethoprim/sulfamethoxazole (TMP-SMX) (used in AIDS patients).

DIAGNOSIS. The histology is nonspecific. Skin biopsy may rule out other diseases. Rechallenge for diagnostic purposes is not a routine practice.

MANAGEMENT. Stop the offending drug and provide symptomatic relief. Group V topical corticosteroid creams and cool compresses are soothing and control itching. Treat severe itching or an extensive eruption with prednisone (0.5 to 1.0 mg/kg/day) for 7 to 10 days. Antihistamines provide sedation but are usually not effective at controlling itching because histamine does not cause maculopapular lesions. Stop treatment of any drug causing a generalized, symmetric, maculopapular rash, and do not retreat with the same drug. Skin-test patients who require ampicillin if the nature of a previous reaction is unknown and there is no adequate substitute drug.

MACULOPAPULAR DRUG ERUPTIONS

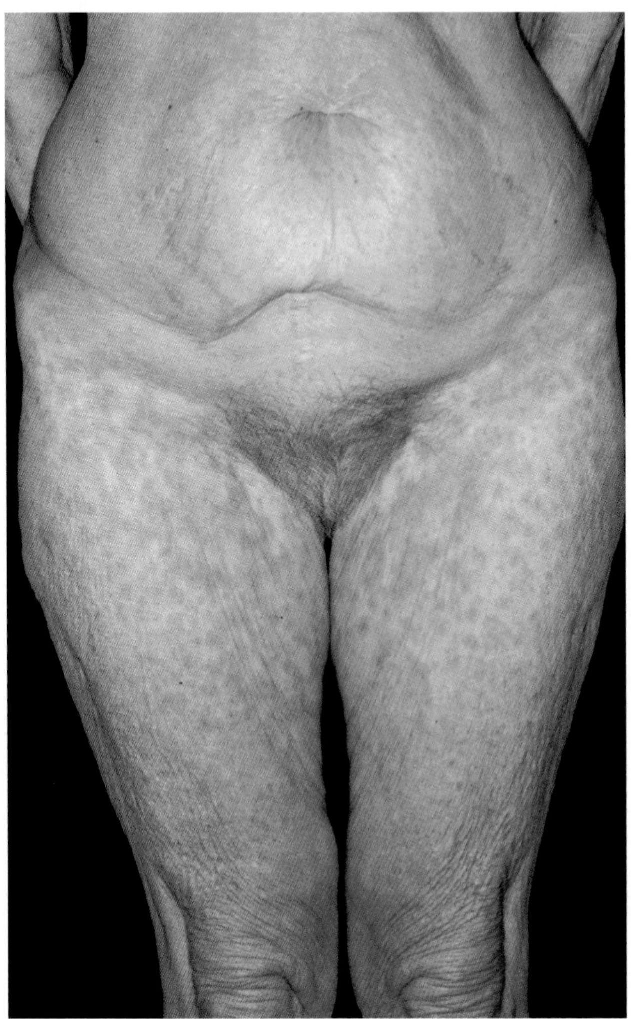

Figure 14-33 Maculopapular exanthems are the most common drug eruption pattern. They occur 7 to 10 days after starting the drug. Exanthems are often widespread and symmetric and spare the face, palms, and soles.

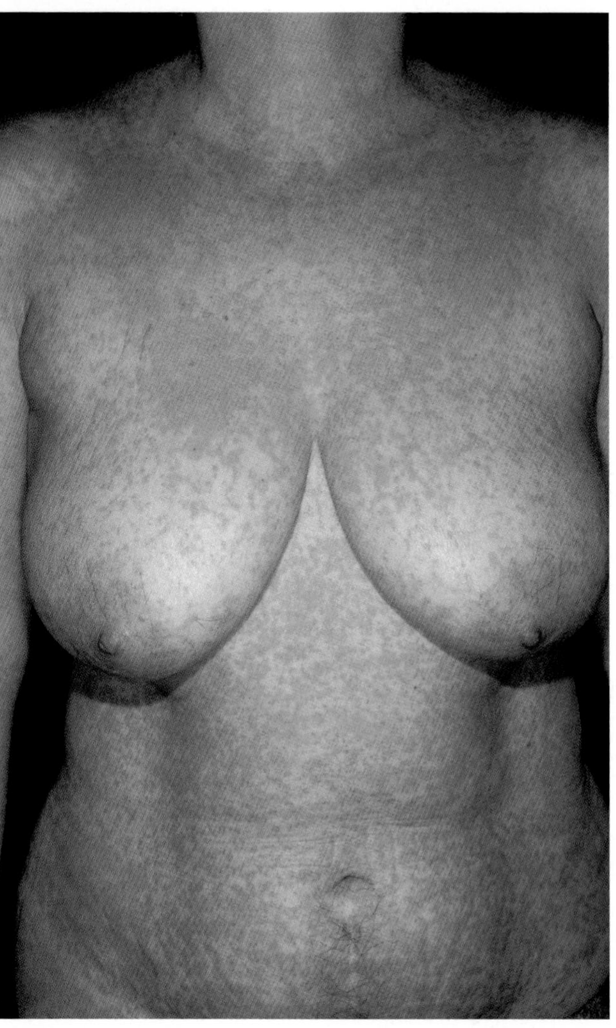

Figure 14-34 Drug eruption (ampicillin). Asymmetric, confluent maculopapular eruption.

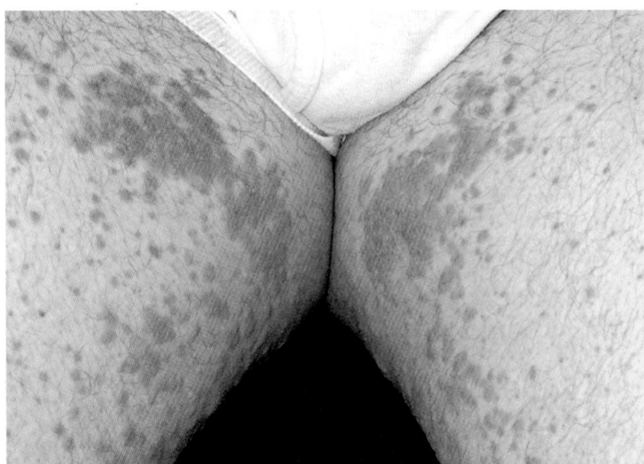

Figure 14-35 Maculopapular exanthems are often symmetric and present with confluent erythematous macules and papules.

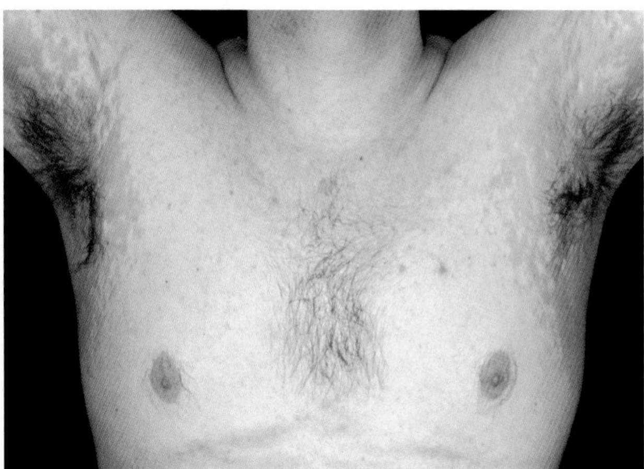

Figure 14-36 Symmetric distribution of a confluent maculopapular drug eruption.

Box 14-6 Drug Reactions and the Drugs That Cause Them

Maculopapular (exanthematous) eruptions

Allopurinol
Amoxicillin
Amphotericin B
Ampicillin
Barbiturates
Captopril
Carbamazepine
Chlorpromazine
Diflunisal (Dolobid)
Enalapril
Gentamicin
Gold salts
Isoniazid
Lithium
Meclofenamate
Naproxen
Oral hypoglycemic agents
Penicillin
Phenothiazines
Phenylbutazone
Phenytoin (5% of children—dose dependent)
Piroxicam
Quinidine
Sulfonamides
Thiazides
Thiouracil
Trimethoprim-sulfamethoxazole (in patients with AIDS)

Anaphylactic reactions

Aspirin
Penicillin
Radiographic dye
Sera (animal derived)
Tolmetin (Tolectin)

Serum sickness

Aspirin
Penicillin
Streptomycin
Sulfonamides
Thiouracils

Acneiform (pustular) eruptions

ACTH
Androgens
Bromides
Corticosteroids
Hormones
Iodides
Isoniazid
Lithium
Oral contraceptives
Phenobarbital (aggravates acne)
Phenytoin

Alopecia

Alkylating agents
Allopurinol
Anticoagulants
Antimetabolites
Antithyroid drugs
Chemotherapeutic agents
Colchicine
Cytotoxic agents
Hypocholesterolemic drugs
Indomethacin
Levodopa
Oral contraceptives
Propanolol
Quinacrine
Retinoids
Thallium
Vitamin A

Erythema nodosum

Iodides
Oral contraceptives
Sulfonamides

Exfoliative erythroderma

Allopurinol
Arsenicals
Barbiturates
Captopril
Cefoxitin
Chloroquine
Cimetidine
Gold salts
Hydantoins
Isoniazid
Lithium
Mercurial diuretics
para-Aminosalicylic acid
Phenylbutazone
Sulfonamides
Sulfonylureas

Fixed drug eruptions

Aspirin
Barbiturates
Methaqualone
Phenazones
Trimethoprim-sulfamethoxazole
Phenolphthalein
Many others reported
Phenylbutazone
Sulfonamides
Tetracyclines

Erythema multiforme–like eruptions

Allopurinol
Barbiturates
Carbamazepine
Hydantoins
Minoxidil
Nitrofurantoin
Nonsteroidal anti-inflammatory drugs
Penicillin
Phenolphthalein
Phenothiazines
Rifampin
Sulfonamides
Sulfonylureas
Sulindac agents

Lupus-like eruptions

Anti–tumor necrosis factor-α agents
Carbamazepine
Chlorpromazine
D-Penicillamine
Hydralazine

Lupus-like eruptions—cont'd

Isoniazid
Methyldopa
Minocycline
Procainamide
Propylthiouracil
Quinidine
Sulfasalazine

Photosensitivity

Amiodarone
Carbamazepine
Chlorpropamide
Demeclocycline
Doxycycline (less frequently with tetracycline and minocycline)
Furosemide
Griseofulvin
Lomefloxacin
Methotrexate (sunburn reactivation)
Nalidixic acid
Naproxen
Phenothiazines
Piroxicam (Feldene)
Psoralens
Quinine
Sulfonamides
Tetracyclines
Thiazides
Tolbutamide

Skin pigmentation

ACTH (brown as in Addison's disease)
Amiodarone (slate-gray)
Anticancer drugs
Antimalarials (blue-gray or yellow)
Arsenic (diffuse, brown, macular)
Bleomycin (30%—brown, patchy, linear)
Busulphan (diffuse as in Addison's disease)
Cyclophosphamide (nails)
Doxorubicin (nails)
Chlorpromazine (slate-gray in sun-exposed areas)
Clofazimine (red)
Heavy metals (silver, gold, bismuth, mercury)
Methsergide maleate (red)
Minocycline (patchy or diffuse blue-black)
Oral contraceptives (chloasma—brown)
Psoralens
Rifampin—very high dose (red man syndrome)

Box 14-6 **Drug Reactions and the Drugs That Cause Them—cont'd**

Pityriasis rosea–like eruptions
Arsenicals
Barbiturates
Bismuth compounds
Captopril
Clonidine
Gold compounds
Methoxypromazine
Metronidazole
Pyribenzamine

Vesicles and blisters
Barbiturates (pressure areas—comatose patients)
Bromides
Captopril (pemphigus-like)
Cephalosporins (pemphigus-like)
Clonidine (cicatricial pemphigoid-like)
Furosemide (phototoxic)
Iodides
Nalidixic acid (phototoxic)
Naproxen (like porphyria cutanea tarda)
Penicillamine (pemphigus foliaceus-like)
Phenazones
Piroxicam (Feldene)
Sulfonamides

Chemotherapy-induced acral erythema
Bleomycin
Cyclophosphamide
Cytarabine
Cytosine arabinoside
Doxorubicin
Fluorouracil
Hydroxyurea
Mercaptopurine
Methotrexate
Mitotane

Phototoxic drugs
Amiodarone
Chlorpromazine
Ciprofloxacin
Demeclocycline
Doxycycline
Furosemide
Lomefloxacin
8-Methoxypsoralen
Nabumetone
Nalidixic acid
Naproxen
Piroxicam
Prochlorperazine
Quinidine
Sparfloxacin
St. John's wort
Tar (topical)
Tetracycline
Thiazides
Voriconazole

Photoallergic drugs
Griseofulvin
Ketoprofen
Piroxicam
Quinidine
Quinine
Quinolones (e.g., enoxacin, lomefloxacin)
Sulfonamides

Hypertrichosis
Cyclosporine
Minoxidil
Phenytoin
Many others reported

Drug-induced pseudoporphyria
Amiodarone
Ampicillin/sulbactam combined with cefepime
Bumetanide
Carisoprodol/aspirin
Celecoxib
Chlorthalidone
Cola beverages
Cyclosporine
Dapsone
Diflunisal
Etretinate
5-Fluorouracil (intravenous)
Flutamide
Furosemide
Hydrochlorothiazide/triamterene
Isotretinoin
Ketoprofen
Leflunomide
Mefenamic acid
Nabumetone
Nalidixic acid
Naproxen (most common)
Oral contraceptives
Oxaprozin
Pyridoxine (vitamin B_6)
Tetracycline
Voriconazole

Erythroderma
Allopurinol
Beta-lactam antibiotics
Captopril
Carbamazepine/oxcarbazepine
Gold
Phenobarbital
Phenytoins
Sulfasalazine
Sulfonamides
Zalcitabine
Many others reported

Lichenoid drug eruptions
Chloroquine
Chlorothiazide
Enalapril
Gold salts
Hydrochlorothiazide
Hydroxychloroquine
Labetalol
Methyldopa
Penicillamine
Propranolol
Quinacrine
Quinidine
Many others reported

Stevens-Johnson syndrome/Toxic epidermal necrolysis
Allopurinol
Aminopenicillins
Amithiozone (thiacetazone)
Antiretroviral drugs
Barbiturates
Carbamazepine
Chlormezanone
Lamotrigine
Phenylbutazone
Phenytoin antiepileptics
Piroxicam
Sulfadiazine
Sulfadoxine
Sulfasalazine
Trimethoprim-sulfamethoxazole
Many others reported

Vasculitis (cutaneous)
Anti-TNF (tumor necrosis factor) agents
COX-2 inhibitors
Granulocyte colony–stimulating factor
Leukotriene inhibitors
Minocycline
NSAIDs (nonsteroidal antiinflammatory drugs)
Penicillins
Propylthiouracil/other antithyroid agents
Quinolones
Serum
Streptokinase

Urticaria

Urticaria is frequently caused by drugs, and most drugs can induce hives. Aspirin, penicillin, and blood products are the most frequent causes of urticarial drug eruptions, but almost any drug can cause hives. Hives are itchy, red, edematous plaques that are usually generalized and symmetric. There is no scaling or vesiculation. Wheals vary in size from small papules to huge plaques. The hives typically fade in less than 24 hours only to recur in another area. Angioedema refers to urticarial swelling of deep dermal and subcutaneous tissues and mucous membranes; the reaction may be life-threatening. There are three mechanisms of drug-induced urticaria: anaphylactic and accelerated reactions (immunologic histamine release), nonimmunologic histamine release, and serum sickness.

ANAPHYLACTIC AND ACCELERATED REACTIONS. These IgE-dependent reactions occur within minutes (immediate reactions) to hours (accelerated reactions) of drug administration. Penicillin and its derivatives are the most common causes.

IgE-induced mast cell degranulation (anaphylaxis) occurs within minutes of exposure. From 1% to 5% of patients treated with beta-lactam antibiotics (penicillin, semisynthetic penicillins such as amoxicillin, cephalosporins, carbapenems) develop hives.

Most patients who give a history of allergy to penicillin do not have evidence of allergy when skin-tested. Patients with a history of a reaction with past penicillin treatment and who require penicillin treatment should be skin-tested within days of a planned therapeutic course of penicillin. Radioallergosorbent (RAST) testing is not reliable to rule out allergy. Patients with a positive skin test have a 50% chance of developing an immediate reaction if given penicillin. From 97% to 99% of patients with a negative test will tolerate penicillin. Many patients with documented allergy to penicillin lose it with time; about 25% may maintain the allergy indefinitely.

Both cephalosporins and penicillins have a beta-lactam ring. Clinically significant cross-reactivity occurs in less than 5% or less of patients with positive skin tests to penicillin who are subsequently given cephalosporins. Most cross-reactions involve first- and second-generation cephalosporins. Patients allergic to cephalosporins may have antibodies directed to side chain structures rather than to the beta-lactam ring; therefore patients who develop an urticarial reaction to cephalosporin rarely react to penicillin. Cephalosporin skin testing is not a standard practice.

SERUM SICKNESS. Circulating immune complexes cause serum sickness. Urticaria occurs 4 to 21 days after drug ingestion. The drug is ingested, antibody is formed over the next few days, and drug and antibody combine to form circulating immune complexes. Fever, hematuria, lymphadenopathy, and arthralgias follow (see Chapter 6).

NONIMMUNOLOGIC HISTAMINE RELEASERS. Reaction can occur in minutes. The drug may exert a direct action on the mast cell or on other pathways.

NON–IgE-INDUCED (ASPIRIN AND NSAIDS) URTICARIA. Nonimmunologic anaphylactoid reactions usually have a latency of 30 minutes to 24 hours. Angioedema or urticaria may occur. Urticaria frequently appears on the face and spreads caudadally. Reactions may be dose dependent; small doses may be tolerated.

Aspirin (ASA) and nonsteroidal antiinflammatory drug (NSAID) induced urticaria occurs in 25% to 50% of patients with chronic idiopathic urticaria. Fifty percent of patients with ASA- or NSAID-induced urticaria are atopic. The mechanism of these reactions is thought to be cyclooxygenase inhibition, which results in the augmented production of leukotrienes. Therefore antihistamines are less effective for ASA-induced urticaria or angioedema. Preservatives (benzoic acid) and dyes (tartrazine) produce the same effect. ASA desensitization is not recommended.

Patients with ASA or NSAID hypersensitivity may use acetaminophen, disalicylic acid (e.g., salsalate, Disalcid), or choline magnesium trisalicylate (Trilisate).

RADIOCONTRAST MEDIA REACTIONS. Reaction rates to radiocontrast media (RCM) range from 4% to 12%. The histamine release is slower than that produced by IgE activation, begins 10 minutes after exposure, and peaks at 45 minutes. Most reactions occur from the hyperosmolar agents. Patients who have had a past reaction to RCM have a 20% to 30% chance of a repeat reaction with subsequent exposure. Non–IgE-induced urticaria with histamine release from both basophils and mast cells occurs in 3%, itching in 3%, and flushing in 1% of patients receiving the hyperosmolar agents. Patients at risk of RCM reactions may be given doxepin (an H_1/H_2 antagonist) 10 to 25 mg 1 to 2 hours before administration of RCM to prevent an anaphylactoid reaction.

OPIATES. Opiates induce mast cells of the skin (not mucosal surfaces) to degranulate by a direct effect on the cell and release histamines. Pretreatment with antihistamines prevents pruritus, urticaria, and flushing that occur with morphine infusion.

Other nonimmunologic histamine releasers include polymyxin B, lobster, and strawberries.

Pruritus

Most drug eruptions itch but itching can be the only manifestation of a drug reaction (e.g., gold, sulfonamides). Histamine in the skin almost always results in a urticarial reaction or, at lower concentrations, flushing. Histamine is the predominant mediator of IgE-induced reactions (with greater potential for life-threatening anaphylaxis), and these are more responsive to antihistamine (an H_1 and, at times, concomitant administration of an H_2 antagonist may be rewarding) therapy. Histamine is not the only mediator of itch released during inflammatory reactions. Kinins, leukotrienes, prostaglandins, and serotonin are also mediators of itching, and itching induced by these mediators would not respond to antihistamines. Oral contraceptives can produce itching similar to pruritus gravidarum.

DRUG ERUPTIONS

Acute generalized exanthematous pustulosis

Acute generalized exanthematous pustulosis (AGEP) is characterized by acute onset often following drug intake; it presents with fever; numerous nonfollicular, sterile pustules on an erythematous background predominantly in the folds and/or on the face; and elevated levels of blood neutrophils (Figure 14-37). Most cases of AGEP are drug induced. The most frequently implicated agents are calcium channel blockers, NSAIDs, anticonvulsants, and antimicrobials, particularly those with beta-lactam and macrolide properties. Acute infections with enteroviruses are also a reported cause. Pustules resolve spontaneously in less than 15 days. Withdraw the drug and consider treatment with systemic steroids. Distinction from generalized pustular psoriasis is important. AGEP has a more acute course with fever, relationship to drug therapy, and rapid spontaneous resolution following drug withdrawal. The biopsy shows subcorneal pustules that resemble those of pustular psoriasis.

Acneiform (pustular) eruptions

These pustular eruptions mimic acne but comedones are absent. Treatment with oral corticosteroids and abuse of anabolic steroids are possible causes (see Box 14-6 and Figure 14-38).

Eczema

A patient who acquires contact dermatitis with a topical agent develops either a focal flare at sites of previous inflammation or a generalized cutaneous eruption if exposed orally or by inhalation to the same or chemically related medication (the so-called external-internal sensitization). The symptoms develop within 2 to 24 hours after ingestion of the drug. Continued use of the medication can intensify the reaction and lead to generalization of the eruption. Antibiotics and oral hypoglycemic agents are most commonly implicated. The term "baboon syndrome" describes a distinctive form of systemic contact dermatitis with symmetric erythema in flexural areas including the elbows, axilla, eyelids, and sides of the neck accompanied by bright red anogenital lesions.

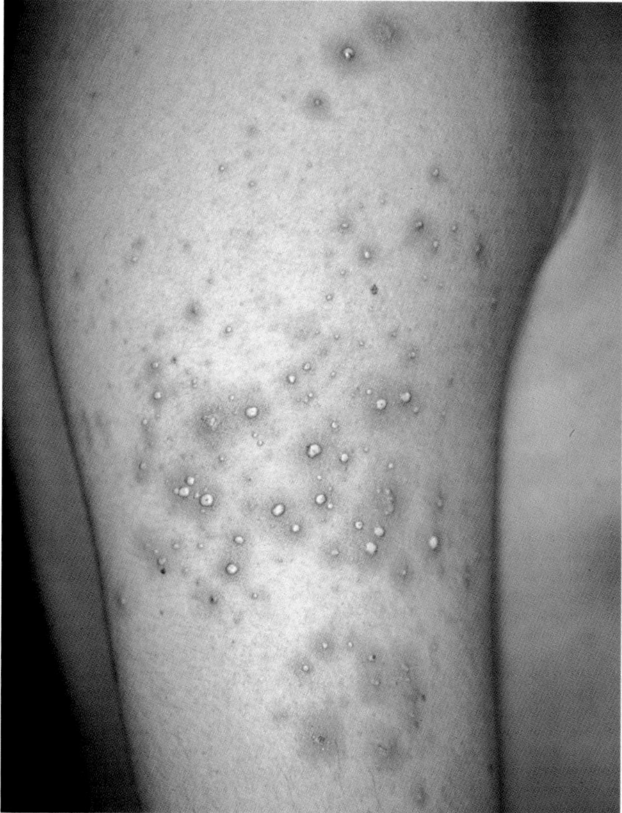

Figure 14-37 Acute generalized exanthematous pustulosis is characterized by the acute onset of fever and generalized erythema with numerous, small, discrete, sterile, nonfollicular pustules. Pustules may appear in a few days of starting the drug. Pustules resolve in less than 15 days followed by desquamation.

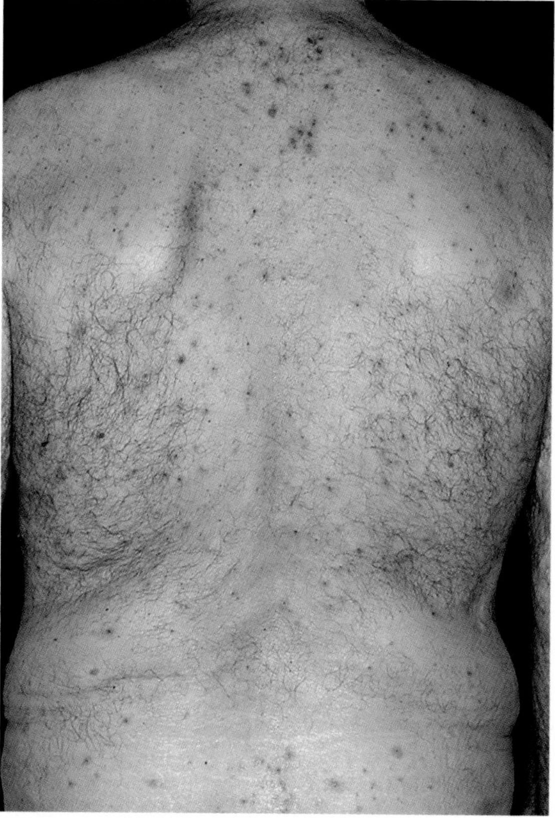

Figure 14-38 Acneiform (pustular) drug eruptions occur on the upper body. In contrast to acne vulgaris, comedones are absent.

Fixed drug eruptions

Fixed drug eruptions are a unique form of drug allergy that produce red plaques or blisters that recur at the same cutaneous or mucosal site each time the drug is ingested (see Box 14-6). The clinical pattern and distribution of lesions may be influenced by the drug in question, and the study of the pattern may provide useful information in selecting the most likely causative drug. Tetracycline and co-trimoxazole commonly cause lesions limited to the glans penis. Cases of familial occurrence suggest that a genetic predisposition might be an important causal factor.

CLINICAL MANIFESTATIONS. Single or multiple, round, sharply demarcated, dusky red plaques appear soon after drug exposure and reappear in exactly the same site each time the drug is taken (Figures 14-39 to 14-41). Lesions may be generalized but typically only a single lesion is present. The lesions are generally preceded or accompanied by itching and burning, the intensity of which is usually proportionate to the severity of the inflammatory changes. Pruritus and burning may be the only manifestations of reactivation in an old patch. The area often blisters and then erodes; desquamation or crusting (after bullous lesions) follows, and brown pigmentation forms with healing. Blistering can be confined to the center of the lesion, resulting in the so-called targetoid appearance (Figure 14-42). Nonpigmenting reactions have been documented. Pseudoephedrine classically causes a nonpigmenting fixed drug eruption. Lesions can occur on any part of the skin or mucous membrane. Lips, hands, genitalia (especially male genitalia), and occasionally oral mucosa are favored sites (Figure 14-43). Regional lymphadenopathy is absent.

REACTIVATION AND REFRACTORY PHASE. The length of time from the reexposure to a drug and the onset of symptoms is 30 minutes to 8 hours (mean, 2.1 hours). Following each exacerbation, some patients demonstrate a refractory period (weeks to several months), during which the offending drug does not activate the lesions.

CROSS-SENSITIVITY. Ingestion of a drug with a similar chemical structure may precipitate exacerbations. This phenomenon has been reported with tetracycline derivatives and sulfonamides. There is greater cross-reactivity between tetracycline and doxycycline, both of which have one methylamino group at the fourth carbon position, than between those two antibiotics and minocycline, which has two methylamino groups at the fourth and seventh carbon positions. Drugs of different chemical structures also can precipitate exacerbations. Three different, pharmacologically unrelated anticonvulsants evoked an eruption at the same site. Sometimes several drugs can induce fixed drug eruptions in the same patient (multisensitivity). The most common reason for multisensitivity is cross-sensitivity between chemically related drugs such as tetracyclines.

DIAGNOSIS. Taking a careful history is important because patients often do not relate their complaints to the use of a drug that they may be taking such as a laxative (phenolphthalein) or headache remedy. Provoking the lesion with the suspected drug confirms the diagnosis, prevents recurrences, and allays the anxiety of the patient regarding venereal origin of the disease. The challenge dose should be smaller than the normal therapeutic dose, but it can be cautiously increased up to the normal therapeutic dose until the reaction is elicited. In some cases two to three times the original dose may be required to elicit a repeat reaction. Some authors do not recommend these tests because of the possible risk of generalized bullous eruptions. Topical and intradermal provocation tests have been used as an alternative to systemic provocation tests. Patch tests are performed on the patient's normal and perilesional skin with the drug in a petrolatum base. In one study, a positive reaction occurred only at the previous lesional site.

A biopsy shows hydropic degeneration of the epidermal basal cells and pigmentary incontinence.

TREATMENT. Group II to V topical steroids are effective. Erosive lesions can be treated with wet compresses. Drug avoidance prevents recurrence.

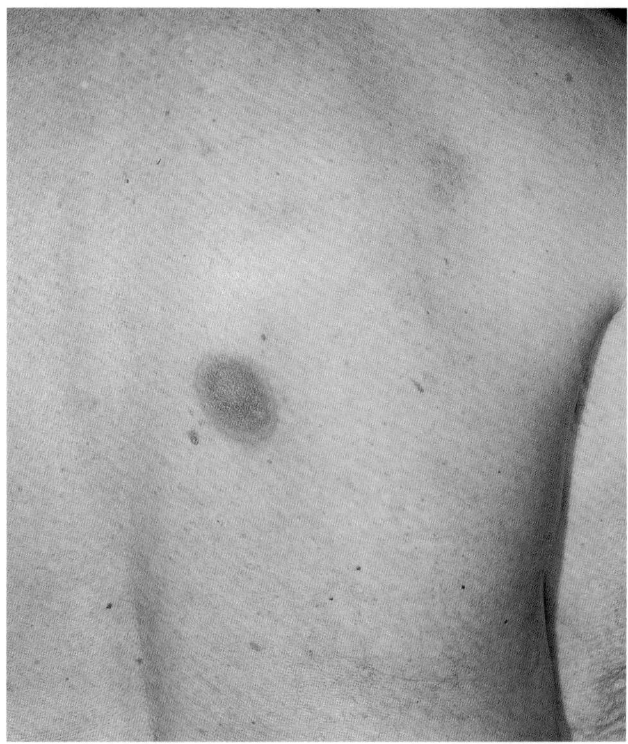

Figure 14-39 Fixed drug eruption. A single, sharply demarcated, round plaque appeared shortly after trimethoprim was taken.

FIXED DRUG ERUPTIONS

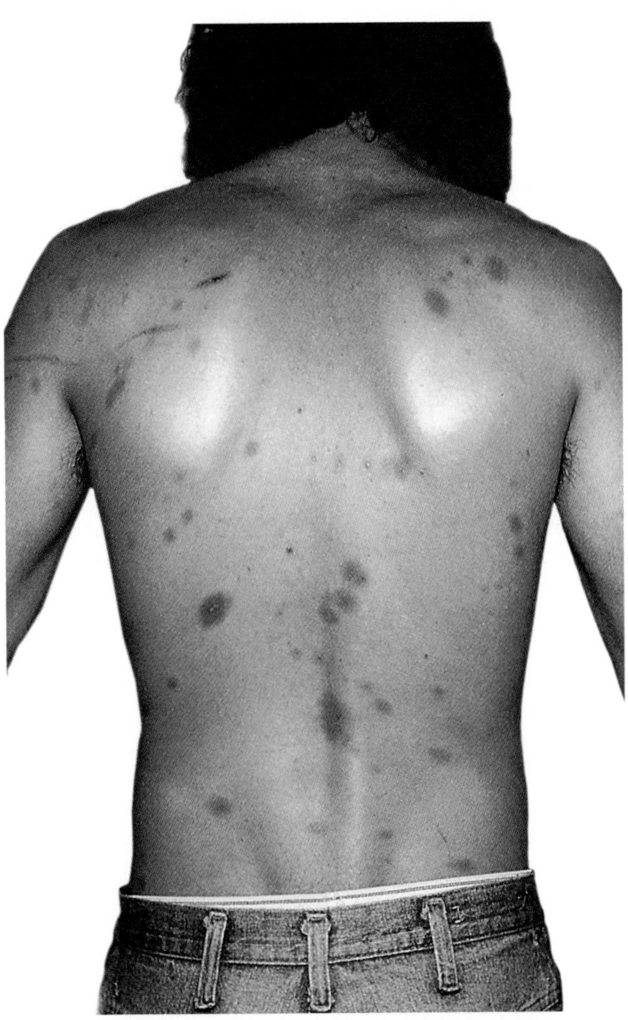

Figure 14-40 Fixed drug eruption. Multiple round, sharply demarcated plaques appeared shortly after methaqualone (Quaalude) was taken. The plaques healed with brown hyperpigmentation. (Courtesy David W. Knox, MD.)

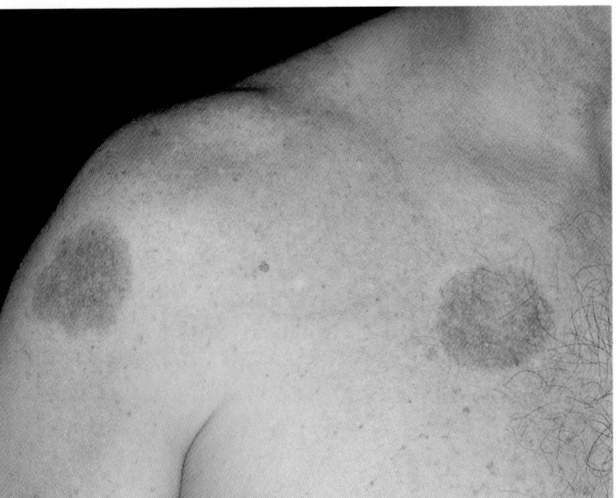

Figure 14-41 Fixed drug eruption. One or several plaques may appear and return in the exact location with future exposure to the same drug.

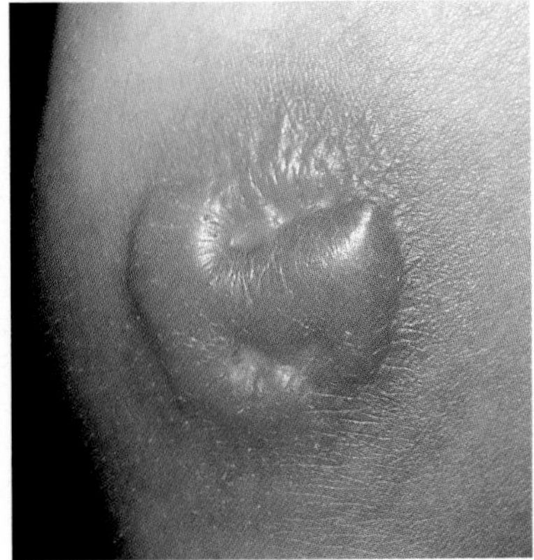

Figure 14-42 Early lesions may have a central blister.

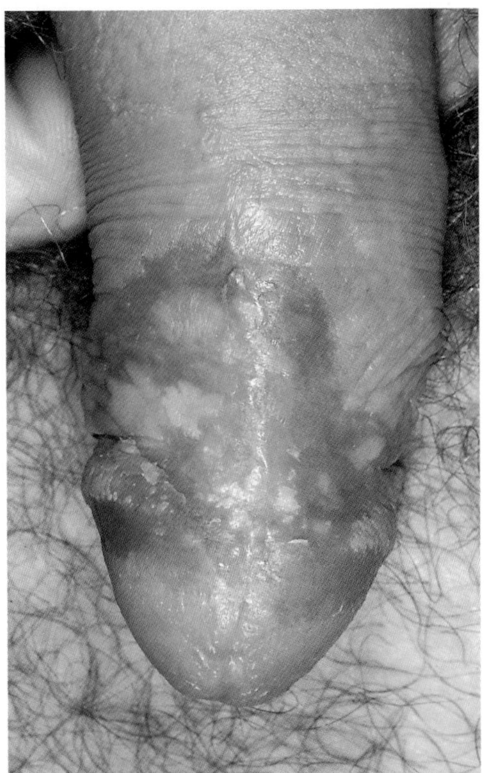

Figure 14-43 Fixed drug eruption. The glans penis is the most common site.

Blistering drug eruptions

Blisters may develop alone, as part of other eruptions (e.g., erythema multiforme, toxic epidermal necrolysis, and fixed drug eruptions), or with exanthemic drug eruptions (see Box 14-6). Drug-induced linear IgA dermatosis presents as a papulovesicular eruption, but mucosal and conjunctival lesions are absent. Drugs may cause a blistering eruption that mimics superficial pemphigus (pemphigus foliaceus). A morbilliform or urticarial eruption precedes the blisters. Direct and indirect immunofluorescence findings resemble non–drug-induced pemphigus. Bullous pemphigoid, an autoimmune blistering dermatosis usually seen in the elderly, presents with tense blisters on a urticarial base. Circulating antibodies are present in most cases. Direct immunofluorescent testing shows linear IgG and C3 along the dermoepidermal junction. Pseudoporphyria resembles porphyria cutanea tarda at a clinical, light microscopic, and direct immunofluorescent level, but porphyrin tests are normal. NSAIDs are the most common cause.

Erythema multiforme and toxic epidermal necrolysis

Reactions occur on the skin and mucous membranes; they include multiple, symmetric, persistent macules, papules, vesicles, and bullae. The iris or target lesion is the classic presentation for erythema multiforme, which presents with central duskiness in an expanding erythematous macule or papule. Severe forms are often caused by medications. Less severe forms are caused by mycoplasmal pneumonia, herpes simplex infections, and medication. Loss of a major portion of the cutaneous surface (toxic epidermal necrolysis) is severe and fatal in up to 30% of cases. The cause of death is loss of large areas of skin, resulting in fluid loss and sepsis. The drugs most often involved are long-acting sulfonamides, NSAIDs, and anticonvulsants. Toxic metabolites (i.e., circulating immune complexes) in predisposed individuals may be the cause of a cell-mediated cytotoxic reaction. Readministration of the responsible drug produces a recurrence. See Box 14-6 and Chapter 18.

Exfoliative erythroderma

Patients may develop erythema involving the entire skin surface from drug therapy (see Box 14-6 and Figure 14-44). Erythroderma may also occur in pityriasis rubra pilaris, psoriasis, and cutaneous T-cell lymphoma. Generalized erythema and scaling may occur if an offending agent is not withdrawn. The reaction is potentially life-threatening.

Lichenoid (lichen planus–like drug eruptions)

Clinically and histologically these eruptions mimic generalized lichen planus. There are multiple, flat-topped, itchy, violaceous papules; oral lesions may be present. The mean age of patients with lichen planus is approximately 50 years; the mean age for lichenoid drug eruptions is approximately 60 years. The latent period between the beginning of administration of a drug and the eruption is between 3 weeks and 3 years. The lesions are chronic and persist for weeks or months after the offending drug is stopped. Lesions heal with brown pigmentation. Gold and antimalarials are most often associated with drug-induced lichen planus (see Box 14-6).

Lupus erythematosus–like drug eruptions

Drug-induced lupus (DIL) is a rare adverse reaction to a large variety of drugs. Older patients are more likely to suffer from DIL than from idiopathic systemic lupus erythematosus (SLE). DIL occurs more frequently in females, with a 4:1 ratio of females to males. Minocycline-induced lupus occurs in young patients (median age, 21 years) and $\geq$80% of patients with minocycline-induced lupus are women. Over 80 drugs have been implicated; the most common are hydralazine, procainamide, isoniazid, methyldopa, quinidine, minocycline, and chlorpromazine. Drug-induced lupus caused by anti-tumor necrosis factor-α agents (TNF-α) (infliximab, etanercept, adalimumab) is reported. There is controversy over whether anti-TNF-α

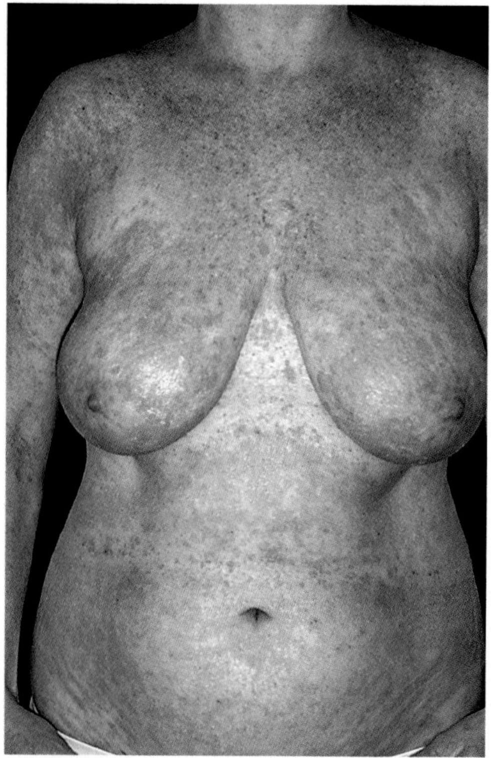

Figure 14-44 Exfoliative erythroderma. Erythroderma (red skin) may be caused by drugs, malignancy, psoriasis, and other conditions.

therapy triggers DIL or unmasks preexisting SLE. Procainamide and hydralazine induces lupus in 15% to 20% and 7% to 13% of patients, respectively. Minocycline-induced DIL has an incidence of only 53 per 100,000 prescriptions for women (who represented 93% of minocycline-induced lupus cases).

CLINICAL SIGNS. The clinical abnormalities in DIL are usually milder than those seen in idiopathic SLE (Box 14-7). Only a few mild symptoms present initially, with gradual worsening over a period of weeks or even months. Arthralgia, myalgia, arthritis, fever, malaise, anorexia, and weight loss are the most frequent. Cutaneous manifestations are much less common than in SLE, with rash (erythematosus, macular, maculopapular, urticarial, or vasculitic) being seen in 5% to 40% of DIL patients. The reaction is dose related. Renal involvement and central nervous system (CNS) disease are rare.

LABORATORY. Antinuclear antibodies (ANAs), antihistone antibodies, and anti–single-stranded DNA antibodies are markers for lupus-like drug eruptions. Antihistone antibodies are found in up to 95% of cases of drug-induced systemic lupus erythematosus (SLE) but are sometimes present in idiopathic SLE. DIL is characterized by the presence of ANAs, but in some cases they are absent. Seroconversion from negative to positive for antinuclear antibodies is not justification to stop medication. The drug is stopped if symptoms develop. Symptoms resolve in 4 to 6 weeks, but ANA remains positive for 6 to 12 months. The ANA fluorescence pattern is most commonly homogeneous. Antihistone antibodies are present in >90% of DIL patients overall but in only 32%, 42%, and <50% of DIL cases associated with minocycline, propylthiouracil, and statins, respectively.

Anti–double-stranded DNA antibodies are rare in DIL but common in SLE. Anti-dsDNA antibodies have been reported in minocycline-, propylthiouracil-, quinidine-, and anti-TNF therapy-induced lupus. Dermoepidermal junction immunofluorescence "lupus-band test" occurs in less than 10% of cases.

Elevated erythrocyte sedimentation rate occurs in up to 80% of patients. Leukopenia and cytopenia are present in 5% to 25% of DIL cases. Low C3 and/or C4 occasionally occurs in DIL. Anemia occurs in 35% and 20% of patients with hydralazine- and procainamide-induced lupus, respectively, and in 33% of quinidine-induced cases. Between 10% and 50% of DIL patients have hypergammaglobulinemia. Perinuclear antineutrophil cytoplasmic antibody (p-ANCA) is reported in 50% of propylthiouracil-induced cases and in 67% to 100% of patients with lupus attributable to minocycline.

Other autoantibodies in DIL include rheumatoid factor (20% to 50%), anticardiolipin (5% to 20% of procainamide- and hydralazine-induced cases and 26% to 33% of minocycline-induced cases), and anti-Sm antibodies (41% of patients with minocycline-induced lupus).

Box 14-7 Diagnostic Criteria for Drug-Induced Lupus

1. Sufficient and continuing exposure to a specific drug
2. At least one symptom compatible with SLE
3. No history suggestive of SLE before starting the drug
4. Resolution of symptoms within weeks (sometimes months) after discontinuation of the drug
5. Positive ANA; negative ANA tests may occur

Adapted from *Ann NY Acad Sci* 1108:166-182, 2007.
PMID: 17893983

MANAGEMENT. DIL resolves within weeks or months after stopping the drug. Irreversibility indicates that the drug unmasked underlying idiopathic SLE. Resolution of signs and symptoms is highly variable and seems to depend both on the agent and on patient and disease characteristics. Severe cases of DIL may require corticosteroids but this is rare. Serologic abnormalities may persist. Rechallenge with the offending agent may induce symptoms within 1 to 2 days.

DRUG-INDUCED SUBACUTE CUTANEOUS LUPUS ERYTHEMATOSUS. Drug-induced subacute cutaneous LE presents with annular or psoriasiform lesions on the upper trunk and extensor surfaces of the arms. They are clinically and histologically identical to those of subacute cutaneous lupus erythematosus. Anti-Ro and anti-La antibodies may be found. Drugs implicated are hydrochlorothiazide, calcium channel blockers, terbinafine, NSAIDs, griseofulvin, docetaxel, psoralen plus ultraviolet A (PUVA), and interferon. The eruption may persist after stopping the drug.

Chemotherapy-induced acral erythema

Chemotherapy-induced acral erythema or palmoplantar erythrodysesthesia syndrome is a well-defined reaction to some of the chemotherapeutic agents such as methotrexate, cytarabine, doxorubicin, fluorouracil, cytosine arabinoside, and bleomycin. This reaction is characterized by symmetric, well-demarcated, painful erythema of the palms and soles, which may progress to desquamation or blisters (see Box 14-6). It appears to be dose dependent, and a direct toxic effect of the drug is likely. Tingling on the palms and soles is followed in a few days by painful, symmetric, well-defined swelling and erythema. Treatment is supportive, with elevation and cold compresses. Systemic steroids have been used with variable success. Cooling the hands and feet during treatment to decrease blood flow may attenuate the reaction. Modification of the dosage schedule may also help.

Pigmentation

Pigmentation can result from drugs that increase production of melanin, causing pigment incontinence by damaging epidermal keratinocytes or melanocytes in the basal layer or by deposition (see Box 14-6).

Photosensitivity

Photosensitivity eruptions represent 8% of all adverse cutaneous drug reactions. Both systemic and topical medications can induce photosensitivity. There are two main types: phototoxicity and photoallergy.

Phototoxic reactions are related to drug concentration and can occur in anyone. The drug absorbs radiation and enters an excited state, producing species including reactive oxygen radicals that react with other cellular constituents. The rash occurs within a few hours following the first exposure to a drug and resembles an exaggerated sunburn with blistering, desquamation, and hyperpigmentation. The eruption is confined to sun-exposed areas (Figure 14-45). The reaction can occur on first administration and subsides when the drug is stopped.

Photoallergic reactions are less common and are not concentration related. They occur in only a small fraction of people exposed and may spread to involve areas that have not been exposed to the sun, possibly from an autosensitization phenomenon. They are a form of delayed hypersensitivity reaction and appear within 24 to 48 hours of antigenic challenge. They occur in sun-exposed areas, sparing the submental and retroauricular areas and upper eyelids. On rare occasions, the reaction can persist for years, even without further drug exposure.

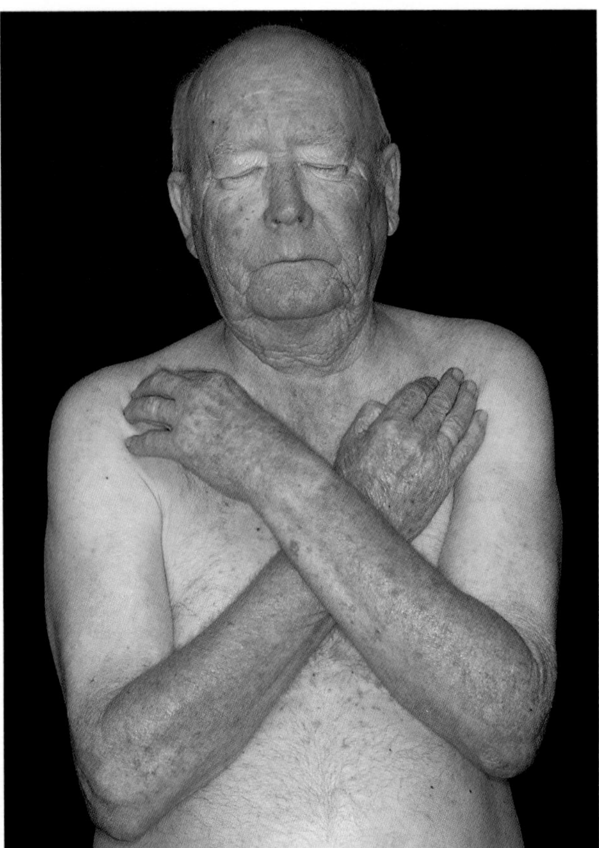

Figure 14-45 Phototoxic eruption. Exposure to sun light after starting hydrochlorothiazide resulted in this intense eruption localized to sun-exposed area.

Onycholysis (separation of the nail plate from the nail bed) may occur from drug photosensitivity and has occurred with tetracyclines, psoralens, and fluoroquinolones.

Vasculitis

Small vessel necrotizing vasculitis (palpable purpura) may be precipitated by drugs (see Box 14-6). Lesions are most often concentrated on the lower legs but may be generalized and involve the kidneys, joints, and brain. Any drug can evoke vasculitis in a predisposed patient.

Lymphomatoid drug eruptions

Any patient who develops an atypical lymphoid infiltrate should have a drug-based etiology excluded before the diagnosis of cutaneous lymphoma is made. Lesions that resemble mycosis fungoides have been reported with phenytoin (Dilantin), phenothiazines, barbiturates, beta-blockers, angiotensin-converting enzyme inhibitors, calcium channel blockers, H_1 and H_2 antagonists, benzodiazepines, and antidepressants.

Skin eruptions associated with specific drugs

CUTANEOUS COMPLICATIONS OF CHEMOTHERAPEUTIC AGENTS. Cancer chemotherapeutic agents adversely affect rapidly dividing cells. Stomatitis, alopecia, onychodystrophy, chemical cellulitis, phlebitis, and hyperpigmentation occur with several agents. Self-limited palmoplantar erythema, occasionally with bulla formation, has been reported (see earlier).

DRUG HYPERSENSITIVITY SYNDROME. This syndrome has a variable spectrum of clinical and laboratory findings: fever, rash, lymphadenopathy, and hepatitis (hepatomegaly and increase in serum aminotransferase level), with leukocytosis and eosinophilia. The three most commonly used anticonvulsants—phenytoin, phenobarbital, and carbamazepine—can each produce the reaction. Other drugs are also reported. Cutaneous reactions to phenytoin occur in up to 19% of patients. These vary from morbilliform eruptions to erythroderma, erythema multiforme, and toxic epidermal necrolysis. A small percentage of patients develop a hypersensitivity syndrome that presents with a macular or papular rash or erythroderma and, rarely, pustules. The outcome depends on the severity of the hepatic injury and the presence of other complications. The reaction is serious and may result in death. This syndrome may possibly be a reaction induced by a complex interplay among several herpesviruses (Epstein-Barr [EB] virus, HHV-6, HHV-7, and cytomegalovirus), antiviral immune responses, and drug-specific immune responses.

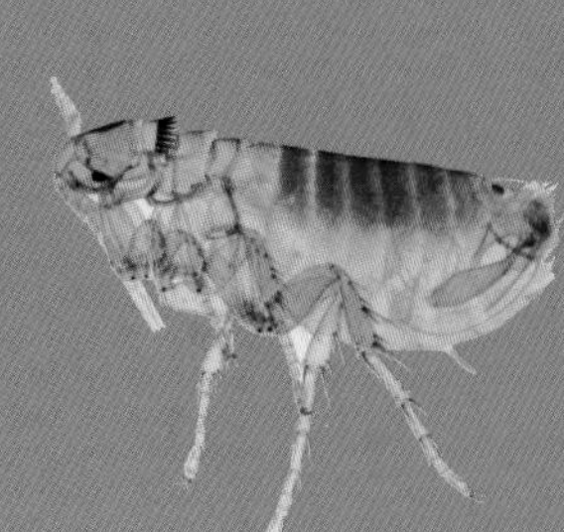

Chapter 15

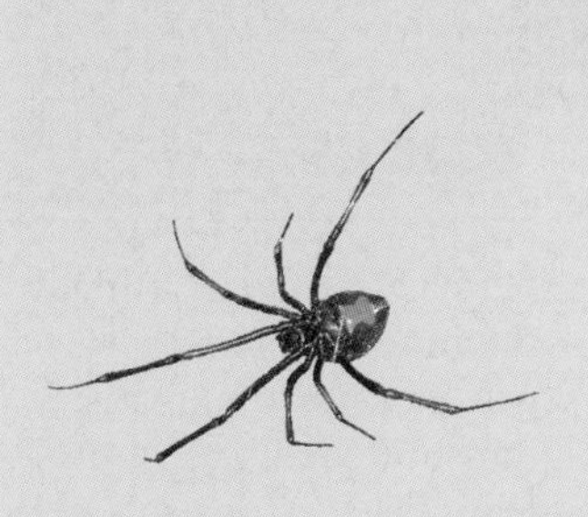

Infestations and Bites

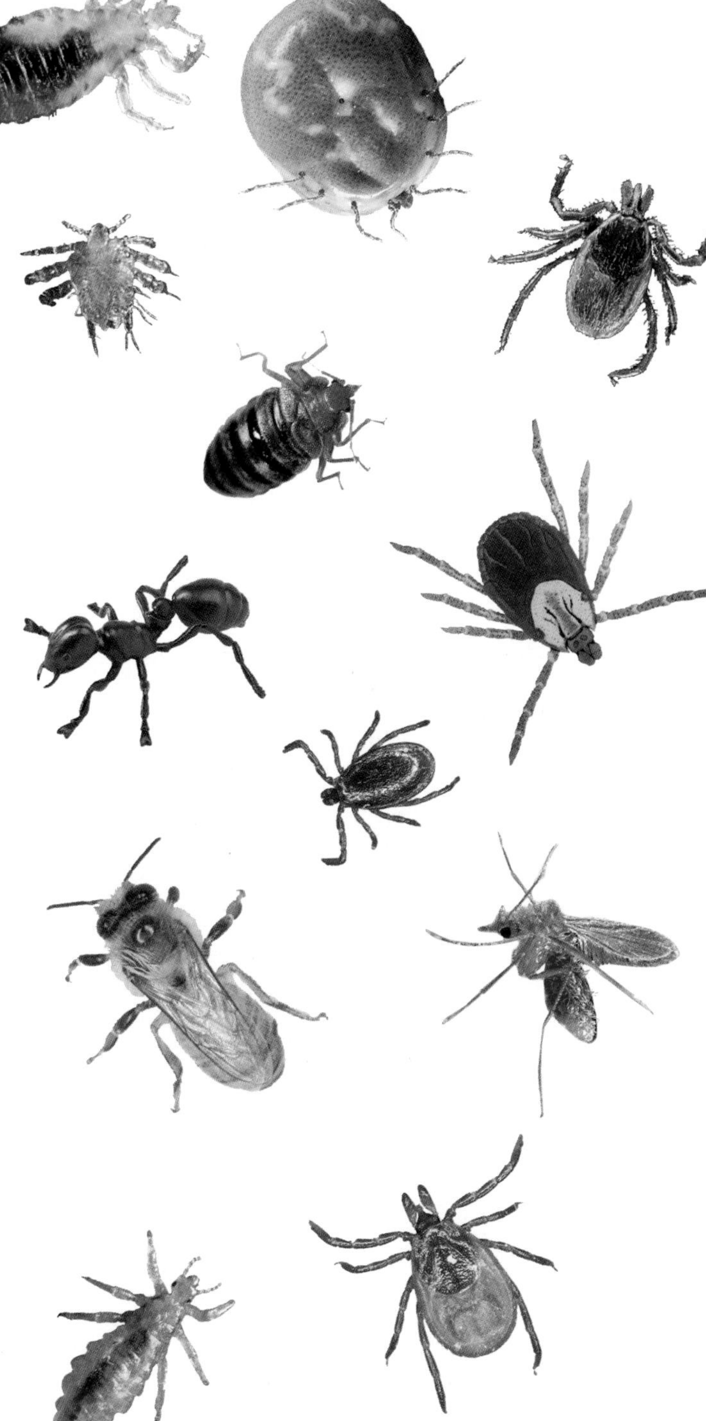

CHAPTER CONTENTS

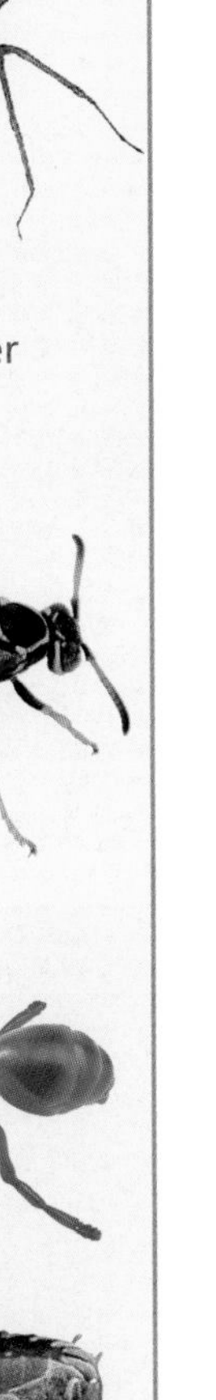

SCABIES

Human scabies is a highly contagious disease caused by the mite *Sarcoptes scabiei* var. *hominis*. The mite is an obligate parasite to humans. Scabies is not primarily a sexually transmitted disease but sexual transmission does occur. High-risk persons include men who have sex with men. *PMID: 15608592* There is no evidence that mites can transmit infection with the human immunodeficiency virus.

Scabies spreads in households and neighborhoods in which there is a high frequency of intimate personal contact or sharing of inanimate objects, and fomite transmission is a major factor in household and nosocomial passage of scabies. Dogs and cats may be infested by almost identical organisms; these sometimes may be a source for human infestation. In the past, scabies was attributed to poor hygiene. Most contemporary cases, however, appear in individuals with adequate hygiene who are in close contact with numbers of individuals, such as schoolchildren. Blacks rarely acquire scabies; the reason is unknown. Scabies is endemic in many developing countries and is usually associated with overcrowding, low socioeconomic standards, and poor hygiene.

Figure 15-1 *Sarcopte's scabiei* in a potassium hydroxide wet mount (×40).

Anatomic features, life cycle, and immunology

ANATOMIC FEATURES

The adult mite is $^{1}/_{3}$-mm long and has a flattened, oval body with wrinklelike, transverse corrugations and eight legs (Figure 15-1). The front two pairs of legs bear claw-shaped suckers and the two rear pairs end in long, trailing bristles. The digestive tract fills a major portion of the body and is readily observed when the mite is seen in cross-section of histologic specimens (Figure 15-2, *A*).

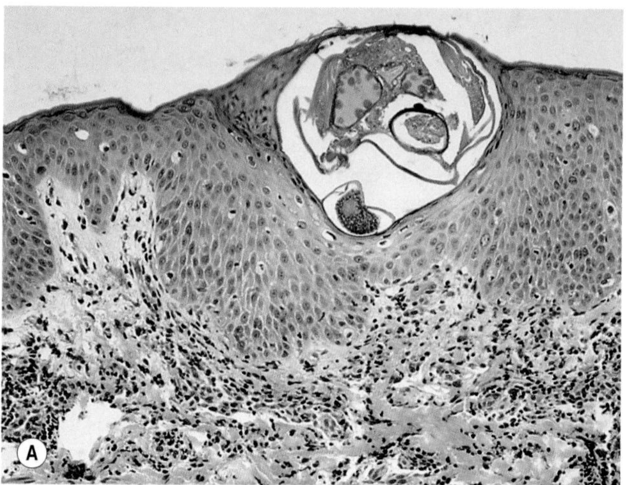

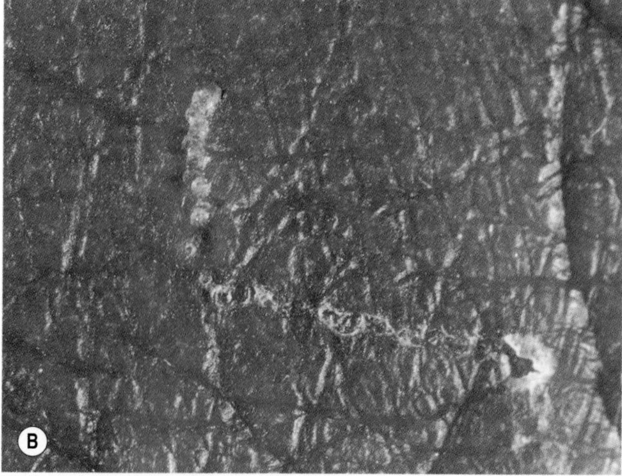

Figure 15-2 A, Cross-section of a mite in the stratum corneum. **B,** Burrow. The mite excavates a burrow in the stratum corneum (the dead, horny layer of the epidermis).

INFESTATION AND LIFE CYCLE. Infestation begins when a fertilized female mite arrives on the skin surface. Within an hour, the female excavates a burrow in the stratum corneum (dead, horny layer) (Figure 15-2, *B*). During the mite's 30-day life cycle, the burrow extends from several millimeters to a few centimeters in length. The burrow does not enter the underlying epidermis except in the case of hyperkeratotic Norwegian scabies, a condition in which scaly, thick skin develops in retarded, immunosuppressed, or elderly patients in the presence of thousands of mites. Eggs laid at the rate of two or three a day (Figure 15-3) and fecal pellets (scybala) are deposited in the burrow behind the advancing female. Scybala are dark, oval masses that are seen easily with the eggs when burrow scrapings are examined under a microscope. Scybala may act as an irritant and may be responsible for some of the itching. The larvae hatch, leaving the egg casings in the burrow, and reach maturity in 14 to 17 days. The adult mites copulate and repeat the cycle. Therefore, 3 to 5 weeks after infestation, there are only a few mites present. This life cycle explains why patients experience few if any symptoms during the first month after contact with an infested individual. After a number of mites (usually less than 20) have reached maturity and have spread by migration or the patient's scratching, the initial, minor, localized itch evolves into intense, generalized pruritus.

IMMUNOLOGY. A hypersensitivity reaction rather than a foreign-body response may be responsible for the lesions, which may delay recognition of symptoms of scabies. Elevated immunoglobulin E (IgE) titers develop in some patients infested with scabies, along with eosinophilia and an immediate-type hypersensitivity reaction to an extract prepared from female mites. IgE levels fall within a year after infestation. Eosinophilia returns to normal shortly after treatment. The fact that symptoms develop much more rapidly when reinfestation occurs supports the claim that the symptoms and lesions of scabies are the result of a hypersensitivity reaction.

Clinical manifestations

Transmission of scabies occurs during direct skin contact with an infected person.

A mite can possibly survive for days in normal home surroundings after leaving human skin. Mites survive up to 7 days in mineral oil microscopic slide mounts.

The disease begins insidiously. Symptoms are minor at first and are attributed to a bite or dry skin. Scratching destroys burrows and removes mites, providing initial relief. The patient remains comfortable during the day but itches at night. Nocturnal pruritus is highly characteristic of scabies. Scratching spreads mites to other areas and after 6 to 8 weeks the once localized area of minor irritation has become a widespread, intensely pruritic eruption.

The most characteristic features of the lesions are pleomorphism and a tendency to remain discrete and small. Primary lesions are soon destroyed by scratching.

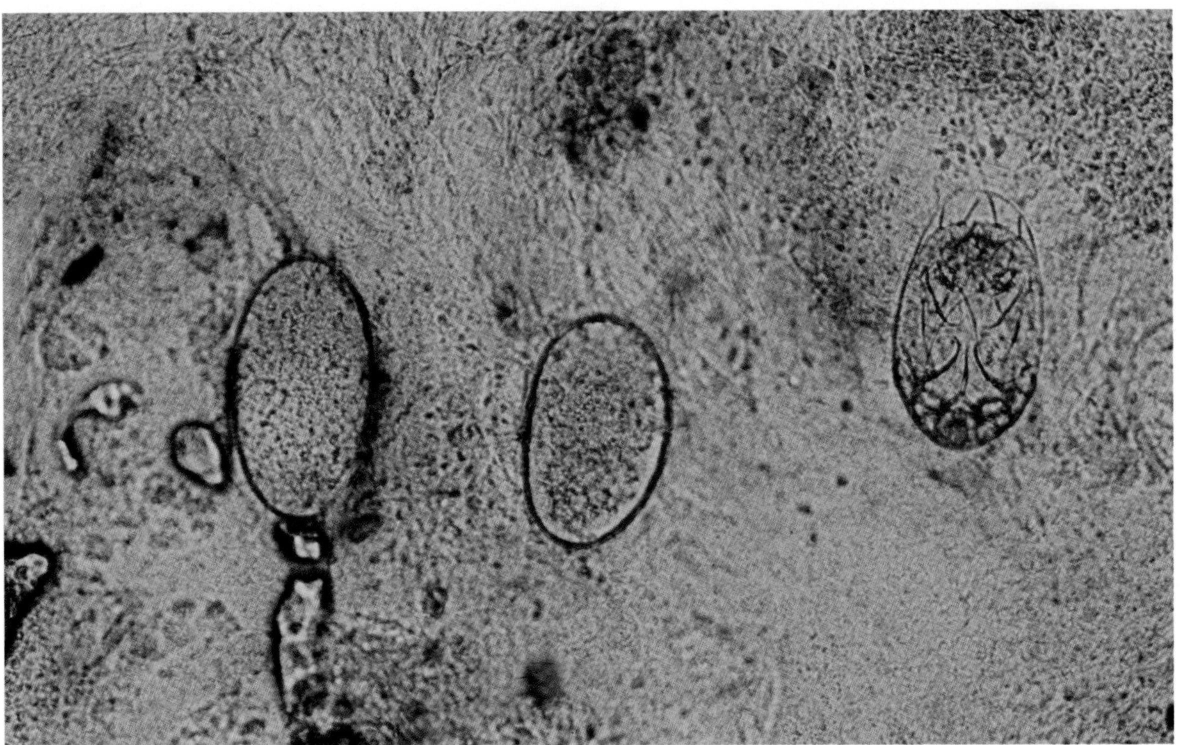

Figure 15-3 *Sarcoptes scabiei.* Eggs containing mites. A potassium hydroxide wet mount (×40).

PRIMARY LESIONS

Mites are found in burrows and at the edge of vesicles but rarely in papules.

BURROW. The linear, curved, or S-shaped burrows are approximately as wide as #2 suture material and are 2 to 15 mm long (see Figure 15-4). They are pink-white and slightly elevated. A vesicle or the mite, which may look like a black dot at one end of the burrow, often may be seen.

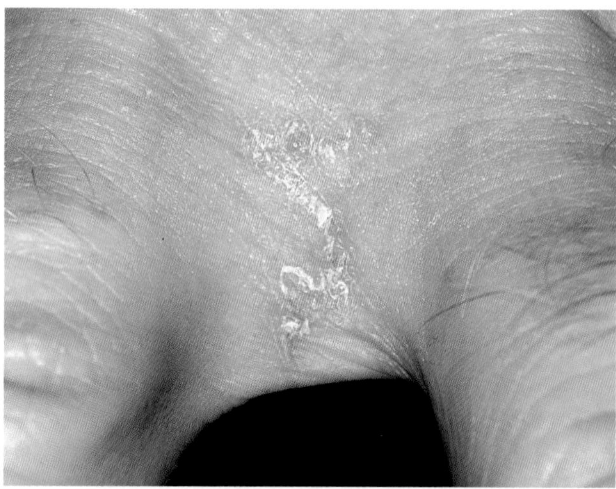

Figure 15-4 Scabies burrows appear as curved tracks and are most often found in the finger webs and on the wrists.

Scratching destroys burrows; therefore they do not appear in some patients. Burrows are most likely to be found in the finger webs, wrists, sides of the hands and feet, penis, buttocks, scrotum, and the palms and soles of infants.

VESICLES AND PAPULES. Vesicles are isolated, pinpoint, and filled with serous rather than purulent fluid. The fact that they remain discrete is a key point in differentiating scabies from other vesicular diseases such as poison ivy. The finger webs are the most likely areas to find intact vesicles (Figure 15-5). Infants may have vesicles or pustules on the palms and soles. Small, discrete papules may represent a hypersensitivity reaction and rarely contain mites.

SECONDARY LESIONS

Secondary lesions result from infection or are caused by scratching. They often dominate the clinical picture. Pinpoint erosions are the most common secondary lesions (Figure 15-6). Pustules are a sign of secondary infection. Scaling, erythema, and all stages of eczematous inflammation occur as a response to excoriation or to irritation caused by overzealous attempts at self-medication. Nodules occur in covered areas such as the buttocks, groin, scrotum, penis, and axillae. The 2- to 10-mm indolent, red papules and nodules sometimes have slightly eroded surfaces, especially on the glans penis (Figure 15-7). Nodules may persist for weeks or months after the mites have been eradicated. They may result from persisting antigens of mite parts.

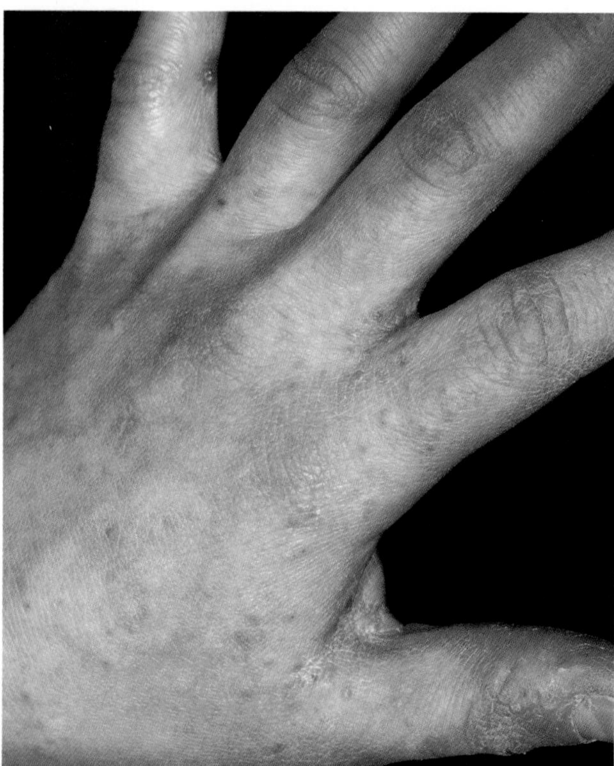

Figure 15-5 Scabies. Tiny vesicles and papules in the finger webs and on the back of the hand.

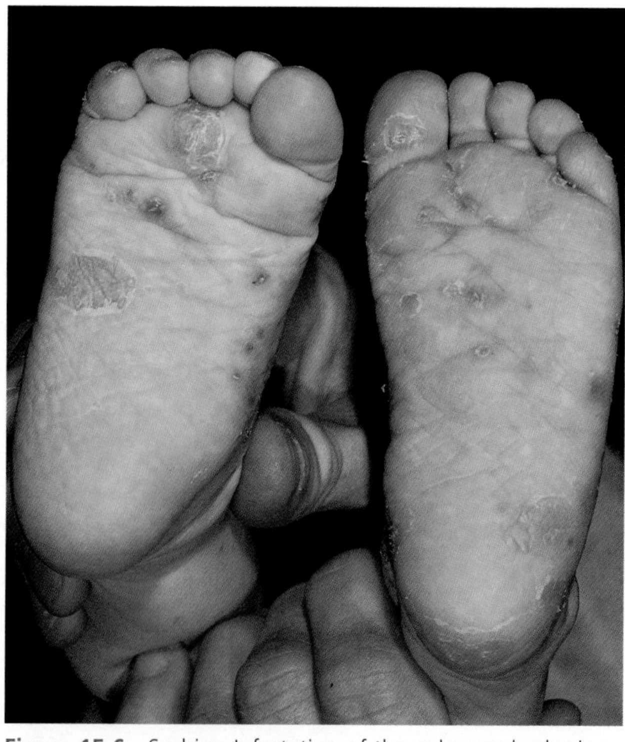

Figure 15-6 Scabies. Infestation of the palms and soles is common in infants. The vesicular lesions have all ruptured.

SCABIES—GENITAL LESIONS

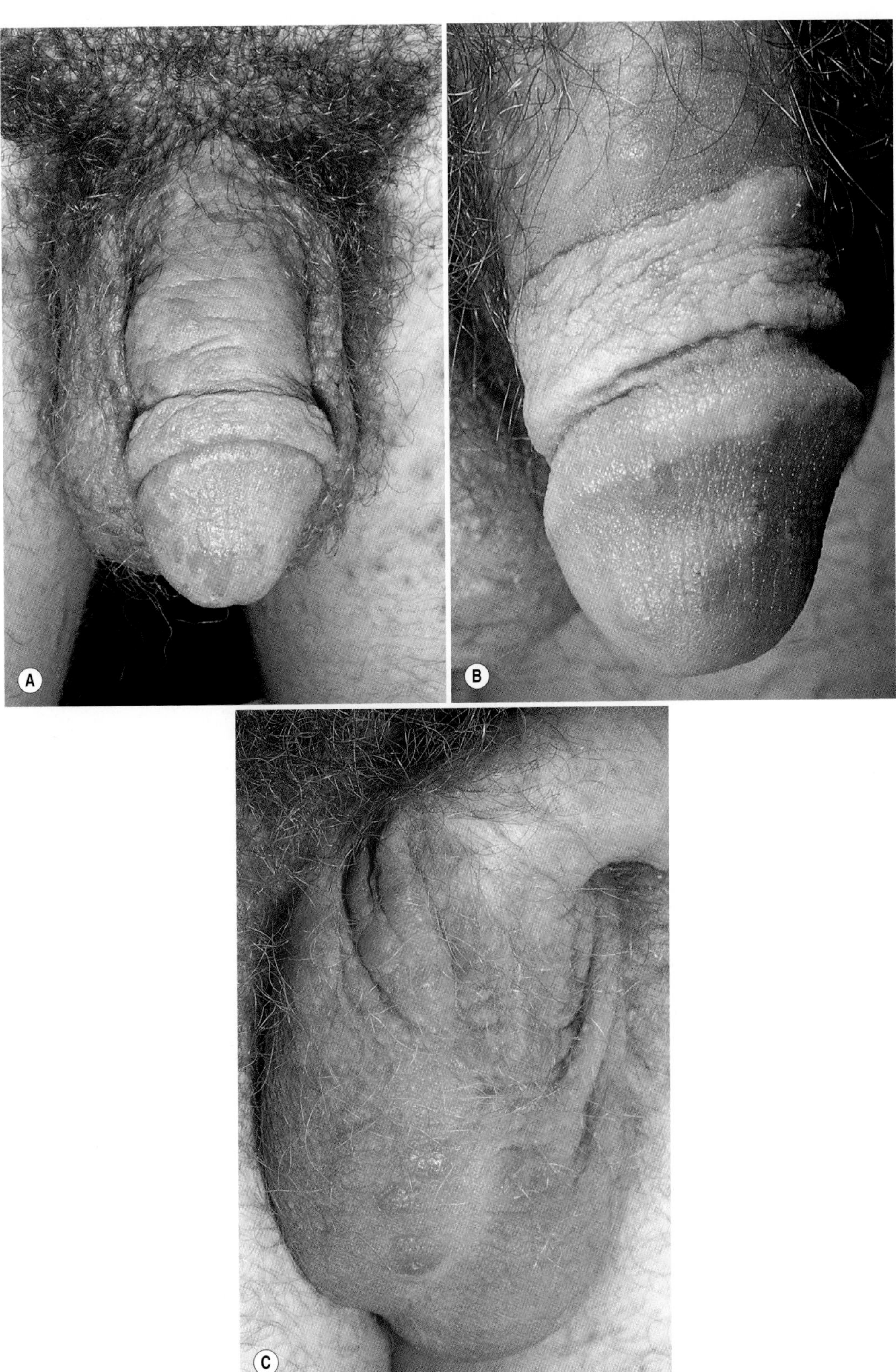

Figure 15-7 **A,** The genitals and groin are acutely inflamed with a widespread infestation. **B,** Eroded papules on the glans is a highly characteristic sign of scabies. **C,** An established infestation of the penis and scrotum. Large papules may remain after appropriate therapy and sometimes require treatment with intralesional steroids.

DISTRIBUTION

Lesions of scabies are typically found in the finger webs, wrists, extensor surfaces of the elbows and knees, sides of the hands and feet, axillary areas, buttocks, waist area, and ankle area (Figures 15-8 and 15-9). In men, the penis and scrotum are usually involved; in women, the breast, including the areola and nipple, may be infested. Lesions, often vesicular or pustular, may be most numerous on the palms and soles of infants. The scalp and face, rarely involved in adults, occasionally are infested in infants.

The number and type of lesions and the extent of involvement vary greatly among patients. Some patients have a few itchy vesicles in the finger webs early in the course of their disease. Many patients in these early stages attempt self-treatment and are encouraged by the relief obtained from over-the-counter, antipruritic lotions. Topical steroids offer greater relief but mask the progressive disease by suppressing inflammation. Delay of proper treatment allows the eruption to extend into all of the characteristic areas, as well as onto the trunk, arms, legs, and occasionally the face. Extensive involvement is often accompanied by erythema, scaling, and infection. Infants and children have diffuse scabies more often than do adults. Symptoms vary from periods of nocturnal pruritus to constant, frantic itching. Untreated scabies can last for months or years.

INFANTS

Infants, more frequently than adults, have widespread involvement. This may occur because the diagnosis is not suspected and proper treatment is delayed while medication is given for other suspected causes of itching, such as dry skin, eczema, and infection. Infants occasionally are infested on the face and scalp, something rarely seen in adults. Vesicles are common on the palms and soles; this is a highly characteristic sign of scabies in infants (see Figure 15-6). Secondary eczematization and impetiginization are common, but burrows are difficult to find. Nodules may be seen in the axillae and diaper area.

THE ELDERLY

Elderly patients may have few cutaneous lesions but itch severely. The decreased immunity associated with advanced age may allow the mites to multiply and survive in great numbers. These patients have few cutaneous lesions other than excoriations, dry skin, and scaling, but they experience intense itching. Eventually papules and nodules appear and may become numerous. Entire nursing home populations may be infested (see Treatment and Management section). A skin scraping from any scaling area may show numerous mites at all stages of development.

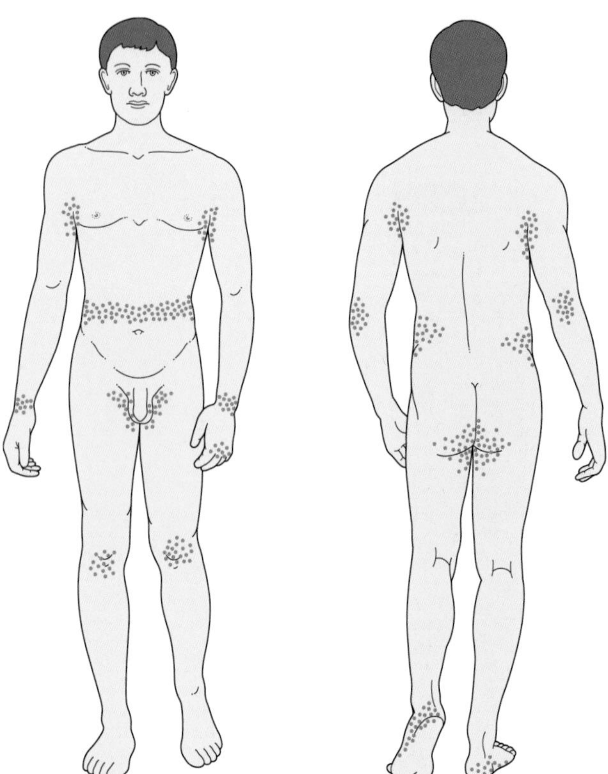

Figure 15-8 Scabies. Distribution of lesions.

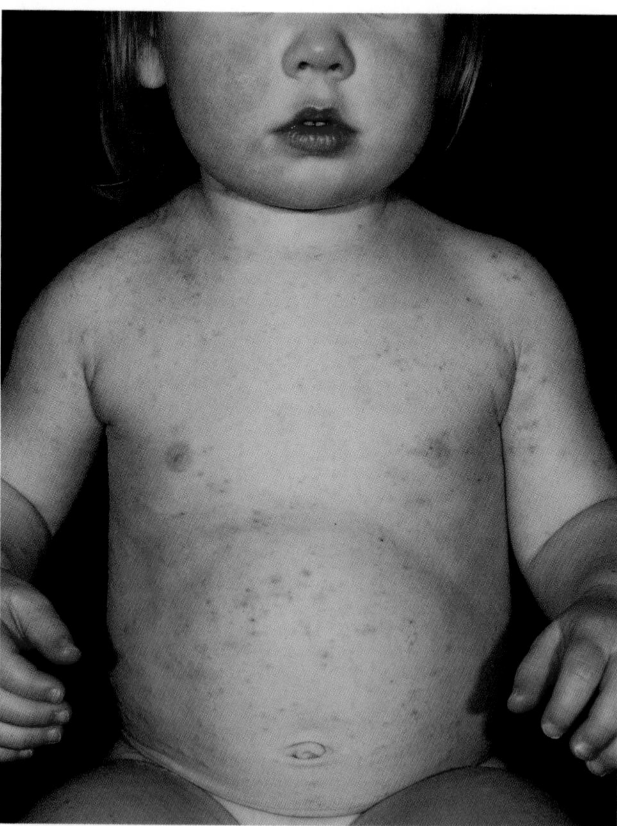

Figure 15-9 Diffuse scabies on an infant. The face is clear. The lesions are most numerous around the axillae, chest, and abdomen.

CRUSTED (NORWEGIAN) SCABIES

The term Norwegian scabies was first used in 1848 to describe an overwhelming scabies infestation of patients with Hansen's disease. In patients with crusted scabies, lesions tend to involve hands and feet with asymptomatic crusting rather than the typical inflammatory papules and vesicles (Figure 15-10). There is thick, subungual, keratotic material and nail dystrophy. Digits and sites of trauma may show wartlike formations. Gray scales and thick crusts may be present over the trunk and extremities. Desquamation of the facial skin may occur. The hair may shed profusely. Crusted scabies occurs in people with neurologic or mental disorders (especially Down syndrome), senile dementia, nutritional disorders, infectious diseases, leukemia, and immunosuppression (such as patients with acquired immunodeficiency syndrome). Itching may be absent or severe. A lack of immunity and indifference to pruritus have been suggested as reasons for the development of this distinct clinical picture. A mineral oil or potassium hydroxide examination of crusts shows numerous mites at all stages of development.

Diagnosis

The diagnosis is suspected when burrows are found or when a patient has typical symptoms with characteristic lesions and distribution (Box 15-1). In a report from a sub-Saharan region, the presence of diffuse itching and visible lesions associated either with at least two typical locations of scabies or with a household member with itching had 100% sensitivity and 97% specificity for the diagnosis. *PMID: 15550260*

A definite diagnosis is made when any of the following products are obtained from burrows or vesicles and identified microscopically: mites, eggs, egg casings (hatched eggs), or feces (scybala). About 5 to 15 female mites live on a person infected with classic scabies. Failure to find a mite is common and does not rule out the diagnosis of scabies.

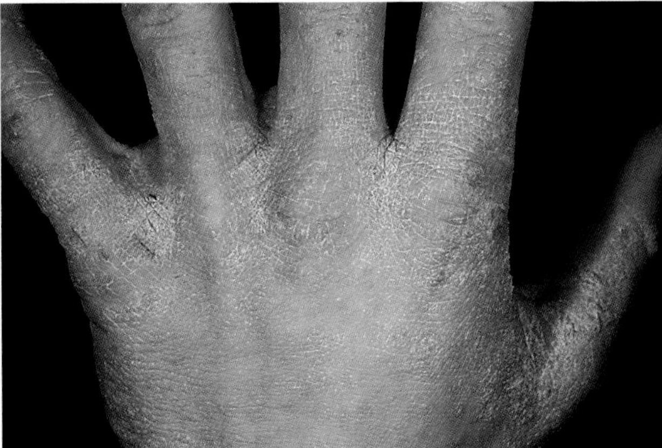

Figure 15-10 Crusted or Norwegian scabies is a variant of scabies in which there are thousands of mites but little itch.

Hundreds or thousands of mites can occur in cases of crusted scabies. Mites are easily demonstrated in such patients.

BURROW IDENTIFICATION

Initially, the areas most apt to contain burrows are observed. To enhance burrows for better viewing, the surface should be touched with a drop of mineral or immersion oil or a blue or black fountain or felt-tip pen (the ink method dyes the burrow; surface ink may be removed with an alcohol swab). The burrow absorbs the ink and is highlighted as a dark line (Figure 15-11). The accentuated lesions are smoothly scraped away with a curved #15 scalpel blade and transferred to a glass microscope slide for examination.

Box 15-1 Signs and Symptoms of Scabies

- Nodules on the penis and scrotum
- Rash present for 4 to 8 weeks has suddenly become worse
- Pustules on the palms and soles of infants
- Nocturnal itching
- Generalized, severe itching
- Pinpoint erosions and crusts on the buttocks
- Vesicles in the finger webs
- Diffuse eruption sparing the face
- Patient becomes better, then worse, after treatment with topical steroids
- Rash is present in several members of the same family
- Patient (especially an infant) develops more extensive rash despite treatment with antibiotics and topical medications

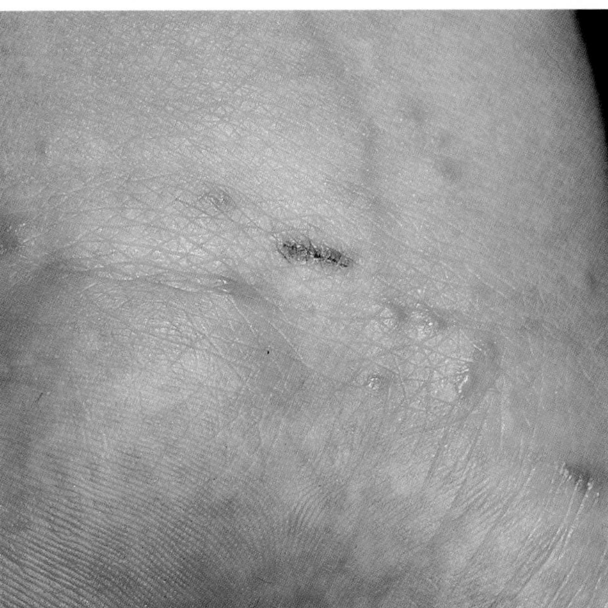

Figure 15-11 Felt-tipped ink pen has penetrated and highlighted a burrow. The ink is retained after the surface is wiped clean with an alcohol swab.

SAMPLING TECHNIQUES AND SLIDE MOUNT PREPARATION

Various techniques are available for obtaining diagnostic material. In most cases the suspected lesion can be sampled easily if it is shaved or scraped with a #15 surgical blade and the material is transferred to a microscope slide for direct examination.

MINERAL OIL MOUNTS. A drop of mineral oil may be placed over the suspected lesion before removal. Skin scrapings adhere, feces are preserved, and the mite remains alive and motile in clear oil. Squamous cells do not separate when heated in a clear oil mount, and mites under a clump of squamous cells may be missed.

POTASSIUM HYDROXIDE WET MOUNTS. The scrapings are transferred directly to a glass slide, a drop of potassium hydroxide is added, and a coverslip is applied. If diagnostic material is not found, the preparation is gently heated and the coverslip is pressed to separate squamous cells. Feces remain intact for short periods but may be dissolved quickly when the mount is heated. Skin biopsy is rarely necessary to make the diagnosis.

ADHESIVE TAPE. Firmly apply the adhesive side of tape onto a skin lesion. The tape is then pulled off and transferred directly onto a slide for microscopy, affixing the adhered separated part of the corneal skin to the slide.

This method is simple and useful for diagnosis of severe scabies infestation in long-term nursing units where scraping lesions is sometimes not practical. *PMID: 16908942*

Treatment and management

PERMETHRIN

Permethrin (Elimite cream) is a synthetic pyrethrin that demonstrates extremely low mammalian toxicity. It is the drug of choice for the treatment of scabies in children and adults of all ages including pregnant and lactating women. Studies show that cure rates are similar or better than those for lindane. A diminished sensitivity to permethrin has been documented. One application is said to be effective but a second treatment 1 week after the first application is standard practice. The over-the-counter permethrin preparation Nix is lower in strength (1%) and ineffective against scabies. Unlike lindane, permethrin undergoes insignificant absorption (2%), after which it is rapidly degraded.

LINDANE

Lindane is the generic name for the chemical γ-benzene hexachloride, a compound chemically similar to an agricultural pesticide also referred to as lindane. It is a central nervous system stimulant that produces seizures and death in the scabies mite. Kwell is one brand name for lindane. Generic lindane is available. Lindane is available as a cream, shampoo, and lotion. Lotion dispensed from bulk containers may not be agitated; therefore the concentration of lindane may be inadequate. Reports of lindane resistance have appeared. A second treatment 1 week after the first application is standard practice. A follow-up examination at 2 to 4 weeks is recommended. Approximately 10% of lindane is absorbed through intact skin. Lindane accumulates in fat and binds to brain tissue. Pruritus may persist for weeks. Additional, unprescribed applications, without documented evidence of persistent infestation, may be dangerous. Lindane should be avoided in children younger than 2 years of age, pregnant or nursing women, and patients with human immunodeficiency virus or acquired immunodeficiency syndrome. Children with severe, underlying, cutaneous disease may be at greater risk for toxicity. This is also true for premature, emaciated, or malnourished children and those with a history of seizure disorders. Lindane is no longer available in the United Kingdom or Australia.

APPLICATION TECHNIQUE FOR PERMETHRIN AND LINDANE. The cream or lotion is applied to all skin surfaces below the neck and the face in children. Patients with relapsing scabies and the elderly should be treated from head (including the scalp) to toe. One ounce is usually adequate for adults. Reapply medicine to the hands if hands are washed. The nails should be cut short and medication applied under them vigorously with a toothbrush. A hot, soapy bath is not necessary before application. Moisture increases the permeability of the epidermis and increases the chance for systemic absorption. If a patient has bathed before lindane administration, the skin must be allowed to completely dry to prevent excessive absorption. Adults should wash 12 hours after application, and infants should be washed 8 to 12 hours after application. One application of either medicine is considered adequate. Many clinicians prefer two applications 1 week apart. Patients should be told that it is normal to continue to itch for days or weeks after treatment and that further application of medication is usually not necessary and worsens itching by causing irritation. Bland lubricants may be applied to relieve itching.

BENZYL BENZOATE

The 25% lotion is the most common preparation. A standard program in developing countries consists of a bath with monosulfiram soap followed by application of benzyl benzoate lotion to the entire body below the neck, repeated daily for 3 to 5 consecutive days. Reported cure rates vary from 50% to over 80%. It may cause irritant dermatitis especially in the genital area and on the face. There is no evidence for adverse effects on pregnancy outcome. It is not avaliable in the United States.

CROTAMITON (EURAX LOTION)

The toxicity of crotamiton is unknown. Reported cure rates for once-a-day application for 2 to 5 days range from 50% to 100%. Crotamiton may have antipruritic properties, but this has been questioned.

SULFUR

Sulfur has been used to treat scabies for more than 150 years. The pharmacist mixes 6% (5% to 10% range) precipitated sulfur in petrolatum or a cold cream base. The compound is applied to the entire body below the neck once each day for 3 days. The patient is instructed to bathe 24 hours after each application. Sulfur applied in this manner is highly effective, but these preparations are messy, have an unpleasant odor, stain, and cause dryness. Sulfur in petrolatum is thought to be safe for infants less than 2 months old and pregnant and nursing women.

IVERMECTIN (STROMECTOL)

Ivermectin is used for patients who fail topical therapy, the elderly, patients with generalized eczema, or those who cannot tolerate or comply with topical therapy. Cure rates increase when ivermectin is used in combination with topical scabicides. A single dose of ivermectin (200 mcg/kg) is reported to be 70% to 80% effective for the treatment of scabies. The cure rate increases to 95% if a second ivermectin dose is taken 2 weeks later. The standard single dose is two Stromectol 6 mg tablets for a 70-kg person. It is important to dose by weight and increase the dose for heavier patients.

ERADICATION PROGRAM FOR NURSING HOMES

Scabies is a problem in nursing homes. The severity is greater than that in an ambulatory population. The face and scalp can be involved, and multiple treatments may be necessary. The first problem is proper diagnosis. The elderly have an atypical presentation with few lesions other than excoriations, dry skin, and scaling, but they experience intense itching. Lesions are located on the back and buttocks rather than the web spaces, axilla, and groin. A plan for eradication of scabies in nursing homes is outlined in Box 15-2.

Box 15-2 **Management of Scabies Epidemic in an Extended-Care Facility**

1. Educate patients, staff, family, and frequent visitors about scabies and the need for cooperation in treatment.
2. Apply scabicide to all patients, staff, contact staff, and frequent visitors, symptomatic or not. Treat symptomatic family members of staff and visitors.
3. Launder in hot water all bedding and clothes worn in the last 48 hours (or dry clean).
4. Clean beds and floors with routine cleaning agents just before scabicide is removed.
5. Reexamine for treatment failures in 1 and 4 weeks.

MANAGEMENT OF COMPLICATIONS

ECZEMATOUS INFLAMMATION AND PYODERMA. Patients with signs of infection should be prescribed systemic antibiotics that treat *Staphylococcus aureus* and *Streptococcus pyogenes*. A group V topical steroid may be applied three times a day to all red, scaling lesions for 1 or 2 days before the application of lindane.

POST-SCABIETIC PRURITUS. Pruritus may persist for weeks after treatment and may be attributed to a hypersensitivity response to remaining dead mites and mite products.

Itching usually decreases substantially 24 hours after treatment and then gradually decreases during the following week or two. Patients with persistent itching may be treated with oral antihistamines, and, if inflammation is present, they may be treated with topical steroids. Intractable itching responds to a short course of systemic corticosteroids.

NODULAR SCABIES. Persistent nodular lesions, most commonly found on the scrotum, are treated with intralesional steroids (e.g., triamcinolone acetonide [Kenalog] 10 mg/ml).

ENVIRONMENTAL MANAGEMENT. Intimate contacts and all family members in the same household should be treated. The spread of scabies via inanimate objects occurs. Live mites have been recovered from dust samples, chairs, and bed linens in the homes of patients with scabies up to 96 hours after being isolated from the host. Clothing that has touched infected skin should be washed. Wash all clothing, towels, and bed linen (in a normal washing machine cycle) that have touched the skin. It is not necessary to rewash clean clothing that has not yet been worn. Bed linens, floors, and chairs should be vacuumed and cleaned. It is especially important to thoroughly clean the rooms of patients who are confined in single rooms in long-term care facilities.

Scabies in long-term care facilities

Scabies in a nursing home can be highly disruptive. The staff, families, and patients become anxious about issues of treatment, origin of infestation, hygiene, and communicability. Everyone has a sense of urgency. Diagnosis is often a problem.

DIAGNOSIS. It is important to confirm the diagnosis microscopically before committing large financial resources to treatment. The diagnosis of scabies should be considered in any nursing home resident with an unexplained generalized rash. The clinical presentation may vary in older, immunocompromised, or cognitively impaired persons. Erythematous, papulosquamous lesions are predominantly truncal. Pruritus is often absent.

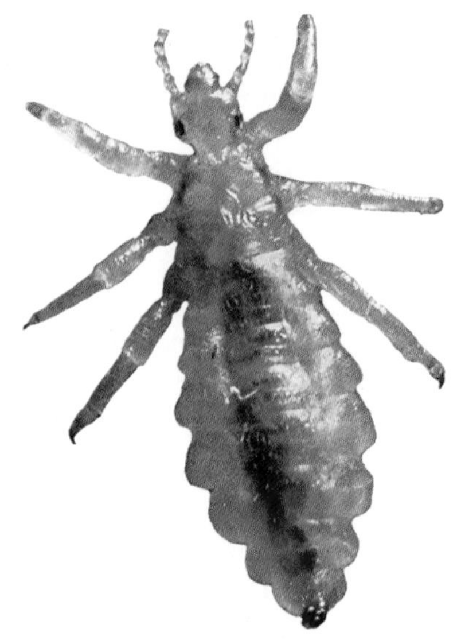

Figure 15-12 Body louse. The largest of three lice infesting humans.

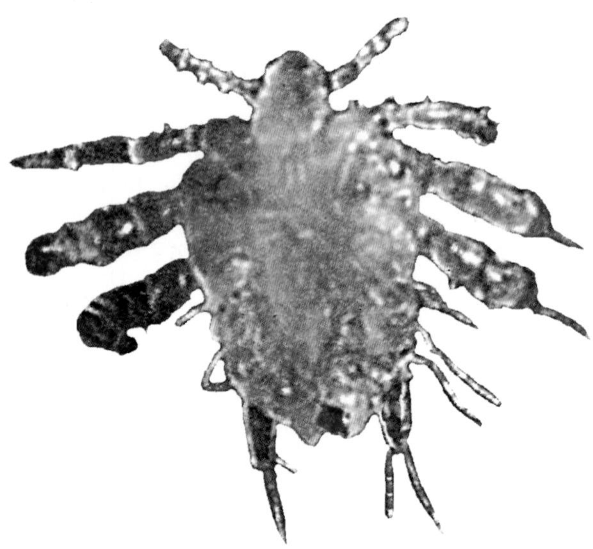

Figure 15-13 Crab louse has a short body and large claws used to grasp hair.

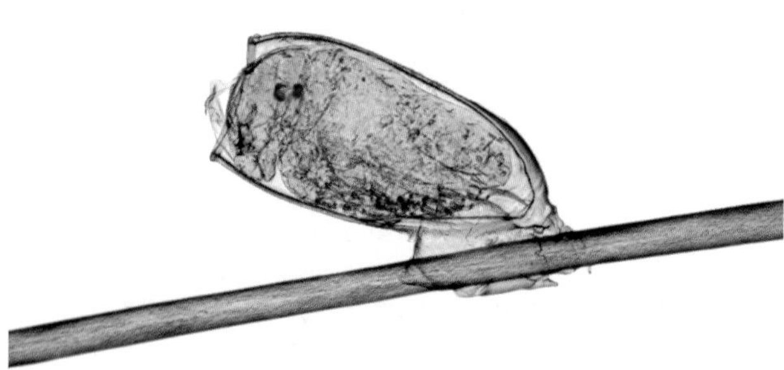

Figure 15-14 Louse egg (nit) is cemented to a hair shaft.

PEDICULOSIS

Infestation with lice is called pediculosis. Lice are transmitted by close personal contact and contact with objects such as combs, hats, clothing, and bed linen. Infestation is usually symptomless and is not associated with serious disease. Lice cannot jump or fly. Pets are not vectors. Diagnosis is made by seeing the lice or their eggs. Treatment with lindane, permethrin, pyrethrins, and malathion is used, but resistance to all medications has been documented in various countries.

Biology and life cycle

Lice are obligate human parasites that cannot survive off their host for more than 10 days (adults) to 3 weeks (fertile eggs). Actual survival rates may be shorter than this. Lice are called ectoparasites because they live on, rather than in, the body. They are classified as insects because they have six legs. Three kinds of lice infest humans: *Pediculus humanus* var. *capitis* (head louse), *Pediculus humanus* var. *corporis* (body louse), and *Phthirus pubis* (pubic or crab louse). All three have similar anatomic characteristics. Each is a small (less than 2 mm), flat, wingless insect with three pairs of legs located on the anterior part of the body directly behind the head. The legs terminate in sharp claws that are adapted for feeding and permit the louse to grasp and hold firmly onto hair or clothing. The body louse is the largest and is similar in shape to the head louse (Figure 15-12). The crab louse is the smallest, with a short, oval body and prominent claws resembling sea crabs (Figure 15-13).

Lice feed approximately five times each day by piercing the skin with their claws, injecting irritating saliva, and sucking blood. They do not become engorged like ticks, but after feeding they become rust colored from the ingestion of blood; their color is an identifying characteristic. Lice feces can be seen on the skin as small, rust-colored flecks. Saliva and, possibly, fecal material can induce a hypersensitivity reaction and inflammation. Lice are active and can travel quickly, which explains why they can be transmitted so easily. The life cycle from egg to egg is approximately 1 month.

NITS

The female lays approximately six eggs, or nits, each day for up to 1 month, and then dies. The louse incubates, hatches in 8 to 10 days, and reaches maturity in approximately 18 days. Nits are 0.8 mm long and are firmly cemented to the bases of hair shafts close to the skin to acquire adequate heat for incubation (Figure 15-14). Nits are very difficult to remove from the hair shaft.

Clinical manifestations

PEDICULOSIS CAPITIS

The head louse effectively infests only the human head and is distinct from body and pubic lice. Lice infestation of the scalp is most common in children. More girls than boys are afflicted and American blacks rarely have head lice. Head lice can be found anywhere on the scalp, but are most commonly seen on the back of the head and neck and behind the ears (Figure 15-15). The average patient carries less than 20 adult lice. Less than 5% of patients will have more than 100 lice in the scalp. Scratching causes inflammation and secondary bacterial infection, with pustules, crusting, and cervical adenopathy. Sensitization to the lice toxin, feces, or body parts takes 3 to 8 months and is a cause of pruritus. Posterior cervical adenopathy without obvious disease is characteristic of lice. The eyelashes may be involved, causing redness and swelling. Examination of the posterior scalp shows few adult organisms but many nits. Nits are cemented to the hair, whereas dandruff scale is easily moved along the hair shaft. Head lice can survive away from the human host for about 3 days, and nits can survive for up to 10 days. The primary source of transmission is direct contact with an infested person but fomite transmission (hats, brushes, combs, earphones, bedding, furniture) is common. Head lice do not carry or transmit any human disease.

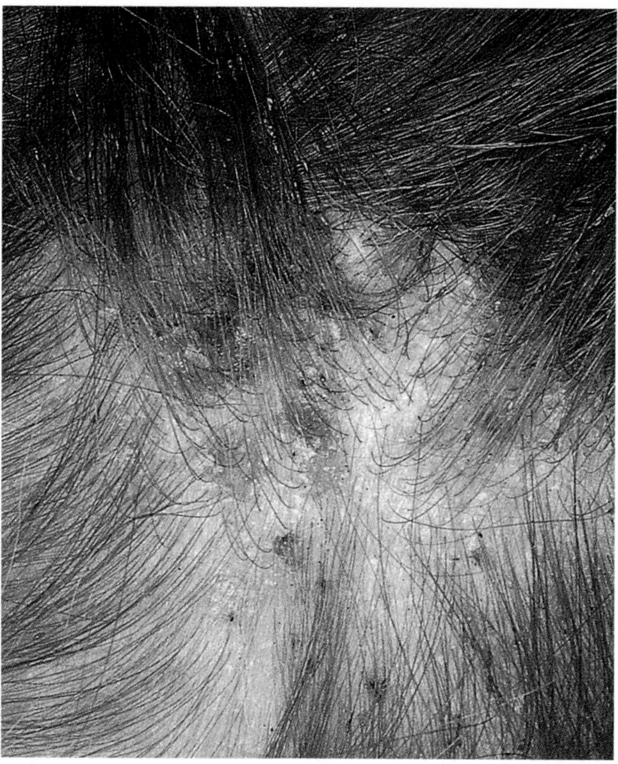

Figure 15-15 Pediculosis capitis. A heavy infestation with secondary pyoderma.

PEDICULOSIS CORPORIS

Infestation by body lice is uncommon. Typhus, relapsing fever, and trench fever are spread by body lice during wartime and in underdeveloped countries. Pediculosis corporis is a disease of the unclean. Body lice live and lay their nits in the seams of clothing and return to the skin surface only to feed. They run and hide when disturbed and are rarely seen. Body lice induce pruritus that leads to scratching and secondary infection.

EYELASH INFESTATION. Infestation of the eyelashes is seen almost exclusively in children. The lice are acquired from other children or from an infested adult with pubic lice. Eyelash infestation may induce blepharitis with lid pruritus, scaling, crusting, and/or purulent discharge. Eyelash infestation may be a sign of childhood sexual abuse (Figure 15-16).

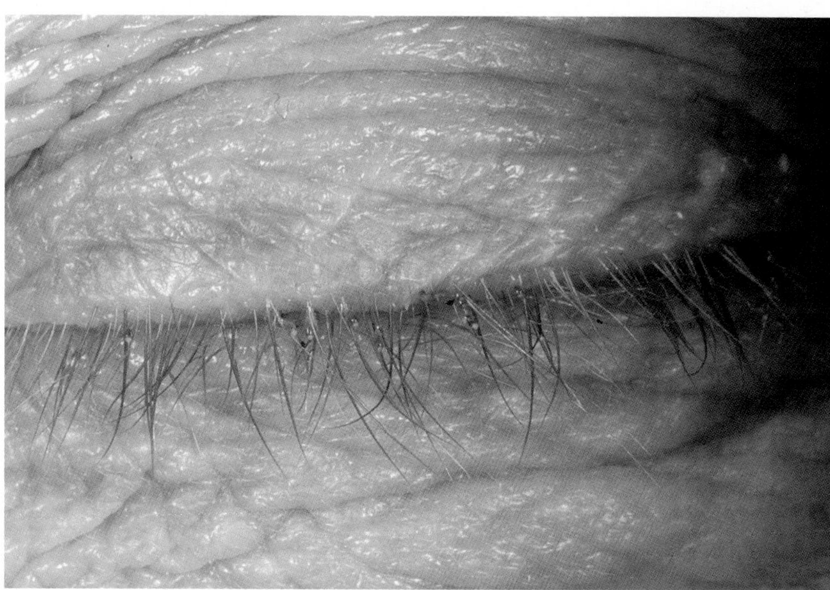

Figure 15-16 Eyelash infestation. *P. pubis* infestation may be found with both parasites and their nits attached to the eyelashes.

PEDICULOSIS PUBIS

Pubic lice are the most contagious sexually transmitted problem known. Up to 30% of patients infested with pubic lice have at least one other sexually transmitted disease. The chance of acquiring pubic lice from one sexual exposure with an infested partner is more than 90%, whereas the chance of acquiring syphilis or gonorrhea from one sexual exposure with an infected partner is approximately 30%. Blacks are affected with the same frequency as whites. The pubic hair is the most common site of infestation (Figure 15-17), but lice frequently spread to the hair around the anus. On hairy persons, lice may spread to the upper thighs, abdominal area, axillae, chest, and beard. Infested adults may spread pubic lice to the eyelashes of children.

The majority of patients complain of pruritus. Many patients are aware that something is crawling on the groin, but are not familiar with the disease and have never seen lice. Approximately 50% of patients have little inflammation, but those who delay seeking help may develop widespread inflammation and infection of the groin with regional adenopathy. Occasionally, gray-blue macules (maculae ceruleae) varying in size from 1 to 2 cm are seen in the groin and at sites distant from the infestation. Their cause is not known, but they may represent altered blood pigment.

Diagnosis

Lice are suspected when a patient complains of itching in a localized area without an apparent rash. Scalp and pubic lice will be apparent to those who carefully examine individual hairs; they are not apparent with only a cursory examination. Finding nits does not indicate active infestation. Nits may persist for months after successful treatment. Live eggs reside within a quarter inch of the scalp.

COMBING

Combing the hair with a fine-toothed "nit," or detection, comb is effective for detecting and removing live lice. The comb is inserted near the crown until it touches the scalp, and then drawn firmly down. The teeth of the comb should be 0.2 to 0.3 mm apart to trap lice. The entire head of hair should be combed at least twice; the comb should be examined for lice after each stroke. It usually takes 1 minute to find the first louse.

Lice and nits can be seen easily under a microscope. Live nits fluoresce and can be detected easily by Wood's light examination, a technique that is especially useful for rapid examination of a large group of children. Nits that contain an unborn louse fluoresce white. Nits that are empty fluoresce gray.

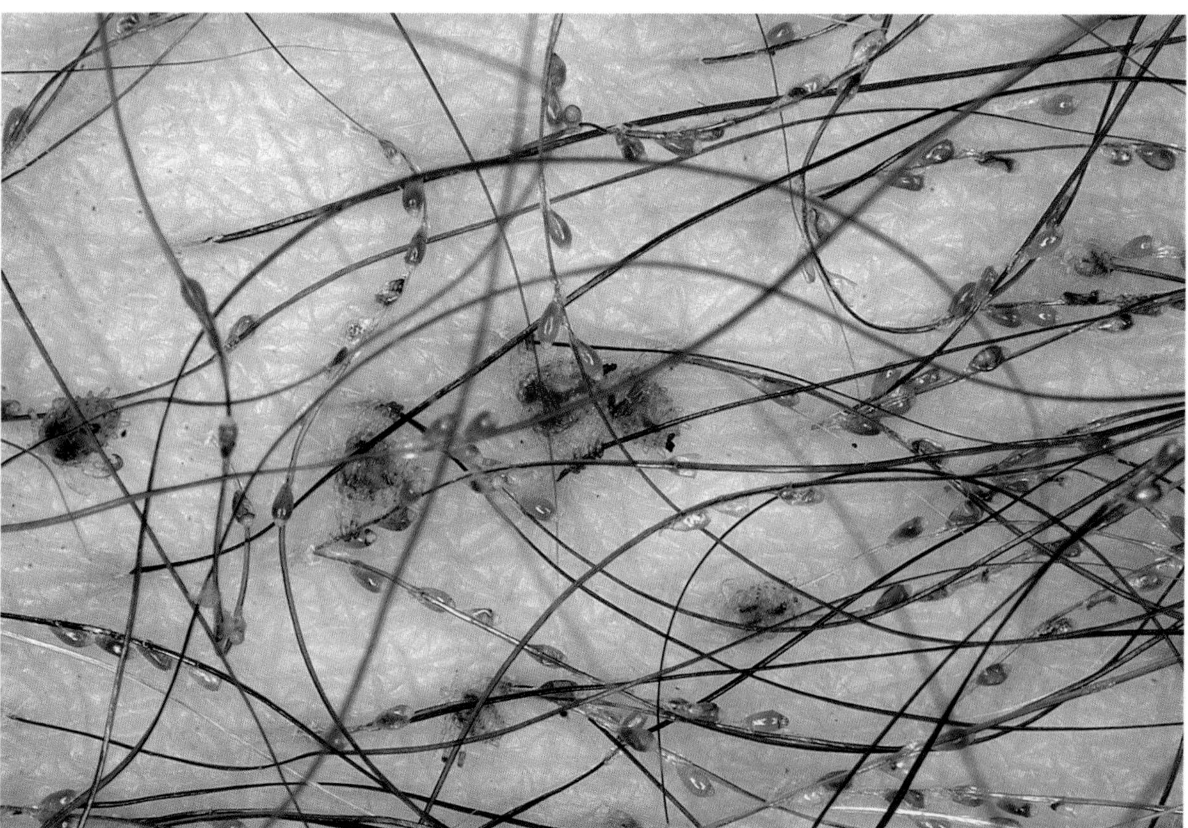

Figure 15-17 Pediculosis pubis. A very heavy infestation with numerous nits and lice in the pubic area. The patient was unaware of the infestation.

Treatment

HEAD, BODY, AND PUBIC LICE

Permethrin 1% or malathion is first-line treatment.

Resistance to all topical medications has been documented. Some head lice in the United States have become resistant to 1% lindane, Nix, and pyrethrins. Ovide was the only pediculicide in the United States that had not become less effective. Insecticides kill both lice and eggs. A fine-toothed comb should be used a day or two after the final application of insecticide to confirm that the treatment has been successful. The presence of live (moving) lice of all sizes suggests resistance to treatment, whereas finding only one adult-sized louse suggests reinfestation. Regular weekly detection combing is recommended for several weeks after cure. Household members and those in close contact with the patient should be screened and treated as necessary. Environmental cleaning is probably unwarranted, although combs and brushes should be washed in hot water.

PERMETHRIN. Permethrin is the most effective over-the-counter treatment. It paralyzes the nerves that allow the lice to breathe. Lice can close their respiratory airways for 30 minutes when immersed in water. Therefore all insecticides are put on dry hair. The cream rinse (Nix) is applied to the scalp after the hair is shampooed and dried. The medication is rinsed out with water after 10 minutes. Permethrin is not 100% ovicidal, and higher cure rates may be obtained by a second application 1 week after the first treatment. Developing eggs have no central nervous system during the first 4 days of life. Insecticides that act on the metabolism of neural tissue must have residual activity to be ovicidal. Permethrin has a clinical efficacy of 95%. Lindane and pyrethrin have cure rates less than 90%. Permethrin, unlike pyrethrin and all other topical insecticides, remains active for 2 weeks and is detectable on the hair for 14 days. Cream rinses and conditioning shampoos coat the hairs and protect the lice from the insecticide. Do not use these products for 2 weeks after permethrin treatment. Patients who fail to respond may respond to the prescription strength cream (5% permethrin; Elimite). The medication is left on overnight under a shower cap.

PYRETHRIN. Pyrethrin (RID, A-200, R & C) is available as a liquid, gel, and shampoo. The shampoos are applied, lathered, and washed off in 5 minutes. Lotions are used for treating body and pubic hair infestation. They are applied over the entire affected area and washed off in 10 minutes. Treatment should be repeated in 7 to 10 days. It does not kill all nits and has no residual activity. It is used a second time 1 week after the initial application.

MALATHION (OVIDE). Malathion is rapidly pediculicidal and ovicidal and is useful for lice resistant to pyrethrins and permethrin. It binds to hair and has residual activity. One treatment is usually sufficient. The lotion is applied to dry hair until the hair and scalp are wet. It need not be applied to the ends of long hair below the level of the shirt collar. It is left on for 8 to 12 hours and then washed out. Nits are removed with a comb. The treatment is repeated in 7 to 9 days if lice are still present. The alcoholic preparation Ovide is flammable until dry. Malathion is available by prescription in the United States but is over-the-counter in the United Kingdom. A 1% shampoo is available outside of the United States. It is applied to the scalp and washed out 10 minutes later and repeated in 1 week. It is not recommended for infants and neonates.

OTHERS. Phenothrin, dimethicone, and carbaryl are other effective topical medications.

LINDANE. Lindane 1% shampoo is indicated for patients who have failed to respond to the previously listed medications or who are intolerant to other lice therapies. Resistance of the louse to lindane is reported.

IVERMECTIN. Ivermectin causes paralysis and death of lice. The drug has selective activity against parasites, without systemic effects in mammals. A single, oral dose of ivermectin (Stromectol) 200 mcg/kg repeated in 10 days is effective. A single dose of 12 mg (two 6-mg pills) is generally used for an average-sized adult. The efficacy is 73% after a single dose. Results were more favorable when ivermectin was used in combination with the LiceMeister comb (www.licemeister.org).

TRIMETHOPRIM/SULFAMETHOXAZOLE (BACTRIM, SEPTRA). A rare patient with severe hair matting and dense infestation may not respond to conventional treatment. The two remaining options are shaving the head or treatment with trimethoprim/sulfamethoxazole (TMP/SMX). One study of 20 females with pediculosis capitis showed that one tablet of Bactrim or Septra (80 mg of trimethoprim plus 400 mg of sulfamethoxazole) twice daily for 3 days resulted in a cure. Within 12 to 48 hours after treatment, the lice migrated to the bed linen and died. *PMID: 678457* Trimethoprim/sulfamethoxazole probably works by killing essential bacteria in the louse's gut. Cotrimoxazole has no effect on nits; therefore a second course must be given 7 to 10 days later.

A combination of 1% permethrin creme rinse (two weekly applications) and TMP/SMX (10-day course) was effective in one study for treating children from 2 to 13 years old. Dual therapy can be reserved for cases of multiple treatment failures or suspected cases of lice-related resistance to therapy. *PMID: 11230611*

NIT REMOVAL

All preparations kill lice, but some nits may survive. Even dead nits remain attached to the hair until removed. Nits are difficult to remove. Over-the-counter "nit looseners" or "nit removers" are probably not very effective. Applying hair conditioner and then gripping the hair with the index finger and thumb and sliding the nits off is effective.

A special comb, the LiceMeister (www.licemeister.org), has 1½-inch-long metal teeth that go through more hair with each pass, collecting both lice and nits. It is available online and at pharmacies. As many nits as possible should be removed to prevent reinfestation. A close haircut may be considered for patients with hundreds of nits.

WET COMBING (BUG BUSTING). Special busting kits are sold with a comb in which the spacing between the teeth is narrow enough to trap the smallest lice but wide enough to pass easily through the hair. Mechanical removal of lice with a wet comb is an alternative to insecticides. The combing procedure is the same as that followed for diagnosis but is done on wet hair with added lubricant (hair conditioner or olive oil) and continued until no lice are found (15 to 30 minutes per session or longer for long, thick hair). Combing is repeated once every 3 to 4 days for several weeks and should continue for 2 weeks after any session in which an adult louse is found. Reported cure rates vary from 38% to 57%.

POMADES. Petrolatum, mayonnaise, and pomades immobilize lice and kill them in about 10 minutes. Copious amounts must be used to ensure inundation of the adult lice in the scalp hair. These noninsecticidal therapies do not kill the eggs (nits), which take 8 to 10 days to hatch. These therapies must be repeated weekly for 4 weeks unless one is able to remove all the nits by combing.

HOT AIR. One 30-minute application of hot air has the potential to eradicate head lice infestations. A custom-built machine called the LouseBuster was effective in killing lice and their eggs when operated at a comfortable temperature, slightly cooler than a standard blow-dryer. *PMID: 17079567*

FOMITE CONTROL. Fomite control is important to prevent reinfestations. Clean bed linens, pillows, towels, clothing, and hats. Rugs, furniture, mattresses, and car seats should be thoroughly vacuumed.

"NO NIT" POLICIES

Exclusion from school for head lice is a common practice. Three fourths of children with nits alone are not infested, and no-nit policies are therefore excessive. Exclusion from school based on the presence of lice or nits is not recommended by the American Public Health Association. A child can return to school immediately after completion of the first application of a normally effective insecticide or the first wet combing session, regardless of the presence of nits. It would be useful to provide a letter of explanation to the school nurse.

EYE INFESTATION

Several methods are used for treating eye infestation. The most practical and effective method is to place petrolatum (Vaseline) on the fingertips, close the eyes, and rub the petrolatum slowly into the lids and brows three times each day for 5 days. A simple alternative is to close the eyes and apply baby shampoo to the lashes and brows with a cotton swab three times each day for 5 days. Some patients are so mortified by the presence of lice close to their eyes that they demand immediate removal. To do so, the reclining patient closes the eyes and the lice are plucked from the eyelashes with forceps. Older children tolerate this simple procedure. Fluorescein drops (10% to 20%) applied to the lids and lashes produce an immediate toxic effect on the lice. Oral ivermectin should be considered for resistant cases.

CATERPILLAR DERMATITIS

Lepidopterism refers to the adverse effects of contact with insects of the order Lepidoptera, which includes moths and butterflies. These effects result from contact with the insects' caterpillar (larval) stage. Of the more than 165,000 species in this order, approximately 150 are medically important. Caterpillars cause illness through urticating setae (hairs) or poisonous spines. Lepidopterism involves multiple pathologic mechanisms, including direct toxicity of venom and mechanical irritant effects. Lepidopterism usually refers to Lepidoptera-associated illness involving systemic reactions, such as generalized pruritus and wheezing. The term *erucism* is used when the condition is limited to contact dermatitis and local urticaria. *PMID: 17368636*

Caterpillars are the larvae of butterflies or moths. Many species of caterpillars possess short hairs (setae) that can irritate the skin (Figure 15-18). Outbreaks of caterpillar dermatitis are seasonal; they occur shortly after the young caterpillars have appeared. Contact with the setae occurs by direct exposure to the caterpillar or windblown setae. Whether the pruritic cutaneous reaction that follows contact is secondary to mechanical irritation, the injection of vasoactive substances, or a hypersensitivity reaction remains unclear.

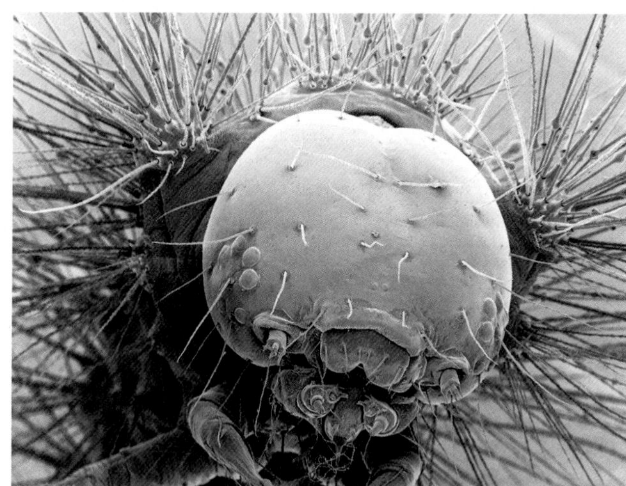

Figure 15-18 Gypsy moth caterpillar. The caterpillar is covered with numerous hairlike structures. (Courtesy Kathleen Shields, PhD, United States Department of Agriculture, Hamden, Conn.)

The brown tail moth and the gypsy moth are found in the northeastern states. Gypsy moth caterpillars hang from trees on long threads. Suspension in the air allows setae to float away on the wind and land on skin or clothing hung out to dry. The puss caterpillar, also known as the wooly slug, is found in the southeastern states. It is approximately 1 inch long and its back and sides are completely covered with fine bristles. The Io moth caterpillar is found east of the Rocky Mountains. It is 2 to 3 inches long and pale green with reddish stripes. Each body segment is armed with tufts of spines. The saddleback caterpillar is found east of Texas and south of Massachusetts. It is approximately 1 inch long, green, and fleshy. The characteristic marking is a brown or purple saddle-shape on the mid-back. Stout spines are located at each end and along the sides; these spines are hollow and contain a toxin. The oak processionary caterpillar is found in several European countries. The larva of *Thaumetopoea processionea* Lepidoptera (oak processionary caterpillar) develops poisonous hair (setae), filled with a urticating toxin that could lead to serious dermatitis, conjunctivitis, and pulmonary problems (lepidopterism) on contact.

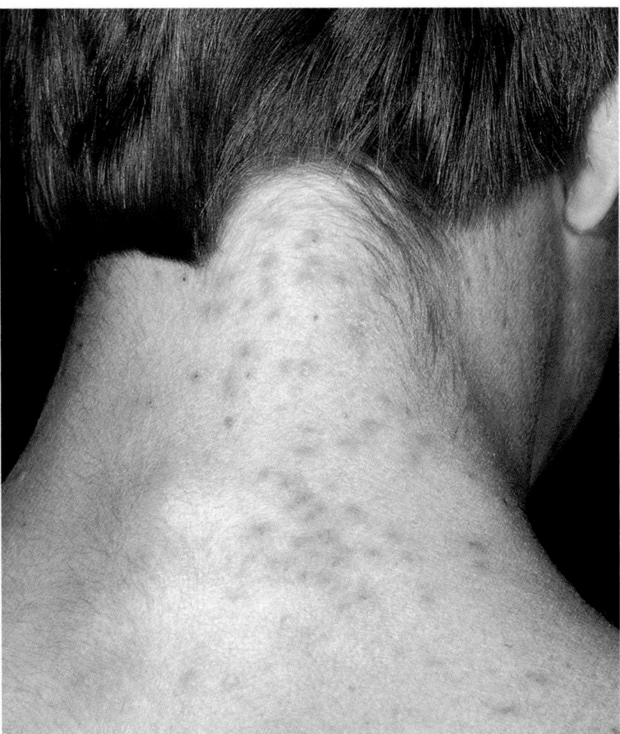

Figure 15-19 Gypsy moth dermatitis. A group of papules and vesicles occurred shortly after a gypsy moth caterpillar was dropped on the neck of this young boy.

Clinical manifestations

Erythema, papules, and vesicles may appear shortly after contact. Irritation may result from mechanical stimulation or from release of irritating substances on the hairs (Figure 15-19). The sting of the puss caterpillar produces an immediate, severe, shooting, burning pain in practically all cases. Some patients experience delayed symptoms such as itching and may develop papules and vesicles similar to those from insect bites 12 hours after exposure. Closed patch testing with gypsy moth caterpillar hairs has revealed that a delayed hypersensitivity response develops in these patients, similar to that in poison ivy contact dermatitis.

DISTRIBUTION

Linear lesions are noted where caterpillars crawl on the skin. Eruptions secondary to windblown hairs that become embedded in clothing are localized around the collar region, the inside surfaces of the arms and legs, the abdominal flank, and the feet. A unique, gridlike track may be left on the skin after contact with the puss caterpillar. In addition to cutaneous signs, some patients develop rhinitis, conjunctivitis, and wheezing. No deaths from caterpillar contact have been reported in the United States.

Diagnosis

The diagnosis is suspected when a rash of the preceding description is seen in the early spring. The diagnosis can be confirmed by demonstrating caterpillar hairs on the skin surface. The technique is as follows. The sticky side of a strip of clear tape is applied to the affected area of skin. The tape is then turned sticky side down onto a microscope slide and observed under low power. Short, straight, threadlike hairs are diagnostic of caterpillar dermatitis.

Treatment

Most cases resolve spontaneously within a few days to 2 weeks. For puss caterpillar stings, the immediate, gentle application of adhesive or clear tape helps to remove remaining spines. Calamine lotion may be helpful, and antihistamines sometimes bring relief if used immediately. Group V topical steroids are useful for persistent or pruritic lesions. Puss caterpillar stings often produce severe pain, which may require potent analgesics. Clothing should not be hung out to dry when thread-suspended caterpillars such as the gypsy moth caterpillar appear in the spring.

SPIDERS

Spiders are carnivorous arthropods that have fangs and venom, which they use to catch and immobilize or kill their prey. Most spiders are small and their fangs are too short to penetrate human skin. Spiders are not aggressive and bite only in self-defense. Spider bites may not be felt at the instant they occur. Localized pain, swelling, itching, erythema, blisters, and necrosis may occur. Most spider venoms are composed of the harmless, enzyme-spreading factor hyaluronidase and a toxin that is distributed by the spreading factor. Most toxins simply cause pain, swelling, and inflammation; however, brown recluse spider toxin causes necrosis, and black widow spider toxin causes neuromuscular abnormalities. Spider bites are common, but of the 50 species of spiders in the United States that have been known to bite humans, only the black widow and the brown recluse spiders are capable of producing severe reactions. The diagnosis of a spider bite cannot be made with certainty unless the act is witnessed or the spider is recovered.

Most spider bites cause pain at the instant they occur. A hivelike swelling appears at the bite site and expands radially, usually for just a few centimeters (Figure 15-20); however, the swelling can sometimes reach gigantic proportions. Occasionally, two puncta or fang marks can be found on the skin surface. The warmth and deep erythema of a bite may resemble bacterial cellulitis, but the hivelike swelling and small, satellite hives are not characteristic of bacterial infection. A biopsy, although usually not necessary for diagnosis, may show mouth parts and intense inflammation. The lesion resolves spontaneously, but itching and swelling can be controlled with cool compresses and antihistamines.

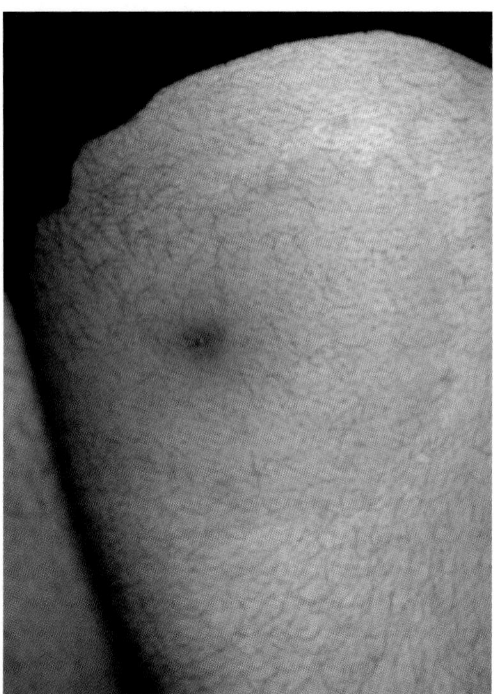

Figure 15-20 Spider bite. An area of erythema may form around the bite site.

Black widow spider

Black widow spider envenomation is commonly associated with severe abdominal pain, muscle cramping, and hypertension. Treatment is primarily symptomatic with the use of opiates and benzodiazepines.

The black widow spider, *Latrodectus mactans* ("shoe-button spider"), is so named because the female attacks and then consumes her mate shortly after copulation. The black widow is found in every state except Alaska and is especially numerous in the rural South. Several species are found in Europe.

Black widow spiders have a shiny, fat abdomen that looks like a big black grape or shoe button, with the longest legs extending out in front. There is a red hourglass marking on the underside of the abdomen. This marking may appear as triangles, spots, or an irregular blotch. Adult females have a total length of 4 cm (Figure 15-21) and are the only spiders capable of envenomation. The venom contains a neurotoxin, alpha-latrotoxin. It binds to specific receptors at the neuromuscular motor end plate of both sympathetic and parasympathetic nerves, resulting in increased synaptic concentrations of catecholamines. This results in clinically migratory muscle cramps and spasm, with nausea, vomiting, hypertension, weakness, malaise, and tremors, usually lasting from days to a week. Normally shy, black widow spiders are found in woodpiles, barns, and garages, but they migrate indoors, into closets and cupboards, during cold weather. They usually do not bite when away from the web because they are clumsy and need the web for support. The web has an unmistakable crinkling, crackling sound when it is disrupted.

CLINICAL MANIFESTATIONS

The bite may produce an immediate, sharp pain or may be painless. The subsequent reaction is minimal, with slight swelling and the appearance of a set of small, red fang marks. The symptoms that follow are caused by lymphatic absorption and vascular dissemination of the neurotoxin and are collectively known as latrodectism. The most com-

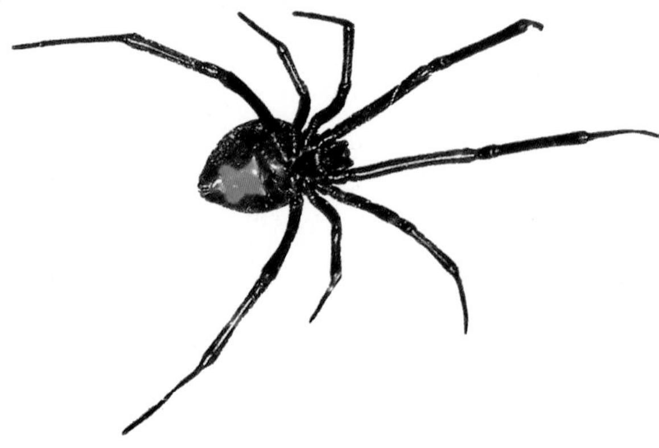

Figure 15-21 Female black widow spider with a red hourglass marking on the underside of her abdomen.

mon presenting complaints are generalized abdominal, back, and leg pain. Fifteen minutes to 2 hours after the bite, a dull muscle cramping or severe pain with numbness gradually spreads from the inoculation site to involve the entire torso but is usually more severe in the abdomen and legs. Any or all of the skeletal muscles may be involved. Severe abdominal pain and spasm simulating a surgical abdomen are the most prominent and distressing features of latrodectism (Figure 15-22). The abdominal muscles assume a boardlike rigidity, but tenderness and distention usually do not occur. There is a generalized increase in the deep tendon reflexes. Other symptoms include dizziness, headache, sweating, nausea, and vomiting. The symptoms increase in severity for several hours (up to 24 hours), slowly subsiding and gradually decreasing in severity in 2 or 3 days. Residual symptoms such as weakness, tingling, nervousness, and transient muscle spasm may persist for weeks or months after recovery from the acute stage. Recovery from one serious attack usually offers complete systemic immunity to subsequent bites. Convulsions, paralysis, shock, and death occur in approximately 5% of cases, usually in the young or the debilitated elderly. There are reports of priapism from widow spider bites that implicate direct venom action on blood vessels, leading to venous engorgement of the penis.

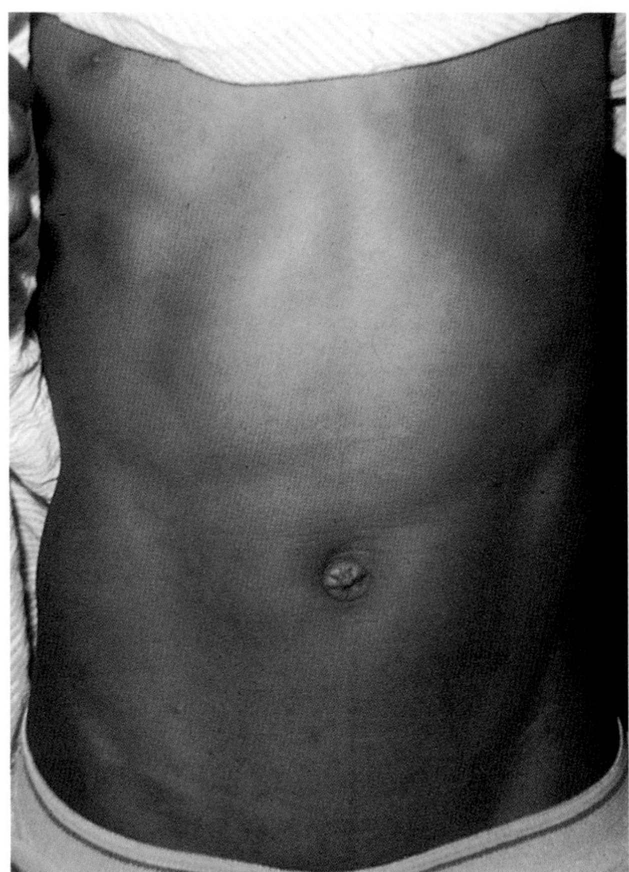

Figure 15-22 Latrodectism. Severe abdominal muscle spasms occurring hours after a black widow spider bite.

TREATMENT

IMMEDIATE FIRST AID. If the patient is seen within a few minutes of being bitten, ice may be applied to the bite site to help restrict the spread of venom. Pain relief is achieved either with black widow spider–specific antivenin alone or with a combination of intravenous opioids and muscle relaxants.

ANTIVENIN. Antivenin (*L. mactans*) has risks, including anaphylaxis and serum sickness. Antivenom is usually reserved for envenomations that cause intractable pain refractory to treatment with opioid analgesia and benzodiazepines or for potentially life-threatening symptoms induced by the envenomation, such as uncontrolled hypertensive emergencies or premature labor. Latrodectus mactans or black widow spider antivenin (Merck & Co., Inc.) is effective regardless of which species of *Latrodectus* causes the bite. The dose consists of the entire contents of one vial (2.5 ml) given intramuscularly or, in severe cases when the patient is under 12 years old or in shock, intravenously in 10 to 100 ml of saline over 15 to 50 minutes. Antivenin may be given intramuscularly for 1 or 2 days. The antivenin is prepared from horse serum and is therefore supplied with a 1-ml vial of normal horse serum for eye-sensitivity testing. The symptoms usually subside in 30 minutes to 3 hours after treatment; occasionally, a second dose is necessary. Hospitalization and treatment with antivenin are indicated for patients who are less than 16 years of age, are older than 60 to 65 years of age, are pregnant, or have hypertensive heart disease, respiratory distress, or symptoms and signs of severe latrodectism. One ampule is sufficient and relieves most of the symptoms within 1 to 2 hours. The administration of antivenin to patients with prolonged or refractory symptoms of latrodectism, even after 90 hours after a bite, may alleviate discomfort and weakness.

Healthy patients between ages 16 and 60 years usually respond to muscle relaxants and recover spontaneously. In emergencies, the local or state poison center or the Department of Public Health may be called for information about the closest source of antivenin.

MUSCLE RELAXANTS. Although calcium gluconate was once the first-line treatment of severe envenomations, it was found in one large series to be ineffective for pain relief compared with a combination of IV opioids and benzodiazepines. Calcium gluconate (10%; 10 ml given intravenously) acts as a muscle relaxant. The administration is repeated only once if pain persists or recurs after 1 to 2 hours. Intravenous Valium may be used and later replaced with Valium pills. Alternatively, diazepam or 1 or 2 gm of methocarbamol (100 mg/ml Robaxin in 10-ml vials) may be administered undiluted over 5 to 10 minutes. Oral doses may be used thereafter, and they usually sustain the relief initiated by the injection.

ANALGESICS. Aspirin or, if pain is severe, intravenous morphine may be given. Morphine should be used with caution, since the venom is a neurotoxin and may cause respiratory paralysis.

Brown recluse spider

The brown recluse spider, *Loxosceles reclusus* ("fiddle-back spider"), is small, approximately 1.5 cm in overall length. Its color ranges from yellowish tan to dark brown. A characteristic, dark, violin- or fiddle-shaped marking is located on the spider's back. The broad base of the violin is near the head and the violin stem points toward the abdomen (Figure 15-23). The spider is a timid recluse, avoiding light and disturbances and living in dark areas (under woodpiles and rocks and inside human habitations, often in closets, behind picture frames, under porches, and in barns and basements). Its web is small, haphazard, and woven in cracks, crevices, or corners. It bites only when forced into contact with the skin, such as when a person puts on clothing in which the spider is residing or rummages through stored material harboring the spider. The brown recluse is usually found in the southern half of the United States, but some have been found as far north as Connecticut. The hobo spider, *Tegenaria agrestis,* has been implicated in necrotic lesions in the Pacific Northwest of the United States (Figure 15-24).

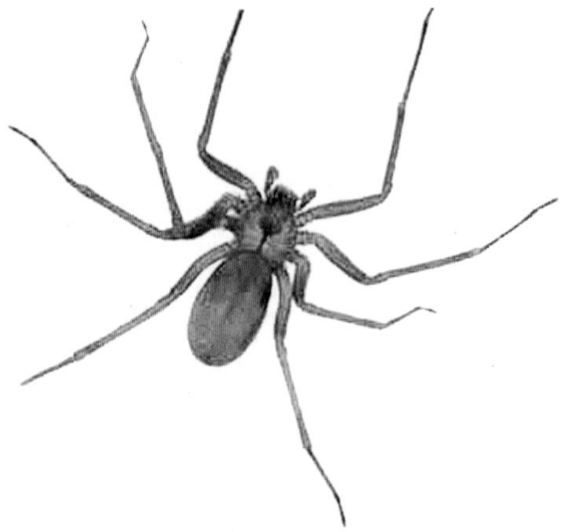

Figure 15-23 The brown recluse spider. A dark, violin-shaped marking is located on the spider's back.

CLINICAL MANIFESTATIONS

Patients infrequently present with a spider for positive identification. Overdiagnosis of brown recluse spider bites has led to harmful sequelae and misdiagnosis. Many patients currently present with a "spider bite," but on investigation they have community-acquired methicillin-resistant *Staphylococcus aureus* (MRSA). There is no laboratory test for diagnosis. A summary of bite severity and treatment is found in Table 15-1. Brown recluse spider bites frequently induce necrotic, slowly healing lesions. Maximum lesion severity is a predictor of time to complete healing. Most bites are on an extremity. The bite produces a minor stinging or burning or an instantaneous sharp pain resembling a bee sting. Most bite reactions are mild and cause only minimal swelling and erythema. Site location seems to be a factor in the severity of the local bite reaction; fatty areas such as the proximal thigh and buttocks show more cuta-

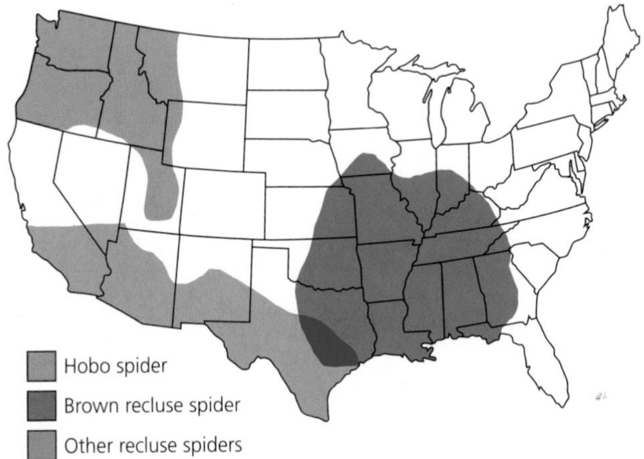

Figure 15-24 Range of the recluse (genus *Loxosceles*) spiders in the United States.

Table 15-1 *L. reclusa* Bite Severity and Treatment

Severity	Clinical appearance/signs	Symptoms	Treatment
Mild	Erythema, punctum, no necrosis	Pruritus	RICE, antihistamine, aspirin, tetanus vaccine
Moderate	Erythema, mild edema, vesicle, necrosis <1 cm^2	Pain, other	Add analgesic, antibiotic; consider dapsone
Severe	Erythema, edema, (hemorrhagic) bullae, ulcer, necrosis >1 cm^2	Pain, other	Add dapsone 50 mg PO daily, then 50 mg bid Order G6PD
Systemic*	Rash, fever, hemolysis, thrombocytopenia, DIC	Myalgia, headache, malaise, nausea	Support; serial CBC and U/A, vigorous hydration, systemic steroids, transfusion

Adapted from Sams HH et al: *J Am Acad Dermatol* 44:561, 2001. *PMID: 11260528*

*Systemic symptoms are possible with bites of all cutaneous severity.

CBC, complete blood cell count; *DIC,* disseminated intravascular coagulation; *G6PD,* glucose-6-phosphate dehydrogenase; *RICE,* rest, ice compresses, elevation; *U/A,* urinalysis.

neous reaction. Severe bites may become necrotic within 4 hours.

The first and most characteristic cutaneous change in necrotic arachnidism, or loxoscelism, is the development and rapid expansion of a blue-gray, macular halo around the puncture site; this halo represents local hemolysis. Violaceous skin discoloration is an indication of incipient necrosis and can be used as a guide to early initiation of therapy, when it is most effective. A cyanotic pustule or vesicle/bulla may also appear at the bite site. The lesion may have an oblong, irregular configuration area at the bite site and a sudden increase in tenderness. At this stage, the superficial skin may be rapidly infarcting and the pain is severe. The necrotizing, blue macule widens and the center sinks below the normal skin surface ("sinking infarct") (Figure 15-25). The extent of the infarct is variable. Most patients experience localized reactions, but the depth of the necrotic tissue may extend to the muscle and over broad areas of skin, sometimes involving most of an extremity. The dead tissue sloughs, leaving a deep, indolent ulcer with ragged edges. Ulcers take weeks or months to heal; scarring is significant.

A severe, progressive reaction that begins with moderate to severe pain at the bite site develops in a few people. Within 4 hours, the pain is unbearable and the initial erythema gives way to pallor. Within 12 to 14 hours after the bite, the victims often experience fever, chills, nausea, vomiting, weakness, joint and muscle pains, and hives or measle-like rashes. The toxin may produce severe systemic reactions such as thrombocytopenia or hemolytic anemia with generalized hemolysis, disseminated intravascular coagulation, renal failure, and sometimes death. Severe systemic reactions are rare and occur most frequently in children. Serial complete blood cell counts should be analyzed for hemolysis, thrombocytopenia, and leukocytosis. Serial urinalyses evaluate the possibility of hemoglobinuria.

A bite during pregnancy does not appear to lead to unusual risks to mother or fetus.

MANAGEMENT

Experience has shown that most bites are mild and should be treated conservatively with the following measures:

1. Bite sites are treated with RICE (Rest, Ice bag Compresses [15 minutes each hour], Elevation).
2. An aspirin a day helps counteract platelet aggregation and thrombosis.
3. Tetanus toxoid is given if necessary.

The application of cold packs to bite sites markedly reduces inflammation, slows lesion evolution, and improves all other combinations of therapy. The application of heat to brown recluse bite sites makes lesions much worse. Immediate surgery is avoided.

MODERATE TO SEVERE SKIN NECROSIS. Serious bites are usually obvious within the first 24 to 48 hours and need medical, but not surgically aggressive, treatment.

- Antibiotics (e.g., cephalosporins) should be used as infection prophylaxis in ulcerating lesions. Secondary infection increases localized skin temperature that increases enzymatic activity and leads to further tissue damage; therefore routine use of antibiotics is suggested.
- Analgesics are usually required.

DAPSONE. Immediate surgical excision of brown recluse bite sites induced more complications than did the use of dapsone with or without delayed excision and/or repair. Dapsone 50 to 200 mg/day may be helpful in severe cutaneous reactions to prevent extensive necrosis, even if it is administered 48 hours after the bite. Dapsone may help prevent the venom-induced perivasculitis with polymorphonuclear leukocyte infiltration that occurs with extensive cutaneous necrosis. Order a glucose-6-phosphate dehydrogenase level and complete blood cell count.

STEROIDS. There is little evidence that oral and intralesional steroids decrease the severity of the progressive reaction. Patients with necrosis greater than 1 cm should be tested to see if progressive hemolytic anemia, manifested by an increasing level of free serum hemoglobin or thrombocytopenia, has developed. Severe systemic loxoscelism may be treated with prednisone (1 mg/kg) given as early as possible in the development of systemic symptoms to treat hematologic abnormalities.

SURGERY. Early excision of necrotic areas was once thought to help prevent the spread of the toxin and further necrosis. This practice is probably ineffective and should be discouraged. If a proven or suspected brown recluse spider bite does not become clinically necrotic within 72 hours, a serious wound healing problem rarely develops.

Sharp debridement or excision of spider bite lesions should be vigorously discouraged. Gentle eschar removal may be performed after the wound has stabilized and inflammation has subsided (approximately 6 to 10 weeks). Surgery is reserved for debridement of necrotic lesions.

ANTIVENIN. An antivenom has been developed. Inquire about availability.

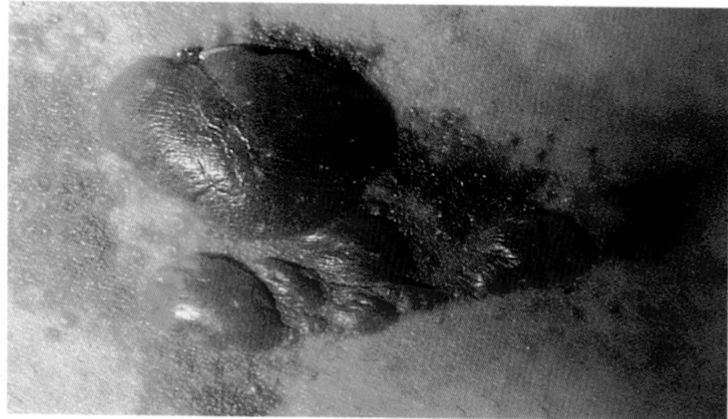

Figure 15-25 Brown recluse spider bite. A severe reaction in which infarction, bleeding, and blistering have occurred.

TICKS

Ticks are blood-sucking ectoparasites that act as vectors for rickettsial, spirochetal, bacterial, and parasitic infections. Adult ticks of some species can reach 1 cm in length; they have eight legs, and the front two are curved forward, as in crabs. The large oval or teardrop-shaped body is flat and saclike and has a leathery outer surface. There are two families of ticks: hard-bodied ticks (Ixodidae) and soft-bodied ticks (Argasidae). They are distinguished by the consistency of their bodies. Hard (ixodid) ticks are of greatest concern because they are vectors for most of the serious tickborne diseases. They can inflict local reactions such as pain, erythema, and nodules, and they are more difficult to remove than the soft (argasid) ticks. Ticks should be removed from the host as soon as possible after they are discovered to reduce the chance of infection. Proper removal of the tick, however, is just as important in reducing the chance of infection as timely removal.

Ticks perch on grass tips and bushes and wait for a warmblooded host to pass by. They insert their recurved teeth into the skin, produce a gluelike secretion that tightens their grip, suck blood (Figure 15-26), and become engorged, sometimes tripling in size. Hard ticks may remain attached to the host for up to 10 days, whereas soft ticks release in a few hours. The bite itself is painless, but within hours an urticarial wheal appears at the puncture site and may cause itching. Ticks may go unnoticed, particularly in children, for several hours after attachment to an inconspicuous area such as the scalp.

Ticks and their associated diseases are listed in Table 15-2.

The deer tick (*Ixodes dammini*) transmits human babesiosis and Lyme disease; it is found in areas such as Massachusetts, Connecticut, New Jersey, and the islands of coastal New England. This tick is common in many areas of southern Connecticut, where it parasitizes three different host animals during its 2-year life cycle. Larval and nymphal ticks have parasitized 31 different species of mammals and 49 species of birds. White-tailed deer appear to be crucial hosts for adult ticks. All three feeding stages of the tick parasitize humans, although most infections are acquired from feeding nymphs in May through early July. Reservoir hosts for the spirochete include rodents, other mammals, and even birds. White-footed mice are particularly important reservoirs, and, in parts of southern Connecticut where Lyme disease is prevalent in humans, *Borrelia* are universally present during the summer in these mice. Prevalence of infected ticks has ranged from 10% to 35%. Isolates of *Borrelia burgdorferi* from humans, rodents, and *I. dammini* are usually indistinguishable, but strains of *B. burgdorferi* with different major proteins have been identified. The recent expansion of the geographic range has been attributed to the proliferation of deer in North America. The spotted fever tick (*Dermacentor variabilis*) is found in sections of the United States other than the Rocky Mountain region. Most *Dermacentor* ticks have white anterodorsal ornamentation. The Rocky Mountain wood tick (*Dermacentor andersoni*) is the vector for Rocky Mountain spotted fever in the west.

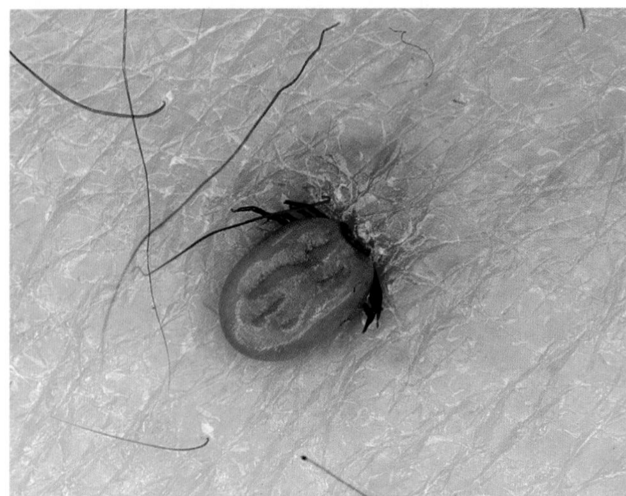

Figure 15-26 Tick. Mouth parts are deeply imbedded in the skin, and the tick is fully engorged with blood.

Lyme disease and erythema migrans

Currently, approximately 15,000 cases of Lyme disease are reported each year. Lyme disease and erythema migrans (EM), which means "chronic migrating red rash," are caused by the spirochete *Borrelia burgdorferi* and are transmitted by the bite of certain *Ixodes* ticks of the *Riricinus* complex and possibly by other ticks. There are at least three different species of *B. burgdorferi* and this may explain why there are differences in the clinical spectrum of Lyme disease in Europe and the United States. *Ixodes* ticks have *B. burgdorferi* in their gastrointestinal systems. Lyme disease is named after Lyme, Connecticut, where the initial cluster of children with arthritis (brief but recurrent attacks of asymmetric swelling and pain in a few large joints, especially the knee, over a period of years) was reported in 1975. Like syphilis, the disease affects many systems, occurs in stages, and mimics other diseases. Cases have since been reported from all parts of the country, and people of all ages are affected. A disproportionate number of children contract Lyme disease because they spend more time in wooded areas than adults. The rapid emergence of focal epidemics is possible. Antigenic differences between European and American strains of the organism may explain some of the minor differences in the clinical presentation of the disease, such as the more prominent skin involvement in European cases.

GEOGRAPHIC DISTRIBUTION

Lyme disease is now recognized on 6 continents and in at least 20 countries. Most cases in the United States are clustered in three regions (Figure 15-27): the Northeast coastal regions; Minnesota and Wisconsin; and parts of California, Oregon, Utah, and Nevada.

REPORTED CASES OF LYME DISEASE
United States, 2007
1 dot placed randomly within county of residence for each reported case

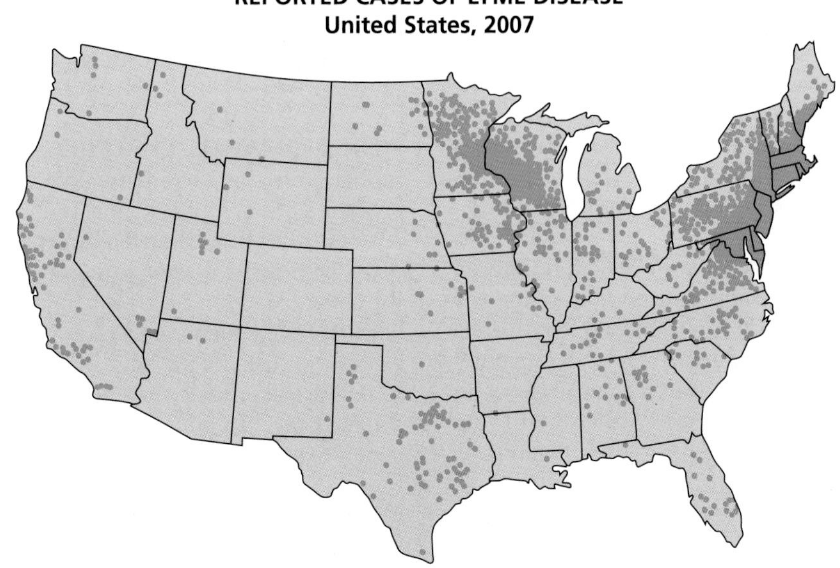

Figure 15-27

Table 15-2 Major Tickborne Diseases in the United States				
Disease	**Causative agent**	**Classification**	**Major vector**	**Region**
Lyme disease	*Borrelia burgdorferi*	Bacteria (spirochete)	*Ixodes*	Northeast, Wisconsin, Minnesota, California
Relapsing fever	*Borrelia* species	Bacteria (spirochete)	*Ornithodoros*	West
Tularemia	*Francisella tularensis*	Bacteria	*Dermacentor, Amblyomma*	Arkansas, Missouri, Oklahoma
Rocky Mountain spotted fever	*Rickettsia rickettsii*	Rickettsia	*Dermacentor*	Southeast, West, South central
Ehrlichiosis	*Ehrlichia chaffeensis*	Rickettsia	*Dermacentor, Amblyomma*	South central, south Atlantic
Colorado tick fever	*Coltivirus* species	Virus	*Dermacentor*	West
Babesiosis	*Babesia* species	Protozoa	*Ixodes*	Northeast
Tick paralysis	Toxin	Neurotoxin	*Dermacentor, Amblyomma*	Northwest, South

From Spach DH et al: *New Engl J Med* 329:936, 1993. *PMID: 8361509*

Eight states (Connecticut, Rhode Island, New York, New Jersey, Delaware, Pennsylvania, Maryland, and Wisconsin) account for 90% of the cases reported. The geographic distribution suggests that *Borrelia* spreads when infested ticks are transported by migratory birds. *Ixodes dammini* (Figure 15-28) is the vector of disease in the Northeast and Midwest, and *Ixodes pacificus* in the West. The disease is reported throughout Europe. Most cases occur in the summer or early fall when people are outdoors, wearing shorts, and walking barefoot through the woods and grass. In the Northeast, they infest the white-tailed deer and white-footed mouse.

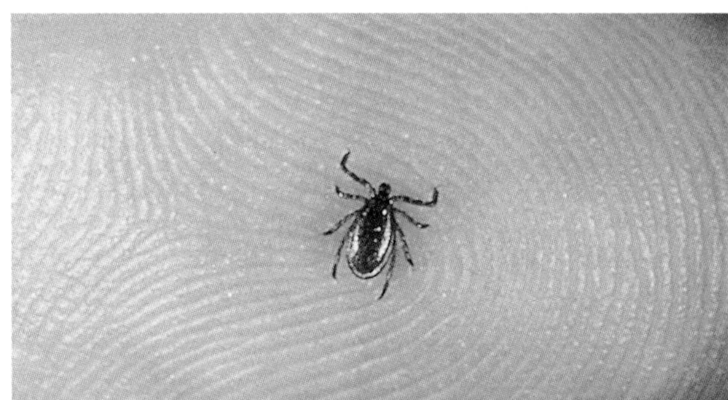

Figure 15-28 The deer tick (*Ixodes dammini*), one of the vectors for transmitting Lyme disease. This tick is very small and can easily go unnoticed when fixed to the skin in an unengorged state.

CUTANEOUS MANIFESTATIONS

The CDC case definition is in Box 15-3. There are three cutaneous lesions associated with Lyme disease: erythema migrans (formally referred to as erythema chronicum migrans), *Borrelia* lymphocytoma, and acrodermatitis chronica atrophicans. There is some evidence that several other cutaneous diseases are associated with *B. burgdorferi* infection.

***BORRELIA* LYMPHOCYTOMA.** *Borrelia* lymphocytoma (BL) generally presents as a bluish-red nodule during the early stages of infection. It most commonly appears on the earlobe or nipple. Histologically there is a dense polyclonal lymphocytic infiltrate, which may appear after erythema migrans (EM) or as the first manifestation of Lyme borreliosis. EM and BL are early, localized cutaneous manifestations, but sometimes extracutaneous signs or symptoms of disseminated disease may appear simultaneously with either of these lesions. BL is rare; the prevalence ranges from 0.6% to 1.3% of cases of Lyme disease.

ACRODERMATITIS CHRONICA ATROPHICANS. During late infection, acrodermatitis chronica atrophicans, an erythematous, atrophic plaque unique to Lyme disease, may appear. It has been described in approximately 10% of patients with Lyme disease in Europe, but it is rarely seen in the United States. It starts with an early inflammatory phase with localized edema and bluish-red discoloration on the extensor surfaces of the hands, feet, elbows, and knees. Years to decades later there may be an atrophic phase where the skin becomes atrophic and dull red and may have a cigarette paper–like appearance.

ERYTHEMA MIGRANS. The skin lesion erythema migrans (EM) is the most characteristic aspect of Lyme disease. It is described in detail in the following paragraphs.

EARLY AND LATE DISEASE. Early Lyme borreliosis includes localized infection, entailing erythema migrans and *Borrelia* lymphocytoma without signs or symptoms of disseminated infection; regional lymphadenopathy and/or minor constitutional symptoms; and/or early disseminated infection, entailing multiple erythema migrans–like skin lesions and early manifestations of neuroborreliosis, arthritis, carditis, or other organ involvement. Late Lyme borreliosis includes chronic infection, entailing acrodermatitis chronica atrophicans, and neurologic, rheumatic, or other organ manifestations that are persistent or remit for at least 12 (or 6) months. The presenting manifestations in symptomatic Lyme disease are listed in Box 15-4.

THREE STAGES OF INFECTION

Lyme disease is divided into three stages that are determined by the duration of the infection from the time of the tick bite (Figure 15-29).

Box 15-3 **CDC Case Definition of Lyme Disease**

Erythema migrans (EM) and early manifestations

EM is defined as a skin lesion that typically begins as a red macule or papule and expands over a period of days to weeks to form a large round lesion, often with partial central clearing. A single primary lesion must reach greater than or equal to 5 cm in size. Secondary lesions also may occur. Annular erythematous lesions occurring within several hours of a tick bite represent hypersensitivity reactions and do not qualify as EM. For most patients, the expanding EM lesion is accompanied by other acute symptoms, particularly fatigue, fever, headache, mildly stiff neck, arthralgia, or myalgia. These symptoms are typically intermittent. The diagnosis of EM must be made by a physician. Laboratory confirmation is recommended for persons with no known exposure.

Late manifestations

Late manifestations include any of the following when an alternate explanation is not found:

Musculoskeletal system

Recurrent, brief attacks (weeks or months) of objective joint swelling in one or a few joints, sometimes followed by chronic arthritis in one or a few joints. Manifestations not considered as criteria for diagnosis include chronic progressive arthritis not preceded by brief attacks and chronic symmetric polyarthritis. Additionally, arthralgia, myalgia, or fibromyalgia syndromes alone are not criteria for musculoskeletal involvement.

Nervous system

Any of the following, alone or in combination: lymphocytic meningitis; cranial neuritis, particularly facial palsy (may be bilateral); radiculoneuropathy; or, rarely, encephalomyelitis. Encephalomyelitis must be confirmed by demonstration of antibody production against *B. burgdorferi* in the CSF, evidenced by a higher titer of antibody in CSF than in serum. Headache, fatigue, paresthesia, or mildly stiff neck alone are not criteria for neurologic involvement.

Cardiovascular system

Acute onset of high-grade (second-degree or third-degree) atrioventricular conduction defects that resolve in days to weeks and are sometimes associated with myocarditis. Palpitations, bradycardia, bundle branch block, or myocarditis alone are not criteria for cardiovascular involvement.

Box 15-4 **Presenting Manifestations in Symptomatic Lyme Disease**

78% presented with erythema migrans.

19% presented with systemic symptoms without erythema migrans; headache and arthralgia were the most common systemic symptoms; sometimes fever; no upper respiratory tract or gastrointestinal symptoms.

3% presented with late systemic involvement (e.g., cranial neuropathy, arthritis).

36% recalled tick bite within preceding month.

There is a 20% risk of Lyme disease after 72 hours of tick feeding vs. 1% with tick feeding <72 hours.

Adapted from *New Engl J Med* 348(24):2472, 2003.
PMID: 12802042

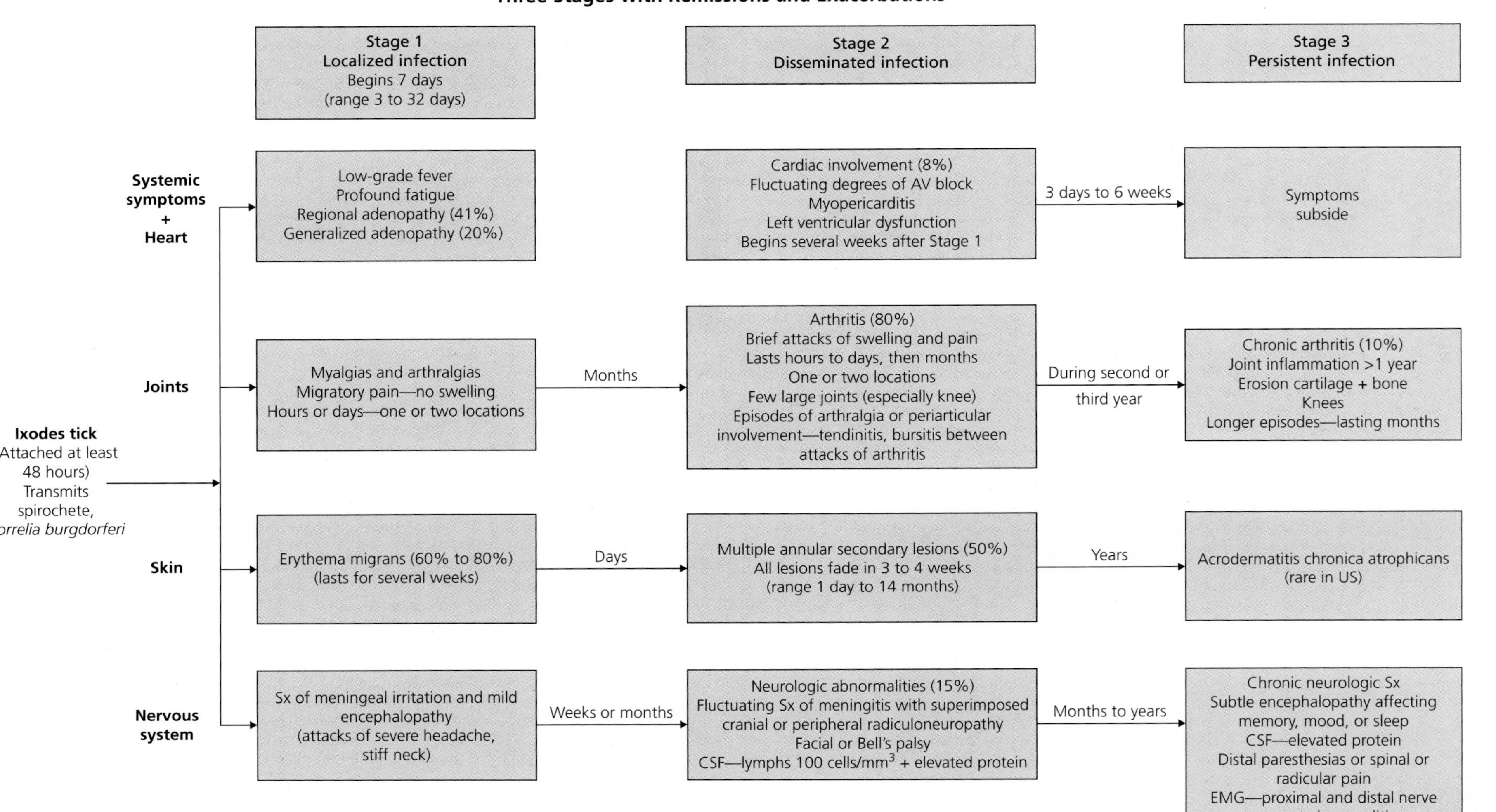
LYME BERRELIOSIS
Three Stages with Remissions and Exacerbations
Stage 1
Localized infection
Begins 7 days
(range 3 to 32 days)
Stage 2
Disseminated infection
Stage 3
Persistent infection
Ixodes tick
(Attached at least 48 hours)
Transmits spirochete, Borrelia burgdorferi
Systemic symptoms + Heart
Low-grade fever
Profound fatigue
Regional adenopathy (41%)
Generalized adenopathy (20%)
Cardiac involvement (8%)
Fluctuating degrees of AV block
Myopericarditis
Left ventricular dysfunction
Begins several weeks after Stage 1
3 days to 6 weeks
Symptoms subside
Joints
Myalgias and arthralgias
Migratory pain—no swelling
Hours or days—one or two locations
Months
Arthritis (80%)
Brief attacks of swelling and pain
Lasts hours to days, then months
One or two locations
Few large joints (especially knee)
Episodes of arthralgia or periarticular involvement—tendinitis, bursitis between attacks of arthritis
During second or third year
Chronic arthritis (10%)
Joint inflammation >1 year
Erosion cartilage + bone
Knees
Longer episodes—lasting months
Skin
Erythema migrans (60% to 80%)
(lasts for several weeks)
Days
Multiple annular secondary lesions (50%)
All lesions fade in 3 to 4 weeks
(range 1 day to 14 months)
Years
Acrodermatitis chronica atrophicans
(rare in US)
Nervous system
Sx of meningeal irritation and mild encephalopathy
(attacks of severe headache, stiff neck)
Weeks or months
Neurologic abnormalities (15%)
Fluctuating Sx of meningitis with superimposed cranial or peripheral radiculoneuropathy
Facial or Bell's palsy
CSF—lymphs 100 cells/mm^3 + elevated protein
Months to years
Chronic neurologic Sx
Subtle encephalopathy affecting memory, mood, or sleep
CSF—elevated protein
Distal paresthesias or spinal or radicular pain
EMG—proximal and distal nerve segment abnormalities

Figure 15-29

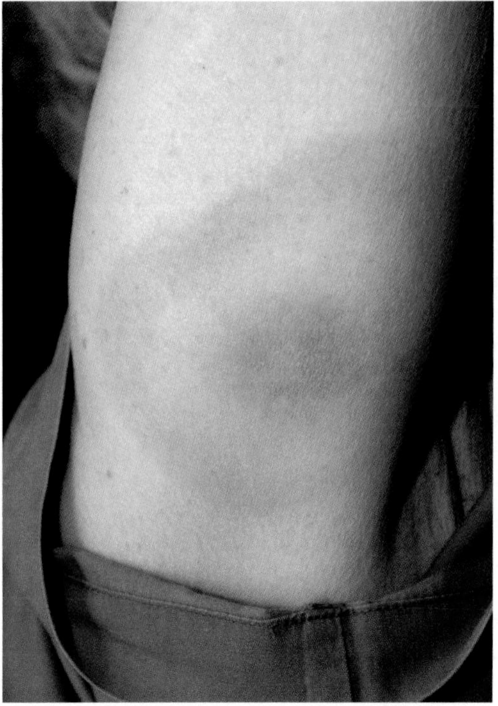

Figure 15-30 Erythema migrans. Broad oval area of erythema has slowly migrated from the central area.

EARLY LOCALIZED DISEASE (ERYTHEMA MIGRANS AND FLULIKE SYMPTOMS). Up to 90% of patients have the pathognomonic rash. It is a spontaneously healing red lesion occurring at the site of *Borrelia* inoculation. The average interval between the infectious bite and the appearance of the skin lesion is approximately 7 days (with a range of 3 to 30 days). The lesion begins as a small papule at the bite site. The papule forms into a slowly enlarging ring, while the central erythema gradually fades and leaves a surface that is usually normal but may be slightly blue. The ring remains flat, blanches with pressure, and does not desquamate, vesiculate, or have scale at the periphery, as ringworm does. The most common configuration of the lesion is circular, but as migration proceeds over skin folds, distortions of the configuration occur. The border of the lesion may be slightly raised. Some patients complain of burning or itching. Over several days, the erythema expands rapidly away from the central bite puncture, centrifugally forming a broad, round-to-oval area of erythema measuring 5 to 10 cm (Figure 15-30). Within 1 week, it clears centrally, leaving a red, 1- to 2-cm ring that advances for days or weeks and may reach a diameter of 50 cm; 20% to 50% of cases have multiple concentric rings (Figures 15-31 and 15-32). Tenderness is present and itching is minimal. Even in untreated patients, lesions usually fade within 3 to 4 weeks. Within days or weeks, the spirochete may spread in the blood or lymph (stage 2). Second-

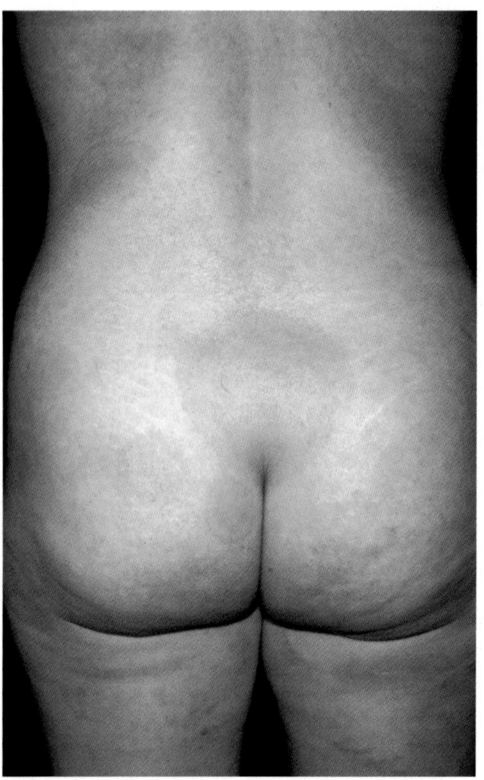

Figure 15-31 Erythema migrans. Most cases in the United States do not exhibit central clearing with a bull's eye. Rings are homogeneous in color and pattern and are frequently multiple.

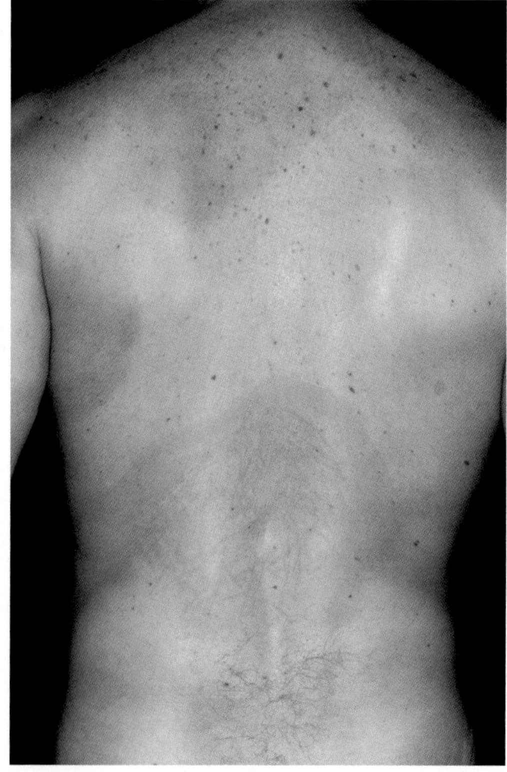

Figure 15-32 Erythema migrans. Lesions are multiple and may exhibit large areas of irregular erythema rather than uniform circles.

ary lesions or *Borrelia* lymphocytoma may occur. Multiple lesions, occurring as a result of hematogenous spread, are the cutaneous markers of disseminated spirochetal disease. A transient erythema may develop after an uninfected tick bite. It does not expand more than 1 cm in diameter and resolves in 1 or 2 days. Spider bites may also cause painful, expanding, red lesions.

The acute illness begins with malaise, fatigue, temperature as high as 105° F, headache, stiff neck, myalgias, and arthralgias. Influenza will be suspected at this stage if the rash is absent. The complete blood count and erythrocyte sedimentation rate are normal. The electrocardiogram may show signs of carditis.

EARLY DISSEMINATED DISEASE (CARDIAC AND NEUROLOGIC DISEASE). Early disseminated Lyme disease develops within 1 to 9 months of infection and can occur without EM.

Cardiac disease. Cardiac manifestations occur in 8% of untreated adults. They include fluctuating degrees of atrioventricular nodal block, mild pericarditis, and mild left ventricular dysfunction. Syncope, dizziness, shortness of breath, chest pain, or palpitations occur with higher degrees of block. Conduction block may resolve without antibiotics. The prognosis is excellent with treatment.

Neurologic disease. Within weeks, signs of acute neuroborreliosis develop in approximately 15% of untreated patients. These include lymphocytic meningitis with episodic headache and mild neck stiffness, subtle encephalitis with difficulty with mentation, cranial neuropathy (particularly unilateral or bilateral facial palsy), motor or sensory radiculoneuritis, mononeuritis multiplex, cerebellar ataxia, or myelitis. Spinal fluid examination may reveal lymphocytic pleocytosis and elevated levels of protein with oligoclonal immunoglobulins.

Acute neurologic abnormalities typically improve or resolve within weeks or months, even in untreated patients.

LATE DISEASE (ARTHRITIS AND CHRONIC NEUROLOGIC SYNDROMES). Late Lyme disease may occur without evidence of early disease.

Joint disease. Months after the onset of illness, approximately 80% of untreated patients begin to have intermittent attacks of joint swelling and pain, primarily in large joints, especially the knee. The joints are warm but not red. After several brief attacks of arthritis, some patients may have persistent joint inflammation. In about 10% of patients, particularly those with HLA-DRB1, the arthritis persists in the knees for months or several years, even after 30 days of intravenous antibiotic therapy or 60 days of oral antibiotic therapy.

The joint fluid contains 10,000 to 25,000 white blood cells/mm^3 (predominately neutrophils); most patients with Lyme arthritis are seropositive for anti–*B. burgdorferi* (by enzyme-linked immunosorbent assay [ELISA]). False-positive test results occur. Specific antibodies in the synovial fluid help confirm that the synovitis is due to *B. burgdorferi*. Patients with Lyme arthritis usually have higher *Borrelia*-specific antibody titers than patients with any other manifestation of the illness, including late neuroborreliosis. The infection can persist for years in areas such as the joints and nervous system.

Neurologic disease. In up to 5% of untreated patients, *B. burgdorferi* may cause chronic neuroborreliosis, sometimes after long periods of latent infection. A chronic axonal polyneuropathy may develop, manifested as spinal radicular pain or distal paresthesias. Lyme encephalopathy, manifested primarily by subtle cognitive disturbances, is a possible late manifestation. There are no inflammatory changes in the cerebrospinal fluid. Computed tomography of the brain is not helpful. In patients with central nervous system involvement, the most sensitive diagnostic test is the demonstration of production of anti–*Borrelia burgdorferi* antibody in the spinal fluid. Lyme encephalopathy may be treated successfully with a 1-month course of intravenous ceftriaxone therapy.

PERSISTENT INFECTION

Some authors have documented persistent infection after treatment with currently recommended schedules. Approximately half the patients continue to experience minor symptoms, such as headache, musculoskeletal pain, and fatigue, after antibiotic treatment. Patients with severe cardiac involvement who do not respond quickly to antibiotic therapy may respond to steroids.

The Lyme disease spirochete may spread transplacentally to organs of the fetus. Women who acquire Lyme disease while pregnant should be treated promptly.

LABORATORY DIAGNOSIS

Diagnosis without the rash may be difficult. Routine laboratory studies are not helpful in confirming the diagnosis.

SEROLOGY. Serology is the only practical laboratory aid in diagnosis (Box 15-5). Tests are insensitive during the first several weeks of infection; 20% to 30% of patients have positive responses, usually of the IgM isotype during this period, but by convalescence 2 to 4 weeks later, approximately 70% to 80% have seroreactivity, even after antibiotic treatment. After antibiotic treatment, antibody titers fall slowly, but IgG and even IgM responses may persist for many years after treatment.

Examination of a single specimen does not discriminate between previous and ongoing infection. Because of a background false positivity even among healthy populations of nonendemic regions, serologic testing is recommended only when there is at least a one in five chance, in the physician's estimation, that the patient has active Lyme disease.

Cultivation of *B. burgdorferi* from a skin lesion or blood is expensive and lacks sensitivity.

False-positive test results. False-positive ELISA titer levels occur with syphilis, infectious mononucleosis, Rocky Mountain spotted fever, rheumatoid arthritis, and systemic lupus erythematosus, and in 7% of normal blood bank donors. Syphilis serologic test results for *Treponema pallidum* (such as rapid plasma reagin, Venereal Disease Research Laboratory [VDRL], or microhemagglutination assays) are usually negative in Lyme disease, but the fluorescent *Treponema* antibody absorption test result may be frequently positive (see Box 15-5). Some false-positive results may be due to prior subclinical infections with *B. burgdorferi* (Figure 15-33).

CULTURE AND BIOPSY. The culture or direct visualization of *B. burgdorferi* from patient specimens is possible but difficult. With Warthin-Starry silver stain, the *Ixodes dammini* spirochete was found, usually in the papillary dermis, in 86% of erythema migrans lesions.

THE OVERDIAGNOSIS OF LYME DISEASE. In areas where anxiety about the disease is high, patients and physicians often ascribe clinical concerns to Lyme disease. Incorrect diagnosis often leads to unnecessary antibiotic treatment. Anxiety about possible late manifestations of Lyme disease has made Lyme disease a "diagnosis of exclusion" in many endemic areas. Persistence of mild to moderate symptoms after adequate therapy and misdiagnosis of fibromyalgia and fatigue may incorrectly suggest persistence of infection, leading to further antibiotic therapy. Attention to patients' anxiety and increased awareness of these musculoskeletal problems after therapy should decrease unnecessary therapy of previously treated Lyme disease.

Box 15-5 **CDC's Two-Step Process for Lyme Disease Testing***

1. The first step uses an ELISA or IFA test. These tests are very sensitive. If the ELISA or IFA is negative, it is highly unlikely that the person has Lyme disease, and no further testing is recommended. If the ELISA or IFA is positive or indeterminate, a second step should be performed to confirm the results.
2. The second step uses a Western blot test that is highly specific for Lyme disease, meaning that it will usually be positive only if a person has been truly infected. If the Western blot is negative, it suggests that the first test was a false positive. Sometimes two types of Western blot are performed, "IgM" and "IgG." Patients who are positive by IgM but not IgG should have the test repeated a few weeks later if they remain ill. If they are still positive only by IgM and have been ill longer than 1 month, this is likely a false positive.

CDC does not recommend testing blood by Western blot without first testing it by ELISA or IFA. Doing so increases the potential for false-positive results. Such results may lead to patients being treated for Lyme disease when they do not have the disease and consequently not receiving appropriate treatment for the true cause of their illness.

*CDC recommends a two-step process when testing blood for evidence of Lyme disease. Both steps can be done using the same blood sample.

THE UNDERDIAGNOSIS OF LYME DISEASE. Most symptoms of *B. burgdorferi* infection are not pathognomonic. Nonspecific symptoms may persist for months even after treatment and it may take months or years for the late features of Lyme disease to resolve. Expanding erythema of EM resembles a spider bite. Radiculoneuropathy is diagnosed as a herniated cervical disk. Lymphocytic meningitis is misdiagnosed as viral meningitis. Monarthritis may be diagnosed as atypical rheumatoid arthritis or septic arthritis. Physicians in endemic areas must have a high index of suspicion for this confusing disease that can mimic so many other diseases.

TREATMENT

RISK OF INFECTION. The risk of Lyme disease after a deer-tick bite in areas with a high incidence of Lyme disease is 3.2%. Ticks must become at least partially engorged with blood (i.e., they must feed for many hours) (Figure 15-34) before *B. burgdorferi* is transmitted. Erythema migrans developed more frequently after untreated bites from nymphal ticks than after bites from adult female ticks (8 of 142 bites [5.6%] vs. 0 of 97 bites [0%]), and particularly after bites from nymphal ticks that were at least partially engorged with blood (8 of 81 bites [9.9%]), as compared with 0 of 59 bites from unfed, or flat, nymphal ticks (0%). Among subjects bitten by nymphal ticks, the risk of Lyme disease was 25% if the tick had fed for 72 hours or longer and 0% if it had fed for less than 72 hours. *PMID: 11450675*

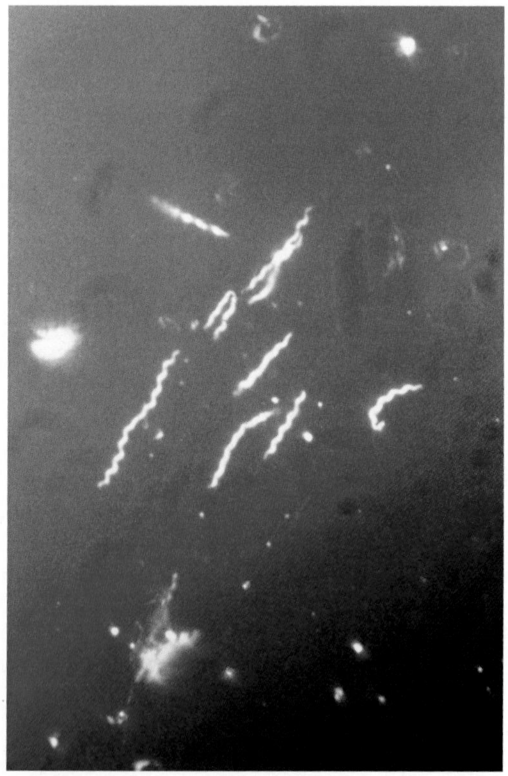

Figure 15-33 *Borrelia burgdorferi.* The tick-borne spirochete *B. burgdorferi* causes Lyme disease (shown here under dark field examination).

PROGNOSIS

The outcome for untreated Lyme disease is summarized in Box 15-6.

PROPHYLACTIC DOXYCYCLINE. A single 200-mg dose of doxycycline given within 72 hours after an *I. scapularis* tick bite can prevent the development of Lyme disease (Box 15-7). Anxiety about Lyme disease may be the most potent factor that drives decision making about chemoprophylaxis. Educating patients with tick bites about the excellent prognosis even if Lyme disease develops may be a better solution for anxiety than doxycycline.

It may be reasonable to administer doxycycline to persons bitten by ticks in areas where the incidence of Lyme disease is high and when the tick is a nymphal deer tick that is at least partially engorged with blood.

ACTIVE DISEASE. Serologic testing has poor sensitivity in early disease. The presence of erythema migrans offers physicians the best opportunity for diagnosis. Aggressive antibiotic treatment may be initiated solely on the basis of this early clinical finding. The most recent recommendations are listed in Table 15-3 and Table 15-4.

ERYTHEMA MIGRANS. Oral antibiotic therapy shortens the duration of the rash and usually prevents development of late sequelae. The duration of therapy is guided by the clinical response. Relapse has occurred with all of the recommended regimens; patients who relapse may need a second course of treatment. Recommended treatment schedules are successful in preventing late sequelae in children; new episodes of erythema migrans were, however, reported in 11% of those patients 1 to 4 years after the initial episode. Other studies show that major late manifestations of Lyme disease are unusual after appropriate early antibiotic therapy (see Table 15-4).

Box 15-6 **Outcome of Lyme Disease without Treatment**

Rash resolves in 3-4 weeks.
Arthritis is common; chronic, disabling arthritis is rare.
20% had no subsequent manifestations of Lyme disease.
18% had arthralgias but no arthritis; symptoms lasted 1 month to 6 years (mean, 3 years).
51% had one or more episodes of arthritis within 2 years (mean, 6 months) but did not develop chronic synovitis; 50% had involvement of the knee.
11% developed chronic synovitis within 4 years (mean, 12 months); 8% had knee involvement.
2% had permanent joint disability.
11% developed neurologic abnormalities.
4% had cardiac involvement.

Adapted from *Ann Intern Med* 107(5):725, 1987. *PMID: 3662285*

JARISCH-HERXHEIMER–LIKE REACTION. Fourteen percent of patients, generally those with more severe disease, have an intensification of symptoms during the first 24 hours after the start of therapy. This Jarisch-Herxheimer–like reaction (severe chills, myalgias, headache, fever, increased heart and respiratory rates lasting for hours, and increased visibility of the rash) usually occurs a few hours after treatment is begun. Regardless of the antibiotic agent given, nearly half of the patients experience minor late complications—recurrent episodes of lethargy and headache or pain in joints, tendons, bursae, or muscles.

PREVENTION

Tick repellents are divided into those applied to the skin and those applied to clothing. The insect repellent *N,N*-diethyl-*meta*-toluamide (DEET) used on the skin repels a variety of insects, including ticks. Permethrin spray applied to clothing appears to be a safe and effective tick repellent. It is especially important to detect and to remove ticks as soon as possible, since transmission of *B. burgdorferi* is unlikely if a deer tick is removed within 48 hours of attachment.

LYME DISEASE VACCINE. The human recombinant outer-surface-protein vaccine (LYMErix, SmithKline Beecham) was licensed in 1998 for persons 15 to 70 years of age who live or work in moderate- to high-risk areas. The vaccine was withdrawn because of lack of use.

Box 15-7 **Prophylaxis of Lyme Disease**

A single dose of doxycycline may be offered to adult patients (200-mg dose) and to children at least 8 years of age (4 mg/kg up to a maximum dose of 200 mg) when all of the following circumstances exist:

1. The attached tick can be reliably identified as an adult or nymphal *I. scapularis* tick that is estimated to have been attached for 36 hours on the basis of the degree of engorgement of the tick with blood or certainty about the time of exposure to the tick.
2. Prophylaxis can be started within 72 hours of the time that the tick was removed.
3. Ecologic information indicates that the local rate of infection of these ticks with *B. burgdorferi* is 20%. Infection of 20% of ticks with *B. burgdorferi* occurs in parts of New England, in parts of the mid-Atlantic states, and in parts of Minnesota and Wisconsin.
4. Doxycycline treatment is not contraindicated. (Doxycycline is relatively contraindicated in pregnant women and children <8 years old.)

From *Clin Infect Dis* 43:1089-1134, 2006. *PMID: 17029130*

Table 15-3 Recommended Antimicrobial Regimens for Treatment of Patients with Lyme Disease (see Table 15-4 for duration)		
Drug	**Dosage for adults**	**Dosage for children**
Preferred Oral Regimens		
Amoxicillin	500 mg three times per day*	50 mg/kg per day in 3 divided doses (maximum, 500 mg per dose)*
Doxycycline	100 mg twice per day†	Not recommended for children aged <8 years For children aged ≥8 years, 4 mg/kg per day in 2 divided doses (maximum, 100 mg per dose)
Cefuroxime axetil	500 mg twice per day	30 mg/kg per day in 2 divided doses (maximum, 500 mg per dose)
Alternative Oral Regimens		
Selected macrolides‡	For recommended dosing regimens, see footnote *d* in Table 15-4	For recommended dosing regimens, see footnote *d* in Table 15-4
Preferred Parenteral Regimen		
Ceftriaxone	2 gm intravenously once per day	50-75 mg/kg intravenously per day in a single dose (maximum, 2 gm)
Alternative Parenteral Regimens		
Cefotaxime	2 gm intravenously every 8 hr§	150-200 mg/kg per day intravenously per day in 3-4 divided doses (maximum, 6 gm per day)§
Penicillin G	18-24 million units per day intravenously, divided every 4 hr§	200,000-400,000 units/kg per day divided every 4 hr§ (not to exceed 18-24 million units per day)

*Although a higher dosage given twice per day might be equally as effective, in view of the absence of data on efficacy, twice-daily administration is not recommended.
†Tetracyclines are relatively contraindicated in pregnant or lactating women and in children <8 years of age.
‡Because of their lower efficacy, macrolides are reserved for patients who are unable to take or who are intolerant of tetracyclines, penicillins, and cephalosporins.
§Dosage should be reduced for patients with impaired renal function.
From Infectious Diseases Society of America (IDSA): Guidelines for Lyme disease 2006, *Clin Infect Dis* 43:1089-1134, 2006. *PMID: 17029130*

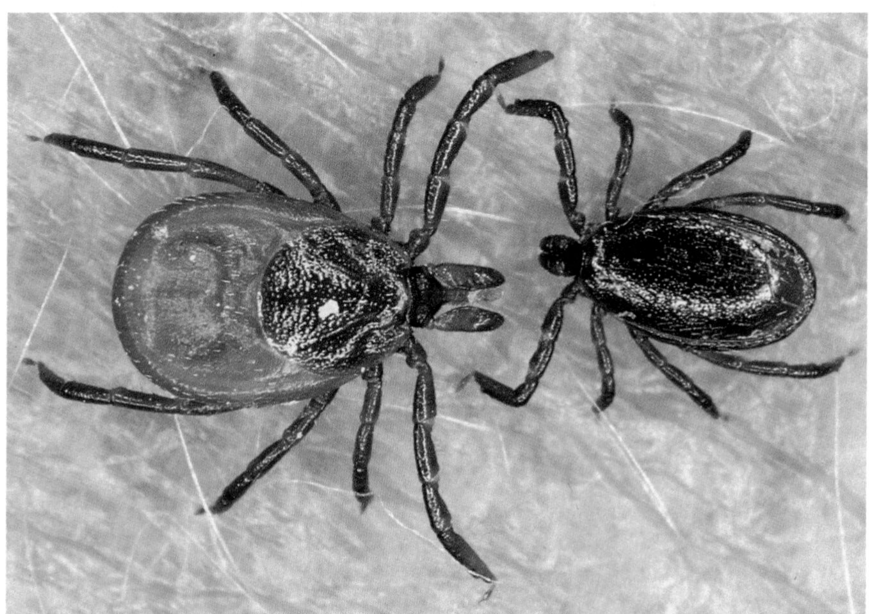

Figure 15-34 The deer tick (*Ixodes dammini*), partly engorged (left) and unengorged (right).

Table 15-4 Recommended Therapy for Patients with Lyme Disease*		
Indication	**Treatment**	**Duration, days (range)**
Tick bite in United States	Doxycycline 200 mg in single dose[a,b] (4 mg/kg in children ≥8 years of age) and/or observation	—
Erythema migrans	Oral regimen[c,d]	14 (14-21)[e]
Early neurologic disease		
Meningitis or radiculopathy	Parenteral regimen[c,f]	14 (10-28)
Cranial nerve palsy[a,g]	Oral regimen[c]	14 (14-21)
Cardiac disease	Oral regimen[a,c,h] or parenteral regimen[a,c,h]	14 (14-21)
Borrelia lymphocytoma	Oral regimen[c,d]	14 (14-21)
Late disease		
Arthritis without neurologic disease	Oral regimen[c]	28
Recurrent arthritis after oral regimen	Oral regimen[a,c]	28
	Parenteral regimen[a,c]	14 (14-28)
Antibiotic refractory arthritis[i]	Symptomatic therapy[j]	—
Central or peripheral nervous system disease	Parenteral regimen[c]	14 (14-28)
Acrodermatitits chronica atrophicans	Oral regimen[c]	14 (14-28)
Post-Lyme disease syndrome	Consider and evaluate other potential causes of symptoms; if none is found, then administer symptomatic therapy[a]	—

*NOTE: Regardless of the clinical manifestation of Lyme disease, complete response to treatment may be delayed beyond the treatment duration. Relapse may occur with any of these regimens; patients with objective signs of relapse may need a second course of treatment.

[a]See text.

[b]A single dose of doxycycline may be offered to adult patients and to children ≥8 years of age when *all* of the following circumstances exist: (1) the attached tick can be reliably identified as an adult or nymphal *Ixodes scapularis* tick that is estimated to have been attached for ≥36 h on the basis of the degree of engorgement of the tick with blood or of certainty about the time of exposure to the tick; (2) prophylaxis can be started within 72 h after the time that the tick was removed; (3) ecologic information indicates that the local rate of infection of these ticks with *Borrelia burgdorferi* is ≥20%; *and* (4) doxycycline is not contraindicated. For patients who do not fulfill these criteria, observation is recommended.

[c]See Table 15-3.

[d]For adult patients intolerant of amoxicillin, doxycycline, and cefuroxime axetil, azithromycin (500 mg orally per day for 7 to 10 days), clarithromycin (500 mg orally twice per day for 14 to 21 days, if the patient is not pregnant), or erythromycin (500 mg orally four times per day for 14 to 21 days) may be given. The recommended dosages of these agents for children are as follows: azithromycin, 10 mg/kg per day (maximum of 500 mg per day); clarithromycin, 7.5 mg/kg twice per day (maximum of 500 mg per dose); and erythromycin, 12.5 mg/kg four times per day (maximum of 500 mg per day). Patients treated with macrolides should be closely observed to ensure resolution of the clinical manifestations.

[e]Ten days of therapy is effective if doxycycline is used; the efficacy of 10-day regimens with the other first-line agents is unknown.

[f]For nonpregnant adult patients intolerant of beta-lactam agents, doxycycline (200 to 400 mg/day orally [or intravenously, if the patient is unable to take oral medications]) in two divided doses may be adequate. For children ≥8 years of age, the dosage of doxycycline for this indication is 4 to 8 mg/kg per day in two divided doses (maximum daily dosage of 200 to 400 mg).

[g]See text. Patients without clinical evidence of meningitis may be treated with an oral regimen. Parenteral antibiotic therapy is recommended for patients with both clinical and laboratory evidence of coexistent meningitis. Most of the experience in the use of oral antibiotic therapy is for patients with seventh cranial nerve palsy. Whether oral therapy would be as effective for patients with other cranial neuropathies is unknown. The decision between oral and parenteral antimicrobial therapy for patients with other cranial neuropathies should be individualized.

[h]A parenteral antibiotic regimen is recommended at the start of therapy for patients who have been hospitalized for cardiac monitoring; an oral regimen may be substituted to complete a course of therapy or to treat ambulatory patients. A temporary pacemaker may be required for patients with advanced heart block.

[i]Antibiotic refractory Lyme arthritis is operationally defined as persistent synovitis for at least 2 months after completion of a course of intravenous ceftriaxone (or after completion of two 4-week courses of an oral antibiotic regimen for patients who are unable to tolerate cephalosporins). In addition, PCR of synovial fluid specimens (and synovial tissue specimens, if available) is negative for *B. burgdorferi* nucleic acids.

[j]Symptomatic therapy might consist of nonsteroidal antiinflammatory agents, intraarticular injections of corticosteroids, or other medications; expert consultation with a rheumatologist is recommended. If persistent synovitis is associated with significant pain or if it limits function, arthroscopic synovectomy can reduce the period of join inflammation.

From Infectious Diseases Society of America (IDSA): Guidelines for Lyme disease 2006, *Clin Infect Dis* 43:1089-1134, 2006. *PMID: 17029130*

Rocky Mountain spotted and spotless fever

The name Rocky Mountain spotted fever (RMSF) was coined to describe a disease that was first observed in the Bitter Root Valley of western Montana. The disease occurs in many areas of the United States (Figure 15-35).

Four states (North Carolina, Oklahoma, Tennessee, and South Carolina) account for 48% of the reports.

RICKETTSIA RICKETTSII AND TICKS

Rocky Mountain spotted fever (RMSF) is caused by *R. rickettsii* and is transmitted by tick bites. *Rickettsiae* are released from tick salivary glands during the 6 to 10 hours they are attached to the host.

Not all tick species are effective vectors of *Rickettsia,* and even in the vector species, not all ticks are infected. Generally, only 1% to 5% of vector ticks in an area are infected. Several tick vectors may transmit RMSF organisms, but the primary ones are the American dog tick, *Dermacentor variabilis,* in the eastern United States and the Rocky Mountain wood tick, *Dermacentor andersoni,* in the West. Most cases occur in eastern states such as Tennessee and North Carolina. Adults of both tick species feed on a variety of medium-to-large mammals and on humans. Ticks are often brought into close contact with people via pet dogs or cats (dog ticks may also feed on cats).

INCIDENCE

The highest incidence of disease is found in the age group 5 to 9 years. Ninety-five percent of patients report onset of illness between April 1 and September 30, the period when ticks are most active.

PATHOLOGY

Rickettsia infect the endothelium and vessel wall, not the cerebral tissue. RMSF is a rickettsial infection primarily of endothelial cells that normally have a potent anticoagulant function. As a result of endothelial cell infection and injury, the hemostatic system shows changes that vary widely from a minor reduction in the platelet count (frequently) to severe coagulopathies, such as deep venous thrombosis and disseminated intravascular coagulation (rarely). After the tick bites, organisms disseminate via the bloodstream and multiply in vascular endothelial cells, resulting in multisystem manifestations. The effects of disseminated infection of endothelial cells include increased vascular permeability, edema, hypovolemia, hypotension, prerenal azotemia, and, in life-threatening cases, pulmonary edema, shock, acute tubular necrosis, and meningoencephalitis.

CLINICAL MANIFESTATIONS

One week (with a range of 3 to 21 days) after the bite, there is abrupt onset of fever (94%), severe headache (88%), myalgia (85%), and vomiting (60%). The signs at onset of infection are difficult to distinguish from those of self-limited viral infections.

The rash is reported in 83% of cases and typically begins on the fourth day. It progresses through a sequence of stages and distribution that are never pathognomonic. It erupts first on the wrists and ankles. In hours it involves the palms and soles (73%) (Figures 15-36 and 15-37); then it becomes generalized. The rash is discrete, macular, and blanches with pressure at first; it becomes petechial in 2 to 4 days (Figure 15-38). The rash is very difficult to see in blacks, which may explain the higher fatality rate for blacks (16%) as compared with whites (3%). In approximately

CDC ROCKY MOUNTAIN SPOTTED FEVER INCIDENCE RATES, 2002

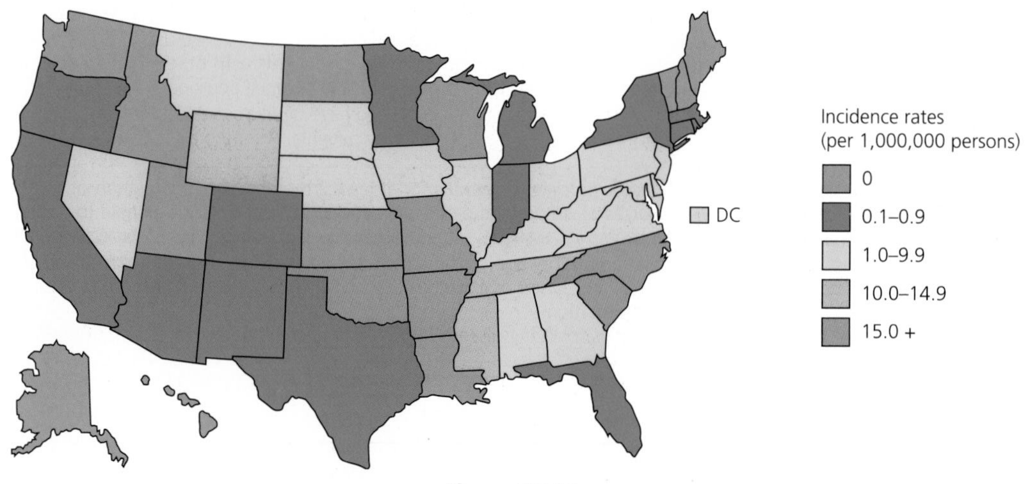

Figure 15-35

ROCKY MOUNTAIN SPOTTED FEVER

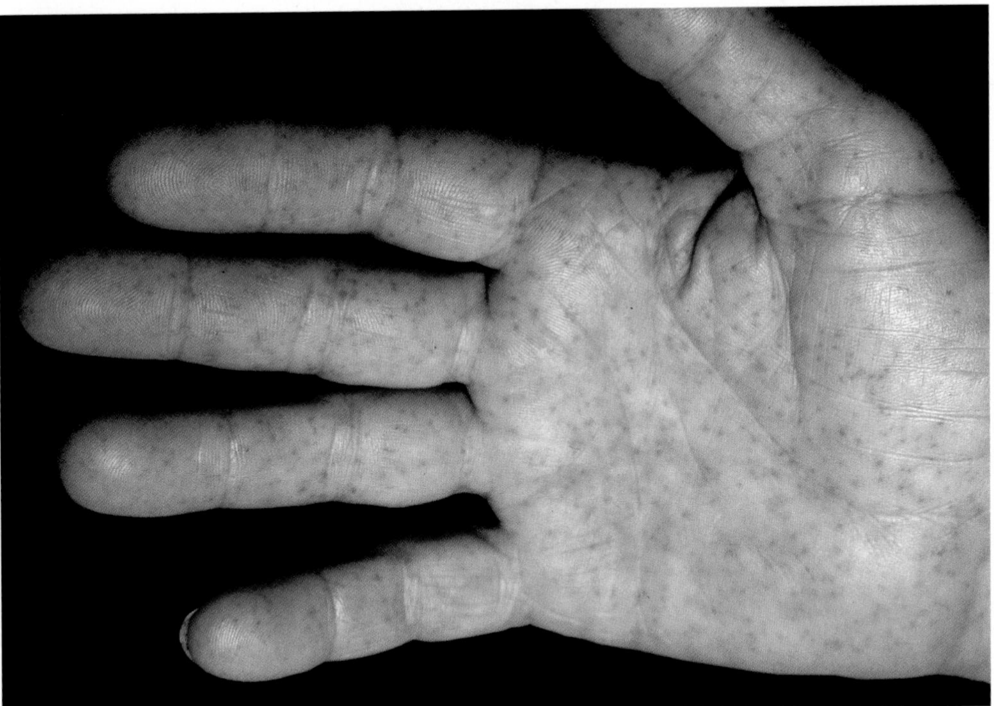

Figure 15-36 Classic distribution of rash on the palms (shown) and soles occurs relatively late in the course. Some reports have documented 36%-80% of patients with RMSF lack the classic distribution of rash on the palms and soles.

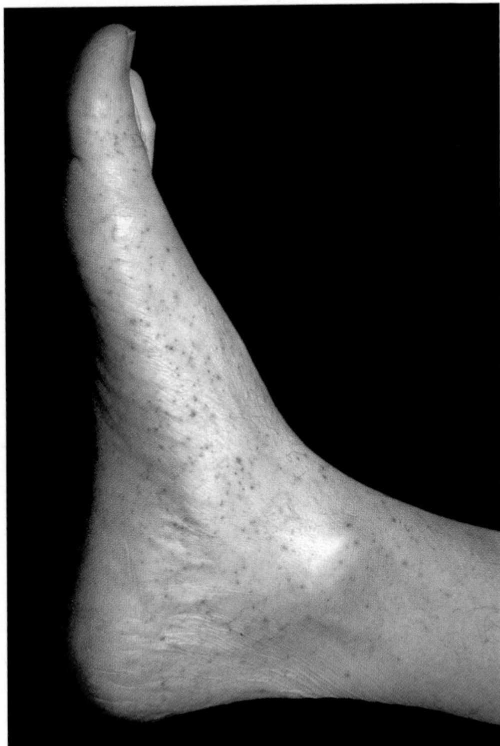

Figure 15-37 The characteristic petechial eruption involves the palms or soles in as many as 50%-80% of patients. 10%-15% of patients may never develop a rash.

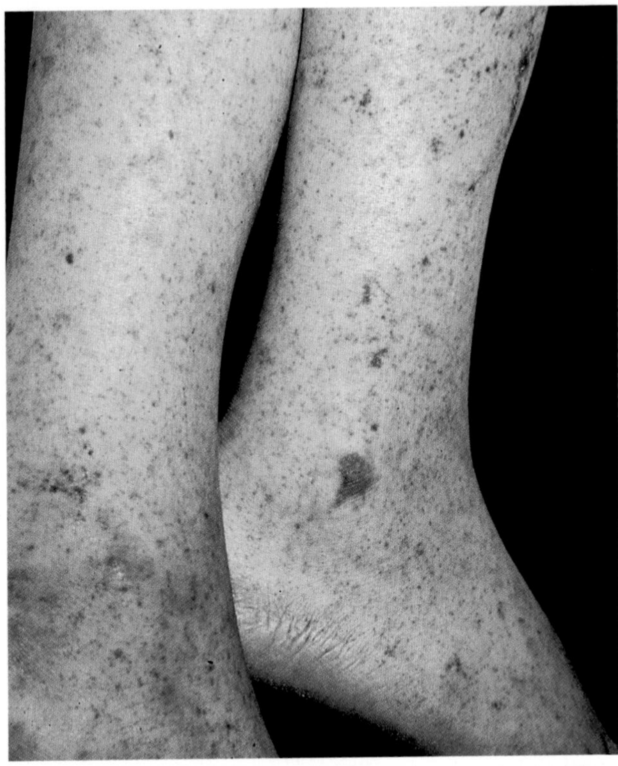

Figure 15-38 A generalized petechial eruption that involves the entire cutaneous surface, including the palms and soles.

15% of cases, the rash does not appear; the disease is then referred to as Rocky Mountain spotless fever. Rashless disease is much more common in adults. Splenomegaly is present in half of the cases. The fever subsides in 2 to 3 weeks, and the rash, if present, fades with residual hyperpigmentation. Although the overall death rate fluctuates between 3% and 7%, the death rate for untreated persons may exceed 30%.

Death usually results from visceral and central nervous system (CNS) dissemination leading to irreversible shock. Many of those who die have a fulminant course and are dead in 1 week. Interstitial nephritis is found at autopsy in most cases. The presence of acute renal failure is strongly associated with death. Significant long-term morbidity (e.g., paraparesis; hearing loss; peripheral neuropathy; bladder and bowel incontinence; cerebellar, vestibular, and motor dysfunction; language disorders) is common in patients with severe illness caused by RMSF.

In its early stages, RMSF may resemble other diseases. Only 3% to 18% of patients present with rash, fever, and a history of tick exposure on their first visit. RMSF should be suspected in patients in endemic areas who report fever, headache, and myalgias without a rash. Cough, rales, nausea, vomiting, abdominal pain, stupor, and meningismus are also RMSF symptoms. Thrombocytopenia and hyponatremia should raise the possibility of RMSF.

DIAGNOSIS

Delayed diagnosis and late initiation of specific antirickettsial therapy (e.g., on or after day 5 of the illness) is associated with substantially greater risk for a fatal outcome. The diagnosis must rely on clinical (fever, headache, rash, myalgia) and epidemiologic (tick exposure) criteria because laboratory confirmation cannot occur before 10 to 14 days after the onset of illness.

LABORATORY. The white blood cell (WBC) count is typically normal, but increased numbers of immature bands are generally observed. Thrombocytopenia, mild elevations in levels of hepatic transaminases, and hyponatremia might be observed.

When CSF is evaluated, a pleocytosis (usually <100 cells/μL) is typically observed (with either a polymorphonuclear or a lymphocytic predominance). Moderately elevated protein levels (100 to 200 mg/dl) and normal glucose levels also are commonly observed in patients with RMSF. A Gram stain indicating gram-negative diplococci, very low glucose levels (i.e., <20 to 30 mg/dl), or neutrophilic pleocytosis is more suggestive of meningococcal meningitis. Reliably distinguishing between RMSF and meningococcal infection based on laboratory testing is difficult (unless a pathogen is cultured). Therefore empiric treatment for both RMSF and meningococcemia is necessary for ill patients with fever and rash and for patients in whom neither disease can be ruled out.

The clinical diagnosis, which is difficult, is rarely assisted by laboratory findings because antibodies are usually detected only in convalescence. Serologic evaluations use the indirect immunofluorescence antibody (IFA) assay.

The sensitivity of the IFA assay is dependent on the timing of collection of the sample. Serologic tests will be negative in the first few days. As the illness progresses to 7 to 10 days, the sensitivity of IFA serology increases. The IFA assay is estimated to be 94% to 100% sensitive after 14 days. Testing two sequential serum or plasma samples together to demonstrate a rising IgG or IgM antibody level is essential to confirm acute infection. Specimens should be taken at least 2 to 3 weeks apart to examine for a fourfold or greater increase in antibody titer.

TREATMENT

Until reliable early diagnostic tests become available, a therapeutic trial of a tetracycline should be considered for any patient in an endemic geographic area during the summer months who has fever, myalgia, and headache. Most broad-spectrum antibiotics, including penicillins, cephalosporins, and sulfa-containing antimicrobials, are ineffective treatments for RMSF.

Doxycycline is the drug of choice for children and adults. The dose is 100 mg administered twice daily (orally or intravenously) for adults or 2.2 mg/kg body weight per dose administered twice daily (orally or intravenously) for children weighing <100 lb (45.4 kg). Treat for at least 3 days after the fever subsides, which is typically for a minimum total course of 5 to 7 days. Limited use of this drug in children during the first 6 to 7 years of life has a negligible effect on the color of permanent incisors. Beyond ages 6 to 7 years, the risk for tetracycline staining is of minimal consequence because visible tooth formation is complete. For patients with RMSF reinfection, up to five courses of doxycycline may be administered with minimal risk of dental staining.

The use of tetracyclines might be warranted during pregnancy in life-threatening situations. Tetracycline use during pregnancy is associated with fluorescent yellow discoloration of the teeth and with maternal hepatotoxicity. Chloramphenicol may be the preferred treatment during pregnancy, but care must be used when administering chloramphenicol late during the third trimester of pregnancy because of risks associated with gray baby syndrome. The recommended dosage is 50 to 75 mg/kg per day in four divided doses. There is no oral preparation.

Other causes of central nervous system infections such as *Neisseria meningitidis* or *Haemophilus influenzae* should be considered in the differential diagnosis, especially in the young. In these cases when diagnosis is uncertain, initial empiric therapy with chloramphenicol may be indicated.

PROGNOSIS

Patients with RMSF who received antirickettsial therapy within 5 days of the onset of symptoms were significantly less likely to die than those who received treatment after the fifth day of illness. Predictors of failure by the physician to initiate therapy the first time a patient was seen were absence of a rash and presentation within the first 3 days of illness. In severe cases, fluid management is a challenge.

Tick bite paralysis

Tick paralysis is a rare disease characterized by acute, ascending, flaccid paralysis that is often confused with other acute neurologic disorders or diseases (e.g., Guillain-Barré syndrome or botulism).

Tick bite paralysis probably results from a neurotoxin in tick saliva that is injected while the tick is feeding. The disease is most common in children, especially girls with long, thick hair. The tick, which hides on the scalp, groin, or other inconspicuous areas, must be attached for approximately 5 to 7 days before symptoms appear. It usually begins with weakness of the lower limbs, progressing in hours to falls and incoordination, which are due to muscle weakness. Then, cranial nerve weakness with dysarthria and dysphagia leads to bulbar paralysis, respiratory failure, and death. Children may present with restlessness, irritability, and malaise. The patient complains of fatigue, irritability, and leg paresthesias, followed by loss of coordination and an ascending paralysis within 24 hours. There is no pain or fever in the early stages. Death from respiratory failure can occur if the tick is not found and removed. Recovery occurs 24 hours after the tick is detached.

The species most often associated with tick paralysis in the United States and Canada are the Rocky Mountain wood tick (*D. andersoni*) and the American dog tick (*D. variabilis*). Most North American cases occur during April to June, when adult *Dermacentor* ticks emerge from hibernation and actively seek hosts.

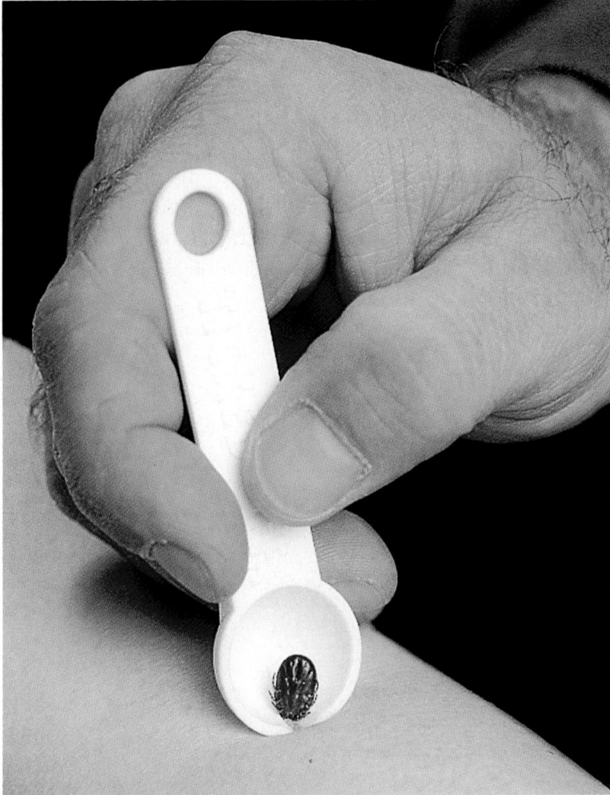

Figure 15-39 TICKED OFF. A plastic tool used to extract ticks. The entire tick, including the mouth parts, is removed.

Removing ticks

A simple plastic tool called TICKED OFF removes ticks, including the mouth parts (Figure 15-39). Embedded ticks are removed completely, in one motion, while the bowl contains the tick for disposal. The tool can be used in any direction to remove ticks from the front, back, or side. TICKED OFF is held vertically. Applying slight pressure downward on the skin pushes the tick remover forward so it surrounds the tick on three sides, the small part of the "V" framing the tick. Continuous sliding motion of the notched area releases the tick. These inexpensive tools are now generally available.

Ixodid ticks are difficult to remove because they cement their mouth parts into the skin. Mechanical removal may or may not remove the cement. If no cement, or "fleshlike" material, is attached to the mouth parts after extraction, the cement is still in the skin, and attempts should be made to remove it to prevent subsequent irritation and infection. Ticks continue to salivate after extraction and must be disposed of immediately. In one study the application of petroleum jelly, fingernail polish, isopropyl alcohol, or a hot kitchen match failed to induce detachment of ticks. Hot objects may induce the ticks to salivate or regurgitate infected fluids into the wound.

Ticks should not be removed by direct finger contact because of the danger of contracting a rickettsial infection. *Dermacentor* ticks are removed by gentle, steady, firm traction; the mouth parts usually separate from the skin still attached to the tick. *Ixodes dammini* can rarely be removed intact by manual extraction. If detached, the mouth parts remain below the skin surface. The residual parts may be walled off and cause little harm or they may produce chronic irritation or stimulate a foreign-body reaction, resulting in a nodule known as a tick-bite granuloma (Figure 15-40). Twisting or jerking the tick during removal may break off the mouth parts. Manipulating a tick's body may cause infectious fluids to escape and enter the skin of the host or of the person removing the tick. The body of the tick should not be squeezed because additional fluid may be injected into the skin.

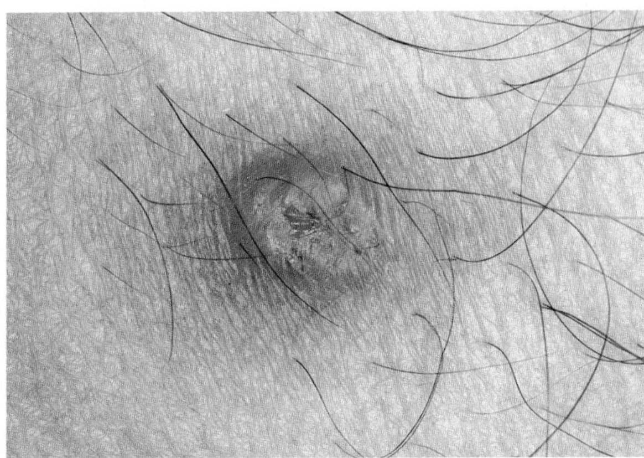

Figure 15-40 Tick-bite granuloma. A nodular reaction that varies in size from 0.5 to 2 centimeters. This nodule develops and progresses from days to months after the bite.

CAT-SCRATCH AND RELATED DISEASES

Cat-scratch disease is caused by the organism *Bartonella henselae*. There are approximately 22,000 cases of cat-scratch disease in the United States every year.

Cat-scratch disease is usually a benign, self-limited disease. Cat contact is documented in 99% of cases, and in most cases the cat is immature. Cat-scratch disease is not easily acquired. Usually just one member of a family is affected, and adults rarely show symptoms, even when all family members are exposed to the same animal. The bacterium is transmitted to humans by scratches or bites. Cats do not have to scratch to transmit the disease. In immunocompetent patients, that bacterium is responsible for cat-scratch disease, characterized by localized lymph node enlargement in the vicinity of the entry site of the bacteria. In 5% to 13% of cases, the disease is more severe, including hepatitis, Parinaud's oculoglandular syndrome, neurologic complications, or stellate retinitis. In immunocompromised patients, *B. henselae* is responsible for bacillary angiomatosis, bacillary peliosis hepatitis and splenitis, acute and relapsing bacteremia, or endocarditis.

BARTONELLA HENSELAE

The causative agent is the pleomorphic, gram-negative bacillus *Bartonella* (formerly *Rochalimaea*) *henselae* carried by cats. Cats are healthy, asymptomatic carriers and can be bacteremic for months or years. *B. henselae* can be transmitted from cat to cat by the cat flea. Approximately 10% to 16% of pet cats and 33% to 50% of stray cats carry this bacterium in their blood. This disease is more likely to occur in pet cats less than 1 year old that are infested with fleas.

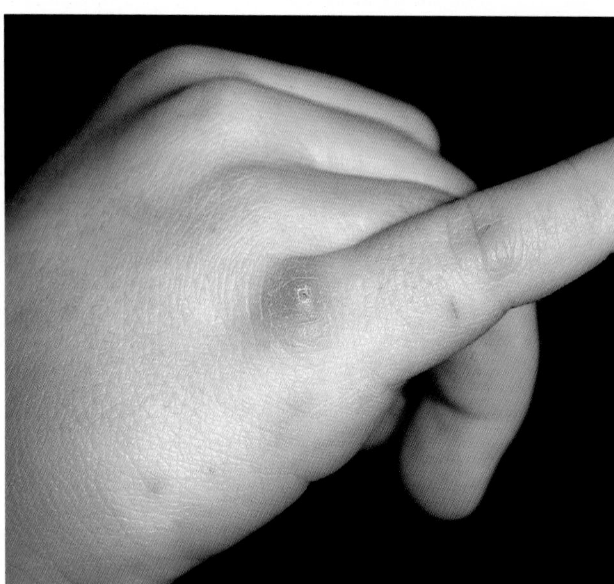

Figure 15-41 Cat-scratch disease. A red, tender papule or pustule occurs at inoculation site.

Clinical manifestations

In one study, the primary inoculation site was observed in 93% of cases. A red macule appears at the contact site and evolves into a nonpruritic papule (insect bites itch, but the papule of cat-scratch disease does not) 3 to 5 days after exposure to a cat; later the papule evolves into a vesicle filled with sterile fluid. The papule progresses through the vesicular and crust stages in 2 to 3 days (Figure 15-41).

Regional lymphadenopathy appears in 1 or 2 weeks. The location of lymphadenopathy depends on the site of inoculation and is seen most often in the axilla, neck, jaw, and groin. The papule may go unnoticed or be attributed to injury, and lymphadenopathy may not be appreciated. The lesion persists for 1 to 3 weeks, with a few persisting for 3 months, and ends with a scar resembling that from chickenpox. The enlarged nodes may persist for months with gradual resolution. In 12% of the cases, the lymph nodes undergo focal necrosis within 5 weeks. Consider the possibility of cat-scratch disease in adults with chronic lymphadenopathy who own cats (Box 15-8).

Most patients experience mild symptoms of generalized aching, malaise, and anorexia. The temperature is usually normal, but in approximately one third of cases it is above 39° C (102° F). Inoculation within the confines of the eyelids or on the lids themselves causes a nonpainful palpebral conjunctivitis, preauricular lymphadenopathy, and fever, which characterizes the most common variant of cat-scratch disease (the oculoglandular syndrome of Parinaud).

Severe systemic diseases—including hepatosplenomegaly, osteolytic lesions, splenic abscesses and granulomas, mediastinal masses, encephalopathy, and neuroretinitis—are uncommon.

OPHTHALMIC MANIFESTATIONS. Ophthalmic manifestations of bartonellosis may occur in up to 13% of patients with systemic cat-scratch disease, including Parinaud's oculoglandular syndrome: granulomatous conjunctivitis with associated preauricular lymphadenopathy, neuroretinitis, and focal chorioretinitis. The majority of patients recover without sequelae.

Box 15-8 Criteria for the Diagnosis of Cat-Scratch Disease

Diagnosis requires three of the following four criteria:

- Lymphadenopathy in the absence of other reason (can be missed because it is not present yet or subclinical)
- Positive *Bartonella henselae* titer or skin test
- Known cat contact, preferably with pustule or papule at the site
- Lymph node biopsy with bacilli present, necrosis

NEUROLOGIC COMPLICATIONS. A large study characterized the neurologic complications of cat-scratch disease. Encephalopathy occurred in 80% of patients; 20% had cranial and peripheral nerve involvement with facial nerve paresis, neuroretinitis, or peripheral neuritis. The average age of encephalopathy patients was 10.6 years (range, 1 to 66 years). Almost twice as many males as females were affected. Fifty percent of patients were afebrile and only 26% had temperatures higher than 39° C. Convulsions occurred in 46% of patients and combative behavior in 40%. Lethargy with or without coma was accompanied by variable neurologic signs. Results of laboratory studies, including imaging of the CNS, were inconsistent and nondiagnostic. All patients recovered within 12 months; 78% recovered within 1 to 12 weeks. There were no neurologic sequelae. Treatment consisted of control of convulsions and supportive measures.

Bacillary angiomatosis

Bacillary angiomatosis is a vascular proliferative disease most commonly associated with long-standing human immunodeficiency virus (HIV) infection or other significant immunosuppression. There is prolonged fever, arthralgia, weight loss, and splenomegaly of 2 or more weeks' duration. Multiple and widely distributed angiomatous nodules resembling Kaposi's sarcoma accompanied by symptoms of systemic cat-scratch disease were first reported in patients with acquired immunodeficiency syndrome (AIDS). There are three characteristic lesions: pyogenic granuloma-like papules (Figure 15-42), erythematous indurated plaques, and subcutaneous nodules. They vary from 1 mm to several centimeters in diameter and may be painful. The pyogenic granuloma-like papules bleed easily. Cutaneous and parenchymal lesions also occur in immunocompromised cardiac and renal transplant recipients. Immunocompetent persons can also develop cutaneous bacillary angiomatosis. Diagnosis often remains solely based on histologic findings. Lobular capillary hemangioma (pyogenic granuloma) is not associated with *Bartonella spp.* infection. *PMID: 16310070*

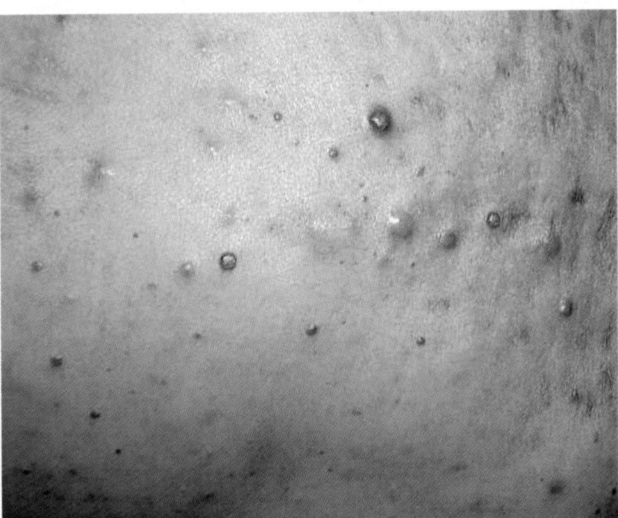

Figure 15-42 Bacillary angiomatosis. The typical lesion is a reddish-purple papule about 0.5-1 cm in diameter.

On the basis of case reports and small series, either erythromycin (500 mg four times per day) or doxycycline (100 mg twice per day) appears to be effective. The duration of initial therapy should be at least 4 weeks. With relapses, retreatment with prolonged therapy (lasting several months) should be considered until immunocompetence returns. Rifampin, trimethoprim-sulfamethoxazole, and ciprofloxacin may also be effective.

Diagnosis of cat-scratch disease

The diagnosis can be established by finding a primary lesion site in the presence of lymphadenopathy and a history of intimate exposure to cats. Lymph node biopsy may not be necessary if these conditions are present.

Serologic diagnosis using indirect fluorescence antibody (IFA) methods is made in elevated titers of either IgM (≥1:20) or IgG (≥1:256) antibodies or a fourfold increase in IgG titer between acute and convalescent sera.

LYMPH NODE HISTOPATHOLOGY VARIES WITH TIME

A Warthin-Starry silver stain of lymph nodes and skin at the primary site of inoculation shows small pleomorphic bacilli. The gram-negative pleomorphic bacilli are found within cells and are most abundant in areas of necrosis in skin and lymph nodes. The primary lesion should be carefully sought in young patients experiencing unilateral lymphadenopathy. It may be remembered as a bump or pimple, or it may be hidden on the scalp, within the earlobe, or between the fingers.

The bacillus can be cultured, but this is not routinely performed. The differential diagnosis includes nontuberculous mycobacterial disease.

Treatment

The majority of cases occurring in normal hosts do not require antibiotics. By contrast, in immunocompromised patients, these infections are successfully treated with ciprofloxacin, trimethoprim-sulfamethoxazole, doxycycline, azithromycin, erythromycin, rifampin, and gentamycin. Treatment of cat-scratch disease with antimicrobial agents has had variable results. Treatment with azithromycin results in regression of lymph node size 30 days after treatment. If antimicrobial therapy is used, patients weighing >45.5 kg (>100 lb) should receive 500 mg of azithromycin orally on day 1, followed by 250 mg once daily for 4 additional days. Those weighing <45.5 kg (<100 lb) should receive 10 mg/kg orally on day 1, followed by 5 mg/kg on days 2 to 5. Resistance to first-generation cephalosporins correlated with clinical failure of therapy. Many other commonly used antibiotics are not effective. Suppurating lymph nodes should be aspirated with a 16- to 18-gauge needle.

ANIMAL AND HUMAN BITES

Animal bites, especially from dogs and cats, are common injuries (Figure 15-43). Most wounds heal with conservative therapy designed to cleanse and disinfect the bite site. Some animal bites are serious or fatal.

Pasteurella species are the most common pathogen in dog and cat bites. *Streptococci, Staphylococci, Moraxella, Corynebacterium,* and *Neisseria* are the next most common aerobic isolates. *Staphylococcus aureus* and *Streptococcus pyogenes* are found relatively infrequently. Anaerobes are rarely present alone; the majority of infections are mixed infections. *Fusobacterium, Bacteroides, Porphyromonas,* and *Prevotella* species are the predominant anaerobic isolates. Anaerobes were more often isolated from cat bites than from dog bites, and from puncture wounds of the arms than from other parts of the body.

Anaerobic and aerobic bacteria infect human bite wounds. Humans harbor more pathogens than animals. Human bites have a higher incidence of serious infections and complications. There are two types of human bites. Occlusional wounds occur when the teeth are sunk into the skin. Clenched-fist injuries occur when a tooth penetrates the hand. These require radiographic and surgical evaluation because severe complications result if a joint or bone is penetrated. Bacteria are carried beyond the penetration site beneath the skin when tendons are moved. The wound is usually 5 mm long. The hand becomes painful and swollen in 6 to 8 hours. *S. aureus, Eikenella corrodens, Haemophilus* species, and (in more than 50% of cases) anaerobic bacteria infect human bites. Residual disability and complications are frequent after clenched-fist injuries. Abscesses, osteomyelitis, tendinitis, tendon rupture caused by infection, and residual stiffness of the joint may occur.

Management

EXAMINATION, IRRIGATION, AND DEBRIDEMENT

Carefully examine all injuries. Bites that appear to be superficial may overlie fractures; involve lacerated tendons, vessels, or nerves; extend into body cavities; or penetrate joint spaces. Cultures taken at the time of injury are of little value because they cannot predict whether infection will develop or, if it does, the causative pathogens.

Copious irrigation at high pressure markedly decreases the concentration of bacteria in contaminated wounds.

Irrigation of the wound decreases the risk of infection. Tear wounds are copiously irrigated with sterile normal saline solution. Puncture wounds are irrigated using normal saline solution in a 20-ml syringe with an 18-gauge needle as a high-pressure jet.

Devitalized tissue in human bite wounds predisposes to infection. Elimination of the crushed devitalized tissue by debridement of wound edges is the key to control infection and to ensure a successful outcome following surgical reconstruction.

HUMAN BITE

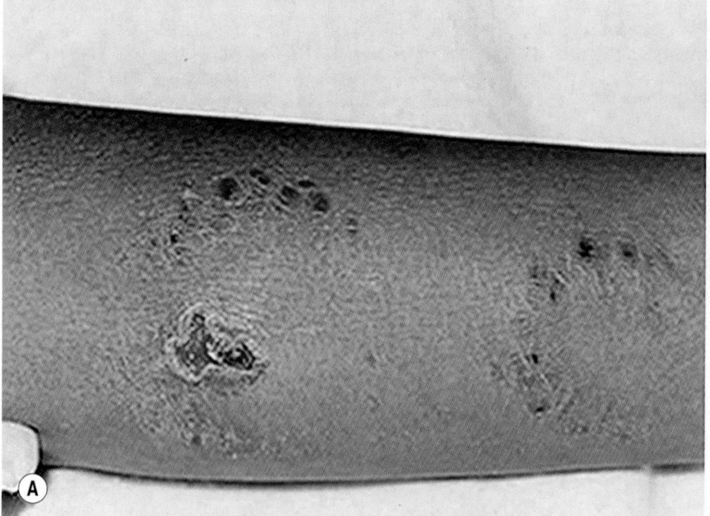

DOG BITE

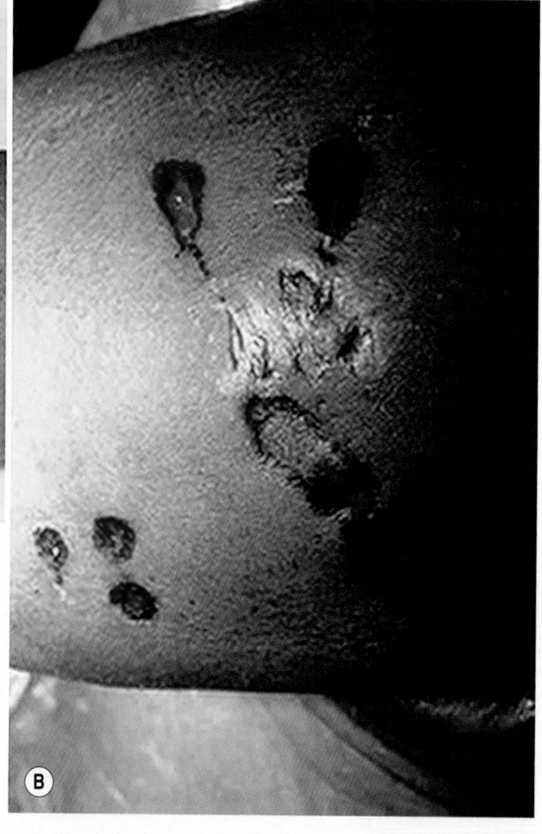

Figure 15-43 **A,** Human bite marks are usually superficial abrasions or contusions. Humans have four incisors in each dental arch and short canines. The incisors leave rectangular marks, and the canines leave triangular marks. The arch is elliptical or oval. **B,** Dogs have six incisors and long, curved canines. Their arch is long, with a short, straight anterior segment. The bite configuration is not oval. Dogs' canines can leave deep punctures, with tissue tearing. (Courtesy Fischer ET al: *NEJM Images in Clinical Medicine* 349 [11]:e11, 2003.)

IMMUNIZATION FOR TETANUS AND RABIES

Tetanus immunoglobulin and tetanus toxoid should be given to patients who have had two or fewer primary immunizations. Tetanus toxoid alone can be given to those who have completed a primary immunization series but who have not received a booster for more than 5 years.

The bite of any mammal can transmit rabies. Rat bites pose a minimal risk. Cleaning a bite with soap is as effective as cleaning with quaternary ammonium compounds in lowering the risk of transmission of rabies.

Rabies prophylaxis is indicated for bites by carnivorous wild animals (skunks, raccoons), bats, and unvaccinated domestic dogs and cats. Vaccination is prophylactic, not therapeutic. Once signs of rabies occur, survival is rare.

All animals that behave wildly or erratically should be killed so that their brains can be evaluated for rabies. Quarantine healthy-appearing dogs, cats, and ferrets for 10 days and kill them if signs of illness occur. Rabies prophylaxis is indicated if laboratory tests confirm rabies in the dead animal or if the animal was not captured.

Patients who have not been vaccinated previously should receive both human rabies vaccine (a series of five doses administered intramuscularly in the deltoid area) and rabies immune globulin (20 international units/kg of body weight, with as much as possible infiltrated in and around the wound and the remainder administered intramuscularly at a site distant from that used for vaccine administration). Rabies prophylaxis is recommended after exposure to bats in a confined setting, particularly for children, even when no bites are visible.

WHEN TO SUTURE THE BITE WOUND

Proper wound preparation with irrigation and debridement of devitalized tissue is the key to success. Wounds should be irrigated and left open if they are punctures rather than lacerations, are not potentially disfiguring, are inflicted by humans, involve the legs and arms (particularly the hands) as opposed to the face, or occurred more than 6 to 12 hours earlier in the case of bites to the arms and legs and 12 to 24 hours earlier in the case of bites to the face.

Facial lacerations from dog bites or cat bites are almost always closed. Foreign material in a contaminated wound increases the risk of infection; therefore subcutaneous sutures should be used sparingly. After 72 hours consider reevaluating wounds that were initially left open to determine whether delayed primary closure is indicated.

ANTIBIOTICS

Antibiotics are not given routinely. Low-risk bites penetrating only the epidermis and not involving the hands, feet, or skin overlying joints or cartilaginous structures do not need to be treated with oral antibiotics. *PMID: 14724871* Oral antibiotics are recommended for deep punctures (particularly if infected by cats), those that require surgical repair, wounds to the hands or near a bone, all moderate to severe wounds, crush injuries, and wounds that may have penetrated a joint. Cat bite wounds are often more severe and have a higher proportion of osteomyelitis and septic arthritis. Empiric therapy for dog and cat bites should be directed against *Pasteurella*, streptococci, staphylococci, and anaerobes. *Pasteurella* species are usually susceptible to ampicillin, penicillin, second-generation and third-generation cephalosporins, doxycycline, trimethoprim-sulfamethoxazole, fluoroquinolones, clarithromycin, and azithromycin. Antibiotics typically used for routine infections of skin and soft tissue, such as antistaphylococcal penicillins, first-generation cephalosporins, clindamycin, and erythromycin, are less active against *Pasteurella*.

Empiric treatment of dog and cat bites is similar (Table 15-5). Cat bites have a greater prevalence of anaerobes and *Pasteurella multocida*. Oral amoxicillin-clavulanate is recommended first-line treatment. Alternative oral agents include doxycycline, or penicillin VK plus dicloxacillin. Other options, including fluoroquinolones, trimethoprim-sulfamethoxazole, and cefuroxime, may require an additional agent active against anaerobes, such as metronidazole or clindamycin. First-generation cephalosporins—such as cephalexin, penicillinase-resistant penicillins (e.g., dicloxacillin), macrolides (e.g., erythromycin), and clindamycin—all have poor in vitro activity against *P. multocida* and should be avoided.

Intravenous options, such as cefuroxime, ceftriaxone, and cefotaxime, may be used but may require the addition of an antianaerobic agent.

Penicillin-allergic pregnant women and children are treated with macrolides (e.g., azithromycin 250 to 500 mg every day or telithromycin 400 mg, two tablets by mouth every day). There is a potential risk of failure with these antibiotics. The duration of therapy varies by the severity of the injury and infection. Cellulitis and abscess are treated for 5 to 10 days. Wounds that are moderate to severe, have crush injury or edema, are on the hands or near a bone or a joint, or are in compromised hosts should receive 3 to 5 days of "prophylactic" antimicrobial therapy.

Table 15-5 Recommended Therapy for Infections following Animal or Human Bites*

Antimicrobial agent, by type of bite	ROUTE OF DRUG ADMINISTRATION Oral	 Intravenous	Comment
Animal bite			
Amoxicillin/clavulanate	500-875 mg twice per day†	—	Some gram-negative rods are resistant; misses MRSA
Ampicillin-sulbactam	—	1.5-3.0 gm every 6-8 hr	Some gram-negative rods are resistant; misses MRSA
Piperacillin/tazobactam	—	3.37 gm every 6-8 hr	
Carbapenem			Misses MRSA
Ertapenem	—	1 gm every day	
Imipenem	—	1 gm every 6-8 hr	
Meropenem	—	1 gm every 8 hr	
Doxycycline	100 mg twice per day	—	Excellent activity against *Pasteurella multocida;* some streptococci are resistant
Penicillin	500 mg four times per day	—	
plus			
Dicloxacillin	500 mg four times per day		
TMP-SMZ	160-800 mg twice per day	—	Good activity against aerobes; poor activity against anaerobes
Metronidazole	250-500 mg four times per day	—	Good activity against anaerobes; no activity against aerobes
Clindamycin	300 mg three times per day	—	Good activity against staphylococci, streptococci, and anaerobes; misses *P. multocida*
First-generation cephalosporin			Good activity against staphylococci and streptococci; misses *P. multocida* and anaerobes
Cephalexin	500 mg three times per day	—	
Cefazolin	—	1 gm every 8 hr	
Second-generation cephalosporin			Good activity against *P. multocida;* misses anaerobes
Cefuroxime	500 mg twice per day	1 gm every day	
Cefoxitin	—	1 gm every 6-8 hr	
Third-generation cephalosporin			
Ceftriaxone	—	1 gm every 12 hr	
Cefotaxime	—	2 gm every 6 hr	
Fluoroquinolones‡			Good activity against *P. multocida;* misses MRSA and some anaerobes
Ciprofloxacin	500-750 mg twice per day	400 mg every 12 hr	
Gatifloxacin	400 mg every day	—	
Moxifloxacin	400 mg every day	400 mg every day	

Table 15-5 Recommended Therapy for Infections following Animal or Human Bites—cont'd

Antimicrobial agent, by type of bite	ROUTE OF DRUG ADMINISTRATION		Comment
	Oral	Intravenous	
Human bite			
Amoxicillin/clavulanate	500 mg every 8 hr†	—	Some gram-negative rods are resistant; misses MRSA
Ampicillin/sulbactam	—	1.5-3.0 gm every 6 hr	Some gram-negative rods are resistant; misses MRSA
Carbapenem			Misses MRSA
Ertapenem	—	1 gm every day	
Imipenem	—	1 gm every day	
Meropenem	—	1 gm every day	
Doxycycline	100 mg twice per day	—	Good activity against *Eikenella* species, staphylococci, and anaerobes; some streptococci are resistant
TMP-SMZ	160-800 mg twice per day	—	Good activity against aerobes; poor activity against anaerobes
Metronidazole	250-500 mg four times per day	—	Good activity against anaerobes; poor activity against aerobes
Clindamycin	300 mg three times per day	—	Good activity against staphylococci, streptococci, and anaerobes; misses *Eikenella corrodens*
Cephalosporin			Good activity against staphylococci and streptococci; misses *E. corrodens* and gram-negative anaerobes
Cephalexin	500 mg four times per day	—	
Cefazolin	—	1 gm every 8 hr	
Fluoroquinolones‡			Good activity against *E. corrodens;* misses MRSA and some anaerobes
Ciprofloxacin	500-750 mg twice per day	400 mg every 12 hr	
Gatifloxacin	400 mg every day	400 mg every day	
Moxifloxacin	400 mg every day	400 mg every day	

Adapted from Practice guidelines for the diagnosis and management of skin and soft-tissue Infections, *Clin Infect Dis* 41:1373-1406, 2005. *PMID: 16231249*

*Duration of therapy: The duration of therapy varies by the severity of the injury/infection. Cellulitis and abscess often respond to 5-10 days of therapy. The therapy for early presenting, noninfected wounds remains controversial. Wounds that are moderate to severe, have associated crush injury, have associated edema (either preexisting or subsequent) that are on the hands or in proximity to a bone or a joint or that are in compromised hosts should receive 3-5 days of "prophylactic" antimicrobial therapy. These wounds are often colonized with potential pathogens (85% of cases), and it is difficult to determine whether the wound will become infected.

†Should be given with food.

‡NOTE: As a rule, the use of fluoroquinolones is contraindicated by the U.S. Food and Drug Administration for children and adolescents <18 years of age. It should also be noted that tetracyclines are rarely used in children younger than 8 years of age. Alternatives should be strongly considered for these two antibiotics.

MRSA, methicillin-resistant *Staphylococcus aureus; TMP-SMZ,* trimethoprim-sulfamethoxazole.

STINGING INSECTS

Honeybees, wasps, hornets, and yellow jackets sting when confronted. A wasp, for example, will vigorously pursue nest intruders. Insect repellents (e.g., DEET) offer no protection. A firm, sharp stinger is imbedded in the skin, followed immediately by secretion of venom. The honeybee stings once and dies. Its barbed stinger, glands, and viscera remain in the victim. Imbedded honeybee stingers should be flicked away with a knife or fingernail. If the stinger is grasped with fingertips, the venom glands will compress and make the sting worse. Stingers of other stinging insects are not barbed and remain intact, ready to be used again. The injected venom can cause a localized or generalized reaction. Reactions are classified as toxic or allergic.

Toxic reactions

Hymenoptera stings cause cutaneous local reactions of limited size and duration in most individuals. This nonallergic local reaction is a toxic response to venom constituents. There is a sharp, pinprick sensation at the instant of stinging, followed by moderate burning pain at the site. A red papule or wheal appears and enlarges if scratched (Figure 15-44). The reaction subsides in hours. Multiple stings can produce a systemic toxic reaction with vomiting, diarrhea, headache, fever, muscle spasm, and loss of consciousness. More than 500 stings at one time may be fatal.

Allergic reactions

Allergic reactions are mediated by IgE antibodies directed at venom constituents. Reactions are localized or generalized.

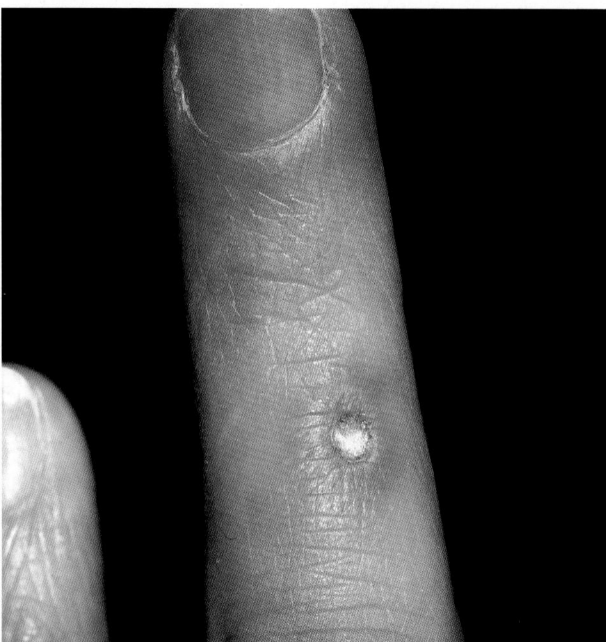

Figure 15-44 Bee sting. Severe local reaction with necrosis and ulceration at the sting site.

LOCALIZED ALLERGIC REACTIONS

Like the toxic reaction, the local allergic reaction begins with immediate pain, but the urticarial response is exaggerated. Swelling is thick and hard, as in angioedema. The urticarial plaque may be small or huge (Figure 15-45). Swelling lasts 1 to several days. Allergic local reactions greater than 10 cm in diameter are called large local reactions. They last for up to 5 days. Forty percent of patients with generalized allergic reactions have had large localized reactions.

GENERALIZED REACTIONS

The prevalence of generalized reactions to stings is approximately 0.4%. There are 40 fatalities from stings each year in the United States. Generalized reactions begin 2 to 60 minutes after the sting. Reactions vary from generalized itching with a few hives to anaphylaxis. Anaphylactic symptoms are typical of those occurring from any cause. They include generalized itching and hives, followed by shortness of breath, wheezing, nausea, and abdominal cramps. The reaction usually subsides spontaneously, but in the unfortunate few it progresses, with edema of the upper airway causing obstruction and death. Following sting anaphylaxis, approximately 50% of patients continue to have allergic reactions to subsequent stings, but up to 42% have an improved response.

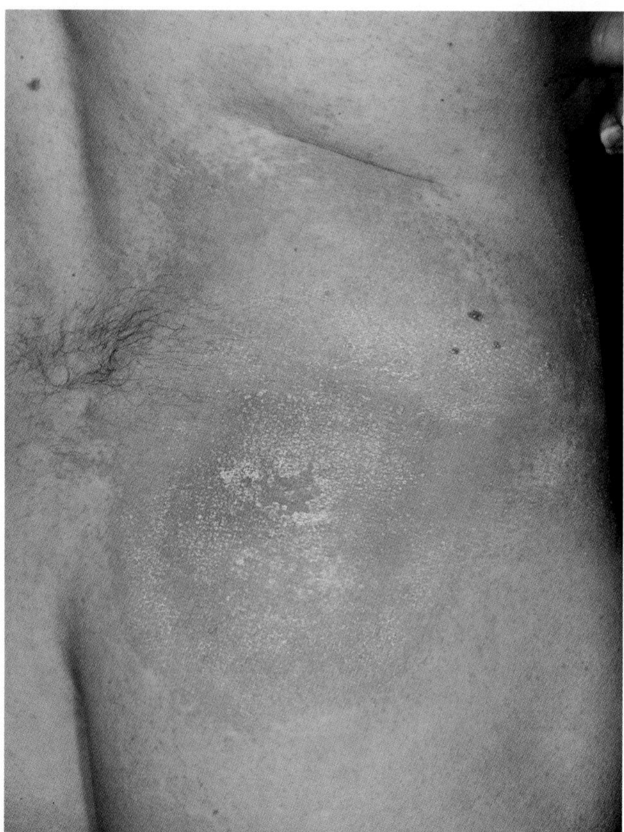

Figure 15-45 Bee sting. A huge, urticarial plaque occurred within hours in this patient with a known history of bee sting allergy.

Most reactions in children are mild, with just hives. Children with dermal reactions have only a benign course and are unlikely to have recurrent reactions. The more severe reactions, such as shock and loss of consciousness, are more common in adults. Adults whose reactions include urticaria, obstruction of the upper or lower airway, or hypotension and children whose reactions include obstruction of the upper or lower airway or hypotension have an increased risk of future systemic reactions to stings. Patients may develop delayed-onset allergic symptoms up to 1 week after the sting that range from typical anaphylaxis to serum sickness and are mediated by venom-specific IgE. Immunotherapy is recommended for patients with these reactions. The possibility of a fatal insect sting should be considered in unwitnessed deaths occurring outdoors in summer.

Diagnosis

The diagnosis of Hymenoptera venom allergy is based on history, skin tests, and determination of venom-specific IgE antibodies in the serum. Only rarely are other tests needed (specific IgG antibodies). To achieve a definite diagnosis, all findings have to be considered carefully, as "false-positive" and "false-negative" results can occur in all test systems. A diagnostic workup is not recommended for local reactions or for persons who have not experienced a systemic reaction. Patients who have large localized or generalized eruptions should be tested with venom extracts from honeybees, yellow jackets, yellow hornets, white-faced hornets, or wasps.

Treatment

Localized nonallergic stings are treated with ice or a paste made by mixing 1 teaspoon of meat tenderizer with 1 teaspoon of water. Localized allergic reactions are treated with cool, wet compresses and antihistamines.

Treatment of severe generalized reactions for adults includes aqueous epinephrine 1:1000 in a dosage of 0.3 to 0.5 ml administered subcutaneously and repeated once or twice at 20-minute intervals if needed. Epinephrine may be given intramuscularly if shock is imminent. If the patient is hypotensive, intravenous injections of 1:10,000 dilution may be necessary. If a severe reaction is feared, epinephrine should be administered immediately; waiting for symptoms to develop can be a dangerous practice.

Kits with preloaded epinephrine syringes are available (e.g., EpiPen Auto-Injector, Ana-Kit). Highly sensitive patients should have these kits available at home and during travel. For practice, one injection of physiologic saline should be self-administered under the supervision of a physician. Shortly after administration of epinephrine, antihistamines such as diphenhydramine (Benadryl 25 to 50 mg) are given orally or intramuscularly, depending on the severity of the reaction.

Patients with a history of insect sting anaphylaxis and positive venom skin test results should have epinephrine available.

BITING INSECTS

Biting insects such as fleas, flies, and mosquitoes do not bite in the literal sense; rather, they stab their victims with a sharp stylet covered with saliva. The sharp pain is caused by the stab; the reaction depends on the degree of sensitivity to the saliva. All of these insects are capable of transmitting infectious diseases. Biting insects seem to prefer some individuals to others. They are attracted by the warmth and moisture of humans. The patient's individual sensitivity determines the type and severity of the bite reaction. Patients who have not had previous exposure or those who have had numerous bites may show little or no response. Those who are sensitive develop localized urticarial papules and plaques immediately following the bite. The papules and plaques proceed to fade in hours and are replaced by red papules that last for days.

Papular urticaria

Papular urticaria refers to hypersensitivity bite reactions in children. Young children who are left outside unattended in the summer months may receive numerous bites. They soon become sensitized, and subsequent bites show red, raised, urticarial papules that itch intensely (Figure 15-46). The young child who was initially indifferent to bites may habitually excoriate newly evolved lesions, creating crusts and infection. Chronically excoriated lesions may last for months, eventually leaving white, round scars.

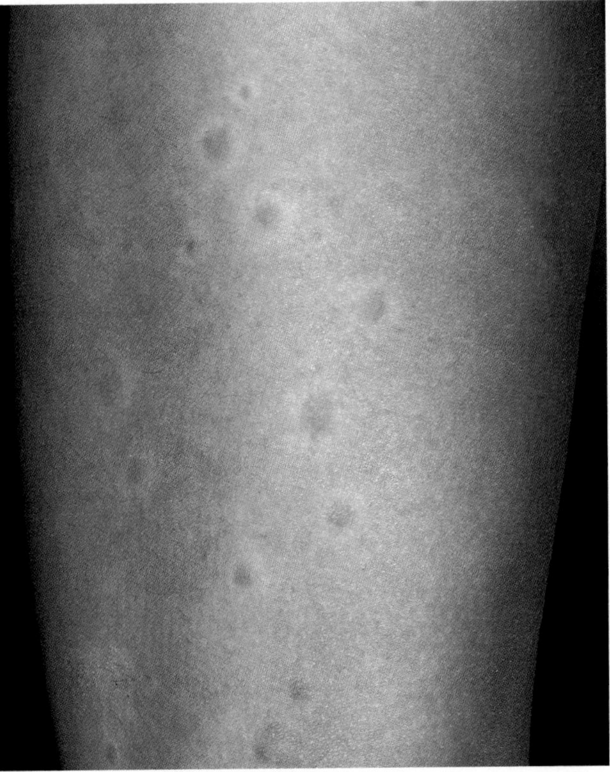

Figure 15-46 Papular urticaria. A hypersensitivity reaction to insect bites seen in children. A wheal develops at the site of each bite.

Fleas

Fleas are tiny, red-brown, hard-bodied, wingless insects that are capable of jumping approximately 2 feet. They have distinctive, laterally flattened abdomens that allow them to slip between the hairs of their hosts (Figure 15-47). They live in rugs and on the bodies of animals and may jump onto humans. Bubonic plague was spread throughout Europe in the Middle Ages by fleas that had fed on infected rats.

Flea bites occur in a cluster or group (Figure 15-48). A tiny, red dot or bite punctum may be seen at times. Most lesions are grouped around the ankles or lower legs, areas within easy leaping distance of the floor. Adult men are infrequently affected because their socks and pants protect them.

CONTROL, ELIMINATION, AND TREATMENT

Fleas reside on cats, dogs, the animal's bedding, and in the entire house. All sources must be treated for effective flea control. Flea control involves eliminating the adult fleas on animals in the house and immature fleas in the environment. Carpets, pet bedding, and resting areas should be aggressively vacuumed. Wash pet bedding. Remove dead vegetation from animal resting areas outside. Many chemicals are available for control. There is no one best chemical.

Myiasis

The invasion of live human or animal tissue by fly larvae (maggots) is termed *myiasis*. Many organs can be involved but the skin is the most common site.

LARVAE SPECIES

Many species of flies around the world cause myiasis. Most cases are seen in returning travelers from Central or South America (*Dermatobia hominis*, the human botfly, a nonbiting insect) or from Africa (*Cordylobia anthropophaga*, the tumbu fly).

INFESTATION

Females do not lay their eggs directly on their host but on the underside of a blood-sucking insect, such as a mosquito, biting fly, or tick. These insects transmit the larvae of the botfly via phoresis, a unique mechanism of egg deposition. Infection with the tumbu fly larvae occurs after direct contact with the eggs that are often deposited in clothes and towels. Young children who fall asleep outside are likely victims. Larvae may be acquired from petting or kissing dogs or cats contaminated with larvae. Larvae adhere and enter the nose, eyes, mouth, or anus, or they penetrate skin. Larvae in the eyes, nose, or trachea of humans may attempt migration through deep organs. Those that penetrate skin develop at the site of penetration. Larvae enter the skin and reach the underlying subcutaneous tissue, where they feed and grow. The time required for mature larvae to develop is species-specific (approximately 7 weeks). At maturity they enlarge the central pore and prepare to exit.

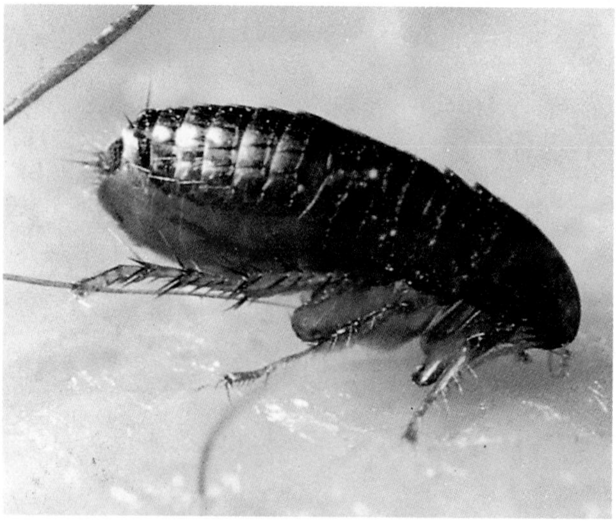

Figure 15-47 Flea. Thin wingless insects with very hard bodies and large hind legs adapted for jumping. (Courtesy Ken Gray, Oregon State University Extension Services.)

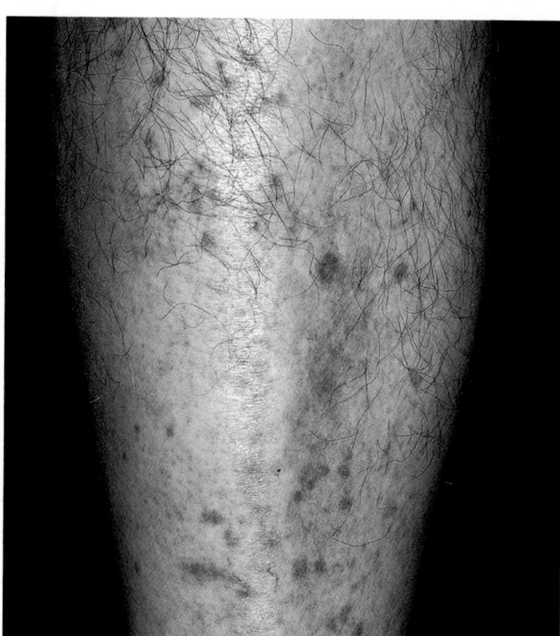

Figure 15-48 Flea bites. A cluster of bites below the knee. This is a common site because a flea can jump no higher than approximately 2 feet.

CLINICAL PRESENTATION

Most patients present in late August or early September. Lesions are found on the face, scalp, chest, arms, or legs. Clinically an abscess-like lesion develops. A red papule 2 to 4 mm in diameter appears (Figure 15-49). The lesion resembles a furuncle or inflamed cyst and is called a warble; the maggot is called a bot. Flies that cause furuncular myiasis are called botflies. The head of the larva rises to the surface for air about once a minute through a small central pore. Movement of the larval spiracle (respiratory apparatus) may be observed. Serous or seropurulent exudate flows from the central punctum. Symptoms range from a mild itching or stinging to intense pain leading to agitation and insomnia. Sensation of movement in the lesion supports the diagnosis. An intense inflammatory reaction occurs in the tissue surrounding the larvae. Infection by *Tunga penetrans* may resemble myiasis. *T. penetrans* is a flea that invades the skin and produces a furuncular nodule. Tungiasis is almost always on the feet, whereas myiasis on the feet is rare. Tungiasis is acquired in South America and Africa.

TREATMENT

Correct diagnosis will prevent unnecessary treatment with antibiotics. In most cases the larva can be forced through the central hole with manual pressure. *D. hominis* is attached to the skin by hooklets. The larva's survival within its host is dependent upon the availability of oxygen. Obstruction of the breathing orifice with occlusive elements is effective. Apply an adhesive dressing such as tape and the larva becomes enmeshed within the dressing when it migrates toward the skin to get oxygen. Application of petroleum jelly over the pore may force the larva out for air. Another method involves the injection of lidocaine hydrochloride under the nodule. The pressure of the injection is sufficient to push the larva out. Bacon therapy is another noninvasive technique. The fatty parts of raw bacon are placed over the opening of the skin lesion. The fly larva crawls far enough into the bacon and can be removed with forceps within 3 hours. It is usually not necessary to enlarge the hole, but if the larva does not emerge, a no. 11 blade may be used to enlarge the hole slightly (Figure 15-49, *B-C*). There is usually only one maggot in each mass. Rarely, a generalized reaction to fly bites may develop. Extracts are available for desensitization for a generalized reaction to fly bites.

MYIASIS

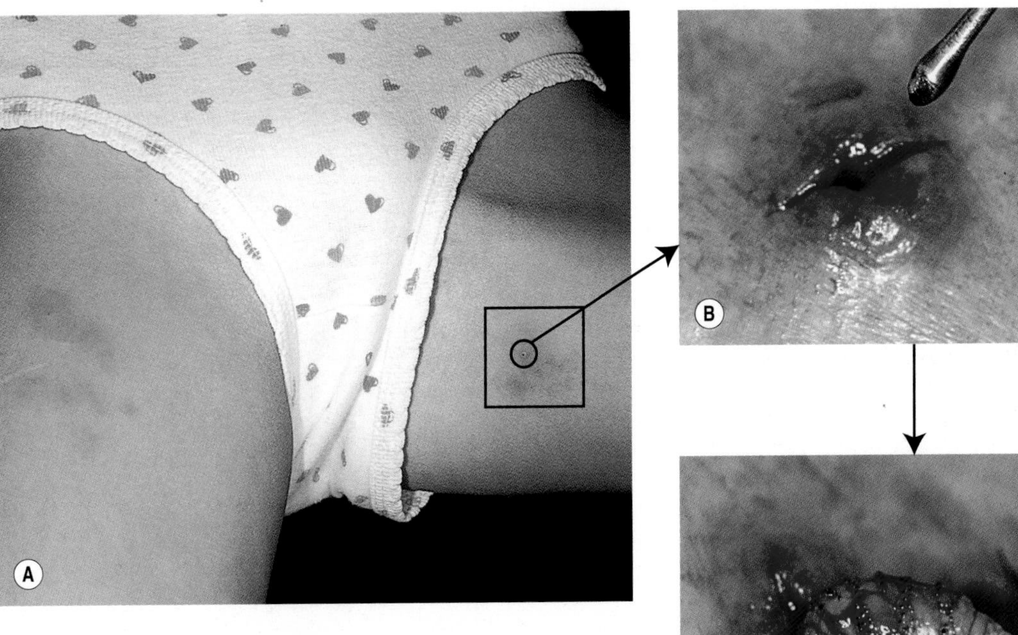

Figure 15-49 **A,** Fly larvae may be deposited on the skin and burrow into the host. They mature, induce skin surface erythema, and rhythmically oscillate by rising to the surface to breathe and then retracting back through the small orifice. Patients can feel this movement and may even see the worm as it rises through the orifice. **B,** An incision is made across the central hole. **C,** The larva is extracted intact with forceps.

Mosquitoes

Mosquito saliva is the source of antigens that produce the bite reactions in humans. Cutaneous reactions to mosquito bites are usually pruritic wheals and delayed papules. The rate of immediate reaction increases from early childhood to adolescence and decreases with age from adulthood. The appearance and intensity of the delayed reaction decrease with age. Arthus-type local and systemic symptoms can occur, but anaphylactic reactions are very rare.

A characteristic sequence of events takes place in all subjects exposed to mosquito bites over time. The initial bite causes no reaction, but with subsequent bites a delayed cutaneous lesion appears several hours after the bite and lasts 1 to 3 days or longer. After repeated bites for approximately 1 month, an immediate wheal develops that varies from 2 to 10 mm in diameter. Then, with further exposure for several months, the delayed reaction disappears. After repeated bites, the old bite sites may show flare-ups. Blisters can occur on the lower legs. In England, the condition known as seasonal bullous eruption was shown to be caused by mosquitoes. Patients with chronic lymphocytic leukemia may exhibit severe, delayed bite reactions that can appear before the malignancy has been diagnosed. Patients with acquired immunodeficiency syndrome who had pruritus and chronic, nonspecific-appearing skin eruptions showed increased antibody titers to mosquito salivary gland antigens. This represents a form of chronic "recall" reaction. The increase may be a consequence of nonspecific B-cell activation, a feature of AIDS.

No desensitization treatment is generally available for mosquito allergy.

PREVENTION AND MANAGEMENT

Biting insects are attracted to human body odor.

DEET. *N,N*-Diethyl-*meta*-toluamide (DEET) is the most effective and best studied insect repellent currently on the market. This substance has a remarkable safety profile after 40 years of worldwide use. DEET is especially active against mosquitoes, but it also repels biting flies, gnats, chiggers, ticks, and other insects. It does not repel stinging insects.

ANTIHISTAMINES. In mosquito-sensitive subjects, a prophylactically administered nonsedating antihistamine (e.g., Allegra 180 mg once daily, Zyrtec 10 mg) is an effective drug against both immediate and delayed mosquito bite symptoms.

PERMETHRIN. Permethrin, a pesticide used for the treatment of lice, is also effective as a clothing spray for protection against mosquitoes and ticks.

THIAMINE. A few reports claim that 75 to 150 mg of thiamine hydrochloride (vitamin B_1) taken orally each day during the summer months protects against insect bites. Others think that it is not effective. Thiamine hydrochloride is safe and may be worth trying, especially for children who are bitten often.

Insect bite symptoms are treated with cool, wet compresses, topical steroids, and oral antihistamines. A paste made of 1 teaspoon of meat tenderizer and 1 teaspoon of water provides symptomatic relief and discourages children from excoriating bites.

Bed bugs

The common bed bug *Cimex lectularius* is a wingless, red-brown, blood-sucking insect that grows up to 7 mm in length and has a lifespan from 4 months up to 1 year. Bed bugs hide in cracks and crevices in beds, wooden furniture, floors, and walls during the daytime and emerge at night to feed on their preferred host, humans.

C. lectularius inject saliva into the blood stream of their host to thin the blood, and to prevent coagulation. It is this saliva that causes the intense itching and welts. The delay in the onset of itching gives the feeding bed bug time to escape into cracks and crevices. In some cases, the itchy bites can develop into painful welts that last several days. Figure 15-50 shows an adult bed bug, *C. lectularius,* as it was in the process of ingesting a blood meal from the arm of a "voluntary" human host.

Bed bug bites are difficult to diagnose due to the variability in bite response between people, and due to the change in skin reaction for the same person over time. It is best to collect and identify bed bugs to confirm bites. Bed bugs are responsible for loss of sleep, discomfort, disfiguring from numerous bites and occasionally bites may become infected.

Bed bugs are not vectors in nature of any known human disease. Although some disease organisms have been recovered from bed bugs under laboratory conditions, none have been shown to be transmitted by bed bugs outside of the laboratory.

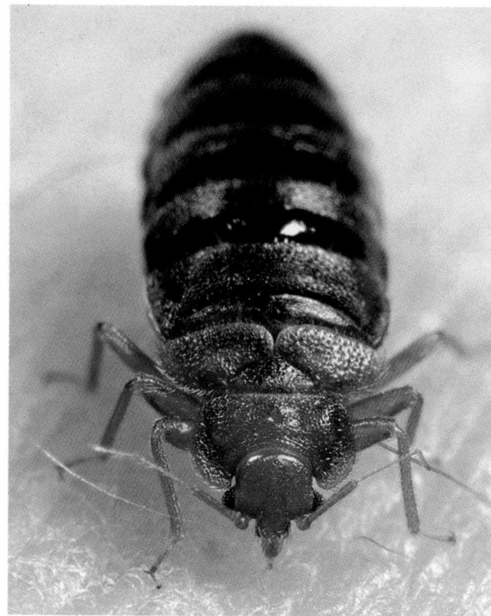

Figure 15-50 The common bed bug feeds on human blood.

CREEPING ERUPTION

Creeping eruption (cutaneous larva migrans) is a unique cutaneous eruption caused by the aimless wandering of the dog or cat hookworm larvae through the skin. It is the most frequent skin disease among travelers returning from tropical countries. There was a history of exposure to a beach in 95% of patients. *Ancylostoma braziliense* is the most common species. Infection is most frequent in warmer climates such as the Caribbean (especially Jamaica), Africa, Central and South America, Southeast Asia, and the Southeastern United States. Exposure to cat feces in a playground sandbox was the source of infection in a reported outbreak in Florida. *PMID: 18075486*

Less frequent use of protective footwear while walking on the beach is significantly associated with a higher risk.

Adult nematodes thrive in the intestines of dogs and cats, where they deposit ova that are carried to the ground in feces. The ova hatch into larvae and lie in ambush in the soil waiting for a cat or dog. In their haste to complete their growth cycle, these indiscriminate parasites may penetrate the skin of a human at the point where skin touches the soil. Workers who crawl on their backs under houses may acquire a diffuse infiltration with numerous lesions. The hookworms soon learn that they have preyed on the wrong host. The larva penetrates the skin in hopes of eventually reaching the intestines; however, physiologic limitations in humans prevent invasion deeper than the basal area of the epidermis. The trapped larva struggles forward 2.7 mm per day laterally through the epidermis in a random fashion, creating a track reminiscent of the trail of a sea snail wandering aimlessly over the sand at low tide (Figure 15-51). The length of the track can be used to estimate the duration of infestation. Many larvae may be present in the same area, creating several closely approximated wavy lines.

Lesions are found on the feet in more than 50% of individuals, followed by the buttocks and thighs. Other sites may include the elbow, breast, legs, and face.

Symptoms begin days to 3 weeks and sometimes months after exposure to infested soil. During larval migration, a local inflammatory response is provoked by release of larval secretions consisting largely of proteolytic enzymes. Itching is moderate to intense and secondary infection or eczematous inflammation occurs. Eosinophilia may approach 30% in some cases. The 1-cm larva stays concealed directly ahead of the advancing tip of the wavy, twisted, red-to-purple, 3-mm track. If untreated, larvae usually die within 2 to 8 weeks, but occasionally persist for up to 1 year or more. The dead worm is eventually sloughed away as the epidermis matures. Löffler's syndrome, which is a transitory, patchy infiltration of the lung, may develop with an accompanying eosinophilia of the blood and sputum. This occurs with dermal penetration and subsequent larval invasion of the bloodstream. This is most common in patients with severe cutaneous infestation.

MANAGEMENT

Children are advised not to sit, lie, or walk barefoot on wet soil or sand. The ground should be covered with impenetrable material when sitting or lying on the ground. Complications (impetigo and allergic reactions), together with the intense pruritus and the significant duration of the disease, make treatment mandatory. Freezing the leading edge of the skin track rarely works and causes unnecessary tissue destruction.

Oral ivermectin and albendazole are first-line treatments. Ivermectin is taken in a single dose (200 mcg/kg, average dose 12 mg). It is well tolerated and highly effective. Symptoms disappear within 1 week. One or two repeated courses are used for resistant cases. Albendazole is also effective and well tolerated (400 to 800 mg/day, according to weight, for 3 days); 10% albendazole ointment, twice a day for 10 days, is a safe and effective alternative for small children (three 400-mg tablets of albendazole in 12 g of petroleum jelly).

PREVENTION

Tropical beaches are often frequented by dogs and cats.

Wear protective footwear when walking on the beach. Lye on sand washed by the tides and avoid dry sand. Mattresses are preferable to towels.

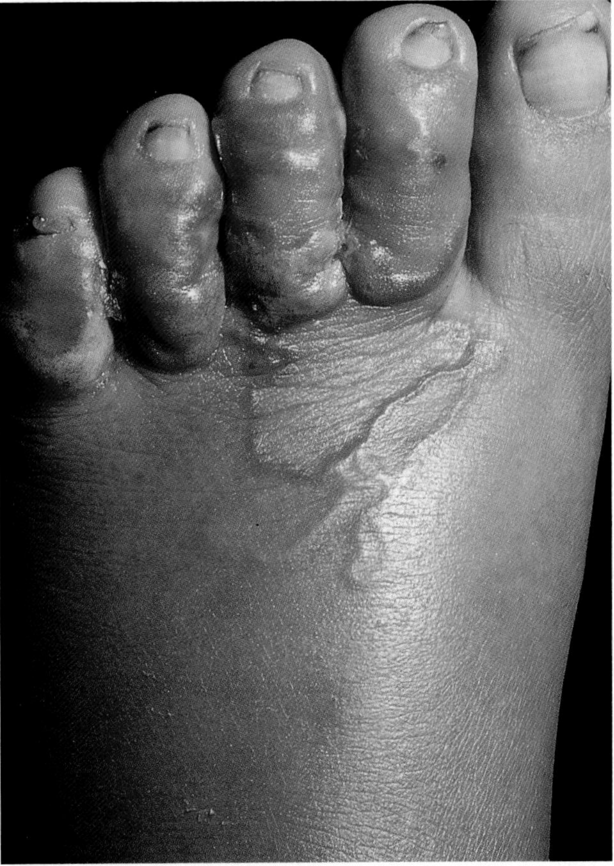

Figure 15-51 A severe infestation with multiple tracks and secondary infection of the toe webs.

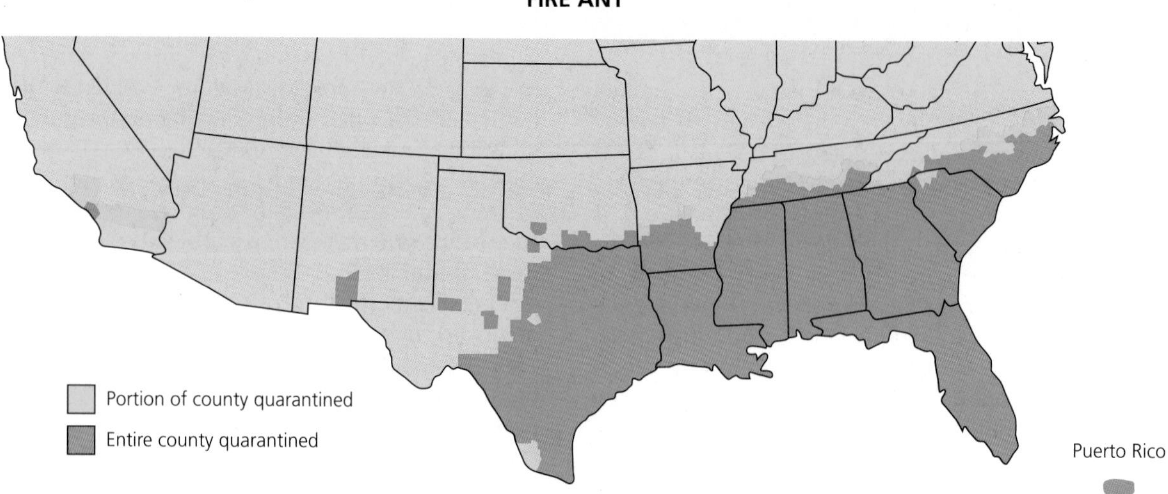

Figure 15-52

ANTS

Fire ants

The fire ant entered the United States from South America circa 1920 and spread quickly to several states in the southeast. There are four species of fire ants found in the United States in addition to the most common, *Solenopsis invicta*. Colonies have been found in Arizona, California, New Mexico, Virginia, and Puerto Rico (Figure 15-52). Invasions of buildings with sting attacks inside occupied dwellings, including health care facilities, have been reported. Fire ants can overwhelm their environment, causing destruction of land and animals. They cause a variety of health problems in humans, ranging from simple stings to anaphylaxis and death.

Between 30% and 60% of the population in infested areas are stung each year. Stings are most frequent during the summer; the legs of children are the most common target.

Fire ants are small (1/16- to 1/4-inch long) and yellow-to-red or black with a large head containing prominent incurved jaws and a beelike stinger on the tail (Figure 15-53).

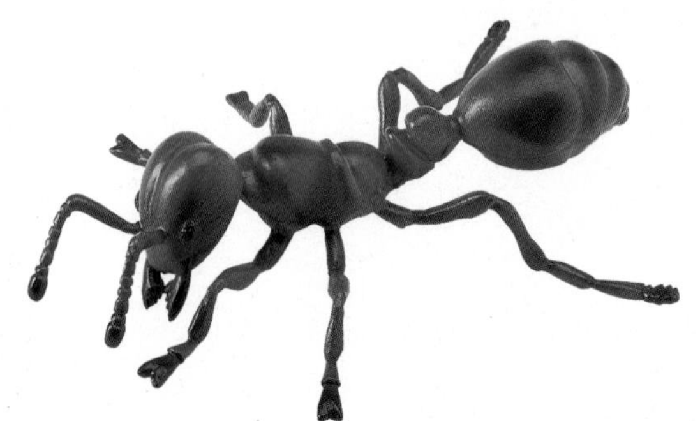

Figure 15-53 The Red imported fire ant has a 10-segmented antennae with a 2-segmented club.

They build large mounds (1 to 3 feet in diameter) in playgrounds, yards, and open fields in concentrations as high as 200 per acre. Colonies are formed at ground level in sandy areas. The grass at the periphery of the mound remains undisturbed and unharvested, unlike the mound of the harvester ant. The venom consists almost entirely of piperidine alkaloids, in contrast to the venoms of other Hymenoptera, such as the wasp, that is up to half polypeptide proteins, measured by weight. The small fraction of proteins in fire ant venom induces the IgE response. They have no natural enemies and may ultimately infest one quarter of the United States.

THE STING REACTION

Sting reactions range from local pustules and large, late-phase responses to life-threatening anaphylaxis. The fire ant is aggressive and vicious. When provoked, they attack in numbers. In an instant, the fire ant grasps the skin with its jaws, which establishes a pivot point. It arches its body, injects venom through a distal abdominal stinger, and then, if undisturbed, rotates and stings repeatedly, inflicting as many as 20 stings. This often results in a circle of stings with two tiny, red dots in the center where the jaws were attached. The pain is immediate and sharp, like a bee sting. Pain subsides in minutes and is replaced by a wheal and flare that resolves in 30 to 60 minutes; 8 to 24 hours later a sterile vesicle forms and later becomes umbilicated. The contents of the vesicle rapidly become purulent (Figure 15-54). Pustules resolve in approximately 10 days. A large, local, late-phase reaction occurs in 17% to 56% of patients and lasts 24 to 72 hours. The plaque is red, edematous, indurated, and extremely pruritic. Eosinophils, neutrophils, and fibrin are present. Edema may be severe and compress nerves and blood vessels.

Patients who are allergic to fire ants may present with anaphylaxis. This life-threatening reaction may occur hours after a sting. Check for stings on the lower extremity, especially between the toes, when a patient presents with anaphylaxis.

TREATMENT

The bite is treated with cool compresses, followed by application of a paste made with baking soda. Sarna lotion (0.5% camphor, 0.5% menthol) is soothing, especially if it is refrigerated. Application of meat tenderizer is of no value. Oral antihistamines provide some relief. A short course of prednisone is used for severe local reactions.

IMMUNOTHERAPY. Sting reactions range from local pustules and large, late-phase responses to life-threatening anaphylaxis. Fire ant allergen-specific immunotherapy can reduce the risk of subsequent systemic reactions. Conventional and rush immunotherapy with fire ant whole body extract is effective, safe, and efficacious; the rate of mild systemic reactions is low. Premedication is not necessary. Consider immunotherapy for patients with severe hypersensitivity to the venom or those who have had a previous anaphylactic reaction. Skin-test with whole body extract.

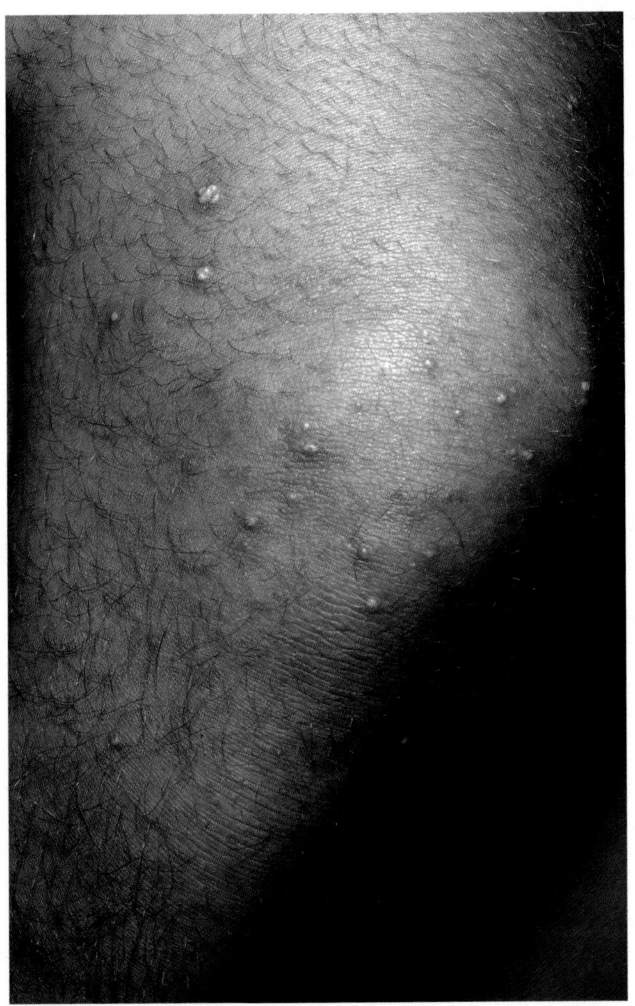

Figure 15-54 Fire ant stings. Multiple pustules in a cluster.

DERMATITIS ASSOCIATED WITH SWIMMING

There is increasing human contact with marine life. As more people travel to oceans for sports diving and other marine-related activities, the incidence of marine envenomations rises. Serious injury from a number of common sea creatures is possible.

Swimmer's itch (freshwater)

Swimmer's itch (schistosome cercarial dermatitis) occurs on uncovered skin and is a transient, pruritic dermatitis caused by the epidermal penetration of cercariae, a larval form of animal schistosome. The microscopic larvae of the parasitic flatworm schistosomes, after being released from snails, swim in the water seeking a warm-blooded host, such as a duck. The indiscriminate larvae may accidentally penetrate a human and do not develop further. Schistosomes of humans cause systemic disease, but animal schistosome cercariae die after epidermal penetration, resulting in a rash. The disease is found throughout the world and is restricted primarily to freshwater, although saltwater infestations have been reported. In the United States, this disease is most common along bird migratory flyways, such as the Great Lakes or Long Island sound regions. Outbreaks are episodic and determined by snail maturation. Shedding occurs on bright, warm days in early or midsummer, with the highest incidence of infestation occurring near the shore.

SYMPTOMS

The intensity of the eruption depends on the degree of sensitization. Some people do not develop a rash, whereas others swimming in the same water develop intense eruptions. Initial symptoms are minor after the first exposure, and papules occur only after sensitization is acquired, approximately 5 to 13 days later. The typical eruption occurs with subsequent exposures. It begins as bathing water evaporates from the skin surface and cercariae begin penetrating the skin. Itching occurs for approximately 1 hour and is followed hours later by the development of discrete, highly pruritic papules and, occasionally, pustules surrounded by erythema at the points of contact. They reach maximum intensity in 2 to 3 days and subside in 1 week. Secondary infection occurs following excoriation.

TREATMENT

Treatment consists of relieving symptoms while the eruption fades. Itching is controlled with antihistamines, cool compresses, and shake lotions such as calamine lotion. Intense inflammation may be suppressed with group II through V topical steroids. Towel drying immediately after leaving the water is an effective preventive measure, since most larvae penetrate the skin as water is evaporating.

Nematocyst stings

Nematocysts are unique structures found on animals in the phylum Cnidaria. Nematocyst stings are responsible for the vast majority of skin problems in people who visit the reefs. Nematocysts are microscopic capsules used both for capturing prey and for defense. They contain a toxin-covered, flexible, barbed whip that is uncoiled and discharged when touched (Figure 15-55).

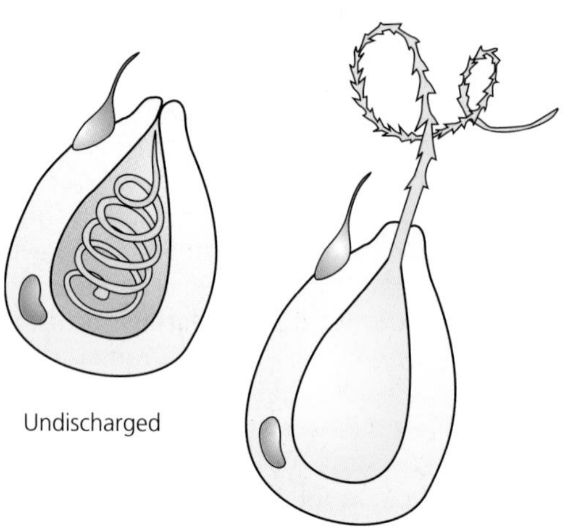

Figure 15-55 Nematocyst capsules.

Cnidarians are either fixed to the reef or free-swimming. Most are tiny individual animals that group together by the thousands to form fixed colonies, such as the corals and hydroids that make up most of a coral reef's structure. Jellyfish and anemones live as individuals. All of these animals have tentacles that contain nematocysts on their surfaces. The stings of most cnidarians are not harmful, but a few are quite toxic.

SAFE SEA AND OTHER CREAM FORMULATIONS

Safe Sea sting lotion protects against most common marine stingers including jellyfish, sea lice, fire coral, and sea nettle. Safe Sea has a waterproof, slippery texture that makes it difficult for the stinging tentacles to attach to the skin. It absorbs secretions from the skin that would tell the jellyfish that it is in contact with prey or predator. Chemicals in Safe Sea block the chemical pathways where the stinging process is activated. Safe Sea reduces the pressure in stinging cells so that they cannot fire, effectively disarming them. Higher (1%) niclosamide cream formulations are very effective. These must be compounded by the pharmacist.

VINEGAR

It is advisable to bring a plastic bottle of vinegar to the beach, because rubbing the affected area or washing with freshwater can cause nematocysts to discharge. Saturating the area with vinegar immobilizes unspent nematocysts.

SEABATHER'S ERUPTION

Seabather's eruption occurs under bathing suits and is predominant in Mexico (Cancun and Cozumel), Bermuda, Florida, the Gulf states, and as far north as Long Island, New York. Larvae of members of the phylum Cnidaria (formerly Coelenterata), such as jellyfish and sea anemones, have been implicated. Outbreaks occur when jellyfish or anemone larvae are transported to shore by ocean currents. The sea thimble (*Linuche unguiculata*) is the jellyfish responsible for seabather's eruption in the Caribbean (Figure 15-56). Each sea thimble larva has more than 200 nematocysts—tiny organs that uncoil a threadlike, hollow stinger. When activated by skin contact, pressure, or contact with freshwater, the nematocysts are activated and toxin is forcefully injected into the swimmer's skin. Larvae are trapped under the bathing suit. Stinging is noted when the bather comes into shallow water or leaves the water. Prolonged wearing of a contaminated suit, strenuous exercise, and exposure to showers or freshwater pools activate nematocysts and make the symptoms much worse. Red, itchy papules or wheals resembling insect bites occur minutes to several hours later. The papules may coalesce to cover wide areas (Figure 15-57). The rash lasts for 3 to 7 days; severe cases last 6 weeks. Headache, chills, and fever are present in extensive cases. The rash may recur if a suit contaminated with nematocysts is reworn.

When the seasonal risk of seabather's eruption is present, children, people with a history of seabather's eruption, and surfers are at greatest risk. Many patients with seabather's eruption have specific IgG antibodies against thimble jellyfish antigen. The extent of the cutaneous eruption or sting severity correlates with antibody titer. This may explain why patients with a history of seabather's eruption are at greatest risk. Length of time spent in the water is not significantly associated with seabather's eruption.

Treatment is symptomatic, with cooling lotions (e.g., Sarna), antihistamines, topical steroids, and, in severe cases, prednisone. During the sea lice season, seabathers can minimize their risk by showering with their bathing suits off after seabathing.

Florida, Caribbean, Bahamas

Seabather's eruption (sea itch) is the most common marine-related problem in the waters south of the United States. Swimmers and divers are affected by the nematocyst-bearing tiny larvae of the sea thimble (jellyfish). Itchy papules occur under or at the edge of bathing suits and wet suits. The eruption used to be seasonal but is now reported year-round. Areas with a high concentration of larvae change with the wind and tides.

Most sea animals are defensive. Divers who do not touch the fragile reef or handle fish are safe. Some of the sponges, corals, and anemones are toxic. Injuries to the feet caused by sea urchin spines are now uncommon because divers wear protective foot gear. Shuffling the feet in the water, rather than walking as on land, alarms stingrays buried in the sand. Stingrays are not aggressive, but stepping on a submerged

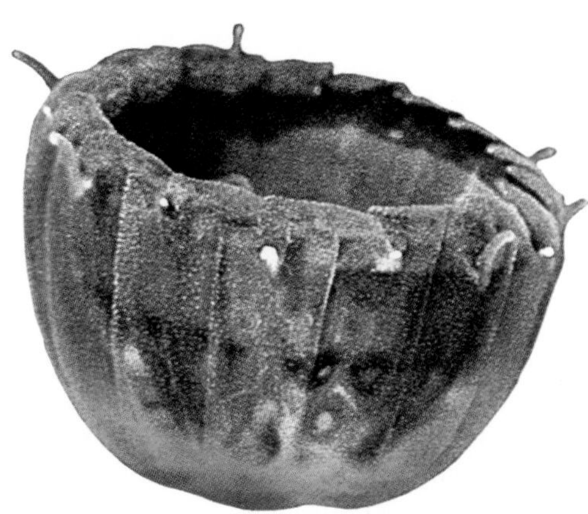

Figure 15-56 Sea thimble. The larva of this tiny jellyfish (½ to ¾ inch) is responsible for most cases of seabather's eruption in the Caribbean. (Courtesy Reid E. McNeal, Grand Cayman, BWI.)

Figure 15-57 Seabather's eruption. A common problem in the Caribbean. Nematocyst-bearing larvae may be trapped under the bathing suit and produce an intensely itching and painful papular eruption.

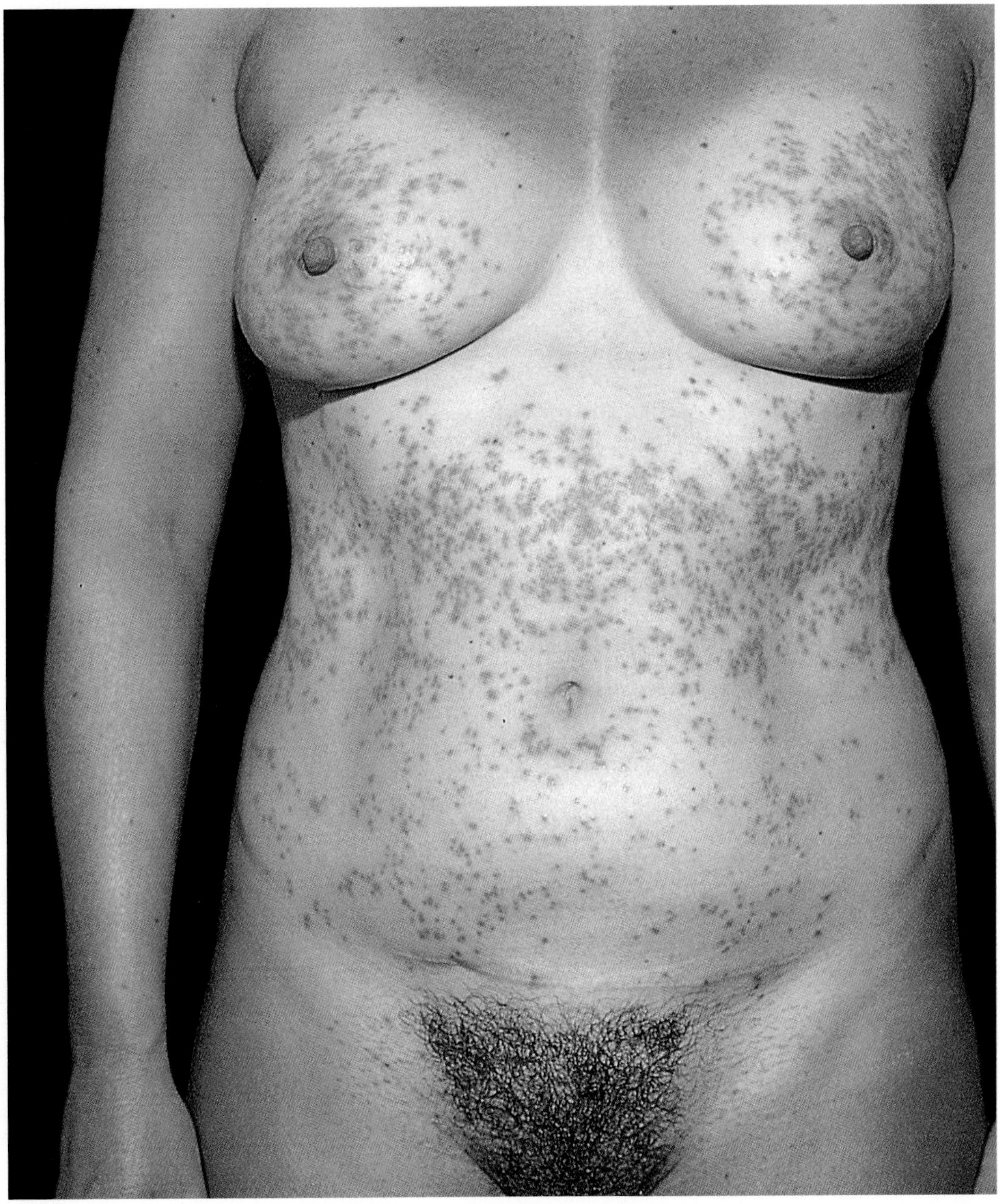

ray's back can result in a deep, gaping wound. The floating Portuguese man-of-war is seen in Florida but is not common in the Caribbean. Becoming wrapped in its tentacles can result in severe swelling and blistering of an entire extremity. Box jellyfish (sea wasps) have a 2- to 3-inch cuboidal dome with 3-inch tentacles. These small creatures are occasionally seen in shallow water at night and are attracted to light. They are one of the most toxic animals on earth and can produce severe stings and shock. The erect dorsal spines of the odd-shaped, bottom-dwelling spotted scorpion fish are covered with a toxin that can penetrate rubber and skin.

JELLYFISH AND PORTUGUESE MAN-OF-WAR

There are two groups of stinging jellyfish found in the coastal waters of North America: the Portuguese man-of-war and the sea nettle (Figure 15-58). The dreaded Portuguese man-of-war has a large, purple air float up to 12 cm long that rides high out of the water and is carried by the wind across the ocean. Tentacles, with their attached stinging structure, the nematocysts, trail out several feet into the water. Red or white jellyfishes seen floating in large groups or washed up on the beaches of the Atlantic coast are called sea nettles. They also have nematocyst-bearing tentacles, which measure up to 4 feet in length. Nematocysts are also found on the inferior surface of the body of the jellyfish. The Southeast Pacific box jellyfish contains the most potent marine venom known.

THE STING. When a small organism or a human brushes against an outstretched tentacle, the object is stung. Each tentacle has numerous rings of projecting stinging cells, and each cell contains a shiny oval body, the nematocyst. A tiny projecting trigger is on the outer surface of each nematocyst. On tactile stimulation, the nematocyst fires a threadlike whip with a hollow poisonous tip and recurved hooks on a nodelike swelling at the base. The hooks hold the prey while the poisonous contents of the nematocyst are discharged through the thread into the body. The force of discharge is great enough to penetrate the upper dermis, where the venom diffuses to enter the circulation.

Stings produce immediate burning, numbness, and paresthesias. Linear papules or wheals occur where a tentacle has brushed against the skin (Figure 15-59). Lesions either fade in hours or blister and become necrotic. Systemic toxic reactions (e.g., nausea, vomiting, headache, muscle spasms, weakness, ataxia, dizziness, low-grade fever) occur with severe or widespread stings. Movement of the envenomated part, such as a limb, leads to increased mobilization of the venom from the inoculation site. Fatalities may occur. It has been estimated that at least 50 feet of box jellyfish tentacles must touch the skin of an adult to deliver a fatal dose. Anaphylactic reactions may occur in victims who are allergic to jellyfish venom.

Recurrent linear eruptions after a sole primary envenomation have been reported. Most patients have only one recurrence, which takes place 5 to 30 days later, but some have multiple recurrences. In multiple recurrences, the duration of succeeding episodes becomes shorter, and the symptom-free intervals lengthen with successive recurrences. The recurrent eruption may be more severe. An immunologic reaction to intracutaneous sequestered antigen may explain this phenomenon.

TREATMENT. The envenomated part is immobilized to prevent mobilization of the venom. It is important to remove or inactivate the nematocysts as rapidly as possible. As long as the tentacles remain in contact with the skin, the nematocysts continue to discharge venom. If washed with freshwater or towel dried, unfired nematocysts on tentacles are activated. Tentacles and toxin are washed off by gently pouring seawater over the affected area. Remaining nematocysts and toxin on the skin are inactivated with alcohol (rubbing alcohol or liquor) or hot seawater. Any remaining tentacles are gently lifted off with a gloved hand. Remaining structures are removed after covering the area with a paste made of baking soda, flour, or talcum and seawater; this paste coalesces the tentacles. The dried paste is scraped off with a knife. Nematocysts of the Portuguese man-of-

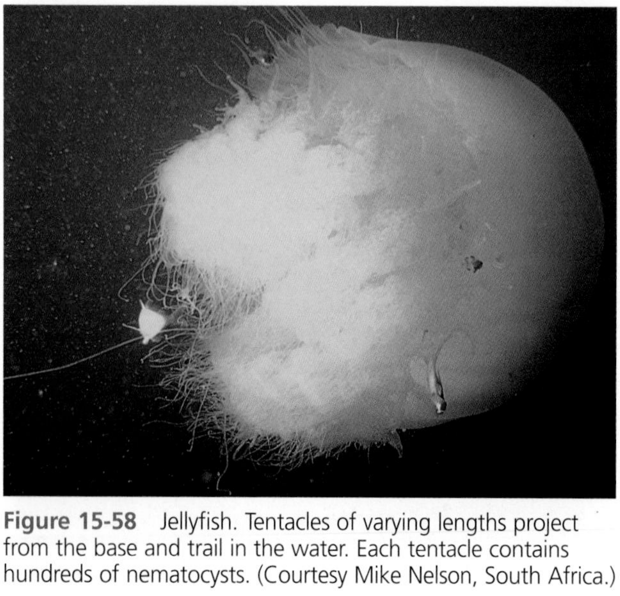

Figure 15-58 Jellyfish. Tentacles of varying lengths project from the base and trail in the water. Each tentacle contains hundreds of nematocysts. (Courtesy Mike Nelson, South Africa.)

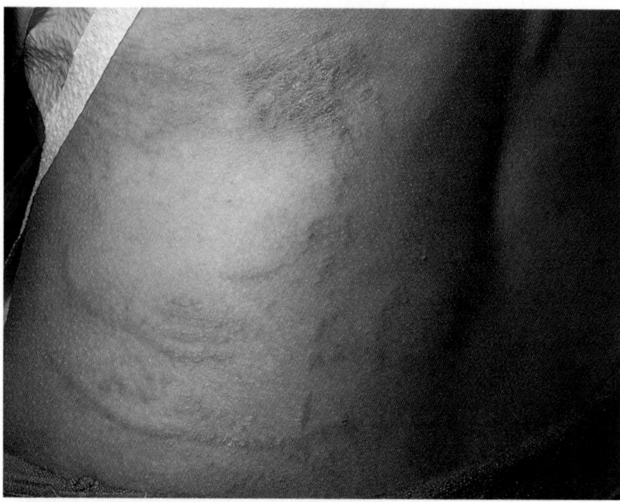

Figure 15-59 Portuguese man-of-war stings. Linear papules produced by nematocysts on tentacles that brushed against the skin.

war can also be deactivated with vinegar. A good general rule for treatment is as follows: for areas on the East Coast north of North Carolina, baking soda should be used; for all other coastal areas of the continental United States, vinegar should be used. Moist beach sand is applied to soothe the irritation. Cool compresses and topical steroid creams suppress inflammation.

CORAL, HYDROIDS, AND ANEMONES

CORAL. Coral is formed by limestone-secreting polyps that become fused, forming sharp, stonelike structures of various shapes and sizes. Coral is encountered in the Caribbean area, including Florida, Bermuda, the Bahamas, the West Indies, and in the Coral Sea extending from Australia to Hawaii and the Philippines. Like jellyfish, coral has nematocysts, but these are few and produce minor symptoms. The most important injuries are cuts (Figure 15-60). Itchy, red wheals ("coral poisoning") occur around the wound. Minor wounds are painful, are slow to heal, and often become infected. Retained bits of calcium may cause a delayed, foreign-body reaction. Wounds should be cleansed thoroughly to remove bits of debris and treated with hydrogen peroxide.

Echinoderms (sea urchins and starfish)

Sea urchins are attached to rocks on the ocean floor. They are encased in a spheric hard shell with numerous brittle, sharp, calcified spines projecting from their surface (Figure 15-61). Pedicellaria are triple-jawed, pincerlike structures that are intermingled with the spines of some tropical species. Stepping or falling on the urchin results in penetrating wounds from spines or pedicellaria. The spines may break off and become imbedded in the wound. The spines or pedicellaria are venomous in some species (e.g., *Toxopneustes pileolus*). Venom-bearing spines are long, slender, and sharp, and are covered with a thin skin. Certain starfish produce wounds similar to those of sea urchins. Glandular tissue located beneath the skin produces slime that is released when the epidermal sheath is torn.

Reactions are immediate and delayed. Contact with spines produces an immediate burning sensation with redness and edema that may persist for hours. Wounds from venomous urchins cause immediate, excruciating pain and severe muscle aching. The wound area may be violet-black because of pigments located in the spines. Venomous species may cause the rapid onset of systemic symptoms such as paresthesias, muscular cramps and paralysis, hypotension, nausea, syncope, ataxia, and respiratory distress. Spines that enter joints may induce severe synovitis. Penetration over a metacarpal bone can cause a severe fusiform, reactive, distal swelling of the finger. Retained spines, if not spontaneously discharged or easily removed, may be dissolved with ammonia. An old native treatment is to pour hot wax on the skin and allow it to cool. The wax is then peeled off with the spines in it. Deep spines may have to be surgically excised. Radiographic examination is important before surgical exploration. Delayed reactions are most commonly foreign-body granulomatous nodules that occur weeks or months later. They are less than 5 mm in diameter and are pink to purple. These may represent a hypersensitivity reaction. They respond to intralesional injections of triamcinolone acetonide (10 mg/ml) and to the surgical removal of spines. Chemicals present on the sea urchin's spines are apparently responsible for a delayed reaction that occurs in some individuals; this reaction consists of induration around the fingers and toes. It lasts for weeks, may cause joint deformity, and responds to systemic antibiotics and corticosteroids.

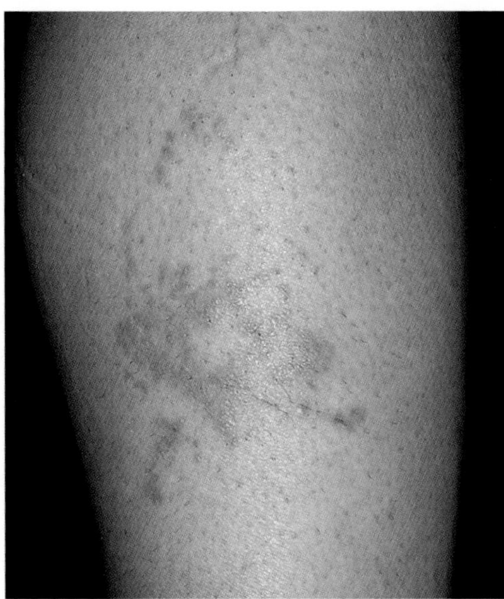

Figure 15-60 Coral poisoning. Calcareous material and protein may be forced into the skin after scraping against coral. Reaction to this foreign material may be intense and long-lasting. Wounds become red and tender and may ulcerate. Linear streaks are characteristic.

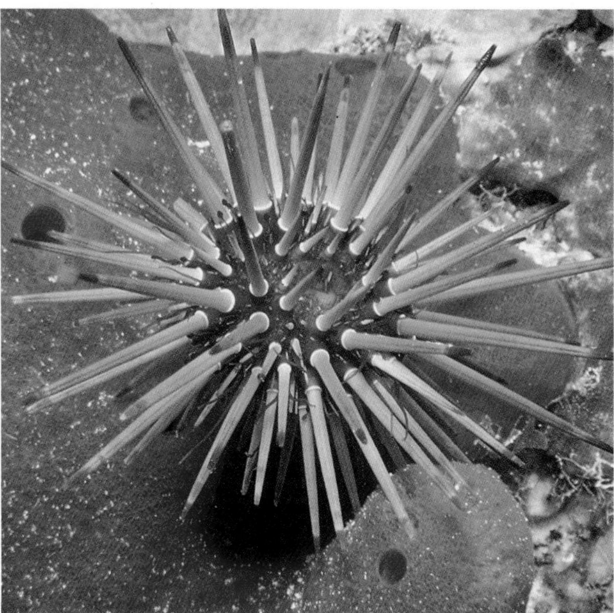

Figure 15-61 Reef urchin; body 1½ to 2 inches, spines 1 to 1½ inches. Pointed spines can cause puncture wounds. The spines crumble and remain lodged in the wound. (Courtesy Steven F. Bennett, Grand Cayman, BWI.)

LEISHMANIASIS

Leishmaniasis is a protozoan disease caused by any of several species of *Leishmania* parasites. It is transmitted to humans and other mammals by the 2- to 3-mm blood-sucking phlebotomine sandfly. A spectrum of clinical presentations exists ranging from small nodules to mucosal tissue destruction. Parasite, host, and other factors affect whether the infection becomes symptomatic and whether cutaneous or visceral leishmaniasis results. It is endemic in the tropics. The diagnosis is made clinically and may be confirmed with smears and biopsy. Cutaneous leishmaniasis may be treated with pentavalent antimonials and other drugs. Immunity to a specific species is acquired after infection.

CAUSAL AGENT

Leishmaniasis is transmitted by sandflies (Figure 15-62) and caused by obligate intracellular protozoa of the genus *Leishmania*. Human infection is caused by about 21 of 30 species. The different species are morphologically indistinguishable, but they can be differentiated by isoenzyme analysis, molecular methods, or monoclonal antibodies. *Leishmania donovani* migrates to the liver and spleen, causing visceral leishmaniasis, which is fatal. *Leishmania brasiliensis* spreads to the lining of the nose and throat, causing the destructive mucocutaneous disease. *Leishmania major* remains in the skin, causing skin ulcers (cutaneous leishmaniasis).

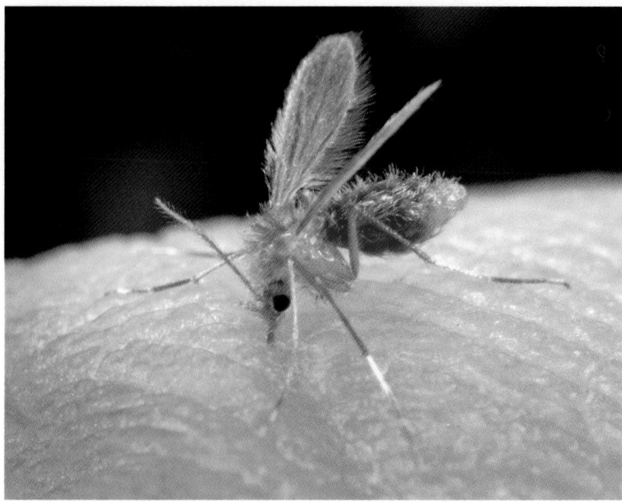

Figure 15-62 Sandflies transmit the disease while taking a blood meal. They do not make noise when they fly. They are one third the size of a mosquito. Sandflies are most active from dusk to dawn.

When biting their hosts, the infected blood-sucking *Phlebotomus* sandflies regurgitate *Leishmania* promastigotes (flagellated form of the parasite) into the skin, which are phagocytosed by macrophages. Promastigotes fuse to lysosomes to form the phagolysosome. Within the phagolysosomes of macrophages, promastigotes evolve into the obligatory tissue-stage intracellular form of the parasite, the amastigote. Amastigotes replicate and may then infect additional macrophages, either locally or in distant tissues after dissemination. When blood-feeding on an infected

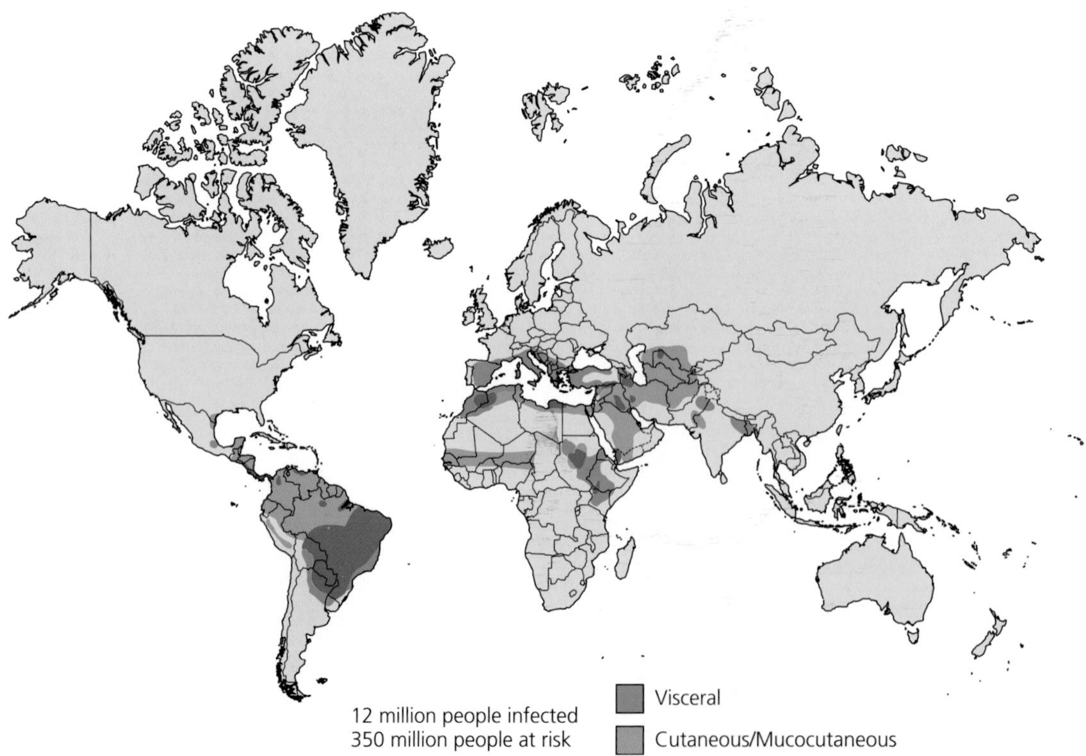

Figure 15-63 Distribution of Old World and New World cutaneous leishmaniasis.

host, sandflies ingest infected macrophages and become infected with amastigotes, which transform back into promastigotes in the sandfly's gut (depending on *Leishmania* spp., different regions of the gut will be parasitized). The parasites then migrate to the sandfly's proboscis, thus completing the *Leishmania* life cycle.

Leishmaniasis is found in about 88 countries (Figure 15-63). Most of the affected countries are in the tropics and subtropics. Cutaneous leishmaniasis is endemic in more than 70 countries, and 90% of cases occur in Saudi Arabia, Syria, Afghanistan, Algeria, Pakistan, Brazil, and Peru. Old World cutaneous leishmaniasis (i.e., Africa, Europe, and Asia) usually occurs in open semiarid or desert conditions; New World cutaneous leishmaniasis (i.e., the Americas) is associated with forests. More than 90% of the world's cases of visceral leishmaniasis are in India, Bangladesh, Nepal, Sudan, and Brazil.

CLINICAL FEATURES

There are two forms of leishmaniasis disease: cutaneous leishmaniasis and visceral leishmaniasis (kala-azar). The form of disease is determined by species, geographic distribution, and immune response. Cutaneous disease presents with one or more lesions at the bite sites. Lesions can change in size and appearance over time. They often look like a volcano, with raised edges and a central crater with or without a crust. Lesions are often painless. Regional adenopathy may occur.

Persons who have visceral leishmaniasis usually have fever, weight loss, and an enlarged spleen and liver (usually the spleen is bigger than the liver). Some patients have generalized adenopathy. Low red blood cell count, low white blood cell count, and low platelet count occur. Some patients develop post–kala-azar dermal leishmaniasis. Visceral leishmaniasis is becoming an important opportunistic infection in areas where it coexists with HIV.

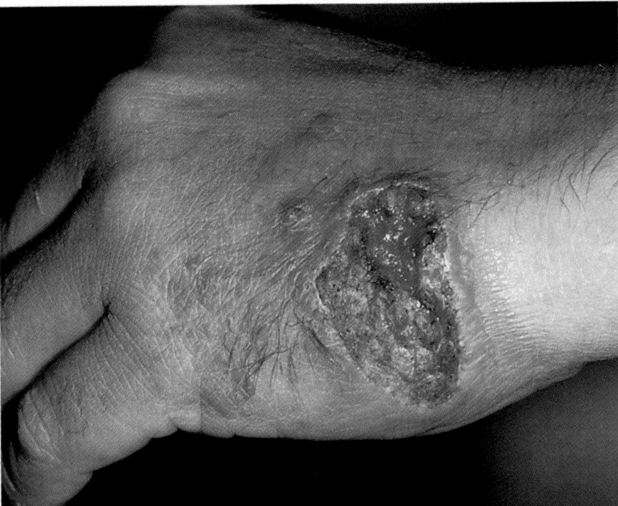

Figure 15-64 Cutaneous leishmaniasis. A red papule eventually ulcerates and forms raised edges with surrounding dusky red skin.

Cutaneous disease (Oriental sore)

Lesions appear on exposed skin surfaces, especially on the extremities and face. Old World cutaneous leishmaniasis is caused by *L. major, L. tropica, L. aethiopica, L. infantum,* and *L. chagasi*. New World cutaneous leishmaniasis is caused by *L. mexicana, L. amazonensis, L. brasiliensis, L. panamensis, L. peruviana,* and *L. guyanensis*. There is a broad spectrum of presentations. The incubation period is variable. Lesions typically appear several weeks after a fly bite but lesions may appear days or months later. A painless papule forms at the bite site, enlarges to a nodule, crusts in the center, and ulcerates over 1 to 3 months. The ulcer has raised edges and the surrounding skin is dusky red (Figure 15-64). Flat plaques or hyperkeratotic or wartlike lesions also develop in Old World disease. Ulcers are either moist with exudate, "wet ulcer," or dry with crust, "dry ulcer." One, two, or sometimes several nonhealing skin lesions may occur. Multiple lesions are more often seen in Old World disease. Ulcerative lesions are most common in New World cutaneous leishmaniasis. Secondary infection may complicate the picture. Regional adenopathy may develop. Disseminated lesions and localized lymphadenopathy preceding skin ulcers occur in Brazil. Lesions heal with depigmented scars.

DIFFUSE CUTANEOUS DISEASE

In diffuse cutaneous leishmaniasis, seen rarely in Ethiopia and Latin America, parasite-laden nodules are widespread and do not ulcerate (Figure 15-65).

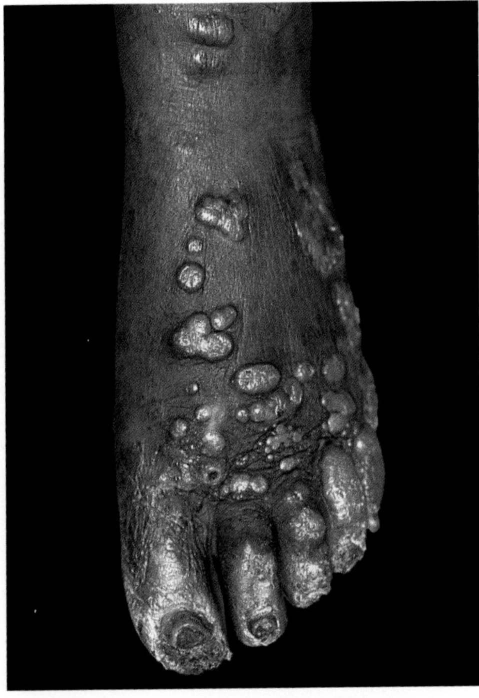

Figure 15-65 Diffuse cutaneous leishmaniasis.

LEISHMANIASIS RECIDIVANS (CHRONIC RELAPSING CUTANEOUS LEISHMANIASIS)

This relapsing form of the disease is usually caused by *Leishmania tropica*. It generally occurs within 2 years after the initial infection. A common presentation is recurrent disease on the face in children. New papules and ulcers form over the edge of an old scar and may spread inward to form a psoriasiform lesion. Infection may be from reactivation of dormant parasites or new infection from a different species. It is difficult to treat.

MUCOCUTANEOUS LEISHMANIASIS (ESPUNDIA)

Mucocutaneous leishmaniasis is caused by *L. brasiliensis* in the Americas. *L. aethiopica* has been reported to cause this disease in the Old World. Mucosal dissemination occurs in 1% to 10% of infections, developing 1 to 5 years after cutaneous leishmaniasis lesions have healed, but sometimes coincident with active skin lesions. About 90% of patients have a preceding cutaneous scar. As many as 30% of patients report no prior evidence of leishmaniasis. Mucosal disease begins with erythema and ulcerations at the nares and progresses to nasal septum perforation with mutilation of the nose, mouth, oropharynx, and trachea (Figure 15-66). Mucosal disease is rarely seen outside of Latin America.

Visceral infection (kala-azar)

Visceral leishmaniasis is caused by *L. donovani* in India and Kenya, *L. infantum* in South Europe and North Africa, and *L. chagasi* in the Americas. Clinical expression varies from no signs or symptoms to fully established (kala-azar). Visceral leishmaniasis may also represent relapse. Reactivation is often provoked by an insult to T cell (CD4) number or function, such as from corticosteroid or cytotoxic therapy, anti-rejection treatment in transplant recipients, or advanced HIV disease. *PMID: 16257344* Fever, weakness, night sweats, anorexia, and weight loss are common and progress over weeks to months. Children can develop diarrhea and growth retardation. Hepatomegaly and splenomegaly are typical. Darkening of the skin (kala-azar means black fever in Hindi) is infrequent. Anemia, leukopenia or thrombocytopenia, and hypergammaglobulinemia are characteristic. Untreated disease results in profound cachexia, bleeding from thrombocytopenia, susceptibility to secondary infections, and death.

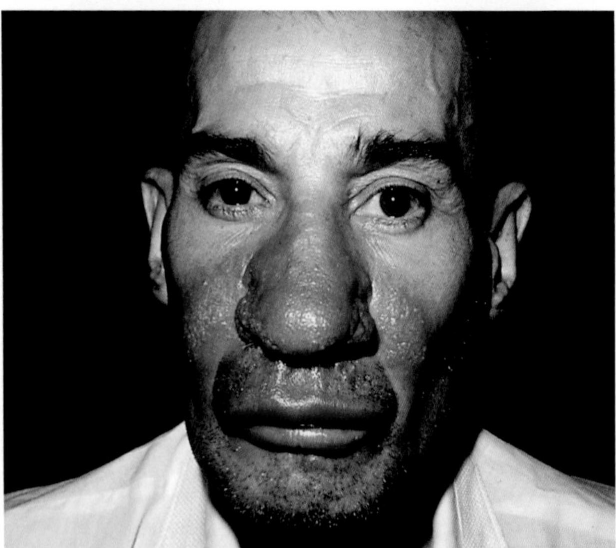

Figure 15-66 Mucocutaneous leishmaniasis.

LABORATORY

Touch preparations and aspirations are stained with Giemsa. Examination of Giemsa-stained slides of tissue is the most commonly used diagnostic technique. Punch and wedge biopsies from the raised edge of a lesion are sent for hematoxylin and eosin staining. Direct visualization of amastigotes with their red, rodlike cytoplasmic kinetoplast is diagnostic.

Isolation of the organism in culture (using, for example, the diphasic NNN medium) is another method of parasitologic confirmation.

Polymerase chain reaction (PCR) techniques provide rapid diagnosis of *Leishmania* species. The test is becoming more widely available.

TREATMENT

Consult the Centers for Disease Control and Prevention (CDC) to obtain information on how to treat leishmaniasis. The drug pentavalent antimony (sodium stibogluconate) is available from the CDC Drug Service. This drug is toxic and is administered intravenously or intramuscularly for 20 to 28 days. Amphotericin B or liposomal amphotericin B and other drugs are alternatives. *PMID: 17448941* Treatment varies depending on region, form and severity of disease, and species of parasite.

Cutaneous disease heals by reepithelialization with scarring. Most Old World lesions self-heal within 2 to 4 months (*L. major*) or 6 to 15 months (*L. tropica*). In New World cutaneous leishmaniasis, self-healing after 3 months is rapid in *L. mexicana* (>75%), but slow in *L. braziliensis* (about 10%) and *L. panamensis* infections (about 35%). *L. mexicana* infection never affects the mucosa. *L. braziliensis* can progress to mucocutaneous disease and is treated.

Cutaneous leishmaniasis is treated to accelerate cure, to reduce scarring, and to attempt to prevent dissemination (e.g., mucosal disease) or relapse. Treatment is given for persistent lesions (6 months), for lesions that are located over joints, or for multiple (5 to 10 or more) or large (4 to 5 cm in diameter) lesions.

Chapter | 16 |

Vesicular and Bullous Diseases

CHAPTER CONTENTS

BLISTERS

Vesicles and bullae are the primary lesions in many diseases. Some are of short duration and are quite characteristic, such as those in poison ivy and herpes zoster. In other diseases, such as erythema multiforme and lichen planus, a blister may or may not occur during the course of the disease. Finally, there is a group of disorders in which bullae are present almost continuously during the period of active disease. These autoimmune blistering diseases tend to be chronic, and many are associated with tissue-bound or circulating antibodies. This chapter deals with those disorders.

Autoimmune blistering diseases

Autoimmune blistering diseases cause impaired adhesion of the epidermis to the epidermal basement membrane (e.g., the pemphigoid group of disorders [bullous, gestational, and mucous membrane]) or impaired adhesion of epidermal cells to each other (e.g., the pemphigus group of disorders). The autoantibodies target structural proteins that promote cell matrix (e.g., pemphigoid) or cell-to-cell (e.g., pemphigus) adhesion in skin. Autoimmune blistering diseases are characterized by substantial morbidity (pruritus, pain, disfigurement), and in some instances, mortality (secondary to loss of epidermal barrier function). Bullous pemphigoid is the most common autoimmune blistering disease. Treatment with systemic immunosuppressives has reduced morbidity and mortality in patients with these diseases.

Major blistering diseases

An overview of the major bullous diseases is presented in Figure 16-1. The differential diagnosis of all blistering diseases and the anatomy of the epidermis and epidermal basement membrane are shown in Figure 16-2.

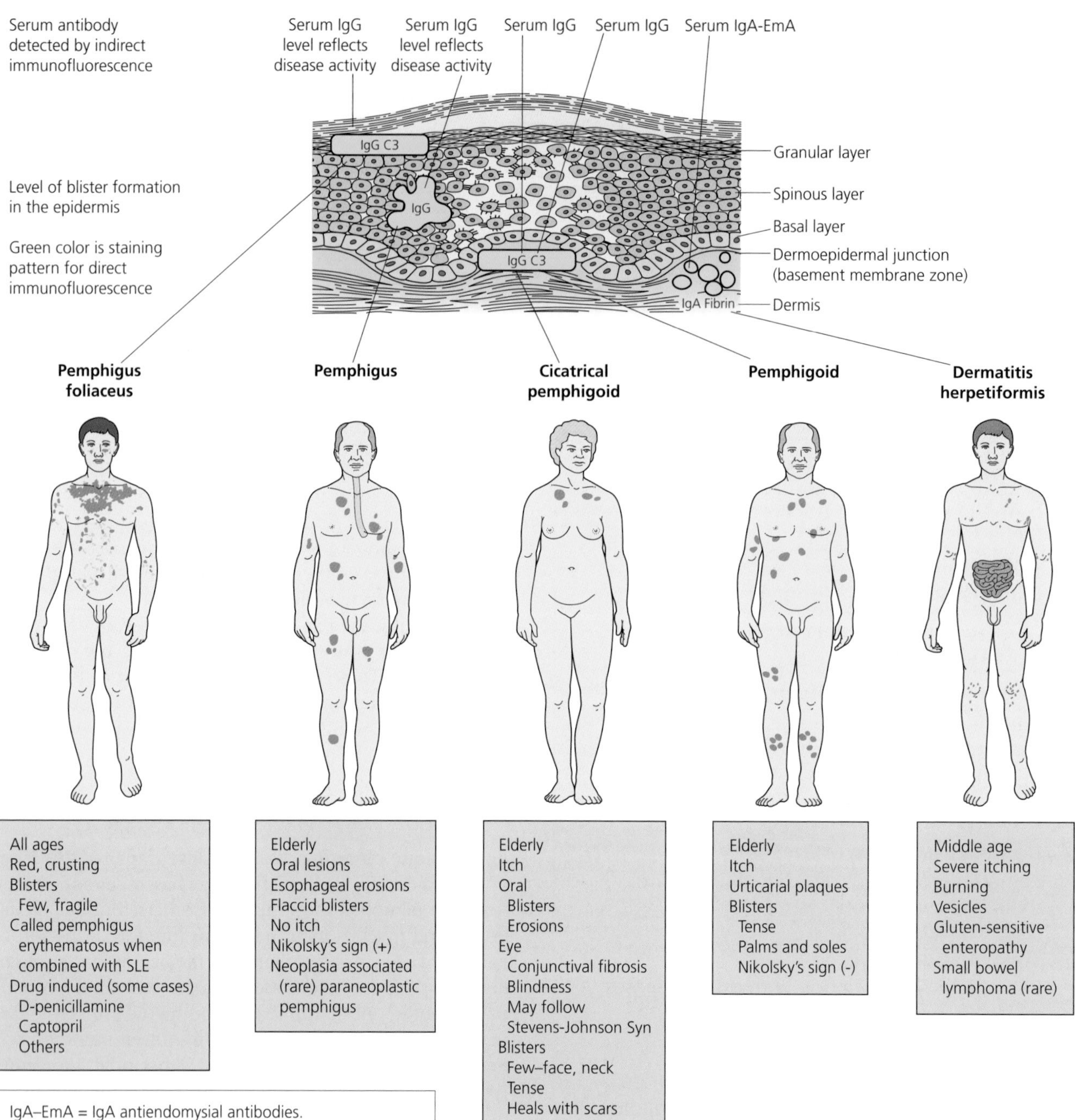

Pemphigus foliaceus	Pemphigus	Cicatrical pemphigoid	Pemphigoid	Dermatitis herpetiformis
All ages Red, crusting Blisters Few, fragile Called pemphigus erythematosus when combined with SLE Drug induced (some cases) D-penicillamine Captopril Others	Elderly Oral lesions Esophageal erosions Flaccid blisters No itch Nikolsky's sign (+) Neoplasia associated (rare) paraneoplastic pemphigus	Elderly Itch Oral Blisters Erosions Eye Conjunctival fibrosis Blindness May follow Stevens-Johnson Syn Blisters Few–face, neck Tense Heals with scars	Elderly Itch Urticarial plaques Blisters Tense Palms and soles Nikolsky's sign (-)	Middle age Severe itching Burning Vesicles Gluten-sensitive enteropathy Small bowel lymphoma (rare)

IgA–EmA = IgA antiendomysial antibodies.
Serum antibody–detected by indirect immunofluorescence.

Figure 16-1

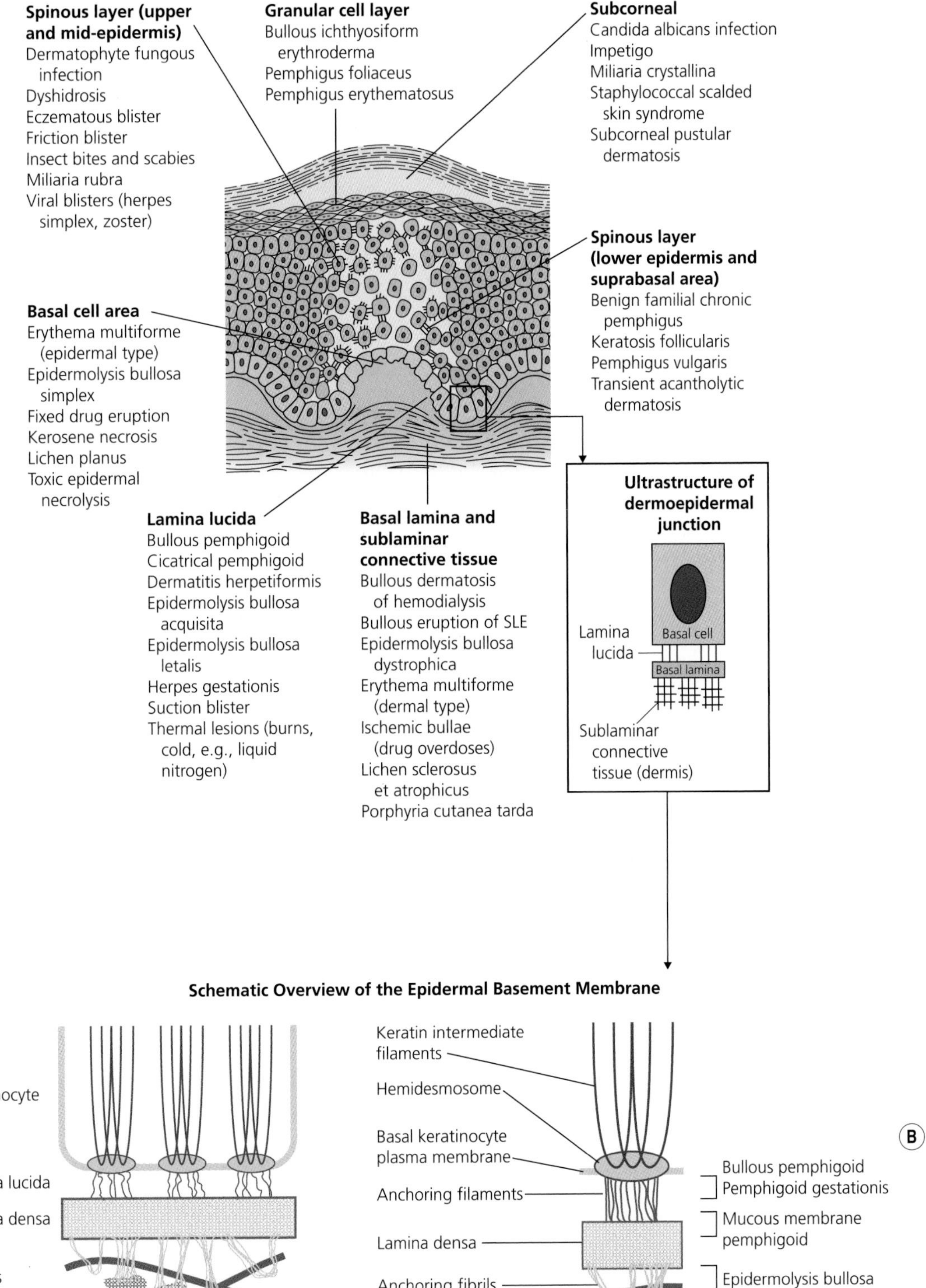

Figure 16-2 **A,** Electron microscopy studies of skin demonstrate that basal keratinocytes overlie the lamina lucida, which is in turn positioned just above the lamina densa (i.e., the basement membrane proper) and superficial dermis. **B,** Ultrastructurally, hemidesmosome-anchoring filament-attachment complexes bind the cytoskeleton of basal keratinocytes to the underlying lamina densa, anchoring fibrils, and fibrillar elements (e.g., interstitial collagen and elastin fibers) within the superficial dermis. The dominant regions within epidermal basement membrane that are targeted by IgG autoantibodies in patients with pemphigoid diseases and epidermolysis bullosa acquisita are indicated by brackets. (Adapted from KB Yancey, CA Egan: *JAMA* 284[3], 350-356, 2000.)

Classification

A blister occurs when fluid accumulates at some level in the skin. The histologic classification of bullous disorders is based on the level in the skin at which that separation occurs (Figures 16-1 and 16-2). Subcorneal blisters are not commonly seen intact; the very thin roof has little structural integrity and collapses. Intraepidermal blisters have a thicker roof and are more substantial, whereas subepidermal blisters have great structural integrity and can remain intact even when firmly compressed.

EPIDERMIS

Desmosomes contribute to epidermal cell-cell adhesion. Desmosomal proteins (desmoglein 1, desmoglein 3) are the autoantigens of pemphigus foliaceus and pemphigus vulgaris (Table 16-1), respectively. Paraneoplastic pemphigus (PNP) is associated with autoantibodies to the desmosomal plaque protein desmoplakin. These diseases have intraepidermal blistering.

THE BASEMENT MEMBRANE ZONE (see Figure 16-2)

The hemidesmosome is a membrane-associated protein complex that extends from the intracellular area of basal keratinocytes to the extracellular area. It links the cytoskeleton of the basal keratinocyte to the dermis. Hemidesmosomes are associated with anchoring filaments, threadlike structures traversing the lamina lucida. Anchoring fibrils, which consist of type VII collagen, extend from the lower portion of the lamina densa to anchoring plaques within the papillary dermis.

BASEMENT MEMBRANE ANTIGENS AND DISEASES. Different components of the basement membrane contain the autoantigens of several autoimmune bullous diseases (Table 16-2). Diseases of hemidesmosomes show subepidermal blisters and, by direct immunofluorescence, linear deposits of IgG, C3, or IgA at the dermoepidermal junction. Bullous pemphigoid (BP) is a disease of hemidesmosomes. Two proteins, BP180 and BP230, are the targets of autoantibodies in BP. BP180 is the target of autoantibodies in herpes gestationis, cicatricial pemphigoid, and linear IgA disease. Laminin 5 is an anchoring filament-lamina densa component of hemidesmosomes. Autoantibodies to laminin 5 cause mucous membrane pemphigoid (cicatricial pemphigoid). Type VII collagen is the major structural component of anchoring fibrils. Type VII collagen is the autoantigen of epidermolysis bullosa acquisita.

Table 16-1 Molecular Classification of Pemphigus

Pemphigus type	Target desmosomal protein
Pemphigus vulgaris	Desmoglein 3 (and desmoglein 1)
Pemphigus foliaceus	Desmoglein 1
Paraneoplastic pemphigus	Desmoglein 3, desmoplakin 1, desmoplakin 2, BP230, envoplakin, periplakin, others
IgA pemphigus	Desmocollin 1

From Mutasim DF et al: *J Am Acad Dermatol* 45:803, 2001. *PMID: 11712024*

DIAGNOSIS OF BULLOUS DISORDERS

The diagnosis of many chronic bullous disorders can often be made clinically. These diseases have such important implications that the diagnosis should be confirmed by histology and, in many instances, immunofluorescence (see Tables 16-3, 16-4, and Figure 16-3).

BIOPSY

For light microscopy. A biopsy specimen must be taken from the proper area to demonstrate the level of blister formation and the nature of the inflammatory infiltrate (see Figure 16-2 and Table 16-3). Small, early vesicles or inflamed skin provides the most diagnostic features. Ruptured or excoriated lesions are of little value and should not be sampled. A small portion of the intact skin should be included in the biopsy specimen. Punch biopsies done through the center of a large blister are of little value.

For immunofluorescence. In most cases, the first biopsy specimen should be taken from the edge of a fresh lesion. A second biopsy is often desirable to establish the diagnosis. One should sample skin near the lesion, preferably from a nonedematous, normal, or red area. The best site for obtaining a biopsy specimen is shown in Table 16-4 and Figure 16-3.

Table 16-2 Molecular Classification of Subepidermal Bullous Diseases

Bullous disease	Targeted molecule
Bullous pemphigoid (BP)	BP180, BP230 (hemidesmosome and lamina lucida)
Herpes gestationis	BP180, BP230 (hemidesmosome and lamina lucida)
Cicatricial pemphigoid	BP180, laminin V (hemidesmosome and lamina lucida)
Epidermolysis bullosa acquisita	Type VII collagen (anchoring fibrils)
Bullous SLE	Type VII collagen (anchoring fibrils)
Linear IgA disease (adults and children)	LAD antigen (BP180) (hemidesmosome and lamina lucida)
Dermatitis herpetiformis	Unknown

From Mutasim DF et al: *J Am Acad Dermatol* 45:803, 2001. *PMID: 11712024*

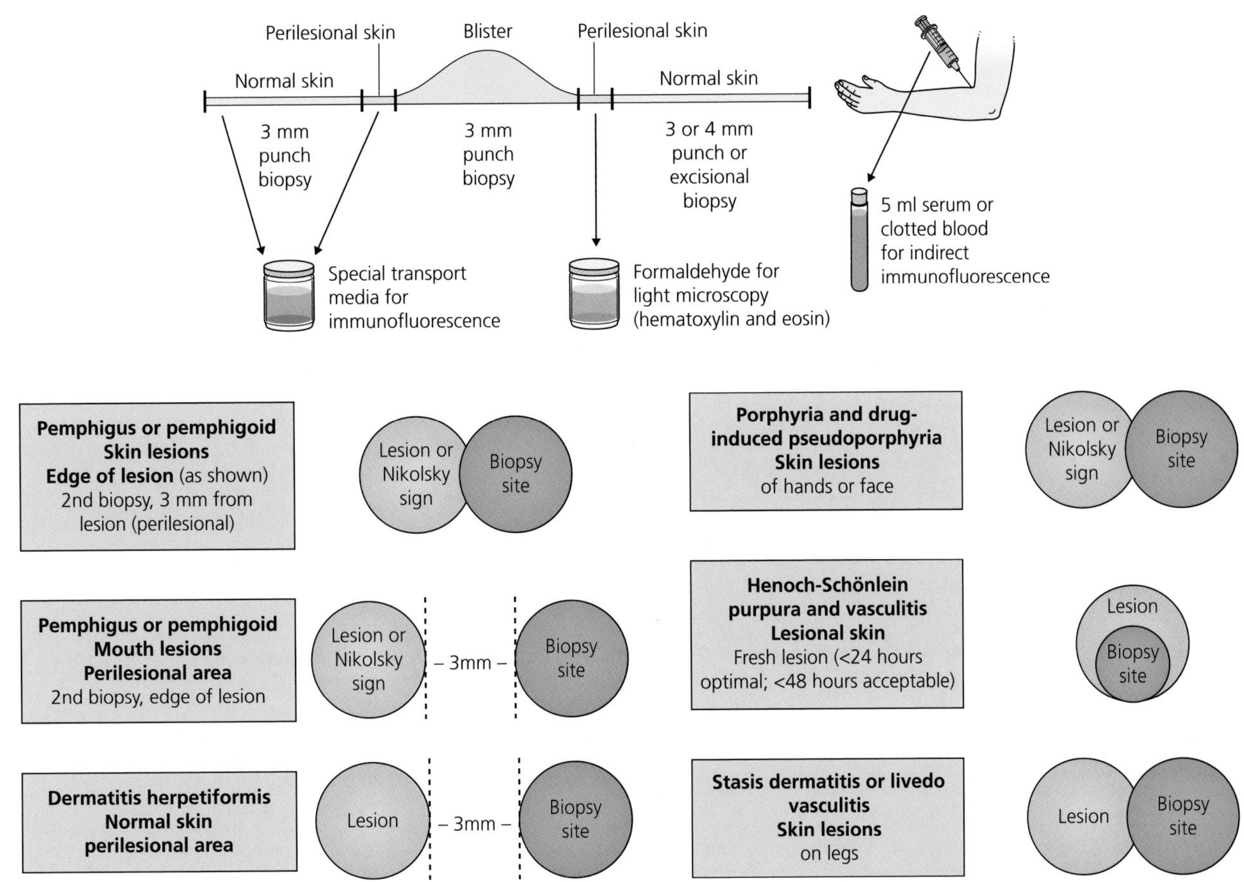

Figure 16-3 Collecting biopsy specimens for direct immunofluorescence. (Beutner Laboratories, Buffalo, NY.)

Table 16-3 Diagnosis of Autoimmune Bullous Diseases

Histopathology	Direct immunofluorescence	Indirect immunofluorescence	Diagnosis
Suprabasal	1. IgG ± C3 at ICS 2. IgG ± C3 at ICS + BMZ	IgG at ICS, monkey esophagus IgG at ICS, rat bladder	Pemphigus vulgaris > paraneoplastic pemphigus
Subcorneal	1. IgA at ICS 2. IgG ± C3 at ICS 3. IgG ± C3 at ICS, Ig ± C3 at BMZ	IgA at ICS IgA at ICS IgG at ICS ± ANA	IgA pemphigus Pemphigus foliaceus Pemphigus erythematosus
Subepidermal noninflammatory	1. IgG, C3 ± IgM, IgA at BMZ 2. IgG, IgA ± IgM, C3 in blood vessel walls	1. Dermal side of SSS 2. Epidermal side of SSS negative	Epidermolysis bullosa acquisita Bullous pemphigoid Porphyria cutanea tarda, pseudo-PCT
Subepidermal with eosinophil-rich infiltrate	C3, IgG at BMZ	Epidermal side of SSS	Bullous pemphigoid Herpes gestationis Mucosal pemphigoid
Subepidermal with neutrophil-rich infiltrate	1. Granular IgA in dermal papillae and BMZ 2. Linear IgA ± C3, BMZ 3. IgG, IgM, C3, IgA, fibrinogen	Negative on epithelium (+ antiendomysial antibodies) IgA at BMZ 1. Dermal side of SSS 2. Dermal side of SSS and positive lupus serology	Dermatitis herpetiformis Linear IgA disease Epidermolysis bullosa acquisita, rare antiepiligrin disease Bullous systemic lupus erythematosus

From Mutasim DF et al: *J Am Acad Dermatol* 45:803, 2001. PMID: 11712024
BMZ, Basement membrane zone; *ICS,* intercellular space; *SSS,* salt split skin; ±, with or without; >, more likely than.

Table 16-4 Immunofluorescence Tests*

Disorder	Selection of biopsy site for direct immunofluorescence*	Biopsy findings: direct immunofluorescence	Serum findings: circulating antibody detected by indirect immunofluorescence
Bullous lupus erythematosus	Involved areas of skin such as erythematous or active borders	BMZ: linear/bandlike IgG and C3 (>90%); IgM and IgA also (50-60%); occasionally granular or fibrillar pattern	ANA Rarely BMZ (IgG) antibodies on split-skin substrate (dermal or combined pattern)
Bullous pemphigoid	Erythematous perilesional skin or mucosa	BMZ: linear IgG and C3; occasionally IgM and/or IgA	BMZ antibodies (IgG) in 75% of patients; application of BMZ-positive serum on split-skin substrate results in staining of epidermal side of separated skin in most cases of BP as compared with dermal side in EBA; dermal or combined pattern also seen rarely in bullous LE ELISA for BP180 autoantibodies
Chronic cutaneous (discoid) lupus erythematosus	Involved areas of skin such as erythematous or active borders	BMZ: granular IgM, IgG, C3 (involved skin >90%, uninvolved negative)	None (ANA rarely)
Cicatricial pemphigoid	Erythematous perilesional skin or mucosa	BMZ: linear IgG and C3; occasionally linear IgA; nonspecific linear fibrinogen	BMZ (IgG) antibodies in <25% of patients
Epidermolysis bullosa acquisita†	Erythematous perilesional skin or mucosa	BMZ: linear IgG, usually also C3; occasionally IgA and/or IgM	BMZ antibodies (IgG) in 25-50% of cases; may be distinguished from BP by dermal pattern on split-skin substrate
Dermatitis herpetiformis classic	Perilesional skin: normal-appearing skin, 0.5-1.0 cm away from lesion	Dermal papillae and/or BMZ: granular or fibrillar IgA; other Igs or C3 may be present	IgA class antiendomysial antibodies in 70% of patients with DH or celiac disease; increased incidence of positive results in patients with gluten-sensitive enteropathy who are not following gluten-free diet ELISA for IgA tissue transglutaminase autoantibodies
Drug reactions		Dermal vessels, cytoids: IgG and/or IgM, C3	None
Linear IgA bullous dermatosis	Perilesional skin	BMZ: linear IgA essential for diagnosis; linear C3 in some cases	BMZ antibodies (IgA) in 30% of patients
Henoch-Schönlein purpura	Lesions no older than 24-48 hr	Granular IgA in vessels	None
Herpes gestationis	Erythematous perilesional skin	BMZ: linear C3 (100%); IgG (10%); rarely IgA/IgM	HG IgG (HG factor) in most patients; BMZ (IgG) in 25% of cases

Modified from *Handbook of clinical relevance of tests,* IMMCO Diagnostics, Buffalo, NY, and Mayo Clinic Test Catalog.

AGA, antigliadin antibodies; *ARA,* antireticulin antibodies; *BMZ,* basement membrane zone; *C,* complement; *CS,* cell surface; *DH,* dermatitis herpetiformis; *EBA,* epidermolysis bullosa acquisita; *ELISA,* enzyme-linked immunosorbent assay; *EMA,* endomysial antibodies; *F,* fibrin or fibrinogen; *HG,* herpes gestationis; *IC,* intercellular area of stratum spinosum; *ICS,* intercellular substance; *Ig,* immunoglobulin; *Igs,* immunoglobulins; *LE,* lupus erythematosus; *SLE,* systemic *LE.*

*Immunofluorescence (IF) tests are performed on sera or tissues. The direct IF test is performed on skin or mucosal biopsy specimens. Specimens are examined for immunoglobulins (IgG, IgM, IgA), complement C3, and fibrinogen. The indirect IF test is performed on serum to detect circulating autoantibodies.

†To differentiate epidermolysis bullosa acquisita from bullous pemphigoid, further direct immunofluorescence studies on lesional biopsy specimens and on normal skin split at the lamina lucida by NaCl are required to demonstrate the location of immunoreactants, laminin, and type IV collagen.

Table 16-4 Immunofluorescence Tests*—cont'd

Disorder	Selection of biopsy site for direct immunofluorescence*	Biopsy findings: direct immunofluorescence	Serum findings: circulating antibody detected by indirect immunofluorescence
Pemphigus, all forms (e.g., vulgaris, foliaceus, paraneoplastic) except Hailey-Hailey disease	Erythematous perilesional skin	CS: IgG, C3; BMZ: granular to linear C3, characteristic of paraneoplastic	CS antibodies (IgG) CS antibodies bind to simple, columnar, and transitional epithelia; BMZ: antibodies may be present, characteristic of paraneoplastic ELISA for desmoglein 1 and 3 autoantibodies
Erythema multiforme	Edge of involved skin Lesions no older than 24-48 hr	Dermal vessels, cytoid bodies; IgM, C3; also IgG, rarely IgA	None
Leukocytoclastic vasculitis, urticarial vasculitis, rheumatoid	Lesions no older than 24-48 hr	Dermal vessels: IgG and/or IgM and/or IgA and/or C3 in early lesions	None
Lichen planus	Edge of involved skin; avoid old lesions or ulcers	Cytoid bodies: IgM characteristically; also IgG, C3, fibrinogen; BMZ: shaggy fibrinogen	None
Lichen planus pemphigoides	Erythematous perilesional skin or mucosa	Changes of lichen planus with linear IgG and/or C3	BMZ antibodies (IgG) in 50% (epidermal side of split-skin substrate)
Mixed connective tissue	Involved areas of skin such as erythematous or active borders For sclerodermoid features, biopsy inflamed area	Varies with clinical presentation; as in LE or vasculitis; ANA in epidermis	ANA
Other pemphigoid diseases (desquamative gingivitis, Brunsting-Perry pemphigoid, localized pemphigoid)	Erythematous perilesional skin or mucosa	BMZ: linear IgG, C3; sometimes IgA and/or IgM	BMZ antibodies (IgG) uncommonly present
Porphyria cutanea tarda and other forms of porphyria	Edge of involved skin, sun-exposed	Strong, homogeneous IgG in and around vessel walls, also immunofluorescent band at BMZ	None
Chronic bullous dermatosis of childhood	Erythematous perilesional skin	BMZ: linear IgA	BMZ antibodies (IgA) in 70% of cases
Subacute cutaneous lupus erythematosus	Involved areas of skin such as erythematous or active borders	Particulate intercellular substance IgG, IgM, IgA, C3, 1 or more conjugate 30%; BMZ: granular IgM or IgG (40% lesional, 10% normal)	ANA
Systemic lupus erythematosus	Involved areas of skin such as erythematous or active borders	BMZ: granular IgM and/or IgG, C3, sometimes IgA (>90% positive involved skin) (50% positive sun exposed, uninvolved) (30% positive unexposed, uninvolved)	ANA
Urticaria	Involved areas of skin such as erythematous or active borders	Patchy staining of connective tissue fibers in dermis with fibrinogen and variable number of eosinophils; dermal vessels (in cases of urticarial vasculitis) as noted below	None

LEVEL OF BLISTER FORMATION. For blisters occurring above the basement membrane zone, the level of blister formation can be determined easily with routine studies. Blisters occurring in the dermoepidermal junction (basement membrane zone) area (see Figure 16-1) were once considered subepidermal in location. With the electron microscope, it has been shown that blisters may occur at different levels in that complex area. Electron microscopy is not routinely used; adequate diagnostic information can be obtained from sections stained with hematoxylin and eosin and from immunofluorescence studies.

IMMUNOFLUORESCENCE. Immunofluorescence is a laboratory technique for demonstrating the presence of tissue-bound and circulating antibodies. Most chronic bullous disorders have specific antibodies that either are fixed to some component of skin or are circulating. Many laboratories around the country provide this testing service and supply transport media and mailing containers for tissue specimens. (Examples are Beutner Laboratories, Buffalo, NY, IMMCO Diagnostics, Buffalo, NY, and Mayo Medical Laboratories, Rochester, MN.) Freezing of specimens is no longer required.

Direct immunofluorescence (skin). Direct immunofluorescence is designed for demonstration of tissue-bound antibody and complement. Sectioned biopsy specimens are treated with fluorescein-conjugated antisera to human immunoglobulins (IgG, IgA, IgM, IgD, and IgE), C3, and fibrin; they are then examined with a microscope equipped with a special light source.

Indirect immunofluorescence (serum). Indirect immunofluorescence is used for demonstration of circulating antibodies directed against certain skin structures. Thin sections of animal squamous epithelium (e.g., monkey esophagus) are first incubated with the patient's serum. Skin-reacting antibodies in the serum attach to specific components of the animal epithelium. Fluorescein-labeled anti–human IgG antiserum is then added for specific identification of the circulating antibody. The circulating antibody responsible for the IgA deposition has not yet been identified, and indirect immunofluorescence is negative.

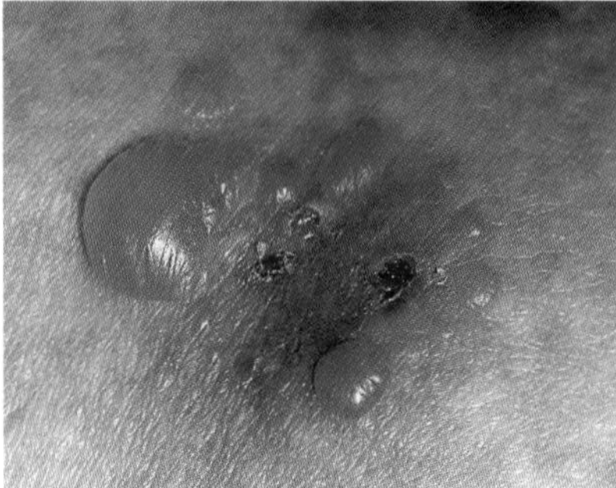

Figure 16-4 Dermatitis herpetiformis. Vesicles arise from an inflamed base and resemble a herpes simplex virus infection.

DERMATITIS HERPETIFORMIS AND LINEAR IgA BULLOUS DERMATOSIS

Dermatitis herpetiformis (DH) is a rare, chronic, intensely burning, pruritic vesicular skin disease associated in most instances with a subclinical gluten-sensitive enteropathy and IgA deposits in the upper dermis. The reported prevalence in northern Europe is 1.2 to 39.2 per 100,000 patients. The prevalence in patients in Utah in 1987 was 11.2 per 100,000. The average age of onset was 41.8 years, with patients having symptoms for an average of 1.6 years before diagnosis.

Dermatitis herpetiformis is rare in children. There is a strong association with specific human histocompatibility leukocyte antigens: HLA-B8 (60%), HLA class II antigens HLA-DR3 (95%), and HLA-DQw2 (100%).

Linear IgA bullous dermatosis has clinical features similar to those of dermatitis herpetiformis, but has a different histologic and immunofluorescence pattern and there is no associated small bowel disease. Drug-induced linear IgA bullous dermatosis is rare but increasing in frequency.

Sulfones produce a dramatic response within hours, but without drugs, some patients have chosen suicide as the only means of relief.

MAYO CLINIC EXPERIENCE

A series of 270 patients were seen at the Mayo Clinic in one study. The mean age at diagnosis was in the fifth decade. The familial incidence was 2.3%. The prevalence of celiac disease was 12.6% in the patients with DH; diagnosis of celiac disease was made either before the study or during follow-up. The true incidence would need to be determined by conducting small bowel biopsies in all patients with DH. A high incidence of autoimmune systemic disorders (22.2%) and malignant neoplasms (10.4%) was found. The risk of lymphoproliferative disorders was less than 2%. Histopathologic findings in biopsies of patients with DH were nonspecific in 22% of patients. Endomysial antibodies were present in 63.5%. *PMID: 17822491*

CLINICAL PRESENTATION. Dermatitis herpetiformis usually begins in the second to fifth decade, but many cases have been reported in children. The disease is rarely seen in blacks or Asians. Dermatitis herpetiformis presents initially with a few itchy papules or vesicles that are a minor annoyance; they may be attributed to bites, scabies, or neurotic excoriation, and they sometimes respond to topical steroids. In time the disease evolves into its classic presentation of intensely burning urticarial papules, vesicles, and, rarely, bullae, either isolated or in groups such as in herpes simplex or zoster (therefore the term *herpetiformis*) (Figure 16-4).

The vesicles are symmetrically distributed and appear on the elbows, knees, scalp and nuchal area, shoulders, and buttocks (Figures 16-5 to 16-8).

The distribution may be more generalized. Destruction of the vesicles by scratching provides relief but increases the difficulty of locating a primary lesion for biopsy. Intact lesions for biopsy may be found on the back.

DERMATITIS HERPETIFORMIS

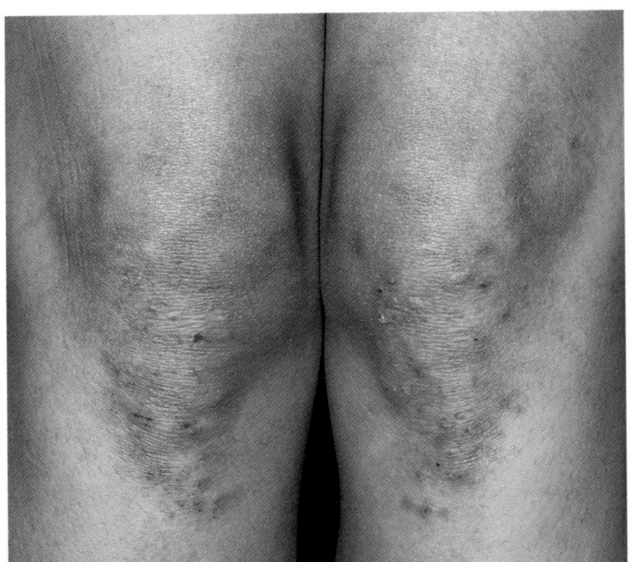

Figure 16-5 Vesicles are symmetrically distributed on the knees. Most have been excoriated.

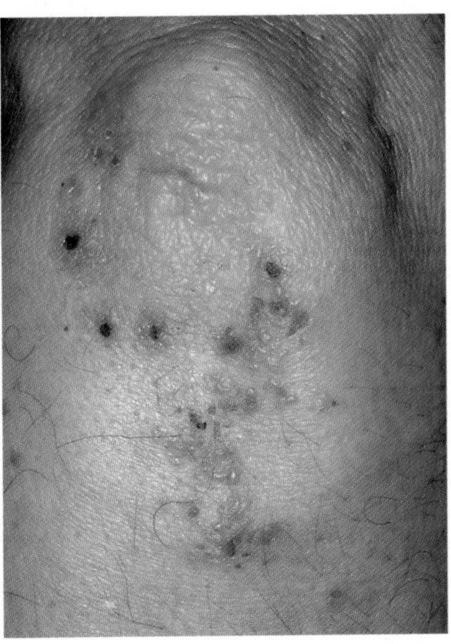

Figure 16-6 Lesions typically occur on the elbows and knees. Blisters have been replaced with crusts.

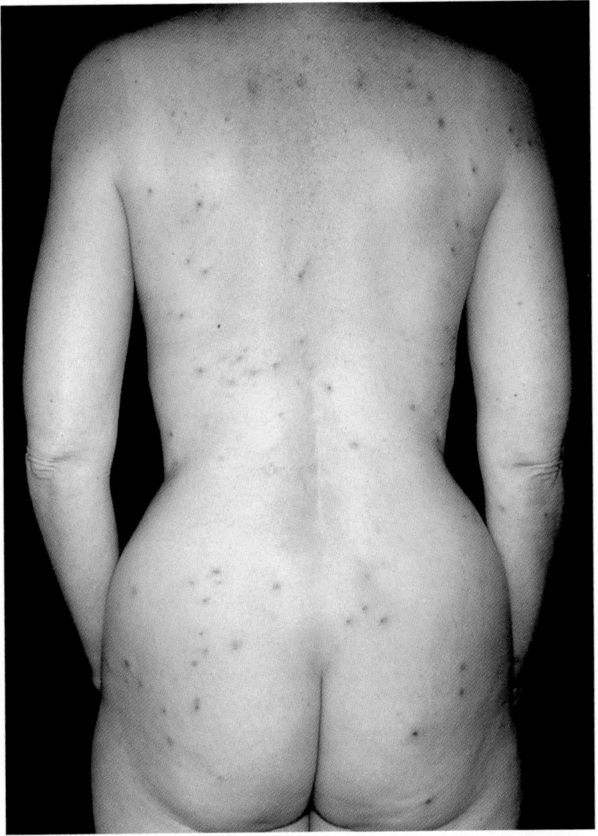

Figure 16-7 The number of lesions is usually small compared to bullous pemphigoid.

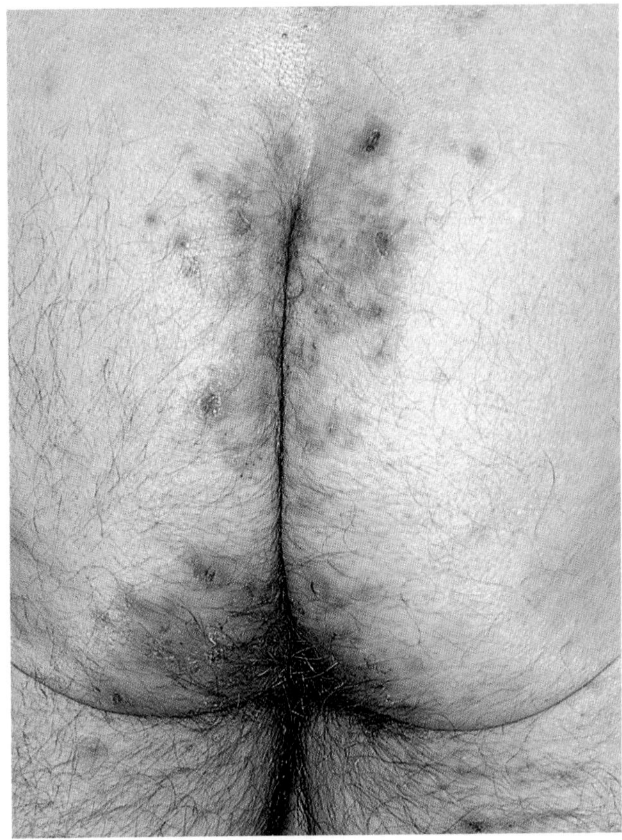

Figure 16-8 Vesicles and erosions are commonly found on the buttocks.

The symptoms vary in intensity, but most people complain of severe itching and burning. One should always think of dermatitis herpetiformis when the symptom of burning is volunteered. The symptoms may precede the onset of lesions by hours, and patients can frequently identify the site of a new lesion by the prodromal symptoms. Treatment does not alter the course of the disease. Most patients have symptoms for years, but approximately one third are in permanent remission.

The vesicular-bullous form is confused with bullous erythema multiforme and bullous pemphigoid. A strong association between dermatitis herpetiformis and diverse thyroid abnormalities has been reported and most likely represents a grouping of immune-mediated disorders. Hypothyroidism was the most common, occurring in 14% of patients. There were clinical or serologic abnormalities in 50% of patients with dermatitis herpetiformis.

Oral symptoms occur in 63% of patients. Oral dryness and recurrent oral mucosal ulceration are the most commonly reported findings.

Celiac-type dental enamel defects. Celiac-type permanent-tooth enamel defects were found in 53% of patients with dermatitis herpetiformis. The grades of these defects were milder than those described for severe celiac disease. This finding suggests that these patients were already suffering from subclinical gluten-induced enteropathy in early childhood, when the crowns of permanent teeth develop.

Linear IgA bullous dermatosis. Linear IgA bullous dermatosis (LABD) may present clinically as typical dermatitis herpetiformis, typical bullous pemphigoid, cicatricial pemphigoid, or in an atypical morphologic pattern, and it has histologic features similar to those of dermatitis herpetiformis. Drugs such as vancomycin are responsible for some cases. Lesions develop within 24 hours to 15 days after the first dose. The diagnosis of LABD is confirmed by direct immunofluorescence, which shows the presence of linear deposition of IgA at the epidermal basement membrane zone (BMZ). Some patients demonstrate both IgA and IgG BMZ autoantibodies. There is no gluten-sensitive enteropathy. Some patients have a circulating-IgA class anti-BMZ antibody on indirect immunofluorescence. Circulating IgA autoantibodies to tissue transglutaminase are detectable in DH but not in linear IgA disease or other subepidermal autoimmune bullous diseases.

Gluten-sensitive enteropathy

A gluten-sensitive enteropathy with patchy areas of villous atrophy and mild intestinal wall inflammation is found in the majority of patients with dermatitis herpetiformis. The changes in the small intestine are similar to but less severe than those found in ordinary gluten-sensitive enteropathy; symptoms of malabsorption are rarely encountered. Fewer than 20% of patients have malabsorption of fat, D-xylose, or iron. A significant correlation was found between IgA antiendomysial antibodies (IgA-EmA) and the severity of gluten-induced jejunum damage. Serum IgA-EmA was present in approximately 70% of patients with dermatitis herpetiformis on a normal diet. IgA-EmA was positive in 86% of dermatitis herpetiformis patients with subtotal villous atrophy, and 11% of dermatitis herpetiformis patients with partial villous atrophy or mild abnormalities. IgA-EmA antibodies disappear after 1 year of a gluten-free diet with the regrowth of jejunal villi. The relationship between IgA-EmA and villous atrophy is a useful diagnostic marker because the enteropathy present in dermatitis herpetiformis is usually without symptoms and therefore difficult to identify.

Lymphoma

Small bowel lymphoma and nonintestinal lymphoma have been reported in patients with dermatitis herpetiformis and celiac disease. All lymphomas occurred in patients whose dermatitis herpetiformis had been controlled without a gluten-free diet (GFD) or in those who had been treated with a GFD for less than 5 years. Therefore patients are advised to adhere to a strict GFD for life.

The incidence of lymphoproliferative disorders is less than 2%.

Diagnosis of dermatitis herpetiformis

SKIN BIOPSY. Figure 16-9 is an example of new red papular lesions that have not blistered. Subepidermal clefts of evolving vesicles, and neutrophils and eosinophils in microabscesses within dermal papillae, are demonstrated. Linear IgA bullous dermatosis histologically resembles dermatitis herpetiformis or bullous pemphigoid.

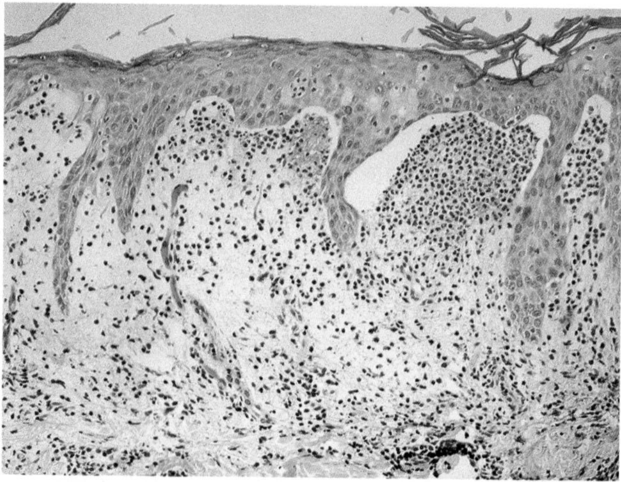

Figure 16-9 Dermatitis herpetiformis. Subepidermal clefts with microabscesses of neutrophils and eosinophils in the dermal papillae.

IMMUNOFLUORESCENCE STUDIES. IgA is not uniformly distributed throughout the skin, and IgA is present in greater amounts near active lesions. Therefore the preferred biopsy site for immunofluorescence studies is normal appearing or faintly erythematous skin that is adjacent to an active lesion. The diagnostic Ig deposits are usually destroyed in an active lesion during the blistering process. More than 90% of patients with dermatitis herpetiformis have granular or fibrillar IgA deposits in the dermal papillae; patients with linear IgA bullous dermatosis have linear deposits of IgA in the BMZ. This includes patients treated with sulfones. Multiple specimens may be needed to obtain positive findings because of the focal nature of deposits. Normal skin sites of more than 3 mm from a lesion or sites in areas not commonly involved may test negative for such IgA deposits. False-negative results may occur (1) if the biopsy is taken from involved skin, (2) if the biopsy is taken from an area never involved, or (3) if the patient has been on a long-term GFD.

IgA ANTIENDOMYSIAL ANTIBODIES (IgA-EmA) and IgA ANTI–TISSUE TRANSGLUTAMINASE (IgA ANTI-tTG). The most sensitive antibody tests for the diagnosis of celiac disease and dermatitis herpetiformis are of the IgA class. The available tests are for connective tissue antibodies (antiendomysial antibodies) and antibodies directed against tissue transglutaminase.

The endomysium is the connective tissue covering the smooth muscle layers of the esophagus, stomach, and small intestine. The endomysial antigen is tissue transglutaminase. Transglutaminase repairs injured tissue. If antibodies to transglutaminase are produced, repair of damaged intestinal mucosa is impaired.

The titers of endomysial antibodies and anti–tissue transglutaminase antibodies correlate with the degree of mucosal damage. Antibody levels indicate the degree of compliance to dietary gluten restriction.

Antiendomysial antibodies are found in approximately 70% of patients with DH and almost 100% of patients with active celiac disease. Either anti–tissue transglutaminase or antiendomysial antibody tests can be ordered to support the diagnosis of DH.

TRIAL OF SULFONES. Patients with a classic history of vesicular eruptions may be given a trial of sulfone therapy if they are very uncomfortable. The dramatic relief of symptoms within hours or a few days supports the diagnosis of dermatitis herpetiformis.

TREATMENT

DAPSONE OR SULFAPYRIDINE. These drugs control but do not cure the disease. Dapsone is more effective than sulfapyridine. The mechanism of action is unknown but is possibly explained by lysosomal enzyme stabilization. For adults, the initial dosage of dapsone is 100 to 150 mg given orally once a day. Itching and burning are controlled in 12 to 48 hours, and new lesions gradually stop appearing. The dosage is adjusted to the lowest level that provides acceptable relief; this is usually in the range of 50 to 200 mg/day. Some patients' symptoms are controlled with 25 mg/day, whereas others may require up to 400 mg/day. Probenecid blocks the renal excretion of dapsone, and rifampin increases the rate of plasma clearance. Dapsone produces dose-related hemolysis, anemia, and methemoglobinemia somewhat in all patients. A leukocyte count and hemoglobin determination should be done weekly when possible for the first month, monthly for 6 months, and semiannually thereafter. Methemoglobinemia, although not usually a significant problem, may cause a blue-gray cyanosis. The coadministration of cimetidine is reported to reduce dapsone-dependent methemoglobinemia in dermatitis herpetiformis patients. Patients with glucose-6-phosphate dehydrogenase (G6PD) deficiency may have profound hemolysis during sulfone or sulfapyridine therapy, and those at risk of having the deficiency (blacks, Asians, and those of Mediterranean descent) should have a G6PD level measurement before starting therapy.

Sulfapyridine, a short-acting sulfonamide (starting dosage, 500 to 1500 mg/day), can be substituted for dapsone and does not cause neuropathy. Consider sulfapyridine for patients who cannot tolerate dapsone.

Sulfapyridine is difficult to obtain. Sulfasalazine (Azulfidine) is metabolized to 5-aminosalicylic acid (5-ASA, mesalamine) and sulfapyridine and may be considered if sulfapyridine cannot be obtained.

Adverse reactions. Peripheral motor neuropathy may develop during the first few months of dapsone therapy. Generally, high dosages from 200 to 500 mg/day or high cumulative doses in the range of 25 to 600 gm have been implicated. Typically, the distal upper and lower extremities, particularly the hand muscles, are involved. Paresthesia and weakness are the most common complaints, and atrophy of interosseus muscles is often found. Patients complain of difficulty with manual tasks and gait disturbance. Footdrop is a common manifestation. Rarely, sensory involvement manifested by paresthesia, diminished pain, and numbness accompanies the motor disorder. Symptoms slowly but invariably improve over months to years when the medication is stopped. Agranulocytosis and aplastic anemia rarely occur but have resulted in death.

Dapsone hypersensitivity syndrome. The dapsone hypersensitivity syndrome (DHS) usually appears 4 weeks or longer after starting the drug. It consists of a mononucleosis-like illness with fever, malaise, and lymphadenopathy. Exanthematous skin eruptions usually resolve within 2 weeks of stopping dapsone. Hypersensitivity hepatitis has been reported as a component of the syndrome. Hypothyroidism may develop 3 months after the onset of DHS. Blood and liver function study results usually become normal within a few months after the patient stops taking dapsone. Prednisone is the preferred treatment. Prednisone is slowly tapered for more than 1 month while the function of affected organs is monitored to minimize recurrences. Dapsone appears to be safe during pregnancy.

GLUTEN-FREE DIET. Strict adherence to a GFD (avoid foods containing wheat, rye, and barley) for at least 6 months allows most patients to begin a decrease in or possibly a discontinuation of sulfone therapy. The diet has to be followed for many months (often 2 years) before medications can be discontinued. Although intestinal villous architecture improves, symptoms and lesions recur in 1 to 3 weeks if a normal diet is resumed. Current evidence indicates that a GFD needs to be continued indefinitely. Patients found to have a linear IgA immunofluorescence pattern do not have villous atrophy and do not respond to a GFD. Oats can be included in a GFD without deleterious effects to the skin or intestine. Wheat starch–based gluten-free flour products were not harmful in the treatment of celiac disease and dermatitis herpetiformis.

Products must be chosen carefully, because some so-called gluten-free foods contain high levels of gliadin, the enterotoxic agent in gluten. Gluten is in all grains except rice and corn. There are many online sources of gluten-free foods such as Ener-G Foods, Inc. (www.ener-g.com). The Gluten Intolerance Group of North America (www.gluten.net) publishes a newsletter and offers other services.

ELEMENTAL DIET. Dietary factors other than gluten may be important in the pathogenesis of dermatitis herpetiformis. Various substances can act as antigens; if the antigens can be eliminated, no new harmful immune complexes are formed. Most antigens that lead to humoral immune responses are proteins; therefore a diet without full proteins (elemental diet) is not likely to contain major antigens. In one study, a diet of amino acids, fat, and carbohydrates produced a rapid benefit and allowed a significant reduction in the dosage of dapsone within 2 weeks. Significant improvements in clinical disease activity, independent of gluten administration, and in small bowel morphology are also seen with an elemental diet.

TETRACYCLINE AND NICOTINAMIDE. Successful treatment of dermatitis herpetiformis and linear IgA bullous dermatosis with tetracycline (500 mg one to three times daily) or minocycline (100 mg twice daily) and nicotinamide (500 mg two or three times daily) is reported. Stopping either nicotinamide or minocycline resulted in a flare-up of the dermatitis herpetiformis. A combination of heparin, tetracycline, and nicotinamide is also reported to be effective.

OTHER TREATMENTS. Prednisone, colchicine, cyclosporine, and heparin have been reported to be effective.

BULLAE IN DIABETIC PERSONS

Crops of bullae may appear abruptly in diabetic persons, usually on the feet and lower legs. They usually develop overnight without preceding trauma. There is little pain or discomfort. Different epidermal split levels and subepidermal separation have been reported. The bullae arise from a noninflamed base, are usually multiple, and vary in size from 1 cm to several centimeters. Occasionally they are huge, involving the entire dorsum of the foot or a major portion of the lower leg (Figure 16-10). The bullae are tense and rupture in approximately 1 week, leaving a deep, painless ulcer that forms a firmly adherent crust. Even if not infected, these large ulcers take many weeks to heal. Many patients never have another episode, whereas others have recurrences.

No immunopathologic features are found. The cause is unknown, but is possibly ischemic.

TREATMENT. Ulcers may be compressed several times a day with tepid Burow's solution. The treatment of deeper erosions and ulcers is described in Chapter 3.

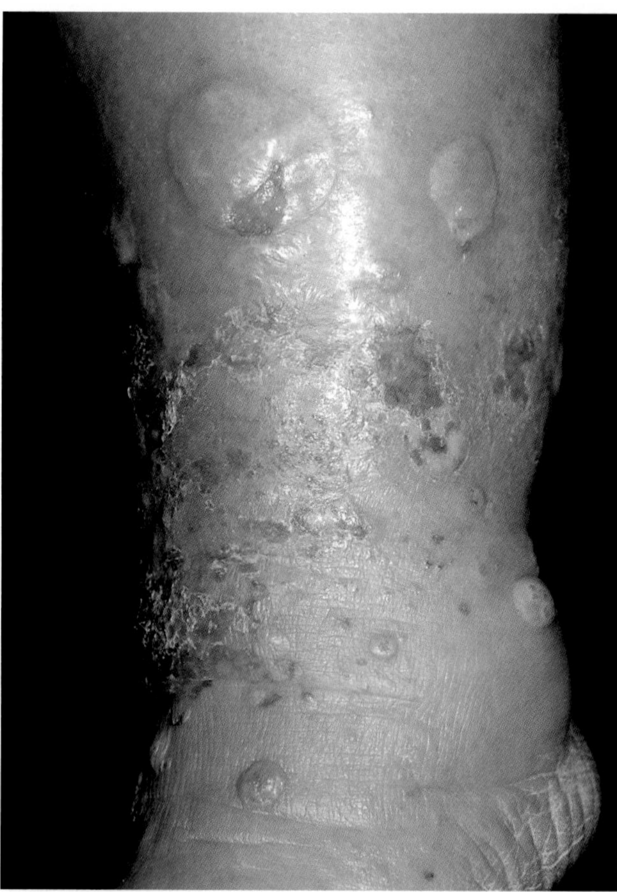

Figure 16-10 Bullosis diabeticorum. Blisters appear spontaneously without any trauma on nonerythematous skin. Blisters usually occur on the lower legs and feet but may occur on the arms. Blisters may be very large. There is little discomfort. Lesions heal spontaneously.

PEMPHIGUS

Pemphigus (from the Greek *pemphix,* meaning bubble or blister) is a rare group of autoimmune, intraepidermal blistering diseases involving the skin and mucous membranes. The group includes pemphigus vulgaris and pemphigus foliaceus. Both were usually fatal before glucocorticoid therapy was used for their treatment. The difference between the two disorders is the level of the epidermis at which acantholysis (loss of cohesion of epithelium) occurs: the suprabasilar level in pemphigus vulgaris and the subcorneal level in pemphigus foliaceus. Other members of the pemphigus group are paraneoplastic pemphigus, which generally occurs in patients with lymphoma, and drug-induced pemphigus, which usually develops after taking penicillamine.

Pathophysiology

Pemphigus is the result of the interaction between genetically predisposed individuals and possibly some exogenous factor. The presence of foci of pemphigus foliaceus (fogo selvagem) in rural South America suggests that the disorder can be triggered in susceptible persons by an environmental agent (probably an unidentified infectious agent), whose antigens mimic those of desmoglein 1, and that clinical disease evolves in the persons who have the most vigorous immune response to desmoglein 1. Both idiopathic pemphigus and induced pemphigus have the same human leukocyte antigen (HLA) pattern.

DESMOGLEIN

The structural integrity of the epidermis depends on the sharing of desmosomes by neighboring keratinocytes. Desmosomal connections are broken and reform as keratinocytes migrates from the basal layer toward the skin surface. Desmoglein is a cell-to-cell adhesion molecule contained in desmosomes that contributes to the strength of the intercellular desmosomal bridge. There are three isotypes of desmoglein, Dsg1, Dsg2, and Dsg3. Dsg2 is expressed in all desmosome-possessing tissues (see Table 16-1); Dsg1 and Dsg3 are restricted to stratified squamous epithelia, where blister formation is found in patients with pemphigus.

DSG1 AND DSG3 AUTOANTIBODIES. Circulating IgG autoantibodies are directed against the normal desmoglein proteins within the desmosomal structure on the cell surface of keratinocytes. The autoantibodies destroy the adhesion between epidermal cells, allowing fluid to accumulate in the gaps in the epidermis to form blisters. The target molecule of pemphigus autoantibodies is a transmembrane desmosomal component—desmoglein 3 (Dsg3) in pemphigus vulgaris (PV) and Dsg1 in pemphigus foliaceus (PF).

Patients with mucosal-dominant PV are negative for anti-Dsg1 antibodies but positive for Dsg3 antibodies. Patients with mucocutaneous PV have both anti-Dsg3 and anti-Dsg1 IgG antibodies. Patients with PF have only anti-Dsg1 IgG.

Pemphigus vulgaris

Pemphigus vulgaris is the most common form of pemphigus. Painful oral erosions usually precede the onset of skin blisters by weeks or months (Figures 16-11 and 16-12). Involvement of other mucosal surfaces occurs in patients with widespread disease. The soft palate was involved in 80% of cases at initial presentation. Nonpruritic flaccid blisters varying in size from 1 cm to several centimeters appear gradually on normal or erythematous skin and may be localized for a considerable time. The most common sites are the scalp, face, axillae, and oral cavity. Blisters invariably become gen-

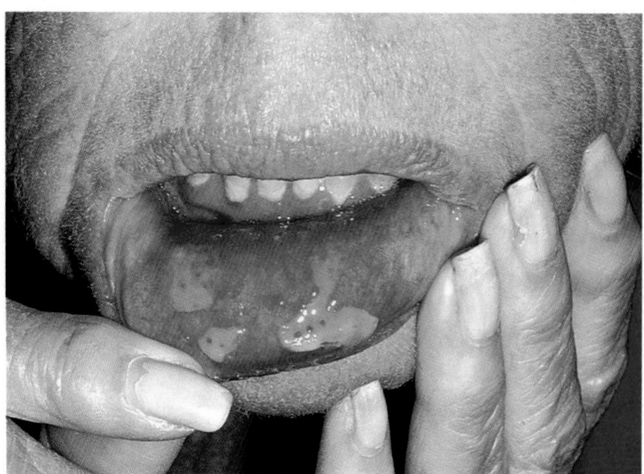

Figure 16-11 Pemphigus vulgaris presents with oral lesions in over 50% of patients. Oral lesions may be the only manifestation of the disease or they may precede the onset of skin lesions by several months.

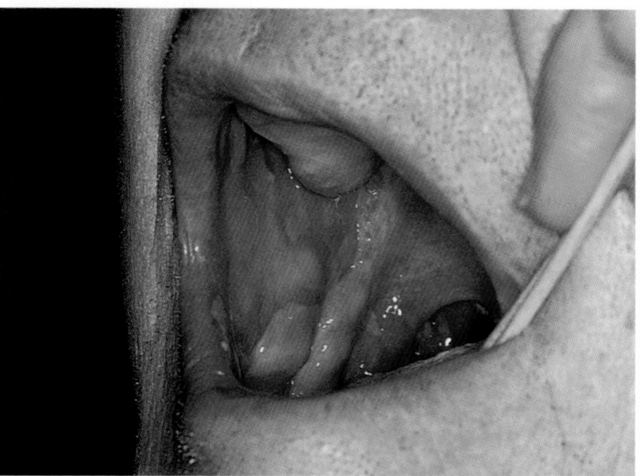

Figure 16-12 Intact bullae are rarely found in the mouth. Painful erosions are the typical finding, and they are slow to heal. Erosions are found in all areas of the oral cavity and may involve the larynx. Pain interferes with eating.

PEMPHIGUS

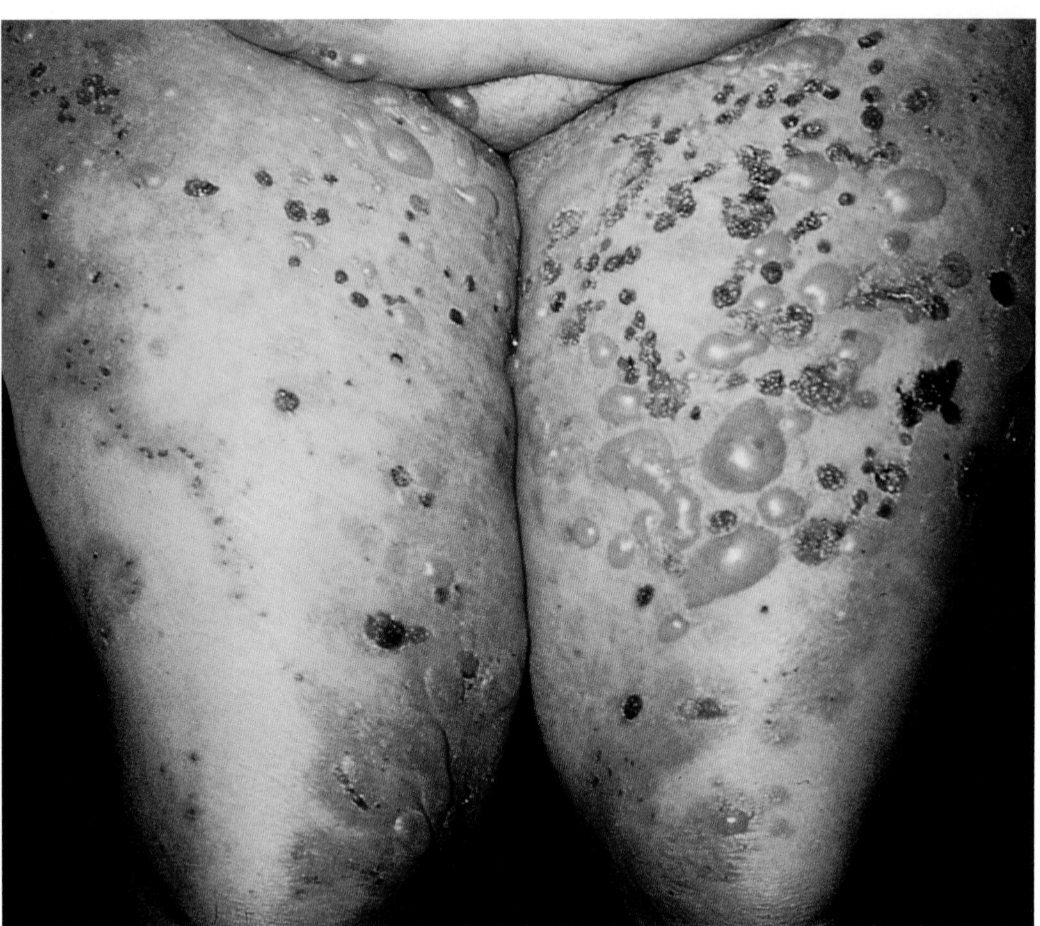

Figure 16-13 Flaccid blisters rupture easily because the roof, which consists of only a thin portion of the upper epidermis, is very fragile. Healing occurs with brown hyperpigmentation, but without scarring.

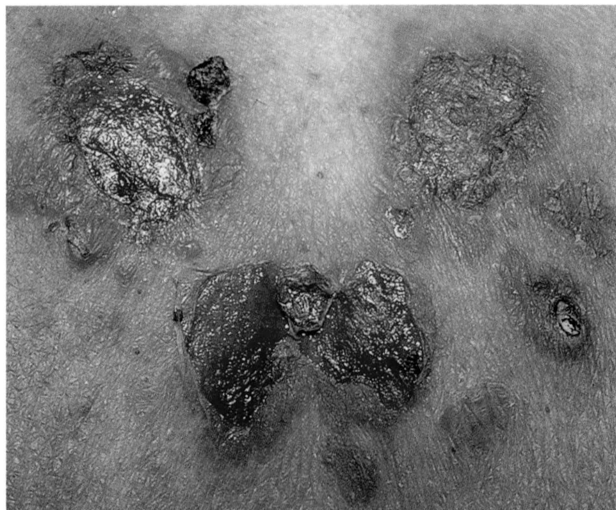

Figure 16-14 Fragile blisters rupture easily to form painful erosions. Finger pressure separates normal-appearing epidermis, producing an erosion (Nikolsky's sign). Pressure on the edge of a blister spreads the blister into unaffected skin.

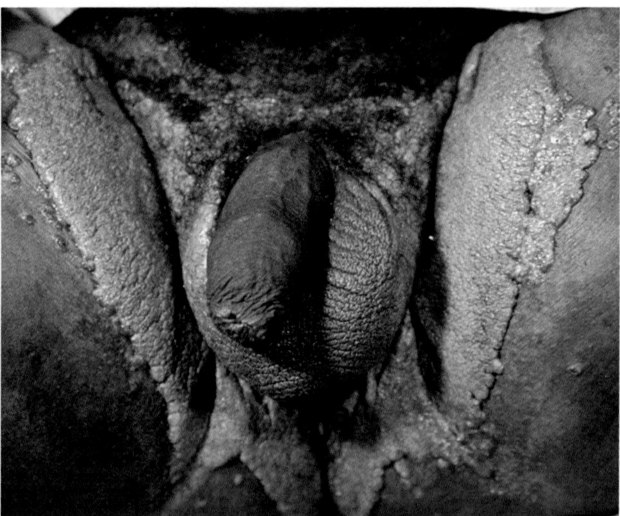

Figure 16-15 Pemphigus vegetans. Intertriginous denuded areas heal with hypertrophic verrucoid granulations.

eralized if left untreated (Figure 16-13). The blisters rupture easily because the vesicle roof, which consists of only a thin portion of the upper epidermis, is fragile (Figure 16-14). Application of pressure to small intact bullae causes the fluid to dissect laterally into the midepidermal areas altered by bound IgG (Nikolsky's sign).

Exposed erosions last for weeks before healing with brown hyperpigmentation but without scarring. Blisters, erosions, and lines of erythema may appear in the esophageal mucosa. Death formerly occurred in all cases, usually from cutaneous infection, but now occurs in only 10% of cases, usually from complications of steroid therapy. Sunlight exposure is harmful.

Pemphigus vegetans is a variant of pemphigus vulgaris that presents with large verrucous confluent plaques and pustules localized to flexural areas in the axillae and groin (Figure 16-15).

Pemphigus foliaceus, IgA pemphigus, and pemphigus erythematosus

The age of onset varies more widely in pemphigus foliaceus and pemphigus erythematosus than in pemphigus vulgaris, and there is no racial prevalence. Oral lesions are rarely present. Pemphigus foliaceus begins gradually on the face (Figures 16-16 and 16-17) in a "butterfly" distribution or first appears on the scalp, chest, or upper back in a seborrheic distribution.

PEMPHIGUS ERYTHEMATOSUS

Pemphigus erythematosus, also known as Senear-Usher syndrome, may actually be a combination of localized pemphigus foliaceus and systemic lupus erythematosus, because many of these patients have a positive antinuclear antibody. If the eruption becomes more diffuse or generalized, the term pemphigus foliaceus is used. The disease may last for years and may be fatal if not treated.

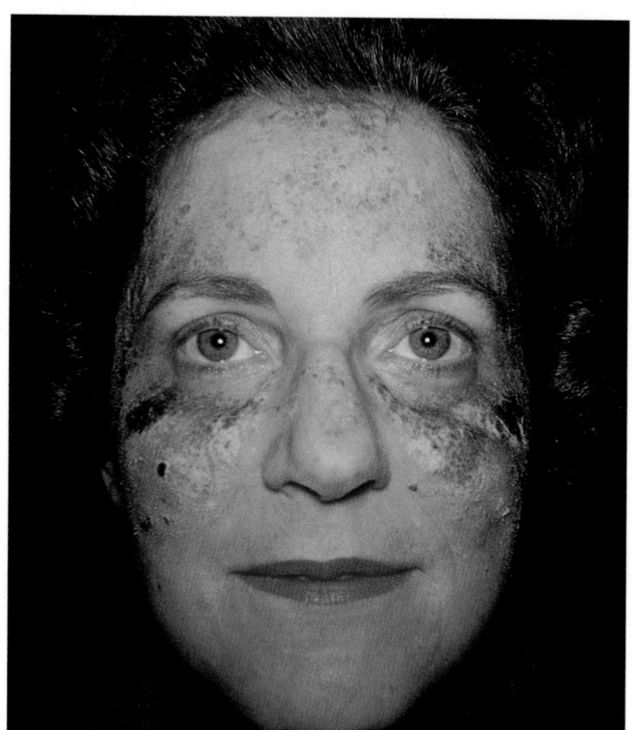

Figure 16-16 Pemphigus foliaceus. Serum and crust with occasional vesicles are present on the face in a butterfly distribution.

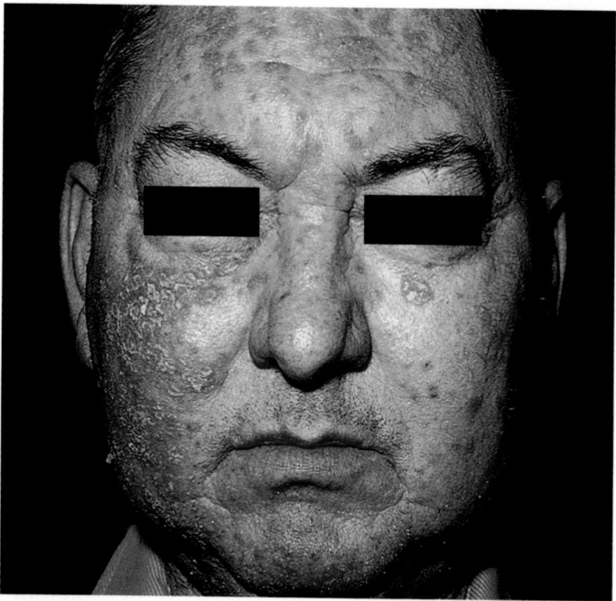

Figure 16-17 Pemphigus foliaceus. Scaly, crusted erosions appear on an erythematous base. They may be confined to seborrheic areas on the face and trunk. The mucous membranes are usually not involved.

PEMPHIGUS FOLIACEUS

Pemphigus foliaceus (superficial pemphigus) presents with recurrent shallow erosions, erythema, scaling, and crusting. Small flaccid blisters may occur but they are superficial, very fragile, and rupture easily. Serum leaks out and desiccates, forming the localized or broad areas of crust (Figures 16-18 and 16-19). Intact thin-walled blisters are sometimes seen near the edge of the erosions. The site of blister formation in the horizontal plane of the stratum corneum can be demonstrated in skin biopsy specimens after the upper portion of the epidermis has been dislodged with lateral finger pressure (Nikolsky's sign). IgA pemphigus has clinical and histologic similarity to subcorneal pustular dermatosis and pemphigus foliaceus. IgA antibodies are bound to the epidermal cell surface, and half of the patients have circulating IgA anti–cell-surface antibodies.

Skin lesions of pemphigus foliaceus are generally well demarcated and do not extend into large eroded areas as those of pemphigus vulgaris. Mucous membrane involvement is uncommon. Pemphigus foliaceus may remain localized for years and it has a better prognosis than pemphigus vulgaris.

FOGO SELVAGEM

Fogo selvagem (Portuguese for "wild fire") is an endemic form of pemphigus foliaceus found in certain rural areas of South America, including Brazil, Colombia, Bolivia, Peru, and Venezuela, as well as in Tunisia. It occurs in jungle areas but the disease disappears when the jungle is cleared. Environmental triggers such as an infectious agent have been proposed to induce fogo selvagem. Fogo selvagem occurs in children and young adults and may affect several family members. This endemic variant is clinically indistinguishable from nonendemic pemphigus foliaceus.

Diagnosis of pemphigus

SKIN BIOPSY FOR LIGHT MICROSCOPY. Histologic studies may yield key findings in cases that are negative by direct immunofluorescence. A small, early vesicle or skin adjacent to a blister biopsied with a 3- or 4-mm punch shows an intraepidermal bulla and acantholysis (separation of epidermal cells near the blister following dissolution of the intercellular cement substance). The basal epidermal cells become detached from each other but remain attached to the basement membrane. There is a mild-to-moderate infiltrate of eosinophils (Figures 16-20 and 16-21).

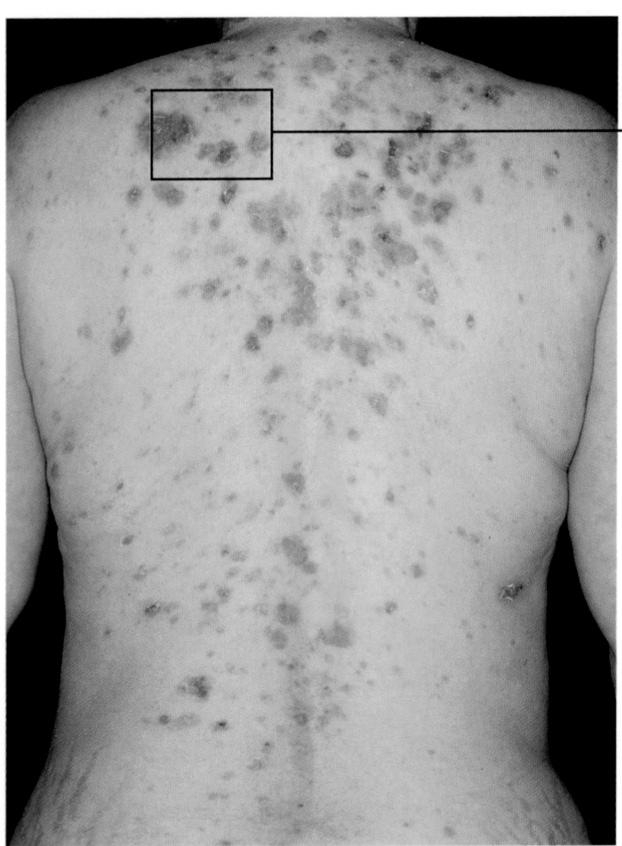

Figure 16-18 Pemphigus foliaceus. The symmetrical distribution of red, eroded, crusted lesions. Occasionally vesicles are seen at the edge of a lesion.

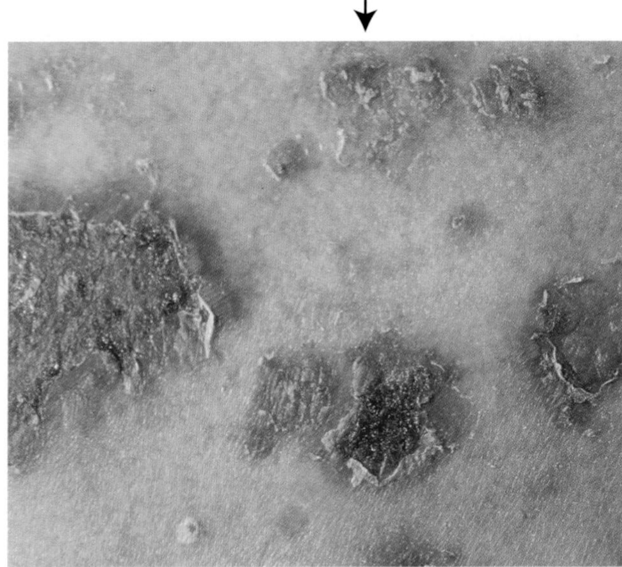

Figure 16-19 Pemphigus foliaceus. The vesicle roof is so thin that it ruptures, leaving erosions with areas of crust.

DIRECT IMMUNOFLUORESCENCE OF SKIN AND MUCOUS MEMBRANES. Two biopsies are recommended. One biopsy specimen should be taken from the edge of a fresh lesion and the second from an adjacent normal area. Two biopsies are especially helpful in evaluation of oral lesions because lesional sites are frequently denuded. Mucosal biopsies should be taken 0.5 cm from a lesion because closer sites may be negative. Perilesional biopsies of skin or mucous membranes usually reveal IgG, strong IgG4, and frequently C3 in the intercellular areas in patients with all clinical variants of pemphigus.

INDIRECT IMMUNOFLUORESCENCE. Serum IgG antibodies directed against the keratinocyte cell surface can be demonstrated by indirect immunofluorescent staining and are present in all forms of true pemphigus in approximately 75% of patients with active disease. Blood should be withdrawn into a red top tube. A combination of indirect immunofluorescence on two substrates (monkey and guinea pig esophagus) and enzyme-linked immunosorbent assay (ELISA) tests for Dsg1 and Dsg3 affords the greatest sensitivity and highest level of confidence in the diagnosis of pemphigus. ELISA for Dsg1 and Dsg3 distinguishes between pemphigus vulgaris and foliaceus. Cases that have both skin and mucosal lesions have both Dsg3 and Dsg1 antibodies (see Table 16-1).

In some cases, the level of circulating intercellular substance IgG antibody reflects the activity of disease, rising during periods of activity and falling or disappearing during times of remission. Many patients show a poor correlation between the titer of circulating antibody and disease activity. Therefore management of pemphigus should be guided by clinical disease activity rather than by the pemphigus antibody titer. In some cases periodic serum tests to detect changes in titers are helpful in evaluating the clinical course. Serum should be tested every 2 to 3 weeks until remission and every 1 to 6 months thereafter.

Treatment

CORTICOSTEROIDS AND IMMUNOSUPPRESSIVE AGENTS. Systemic glucocorticosteroids are still the mainstay of therapy. Very-high-dose regimens (more than 120 mg/day) provide no benefit over the low-dose regimens with respect to the frequency of relapse or the incidence of complications.

The majority of pemphigus vulgaris patients present with oral disease at an early and relatively stable stage. These patients may be controlled by starting prednisone 40 mg on alternate days plus 100 mg azathioprine every day until there is complete healing of all lesions. A gradual monthly and later bimonthly decrease of prednisone was followed by the tapering of azathioprine, in a 1-year period. *PMID: 17958846* The time required for the epithelialization of lesions varies between 4 and 7 months.

TOPICAL STEROIDS. Patients with mild pemphigus vulgaris or pemphigus foliaceus responded to clobetasol propionate 0.05% cream applied to mucosal lesions and involved skin twice a day for at least 15 days, followed by progressive tapering.

ADJUVANTS. Because of the potential toxicity of systemic corticosteroids, another drug may be initiated long term. The adjuvant therapy (corticosteroid-sparing medication) is initiated with or after starting corticosteroids. Although there are no controlled studies most experts believe that immunosuppressive agents have a steroid-sparing effect. They may decrease the side effects of steroid therapy by allowing the use of lower steroid dosages and lead to increased remission rates. Others disagree and feel that the improved prognosis of pemphigus in recent years is due to the use of lower dosages of corticosteroids, and the improved treatment of corticosteroid complications. The most commonly used agents are cyclophosphamide, and azathio-

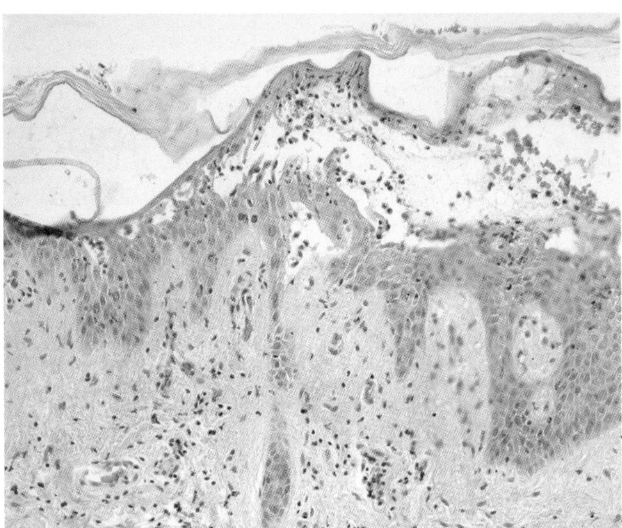

Figure 16-20 Pemphigus foliaceus. The intraepidermal separation appears high in the epidermis.

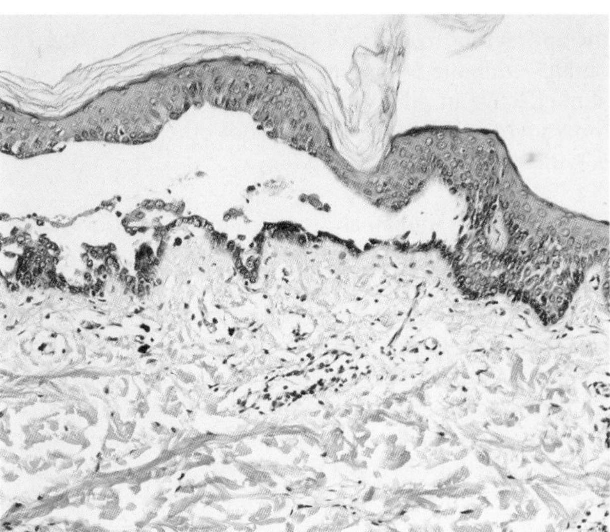

Figure 16-21 Pemphigus vulgaris. The epidermal separation occurs low in the epidermis.

prine and mycophenolate mofetil. Methotrexate is rarely used because of the reported high incidence of severe infections. One study showed that mycophenolate mofetil and azathioprine had similar efficacy, corticosteroid-sparing effects, and safety profiles as adjuvants during treatment of pemphigus vulgaris and pemphigus foliaceus. *PMID: 17116835*

CYCLOPHOSPHAMIDE. Average starting dosage is 100 mg (1.1 to 2.5 mg/kg) per day. Cyclophosphamide may be the most effective drug but it is toxic. Side effects include bone marrow suppression, hemorrhagic cystitis, bladder fibrosis, reversible alopecia, and an increased risk of bladder carcinoma and lymphoma. Monitor urinalysis and blood cell counts. Encourage oral fluid intake to decrease the risk of bladder fibrosis and hemorrhagic cystitis.

AZATHIOPRINE. Average starting dosage is 100 mg (1.1 to 2.5 mg/kg) per day. Azathioprine causes bone marrow suppression, hepatotoxicity, and an increased risk of malignancy that is lower than that of cyclophosphamide. Monitor blood cell counts and liver function tests. Detailed prescribing information for azathioprine is found on p. 302.

MYCOPHENOLATE MOFETIL. Average starting dosage is 1 gm/day. Adverse effects are gastrointestinal disorders (most common), genitourinary complaints, increased incidence of viral or bacterial infection, and neurologic symptoms. Relative contraindications include lactation, peptic ulcer disease, hepatic or renal disease, and concomitant azathioprine or cholestyramine therapy. Detailed prescribing information is found on p. 298.

INTRAVENOUS IMMUNOGLOBULIN. In patients who do not respond to conventional immunosuppressants, intravenous immunoglobulin (IVIG) appears to be an effective treatment alternative. Its early use may be of benefit in patients who may experience life-threatening complications from immunosuppression. IVIG is effective as monotherapy. Several courses of treatment may be required to obtain a durable remission. The treatment is not predictably effective in all patients. Headache is the most common adverse effect. The incidence of other adverse events is low.

RITUXIMAB. Rituximab is a chimeric murine-human monoclonal antibody that targets the CD20 antigen found on B cells and results in rapid depletion of this cell population. It is indicated for patients with relapsed or refractory, low-grade or follicular, CD20-positive, B cell non-Hodgkin's lymphoma. It has been used for refractory pemphigus vulgaris, pemphigus foliaceus, and paraneoplastic pemphigus. Response may be delayed, and prolonged treatment may be required for control. A typical treatment program consists of rituximab 375 mg/m^2 once weekly for 4 weeks administered intravenously. *PMID: 17709662* Infectious adverse events are a risk with use of this biologic agent. The combination of rituximab and intravenous immune globulin is effective in patients with refractory pemphigus vulgaris. *PMID: 17065638.*

Many other agents have been tried alone or as adjuvants. These include chlorambucil, mycophenolate mofetil, dapsone, gold, plasma exchange, extracorporeal photopheresis, and tetracycline 2 gm/day.

APPROACH TO TREATMENT

Therapeutic choices are determined by the patient's age, degree of disease involvement, rate of disease progression, and subtype of pemphigus.

PREDNISONE. Elderly patients with mild to moderate disease can be treated with prednisone, at 40 mg/day, along with cyclophosphamide or azathioprine. Patients with more severe disease may require 60 to 80 mg/day of prednisone. The dosage of prednisone is tapered to a level that controls most disease activity. Attempts are made to use an alternate-day regimen to minimize side effects.

One taper method is to reduce prednisone by 10 mg every week until the daily dose reaches 20 mg. Then the dose is reduced each alternate week until a dose of 20 mg on alternate days is reached. Then the dose reduction is slower until a final dose of 5 mg on alternate days is achieved.

During the prednisone taper, the immunosuppressive agent is continued at full dosage. The speed of the prednisone taper is determined by the level of disease activity. It is not necessary to have the disease totally suppressed before lowering the prednisone dose.

Patients who cannot take steroids may be treated with azathioprine, mycophenolate mofetil, or cyclophosphamide alone. Patients who fail to respond to corticosteroids and immunosuppressive agents can be treated with IVIG, rituximab, plasmapheresis, or extracorporeal photopheresis.

Many patients with pemphigus foliaceus can be treated with potent topical steroids or low doses of corticosteroids. Hydroxychloroquine 200 mg twice a day was reported to be an effective adjuvant in patients with persistent and widespread pemphigus foliaceus. This was especially true when photosensitivity was present. The combination of nicotinamide (1.5 gm/day) and tetracycline (2 gm/day) or minocycline (100 mg twice a day) may be an effective alternative to steroids in pemphigus foliaceus and a steroid-sparing adjuvant, rather than a steroid alternative for pemphigus vulgaris. Dapsone may also be effective.

Sunlight exposure is harmful. Protection from sunlight should be part of the treatment.

COURSE AND REMISSION

It is possible to eventually induce complete and durable remissions in most patients with pemphigus that permit systemic therapy to be safely discontinued without a flare in disease activity. The proportion of patients in whom this can be achieved increases steadily with time, and therapy can be discontinued in approximately 75% of patients after 10 years.

RISK OF RELAPSE

There are three subtypes of pemphigus vulgaris: mucosal, mucocutaneous, and cutaneous. The death rate is higher for the mucocutaneous type. Remission rates vary by subtype. Patients with the three different subtypes were treated with prednisolone 2 mg/kg/day plus azathioprine 2 to 2.5 mg/kg/day. The partial and complete remission rates, at the end of the first and second years of treatment, and the number of relapses were compared in the three patient groups: 71.1% had mucocutaneous involvement, 18.8% had mucosal involvement, and 10.2% had only cutaneous involvement. The mean duration required for the mucocutaneous group to reach a prednisolone dosage of 30 mg/day was significantly longer. Mucocutaneous patients had a significantly lower rate of remission (31.9%) compared with those with only mucosal or cutaneous involvement (48.6%) at the end of the first year of the treatment. After 2 years, mucocutaneous patients again had a lower remission rate (32.9% vs. 44.5%). Relapses were more frequent in this subtype. Those presenting with mucosal or mucocutaneous erosions had a higher rate of active disease after receiving treatment for 1 year compared with those with only cutaneous presentation (66.7% vs. 45%).

CONCLUSIONS

In the mucocutaneous subtype, clinical control is achieved later, and these patients have a lower rate of remission at the end of the first and second years of treatment. They are also prone to relapses. *PMID: 18194237*

The risk of disease relapse after treatment discontinuation in pemphigus vulgaris varies with the treatment regimen. Four therapy regimens were compared: (1) oral prednisone at an initial dose of 100 mg (1.1 to 1.5 mg/kg/day) in monotherapy; (2) prednisone combined with oral azathioprine at a dose of 100 mg (1.1 to 1.5 mg/kg) per day; (3) prednisone combined with cyclosporine A at a dose of 2.5 to 3.0 mg/kg/day; or (4) prednisone combined with cyclophosphamide at a dose of 100 mg (1.1 to 1.5 mg/kg) per day. The risk of relapse was 44%. Treatment with prednisone plus oral cyclophosphamide combination therapy was associated with the lowest relapse rate and longest disease-free period; 54% of patients remained disease free for 5 years after treatment discontinuation.

DETERMINING REMISSION AND WHEN TO STOP TREATMENT. Treatment is stopped when patients are clinically free of disease and when they have a negative finding on direct immunofluorescence. The titers of circulating antibodies have a rough correlation with disease activity, but they are not accurate enough to determine when to stop therapy. A skin biopsy for direct immunofluorescence can predict when a patient is in remission and may be used to predict relapse. A negative direct immunofluorescence finding suggests that there is immunologic remission, and 80% of patients with a negative direct immunofluorescence study remained disease free for the next 5 years.

Pemphigus in association with other diseases

Myasthenia gravis and thymoma have been reported on many occasions in association with pemphigus (usually erythematosus and vulgaris). The clinical course is variable, but myasthenia gravis develops in most patients, followed by the detection of thymus disease, and finally by the appearance of pemphigus. Malignancy, usually of the lymphoid or reticuloendothelial systems, occurs more frequently in patients with pemphigus than in normal persons. Paraneoplastic pemphigus is described in the following sections.

DRUG-INDUCED VERSUS DRUG-TRIGGERED PEMPHIGUS

Drugs implicated in pemphigus can be divided into two main groups according to their chemical structure: those containing a sulfhydryl radical (thiol drugs or SH drugs) and nonthiol drugs. Penicillamine (a thiol drug) was the first drug reported to induce pemphigus (Figure 16-22). Pemphigus foliaceus has been reported in approximately 5% of patients taking 500 to 2000 mg of D-penicillamine or captopril for 2 months to 4 years. Most cases were mild. Patients with pemphigus induced by the SH drugs penicillamine and captopril showed spontaneous recovery in 39.4% and 52.6% of cases, respectively, once the drug was discontinued.

Pemphigus induced by other drugs shows spontaneous recovery in only 15% of cases. This suggests that penicillamine (SH drugs) induces pemphigus, whereas other drugs only trigger the disease in patients with a predisposition.

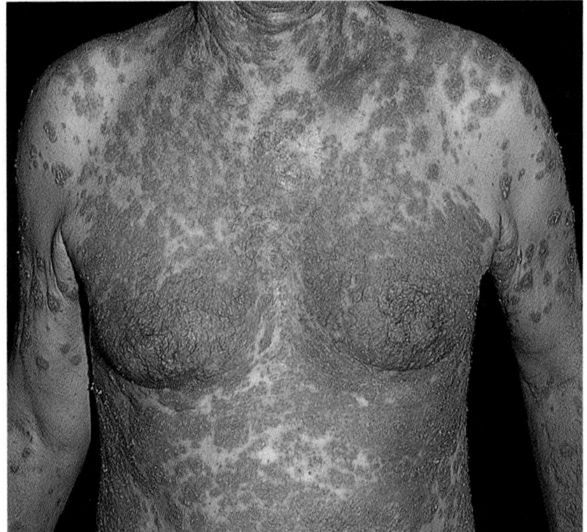

Figure 16-22 Drug-induced pemphigus (penicillamine). The eruption may not develop until months after starting the drug. Lesions produced by the thiol drugs (sulfhydryl radicals) usually present as pemphigus foliaceus with scaling and crusts concentrated on the trunk. Oral lesions do not occur. Non–thiol drugs present with a pemphigus vulgaris pattern with flaccid blisters and oral erosions.

The pemphigus-like eruption is not always limited, and the mortality approaches 10%.

The autoantibody response is similar in both spontaneous and drug-related disease. Therefore a similar molecular mechanism in the two types of pemphigus is suggested.

PARANEOPLASTIC PEMPHIGUS (NEOPLASIA-ASSOCIATED PEMPHIGUS)

Paraneoplastic pemphigus is an autoimmune disease that accompanies an overt or occult neoplasm and causes blisters. It has clinical and histologic features of both Stevens-Johnson syndrome and pemphigus vulgaris. There are painful mucosal ulcerations, conjunctival reactions, and polymorphous skin lesions on the trunk and extremities that usually progress to blisters (Figure 16-23, *A-C* and Box 16-1). Antibodies against epithelial proteins are present in desmosomes and hemidesmosomes in the epidermis and respiratory epithelium. The prognosis is poor except for some patients who undergo total resection of their neoplasm. Progressive respiratory failure with clinical features of bronchiolitis obliterans is frequently the cause of death.

LABORATORY DIAGNOSIS OF PARANEOPLASTIC PEMPHIGUS

HISTOLOGIC STUDIES. The histologic findings show features of pemphigus and erythema multiforme. There are intraepithelial clefts with epidermal acantholysis. In addition, there are dyskeratotic keratinocytes, vacuolar change of the basilar epidermis, and epidermal exocytosis of inflammatory cells.

DIRECT IMMUNOFLUORESCENCE. Testing of mucous membrane and skin biopsies shows cell-surface deposits of IgG and C3 along with granular basement membrane deposits of C3.

INDIRECT IMMUNOFLUORESCENCE. Indirect immunofluorescence with rat bladder substrate is used to differentiate paraneoplastic pemphigoid (PNP) from classic pemphigus. Circulating IgG anti–cell-surface and anticytoplasmic antibodies occur in a pattern and intensity unique to these patients.

Box 16-1 Criteria for the Diagnosis of Neoplasia-Associated Pemphigus

- Severe and painful mucosal involvement and polymorphic cutaneous eruptions
- Intraepidermal acantholysis, keratinocyte necrosis, and vacuolar interface dermatitis
- Indirect immunofluorescence of patient serum with rat bladder epithelia showing intercellular staining
- The presence of neoplasm, especially lymphoproliferative tumors

PARANEOPLASTIC PEMPHIGUS

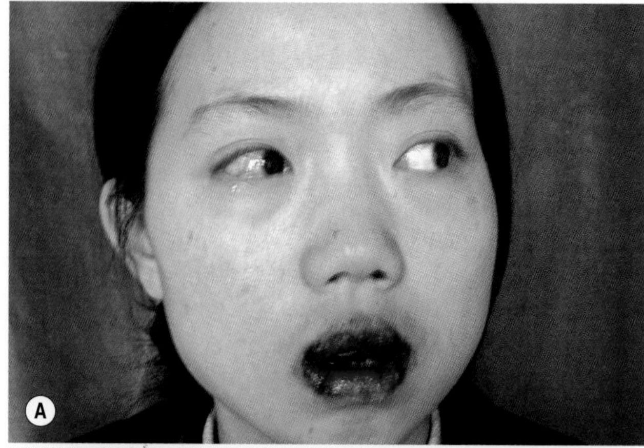

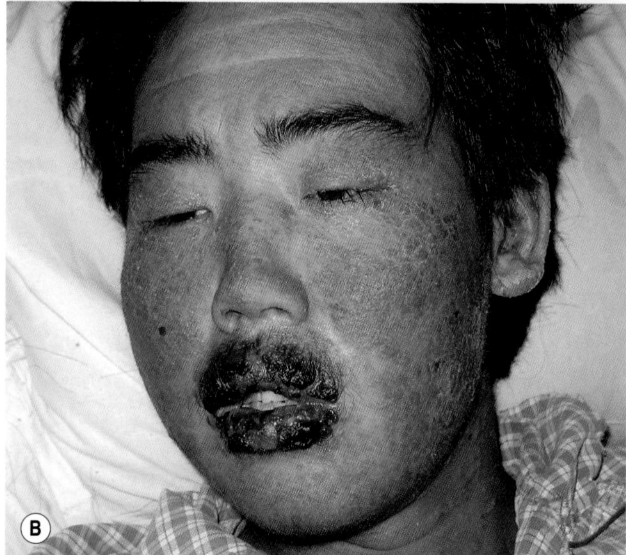

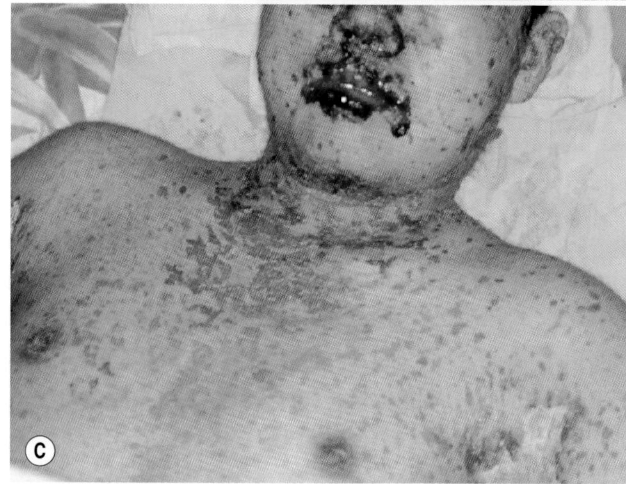

Figure 16-23 Conjunctival reactions, mucosal ulcerations and polymorphous skin lesions on the body are the prominent features. (Courtesy Professor Xuejun Zhu, MD, Department of Dermatology, Peking University First Hospital.)

THE PEMPHIGOID GROUP OF DISEASES

Bullous pemphigoid, herpes gestationis, and cicatricial pemphigoid are autoimmune subepidermal blistering diseases with circulating IgG and basement membrane zone–bound IgG antibodies and C3.

Bullous pemphigoid

Bullous pemphigoid (BP) is a rare, relatively benign, autoimmune subepidermal bullous disease of the elderly. Like patients with other autoimmune diseases, patients with BP have an immune response to constituents of normal tissue. There is no racial or gender prevalence. Pemphigoid is a disease of the elderly, with most cases occurring after age 60, although cases have been reported in children. There have been many reports of the coexistence of bullous pemphigoid with other disorders, but their association is probably coincidental. There is little evidence of an association of bullous pemphigoid with internal malignancy. Drugs are often suspected of causing pemphigoid; stopping medication or changing to a different oral medication may help.

CLINICAL MANIFESTATIONS. Oral blisters are present in 24% of patients. If present, they are mild and transient. Pemphigoid begins with a localized area of erythema or with pruritic urticarial plaques that gradually become more edematous and extensive. A diagnosis of hives is frequently made in this preblistering stage. The amount of itching varies but is usually moderate to severe. A group of elderly patients had pruritus for a mean period of 10 months before the diagnosis was made. In most cases the plaques turn dark red or cyanotic in 1 to 3 weeks, resembling erythema multiforme, as vesicles and bullae rapidly appear on their surface.

The eruption is usually generalized (Figure 16-24, *A-B*). The most common sites are the lower part of the abdomen, the groin, and the flexor surfaces of the arms and legs. The palms and soles are affected. Involvement of genital mucous membranes occurs in 7% of patients. The 1- to 7-cm bullae appear isolated or in clusters and are tense with good structural integrity, in contrast to the large, flaccid, easily ruptured bullae of pemphigus. Firm pressure on the blister will not result in extension into normal skin as occurs in pemphigus; therefore Nikolsky's sign is negative. Most bullae rupture within 1 week, leaving an eroded base that, unlike the situation with pemphigus, does not spread and heals rapidly.

Many localized clinical variants of bullous pemphigoid have been reported (vesicular, vegetating, hyperkeratotic, erythrodermic) that have the same histologic and immunologic characteristics as generalized bullous pemphigoid. Bullous pemphigoid may occur at sites of trauma and with little spread of the condition outside such areas. The diagnosis is confirmed with histologic studies and direct and/or indirect immunofluorescence. See the next section on localized bullous pemphigoid. Ultraviolet light and scratching may induce bullae and should be avoided. One should consider stopping or changing oral medications that are sometimes suspected of causing pemphigoid.

DIFFERENTIAL DIAGNOSIS. The differential diagnosis includes epidermolysis bullosa acquisita, dermatitis herpetiformis, pemphigus, bullous systemic lupus erythematosus, and bullous drug eruptions.

BULLOUS PEMPHIGOID

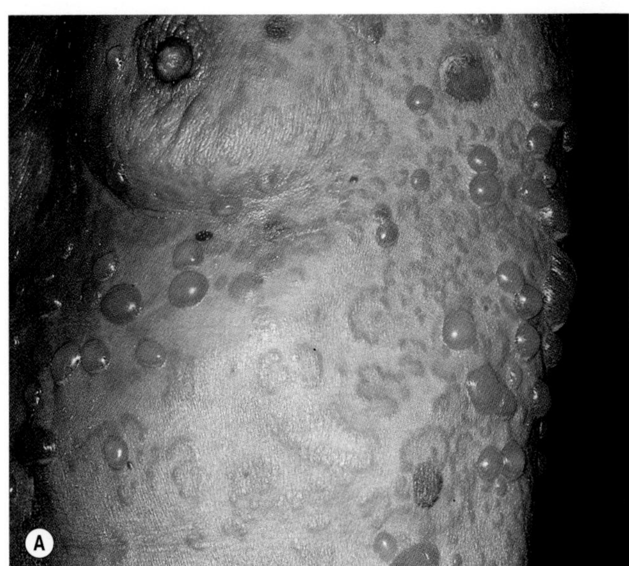

Generalized eruption with tense blisters arising from an edematous, erythematous annular base.

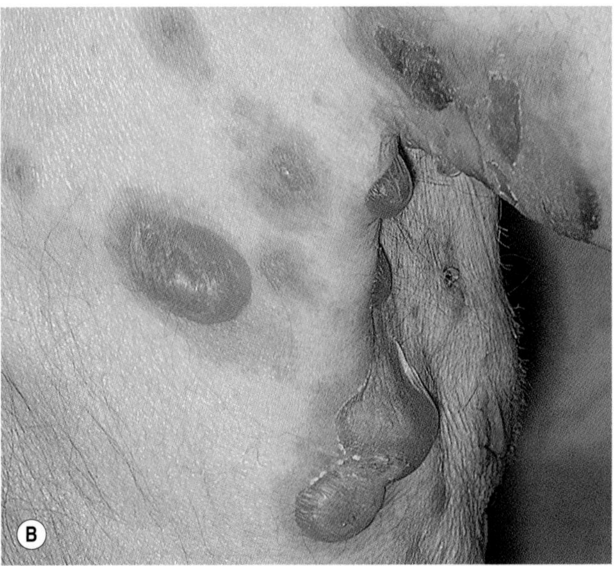

Urticarial lesions may appear weeks or months before the appearance of blisters. Bullae occur on normal-appearing and erythematous skin. They heal without scarring or milia formation.

Figure 16-24

COURSE AND PROGNOSIS. The course is variable. Untreated pemphigoid may remain localized and undergo spontaneous remission, or it may become generalized. Generalized BP has a poor prognosis, especially in older patients and those in poor general condition. The prognosis was documented in 82 bullous pemphigoid patients treated with a variety of medications. The mortality at 1 year was 19%, and treatment was believed to be contributory in seven deaths. The duration varied from 9 weeks to 17 years. The remission rate was 30% at 2 years and 50% at 3 years. Late relapse was observed after disease-free intervals of more than 5 years. Throughout this impressive disease, patients remain afebrile, relatively comfortable, and ambulatory. No clinical, immunologic, or immunogenetic factors are predictive of disease duration.

Of the factors related to bullous pemphigoid activity (duration; pruritus; and number and extent of blisters, eosinophilia, and serum antibodies), only generalized pemphigoid was predictive of death in comparison with localized forms. The presence of circulating autoantibodies against BP180 autoantigen but not autoantibodies against BP230 was found to be significantly more frequent (60% vs. 25%) in BP patients who died within the first year of treatment. Older patients who required a higher dosage of oral glucocorticosteroids at hospital discharge and who had low serum albumin levels were at higher risk of death within the first year after hospitalization.

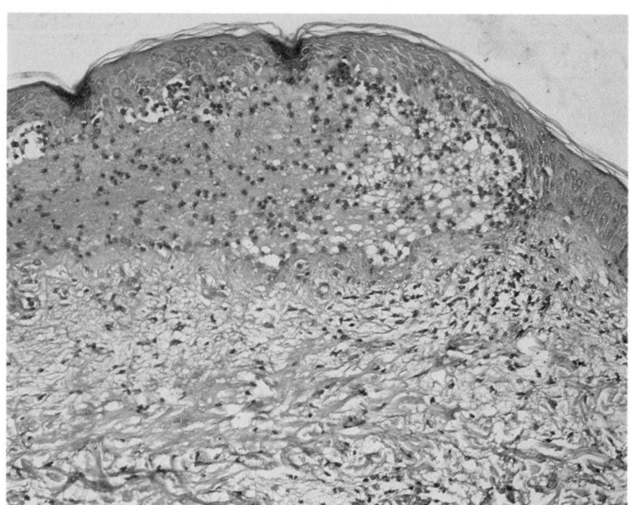

Figure 16-25 Bullous pemphigoid. A subepidermal blister contains numerous eosinophils.

LABORATORY. Peripheral blood eosinophilia occurs in 50% of patients, and elevated levels of serum IgE in 85%. Remission of BP is paralleled by a decrease of serum levels of IgE and the different IgG subclasses reactive with BP180.

Skin biopsy for light microscopy. There are two important features to demonstrate in biopsy specimens of bullous diseases: the level of cleft formation (i.e., intraepidermal or subepidermal) and the presence or absence of an inflammatory infiltrate, as well as the type of cell present (e.g., eosinophils or neutrophils). Bullae in pemphigoid may arise from inflamed (infiltrate-rich) or noninflamed (infiltrate-poor) skin; the most information is provided through a biopsy on an early bulla on inflamed skin. Histologically, there are subepidermal bullae with eosinophils in the dermis and bullae cavities (Figure 16-25).

Direct immunofluorescence of skin. Another 3- or 4-mm punch biopsy specimen is taken and submitted in special transport media. The highest diagnostic yield for direct immunofluorescence (DIF) comes from biopsy specimens of inflamed skin next to a blister. DIF results are positive in a high percentage of patients even after treatment is initiated. The yield is 62% from oral mucosal biopsy specimens.

DIF shows IgG and/or C3 and, sometimes, IgA, IgM, and fibrin in a linear band at the BMZ. Similar findings can be observed in epidermolysis bullosa acquisita, cicatricial pemphigoid, herpes gestationis, and bullous eruption of systemic lupus erythematosus. Therefore indirect immunofluorescence studies are necessary to complete the evaluation. Bullous pemphigoid and epidermolysis bullosa acquisita (EBA) are characterized by linear IgG deposits along the BMZ. Patients with EBA are more likely to have IgG staining without concomitant C3 deposition than are patients with bullous pemphigoid. Biopsy specimens treated with sodium chloride separate through the lamina lucida. The IgG appears in the dermal side of the split specimens in EBA and predominantly or exclusively in the epidermal side in bullous pemphigoid. DIF studies relate to treatment responses. As the disease subsides, complement C3 deposits disappear. Normal skin of the forearm can be used for such studies.

Indirect immunofluorescence. Most cases of BP can be diagnosed with serologic studies. By indirect immunofluorescence microscopy using NaCl-separated human skin, 87% of cases reveal circulating serum IgG antibodies.

These antibodies detect the 230-kilodalton (230-kDa) major or the 160- to 180-kDa minor bullous pemphigoid antigens synthesized by keratinocytes. Some BP sera recognize both antigen proteins, while others detect only BP230 or BP180 or none. Their level does not correlate with disease activity as it does in pemphigus. In sera analyzed for reactivity with BP180, autoantibodies are detected in 90% by immunoblot analysis or by ELISA. In contrast to indirect immunofluorescence reactivity that reflects reactivity to both BP180 and BP230, serum levels of autoantibodies to BP180 correlate with disease activity in BP. Therefore assaying reactivity to BP180 may be a helpful guide for disease management.

Approximately 10% to 15% of patients may not have detectable circulating autoantibodies using salt-split skin indirect immunofluorescence studies; these patients should be evaluated using the salt-split skin direct immunofluorescence assay.

TREATMENT. The degree of involvement and the rate of disease progression dictate treatment.

Itching is controlled with hydroxyzine (Atarax) 10 to 50 mg every 4 hours as needed. Systemic steroids combined with immunosuppressive agents such as azathioprine, cyclophosphamide, methotrexate, or chlorambucil have been the mainstay of therapy. Antibiotics, dapsone, and topical steroids may be a safe and effective alternative for some patients. For more information, see the treatment section for cicatricial pemphigoid.

Topical steroids. A study showed that topical corticosteroid therapy is effective for limited, moderate, and severe bullous pemphigoid and is superior to oral corticosteroid therapy for extensive disease. Patients received either topical clobetasol propionate cream (40 gm per day) or oral prednisone (0.5 mg/kg of body weight per day for those with moderate disease, and 1 mg/kg per day for those with extensive disease). Disease was controlled at 3 weeks in the entire topical corticosteroid group. Severe complications occurred in 29% of the topical corticosteroid group and in 54% in the oral prednisone group. *PMID: 11821508*

Antibiotics. Studies have reported an excellent clinical response when localized or generalized bullous pemphigoid was treated with tetracycline, minocycline, or erythromycin, with or without niacinamide. The recommended schedules are tetracycline or erythromycin 1.0 to 2.5 gm/day, or minocycline 200 mg/day and niacinamide 1.5 to 2.5 gm/day. Patients with generalized bullous pemphigoid were treated with tetracycline (2 gm daily) without niacinamide. Bulla formation was significantly reduced within 1 week and stopped within 1 to 3 weeks. The 2-gm dosage was maintained for 1 to 2 months, decreased by 500-mg decrements every month, and then stopped. These drugs may suppress the inflammatory response at the BMZ, inhibit neutrophil chemotaxis, and increase cohesion of the dermoepidermal junction. The effect may be enhanced by the synergetic effect of niacinamide.

***Sulfones*.** The efficacy of dapsone is limited. Patients who have a neutrophil-predominant infiltrate may be the best candidates for this drug. The response occurs within 2 weeks; the dosage of dapsone is usually 100 mg/day. The dosage is regulated according to the patient's response. Dapsone therapy is described in detail under the Dermatitis Herpetiformis and Linear IgA Bullous Dermatosis sections earlier in this chapter.

Prednisone and immunosuppressive drugs (adjuvant therapy). The mainstay of therapy in past years has been systemic corticosteroids. Patients who do not respond to attempts to control their conditions with topical steroids, antibiotics, and dapsone and require suppression may be treated with prednisone or prednisolone. Most authorities recommend an initial dosage of 0.75 to 1 mg/kg per day divided in two daily doses. Most patients are controlled in 28 days. As the disease comes under control the prednisone therapy is tapered to every other day and then stopped. The time required for resolution with prednisone depends on the number of blisters on day 1. The addition of dapsone to the existing regimen of corticosteroids may help to produce a clinical remission, to lower the dosage of prednisone, and to taper off prednisone more easily.

Noncontrolled trials have reported the use of adjuvant therapies with steroid-sparing effects. These have included methotrexate, mycophenolate mofetil, azathioprine, cyclophosphamide, and chlorambucil.

Consider adjuvant immunosuppressive therapy with azathioprine if dapsone and prednisone fail. Azathioprine is continued for another 3 to 6 months and stopped when the disease has cleared. Cyclophosphamide is also used as a steroid-sparring drug. It is more toxic than azathioprine and is reserved for elderly patients who have extensive disease and who do not tolerate azathioprine.

Methotrexate. Low-dose oral pulse methotrexate may be an effective alternative in patients with generalized bullous pemphigoid. Initiate treatment with oral methotrexate (10 mg/week). The methotrexate treatment is modified according to the following responses: (1) if the number of blisters increases, the dosage is increased by 2.5 mg/week; (2) if severe itching is present, a potent topical corticosteroid (0.5% clobetasol) is added, to a maximum of 20 gm/day, and its use is discontinued if the itching stops; and (3) if a positive response appears to be permanent, the dosage is reduced by 2.5 mg/week every 2 months, and then discontinued. *PMID: 14623719*

Mycophenolate mofetil. One study showed that mycophenolate mofetil and azathioprine demonstrate similar efficacy during treatment of bullous pemphigoid, and similar cumulative corticosteroid doses were given in both treatment arms to control disease. Mycophenolate mofetil showed a significantly lower liver toxicity profile than azathioprine therapy (see p. 298). *PMID: 18087004*

Azathioprine. Azathioprine as a single agent may be considered for older patients with more significant disease who do not respond to dapsone or antibiotics and who do not tolerate prednisone. Younger patients are usually not treated with azathioprine because of the increased risk of malignant neoplasms. Patients respond within 3 to 6 months of treatment. Treatment may then be stopped and restarted with disease flares (see p. 302).

The risk of azathioprine-induced myelosuppression can be predicted by detecting patients with intermediate or low thiopurine methyltransferase (TPMT) activity.

TPMT levels are evaluated to ensure the patient receives adequate levels of azathioprine.

OTHER TREATMENTS. Cyclosporine, plasmapheresis, and intravenous immunoglobulin (IVIG) have been used in patients with severe progressive disease. IVIG is reported to have a low rate of efficacy.

Localized pemphigoid

Cicatricial pemphigoid (mucosal surfaces), localized childhood vulvar pemphigoid, pretibial pemphigoid (nonscarring bullous lesions predominantly on the legs of women), localized chronic pemphigoid of Brunsting-Perry (crops of grouped blisters on the head and neck that heal with atrophic scars), dyshidrosiform pemphigoid (vesiculobullous hemorrhagic lesions of the palms and soles), and pemphigoid vegetans (erosive and vegetating plaques) are variants of localized pemphigoid. These patients possess the same circulating IgG autoantibodies as patients with generalized bullous pemphigoid. Direct immunofluorescence is, however, a less useful diagnostic test in localized bullous pemphigoid; the intensity of the reaction correlates roughly with the extent of disease.

MUCOUS MEMBRANE PEMPHIGOID. Cicatricial pemphigoid, or mucous membrane pemphigoid (MMP), is a rare, chronic, subepidermal blistering and scarring disease. It is characterized by the production of autoantibodies against BMZ antigens (lamina lucida proteins involved in human keratinocyte adhesion to extracellular matrix). MMP affects persons older than 40 years of age and has a 2:1 predilection for women. Any mucous membrane can be involved, but the most commonly involved sites in decreasing frequency include the oral mucosa (85%), conjunctiva (64%), skin (24%), pharynx (19%), external genitalia (17%), nasal mucosa (15%), larynx (8%), anus (4%), and esophagus (4%). Unlike bullous pemphigoid, there are few remissions.

Oral disease. The mouth is involved in 85% of cases. Desquamative gingivitis is the most frequent manifestation. The gingiva appears red with diffuse or patchy involvement (Figure 16-26). Oral vesiculobullous lesions form, and then rupture, leaving clean, noninflamed erosions that are relatively painless and do not interfere with eating. The vermilion border of the lips is spared, in contrast to the situation with pemphigus. Hoarseness is a sign of laryngeal involvement (8% of cases). A subset of patients have only oral disease, which has a relatively benign course compared with patients with oral cavity and other mucosae and skin involvement.

Ocular disease. The eye is involved in 65% of cases. Unilateral conjunctivitis is often the initial presentation; within 2 years the disease is usually bilateral. Fibrosis beneath the conjunctival epithelium is the primary destructive process. Gradual shrinkage of the conjunctiva leads to obliteration of the conjunctival sac (Figure 16-27). Reduced tearing with erosion and neovascularization of the cornea leads to corneal opacification and perforation. Fibrous conjunctival adhesions become more numerous; the disease leads to blindness in approximately 20% of cases. Prolonged periods of remission after stopping therapy occur in one third of patients. Follow-up must be continued for life, because relapse occurs in 22% of those who were in remission and not undergoing therapy.

Other mucous membranes. Nasopharyngeal involvement can lead to ulcerations of the septum, stenosis, and obstruction necessitating a tracheostomy. Esophageal disease may manifest with ulcerations, dysphagia, odynophagia, strictures, and stenosis. Urethral stenosis, vaginal orifice stenosis, and rectal stenosis have also resulted from chronic inflammation and scarring attributable to MMP.

Skin disease. Approximately 25% of patients develop cutaneous lesions, consisting of scattered tense vesicles or bullae that arise from a red base, usually on the face, neck, and scalp (Figure 16-28). Vesicles rupture and leave an erosion that eventually heals with or without atrophic scars. Fibrous adhesions and atrophy can occur on the penis,

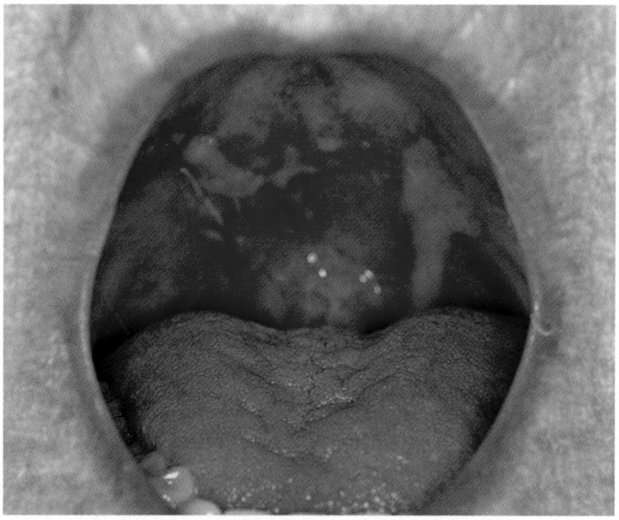

Figure 16-26 Cicatricial pemphigoid. Recurrent, painful erosions occur in the mouth. Scarring may lead to esophageal stenosis.

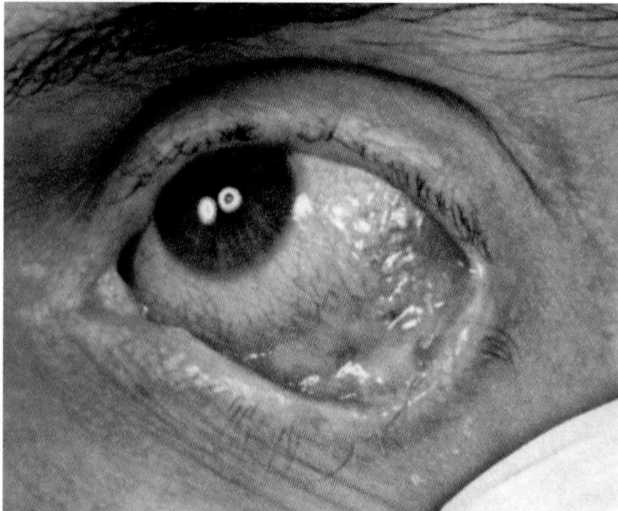

Figure 16-27 Cicatricial pemphigoid. Patients with ocular involvement present with pain, conjunctivitis, and conjunctival erosions, which lead to development of entropion and many other ocular changes, including opacification and blindness.

vulva, vagina (17% of cases), and anus. When there is involvement of the head and neck but not the mucous membrane, the disease is known as the Brunsting-Perry type of cicatricial pemphigoid.

DIAGNOSIS

The biopsy shows a subepidermal bulla with little inflammation. Direct immunofluorescence of lesional, perilesional, and normal mucous membrane biopsy specimens shows linear deposition of complement and IgG and, less often, IgA. Circulating IgG and IgA antibodies are found in 10% of cases with routine techniques and up to 82% when salt-split human skin is used as a substrate. The autoantibodies bind to the epidermal roof in most cases.

TREATMENT

Patients with MMP are treated like those with bullous pemphigoid (see the Treatment section under Bullous Pemphigoid). Treatment is guided by the extent of disease and the site of involvement. Ocular, laryngeal, esophageal, and genital involvement are treated aggressively.

PLAN OF THERAPY. Treat localized disease with topical therapy and use intralesional steroids if that fails. Start dapsone if topical therapy is ineffective. Patients not responsive to dapsone after 12 weeks are treated with prednisone with or without dapsone. Immunosuppressive agents and prednisone are used if dapsone fails. Cyclophosphamide is tried first; azathioprine is the alternate choice. The response is slow. The skin and oral lesions respond more quickly and predictably than the eye lesions. Most patients require long-term suppression. Taper and withdraw drugs when a remission is achieved.

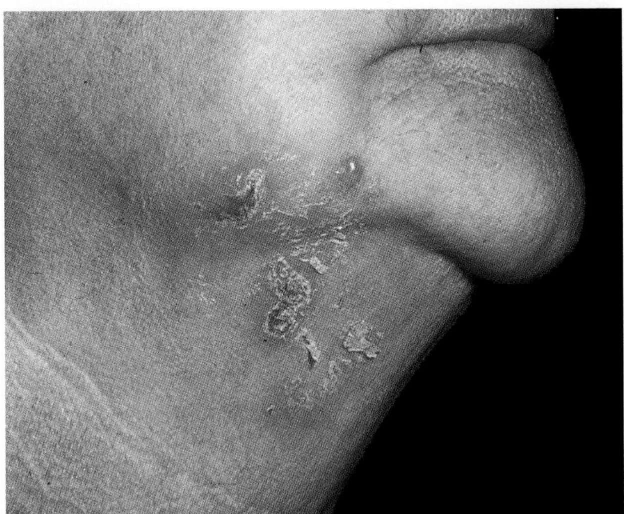

Figure 16-28 Cicatrical pemphigoid. Blisters or erosions appear on normal skin or red plaques. Common sites include the head and neck. Lesions heal with scarring and milia.

TOPICAL THERAPY

Oral cavity. Debride dead tissue from the oral mucosa. Hydrogen peroxide, elixir of dexamethasone, and elixir of diphenhydramine are each diluted with tap water to a concentration of 1:4 or 1:6, as tolerated. They are not swallowed. Before meals, patients rinse with hydrogen peroxide and diphenhydramine (reduces pain, does not suppress taste completely as does viscous lidocaine). After meals, patients rinse with hydrogen peroxide to remove food particles and debris, and then with dexamethasone for its antiinflammatory effect. Between meals and before bedtime, patients rinse with hydrogen peroxide and then with dexamethasone. This schedule is demanding but effective. Treat oral lesions with fluocinonide gel, which is more adherent and results in better patient compliance than triamcinolone acetonide in Orabase. Food can be puréed in a blender if eating is painful.

Eyes. Lubricate frequently with artificial tears and ointments. Infection of the lids is treated with topical or systemic antibiotics. Topical steroids are not effective.

Intralesional therapy. Lesions of the skin, oral cavity, nose, genitalia, and anus respond to intralesional steroids. Inject high in the dermis to avoid atrophy. Use triamcinolone acetonide (dilution of 5 to 10 mg/ml); repeat every 2 to 4 weeks.

SYSTEMIC THERAPY

Dapsone. Dapsone (75 to 200 mg/day) is the drug of first choice; it controls the inflammation in most patients and achieves a remission in others.

Corticosteroids. Prednisone (0.75 to 1 mg/kg per day) is used. The initial dose depends on the severity of the disease. A twice-daily dosage is used during the acute stage and changed to a single daily morning dose after new blister formation stops. Taper dosage slowly to avoid a relapse.

Immunosuppressive agents (adjuvant therapy). Immunosuppressive agents have a corticosteroid-sparing effect. They are started when corticosteroids are initiated or shortly afterward. Cyclophosphamide (1.5 to 2.5 mg/kg/day) is superior to azathioprine but is more toxic. Azathioprine is the alternate choice. A significant response requires 8 to 12 weeks.

Etanercept. Chronic overproduction of tumor necrosis factor-α (TNF-α) has been implicated in the pathogenesis of MMP. Case reports have documented the effectiveness of etanercept in patients recalcitrant to prednisone.

Antibiotics. Infections of the mucous membranes and skin are treated with systemic antibiotics (e.g., doxycycline 200 mg/day).

SURGICAL THERAPY. Surgery to deal with scarring and to prevent blindness, upper airway stenosis, or esophageal stricture is performed after disease activity has stopped.

LOCALIZED VULVAR PEMPHIGOID

Childhood localized vulvar pemphigoid is a morphologic variant of bullous pemphigoid. Patients present with recurrent vulvar vesicles and ulcers. Scarring may or may not occur. As with generalized pemphigoid, direct immunofluorescence shows linear IgG and C3 at the basement membrane, and indirect immunofluorescence is positive in some cases. Lesions may be treated with a group III through V topical steroid. Oral erythromycin may be effective, as is reported for generalized pemphigoid. Periodic outbreaks have been reported to occur for 3 years. Cases have been misdiagnosed as child abuse.

Benign chronic bullous dermatosis of childhood

Chronic bullous dermatosis of childhood is a rare, nonhereditary, subepidermal blistering disease with clinical features similar to those of bullous pemphigoid and dermatitis herpetiformis except that there is only moderate itching. Large, tense subepidermal bullae appear in clusters on the face (particularly around the mouth), lower trunk, inner thighs, and genitalia. A significant number of patients have linear IgA deposits at the BMZ, circulating IgA anti-BMZ antibodies, and normal jejunal biopsy results. The prognosis is good: the disease eventually clears after remissions and exacerbations, and always before puberty. Corticosteroids are used only if dapsone fails.

Herpes gestationis (pemphigoid gestationis)

Herpes gestationis (HG), an intensely pruritic, blistering disease of pregnancy, occurs in fewer than 1 in 50,000 pregnancies. There is a genetic predisposition; 90% of patients express class II antigens (HLA-DR3 and HLA-DR4) and a class III antigen (C4). HG appears to be mediated by an IgG1 specific for a 180-kDa component of hemidesmosomes. The disease may appear for the first time during any pregnancy, but once it has occurred, it tends to reappear earlier and be more severe during any subsequent pregnancy. The disorder usually appears during the second or third trimester but may occur from the second week to the early postpartum period. It disappears 1 or 2 months after delivery and recurs with subsequent pregnancies. The newborn fetus has cutaneous involvement 10% of the time. HG is associated with an increase in prematurity.

CLINICAL PRESENTATION. The intensity of disease varies. HG may be subclinical or mild and nonvesicular during one pregnancy, and explosive and vesiculobullous during another. Edematous plaques occur in crops on the abdomen and extremities and coalesce into bizarre polycyclic rings covering wide areas of the skin (Figure 16-29). As with pemphigoid, within days to weeks the tense blisters evolve from the edematous plaques, rupture to leave slowly healing denuded areas, and heal without scarring; they do cause postinflammatory hyperpigmentation. Spontaneous clearing may be seen during the latter period of the pregnancy, but flares are seen at the time of delivery in 75% to 80% of cases. Mild recurrences may occur with menstruation and the use of oral contraceptives. Mucous membrane involvement is rare.

DIAGNOSIS. Biopsy specimens taken from inflamed skin adjacent to a blister exhibit histologic features similar to those of pemphigoid. A bandlike deposit of C3 in most cases and IgG in 10% of cases can be demonstrated at the BMZ by direct immunofluorescence. Antibodies to the 180-kDa bullous pemphigoid (BP) antigen (BP180), which is type 17 collagen contained in the hemidesmosomal components, are present.

The herpes gestationis antibody can pass through the placenta and may be responsible for the transient pemphigoid-like skin lesions present in some newborns of affected mothers. Peripheral eosinophilia is the only other common laboratory abnormality.

TREATMENT. Mild cases of pemphigoid gestationis may respond to topical corticosteroid therapy with or without orally administered antihistamines Most patients require prednisone (0.5 to 1.0 mg/kg per day) in divided doses. There appears to be no difference in the frequency of uncomplicated live births in patients with pemphigoid gestationis treated with systemic glucocorticoids versus those treated with topical agents. If systemic glucocorticoids are administered during pregnancy, newborns are at risk for development of reversible adrenal insufficiency. As with pemphigoid, the dosage is adjusted to disease response.

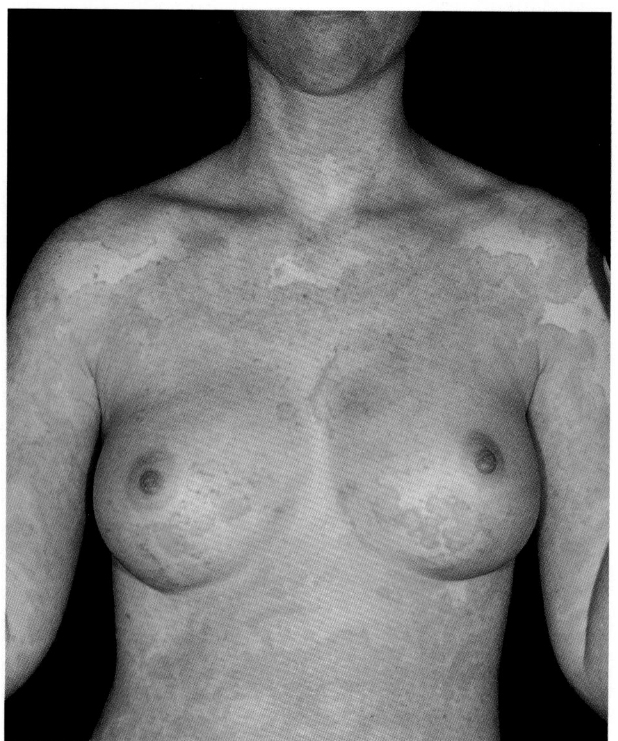

Figure 16-29 Herpes gestationis. Blisters arise from erythematous, edematous polycyclic rings.

PEMPHIGOID-LIKE DISEASE

Epidermolysis bullosa acquisita

Epidermolysis bullosa acquisita (EBA) is a rare, chronic, subepidermal, mucocutaneous blistering disease characterized by skin fragility and spontaneous, trauma-induced blisters that heal with scar formation and milia.

The clinical and histologic picture may mimic bullous or cicatricial pemphigoid and bullous systemic lupus erythematosus. It is characterized by a chronic course, poor response to therapy, and occasional remissions. It is seen in children and adults. There are two distinctive clinical presentations that are not mutually exclusive. Diagnosis requires immunofluorescence studies of serum and biopsy specimens.

TYPE VII COLLAGEN. EBA is associated with autoimmunity to type VII collagen. Type VII collagen (the protein component of anchoring fibrils that fortify the attachment of the epidermis to the dermis) is the target molecule in EBA. Autoantibodies interfere with type VII collagen function and are believed to play an important role in the pathogenesis of sublamina densa blister formation in this disease.

CLASSIC EPIDERMOLYSIS BULLOSA ACQUISITA. The classical or mechanobullous form of EBA is characterized by skin fragility and trauma-induced blisters and erosions with mild mucous membrane involvement and healing with dense scars. It resembles the dystrophic forms of inherited epidermolysis bullosa. Classic EBA presents with tense blisters on a noninflammatory base. They appear in trauma-prone areas of the palms, soles, elbows, and knees. The lesions heal with scarring and milia formation that resembles porphyria cutanea tarda (Figure 16-30). Some of these patients may have scarring alopecia and nail dystrophy.

EBA may extensively (or predominantly) affect mucosal epithelia in a manner resembling cicatricial pemphigoid. Ocular involvement is common, but visual loss is rare.

BULLOUS PEMPHIGOID-LIKE EPIDERMOLYSIS BULLOSA ACQUISITA. Approximately 50% of patients with EBA present this type of clinical picture early in the course of their disease. Tense blisters on an inflammatory base are widely distributed on the trunk and flexural surfaces. There is pruritus, minimal skin fragility, and healing of some of the lesions without scarring and milia (Figure 16-31).

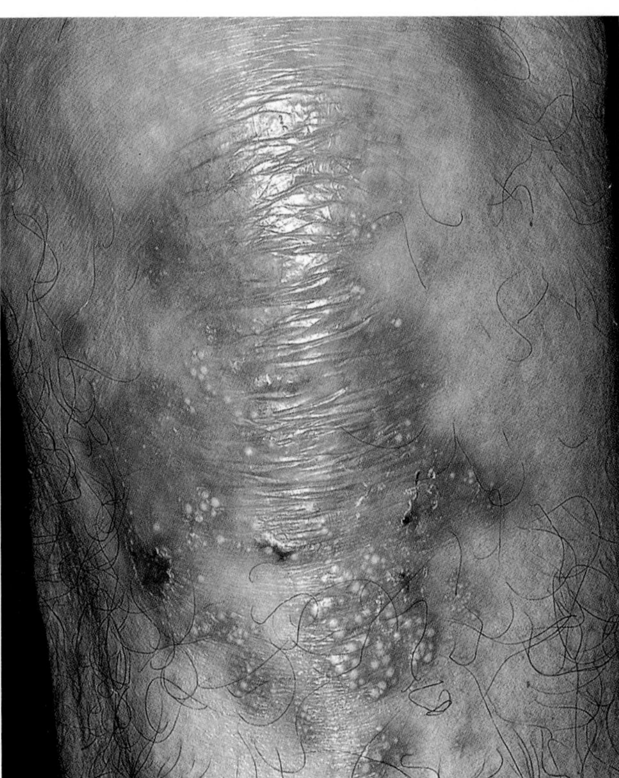

Figure 16-30 Epidermolysis bullosa acquisita. There are several forms of the disease. The mildly inflammatory form is the most common and presents with vesicles and bullae on the extensor surfaces of the hands, elbows, and knees. This form resembles the dominantly inherited form of epidermolysis bullosa dystrophica and heals with scar and milia formation.

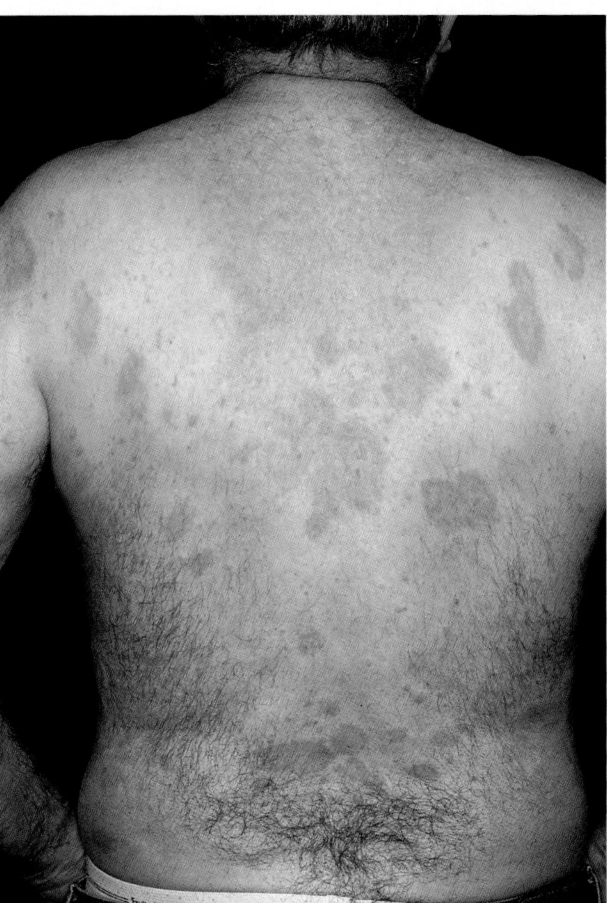

Figure 16-31 Bullous pemphigoid-like epidermolysis bullosa acquista. This generalized form presents with bullae and resembles bullous pemphigoid. Lesions heal with little or no scarring.

DIAGNOSIS. Special immunofluorescence tests are required to differentiate EBA from bullous pemphigoid (see Table 16-5). Direct immunofluorescence of perilesional skin shows linear and homogeneous deposits of IgG and C3 in the BMZ; bullous pemphigoid shows the same picture. These two diseases can be distinguished by studies of serum tested by indirect immunofluorescence on salt-split normal skin or by obtaining a fresh perilesional skin biopsy, inducing a split at the lamina lucida, and testing for the site of IgG deposition by direct immunofluorescence. Deposition of IgG on the dermal side of the separation differentiates EBA from bullous pemphigoid, which shows IgG on the epidermal side of the separation. Indirect immunofluorescence studies of serum with 1 mol/L NaCl-separated human skin shows IgG anti-BMZ autoantibody (anti–type VII collagen antibodies) bound to the dermal side of the separation.

TREATMENT. Most patients respond poorly to topical and systemic therapy. Some patients respond to high-dose prednisone therapy. Dapsone, azathioprine, colchicine (0.6 to 1.5 mg a day for up to 4 years), cyclosporine (6 mg/kg/day), and rituximab may be effective. Response to intravenous immunoglobulins is documented in case reports. *PMID: 11952298*

BENIGN FAMILIAL CHRONIC PEMPHIGUS

Benign familial chronic pemphigus (Hailey-Hailey disease) is a rare, autosomal dominant, intraepidermal (Figure 16-32), nonscarring bullous disease characterized by erosions, blisters, and warty papules. The disease first appears in adolescence or early adult life, usually during the summer; it is characterized by remissions and exacerbations. Lesions develop on areas exposed to ultraviolet light (nape of the neck and back) and on areas subjected to friction and maceration (axillae and groin). Friction, heat, and sweating exacerbate the lesions, and pain may limit physical activities. Infection with staphylococci, herpes simplex virus, or *Candida* may also precipitate the disease. Longitudinal white bands are present in the fingernails in 71% of patients. Suction tests on clinically normal skin demonstrate a widespread subclinical abnormality in keratinocyte adhesion. An ultraviolet provocation test has been used to identify genetic carriers of Hailey-Hailey disease.

NONINTERTRIGINOUS LESIONS. The eruption begins with a group of pruritic vesicles arising from a red or noninflamed base; they are grouped in an annular or serpiginous pattern (Figure 16-33). The vesicles rupture quickly and are replaced by an advancing rim of scale and crust similar to that seen in impetigo and tinea. The active border extends peripherally, leaving a pale, hypopigmented center. New crops of vesicles appear on the border but rupture so quickly that they may not be appreciated. These moist, indurated plaques ooze serum. Lesions may heal spontaneously in colder weather.

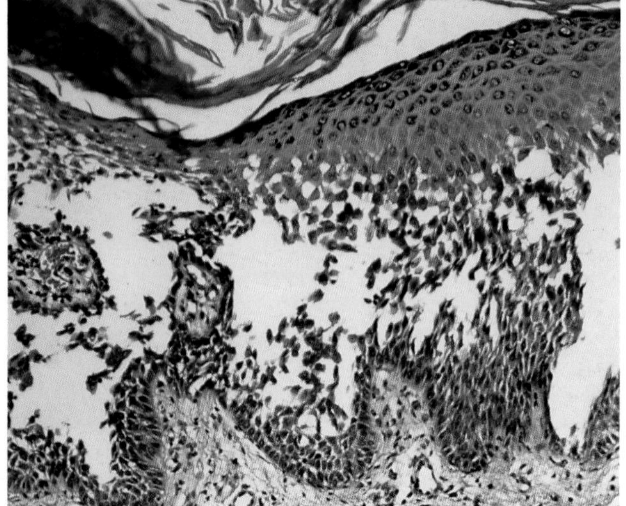

Figure 16-32 Benign familial chronic pemphigus. Intraepidermal acantholysis (separation of keratinocytes) is seen.

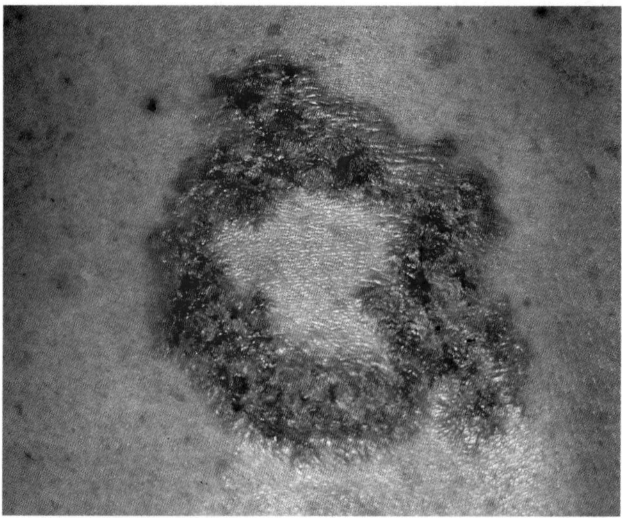

Figure 16-33 Benign familial chronic pemphigus. Vesicles and red plaques with crusts occur in the genital area, on the chest, and axillae.

INTERTRIGINOUS LESIONS (Figures 16-34 and 16-35). Vesicles sometimes appear in intertriginous lesions, but most often the patient has broad, moist, red, fissured areas or vegetating warty papules and plaques that do not extend beyond the opposing skin surfaces of the groin or axillae. Intertriginous lesions are chronic and respond slowly to therapy, especially in obese patients.

TREATMENT

Nonintertriginous lesions. Oral antibiotic therapy (e.g., erythromycin, dicloxacillin, or a cephalosporin) should be started, followed in 3 or 4 days by administration of a group III through V topical steroid. Most lesions of the back and neck respond quickly to this simple program, and treatment is stopped when the lesions have healed. Sunscreens should be worn on exposed surfaces in the summer.

Intertriginous lesions. Groin and axillary lesions may be infected with bacteria and yeast. Therapy with one of the previously listed oral antibiotics is started, and anti-yeast creams (e.g., ketoconazole) are applied. Cream is applied to moist lesions and compressed with cool Burow's or silver nitrate solution. Compressing is discontinued once the surfaces are dry, and group V topical steroid creams are applied twice a day until lesions have healed. Chronic and unresponsive lesions have been treated successfully by excision, topical cyclosporine, carbon dioxide laser, split-thickness skin grafting, and dermabrasion.

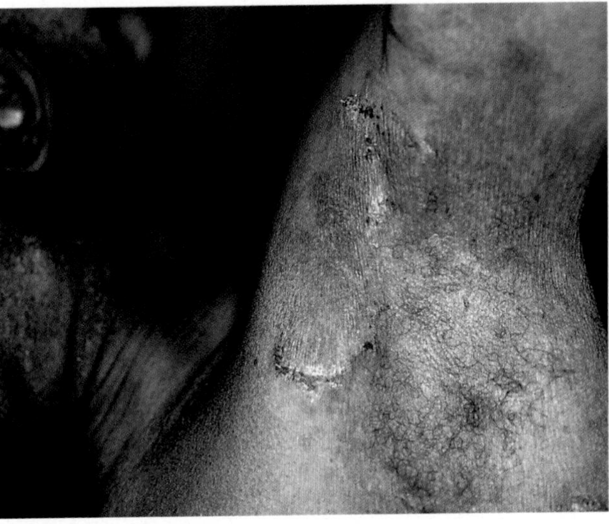

Figure 16-34 Benign familial chronic pemphigus. The axilla is a common site.

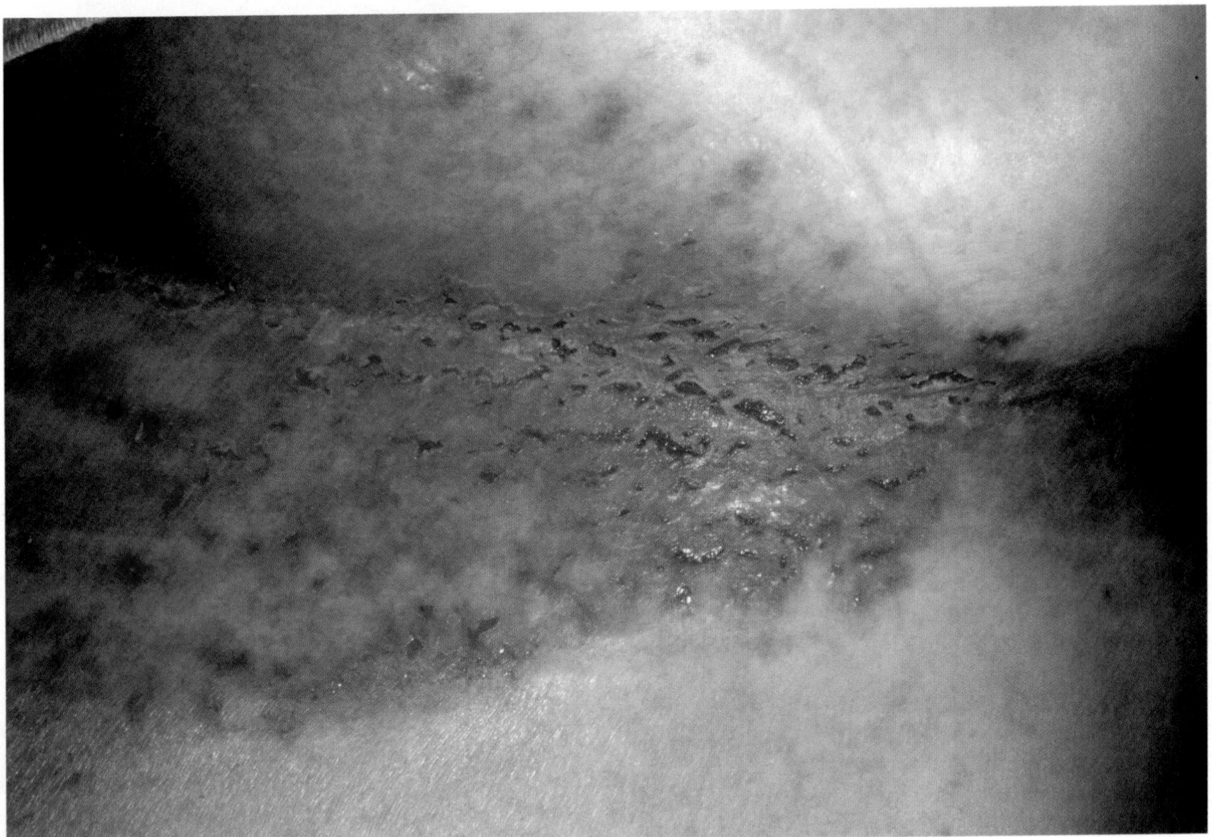

Figure 16-35 Benign familial chronic pemphigus. Chronic, recurrent blistering with erosions occurs primarily in intertriginous regions.

EPIDERMOLYSIS BULLOSA

Epidermolysis bullosa is a term given to three major groups and approximately 16 variants of rare dominant and recessive genetic diseases in which minor trauma causes noninflammatory blistering (mechanobullous diseases). These diseases are classified as scarring or nonscarring and histologically by the level of blister formation.

The National Epidermolysis Bullosa Registry assists patients and physicians in determining what form of epidermolysis they have and advises them on treatment, medical management, and genetic counseling. Approximately 50 epidermolysis cases occur per 1 million live births in the United States. Of these cases, approximately 92% are epidermolysis bullosa simplex, 5% are dystrophic epidermolysis bullosa, and 1% are junctional epidermolysis bullosa.

CLINICAL CLASSIFICATION (SCARRING VS. NONSCARRING). The clinical classification is based on the presence or absence of dystrophic changes and scarring. The intraepidermal forms (epidermolysis bullosa simplex) do not scar. Junctional forms (junctional epidermolysis bullosa) manifest as atrophy. Dermal forms (dystrophic epidermolysis) result in atrophy and scarring.

HISTOLOGIC CLASSIFICATION (LEVEL OF BLISTER FORMATION). Classification is based on light and electron microscopic levels of separation:

- Split-through epidermal basal cells—intraepidermal types
- Split-through basement membrane area—junctional types
- Split-through upper dermis—dermal forms

Epidermolysis bullosa simplex. The disease is autosomal dominant. The cleavage plane is in epidermis. Sporadic cases may arise by new mutation. Blistering begins in infancy or childhood, especially on the hands and feet or any other point of trauma, and heals without scarring (Figure 16-36). The mucosa, nails, and teeth are usually not affected. The major complication is infection.

Junctional epidermolysis bullosa. The disease is autosomal recessive. In most cases severe, generalized blistering of the skin with the exception of the palms and soles begins in infancy. There is scarring in some variants. Extensive involvement of the mouth, larynx, eyes, and esophagus is often present. The dentition may become defective. Most patients die in early childhood.

Dystrophic epidermolysis bullosa. This disease may be either autosomal dominant or autosomal recessive. There is great variation in the severity of the several forms of dystrophic epidermolysis bullosa. The severe, recessive form exhibits repeated cycles of blistering and scarring that lead to fusion of the digits, producing the so-called mitten deformity (Figure 16-37).

DIAGNOSIS. Electron microscopic examination of the skin is the standard for diagnosis. Monoclonal antibodies have recently been used for diagnosis. Immunofluorescence tests for localization of type IV collagen, laminin, and pemphigoid antibodies in the roof or floor of bullae help differentiate the forms of epidermolysis bullosa.

MANAGEMENT. Patients must avoid trauma. Dilantin, a known collagenase inhibitor, is not an effective treatment for recessive dystrophic epidermolysis bullosa. Genetic counseling is essential, and fetal skin biopsy techniques have been developed for prenatal diagnosis. Additional information can be obtained from the Dystrophic Epidermolysis Bullosa Research Association of America (D.E.B.R.A.) (www.debra.org/).

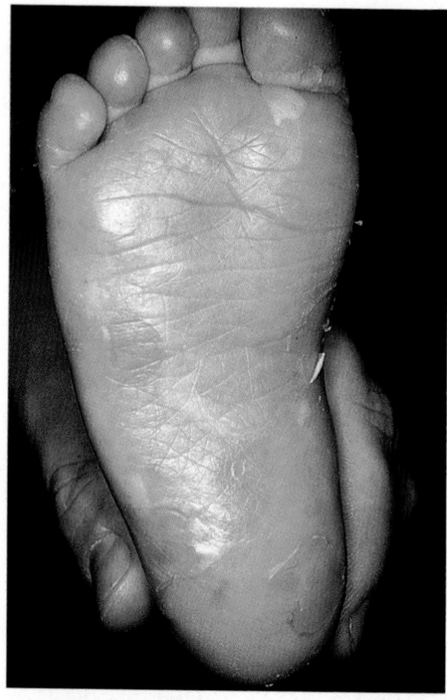

Figure 16-36 Epidermolysis bullosa simplex. Fragility of the skin results in nonscarring blisters caused by little or no trauma. There are several subtypes. Mild blistering of the hands and feet is called Weber-Cockayne syndrome. The inheritance is autosomal dominant.

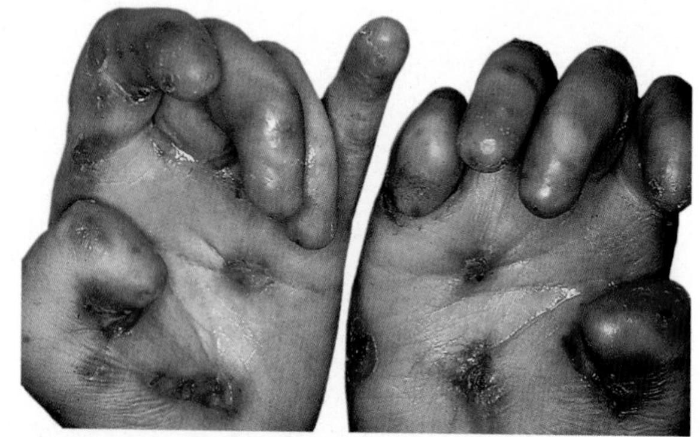

Figure 16-37 Dystrophic epidermolysis bullosa is characterized by blistering in response to the slightest trauma. Repetitive trauma leads to a mitten-like deformity with digits encased in an epidermal "cocoon."

THE NEWBORN WITH BLISTERS, PUSTULES, EROSIONS, AND ULCERATIONS

There are more than 30 diseases in the newborn that can present with blisters, pustules, erosions, and ulcerations (Boxes 16-2 to 16-4). For diagnostic purposes they are divided into infectious causes, common transient skin lesions, and uncommon and rare causes (Table 16-5). The most common transient diseases are described in the following section. The following laboratory tests may be helpful: bacterial, viral, or fungal cultures; Gram stain; Wright's stain; Tzanck smears; potassium hydroxide (KOH) preparations; and skin biopsies.

DIAGNOSIS. The diagnosis is usually based on clinical findings. The Tzanck smear should be the first test performed. It detects herpes infection (multinucleated giant cells) and noninfectious pustular eruptions (eosinophils, neutrophils). Gram stain and potassium hydroxide preparation detect bacterial and fungal infections.

The main benign transient neonatal types of pustulosis are erythema toxicum neonatorum, transient neonatal pustular melanosis, and neonatal acne.

Box 16-3 Conditions Where Bullae May Predominate

Common causes

Bullous impetigo
Sucking blisters

Uncommon causes

Epidermolysis bullosa
Staphylococcal scalded skin syndrome

Rare causes

Acrodermatitis enteropathica
Aplasia cutis congenita
Chronic bullous dermatosis of childhood
Congenital protein C or S deficiency
Congenital syphilis
Diffuse cutaneous mastocytosis
Ectodermal dysplasias
Epidermolytic hyperkeratosis
Erythropoietic porphyria
Maternal bullous disease
Neonatal varicella
Perinatal gangrene of the buttock
Pseudomonal infection
Toxic epidermal necrolysis

From Frieden IJ: *Curr Probl Dermatol* 4:123, 1992.

Box 16-2 Conditions Where Pustules or Vesicles Predominate

Common causes

Erythema toxicum neonatorum
Miliaria
Neonatal acne
Neonatal candidiasis
Neonatal pustular melanosis
Staphylococcal pyoderma

Uncommon causes

Acropustulosis of infancy
Congenital candidiasis
Herpes simplex
Incontinentia pigmenti
Scabies

Rare causes

Acrodermatitis enteropathica
Congenital self-healing histiocytosis
Cytomegalovirus
Eosinophilic pustular folliculitis
Hyperimmunoglobulin E syndrome
Listeria monocytogenes
Neonatal Behçet's syndrome
Varicella

From Frieden IJ: *Curr Probl Dermatol* 4:123, 1992.

Box 16-4 Conditions Where Erosions or Ulcerations May Predominate

Common causes

Skin changes attributable to perinatal or neonatal trauma
Sucking blisters

Uncommon causes

Aplasia cutis congenita
Epidermolysis bullosa
Herpes simplex, especially congenital
Staphylococcal scalded skin syndrome

Rare causes

Aspergillus infection
Congenital erosive and vesicular dermatosis
Congenital protein C deficiency
Ectodermal dysplasias
Group B streptococcal infection
Hemangiomas and vascular malformations
Intrauterine varicella infection
Neonatal Behçet's syndrome
Neonatal lupus erythematosus
Pseudomonas aeruginosa (ecthyma gangrenosum)
Perinatal gangrene of the buttock
Toxic epidermal necrolysis

From Frieden IJ: *Curr Probl Dermatol* 4:123, 1992.

Table 16-5 Differential Diagnosis: Blisters and Pustules in the Newborn

Disease	Usual age	Skin: Morphology
Infectious causes		
Staphylococcal pyoderma	A few days to weeks	Pustules, bullae, occasional vesicles
Staphylococcal scalded skin syndrome	3-7 days; occasionally older	Erythema, cutaneous tenderness, superficial blisters, erosions
Group A streptococcal disease	A few days to weeks	Isolated pustules, honey-crusted areas
Group B streptococcal disease	At birth or first few days	Vesicles, bullae, erosions, honey-crusted lesions
Listeria monocytogenes	Usually at birth	Hemorrhagic pustules and petechiae
Haemophilus influenzae	Birth or first few days	Vesicles and crusted areas
Pseudomonas aeruginosa	Days to weeks	Erythema, pustules, hemorrhagic bullae, necrotic ulcerations
Congenital syphilis	Usually at birth	Blisters or erosions on dusky or hemorrhagic base
Congenital candidiasis	At birth or first week	Erythema and fine papules evolve into vesicles and pustules
Neonatal candidiasis	Weeks to months	Scaly red patches with satellite papules and pustules
Aspergillus	5+ days	Morphology: pustules rapidly evolve to other ulcers
Neonatal herpes simplex	Usually 5-14 days	Vesicles, crusts, erosions may be grouped or not; may follow dermatome
Intrauterine herpes simplex	At birth	Vesicles, widespread bullae, erosions, scars, missing skin
Fetal varicella infection	At birth	Usually scarring, limb hypoplasia, erosions
Neonatal varicella	0-14 days	Vesicles on an erythematous base; may be very numerous
Scabies	3-4 weeks or later	Papules, nodules, crusted area
Transient skin lesions		
Erythema toxicum neonatorum	Usually 24-48 hr	Erythematous macules, papules, and pustules
Neonatal pustular melanosis	At birth	Pustules without erythema; hyperpigmented macules; some have collarette of scale
Miliaria crystallina	Usually first week of life	Dewdrop-like vesicles, very superficial, no erythema
Miliaria rubra	Days to weeks	Erythematous papules with superimposed pustules
Sucking blisters	At birth	Flaccid bulla or bullae on nonerythematous base
Neonatal acne	3-4 weeks	Comedones, papules, pustules
Skin changes of perinatal/neonatal trauma	Birth to few days	Erosions on scalp, perineal or scalp gangrene (rare)

Skin: Usual distribution	Clinical: Other	Diagnosis/Findings
Mainly diaper area, periumbilical	Boys more than girls; may be in epidemic setting	Gram stain: polymorphonuclear neutrophilic leukocytes, gram + cocci in clusters Bacterial culture
Generalized, begins on face; blistering and erosions in areas of mechanical stress	Irritability, fever	Skin biopsy: separation from upper epidermis Bacterial cultures: blood, urine, etc.
No specific area predisposed	Moist umbilical stump; occasional cellulitis, meningitis, pneumonia	Gram stain: gram + cocci in chains; bacterial l cuture
No specific area predisposed	Pneumonia, bacteremia	Gram stain: gram + cocci chains; bacterial culture
Generalized, especially trunk and extremities	Septic; respiratory distress; maternal	Gram stain: gram + rods; bacterial culture
No specific area predisposed	Bacteremia, meningitis may be present	Gram stain: small gram-bacilli; bacterial culture
Any area; may concentrate in diaper area	Prematurity, history of surgery, GI or pulmonary anomalies are risk factors	Skin or tissue Gram stain: gram-negative rods; cultures of skin, blood, etc.
Palms, soles, knees, abdomen	Low birth weight, hepatosplenomegaly, metaphyseal dystrophy	Dark field of involved skin; incompletely treated maternal syphilis
Any part of body; palms and soles often involved	Prematurity and foreign body in cervix or uterus are risk factors	KOH: hyphae, budding yeast
Diaper area or intertriginous areas	Usually none; previous antibiotic prescribed	KOH: hyphae, budding yeast
Any area	Extreme prematurity/immunocompromised host	Skin biopsy: septate hyphae; tissue fungal culture
Anywhere; scalp monitor site, torso, oral lesions are most frequent sites	Signs of sepsis; irritability and lethargy; eye, CNS* are frequent sites of disease	Tzanck smear viral culture
Anywhere on body	Low birth weight; microcephaly, chorioretinitis	Tzanck smear viral culture
Anywhere; usually extremities	Maternal varicella first trimester	Tzanck smear viral culture
Generalized distribution	Maternal varicella 7 days before to 2 days after delivery	Tzanck smear viral culture
Generalized, palms, soles	Others in family with itching or rash	Scabies prep: mites (eggs, feces)
Buttocks, torso, proximal extremities; no palms, soles	Usually term infants over 2500 gm	Wright's stain: eosinophils
Anywhere; most common on forehead, behind ears, neck, back, fingers, toes	Term infants; more common in black infants	Wright's stain: PMNs, occasional eosinophils
Forehead, upper trunk, volar forearms most common sites	May be history of warm incubator, occlusive clothing, dressings	Usually clinical; Wright's Gram stain negative
Same as miliaria crystallina	Same as miliaria crystallina	Usually clinical; skin biopsy if doubt
Radial forearm, wrist, hand, dorsal, thumb, index finger	Infants sucks vigorously on affected areas	Clinical diagnosis
Mainly cheeks, forehead	Comedones clue to diagnosis	Clinical diagnosis
Scalp, perineum, heels	History of fetal monitoring, vacuum extraction, neonatal intensive care	Usually clinical diagnosis

Continued

Table 16-5 Differential Diagnosis: Blisters and Pustules in the Newborn—cont'd

Disease	Usual age	Skin: Morphology
Uncommon and rare causes		
Perinatal gangrene of buttock	First few hours to days of life	Erythema or blanching, then localized gangrene, hemorrhagic bulla
Acropustulosis of infancy	Birth or first days or weeks	Vesicles and pustules
Congenital self-healing histiocytosis	Usually at birth	Erythematous papules, pustules, vesicles, crusting
Diffuse cutaneous mastocytosis	Birth, first weeks of life	Bullae, infiltrated skin, hives, dermographism
Maternal bullous disease	At birth	Tense or flaccid bullae or erosions
Neonatal lupus erythematosus	Birth, first few days	Erosions, other scaly or atrophic plaques
Neonatal Behçet's syndrome	Congenital or first few days	Mucous membrane erosions, pustules, and necrotic ulcers
Chronic bullous dermatosis of childhood	One congenital case	Tense blisters, often grouped with rosettes, sausage-shaped
Toxic epidermal necrolysis	Birth to few weeks of age	Diffuse skin erythema, tenderness, erosions
Erosive and vesicular dermatosis	Birth	Vesicles and erosions
Hemangiomas and vascular malformations	Birth or first few weeks	Ulcerations overlie macular erythema or obvious vascular anomaly
Eosinophilic pustular folliculitis	Birth or later	Multiple pustules, crusted area
Acrodermatitis enteropathica	Weeks to months	Sharply demarcated psoriasiform plaques, sometimes vesicles and bullae
Epidermolysis bullosa (EB)	Birth, rarely later	Bullae or erosions, milla nail dystrophy in dystrophic EB, occasional aplasia cutis
Epidermolytic hyperkeratosis	Birth	Bullae, erosions, ichthyotic areas of skin
Incontinentia pigmenti	Birth or first weeks	Linear streaks of erythematous papules and vesicles
Hyperimmunoglobulin E syndrome	Days to weeks	Multiple vesicles, grouped and individual
Aplasia cutis congenital	Birth	One or multiple membrane-covered, depressed areas of skin or raw, ulcerated areas
Ectodermal dysplasias (ED)	Congenital or early infancy	Vesicles or bullae
Erythropoietic porphyria	Early infancy	Vesicles or bullae
Protein C or S deficiency	Birth or first days of life	Hemorrhagic bullae and cutaneous infarctions

From Frieden IJ: *Curr Probl Dermatol* 4:123, 1992.
CNS, central nervous system; *GI,* gastrointestinal.

Skin: Usual distribution	Clinical: Other	Diagnosis/Findings
Buttock, perineal area; unilateral	Variable history, umbilical artery catheterization	Clinical diagnosis
Hands and feet, especially medial	Severe pruritus; lesions come in crops on palms and soles	Clinical; skin biopsy: intraepidermal pustule
Generalized distribution	Check lymph nodes, liver, spleen, blood, bones	Skin biopsy: large histiocytes
Generalized distribution, bleeding, diatheses	Wheezing, diarrhea	Skin biopsy: infiltrate of mast cells
Generalized distribution	Maternal history of blistering disease	Maternal history, direct immunofluorescence
Face, upper torso	Occasional pancytopenia; heart block	Skin biopsy: epidermal atrophy and vascular interface dermatitis; positive maternal neonatal serology (anti-SSA, SSB)
Oral, genital mucosa; extremities, especially periungual	Maternal history of Behçet's syndrome	Circulating immune complexes; elevated IgG, decreased total hemolytic complement
Generalized; may concentrate in perineum	Neonatal case: severe eye involvement, milia	Skin biopsy: subepidermal bulla; direct immunofluorescence: linear IgA
Generalized distribution	Graft-vs.-host disease, *Klebsiella* sepsis, etc.	Skin biopsy: full-thickness necrosis
Generalized, over 75% of body	? infection or placental infarctions	? Clinical
Ear, lip, perineum, extremities	Contiguous vascular anomaly usually evident	Clinical
Scalp, hands, feet	Frequent eosinophilia	Skin biopsy: folliculitis with eosinophils
Periorificial and acral	Diarrhea, irritability, alopecia, history of hyperalimentation	Serum zinc level < 50
Anywhere, especially extremities, mucosa	Other epithelial tissues (i.e., GI, genitourinary, cornea, trachea) may be affected	Skin biopsy for electron microscopy or immunofluorescence mapping
Generalized; blisters more on hands and feet	Family history may be positive	Skin biopsy: big keratohyaline granules
Generalized following Blaschko's lines	Family history may be positive; eye, CNS, and other abnormalities	Skin biopsy: eosinophilic spongiosis and dyskeratosis
Generalized distribution	Recurrent *S. aureus* infection, eosinophilia	? Clinical (IgE not high in newborn period)
Usually scalp, may be elsewhere	May be associated with epidermal nevus, placental infarctions, etc.	Clinical or skin biopsy
Depends on specific kind; acral in some; Blaschko's lines in Goltz syndrome	Sweating, limb, oral abnormalities, varies with specific kind of ED	Usually clinical diagnosis
Photodistribution	Hemolytic anemia, pink urine	High porphyrins in blood, urine
May be focal or generalized	Blood picture consistent with disseminated intravascular coagulation	Absent protein C or S in blood

COMMON TRANSIENT SKIN LESIONS

Erythema toxicum neonatorum. Lesions are not present at birth. Erythema toxicum neonatorum (ETN) (toxic erythema of the newborn) occurs in 20% to 50% of term infants—usually second and later deliveries—who are otherwise healthy. It is rare in premature infants and in those weighing less than 2500 gm. Most cases occur between 24 and 48 hours of age.

The rash often begins on the face; the trunk, proximal extremities, and buttocks are commonly involved. Palms and soles are not affected. Lesions may localize at pressure sites. Four types of lesions occur: macules, wheals, papules, and pustules. Tiny papules and pustules are superimposed on macules or wheals. New lesions appear as older lesions resolve. Wright's stain of a pustule shows numerous eosinophils. Peripheral eosinophilia is unusual.

Transient neonatal pustular melanosis. Lesions are present at birth but may be overlooked for 1 or 2 days. Transient neonatal pustular melanosis (TNPM) occurs in 2% to 5% of term black infants or neonates and 0.6% of whites infants or neonates who are otherwise healthy. Vesiculopustules, with no underlying erythema, rupture and form a hyperpigmented macule with a collarette of scale. Lesions may be solitary or grouped; most are 2 to 3 mm in diameter. They are located on the forehead, behind the ears, under the chin, on the neck and back, and on the hands and feet. The palms and soles may be affected. Lesions are very superficial, located within or just beneath the stratum corneum. Wright's stain shows polymorphonuclear neutrophilic leukocytes (PMNs); eosinophils may predominate. No treatment is necessary. Pustules resolve in a few days; pigmented macules may last for several weeks to months.

A clear-cut differentiation between TNPM and ETN is not always possible. The name sterile transient neonatal pustulosis has been proposed to unify these conditions.

Neonatal acne. Lesions occur 1 to 2 weeks after birth in approximately 20% of newborns. Comedones, papules, and pustules occur in the same distribution as in adolescent acne. Lesions resolve spontaneously.

Miliaria. Lesions occur approximately 1 week after birth. Miliaria, or heat rash, occurs in warm climates, while warming in an incubator, during a fever, or from wearing occlusive dressings or warm clothing. Eccrine sweat duct occlusion is the initial event. The duct ruptures, leaks sweat into the surrounding tissues, and induces an inflammatory response. Occlusion occurs at two different levels to produce two distinct forms of miliaria. In miliaria crystallina, occlusion of the eccrine duct at the skin surface results in accumulation of sweat under the stratum corneum. The lesion appears as a clear dewdrop. There is little or no erythema. The vesicles appear individually or in clusters. Miliaria rubra results from occlusion of the intraepidermal section of the eccrine sweat duct. Papules and vesicles surrounded by a red halo or diffuse erythema develop as the inflammatory response develops. A cool water compress and proper ventilation are all that is necessary to treat this self-limited process.

Chapter 17

Connective Tissue Diseases

CHAPTER CONTENTS

AUTOIMMUNE DISEASES

Diseases that result from attack by one's own immune system are called autoimmune diseases. Autoimmune disease are organ-specific illnesses or systemic illnesses such as systemic lupus erythematosus (Table 17-1). Autoimmune diseases are associated with circulating autoantibodies, which bind self-protein. Pathogenesis may be then mediated by autoimmune T lymphocytes and other immune mechanisms. Autoantibodies either are responsible for the manifestations of autoimmune disease or are markers of future disease. Autoantibodies may be found in serum samples many years before disease onset in several of these diseases. Autoimmunity is common in the population, but systemic autoimmune diseases, such as the connective tissue diseases, are relatively rare. Many people show some serologic evidence of autoimmunity but few have the signs and symptoms and disease-specific autoantibodies to make a diagnosis of a connective tissue disease.

Table 17-1 Autoimmune Diseases and Autoantigens*

	Known antigens
Organ-specific diseases	
Addison's disease	21-Hydroxylase
Celiac disease	Tissue transglutaminase
Type 1 diabetes	GAD-65, insulin, IA-2A
Graves' hyperthyroidism	Thyroid-stimulating-hormone receptor
Hashimoto's thyroiditis	Thyroid peroxidase, thyroglobulin
Myasthenia gravis	Acetylcholine receptor
Goodpasture's syndrome	Type IV collagen
Pemphigus vulgaris	Desmoglein 3
Pernicious anemia	H^+/K^+-ATPase, intrinsic factor
Primary biliary cirrhosis	E2 PDC
Vitiligo	Tyrosinase, SOX-10
Multiple sclerosis	Myelin basic protein, myelin oligodendritic glycoprotein
Systemic diseases	
Systemic lupus erythematosus	Spliceosomal snRNP, Ro/La (SS-A/SS-B) particle, histone and native DNA
Sjögren's syndrome	Ro/La ribonuclear particle, muscarinic receptor
Rheumatoid arthritis	Citrullinated cyclic peptide, IgM
Dermatomyositis/polymyositis	t-RNA synthetases
Diffuse systemic sclerosis	Topoisomerase
Limited systemic sclerosis (CREST)	Centromere proteins

From Scofield RH: *Lancet* 363(9420):1544-1546, 2004.
PMID: 15135604
*Autoantibodies as predictors of disease.

CONNECTIVE TISSUE DISEASES

Connective tissue diseases (rheumatoid arthritis, lupus, dermatomyositis, scleroderma, overlap syndromes) are a group of multisystem illnesses of unknown etiology. They have no typical pattern of onset, duration, or organ involvement. This variability makes classification and diagnosis difficult; therefore a list of clinical diagnostic criteria has been established for each entity and is tabulated in the text.

Connective tissue diseases can be more accurately described as autoimmune diseases. Many serum antibodies directed at cellular components (autoantibodies) have been found in each disease and are probably responsible for the clinical manifestations (Figure 17-1).

Diagnosis

The diagnosis of connective tissue disease is made by the clinical picture. Antibodies to cell components (typically nuclear antigens) are present in these multisystem disorders. Detecting and defining them helps support the clinical diagnosis and provides information about subsets of disease and prognosis. A large number of antibodies are reported in the literature. Each systemic autoimmune disease has a characteristic antinuclear antibody (ANA) spectrum. Patients often produce multiple autoantibodies. The problem is knowing which tests to order and how to interpret them. An approach to the diagnosis of connective tissue diseases is shown in Figure 17-2.

SEROLOGIC PROFILES IN CONNECTIVE TISSUE DISEASES

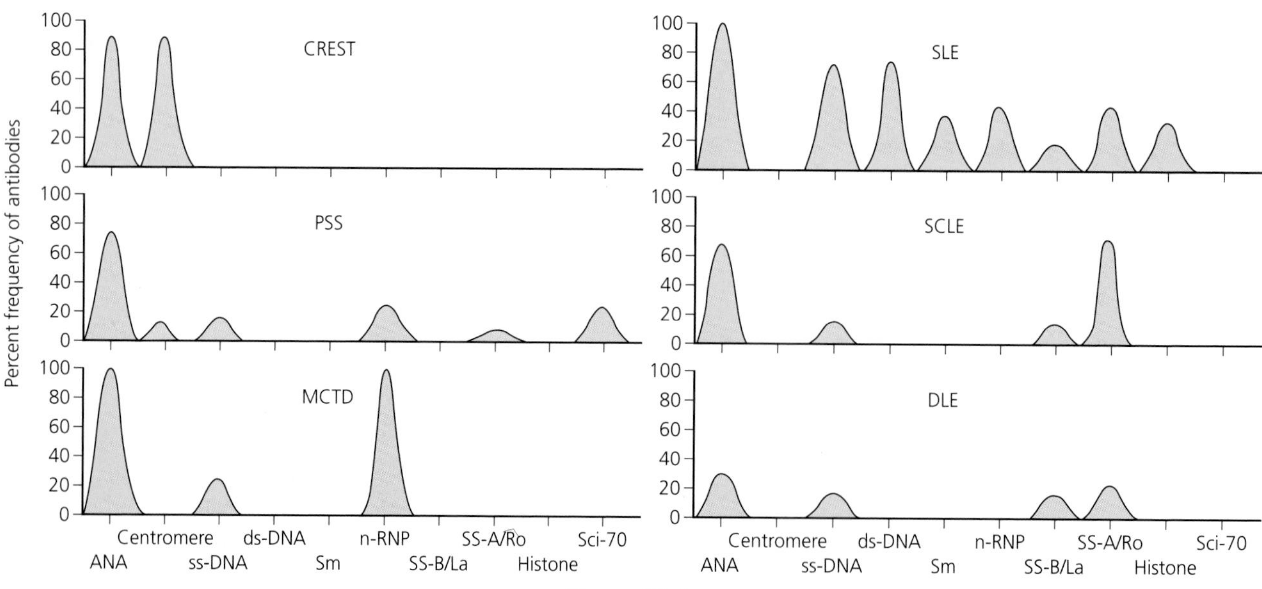

Figure 17-1

APPROACH TO THE DIAGNOSIS OF CONNECTIVE TISSUE DISEASES*

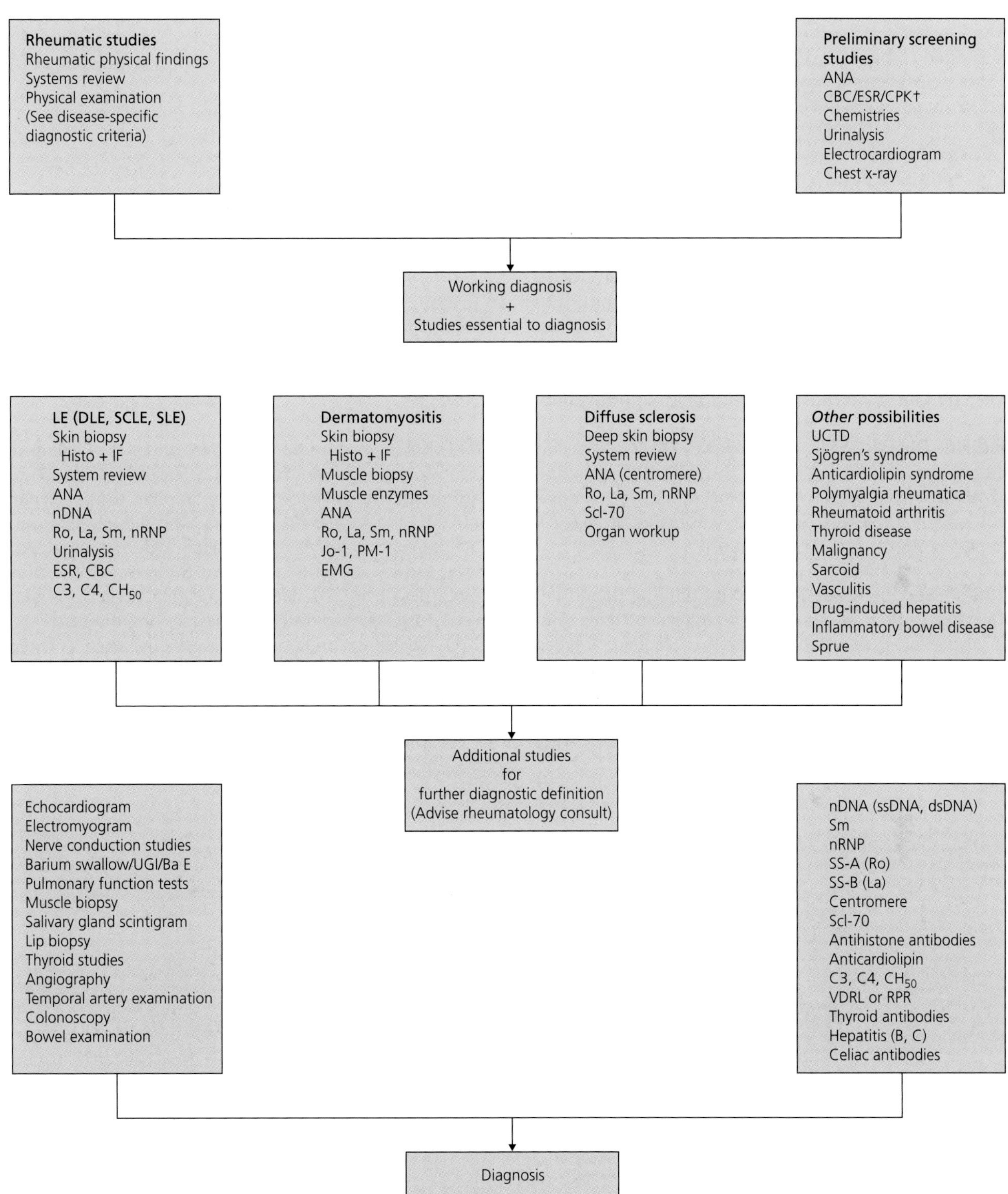

*Flow sheet designed by Constance Passas, M.D. (rheumatologist).
†*CBC,* Complete blood count; *ESR,* erythrocyte sedimentation rate; *CPK,* creatine phosphokinase; *IF,* immunofluorescence; *UCTD,* undifferentiated connective tissue disease (formerly mixed CTD); *EMG,* electromyogram; *ENA,* extractable nuclear antigens; *SLE,* systemic lupus erythematosus; *PSS,* progressive systemic sclerosis; *SCLE,* subacute cutaneous lupus erythematosus; *DLE,* discoid lupus erythematosus.

Figure 17-2

Antinuclear antibody screening

ANA is the first test to order when collagen vascular disease is suspected (Table 17-2).

ANA tests identify antibodies present in serum that bind to autoantigens present in the nuclei of mammalian cells.

A negative result suggests that a connective tissue disease is unlikely; a positive result, especially a high titer in a patient with appropriate clinical findings, supports a diagnosis of a connective tissue disease.

FALSE-POSITIVE TEST RESULTS. Positive results occur in normal blood donors and in patients with chronic liver disease, neoplasms, or active chronic infections. These patients usually have lower titers than those in patients with autoimmune diseases. Any autoantibody test must be interpreted in the context of available clinical information.

SPECIFIC DIAGNOSTIC ANTIBODY TESTS. Specific antibody tests should be ordered. The clinical presentation and ANA pattern help to determine which test to order (Tables 17-3 and 17-4). Some laboratories offer tests for groups of antigens (i.e., ANA profiles).

TITERS. Specimens are screened by diluting them 1:40 with saline. If there is no nuclear fluorescence at this dilution, the result is reported as "negative." If there is green fluorescence, the level of ANA present is determined by repeating the test after serially diluting the specimen. ANA results are now reported by many laboratories using the international unit system (e.g., 1 international unit rather than a titer of 160).

Table 17-2 ANA Screening Test

ANA (on Hep-2 cells)	Frequency of ANA positivity (%)
Systemic lupus erythematosus	95-100
Drug-induced lupus erythematosus	100
Scleroderma	60-95
Sjögren's syndrome	80
Polymyositis-dermatomyositis	49-74
Rheumatoid arthritis	40-60
Mixed connective tissue disease	100
Normal	<4

Modified from Harmon CE: *Med Clin North Am* 69:547, 1985. *PMID: 3892191*

PATTERNS. Antibodies to nuclear antigens attach to the various components of the nucleus. The fluorescein-labeled antihuman immunoglobulins are applied to the preparation and react with ANAs that have attached to the nucleus. The preparation is visualized with a fluorescent microscope. Diverse patterns of nuclear fluorescence (homogeneous, peripheral, speckled, or nucleolar) reflect the binding of antibodies to different nuclear components (Figure 17-3). Nuclear staining patterns were once used as criteria for subsetting, but, with the availability of direct measurements for specific autoantibodies, pattern identification has become less important. The test requires interpretation by visual inspection and consequently lacks a high degree of specificity.

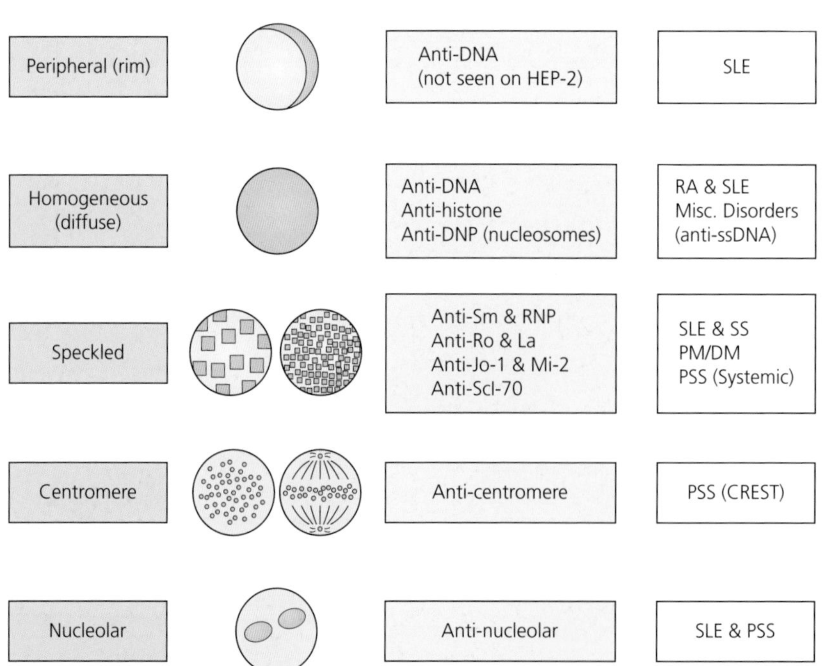

Figure 17-3

Table 17-3 Autoantibody Tests for Connective Tissue Diseases

Antibody	Clinical significance
Antinuclear antibodies	Screening for SLE and PSS
Centromere antibodies	Marker for CREST
Histone antibodies	To exclude drug-induced LE
ENA: Sm antibodies	Marker for SLE
RNP antibodies	SLE, MCTD, scleroderma
SS-A (Ro)/SS-B (La) antibodies	SLE, Sjögren's syndrome, SCLE, and others
Scl-70 antibodies	Marker for scleroderma
Jo-1 antibodies	Marker for polymyositis
Ku (Ki) antibodies	Polymyositis/scleroderma overlap, SLE
Phospholipid antibodies (lupus anticoagulant)	Marker for SLE subset with thrombosis: frequent aborters

Modified from Handbook: clinical relevance of tests, Buffalo, NY: IMMCO Diagnostics, 1993.
ENA, Extractable nuclear antigen; *LE,* lupus erythematosus; *MCTD,* mixed connective tissue disease; *PSS,* progressive systemic sclerosis; *SCLE,* subacute cutaneous lupus erythematosus; *SLE,* systemic lupus erythematosus.

Table 17-4 Diagnostic Significance of Immunologic Findings in Serum and Skin Biopsies in Connective Tissue Diseases

Disease	Biopsy findings: Direct immunofluorescence	Serum findings	Relevance
Systemic LE	LE band (granular immune deposits, IgG, and/or IgM) IgA, C3 at DEJ in lesional and/or normal skin (over 90% in sun-exposed skin)	ANA elevated titers (about 95%-99%); nDNA antibodies about 50%-75%; DNP antibodies <50%; Sm antibodies in about 20%; RNP antibodies in about 5%-30%; SS-A antibodies in about 30%-40%; SS-B antibodies in about 1%-15%; phospholipid antibodies in about 30%-50%; PCNA antibodies in about 2%-10%; Ku(Ki) antibodies in about 10%	DIF, ANA, and ENA usually diagnostic; nDNA and Sm antibodies are diagnostic markers
Discoid LE	LE band, mostly IgG and C in lesion ONLY	Essentially negative; ANA titers usually in normal range	LE band highly characteristic
Subacute, cutaneous LE	LE band in lesion	ANA positive in 70%; SS-A (Ro) antibodies positive in more than 60%	DIF and anti–SS-A (Ro) highly characteristic
Neonatal LE	LE band in lesion (about 50%)	ANA positive in 30%; antibodies to SS-A (Ro) in 100%; antibodies to SS-B (La) in about 60%	DIF and anti–SS-A (Ro) highly characteristic
Drug-induced LE	LE band in lesion (rare)	ANA positive in more than 90%; histone positive about 90%; other antibodies to nDNA and ENA negative	DIF and histone antibodies in absence of other nuclear antibodies highly characteristic
Mixed connective tissue disease	Nuclear IgG or LE band in normal and/or lesional epidermis	Speckled ANA antibodies in more than 95% and RNP antibodies in more than 90%	Serology and/or DIF of nuclei diagnostic for MCTD, SLE, or PSS
Sjögren's syndrome	Negative	ANA positive in about 55%; antibodies to SS-A (Ro) in 43%-88%; SS-B (La) in 14%-60%; RF positive	Positive serum results support diagnosis
Progressive systemic sclerosis (scleroderma)	Nucleolar IgG in epidermis in few cases; most negative	ANA (about 85%) speckled or nucleolar; centromere antibody in CREST (70%-90%); Scl-70 antibodies in diffuse sclerosis (45%) and in acrosclerosis (15%-20%)	DIF limited value; centromere antibodies are diagnostic marker in CREST; Scl-70 antibodies are diagnostic marker in scleroderma
Polymyositis/ dermatomyositis	Negative	ANA usually positive (more than 80%); Jo-1 antibodies in 30% PM, 10% DM; SS-A (Ro) antibodies in 55% PM/scleroderma overlap; Ku (Ki) antibodies in 10% PM/scleroderma overlap	Limited value, but positive serum results support diagnosis
Rheumatoid arthritis	Negative	ANA usually negative or low titer; RF positive in about 90%; RNA positive in about 70%-90% and 95% of RF-negative cases	Positive serum results support diagnosis

DEJ, Dermal-epidermal junction; *DIF,* direct immunofluorescence; *DM,* dermatomyositis; *DNP,* deoxyribonuclear protein; *ENA,* extractable nuclear antigen; *LE,* lupus erythematosus; *MCTD,* mixed connective tissue disease; *PCNA,* proliferating cell nuclear antigen; *PM,* polymyositis; *PSS,* progressive systemic sclerosis; *RNA,* antibodies to rheumatoid arthritis–associated nuclear antigen; *RF,* rheumatoid factor; *SLE,* systemic lupus erythematosus.

Connective tissue laboratory screening tests

The signs and symptoms often associated with connective tissue disease (fatigue, arthralgias, fever, and weight loss) are not specific for autoimmune disease and occur in many other diseases. This makes early and accurate diagnosis difficult. The Mayo Medical Laboratories developed a Connective Tissue Diseases Cascade of tests for the primary care physician to evaluate patients with signs and symptoms compatible with a connective tissue disease in a setting of low disease prevalence. It provides immediate disease-specific, follow-up tests in those patients with presumptive serologic evidence of disease.

This algorithmic approach (Figure 17-4) is more efficient than a panel of tests that can result in unnecessary testing for specific autoantibodies in ANA-negative or low-titer ANA samples. Panel testing carries an increased potential to overdiagnose patients with benign autoimmunity.

FIRST-ORDER TESTS. The Connective Tissue Diseases Cascade begins with the following two tests that are done in all cases:

1. **Cyclic citrullinated peptide antibodies**—Serum autoantibodies to cyclic citrullinated peptide (CCP) are quite specific for rheumatoid arthritis (RA), the most common connective tissue disease. Unlike the test for rheumatoid factor, which has poor specificity for

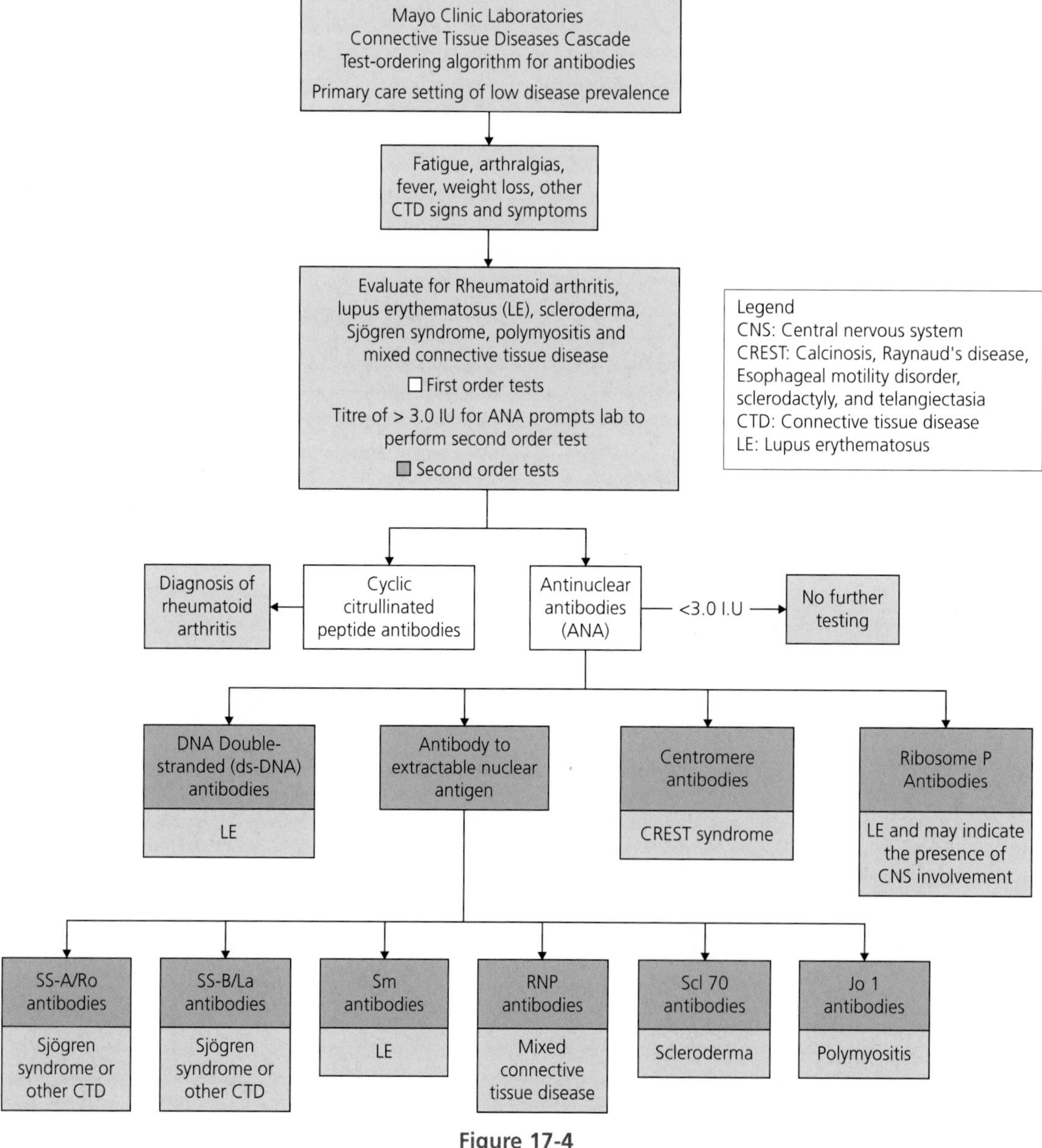

Figure 17-4

RA, the test for CCP antibodies has proven to be reliable for differentiating RA from other connective tissue diseases. This test is not an ideal screening test since it is positive in fewer than 80% of patients with RA and negative test results do not conclusively exclude RA. Strongly positive tests for CCP antibodies have a very high positive predictive value for this disease.

2. **Antinuclear antibodies (ANAs)**—A negative ANA test result is useful for excluding lupus erythematosus and scleroderma, the two most commonly encountered connective tissue diseases other than RA. Other disease-specific autoantibodies rarely occur in sera that test negative or have low levels of reactivity for ANA. Using a cutoff level of 3.0 units for ANA permits detection of >90% of sera with an identifiable specific autoantibody on follow-up testing. If the screening test for ANA is >3.0 units, second-order testing is performed for additional disease-specific autoantibodies.

SECOND-ORDER TESTS. The second level of testing includes the following four components:

1. **Double-stranded DNA (dsDNA) antibody, IgG, serum (anti-dsDNA)**—A positive test result for anti-dsDNA antibodies is found in up to 82% of patients with active lupus erythematosus (LE). Anti-dsDNA antibodies are highly specific for LE, making this test useful for confirming the diagnosis. Low levels may account for false-positive reactivity. The levels of anti-dsDNA correlate with disease activity. Order this as a stand-alone test to monitor disease activity. dsDNA antibodies are also found in 20% to 30% of patients with Sjögren's syndrome, 20% to 25% of patients with mixed connective tissue disease (MCTD), and less than 5% of patients with progressive systemic sclerosis (PSS).
2. **Antibodies to extractable nuclear antigens, serum (ENA)**—The antibodies to the ENA group are comprised of six autoantibodies directed against small nuclear ribonucleoproteins (snRNPs) and enzymes. Autoantibodies to these individual antigens are important serologic markers of particular connective tissue diseases.
   - A. **Autoantibodies to SS-A/Ro, serum (SS-A):** SS-A antibodies occur with variable frequencies in several connective tissue diseases including Sjögren's syndrome, LE, and RA. When present in isolation or with SS-B antibodies, the finding of this autoantibody is consistent with Sjögren's syndrome. SS-A antibodies are found in approximately 60% of patients with Sjögren's syndrome and 35% of patients with LE.
   - B. **Autoantibodies to SS-B/La, serum (SS-B):** SS-B antibodies rarely occur in isolation and are most often encountered in sera that contain SS-A antibodies. SS-B (La) antibody is seen in 50% to 60% of Sjögren's syndrome cases and is specific if it is the only ENA antibody present; 15% to 25% of patients with systemic lupus erythematosus and 5% to 10% of patients with progressive systemic sclerosis also have this antibody.
   - C. **Autoantibodies to Sm, serum (Sm):** Sm antibodies are highly specific for LE. The test for Sm antibodies lacks sensitivity; and this autoantibody is detectable in only approximately 30% of patients with documented LE. The presence of antibodies to Smith (Sm) is often associated with renal disease.
   - D. **Autoantibodies to U(1) RNP, serum (U1RNP):** Antibodies to U1RNP occur in several different connective tissue diseases including mixed connective tissue disease and LE. The finding of U1RNP antibodies in the absence of anti-dsDNA antibodies and antibodies to other ENAs is consistent with the diagnosis of mixed connective tissue disease. U1RNP antibodies have been reported in 71% to 100% of patients with mixed connective tissue disease.
   - E. **Autoantibodies to Scl-70, serum (Scl-70):** Scl-70 antibodies react with the enzyme DNA topoisomerase I and are highly specific for scleroderma. Scl-70 antibodies have been reported in approximately 40% of patients with scleroderma. The presence of Scl-70 antibodies is consistent with the diagnosis of scleroderma and indicates an increased risk for systemic involvement including pulmonary fibrosis.
   - F. **Autoantibodies to Jo-1, serum (Jo-1):** Jo-1 antibodies are highly specific for polymyositis but occur in only approximately 20% of polymyositis patients. The presence of Jo-1 antibody is also found in patients with dermatomyositis, or myositis associated with another rheumatic disease. The finding of Jo-1 antibodies indicates an increased risk for severe disease with pulmonary involvement and fibrosis.
3. **Centromere antibodies, IgG, serum**—Centromere antibodies demonstrate a specific ANA pattern, which is present in 80% to 90% of individuals with CREST variant scleroderma. The pattern is also seen in 30% of patients with Raynaud's phenomenon; 12% of patients with mixed connective tissue disease, diffuse scleroderma, interstitial pulmonary fibrosis, and primary biliary cirrhosis; and in a smaller percent of patients with SLE and RA.
4. **Ribosome P antibodies, IgG, serum**—Autoantibodies reacting with cytoplasmic ribosomes are highly specific for systemic lupus erythematosus. Ribosomal P antibodies are found in approximately 12% of patients with SLE and in 90% of patients with lupus psychosis; titers often increase more than fivefold during and before active phases of psychosis.

LUPUS ERYTHEMATOSUS

Clinical classification (Tables 17-5 and 17-6)

Systemic lupus erythematosus (SLE) is a multisystem disease of unknown origin characterized by the production of numerous diverse types of autoantibodies that, through immune mechanisms in various tissues, cause several combinations of clinical signs, symptoms, and laboratory abnormalities. The natural history of SLE is characterized by episodes of relapses, flares, and remissions. The outcome is highly variable, ranging from remission to death.

The prevalence of LE in North America and northern Europe is about 40 per 100,000 population. There appears to be a higher incidence in blacks and Hispanics. More than 80% of cases occur in women during childbearing years.

Table 17-5 American College of Rheumatology: The 1997 Revised Criteria for Classification of Systemic Lupus Erythematosus*

Definition	Criterion
1. Malar rash	Fixed erythema, flat or raised, over malar eminences, tending to spare nasolabial folds
2. Discoid rash	Erythematous raised patches with adherent keratotic scaling and follicular plugging; atrophic scarring may occur in older lesions
3. Photosensitivity	Skin rash as a result of unusual reaction to sunlight, by patient history or physician observation
4. Oral ulcers	Oral or nasopharyngeal ulceration, usually painless, observed by physician
5. Arthritis	Nonerosive arthritis involving 2 or more peripheral joints, characterized by tenderness, swelling, or effusion
6. Serositis	(a) Pleuritis—convincing history of pleuritic pain or rubbing heard by a physician or evidence of pleural effusion **or** (b) Pericarditis—documented by ECG or rub or evidence of pericardial effusion
7. Renal disorder	(a) Persistent proteinuria greater than 0.5 gm per day or greater than 3+ if quantitation not performed **or** (b) Cellular casts—may be red cell, hemoglobin, granular, tubular, or mixed
8. Neurologic disorder	(a) Seizures—in absence of offending drugs or known metabolic derangements (e.g., uremia, ketoacidosis, or electrolyte imbalance) **or** (b) Psychosis—in absence of offending drugs or known metabolic derangements (e.g., uremia, ketoacidosis, or electrolyte imbalance)
9. Hematologic disorder	(a) Hemolytic anemia—with reticulocytosis **or** (b) Leukopenia—less than 4000/mm^3 total on 2 or more occasions **or** (c) Lymphopenia—less than 1500/mm^3 on 2 or more occasions **or** (d) Thrombocytopenia—less than 100,000/mm^3 in absence of offending drugs
10. Immunologic disorder	(a) Anti-DNA: antibody to native DNA in abnormal titer **or** (b) Anti-Sm: presence of antibody to Sm nuclear antigen **or** (c) Positive finding of antiphospholipid antibodies based on (1) an abnormal serum level of IgG or IgM anticardiolipin antibodies, (2) a positive test result for lupus anticoagulant using a standard method, or (3) A false-positive serologic test for syphilis known to be positive for at least 6 months and confirmed by *Treponema pallidum* immobilization or fluorescent treponemal antibody absorption test; standard methods should be used in testing for presence of antiphospholipid
11. Antinuclear antibody	An abnormal titer of antinuclear antibody by immunofluorescence or an equivalent assay at any point in time and in absence of drugs known to be associated with "drug-induced lupus" syndrome

From Hochberg MC: *Arthritis Rheum* 40:1725, 1997. *PMID: 9324032*

*The proposed classification is based on 11 criteria. For the purpose of identifying patients in clinical studies, a person shall be said to have systemic lupus erythematosus if any 4 or more of the 11 criteria are present, serially or simultaneously, during any interval of observation.

The American College of Rheumatology classification criteria for SLE were updated in 1997 (www.rheumatology.org) (see Table 17-5). The presence of 4 or more of the 11 parameters, serially or simultaneously, is believed to be compatible with the diagnosis of LE. Those criteria in a modified form are illustrated in Figure 17-5.

There are several forms (subsets) of cutaneous erythematosus (see Table 17-6).

Table 17-6 Classification of Cutaneous Lupus Erythematosus

Type	Clinical forms	Clinical and laboratory features	Histologic features
DLE, 15%-20%*	Localized Generalized (lesions above and below neck) Hypertrophic	Usually localized, chronic, scarring lesions of head or neck region or both lasting months to years Usually no extracutaneous disease (5% of patients develop SLE) Antinuclear antibodies occasionally present in low titer; anticytoplasmic antibodies not present Anti-dsDNA antibodies rarely present Subepidermal immunoglobulin deposits commonly found in lesions (75%) but rarely present in uninvolved skin Simultaneous occurrence of severe systemic lupus erythematosus with nephritis is rare	Hydropic degeneration of epidermal basal cell layer with focal epidermal atrophy Heavy mononuclear cell infiltrate in upper dermis, periappendiceal, and perivascular regions, extending into deep dermis
SCLE, 10%-15%*	Papulosquamous (psoriasiform), 8% Annular-polycyclic, 5%*	Usually widespread, nonscarring lesions with associated scaling, depigmentation, and telangiectasias on face, neck, upper and extensor arms (photosensitive distribution) lasting weeks to months; lesions often exacerbated by exposure to sun Usually associated with extracutaneous disease, but severe renal or central nervous system disease uncommon Antinuclear and anticytoplasmic antibodies frequently present (60% of patients) Anti-dsDNA antibodies present in low serum concentrations in 30% of patients; hypocomplementemia rare HLA-A1, HLA-B8, and HLA-DR3 significantly increased Subepidermal immunoglobulin deposits present in only 50% of lesions and 30% of uninvolved skin	Marked hydropic changes along epidermal basal cell layer Moderate mononuclear cell infiltrate in superficial dermis only Pilosebaceous atrophy, hyperkeratosis; direct IF staining reveals discrete, speckled IgG deposits in basal cell cytoplasm associated with Ro/SS-A antibodies
Acute cutaneous LE, 30%-50%*	Localized, indurated erythematous lesions (malar areas of face—butterfly rash) Widespread indurated erythema (face, scalp, neck, upper chest, shoulders, extensor arms, backs of hands)	Transient (hours to days) Multisystem disease usually present; renal disease common Antinuclear antibodies usually present Anti-dsDNA antibodies present in 60%-80% of patients, often in high concentration; hypocomplementemia common Subepidermal immunoglobulin deposits commonly found in lesional (>95%) and exposed nonlesional (75%) skin	Hydropic changes along epidermal basal layer Sparse mononuclear cell infiltrate and upper dermal edema

Modified from Gilliam JN, Sontheimer RD: *J Am Acad Dermatol* 4:471, 1981 *PMID: 7229150*; and Valesk JE et al: *J Am Acad Dermatol* 27:194, 1992.
*Estimated percentage incidence in systemic lupus erythematosus.
dsDNA, Double-stranded DNA.

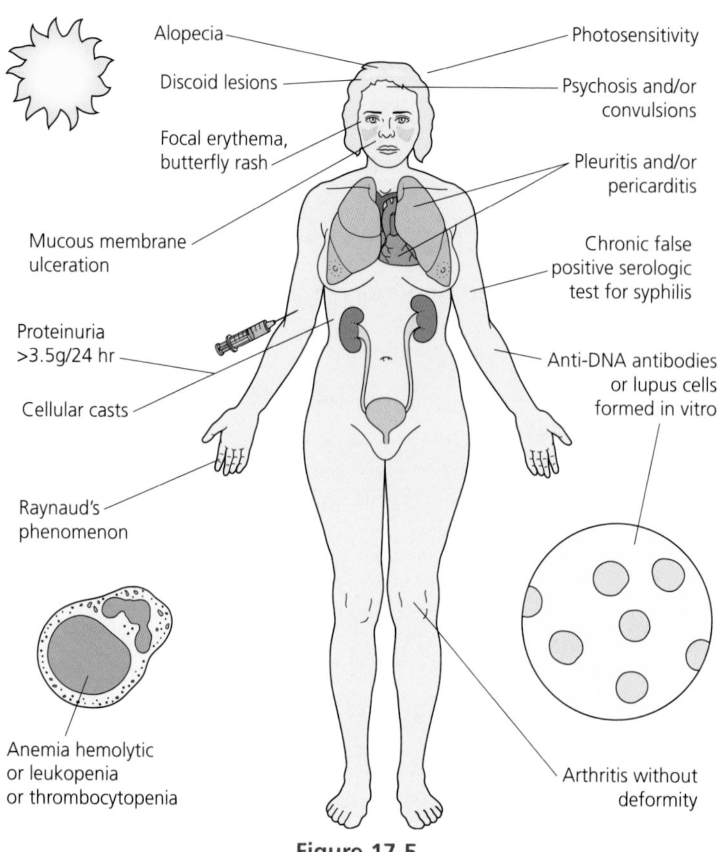

Figure 17-5

Subsets of cutaneous lupus erythematosus

Attempts have been made to group patients into subsets to define more homogeneous groups with a predictable course or response to treatment. Subsets of LE have been defined by cutaneous manifestations present in some form in most patients with lupus. The classification in Table 17-5 divides cutaneous LE into three types on the basis of the clinical appearance of the skin lesion: chronic cutaneous LE (scarring, discoid LE [DLE]), subacute cutaneous LE (SCLE), and acute cutaneous LE (ALE). A comparison of laboratory findings in these subsets is shown in Table 17-7.

An overview of the lupus syndromes appears in Figure 17-6.

Table 17-7 Comparison of Laboratory Findings in the Cutaneous Subsets of Lupus Erythematosus

Finding	DLE (%)	SCLE (%)	ALE (%)
ANA titer (≥1:160)	4	63	98
Anti-dsDNA	Rare	30	60-80
ESR greater than 30	Few	59	90
LE cell preparation	2	55	80
Low C3 or CH50	Rare	Rare	90
WBC count less than 4000/mm^3	7	19	17
Rheumatoid factor latex test positive	15	19	37
Low hemoglobin level	Few	15	50
VDRL biologic false-positive	Few	7	22
Direct immunofluorescence and the lupus band test			
Lesion	90	60	95
Normal sun-exposed	0	46	75
Normal nonexposed	0	26	50

ANA, Antinuclear antibody; *ESR,* erythrocyte sedimentation rate; *LE,* lupus erythematosus; *VDRL,* Venereal Diseases Research Laboratories (test); *WBC,* white blood cell.

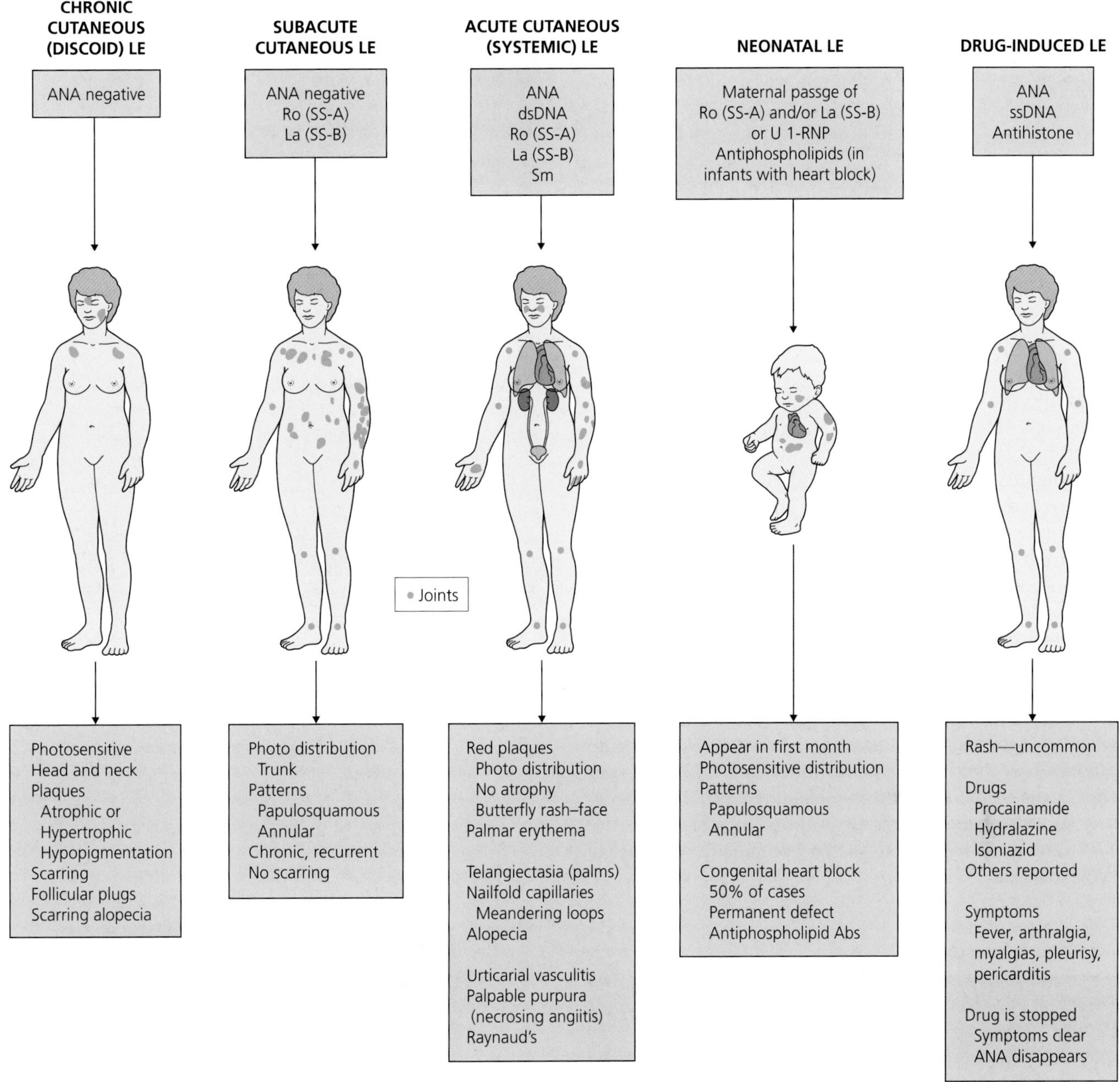
OVERVIEW OF LUPUS SYNDROMES:
AUTOANTIBODY PROFILES AND CUTANEOUS MANIFESTATIONS
CHRONIC CUTANEOUS (DISCOID) LE
ANA negative
Photosensitive
Head and neck
Plaques
Atrophic or
Hypertrophic
Hypopigmentation
Scarring
Follicular plugs
Scarring alopecia
SUBACUTE CUTANEOUS LE
ANA negative
Ro (SS-A)
La (SS-B)
Photo distribution
Trunk
Patterns
Papulosquamous
Annular
Chronic, recurrent
No scarring
ACUTE CUTANEOUS (SYSTEMIC) LE
ANA
dsDNA
Ro (SS-A)
La (SS-B)
Sm
• Joints
Red plaques
Photo distribution
No atrophy
Butterfly rash–face
Palmar erythema
Telangiectasia (palms)
Nailfold capillaries
Meandering loops
Alopecia
Urticarial vasculitis
Palpable purpura
(necrosing angiitis)
Raynaud's
NEONATAL LE
Maternal passge of
Ro (SS-A) and/or La (SS-B)
or U 1-RNP
Antiphospholipids (in
infants with heart block)
Appear in first month
Photosensitive distribution
Patterns
Papulosquamous
Annular
Congenital heart block
50% of cases
Permanent defect
Antiphospholipid Abs
DRUG-INDUCED LE
ANA
ssDNA
Antihistone
Rash—uncommon
Drugs
Procainamide
Hydralazine
Isoniazid
Others reported
Symptoms
Fever, arthralgia,
myalgias, pleurisy,
pericarditis
Drug is stopped
Symptoms clear
ANA disappears

Figure 17-6

Chronic cutaneous lupus erythematosus (discoid lupus erythematosus)

Patients with discoid lupus erythematosus (DLE) have a low incidence of systemic disease. The disease is more common in females, and it has a peak incidence in the fourth decade. Less than 2% of patients with DLE develop the disease before 10 years of age. Trauma and ultraviolet light exposure (UVB) may initiate and exacerbate lesions. There are several clinical variations (see Table 17-6).

The most common manifestation is the DLE lesion. Lesions are sharply demarcated and can be round, thus giving rise to the term *discoid* (or disclike). The face and scalp are the most commonly affected areas, but lesions may occur on any body surface. Lesions are usually asymmetrically distributed and begin as asymptomatic, well-defined, elevated, red-to-violaceous, 1- to 2-cm, flat-topped plaques with firmly adherent scale (Figure 17-7). The scale penetrates into the orifices of the hair follicle. Peeling the scale reveals an undersurface that has the appearance of a carpet penetrated by several carpet tacks; it is called carpet tack scale (Figure 17-8). Carpet tack scale is most apparent on the face and scalp where the follicular orifices are larger.

Atrophy occurs in both the epidermis and the dermis. Epidermal atrophy occurs early and gives the surface either a smooth white or a wrinkled appearance. Hypopigmentation is particularly disfiguring for blacks (Figure 17-9). Follicular plugs may be prominent (Figures 17-10 and 17-11). These lesions endure for months and either resolve spontaneously or progress with further atrophy, ultimately forming smooth white or hyperpigmented depressed scars with telangiectasia and scarring alopecia. Occasionally plaques become thick (hypertrophic DLE). DLE can cover wide areas of the face, causing disfigurement. The laboratory and histologic features are outlined in Tables 17-6 and 17-7. The presence of anti-ssDNA occurs with widespread active disease.

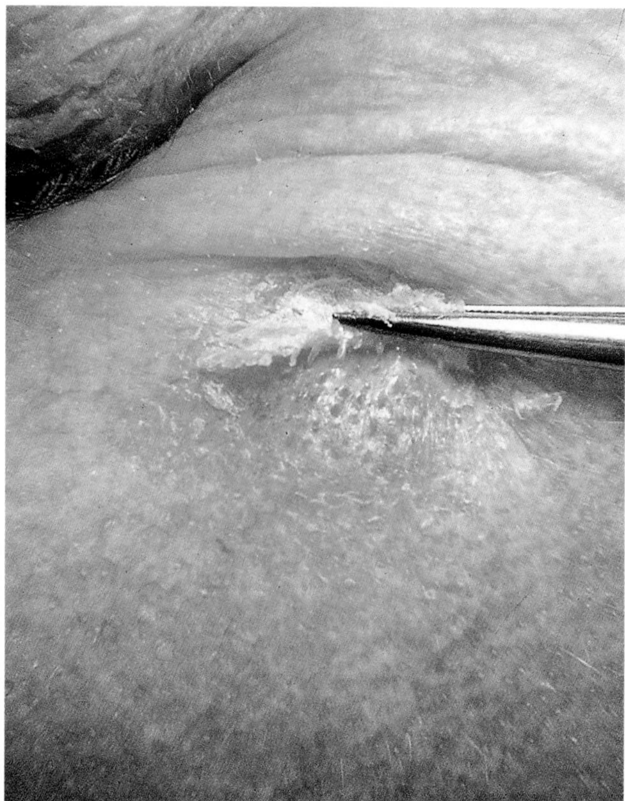

Figure 17-8 Chronic cutaneous LE (discoid LE). Carpet tack scale created by keratin plugs that penetrate deep into the hair follicle.

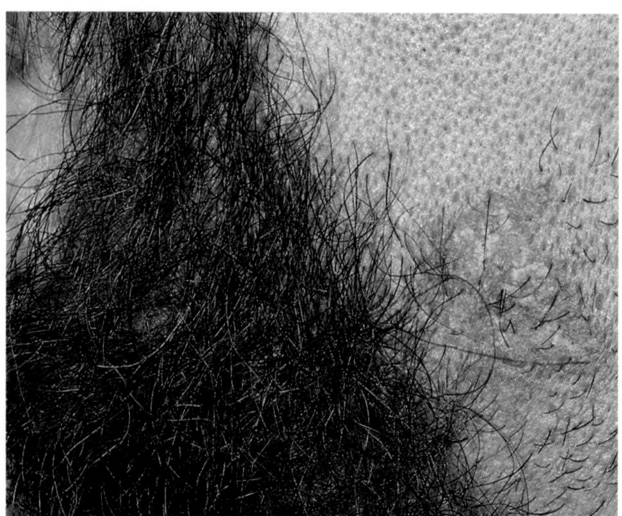

Figure 17-7 Chronic cutaneous LE (discoid LE). An early lesion. Well-defined, elevated, flat-topped plaques with adherent scale.

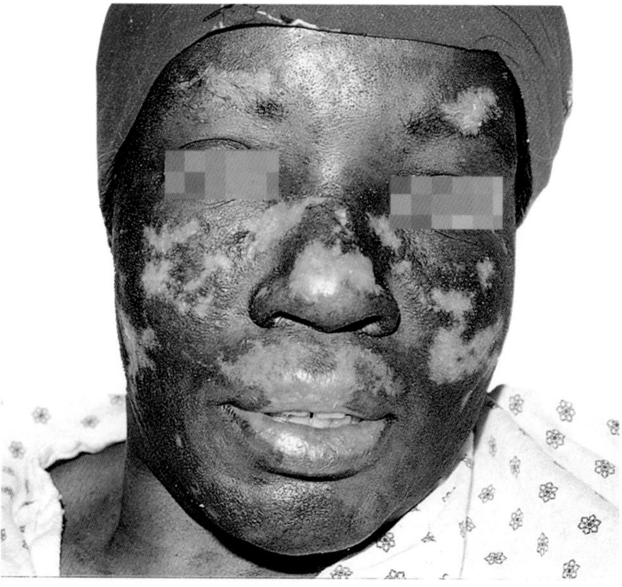

Figure 17-9 Discoid LE is more common in blacks. The typical hypopigmented lesions are disfiguring.

CHRONIC CUTANEOUS LE (DISCOID LE)

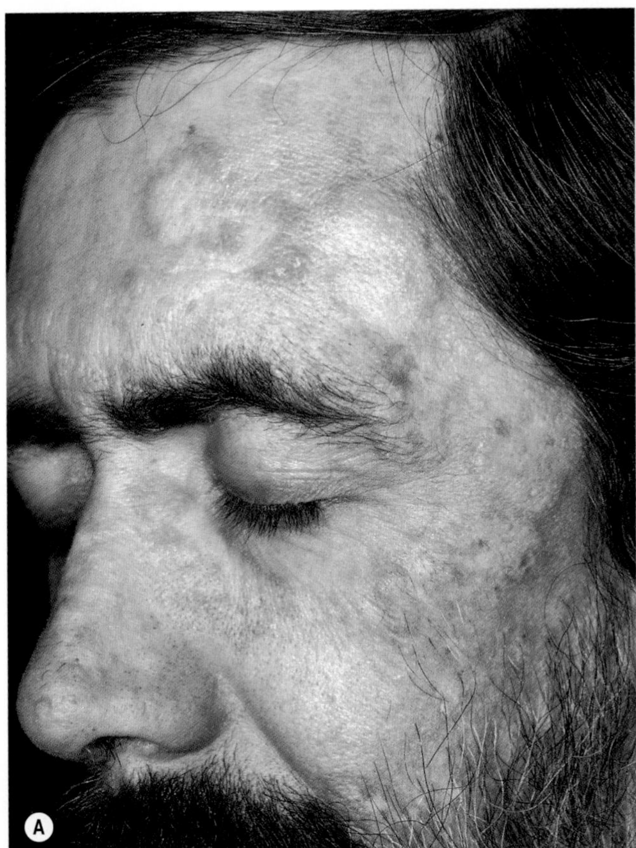

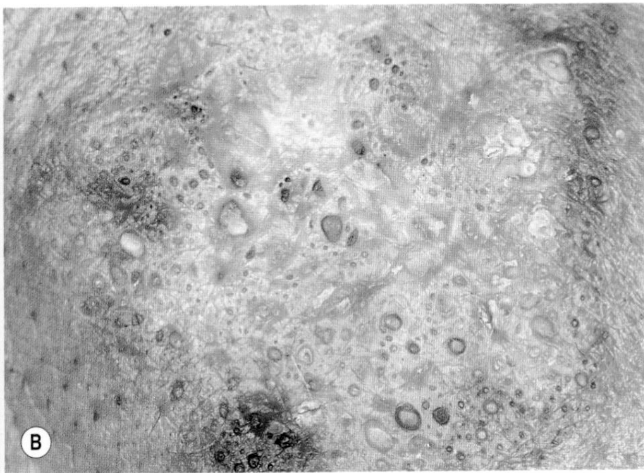

Figure 17-10 **A,** Lesions that are several months old are hypopigmented and atrophic. **B,** Close-up of a lesion from patient in **A.** The plaque has been present for months. There is hypopigmentation and prominent follicular plugging.

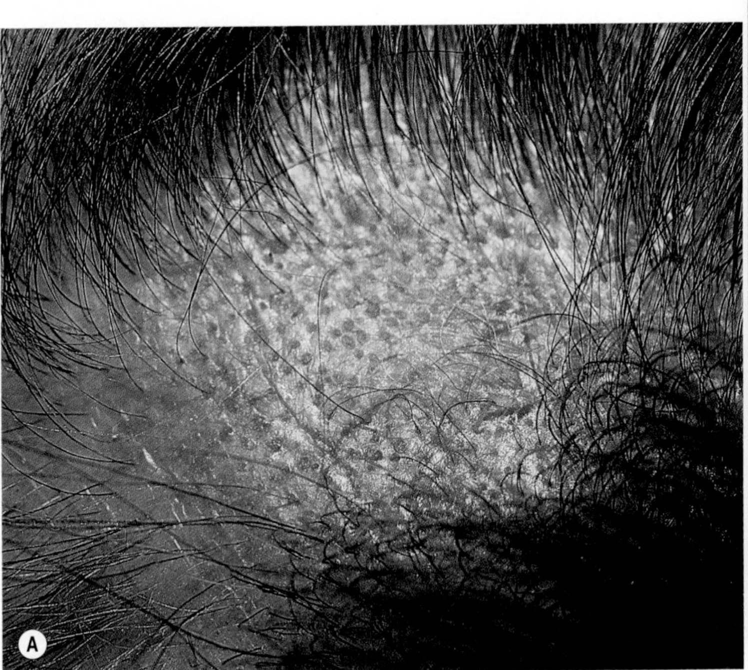

Prominent follicular plugging in a plaque of discoid LE located in the scalp.

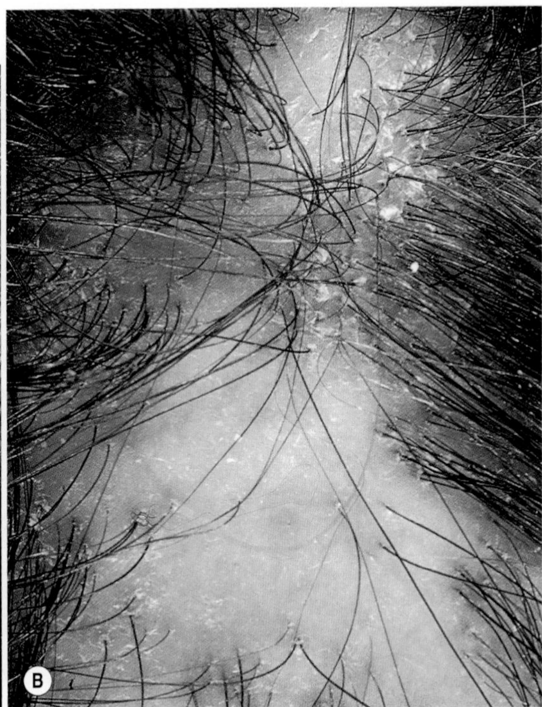

Scarring alopecia of the scalp; end-stage disease. Follicular structures have been replaced by scar tissue.

Figure 17-11

Subacute cutaneous lupus erythematosus

Subacute cutaneous lupus erythematosus (SCLE) encompasses the clinical spectrum of cutaneous LE between the chronic, destructive DLE and the erythema of acute cutaneous LE. However, SCLE can be associated with the full spectrum of LE-associated phenomena (Table 17-6). Like DLE, the individual lesions of SCLE may last for months; in contrast to DLE, they heal without scarring. Most patients with SCLE are white females. SCLE may be induced by a variety of drugs, most notably hydrochlorothiazide and calcium channel blockers.

Two morphologic varieties are a papulosquamous pattern (Figure 17-12) and an annular-polycyclic pattern (Figure 17-13). Both occur most often on the trunk; one predominates. The lesions spare the knuckles, the inner aspects of the arms, the axillae, and the lateral part of the trunk. They are rarely seen below the waist. A subtle gray hypopigmentation and telangiectasia are frequently seen in the center of annular lesions, bordered by erythema and a superficial scale. Follicular plugging, adherent hyperkeratosis, scarring, and dermal atrophy that are characteristic of DLE are not prominent features of SCLE. Hypopigmentation and telangiectasia become more evident as individual lesions resolve. The hypopigmentation fades after several months, but the telangiectasia may persist. The disease tends to be chronic and recurrent, lasting for years. SCLE and antibodies to Ro/SS-A have been associated with hydrochlorothiazide therapy.

Other dermatologic manifestations are photosensitivity (52% to 85%), periungual telangiectasia (22% to 51%), discoid LE (19% to 35%), and vasculitis (12%). Systemic manifestations (arthritis/arthralgia [43% to 74%], renal disease [11% to 19%], serositis [12%], and central nervous system [CNS] symptoms [6% to 19%]) are not severe and follow a benign course.

The laboratory and histologic features of SCLE are outlined in Tables 17-6 and 17-7. Antibodies to Ro/SS-A are present in 29% of patients.

SUBACUTE CUTANEOUS LUPUS ERYTHEMATOSUS

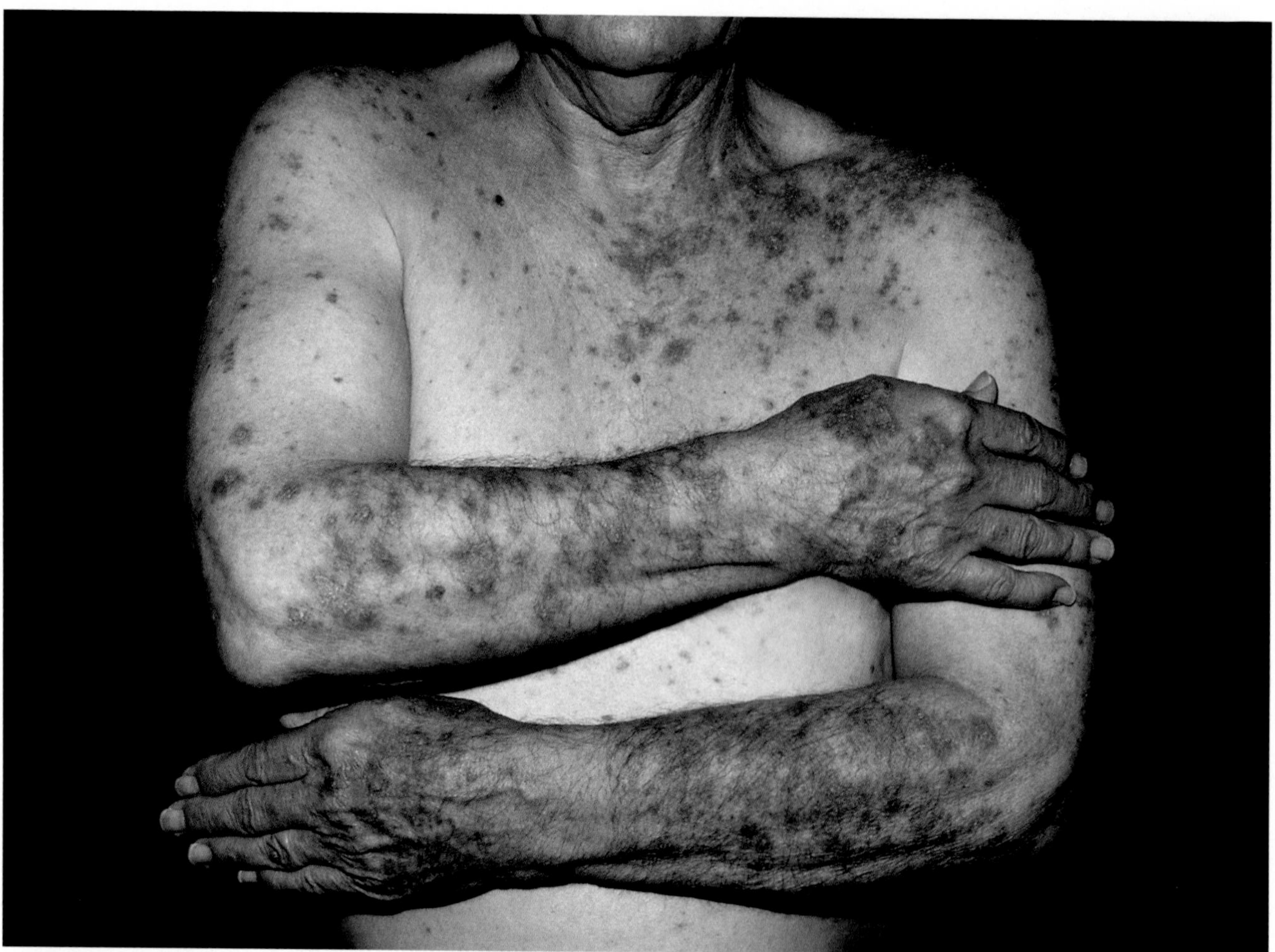

Figure 17-12 Papulosquamous pattern. Lesions are confined to exposed areas on the upper half of the body.

SUBACUTE CUTANEOUS LUPUS ERYTHEMATOSUS

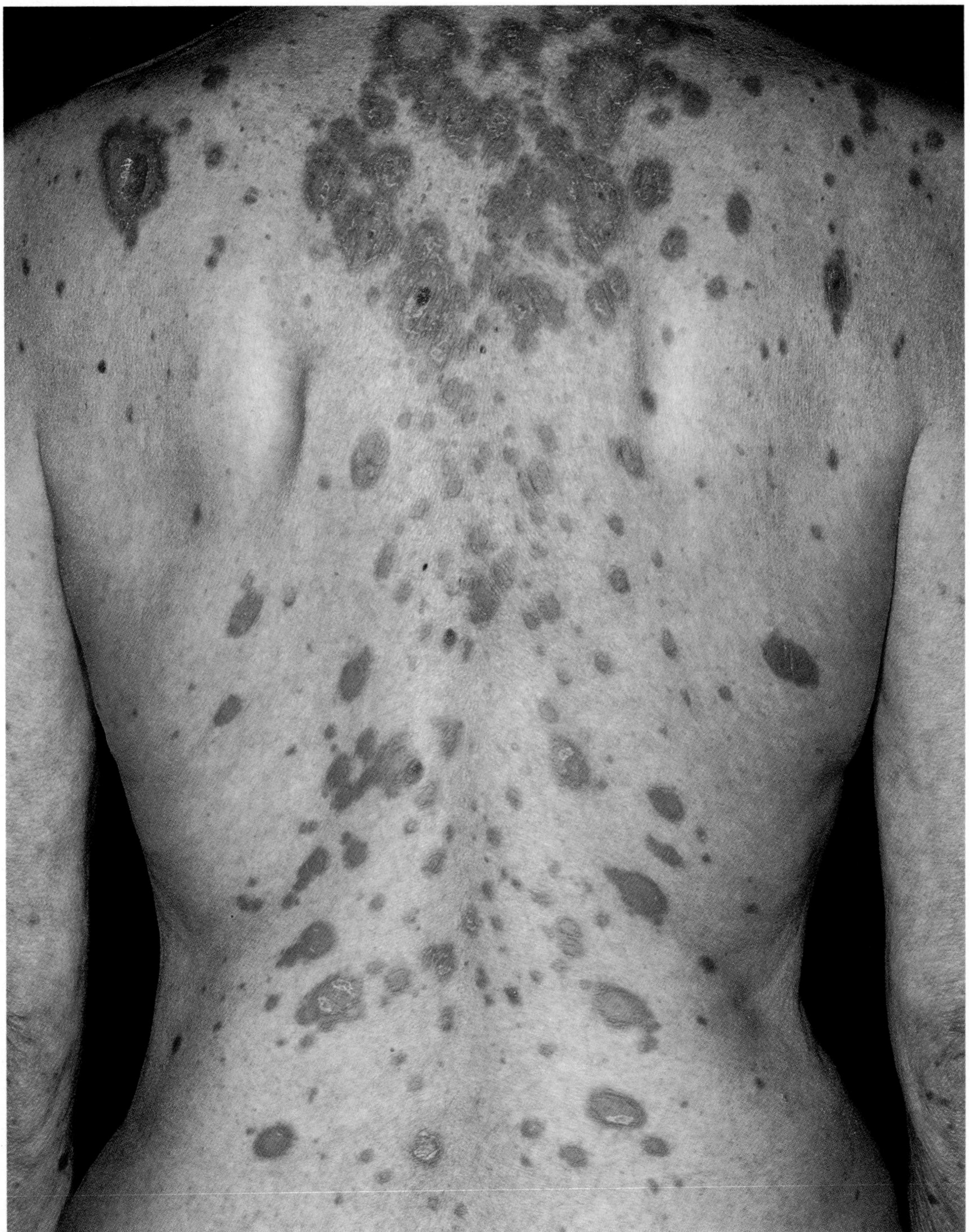

Figure 17-13 Annular-polycyclic pattern. The annular plaques have an erythematous scaly border, the central area is hypopigmented, and the eruption is confined to the back and hands.

Systemic lupus erythematosus

OVERVIEW OF SLE

An overview of SLE can be accessed at the National Guideline Clearinghouse (www.guideline.gov).

DEFINITION. Systemic lupus erythematosus is a syndrome characterized by clinical diversity, by changes in the disease activity over time, and by aberrant immunologic findings and especially the presence of antinuclear antibodies.

EPIDEMIOLOGY. The prevalence of SLE worldwide is 4 to 250 per 100,000. About 90% of the patients are female. The incidence is most frequent in women aged 15 to 25 years.

CLINICAL PRESENTATION. The clinical presentation varies between different patients, and in a single patient the disease activity varies over time. General symptoms such as fatigue and fever are common. A vast majority of the patients have arthralgia, mostly of the hands. About half of the patients have cutaneous features, such as butterfly rash and discoid lupus as well as photosensitivity, while one third of the patients have oral ulcerations. Approximately 50% of the patients have nephropathy, which varies from mild proteinuria and microscopic hematuria to end-stage renal failure. About 20% to 40% of the patients have pleurisy. Acute pneumonitis and chronic fibrosing alveolitis are relatively rare.

Pericarditis is somewhat more uncommon than pleuritis. T-wave changes in the electrocardiogram (ECG) are usual. Depression and headache are the most common of the neuropsychiatric symptoms. Generalized tonic-clonic seizures and organic psychoses are rare. Peripheral neuropathy is observed in about 10% of the patients, and approximately 10% of patients have a thromboembolic or hemorrhagic complication of the brain. The lymph nodes may enlarge, especially when the disease is active. There is a risk of first- and second-trimester fetal losses and of premature birth.

LABORATORY FINDINGS. Laboratory findings are diverse and may include the following:

- Erythrocyte sedimentation rate (ESR) is usually elevated; the C-reactive protein (CRP) value is often normal.
- Mild or moderate anemia is common. A clear-cut hemolytic anemia is seen in less than 10% of patients.
- Leukocytopenia (lymphocytopenia) is usually present.
- Mild thrombocytopenia is typically present.
- Antinuclear antibodies are found in more than 90% of patients.
- Anti–deoxyribonucleic acid (DNA) antibodies are found in 50% to 90% of patients.
- Polyclonal hypergammaglobulinemia is usually present.
- Decreased complement values (C3 and C4) are found.
- Antiphospholipid antibodies are present.
- Proteinuria, microscopic hematuria, and decreased creatinine clearance are present.

DIAGNOSIS. There is no single symptom or finding that is sufficient in itself for making the diagnosis. When SLE is suspected the basic laboratory investigations are as follows:

- Blood count
- Platelet count
- Erythrocyte sedimentation rate
- Measurement of antinuclear antibodies
- Dipstick test of the urine and urinalysis

The diagnosis is based on the clinical symptoms and the laboratory findings and on the American Rheumatism Association (ARA) classification criteria, 1997 (see Table 17-5). The patient should be referred to a specialist for confirmation of the diagnosis.

TREATMENT. The treatment is always individual and depends on the manifestations and activity of the disease. There is no need for treatment solely on the basis of the immunologic findings. Patients should be encouraged to restrain from sunbathing and to use sunscreens.

The most important drugs used for treatment of SLE are the following:

- Nonsteroidal antiinflammatory drugs
- Hydroxychloroquine
- Corticosteroids
- Immunosuppressive drugs (e.g., azathioprine, cyclophosphamide, methotrexate, mycophenolate)

Hydroxychloroquine and nonsteroidal antiinflammatory drugs are used in the treatment of mild symptoms such as cutaneous manifestations and arthralgia. When the response is insufficient or when the patient has fatigue or fever, a low dose of corticosteroids (prednisolone 5 to 7.5 mg/day) can be added. In the treatment of pleuritis or pericarditis, larger amounts of corticosteroids (about 30 mg of prednisolone per day) are used. For the treatment of severe central nervous system (CNS) symptoms and severe glomerulonephritis, thrombocytopenia, and hemolytic anemia, large corticosteroid doses and other immunosuppressive drugs are used.

The differential diagnosis between an infection and a flare of SLE is of utmost importance. Other drugs that the patient might need, such as antihypertensive treatment, should be remembered.

If there are signs of renal manifestations, the patient should be referred to a nephrologist for a renal biopsy. SLE patients are often allergic to a variety of antibiotics, especially sulfonamides.

The main causes of morbidity and mortality and the main immunologic parameters in SLE were analyzed for 1000 patients (female to male ratio, 10:1) in a 5-year multicenter study. Table 17-8 shows the frequencies of the main SLE clinical manifestations during the 5-year study.

Oral steroids were used in 65.2% of patients, antimalarial agents in 40.2%, nonsteroidal antiinflammatory drugs in 28.4%, antiaggregants (mainly aspirin) in 13.6%, azathioprine in 13.1%, pulse cyclophosphamide in 8.5%, oral cyclophosphamide in 7.4%, and anticoagulants (heparin, warfarin, or Coumadin) in 6.9% of patients.

The most frequent causes of death were active SLE (28.9%), infections (28.9%), and thromboses (26.7%). Most patients who died of active SLE had progressive frequent multisystemic disease. The most frequent infections were bacterial sepsis of pulmonary (8.9%), abdominal (8.9%), and urinary (6.7%) origin. A survival probability of 95% at 5 years was found.

Table 17-8 Clinical Manifestations Related to SLE

SLE manifestation	Percent
Arthritis	41.3
Malar rash	26.4
Nephropathy	22.2
Photosensitivity	18.7
Fever	13.9
Neurologic involvement	13.6
Raynaud's phenomenon	13.2
Serositis	12.9
Thrombocytopenia	9.5
Oral ulcers	8.9
Thrombosis	7.2
Livedo reticularis	5.5
Discoid lesions	5.4
Subacute cutaneous lesions	4.6
Myositis	4
Hemolytic anemia	3.3

Adapted from Cervera R: *Medicine* 78(3):167-175, 1999.
PMID: 10352648

CUTANEOUS DISEASE

The rash of SLE consists of superficial-to-indurated, nonpruritic, erythematous-to-violaceous plaques; these occur primarily on sun-exposed areas of the face, chest, shoulders, extensor arms, and backs of the hands (Figure 17-14). There may be fine scaling on the surface, but atrophy does not occur. Superficial erythematous plaques may last for a few days, becoming more intense as disease activity increases and fading with improvement in systemic symptoms. The most indurated hivelike plaques remain relatively fixed in shape and may persist for months. The classic butterfly rash (Figure 17-15) over the malar and nasal area occurs in 10% to 50% of patients with SLE, but it is not the most common cutaneous presentation.

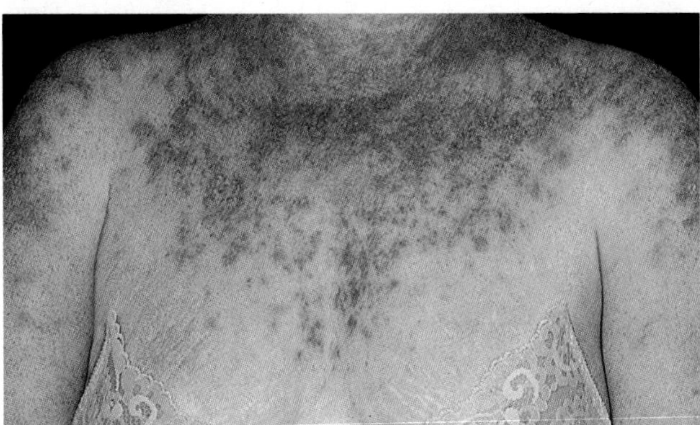

Figure 17-14 Exposure to sun produces a nonpruritic, scaling eruption that does not become atrophic.

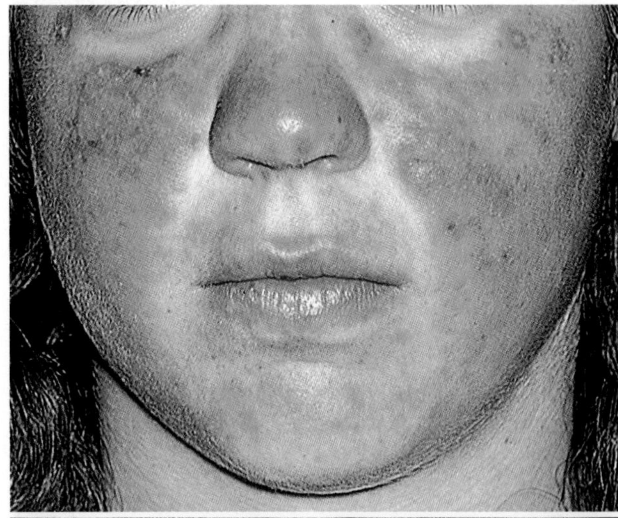

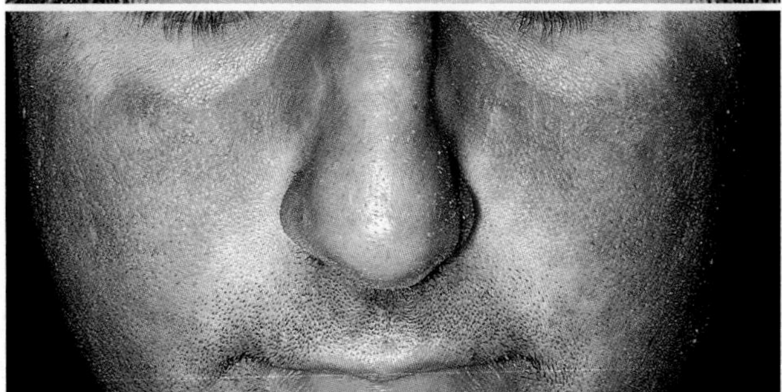

Figure 17-15 Acute cutaneous LE (systemic LE). The classic butterfly rash occurs in 10% to 50% of patients with acute LE.

Other cutaneous signs of lupus erythematosus

TELANGIECTASIA. Telangiectasia is a prominent feature of connective tissue disease. Telangiectasia occurs on the palms and fingers in association with palmar erythema; it resembles that observed in liver disease and pregnancy (Figures 17-16 and 17-17). Short, linear telangiectasias are a frequent finding in SLE. Using the ophthalmoscope technique described later in this chapter, nailfold capillary microscopy reveals tortuous, "meandering" capillary loops in 53% of patients with SLE. Usually some disorganization of the capillary pattern is present, but avascular areas are rare, and the capillaries are not widened (see Figure 17-31).

ALOPECIA. Alopecia is one of the major features of SLE and occurs in more than 20% of cases. Both scarring and nonscarring alopecia occur. Nonscarring hair loss occurs more frequently in SLE, and scarring alopecia is more common in DLE. In nonscarring alopecia the scalp may show focal or diffuse areas of erythema and scale similar to that seen with seborrheic dermatitis. The hair, especially in the frontal areas, becomes coarse and dry. The fragile, poorly formed shafts break, leaving patches of short, unmanageable hair, called lupus hair. The scalp and hair eventually become normal as disease activity wanes.

URTICARIA. The reported incidence of urticaria or urticaria-like lesions with LE varies between 7% and 28%. Urticaria is the presenting sign in approximately 5% of cases. Clinically, lesions may be indistinguishable from typical hives; but unlike hives, they are usually nonpruritic, persist for days, and remain relatively fixed in position. This clinical presentation is typical of urticarial vasculitis. In most cases a biopsy reveals necrotizing vasculitis, and the lupus band test is generally positive. Therefore the hive-like lesions are probably a result of immune complex deposition rather than a manifestation of allergy.

RAYNAUD'S PHENOMENON. Raynaud's phenomenon is another major diagnostic criterion for SLE. It occurs in 20% or more of SLE patients and may precede other signs and symptoms of SLE by months or years. Progression to digital ulceration is more common in scleroderma.

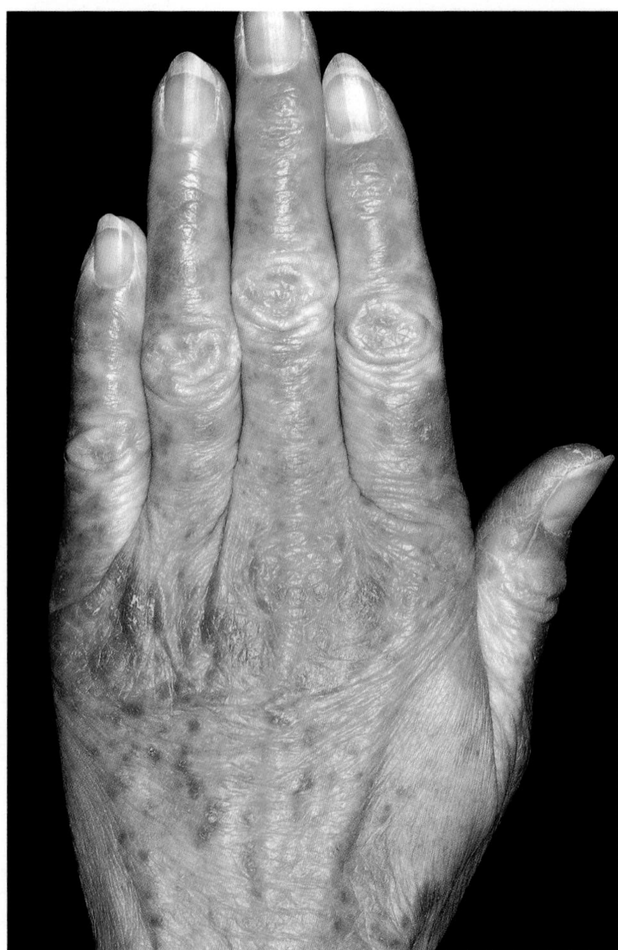

Figure 17-16 Systemic LE. In contrast to dermatomyositis, erythema and telangiectasia spare the knuckles.

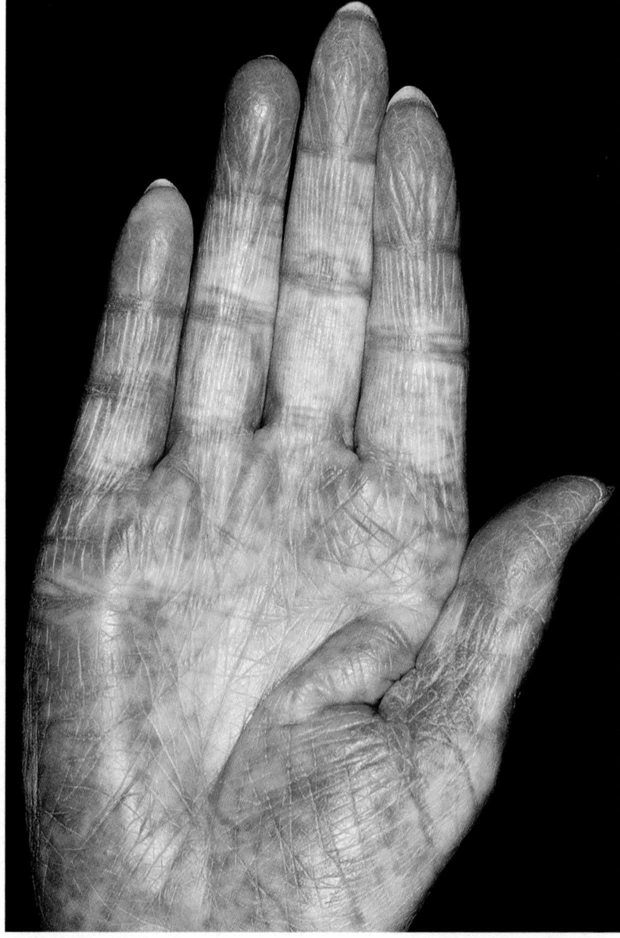

Figure 17-17 Systemic LE. Erythema and telangiectasia may appear on the palms.

Diagnosis and management of cutaneous lupus erythematosus

Lupus is an uncommon disease that has been described extensively in the medical literature and in the lay press. Some patients are familiar with the term and fear the worst when informed of their diagnosis. They should be assured that the disease in the majority of patients can be controlled with existing therapy, but that periodic clinical and laboratory evaluations are necessary to monitor disease activity.

Management consists of defining the type of cutaneous subset, performing a physical examination to document systemic symptoms, obtaining a battery of relevant blood studies as a baseline for diagnosis and later comparison as disease activity changes, obtaining a biopsy specimen of lesional skin for routine histologic studies and immunofluorescence, and, if appropriate, obtaining a biopsy specimen of nonlesional skin for immunofluorescence and topical and/or systemic treatment. A discussion of systemic symptom management is beyond the scope of this book.

LABORATORY STUDIES. A compilation of some of the studies used for the evaluation of LE is listed in Box 17-1. Patients with chronic cutaneous LE but without evidence of systemic disease should have a similar evaluation for documentation, because a few of these patients may later develop SLE. A comparison of the laboratory findings in the cutaneous subsets of LE is found in Table 17-7. Changes in values of some of these tests may reflect changes in disease activity.

ANTINUCLEAR AND ANTICYTOPLASMIC ANTIBODIES. The production of antinuclear and anticytoplasmic antibodies is a fundamental characteristic of LE. Numerous diverse antibodies are produced, and most laboratories have access to facilities that can measure the antibodies listed in Table 17-3. Measurement of these antibodies provides valuable information for diagnosis and prognosis. Quantitative measurement of some of these antibodies, such as anti–double-stranded DNA, can be made, and changes in levels assist in determining disease activity.

Measurement of ANA was the first test available for directly measuring antinuclear antibodies in a qualitative and quantitative manner. The test is positive in the vast majority of patients with LE (see Tables 17-2, 17-4, and 17-6) and is an important screening test.

The ANA test is a nonspecific test that detects many types of antinuclear antibodies. The significance of titers varies with different laboratories, but generally titers below 1:16 are believed to be negative, whereas titers above 1:64 indicate possible SLE. Extremely high titers such as 1:32,000 may be found. Unfortunately the titer level or change of titer has not been a reliable indicator of disease activity.

ANTINUCLEAR ANTIBODY PATTERNS. The pattern of the ANA may correlate with specific antibodies, but interpretation of patterns should be attempted only by experts (see Figure 17-3).

SKIN BIOPSY. A biopsy of skin lesions provides important diagnostic information. The histologic characteristics are listed in Table 17-6.

Lupus band test. The term lupus band test (LBT) refers to direct immunofluorescence examination of normal sun-protected, normal sun-exposed, or lesional skin. Deposits of one or more immunoglobulins are found at the dermoepidermal junction and in the walls of dermal vessels in patients with DLE, SCLE, and SLE. Immunofluorescence may be helpful when the diagnosis is in question. Antibody testing has reduced the need for immunofluorescence testing.

SUNSCREENS. Photosensitivity is a major factor in all types of cutaneous LE. Sunlight in the ultraviolet B (UVB) and ultraviolet A (UVA) regions can induce and exacerbate all forms of lupus erythematosus. Patients should avoid direct exposure to sunlight, particularly during the summer and between the hours of 10 AM and 3 PM, and exposure through window glass. Broad-spectrum sunscreens with a sun protection factor of maximum value (greater than 15) that block UVB and UVA light should be applied if sun exposure is anticipated. Zinc oxide and titanium dioxide containing sunscreen block UVA and UVB light. Patients should be encouraged to apply sunscreens as a routine procedure after morning washing during the summer months.

TOPICAL CORTICOSTEROIDS. Topical corticosteroids are the agents of first choice for all forms of cutaneous LE. Groups I through V topical steroids are required to control DLE. They may be applied three times a day to all active lesions, including those on the face. Patients should be

Box 17-1 **Workup for Suspected Cutaneous Lupus Erythematosus (DLE, SCLE, SLE)**

History and physical examination
Skin lesion biopsy for histologic studies
CBC, ESR, platelet count
ANA
Anti-nDNA
Anti-RNP (U1-RNP)
Anti-Ro (SS-A), anti-La (SS-B), SM
Serologic tests
Urinalysis

Optional tests

Serum protein electrophoresis
Circulating immune complexes
Immunofluorescence skin biopsy
Antiphospholipid antibodies
Total hemolytic complement (if abnormal, C2, C3, C4 levels)
Creatinine clearance

encouraged to restrict application to the active lesion and to avoid normal surrounding skin. Lesions of SCLE and SLE may be treated with groups III through V topical steroids applied three times a day. Those who do not respond should be advanced to group II topical steroids. Discontinue treatment when lesions have cleared.

INTRALESIONAL CORTICOSTEROIDS. DLE lesions that are resistant to topical steroids may be managed well with periodic intralesional injections of steroids (e.g., equal parts of 1% Xylocaine or saline and triamcinolone acetonide [Kenalog] 10 mg/ml). Lesions frequently become inactive after a single injection and may remain in remission for months. The steroid should be injected with a 27- or 30-gauge needle with sufficient solution to blanch the lesion—approximately 0.1 ml for a 1.0-cm lesion.

ANTIMALARIAL AGENTS. The antimalarial agents remain the cornerstone of treatment because of their effectiveness and safety. They are effective in the treatment of all forms of cutaneous LE. Hydroxychloroquine or chloroquine also reduces arthritis, arthralgia, and joint pain in persons with mild SLE. These patients may also benefit from the simultaneous use of oral corticosteroids.

The recommended safe and effective dosage for an individual weighing 150 pounds is 200 mg of hydroxychloroquine (Plaquenil) twice a day. Patients can be maintained on this dosage as long as needed, but they should have periodic eye evaluations. Antimalarial agents are maintained at the recommended dosages until the lesions resolve. They are then reduced to the lowest possible dosage to maintain control. Patients with quiescent SLE who are taking hydroxychloroquine are less likely to have a clinical flare-up if they are maintained on the drug. The discontinuation of treatment in patients with quiescent disease is associated with a 2.5-fold increase in the risk of new clinical manifestations or, in the case of previous manifestations, a recurrence or an increase in severity.

Patients with cutaneous LE who smoke are significantly less likely to respond to antimalarial therapy.

Antimalarial ocular toxicity. Fear of retinal toxicity resulted in a substantial reduction in the use of antimalarial drugs, but it was later discovered that excessive daily dosages influenced retinal damage. No cases of retinopathy have been reported when the dose of hydroxychloroquine did not exceed 6.5 mg/kg/day and with therapy that did not extend longer than 10 years. By performing serial testing of the foveal reflex and of the reaction of visual fields to red targets, the ophthalmologist can detect a state of "premaculopathy." While the patient is receiving therapy, premaculopathy is defined as the loss of foveal reflex or the development of paracentral scotomata to red test objects. It is a state of functional loss that is reversible by discontinuation of the drug. Testing is done before treatment and every 12 to 18 months during therapy. The package insert recommends baseline screening and follow-up eye examinations every 3 months. Screening at such intervals is unlikely to be cost-effective at the recommended dosage when a patient has had less than 10 years of therapy. Patients taking high doses of antimalarial agents or with decreased renal function need more frequent examinations. Visual field testing can be performed by Amsler grid. It is simple and inexpensive and is easily administered at home by the patient, and it can screen for shallow relative paracentral scotomata.

DAPSONE. Antimalarial agents are the drugs of first choice for cutaneous LE when topical steroids have failed. Dapsone (initial dosage 100 mg/day) is an effective alternative for all forms of cutaneous LE. The dosage is adjusted after evaluation of clinical response and side effects. Dapsone therapy is described on p. 645.

ORAL CORTICOSTEROIDS. Occasionally patients with cutaneous LE do not respond to topical steroids, antimalarial agents, or dapsone. Such patients should discontinue other forms of therapy and begin prednisone at dosages high enough to control the disease (e.g., 20 mg twice a day), until control is obtained. Oral steroids are then tapered and discontinued; the patient is once more given a trial of conventional therapy. Oral corticosteroids are effective in the management of joint symptoms, fatigue, and serositis in persons with SLE.

OTHER TREATMENTS. Azathioprine (100 to 150 mg/day), methotrexate, thalidomide (50 to 300 mg/day), and acitretin (50 mg/day) are effective for severe, chloroquine-resistant DLE. Isotretinoin (1 mg/kg/day) is reported to be effective for patients with DLE and SCLE. Mycophenolate mofetil may be effective in refractory dermatologic manifestations of SLE.

Neonatal lupus erythematosus

Neonatal LE (NLE) is a rare disorder caused by the transfer of transplacental autoantibodies from the mother to the fetus. This syndrome is characterized by one or more of the following findings: subacute cutaneous lupus–like annular and polycyclic lesions, congenital heart block, cardiomyopathy, cholestatic hepatitis, and thrombocytopenia. Connective tissue disease may develop in adulthood. NLE is caused by the transplacental passage of maternal IgG anti–Ro/SS-A and/or anti–La/SS-B or anti-U1RNP. Most babies of mothers with anti–Ro/SS-A, anti–La/SS-B, or anti-U1RNP autoantibodies do not develop NLE. There is no way to determine which fetus or infant will be affected. The predominant autoantibodies are anti–Ro/SS-A, and are found in approximately 95% of cases.

The skin lesions (present in approximately 50% of affected infants) usually appear within the first month of life and may be initiated by sun exposure. Lesions present with plaques of erythema with central atrophy. A periorbital "owl-eye" or "eye mask" facial rash is common. Lesions appear on the scalp (Figure 17-18), arms and legs, trunk, and groin. Crusted lesions predominate in male infants. The lesions heal without scarring or atrophy within 6 months. The autoantibodies disappear with the rash. The congenital

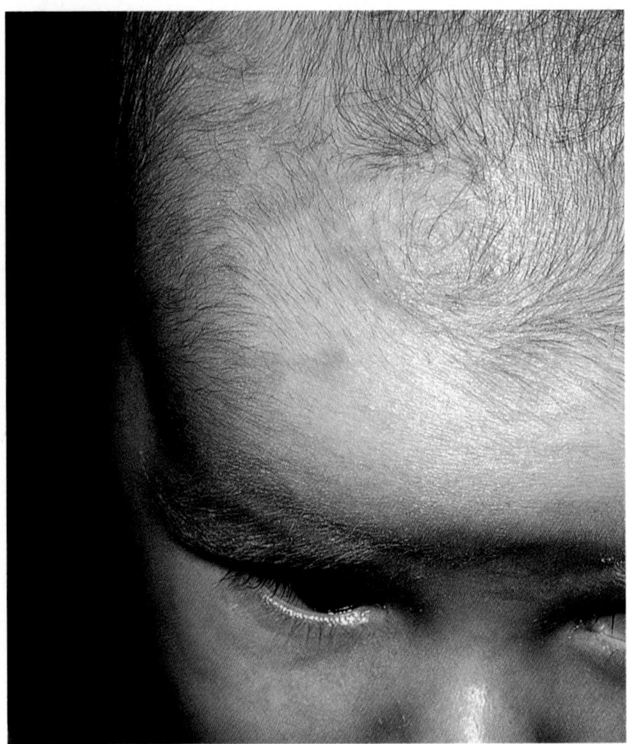

Figure 17-18 Neonatal lupus. Annular erythematous plaques with a slight scale usually appear on the head slightly after birth. Sun-exposed areas of the arms and trunk may also be involved. Telangiectasia is often prominent. Skin lesions resolve with time.

heart block (present in approximately 50% of affected infants) is a permanent defect that develops in utero during the late second and the third trimesters of pregnancy. Many babies require pacemakers, and approximately 10% die of complications related to cardiac disease. The proposed cause is that the anti–Ro/SS-A antibody binds with an autoantigen in the heart and produces an inflammatory process, resulting in fibrotic replacement and destruction of one or more of the following: the sinoatrial bundle, the atrioventricular bundle, or the bundle of His.

Approximately 50% of mothers have clinical features of either Sjögren's syndrome or LE at the time of birth, but more than 85%, with time, demonstrate the onset of Sjögren's symptoms (dry eyes, dry mouth) and/or joint stiffness, arthralgias, or swelling. Of anti–Ro/SS-A-positive patients, 90% to 95% possess either the HLA-DR2 or the HLA-DR3 phenotype. Of lupus patients with abnormal fetal heart rate, 100% have antibodies to phospholipids (lupus anticoagulant).

MANAGEMENT. Two lesional skin biopsies are taken: one for hematoxylin and eosin and the other for immunofluorescence. The finding of anti–Ro/SS-A antibody in the infant and mother confirms the diagnosis. Mothers are advised that the risk of a similarly affected infant in subsequent pregnancies is approximately 25%. Patients with heart block may be asymptomatic or require pacemakers.

Drug-induced lupus erythematosus

Many drugs have been reported to cause a syndrome similar to systemic lupus erythematosus. Many patients with probable drug-induced lupus erythematosus (DILE) have the clinical picture and serologic findings typical for lupus.

Diagnostic criteria for DILE include the following:

1. Exposure (3 weeks to 2 years) to a drug suspected to induce DILE
2. No history for SLE before the use of the drug therapy
3. Detection of positive ANA with at least one clinical sign of SLE
4. Rapid improvement and gradual fall in the ANA and other serologic findings upon withdrawal of the drug

More than 80 drugs have been associated with DILE. Drugs responsible for the development of DILE can be divided into four groups.

1. Drugs for which there are well-controlled studies and their role for inducing DILE has been documented (e.g., hydralazine, procainamide, isoniazid, methyldopa, chlorpromazine, and quinidine)
2. Drugs possibly related to DILE (e.g., anticonvulsant agents, antithyroid drugs, penicillamine, sulfasalazine, beta-blockers, and lithium)
3. Drugs suggested as causes for DILE but lacking well-controlled studies (e.g., gold salts, penicillin, tetracycline, phenylbutazone, estrogens and oral contraceptives, griseofulvin)
4. Drugs recently reported to induce DILE (e.g., minocycline, valproate, calcium-channel blockers, interferon, interleukin-2 [IL-2])

DRUGS. Procainamide is the most common cause of drug-related lupus in the United States. Up to 80% of patients taking procainamide have a positive ANA test result. Approximately 30% of that group have clinical symptoms. Patients treated with the usual doses of hydralazine have a relatively low incidence of positivity for ANAs and a very low rate of occurrence of the clinical syndrome.

CLINICAL PRESENTATION. Most commonly the onset of symptoms occurs many months after the drug has been initiated. DILE resembles mild SLE. It usually occurs in older age groups; SLE commonly occurs in young women. DILE is characterized by arthralgia and/or arthritis (80% to 90%), myalgia (up to 50%), serositis (pleurisy and pericarditis), fever, hepatomegaly, splenomegaly, and skin manifestation. Arthralgia or arthritis is sometimes the only clinical symptom. The small joints are usually affected. There is no central nervous system involvement.

SKIN MANIFESTATIONS. Skin manifestations appear in 25% to 53% of patients and include lesions compatible with the typical lesions of SLE. Butterfly rash, alopecia, discoid lesions, and mucosal ulcers are usually absent. Some drugs (e.g., hydrochlorothiazide, captopril, calcium channel blockers, terbinafine) induce skin and clinical symptoms compatible with the diagnosis of subacute cutaneous LE. These include photosensitivity, annular or squamous lesions, and Ro/SS-A antibodies.

LABORATORY FINDINGS. ANA is an important marker for DILE. The incidence ranges up to 90% in hydralazine-related DILE, but ANA may be absent. The pattern of ANA is homogeneous or speckled. ANA may persist in falling titers for a long period after discontinuing the implicated drug. Antinuclear antibodies in DILE are fairly specific and mainly directed against histones or single-stranded DNA (ssDNA). The histone antibodies are specific for DILE, but they might be detected in 20% of the patients with SLE. Anemia, leukocytopenia, and thrombocytopenia are rarely reported. Involvement of the kidney has been reported in cases treated with D-penicillamine, hydralazine, griseofulvin, procainamide, and anticonvulsants. Acute hepatitis accompanies DILE associated with minocycline. Anti-dsDNA antibodies are absent and serum complement levels are normal. The histologic picture is not specific.

GENETIC FACTORS. A liver acetyltransferase enzyme inactivates some of these drugs. Patients can be categorized as either slow or fast acetylators. The rate of drug acetylation is genetically determined. Rapid acetylators have a much lower incidence of hydralazine-induced DILE. Slow acetylators are at high risk for developing DILE. Acetylation patterns are important for patients treated with hydralazine, procainamide, isoniazid, and sulfonamides. HLA-DR4 and DILE are closely related. Seventy-three percent of patients with hydralazine-related DILE have HLA-DR4.

PROGNOSIS. DILE is a mild form of SLE. DILE resolves in weeks and rarely in years after drug withdrawal. The ANA level typically remains elevated after symptoms have resolved (an average of 4 months). Acute, severe hepatitis sometimes occurs in patients with DILE secondary to minocycline.

TREATMENT. DILE does not usually require treatment. Patients with pericarditis, pleural effusions, or pulmonary infiltrates often require prednisone. They respond quickly, and prednisone can be tapered and then discontinued over a few months. Symptomatic patients may also respond to anti–malarial agents.

DERMATOMYOSITIS AND POLYMYOSITIS

Dermatomyositis (DM) and polymyositis (PM) are rare inflammatory muscle diseases. The term polymyositis is reserved for cases in which skin inflammation is absent. Although patients of any age may be affected, most patients are either children or adults older than 40 years of age. Adult DM is a multisystem disease that can be associated with malignancy and collagen vascular diseases. The clinical picture varies considerably, and the following classification and diagnostic criteria (Box 17-2) of the idiopathic inflammatory myopathies have been suggested. Newer classifications have been proposed that have diagnostic, prognostic, and therapeutic value. *PMID: 16010208*

Original Bohan and Peter Classification of Idiopathic Inflammatory Myopathies

Group I	PM
Group II	DM
Group III	PM or DM with malignancy
Group IV	Childhood PM or DM
Group V	PM or DM associated with collagen vascular disease

Polymyositis

Symmetric proximal muscular weakness, especially of the hips and thighs, is characteristic of PM. The onset is insidious; patients first note difficulty rising from a chair. Neck muscles are commonly involved, leading to weakness in raising the head ("drooped head"). Dysfunction of the pharyngeal muscles may lead to dysphagia and aspiration pneumonia. Respiratory muscles of the chest wall can be involved. Distal strength is usually preserved. Myalgias can occur, and tenderness is uncommon. Arthralgias are a pre-

Box 17-2 **Diagnostic Criteria for Dermatomyositis and Polymyositis**

Major criteria

Proximal symmetric muscle weakness
Compatible muscle biopsy
Myopathy or inflammatory myositis
Elevated skeletal muscle enzymes (e.g., CPK, aldolase, SGOT)
Compatible dermatologic features

Exclusion of other disorders causing myopathy

Neurologic disease
Muscular dystrophies
Infections
Toxins
Endocrinopathies

Confidence limits

Definite PM: three or four criteria (DM + rash)
Probable PM: two criteria (DM + rash)
Possible PM: one criterion (DM + rash)

Modified from Bohan A et al: *Medicine* 56:255, 1977 *PMID: 327194*; and Callen JP: *Dis Mon* 33:237, 1987. *PMID: 3556110*

senting sign in 41% of patients. Weakness progresses over weeks to months; spontaneous remission may occur. Deep tendon reflexes remain normal, and atrophy occurs late in the course of the disease. The muscle changes are indistinguishable from those seen in DM.

Dermatomyositis

The associated features of PM may precede by months, accompany, or follow the skin signs. Proximal muscle weakness is the most common presenting manifestation; the rash is present in 40% of patients when they are first evaluated. The cutaneous changes sometimes precede the onset of muscle weakness by more than 1 year. The course of adult DM may be acute, chronic, recurrent, or cyclic. DM tends to be a more severe disease than PM, with a more severe myopathy. DM occurs in all age groups and equally in males and females. Malignancy seems to be associated with skin disease. Malignancy occurs in patients with dermatomyositis who do not have muscle disease, but the incidence of malignancy is not increased in patients with the muscle disease alone (i.e., polymyositis).

SYSTEMIC DISEASE. Arthralgias and/or arthritis may be present with generalized arthralgias and morning stiffness. The small joints of the hands, wrists, and ankles may be involved with symmetric nondeforming arthritis that is nonerosive.

Esophageal disease with proximal or distal dysphagia occurs in up to 50% of patients. Pulmonary disease occurs in up to 50% of patients. Nonspecific interstitial pneumonitis or diffuse alveolar damage is the most common presentation. Cardiac involvement is uncommon. Calcinosis of the skin or muscle is unusual in adults, but occurs in up to 40% of children. Nodules are seen over bony prominences.

AMYOPATHIC DERMATOMYOSITIS. The term *amyopathic dermatomyositis* has been applied to three groups of patients: those with cutaneous changes only, those with cutaneous changes only at baseline with subsequent development of myositis, and those with cutaneous changes with normal muscle enzyme serum levels at baseline but with myositis demonstrated by electromyography and/or muscle biopsy specimens.

DERMATOLOGIC MANIFESTATIONS. There are six dermatologic features of DM. The heliotrope rash and Gottron's papules are pathognomonic signs. The other features are a photosensitive violaceous eruption, periungual telangiectasia, poikiloderma, and scaly red scalp.

Heliotrope rash. Heliotrope erythema of the eyelids (heliotrope: violet color) is a term used to describe the violaceous discoloration around the eyes (Figure 17-19). It is a pathognomonic sign of DM. Periorbital edema and violet discoloration may be either the earliest cutaneous sign or a residual finding as diffuse erythema fades. There is a violaceous to dusky red rash with or without edema in a symmetric distribution involving periorbital skin. Scaling and desquamation may occur.

Figure 17-19 Dermatomyositis. Heliotrope (violaceous) discoloration around the eyes and periorbital edema.

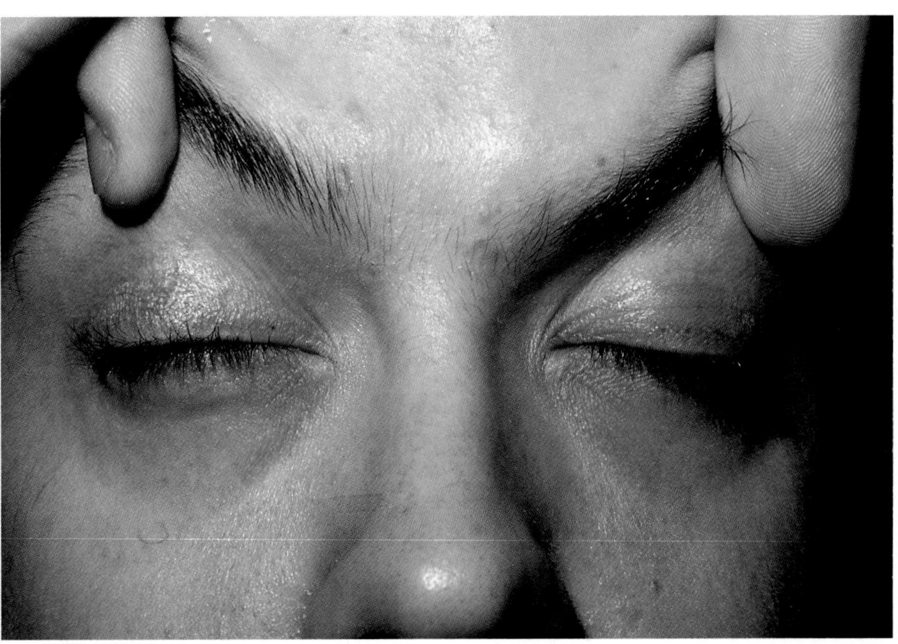

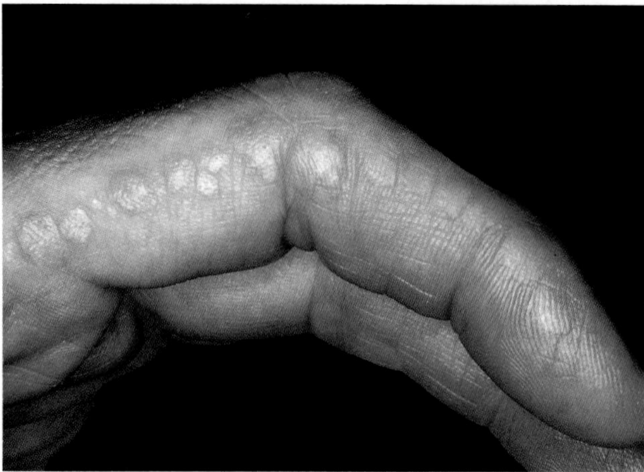

Figure 17-20 Gottron's papules, a pathognomonic sign of dermatomyositis, are round, smooth, violaceous-to-red, flat-topped papules that occur over the knuckles and along the sides of the fingers.

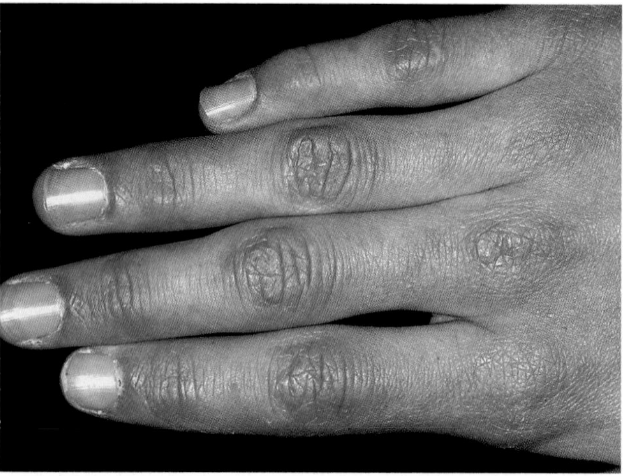

Figure 17-21 Gottron's papules are found over bony prominences, finger, elbows and knees. The lesions are slightly elevated, violaceous papules with slight scale.

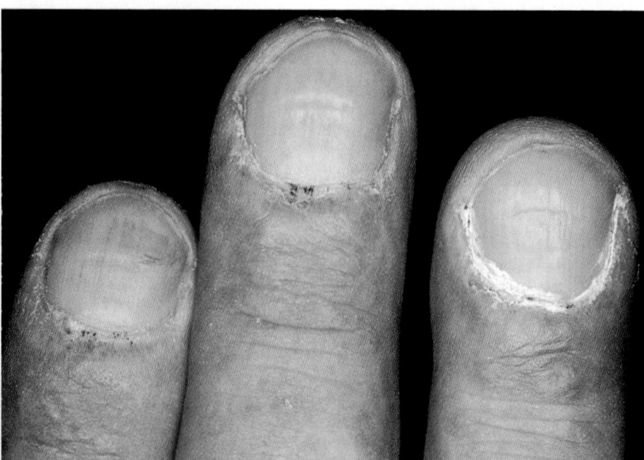

Figure 17-22 Dermatomyositis. Periungual erythema and telangiectasia similar to that seen in other connective tissue diseases.

Gottron's papules. Gottron's papules, a pathognomonic sign of DM, are round, 0.2- to 1-cm, smooth, violaceous-to-red, flat-topped papules that occur over bony prominences, particularly the knuckles, along the sides of the fingers (Figures 17-20 and 17-21), and sometimes over the knees and elbows. There may be a slight scale and sometimes a thick psoriasiform scale. Telangiectasia may be present in the lesions. Lupus of the back of the hand usually spares the knuckles. Biopsy cannot distinguish the cutaneous lesions of DM from those of LE. Several lesions appear simultaneously any time during the course of the disease; they tend to remain fixed in position. Approximately 60% to 80% of DM patients have Gottron's papules sometime during the course of the disease.

Periungual erythema and telangiectasia. Clinically these are similar to those seen in other connective tissue diseases. The telangiectasia is most prominent on the proximal nailfold and appears as irregular, red, linear streaks (Figure 17-22). Nailfold capillary microscopy using the ophthalmoscope (see Figure 17-31) reveals a pattern identical to that seen in scleroderma but quite different from that seen in SLE. Therefore this technique may help to distinguish DM from SLE. The cuticles are thick, rough, hyperkeratotic, and irregular (moth-eaten appearance).

Violaceous scaling patches. A characteristic violet erythema with or without scaling occurs in a localized or diffuse distribution. The localized eruption appears symmetrically over bony prominences such as the knees, elbows, and interphalangeal joints (Figure 17-23). DM typically involves the knuckles and spares the skin over the phalanges. The distribution is reversed in SLE when the skin over the phalanges is involved and the knuckles are spared (see Figure 17-16). The diffuse form begins as a patchy, diffuse, dusky-red or violet erythema of the sun-exposed areas of the face, neck, back, and arms and later may involve the buttocks and legs. Over time the rash becomes confluent, and involved areas become minimally raised and slightly scaly. A diffuse, deep red erythema (malignant erythema) may appear superimposed on the existing eruption in patients with an evolving malignancy. Photosensitivity is common. The rash tends to be confined to sun-exposed areas and is worse after sun exposure.

Poikiloderma. Late in the course of the disease, as the erythema fades, a highly characteristic pattern may occur in the same sun-exposed areas occupied by the diffuse erythema. Poikiloderma is a descriptive term for the pattern that consists of finely mottled white areas and brown pigmentation, telangiectasia, and atrophy. Poikiloderma also occurs as an isolated phenomenon with mycosis fungoides and other rare dermatologic conditions.

Scaly red scalp. Scalp scaling is a relatively common sign of DM. Erythematous to violaceous, scaly, atrophic scalp lesions may be initially diagnosed as psoriasis, seborrheic dermatitis, or lupus erythematosus (Figure 17-24).

DIFFERENTIAL DIAGNOSIS. A diagnosis of psoriasis might be made if scale forms on poikilodermatous patches, especially if there is no photodistribution. T-cell lymphoma or lupus might be confused with poikiloderma. Differential diagnoses of early skin lesions include polymorphic light eruption, contact dermatitis, and atopic dermatitis.

DERMATOMYOSITIS WITH MALIGNANCY. There is an increased incidence of malignancy in adult DM and PM. Therefore PM/DM may occur as a paraneoplastic syndrome. This association appears to correspond most closely with the dermatologic manifestations, as it occurs in patients with dermatomyositis who do not have muscle disease, but the incidence of malignancy is lower in patients with the muscle disease alone (i.e., polymyositis). The incidence of malignancy in patients with dermatomyositis without myositis corresponds to that seen in patients with fully developed dermatomyositis. The association is largely with malignant neoplasms diagnosed at or before the time of diagnosis of PM and DM. Therefore steps aimed at early cancer detection and treatment must be taken. Patients older than 50 years are at greatest risk. The cancer incidence declines steadily with increasing years since initial diagnosis of PM/DM. The cancer risk is increased approximately sixfold during the first year, but is lower during the second year, with no significant excesses in subsequent years of follow-up. Therefore among long-term survivors of PM/DM, there is little evidence to warrant extensive preventive and screening measures after 2 years. Tumors may appear at any site, but significant excesses are observed for cancers of lung, ovary, lymphatic and hematopoietic systems, and nasopharyngeal areas. In 30% of patients the tumor appeared first, and symptoms of DM subsequently appeared, with a mean interval of 16 months. The rash and symptoms of DM may clear following resection of the tumor. Recurrence of dermatomyositis may indicate the occurrence of a second primary malignancy or recurrent cancer.

CHILDHOOD DERMATOMYOSITIS. Juvenile dermatomyositis is characterized by a nonsuppurative myositis that causes symmetric weakness, rash, and vasculitis affecting the gastrointestinal tract and the myocardium. Skin lesions are similar to those in adult dermatomyositis. The female-to-male ratio is 2:1. The average age of onset is 7.8 years.

Calcinosis of subcutaneous tissue (Figure 17-25) occurs in approximately two thirds of patients and is complicated by recurrent infections, muscle atrophy, residual proximal weakness, contractures, Raynaud's phenomenon, and arthritis are possible late sequelae. Approximately 50% of children have a very acute, rapidly progressive disease, whereas the remainder present subacutely with rash and a gradually progressive weakness of muscles, joint contractures, and, very infrequently, calcinosis. The course of treated patients is variable: 25% are well in 2 years, 31% experience recurrences when steroids are stopped after remission, and 44% have continuous disease for more than 2 years despite continual corticosteroid therapy.

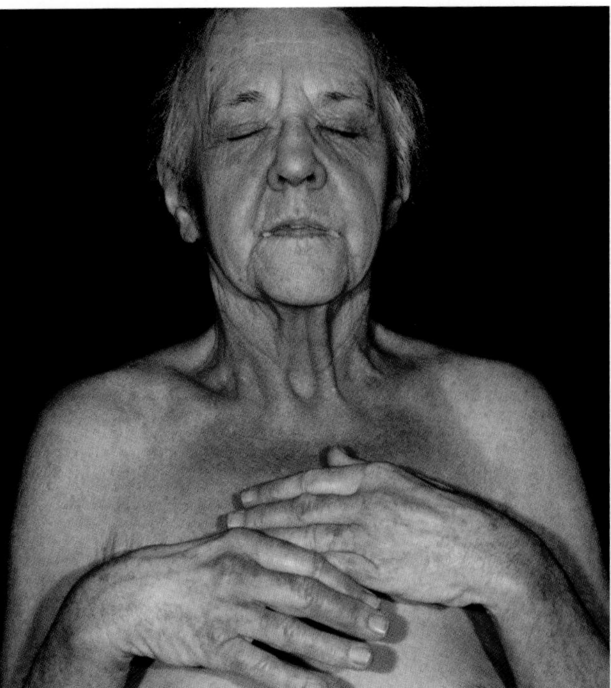

Figure 17-23 Violaceous scaling patches on the face and dorsal interphalangeal joints. The knuckles are involved; they are spared in SLE.

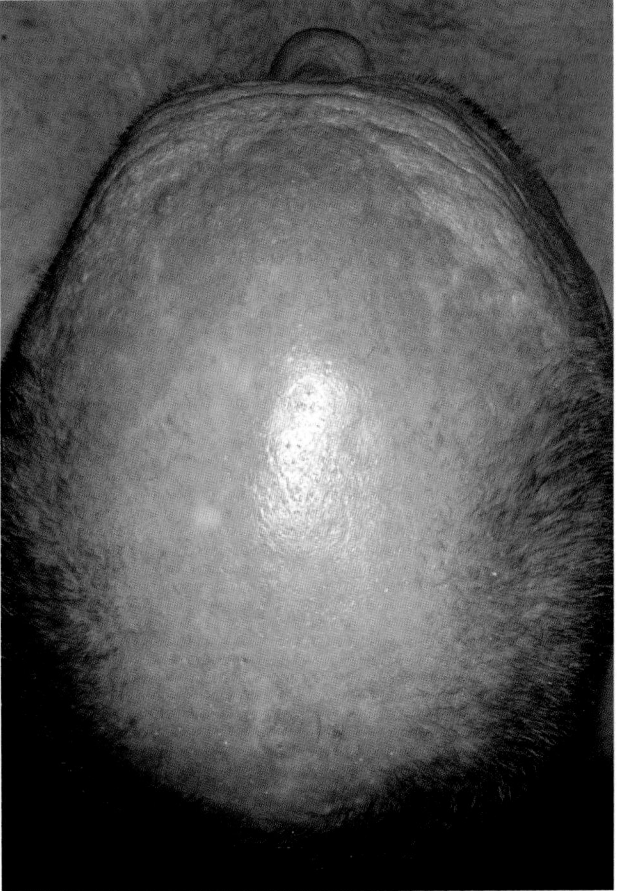

Figure 17-24 A red-to-violaceous, psoriasiform dermatitis with alopecia may appear on the scalp.

Elevations in erythrocyte sedimentation rate, lactate dehydrogenase level, and aspartate aminotransferase (AST) level occur commonly. Elevations in creatine kinase (CK) and aldolase levels may be delayed, especially in patients who demonstrate gradual onset of disease. Therefore serial laboratory values are recommended. The creatine phosphokinase concentration is elevated when there is acute muscle damage; antinuclear antibodies are usually present. The clinical course, incidence of calcinosis, and survival improve significantly with intensive early therapy with corticosteroids and physical therapy; as many as 92% survive and as many as 85% are functionally normal after 5 years. The incidence of cancer is low. Death can occur in the acute phase as a result of myocarditis, progressive unresponsive myositis, perforation of the bowel as a sequel to vasculitis ulceration, or, occasionally, lung involvement. Muscle biopsy specimens studied by electron microscopy show tuboreticular inclusions.

DRUG-INDUCED DM. The cutaneous manifestations of DM may in a small number of cases be caused by or exacerbated by drugs. Hydroxyurea, nonsteroidal antiinflammatory drugs, quinidine, D-penicillamine, and tumor necrosis factor (TNF) antagonists have been implicated.

OVERLAP SYNDROMES. Myositis may occur during the course of other connective tissue diseases such as scleroderma, rheumatoid arthritis, and LE. The most common

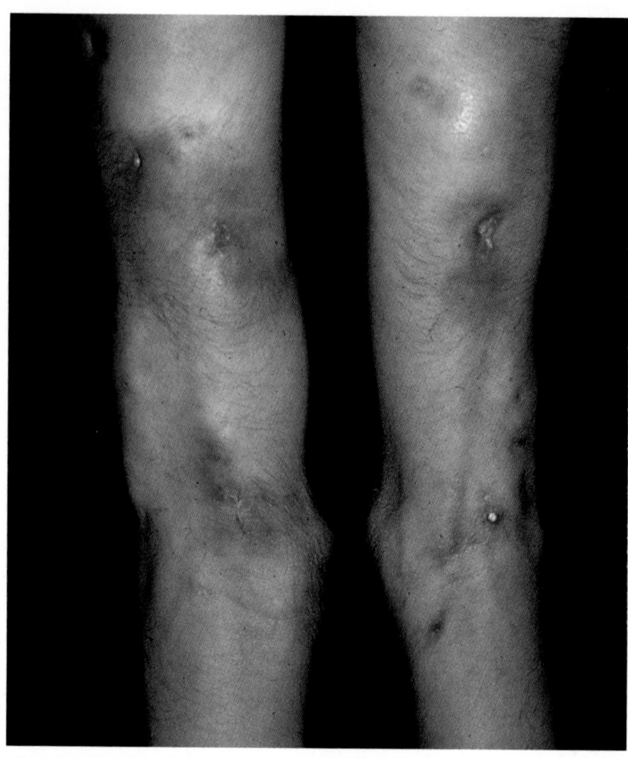

Figure 17-25 Calcinosis of the skin or muscle is found in about 50% of children or adolescents with dermatomyositis. There are firm yellow nodules, often over bony prominences. They can extrude through the skin and cause infection.

Table 17-9 Dermatomyositis: Clinical and Laboratory Evaluation

Test	Significance
Skin exam and skin biopsy	Establish diagnosis with high degree of certainty
Strength of proximal extensor muscles	Especially the extensor groups (triceps and quadriceps)
MRI or ultrasound of proximal muscles	Obtain before, or instead of, a muscle biopsy (especially patients with classic cutaneous lesions)
Triceps muscle biopsy	Only for difficult diagnostic cases
Electromyogram	Only for difficult diagnostic cases
Muscle enzymes	Creatine kinase, aldolase, lactate dehydrogenase, alanine aminotransferase
Muscle enzymes at regular intervals	Creatine kinase and lactate dehydrogenase are used to follow response to therapy
Chest x-ray or high-resolution CT scan	Investigations for interstitial pulmonary disease Often predicted by anti–Jo-1 antibodies
Pulmonary function studies	Demonstrate degree of diffuse interstitial fibrosis
Diffusion studies (pulmonary)	Demonstrate degree of diffuse interstitial fibrosis
Esophageal motility studies	For those with an inability to swallow and symptoms of aspiration
Occult malignancy evaluation	Repeated every 4-6 months for at least 2 years
Electrocardiogram	Cardiac disease is not usually symptomatic Cardiac involvement is the major prognostic factor for death in patients with DM not associated with malignancy
ANA	Frequently positive in patients with DM
Anti–Jo-1 antibody	Predictive of pulmonary involvement and is much more common in patients with PM
Anti–Mi-2 antibody	25%-30% of patients with DM; presence indicates best prognosis
PM-SCL or U1-RNP antibody	If present, overlap syndrome is suggested

association is with scleroderma and is termed sclerodermatomyositis. Sclerodermatomyositis is a distinct overlap syndrome, with features of SLE, scleroderma, and PM; it is called mixed connective tissue disease. Of these patients, 80% are females, and the peak age of onset is 35 to 40 years of age. Clinically, females come to the physician with swollen hands and tapered fingers, Raynaud's phenomenon, abnormal esophageal motility, myositis, and lymphadenopathy. High titers of antibody (anti-RNP) to an extractable nuclear antigen called ribonucleoprotein (RNP) occur in all such patients but are not unique to mixed connective tissue disease. ANA is present, but Sm is absent.

DIAGNOSIS. Diagnostic measures include muscle biopsy from weak muscles, skin biopsy of involved skin, and electromyography and measurement of muscle enzymes (Table 17-9). One or more of these parameters may be normal at the time of diagnosis or during the course of the disease; therefore a complete evaluation is needed in all cases. Patients with a rash suggestive of DM should have the diagnosis confirmed by skin biopsy. Patients with a confirmed diagnosis of cutaneous disease then need an evaluation for muscle disease. Therapeutic decisions are based on the presence or absence of myositis.

Muscle enzymes. Muscle enzymes are released when muscle cell damage occurs. The following serum muscle enzymes may be elevated: creatine kinase (CK), serum glutamic-oxaloacetic transaminase (SGOT), alanine aminotransferase (ALT), lactate dehydrogenase (LDH), AST, or aldolase. Measure all muscle enzymes (CK, aldolase, LDH, ALT, AST) because elevation of only one enzyme can occur. Serum muscle enzymes are measured for diagnostic purposes and to monitor disease activity. Although some patients with myositis have normal CK levels, most experts use the CK level as a guide to clinical response or reactivation of the myositis. These changes can occur months before or after a change in clinical course, predicting improvement or therapy failure. Measuring urinary creatine concentration (not creatinine) in a 24-hour collection is an early and sensitive indicator of muscle injury and a better indicator of activity than the serum creatine kinase concentration. The test is especially useful when serum creatine level is normal.

Histology of skin lesions. Histopathologic findings are similar to those for cutaneous lupus erythematosus with hyperkeratosis, vacuolization of the basal keratinocytes, melanin incontinence, perivascular lymphocytic infiltrate, and epidermal atrophy.

Muscle biopsy. Muscle biopsies from the same patient may vary. Several specimens may have to be taken to demonstrate an abnormality. A weak muscle should be sampled, usually from a proximal muscle group such as the biceps or quadriceps. Magnetic resonance imaging (MRI) can be used to accurately localize an affected area for biopsy. Avoid muscles where electromyography has already been done or where injectable anesthetics have been used. Dermatomyositis is a complement-mediated microvasculopathy and will show muscle fiber and capillary damage. Lymphocytes and macrophages partially invade non-necrotic fibers.

Electromyographic studies. These studies are indicated to diagnose the disease but not to follow disease activity.

Magnetic resonance imaging. MRI may help to establish the diagnosis, to find an appropriate muscle biopsy site, and to monitor the progress of the disease. MRI findings include subcutaneous edema, increased water content of the muscle, intramuscular calcium deposits, and fatty infiltration or atrophy of the muscle.

Antibody tests. Specific autoantibody tests (ANA, Jo-1, SS-A [Ro], Ku [Ki]) should be ordered (see Tables 17-2 to 17-4, Tables 17-9 and 17-10). These tests are of limited value in making the diagnosis, but positive serum results help to support it. Serologic studies such as rheumatoid factor, ANA, anti–Ro/SS-A, anti–La/SS-B, and anti-RNP are performed to rule out associated collagen vascular diseases. Positive low-titer ANA occurs in most cases, even in the absence of connective tissue disease. Anti-Ku antibodies are associated with myositis overlap with scleroderma or systemic lupus erythematosus.

EVALUATION FOR POSSIBLE MALIGNANCY. Patients with DM should be evaluated for internal malignancy (see Box 17-3). Complete history and physical examination in a search for malignancy should be repeated at certain intervals (e.g., every 4 to 6 months, particularly in patients older than 50 years). All unusual signs, symptoms, and laboratory values should be pursued. The cancer risk is increased about sixfold during the first year, but is lower during the second year, with no significant excesses in subsequent years of follow-up. Therefore among long-term survivors of PM/DM, there is little evidence to warrant extensive preventive and screening measures after 2 years. Tumors may appear at any site but significant excesses are observed for cancers of lung, ovary, pancreas, stomach, colorectal, non-Hodgkin's lymphoma, and nasopharyngeal areas. The signs and symptoms of DM often clear shortly after the removal of a malignancy.

Box 17-3 **Initial Evaluation for Malignancy**
History and physical examination
Complete blood count
Comprehensive metabolic panel
Tests for blood in stool
CT scans of chest and abdomen
Ultrasound pelvis (women)
Mammography
Endoscopic studies of upper and lower GI tract (according to patient's age)
ENT evaluation (especially for Southeast Asia patients)

Adapted from Sparsa A et al: *Arch Dermatol* 138:885, 2002. *PMID: 12071815*

TREATMENT. Untreated patients die, are crippled, or survive without sequelae. Oral corticosteroids are the treatment of first choice for most adults who have skin and muscle symptoms. Adjuvant immunosuppressive drugs are used if muscle symptoms do not respond to oral steroids. Physical therapy is essential to prevent joint contractures and muscle atrophy. Skin disease is treated with group I to V topical steroids, sunscreens, and other agents.

Treating cutaneous disease. The cutaneous eruption often resists systemic therapy. Group I to V topical steroids reduce the erythema but do not clear the eruption. Nonsteroidal immunomodulators such as tacrolimus ointment (0.1%) or pimecrolimus cream (1%) may be effective and may be used intermittently as steroid-sparing agents. Most patients with cutaneous lesions are photosensitive; therefore exposure to sunlight should be minimized; broad-spectrum sunscreens are important. Antimalarials are sometimes effective in treating the cutaneous lesions. Hydroxychloroquine sulfate (200 to 400 mg/day) is prescribed. Add quinacrine (100 mg twice a day) if response is slow. Switch to chloroquine phosphate (250 to 500 mg/day) if hydroxychloroquine is not effective. Add quinacrine 100 mg twice a day if the response to chloroquine is not adequate. Antimalarial drugs have no effect on muscle disease. Non–life-threatening cutaneous reactions (generalized morbilliform eruptions) may occur in one third of patients. Add other systemic agents such as low-dose methotrexate (5 to 15 mg weekly) or mycophenolate mofetil. Start mycophenolate mofetil at 1 gm two times a day and increase to 1.5 gm twice a day as tolerated during the first several weeks. The onset of action is slow and other treatments are continued at reduced dosages; after 4 to 8 weeks the disease begins to respond.

Calcinosis. Calcinosis occurs in some children and adolescents. Early aggressive treatment may prevent this complication. Calcinosis is difficult to treat once it is established. Reports suggest that diltiazem may be effective.

Treating cutaneous and systemic disease. Systemic corticosteroids are the mainstay of treatment. Approximately 25% of patients will not respond and others will develop side effects. Early intervention with steroid-sparing agents may help to induce and maintain a remission. Methotrexate, mycophenolate mofetil, azathioprine, cyclophosphamide, chlorambucil, or cyclosporine have all been reported as effective.

Table 17-10 Autoantibodies Commonly Present in Sera of Patients with Idiopathic Inflammatory Myopathies

Autoantibody	Frequency of occurrence	FANA pattern in Hep-2 cells	Clinical associations
Myositis specific anti-synthetase antibodies		35%-40%	Found exclusively or most commonly in PM-DM or PM-DM overlap
Jo-1	20% PM-DM	Speckled cytoplasmic	Interstitial lung disease, arthritis, Raynaud's phenomenon, and mechanic's hands = "antisynthetase syndrome"
PL-7	3%-5% PM-DM	Speckled cytoplasmic	Antisynthetase syndrome
PL-12	3% PM-DM	Speckled cytoplasmic	Antisynthetase syndrome
EJ	<3% PM	Cytoplasmic	Antisynthetase syndrome
OJ	<3% PM/DM	Undescribed	Antisynthetase syndrome
SRP	4%-5% PM-DM	Nucleolar and speckled cytoplasmic	Severe disease, poor prognosis
KJ	<1% PM	Dense speckled cytoplasmic	ILD, PM, Raynaud's phenomenon
Mas	<1% PM	Not described	? History of alcohol abuse
Fer	<1% PM	Not described	Localized myositis
Mi-2	5%-35% PM-DM	Fine speckled nuclear	V-sign rash, nailfold changes
Other autoantibodies			
Ku	5%-12% PM-DM	Homogenous nuclear and nucleolar	Overlap syndrome
PM-Scl	8%-25% PM/overlap	Homogenous nuclear and nucleolar	Overlap syndrome
Ro/SS-A	5%-10% PM-DM	Fine speckled nuclear	Sicca symptoms, overlap syndrome
U1-RNP	12% PM-DM	Coarse speckled	Overlap syndrome

DM, Dermatomyositis; *ILD,* interstitial lung disease; *PM,* polymyositis; *RNP,* ribonucleoprotein; *RP,* Raynaud's phenomenon; *SRP,* signal recognition particle.

Corticosteroids. Patients respond better if treatment is started as soon as possible after diagnosis. Oral prednisone (0.5 to 1.5 mg/kg) is given in a single daily dose (not every-other-day dosing) until serum CK level is normal. Most patients begin to improve after the first month. Muscle strength improvement usually lags behind decreasing CK values. The dosage is lowered over a 12- to 24-month period as disease activity improves, as indicated by improving clinical signs and decreasing levels of muscle enzymes. Another regimen involves the following steps: (1) administration of oral prednisone in a divided daily dose of 40 to 60 mg/day (1 to 2 mg/kg in children) until the CK level has normalized; (2) consolidation of the prednisone into a single daily dose, which is then reduced by one fourth every 3 to 4 weeks only if the CK value is still normal; and (3) continuation of the prednisone until a maintenance dose of 5 to 10 mg/day is reached, at which time this dosage is continued for 1 year. Progressive weakness with normal or no increase in CK values suggests steroid myopathy. Reduction of neck flexor strength is seen with dermatomyositis. Neck flexor strength is unchanged if steroid myopathy is developing.

Consider adjunctive therapy if there is no improvement in muscle strength after 3 months of therapy.

Methotrexate. Methotrexate is a first-line adjuvant therapy in patients unresponsive to steroids (see p. 288). Start oral methotrexate at 7.5 to 10 mg per week, increased by 2.5 mg per week to a total dosage of 35 mg per week. Intravenous dosage is 10 mg per week, increased by 2.5 mg per week to a total dosage of 0.5 to 0.8 mg/kg. Taper steroid dose as dosage increases. Side effects occur frequently and include stomatitis, gastrointestinal symptoms, pneumonitis, pruritus, fever, neutropenia, hepatic fibrosis, and cirrhosis. Taking 1 to 3 mg of folic acid daily minimizes side effects. A pretreatment liver biopsy is performed for patients with liver disease. Patients who do not drink excessively, are not obese, do not have diabetes, and have normal liver function tests probably do not require periodic liver biopsies.

Mycophenolate mofetil. Mycophenolate mofetil (MMF) may be effective for recalcitrant cutaneous disease (see p. 298). Add MMF without changing other therapies in a dose of 1 gm twice daily and advance to 1.5 gm twice daily. The onset of action is slow. Reduce other therapies after 4 to 8 weeks. Mycophenolate mofetil may be used alone or in combination with methotrexate.

Azathioprine (Imuran). Start oral medication with 2 to 3 mg/kg per day (usually 100 to 200 mg/day) tapered to 1 mg/kg per day once steroid is tapered to 15 mg per day (see p. 302). Reduce dosage monthly by 25-mg intervals. Maintenance dosage is 50 mg per day. Screen patients for thiopurine methyltransferase deficiency before treatment. Adverse effects include gastrointestinal symptoms, leukopenia from bone marrow suppression, and increased risk of lymphoma and hepatotoxicity.

Cyclophosphamide (Cytoxan). The drug is less effective than azathioprine. Start oral medication at 1 to 3 mg/kg per day or intravenous dose at 2 to 4 mg/kg per day, with prednisone. There is an increased risk of malignancy. Cyclosporine (3 to 5 mg/kg/day) is a very effective alternative treatment. Intravenous immune globulin (2 gm/kg/month) administered monthly can result in the clearing of cutaneous lesions. It is very expensive.

Physical therapy. Bed rest is essential for patients with active muscle disease. Physical therapy is very important in the management of DM to prevent atrophy and contractures. Prednisone and immunosuppressive agents treat inflammation, but they do not make muscles strong. An aggressive-passive physical therapy program should be started, and as muscle pain decreases an active exercise program should begin. Patients with dysphagia should elevate the head of their bed and avoid eating before bedtime.

PROGNOSIS. There is a poor prognosis when muscle weakness has existed for more than 4 months before diagnosis, with dysphagia, pulmonary disease and malignancy, and for DM patients with a lack of creatine kinase elevation. The cumulative survival rate is as high as 73% after 8 years. Polymyositis is almost always chronic and has the highest level of refractoriness to corticosteroid therapy. Dermatomyositis is chronic, but is usually responsive to corticosteroid therapy. *PMID: 16010208*

SCLERODERMA

Scleroderma is a disease characterized by sclerosis of the skin and visceral organs, vasculopathy (Raynaud's phenomenon), and the presence of autoantibodies. The spectrum of disease is wide, with systemic and localized forms (Box 17-4).

Systemic sclerosis

Systemic sclerosis has a reported incidence of 2 to 12 cases per million people per year. There are two major subsets of the systemic form: diffuse scleroderma and CREST syndrome. The criteria for the diagnosis of scleroderma are listed in Box 17-5. CREST (**c**alcinosis cutis, **R**aynaud's phenomenon, **e**sophageal involvement, **s**clerodactyly, **t**elangiectasia) syndrome is slowly progressive. Diffuse scleroderma can be rapidly progressive and potentially fatal; there is symmetric fibrous thickening and hardening (sclerosis) of the skin and fibrous and degenerative changes in synovium, digital arteries, and certain internal organs, most notably the esophagus, intestinal tract, heart, lungs, and kidneys (Tables 17-11 and 17-12).

Overlap syndromes exist in which typical scleroderma skin changes accompany a variety of other skin and internal diseases.

Localized scleroderma is restricted to the skin in an asymmetric manner. The other forms are rare and are not discussed here. Raynaud's phenomenon precedes or is an early manifestation in the majority of cases. All forms of scleroderma are more common in females.

Chemically induced scleroderma

Scleroderma-like diseases can be induced by a number of chemical compounds, such as plastics, solvents, and drugs. Contaminated rapeseed oil is the cause of toxic oil syndrome, and L-tryptophan induces eosinophilia-myalgia syndrome. Paraffin and silicon can trigger so-called adjuvant disease. Long-term exposure to silica can lead to idiopathic scleroderma. This supports the hypothesis that collagen disease may be attributable to the occupations of hypersusceptible persons.

Box 17-4 **Classification of Scleroderma and Scleroderma-like Disorders**

Systemic sclerosis

Diffuse scleroderma (10% of cases of systemic sclerosis)
- Skin—bilateral symmetric fibrosis of skin, face, proximal and distal portions of the extremities
- Visceral disease—relatively early appearance

CREST syndrome (90% of cases of systemic sclerosis)
- Skin—relatively limited involvement, often confined to fingers and face
- Visceral disease—delayed appearance

Overlap syndromes
- Sclerodermatomyositis
- Mixed connective tissue diseases

Localized scleroderma

Morphea
- Plaquelike
- Guttate
- Generalized
- Subcutaneous and keloid morphea

Linear scleroderma

En coup de sabre (with or without facial hemiatrophy)

Chemical-induced scleroderma-like conditions

Vinyl chloride disease

Pentazocine-induced fibrosis

Bleomycin-induced

Eosinophilic fasciitis pseudoscleroderma

Edematous (scleroderma, scleromyxedema)

Indurative (amyloidosis, porphyria cutanea tarda, carcinoid syndrome, phenylketonuria)

Atrophic (progeria, Werner's syndrome, lichen sclerosis et atrophicus)

Adapted from Masi AT et al: *Bull Rheum Dis* 3:1, 1981.

DIFFUSE SCLERODERMA

INITIAL SIGNS AND SYMPTOMS. Presenting signs are skin thickening of the hands and/or Raynaud's phenomenon (64%); rheumatic complaints, including arthralgias and stiffness of the knees (30%); or weakness, weight loss, easy fatigability, stiffness, edema, and diffuse musculoskeletal aching.

SKIN. The disease typically remains confined to the fingers, hands, and face for months or years but may progress to involve the forearms, legs, and eventually the entire body (Figure 17-26). In both systemic sclerosis and CREST syndrome there are three stages of skin disease: (1) edematous, (2) indurative or sclerotic, and (3) atrophic.

Box 17-5 **Scleroderma Criteria**

Major criteria

Proximal sclerosis—single major criterion (91% sensitivity and greater than 99% specificity)*

Minor criteria

Sclerodactyly

Digital pitting scars of fingertips or loss of substance of the finger pad

Pulmonary fibrosis-bibasilar

One major criterion or two or more minor criteria were found in 97% of patients with definite systemic sclerosis, but in only 2% of the comparison patients with SLE, PM/DM, or Raynaud's phenomenon†

*From American Rheumatism Association: *Arthritis Rheum* 23:581, 1980. *PMID: 7378088*

†Excludes localized scleroderma and pseudoscleroderma.

Table 17-11 Organ Involvement in Progressive Systemic Sclerosis

Organ	Involvement (%)
Skin	98
Esophageal atrophy or fibrosis	74
Small intestinal atrophy or fibrosis	48
Large intestinal atrophy or fibrosis	39
Myocardial fibrosis	81
Pericardium*	53
Pericardial effusion	35
Pulmonary interstitial fibrosis	74
Pleural disease	81
Kidneys†	58
Skeletal muscle atrophy	41
Skeletal muscle round cell infiltration	8
Thyroid (fibrosis)	24
Adrenal atrophy	26
Cancer	2

Adapted from D'Angelo WA et al: *Am J Med* 46:428, 1969. *PMID: 5780367*

*Pericarditis (fibrous or fibrinous) or pericardial adhesions.

†Any of the following: (1) fibrinoid necrosis of afferent arterioles or glomeruli; (2) hyperplasia of interlobular artery; or (3) thickening of basement membrane or wire-loop.

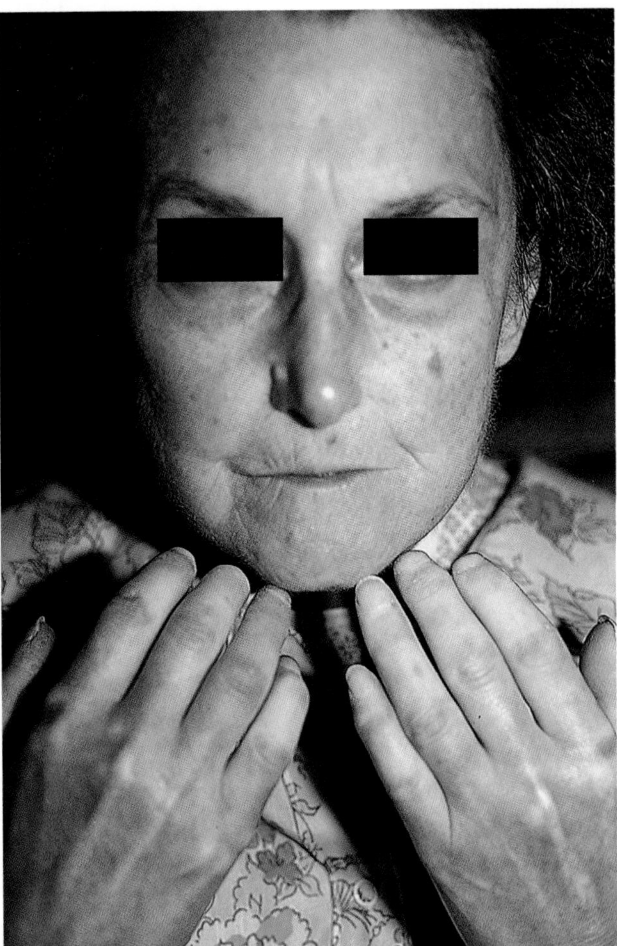

Figure 17-26 Scleroderma. The hands may be edematous and swollen early in the disease. These changes progress to other areas including the face. This edematous stage precedes the sclerotic stage.

Table 17-12 Signs of Visceral Involvement in Systemic Sclerosis

	Mild	Severe
Raynaud's phenomenon	Less than 5 times/day	More than 15 times/day, or digital ulcerations, or both
Esophagus	Dysphagia to solid foods; normal barium swallow	Dysphagia to solid and soft foods and weight loss (>10%); abnormal barium swallow with dilation of lower two thirds of esophagus
Lung	No symptoms: vital capacity >70% predicted and CO_2-diffusing capacity between 50% and 75% of predicted, PO_2 >69 mm Hg	Dyspnea + vital capacity <50% of predicted or CO_2-diffusing capacity <33% of predicted, PO_2 <69 mm Hg
Heart	Nonspecific ST	T changes; angina; definite ischemic changes by ECG; hypokinesis by MUGA scan or an ejection fraction <30%
Muscle	Mild EMG or CK abnormalities	Definite myositis clinically, biochemically, by EMG, or by muscle biopsy
Kidney	Mild hypertension or serum creatine level 1.5 times normal, or creatine clearance <80%, or 24-hour protein <500 mg	Refractory hypertension, or serum creatine level 4 times normal, or creatine clearance <20%, or 24-hour protein <3 gm

CK, Creatine kinase; *ECG,* electrocardiogram; *EMG,* electromyogram; *MUGA,* multiunit gated acquisition.

SCLERODERMA

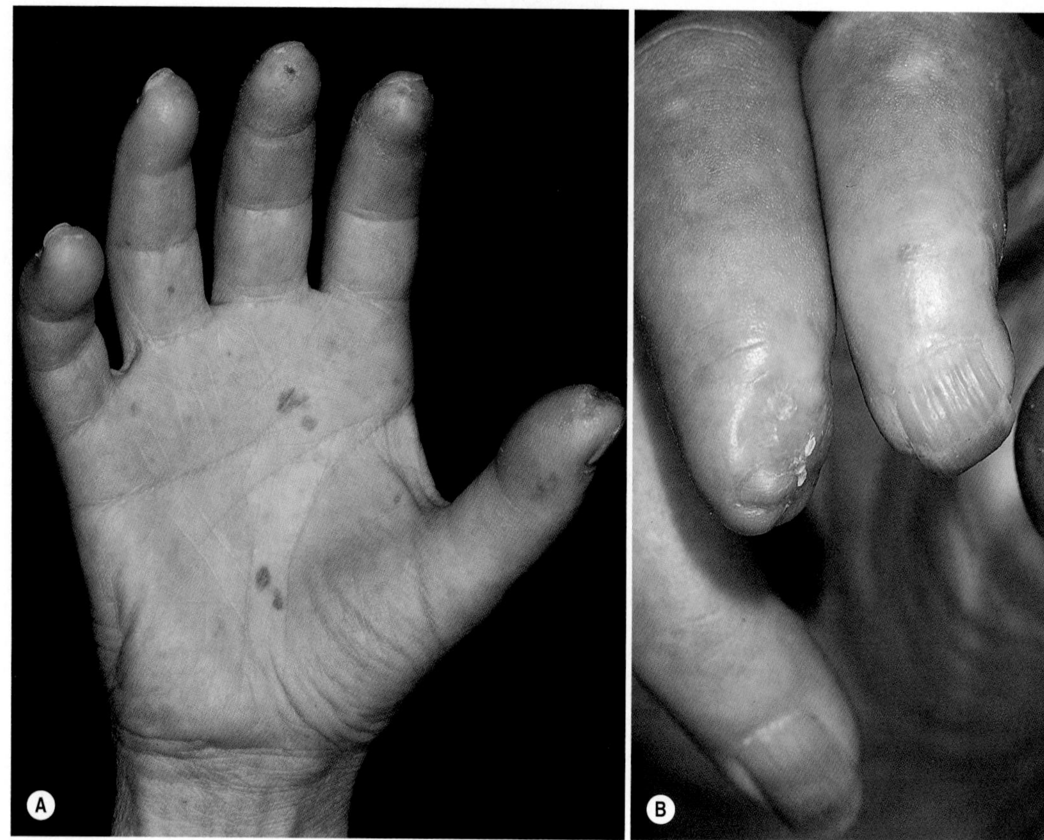

A: The skin is tightly bound down. The fingers are contracted. Telangiectatic mats are evident on the palms. There are fingertip ulcerations.

B: Fingertips are narrowed, and the fingers are shortened as a result of distal bone resorption.

Figure 17-27

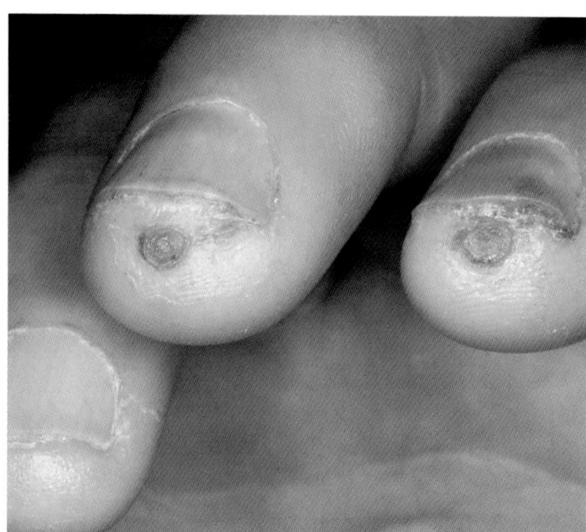

Figure 17-28 Repeated and increasingly severe attacks of Raynaud's phenomenon lead to fingertip ulcerations that leave pitted or star-shaped scars.

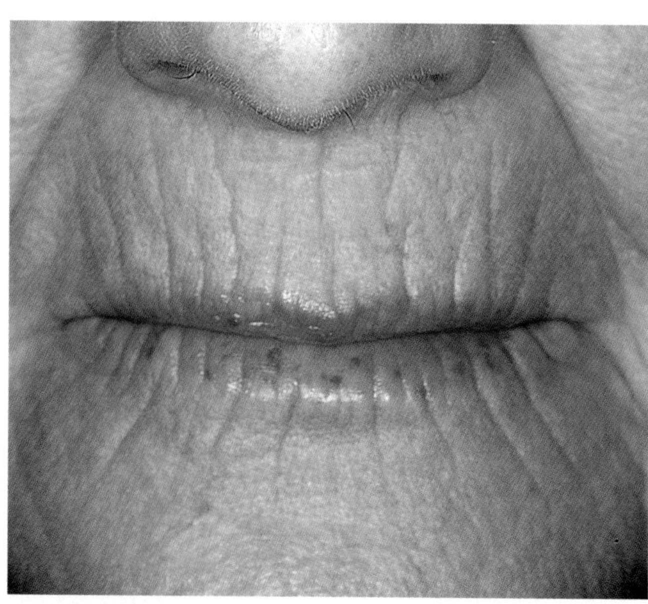

Figure 17-29 Telangiectasias are most obvious in the perioral area and neck. The skin about the mouth is drawn into furrows that radiate from the mouth.

In the edematous phase the skin is thickened and swollen and appears tense, with nonpitting edema producing the classic early signs of a masklike facies and "sausaging" of the fingers (Figure 17-26). Hand motion is restricted. The disease progresses to the indurative phase, and skin becomes hard, stiff, and bound down. Hand motion is further restricted. Hair loss and anhidrosis reflect fibrosis and degeneration of appendages. Mottled brown pigmented and hypopigmented areas occur on the forearms, upper thorax, chest, and scalp. Ulcerations, telangiectasia, and atrophy gradually appear. The skin of the fingers and hands becomes thin, shiny, smooth, and tightly bound down with the fingers contracted (sclerodactyly: "claw deformity") (Figure 17-27, *A*). The fingers narrow or taper distally, and the terminal phalanges become shortened as a result of distal bone resorption (Figure 17-27, *B*).

Repeated and increasingly severe attacks of Raynaud's phenomenon lead to fingertip ulcerations that leave pitted or star-shaped scars (Figure 17-28). Facial skin contracts and appears fixed to bone. The nose becomes beak shaped, and the skin about the mouth is drawn into furrows that radiate from the mouth (Figure 17-29). The curvature of the mouth becomes smaller, and the lips are thinned. Telangiectatic mats appear on the hands, face, and trunk, and dilated capillary loops are found at the proximal nailfold. Atrophy and softening of the dermis eventually make the skin more pliable.

RAYNAUD'S PHENOMENON. Raynaud's disease is a vasospastic disorder precipitated by temperature changes. The term Raynaud's phenomenon is used when the changes occur in scleroderma or other connective tissue diseases, and the term Raynaud's disease is used when the syndrome occurs in the absence of other conditions. Raynaud's phenomenon is the first symptom of systemic sclerosis in 47% of patients, preceding the onset of sclerodermatous skin changes by several months or years. It occurs during the course of the disease in 90% to 95% of patients. One study showed that 18% of patients with Raynaud's syndrome had systemic sclerosis. The phenomenon does not commonly occur with morphea or other localized forms of scleroderma.

Raynaud's phenomenon represents an episodic vasoconstriction of the digital arteries and arterioles that is precipitated by cold or stress. It is much more common in women. There are three stages during a single episode: pallor (white), in which vasospasm causes the fingers to turn white, cold, numb, and painful; cyanosis (blue), in which relaxation of vasospasm occurs; and hyperemia (red), in which relaxation results in reactive hyperemia and the fingers turn red.

Nailfold capillary patterns as detected by nailfold capillary microscopy may help distinguish Raynaud's disease (no scleroderma) from Raynaud's phenomenon (associated with scleroderma). A decrease in capillary loops occurs in Raynaud's phenomenon. This fact may help to predict which cases of Raynaud's disease will evolve into systemic sclerosis.

TELANGIECTASIAS. The telangiectasias of CREST syndrome and scleroderma have a unique morphology. They occur as flat (macular), 0.5-cm, rectangular collections of uniform, tiny vessels; these are the so-called telangiectatic mats (see Figure 17-27, *A*). These mats are most commonly found on the face, lips, palms, and backs of the hands. Telangiectasias may be present around the lips, tongue, and mucous membranes. Involvement of the oral mucosa also suggests Rendu-Osler-Weber syndrome (hereditary hemorrhagic telangiectasia).

GASTROINTESTINAL TRACT. Fibrosis and atrophy of smooth muscle can occur in any part of the gastrointestinal (GI) tract. Approximately 10% of patients may have GI symptoms before the appearance of skin changes. Dysphagia is the most common sign of GI involvement.

Esophageal dysfunction with hypomotility, dysphagia, reflux esophagitis, and fibrotic strictures occurs in approximately 90% of patients. Gastroesophageal reflux rather than impaired motility is the major cause of esophageal symptoms. Cinefluoroscopic and manometric studies disclose reduced or absent peristalsis of the lower third of the esophagus. Extremely sensitive, noninvasive scintigraphic procedures are available for quantitative assessment of esophageal function. There is no increased frequency of esophageal carcinoma.

Intestinal dilation and hypoperistalsis are the most common small bowel abnormalities. They lead to a "stagnant loop" syndrome with bacterial overgrowth, malabsorption, and steatorrhea. A characteristic mucosal fold pattern is called the hide-bound small bowel of scleroderma. Bleeding gastric telangiectasias located primarily in the upper part of the GI tract can result in severe blood loss. Wide-mouthed sacculations, loss of colonic haustration, and constipation occur with colonic involvement.

LUNGS. Lung disease is a frequent cause of death. Abnormal pulmonary function studies with reduced vital and total lung capacities are usually the first signs of lung disease. Dyspnea is the most common symptom; moist basilar rales are the most frequent sign. Interstitial fibrosis and thickening of the alveolar septa are the most common histologic changes. Fibrotic changes typically involve the lower lung fields, and pleural effusions are unusual. A diffuse reticulonodular interstitial pattern in a basilar distribution may be seen in the chest radiograph. Pulmonary hypertension occurs in 33% of patients.

KIDNEYS. Renal disease and hypertension are the major causes of death in patients with systemic scleroderma. Proteinuria, hypertension, and azotemia are poor prognostic signs, and death usually occurs in less than 1 year.

OTHER ORGANS. Myocardial fibrosis results in arrhythmias, and pulmonary fibrosis leads to pulmonary hypertension and right-sided heart failure. Polyarthralgia or arthritis was among the initial symptoms in 41% of patients. Sclerosis of the frenulum may immobilize the tongue. Fibrosis of the minor salivary glands may cause the clinical features of Sjögren's syndrome.

PROGNOSIS. Baseline factors that are most predictive of a poor outcome (rapidly progressive disease and early death) included the presence of abnormal cardiopulmonary signs and abnormal urine sediment (pyuria, hematuria). Subsets of patients with scleroderma with antibodies to centromere and histone have severe pulmonary or vascular disease.

Box 17-6 **Workup for Diffuse Sclerosis**

- Deep skin biopsy
- System review
- Office nailfold capillary microscopy
- ANA (centromere)
- Antibodies: SS-A (Ro), SS-B (La), Sm, nRNP Scl-70
- Organ workup

CREST syndrome

A more benign, chronic, and localized variant of scleroderma is called CREST syndrome (formerly known as acrosclerosis). The five clinical features of this disease (**c**alcinosis cutis, **R**aynaud's phenomenon, **e**sophageal involvement, **s**clerodactyly, and **t**elangiectasia) (Figure 17-30) are discussed in the section on systemic sclerosis. Calcinosis is a unique feature of CREST.

CALCINOSIS. Subcutaneous calcinosis occurs most commonly on the palmar aspects of the tips of the fingers. Calcinosis also occurs over the bony prominences of the knees, elbows, spine, and iliac crests. The deposits appear as firm, subcutaneous nodules that may eventually rupture at the surface, discharging fragments of calcium. In response to this foreign material, the skin surrounding the calcium becomes painful, red, and sometimes chronically infected, requiring courses of oral antibiotics.

Although patients with CREST syndrome can progress to more involved systemic disease, those with the clinical and serologic markers of the syndrome have a more benign course than patients with diffuse scleroderma.

The clinical differentiation between CREST syndrome and Osler's disease (telangiectasia hereditaria hemorrhagica) is difficult because telangiectasia may be the most prominent clinical feature in both disorders. However, patients with CREST syndrome usually have anticentromere antibodies in the serum.

DIAGNOSIS OF DIFFUSE SCLERODERMA

Specific circulating antibodies are useful in establishing the diagnosis. Most other laboratory studies are nonspecific (Box 17-6).

AUTOANTIBODIES. Antinuclear antibodies can be detected in more than 85% to 95% of patients with systemic sclerosis. Centromere antibody is found most frequently in patients with limited disease; autoantibodies are found in as many as 96% of patients with CREST or acroscleroderma and sclerosis limited to the digits, and in only 21% of patients with diffuse sclerosis (Table 17-13).

Table 17-13 Autoantibodies Commonly Present in Sera of Patients with Scleroderma

Autoantibody	Frequency of occurrence	FANA pattern in Hep-2 cells	Clinical associations
ACA	20%-59% scleroderma	Diffuse punctate speckled nuclear metaphase plate in dividing cells	Limited scleroderma, Raynaud's phenomenon, less pulmonary fibrosis, and renal crisis
Scl-70	20%-30% scleroderma	Homogeneous nuclear and speckled nucleolar	Diffuse skin involvement, pulmonary interstitial fibrosis, peripheral vascular disease, ? association with cancer
Th/To	4%-10% scleroderma	Homogeneous nucleolar	? Association with puffy fingers, small bowel involvement, low thyroid hormone levels, less arthritis
Fibrillarin (U3-RNP)	6%-8% scleroderma	Clumpy nucleolar	More common in patients of African descent and with diffuse disease, more severe disease
RNA polymerase I	4%-20% scleroderma	Speckled nucleolar	Diffuse disease
RNA polymerase II	4% scleroderma	Speckled nucleolar	Diffuse disease, also found in patients with SLE and overlap
RNA polymerase III	23% scleroderma	Nuclear speckled	Diffuse disease
PM-Sc-1	2%-5% scleroderma	Homogeneous nucleolar	Overlap with PM-DM

ACA, anticentromere antibody; *PM-DM,* polymyositis-dermatomyositis; *SLE,* systemic lupus erythematosus.

The frequency of antibodies in patients with systemic sclerosis is as follows: centromere (21% to 32%), Scl-70 (45%), and nucleolar (15%). More than one of the three antibodies is rarely demonstrated in any one serum. One of the three antibodies is found in two thirds of sera from patients with systemic sclerosis (SSc). Scl-70 antibody is found almost exclusively in sera from patients with extensive SSc (involving the skin of the trunk).

A subset of patients with antibodies to centromere and histone have severe pulmonary or vascular disease.

OTHER STUDIES. Hypergammaglobulinemia (most often IgG) occurs in approximately 50% of patients. The ESR is elevated (20 to 80 mm/hr) in 60% of cases. There are many other nonspecific findings.

CREST SYNDROME

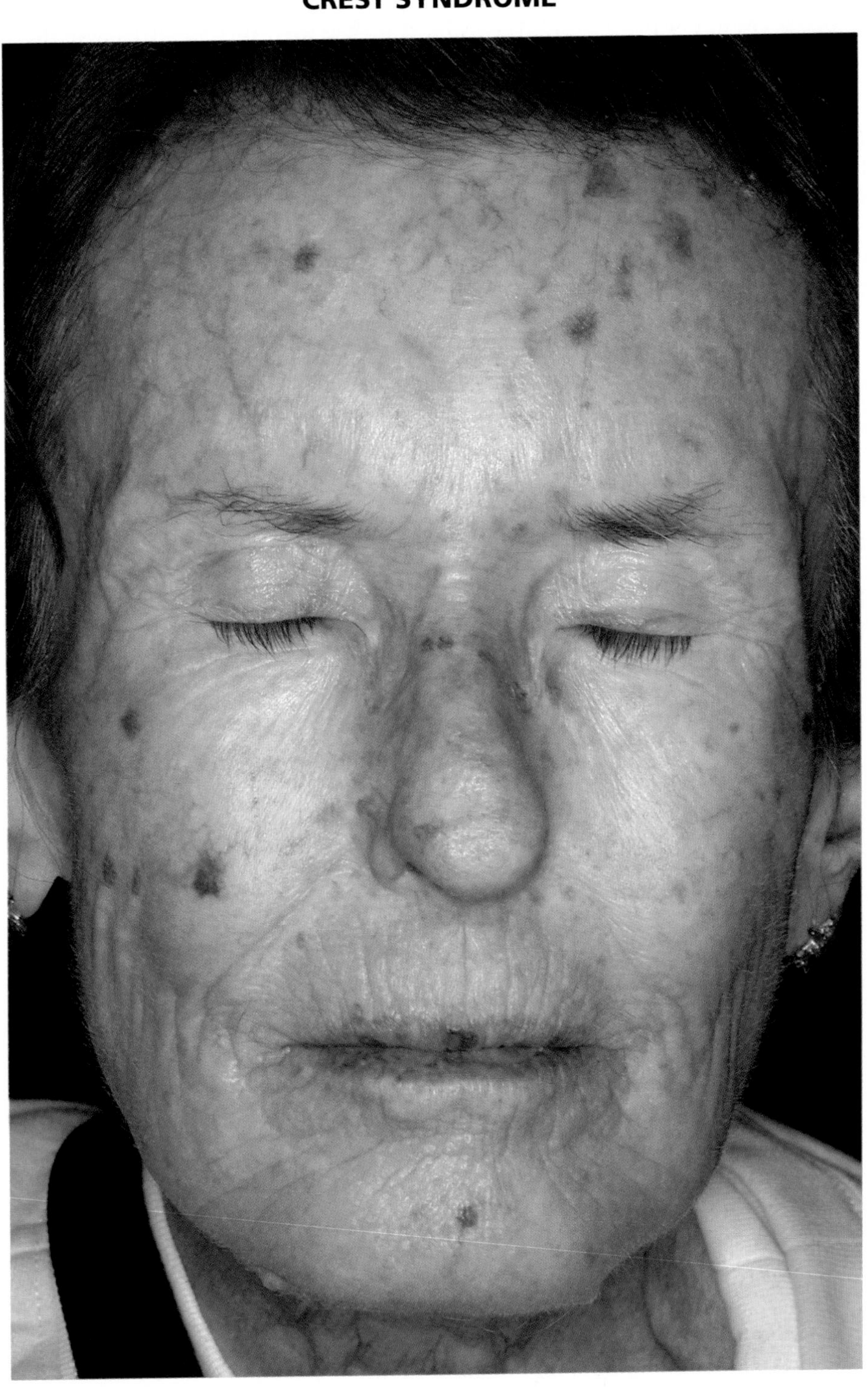

Figure 17-30 Telangiectases are flat, nonpulsatile, and appear in close groups called mats. Sclerodactyly means thickening of the skin of the digits of the hands and feet. In this limited form of scleroderma, skin involvement typically remains distal to the elbows and knees. It begins in the distal fingers and advances proximally. The process may also occur on the face, over the forehead (diminished wrinkles), and around the mouth (radial furrowing). Lips become thinner. The mouth opening is reduced in size. Sclerodactyly evolves through three phases: the edematous phase, indurative phase, and atrophic phase. The edematous phase begins with finger swelling, morning stiffness, and arthralgias. This phase lasts months to years. The skin becomes thickened, shiny, and tight in the indurative phase. This phase lasts for years. Finally the skin becomes fragile and lax.

OFFICE NAILFOLD CAPILLARY MICROSCOPY

A technique has been described for characterizing the telangiectasias seen in the proximal nailfold of the various connective tissue diseases. The scleroderma pattern is distinctive and is also seen in dermatomyositis. Familiarity with this technique may help to differentiate patients with lupus and dermatomyositis from patients who have cutaneous eruptions that appear to be similar. The technique used by Minkin and Rabhan is as follows:

A drop of mineral oil is placed on each nailfold. The ophthalmoscope is set at 40×, resulting in a 10× magnification. The instrument is placed close to, but not in touch with, the oil. Generally the capillaries are best seen in the nailfold of the fourth finger. Because the field of observation is smaller than in wide-field microscopy, the ophthalmoscope must be moved over the entire nailfold. A technique for using a television camera to record nailfold capillary characteristics has been described.

NORMAL. In normal people the capillaries are seen as fine, regular loops with a small, even space between the afferent and efferent limbs, in a row perpendicular to the nail (Figure 17-31).

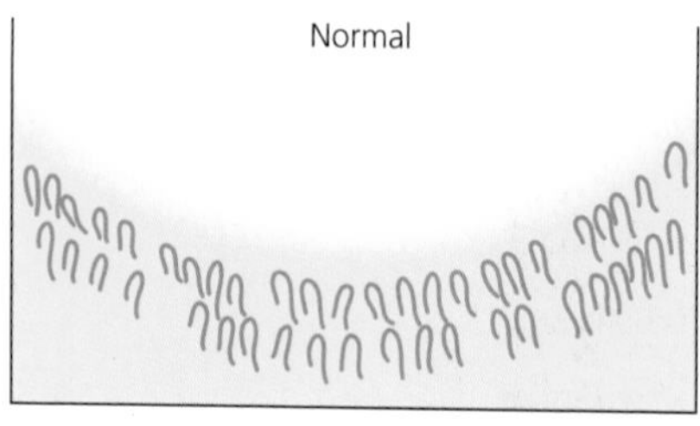

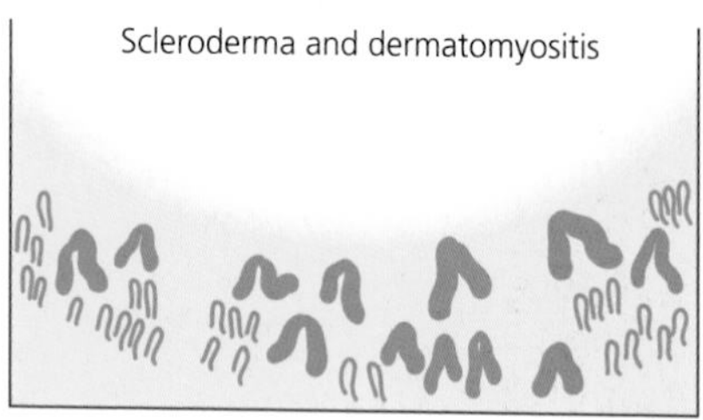

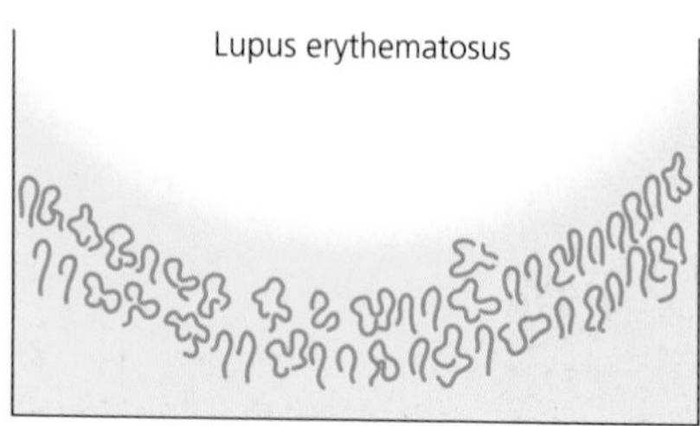

Figure 17-31 Office nailfold capillary microscopy. In normal people the capillaries are seen as fine, regular loops. In scleroderma and dermatomyositis the capillary loops are enlarged, deformed, and dilated. Many capillary loops have been lost. In lupus the capillaries are tortuous but there is little dilation of capillary loops. (From Minkin W, Rabhan NB: *J Am Acad Dermatol* 7:190, 1982.)

OVERLAP SYNDROMES (SCLERODERMA, DERMATOMYOSITIS). The scleroderma pattern (megacapillaries and/or avascularity) (see Figure 17-31) seen in 74% of patients with scleroderma consists of enlarged and deformed capillaries with dilation of both limbs of the loop, which is often engorged with blood ("sausage loop"). There is marked disorganization of the loop arrangement. Loss of capillaries produces many avascular areas and disruption of the orderly appearance of the capillary bed. Patients with Raynaud's phenomenon who present with avascularity and/or a mean of more than two megacapillaries per digit are likely to progress to a scleroderma spectrum disorder. The same pattern is seen in 82% of patients with dermatomyositis.

MIXED CONNECTIVE TISSUE DISEASE. The scleroderma pattern is present in 63%, the lupus pattern in 22%; 73% have bushy capillary formation. The presence of bushy capillaries suggests mixed connective tissue disease (Figure 17-32).

LUPUS. In lupus there are tortuous, "meandering" capillary loops, but there is relatively little dilation of the capillary limbs. At times the loop length is increased and may resemble a renal glomerulus. There is usually some disorganization of the capillary pattern, but only rarely are avascular areas seen.

The changes are distinctive enough that a relatively inexperienced observer can accurately distinguish between patients with scleroderma and those with systemic LE or rheumatoid arthritis. There is a close association between the degree of visible capillary abnormalities and organ involvement.

TREATMENT

SYSTEMIC THERAPY. Penicillamine, methotrexate, photopheresis, relaxin, interferons, and cyclosporine have all been studied in controlled trials with variable out-

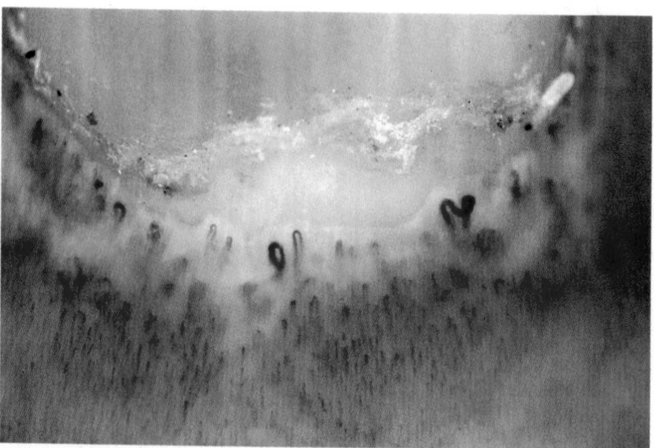

Figure 17-32 Nailfold capillary microscopy. Mixed connective tissue disease. Presence of bushy capillaries is suggestive of mixed connective tissue disease.

comes. Many other case reports for other drugs exist. There is no overall effective therapy.

Penicillamine (500 to 1500 mg/day) is often the treatment of choice for progressive systemic sclerosis. The clinical response to this agent is variable. There is no advantage to using penicillamine in doses higher than 125 mg every other day.

MANAGEMENT OF CUTANEOUS DISEASE. Cutaneous ulcers are protected with an occlusive dressing such as DuoDerm. Ischemic digital-tip ulcers may be protected with a small plastic "cage." Infection is signaled by abrupt erythema, swelling, and increased pain and is usually due to *Staphylococcus*. Adequate skin lubrication is difficult to maintain. Patients should bathe less and use moisturizers. Pruritus tends to occur early in the course of diffuse disease, especially over the forearms, and disappears after months or several years. Antipruritic moisturizers such as Sarna lotion may help.

No satisfactory medical approaches to calcinosis have yet been developed. Simple surgical excision may be performed if the overlying skin is intact and is not infiltrated with calcium, which may interfere with wound healing. When skin breakdown and draining fistulous tracts occur from deeper deposits in deeper levels, primary wound closure is not possible. Intense, sterile, inflammatory reactions surrounding hydroxyapatite deposits, along with constitutional symptoms such as low-grade fever, may be dramatically improved by a course of oral colchicine 0.5 mg once or twice daily for 7 to 10 days.

A daily physical therapy program emphasizing full range of motion of all large joints is important.

Therapies for scleroderma target the immune system, with the goal of reducing inflammation and secondary tissue injury and fibrosis. Therapy targeting underlying vascular disease is designed to improve the symptoms of Raynaud's phenomenon and to reduce ischemic injury to involved organs. Few controlled trials of therapy exist. Recent trials demonstrate promising results in the treatment of interstitial lung disease with cyclophosphamide, and treatment of vascular disease of the lungs and digits with endothelin receptor antagonists, the phosphodiesterase inhibitor sildenafil, and prostacyclins. Trials with methotrexate show only modest benefit in controlling scleroderma-associated skin disease. Prostacyclins are a therapeutic option in patients with secondary Raynaud's phenomenon. *PMID: 17917543*

Localized scleroderma

Raynaud's phenomenon, acrosclerosis, or involvement of internal organs does not occur in localized scleroderma. There are several variants (Box 17-7).

MORPHEA (Figure 17-33)

Morphea is more common in females; it can occur at any age but is more common after age 30. Like scleroderma, morphea begins spontaneously and involves thickening or sclerosis of the skin. The two diseases differ in appearance, in the extent of the lesions, and in evolution. Scleroderma appears as a bound-down skin thickening with minor skin color change, progresses to involve large contiguous areas of skin, and does not improve with time. The lesions of morphea begin as one-to-several circumscribed areas of purplish induration.

After weeks or months, the major portion of the central region of discoloration becomes thickened, firm,

Box 17-7 **Classification of Juvenile Localized Scleroderma**

Circumscribed morphea	Superficial	Oval or round, circumscribed areas of induration limited to epidermis and dermis, often with altered pigmentation and violaceous, erythematous halo (lilac ring). They can be single or multiple.
	Deep	Oval or round, circumscribed deep induration of skin involving subcutaneous tissue extending to fascia and may involve underlying muscle. Lesions can be single or multiple. Sometimes primary site of involvement is in subcutaneous tissue without involvement of skin.
Linear scleroderma	Trunk/limbs	Linear induration involving dermis, subcutaneous tissue, and, sometimes, muscle and underlying bone; affects limbs and trunk.
	Head	En coup de sabre. Linear induration that affects face and scalp and sometimes involves muscle and underlying bone.
		Parry-Romberg syndrome or progressive hemifacial atrophy: loss of tissue on one side of face that may involve dermis, subcutaneous tissue, muscle, and bone. Skin is mobile.
Generalized morphea		Induration of skin starting as individual plaques (4 or more and larger than 3 cm) that become confluent and involve at least 2 out of 7 anatomic sites (head and neck, right upper extremity, left upper extremity, right lower extremity, left lower extremity, anterior trunk, posterior trunk).
Pansclerotic morphea		Circumferential involvement of limb(s) affecting skin, subcutaneous tissue, muscle, and bone. Lesion may also involve other areas of body without internal organ involvement.
Mixed morphea		Combination of two or more of previous subtypes. Order of concomitant subtypes, specified in bracket, will follow their predominant representation in individual patient (e.g., mixed morphea [linear-circumscribed]).

Adapted from Laxer RM: *Curr Opin Rheumatol* 18(6):606-613, 2006. *PMID: 17053506*

MORPHEA

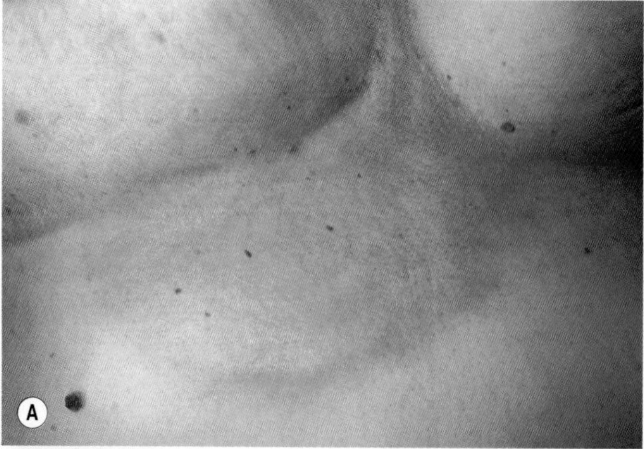

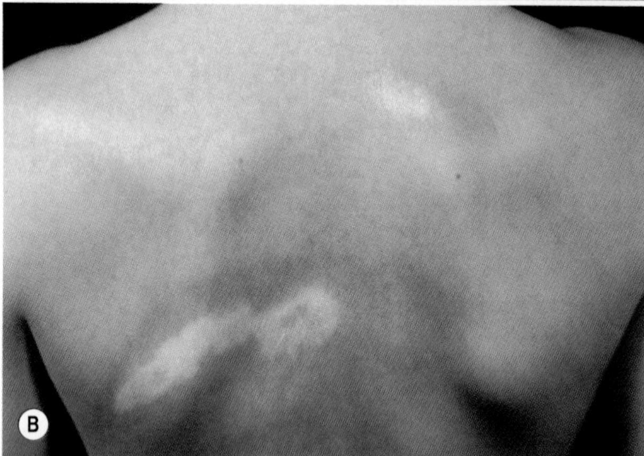

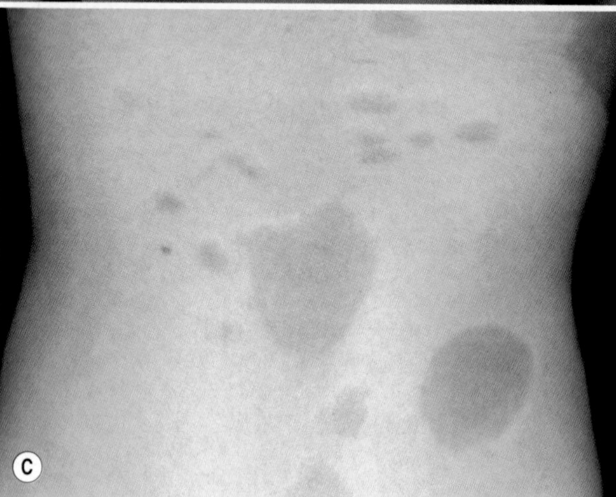

Figure 17-33 A single or few oval areas of nonpitting erythema and edema typically appear on the trunk. A violaceous border (lilac ring) surrounds the indurated area. The center of the lesion then develops smooth, ivory-colored hairless or hyperpigmented plaques, and the ability to sweat is lost.

hairless, and ivory-colored. The smooth, dull, white, waxy surface is elevated, in contrast to the diffusely bound-down skin of scleroderma. The violaceous or lilac-colored active inflammatory border is a highly characteristic feature of morphea. During the active stage, the round-to-oval plaques slowly extend peripherally but do not increase very much in size. Active lesions persist for 1 to 25 years. Inactive lesions leave their mark. Although much of the induration and skin thickening disappear, previously involved sites may exhibit atrophy and a mottled brown hyperpigmentation at the border and in the previously thickened plaque area. The remainder of the lesion becomes hypopigmented.

Multiple small, white plaques (guttate morphea) are a rare form of morphea. Most reported cases are probably cases of lichen sclerosis et atrophicus; in fact, the two diseases may appear simultaneously in the same patient.

LABORATORY DIAGNOSIS. Anti-DNA antibodies have been reported in some children. The presence of antihistone antibodies (AHAs) has been demonstrated in localized scleroderma. AHAs were detected in 42% of patients with localized scleroderma and in 87% of patients with generalized morphea. The presence of AHAs strongly correlated with the number of morphea lesions, the total number of lesions, and the number of involved areas of the body. ANAs did not correlate with the presence or number of linear lesions. The relationship of morphea to *Borrelia* infection remains undetermined.

BIOPSY. The histopathologic features vary with the course of the disease. Early active lesions show inflammatory cells in the dermis and subcutaneous tissue. Inflammation is most marked at the violaceous border. The collagen becomes eosinophilic and increases to occupy portions of the subcutaneous fat. Inflammation and sclerosis diminish with time.

TREATMENT. Asymptomatic plaques should probably be left alone to resolve spontaneously. Topical steroids and occlusion may induce slight improvement.

Inducing atrophy by infiltrating with triamcinolone acetonide (10 mg/ml) may be useful in areas where skin thickening has resulted in discomfort or limitation of motion. Thickened tissue offers great resistance to infiltration, and scattered pitted areas of atrophy rather than a uniform decrease in plaque thickness may result.

Hydroxychloroquine sulfate (200 mg) may be considered for patients who have multiple lesions that on skin biopsy are shown to be in an active inflammatory stage. The adult dosage is 200 mg of hydroxychloroquine twice a day. Induration may be markedly reduced or disappear in 2 to 4 months. The medication should be discontinued after lesions improve. The fundi should be examined by an ophthalmologist before antimalarials are started and should be monitored periodically.

Calcipotriene cream (Dovonex) 0.005% may be an effective treatment for localized scleroderma. Calcipotriene ointment 0.005% was applied without occlusion in the morning but with occlusion at night. The effects of the application are evident by 1 month.

LINEAR SCLERODERMA

Lesions of linear scleroderma have bands of sclerotic skin that often cross joint lines and lead to mild, but occasionally severe and disabling, joint contractures. Unlike oval plaque morphea, the inflammatory and fibrotic process may involve the underlying subcutaneous tissue and muscle, causing the fibrotic band to be more firmly anchored (Figure 17-34). One large study provides the following data. The female-to-male ratio is 4:1, and 83% of patients are younger than 25 years old when the disease begins. Trauma to the involved site precedes the lesions in 23% of cases. The onset is usually slow and insidious. Most lesions occur on the extremities, and two or more lesions appear simultaneously (61%), often bilaterally (46%). Joint contractures occur in 56% of patients. The typical patient has active disease for 2 to 3 years. It remains controversial whether linear scleroderma follows Blaschko's lines.

LABORATORY. In one study, peripheral blood eosinophilia (200 to 2500 cells/mm^3) occurred in 50% of patients with early active disease and declined with time. The frequency of antinuclear antibodies (Hep-2 cells) was 46%. Antibodies to single-stranded DNA were present in 50% of patients and were more common in those with joint contractures and disease duration of greater than 2 years, but the level of antibody does not correlate with extent of disease. Morphea occurred in 50% of patients.

TREATMENT. Early and continued physical therapy is crucial to maintain adequate joint motion. Methotrexate (MTX) 0.3 to 0.6 mg/kg per week and pulse intravenous methylprednisolone 30 mg/kg for 3 days monthly for 3 months were effective after 3 months of treatment. Low-dose UVA1 phototherapy can be highly effective for sclerotic plaques, even in patients with advanced localized scleroderma and with lesions rapidly evolving. Psoralen cream plus ultraviolet A (PUVA) therapy may be effective.

EN COUP DE SABRE

The most distinct form of localized scleroderma is morphea of the frontoparietal face and scalp regions, called en coup de sabre, so named because it appears that the blade of a sabre has struck a sharp, deep, vertical line on the face (Figure 17-35). The involved site may show all of the features of morphea. In time, atrophy of one side of the face may occur, giving the impression that a blade was turned to the side to remove a thickness of skin after landing vertically. Frontoparietal scleroderma may occur along the lines of Blaschko.

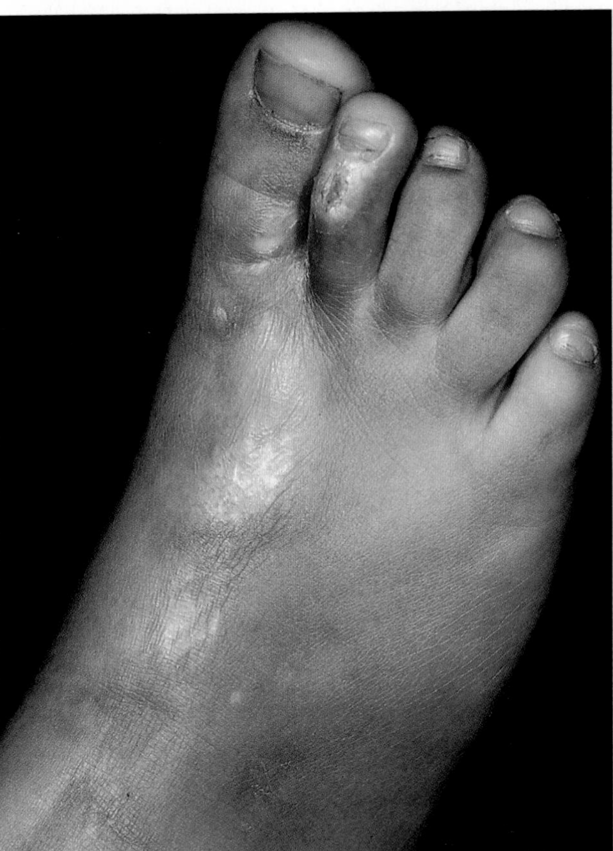

Figure 17-34 Linear morphea occurs as a single linear band, usually along the length of a limb. The deep fascia is closer to the dermis than on the trunk. This may explain why lesions may be fixed to underlying structures and extend to muscle or bone.

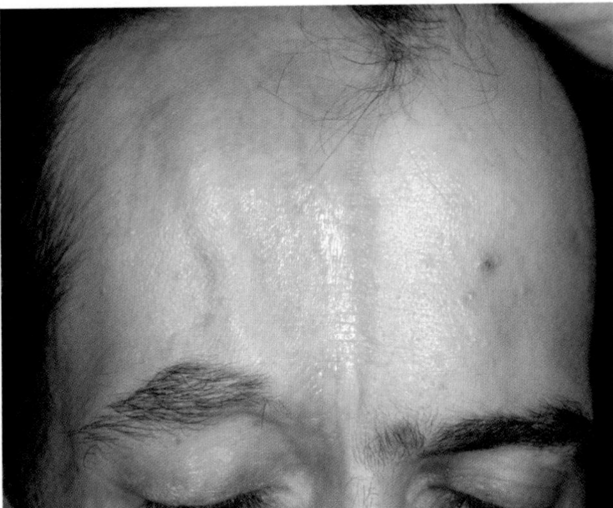

Figure 17-35 Frontoparietal linear morphea (en coup de sabre) is a depression suggestive of a stroke from a sword. Extensive lesions may cause hemifacial atrophy.

Chapter 18

Hypersensitivity Syndromes and Vasculitis

CHAPTER CONTENTS

HYPERSENSITIVITY SYNDROMES

Hypersensitivity syndromes are displayed in Figure 18-1.

ERYTHEMA MULTIFORME

Erythema multiforme (EM) is a relatively common, acute, often recurrent inflammatory disease. Many factors have been implicated in the etiology of EM, including numerous infectious agents, drugs, physical agents, x-ray therapy, pregnancy, and internal malignancies (Box 18-1). In approximately 50% of cases no cause can be found. EM is commonly associated with a preceding acute upper respiratory tract infection, herpes simplex virus (HSV) infection, or *Mycoplasma pneumoniae* infection such as primary atypical pneumonia.

Box 18-1 **Erythema Multiforme**

Etiology

Infections (viral, bacterial, fungal, protozoal)
Herpes simplex virus 1 and 2
Mycoplasma pneumoniae
Fungal infections
Medications

Management

Acute EM
- Observation
- Oral antihistamines
- Topical steroids
- Acyclovir
- Prednisone

Recurrent erythema multiforme
- Oral acyclovir
- Valacyclovir
- Famciclovir
- Dapsone
- Hydroxychloroquine
- Azathioprine
- Cyclosporine
- Thalidomide

HYPERSENSITIVITY SYNDROMES

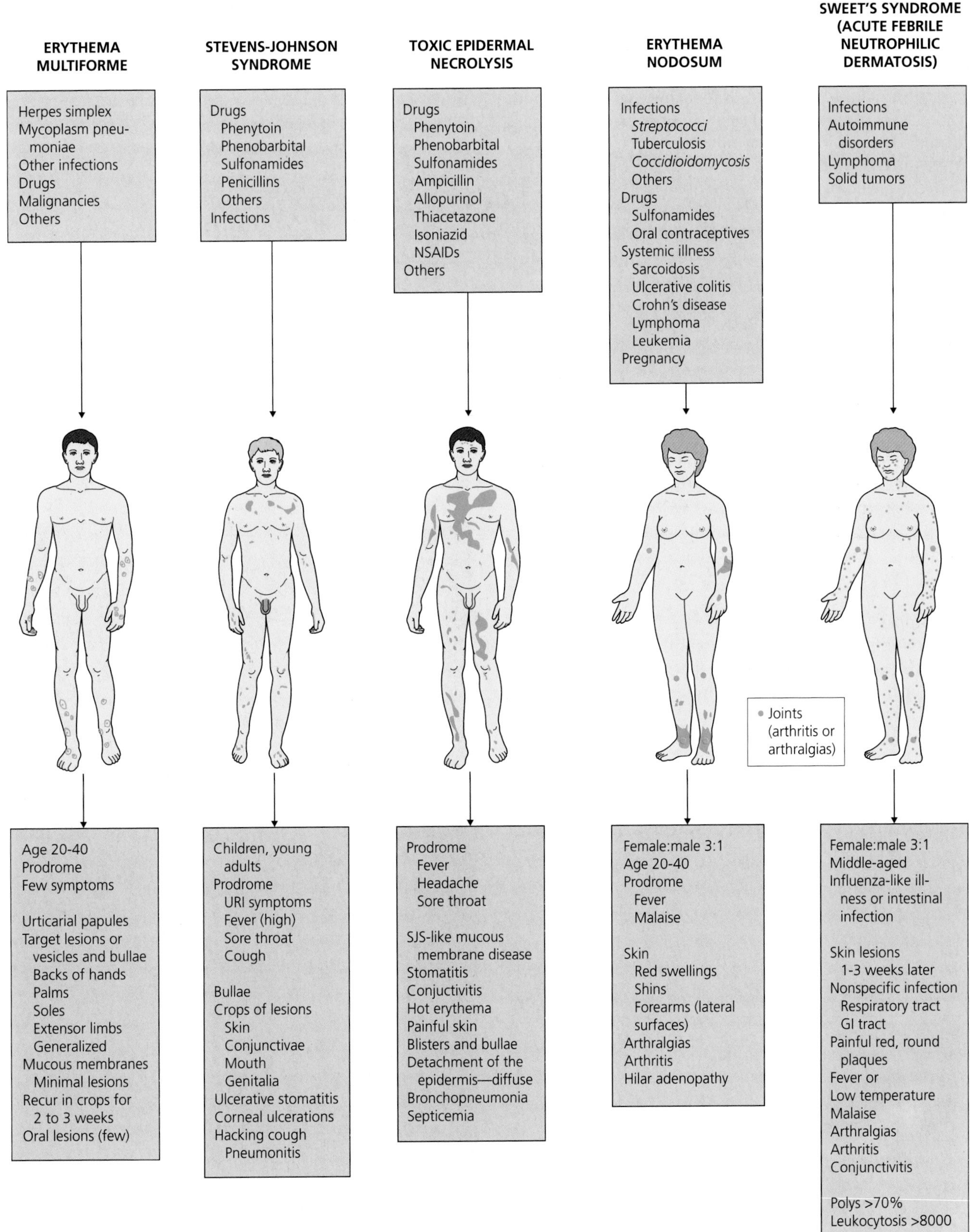

Figure 18-1

CLASSIFICATION. A new classification, based on the pattern and distribution of cutaneous lesions, separates erythema multiforme major from Stevens-Johnson syndrome (SJS) and toxic epidermal necrolysis (TEN) (see the section on Stevens-Johnson syndrome). Erythema multiforme differs from Stevens-Johnson syndrome and toxic epidermal necrolysis by occurrence in younger males, frequent recurrences, less fever, milder mucosal lesions, and lack of association with collagen vascular diseases, human immunodeficiency virus infection, or cancer. Recent or recurrent herpes is the principal risk factor for EM. Drugs have higher etiologic fractions for SJS and TEN.

HERPES ASSOCIATED WITH RECURRENT EM. Herpes-associated EM develops in only a few of the many individuals who experience recurrent herpes simplex virus infection. EM develops in some adults and children after each episode of herpes simplex. Skin biopsy specimens of EM lesions from patients with recurrent disease show HSV-specific DNA in most cases.

PATHOGENESIS

Studies suggest that immune complex formation and subsequent deposition in the cutaneous microvasculature may play a role in the pathogenesis of EM. Circulating complexes and deposition of C3, immunoglobulin M (IgM), and fibrin around the upper dermal blood vessels have been found in the majority of patients with EM. Histologically, a mononuclear cell infiltrate is present about these same upper dermal blood vessels; in the other immune complex–mediated cutaneous vasculitis (leukocytoclastic vasculitis), polymorphonuclear leukocytes are present. EM shows lichenoid inflammatory infiltrate and epidermal necrosis that mainly affects the basal layer. Necrotic keratinocytes range from individual cells to confluent epidermal necrosis. The epidermodermal junction shows changes ranging from vacuolar alteration up to subepidermal blisters. The dermal infiltrate is mostly perivascular. SJS has a predominantly necrotic pattern in which major epidermal necrosis and minimal inflammatory infiltration are found. Acrosyringeal concentration of keratinocyte necrosis in EM occurs in drug-related cases and is more likely to be accompanied by a dermal inflammatory infiltrate containing eosinophils. Drug concentration in sweat may explain this pattern with subsequent toxic and immunologic mechanisms leading to the fully evolved lesion. Erythema multiforme has a high-density cell infiltrate rich in T lymphocytes. In contrast, toxic epidermal necrolysis is characterized by a cell-poor infiltrate in which macrophages and dendrocytes predominate.

CLINICAL MANIFESTATIONS

The prodromal symptoms, morphologic configuration of the lesions, and intensity of systemic symptoms vary. Milder forms of the disease may be preceded by malaise, fever, or itching and burning at the site where the eruption will occur. The cutaneous eruptions are most distinctive, and classification is based on their form. Mucosal lesions may occur in up to 70% of cases. The most common sites are the lips and buccal mucosa. The differential diagnosis is listed in Box 18-2.

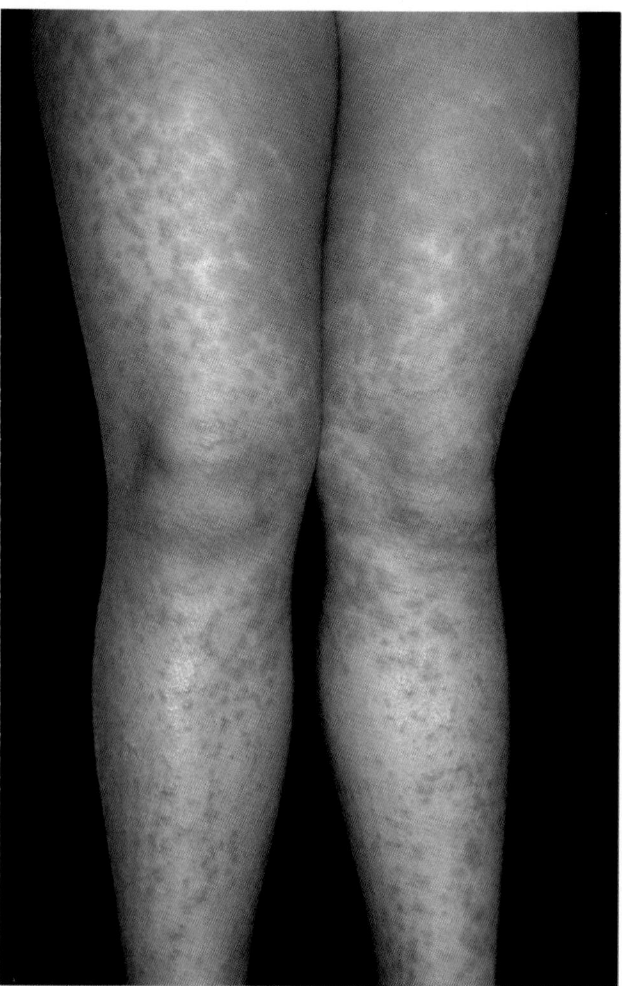

Figure 18-2 Erythema multiforme. Lesions may be concentrated on the extremities.

Box 18-2 **Differential Diagnosis of Erythema Multiforme**

- Bullous pemphigoid
- Dermatitis herpetiformis
- Drug eruptions
- Leukocytoclastic vasculitis
- Lupus erythematosus
- Pityriasis rosea
- Polymorphic light eruption
- Stevens-Johnson syndrome
- Toxic epidermal necrolysis
- Urticaria
- Urticarial vasculitis
- Viral exanthems

TARGET LESIONS AND PAPULES. Target lesions and papules are the most characteristic eruptions. Dusky red, round maculopapules appear suddenly in a symmetric pattern on the backs of the hands and feet and the extensor aspect of the forearms and legs. The trunk may be involved in more severe cases. Early lesions itch, burn, or are asymptomatic. The diagnosis may not be suspected until the nonspecific early lesions evolve into target lesions during a 24- to 48-hour period (Figures 18-2 to 18-4). The classic "iris" or target lesion results from centrifugal spread of the red maculopapule to a circumference of 1 to 3 cm as the center becomes cyanotic, purpuric, or vesicular. The mature target lesion consists of two distinct zones: an inner zone of acute epidermal injury with necrosis or blisters and an outer zone of erythema. There may be a middle zone of pale edema. Partially formed targets with annular borders or target lesions on the palms and soles are less distinctive and clinically resemble urticaria. Individual lesions heal in 1 or 2 weeks without scarring but with hypopigmentation or hyperpigmentation, while new lesions appear in crops.

Bullae and erosions may be present in the oral cavity. The entire episode lasts for approximately 1 month.

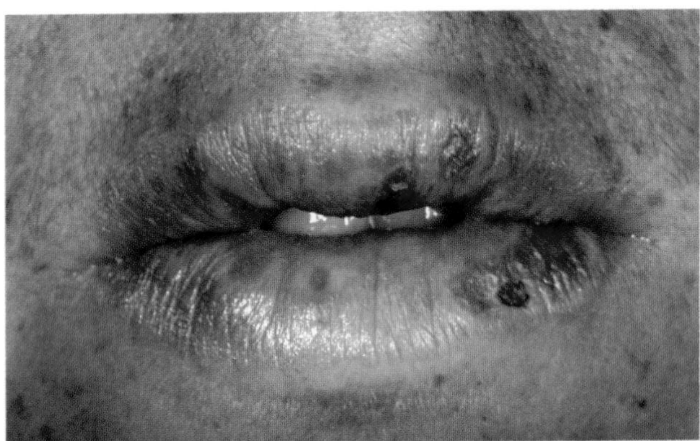

Figure 18-3 Erythema multiforme. The lips, palate, and gingiva are often affected. Inflammation is usually mild and lesions heal without scarring.

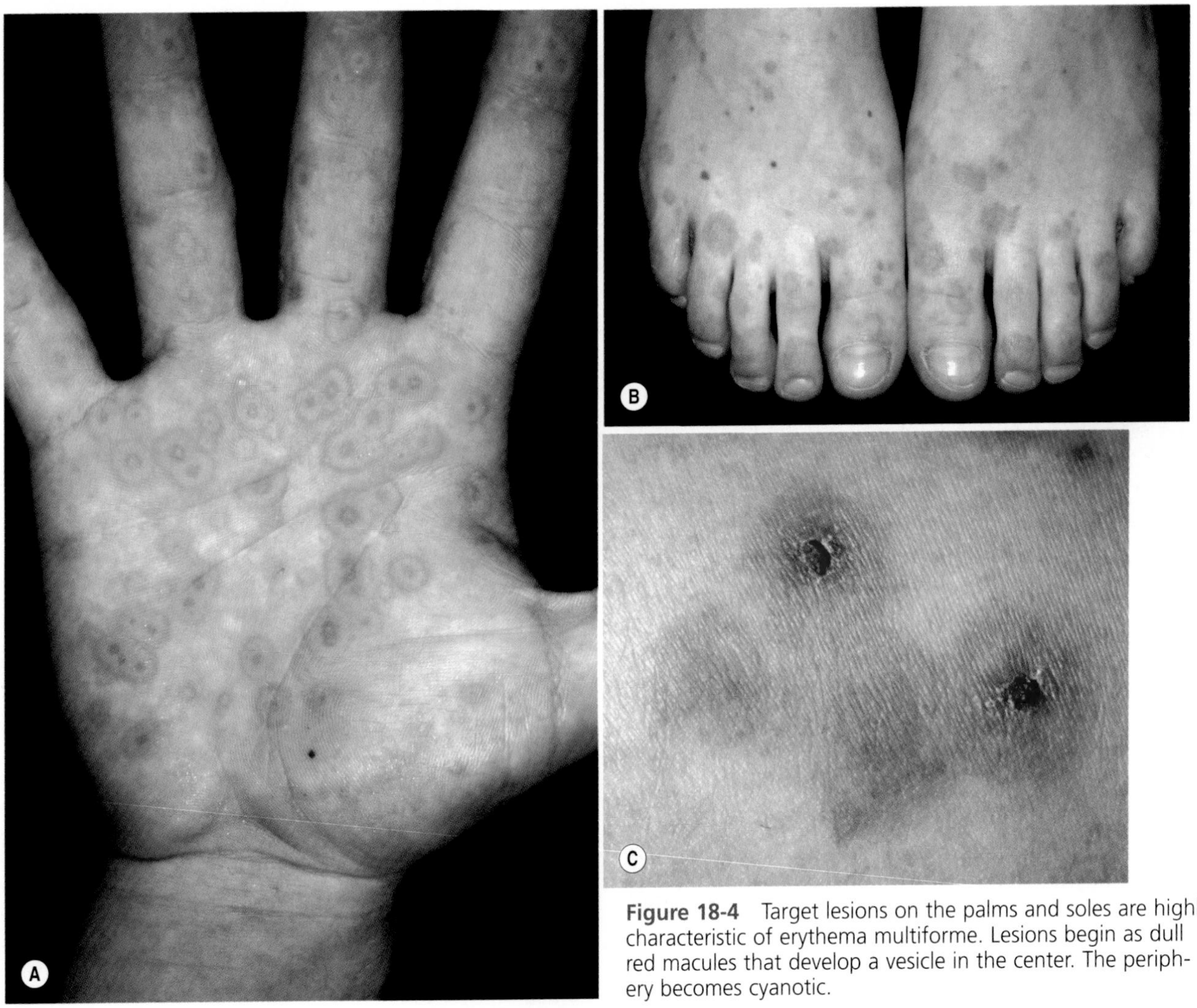

Figure 18-4 Target lesions on the palms and soles are highly characteristic of erythema multiforme. Lesions begin as dull red macules that develop a vesicle in the center. The periphery becomes cyanotic.

LABORATORY INVESTIGATIONS. Elevated erythrocyte sedimentation rate and moderate leukocytosis are found in the more severe cases. Biopsy is performed for atypical cases. Direct immunofluorescence may be needed to exclude other bullous diseases.

TREATMENT. Mild cases are not treated. Patients with many target lesions respond rapidly to a 1- to 3-week course of prednisone. Prednisone (40 to 80 mg/day) is continued until control is achieved and is then tapered rapidly in 1 week. Treatment with prednisone can successfully abort a recurrence. Oral acyclovir (400 mg twice a day) used continually prevents herpes-associated recurrent EM in many cases (Figure 18-5). Herpes-associated EM is not prevented if oral acyclovir is administered after a herpes simplex recurrence is evident, and it is of no value after EM has occurred. Acyclovir has been used by some patients continually for years without any apparent ill effects. Recurrent erythema multiforme patients should receive oral acyclovir (where HSV is not an obvious precipitating factor) for 6 months. Valacyclovir and famciclovir are absorbed better than acyclovir and may be used for patients who do not respond to acyclovir. If these treatments fail, dapsone or antimalarial drugs may be tried. Partial or complete suppression was evident in patients treated with dapsone (100 to 150 mg daily). Azathioprine was used successfully in patients with severe disease for whom all other treatments had failed. The response to treatment was dose-dependent (100 to 150 mg daily). The condition recurred on discontinuation of therapy.

Patients with chronic recurrent EM were given thalidomide 100 mg/day after other treatments had failed, particularly acyclovir and prednisone. Thalidomide was given at the beginning of an episode. The duration of the episodes was reduced by 11 days on average. Patients with frequent recurrent EM were given continuous treatment. Lesions disappeared within 5 to 8 days, and remission was maintained with low-dose treatment.

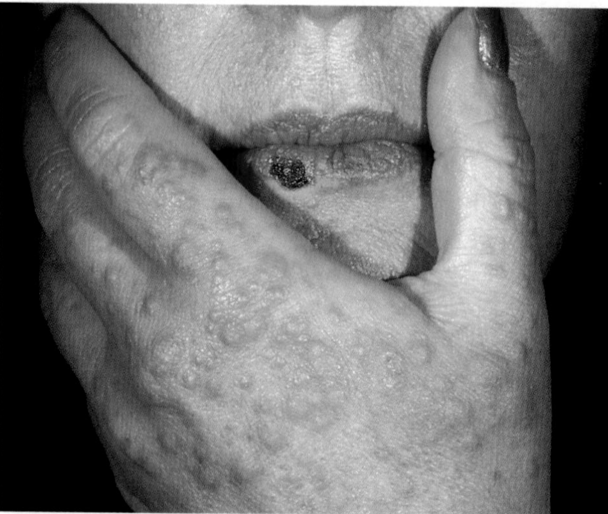

Figure 18-5 Erythema multiforme. An episode may be precipitated by herpes simplex infection.

STEVENS-JOHNSON SYNDROME/ TOXIC EPIDERMAL NECROLYSIS SPECTRUM OF DISEASE

INTRODUCTION. SJS and TEN are rare diseases with an annual incidence of 1.2 to 6 and 0.4 to 1.2 per million persons, respectively. Patients at greatest risk are those with slow acetylator genotypes, immunocompromised patients (e.g., HIV infection, lymphoma), and patients with brain tumors who are undergoing radiotherapy and receiving antiepileptics. Drugs are implicated in over 95% of patients with TEN. The etiology of SJS is less well-defined as about 50% of reported SJS cases are claimed to be drug related. The most frequently implicated drugs are shown in Box 18-3.

Stevens-Johnson syndrome and toxic epidermal necrolysis have traditionally been considered the most severe forms of erythema multiforme (EM). It was proposed that EM major is distinct from SJS and TEN on the basis of clinical criteria. The proposed concept is to separate an EM spectrum from an SJS/TEN spectrum. EM, characterized by typical target lesions, is a postinfectious disorder, often recurrent but with low morbidity. The second spectrum (SJS/TEN), characterized by widespread blisters and purpuric macules, is usually a severe drug-induced reaction with high morbidity and a poor prognosis. In this concept, SJS and TEN might be only types of the same drug-induced process that vary in severity.

A three-grade classification has been proposed and the degree of cutaneous involvement in TEN and SJS is shown in Box 18-4.

Box 18-3 **Drugs That Cause Toxic Epidermal Necrolysis and Stevens-Johnson Syndrome**

- Allopurinol
- Antibiotics
  - Chloramphenicol
  - Macrolides
  - Penicillin
  - Quinolones
  - Sulfonamides
- Anticonvulsants
  - Carbamazepine
  - Lamotrigine
  - Phenobarbital
  - Phenytoin
  - Valproate
- NSAIDs (nonsteroidal antiinflammatory drugs)

Box 18-4 **Classification of SJS/TEN**

Grade 1: SJS mucosal erosions and epidermal detachment below 10%

Grade 2: Overlap SJS/TEN epidermal detachment between 10% and 30%

Grade 3: TEN epidermal detachment more than 30%

PREDICTING PATIENT OUTCOME. A scoring system for TEN named the SCORTEN severity of illness score was developed to predict patient mortality (Box 18-5). Seven parameters are given one point if positive and zero if negative. Computing the sum of the scores results in a "SCORTEN" ranging from 0 to 7, with a score of 0 or 1 predicting a mortality of 3.2%, and a score of 5 or above predicting a mortality of greater than 90%.

EVOLUTION OF LESIONS IN SJS AND TEN. Skin lesions appear on the trunk first and then spread to the neck, face, and proximal upper extremities. The distal portions of the arms are usually spared, but the palms and soles can be an early site of involvement. Erythema and erosions of the buccal, ocular, and genital mucosa are present in more than 90% of patients. The epithelium of the respiratory tract is involved in 25% of cases of TEN, and gastrointestinal lesions can also occur. Skin lesions are tender, and mucosal erosions are painful. First, lesions appear as dusky-red or purpuric macules that have a tendency to coalesce. The macular lesions assume a gray hue. This process can occur in hours or take several days. The necrotic epidermis then detaches from the dermis and fluid fills the space to form blisters. The blisters break easily (flaccid) and extend sideways with slight thumb pressure as more necrotic epidermis is displaced laterally (Nikolsky's sign). The skin looks like wet cigarette paper as it is slid away by pressure to reveal large areas of bleeding dermis.

Stevens-Johnson syndrome

Vesiculobullous disease of the skin, mouth, eyes, and genitals is called Stevens-Johnson syndrome. The disease occurs most often in children and young adults. The cutaneous eruption is preceded by symptoms of an upper respiratory tract infection. A harsh, hacking cough and patchy changes on chest radiograph examination indicate pulmonary involvement. Patients with limited disease may be weak and lethargic, but the prognosis is good with conservative treatment. Mortality approaches 10% for patients with extensive disease. Fever is high during the active stages. Oral lesions may continue for months.

Box 18-5 **Scoring System for Predicting Patient Outcome in Toxic Epidermal Necrolysis**

SCORTEN variables*

- Extent of epidermal detachment >10%
- Age >40 years
- History of malignancy
- Heart rate >120 bpm
- Urea >10 mmol/L
- Glucose >14 mmol/L
- Bicarbonate <20 mmol/L

SCORTEN total	Predicted mortality rate (%)
0-1	3.2
2	12.1
3	35.3
4	58.3
≥5	90

*One point is scored for each variable in the left column present in the first 24 hours after admission. Cartotto R, et al: *J Burn Care Res* 29(1):141 2008. *PMID: 18182912*

INITIAL SYMPTOMS. Initial symptoms are fever, stinging eyes, and pain with swallowing. They precede cutaneous manifestations by 1 to 3 days.

SKIN LESIONS. Skin lesions in SJS are flat, atypical targets, or purpuric maculae that are widespread or distributed on the trunk first and then spreading to the neck, face, and proximal upper extremities. The palms and soles may be an early site of involvement (Figures 18-6 and 18-7).

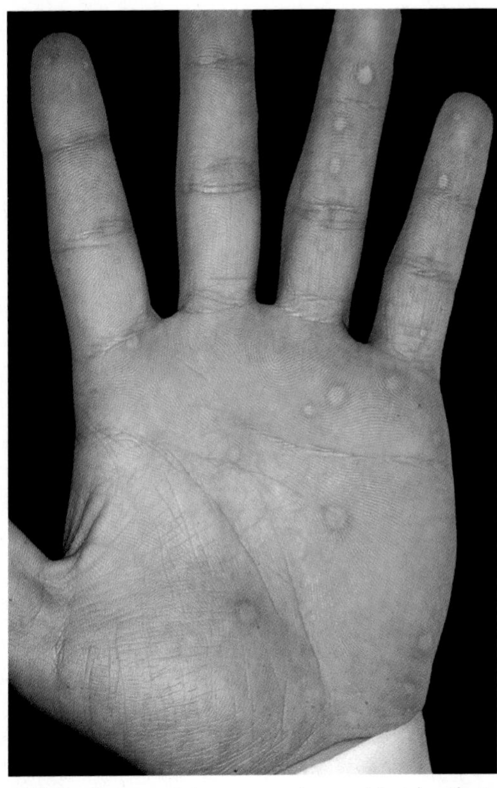

Figure 18-6 Stevens-Johnson syndrome. Vesicles that do not form the typical target of erythema multiforme may appear on the palms and soles.

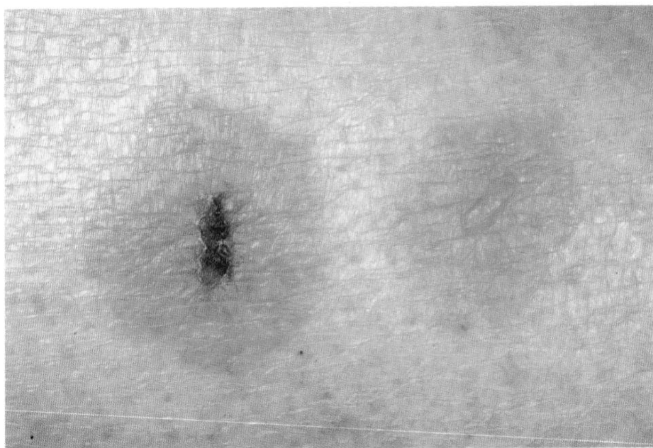

Figure 18-7 Stevens-Johnson syndrome. Atypical target lesions consist of round red macules, some of which have a central vesicle.

STEVENS-JOHNSON SYNDROME

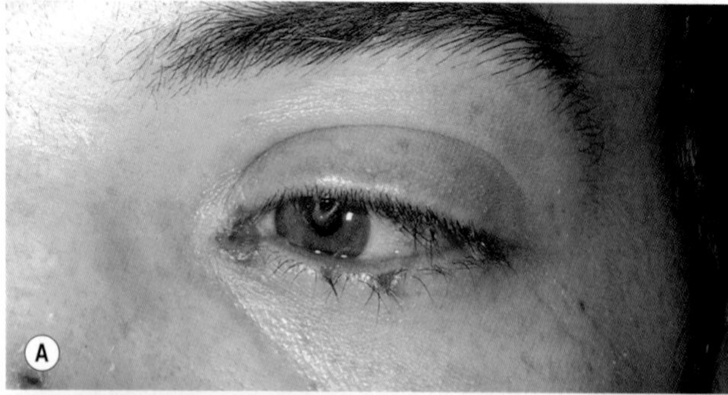

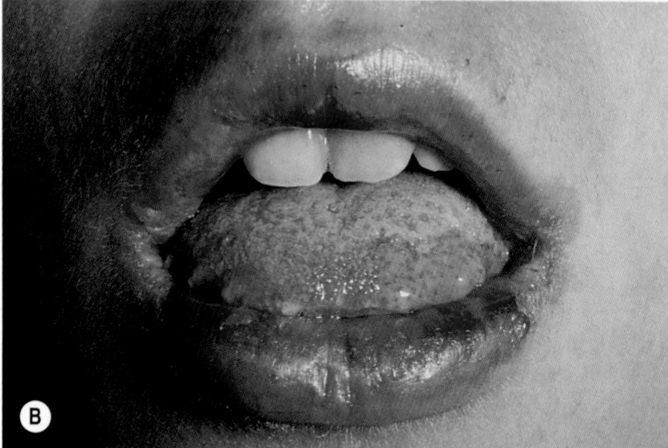

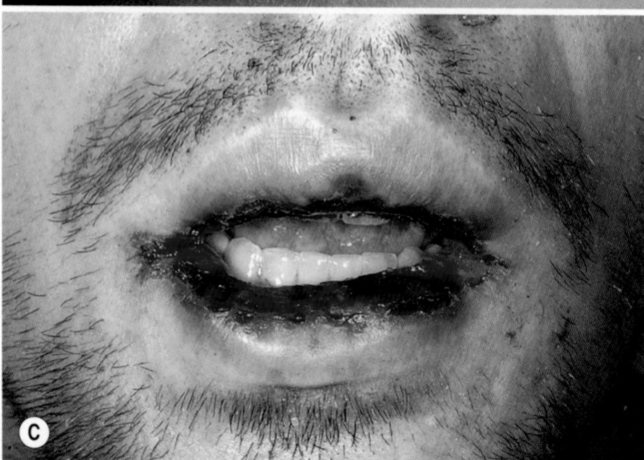

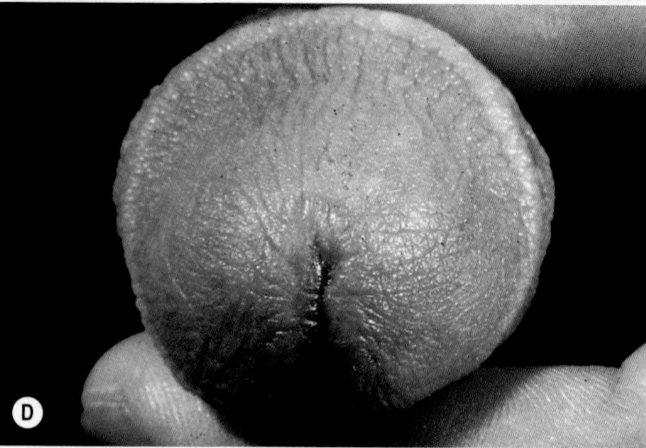

Figure 18-8 Bullae are present on the conjunctivae **(A)** and in the mouth (**B** and **C**). Sloughing, ulceration, and necrosis in the oral cavity interfere with eating. Genital lesions **(D)** cause dysuria and interfere with voiding.

This is in contrast to the lesions in erythema multiforme, which consist of typical or raised atypical targets or raised edematous papules that are located on the extremities and/or the face. New crops of lesions appear, but the disease is self-limited and resolves in approximately 1 month if there are no complications.

MUCOSAL LESIONS. Bullae occur suddenly 1 to 14 days after the prodromal symptoms, appearing on the conjunctivae and mucous membranes of the nares, mouth (Figure 18-8), anorectal junction, vulvovaginal region, and urethral meatus. Ulcerative stomatitis leading to hemorrhagic crusting is the most characteristic feature.

OCULAR SYMPTOMS. Corneal ulcerations may lead to blindness. Severe ocular mucosal injury that occurs in Stevens-Johnson syndrome may be a precipitating factor in the development of ocular cicatricial pemphigoid, a chronic, scarring inflammation of the ocular mucosae that can lead to blindness. The time between the onset of Stevens-Johnson syndrome and cicatricial pemphigoid ranges from a few months to 31 years.

ETIOLOGY. Drugs are the most common cause (see Box 18-3). The disease occurs most often in patients treated for seizure disorders. Upper respiratory tract infection, *Mycoplasma pneumoniae* infection, gastrointestinal (GI) disorders, and herpes simplex virus infection are all implicated. Possible causes should be sought diligently so that recurrences can be avoided.

DIAGNOSIS. A skin biopsy should be performed if the classic lesions are not present. Direct immunofluorescence may be helpful in nontypical cases.

TREATMENT. The use of corticosteroids remains controversial. A study of children suggests that treatment with systemic corticosteroids may be associated with delayed recovery and significant side effects. Other studies conclude that corticosteroids are beneficial and may be lifesaving. Many physicians presented with a sick child who has extensive cutaneous, ocular, and oral lesions elect to treat with oral steroids; most often prednisone (20 to 30 mg twice a day) is given until new lesions no longer appear; it is then tapered rapidly.

Itching can be controlled with antihistamines. Cutaneous blisters are treated with cool, wet Burow's compresses. Topical steroids should not be applied to eroded areas. Papules and plaques may respond to group II to V topical steroids. Frequent rinsing with lidocaine hydrochloride (Xylocaine Viscous) may relieve oral symptoms. Patients may tolerate only a liquid or soft diet. Ocular involvement is monitored by an ophthalmologist to minimize conjunctival scarring. Antiseptic eye drops and separation on synechiae are required. Vitamin A administered topically and systemically was reported to be effective for lacrimal hyposecretion. Secondary infection is treated with oral antibiotics. Stevens-Johnson syndrome associated with herpes simplex virus may be prevented by early use of acyclovir and prednisone.

Toxic epidermal necrolysis

Toxic epidermal necrolysis (TEN) is initially seen with Stevens-Johnson-like mucous membrane disease and progresses to diffuse, generalized detachment of the epidermis through the dermoepidermal junction. This full-thickness loss of the epidermis results in a high death rate. Fluid loss is not a major problem; death is usually caused by overwhelming sepsis originating in denuded skin or lungs. TEN is rare, occurring in 1.3 cases per million persons per year.

The death rate is 1% to 5% for Stevens-Johnson syndrome, and 34% to 40% for TEN. Mortality is not affected by the type of drug responsible. In contrast to previous series, today there is a high prevalence of human immunodeficiency virus infection among patients with TEN. This high rate of HIV infection is linked to an increased use of sulfonamides—mainly sulfadiazine—in these patients. TEN may occur after bone marrow transplantation. It seems to be related to a drug reaction to sulfonamides as often as to acute graft-versus-host disease.

TOXIC EPIDERMAL NECROLYSIS VS. STAPHYLOCOCCAL SCALDED SKIN SYNDROME. This life-threatening disease is similar in appearance to staphylococcal scalded skin syndrome (SSSS), which is induced by a staphylococcal toxin. The split in SSSS, however, is high in the epidermis, just below the stratum corneum, permitting rapid healing of the epidermis without danger of infection. The diagnosis of either TEN or SSSS can be made rapidly by examination of a skin biopsy by frozen section technique.

PATHOLOGY AND PATHOGENESIS. Histologically there is an early mild interface dermatitis that evolves into full-thickness necrosis of the epidermis. Keratinocytes from patients with TEN were found to undergo extensive apoptosis. There is subepidermal blister formation, keratinocyte necrosis, and a sparse lymphohistiocytic infiltrate around superficial dermal blood vessels. Lymphopenia is frequently documented. Cytotoxic T cells may contribute to the pathogenesis of blister formation by causing degeneration and necrosis of drug-altered keratinocytes.

ETIOLOGY. The causes of TEN are the same as those of Stevens-Johnson syndrome, but drugs are most frequently implicated in TEN. The reaction is independent of dosage. Culprit drugs include antibiotics (40%), anticonvulsants (11%), and analgesics (5% to 23%). Developing countries have a higher incidence of reactions to antituberculous drugs. The most frequent underlying diseases justifying drug treatment are infections (52.7%) and pain (36%). Challenge tests are absolutely contraindicated in Stevens-Johnson syndrome and toxic epidermal necrolysis. TEN and other severe cutaneous adverse drug reactions may be linked to an inherited defect in the detoxification of drug metabolites. In a few predisposed patients, a drug metabolite may bind to proteins in the epidermis and trigger an immune response, leading to immunoallergic cutaneous adverse drug reaction.

MEDICATIONS. The use of antibacterial sulfonamides, anticonvulsant agents, oxicam NSAIDs, allopurinol, chlormezanone, and corticosteroids is associated with large increases in the risk of Stevens-Johnson syndrome or toxic epidermal necrolysis (see Box 18-3). The excess risk of these drugs does not exceed 5 cases per million users per week. The risk of developing TEN from antiepileptic drugs is highest in the first 8 weeks after onset of treatment.

The following drugs are most commonly implicated:

Acetaminophen
Allopurinol
Aminopenicillins
Carbamazepine
Cephalosporins
Chlormezanone
Corticosteroids
NSAIDs
Phenobarbital
Phenytoin
Quinolones
Sulfonamides
Trimethoprim-sulfamethoxazole
Valproic acid

PRODROMAL SYMPTOMS. Fever is the most frequent prodromal symptom. Symptoms suggestive of an upper respiratory tract infection, such as headache and sore throat, usually precede the appearance of skin lesions by 1 or 2 weeks. Stomatitis, conjunctivitis, and pruritus occur 1 to 2 days before the onset of the rash.

SKIN. TEN begins with diffuse, hot erythema covering wide areas. In hours the skin becomes painful, and with slight thumb pressure the skin wrinkles, slides laterally, and separates from the dermis (Figures 18-9 and 18-10). This ominous sign (Nikolsky's sign) heralds the onset of a life-threatening event. Small blisters and large bullae may appear. Nonerythematous skin usually remains intact, and the scalp is spared.

MUCOUS MEMBRANES. Inflammation, blistering, and erosion of the mucosal surfaces, especially the oropharynx, are early and characteristic findings. The vaginal tract epithelium frequently blisters and erodes. Pain and erosion of oral mucous membranes interfere with oral intake, and nasogastric or duodenal tube feeding is often required. The rest of the gastrointestinal tract functions normally if sepsis does not occur.

EYES. Severe eye involvement is a constant feature. Purulent conjunctivitis leads to swelling, crusting, and ulceration with pain and photophobia. Complications include conjunctival erosions with subsequent revascularization, fibrous adhesions, and corneal ulceration and blindness. Photophobia, mucinous discharge, and decreased visual acuity may last for years.

TOXIC EPIDERMAL NECROLYSIS

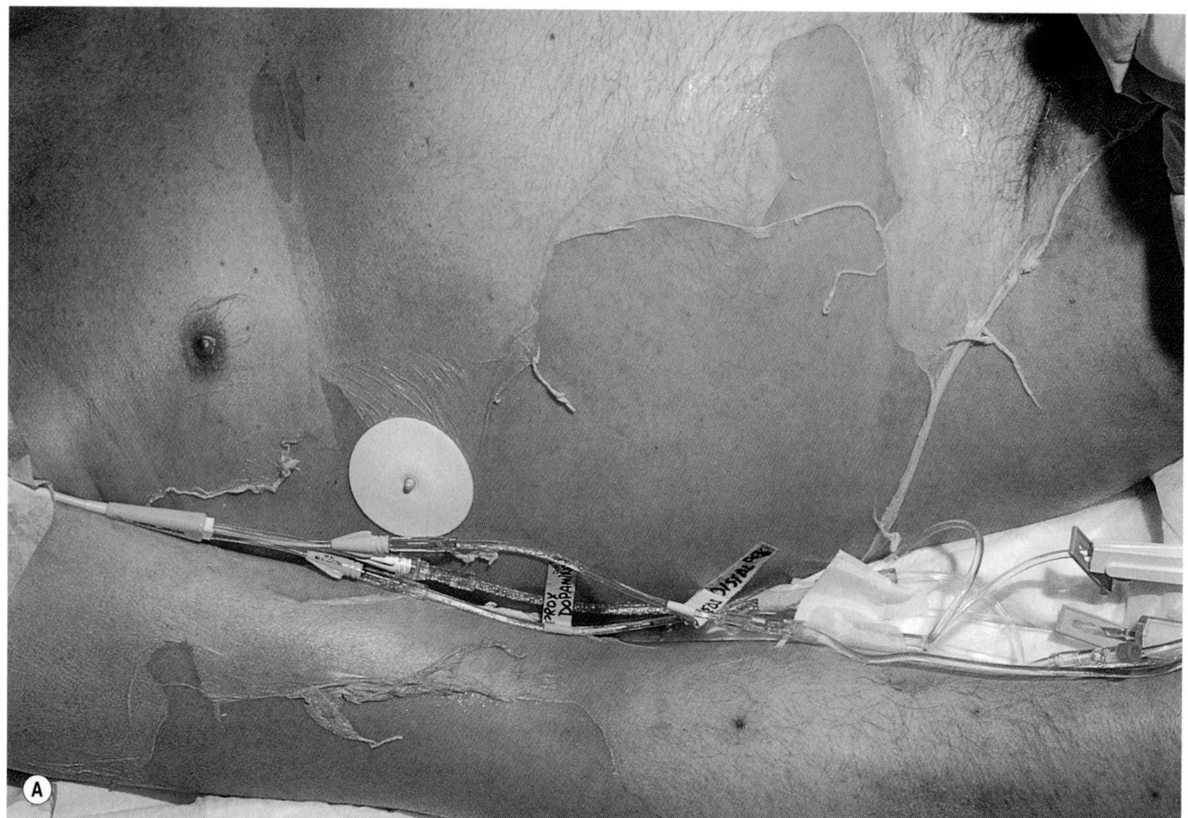

Large sheets of full-thickness epidermis are shed.

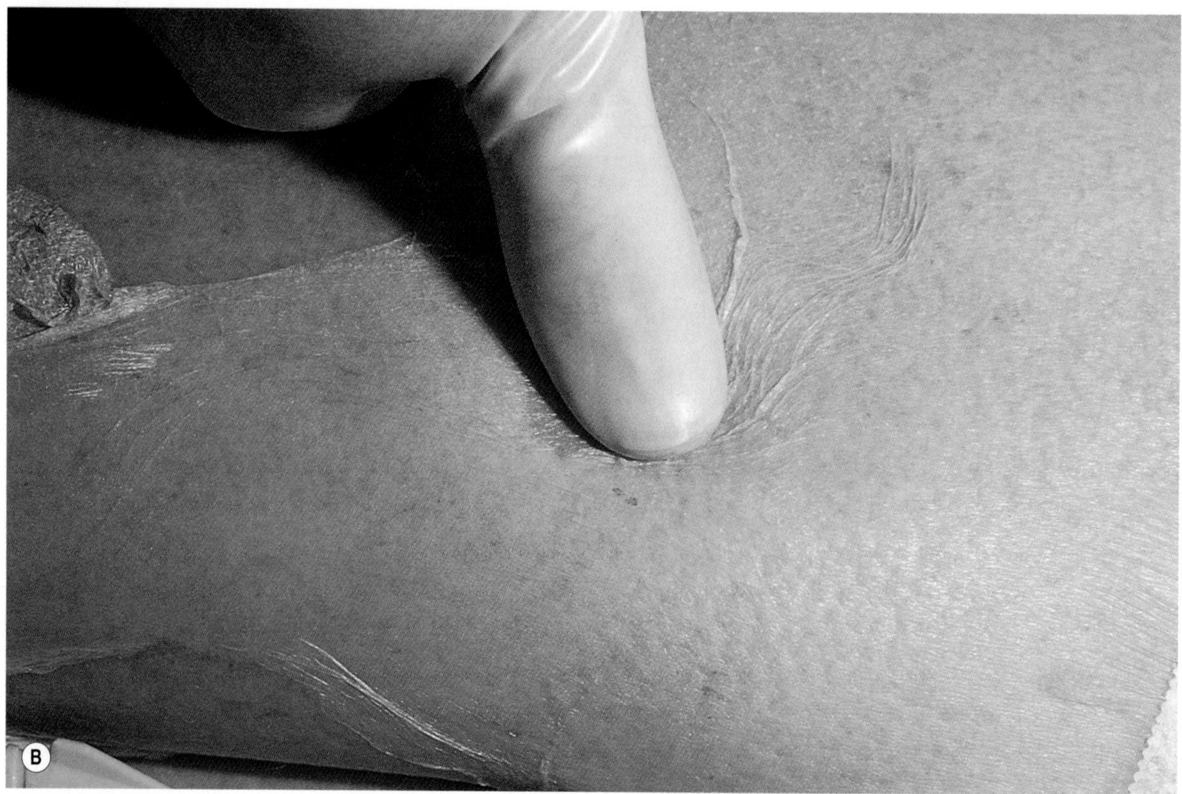

Toxic epidermal necrolysis begins with diffuse, hot erythema. In hours the skin becomes painful, and with slight thumb pressure the skin wrinkles, slides laterally, and separates from the dermis (Nikolsky's sign).

Figure 18-9

RESPIRATORY TRACT. Involvement of bronchial epithelium was noted in 27% of cases and must be suspected when dyspnea, bronchial hypersecretion, normal chest radiograph, and marked hypoxemia are present during the early stages of toxic epidermal necrosis. Bronchial injury indicates a poor prognosis. Life-threatening acute respiratory decompensation requiring ventilatory support and long-term pulmonary function abnormalities may occur. Patients should be closely monitored for pulmonary complications. Bronchopneumonia occurs in 30% of reported cases and is the cause of death in many cases. Many patients require intubation or ventilatory support. Respiratory failure can occur, with mucus retention and sloughing of the tracheobronchial mucosa.

INFECTION. Septicemia and gram-negative pneumonia are the most common causes of death. The lungs and denuded skin are the common portals of entry. The incidence of positive blood culture results is very high when central venous lines are used. Intravenous lines are changed or discontinued if it is probable that they are the source of positive blood culture findings. The urethra is often involved, but the use of Foley catheters can be avoided in many cases.

FLUID AND ELECTROLYTE LOSS. Fluid loss in TEN is not as severe as it is in burn patients, but significant losses can occur if grafts are not applied. Apparently, the acute-phase reactants that create massive edema after thermal injury are not released in TEN.

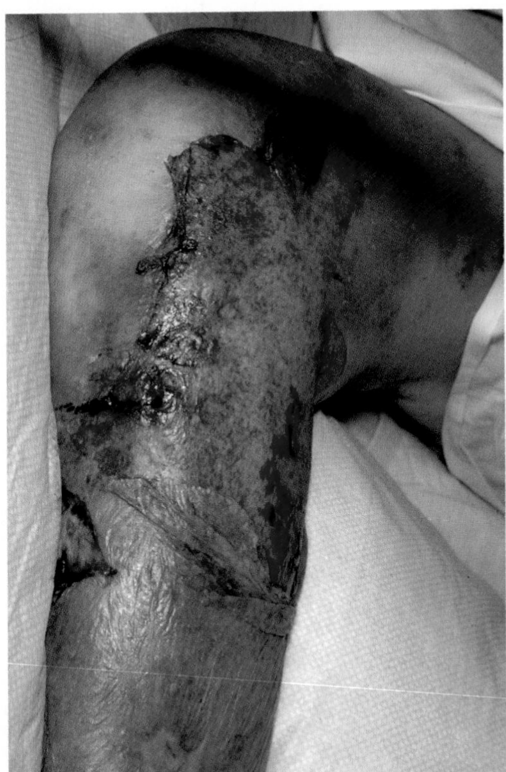

Figure 18-10 Toxic epidermal necrolysis. Denuded epidermis becomes dark red with an oozing surface.

OTHER COMPLICATIONS. Leukopenia of uncertain cause may occur. Toxins (e.g., from absorbed silver sulfadiazine) or immune complexes may be the cause. In one series, renal involvement consisting of hematuria, proteinuria, and elevated serum creatine level occurred in 50% of patients with Stevens-Johnson syndrome.

TREATMENT

Systemic steroids. The use of systemic steroids is still controversial, but most authors recommend that steroids not be used.

Steroids cannot prevent the occurrence of TEN, even in high dosages. Patients treated for other diseases with glucocorticosteroids for at least 1 week before the first dermatologic sign of TEN showed no difference in mortality compared with untreated patients. This suggests that steroids do not protect the epidermis from drug-induced keratolysis. Improved survival rates have been reported when patients with TEN have been treated without steroids.

Cyclosporine. Patients with TEN treated with cyclosporin A (3 to 4 mg/kg per day) without other immunosuppressive agents experienced rapid reepithelialization and a low death rate. This regimen was more effective than a series of patients previously treated with cyclophosphamide and corticosteroids.

Cyclophosphamide. In one study, cyclophosphamide (100 to 300 mg/day intravenously for 5 days) stopped the blistering, pain, and erythema in a few days. Reepithelialization rapidly occurred in 4 to 5 days. Cyclophosphamide inhibits cell-mediated cytotoxicity.

Plasma exchange and immunoglobulins. Plasma exchange resulted in complete remission in two series. Plasmapheresis is a safe intervention in extremely ill patients and may reduce the death rate. The efficacy of IV immunoglobulin (IVIG) is yet to be defined.

Burn center treatment. TEN has pathophysiologic similarities to partial-thickness burn injury. The management of major fluid and electrolyte derangements, the intensive nutritional support, and the management of extensive cutaneous injuries with ready access to biologic and semisynthetic wound dressings are best accomplished in a multidisciplinary burn center.

The current trend toward prolonged treatment in outside facilities before referral to a burn center is detrimental to the care of patients with TEN. The overall rate of bacteremia, septicemia, and mortality is significantly reduced with early ($\leq$7 days) referral to a regional burn center.

Separation at the junction of the dermis and epidermis leaves totally viable dermis and intact skin appendages. If the dermis can be protected from toxic detergents, salves, or desiccation, rapid resurfacing by proliferation of epithelium from the skin appendages will occur in approximately 14 days without scarring. Silver sulfadiazine and mafenide acetate (Sulfamylon) delay epithelialization.

ERYTHEMA NODOSUM

Erythema nodosum (EN) is a nodular erythematous eruption that is usually limited to the extensor aspects of the extremities. EN represents a hypersensitivity reaction to a variety of antigenic stimuli and may be observed in association with several diseases (infections, immunopathies, malignancies) and during drug therapy (with halides, sulfonamides, oral contraceptives). Approximately 55% of cases are idiopathic. Laboratory tests show no specific abnormalities except those related to an underlying disease. Familial EN is reported, with affected family members showing a common haplotype. The incidence has decreased in the antibiotic era. EN is seen more frequently in females. The peak incidence occurs between the ages of 18 and 34 years. The female to male ratio is 5:1.

CLINICAL MANIFESTATIONS AND COURSE. Prodromal symptoms of fatigue and malaise or symptoms of an upper respiratory tract infection precede the eruption by 1 to 3 weeks. The clinical picture is that of a nonspecific systemic illness, with low-grade fever (60%), malaise (67%), arthralgias (64%), and arthritis (31%). Pulmonary hilar adenopathy may develop as part of the hypersensitivity reaction of EN and is seen in cases with diverse causes.

JOINT SYMPTOMS. Arthralgia occurs in more than 50% of patients and begins during the eruptive phase or precedes the eruption by 2 to 8 weeks. Symptoms may disappear in a few weeks or persist for 2 years, but they always resolve without destructive joint changes. Testing for rheumatoid factor is negative. Joint symptoms consist of erythema, swelling, and tenderness over the joint, sometimes with effusions; arthralgia and morning stiffness, most commonly in the knee, but any joint may be affected; and polyarthralgia lasting for days.

SKIN ERUPTION. The eruptive phase begins with flulike symptoms of fever and generalized aching. The characteristic lesions begin as red, nodelike swellings over the shins; as a rule, both legs are affected. Similar lesions may appear on the extensor aspects of the forearms, thighs, and trunk (Figure 18-11). The border is poorly defined, with size varying from 2 to 6 cm. Lesions are oval, and their long axis corresponds to that of the limb. During the first week the lesions become tense, hard, and painful; during the second week they become fluctuant, as in an abscess, but never suppurate. The color changes in the second week from bright red to bluish or livid; as absorption progresses, it gradually fades to a yellowish hue, resembling a bruise; this disappears in 1 or 2 weeks as the overlying skin desquamates. The individual lesions last approximately 2 weeks, but new lesions sometimes continue to appear for 3 to 6 weeks. Aching of the legs and swelling of the ankles may persist for weeks. The condition may recur for months or years.

PATHOGENESIS AND ETIOLOGY. Erythema nodosum is probably a delayed hypersensitivity reaction to a variety of antigens; circulating immune complexes have not been found in idiopathic or uncomplicated cases. EN is a reaction pattern elicited by many different diseases (Box 18-6). In one large series, 32.5% of cases were idiopathic. The most common cause today is streptococcal infection and noninfectious inflammatory diseases in children and streptococcal infection and sarcoidosis in adults. Dental treatment and the possible presence of infectious dental foci should be considered in the differential diagnosis. EN is reported following dental treatment associated with gingival bleeding or because of infectious dental foci. Many other causes of EN have been reported; most consist of single histories. New etiologies continue to be described.

FUNGAL INFECTIONS. Coccidioidomycosis (San Joaquin Valley fever) is the most common cause of EN in the West and Southwest United States. In approximately 4% of males and 10% of females, the primary fungal infection, which may be asymptomatic or involve symptoms of an upper respiratory tract infection, is followed by the devel-

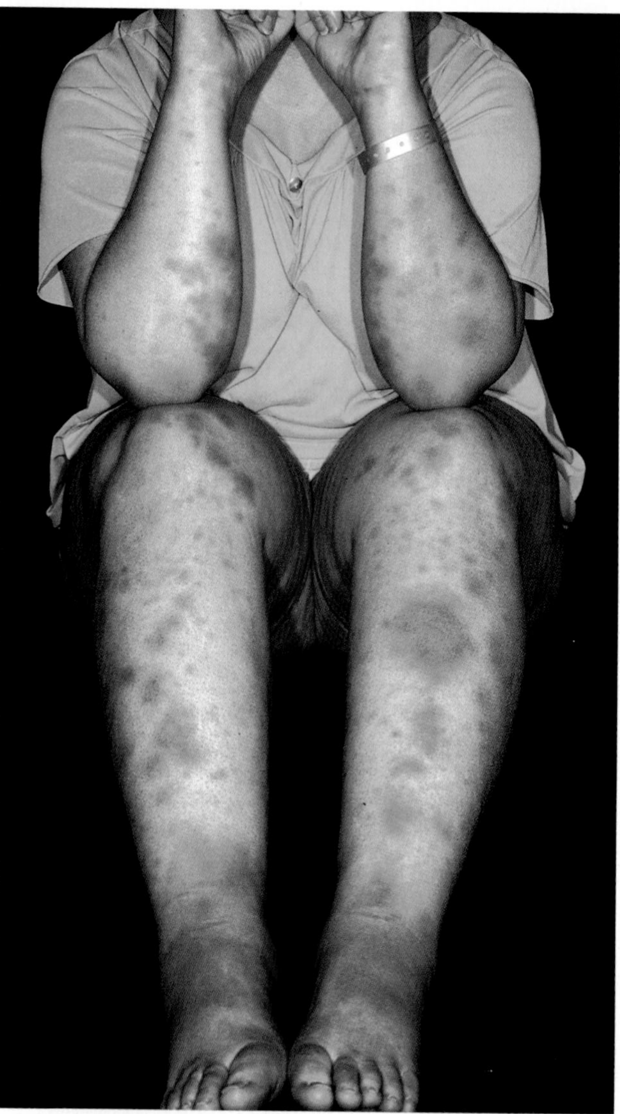

Figure 18-11 Erythema nodosum. Red, nodelike swelling in the characteristic distribution.

Box 18-6 **Erythema Nodosum—The Most Common Causes**

Infections	Drugs
Streptococci	Sulfonamides
Tuberculosis	Bromides
Psittacosis	Oral contraceptives
Yersiniosis	**Systemic Illnesses**
Lymphogranuloma venereum	Sarcoidosis
Cat-scratch disease	Inflammatory bowel disease
Coccidioidomycosis	Hodgkin's disease
Upper respiratory tract infection	**Pregnancy**

opment of EN. The lesions appear when the skin test result becomes positive, 3 days to 3 weeks after the end of the fever caused by the fungal infection. Dissemination and serious disease develop more often in pregnant patients with coccidioidomycosis than in the general population. Erythema nodosum appears to be a salient marker of a positive outcome for pregnant patients, more so than for the general population.

INFLAMMATORY BOWEL DISEASE. Inflammatory bowel diseases such as ulcerative colitis and regional ileitis may trigger EN, usually during active disease with symptoms of abdominal complaints and diarrhea. The mean duration of chronic ulcerative colitis before the onset of EN is 5 years, and the EN is controlled with adequate therapy of the colitis. *Yersinia enterocolitica*, a gram-negative bacillus that causes acute diarrhea and abdominal pain, is a reported cause.

DRUGS. Sulfonamides, bromides, and oral contraceptives have been reported to cause EN. Several other drugs, such as antibiotics, barbiturates, and salicylates, are often suspected but seldom proved causes.

SARCOIDOSIS. EN occurs in up to 39% of cases of sarcoidosis and has also been observed in pregnant women. Seasonal clustering of sarcoidosis presenting with EN has been reported. This suggests a common environmental trigger in the etiology of sarcoidosis.

LÖFGREN'S SYNDROME. Löfgren's syndrome is the association of erythema nodosum or periarticular ankle inflammation with unilateral or bilateral hilar or right paratracheal lymphadenopathy with or without pulmonary involvement. The mean age of onset is 37 years. Löfgren's syndrome, which in most cases represents an acute variant of pulmonary sarcoidosis with benign course, is more frequent in females, especially during pregnancy and puerperium.

LYMPHOMA. EN should be considered as a warning signal of impending relapse in a patient with a history of Hodgkin's disease. Patients in whom erythema nodosum was associated with non-Hodgkin's lymphoma have an extremely protracted course. Erythema nodosum associated with non-Hodgkin's lymphoma may precede the diagnosis of lymphoma by months.

DIAGNOSIS. Initial evaluation should include throat culture, antistreptolysin titer, chest radiograph, purified protein derivative skin test, and erythrocyte sedimentation rate (ESR). The ESR is elevated in all patients with EN. The white blood count is normal or only slightly increased. Patients with GI symptoms should have a stool culture for *Y. enterocolitica*, *Salmonella*, and *Campylobacter pylori*. Bilateral hilar adenopathy on chest radiograph examination does not establish the diagnosis of sarcoidosis, because hilar adenopathy occurs in EN produced by coccidioidomycosis, histoplasmosis, tuberculosis, streptococcal infections, and lymphoma, and as a nonspecific reaction in many cases. When the etiology is in doubt, blood should be serologically investigated from those bacterial, virologic, fungal, or protozooal infections more prevalent in the area.

BIOPSY. The clinical picture is characteristic in most cases, and a biopsy is not required. Histologic confirmation is desirable in atypical cases. An excisional rather than a punch biopsy is necessary to sample the subcutaneous fat adequately. Tissue sections show lymphohistiocytic infiltrate, granulomatous inflammation, and fibrosis in the septa of the subcutaneous fat; these are all features of a septal panniculitis.

DIFFERENTIAL DIAGNOSIS. In Weber-Christian panniculitis, localized areas of subcutaneous inflammation tend to occur on the thighs and trunk rather than on the lower legs. Lesions may suppurate and heal with atrophy and localized depressions. Superficial and deep thrombophlebitis and erysipelas must also be differentiated from EN.

TREATMENT. EN in most instances is a self-limited disease and requires only symptomatic relief with salicylates and bed rest. Indomethacin (250 mg three times daily) or naproxen (250 mg twice daily) may be more effective than aspirin. Cases that are recurrent, unusually painful, or long lasting require a more vigorous approach.

A supersaturated solution of potassium iodide (5 drops three times daily) in orange juice is started. Increase the dose by 1 drop per dose per day until the patient responds. Relief of lesional tenderness, arthralgia, and fever may occur in 24 hours. Most lesions completely subside within 10 to 14 days. However, potassium iodide is not effective for all patients with EN. Patients who receive medication shortly after the initial onset of EN respond more satisfactorily than those with chronic EN. Side effects include nasal catarrh and headache. Hyperthyroidism may occur with long-term use. Potassium iodide is contraindicated during pregnancy, because it can produce a goiter in the fetus.

Corticosteroids are effective but seldom necessary in self-limited diseases. Recurrence following discontinuation of treatment is common, and underlying infectious disease may be worsened.

There is limited experience with colchicine (0.6 to 1.2 mg twice daily), hydroxychloroquine (200 mg twice daily), and dapsone.

VASCULITIS

Cutaneous vasculitis encompasses a highly heterogeneous group of disorders of diverse etiology, pathogenesis, and clinical features (Boxes 18-7 to 18-9 and Table 18-1).

CLASSIFICATION. Vasculitis, or angiitis, defined as inflammation of the vessel wall, is probably initiated by immune complex deposition. The cutaneous vasculitic diseases are classified according to the type of inflammatory cell within the vessel walls (neutrophil, lymphocyte, or histiocyte) and the size and type of blood vessel involved (venule, arteriole, artery, or vein). Some vasculitic diseases are limited to the skin; others involve vessels in many different organs.

Box 18-7 **Major Categories of Noninfectious Vasculitis***

Large vessel vasculitis

- Giant cell arteritis
- Takayasu's arteritis

Medium-sized vessel vasculitis

- Polyarteritis nodosa
- Kawasaki's disease
- Primary granulomatous central nervous system vasculitis

Small vessel vasculitis

- ANCA-associated small vessel vasculitis
  - Microscopic polyangiitis
  - Wegener's granulomatosis
  - Churg-Strauss syndrome
  - Drug-induced ANCA-associated vasculitis
- Immune-complex small vessel vasculitis
  - Henoch-Schönlein purpura
  - Cryoglobulinemic vasculitis
  - Lupus vasculitis
  - Rheumatoid vasculitis
  - Sjögren's syndrome vasculitis
  - Hypocomplementemic urticarial vasculitis
  - Behçet's syndrome
  - Goodpasture's syndrome
  - Serum-sickness vasculitis
  - Drug-induced immune-complex vasculitis
  - Infection-induced immune-complex vasculitis
- Paraneoplastic small vessel vasculitis
  - Lymphoproliferative neoplasm-induced vasculitis
  - Myeloproliferative neoplasm-induced vasculitis
  - Carcinoma-induced vasculitis
- Inflammatory bowel disease vasculitis

From Jennette JC, Falk RJ: *New Engl J Med* (337)21:1512, 1997. *PMID: 9366584*

*Vascular inflammation is categorized as either infectious vasculitis, which is caused by the direct invasion of vessel walls by pathogens (e.g., rickettsial organisms in Rocky Mountain spotted fever), or noninfectious vasculitis, which is not caused by the direct invasion of vessel walls by pathogens (although infections can indirectly induce noninfectious vasculitis, for example, by generating pathogenic immune complexes). ANCA denotes antineutrophil cytoplasmic autoantibody.

Box 18-8 **Names And Definitions of Vasculitis Adopted by the Chapel Hill Consensus Conference on the Nomenclature of Systemic Vasculitis**

Name	Definition
Large vessel vasculitis	
Giant cell (temporal) arteritis	Granulomatous arteritis of the aorta and its major branches, with a predilection for the extracranial branches of the carotid artery; often involves the temporal artery; usually occurs in patients older than 50 yr and is often associated with polymyalgia rheumatica
Takayasu's arteritis	Granulomatous inflammation of the aorta and its major branches; usually occurs in patients younger than 50 yr
Medium-sized vessel vasculitis	
Polyarteritis nodosa (classic PAN)	Necrotizing inflammation of medium-sized or small arteries without glomerulonephritis or vasculitis in arterioles, capillaries, or venules
Kawasaki disease	Arteritis involving the large, medium-sized, or small arteries and associated with mucocutaneous lymph node syndrome; coronary arteries are often involved; aorta and veins may be involved; usually occurs in children
Small vessel vasculitis	
Wegener's granulomatosis	Granulomatous inflammation involving the respiratory tract and necrotizing vasculitis affecting small- to medium-sized vessels (e.g., capillaries, venules, arterioles, and arteries); necrotizing glomerulonephritis is common
Churg-Strauss syndrome	Eosinophil-rich and granulomatous inflammation involving the respiratory tract, necrotizing vasculitis affecting small- to medium-sized vessels, and associated with asthma and eosinophilia
Microscopic polyangiitis	Necrotizing vasculitis, with few or no immune deposits, affecting small vessels (e.g., capillaries, venules, or arterioles); necrotizing arteritis involving small- and medium-sized arteries may be present; necrotizing glomerulonephritis is very common; pulmonary capillaritis often occurs
Henoch-Schönlein purpura	Vasculitis, with IgA-dominant immune deposits, affecting small vessels (e.g., capillaries, venules, or arterioles); typically involves skin, gut, and glomeruli and is associated with arthralgias or arthritis
Essential cryoglobulinemic vasculitis	Vasculitis, with cryoglobulin immune deposits, affecting small vessels (e.g., capillaries, venules, or arterioles), and associated with cryoglobulins in serum; skin and glomeruli are often involved
Cutaneous leukocytoclastic angiitis	Isolated cutaneous leukocytoclastic angiitis without systemic vasculitis or glomerulonephritis

From Jennette JC, Falk RJ: *New Engl J Med* 337(21):1512, 1997, *PMID: 9366584*; and Nataraja A, et al: *Best Pract Res Clin Rheumatol* 21(4):713-732, 2007. *PMID: 17678832*

Box 18-9 **The American College of Rheumatology Classification Criteria for Vasculitis**

Giant cell (temporal) arteritis (GCA)

1. Age >50 yr at onset
2. New type of headache
3. Abnormal temporal artery on clinical examination (tenderness to palpation or decreased pulsation)
4. Elevated erythrocyte sedimentation rate
5. Temporal artery biopsy showing vasculitis

Three criteria classify GCA with sensitivity of 93.5% and specificity of 91.2%.

Takayasu's arteritis (TA)

1. Age less than 40 yr at onset
2. Limb claudication
3. Decreased brachial artery pulses
4. BP >10 mm Hg difference between two arms
5. Bruits
6. Arteriogram normal

Three criteria classify TA with sensitivity of 90.5% and specificity of 97.8%.

Polyarteritis nodosa (PAN)

1. Weight loss >4 kg
2. Livedo reticularis
3. Testicular pain or tenderness
4. Myalgias, myopathy, or tenderness
5. Neuropathy
6. Hypertension (diastolic BP >90 mm Hg)
7. Renal impairment (elevated BUN or creatine)
8. Hepatitis B virus
9. Abnormal arteriography
10. Biopsy of artery showing PAN

Three criteria classify PAN with sensitivity of 82.2% and specificity of 86.6%.

Wegener's granulomatosis (WG)

1. Nasal or oral inflammation
2. Chest x-ray showing nodules, infiltrates (fixed), or cavities
3. Microscopic hematuria or red cell casts in urine
4. Granulomatous inflammation on biopsy (within vessel wall or perivascular)

Two criteria classify WG with sensitivity of 88.2% and specificity of 92.0%.

Churg-Strauss syndrome (CSS)

1. Asthma
2. Eosinophilia (>10%)
3. Neuropathy
4. Pulmonary infiltrates (nonfixed)
5. Sinusitis
6. Extravascular eosinophils on biopsy

Four criteria classify CSS with sensitivity of 85% and specificity of 99.7%.

Hypersensitivity vasculitis

1. Age >16 yr at onset
2. Medications may have precipitated event
3. Palpable purpura
4. Cutaneous eruption
5. Positive biopsy results

Three criteria classify hypersensitivity vasculitis with sensitivity of 71.0% and specificity of 83.9%.

Henoch-Schönlein purpura (HSP)

1. Palpable purpura
2. Age at onset <20 yr
3. Bowel angina
4. Vessel wall granulocytes on biopsy

Two criteria classify HSP with sensitivity of 87% and specificity of 88%.

BP, Blood pressure; *BUN,* blood urea nitrogen; *PMN,* polymorphonuclear cells.

Table 18-1 Comparison of Organ Involvement (Percentage) in Various Vasculitides

Organ system	PAN	WG	MPA	CSS	CV	UV	HSP
Cutaneous	50	40	50	55	90	100	90
Pulmonary	30	90	35	60	<5	10	<5
Renal	30	80	90	35	25	<5	50
Ear, nose, throat	7	90	25	50	<5	<5	<5
Musculoskeletal	70	60	60	50	70	40	75
Neurologic	60	50	35	70	40	<5	10
Gastrointestinal	30	50	40	45	30	15	60

From Fiorentino DF: *J Am Acad Dermatol* 48:311, 2003. *PMID: 12637912*

CSS, Churg-Strauss syndrome; *CV,* cryoglobulinemic vasculitis; *HSP,* Henoch-Schönlein purpura; *MPA,* microscopic polyangiitis; *PAN,* polyarteritis nodosa; *UV,* urticarial vasculitis; *WG,* Wegener's granulomatosis.

VASCULITIC SYNDROMES

Large- to medium-sized artery	Small artery	Arteriole	Capillary	Venule	Vein
Branches directed to extremities, head, neck Main visceral arteries (renal, hepatic, coronary, mesenteric)	Skin nodules		Purpura		
	Distal arterial radicals (subcutaneous and deep dermal arteries)				

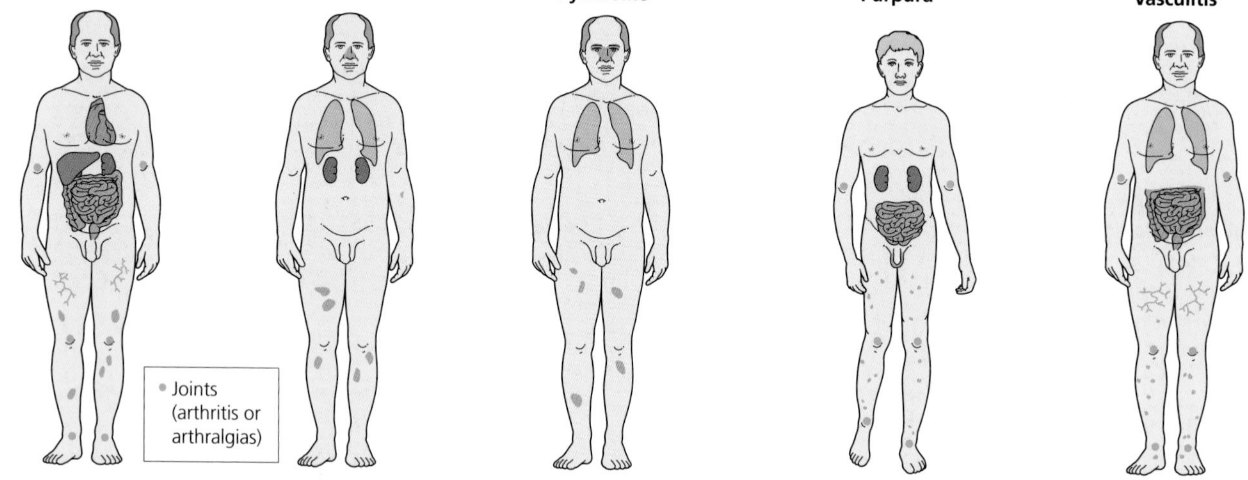

Polyarteritis Nodosa

- * Weight loss
- * Testicular pain
- * Myalgias, weakness, or leg tenderness
- * Mono- or poly-neuropathy
- * Diastolic BP >90

Skin
Livedo reticularis
Nodules
Ulcers

- * Elevated BUN or creatine
- * Hepatitis B surface antigen or antibody
- * Arteriographic abnormality
- * Granulocytes in artery wall

p-ANCA

• Joints (arthritis or arthralgias)

Wegener's Granulomatosis

- * Oral ulcers or nasal discharge (purulent or bloody)
- * Hemoptysis

Skin
Palpable purpura

- * Chest x-ray
  Nodules
  Infiltrates (fixed) or cavities
- * Microhematuria or red cell casts
- * Granulomatous inflammation
  Peri- or extra-vascular area (artery or arteriole)

c-ANCA

Churg-Strauss Syndrome

- * Asthma
- * History of allergy
- * Mono- or poly-neuropathy
- Fever

Skin
Palpable purpura
Nodules
Ulcers

- * Eosinophilia >10%
- * Paranasal sinus abnormality
- * Extravascular eosinophils

Elevated IgE
Pulmonary infiltrates (nonfixed)

p-ANCA

Henoch-Schönlein Purpura

- * Age <20
- * GI bleeding
- Abdominal pain
- Arthralgia
- Scrotal swelling

Skin
Palpable purpura

- * Skin
  Extravascular or perivascular granulocytes
- Hematuria
- Proteinuria
- IgA-glomeruli
- IgA-arterioles (skin)

Hypersensitivity Vasculitis

- * Age >16
- * Medication at onset
- Neuropathy
- Abdominal pain
- Arthralgia
- GI bleeding

Skin
- * Palpable purpura
- * Maculopapular rash

- * Skin—peri- or extravascular granulocytes
- ESR elevated
- Hematuria
- Proteinuria

*1990 American College of Rheumatology criteria of diagnosis.
ANCA, Antineutrophil cytoplasmic autoantibodies.
IC, Immune complex mediate.

Figure 18-12

MULTISYSTEM DISEASE. A broad spectrum of symptoms is seen in the vasculitic syndromes (Box 18-10). These symptoms and signs are suggestive or consistent with a diagnosis of systemic vasculitis. The presence of many symptoms means that there is no single pathognomonic feature of vasculitis. Recognizing patterns is important for early diagnosis. For example, a new-onset headache in a person over the age of 50 years with an elevated erythrocyte sedimentation rate should trigger a suspicion of giant cell arteritis.

Box 18-10 **Signs and Symptoms Found in Patients with Vasculitis**

SYSTEMIC
Malaise
Myalgia
Arthralgia/arthritis
Fever or change in temperature
Weight loss within past month

CUTANEOUS
Infarct
Purpura
Ulcer
Other skin vasculitis
Gangrene
Multiple digit gangrene

MUCOUS MEMBRANES/EYES
Mouth ulcers
Genital ulcers
Conjunctivitis
Episcleritis
Uveitis
Retinal exudates
Retinal hemorrhage

ENT
Nasal discharge/obstruction
Sinusitis
Epistaxis
Crusting
Aural discharge
Otitis media
New deafness
Hoarseness/laryngitis
Subglottic involvement

CHEST
Dyspnea or wheeze
Nodules or fibrosis
Pleural effusion/pleurisy
Infiltrate
Hemoptysis/hemorrhage
Massive hemoptysis

CARDIOVASCULAR
Bruits
New loss of pulses
Aortic incompetence
Pericarditis
New myocardial infarct
CCF/cardiomyopathy

ABDOMINAL
Abdominal pain
Bloody diarrhea
Gall bladder perforation
Gut infarction
Pancreatitis

RENAL
Hypertension (diastolic >90)
Proteinuria (>1 + or >0.2 g/24 h)
Hematuria (>1 + or >10 rbc/ml)
Creatinine elevated or
Rise in creatinine >10%

NERVOUS SYSTEM
Organic confusion/dementia
Seizures (not hypertensive)
Stroke
Cord lesion
Peripheral neuropathy
Motor mononeuritis multiplex

Adapted from Luqmani RA et al: *QJM* 87(11):67, 1994. *PMID: 7820541*

CLINICAL PRESENTATION. The clinical presentation varies with the size of the blood vessel involved and the intensity of the inflammation (see Box 18-8 and Figure 18-12). Small vessel vasculitis—arteriole, capillary, venule—most commonly affects the skin and rarely causes serious internal organ dysfunction, except when the kidney is involved.

There are numerous cutaneous diseases that histologically show some degree of vessel inflammation. Only those diseases that have inflammation severe enough to cause necrosis of vessel walls are discussed here. Necrotizing angiitis is the term given to this group of diseases. These diseases have clinical features that allow one to predict that vessel inflammation and necrosis are taking place and to identify the size of vessel involved (see Table 18-1).

ANTINEUTROPHIL CYTOPLASMIC ANTIBODIES. The diagnosis and classification of vasculitis have been revolutionized by the discovery of serum antineutrophil cytoplasmic autoantibodies (ANCAs) (Table 18-2). ANCAs are a

Table 18-2 Frequency and Type of ANCA Found in Various Vasculitic and Nonvasculitic Disorders

Disease	ANCA (frequency, %)
Wegener's granulomatosis	C-ANCA (75%-80%) P-ANCA (10%-15%) Negative (5%-15%)
Microscopic polyangiitis/ idiopathic crescentic GN	C-ANCA (25%-35%) P-ANCA (50%-60%) Negative (5%-10%)
Churg-Strauss syndrome	C-ANCA (10%-15%) P-ANCA (55%-60%) Negative (30%)
Drug-induced vasculitis	P-ANCA (?)
Rheumatoid arthritis/ Felty's syndrome	P-ANCA (30%-70%), A-ANCA (?)
SLE	P-ANCA (20%-30%) A-ANCA (?)
Ulcerative colitis	P-ANCA (50%-70%)
Crohn's disease	(20%-40%)
Sclerosing cholangiitis	P-ANCA (60%-70%)
Primary biliary cirrhosis	P-ANCA (30%-40%)
Autoimmune hepatitis	C-ANCA (45%) P-ANCA (33%-90%)
Chronic infections	C-ANCA (?) P-ANCA (?) A-ANCA (?)

From Fiorentino DF: *J Am Acad Dermatol* 48:311, 2003. *PMID: 12637912*
GN, Glomerular nephritis; *SLE,* systemic lupus erythematosus.

serologic marker for many forms of necrotizing vasculitis. Use of ANCA testing provides a significant diagnostic advantage over reliance on biopsy findings alone in patients whose differential diagnosis includes any of the vasculitic diseases. Two staining patterns may be identified using immunofluorescence (IFA) on ethanol-fixed neutrophils: either a diffuse granular staining of the cytoplasm (cytoplasmic, or C-ANCA) or concentration of fluorescence around the nucleus (perinuclear, or P-ANCA).

Antineutrophil cytoplasmic autoantibody–associated vasculitis. ANCA-associated small vessel vasculitis is the most common primary systemic small vessel vasculitis in adults and includes three major categories: Wegener's granulomatosis, microscopic polyangiitis, and Churg-Strauss syndrome. Most patients with Wegener's granulomatosis have PR3-ANCA (cytoplasmic ANCA or C-ANCA); most patients with microscopic polyangiitis or Churg-Strauss syndrome have MPO-ANCA (perinuclear ANCA or P-ANCA). Approximately 10% of patients with typical Wegener's granulomatosis or microscopic polyangiitis have negative assays for ANCA; therefore ANCA negativity does not rule out these diseases. The specificity of ANCA positivity is not absolute; a positive result is not diagnostic for an ANCA-associated vasculitis, especially if the result of an indirect immunofluorescence assay has not been confirmed by the more specific enzyme immunoassay (EIA) technique. Patients are usually screened with the indirect immunofluorescence (IFA) test. The EIA is performed when the IFA test result is positive to identify the antigen. A more comprehensive strategy would be to order the IFA and EIA.

A positive test result for C- or P-ANCA predicts a 96% probability that necrotizing vasculitis or crescentic glomerulonephritis will develop; a negative test result portends a 93% probability that the patient does not have these diseases. ANCAs are reliable monitors of disease activity because antibody titers decline when patients go into remission with effective immunosuppressive therapy and increase with relapse.

VASCULITIS OF SMALL VESSELS

Most diseases characterized by necrotizing inflammation of small blood vessels have a number of features in common. Skin lesions reflect various degrees of small vessel necrotizing inflammation; the most common is palpable purpura (Table 18-3).

ETIOLOGY. There is hypersensitivity to various antigens (drugs, chemicals, microorganisms, and endogenous antigens) with formation of circulating immune complexes that are deposited in walls of vessels. Some of the diseases reported to be associated with hypersensitivity vasculitis and the incidence of these diseases are listed in Table 18-4.

In many cases, the cause is not determined.

PATHOGENESIS. The vessel-bound immune complexes activate complement that is chemotactic for neutrophils. Neutrophils adhere to endothelial cells and migrate into the surrounding connective tissue. Activated endothelial cells release inflammatory mediators (cytokines) that attract in-

Table 18-3 Clinical Signs of Necrotizing Vasculitis with Respect to Vessel Size Involved

Signs	Diseases
Small vessels (arteriole, capillary, venule)	
Urticaria reflects minimal vessel inflammation and necrosis.	Hypersensitivity vasculitis
Palpable purpura: exudation and hemorrhage from damaged vessels produce most characteristic lesion of small vessel necrotizing vasculitis. Lesion is a red, slightly elevated papule that does not blanch on application of external pressure.	Henoch-Schönlein purpura Essential mixed cryoglobulinemia Vasculitis associated with connective tissue disease Vasculitis associated with malignancies Serum sickness and serum sickness–like reactions
Nodules, bullae, or ulcers may be present if vessel wall inflammation and necrosis are intense.	Chronic urticaria (urticarial vasculitis) Urticarial prodrome of acute hepatitis type B infection
Large vessels (small- and medium-sized muscular arteries)	
Subcutaneous nodules, ulceration, and ecchymoses result from necrosis and thrombosis of larger vessels, which lead to infarction.	Polyarteritis nodosa Churg-Strauss syndrome Wegener's granulomatosis Giant cell (temporal) arteritis

flammatory cells. There is an inflammatory response in the walls of small vessels in which leukocytes, by release of lysosomal enzymes, damage vessel walls, causing extravasation of erythrocytes. The term leukocytoclastic vasculitis describes the histologic pattern produced when leukocytes fragment (i.e., undergo leukocytoclasis during the inflammatory process, leaving nuclear debris or "dust").

Hypersensitivity vasculitis

Cutaneous small vessel vasculitis (leukocytoclastic vasculitis, hypersensitivity vasculitis) is the most commonly seen form of small vessel necrotizing vasculitis. The disease may be limited to the skin or may involve many different organs and be coexistent with many other diseases. Histologically there is fibrinoid necrosis of small dermal blood vessels, leukocytoclasis, endothelial cell swelling, and extravasation of red blood cells (RBCs).

SKIN LESIONS. Prodromal symptoms include fever, malaise, myalgia, and joint pain. The characteristic lesions are referred to as palpable purpura. The lesions begin as asymptomatic, localized areas of cutaneous hemorrhage that acquire substance and become palpable as blood leaks out of damaged vessels (Figure 18-13). Lesions may coalesce, producing large areas of purpura. Nodules and urticarial lesions may appear. Hemorrhagic blisters and ulcers may arise from these purpuric areas and indicate more severe vessel inflammation and necrosis. A few to numerous discrete, purpuric lesions are most commonly seen on the lower extremities but may occur on any dependent area, including the back if the patient is bedridden, or the arms. Ankle and lower leg edema may occur with lower leg lesions (Figure 18-14, *A-C*).

Small lesions itch and are painful; nodules, ulcers, and bullae may be very painful.

Lesions appear in crops, last 1 to 4 weeks, and heal with residual scarring and hyperpigmentation. Patients may experience one episode if a drug or viral infection is the cause or multiple episodes when the lesions are associated with a systemic disease, such as rheumatoid arthritis or systemic lupus erythematosus. Recurrent crops of new lesions may appear for weeks, months, or years. The disease is usually self-limited and confined to the skin.

Table 18-4 Causal Agents, Associated Conditions, and Vasculitis Syndromes Identified

	% of patients
Cause/association	
Hepatitis C virus	19.0
Hepatitis B virus	5.0
Other infections	4.0
Drug intake	9.6
Underlying malignant neoplasm	10.0
Connective tissue diseases	8.4
Behçet's syndrome	2.0
Rheumatologic disease	2.4
Essential mixed cryoglobulinemia	1.3
Inflammatory bowel disease	2.5
Miscellaneous	3.0
Vasculitic syndrome	
Hypersensitivity vasculitis	64.0
Polyarteritis nodosa	6.0
Pustular vasculitis	6.0
Henoch-Schönlein purpura	5.2
Livedo vasculitis	4.5
Urticarial vasculitis	3.2
Rheumatoid vasculitis	3.2
Erythema elevatum diutinum	2.6
Churg-Strauss vasculitis	2.0

From Sais G: *Arch Dematol* 34:309, 1998. *PMID: 9521029*

DURATION. In one study the disease resolved in less than 6 months in 46.9% of the patients and persisted in 43.8%. The duration of the cutaneous vasculitis ranged from 1 week to 318 months. The average duration of cutaneous lesions was 27.9 months.

SYSTEMIC DISEASE. Hypersensitivity vasculitis has many systemic manifestations; the numbers in parentheses in the following discussion indicate the approximate percentage of involvement.

An analysis of cutaneous hypersensitivity vasculitis in patients seen by two practicing dermatologists showed that the disease has a better prognosis with less systemic involvement than in those patients seen at medical center clinics. *PMID: 6703752*

- *Kidneys (50%):* Kidney disease is the most common systemic manifestation. Mild vasculitis of the kidneys causes microscopic hematuria and proteinuria. Necrotizing glomerulitis or diffuse glomerulonephritis may lead to chronic renal insufficiency and death.
- *Nervous system (40%):* Peripheral neuropathy with hypoesthesia or paresthesia is more common than central nervous system involvement.
- *Gastrointestinal tract (36%):* Vasculitis of the bowel causes abdominal pain, nausea, vomiting, diarrhea, and melena.
- *Lung (30%):* Pulmonary vasculitis may be asymptomatic, detected only as nodular or diffuse infiltrates on chest film; it also may be symptomatic, with cough, shortness of breath, and hemoptysis.
- *Joints (30%):* Symptoms vary from pain to erythema and swelling.
- *Heart (50%):* Myocardial angiitis produces arrhythmias and congestive heart failure.

HYPERSENSITIVITY VASCULITIS

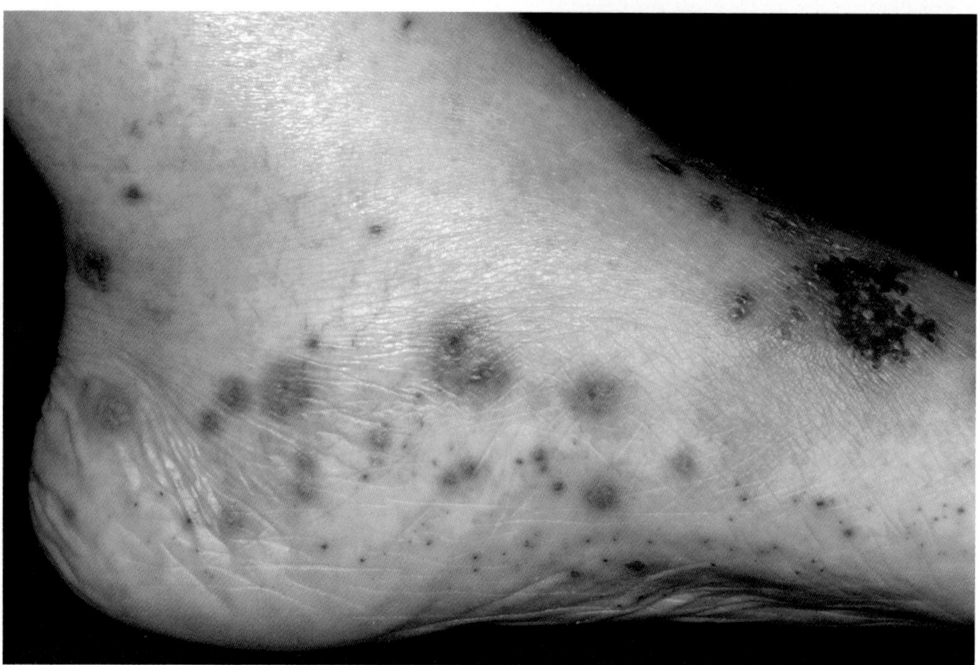

Figure 18-13 The characteristic lesion is palpable purpura. Lesions begin as 1-3 mm papules that increase in size and become palpable. They may coalesce to form plaques; in some instances, they may ulcerate. Palpable purpura is most common on the legs, but any surface can be involved. In some cases, the purpuric lesions are barely palpable.

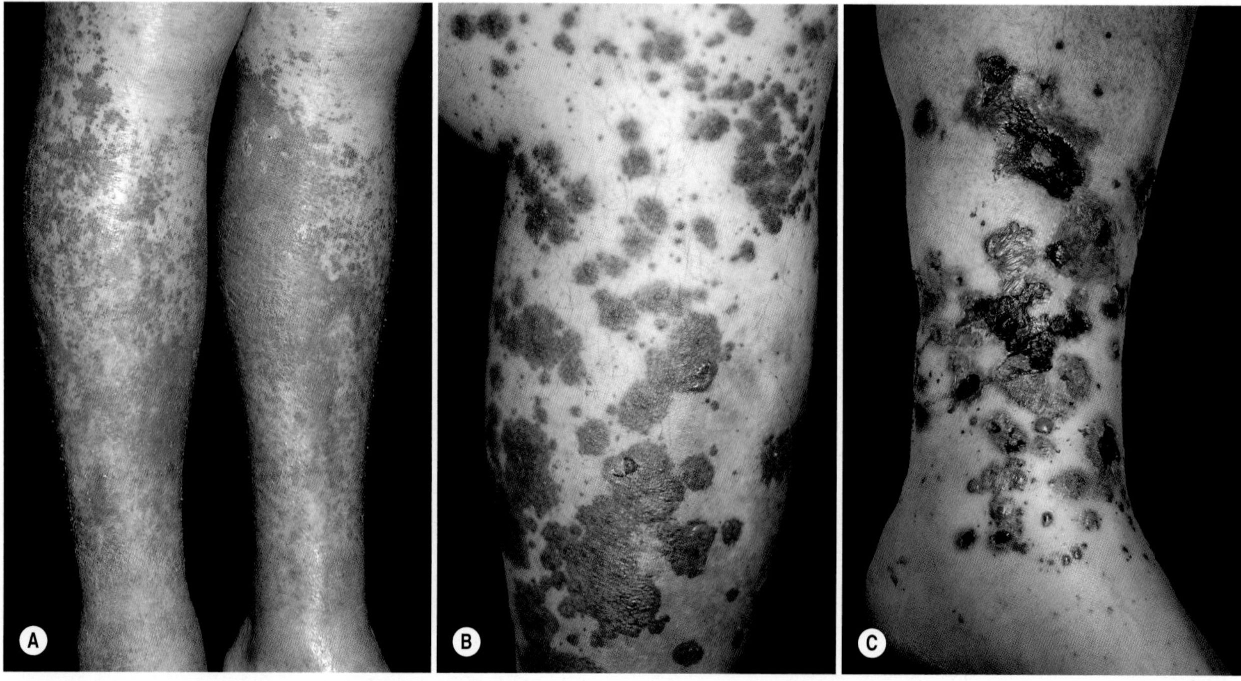

A: Lesions are most often seen on the lower legs. Lesions are numerous and have coalesced. They are superficial and barely palpable.

B: Lesions extend onto the thighs and are confluent and palpable.

C: Thick palpable lesions have ulcerated.

Figure 18-14

PHYSICAL EXAMINATION. Look for systemic disease with a complete history and physical examination. Examine ear, nose, and throat for signs of Wegener's granulomatosis.

LABORATORY STUDIES. Studies to consider are listed in Box 18-11. Decreased levels of complement components are more often present in vasculitis associated with rheumatoid arthritis, systemic lupus erythematosus, cryoglobulinemia, Sjögren's syndrome, or urticarial vasculitis. Every patient should be screened for renal involvement.

Order ANCA tests when systemic vasculitis is suspected. The ESR is almost always increased during active vasculitis. A normal ESR in a patient with purpura suggests that immune complex disease is absent. Low complement levels are associated with other features such as renal disease, arthritis, and the presence of immunoreactants deposited along the basement membrane zone of the epidermis.

Box 18-11 **Tests to Consider for Evaluation of Cutaneous Small-Vessel Vasculitis**

Initial laboratory evaluation

- Complete blood cell count
- Erythrocyte sedimentation rate
- Urinalysis
- Stool guaiac tests
- Serum chemistry profile
- Antinuclear antibodies
- Antineutrophil cytoplasmic autoantibodies
- Chest radiography
- Rheumatoid factor
- Cryoglobulins
- Complement (total)
- Hepatitis B virus
- Hepatitis C virus

Adults with persistent fever, abnormal blood smears, risk for HIV infection, severe vasculitis

- Anticardiolipin
- Antistreptolysin O titer
- Anti-DNA, anti-Ro, anti-La antibodies
- Electrocardiography
- HIV serology
- Platelet counts
- Prothrombin and partial thromboplastin times
- Serum creatine
- Serum immunoglobulin determination
- Serum protein electrophoresis
- Throat culture
- Urinary protein determination (24 hour)

Adapted from Blanco R et al: *Medicine* 77:403, 1998. *PMID: 9854604*

SKIN BIOPSY. The clinical presentation is so characteristic that a biopsy is generally not necessary. In doubtful cases, a punch biopsy should be taken from an early active lesion. The characteristic mixed infiltrate of mononuclear cells and neutrophils, fibrinoid necrosis of blood vessel walls, and nuclear dust from neutrophil fragmentation (leukocytoclasis) will be obscured if ulcerated lesions are sampled. Patients with deeper levels of vasculitis (down to the lower half of the reticular dermis) have evidence of a more severe clinical disease with systemic involvement.

IMMUNOFLUORESCENT STUDIES. Immunofluorescent studies may be done if the diagnosis cannot be determined from the clinical presentation and skin biopsy. Immune complexes are phagocytized rapidly after deposition in the vessels. Therefore the best time for biopsy of a vessel for immunofluorescence is within the first 24 hours after the lesion forms. The most common immunoreactants present in and around blood vessels are IgM, C3, and fibrin. The presence of IgA in blood vessels of a child with vasculitis suggests the diagnosis of Henoch-Schönlein purpura.

TREATMENT. Identify and remove the offending antigen (i.e., drug, chemical, or infection). No other treatment may be necessary, and the disease may clear spontaneously. In other instances the disease persists or becomes recurrent.

Topical corticosteroids and topical antibiotic creams may be helpful. Prednisone, 60 to 80 mg per day, controls systemic symptoms and cutaneous ulceration. Taper slowly (3 to 6 weeks) to prevent rebound. Nonsteroidal antiinflammatory drugs (acetylsalicylic acid, indomethacin) may be used for persistent or necrotic lesions, myalgias, fever, and arthralgia.

Colchicine, which inhibits neutrophil chemotaxis, in doses of 0.6 mg two to three times daily, might be helpful in chronic forms of the disease. Effects are seen in 7 to 10 days, and colchicine is tapered and discontinued when lesions resolve. Treatment can be continued for months if necessary, and side effects are minimal.

Dapsone 100 to 150 mg per day controlled three patients in whom disease was confined to the skin. Potassium iodide (0.3 to 1.5 gm four times daily) is useful in nodular vasculitis. H_1 antihistamines alone or with H_2 antihistamines alleviate pruritus and block histamine-induced endothelial gap formation with resultant trapping of immune complexes. Azathioprine 150 mg/day was used in patients with recalcitrant disease or steroid-induced side effects and produced a good clinical response in 4 to 8 weeks. Cyclophosphamide 2 mg/kg per day induced remissions in patients with multiple-organ involvement who were not controlled with prednisone. Methotrexate (10 to 25 mg/week) or cyclosporine (3 to 5 mg/kg per day) are alternatives for patients with a rapidly progressing course and systemic involvement. Hydroxychloroquine is not effective.

Henoch-Schönlein purpura

Henoch-Schönlein purpura (HSP), or anaphylactoid purpura, is an acute leukocytoclastic vasculitis that occurs mainly in children between the ages of 2 and 10, although adult cases are reported. It is the most common systemic vasculitis in children and is characterized by vascular deposition of IgA-dominant immune complexes, and preferentially involves venules, capillaries, and arterioles. Symptoms include palpable purpura over the legs and buttocks, abdominal pain (63%), GI bleeding (33%), arthralgia (82%), nephritis (40%), and hematuria (Table 18-5), and, histologically, leukocytoclastic vasculitis. It is a self-limited illness, but one third of patients will have one or more recurrences of symptoms.

PROGNOSIS. HSP is usually benign and self-limiting; the degree of renal involvement determines the prognosis. The long-term prognosis is excellent for both adults and children. In 50% of cases, there are recurrences, typically in the first 3 months; these are milder and more common in patients with nephritis.

ADULTS VS. CHILDREN. The frequency of previous drug treatment, primarily antibiotics or analgesics, is similar in both groups, but previous upper respiratory tract infection is more frequent among children. No precipitating event is found in 72% of the adults and 66% of the children. Adults have a lower frequency of abdominal pain and fever and a higher frequency of joint symptoms. Adults have more frequent and severe renal involvement. An increased erythrocyte sedimentation rate is more frequent in adults. Complete recovery occurs in 93.9% of children and in 89.2% of adults. Adults required more aggressive therapy, consisting of steroids and/or cytotoxic agents. However, the final outcome of HSP is equally good in adults and children.

Table 18-5 Clinical Features in 25 Patients with Henoch-Schönlein Purpura

Purpura	100%
Arthralgia	84%
Abdominal pain	76%
Gastrointestinal bleeding	30%
Occult bleeding	20%
Gross bleeding	10%
Nephritis	44%
Microscopic hematuria	40%
Gross hematuria	10%
Proteinuria	25%
Nephrotic syndrome	5%
End-stage renal disease	1%
Miscellaneous	
Encephalopathy	8%
Orchitis	4%

Adapted from Saulsbury FT: *Lancet* 369(9566):976-978, 2007. *PMID: 17382810*

ETIOLOGY. HSP tends to occur in the springtime; a streptococcal or viral upper respiratory tract infection may precede the disease by 1 to 3 weeks. A cluster of cases was reported, suggesting that HSP is caused by person-to-person spread of an infectious agent of the respiratory tract to susceptible hosts.

A number of infectious agents and drugs have been implicated, but the etiology of HSP remains unknown.

Immunoglobulin A. IgA plays a critical role in the immunopathogenesis of HSP. There are increased serum IgA concentrations, IgA-containing circulating immune complexes, and IgA deposition in vessel walls and renal mesangium. There are two subclasses of IgA, but HSP is associated with abnormalities involving IgA1 exclusively and not IgA2. All of its features are attributable to the widespread vasculitis believed to be initiated by entrapment of circulating IgA-containing immune complexes in blood vessel walls in the skin, kidneys, and GI tract.

CLINICAL FEATURES. Prodromal symptoms include anorexia and fever. The clinical features of HSP are as follows.

Skin. Nonthrombocytopenic palpable purpura is most common on the lower extremities and buttocks but can appear on the arms, face, and ears; the trunk is usually spared (Figures 18-15 to 18-18). The lesions evolve from urticarial papules into the classic leukocytoclastic vasculitic lesions within 48 hours. The lesions are 2 to 10 mm in diameter and appear in crops among coalescent ecchymoses and pinpoint petechiae. Lesions fade in several days, more rapidly with bed rest, leaving brown macules. New lesions appear with ambulation. Seventy-seven percent of patients present with cutaneous signs; 10% have no leg involvement; 4.5% have edema of the hands, feet, or face.

Abdominal symptoms. GI symptoms occur in 40% to 60% of patients; these include colicky pain, nausea, vomiting, upper GI bleeding, diarrhea, and bloody stool and are potentially the most serious manifestations. Severe abdominal pain was a significant predictor of nephritis in Henoch-Schönlein purpura. Although GI bleeding occurs in 52% of patients, it is self-limiting, and blood transfusions have not been required. Symptoms precede the skin disease by up to 2 weeks and simulate a number of inflammatory or surgically treated bowel diseases. Major complications of abdominal involvement develop in 4.6%, of which intussusception is by far the most common. The intussusceptum is confined to the small bowel in 58% and it is frequently inaccessible to demonstration by contrast enema.

Ultrasound is the imaging modality of choice. It provides an easy, noninvasive, objective method of monitoring patient progress. It allows direct visualization of bowel involvement and detection of complications such as intussusception. It also demonstrates edematous hemorrhagic infiltration of the intestinal wall, which can occur in the duodenal, jejunal, and ileal segments. Ultrasonography complements serial clinical assessment, clarifies the nature of the gastrointestinal involvement, and reduces the likelihood of unnecessary surgery.

Routine abdominal radiographs are not recommended, unless perforation is clinically suspected.

Upper GI endoscopy can be useful. Inflammation of the duodenum, especially of the second part, is characteristic of HSP. Upper GI endoscopy shows redness, swelling, petechiae or hemorrhage, or erosions and ulceration of the mucosa. Histology of mucosal biopsy specimens shows nonspecific inflammation with positive staining for IgA in the capillaries.

Joint symptoms. Arthralgia, probably resulting from painful periarticular edema rather than from inflammatory joint disease, involves the ankles, knees, and dorsum of the hands and feet in more than 80% of patients. It is often incapacitating, but it is self-limiting and nondeforming.

Nephritis. The long-term prognosis of HSP is directly dependent on the severity of renal involvement. Nephritis occurs in 20% to 50% of children. The renal disease is usually milder in children and almost always heals. The onset may be acute or delayed. Acute nephritis occurs from 1 to 12 days after the onset of other signs and symptoms. The onset of renal involvement may be delayed for weeks or months in a substantial proportion of patients. Microscopic hematuria is a constant feature, but episodes of gross hematuria occur in 40% of patients with nephritis. Proteinuria and hematuria are found in about 40% of cases. Urinary abnormalities can persist for 2 to 5 years in patients who develop nephritis in the acute phase of HSP. Progression to nephrotic syndrome and acute and chronic renal failure is possible.

When HSP presents with more than just microhematuria, only 72% of cases proceed to complete recovery. Heavy proteinuria at onset, focal sclerotic and tubulointerstitial changes, and crescents and capsular adhesions are poor prognostic indicators. After a follow-up of at least 8 years, 53% of patients are clinically in remission. Evidence of renal disease may reappear after apparent complete recovery. Childhood HS nephritis requires long-term follow-up, especially during pregnancy. A study of 78 subjects who had HS nephritis during childhood (at a mean of 23.4 years after onset) showed that severity of clinical presentation and initial findings on renal biopsy correlate well with outcome but have poor predictive value in individuals. Forty-four percent of patients who had nephritic or nephrotic syndromes at onset have hypertension or impaired renal function; 82% of those who presented with hematuria (with or without proteinuria) are normal. Of 44 full-term pregnancies, 16 were complicated by proteinuria and/or hypertension, even in the absence of active renal disease.

HENOCH-SCHÖNLEIN DISTRIBUTION

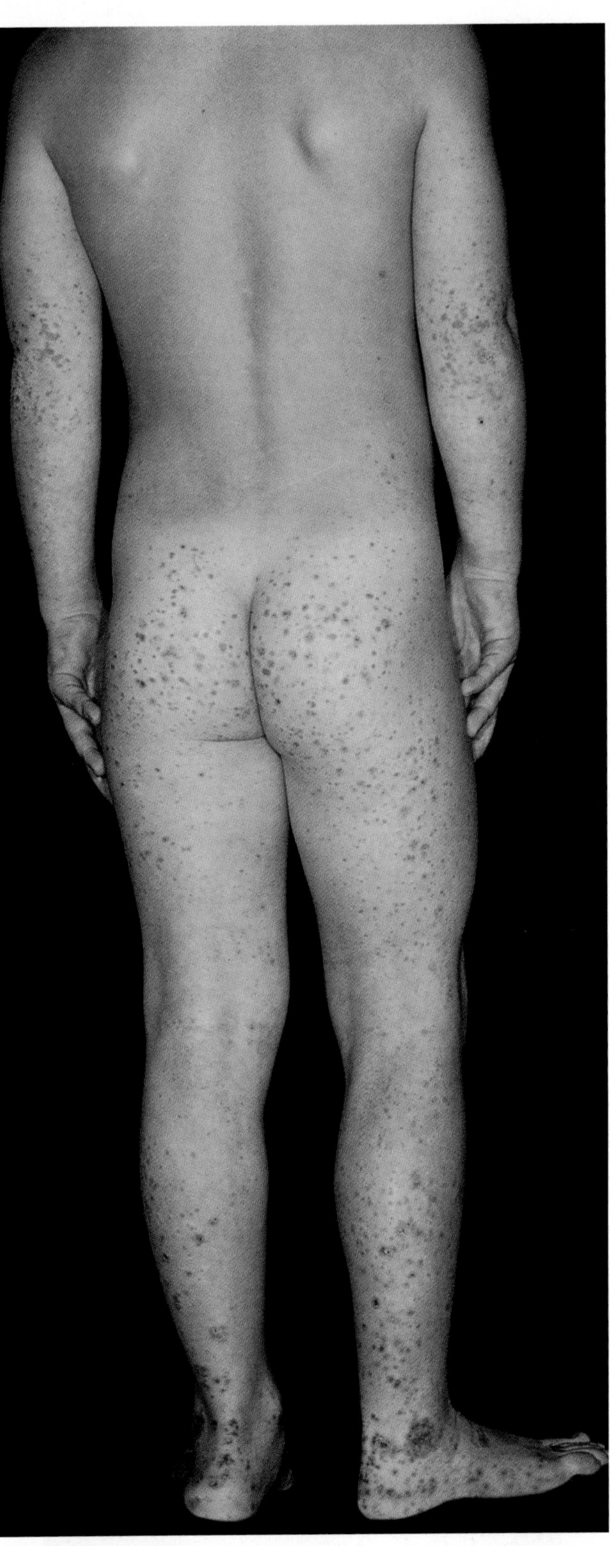

Figure 18-15 Henoch-Schönlein purpura. Palpable purpuric lesions are most common on the lower extremities and buttocks but can appear on the arms, face, and ears; the trunk is usually spared.

HENOCH-SCHÖNLEIN PURPURA

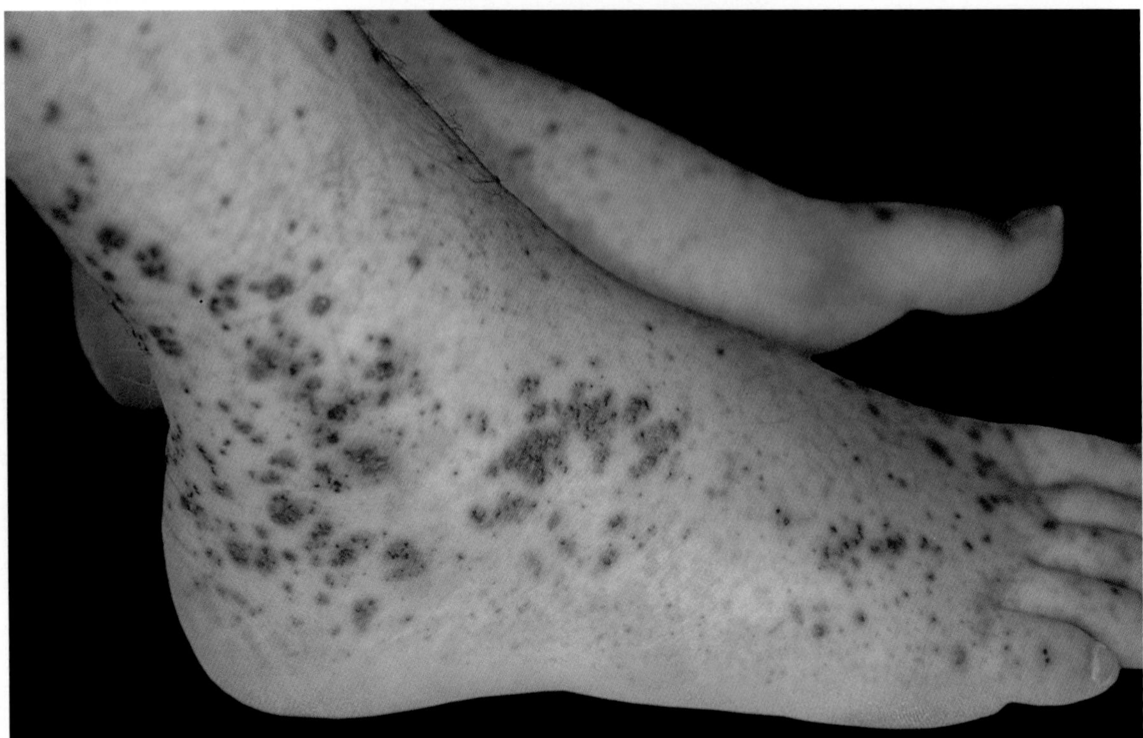

Figure 18-16 The initial presentation is often characterized by an acute onset of purpura, arthralgias, and colicky abdominal pain. Cutaneous lesions usually have a symmetrical distribution and begin as macular erythema or urticarial papules. They subsequently progress to inflammatory purpuric macules and papules that can range in size from pinpoint to several millimeters. Urticaria, vesicles, bullae, and foci of necrosis can also be seen. There is a predilection for the lower extremities and buttocks, but lesions can also occur on the trunk, upper extremities, and face. Individual lesions usually regress within 10 to 14 days, with resolution of skin involvement over a period of several weeks to months, although recurrences are observed in 5%-10% of patients.

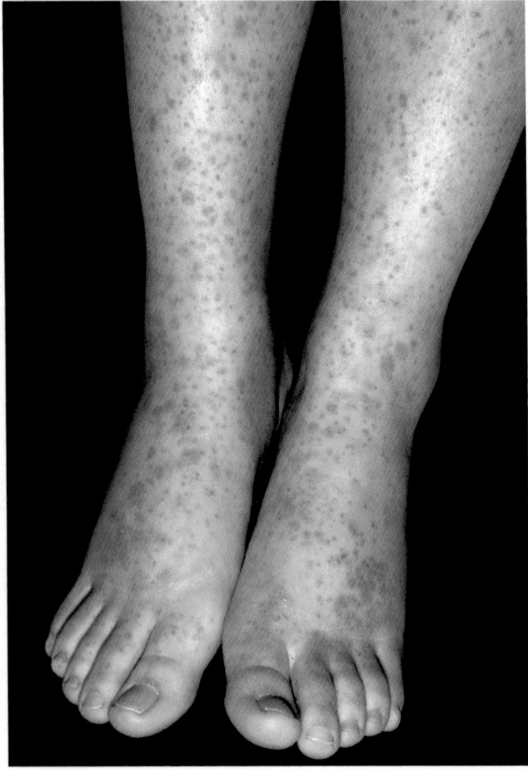

Figure 18-17 Multiple pink papules on the lower extremities are becoming purpuric and more numerous.

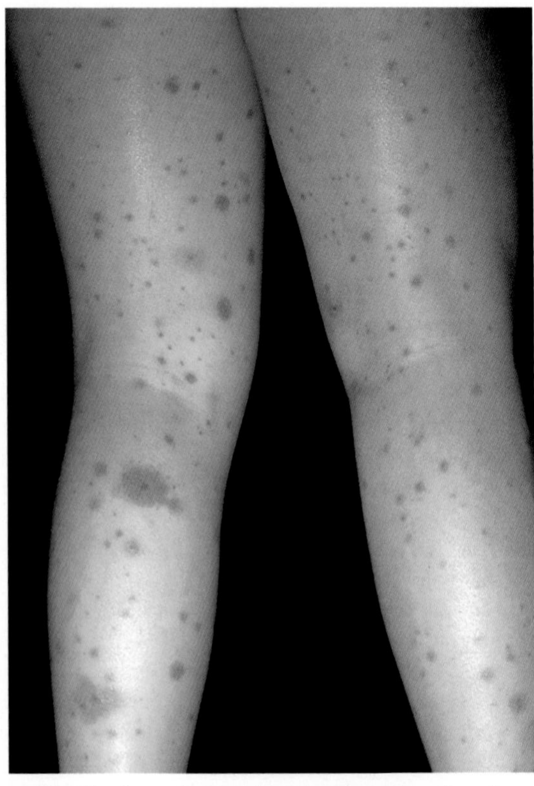

Figure 18-18 Some lesions have coalesced and undergone central necrosis.

The renal pathologic findings present a spectrum from mild focal glomerulitis to necrotizing or proliferative glomerulonephritis with diffuse mesangial proliferation. Diffuse mesangial deposits of IgA are seen on immunofluorescent studies. HS nephritis may be the single most common form of crescentic glomerulonephritis, accounting for 30% of cases.

Adults. A multicenter collaborative study of 152 patients compared the progression of renal disease in children and adults with HPS nephritis. Crescents were found in 36% of adults and 34.6% of children, nephrotic-range proteinuria in 29.5% of adults and 28.1% of children, and functional impairment in 24.1% of adults and 36.9% of children. The outcome was similar for both age groups (remission, 32.5% of adults and 31.6% of children; renal function impairment, 31.6% of adults and 24.5% of children). End-stage renal disease was observed in 15.8% of adults and in 7% of children. None of the children died, and adult survival was 97% at 5 years. In adults at presentation, renal function impairment and also proteinuria greater than 1.5 gm per day and hypertension were negative prognostic factors. In children no definite level of proteinuria, hypertension, or other data were found to be associated with poor prognosis. *PMID: 9394311*

A recent infectious history, pyrexia, the spread of purpura to the trunk, and biologic markers of inflammation are predictive factors for renal involvement.

Acute scrotal swelling. Acute scrotal swelling may be the presenting manifestation and occur in up to 15% of boys with HSP. The vasculitis of HSP may involve the scrotum and clinically mimic diseases requiring surgical intervention, such as testicular torsion or an incarcerated inguinal hernia. Sonographic findings include an enlarged, rounded epididymis, thickened scrotal skin, and a hydrocele with intact vascular flow in the testicles. Nuclear imaging may be used to assess testicular perfusion. The sonographic findings in the scrotum are sufficiently characteristic to allow distinction from torsion in most cases. These findings help prevent unnecessary surgical exploration.

PATHOLOGY. The pathology of HSP is that of an acute vasculitis of arterioles and venules in the superficial dermis and the bowel. Immunofluorescence staining of tissues usually shows the presence of IgA in the walls of the arterioles and in the renal glomeruli. The serum IgA level is frequently higher than normal.

DIAGNOSIS. There are no diagnostic laboratory tests. Complete blood counts (CBCs), antinuclear antibodies (ANAs), platelet counts, and coagulation studies are normal. The ESR may be elevated, and the serum complement level may be depressed. In one study, serum IgA concentrations were increased in 44% of children. Direct immunofluorescent studies show IgA deposition in blood vessels (75% in affected skin and 67% in uninvolved skin) of the superficial dermis. IgA1 is the dominant IgA subclass.

IgA in vessel walls is a sensitive and specific marker that helps to solidify the diagnosis of HSP. This finding should not be used as the sole criterion for making the diagnosis because it is seen in many other disorders, such as venous stasis and erythema nodosum. One study disclosed a significant correlation between plasma levels of anaphylatoxins C3a and C4a and plasma creatine levels in patients with nephritis. The role of IgA ANCA has not been defined.

MANAGEMENT. The offending antigen must be identified and removed. The possibilities include infections, malignancies, foods, and drugs. Patients with ANCA-associated small vessel vasculitis who present with purpura, abdominal pain, and nephritis but do not have IgA immune deposits do not have Henoch-Schönlein purpura and do not have a good prognosis; they should be treated quickly with immunosuppressive therapy.

Corticosteroids. The joint pain, inflammation, and painful cutaneous edema are treated with analgesics, nonsteroidal antiinflammatory agents, and corticosteroids. Corticosteroid therapy may hasten the resolution of arthritis and abdominal pain but does not prevent recurrences. Corticosteroids in usual doses have no effect on established nephritis. The optimal management of HSP-associated gastrointestinal and renal involvement has not yet been determined. Reports favor a short course of oral corticosteroids for severe abdominal pain and immunosuppressive therapy for patients with progressive nephritis. Prednisone in a dose of 1 mg/kg a day for 2 weeks, then tapered over 2 weeks, decreased the intensity and duration of gastrointestinal symptoms and the severity of joint symptoms. *PMID: 16887443*

That study also showed that prednisone hastened the resolution of mild HSP nephritis. The use of corticosteroids early in the course of HSP does not seem to be effective in preventing the development of nephritis, however. Thus corticosteroid therapy is beneficial in ameliorating the gastrointestinal and joint symptoms and perhaps in shortening the duration of mild nephritis, but not in preventing delayed nephritis. There is no evidence that corticosteroid therapy is effective in treating the purpura, shortening the duration of the disease, or preventing recurrences.

Intravenous pulse methylprednisolone (30 mg/kg a day for 3 consecutive days) followed by oral corticosteroids was effective in reversing severe nephritis and preventing progression. Others have reported the benefits of corticosteroids combined with cyclophosphamide, azathioprine, or cyclosporine in severe HSP nephritis and thus early aggressive therapy is warranted in patients with severe nephritis. *PMID: 17382810*

NEUTROPHILIC DERMATOSES

Neutrophilic dermatosis represents a continuous spectrum encompassing five entities: subcorneal pustular dermatosis, Sweet's syndrome, erythema elevatum diutinum, pyoderma gangrenosum, and neutrophilic eccrine hidradenitis. The different neutrophilic dermatoses are manifestations of a potentially multisystemic neutrophilic disease. All may present with pustules, plaques, nodules, and ulcerations. Histologically, a neutrophilic infiltrate appears at variable levels in the epidermis, dermis, and subcutaneous tissue. Systemic manifestations include generalized symptoms and joint, renal, ocular, and lung involvement. There is an overlap in the clinical manifestations of the four entities. Subcorneal pustular dermatosis and neutrophilic eccrine hidradenitis are very rare and not described here.

Sweet's syndrome (acute febrile neutrophilic dermatosis)

Sweet, in 1964, described a disease with four features: fever; leukocytosis; acute, tender, red plaques; and a papillary dermal infiltrate of neutrophils. This led to the name acute febrile neutrophilic dermatosis. Larger series of patients showed that fever and neutrophilia are not consistently present. The diagnosis is based on the two constant features—a typical eruption and the characteristic histologic features; thus the eponym Sweet's syndrome (SS) is used. The criteria of the diagnosis of SS are listed in Box 18-12.

Eighty-six percent of patients are women with a preceding upper respiratory tract infection. The mean age at presentation is 56 years (range, 22 to 82 years). SS is common in Japan. A genetic predisposition is possible; HLA-Bw54 was found to be a risk factor in a series of Japanese patients with SS.

Box 18-12 **Diagnostic Criteria for Sweet's Syndrome***

Major criteria

1. Abrupt onset of tender or painful erythematous plaques or nodules occasionally with vesicles, pustules, or bullae
2. Predominantly neutrophilic infiltration in the dermis without leukocytoclastic vasculitis

Minor criteria

1. Preceded by a nonspecific respiratory or gastrointestinal tract infection or vaccination or associated with:
   - Inflammatory diseases such as chronic autoimmune disorders and infections
   - Hemoproliferative disorders or solid malignant tumors
   - Pregnancy
2. Accompanied by periods of general malaise and fever (>38° C)
3. Laboratory values during onset: ESR, >20 mm/hr; C-reactive protein, positive; segmented-nuclear neutrophils and stabs, >70% in peripheral blood smear; leukocytosis, >8000/mm^3 (three of four of these values necessary)
4. Excellent response to treatment with systemic corticosteroids or potassium iodide

Modified from von den Driesch P: *J Am Acad Dermatol* 31:535, 1994. *PMID: 8089280*

*Both major and two minor criteria are needed for diagnosis.

ETIOLOGY. Sweet's syndrome can be classified based upon the clinical setting in which it occurs: classical or idiopathic Sweet's syndrome, malignancy-associated Sweet's syndrome, and drug-induced Sweet's syndrome.

SYSTEMIC DISEASES. SS is a reactive phenomenon and should be considered a cutaneous marker of systemic disease. Careful systemic evaluation is indicated, especially when cutaneous lesions are severe or hematologic values are abnormal. Approximately 20% of cases are associated with malignancy, predominantly hematologic, especially acute myelogenous leukemia. An underlying condition (streptococcal infection, inflammatory bowel disease, nonlymphocytic leukemia and other hematologic malignancies, solid tumors, pregnancy) is found in up to 50% of cases. Attacks of SS may precede the hematologic diagnosis by 3 months to 6 years, so that close evaluation of patients in the "idiopathic" group is required.

There is now good evidence that treatment with hematopoietic growth factors, including granulocyte colony–stimulating factor (G-CSF), which is used to treat acute myelogenous leukemia, and granulocyte-macrophage colony-stimulating factor, can cause Sweet's syndrome. Lesions typically occur when the patient has leukocytosis and neutrophilia but not when the patient is neutropenic. However, G-CSF may cause SS in neutropenic patients because of the induction of stem cell proliferation, the differentiation of neutrophils, and the prolongation of neutrophil survival.

CLINICAL MANIFESTATIONS. Acute, tender, erythematous plaques; nodes; pseudovesicles; and, occasionally, blisters with an annular or arciform pattern occur on the head, neck, legs, and arms, particularly the back of the hands and fingers (Figures 18-19 to 18-22). The trunk is rarely involved. Fever (50%); arthralgia or arthritis (62%); eye involvement, most frequently conjunctivitis or iridocyclitis (38%); and oral aphthae (13%) are associated features. Differential diagnosis includes erythema multiforme, erythema nodosum, adverse drug reaction, and urticaria. Recurrences are common and affect up to one third of patients.

LABORATORY STUDIES. Studies show a moderate neutrophilia (less than 50%), elevated ESR (greater than 30 mm/hr) (90%), and a slight increase in alkaline phosphatase level (83%). Skin biopsy shows a papillary and mid-dermal mixed infiltrate of polymorphonuclear leukocytes with nuclear fragmentation and histiocytic cells. The infiltrate is predominantly perivascular with endothelial cell swelling in some vessels, but vasculitic changes (thrombosis; deposition of fibrin, complement, or immunoglobulins within the vessel walls; red blood cell extravasation; inflammatory infiltration of vascular walls) are absent in early lesions.

SWEET'S SYNDROME

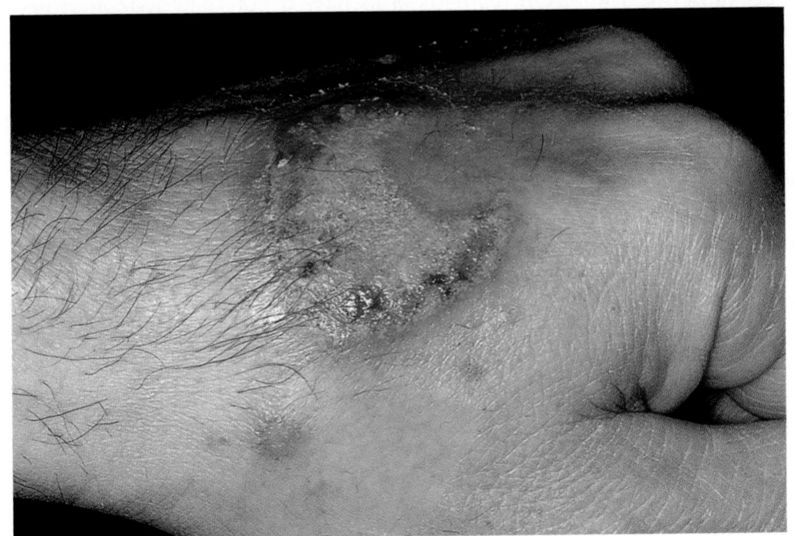

Figure 18-19 Red-blue papules may coalesce into round plaques. The edges are sometimes studded with pustules. Edema at the border of the lesion can produce a vesicular appearance.

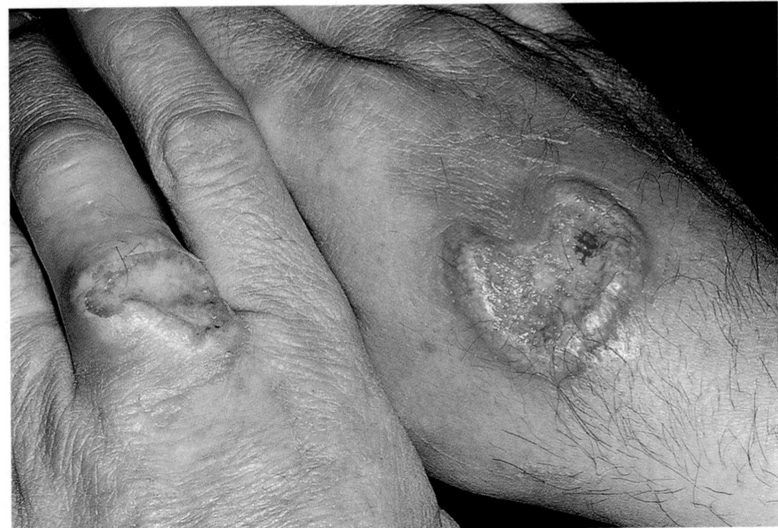

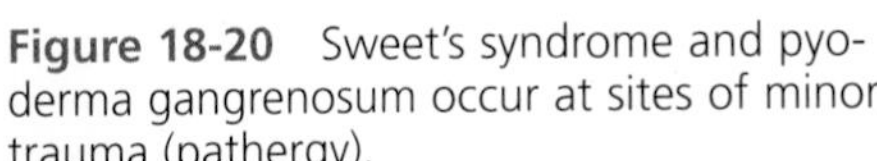

Figure 18-20 Sweet's syndrome and pyoderma gangrenosum occur at sites of minor trauma (pathergy).

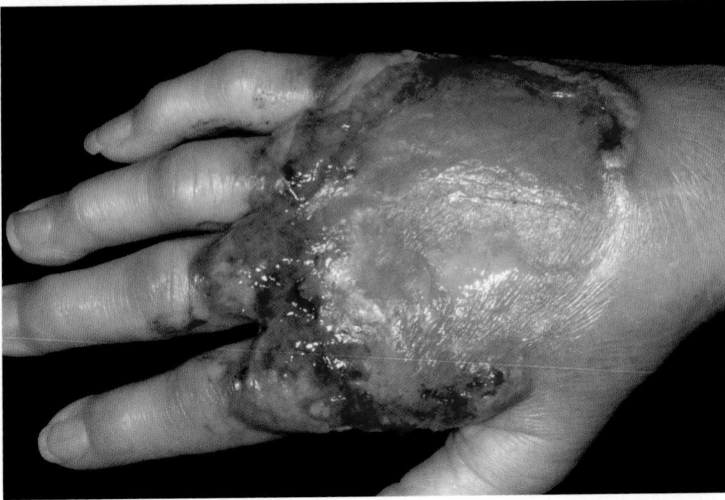

Figure 18-21 Atypical Sweet's syndrome. Neutrophilic dermatosis of the dorsal hands is an evolving disease concept and is felt to be a localized variant of Sweet's syndrome. Most cases occur in women. There is fever, leukocytosis, and/or elevated erythrocyte sedimentation rate. Cases are associated with leukemia, lung carcinoma, and inflammatory bowel disease. Superficially ulcerated plaques with violaceous undermined borders occur on the dorsal hand and fingers. Biopsy shows a dense, dermal neutrophilic infiltrate with small subcorneal pustules, subepidermal vesiculation, papillary dermal edema, and hemorrhage. All respond to systemic corticosteroid therapy. Other treatments include dapsone, methotrexate, and potassium iodide. Postinflammatory hyperpigmentation of dorsal hands persists for months. *PMID 16415387*

Vasculitis occurs secondary to noxious products released from neutrophils. Blood vessels in lesions of longer duration are more likely to develop vasculitis than those of shorter duration because of prolonged exposure to noxious metabolites. Therefore vasculitis does not exclude a diagnosis of Sweet's syndrome.

TREATMENT. Systemic corticosteroids (prednisone 0.5 to 1.5 mg/kg of body weight per day) produce rapid improvement and are the "gold standard" for treatment. The patient's temperature, WBC count, and eruption improve within 72 hours. The skin lesions clear within 3 to 9 days. Abnormal laboratory values rapidly return to normal. There are, however, frequent recurrences. Corticosteroids are discontinued by tapering over 2 to 6 weeks. Resolution of the eruption is occasionally followed by milia and scarring. The disease clears spontaneously in some patients. Topical and/or intralesional corticosteroids may be effective as either monotherapy or adjuvant therapy.

Oral potassium iodide or colchicine may induce rapid resolution. Patients who have a potential systemic infection or in whom corticosteroids are contraindicated can use these agents as a first-line therapy.

In one study, indomethacin 150 mg per day was given for the first week followed by indomethacin 100 mg per day for 2 additional weeks. Of the 18 patients, 17 had a good initial response; fever and arthralgias were markedly attenuated within 48 hours, and eruptions cleared between 7 and 14 days. Patients whose cutaneous lesions continued to develop were successfully treated with prednisone (1 mg/kg per day). No patient had a relapse after discontinuation of indomethacin. *PMID: 9091476*

Other alternatives to corticosteroid treatment include dapsone, doxycycline, clofazimine, and cyclosporine. All of these drugs influence migration and other functions of neutrophils.

SWEET'S SYNDROME

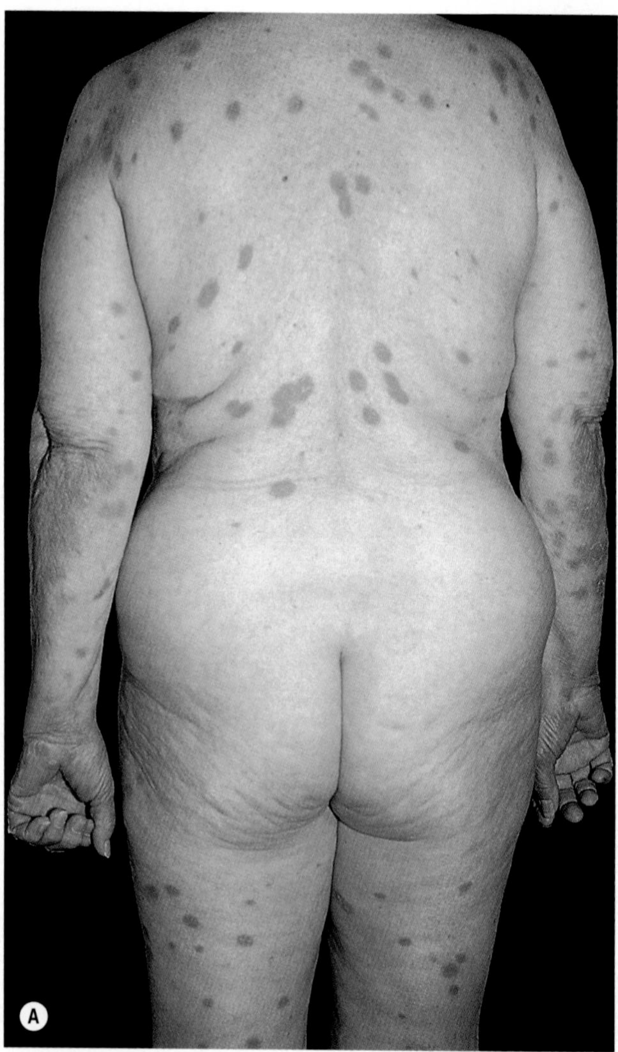

Multiple, painful, sharply demarcated, erythematous plaques occur on the neck, upper chest, back, and extremities.

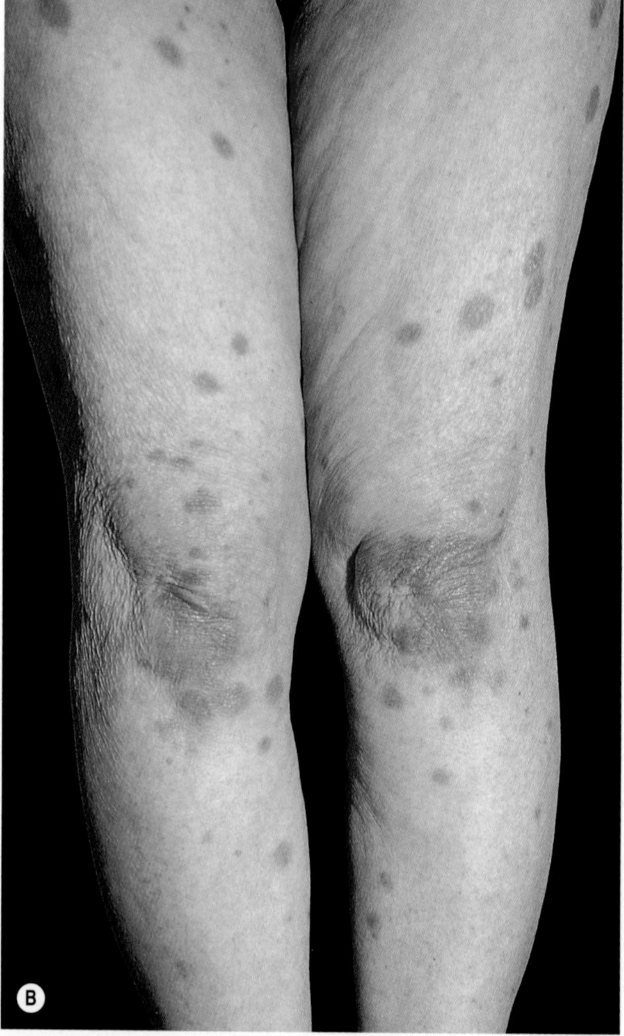

Plaques are painful and burning but not itching. The surface is mammillated (papular) or may contain pustules.

Figure 18-22

Erythema elevatum diutinum

Erythema elevatum diutinum (EED) is a rare skin disease (average age, 53 years; range, 32 to 65 years). There are persistent, nonpurpuric, deep, brown-red to purple papules, nodules, and plaques. Blisters and ulcers can develop. Lesions are symmetrically distributed on extensor surfaces on the extremities with a preference for joint regions. Occasionally lesions are found on the buttocks, face, and torso. EED may be a complication of HIV infection. Cutaneous lesions may closely resemble Kaposi's sarcoma and other malignant neoplasms. The lesions are often accompanied by arthralgias (in approximately 40% of patients) and drug intolerance.

ETIOLOGY. EED is most likely caused by immune complex deposition (Arthus reaction) in the dermal vessels. Excess exposure to antigens (recurrent infections) or situations in which high levels of antibody occur (e.g., paraproteinemias) are likely to result in immune complexes. The cause of this disorder might be an allergic reaction to streptococcal superantigens. Associated medical problems include hypergammaglobulinemia, both monoclonal (IgA clonal gammopathies) and polyclonal; multiple myeloma; and myelodysplasia. EED may precede the myeloproliferative disorders by up to 7.8 years. Chronic infection or recurrent infections (both streptococcal and non-streptococcal) are also reported.

HISTOLOGY. Early lesions show leukocytoclastic vasculitis and a massive dermal infiltrate composed mainly of neutrophils, histiocytes/macrophages, and Langerhans cells. Later lesions contain patterned (storiform or concentric) fibrosis and a dermal infiltrate of lymphocytes and histiocytes/macrophages and Langerhans cells. Lipid material forms in some older lesions. The term extracellular cholesterosis is used to describe this process.

LABORATORY STUDIES. Laboratory studies to consider for patients with EED include skin biopsy, serum protein electrophoresis, quantitative immunoglobulins, immunoelectrophoresis, cryoglobulins, and complement studies (C3, C4, and CH50). Direct immunofluorescence studies are generally nondiagnostic.

TREATMENT. Dapsone (e.g., 100 mg per day) is the treatment of choice. One case of EED that was unresponsive to dapsone was successfully treated with colchicine.

Pyoderma gangrenosum

Pyoderma gangrenosum (PG) is a rare, poorly understood, noninfectious neutrophilic ulcerating skin disease. It often occurs in patients with chronic underlying inflammatory or malignant disease such as ulcerative colitis, rheumatoid arthritis, chronic active hepatitis, Crohn's disease, IgA monoclonal gammopathy, and hematologic and lymphoreticular malignancies, but in 40% to 50% of patients, no associated disease is found. Trauma (pathergy) may precede PG in a few patients. The disease is recurrent in approximately 30% of patients. In rare instances, PG occurs in children; thus it should be considered in the differential diagnosis of pustular disorders in children with underlying conditions such as ulcerative colitis. A seronegative arthritis affecting large joints is present in approximately 40% of cases.

CUTANEOUS MANIFESTATIONS. Lesions are most commonly found on the lower legs, but they may occur on the thighs, buttocks, chest, head, neck, and anywhere on the skin. One study showed that lesions were multiple in 71% of cases, and more than 50% were situated below the knees. The lesion begins as a tender, red macule or papule, pustule, nodule, or bulla. Pustules or vesicles appear on the surface, and the surrounding skin becomes dusky red and indurated. A necrotizing inflammatory process extends peripherally from the primary lesion, resulting in a necrotic ulcer or ulcers with a purulent base with an undetermined purple-to-red margin and a halo of surrounding erythema (Figures 18-23 to 18-26). The fully evolved lesion is generally less than 10 cm, but it may be enormous. The lesions tend to endure, lasting months to years, and heal with cribriform scarring.

BOWEL DISEASE. PG occurs both in ulcerative colitis and in Crohn's disease. Approximately 50% of PG cases occur in association with ulcerative colitis. Approximately 2% of patients with active and extensive ulcerative colitis have PG, and another 4% of patients with active ulcerative colitis have erythema nodosum, which in its early stages can be confused with PG. Males and females are affected equally. The mean duration of chronic ulcerative colitis before the appearance of erythema nodosum and PG is 5 and 10 years, respectively. The lesions generally appear during the course of active bowel disease, but they also occur in inactive colitis or less severe disease and may not appear until after colectomy. Pyoderma resolved without intestinal resection in two thirds of patients. Healing after intestinal resection is unpredictable regarding both timing and extent of resection.

PYODERMA GANGRENOSUM

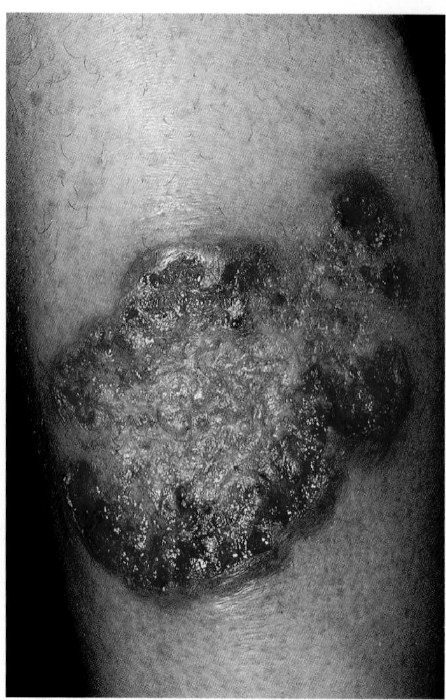

Figure 18-23 The classic presentation of rapidly progressive, painful, suppurative cutaneous ulcers with edematous, boggy, blue, undermined, and necrotic borders.

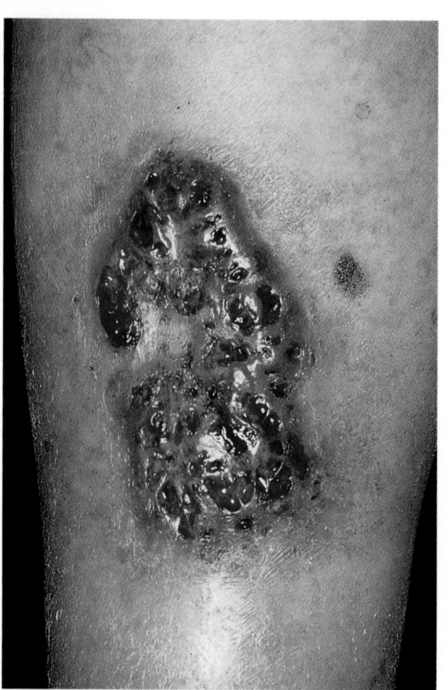

Figure 18-24 Neutrophilic dermatoses inflammatory disorders have in common a tendency for pathergy (induction of the inflammatory process after skin trauma).

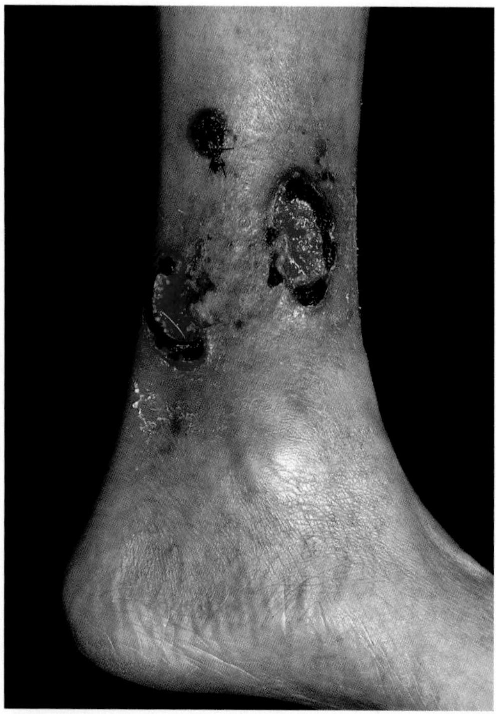

Figure 18-25 Lesions are most often found on the lower extremities, but may occur anywhere. There are large painful ulcerations.

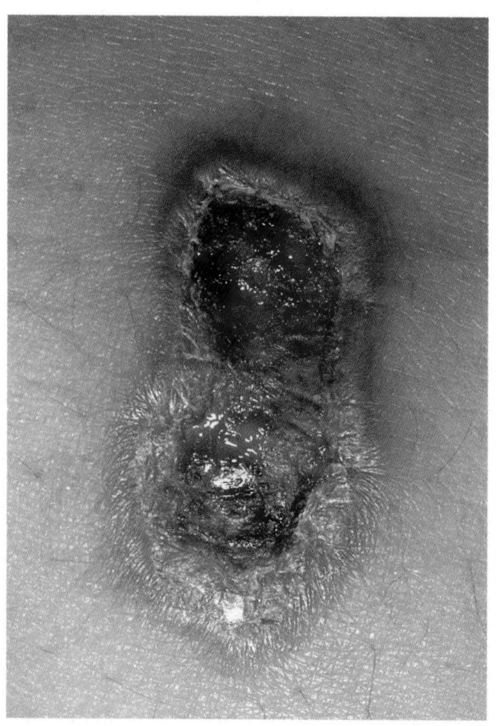

Figure 18-26 Lesions begin as a vesiculopustule that forms an ulcer with deep violaceous overhanging or undermined borders.

DIAGNOSIS. The diagnosis is based on clinical and pathologic features and requires exclusion of conditions that produce ulcerations (Boxes 18-13 and 18-14). The diagnosis is difficult to make because of the condition's ability to mimic other ulcerative lesions and its lack of specific laboratory and pathologic findings. Histopathologically, PG evolves from folliculitis and abscess formation; it may also show leukocytoclastic vasculitis. The lesions then evolve to suppurative granulomatous dermatitis and finally regress with prominent fibroplasia. These changes are nonspecific; therefore biopsy is of little diagnostic value. No specific abnormal laboratory determination has been found that is useful to diagnosis. Serum protein immunoelectrophoresis may be ordered to test for monoclonal gammopathy.

Box 18-13 **Approach to the Patient with Suspected Pyoderma Gangrenosum**

Important historical data

Markedly painful ulcer
Rapid progression of ulceration
Type of skin lesion preceding the ulcer (papule, pustule, or vesicle)
Minor trauma (pathergy) preceding development of the ulcer
Symptoms of an associated disease (e.g., inflammatory bowel disease or arthritis)
Drug history (e.g., bromides, iodide, hydroxyurea, or granulocyte-macrophage colony-stimulating factor)

Characteristic features of ulcer on physical examination

Tenderness
Necrosis
Irregular violaceous border
Undermined, rolled edges

Skin biopsy

Aim: to rule out diagnoses that mimic pyoderma gangrenosum
Protocol:

- Elliptical incisional biopsy preferable to punch biopsy; include inflamed border and ulcer edge at a depth that includes subcutaneous fat
- Specimen from inflamed border—routine histology (hematoxylin and eosin staining) and special staining (Gram's methenamine silver and Fite) to detect microorganisms
- Specimen from edge of ulcer—culture in appropriate culture media (to detect bacteria, fungi, and atypical *Mycobacteria*)

Laboratory investigations

Aims: to identify associated diseases and to rule out diagnoses that mimic pyoderma gangrenosum
Investigations to consider:
  Complete blood count
  Erythrocyte sedimentation rate
  Blood chemistry (liver and kidney function tests)
  Protein electrophoresis
  Chest radiography
  Colonoscopy
  Coagulation panel (including antiphospholipid antibody screening)
  Antineutrophilic cytoplasmic antibodies
  Cryoglobulins
  Venous and arterial function studies
Close, continuous follow-up
  Monitor response to and side effects of therapy
If no response to treatment, reconsider diagnosis and repeat biopsy

From Weenig RH et al: *New Engl J Med* 347:1412, 2002.
PMID: 12409543

Box 18-14 **Ulcers Resembling Pyoderma Gangrenosum**

Cause of cutaneous ulceration

Vascular occlusive or venous disease

Antiphospholipid antibody syndrome
Livedoid vasculopathy
Venous stasis ulceration
Small vessel occlusive artery disease
Type I cryoglobulinemia
Klippel-Trénaunay-Weber syndrome

Vasculitis

Wegener's granulomatosis
Polyarteritis nodosa
Cryoglobulinemic (mixed) vasculitis
Takayasu's arteritis
Leukocytoclastic vasculitis plus secondary infection

Cutaneous involvement of malignant process

Lymphoma
  Angiocentric T-cell lymphoma
  Anaplastic large-cell T-cell lymphoma
  Mycosis fungoides bullosa
  Unspecified lymphomas
Leukemia cutis
Langerhans cell histiocytosis

Primary cutaneous infection

Deep fungal infection
  Sporotrichosis
  Aspergillosis
  Cryptococcosis
  Zygomycosis
  Penicillium marneffei infection
Herpes simplex virus type 2
Cutaneous tuberculosis
Mycobacterium ulcerans (Buruli ulcer)
Amebiasis cutis

Drug-induced or exogenous tissue injury

Munchausen syndrome or factitial disorder
Hydroxyurea-induced ulceration
Contact vulvitis
Injection drug abuse with secondary infection
Bromoderma
Loxoscelism (bite of a brown recluse spider)
Drug-induced lupus

Other inflammatory disorders

Cutaneous Crohn's disease
Ulcerative necrobiosis lipoidica

From Weenig RH et al: *New Engl J Med* 347:1412, 2002.
PMID: 12409543

TREATMENT. Systemic corticosteroids and cyclosporine are common treatments for extensive disease. Prednisolone (60 to 120 mg) is started at high doses. Combinations of corticosteroids with cytotoxic drugs such as azathioprine, cyclophosphamide, or chlorambucil are used in patients with disease that is resistant to corticosteroids. Many other treatments are reported. Trauma must be avoided.

APPROACH TO RAPIDLY ADVANCING DISEASE. Rapidly advancing disease is treated with oral corticosteroids. If response is slow then consider using infliximab IV. An induction dose of 5 mg/kg at weeks 0, 2, and 6 is followed by further treatments as necessary. Another immunosuppressant, such as azathioprine, is given at the same time as infliximab. *PMID: 16858047*

Oral immunosuppressive agents. Immunospressive agents may be the most effective treatment. When corticosteroids fail, the most widely used alternative is cyclosporine. Improvement is seen within 3 weeks with a dose of 3 to 5 mg/kg/day. An intravenous bolus of cyclophosphamide is reported to be effective in inducing a remission. Oral chlorambucil 2 to 4 mg/day in combination with prednisone or used alone is an effective corticosteroid-sparing agent. Mycophenolate mofetil (2 gm/day) or tacrolimus (0.1 mg/kg/day) may be effective.

Anti-tumor necrosis factor agents. Pyoderma is reported to respond to infliximab and etanercept. There is more experience with infliximab.

Localized steroids. The small early lesion may be aborted with an intralesional injection of triamcinolone acetonide (Kenalog 10 mg/ml or 40 mg/ml). Group II to V topical steroids with or without occlusion may be effective.

Topical calcineurin inhibitors. Tacrolimus ointment 0.1% or pimecrolimus cream 1% may be effective for mild or early cutaneous lesions.

SCHAMBERG'S DISEASE

Schamberg's disease (progressive pigmented purpuric dermatosis, purpura simplex) is an uncommon eruption characterized by petechiae and patches of brownish pigmentation (hemosiderin deposits), particularly on the lower extremities. Patients are frightened by this vasculitic-appearing eruption, but there is no hematologic disease, venous insufficiency, or associated internal disease. Males are affected more often than females. Children are also affected. Lesions remain for months or years and present only a cosmetic problem. Histologically, there is inflammation and hemorrhage without fibrinoid necrosis of vessels. The cause is unknown, but a cellular immune reaction may play a role. In some patients, the eruption was related to medications.

CLINICAL MANIFESTATIONS. Asymptomatic, irregular, orange-brown patches of varying shapes and sizes appear (Figure 18-27). The most characteristic feature is orange-brown, pinhead-sized "cayenne pepper" spots. Mild erythema and scaling sometimes cause slight itching. Lesions are most common on the lower legs, but they can appear on the upper body. New spots can appear and older ones can fade. In contrast to hypersensitivity vasculitis (palpable purpura), the lesions are macular.

MANAGEMENT. The patient should be assured that there is no systemic disease. Inform patients that the pigmentation lasts for years. Mild itching and erythema respond quickly to group V topical steroids. Lesions persist, but 67% eventually clear.

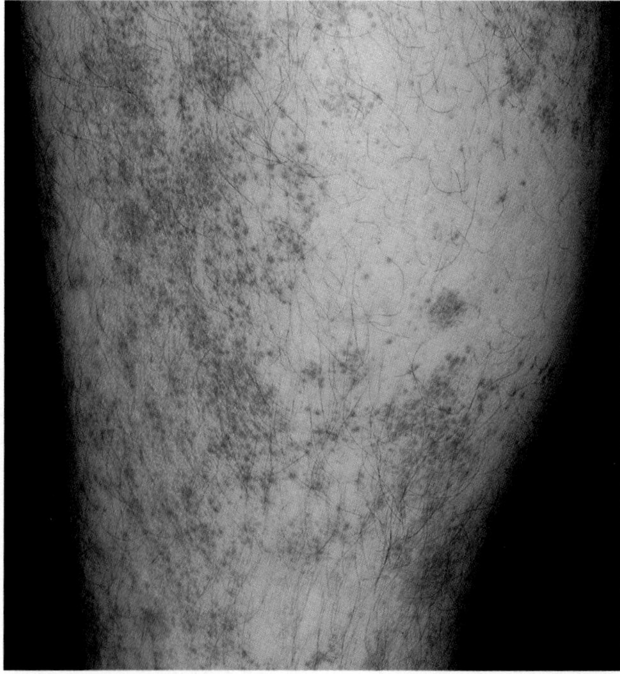

Figure 18-27 Schamberg's disease. Asymptomatic, irregular, orange-brown patches of varying shapes and sizes occur most often on the lower extremities.

Chapter 19

Light-Related Diseases and Disorders of Pigmentation

CHAPTER CONTENTS

PHOTOBIOLOGY

Sunlight has profound effects on the skin and is associated with a variety of diseases (see Boxes 19-1, 19-2, and 19-3). Ultraviolet (UV) light causes most photobiologic skin reactions and diseases. The accepted unit for measurement of the wavelength of light is the nanometer (nm). The solar radiation that reaches the earth is a continuous spectrum consisting of wavelengths of electromagnetic energy above 290 nm. By convention, UV light is divided into UVA (320 to 400 nm; long wave, black light), UVB (290 to 320 nm; middle wave, sunburn), and UVC (100 to 290 nm; short wave, germicidal). UVA is further subdivided into two regions: short-wave UVA, or UVA II (320 to 340 nm); and long-wave UVA, or UVA I (340 to 400 nm). The ratio of UVA to UVB is 20:1, and two thirds of this UVA is UVA I. Eighty percent of UVB and 70% of UVA radiation occur between the hours of 10 AM and 2 PM. More than 90% of UV radiation may penetrate clouds. UV radiation generates reactive oxygen species that damage skin.

UVA. UVA causes immediate and delayed tanning and contributes little to erythema and burning. It is constant throughout the day and throughout the year. The longer wavelengths of UVA can penetrate more deeply, reaching the dermis and subcutaneous fat. Chronic exposure to UVA radiation causes the connective tissue degeneration seen in photoaging, photocarcinogenesis, and immunosuppression. Photocarcinogenesis is augmented in patients who are immunosuppressed for organ transplantation. UVA augments the carcinogenic effects of UVB. UVA penetrates window glass and interacts with topical and systemic chemicals and medication. It produces photoallergic and phototoxic reactions.

Box 19-1 **Photosensitivity Diseases: Diseases Characterized by the Development of a Cutaneous Eruption After Exposure to Light**

Idiopathic

Polymorphous light eruption
Actinic prurigo
Hydroa vacciniforme
Hydroa aestivale
Chronic actinic dermatitis
Solar urticaria

Degenerative and neoplastic

Actinic damage
Actinic keratosis
Basal cell carcinoma
Squamous cell carcinoma
Malignant melanoma
Secondary to exogenous agents
Phototoxicity: Contact and systemic
Photoallergy: Contact and systemic
Drug eruptions

Metabolic

Erythropoietic porphyria
Erythropoietic protoporphyria
Porphyria cutanea tarda
Variegate porphyria

Photoexacerbated dermatoses

Autoimmune diseases

Lupus erythematosus
Dermatomyositis
Pemphigus
Pemphigus foliaceus
Bullous pemphigoid

Genodermatoses

Familial benign chronic pemphigus
Keratosis follicularis (Darier's disease)
Bloom syndrome
Rothmund-Thomson syndrome
Kindler syndrome
Cockayne's syndrome
Xeroderma pigmentosum
Trichothiodystrophy
Hartnup disease

Infectious disease

Herpes simplex labialis

Nutritional deficiencies

Pellagra
Pyridoxine deficiency

Primary dermatologic diseases

Atopic dermatitis
Transient acantholytic dermatosis
Disseminated superficial actinic porokeratosis
Lichen planus actinicus
Psoriasis
Reticular erythematous mucinosis
Acne rosacea
Acne
Darier's disease
Hailey-Hailey disease

Adapted from Lim HW, Epstein J: *J Am Acad Dermatol* 36:84, 1997. *PMID: 8996266*

Box 19-2 **Photosensitivity Skin Disorders**

Disorder	Action spectrum	Protection required
Polymorphous light eruption	290-365 nm	Broad spectrum
Porphyrias	400-410 nm	Physical blocking agent
Solar urticaria	290-515 nm	Broad spectrum
Lupus erythematosus	290-330 nm	UVB most important, also UVA
Xeroderma pigmentosum	290-340 nm	Broad spectrum

Box 19-3 **Most Common Photodermatoses According to Age the Symptoms First Occur**

Childhood

- Juvenile spring eruption (lesions on ears in spring)
- Polymorphous light eruption (itchy lesion in V area of neck and elsewhere)
- Erythropoietic protoporphyria (burning pain, increased protoporphyrin levels in red blood cells)
- Hydroa vacciniforme (very rare, scar formation)

Adulthood

- Polymorphous light eruption (females with itchy lesion in V area of neck and elsewhere)
- Drug-induced photosensitivity (all sun-exposed areas, positive phototest results)
- Solar urticaria (lesions appear within 5-10 min and disappear in 1-2 hr) (urticaria on phototesting)
- Lupus erythematosus (anti–Ro/SS-A antibodies, skin immunofluorescence)
- Porphyria cutanea tarda (porphyrin determinations)

Old age

- Chronic actinic dermatitis (persistent redness of face in elderly man)
- Drug-induced photosensitivity (all sun-exposed areas, positive phototest results)
- Cutaneous T-cell lymphoma (CD4+ cells on histologic examination)
- Dermatomyositis

Adapted from Roelandts R: *Arch Dermatol* 136:1152, 2000. *PMID: 10987875*

UVB. UVB produces the most harmful effects and is greatest during the summer. Snow and ice reflect UVB radiation. UVB delivers a high amount of energy to the stratum corneum and superficial layers of the epidermis and is primarily responsible for sunburn, suntan, inflammation, delayed erythema, and pigmentation changes. It produces tanning more efficiently than does UVA. Chronic effects include photoaging, immunosuppression, and photocarcinogenesis. It is most intense when the sun is directly overhead between 10 AM and 2 PM. UVB is absorbed by window glass. Prior exposure to UVA enhances the sunburn reaction from UVB.

UVC. UVC is almost completely absorbed by the ozone layer and is transmitted only by artificial sources such as germicidal lamps and mercury arc lamps.

SUN-DAMAGED SKIN

SUNLIGHT-SKIN INTERACTION. DNA is mutated by UVB. Absorption of UVA leads to the release of reactive oxygen species that cause oxidation of lipids and proteins that affect DNA repair, produce dyspigmentation, and cause photoaging and carcinogenesis.

AGING VERSUS SUN DAMAGE. Sun exposure is the major cause of the undesirable skin changes often inaccurately perceived as aging. These changes, known as photoaging, are caused primarily by repeated sun exposure and not by the passage of time. Many of the clinical signs attributed to aging are actually manifestations of solar damage. The two processes are biologically different. The difference can best be demonstrated to patients by comparing the appearance of the skin under the arm near the axillae with the sun-exposed surface of the lower arm.

NORMAL AGING. The skin begins to show signs of aging by ages 30 to 35. Aged skin is thin, fragile, and inelastic. The epidermis becomes thin. There is a gradual loss of blood vessels, dermal collagen, fat, and the number of elastic fibers. There is a reduction in the density of hair follicles, sweat ducts, and sebaceous glands, resulting in a reduction in perspiration and sebum production. Potent steroids should not be used on aged skin with few blood vessels because the steroids are not cleared from the skin as easily as in younger persons.

The skin becomes atrophic and fragile when subcutaneous tissue is lost. Elastic fibers are responsible for the elasticity and resilience of the skin. In normal aging, there is loss and fragmentation of elastic fibers, which result in fine wrinkles that resemble crumpled cigarette paper. These shallow wrinkles disappear by stretching. The skin is easily distorted, but it recoils slowly.

PHOTOAGING. Photoaging refers to those skin changes superimposed on intrinsic aging by chronic sun exposure (Box 19-4). Unprotected, chronically exposed children can acquire significant actinic damage by the time they reach age 15. The effects of this damage may become apparent after age 20. Sun-damaged skin is characterized by elastosis (a coarsening and yellow discoloration of the skin), irregular pigmentation, roughness or dryness, telangiectasia, atrophy, deep wrinkling, follicular plugging, and a variety of benign and malignant neoplasms. The epidermis thickens. Although many different cells are affected, it is the elastotic material that accounts for the most striking effects of sun damage.

Solar elastosis is a sign highly characteristic of severe sun damage (Figure 19-1). There is massive deposition in the upper dermis of an abnormal, yellow, amorphous elastotic material that does not form functional elastic fibers. This altered connective tissue does not have the resilient properties of elastic tissue.

Box 19-4 **Sun-Induced Skin Changes**

Texture changes

Solar elastosis
- Thickened, wrinkled, yellowish skin

Atrophy
- Thinning of the skin; fine wrinkling, prominent blood vessels, easy bruising and tearing of the skin, often with many linear scars

Wrinkles
- Deep—do not disappear by stretching
- Posterior neck sun damage (cutis rhomboidalis nuchae)
- Thickened skin is crisscrossed by deep lines creating rhomboidal patterns

Vascular changes

Diffuse erythema
- Most apparent in fair-skinned people

Ecchymoses and stellate pseudoscars
- Bleeding into the skin follows minor trauma—only on exposed surfaces of the back of the hands and arms; associated with atrophy, ease of skin tearing, and linear scars

Telangiectasias
- Cheeks, nose, and ears

Venous lake
- Round, purple, ectatic vessels—lower lips and ears

Pigmentation changes

Freckles
- Small, oval, brown macules—primarily on the face

Lentigo
- Large brown macules—face, back of the hands, arms, chest, upper back

Guttate hypomelanosis
- Discrete, round, white macules—lower legs and arms

Brown and white pigmentation (irregular)
- Deep brown with areas of hypopigmentation

Poikiloderma of Civatte
- Reddish-brown reticulated pigmentation with telangiectasias, atrophy, and prominent hair follicles—chest and neck

Papular changes

Nevi
- More numerous on sun-exposed surfaces in predisposed individuals

Yellow papules (solar elastosis)
- Dull-to-bright-yellow papules that may coalesce to form plaques

Seborrheic keratosis
- Discrete superficial (stuck-on) lesions—more numerous in sun-exposed areas; flat on extremities, elevated on the trunk

Comedones and cysts around the eyes (Favre-Racouchet syndrome)

Wrinkling becomes coarse and deep rather than fine, and the skin is thickened (Figure 19-2). These wrinkles do not disappear by stretching. Sun-induced wrinkling on the back of the neck shows a series of crisscrossed lines (Figure 19-3) that form a rhomboidal pattern (cutis rhomboidalis nuchae).

Reactive hyperplasia of melanocytes causes persistent pigmentation in the form of freckles, lentigines, and irregular hyperpigmentation and hypopigmentation on the hands, forearms, legs, chest, back, and neck (Figures 19-3 and 19-4).

Chronic sun exposure disrupts the maturation of keratinocytes, causing scaling, roughness, seborrheic keratosis (Figures 19-5 to 19-7), actinic keratosis, actinic cheilitis, and squamous cell carcinoma.

Blood vessels diminish in number, and the walls of the remaining vessels become thin. Blood vessels need connective tissue for support. Bleeding occurs with the slightest trauma to the sun-damaged surfaces of the forearms and hands but not to the unexposed surfaces. Haphazard scarring may follow (Figure 19-8). Making patients aware of this difference convinces them that they do not have a platelet abnormality.

Comedones form about the eyes (Figures 19-9 and 19-10).

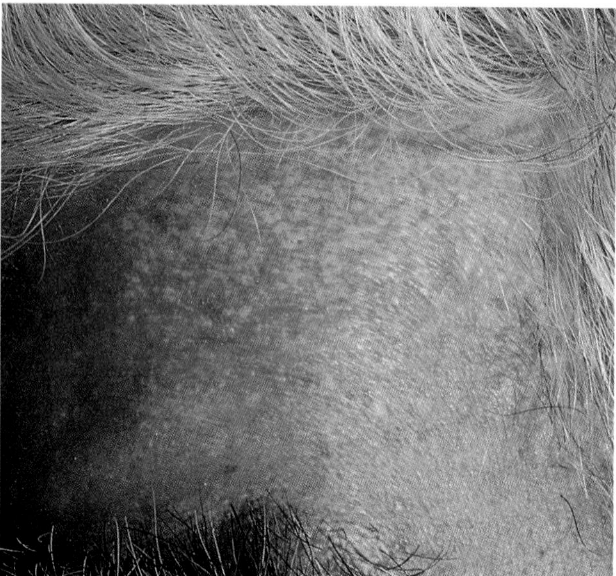

Figure 19-1 Solar elastosis. Numerous yellowish globules in the dermis can be seen through the thin, atrophic epidermis.

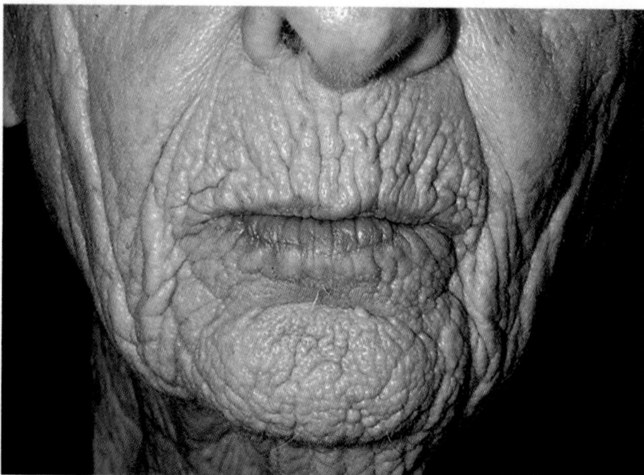

Figure 19-2 Leathered wrinkling is a sign of severe sun damage.

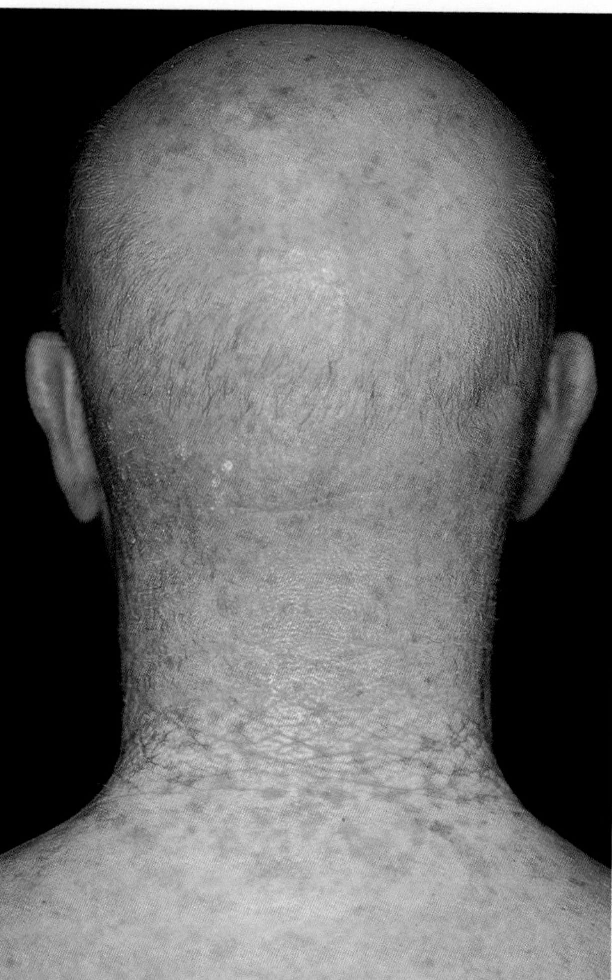

Figure 19-3 Reactive hyperplasia of melanocytes causes lentigines on the upper back. Diffuse persistent erythema is most prominent in fair-skinned people. Sun-induced wrinkling on the back of the neck shows a series of crisscrossed lines.

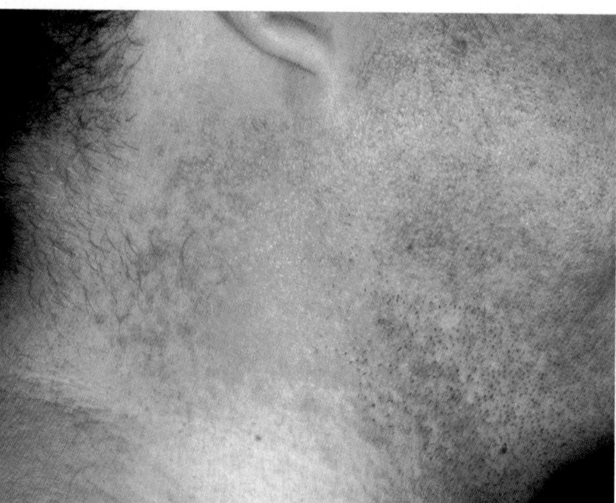

Figure 19-4 Reddish-brown, reticulate pigmentation with atrophy and telangiectasia is seen on the sides of the neck. This is referred to as poikiloderma of Civatte.

SUN DAMAGE

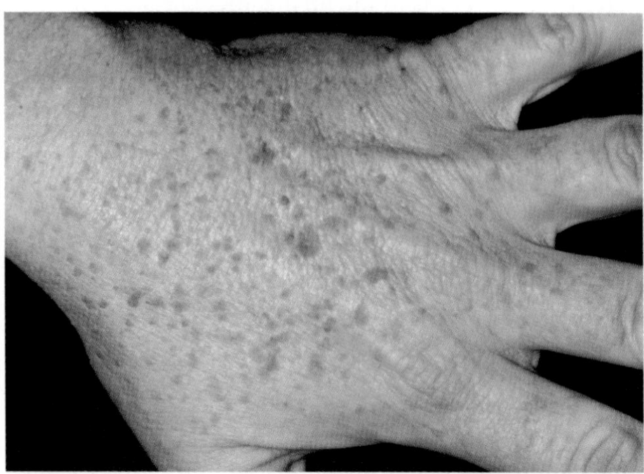

Figure 19-5 Slightly elevated seborrheic keratoses occur on the back of the hands and may be misdiagnosed as solar lentigines.

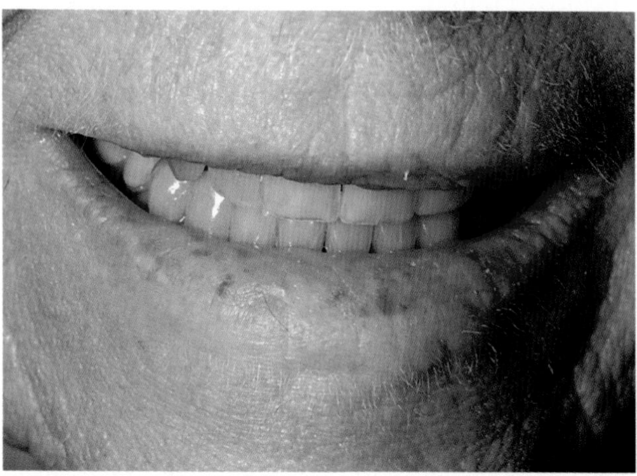

Figure 19-6 Sun damage causes lower lip atrophy with loss of normal skin lines.

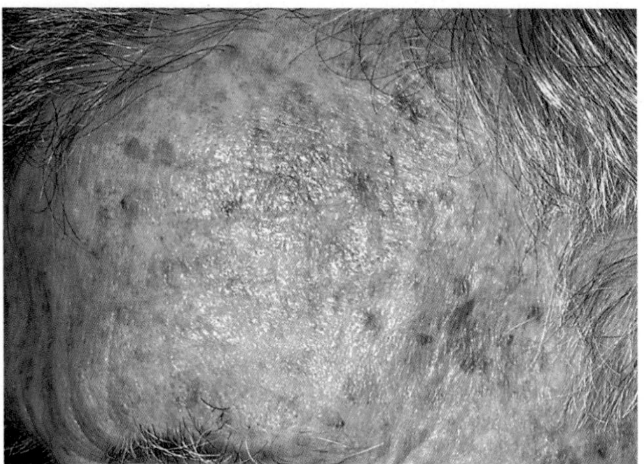

Figure 19-7 Variations in pigmentation and diffuse actinic keratosis may occur after years of sun exposure.

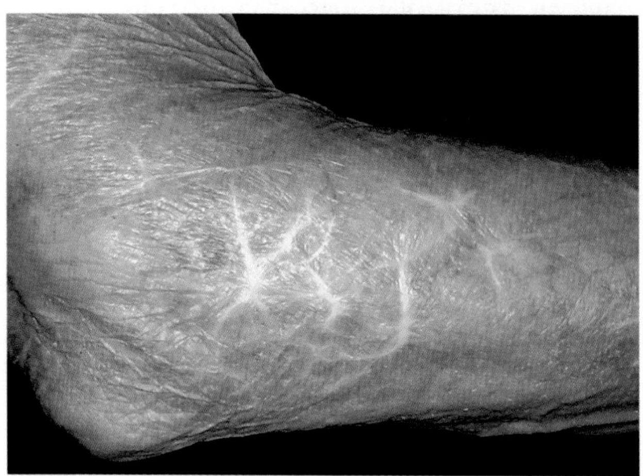

Figure 19-8 Fragile sun-damaged skin is easily torn and heals with haphazard scars called stellate pseudoscars.

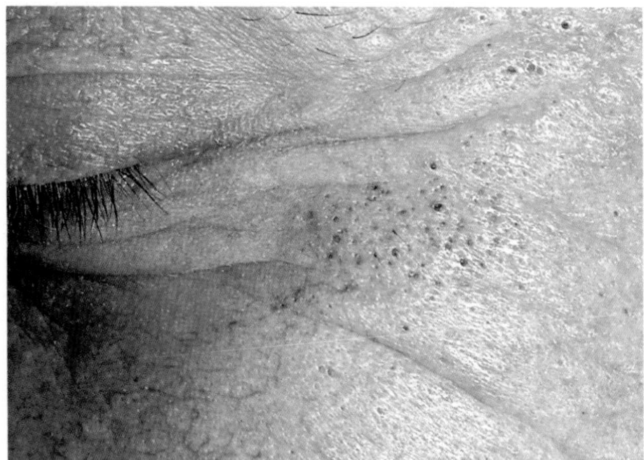

Figure 19-9 Actinic comedones. Open and closed comedones are present in the periorbital areas. Acne-like inflammation does not occur.

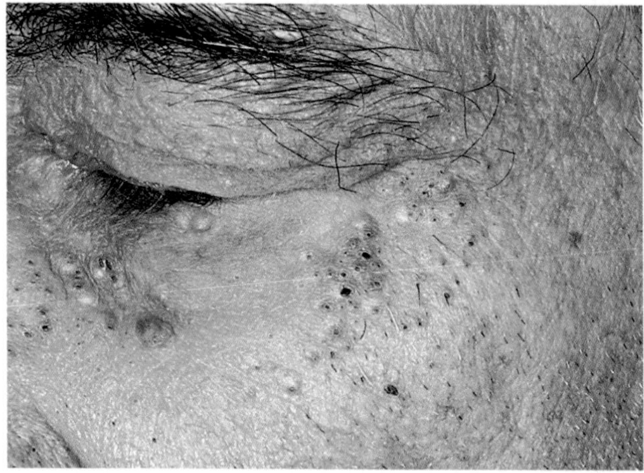

Figure 19-10 Actinic comedones may become very large and can easily be expressed with a comedone extractor.

TREATMENT OF PHOTOAGING

Photoaging is treated with either topical treatments or resurfacing through chemical peels, dermabrasion, or lasers.

TOPICAL TREATMENT. Topical treatments have the following characteristics:

1. Noninvasive
2. Slow to produce changes (latency period is 3 to 6 months)
3. Maintenance of improvements requires continued use
4. Medication is expensive

Photoaging responds to treatment with topical retinoids such as tretinoin and tazarotene. The improvement is retinoid specific and not secondary to irritation. Improvement can be achieved without excessive use of medication, thereby minimizing the occurrence of irritation. Some skin peeling is unavoidable.

TOPICAL TRETINOIN AND TAZAROTENE. Topical retinoids provide some reversal of photodamaged skin (Box 19-5). Objective improvements in wrinkling are seen after 3 to 6 months. Dyspigmentation (brown spots and mottled hyperpigmentation), surface roughness, and fine wrinkles respond best. The greatest response to therapy occurs during the initial 6 to 9 months.

Repeated applications of retinoids produce a skin reaction resembling irritation. This reaction is characterized by redness and desquamation, signs that correspond histologically to alterations in the stratum corneum and epidermal hyperplasia. Initially patients experience skin tightening and a pink glow. This smoothening occurs within 1 to 2 weeks of treatment. It is the first sign of improvement, and it occurs because the stratum corneum is thinner and more compact, and the epidermal layer is thicker and spongiotic. Increased proliferation of basal keratinocytes eventually doubles the epidermal thickness.

Collagen formation is reduced in photoaged skin and is partly responsible for wrinkle formation. Tretinoin and tazarotene increase collagen levels in photoaged skin; the end result is wrinkle effacement. Effacement of fine wrinkles occurs after 3 to 4 months of tretinoin therapy. The deepest, coarse facial wrinkles are still evident. Despite continued improvement in wrinkle effacement, the epidermal histology reverts to the pretherapy state.

Box 19-5 **Topical Tretinoin and Tazarotene—Effects of Treatment**

Fine wrinkling—improved
Coarse wrinkling—improved
Tactile roughness—improved
Lentigines—reduction in number
Freckles—reduction in color
Actinic keratoses—decrease in number
Telangiectasia—did not improve
Cutaneous reaction
Dermatitis—(1 to 10 weeks) xerosis, mild scaling, irritation
Increased pinkness, "rosy glow"
Inflammation—(3+ months) of presumed subclinical actinic keratoses

Hyperpigmented lesions are a predominant component of photoaging in Chinese and Japanese persons; tretinoin cream lightens the hyperpigmentation of photoaging in these patients. Tretinoin therapy for individuals with darker skin pigmentation is safe. Postinflammatory dyspigmentation at sites of retinoid dermatitis does not occur in black and Asian patients.

RETINOID APPLICATION PROCEDURES. The response to retinoids may be dose dependent; higher concentrations in one study were more effective. Many patients experience a "retinoid dermatitis" with erythema and peeling. To achieve maximum clinical improvement of photoaged skin, it is not necessary to push retinoid use to the point that brisk retinoid dermatitis develops. A 48-week regimen of once-daily treatment with medication, followed by treatment 3 times weekly for an additional 24 weeks, maintains and, in some cases, even enhances the improvements in photoaged skin. Treatment on a once-a-week basis with retinoids is less effective in sustaining the clinical improvement achieved by the initial treatment regimen of tretinoin on a once-daily basis. Some reversal of the beneficial effects of tretinoin treatment is observed after discontinuation of therapy for 24 weeks, which indicates the need to continue tretinoin therapy to maintain clinical improvement.

Begin with nighttime application. Start treatment with cream-based tretinoin (0.025%), emollient-based tretinoin (Renova 0.05% or 0.02%), or cream-based tazarotene (AVAGE 0.1%). A gradual introduction to treatment using every-other-day application is appropriate for patients with sensitive skin (usually type I; Table 19-1), followed by more frequent applications when patients accommodate. Apply moisturizing cosmetics or lubricating lotions if dryness occurs. Maximum response occurs after 8 to 12 months of treatment; thereafter application frequency should be reduced to 3 or 4 times a week to maintain improvement.

SUN PROTECTION DURING USE. Encourage the daily use of sunscreens. Increased "photosensitivity" during tretinoin use is not an accelerated sunburn response. No increased risk of photocarcinogenesis has been detected in humans.

TRETINOIN USE AND PREGNANCY. The data on routine clinical use of topical tretinoin indicate that there is no increased risk for pregnant women. However, spontaneous malformation of the fetus occasionally occurs in "normal" pregnancies. It may therefore be prudent to postpone tretinoin therapy for patients who are actively trying to conceive, to avoid wrongful blame for congenital defects that may occur by chance.

ESTROGEN REPLACEMENT. Statistically significant reductions in dry skin and skin wrinkling occur with estrogen replacement.

Table 19-1 Skin Types and Suggested Sunscreen Protection Factors

Type*	Characteristic†	Examples	SUGGESTED SPF	
			Routine day	Outdoor activity (waterproof)
I	Always burns easily, never tans	Celtic or Irish extraction; often blue eyes, red hair, freckles	15	25-30
II	Burns easily, tans slightly	Fair-skinned individuals; often have blond hair; many whites	12-15	25-30
III	Sometimes burns, then tans gradually and moderately	Mediterraneans and some Hispanics	8-10	15
IV	Burns minimally, always tans well	Darker Hispanics and Asians	6-8	15
V	Burns rarely, tans deeply	Middle Easterners, Asians, some blacks	6-8	15
VI	Almost never burns, deeply pigmented	Some blacks	6-8	15

Adapted from *Dermatol Clin* 24(1):9-17, 2006. *PMID: 16311163*

*Reflects color of unexposed buttock skin. Skin types I to III are white, type IV is white or faintly brown, type V is brown, and those with skin type VI have dark brown or black buttock skin.

†Based on first 30 to 45 minutes of sun exposure after winter season or no sun exposure.

SUNTAN AND SUNBURN

Light-induced skin changes depend on the intensity and duration of exposure and genetic factors.

SUNTAN. A tan protects the body from photoinjury, but UV-induced injury must occur to produce a tan. Therefore intentional suntanning is unwise. Repeated brief exposures sufficient to induce tanning add to long-term damage. In general for a given individual, the deeper the tan, the more skin damage is sustained in achieving the tan.

Tanning follows moderate and intense sun exposure and occurs in two stages. The first stage, immediate pigment darkening (IPD), is caused primarily by UVA. The skin becomes brown while exposed but fades rapidly after exposure. IPD is caused by a photochemical change in existing melanin, not by an increase in melanin. A lasting tan requires the synthesis of new melanin; a more lasting tan becomes visible within 72 hours.

TANNING PARLORS. Evidence shows that tans of comparable degrees acquired from different UV sources are similar in the amount of photodamage and skin cancer risk that accompany a tan. Large amounts of radiation are delivered in a short time in commercial tanning parlors. This accelerates photoaging and increases the risk of skin cancer.

SUNBURN. Forty-three percent of white U.S. children experienced one or more sunburns during the year. The sunburn reaction occurs in stages. With sufficient exposure, erythema appears within minutes (immediate erythema), fades, and then reappears and persists for days (delayed erythema). Vascular permeability of varying degrees results in edema and blisters. Desquamation occurs within a week. Systemic and topical corticosteroids have little or no clinically important effect on the sunburn reaction. Systemic and topical nonsteroidal antiinflammatory drugs, when used at dosages to achieve optimal serum levels for antiinflammatory effect, only result in an early and mild reduction of UVB-induced erythema. Sunburn is best treated with cool, wet compresses. Topical anesthetic preparations that contain lidocaine provide some relief. Benzocaine, incorporated into some sunburn preparations, is a sensitizer and should be avoided. Protection with sunscreens can, if used properly, prevent burning in even fair-skinned individuals.

SUN PROTECTION

UV-induced damage to collagen and elastic fibers and a number of skin cancers can be greatly reduced by high *sun protection factor* (SPF; see later) sunscreens and other methods to reduce sun exposure (Box 19-6). Sun protection may allow for repair of damaged skin. New collagen and elastin may form, and precancerous changes may regress.

Box 19-6 **Protection Against UV Damage**

Use a sunscreen SPF of at least 15 to 30 daily.
Apply sunscreen 15 to 30 minutes before going outdoors.
Reapply sunscreen every 2 hours or after exposure to water.
Avoid peak sunlight hours (10 AM to 3 PM).
Wear dark, loose, dry clothing with a tight weave, wide-brim hat, long-sleeved shirt, pants.

Substantial lifetime sun exposure occurs with brief incidental exposures such as working outdoors, participating in recreational activities, and walking outside for lunch; therefore many people need daily protection.

METHODS OF SUN PROTECTION. Natural protection is provided by the stratum corneum and the skin pigment, melanin. People vary widely in their natural ability to tan or burn. A sun-reactive skin typing system has been devised to classify individuals as to their ability to tan or burn. These categories (see Table 19-1) are useful guides for devising programs for sun protection.

Recommendations for minimizing sun exposure are listed (see Box 19-6). Sunburns are particularly harmful, and great emphasis should be placed on preventing burns. Patients frequently relate that permanent freckling occurred on the upper back after one severe burn. People who take short winter vacations in the South are particularly apt to burn. Total sun exposure during a lifetime is greatest on the face, back of the neck, bald head, upper chest, forearms, backs of the hands, and exposed lower legs. The effects of sunlight can readily be appreciated by comparing the lateral (sun-exposed) surfaces with the medial (sun-protected) surfaces of the forearms of older individuals.

Table 19-2 Food and Drug Administration–Approved Sunscreen Ingredients in the United States for 1997

Chemical	Approved (%)
UVA absorbers	
Oxybenzone	2-6
Sulisobenzone	5-10
Dioxybenzone	3
Methyl anthranilate	3.5-5
Avobenzone	2-3
Terephtalylidenedicamphorsulfonic acid	—
Bis(ethylhexyl)oxyphenol methoxyphenyl triazene	—
UVB absorbers	
PABA	1-5
p-Amyldimethyl-PABA (padimate A)	1-3
2-Ethoxyethyl *p*-methoxycinnamate	8-10
Digalloyl trioleate	2-5
Ethyl 4-bis(hydroxypropyl)aminobenzoate	1-5
2-Ethylhexyl 2-cyano-3,3-diphenylacrylate	7-10
2-Ethylhexyl *p*-methoxycinnamate	2-7.5
2-Ethylhexyl salicylate	3-5
Glyceryl-PABA	2-3
Homomenthyl salicylate	4-25
Dihydroxyacetone	0.25-3
Octyldimethyl-PABA (padimate O)	1.4-8
2-Phenylbenzimidazole-5-sulfonic acid	1.4
Triethanolamine salicylate	5-12
Physical blockers	—
Red petrolatum	30-100
Titanium dioxide	—
Sunscreen stabilizers	
Mexoryl SX (Europe)	
Tinosorb (Europe)	
Helioplex	—

CLOTHING. Clothing is the best protection. Weave tightness and fabric type determine the potential for photoprotection. Stretched or wet fabric is less effective. Darker colors provide greater protection than lighter colors. Some manufacturers market special clothing with SPF ratings, including Solumbra (Sun Precautions, Everett, Wash., www.solumbra.com). See the Formulary for a complete list of clothing manufacturers.

PROTECTING THE YOUNG. Significant sun exposure occurs during the early years of life when children spend hours playing outside. A study showed that regular use of a sunscreen with an SPF of 15 during the first 18 years of life reduces the lifetime incidence of basal and squamous cell carcinoma by 78%. All children should be protected with high-number SPF sunscreens. One-piece bathing suits that cover the trunk, upper arms, and legs are ideal for children.

SUNSCREENS. Sunscreens are topical agents that protect the skin from UV light. Guidelines for their application are listed in Box 19-6. Sunscreens should not be used as a means of allowing more time in the sun; this negates their beneficial effects.

Sunscreens are topical agents that absorb, scatter, or reflect ultraviolet radiation (UVR) and visible light. UVA agents absorb radiation in the spectral range of 320 to 400 nm. UVB agents absorb radiation in the range of 290 to 320 nm.

The FDA has issued the final monograph for sunscreen drug products for over-the-counter human use. This establishes conditions for safety, efficacy, and labeling. The regulations reduce the number of allowable sunscreen ingredients (Table 19-2). The monograph specifies an upper limit of SPF 30; any product with an SPF greater than 30 can be labeled only as SPF 30 plus.

The absorption spectra of some of these sunscreens are shown in Figure 19-11.

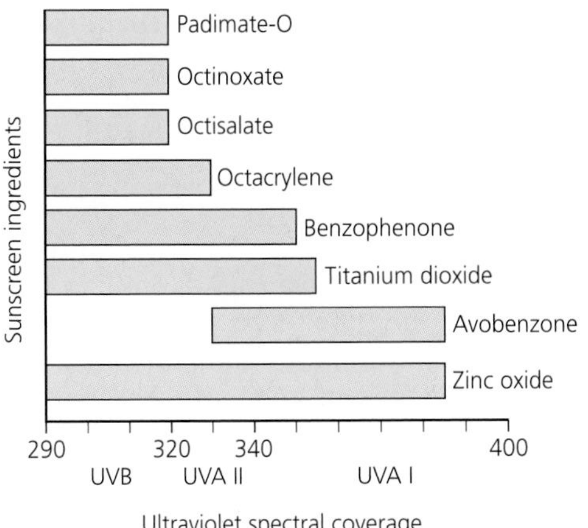

Figure 19-11 Absorption spectra of sunscreen components.

PHYSICAL SUNSCREENS. Physical sunscreens (referred to as inorganic or nonchemical sunscreens) are composed of particles that scatter and reflect light. Physical blocking agents, such as zinc oxide and titanium dioxide, are composed of particles of a size that scatter, reflect, or absorb solar radiation. Twenty percent zinc oxide, or 20% titanium dioxide reduces transmittance in the UVA and visible ranges to a maximum of approximately 20%. Newer micronized preparations that are suspensions are more cosmetically acceptable.

CHEMICAL SUNSCREENS. Chemical sunscreens absorb radiation. Newer broad-spectrum chemical sunscreens include a combination of chemicals that absorb both UVB and UVA radiation.

WATER-RESISTANT SUNSCREENS. Substantivity is the characteristic of a sunscreen that reflects how effectively the advertised degree of protection is maintained under adverse conditions, including repeated water exposure or sweating. According to the FDA, a sunscreen is declared water-resistant if it can maintain its original SPF after two 20-minute immersions. A sunscreen is very water-resistant if it retains its protective integrity after four 20-minute immersions.

SUN PROTECTION FACTOR. The effectiveness of sunscreens is expressed as the SPF. The SPF is defined as the ratio of the least amount of UVB energy (minimum erythema dose) required to produce a minimum erythema reaction through a sunscreen product film to the amount of energy required to produce the same erythema without any sunscreen application. For an individual who wears a sunscreen with an SPF of 15, 15 times longer than usual is required to develop erythema. The SPF for commercially available products is derived from tests with application of a uniform amount of sunscreen that is thicker than most individuals routinely use. A substantial amount of sunscreen must be applied to obtain a full SPF rating.

CHOICE OF SUNSCREEN STRENGTH. A sunscreen with an SPF of 15 or greater is recommended under most conditions. Sun protection does not increase proportionally with the designated SPF. In the higher range of SPFs, the differences become less meaningful. An SPF of 15 indicates 93% protection; an SPF of 34 indicates 97% protection. Newer sunscreens contain Mexoryl or Helioplex. Avobenzone is one of the best UVA absorbers, while oxybenzone is a very good UVB absorber with some UVA absorbency. Together with the Helioplex or Mexoryl SX stabilizing technology, these two sunscreen ingredients complement each other for high, broad-spectrum, and photostable coverage.

FREQUENCY OF USE. The majority of lifetime sun exposure occurs during multiple brief exposures that are not intended to produce tanning; therefore daily sun protection should be encouraged. People who sunburn easily or those who have light complexions or sun-sensitivity disorders should use a high SPF sunscreen every day, all year, particularly if they live in more equatorial latitudes. Sunscreens should be applied once in the morning and reapplied every 2 hours or after swimming and heavy exercise. Encourage people to have sunscreens available in the bathroom and to make morning application part of their daily ritual. Sunscreen may fail to prevent sunburn if it is washed off during swimming or if it is not applied to all exposed skin. The protection against sunburn afforded by a reapplication of sunscreen relative to a single application is significant. Compared with the first application, the second sunscreen application affords 3.1 times more protection against minimal UVR-induced erythema. The combined effect of two sunscreen applications gives 2.5 times better protection from UVR than does a single sunscreen application.

GLASS FILTERS. Glass filters out UVB but transmits UVA. Protective coatings applied to glass can block UVA radiation. Llumar window film (www.llumar.com) is a microthin film that is installed onto home and automobile glass surfaces to provide solar protection. It blocks 99% of the UV rays. Glass filters are indicated for patients with multiple skin cancers, transplant patients with skin cancers, and patients with photosensitive dermatoses.

ADVERSE REACTIONS TO SUNSCREENS. Allergic reactions occur more frequently to preservatives or fragrances than to the active ingredients. Irritation to creams is much more common than allergy to a component. Burning or stinging may be experienced in the eye area. Sunscreen active ingredients may cause photocontact allergic reactions. Most patients who develop photocontact dermatitis to sunscreens are patients with photodermatides.

VITAMIN D LEVELS. Sun protection is important to prevent skin malignancies. Vitamin D is formed in the skin through the action of the sun. Vitamin D deficiency may induce various types of cancer, bone diseases, autoimmune diseases, hypertension, and cardiovascular disease. Strict sun protection can cause vitamin D deficiency. Vitamin D status can be measured. Balanced recommendations on sun protection have to ensure an adequate vitamin D status. Twenty minutes of exposure each day to an area the size of the trunk may be reasonable until guidelines are established.

SUNLESS OR SELF-TANNING LOTIONS. Sunless or self-tanning lotions contain dihydroxyacetone (DHA), which darkens the skin by staining. The preparations are nontoxic. The site of action of DHA is the stratum corneum. Staining of skin occurs when DHA combines with free amino groups in skin proteins (keratin) in the stratum corneum to form brown products called melanoidins. Little to no sunscreen protection is provided by their use. Some products are formulated with standard sunscreens.

The newer preparations are cosmetically acceptable, as opposed to the orange color that was produced by older formulations.

POLYMORPHOUS LIGHT ERUPTION

Polymorphous light (PML) eruption is the most common light-induced skin disease seen by the practitioner. It is a long-standing, slowly ameliorating disease; the risk for lupus erythematosus is not increased. Not only does the clinical picture vary, but also symptoms may vary over the years. There are several morphologic subtypes, but individual patients tend to develop the same type each year. Lesions usually heal without scarring. The eruption appears first on limited areas but becomes more extensive during subsequent summers. Most people with PML eruption have exacerbations each summer for many years; a few have temporary remissions. The disease may begin at any age. The amount of light exposure needed to elicit an eruption varies greatly from one patient to another. Patients can tolerate a certain minimum exposure time, such as 30 minutes, after which the eruption appears. Light sensitivity decreases with repeated sun exposure; this phenomenon is referred to as hardening. The eruption may cease to appear after days or weeks of repeated sun exposure. Those exposed to sunlight all year rarely acquire PML eruption. Most patients have symptoms 2 hours after exposure. In a 7-year follow-up study, 57% of patients reported a decreased sun sensitivity, including 11% in whom the PML eruption totally cleared; none of the patients developed systemic lupus erythematosus. *PMID: 6610391*

HEREDITARY PML ERUPTION (ACTINIC PRURIGO). Hereditary PML eruption occurs in the Inuit of North America and in native Americans of North, Central, and South America. Its transmission appears to be autosomal dominant with incomplete penetrance and variable expressivity. In northern latitudes, the eruption appears on sun-exposed areas of the body as early as March and persists through October. The face is the most commonly involved area. The majority of patients are sensitive to UVA light. The younger ages of onset (up to 20 years of age) are associated with cheilitis and more acute eruptions and are more likely to improve over 5 years. Those who develop actinic prurigo as adults (21 years of age and older) tend to have a milder and more persistent dermatosis.

CLINICAL PRESENTATION. Women are affected more often than are men. The mean age at onset is 34 years (5 to 82 years). For men the mean age is 46 years and for women, 28 years. The most common initial symptoms are burning, itching, and erythema. The eruption usually lasts for 2 or 3 days, but in some cases it does not clear until the end of summer. Many patients experience malaise, chills, headache, and nausea starting approximately 4 hours after exposure but lasting only 1 or 2 hours. The most commonly involved areas are the V of the chest (the area exposed by open-necked shirts), the backs of the hands, extensor aspects of the forearms, and the lower legs of women. Reports vary as to the wavelength of light responsible for inducing lesions. The wavelength of light necessary to elicit the eruption varies with each patient. Many react to UVB, others to UVA, or some to both.

CLINICAL SUBTYPES. There are a number of clinical types of PML eruption.

Papular type. The papular type is the most common form (Figure 19-12). Small papules are disseminated or densely aggregated on a patchy erythema. A pinpoint papular variant has been described.

Plaque type. The plaque type is the second most common pattern. Plaques may be superficial or urticarial. They may coalesce to form larger plaques and at times are eczematous (Figures 19-13 and 19-14).

Papulovesicular type. The papulovesicular type is less common. It occurs primarily on the arms, lower limbs, and V area of the chest and usually begins with urticarial plaques from which groups of vesicles arise (Figure 19-15). Itching is common and is usually moderate or marked. This form occurs almost exclusively in women.

Eczematous type. Erythema, papules, scale, and sometimes vesicles occur. Eczematous lesions occur almost exclusively in men.

Erythema multiforme type. Erythema multiforme–type lesions and distribution are similar to those of classic erythema multiforme, with lesions most frequent on the backs of the hands and extensor forearms.

Hemorrhagic type. The hemorrhagic type may first appear as hemorrhagic papules or purpura. This form is rare.

Differential diagnosis. The papular form resembles atopic dermatitis. PML eruption is less pruritic and occurs in a sun-exposed distribution, not in crease areas, as does atopic dermatitis.

Systemic and discoid lupus erythematosus plaque–like lesions and histology may be identical to those of PML eruptions. The characteristic direct and indirect immunofluorescence patterns of lupus erythematosus clarify the diagnosis.

DIAGNOSIS. The histologic features are not diagnostic. Immunofluorescence is negative. Phototesting is not essential but, when performed, must include both UVB and UVA testing.

TREATMENT

Topical steroids, antimalarial agents, and beta-carotene are often disappointing. Prophylactic therapy with sunscreens is partially effective. In the case of minor complaints, patients can become disease free by using sunscreens and gradually increasing sun exposure in the spring. Phototherapy and photochemotherapy are most effective.

POLYMORPHOUS LIGHT ERUPTION

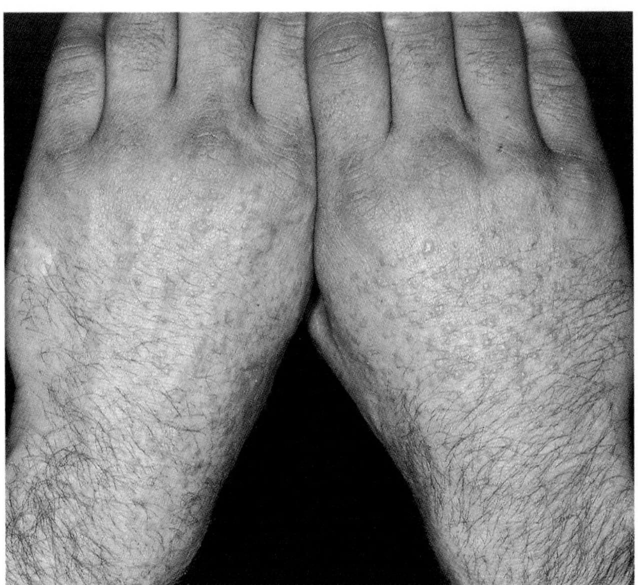

Figure 19-12 Papular type.

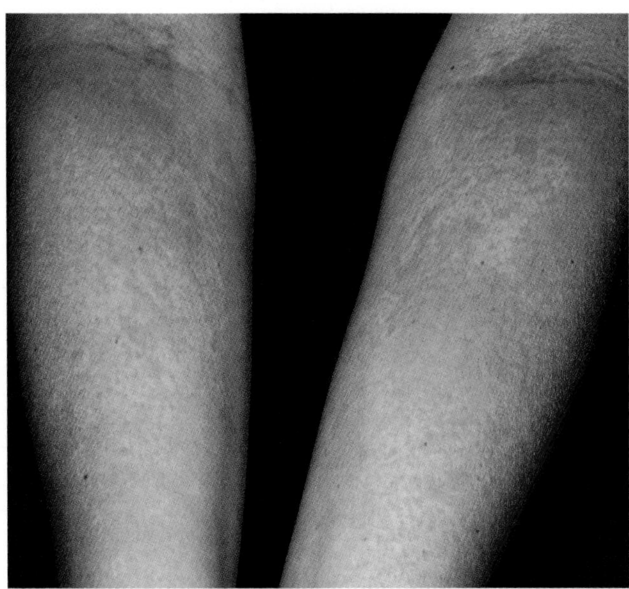

Figure 19-13 Plaque type.

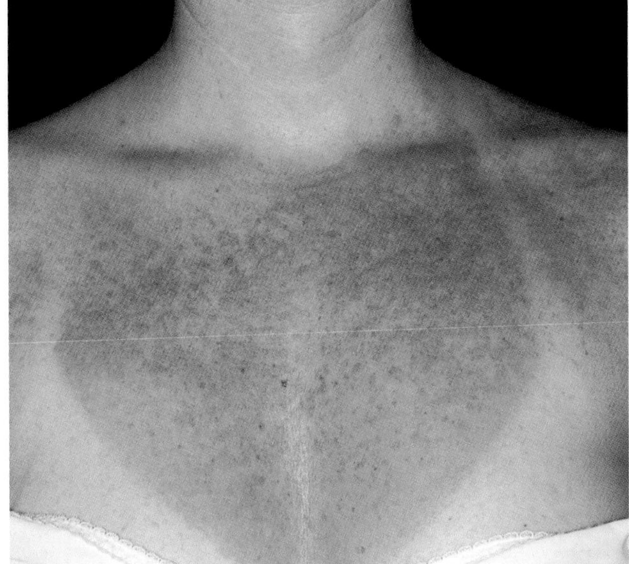

Figure 19-14 Plaque type.

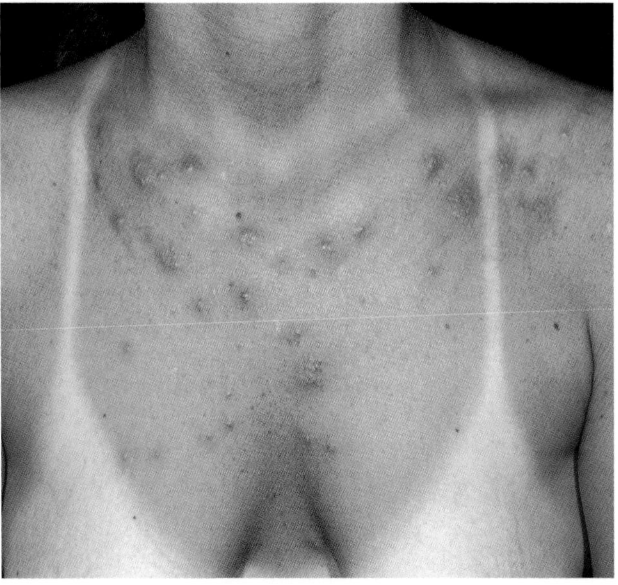

Figure 19-15 Papulovesicular type.

TOPICAL AND ORAL STEROIDS. Short, intermittent 3- to 14-day courses of groups I to V topical steroids are effective. Groups II through V topical steroids reduce pruritus and hasten resolution. Short courses of oral steroids are useful for very itchy, widespread eruptions or for patients who flare during a course of phototherapy or photochemotherapy.

PROTECTION. Sun exposure during times of maximum intensity (between 10 AM and 2 PM) should be avoided. Sunscreens with maximum sun-protecting factors should be used. The most sensitive patients are advised about filters for car windows (Llumar UV shield, www.llumar.com) and fluorescent lighting at home.

DESENSITIZATION WITH PHOTOTHERAPY. The sensitivity of human skin to UV radiation decreases after exposure to UV radiation. Adaptation occurs by exposing patients to small and controlled doses of light. Doses small enough not to cause any abnormal reaction but large enough to increase the tolerance of the skin to light are used. A regular series of such exposures, with small increments in exposure time, can result in an appreciable tolerance. Increments of 10% per exposure are given as long as there are no adverse reactions. This is the so-called phenomenon of hardening. This practice is safe; therefore controlled exposure to sunlight or artificial UV light sources should be the first type of treatment. Patients treated with UVB or narrow-band UVB in the dermatologist's office receive five exposures per week for 3 weeks in the spring, with gradually increasing exposure doses. Hardening may also be accomplished with either UVA (340 to 400 nm) or UVA and UVB (300 to 400 nm) (10 exposures to UV light). Commercial "sun beds" are not recommended because they are most likely to provoke the PML eruption rash. Prophylactic UVB may sometimes trigger the eruption, particularly in severely affected subjects, necessitating concurrent systemic corticosteroid therapy.

PSORALEN UVA (PUVA). Treatment can be acquired in the dermatologist's office using artificial UVA light and 8-methoxypsoralen (PUVA). A remission can be obtained for most patients by treatment two or three times each week for 4 to 12 weeks in the early spring. (See the section on treatment of psoriasis for details.) PUVA therapy protects temporarily, and repeated sun exposures are required to maintain protection. A number of patients remain protected for 2 to 3 months, even after pigmentation has faded. Topical steroids should be applied if the disease is activated by treatment. Maximum protection is reached 3 weeks after a 1-week course of treatment, and a single course offers a minimum of 6 weeks of protection. The course can be repeated each month during the spring and summer months if needed. Protective glasses such as NoIR should be worn for the remainder of the day after taking psoralens.

ANTIMALARIAL DRUGS. Antimalarial drugs may be effective and should be considered for patients who are not protected by sunscreens and do not respond to UVB or PUVA phototherapy. Antimalarials need to be used only during the summer months; therefore the total necessary dose is small. A 3-month trial (hydroxychloroquine 400 mg/day for the first month and 200 mg/day thereafter) has been effective in reducing rash and irritation. Although the risk of eye damage is slight, ophthalmologic examinations should be obtained periodically to monitor for antimalarial toxicity.

OTHER TREATMENTS. Beta-carotene is somewhat effective for prophylactic treatment of PML eruption, but the skin turns yellow-orange. Only 30% of patients responded satisfactorily to a dosage of 3 mg/kg body weight continued throughout the summer.

Cyclosporine or azathioprine may be used for rare severe disabling cases.

HYDROA AESTIVALE AND HYDROA VACCINIFORME

Hydroa aestivale (summer prurigo of Hutchinson) and hydroa vacciniforme are rare but very distinctive light-induced eruptions. They may represent a type of PML eruption that is peculiar to children. The onset is before puberty (average age at onset is about 6 years), and males are affected more frequently than females. It begins with moderate erythema and itching within 1 to 2 hours of sun exposure. The lesions of hydroa aestivale consist of papules with weeping and crusting. The symmetric photodistributed eruption is most prominent on the face, ears, and backs of the hands (Figure 19-16). Involvement of non–sun-exposed areas, especially the buttocks, is not uncommon. The rash fades but may persist through the winter months. There is evidence of genetic transmission. In many cases, UVB light reproduces the lesions.

Hydroa vacciniforme (HV) (Figures 19-17 and 19-18) is similar to hydroa aestivale, except that tense, umbilicated vesicles resembling smallpox appear on the face, ears, chest, and backs of the hands; after they break and form a crust, they may heal with scarring.

Broad-band UVB therapy may be effective for hydroa vacciniforme. UVA light may reproduce the eruption. Both diseases usually clear after puberty. Avoidance of the sun and use of sunscreens, group V topical steroids, and wet compresses and antimalarials can control these diseases. *PMID 1670249*

HYDROA AESTIVALE AND HYDROA VACCINIFORME

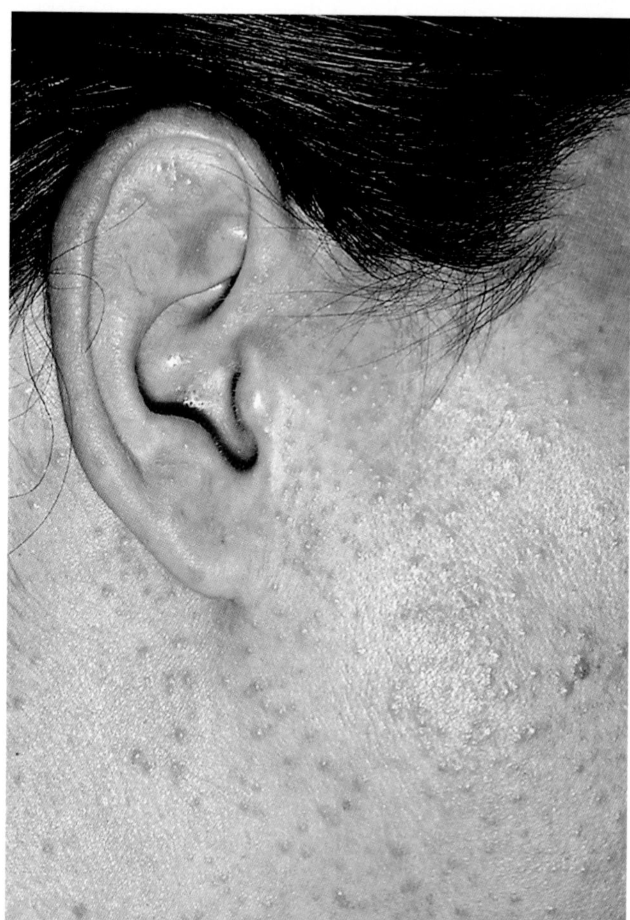

Figure 19-16 Hydroa aestivale. Papules appear on sun-exposed skin and may progress to weeping and crusting.

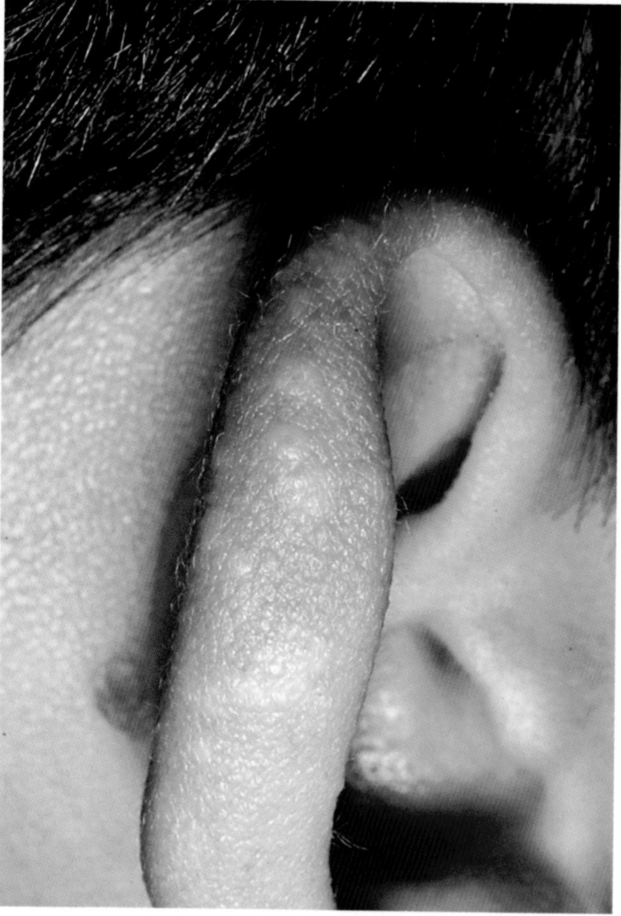

Figure 19-17 Hydroa vacciniforme. Papules and pustules appear on exposed areas of the face and ears. Lesions become umbilicated and sometimes necrotic. They may heal with hypopigmented depressed scars. Broadband UVB therapy may be effective for hydroa vacciniforme. UVA light may reproduce the eruption. Both diseases usually clear after puberty. Avoidance of the sun and use of sunscreens, group V topical steroids, and wet compresses and antimalarials can control these diseases. *PMID 1670249.*

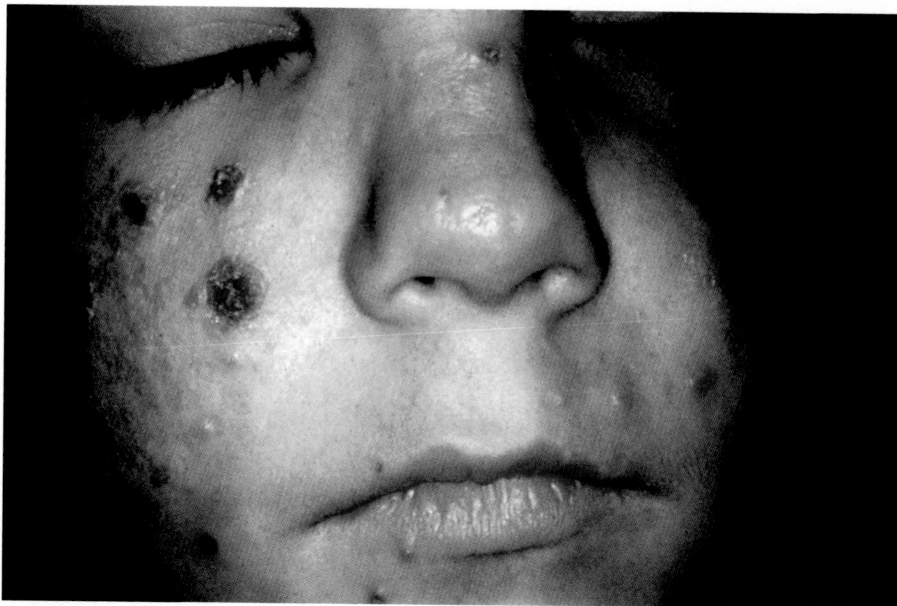

Figure 19-18 Hydroa vacciniforme. This childhood disease begins with the appearance of papules that progress to vesicles on sun-exposed skin of the cheeks. Lesions umbilicate, become necrotic, and heal with hypopigmented depressed (vacciniform or varioliform) scars.

PORPHYRIAS

The porphyrias are a group of diseases caused by inborn enzymatic defects in the heme biosynthetic pathway (Table 19-3). Each type of porphyria is associated with a specific enzymatic defect that results in an excess of a specific porphyrin (see Tables 19-4 and 19-5). The porphyrias are classified into two groups, erythropoietic and hepatic, on the basis of the principal site of the specific enzymatic defect. They are differentiated by measuring levels of heme precursors in urine, feces, erythrocytes, and plasma. Most forms are inherited as mendelian autosomal dominants (Figure 19-19).

Two main types of clinical manifestation occur: life-threatening attacks of acute porphyria and skin

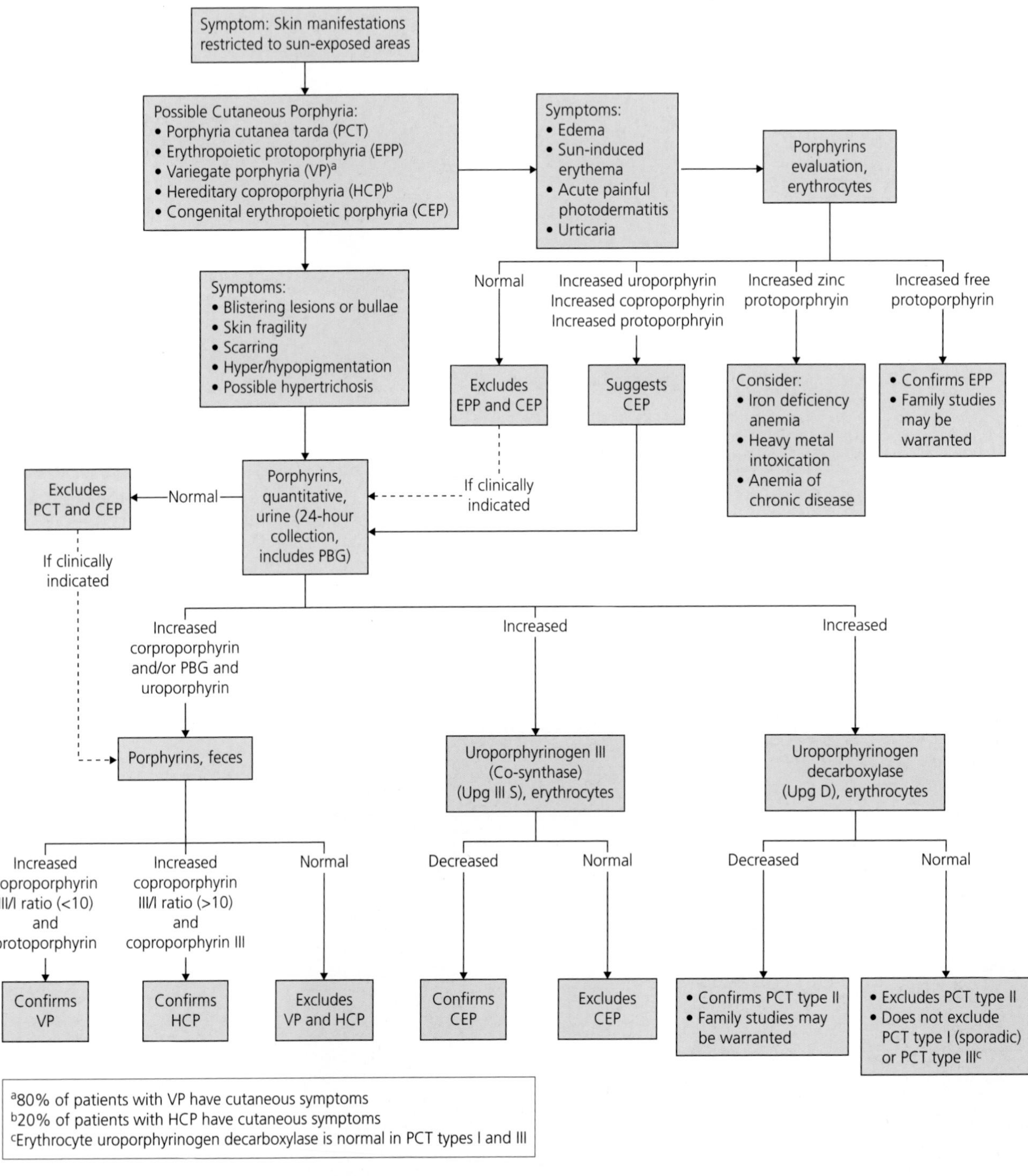

Figure 19-19 Laboratory evaluation of porphyria. (Courtesy Mayo Clinic Laboratories.)

Table 19-3 Porphyrias: Enzyme Defects and Inheritance

Condition	Mode of inheritance	Enzyme defect	Prominent site(s) of metabolic expression
Aminolevulinic acid dehydratase deficiency porphyria (ADP)	Autosomal recessive	Aminolevulinic acid dehydratase	Liver and probably erythroid cells
Acute intermittent porphyria (AIP)	Autosomal dominant	Porphobilinogen deaminase	Liver and probably erythroid cells
Congenital erythropoietic porphyria (CEP)	Autosomal recessive	Uroporphyrinogen III cosynthase	Erythroid cells
Porphyria cutanea tarda (PCT)	Autosomal dominant	Uroporphyrinogen decarboxylase	Liver and possibly erythroid cells
Hereditary coproporphyria (HCP)	Autosomal dominant	Coproporphyrinogen oxidase	Liver and possibly erythroid cells
Variegate porphyria (VP)	Autosomal dominant	Protoporphyrinogen oxidase	Liver and possibly erythroid cells
Erythropoietic porphyria (EPP)	Autosomal dominant	Ferrochelatase	Erythroid cells and probably hepatocytes
Acquired porphyria	Not inherited	Variable and often multiple	Liver and erythroid cells

From *Mayo Clinic Test Catalog,* 2008. www.mayomedicallaboratories.com

Table 19-4 Tests to Establish Diagnoses of Porphyrias and to Establish the Specific Type

Suspected porphyria	Recommended tests
Acute intermittent porphyria (AIP)	During acute episodes, analysis of urine Pbg, urine porphyrins, and urine δ-ALA. Erythrocyte Pbg deaminase (uroporphyrinogen I synthase) and erythrocyte δ-ALA dehydratase may be particularly useful in family studies.
Congenital erythropoietic porphyria (CEP)	Urine porphyrins, erythrocyte porphyrins with fractionation, fecal porphyrins, and uroporphyrinogen III cosynthase in RBCs.
Porphyria cutanea tarda (PCT)	Urine, fecal, and plasma porphyrins; uroporphyrinogen decarboxylase in RBCs.
Coproporphyria (CP)	Fecal porphyrins; urine Pbg, δ-ALA, and porphyrins; erythrocyte Pbg deaminase and δ-ALA dehydratase may be necessary to differentiate from AIP.
Variegate porphyria (VP)	Fecal porphyrins; urine Pbg, δ-ALA, and porphyrins; erythrocyte Pbg deaminase and δ-ALA dehydratase may be necessary to differentiate from AIP.
Erythropoietic porphyria	Erythrocyte porphyrins;* urine Pbg, δ-ALA, and porphyrins; fecal porphyrins; δ-ALA dehydratase, Pbg deaminase, and/or uroporphyrinogen decarboxylase in RBCs may be necessary.

From *Mayo Clinic Test Catalog,* 2008. www.mayomedicallaboratories.com
δ-ALA, Delta-aminolevulinic acid; *Pbg,* porphobilinogen.
*In some cases, the quantitation of erythrocyte zinc protoporphyrin should be included to distinguish acquired porphyria from protoporphyria.

Table 19-5 The Porphyrias: Clinical Characteristics

Type	Prevalence among porphyric persons	Dermopathy	Neuropathy	Other indicators
Acute intermittent porphyria (AIP) RBC Pbg deaminase deficiency	Among most prevalent	None	Mild to severe	Intermittent fever, hypertension
Congenital erythropoietic porphyria (CEP)	Very rare	Very severe, mutilating; evidence in infancy	Possibly	Pink, red, or violet urine staining diapers
Porphyria cutanea tarda (PCT)	Among most prevalent	Mild to severe	Not usually	Siderosis
Coproporphyria (CP)	Among most prevalent	20%-30% of cases; mild to severe	Mild to severe	Intermittent fever, hypertension
Variegate porphyria (VP)	Among most prevalent	Present in 75%-80% of all cases	Mild to severe	Intermittent fever, hypertension
Protoporphyria (PP)	Quite rare	Mild severe	Not usually	Abnormal liver function tests; gallstones
Acquired porphyria	Among most prevalent	In some cases, not in others	Usually	Variable; intermittent fever, hypertension

From *Mayo Clinic Test Catalog,* 2009. www.mayomedicallaboratories.com

photosensitization. Attacks of the acute porphyrias (acute intermittent porphyria, variegate porphyria, and hereditary coproporphyria) are important because they may be life-threatening. The nonacute porphyrias (porphyria cutanea tarda and erythropoietic porphyria) present as skin photosensitization.

The skin lesions in porphyria cutanea tarda (the most common cutaneous porphyria), variegate porphyria, hereditary coproporphyria, and congenital erythropoietic porphyria are similar: mechanical fragility, subepidermal bullae, hypertrichosis, and pigmentation. Erythropoietic protoporphyria (EPP) is characterized by acute photosensitivity without these lesions.

All types show excess porphyrin metabolites in blood, urine, or feces and in various tissues such as skin and liver. Porphyrins are red-brown pigments. Certain porphyrin metabolites (porphyrinogens) accumulate in the skin and are auto-oxidized to become porphyrins. Porphyrins absorb UVA light in the 400- to 410-nm range (Soret band). These excited porphyrins generate peroxides that cause the blisters seen in porphyria cutanea tarda and variegate porphyria.

The porphyrias are potentially lethal. They manifest primarily with neurologic and skin signs and symptoms. Congenital erythropoietic porphyria (CEP) presents in infancy. The other porphyrias become symptomatic in adults.

Porphyria cutanea tarda

Porphyria cutanea tarda (PCT) is the most common type of porphyria. PCT results from a deficiency of hepatic uroporphyrinogen decarboxylase activity. Both acquired and familial forms exist and are commonly associated in adults with liver disease and hepatic iron overload. The acquired ("sporadic") form is most often precipitated by alcohol. Estrogens, oral contraceptives, certain environmental pollutants, and iron overloading may precipitate PCT (Table 19-6). There is also a dominantly inherited form. Most people who consume alcohol or take estrogens do not develop porphyria; therefore it is likely that genetic factors are important in the pathogenesis of nonfamilial cases. This genetic predisposition may explain why some patients on chronic hemodialysis develop PCT. Some of these patients with chronic renal failure have highly increased uroporphyrin concentrations. Photosensitivity results from activation of porphyrins in the skin by long-wave UV light and generation of reactive oxygen species.

HEPATITIS C AND PCT. There is a strong association between hepatitis C virus (HCV) infection and PCT. PCT has also been associated with mutations in the hemochromatosis gene (*HFE*) that are associated with HLA-linked hereditary hemochromatosis. The prevalence of HCV infection (56%) and mutations in *HFE* (73%) are high among North American patients with PCT. Of 39 PCT patients with HCV, 32 were men, all of whom used alcohol. In contrast, 22 of 31 PCT patients without HCV infection were women, 12 of whom had taken estrogens. The HCV-positive group was more likely to have used illicit intravenous drugs and to have had several (more than four) sex partners. All PCT patients should be tested for HCV infection and for HFE mutations. Although HCV infection is a trigger for PCT, preclinical PCT is rare in chronic HCV infection in the United States. *PMID: 9620340*

CLINICAL MANIFESTATIONS. The clinical features in order of frequency are blistering in sun-exposed areas (Figures 19-20 and 19-21), increased skin fragility, facial hypertrichosis, hyperpigmentation, sclerodermoid changes, dystrophic calcification with ulceration, and localized sclerosis of the scalp (alopecia porphyrinica). The milia occur in previously blistered sites on the hand. The classic form of epidermolysis bullosa acquisita has similar features (see Chapter 16).

DIAGNOSIS. The patient's urine may have a red-brown discoloration ("port-wine urine") from high levels of porphyrin pigments, and it may show a bright pink fluorescence under a Wood's light (Wood's light is a blue light with an emission peak of 360 nm). PCT may be confused with other forms of porphyria and other bullous diseases. Assays of

Table 19-6 Prevalence of Established and Suspected Susceptibility Factors in PCT*

Susceptibility factors	Prevalence
Inherited	
Uroporphyrinogen decarboxylase mutations (UROD)	19% (based on erythrocyte UROD activity)
Hemochromatosis gene mutations (*HFE* mutations)	65% (9% CYP282Y/CYP282Y)
CYP1A2 polymorphism	72%
Exposures	
Alcohol	38%-79%
Smoking	86%
Estrogens	55%-73% of females
Infections	
Hepatitis C (male)	29%-74% (all in nonhereditary group)
HIV	15%
Metabolic and nutritional	
Excess iron	>95% (stainable iron in hepatocytes)
Diabetes	17%
Ascorbic acid deficiency	62%

From *Hepatology* 45(1):6-8, 2007; and *Acta Dermatol Venereol* 85(4):337-344, 2005. *PMID: 17187403; PMID: 16191856*
*Multiple factors were assessed in the same patients.

PORPHYRIA CUTANEA TARDA

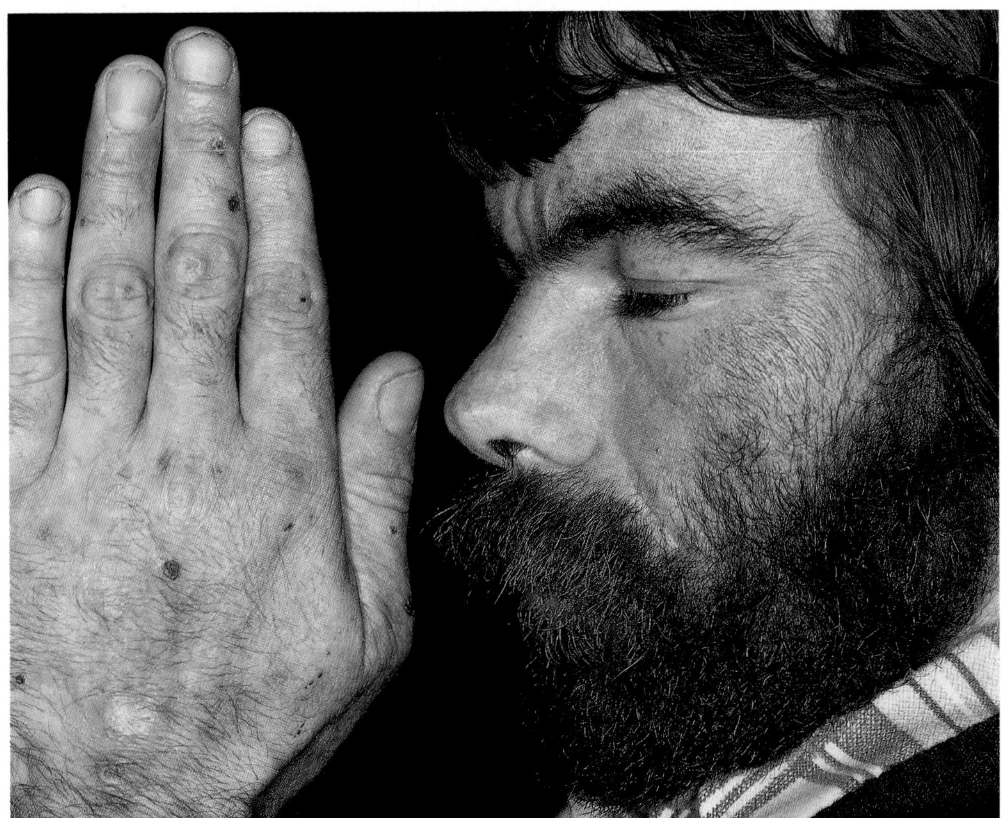

Figure 19-20 There is increased facial hair around the eyes. Chronic sun exposure has resulted in blistering, erosions, and atrophic scars on the backs of the hands.

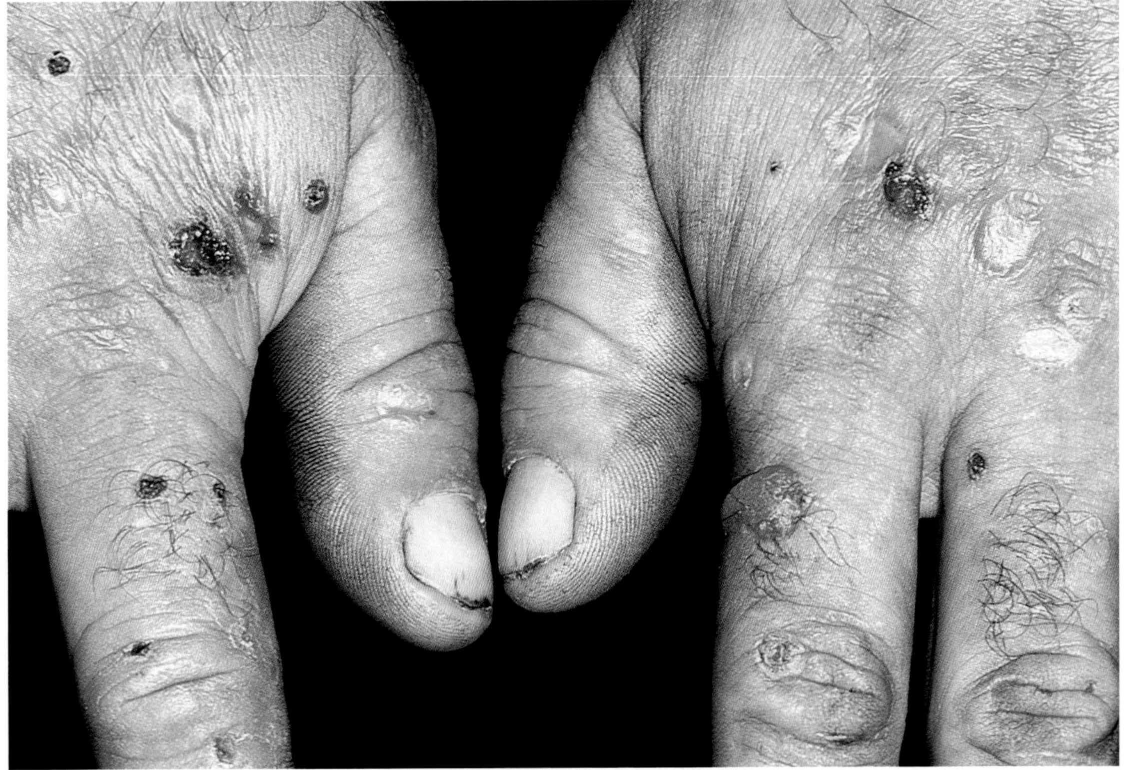

Figure 19-21 Fragile sun-exposed skin develops erosions and bullae after mechanical trauma. This is most commonly seen on the dorsal aspects of the hands and forearms. Healing results in scars, milia, and hyperpigmented and hypopigmented atrophic patches.

fecal, plasma, urinary, and red blood cell porphyrins should be ordered, especially if other forms of porphyria are in the differential diagnosis. The diagnosis is confirmed by demonstrating an elevated urine uroporphyrin level. A 24-hour collection of urine contains different amounts of the various porphyrins in ratios that can be diagnostic. The proportion reported as uroporphyrin dominates the urinary assay in PCT, usually being present in a ratio of 4:1 or more to the coproporphyrin proportion. Quantitative assays of the various porphyrins must be performed to obtain a reliable diagnosis. Biopsy specimens for direct immunofluorescence are taken from the edge of lesions.

HEREDITARY HEMOCHROMATOSIS. PCT can be seen in patients with mutations of the *HFE* gene. *HFE* gene analysis should be done in patients who present with PCT. Polymerase chain reaction analysis of peripheral blood for hemochromatosis gene (*HFE*) mutations is available for clinical use.

TREATMENT

The basis of treatment of PCT consists of three elements: avoidance of triggering factors (alcohol, estrogens), iron depletion (phlebotomy), and porphyrin elimination (low-dose chloroquine therapy). It is important to identify all risks or etiologic factors that contribute to the development of PCT.

PHLEBOTOMY. Iron overload is one of the factors that trigger the disease; iron removal by phlebotomy is the treatment of choice. It reduces hepatic iron stores and produces remissions of several years' duration. One unit of blood should be removed every 2 to 4 weeks until the hemoglobin level drops to 10 gm/dl or until the serum iron level drops to 50 mg/dl. The average number of units required for remission varies between 8 and 14. Measurement of plasma uroporphyrin level is an effective way to monitor the progress of patients with PCT. Treatment should continue until plasma uroporphyrin levels drop under 10 mmol/L. Plasma ferritin levels can also be used as a guide to treatment by venisection. Phlebotomy can be terminated when iron stores, as reflected by plasma ferritin concentration, have fallen to low-normal limits.

CHLOROQUINE. Chloroquine in very low dosages may also be used. Chloroquine causes the release of hepatic tissue-bound uroporphyrin, and subsequently it is rapidly eliminated by the plasma and excreted by the urine. A release of porphyrins that is too rapid might severely affect liver function. Complete clinical and biochemical response has occurred with the use of chloroquine 125 to 250 mg twice weekly for 8 to 18 months. Remission in most patients has been for more than 4 years.

Combined treatment with repeated phlebotomy and chloroquine results in remission in an average of 3.5 months. The time necessary for remission with chloroquine alone is 10.2 months; the time for remission with phlebotomy alone is 12.5 months.

Complete elimination of alcohol and exposure to other hepatotoxins resulted in complete clinical clearing of bullae and skin fragility in 2 months to 2 years.

Sunscreens that block UVA light should be used. Physical sunblockers that contain titanium dioxide are moderately effective. A nutritionally adequate intake of ascorbic acid may be beneficial.

In patients with chronic hemodialysis-associated PCT, chloroquine is ineffective. Erythropoietin, desferrioxamine, and small-volume phlebotomy have been employed to control the disease.

Pseudoporphyria

Pseudoporphyria is a therapy-induced bullous photosensitivity disorder. It is a condition that mimics PCT in almost every aspect, except that porphyrin levels in the urine, plasma, and stools are normal. It has been attributed to drugs, UVA irradiation (tanning beds), excessive sun exposure, and chronic renal failure/dialysis.

CLINICAL MANIFESTATIONS. There is increased skin fragility, easy bruising, and light-provoked bullae on the dorsum of the hand followed by healing with scarring and milia (Figure 19-22). The onset of bullae may occur 1 week after the drug has been initiated or may not occur for months. An important clue to the diagnosis is that few patients with pseudoporphyria have hypertrichosis, hyperpigmentation, or the sclerodermoid changes found in PCT.

DRUGS. Naproxen, a propionic acid derivative, is the nonsteroidal antiinflammatory drug (NSAID) most frequently linked to pseudoporphyria. Most cases of naproxen-induced pseudoporphyria occur in children. Pseudoporphyria was reported in up to 12% of patients with juvenile rheumatoid arthritis who were treated with naproxen. Naproxen-induced pseudoporphyria in adults occurs primarily in women. Patients who require NSAIDs and develop pseudoporphyria should be switched to agents that are less photosensitizing, such as diclofenac, indomethacin, and sulindac. Other drugs, including tetracyclines, furosemide, nalidixic acid, dapsone, oxaprozin, voriconazole, and nabumetone, are implicated.

TANNING BEDS. Most patients are young women with fair skin. Vesicles and bullae occur on the dorsal hands, but other areas may be involved. Skin fragility, scarring, and milia occur. Some patients had been taking medications (NSAIDs, furosemide, tetracycline, oral contraceptives).

CHRONIC RENAL FAILURE/DIALYSIS. Pseudoporphyria has been reported in patients undergoing hemodialysis or peritoneal dialysis and in cases of chronic renal failure without accompanying dialysis. Hemodialysis-related pseudoporphyria has been successfully treated with *N*-acetylcysteine.

LABORATORY FINDINGS. The histologic (subepidermal bullae with no inflammation, thickened dermal capillary walls with deposition of periodic acid/Schiff-positive material) and immunofluorescent (granular deposits of IgG and C3 at the dermoepidermal junction and in the upper dermal vasculature) findings are identical to those found in PCT. Porphyrin levels in the urine, plasma, and stools are normal. Because of difficulties in interpreting urinary testing in the setting of dialysis, levels of plasma porphyrins and fecal porphyrins should also be assayed in the evaluation of patients with chronic renal failure who have bullous dermatoses.

TREATMENT. Stopping the drug is curative in most cases, but remission may not occur for months.

ACUTE INTERMITTENT PORPHYRIA (AIP), COPROPORPHYRIA (CP), AND VARIEGATE PORPHYRIA (VP). These types are the most common forms of porphyria (see Tables 19-3, 19-4, and 19-5). They present with acute episodes of mild-to-severe abdominal pain and depression or psychosis. Less common findings are hypertension, paresthesias, fever, and seizures. Episodes of neuromuscular weakness can progress to whole-body paralysis and life-threatening respiratory paralysis. Acute attacks of AIP, hereditary coproporphyria, and VP can be provoked by medications (barbiturates, antibacterials) and alcohol. Household or industrial chemicals, agricultural pesticides, industrial chemical wastes, garden chemicals, chemicals used in hobby crafts (such as mineral pigments used in ceramics work), and chemicals found in degreasing solvents used in automotive and other mechanical repair work may precipitate an acute attack.

SKIN SIGNS. Up to 30% of CP cases and most cases of VP have increased skin fragility and photosensitivity with erythema, urticaria, blistering, and vesicular lesions. Hypertrichosis and regional alopecia may also occur. AIP does not involve the skin.

LABORATORY STUDIES. Initial screening for suspected cases of AIP should include a 24-hour urine collection for measurement of levels of porphobilinogen and urine porphyrins (see Table 19-4 and Figure 19-19). Urinary delta-aminolevulinic acid (d-ALA) analysis may be helpful. CP and VP can be detected by analysis of levels of fecal porphyrins: coproporphyrin excretion is increased in CP, and excretion of both fecal coproporphyrins and protoporphyrins is increased in VP. During acute episodes, levels of urinary porphobilinogen and porphyrins will be increased.

Acquired porphyria (intoxication porphyria). Accumulation of porphyrins and porphyrin precursors in blood and tissue can be caused by toxic substances such as the ingestion of lead. Heavy metals, halogenated aromatic hydrocarbons, and drugs can suppress enzymes involved in porphyrinogen metabolism, leading to the accumulation of intermediates. Intoxication porphyria can mimic porphyria cutanea tarda in both clinical signs and laboratory findings.

Figure 19-22 Pseudoporphyria. Light-provoked bullae on the back of the hands, followed by healing with scarring, are precipitated by certain drugs such as naproxen.

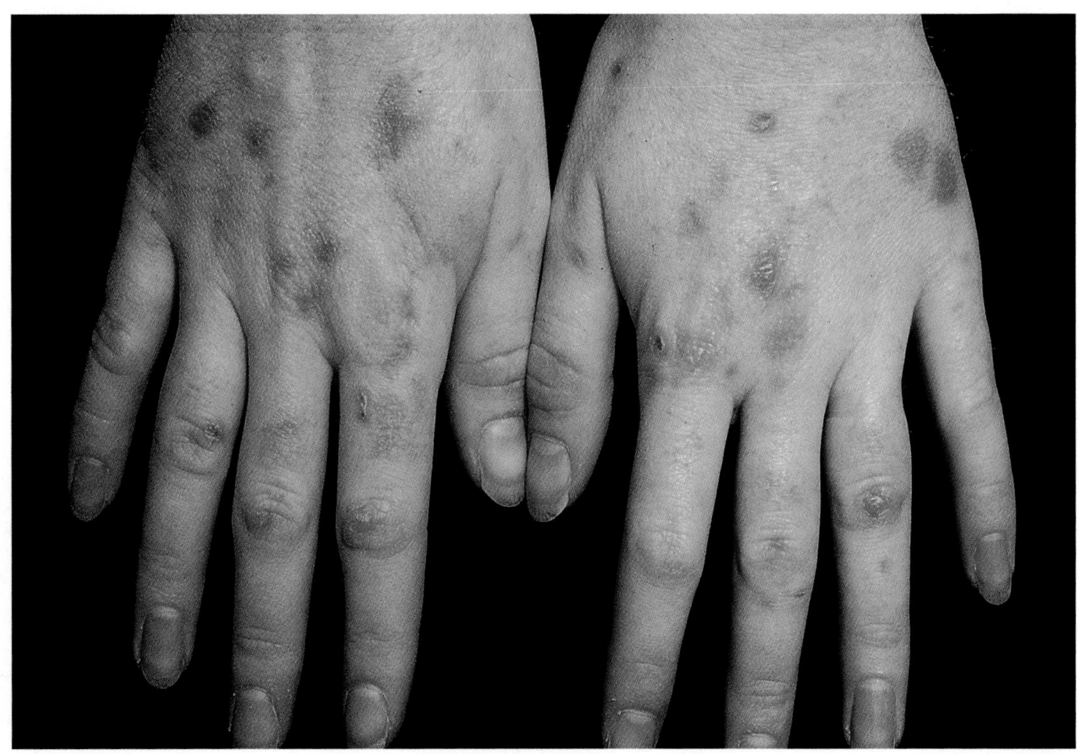

Erythropoietic protoporphyria

Erythropoietic protoporphyria (EPP) differs clinically from PCT. This disease begins in childhood. There are few or no blisters; rather, children complain of burning and redness when exposed to sun or UV light. There are no porphyrins in the urine. EPP is an autosomal dominant hereditary disorder with irregular penetrance. It is characterized by a deficiency of ferrochelatase, the terminal enzyme in the heme biosynthetic pathway that catalyzes the insertion of ferrous iron into protoporphyrin to form heme. The enzyme deficiency causes the accumulation of the photoreactive molecule protoporphyrin in various tissues. Protoporphyrin overproduction occurs mainly in erythroid tissue. Circulating erythrocytes leak protoporphyrin, which accumulates in skin cells. The release of protoporphyrin from erythrocytes is greatly increased if the erythrocytes are exposed to small amounts of light. The cutaneous symptoms are elicited by protoporphyrin-sensitized photodamage of endothelial cells.

CLINICAL MANIFESTATIONS. The disease is often suspected in infancy or childhood when patients cry or complain of burning of the skin on the face and hands within minutes of sun exposure. Exposure through window glass also elicits symptoms. Hours later, diffuse swelling or erythema appears, and burning persists (Figure 19-23). Purpura may occur, but vesiculation is uncommon. Often, acute changes are not seen. The period of sun exposure required to elicit burning varies from day to day. Several hours of exposure may be tolerated. A "priming phenomenon" has been reported. A certain duration of exposure "primes" the skin so that a short period of additional sun exposure in the same area, even the next day, produces symptoms. It may then take several days after symptoms have developed to regain the usual degree of tolerance. Patients may present with a waxy, cobblestone-like induration of the involved skin. When this change occurs over the knuckles and fingers, the hands look old ("old knuckles"). This is a pathognomonic change in children. Depressed scars form on the nose, cheeks, and dorsum of the hands. Large second-degree phototoxic burns of the abdominal wall have occurred after prolonged exposure to light during surgery.

Most treated patients function well and have a normal life span. Protoporphyrins may accumulate in hepatocytes and cause liver disease.

LIVER DISEASE. Excess protoporphyrin affects hepatobiliary structures, and a spectrum of changes, which range from ultrastructural bile canalicular damage to cirrhosis or acute hepatic failure, may occur. The course is unpredictable. Patients may be stable for several years after evidence of liver function abnormalities. Then, within weeks, hepatic failure may develop, requiring urgent orthotopic liver transplantation. Gallstones may occur in young children.

LABORATORY. Erythrocyte and plasma protoporphyrin and fecal protoporphyrin levels are elevated (see Table 19-4). Fluorescence microscopy is a highly reliable screening test for the detection of increased levels of red cell porphyrins. The urine is normal. Levels of red blood cell protoporphyrins are also increased in iron deficiency anemia and lead poisoning, but photosensitivity is absent. Liver biopsy may show periportal fibrosis.

TREATMENT. Oral beta-carotene (Solatene 30 mg) is helpful in treating the skin photosensitivity.

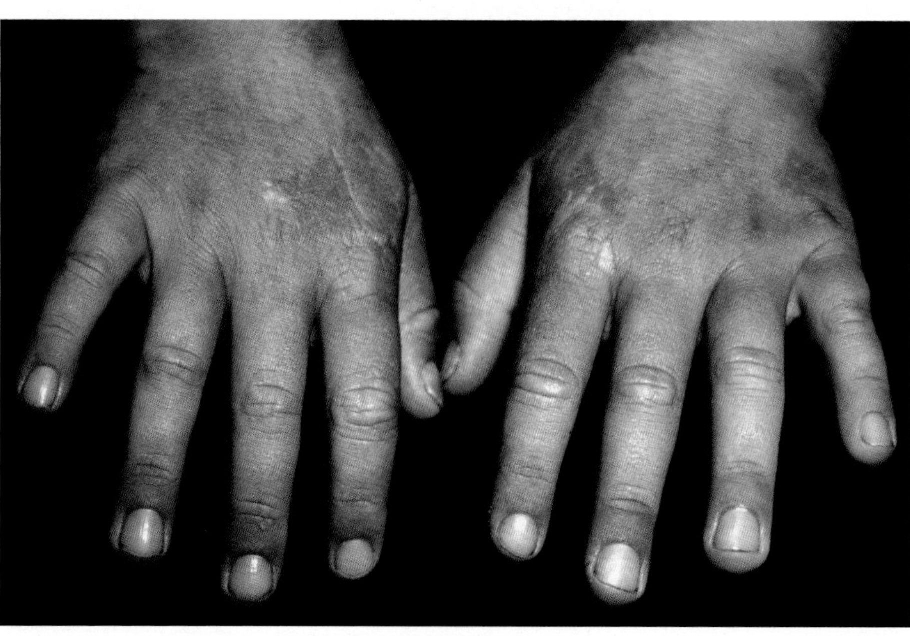

Figure 19-23 Erythropoietic protoporphyria. Pain and burning occur after sun exposure. The skin becomes red, swollen, and sometimes blisters. The skin may become thickened or scarred. When this change occurs over the knuckles and fingers, the hands look old ("old knuckles"). This is a pathognomonic change in children.

PHOTOTOXIC REACTIONS

Phototoxic reactions are nonallergic cutaneous responses induced by a variety of topical and systemic agents (Table 19-7). The frequency of these eruptions has decreased as informed physicians, aware of the photosensitive potential of certain drugs, have chosen alternatives. Phototoxicity occurs when a photosensitizer is absorbed into the skin either topically or systemically in appropriate concentrations and is exposed to adequate amounts of specific wavelengths of light, usually UVA. Theoretically, if sufficient quantities of chemical and light are delivered, the reaction should occur in all exposed individuals. In fact, the response varies.

TOPICAL EXPOSURE. Exposure to plants or chemicals that contain light-sensitizing compounds followed by exposure to certain activating wavelengths of UV light produces a highly characteristic eruption. A minimum response consists of an almost imperceptible erythema, followed by prolonged hyperpigmentation. A maximum response consists of tingling of the exposed skin and erythema that occur shortly after exposure, followed within hours by burning edema and vesiculation at the end of 24 hours. This is followed by a bullous reaction that lasts for days (Figure 19-24). Linear streaks (similar to poison ivy) of erythema and vesicles produced by drawing the offending agent across the skin surface are particularly characteristic of topical exposure (Figure 19-25). Desquamation occurs, and residual hyperpigmentation may persist for 1 year or longer.

Table 19-7 Comparison of Phototoxic and Photoallergic Reactions

Feature	Phototoxic reaction	Photoallergic reaction
Incidence	High	Low
Amount of agent required	Large	Small
Onset of reaction	Minutes to hours	24-72 hours
More than one exposure to agent required	No	Yes
Distribution	Sun-exposed skin only	Sun-exposed skin; may spread to unexposed areas
Clinical characteristics	Resembles exaggerated sunburn or blisters	Dermatitis
Immunologically mediated	No	Yes; type IV

PHYTOPHOTODERMATITIS. Exposure to plants that contain light-sensitizing compounds such as furocoumarin (psoralens) can cause intense reactions (see Box 19-7).

Examples are exposure to celery by salad makers and grocery workers, wild parsnip in meadows, the rind and pulp of limes, berlock dermatitis caused by the psoralen compounds in oil of bergamot (used in some perfumes) (Figure 19-26), and the leaves and young fruits of figs. The furocoumarins most abundant in limes are psoralen and bergapten, with the rind containing higher concentrations than the pulp.

The distribution of phototoxic reactions is sharply limited to areas of sun exposure. Topical exposure to solutions or plants produces bizarre patterns of inflammation, such as streaks from brushing against a plant or haphazard lines from celery juice (see Box 19-7) .

DRUGS. Exposure to certain drugs may result in a generalized intense erythema in sun-exposed skin (Box 19-8). Long lists of drugs reported to cause photosensitivity have been compiled; these are misleading because many are from single case reports. Thiazide diuretics are common offenders. The characteristic areas affected are the forehead, nose, malar eminences, cheeks, upper ears, lateral and posterior neck, V of the chest, extensor surfaces of the forearms, backs of the hands, and prominences of the pretibial and calf areas. The upper eyelids, nasolabial folds, and submental areas are typically spared. Photoonycholysis, which is the separation of the nails from the nail beds, may occur with drugs such as demeclocycline hydrochloride (Declomycin) and tetracycline.

MANAGEMENT. In most instances, withdrawal of the drug results in clearance of the clinical reaction. The patient should never take the offending drug again. In rare instances, photosensitivity persists for months or years. These patients may benefit from treatment with PUVA. Topical steroids provide some relief, but oral steroids are often necessary. When simple elimination fails to establish the offending agent, phototesting by physicians experienced with such procedures should be performed.

Box 19-7 **Agents Causing Phototoxic Reactions**

Topical agents

Perfumes

Plants containing psoralen compounds (phytophotodermatitis)

Celery
Gas plant (burning bush, dittany)
Meadow grass (agrimony)
Parsnip (wild parsnip)
Persian limes
Wild angelica
Angelica
Cow parsley
Carrot (wild)
Fig (wild)
Sweet orange
False bishop's weed
Hogweed
Rue
Many others reported, but rare

PHOTOTOXIC ERUPTION—PHYTOPHOTODERMATITIS

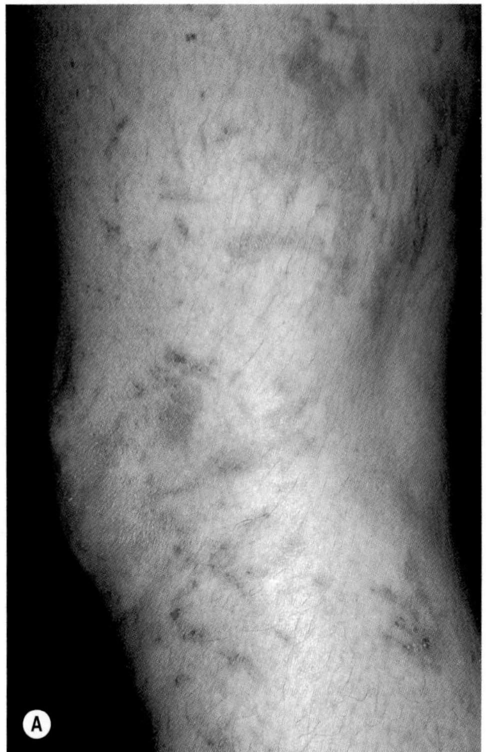

Contact with plants in a field followed by direct sun exposure resulted in this patterned eruption of erythema and vesicles.

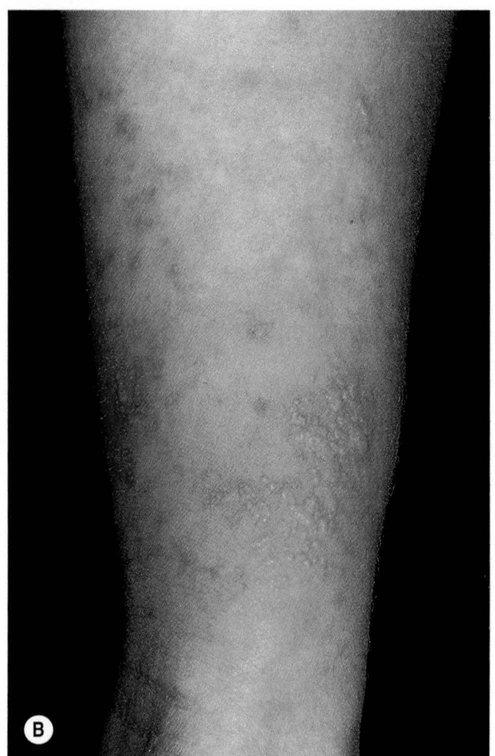

Diffuse erythema and vesiculation occurred 24 hours after contact with celery juice and sun exposure.

Figure 19-24

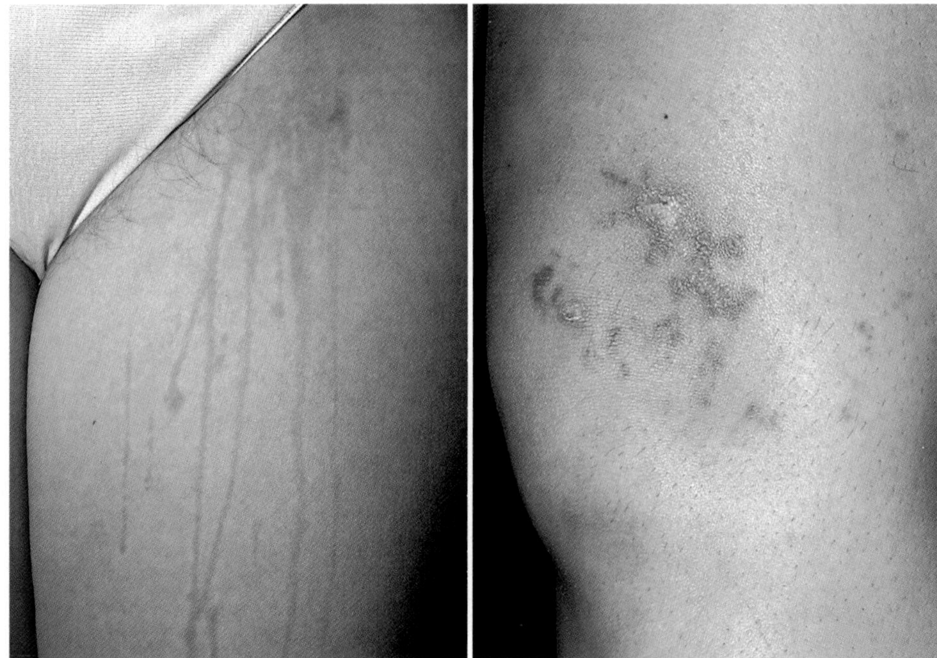

Figure 19-25 Exposure to substances that contain psoralen compounds, such as lime juice followed by sun exposure can cause erythema and vesicles that heal with brown hyperpigmentation.

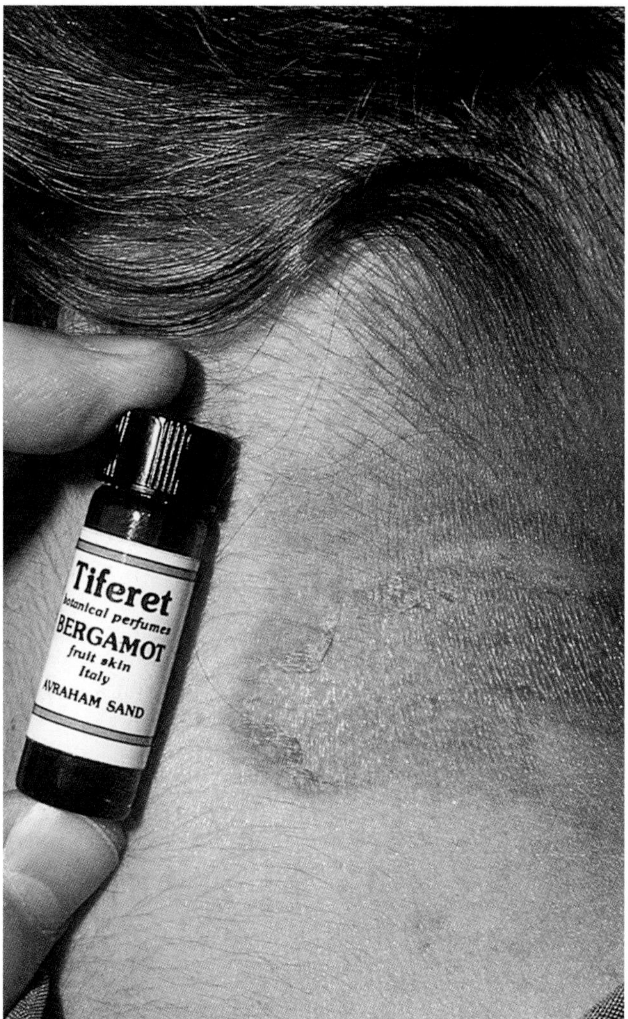

Figure 19-26 Phototoxic reaction (berloque dermatitis). Oil of bergamot (used in some perfumes) contains psoralens, which can cause erythema followed by prolonged hyperpigmentation after exposure to light.

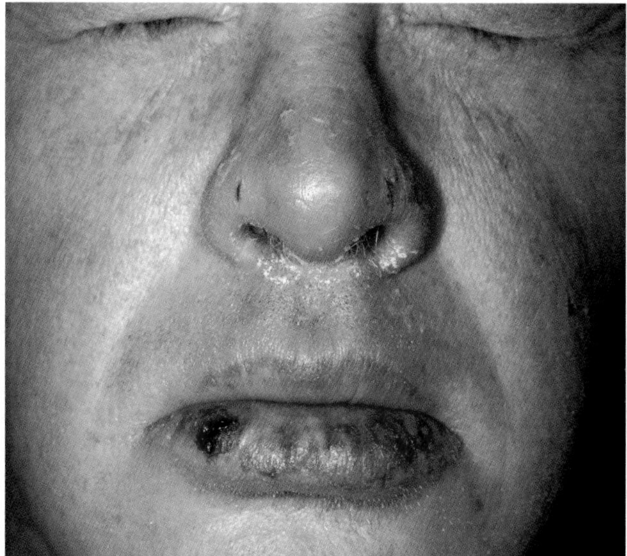

Figure 19-27 Doxycycline-induced phototoxicity. The patient was taking 100 mg doxycycline twice a day for acne. Sun exposure caused burning and erythema on his cheeks, nose and lips.

Box 19-8 **Medications Causing Phototoxic Reactions**

Antibiotics

Tetracyclines (doxycycline [Figure 19-27], tetracycline)
Fluoroquinolones (ciprofloxacin, ofloxacin, levofloxacin)
Sulfonamides

Nonsteroidal antiinflammatory drugs (NSAIDs)

Ibuprofen
Ketoprofen
Naproxen

Diuretics

Furosemide
Hydrochlorothiazide

Retinoids

Isotretinoin
Acitretin
PDT prophotosensitizers
5-Aminolevulinic acid
Methyl-5-aminolevulinic acid
Verteporfin
Photofrin

Neuroleptic drugs

Phenothiazines (chlorpromazine, fluphenazine, perazine, perphenazine, thioridazine)
Thioxanthenes (chlorprothixene, thiothixene)

Antifungals

Itraconazole
Voriconazole

Other drugs

para-Aminobenzoic acid (PABA)
5-Fluorouracil (5-FU)
Amiodarone (Figure 19-28)
Diltiazem
Quinidine
Coal tar

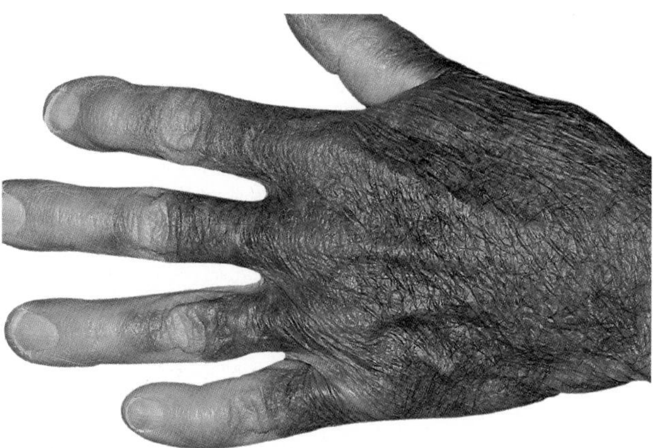

Figure 19-28 Amiodarone toxicity. Severe blue-gray cutaneous discoloration occurs in up to 10% of patients taking amiodarone. Sun exposure induces the discoloration.

PHOTOALLERGY

Photoallergic reactions are uncommon. UV light initiates a reaction between skin protein and a chemical or drug to form an antigen (Box 19-9). A delayed hypersensitivity reaction follows, and the clinical presentation is, like poison ivy, eczematous inflammation. Plant and pesticide allergens should be included in the patch and photo-patch test series used for the evaluation of patients with suspected photoallergy. Photoallergic contact dermatitis to PABA and structurally related PABA sunscreen has been documented. Some patients without additional drug exposure continue to have flares for years when exposed to sunlight; this is termed a *persistent light reaction*.

Box 19-9 **Medications Causing Photoallergic Reactions**
5-FU
Celecoxib
Cinnamates
Dapsone
Hydrochlorothiazide
Itraconazole
Ketoprofen
Oral contraceptives
PABA
Phenothiazines (chlorpromazine, fluphenazine, perazine, perphenazine, thioridazine)
Quinidine
Salicylates
Sulfonylureas (glipizide, glyburide)

DISORDERS OF HYPOPIGMENTATION

Diseases that present with hypopigmentation or hyperpigmentation are listed in Table 19-8. The most common and distinctive are described in the following paragraphs.

Vitiligo

The word *vitiligo* may be derived from the Greek *vitellius,* signifying a "calf's white patches." Vitiligo is an acquired loss of pigmentation characterized histologically by absence of epidermal melanocytes. It may be an autoimmune disease associated with antibodies (vitiligo antibodies) to melanocytes, but the pathogenesis is still not understood. Studies suggest there is some genetic mechanism involved in the etiology of vitiligo and that it is polygenic in nature. There is a positive family history in at least 30% of cases. Both genders are affected equally. Approximately 1% of the population is affected; 50% of cases begin before age 20. The pigment loss may be localized or generalized. Many patients are embarrassed. Physicians should be especially alert to the effects of disfigurement.

CLINICAL MANIFESTATIONS. There are two types of vitiligo (A and B) (Table 19-9). In the more common type A (generalized), there is a fairly symmetric pattern of white macules with well-defined borders. The borders may have a red halo (inflammatory vitiligo) or a rim of hyperpigmentation. The loss of pigmentation may not be apparent in fair-skinned individuals, but it may be disfiguring in blacks. Initially the disease is limited; it then progresses slowly over years. Commonly involved sites include the backs of the hands, the face, and body folds, including axillae and genitalia (Figures 19-29 to 19-32). White areas are common around body openings such as the eyes, nostrils, mouth, nipples, umbilicus, and anus. The palms, soles, scalp, lips, and mucous membranes may be affected. Genital vitiligo-like depigmentation following use of imiquimod 5% cream is reported. Vitiligo occurs at sites of trauma (Koebner phenomenon), such as around the elbows and in previously sunburned skin. Many patients with vitiligo develop halo nevi. An acrofacial or lip-tip type (involving lips and digits) also occurs.

Segmental vitiligo (type B) occurs in an asymmetric distribution. The segments do not correspond to a dermatomal distribution. It is common in segmental forms for

Table 19-8 Disorders of Pigmentation

Hypopigmentation	Hyperpigmentation
Acquired	**Circumscribed brown**
Chemical-induced	Café-au-lait spots
Halo nevus	Diabetic dermopathy
Idiopathic guttate hypomelanosis	Erythema ab igne
Leprosy	Fixed drug eruption
Leukoderma associated with melanoma	Freckles
Pityriasis alba	Lentigo in children
Postinflammatory hypopigmentation	Peutz-Jeghers syndrome
Tinea versicolor	Lentigo in adults
Vitiligo	Melasma
Phytophotodermatitis	
Congenital	**Diffuse brown**
Albinism, partial (piebaldism)	Addison's disease
Albinism, total	Biliary cirrhosis
Nevus anemicus	Hemochromatosis
Nevus depigmentosus	Malignant melanoma (metastatic)
Piebaldism	
Tuberous sclerosis	

VITILIGO

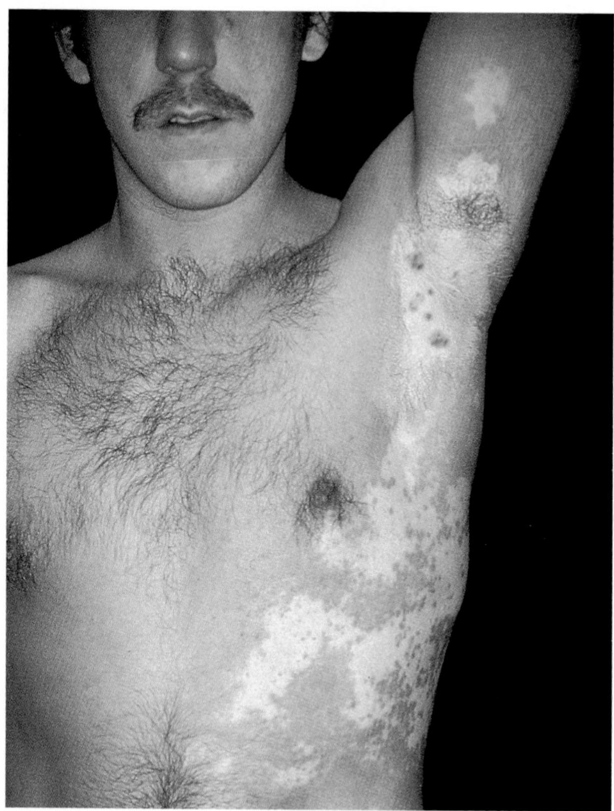

Figure 19-29 Body folds, including the axillae, are commonly involved. Wood's light examination may be necessary to demonstrate this in patients with light skin.

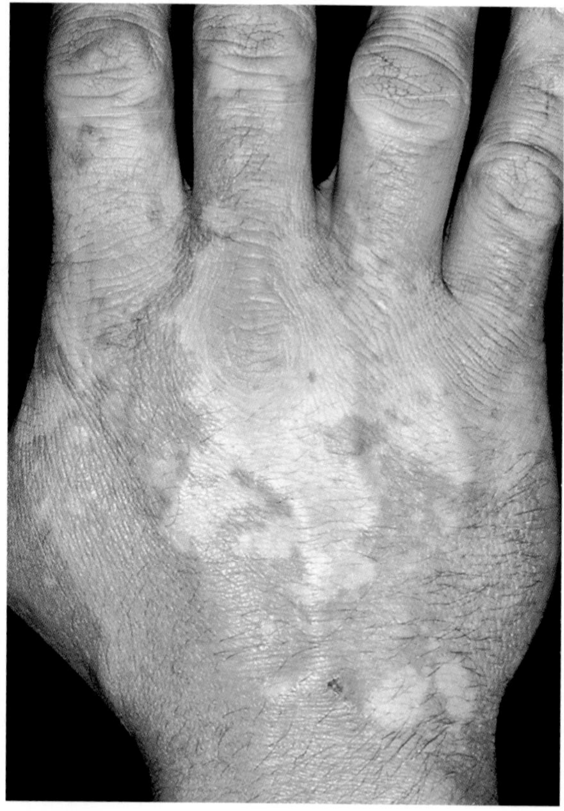

Figure 19-30 The back of the hand is a commonly involved site.

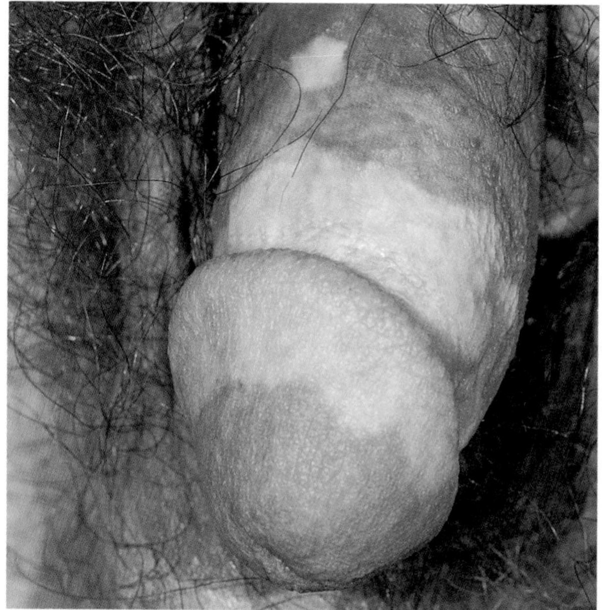

Figure 19-31 The penis is a commonly involved site.

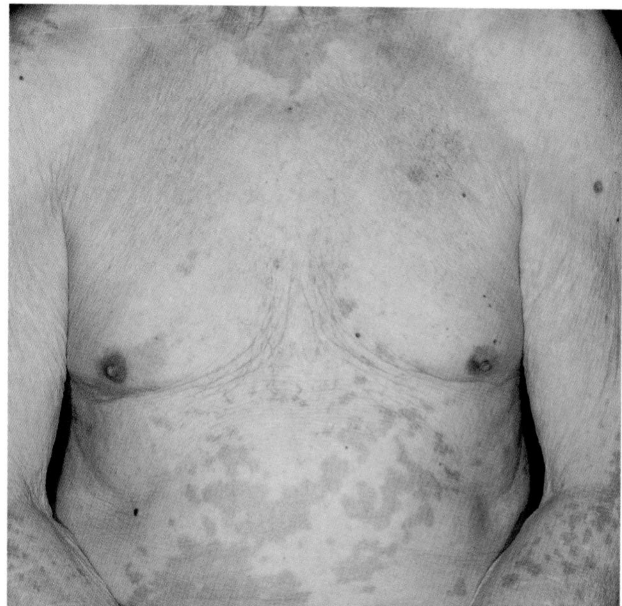

Figure 19-32 There is almost total loss of pigment. Monobenzone (Benoquin), a potent depigmenting agent, could be used for cosmetic purposes to remove the remaining pigment.

Table 19-9 Vitiligo (Types A and B) Clinical Manifestations

	Type A	Type B
Distribution	Nondermatomal	Dermatomal (zosteriform)
Ratio	3	1
Onset	Any age (50% before age 20)	Young
Activity	Lifelong	Rapid spread in 1 year
Associated with halo nevus	Yes	No
Koebner phenomenon	Yes	No
Associated with immunologic diseases	Yes	No

Modified from Koga M, Tango T: *Br J Dermatol* 118:223, 1988.
PMID: 3348967

the hair follicles to be depigmented, indicating an absence of follicular melanocytes. The onset is earlier than the generalized form. There is a decreased association with autoimmune disease.

CHILDHOOD VITILIGO. Childhood vitiligo is a distinct subset of vitiligo. There is an increased incidence of segmental vitiligo (type B vitiligo), of autoimmune and/or endocrine disease, of premature graying in immediate and extended family members, and of organ-specific antibodies, in addition to a poor response to topical PUVA therapy.

PSYCHOLOGIC IMPACT. Vitiligo can have a major impact on personality. Feelings of stress, embarrassment, self-consciousness, and low self-esteem can occur. Patients claim the disease interferes with sexual relationships. The psychologic impact can be profound in deeply pigmented races. The disease can have serious social stigma in some cultures.

EYE, EAR, AND MENINGEAL FINDINGS. Vitiligo affects all melanocytes. Depigmented areas in the pigment epithelium of the retina and choroid occur in up to 40% of vitiligo patients. The incidence of uveitis is elevated. The membranous labyrinth of the inner ear contains melanocytes. Minor hearing problems can occur. The Vogt-Koyanagi-Harada syndrome consists of vitiligo with many other associated findings; the most common are meningismus, hearing loss, alopecia, tinnitus, and poliosis. The aseptic meningitis may be due to destruction of leptomeningeal melanocytes. The disease appears in the fourth to fifth decade and is more common in women and in persons with dark pigmentation.

ASSOCIATED DISEASES. Most patients with vitiligo have no other associated findings; however, vitiligo has been reported to be associated with alopecia areata, hypothyroidism, Graves' disease, Addison's disease, pernicious anemia, insulin-dependent diabetes mellitus, uveitis, chronic mucocutaneous candidiasis, the polyglandular autoimmune syndromes, and melanoma. Thyroid disorders have been reported in as many as 30% of vitiligo patients. Circulating autoantibodies such as antithyroglobulin and antimicrosomal and antiparietal cell antibodies have been found in more than 50% of patients.

WOOD'S LIGHT EXAMINATION. Examination with the Wood's light in a dark room accentuates the hypopigmented areas and is useful for examining patients with light complexions. The axillae, anus, and genitalia should be carefully examined. These areas are frequently involved but often clinically nonapparent without the Wood's light. Vitiligo may be a predictor of metastases in melanoma patients, and a Wood's light examination may show early subtle changes in these patients.

STUDIES. Obtain a thyroid-stimulating hormone level and complete blood count with indices and blood glucose level to rule out thyroid disease, pernicious anemia, and diabetes mellitus.

RESOURCES. The National Vitiligo Foundation provides information and support for patients (www.nvfi.org).

INDICATIONS FOR TREATMENT. Treatment is necessary for patients in whom the disease causes emotional and social distress. Vitiligo in individuals with fair complexions is usually not a significant cosmetic problem. The condition becomes more apparent in the summer months when tanning accentuates normal skin. Tanning may be prevented with sunscreens that have an SPF of 15 or higher. Vitiligo is a significant cosmetic problem in people with dark complexions, and repigmentation with psoralens may be worthwhile.

MECHANISM OF REPIGMENTATION. The goal of treatment is to restore melanocytes to the skin. Therapy involves stimulating melanocytes within the hair follicle to proliferate and migrate back into depigmented skin. Depigmented skin is devoid of melanocytes in the epidermis. Melanotic melanocytes in the bulb and infundibulum of the hair follicle are absent in vitiliginous skin. Repigmentation is caused by activation and migration of melanocytes from a melanocytic reservoir located in the hair follicles. Therefore skin with little or no hair (hands and feet) or with white hair responds poorly to treatment. Inactive amelanotic melanocytes in the middle and lower parts of the follicle and the outer root sheath are still present. These cells can be activated by treatment to acquire enzymes for melanogenesis. They proliferate and mature as they migrate up the hair follicle into the epidermis and spread centrifugally. When a vitiliginous spot repigments, it repigments from the follicle and spreads outward. This process is slow and requires at least 6 to 12 months of treatment. The face, arms, trunk, and legs respond best.

Melanocytes divide rapidly after any inflammatory process or after UV irradiation. PUVA produces inflammation in the skin at the depth of the hair follicle. Cytokines released by the inflammatory process may stimulate melanocytes to proliferate and migrate outward.

TREATMENT PERSPECTIVE. All treatment options have limited success. The face and neck respond best to all therapeutic approaches; the acral areas are least responsive. For generalized vitiligo, phototherapy with narrow-band UVB (NB-UVB) radiation is most effective with the fewest side effects; PUVA is the second best choice. Topical corticosteroids are the preferred drugs for localized vitiligo. They may be replaced by topical immunomodulators, which display comparable effectiveness and fewer side effects. The effectiveness of vitamin D analogues is controversial with limited data but they are felt to be the least effective topical treatment. The excimer laser is an alternative to UVB therapy especially for localized vitiligo of the face. Surgical therapy can be very successful, but requires an experienced surgeon and is very demanding of time and facilities, thus limiting its widespread use. *PMID: 17537039*

GUIDELINES FOR THE TREATMENT OF VITILIGO

Evidence-based guidelines for the treatment of vitiligo in children and in adults have been established. A treatment scheme is found in Table 19-10.

CHILDREN. Vitiligo can be associated with significant psychologic trauma; early treatment is more effective. Early lesions may respond better to therapy. Repigmentation therapies stimulate the melanocytic reserves in the hair follicles. Follicular melanocytes are mostly destroyed in older lesions and response to repigmentation therapy is poor.

For children younger than 12 years, treatment with class 3 topical corticosteroids (e.g., fluticasone propionate or betamethasone valerate) is recommended as the first-choice therapy. This choice is made regardless of the clinical type. When no repigmentation is observed after 6 months, localized UVB therapy or topical PUVA therapy could be prescribed and the "skin-saving principle" applied (i.e., parts of the body where no lesions are present [especially the face] should be shielded during treatments). Parts of the body that have repigmented satisfactorily during the course of the therapy should, if possible, be shielded during subsequent treatments (e.g., trousers should be worn). In children, genital areas should be protected during UV exposures. Treatment with topical corticosteroids may be combined with UVA radiation. Comparative studies have shown that the combined treatment with fluticasone and UVA led to a greater repigmentation than did treatment with either fluticasone or UVA alone. A facial tanner or a sun bed may be used as the UVA source.

ADULTS. Treatment choice is guided by clinical type. Patients with localized vitiligo can be treated with class 3 corticosteroids combined with UVA therapy. If there is no response after 6 months, localized UVB or topical PUVA therapy can be given as an alternative. Narrow-band UVB therapy is recommended as the most effective and safest therapy for generalized vitiligo. A minimum treatment duration of 6 months is recommended. Responsive patients can be given this treatment for a maximum of 24 months. After the first course of 1 year, a resting period of 3 months is recommended to minimize the annual cumulative dose of UVB.

Segmental and lip-tip vitiligo (lips and digits) are best treated with autologous transplantation.

In patients with extensive areas of depigmentation (80%) and/or disfiguring lesions on the face who do not respond to repigmentation therapies, depigmentation of

Table 19-10 Treatment Scheme for Vitiligo

	Clinical type of vitiligo	First-choice therapy*	Alternative therapies*
Children <12 yr	All	Class 3 corticosteroids (and UVA); course, 6-9 mo (aged <6 yr, no UVA)	Local UVB (311 nm); course, 6-12 mo Topical psoralen—UVA; course, 6-12 mo
Adults	Localized (≤2% depigmentation)	Class 3 corticosteroids (and UVA); course, 6-9 mo	Local UVB (311 nm); course, 6-12 mo Topical psoralen—UVA; course, 6-12 mo
	Generalized (>2% depigmentation)	UVB (311 nm); course, 6-24 mo	Oral psoralen—UVA; course, 6-24 mo
	Segmental or stable	Autologous transplantation (until 100% repigmentation)	Class 3 corticosteroids (and UVA); course, 6-9 mo UVB (311 nm); course, 6-24 mo
	Lip-tip (lip-digits)	Autologous transplantation (until 100% repigmentation)	Micropigmentation (until 100% repigmentation)
	Therapy-resistant and/or generalized (>80% depigmentation)	Depigmentation with bleaching cream and/or laser (until 100% depigmentation)	None

From Njoo M et al: *Arch Dermatol* 135:1514,1999. *PMID: 10606057*
*The course is expressed as a range from minimum to maximum.

the residual melanin should be considered. During and on completion of the therapy, patients should minimize sun exposure and apply broad-spectrum sunscreens. The use of a potent bleaching cream and/or laser therapy (e.g., the Q-switched ruby laser) is considered to be the cornerstone of depigmentation therapy for these patients.

In all cases, advice regarding the use of camouflage and sun-blocking agents should always be given. If necessary, psychologic counseling may be recommended.

NARROW-BAND UVB. Current evidence-based guidelines indicate that NB-UVB phototherapy is recommended for generalized vitiligo. Narrow-band (311 nm) UVB radiation provides a new alternative to conventional PUVA therapy without many of the adverse effects associated with PUVA therapy. Narrow-band UVB lamps produce less erythema, and hyperkeratosis is not observed after long-term irradiation. Treatments are given two or three times weekly, and exposure times are usually no longer than 5 minutes. Narrow-band UVB therapy is effective and safe in childhood vitiligo. As with other forms of phototherapy, the face and trunk had better repigmentation than distal extremities

Some patients spontaneously repigment, sometimes after moderate sun exposure. UVB or PUVA can then be used to encourage further repigmentation. Reevaluate patients every 2 or 3 months. Therapy should be stopped if no color returns after this period. Patients who respond usually keep their pigment. Patients who have actively spreading vitiligo should not be treated; treatment does not halt the spread of the disease.

RESPONSE TO TREATMENT. Improvement begins with perifollicular pigmentation, which then enlarges. Repigmentation occurs at the borders but at a slower rate. Best results are obtained on the face and neck. The face begins to respond after 25 treatments; other areas respond after 50 treatments. Results are poor on the hands and feet and over bony prominences. Focal vitiligo responds better than generalized vitiligo (i.e., it responds to 100 treatments or less, whereas generalized vitiligo requires as many as 200 treatments). Most patients who respond do not develop new areas of pigment loss. The appearance of new or enlarged macules indicates the possible beginning of treatment failure. Maintenance therapy is not required. Totally repigmented macules should remain filled with 85% certainty; those incompletely filled in are likely to reverse and depigment.

PHOTOCHEMOTHERAPY. PUVA or combined PUVA and calcipotriol therapy was used as first-line treatment years ago. NB-UVB is safer and possibly more effective. PUVA resulted in greater than 90% repigmentation in only 8% of patients, usually inhomogeneous and weak repigmentation.

TOPICAL THERAPY. Topical psoralens and topical steroids have been used with some success in patients with limited areas of pigmentation (see Box 19-8). Some dermatologists who have years of experience with phototherapy will not use topical psoralens. They believe that the potential for phototoxicity to produce severe burns is too great. The edges where there is residual pigmentation always hyperpigment; this disappears with time.

IMMUNOMODULATORS. Tacrolimus ointment (Protopic) and pimecrolimus (Elidel) have been used to treat vitiligo. These medications are well tolerated and can be used for prolonged periods without steroid-like side effects. Varying degrees of pigmentation have been experienced.

EXCIMER LASER. Targeted therapy of only the affected area with increased intensity is possible with this modality. In several studies excimer laser showed less success than topical corticosteroids and NB-UVB. Repigmentation is inhomogeneous. The excimer laser is best for treating the face.

GRAFTING AND TRANSPLANTATION. Several surgical procedures have been developed for treating depigmented skin; these include grafting suction-blistered epidermis, minigrafts, and transplantation of in vitro–cultured epidermis-bearing melanocytes.

SYSTEMIC STEROIDS. Systemic corticosteroids can arrest the progression of vitiligo and lead to repigmentation in a significant proportion of patients, but they may also produce unacceptable side effects. Oral minipulse therapy with 5 mg of betamethasone/dexamethasone was reported to arrest the progression and induce spontaneous repigmentation in some vitiligo patients. To minimize the side effects, betamethasone as a single oral dose was taken after breakfast on 2 consecutive days per week. The progression of the disease was arrested in 89% of patients with active disease, whereas some patients needed an increase in the dosage to 7.5 mg/day to achieve a complete arrest of lesions. Within 2 to 4 months, 80% of the patients started having spontaneous repigmentation of the existing lesions that progressed with continued treatment.

COSMETICS. For cosmetic purposes, lesions may be temporarily dyed brown with DY-O-Derm or Vita-Dye. Cosmetics that camouflage (e.g., Dermablend and Covermark; see the Formulary) effectively hide the white patches. Each product is available in several shades.

The sunless or self-tanning lotions that contain dihydroxyacetone (DHA) darken the skin by staining. These preparations work best in vitiligo patients with skin phototypes II and III and are particularly useful if their normal skin is already tanned. The major problem is color blending and matching at the border of vitiliginous and normal skin.

DEPIGMENTATION OF REMAINING NORMAL SKIN. Patients with more than 40% involvement of the skin surface may choose to remove the remaining normal skin pigment with 20% monobenzone (Benoquin cream).

It is not always successful in achieving complete depigmentation. Monobenzone destroys melanocytes and can cause contact dermatitis. Therefore, as a test before starting generalized therapy, monobenzone should be applied to a single pigmented spot daily for 1 week. Thereafter larger pigmented areas are treated twice daily for 1 year or longer, not 4 months as is stated in *The Physicians' Desk Reference*. Application for 3 to 4 years may be necessary. Resistant areas such as the hands are treated with monobenzone under Saran Wrap occlusion. Patients may note an inflammatory response within the pigmented skin but not in the white skin. The monobenzone can be diluted to a 10%, 5%, or lower concentration for these patients. A group VI topical steroid may also be used to control inflammation.

Depigmentation is usually done in regions to limit drug absorption. Start with the face and upper extremity areas and then treat lower extremity sites. Truncal areas are last, and many patients choose to leave their trunk its normal color. The rate of depigmentation can vary from weeks to 4 years.

People assisting others with application of monobenzone must wear gloves and use applicators to prevent depigmenting their own skin.

Patients must understand that this is a permanent procedure. They will be sun sensitive for the rest of their lives and must use sunscreen during sun exposure. The results of treatment are usually very gratifying.

Patients who would like some skin color after treatment can use beta-carotene (Solatene) 60 mg three times a day for 10 weeks, followed by 30 mg three times a day for maintenance (www.tishcon.com).

Idiopathic guttate hypomelanosis

Idiopathic guttate hypomelanosis (white spots on the arms and legs) is characterized by 2- to 5-mm white spots with sharply demarcated borders. They are located on the exposed areas of hands, forearms, and lower legs of middle-aged and older people (Figure 19-33). Patients have signs of early aging and sun exposure, including seborrheic keratoses, lentigines, and xerosis in the same areas. A subset of these patients has lesions unrelated to sun exposure. The condition is asymptomatic. Lesions show a decrease in the number of melanocytes. Melanin is absent in basal keratinocytes. Treatment with tretinoin for 4 months restores the elasticity, with a partial restoration of pigmentation. Cryotherapy for 3 to 5 seconds is effective.

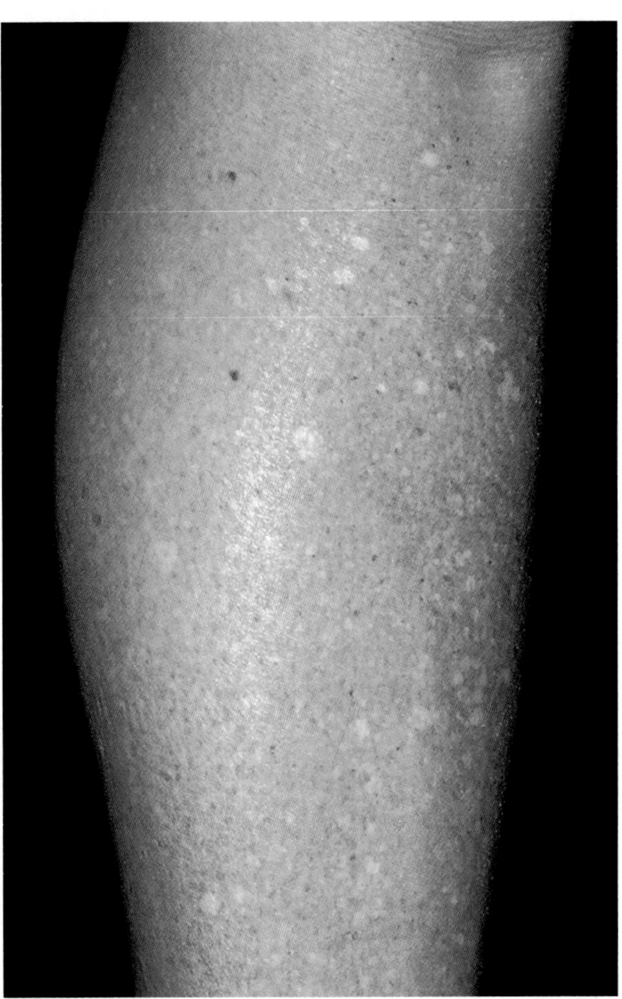

Figure 19-33 Idiopathic guttate hypomelanosis. White spots on the arms and lower legs occur in the middle-aged and the elderly.

Nevus anemicus

Nevus anemicus is a congenital localized pharmacologic cutaneous anomaly most often seen on the trunk. It may be linked with certain genodermatoses, including neurofibromatosis. The lesion usually consists of a well-defined white macule with an irregular border, often surrounded by smaller white macules beyond the border of the major lesion (Figure 19-34). Histologically the skin appears normal; the pale color has been attributed to local blood vessel sensitivity to catecholamines. Hence, it has been called a pharmacologic nevus. Special stains confirm the presence of melanin and melanocytes. There is a lack of dermatitis within the margins of nevus anemicus in generalized contact dermatitis. The lesion is most often confused with tinea versicolor or vitiligo. The white macule lacks the scale of tinea and, during Wood's light examination, does not become as prominent as vitiligo. Friction or cold or heat application fails to induce erythema in the involved areas. Treatment is not required. Camouflage make-up hides the lesion.

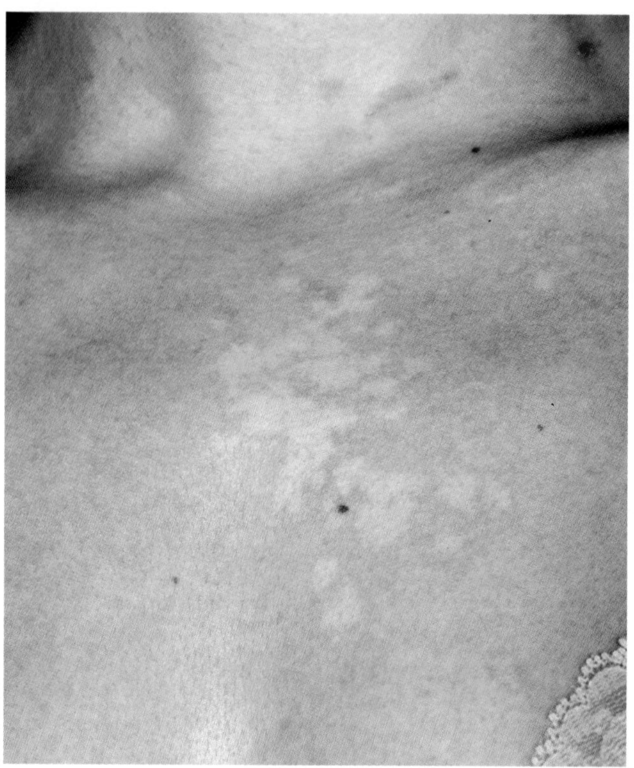

Figure 19-34 Nevus anemicus.

Tuberous sclerosis

Hypopigmented macules (oval, ash leaf–shaped, or stippled) that are concentrated on the arms, legs, and trunk are the earliest signs of tuberous sclerosis (Figure 19-35; see also Chapter 26). They are present in 40% to 90% of patients with the disease, and they number from 1 to 32 in affected individuals. Minimally visible hypopigmented spots are more easily visualized with the Wood's lamp. As noted, Wood's light is a blue light with an emission peak of 360 nm. The blue end of visible light is absorbed by epidermal pigmentation. If there is no epidermal pigmentation in a site, the area will appear nonpigmented compared with the surrounding skin.

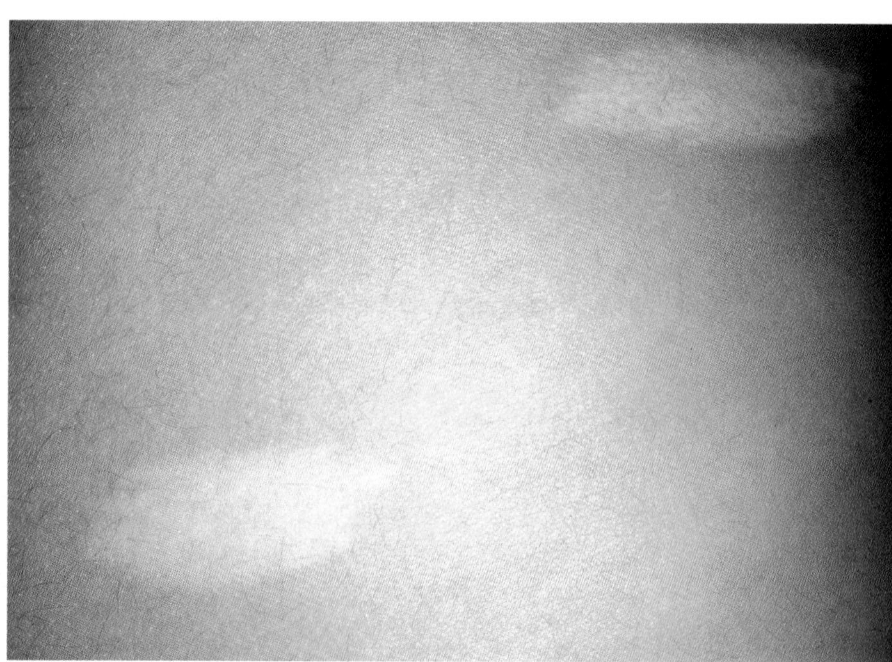

Figure 19-35 Tuberous sclerosis. Ash leaf–shaped hypopigmented macules.

Pityriasis alba

Pityriasis alba is a common finding (5% of children) that is probably more usual in patients with the atopic diathesis (see p. 171). The condition appears in most instances before puberty. The face, neck, and arms are the most common sites. The lesions begin as a nonspecific erythema and gradually become scaly and hypopigmented. The hypopigmentation is transient and caused by mild dermal inflammation and the UV screening effect of the scaly skin. The condition gradually improves after puberty. Treatment consists of lubrication. Mild inflammation responds to group V topical steroids, but the degree of pigmentation is not affected by any treatment. Pimecrolimus cream 1% or tacrolimus ointment 0.03% or 0.1% are nonsteroidal alternatives for treatment. The condition is often confused with vitiligo and tinea versicolor. Vitiligo does not scale. The potassium hydroxide preparation is positive in tinea versicolor.

DISORDERS OF HYPERPIGMENTATION

FRECKLES (EPHELIDES) VS. LENTIGO. Ephelides and solar lentigines are different types of pigmented lesions. Solar lentigines are more prevalent than ephelides, increase in prevalence and number with higher age, are most prevalent on the trunk, and occur more frequently in males. Ephelides loose their prevalence with age; become equally distributed on the face, arms, and trunk; and occur more frequently in females. An intimate association of ephelides, but not solar lentigines, has been found with hair color and skin type.

Freckles

Freckles, or ephelides, are small, red or light brown macules that are promoted by sun exposure and fade during the winter months. They are usually confined to the face, arms, and back. The number varies from a few spots on the face to hundreds of confluent macules on the face and arms. They occur as an autosomal dominant trait and are most often found in individuals with fair complexions. The use of sunscreen prevents the appearance of new freckles and helps prevent the darkening of existing freckles that typically accompanies sun exposure.

Lentigo in children

A lentigo is a small (0.5 to 2 cm) tan, brown, or black oval-to-round macule that is darker than a freckle and is not affected by sunlight. Freckles darken with sun exposure. Lentigines may increase in number during childhood and adult life or fade at any time. The Peutz-Jeghers syndrome refers to mucocutaneous pigmentation consisting of many blue-brown lentigines, less than 0.5 cm in diameter, on the buccal mucosa and other areas of the glabrous skin, accompanied by generalized intestinal polyposis.

Lentigo in adults

Lentigo, or liver spots, occurs in sun-exposed areas of the face, arms, and hands (Figures 19-36 and 19-37). The lesions vary in size from 0.2 to 2 cm and become more numerous with advancing age. Facial solar lentigines frequently lack the rete ridge hyperplasia classically associated with lentigines from other anatomic sites.

A biopsy should be taken from any lentigo that develops a highly irregular border, localized increase in pigmentation, or localized thickening to rule out lentigo maligna melanoma. Cryotherapy is an effective treatment, but hypopigmentation or hyperpigmentation is a possible side effect. Solar lentigines of the back of the hands responds well to cryotherapy. Best results occur in fairer skin types, where postinflammatory hyperpigmentation is not as pronounced as in darker skinned individuals.

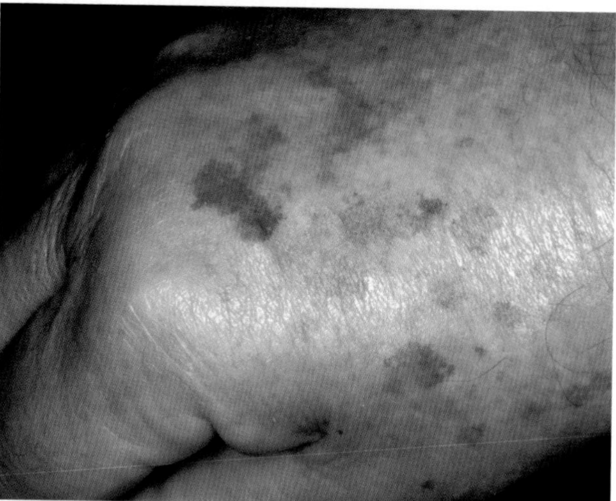

Figure 19-36 Lentigo on the hand. Lesions may be extensive but degeneration to melanoma in this area is very uncommon.

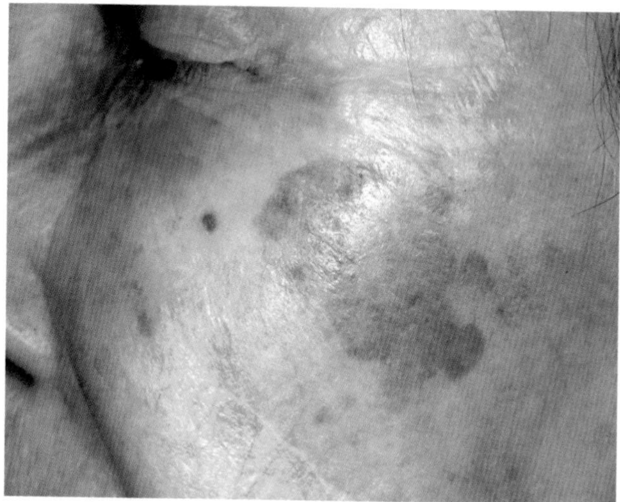

Figure 19-37 Lentigo on the face. Irregular pigmentation is a common finding in adults. Suspect lentigo maligna in lesions that expand and show black irregular pigmentation.

Topical 0.1% tretinoin cream or 0.1% tazarotene cream (AVAGE) significantly improves both clinical and microscopic manifestations of liver spots. After 10 months, 83% of patients with facial lesions who were treated with tretinoin had lightening of these lesions. The lesions do not return for at least 6 months after therapy is discontinued.

A single course of Q-switch ruby laser exposure completely clears lesions on the arms and hands. Peeling solution with glycolic acid is ineffective.

Hyperpigmented lesions are a predominant component of photoaging in Chinese and Japanese persons; 0.1% tretinoin cream significantly lightens the hyperpigmentation of photoaging in these patients. Hydroquinone preparations are occasionally useful for bleaching these lesions.

Melasma

Melasma (chloasma, or mask of pregnancy) is a common acquired symmetric brown hyperpigmentation involving the face and neck in genetically predisposed women and men.

The psychosocial impact can be devastating. The pigmentation develops slowly without signs of inflammation and may be faint or dark. Blacks, Asians, and Hispanics are the most susceptible populations.

ETIOLOGY. Genetic factors and UV radiation are the most important causes. Other causes include pregnancy, oral contraceptives, estrogen-progesterone therapies, thyroid dysfunction, cosmetics, and phototoxic and antiseizure drugs. Melasma may not resolve after delivery or withdrawal of oral contraceptives. Mild subclinical ovarian dysfunction may be present in some patients.

CLINICAL AND HISTOLOGIC PATTERNS. Perform a Wood's lamp examination to identify the depth of the melanin pigmentation.

There are three clinical patterns: centrofacial, malar, and mandibular (Table 19-11). There are four types based on Wood's light examination: (1) The epidermal type has increased melanin in the basal, suprabasal, and stratum corneum layers; the pigmentation is intensified by Wood's light examination. (2) The dermal type does not show enhancement with the Wood's light; melanophages are found in the superficial dermis and in the deep dermis. (3) A mixed-type epidermal and dermal pigment type shows no or slight enhancement with the Wood's light. (4) Darker individuals can show the Wood's lamp inapparent type (Table 19-12). The epidermal type responds to depigmenting agents; the dermal pigmentation resists the action of bleaching agents. Three histologic patterns of pigmentation have been described: epidermal, dermal, and mixed.

Table 19-11 Melasma—Clinical Patterns

Centrofacial (most common)	Cheeks, forehead, upper lip, nose, and chin
Malar	Cheeks and nose
Mandibular pattern	Lesions that occur over ramus of mandible

There is an increased number and activity of melanocytes in the epidermis and an increased number of melanophages in the dermis. The forehead, malar eminences, upper lip, and chin are most frequently affected (Figure 19-38). Melasma occurs during the second or third trimester of pregnancy, gradually fades after delivery, and darkens with subsequent pregnancies. Melasma occurs in some women taking oral contraceptives.

DIFFERENTIAL DIAGNOSIS. The differential diagnoses includes postinflammatory hyperpigmentation, actinic lichen planus, hyperthyroidism-related pigmentation, hydantoin intake pigmentation, HIV infection–related pigmentation, and "pigmented cosmetic dermatitis" (related to photodynamic substances in cosmetics). Pigmented cosmetic dermatitis shows brownish gray to reddish brown pigmentation that is often reticulate, has indefinite margins, and involves rapid development.

TREATMENT. Melasma is difficult to treat. Treatments include hypopigmenting agents, chemical peels, and lasers (Table 19-13). Cosmetics (such as Dermablend) may be used to camouflage the pigmentation. Cosmetics are heavy and objectionable to some patients.

Table 19-12 Melasma—Clinical Types and Patterns

Type	Clinical	Wood's light examination	Histology
Epidermal	Light brown	Enhancement of pigmentation	Melanin increase in basal, suprabasal, and stratum corneum layers
Dermal	Ashen or bluish gray	No enhancement of pigmentation	Melanin-laden macrophages in a perivascular location found in superficial and mid-dermis
Mixed	Dark brown	Enhancement of pigmentation in some places	Melanin deposition found in epidermis and dermis
Indeterminate	Ashen gray or unrecognized	Inapparent (in patients with dark skin)	Melanin deposition found in dermis

MELASMA

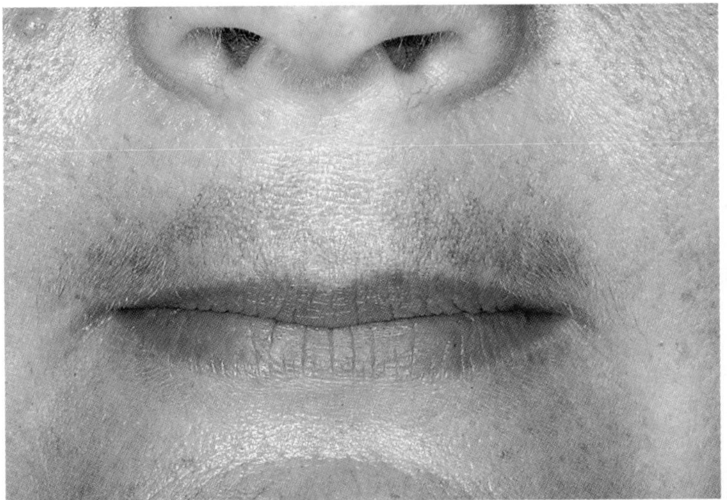
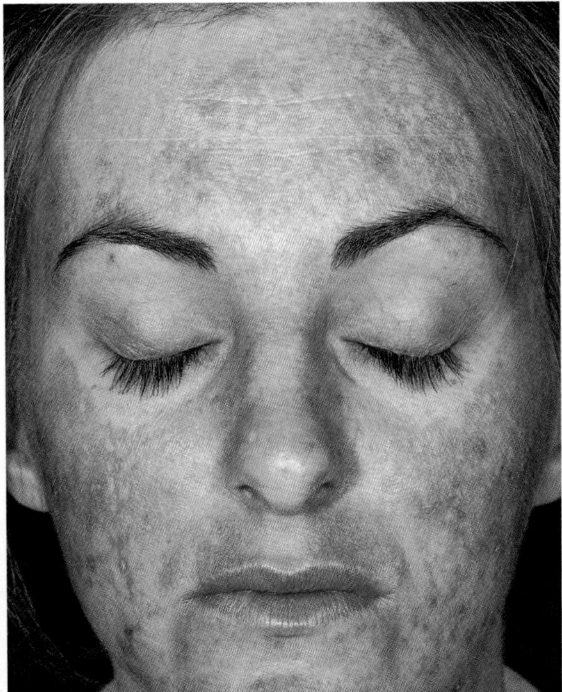
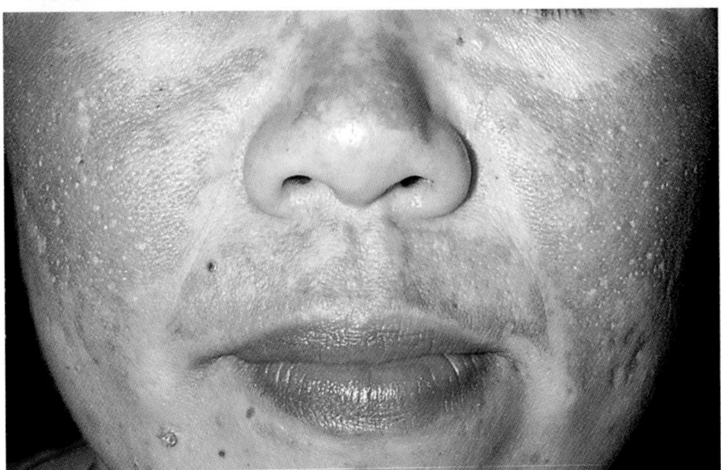

Figure 19-38 Diffuse brown hyperpigmentation may occur during pregnancy or while taking oral contraceptives. The upper lip, malar eminences, and forehead are the most frequently affected.

Table 19-13 Hypopigmenting Agents

Class	Treatment	Mechanism of action
Phenolic hypopigmenting agent	Hydroquinone	Inhibits tyrosinase, leading to decreased conversion of dopa to melanin
Nonphenolic hypopigmenting agent	Glycolic acid (alpha-hydroxy acid)	Thins stratum corneum, disperses melanin in basal layer of epidermis, enhances epidermolysis, increases collagen synthesis in dermis
Nonphenolic hypopigmenting agent	Kojic acid (produced by fungus *Aspergillus oryzae*)	Inhibitor of tyrosinase
Nonphenolic hypopigmenting agent	Azelaic acid (saturated dicarboxylic acid)	Reversible inhibitor of tyrosinase; inhibits mitochondrial respiration
Nonphenolic hypopigmenting agent	Tretinoin (retinoid)	Enhances keratinocyte proliferation and increases epidermal cell turnover
Chemical peel	Glycolic acid peel	Thins stratum corneum, disperses melanin in basal layer of epidermis, enhances epidermolysis, increases collagen synthesis in dermis
Laser	Pulsed CO_2 laser with Q-switch alexandrite laser	Pulsed CO_2 laser; resurfacing of epidermis Q-switch alexandrite laser; photothermolysis of melanosomes
Light	Intense pulsed light	High-intensity pulses of broad-band light that are different from narrow-band light of lasers; causes thermal damage; does not damage surface

Adapted from *J Cutan Med Surg* 8(2):97-102, 2004. Epub 2004 May 4. *PMID: 15685388*

First-line therapy is fixed triple combinations (e.g., Tri-Luma cream [fluocinolone acetonide 0.01%, hydroquinone 4%, tretinoin 0.05%]). Patients who do not tolerate triple combination therapy are treated with single agents (4% hydroquinone, retinoic acid, or azelaic acid) or combinations of these agents. Lasers and intense pulsed light may be of some use in patients who fail topical creams.

SUN PROTECTION. UV radiation has a significant effect on the pathogenesis of melasma. Sun exposure must be minimized. Sunscreens that block both UVA and UVB light should be used. Titanium dioxide–and zinc oxide–containing sunscreens reflect UVA and UVB. There are several brands.

HYPOPIGMENTING AGENTS. Hydroquinone is the most effective topically applied bleaching agent. This agent is available in 2% concentrations without prescription (Porcelana) and by prescription in 3% (Melanex) and 4% (Claripel, Eldoquin Forte, Eldopaque Forte, Solaquin Forte, Lustra, Lustra-AF) concentrations (see the Formulary). Higher extemporaneously compounded concentrations of hydroquinone (as high as 10%) can be prescribed for difficult cases. The medication should be applied twice daily—in the morning and before bedtime. Hydroquinone is an irritant and a sensitizer, and skin should be tested for sensitivity before use by applying a small amount to the cheek or arm once each day for 2 days (open patch testing). The development of erythema or vesiculation indicates an allergic reaction and precludes further use. These preparations must be used for months and in many cases result in gradual depigmentation. Skin must be protected with broad-spectrum sunscreens both during and after treatment. Tretinoin (Retin-A) enhances the epidermal penetration of hydroquinone and is often prescribed to be used at a different time of day. Start with a low concentration of tretinoin. Increase the concentration until slight irritation occurs. Hydroquinones also bleach freckles and lentigines but not café-au-lait spots or pigmented nevi.

TRI-LUMA CREAM. Tri-Luma cream is a combination product containing 4.0% hydroquinone, 0.05% tretinoin, and 0.01% fluocinolone acetonide. The recommended course of therapy is daily for 8 weeks. Significant results have been seen after the first 4 weeks of treatment. After 8 weeks of treatment, 13% to 38% of the patients achieved clearing of melasma. It is more effective than any of the single agent treatments. Treatment may be repeated.

TRETINOIN. Topical tretinoin (several concentrations) used alone produces significant clinical improvement of melasma, mainly as a result of reduction in epidermal pigment. Compared with hydroquinone, tretinoin must be applied for a longer time (up to 1 year). Improvement occurs slowly. Significant lightening becomes evident after 24 weeks. Tazarotene creams or gels may be more effective that tretinoin.

AZELAIC ACID. Azelaic acid (Finacea is 15% azelaic acid) is used to treat acne and melasma. It has selective effects on hyperactive and abnormal melanocytes and minimal effects on normally pigmented human skin, freckles, and senile lentigines. It is reported to be as effective as 4% hydroquinone. Azelaic acid with tretinoin causes more skin lightening after 3 months than azelaic acid alone. Azelaic acid is applied twice daily for several (up to 8) months; lightening starts after 1 to 2 months. Both 20% azelaic acid and 4% hydroquinone are equally effective. There is initial and transitory irritation but the medication is well tolerated and safe for use during pregnancy.

KOJIC ACID. Kojic acid (KA) is an antibiotic produced by many species of *Aspergillus* and *Penicillium* that inhibits tyrosinase. KA is used in 1% to 4% preparations, twice daily for 2 months; higher concentrations do not improve its depigmenting activity. Contact allergy is reported. It is available over-the-counter.

CHEMICAL PEELS. Superficial, medium, and deep chemical peels are used to treat melasma in lighter-complexioned whites. Trichloroacetic acid and glycolic acid have been used; they are somewhat effective. Darker complexioned individuals are poor candidates for chemical peels because postinflammatory hyperpigmentation frequently occurs.

CRYOSURGERY. Cryosurgery is effective in people with light complexions. It works well in localized spots. Hyperpigmentation and hypopigmentation are possible side effects.

LASERS. Best results are obtained through the combination of pulsed CO_2 laser with Q-switch alexandrite laser. The CO_2 laser destroys melanocytes; the alexandrite laser removes pigment left in the dermis.

INTENSE PULSED LIGHT (IPL). IPL treatment is a good option for patients with melasma. Epidermal melasma treated with two pulses of intense pulsed light can reach a clearance of 76% to 100% from baseline. Individuals with deep pigmented lesions (including mixed melasma) show fair or poor clearance.

Café-au-lait spots

Café-au-lait spots are uniformly pale-brown macules that vary in size from 0.5 to 20 cm and can be found on any cutaneous surface (Figure 19-39) (see also Chapter 26, p. 983). They may be present at birth, are estimated to be present in 10% to 20% of normal children, and increase in number and size with age. Six or more spots greater than 1.5 cm in diameter are presumptive evidence of neurofibromatosis (von Recklinghausen's disease) in young children over 5 years of age. In children under 5 years of age, five or more café-au-lait spots greater than 0.5 cm in diameter suggest the diagnosis of neurofibromatosis. Café-au-lait spots are present in 90% to 100% of patients with von Recklinghausen's disease. Smaller spots 1 to 4 cm in diameter in the axillae (axillary freckling or Crowe's sign) are a rare but diagnostic sign of neurofibromatosis. There is no increased incidence of café-au-lait spots in tuberous sclerosis. Lesions that are similar but that have a more irregular border (shaped like "the coast of Maine") are seen in polyostotic fibrous dysplasia (Albright's syndrome). The smooth, regular border of the café-au-lait macules of neurofibromatosis has been compared with "the coast of California."

Macromelanosomes, or larger-than-normal pigment granules, have been detected with the electron microscope in the café-au-lait spots of some patients with neurofibromatosis, but their absence does not rule out the diagnosis. Café-au-lait spots cannot be lightened by hydroquinone bleaching agents. Q-switched laser and erbium:YAG laser treatments have been reported to be effective.

Diabetic dermopathy

Diabetic dermopathy is the most common cutaneous marker of diabetes mellitus and is present in 40% of diabetic patients.

There is an unfavorable association with the three most common microangiopathic complications of diabetes mellitus: neuropathy, nephropathy, and retinopathy. A relationship between diabetic dermopathy and coronary artery disease has also been demonstrated. Diabetic dermopathy is a clinical sign of an increased likelihood of internal complications in diabetic patients, such as retinopathy, neuropathy, and nephropathy.

Lesions are asymptomatic, round, atrophic, hyperpigmented areas on the shins (shin spots). They begin as round-to-oval, flat-topped, red, scaly papules that may become eroded. The lesions eventually clear or heal with epidermal atrophy or hyperpigmentation. They may also appear on the forearms, the anterior surface of the lower thighs, and the sides of the feet. Men are affected twice as often as women. They may be initiated by trauma.

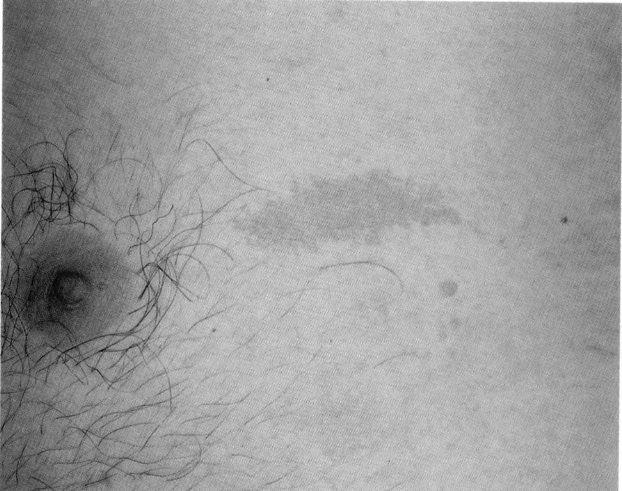

Figure 19-39 Café-au-lait spots. Irregular brown macules that are found in 10% to 20% of normal children. Number and size are increased in neurofibromatosis.

Erythema ab igne

Chronic exposure to heat from a wood stove, fireplace, electric blanket, electric heater, hot water bottle, laptop computer, or hot compress may cause a distinctive cutaneous eruption with a reticular pattern. The eruption initially appears as bands of erythema, but brown hyperpigmentation develops with repeated exposure (Figure 19-40).

Erythema ab igne may develop in patients who apply local heat or hot water bottles to painful metastatic and primary tumors.

The pigmentation, caused by melanin, may fade in time or may be permanent. The eruption must be differentiated from livido reticularis, which occurs with diseases such as leukocytoclastic vasculitis. Livido reticularis is a reddish purple reticular pigmentation, probably caused by restricted blood flow through the horizontal venous plexus. The color persists, but brown hyperpigmentation does not occur.

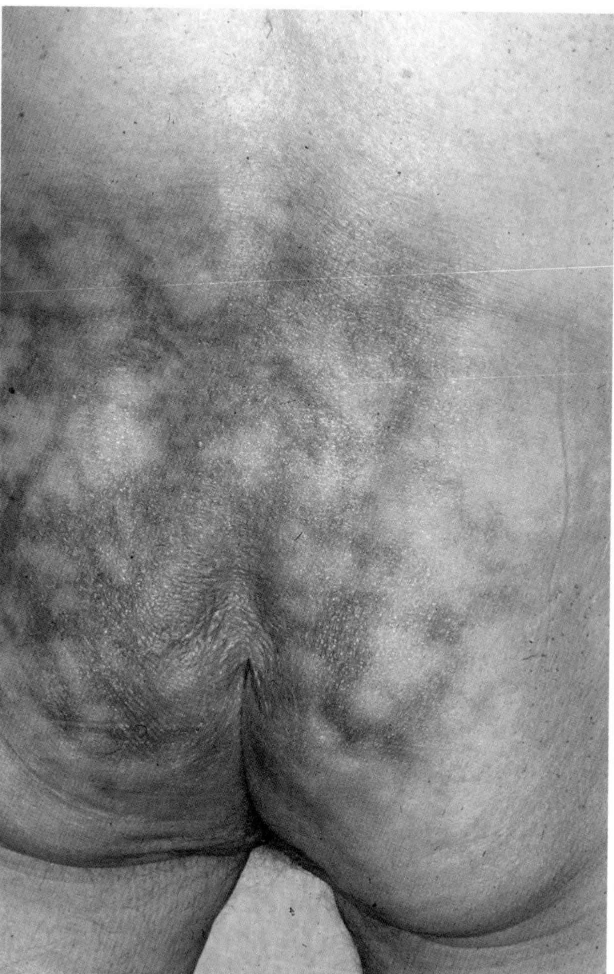

Figure 19-40 Erythema ab igne. Reticular brown hyperpigmentation that develops in areas chronically exposed to heat. A heating pad used for several months produced the eruption depicted here.

Chapter 20

Benign Skin Tumors

CHAPTER CONTENTS

- Seborrheic keratosis
- Stucco keratoses
- Skin tags (acrochordon) and polyps
- Dermatosis papulosa nigra
- Cutaneous horn
- Dermatofibroma
- Hypertrophic scars and keloids
- Keratoacanthoma
- Epidermal nevus
- Nevus sebaceous
- Chondrodermatitis nodularis helicis
- Epidermal cyst
- Pilar cyst (wen)
- Senile sebaceous hyperplasia
- Syringoma

SEBORRHEIC KERATOSIS

Seborrheic keratosis (SK) and nevi are the most common benign cutaneous neoplasms. SKs are of unknown origin and have no malignant potential. One must be familiar with all of the characteristics and variants of these lesions to differentiate them from other lesions and to prevent unnecessary destructive procedures. SKs can be easily and quickly removed and, if the procedure is correctly executed, heal with little or no scarring. Most people develop at least one SK at some point in their lives. SKs appear in a substantial proportion of people younger than 30 years. The term senile keratosis is no longer appropriate for these lesions. The number varies from less than 20 in most individuals to numerous lesions. They can occur on any hair-bearing surface on the face, trunk, extremities, and genitals. They do not occur on the lips, palms, or soles. Patients refer to them as warts, but SKs do not contain human papillomaviruses.

SURFACE CHARACTERISTICS. The surface of SKs is either smooth with tiny, round, embedded pearls or rough, dry, and cracked. SKs are sharply circumscribed and vary from 0.2 cm to more than 3 cm in diameter. They appear to be stuck to the skin surface and, in fact, occur totally within the epidermis. The surface characteristics vary with the age of the lesion and its location. Those on the extremities are often subtle, flat, or minimally raised and are slightly scaly with accentuated skin lines. Lesions on the face and trunk vary considerably in appearance, but the characteristics common to all lesions are the well-circumscribed border, the stuck-on appearance, and the variable tan-brown-black color (Figures 20-1, 20-2, and 20-5 to 20-8). When the border is irregular and notched, the SK resembles a malignant melanoma.

Smooth or rough surfaced. The surface characteristics show considerable variation (see Figures 20-3 and 20-4). Smooth-surfaced, dome-shaped tumors have white or black pearls of keratin, are 1 mm in diameter, and are embedded in the surface. These horn pearls are easily seen with a hand lens. The presence of horn cysts on the surface helps to confirm the diagnosis of an SK. Horn cysts are also found on the surface of some dermal nevi. The rough-surfaced SKs are the most common. They are oval-to-round, flattened domes with a granular or irregular surface that crumbles when picked.

SEBORRHEIC KERATOSIS

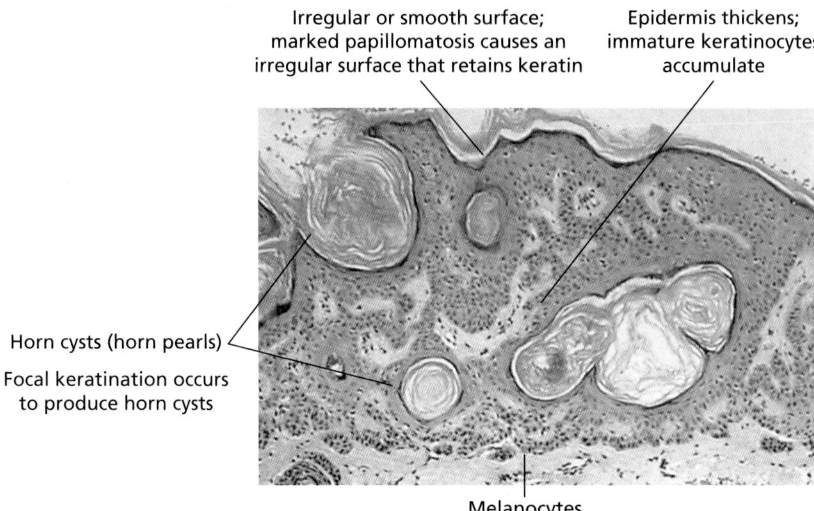

Figure 20-1 Cross-section shows embedded horn cysts.

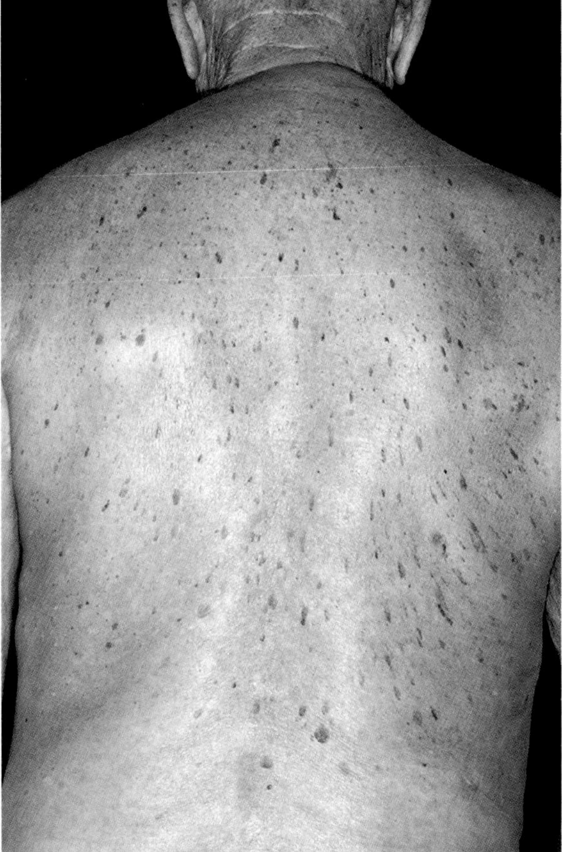

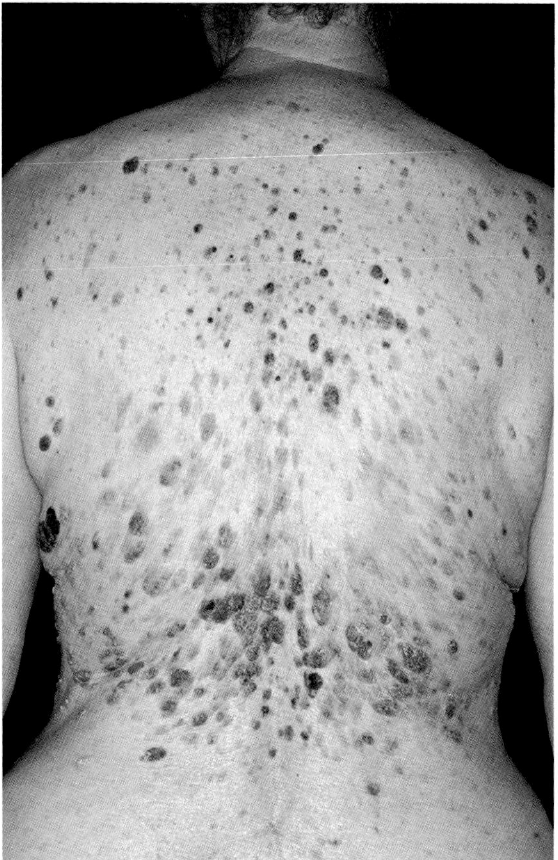

Figure 20-2 Lesions are very common on the back; an individual may have numerous lesions on the sun-exposed back and none on the buttocks.

SEBORRHEIC KERATOSIS—ROUGH SURFACE LESIONS

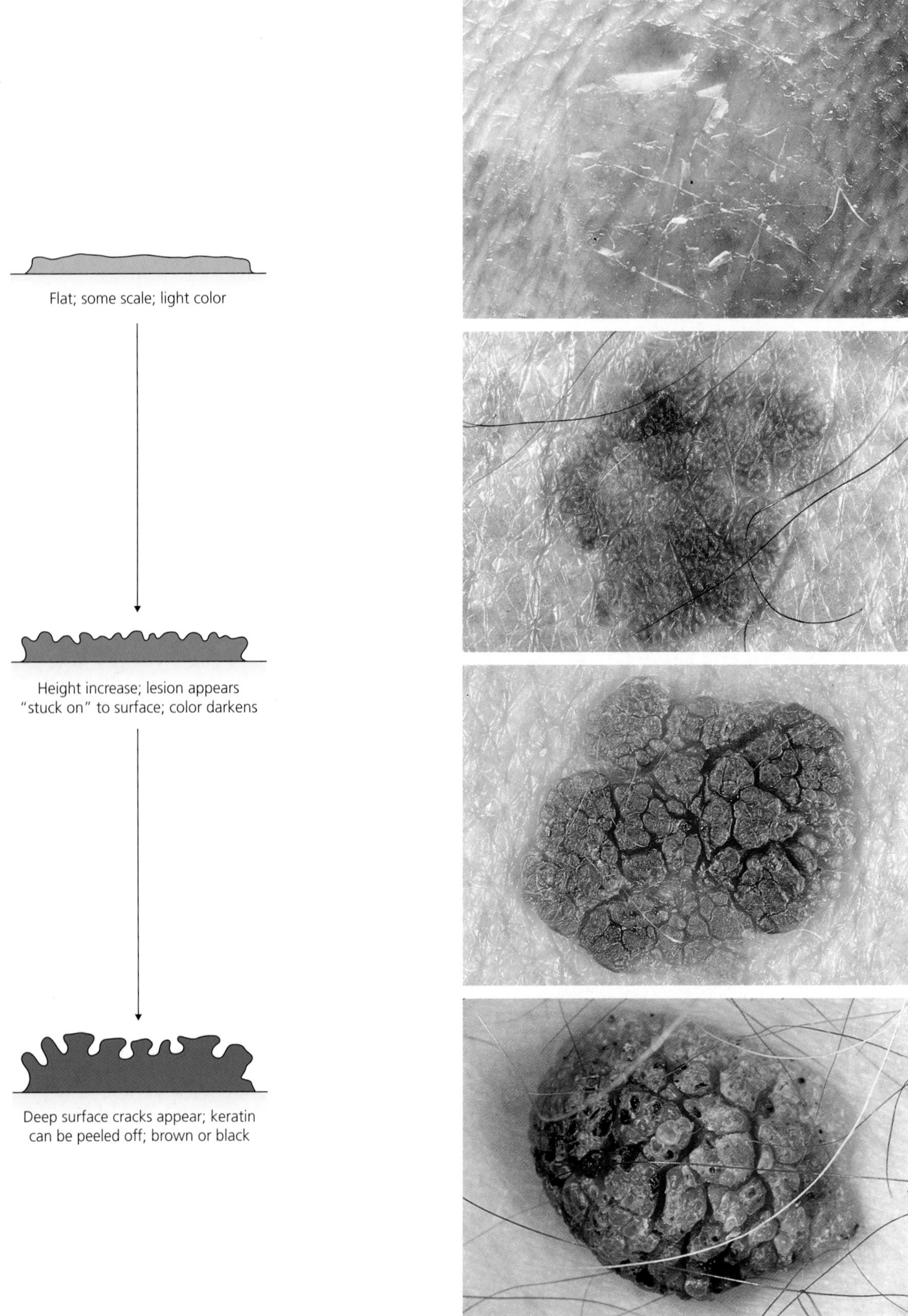

Figure 20-3

SEBORRHEIC KERATOSIS—SMOOTH SURFACE LESIONS

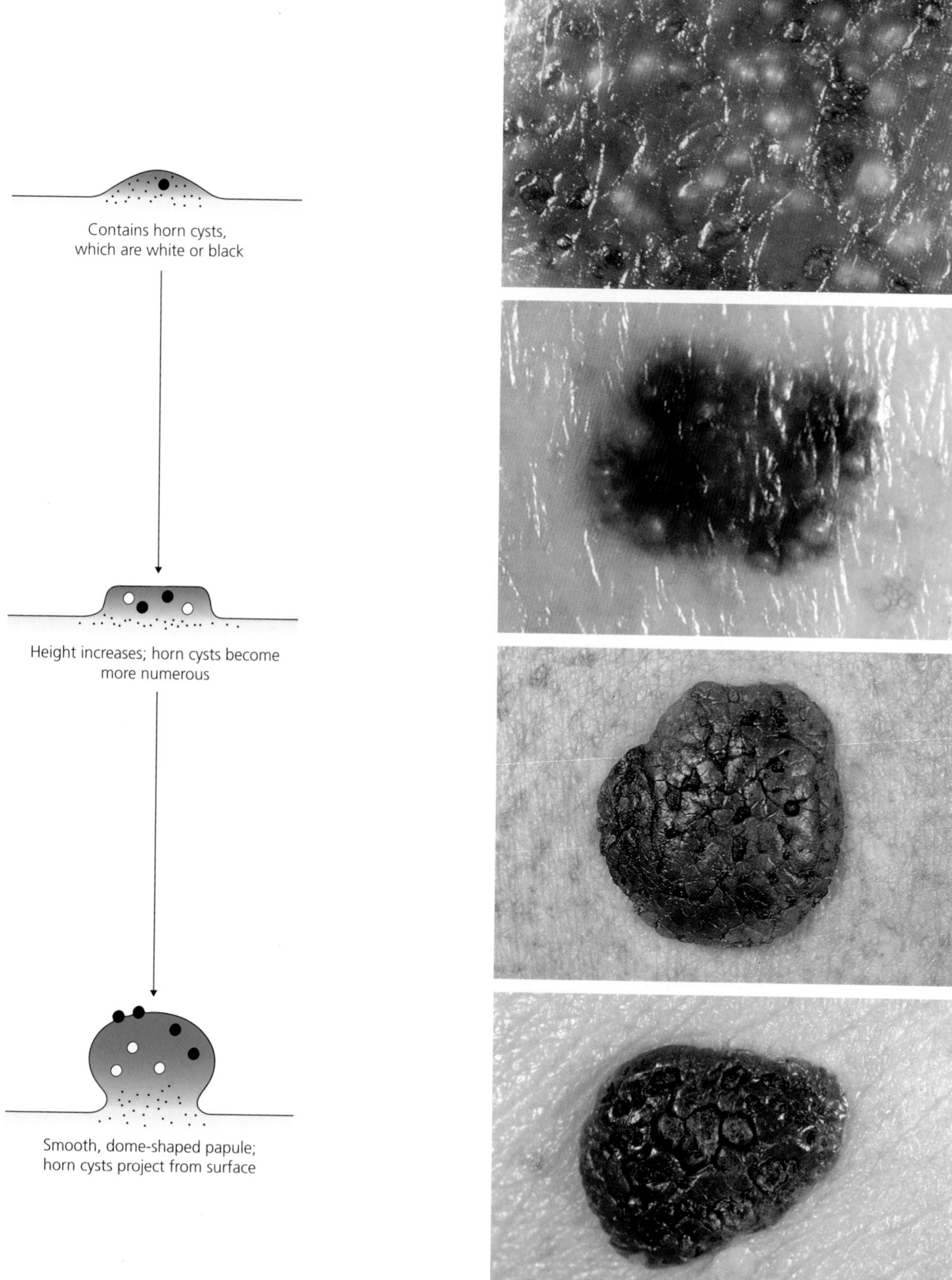

Figure 20-4

SEBORRHEIC KERATOSIS

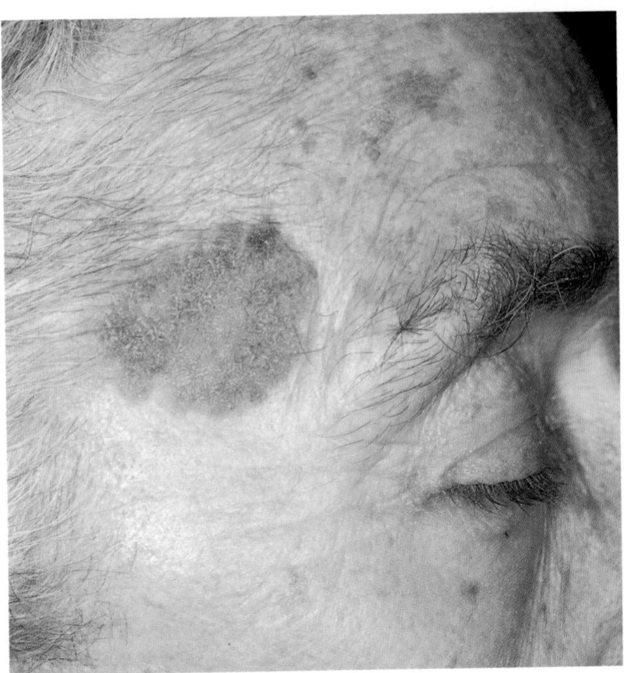

Figure 20-5 Very large lesions may form along the hairline and temple. Flat lesions are usually brown.

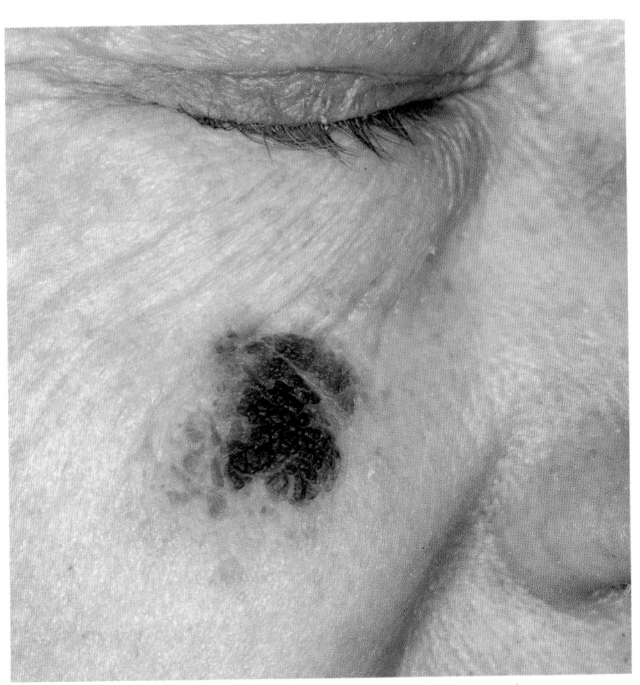

Figure 20-6 Thicker lesions may become dark brown or black.

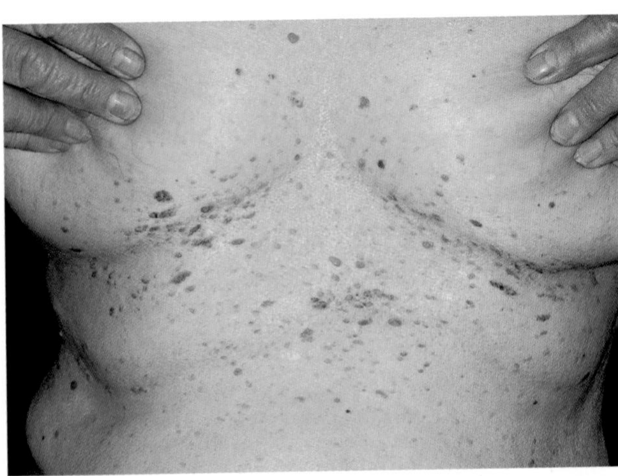

Figure 20-7 Lesions are commonly found under the breasts. Maceration may cause keratosis to become red and irritated.

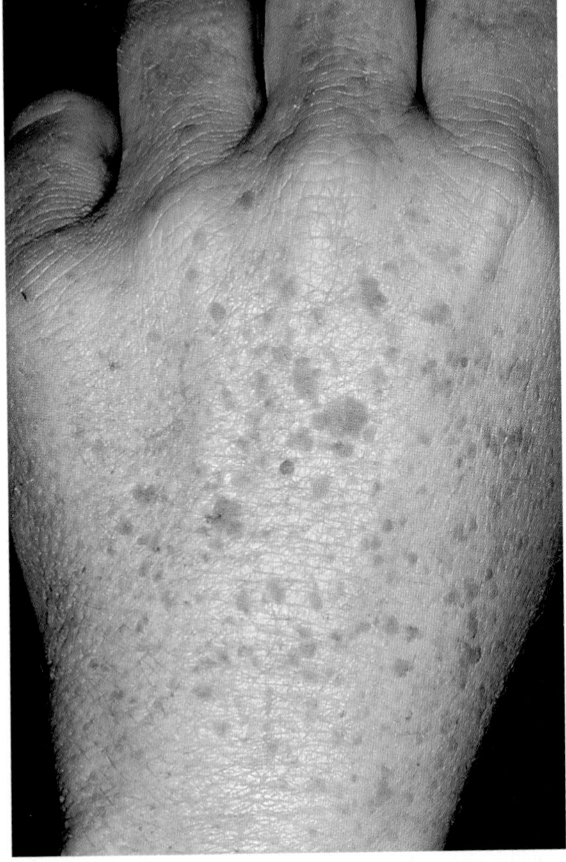

Figure 20-8 Sun exposure causes keratosis on the back of the hand in predisposed individuals.

SEBORRHEIC KERATOSIS VS. MALIGNANT MELANOMA. Many patients present with dark, irregular, sometimes irritated SKs and worry that they are melanomas. SKs can show many of the features of a malignant melanoma, including an irregular border and variable pigmentation (Figures 20-9 to 20-12). The key differential diagnostic features are the surface characteristics. Melanomas have a smooth surface that varies in elevation and in color, density, and shade. SKs preserve a uniform appearance over their entire surface. Examination with a hand lens is very helpful. Many SKs occur in sun-exposed areas.

ACCURACY OF DIAGNOSIS. When a clinical diagnosis of SK is made with confidence, the lesion is often left untreated or a destructive method of removal is used. The diagnostic accuracy must be high to justify such practices, which do not yield material for histopathologic confirmation. A diagnostic accuracy of greater than 99% was established by dermatologists in a study. The extremely high diagnostic accuracy of greater than 99% justifies common clinical practice. A biopsy should be performed in cases of diagnostic doubt. Submit all specimens that have been removed for histologic examination.

MELANOMA MIMICS

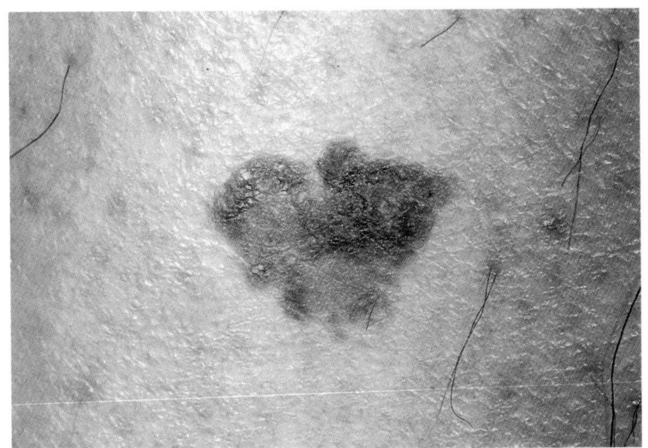

Figure 20-9 There is variation in pigmentation, and the border is irregular and notched, but the surface is regular with dense keratin.

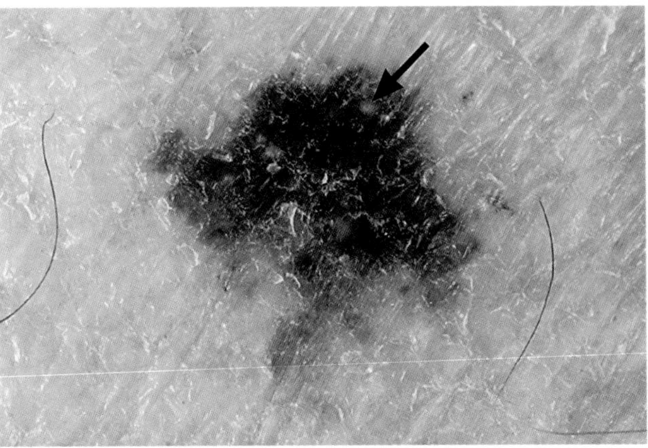

Figure 20-10 This black irregular lesion resembles a melanoma. The white horn pearl imbedded in the surface *(arrow)* supports the diagnosis of seborrheic keratosis.

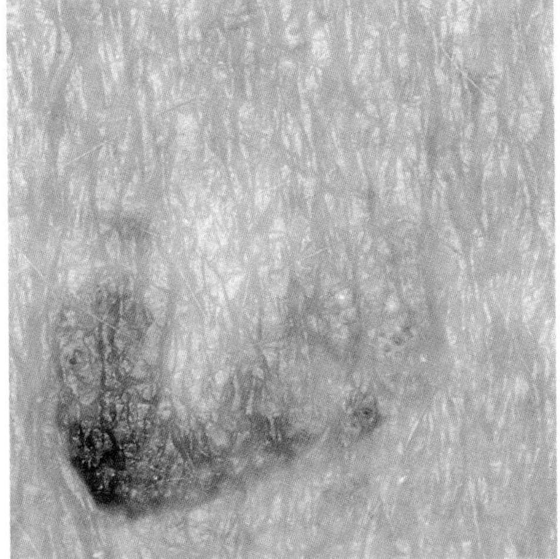

Figure 20-11 This flat lesion has many features of a superficial spreading melanoma. The colors are variable and the white area looks like an area of tumor regression.

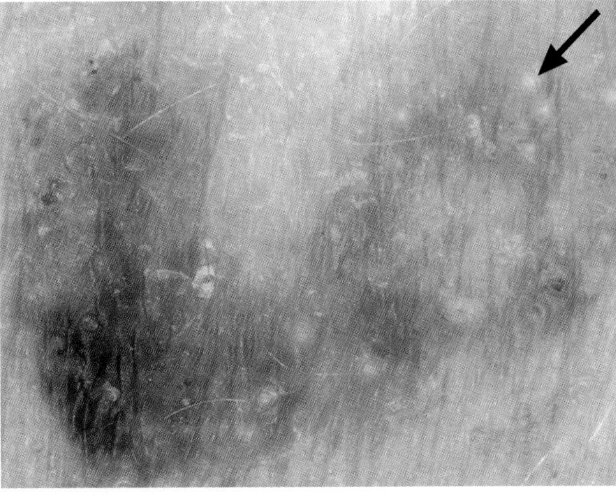

Figure 20-12 A magnified view shows several horn cysts *(arrow)* that are typically found in seborrheic keratosis and rarely present in melanoma.

IRRITATED SEBORRHEIC KERATOSIS. Although generally asymptomatic, SKs can be a source of itching, especially in the elderly, who have a tendency to unconsciously manipulate these protruding growths. Irritation can be aggravated by chafing from clothing or from maceration in intertriginous areas, such as under the breasts and in the groin. When inflamed, SKs become slightly swollen and develop an irregular, red flare in the surrounding skin. Itching and erythema can then appear spontaneously in other SKs that have not been manipulated (Figures 20-13 and 20-14) and in areas without SKs. A halo of eczema can appear around SKs; the inflamed border is red and scaly and may represent a localized form of nummular (coin-shaped) dermatitis. The only treatment is to apply topical steroids or to remove all inflamed lesions. With continued inflammation, the SK loses most of its normal characteristics and becomes a bright red, oozing mass with a friable surface that itches intensely and resembles an advanced melanoma or a pyogenic granuloma.

IRRITATED SEBORRHEIC KERATOSIS—LOCALIZED

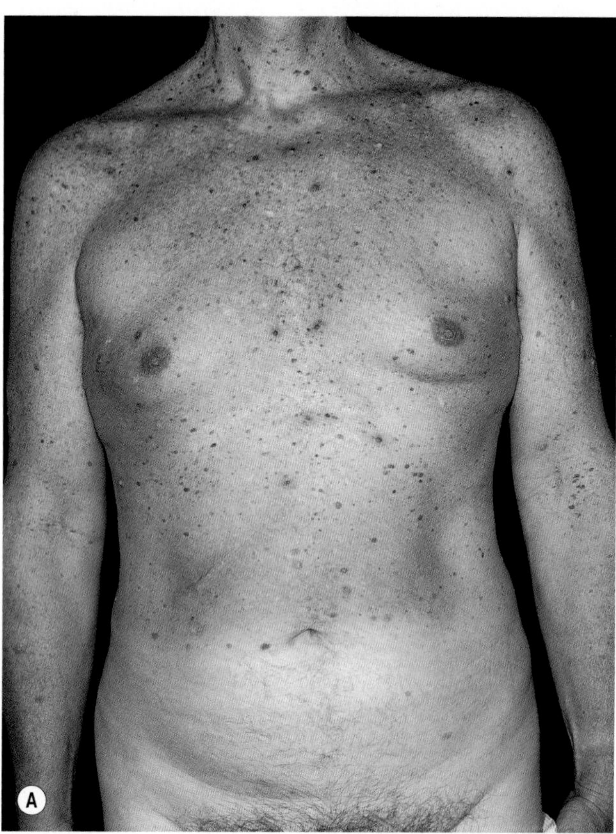

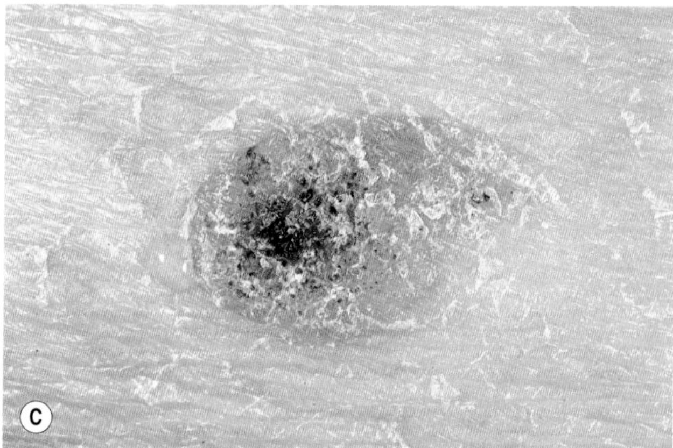

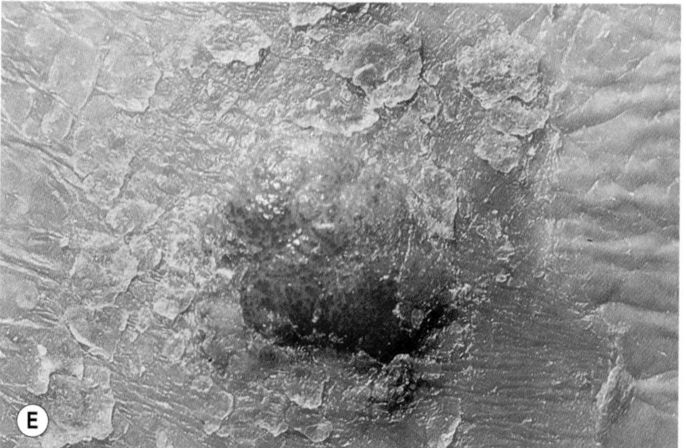

Figure 20-13 Irritated seborrheic keratosis—localized. **A,** Most lesions are solitary but many keratoses may become inflamed at once. **B,** Minimal inflammation at the base. **C,** Surface characteristics are less distinct as inflammation intensifies. **D,** Dense scale and crust obliterate diagnostic features. **E,** This red, oozing mass has lost all diagnostic characteristics and resembles a pyogenic granuloma or melanoma.

IRRITATED SEBORRHEIC KERATOSIS—GENERALIZED

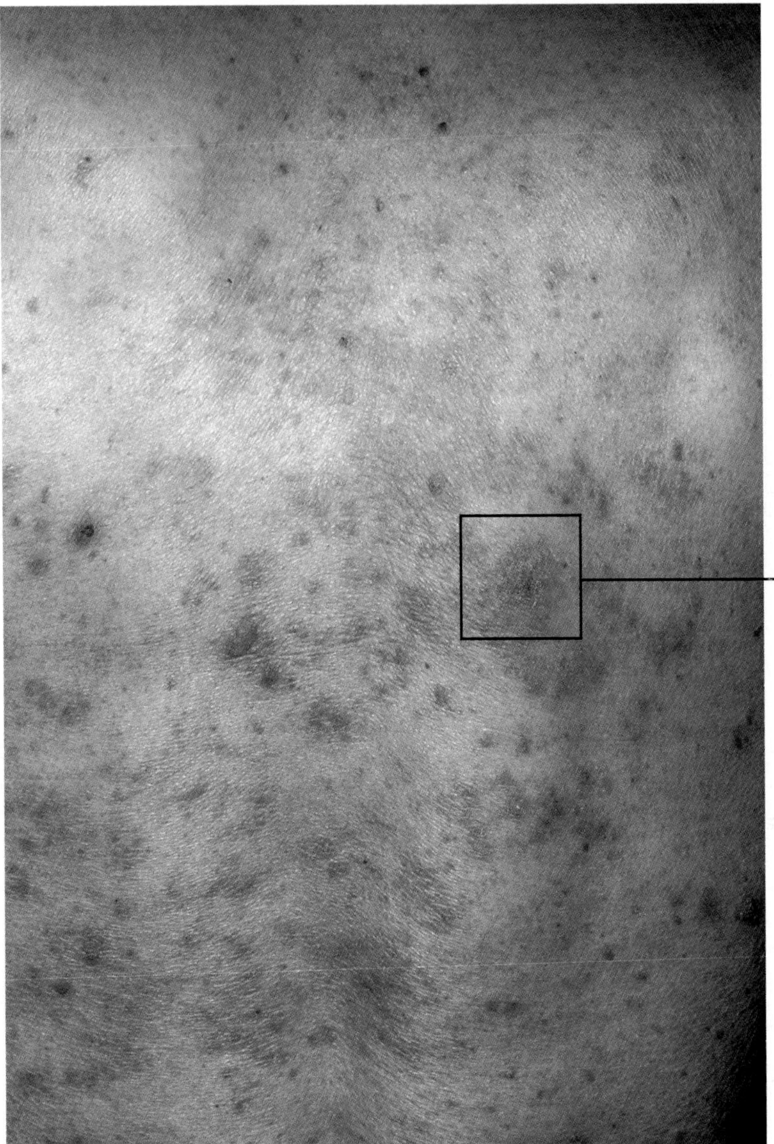

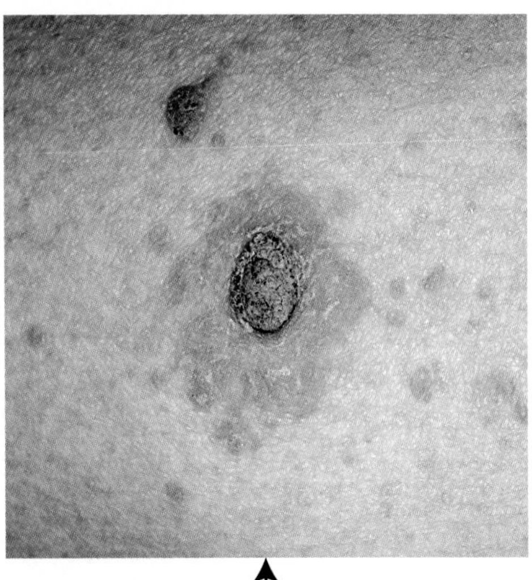

Figure 20-14 Irritated seborrheic keratosis. A single lesion may become inflamed and progress to form a peripheral ring of erythema. A few to numerous other lesions then become inflamed, and redness and swelling may extend to broad areas of the skin surface. Attempts to control the eruption with oral steroids or strong topical steroids are often only partially effective. One approach is to treat with group II topical steroids and exercise suit occlusion (see Chapter 2). Once the inflammation is controlled, the keratosis must be destroyed. Several sessions of cryotherapy are effective.

LESER-TRÉLAT SIGN (ERUPTIVE SEBORRHEIC KERATOSIS AS A SIGN OF INTERNAL MALIGNANCY). The sudden appearance of or sudden increase in the number and size of SKs on noninflamed skin has been reported to be a sign of internal malignancy (see Figure 26-23).

TREATMENT. Lesions are removed for cosmetic purposes or to eliminate a source of irritation. Since these growths appear entirely within the epidermis, scalpel excision is unnecessary. They are easily removed with cryosurgery or curettage. Lesions to be curetted are first anesthetized with Xylocaine introduced with a needle. With multiple strokes, a small curette is smoothly drawn through the lesion (see Chapter 27). SKs on the face or on other areas with inappreciable underlying support can be softened before curettage with the electric needle. Monsel's solution controls bleeding, and the site remains exposed to heal. Some lesions are tenaciously fixed to the skin and resist curettage; others are on sites that are difficult to curette, such as the eyelid. These can be dissected with curved, blunt-tipped scissors. Cryosurgery is effective for thin SKs but posttreatment hyperpigmentation or hypopigmentation is a possible side effect.

STUCCO KERATOSES

Stucco keratoses, sometimes referred to as barnacles, are common, nearly inconspicuous, papular, warty lesions occurring on the lower legs (Figure 20-15), especially around the Achilles tendon area, the dorsum of the foot, and the forearms of the elderly. The 1- to 10-mm, round, very dry, stuck-on lesions are considered by most patients to be simply manifestations of dry skin. The dry surface scale is easily picked intact from the skin without bleeding, but it recurs shortly thereafter. The lesions can be removed with curettage or cryosurgery.

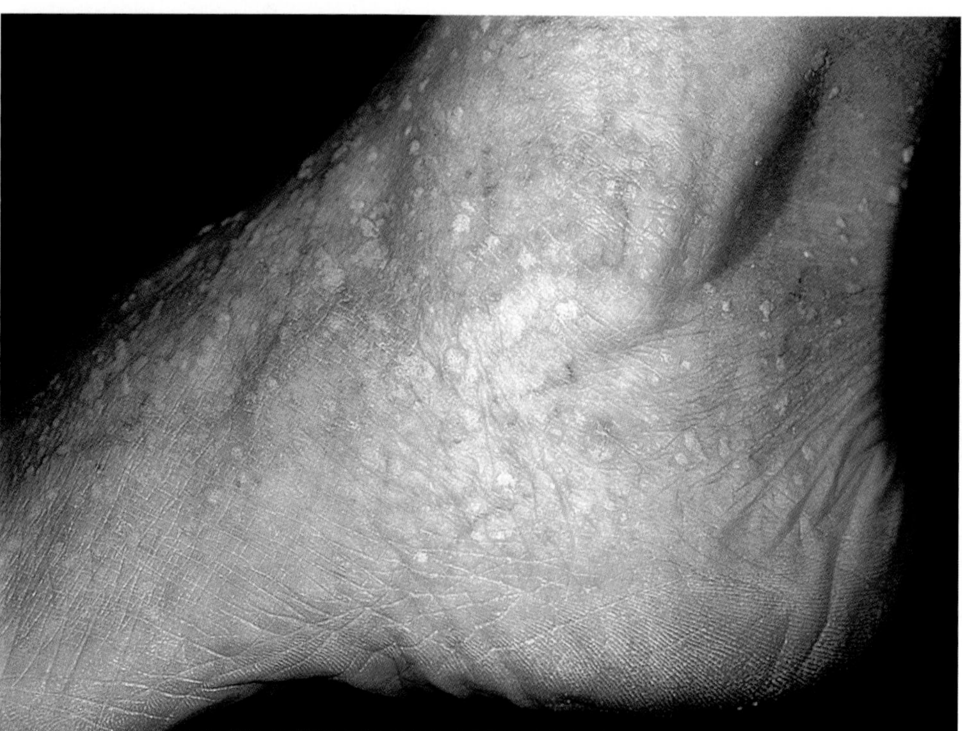

Figure 20-15 Stucco keratoses. Multiple small, scaling lesions in a typical location.

SKIN TAGS (ACROCHORDON) AND POLYPS

SKIN TAGS. Skin tags are common tumors found in approximately 25% of males and females. They occur more often and in greater number in obese patients. The most frequent affected area is the axilla (48%), followed by the neck (35%) and inguinal region. The majority of carriers (71%) have no more than three skin tags per location. They can begin in the second decade, with a steady increase in frequency up to the fifth decade; above this age there is no further growth. The skin tags begin as a tiny, brown or skin-colored, oval excrescence attached by a short, broad-to-narrow stalk (Figures 20-16 to 20-19). With time, the tumor can increase to 1 cm as the stalk becomes long and narrow. Patients complain that when they wear clothing or jewelry, these tumors are annoying. The stalks are easily removed by scissor excision or with a light touch of the electrocautery. Local anesthesia is usually not necessary.

POLYPS. Skin polyps have a long, narrow stalk and a broad tip (Figures 20-20 to 20-22). Sometimes they become twisted and compromise the blood supply. Lesions then turn dark brown or black. This sudden change is alarming to patients (see Figure 20-22). Polypoid growths may be skin tags, nevi, or melanomas. Polyps occur on the eyelids (see Figure 20-16), groin, axilla, or any skin surface except the palms and soles.

SKIN TAGS AND COLONIC POLYPS. A series of articles claimed that there is an association between skin tags and adenomatous polyps. A study of 150 consecutive patients who underwent colonoscopy concluded that skin tags as markers of colon neoplasms are insufficient to warrant endoscopic examination.

SKIN TAGS AND POLYPS

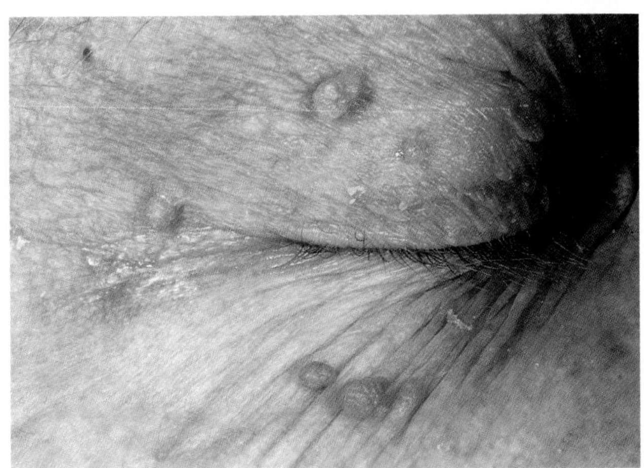

Figure 20-16 Skin tags and polyps are frequently present on the lids.

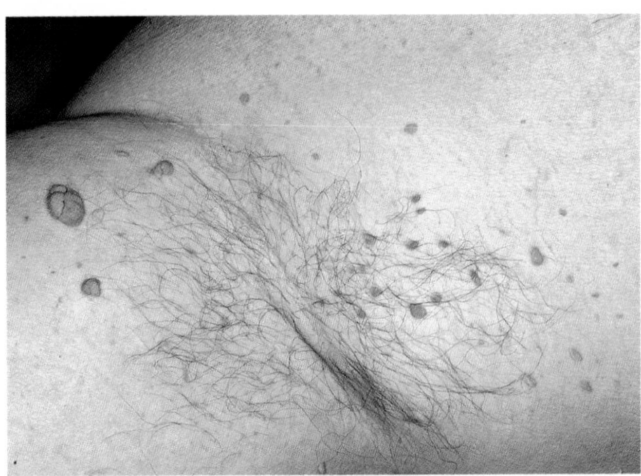

Figure 20-17 Skin tags are commonly found in the axillae. There is great variation in the number of lesions.

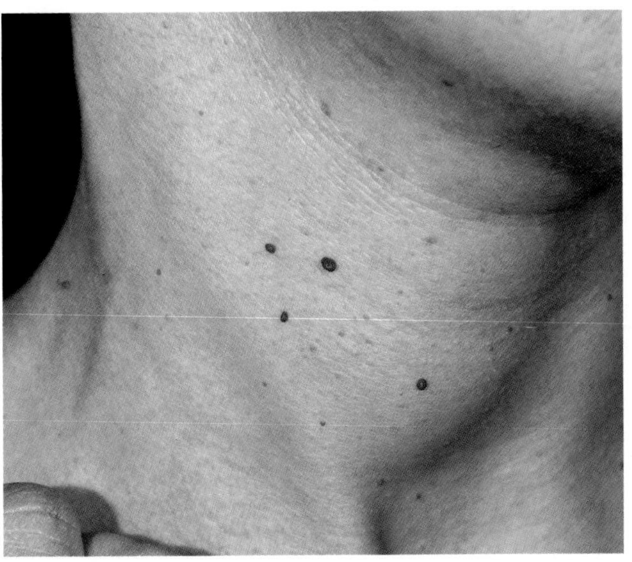

Figure 20-18 Multiple round, black, oval excrescences attached by a short broad-to-narrow stalk.

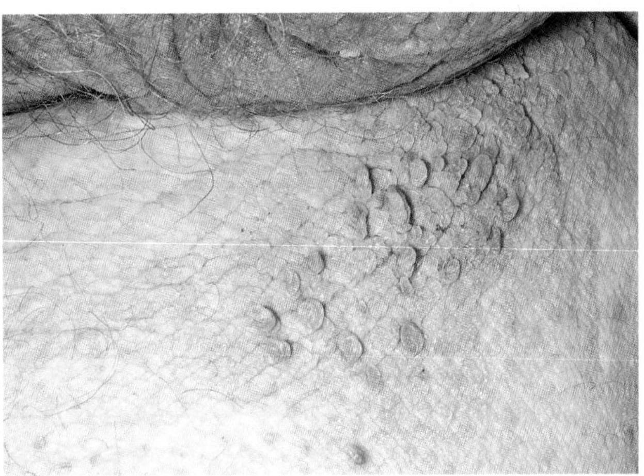

Figure 20-19 Skin tags may be numerous in the groin. Obesity predisposes to this dense clustered pattern.

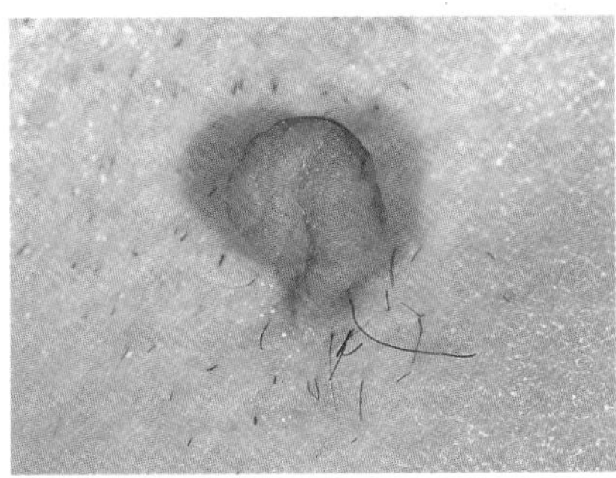

Figure 20-20 A polypoid mass on a long, narrow stalk. Some nevi have an identical appearance.

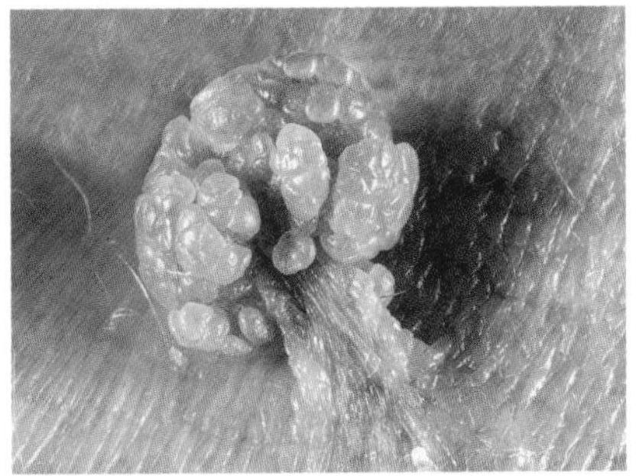

Figure 20-21 Polyps contain a long stalk and a broad tip. A biopsy showed this lesion to be a dermal nevus.

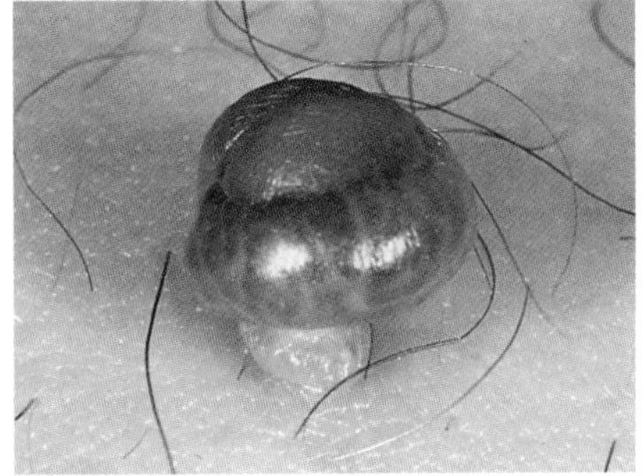

Figure 20-22 Infarcted polyp. Torsion on the stalk can compromise the blood supply. Lesions turn blue-black in hours to days.

DERMATOSIS PAPULOSA NIGRA

Young and middle-aged blacks may develop multiple brown-black, 2- to 3-mm, smooth, dome-shaped papules on the face (Figure 20-23) in a photodistribution. The average age of onset is 22 years. There is a female predominance and family predisposition. They probably represent a type of seborrheic keratosis. Patients who desire removal should be informed that white, hypopigmented scarring may result. The patient's response should be determined by curetting or freezing one or two lesions and permitting them to heal completely. EMLA (a mixture of lidocaine 2.5% and prilocaine 2.5%) may be applied under occlusion for 30 minutes to provide anesthesia before electrodesiccation of the superficial skin lesions.

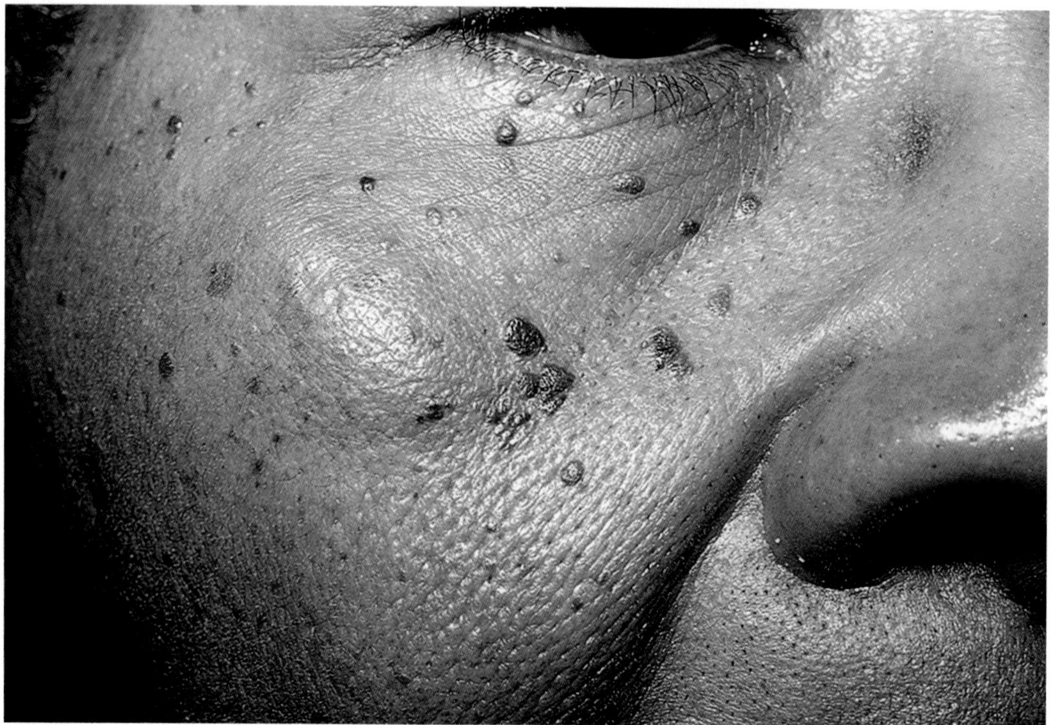

Figure 20-23 Dermatosis papulosa nigra. Lesions begin after puberty in blacks and slowly increase in number. They are smooth, brown-black papules that occur on the malar area of the face and forehead.

CUTANEOUS HORN

Cutaneous horn refers to a hard, conical projection composed of keratin and resembling an animal horn. It occurs on the face, ears, and hands (Figure 20-24) and may become very long. Warts, SKs, actinic keratosis, and squamous cell carcinoma may all retain keratin and produce horns. Cryosurgery, local scissor excision, or surgical excision are forms of treatment.

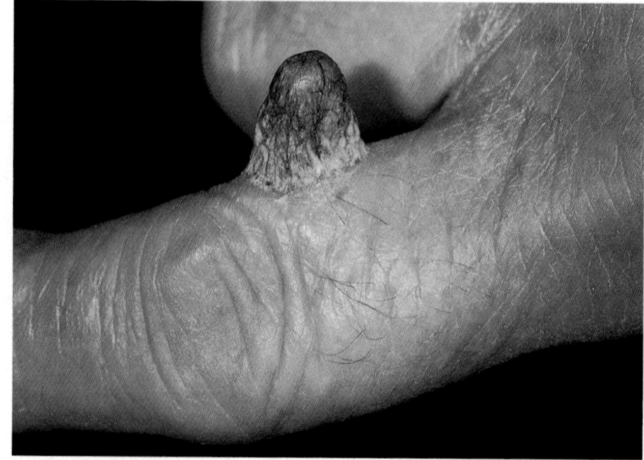

Figure 20-24 Cutaneous horn. A biopsy showed this lesion to be an actinic keratosis.

DERMATOFIBROMA

Dermatofibromas are common, benign, asymptomatic to slightly itchy lesions occurring more frequently in females. They vary in number from 1 to 10 and can be found anywhere on the extremities and trunk, but they are most likely to occur on the anterior surface of the lower legs. Dermatofibromas may not be tumors; rather, they may represent a fibrous reaction to trauma, a viral infection, or an insect bite. They appear as 3- to 10-mm, slightly raised, pink-brown, sometimes scaly, hard growths that retract beneath the skin surface during attempts to compress and elevate them with the thumb and index finger (Figures 20-25 to 20-28). Multiple dermatofibromas (i.e., more than 15) are very rare but have been reported with systemic lupus erythematosus, with and without immunosuppressive therapy. Dermatoscopic examination shows a central, white, scarlike patch and a delicate pigment network at the periphery (see Figure 20-27).

TREATMENT. Some patients object to the color of the lesion and therefore request excision. These lesions are most commonly found on the lower legs, where elliptic excisions closed with sutures may result in wide, unsightly scars. An alternative is to shave the brown surface with a #15 surgical blade and allow the wound to granulate and reepithelialize. The healed area remains hard because a portion of the fibrous tissue has remained. The brown color may reappear in some lesions. Conservative cryosurgery may also eliminate the color and part of the tumor.

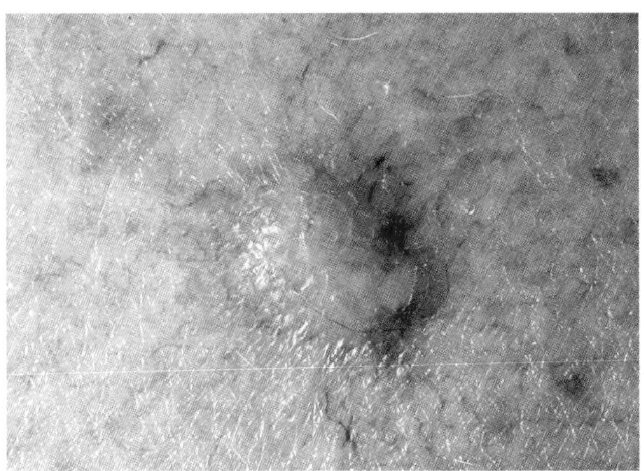

Figure 20-25 Early lesions have a well-defined border with an irregular red surface. Brown pigmentation may occur at the periphery after months or years. Pigmentation may extend onto the lesion but almost never reaches the center. Patients often suspect melanoma at this stage.

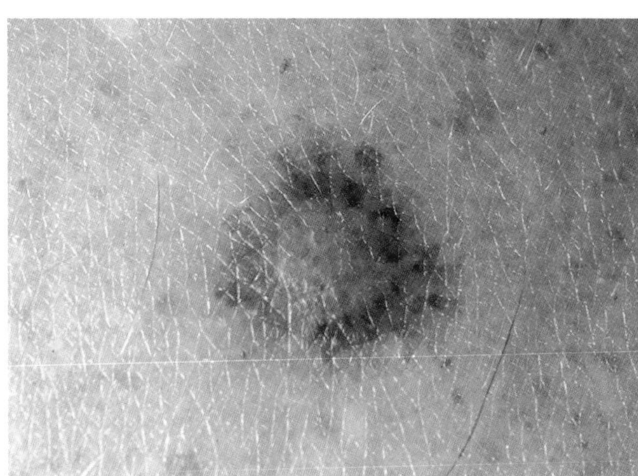

Figure 20-26 A typical lesion on the lower leg that is slightly elevated, round, and hyperpigmented, with a scaling surface.

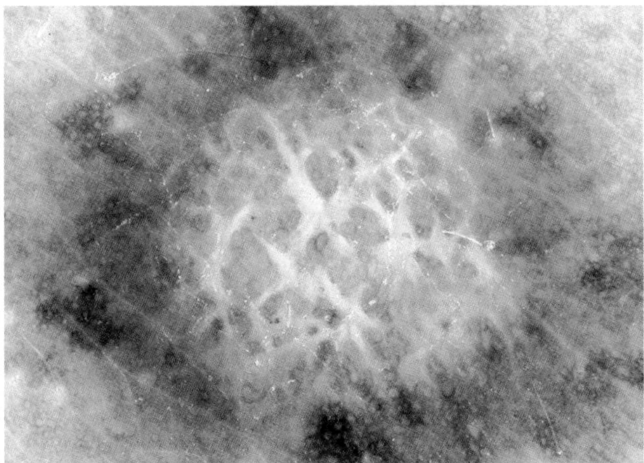

Figure 20-27 Dermoscopy (see Chapter 22) reveals a white lacy center surrounded by a uniform network.

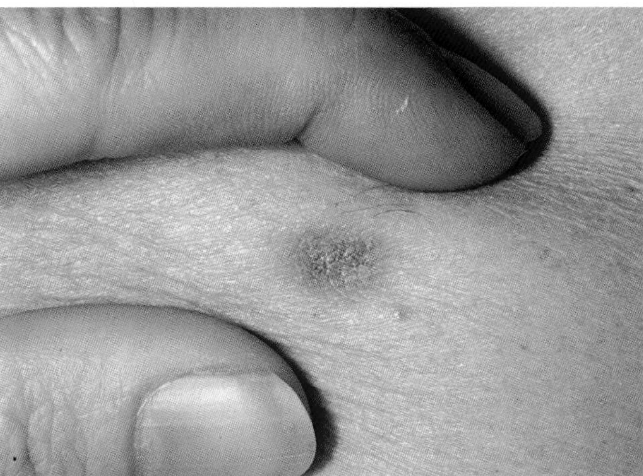

Figure 20-28 Retraction sign. Dermatofibromas retract beneath the skin during attempts to compress and elevate them.

HYPERTROPHIC SCARS AND KELOIDS

Injury or surgery in a predisposed individual can result in an abnormally large scar. A hypertrophic scar is inappropriately large but remains confined to the wound site and in time regresses; a keloid extends beyond the margins of injury (Figures 20-29 to 20-32) and usually is constant and stable without any tendency to subside. Hypertrophic scars may regress with time and occur earlier after injury (usually within 4 weeks); keloidal scars may begin later, even years after the event. There are histologic differences between hypertrophic scars and keloids. Large collagen bundles occur in keloidal scars but not in hypertrophic scars. Keloids are often symptomatic, and complaints arise because of tenderness, pain, and hyperesthesia, particularly in the early stages of development. Keloids are most common on the shoulders and chest, but they may occur on any skin surface. Blacks are more susceptible and sometimes are victims of facial keloids. Some patients with cystic acne of the back and chest form numerous keloidal scars.

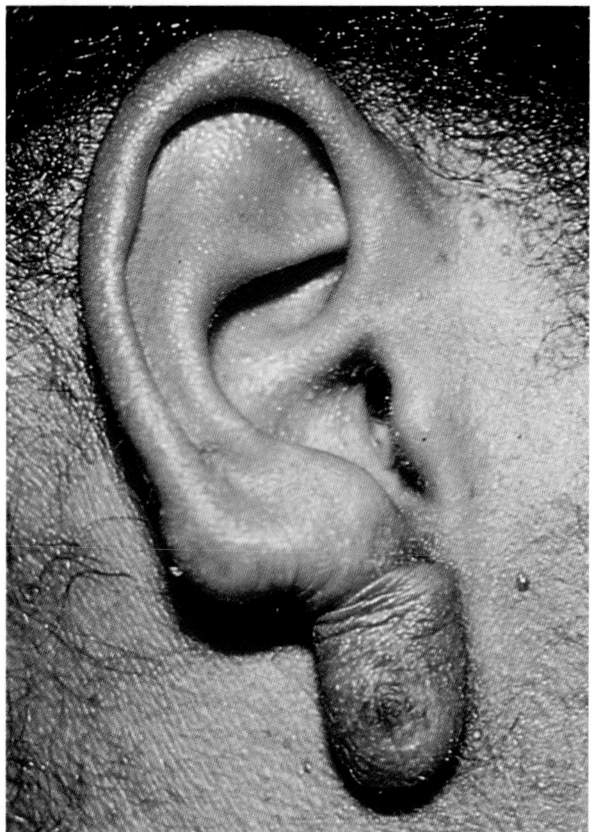

Figure 20-29 Keloid. Huge keloids may form on the earlobes after any surgical procedure.

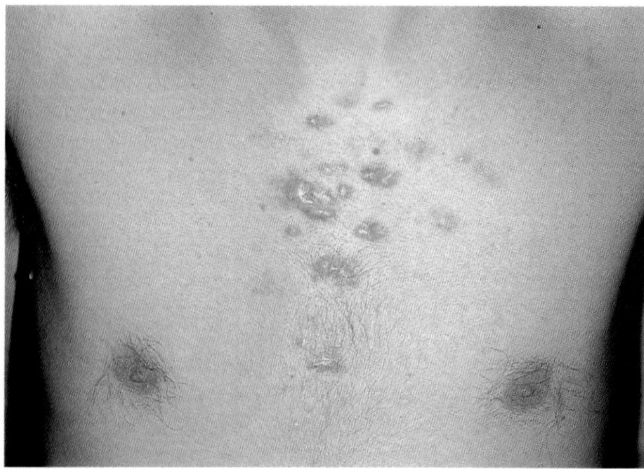

Figure 20-30 Keloids form in predisposed individuals following cystic acne.

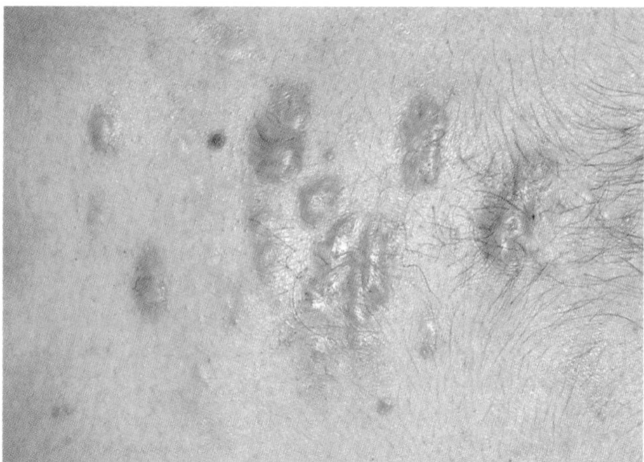

Figure 20-31 Keloids on the chest and extremities are raised with a flat surface. The base is wider than the top.

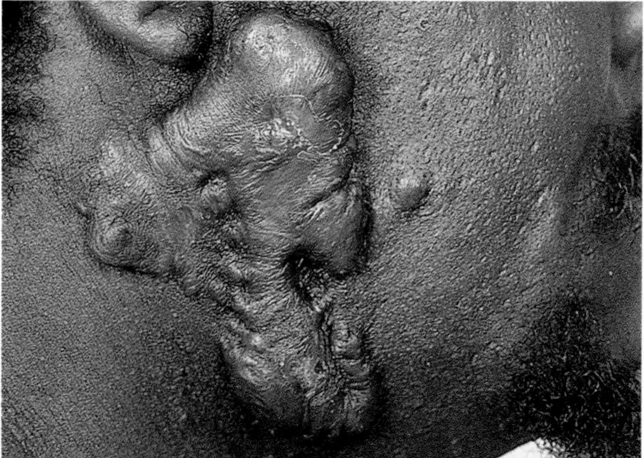

Figure 20-32 Blacks develop keloids most commonly on the earlobes and face.

TREATMENT. There is no routinely effective therapy for all keloids, but a variety of treatment methods exists, including intralesional steroid injection, surgical correction, cryotherapy, compression therapy, and irradiation. High-quality research in evaluating keloid therapy is lacking. *PMID: 17644502*

INTRALESIONAL STEROID INJECTIONS. Proposed mechanisms of action include inhibition of collagen synthesis, inhibition of keloid fibroblast growth, and fibroblast degeneration. Fresh, small, and narrow lesions are treated with intralesional injections of corticosteroids every 2 to 4 weeks. Early keloids have softer proliferating connective tissue and are more inclined to improve with intralesional injections than are older, inactive lesions. When the lesion shrinks to near the skin surface, the frequency and concentration of injections should be decreased to avoid overcompensation and telangiectasia. Inducing atrophy with an intralesional injection of triamcinolone acetonide (Kenalog) 10 to 40 mg/ml is adequate for most small lesions; a 27- or 30-gauge needle is used. The 40 mg/ml concentration is preferred for most patients. A commonly used program is to use triamcinolone acetonide given with four injections at 1- to 4-week intervals, and is dependent on lesion surface area (1 to 2 cm^2, 20 to 40 mg per course; 2 to 6 cm^2, 40 to 80 mg; 6 to 12 cm^2, 80 to 120 mg; with courses repeated if necessary).

To distribute the suspension evenly, the triamcinolone should be injected while continuously advancing the needle. Particles of steroid that have not been properly dispersed remain visible as white flecks in the scar tissue. The pressure of the injection should be firm until the lesion blanches. Light cryosurgery before the injection facilitates the process. Nitrogen is applied briefly for 2 to 4 seconds until the skin frosts. The keloid is injected 10 to 15 minutes later. This allows better dispersal of the steroid and minimizes deposition into surrounding normal tissue. Intralesional steroids also result in symptomatic relief.

SURGERY AND INTRALESIONAL STEROID INJECTIONS. Surgical excision removes the bulk of the scar and has the potential to replace a broad-based scar with a thin scar. Surgical removal alone is associated with a 55% to 100% recurrence rate, but better results are realized when intralesional steroids are used following surgery. A typical treatment program involves injecting triamcinolone acetonide 10 to 40 mg/ml into the wound edges after excision. Treatment of the healed site is repeated at 2- to 4-week intervals for 6 months.

CRYOTHERAPY. Cryotherapy can produce flattening in some patients. Ischemic damage induced by the freeze-thaw cycle leads to cellular anoxia, with subsequent tissue necrosis, and should lead to a reduction in keloid size. Cryosurgery may be more effective in lesions with greater vascularity. Lesions on the back responded better than those on the chest.

Lesions less than 2 years old respond better. At each treatment session, the entire lesion is treated with two or three freeze-thaw cycles. Lesions require 2 to 10 treatment sessions. A topical antibiotic cream and dressing are applied each day during the 1-month healing process. Side effects are limited to hypopigmentation and atrophy. Cryotherapy has been used with corticosteroid injections. Darker skinned patients are at greater risk for hypopigmentation.

SILICONE GEL SHEETING. The effectiveness of silicone gel sheeting (e.g., Epi-Derm, Sil-K, Cica-Care, ReJuveness, DuraSil, Silastic gel sheeting) and other occlusive dressings in treating keloidal and hypertrophic scars is uncertain. Limited studies suggest that some beneficial effect may exist. It is claimed that these dressings can prevent keloids from recurring after surgery. Silicone gel sheeting is soft, self-adhesive, and semi-occlusive. The mechanism of action is unknown; it might act as an impermeable membrane that keeps the skin hydrated. Sheets are used to cover the entire scar for periods of at least 12 hours each day, and ideally 24 hours for at least 2 months. Beneficial effects are not related to pressure.

RADIATION THERAPY WITH SURGERY. Radiation after surgical excision can prevent recurrence. The most frequently used treatment is superficial x-rays of 900 cGy or greater in fractions given within 10 days of surgery. Radiation is usually given within 24 hours after surgery to subdue the second-generation fibroblasts. It should be performed within 10 days of the surgery and is of no additional benefit when performed before surgery. The recurrence rate after combined surgical excision and postoperative electron beam radiation varied from 8% to 71% in a number of reports. First radiation was performed at an average of 2.1 days after surgery. Ear keloids are considered differently from other keloids, because the required dose of radiation seems lower and cellular responsiveness is more prone to normal fibroblasts. Craniofacial locations such as the neck and upper lip also demonstrate no recurrence rate. Therefore postoperative electron beam irradiation is especially effective in these locations. *PMID: 17912105*

5-FLUOROURACIL. 5-Fluorouracil (5-FU) (50 mg/ml) intralesionally is used in the treatment of inflamed hypertrophic scars, both as an individual agent and with low-dose intralesional corticosteroids plus pulsed dye laser therapy. Frequent initial injections (once to three times weekly) were found to be more efficacious with decreasing frequency (weekly to monthly) during a period of stabilization and resolution of the scars. The combination of 5-FU and Kenalog was more effective and less painful. The addition of the pulsed dye laser treatments simultaneously with injection therapy was found to be most effective.

LASERS. The 585-nm pulsed dye laser is effective in reducing symptoms and erythema. Multiple treatment sessions are suggested for achieving greater response.

KERATOACANTHOMA

Keratoacanthoma (KA) is a relatively common, benign, epithelial tumor that was previously considered to be a variant of squamous cell carcinoma. *PMID: 17614793* The etiology is unknown. Human papillomavirus-DNA sequences have been detected in lesions. It is a disease of the elderly (mean age, 64 years) with an annual incidence rate of 104 per 100,000. It is not associated with internal malignancy. There may be a seasonal presentation of keratoacanthoma that suggests that ultraviolet radiation has an acute effect on the development of KA. KAs may develop in sites of previous trauma. There are several reports of KAs occurring in tattoos.

Most cases are the "crateriform" type, which grow rapidly and then undergo spontaneous regression. Less than 2% belong to the rare destructive variants with no regression and persistent invasive growth. These are referred to as keratoacanthoma marginatum centrifugum and mutilating keratoacanthomas and can lead to severe defects; they are very rare.

Muir-Torre syndrome is a rare autosomal dominant genodermatosis that is characterized by the presence of at least one sebaceous gland tumor and a minimum of one internal malignancy. Keratoacanthomas have been noted in 23% of patients. The most commonly associated neoplasms are colorectal (61%) and genitourinary (22%).

Clinical presentation. KA begins as a smooth, dome-shaped, red papule that resembles molluscum contagiosum. In a few weeks the tumor may rapidly expand to 1 or 2 cm and develop a central keratin-filled crater that is frequently filled with crust (Figure 20-33). The growth retains its smooth surface, unlike squamous cell carcinoma. When untreated, growth stops in approximately 6 weeks, and the tumor remains unchanged for an indefinite period. In the majority of cases it then regresses slowly over 2 to 12 months and frequently heals with scarring. The limbs, particularly the sun-exposed hands and arms, are the most common site; the trunk is the second most common site, but KA may occur on any skin surface, including the anal area. On occasion, multiple KAs appear, or a single lesion extends over several centimeters. These variants resist treatment and are unlikely to undergo spontaneous remission.

DIFFERENTIATING SQUAMOUS CELL CARCINOMA FROM KERATOACANTHOMA. Squamous cell carcinoma (SCC) and KA are sometimes difficult to distinguish by histopathologic examination, since cytologic features are similar in both tumors. Many of the criteria commonly used for the differential diagnosis of SCC and KA are not reliable. Atypical or difficult cases should therefore be considered and treated as SCC.

TREATMENT. There is no advantage to waiting for spontaneous regression to occur, since most KAs ultimately heal with scarring. KAs are treated surgically or medically. KAs may recur.

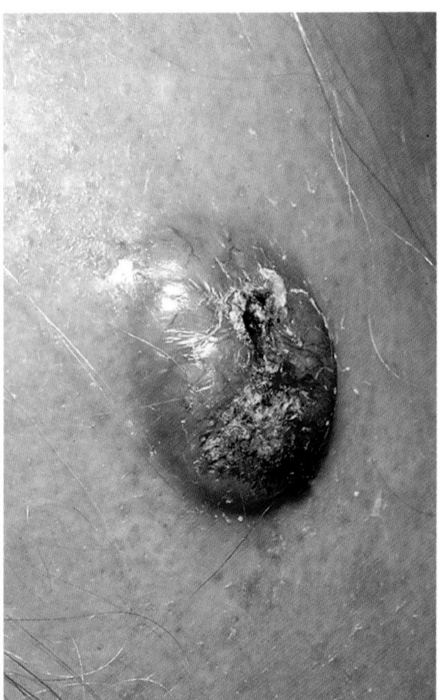
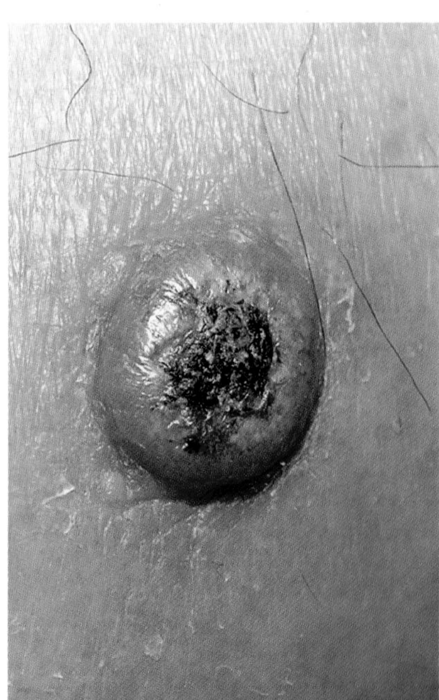
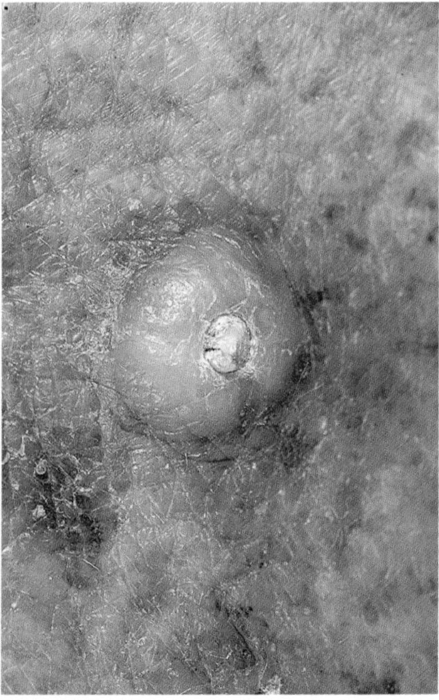

Figure 20-33 Keratoacanthoma. Lesions are solitary, smooth, dome-shaped red papules or nodules. They have a central keratin plug. Most occur on sun-exposed surfaces of the face and dorsum of the upper extremities.

SURGERY. Electrodesiccation and curettage or blunt dissection (Figure 20-34) (see Chapter 27) are efficient and effective for smaller lesions. Excision is effective for large tumors.

METHOTREXATE (INTRALESIONAL INJECTION). After biopsy confirms the diagnosis of KA, approximately 1 ml of methotrexate (MTX) in a concentration of either 12.5 or 25 mg/ml is injected with a 3-gauge needle directly into the remaining tumor at 2- to 3-week intervals, with a total of one to four total injection sessions required for tumor resolution. Small KAs are injected at a single central point at the base of the lesion whereas large KAs are injected into four quadrants and at the central lesion base. MTX is injected until an end point of uniform tumor blanching is achieved. Given the poor cohesion between tumor cells, approximately 50% leakage of the total injected MTX volume typically occurs. A 92% complete response rate for intralesional MTX for primary treatment of KA tumors was achieved. *PMID: 17504715* Perform baseline and postinjection complete blood cell counts to assess for potential MTX-induced cytopenias. Renal failure may be considered a relative contraindication for intralesional MTX therapy. Intralesional MTX may be particularly useful as a treatment in patients who are elderly and debilitated.

KERATOCANTHOMA—SURGICAL SPECIMEN

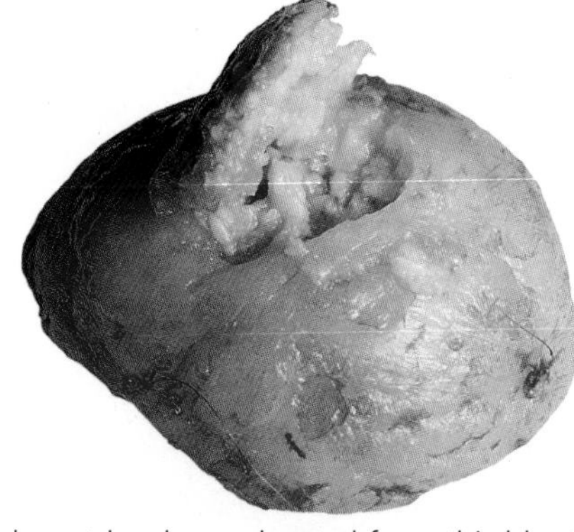

The central crust has been elevated from this blunt dissected lesion.

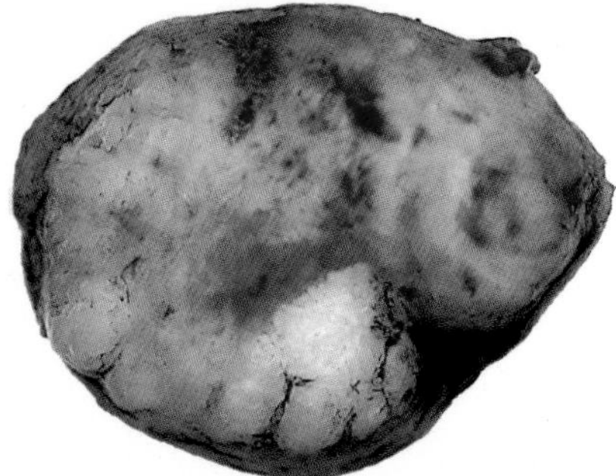

The undersurface is smooth and lobulated like a wart.

Figure 20-34

5-FLUOROURACIL (TOPICAL). Topical 5% fluorouracil cream (Efudex) applied three times a day in the rapid growth phase cured most lesions in 1 to 6 weeks. If possible the central crust should be removed to enhance penetration of medicine. The cream is applied to the lesion and its immediate vicinity, preferably under tape occlusion. Pretreatment with 6% salicylic acid gel (Keralyt) or 40% urea cream for lesions on the forearms, hands, or legs enhances penetration of the 5-fluorouracil cream. Lesions on the face and lips may clear in 1 or 2 weeks, but as long as 6 weeks is required for lesions in other areas to respond.

5-FLUOROURACIL (INTRALESIONAL INJECTION). Excellent results have been reported with 5-fluorouracil injections. The tumor is injected with the undiluted solution of 5-fluorouracil 50 mg/ml (available as fluorouracil injection in 500 mg/10 ml ampules). The usual amount is 0.1 to 2 ml, depending on the size of the tumor, injected tangentially into the slopes and then under the tumor. Extravasation of 5-fluorouracil from the central crater causes the amounts absorbed to be less than the amounts injected. Injections are given at 1- to 4-week intervals, depending on the response to treatment. Repeat injections are postponed if a lesion is undergoing necrosis. Patients should be evaluated at weekly intervals. This technique is especially useful for large KAs in difficult locations. Intralesional 5-fluorouracil may be ineffective for older KAs that are not rapidly proliferating. Reported time for healing varies from 1 to 9 weeks.

IMIQUIMOD. Topical treatment with imiquimod cream every other day for 4 to 12 weeks caused complete regression in six patients in two case reports. No recurrence occurred.

PODOPHYLLUM RESIN. Podophyllum (20%) in compound tincture of benzoin or alcohol may cure KAs. Remove the central crust and apply podophyllum with a cotton swab. Repeat the treatment every 2 weeks until the lesion disappears.

RADIOTHERAPY. KAs that are recurrent after surgical excision or those in which resection would result in cosmetic deformity may benefit from radiotherapy (total doses from 3500 cGy in 15 fractions to 5600 cGy in 28 fractions).

ISOTRETINOIN. Patients with multiple KAs have been treated with oral isotretinoin and oral acitretin. *PMID: 17714527* Patients with a solitary KA may respond to a short course of isotretinoin. Nine of twelve patients achieved complete resolution of the KA. The average duration of isotretinoin therapy was 6.3 weeks (range, 10 days to 12 weeks) in dosages of 0.5 to 1.0 mg/kg/day.

An initial trial of oral isotretinoin is an alternative to immediate surgical excision for the treatment of large keratoacanthomas in instances when tumor removal would cause considerable cosmetic deformity.

EPIDERMAL NEVUS

Epidermal nevi are organoid nevi arising from the pleuripotential germinative cells in the basal layer of the embryonic epidermis, on both the surface epidermis and adnexal structures. PMID: 17651173 The epidermal nevi are classified according to their predominant component: nevus sebaceus (sebaceous glands), nevus comedonicus (hair follicles), nevus syringocystadenoma papilliferum (apocrine glands), and nevus verrucosus (keratinocytes). The term *epidermal nevus* is commonly used to describe a group of cutaneous hamartomas composed of keratinocytes that are linked by common clinical and histologic features. Linear epidermal nevus or nevus unius lateris (a linear, unilateral, wartlike nevus), nevus verrucosus (a localized, wartlike nevus), and ichthyosis hystrix (an irregular, bilateral, truncal nevus) are some of the names given to variants of epidermal nevus. Inflammatory linear verrucous epidermal nevus (ILVEN) is characterized by intensely erythematous, pruritic, inflammatory papules that occur as linear bands along the lines of Blaschko. It has been reported as a cutaneous manifestation in the epidermal nevus syndrome. The term nevus means a congenital defect of the skin characterized by the localized excess of one or more types of cells. Histologically the cells are identical to or closely resemble normal cells.

CLINICAL CHARACTERISTICS. These well-circumscribed growths are present at birth or appear in infancy or childhood. They are round, oval, or oblong; elevated; flat-topped; yellow-tan to dark brown; and have a uniformly warty or velvety surface with sharp borders (Figures 20-35 and 20-37). They appear more commonly on the head and neck; 13% of patients have widespread lesions. Blaschko described a system of lines on the skin that linear nevi follow. These lines represent a developmental growth pattern of the skin (Figures 20-36, 20-38, and 20-39). Epidermal nevi may spread beyond their original distribution; further progression is unlikely after late adolescence. Nevi present at birth and those on the head are less likely to spread. In spite of their unusual appearance and occasional itching, they are generally inconsequential. Occasionally the growths are very large and disfiguring. Patients with epidermal nevi are at significant risk of having other anomalies in other organ systems. Abnormalities are more likely in patients with widespread nevi. The most common systems involved are skeletal, neurologic, and ocular.

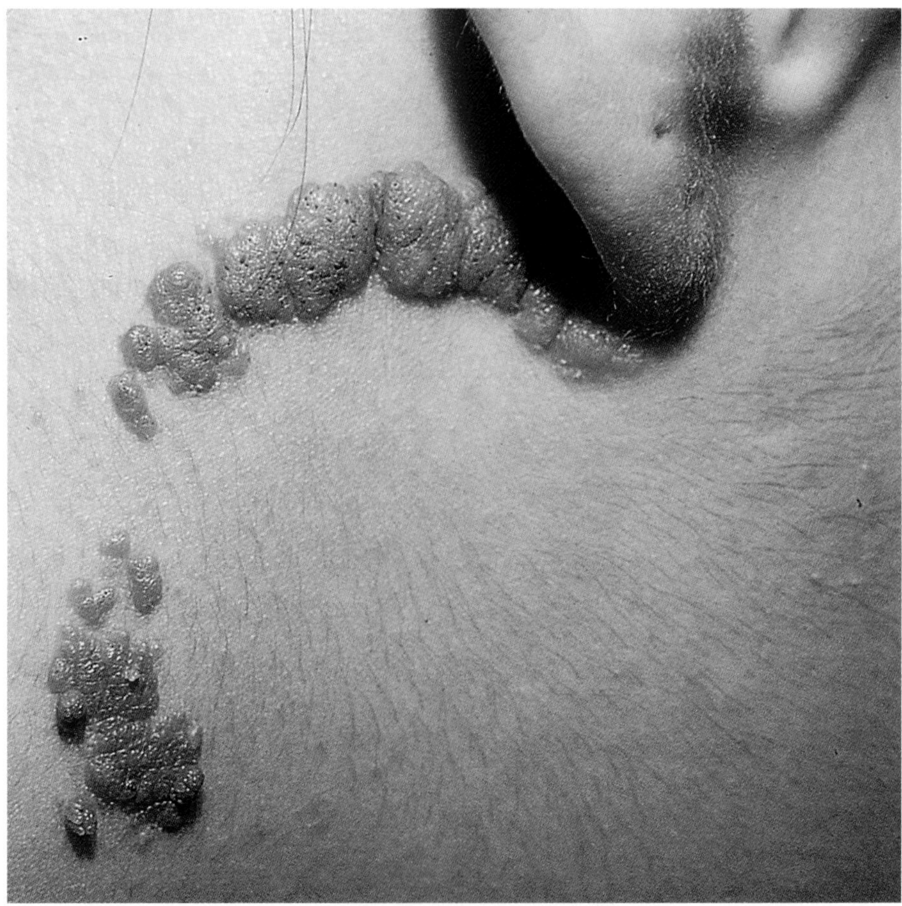

Figure 20-35 Epidermal nevus. A congenital lesion, which is often linear, has a dark brown, warty, or velvety surface.

GENETIC COUNSELING. The very rare epidermal nevus syndrome consists of extensive epidermal nevi associated with skeletal, ocular, cerebral, and sometimes cardiac and renal abnormalities. Small lesions are sporadic. Patients do not have a family history of epidermal nevi. Most cases of epidermal nevus syndrome occur sporadically, but there is some suspicion that an autosomal dominant transmission may be present. Inform patients that genetic transmission is possible with large epidermal nevi but that data are inadequate to make an accurate determination.

The cause of epidermal nevus syndrome is unknown. Possible explanations are faulty migration and development of embryonic tissue or a developmental error in separation of the ectoderm from the neural tube. Treatment may be attempted with cryosurgery or dermabrasion, but the growths may recur; plastic surgery excision produces the most predictable results.

TREATMENT. Inflammatory linear verrucous epidermal nevus (ILVEN) is treated to relieve discomfort and improve cosmetic appearance. Reported therapeutic approaches include dermabrasion, cryotherapy, laser therapy, and partial-thickness excision. Full-thickness surgical excision is effective definitive treatment. Inflamed verrucous epidermal nevus may improve using a program of alternating fluocinonide ointment and tacrolimus 0.1% ointment.

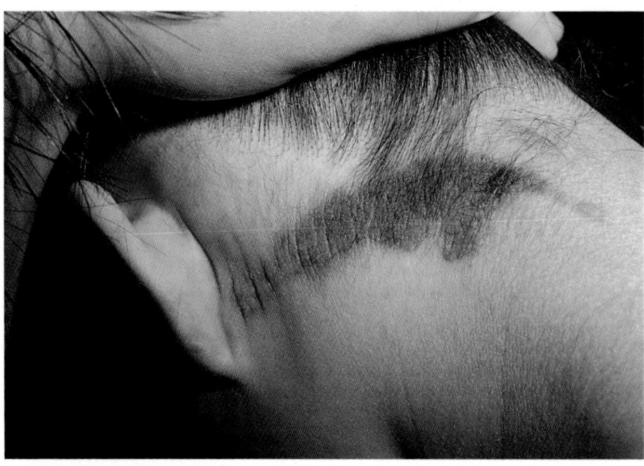

Figure 20-37 Epidermal nevus. A flat, broad lesion that follows Blaschko's lines.

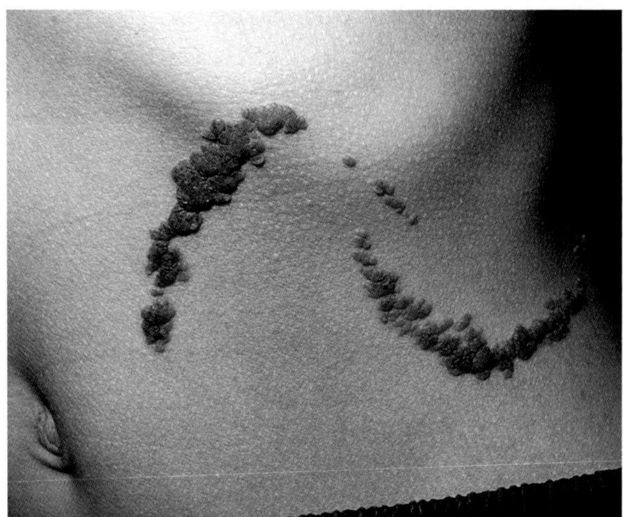

Figure 20-38 Epidermal nevus. A dark segmented lesion on the abdomen and side that follows Blaschko's lines. The umbilicus is on the left lower corner of the picture.

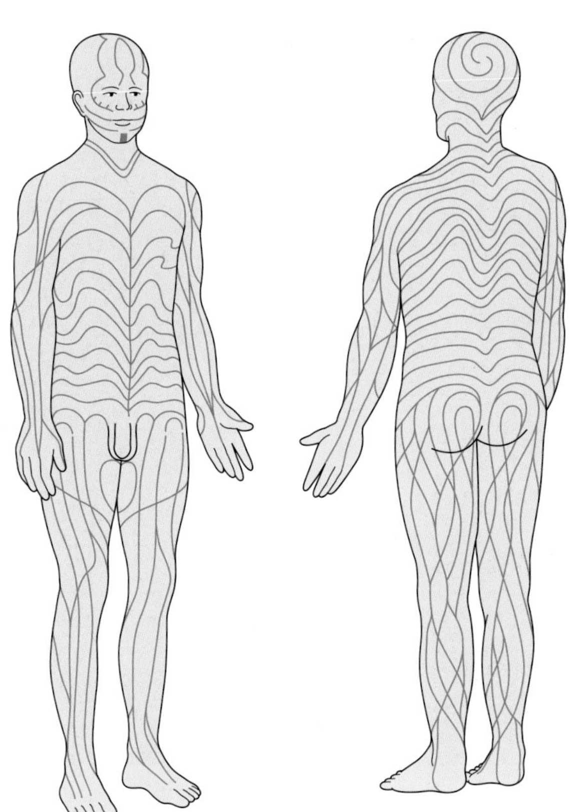

Figure 20-36 Blaschko's lines.

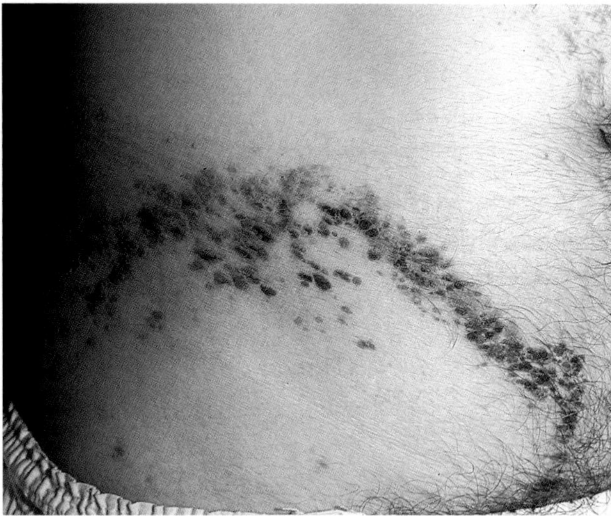

Figure 20-39 Epidermal nevus. A light colored lesion on the abdomen and side that follows Blaschko's lines.

NEVUS SEBACEOUS

Nevus sebaceous is a distinctive growth most commonly found on the scalp, followed by the forehead and retroauricular region. Involvement of the neck and trunk is exceptional. A nevus of epithelial and nonepithelial skin components, nevus sebaceous sustains age-related modifications in morphology. The nevus occurs singly and is asymptomatic. Two thirds of cases are present at birth; the others develop in infancy or early childhood. Males and females are equally affected. The very rare nevus sebaceous of Jadassohn syndrome consists of the triad of a linear sebaceous nevus, convulsions, and mental retardation. A variety of congenital malformations of the ocular, skeletal, vascular, and urogenital systems have been described in association with nevus sebaceous. Neurologic abnormalities have been reported in patients with sebaceous nevi, but the incidence is low. It is recommended that patients with sebaceous nevi have a neurologic assessment and that imaging be performed on all those in whom clinical abnormalities are demonstrated, as well as on those patients with large nevi involving the centrofacial area.

Most lesions are sporadic, but cases of inherited nevus sebaceous have been reported.

EVOLUTION OF LESIONS. Lesions are oval to linear, varying from 0.5 × 1 cm to 7 × 9 cm. The three-stage evolution of the nevoid condition (newborn, puberty, adult) parallels the natural histologic differentiation of normal sebaceous glands. The lesions in infants and younger children are smooth to gently papillated, waxy, hairless thickenings (Figure 20-40). During puberty there is a massive development of sebaceous glands with epidermal hyperplasia within the lesions (Figure 20-41). At this stage they change clinically by developing a verrucous mulberry irregularity of the surface covered with numerous, closely aggregated, yellow to dark brown papules. When this transformation becomes noticeable, parents become worried and seek medical attention. In approximately 20% of the cases, a third phase of evolution involves the development of secondary neoplasia in the mass of the nevus.

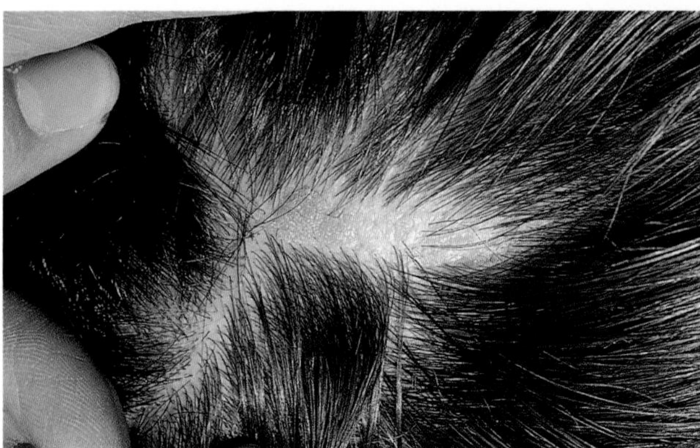

Figure 20-40 Nevus sebaceous. A typical lesion on the scalp of a prepubertal male.

TUMORS ARISING IN NEVUS SEBACEOUS. A number of benign and malignant "nevoid tumors" may occur. Prophylactic surgical excision during childhood is often recommended. The rate of malignant tumors is very low. Benign neoplasms are common. Trichoblastoma, not basal cell carcinoma, is the most frequent follicular tumor, showing a striking female predominance. Most tumors occur in adults older than 40 years; therefore prophylactic surgery in young children is of uncertain benefit. Clinical follow-up is probably sufficient, and even those cases with clinical changes often prove to be benign tumors. The malignant degenerations are relatively low grade; only a few cases of metastasis are reported.

TREATMENT. Most tumors occur in adults older than 40 years. Therefore prophylactic surgery in young children is of uncertain benefit. Clinical follow-up is probably sufficient. Most cases with clinical changes often prove to be benign tumors. Plastic surgical excision is the most effective treatment. Attempts at local destruction with electrocautery or cryosurgery may lead to recurrence.

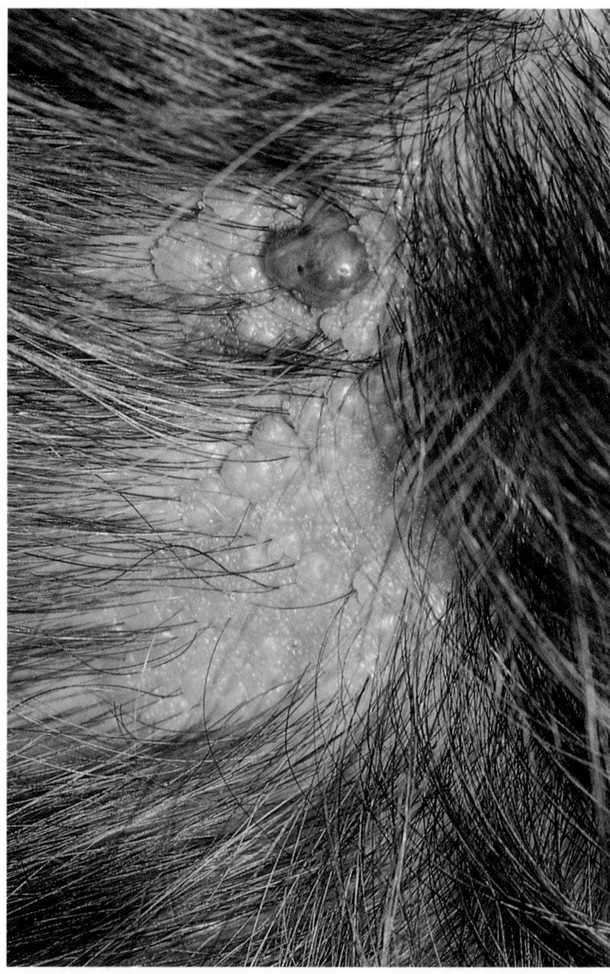

Figure 20-41 Nevus sebaceous. A white globular surface indicative of sebaceous gland hyperplasia that occurs after puberty.

CHONDRODERMATITIS NODULARIS HELICIS

This uncommon disorder occurs on the lateral surface of the helix (Figure 20-42) and occasionally on the antihelix, a site rarely occupied by other growths. One (occasionally more) firm, 2- to 6-mm nodule appears spontaneously. It subsequently develops a central scale that lacks the keratinous plug of a keratoacanthoma (Figure 20-43). Removal of the scale reveals a small central erosion. Unlike the full, distended margins of a squamous or basal cell carcinoma, the sides of this mass slope down from the center (Figure 20-44). The small mass is dull red to white and is painful. During the active stage, the base may become red and swollen; pain is constant. Pressure of any type becomes intolerable. As the mass attains its maximum size, it becomes lighter in color but remains symptomatic. The cause of this disorder is unknown, but chronic sun exposure may be a factor. Men over the age of 40 account for 90% of the patients.

Histologically the dermis shows collagen degeneration with granulation tissue, edema, and inflammation.

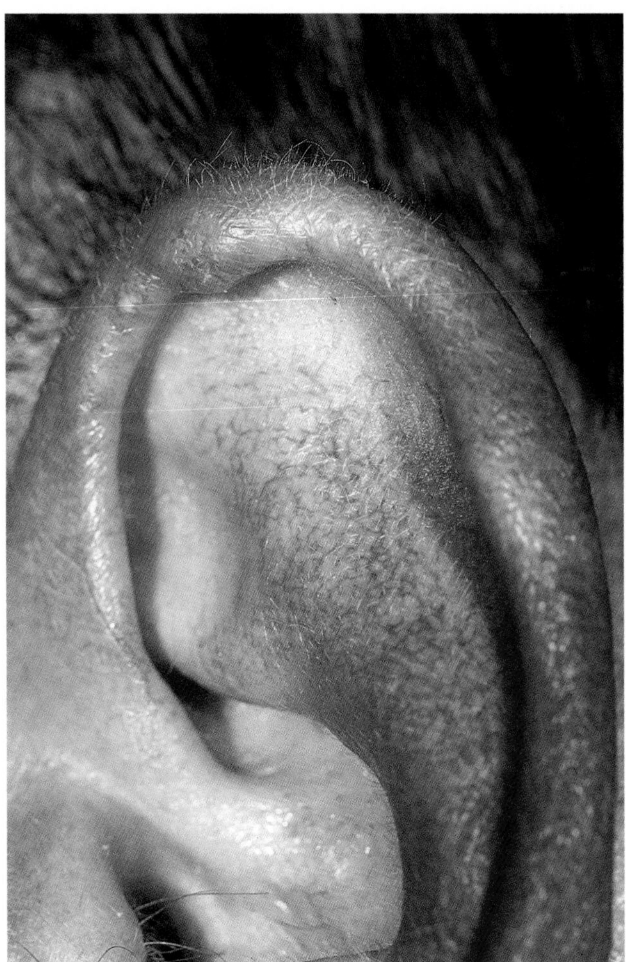

Figure 20-42 Chondrodermatitis nodularis helicis. A painful, firm nodule with scaling in the center, occupying a commonly observed site on the lateral surface of the helix.

TREATMENT

Medical management. Medical management is often unsatisfactory. A special pillow relieves pressure (CNH Pillow, Abilene, TX). Intralesional triamcinolone acetonide (10 to 40 mg/ml) once every 2 to 3 weeks until clear may be sufficient. There is some degree of persistent pain throughout treatment. The CO_2 laser may be used to vaporize the cutaneous nodules and involved cartilage. Cryotherapy also has been used.

Surgical management. A simple and effective treatment is to excise the nodule with scissors, curette the base, and gently electrodesiccate to eradicate all foci of inflammation. Bleeding is controlled with Monsel's solution. The wound granulates and heals with a defect (see Chapter 27). Recurrences are common if all sites of inflammation have not been eradicated. Several other techniques have been described.

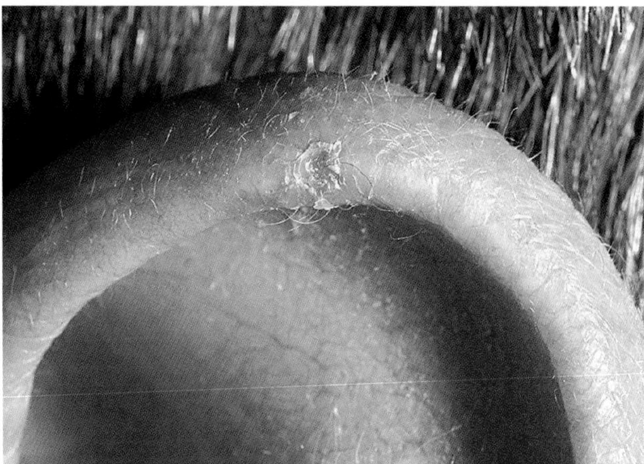

Figure 20-43 Chondrodermatitis nodularis. Shown is an early lesion with a central crust on the most common site, the apex of the helix.

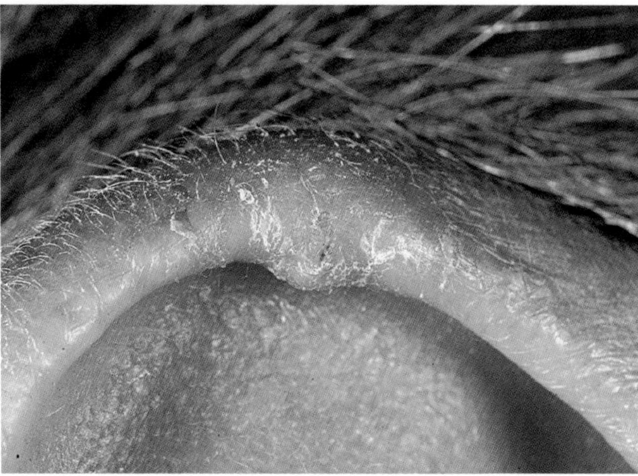

Figure 20-44 Chondrodermatitis nodularis. A long-standing lesion with a dense rolled edge and a central crust.

EPIDERMAL CYST

The common epidermal or sebaceous cyst occurs primarily on the face, back or base of the ears, chest, and back, or on almost any skin surface (Figures 20-45 to 20-48). Children with epidermal cysts or patients with epidermal cysts in unusual areas such as the legs should be suspected of having Gardner's syndrome (see Chapter 26). The cyst wall is lined with stratified squamous epithelium, which produces keratin. The round, protruding, smooth-surfaced mass is movable and varies in size from a few millimeters to several centimeters. The cyst communicates with the surface through a narrow channel, and the surface opening appears as a small, round, sometimes imperceptible, keratin-filled orifice (i.e., a blackhead) (see Figure 20-46). Epidermal cysts may originate from comedones; such lesions are superficial, with a large, black, keratinous plug on the surface. They are referred to as giant comedones and are commonly found on the back. Cysts may remain small for years or may progressively develop. Spontaneous rupture of the wall results in discharge of the soft, yellow keratin into the dermis. A tremendous inflammatory response ensues, and the sterile purulent material either points and drains through the surface or is slowly reabsorbed (Figures 20-45 and 20-49). If the wall is destroyed during the inflammatory process, the cyst will not recur.

TREATMENT. Like boils, fluctuant, inflamed cysts must be drained and evacuated. Small cysts are removed by making a linear incision with a #11 blade over the surface and, if possible, through the orifice. The soft keratinous material is expressed through the incision, and the remaining material is dislodged with a #1 curette. After total evacuation, firm pressure generally forces the cyst wall through the incision, where it can be grasped with the forceps and separated from connective tissue with scissors (this technique is illustrated in Chapter 27). To absorb blood and serum, the wound is compressed for several minutes. If necessary, the wound edges may be supported with Steri-Strips. Excision is the procedure of choice for large cysts. Cysts may also be excised and sutured or dissected (Figure 20-50). Most clinicians prescribe oral antibiotics for ruptured epidermal cysts but this practice is unnecessary in most cases.

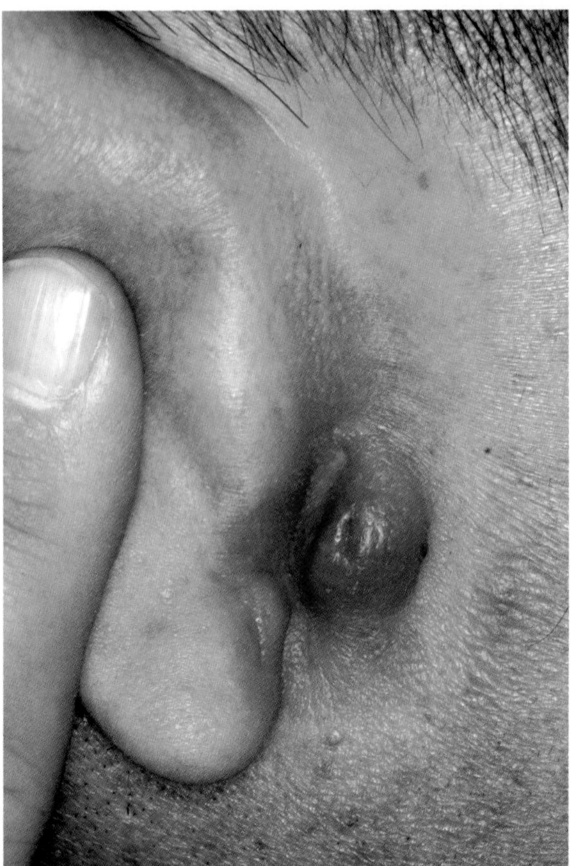

Figure 20-45 The posterior auricular fold is a common place to find one or many epidermal cysts. This lesion has ruptured and is inflamed.

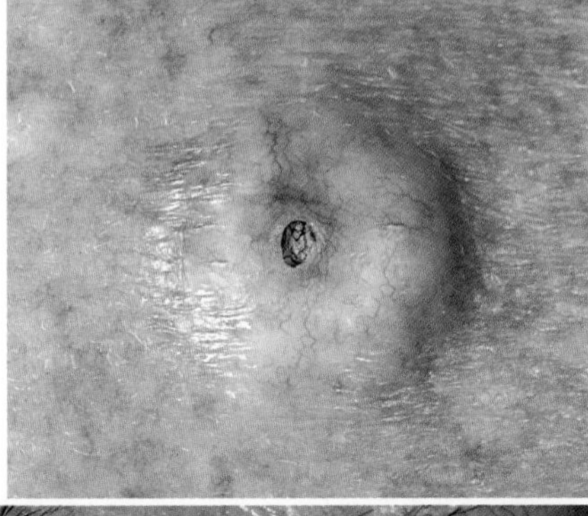

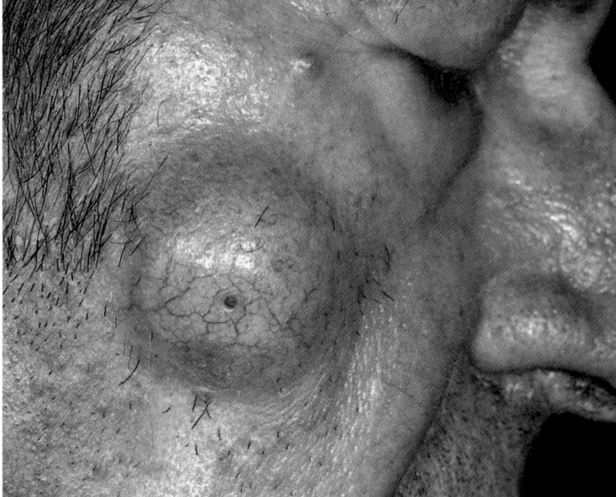

Figure 20-46 The keratin-filled orifice (blackhead) communicating with the surface is not usually as prominent as illustrated here.

EPIDERMAL CYSTS

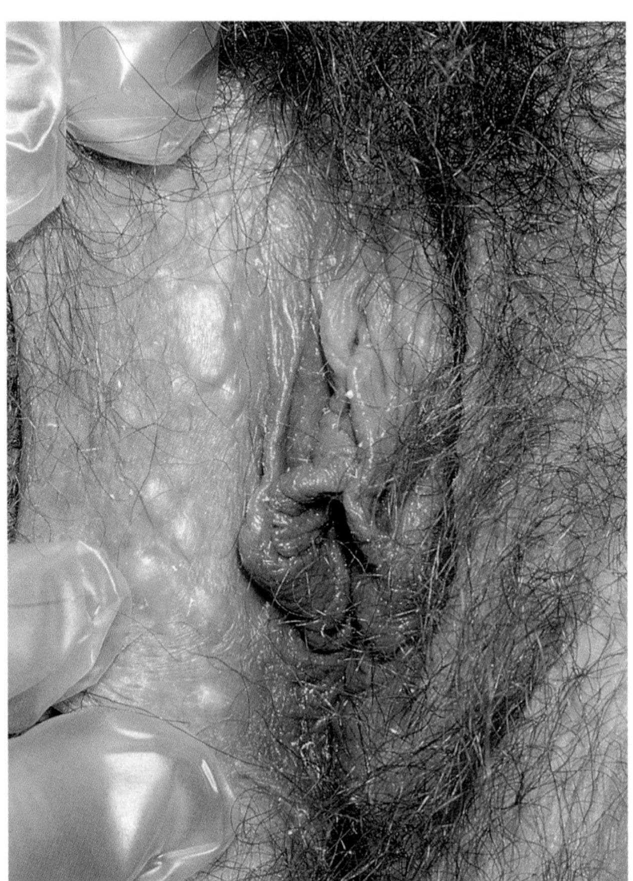

Figure 20-47 Epidermal cysts occur in areas where sebaceous glands are large and numerous, such as on the labia.

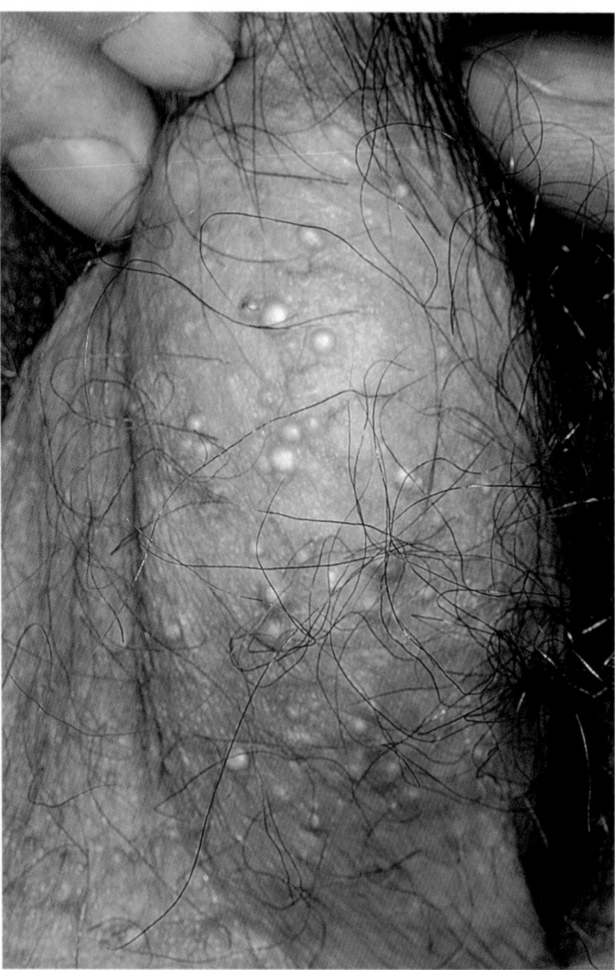

Figure 20-48 Epidermal cysts are common on the scrotum. Lesions may be few or numerous and vary in size. Some are larger than 1 cm.

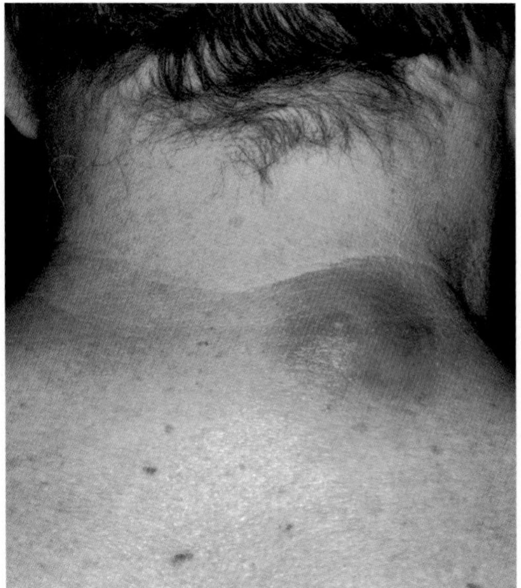

Figure 20-49 A ruptured epidermal cyst results in intense inflammation and resembles a furuncle.

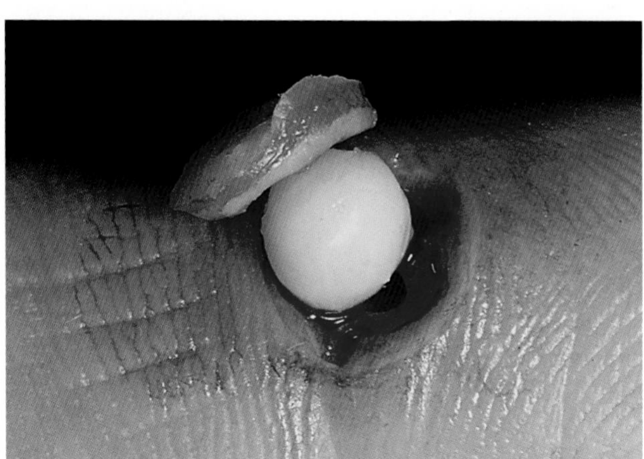

Figure 20-50 An epidermal cyst that has been dissected intact.

PILAR CYST (WEN)

Pilar cysts occur in the scalp and, like epidermal cysts, are freely movable. They are frequently multiple and may become large masses (Figures 20-51 and 20-52). The epithelial-lined wall produces keratin of a different quality than that of the epidermal cyst, but rupture of the wall creates the same intense reaction. The cyst contains concentric layers of dry keratin, which over time may become macerated, soft, and cheesy (Figure 20-53).

TREATMENT. Except for the largest structures, pilar cysts can be satisfactorily removed through a linear excision, avoiding suture closure. The following procedure should be used (this procedure is illustrated in Chapter 27):

1. Cut the hair over the cyst and make a 3- to 10-mm linear incision.
2. With firm pressure, express the contents and dislodge remaining fragments with a #1 curette.
3. Firmly press the curette against the inner wall of the cyst and move it back and forth to dislodge the cyst from its surroundings. The wall is firm and has a smooth, glazed surface that is easily separated from connective tissue.
4. Hold the cut edge of the cyst with forceps and, while applying continuous pressure to the sides of the wound, separate the cyst from the supporting connective tissue with a blunt dissecting instrument such as a Schamberg or blunt-tipped scissors. The cyst will literally pop out of the wound.
5. To control bleeding, apply firm pressure for 5 minutes. Dressings or bandages are unnecessary.

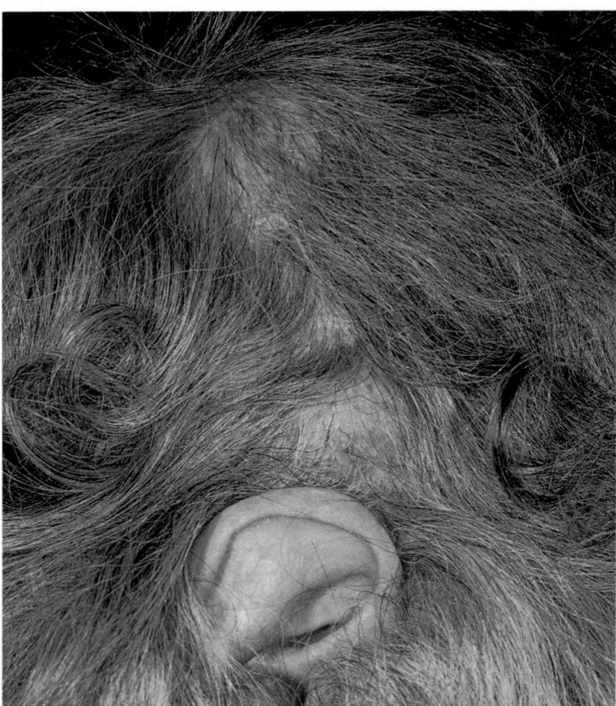

Figure 20-51 Pilar cyst. A freely movable cystic mass found on the scalp. Communication with the surface is rarely observed.

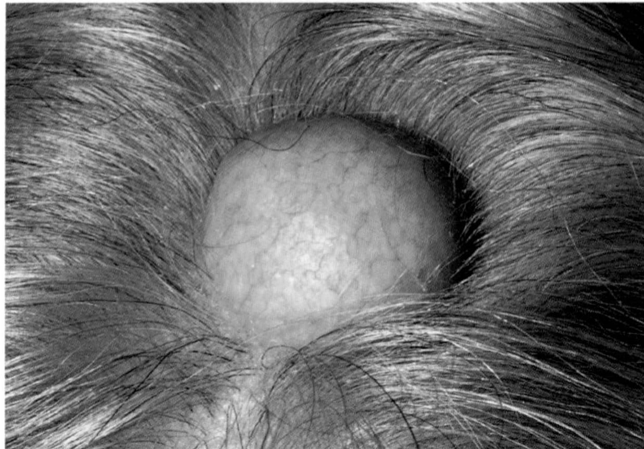

Figure 20-52 Pilar cyst. This very large cyst is more prominent than most lesions. Expansion of the cyst has destroyed hair follicles.

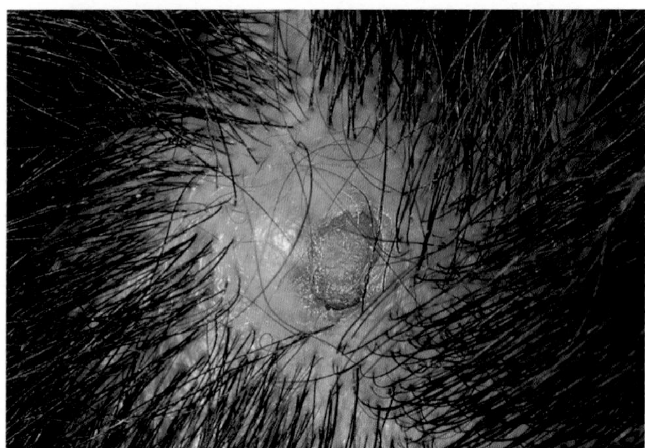

Figure 20-53 Pilar cyst. The cyst has spontaneously ruptured and is discharging amorphous cyst contents onto the skin surface.

SENILE SEBACEOUS HYPERPLASIA

Senile sebaceous hyperplasia consists of small tumors composed of enlarged sebaceous glands. They begin as pale yellow, slightly elevated papules; with time they become yellow, dome-shaped, and umbilicated (Figure 20-54). Senile sebaceous hyperplasia with telangiectasia may be mistaken for a basal cell carcinoma. However, close examination of the surface with a hand lens shows a haphazard distribution of vessels on the surface of basal cell carcinoma, whereas the vessels in sebaceous hyperplasia occur only in the valleys between the small yellow lobules. The lesions occur after age 30 in 25% of the population and gradually become more numerous. There is no relationship between skin type and the occurrence of these lesions. They are commonly found on the forehead, cheeks, lower lid, nose, and rarely on the vulva. The etiology remains unclear; chronic solar exposure is not a likely cause.

TREATMENT. Treatment consists of removal of the elevated portion of the papule. A pitted scar results if the entire structure is removed with a curette. The superficial portion of the lesion may be removed by shave excision or destroyed with conservative surface or intralesional electrosurgery. Bichloracetic acid can be used for treatment. A tiny amount of acid is carefully applied to the surface with a wooden applicator stick. A stinging sensation occurs and lasts for 24 hours. Polysporin ointment is applied twice a day for 1 week. The treated area forms a crust, heals with residual erythema, and fades over time. Patients with numerous lesions have been reported. Most lesions regress after one treatment with three stacked pulses of the 585-nm pulsed dye laser.

Oral isotretinoin in very low dosages (10 to 20 mg daily) is dramatically effective for patients with numerous lesions. All lesions clear within 2 weeks but recur after the medication is stopped. Patients can often maintain control with low dosages of isotretinoin (e.g., 10 mg once or twice each week). It has been speculated that longer treatment (more than 12 weeks) may result in perifollicular fibrosis in the region formerly occupied by the sebaceous gland and may offer a long-term remission. Optimum treatment and dosage schedules have not been established. Intermittent low-dose isotretinoin may be the best approach. Long-term isotretinoin therapy may be associated with many side effects.

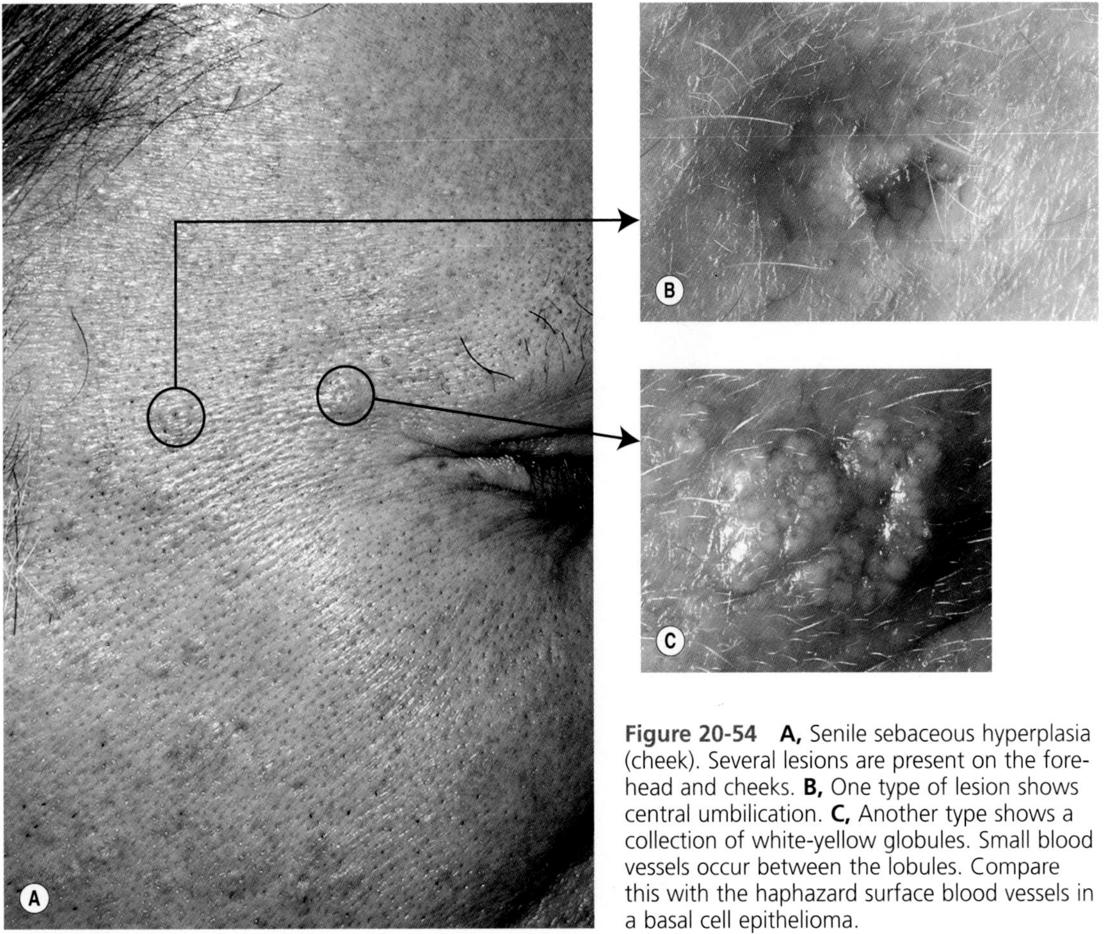

Figure 20-54 **A,** Senile sebaceous hyperplasia (cheek). Several lesions are present on the forehead and cheeks. **B,** One type of lesion shows central umbilication. **C,** Another type shows a collection of white-yellow globules. Small blood vessels occur between the lobules. Compare this with the haphazard surface blood vessels in a basal cell epithelioma.

SYRINGOMA

Syringomas are sweat duct tumors composed of small, firm, flesh-colored dermal papules (Figures 20-55 to 20-57) that occur on the lower lids and, less commonly, on the forehead, chest, abdomen, and vulva. Lesions may develop at any age, but they initially appear most frequently during the third and fourth decades; they then slowly become more numerous. The tumors have no malignant potential. They may be removed for cosmetic purposes by electrodesiccation and curettage or excised by gently elevating the small mass with forceps or the curved bevel of a 25-gauge needle and cut out with curved scissors or shaved with a #11 scalpel blade. The oval wound is left to heal by secondary intention.

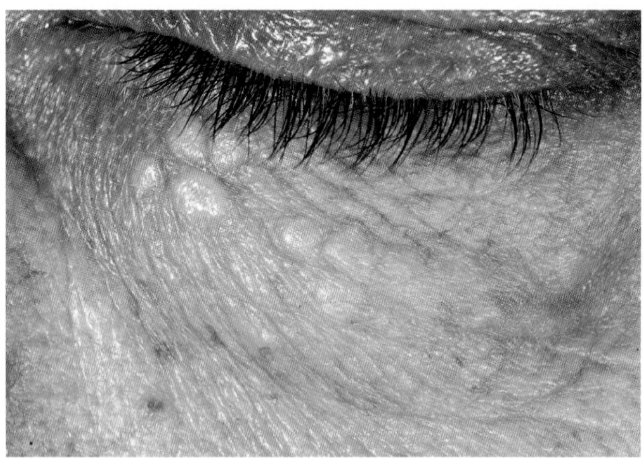

Figure 20-55 Syringoma. Yellow-white round and flat-topped papules are most commonly found on the lower lids.

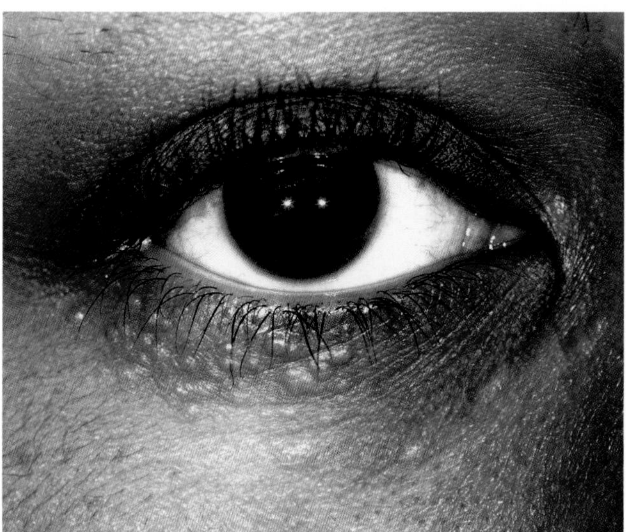

Figure 20-56 Syringoma on the lower lid of a young woman.

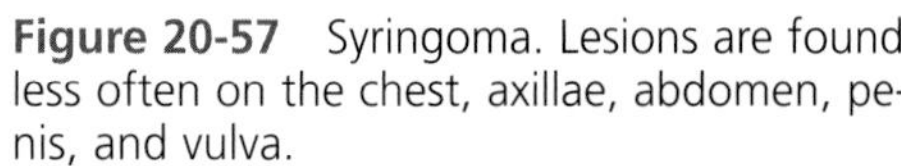

Figure 20-57 Syringoma. Lesions are found less often on the chest, axillae, abdomen, penis, and vulva.

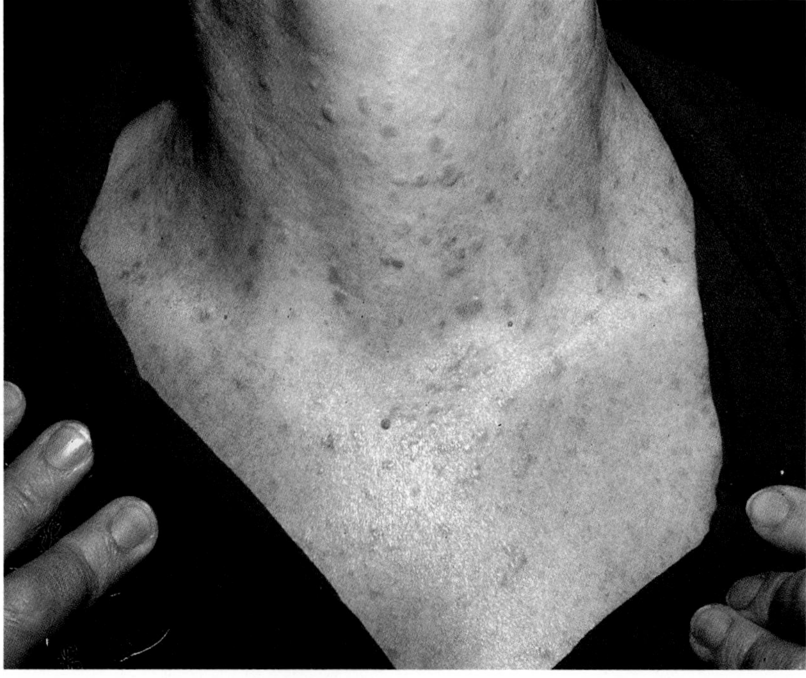

Chapter 21

Premalignant and Malignant Nonmelanoma Skin Tumors

CHAPTER CONTENTS

- Basal cell carcinoma
- Actinic keratosis
- Squamous cell carcinoma in situ
- Bowen's disease
- Erythroplasia of Queyrat
- Arsenical keratoses and other arsenic-related skin diseases
- Squamous cell carcinoma
- Leukoplakia
- Verrucous carcinoma
- Primary cutaneous lymphomas
- Cutaneous T-cell lymphoma
- Paget's disease of the breast
- Extramammary Paget's disease
- Cutaneous metastasis

BASAL CELL CARCINOMA

Basal cell carcinoma (BCC) is the most common invasive malignant cutaneous neoplasm found in humans. The most common presenting complaint is a bleeding or scabbing sore that heals and recurs. Unfortunately, there is a tendency to regard BCC as nonmalignant because the tumor rarely metastasizes. BCC advances by direct extension and destroys normal tissue. Left untreated or inadequately treated, the cancer can destroy the whole side of the face or penetrate subcutaneous tissue into the bone and brain.

BASAL CELL CARCINOMA VS. SQUAMOUS CELL CARCINOMA. BCC and squamous cell carcinoma (SCC) are referred to as nonmelanoma skin cancers. A number of differences between these two tumors exist (Table 21-1). The relationship with ultraviolet (UV) radiation is stronger for SCC. SCCs of the head and neck occur on areas receiving maximal irradiation. The distribution of BCC on the face does not correspond well with areas of maximal sun exposure. Many BCCs occur on sun-protected sites, such as the inner canthus and behind the ears. Approximately one third of all BCCs occur on areas of the skin that receive little or no UV radiation and, unlike SCCs, they are uncommon on the back of the hands and on the forearms. Increasing grade of wrinkling is associated with a progressive reduction in risk of a BCC.

LOCATION. Eighty-five percent of all BCCs appear on the head and neck region; 25% to 30% occur on the nose alone, the most common site. BCC is rarely found on the backs of the hands, although this site receives a significant amount of solar radiation. Tumors also occur in sites protected from the sun, such as the genitals and breasts. BCC in blacks is rare.

Table 21-1 Basal Cell Carcinoma vs. Squamous Cell Carcinoma

Incidence	Basal cell carcinoma	Squamous cell carcinoma
Males	175 per 100,000 Minnesota 849 per 100,000 Australia	106 per 100,000 in Pacific Northwest 166 per 100,000 in Australia
Females	124 per 100,000 Minnesota 605 per 100,000 Australia	30 per 100,000 in Pacific Northwest
United States 1999	800,000	200,000
United States 1978 Number per 100,000 person-years	247 (males) 150 (females)	65 (males) 24 (females)
Distribution	Face, head, neck: distribution does not correspond well with areas of maximal sun exposure Occurs on relatively sun-protected sites, such as inner canthus and behind ears One third occur on areas that receive little or no UV radiation Uncommon on back of hands and on forearms	Head, neck: areas of maximal irradiation
Age	20% occur in patients younger than 50 yr	Uncommon in the young
Celtic ancestry: fair skin, blue eyes, red or fair hair, inability to tan	Risk low: patients do not have phenotypic markers of high risk	High risk
Most important risk factor	Inability to tan	Cumulative sun exposure; increasing age more important than tanning ability
UV exposure patterns	Intermittent sun exposure Childhood and adolescent sun exposure	Cumulative exposure; childhood and adolescent sun exposure
Other environmental exposures		Chronic ulceration and inflammation, scarring dermatosis, immunosuppressed states, human papillomavirus infection, chemical carcinogens (coal-tar products), psoralens and UVA, arsenic, cigarette smoking
Risk of developing a subsequent nonmelanoma skin cancer of same type	3-year cumulative risk of a subsequent BCC after an index BCC is 44% BCC patients are 8 times more likely to develop another BCC than a first SCC 3-year cumulative risk of developing a BCC for patients with a history of an SCC is 43%	3-year cumulative risk of a subsequent SCC after an index SCC is 18% Risk of developing an SCC in patients with a prior BCC is 6%
Genodermatoses	Xeroderma pigmentosum Nevoid BCC syndrome	Xeroderma pigmentosum Epidermodysplasia verruciformis

Adapted from Leman JA et al: *Arch Dermatol* 137:1239, 2001 *PMID: 11559224*; and Marcil I, Stern RS: *Arch Dermatol* 136:1524, 2000. *PMID: 11115165*

EPIDEMIOLOGY. The average lifetime risk for Caucasians to develop BCC is 30%. BCC most commonly occurs in adults, especially in the elderly population. Individuals with fair skin, blond or red hair, light eye color, poor tanning ability (skin type I), and sun-damaged skin are at greatest risk. The male-to-female ratio is 2:1. Women younger than 40 years of age outnumber men in this age group. The closer Caucasians live to the equator, the greater is their risk for developing BCC.

PATHOGENESIS. The main risk factor for the development of BCC is ultraviolet light exposure. UVB radiation (290 to 320 nm, sunburn rays) plays a greater role in BCC development than UVA radiation (320 to 400 nm, tanning rays). UVA and UVB damage DNA. Light exposure is not the only factor; 20% of BCCs arise on non–sun-exposed skin. Individuals with fair skin, blond or red hair, and light-colored eyes (skin type I) who are susceptible to sunburn have the highest risk. This increases with intense, intermittent amount of sun exposure when compared to an equal dose of continuous exposure. The incidence in people with dark skin is much lower.

The incidence of developing BCC in transplant patients is 10 to 100 times higher than in the general population.

There is a 10-fold increased risk of developing a subsequent BCC 3 years after the first diagnosis of BCC. BCC occurs at the site of previous trauma, such as scars, thermal burns, and injury. BCC occurs years later at sites treated with ionizing radiation. The tumor appears 3 months to 7 or more years later at the site of a previous injury.

Pathophysiology

BCCs arise from basal keratinocytes of the epidermis and adnexal structures (e.g., hair follicles, eccrine sweat ducts). UVB radiation damages DNA and its repair system and alters the immune system. BCC grows by direct extension and appears to require the surrounding stroma to support its growth. This may explain why the cells are not capable of metastasizing through blood vessels or lymphatics. The course of BCC is unpredictable. BCC can remain small for years with little tendency to grow, particularly in the elderly, or it may grow rapidly or proceed by successive spurts of extension of tumor and partial regression.

Histologic characteristics

The cells of BCC resemble those of the basal layer of the epidermis. They are basophilic, have a large nucleus, and appear to form a basal layer by developing an orderly line around the periphery of tumor nests in the dermis, a feature referred to as palisading (Figure 21-1).

There are five major histologic patterns:

1. Nodular (21%): a rounded mass of neoplastic cells with well-defined peripheral contours. Peripheral palisading is well developed (see Figure 21-1).
2. Superficial (17%): contains buds of atypical basal cells extending from the basal layer of the epidermis (Figure 21-2).
3. Micronodular (15%): small, rounded nodules of tumor about the size of hair bulbs. Tumor islands are rounded and well demarcated, and demonstrate peripheral palisading.
4. Infiltrative (7%): tumor islands vary in size and show a jagged configuration.
5. Morpheaform (1%): numerous small, elongated islands containing a few cells that appear as strands or cords in a fibrous stroma.

A mixed pattern (two or more major histologic patterns) is present in 38.5% of cases.

Clinical types

BCC occurs in many different clinical forms, which vary in appearance and malignant potential.

NODULAR BASAL CELL CARCINOMA. Nodular BCC is the most common form of BCC. The lesion begins as a pearly white or pink, dome-shaped papule resembling a molluscum contagiosum or dermal nevus (Figures 21-3 and 21-4). The mass extends peripherally. The lesion may remain flat. Traction on the surrounding skin accentuates the pearly border. Telangiectatic vessels become prominent and easily recognizable through the thin epidermis as the lesion enlarges. The growth pattern is irregular, forming an oval mass whereby the surface may become multilobular. The center frequently ulcerates and bleeds and subsequently accumulates crust and scale (see Figure 21-4). Ulcerated BCCs were formerly termed rodent ulcers.

Ulcerated areas heal with scarring, and patients often assume their conditions are improving. This cycle of growth, ulceration, and healing continues as the mass extends peripherally and deeper; masses of enormous size may be attained. BCCs may present as nonhealing leg ulcers. Biopsy specimens should be taken of leg ulcers that do not respond to treatment. The tissue mass of a nodular BCC has a distinctive consistency that can be appreciated during curettage or biopsy. It has poor cohesive forces and collapses or breaks down when manipulated with a curette. This is an important diagnostic feature that supports the clinical impression during the biopsy procedure.

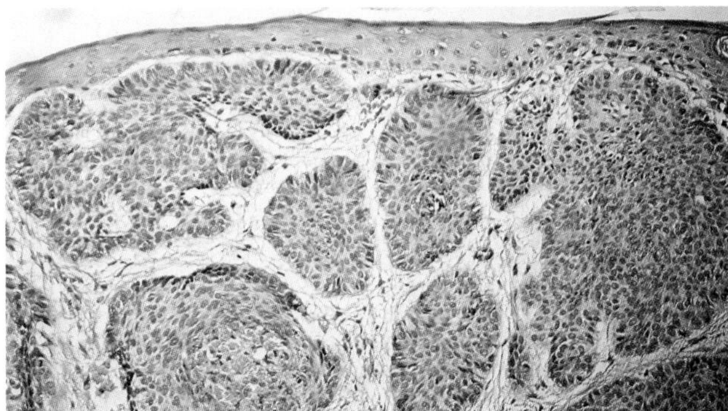

Figure 21-1 Nodular basal cell carcinoma. Nests of atypical basal cells are found in the dermis.

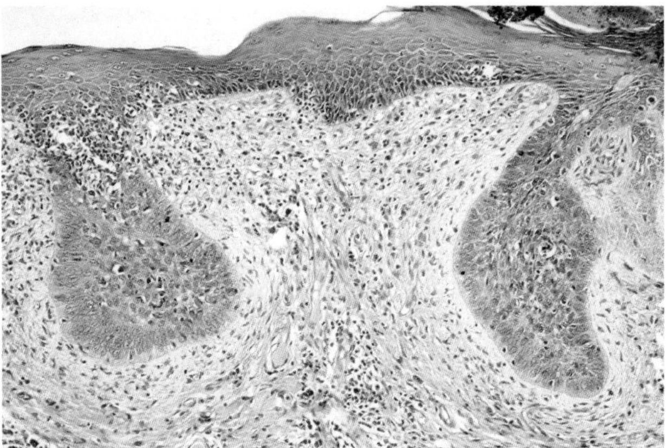

Figure 21-2 Superficial basal cell carcinoma. Buds of atypical basal cells extending from the basal layer of the epidermis.

NODULAR BASAL CELL CARCINOMA

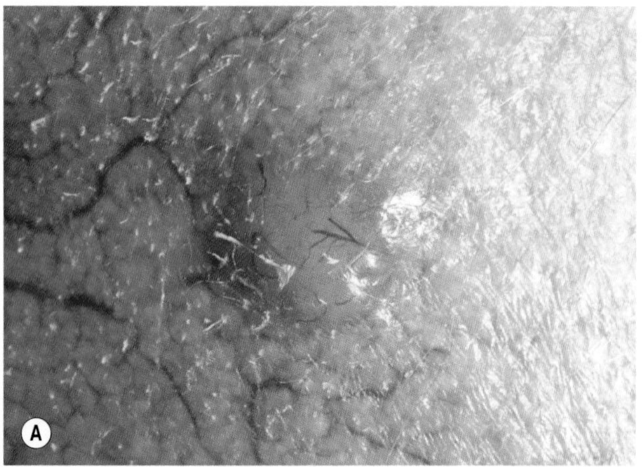

Classic presentation. A pink, pearly-white papule with prominent telangiectatic vessels.

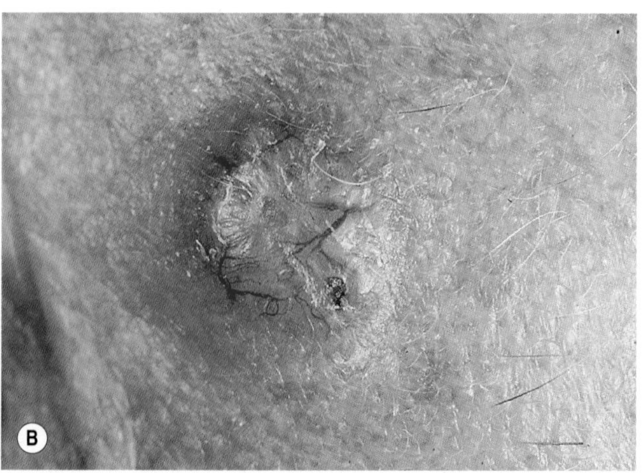

Lesion is not pearly white and resembles a dermal nevus.

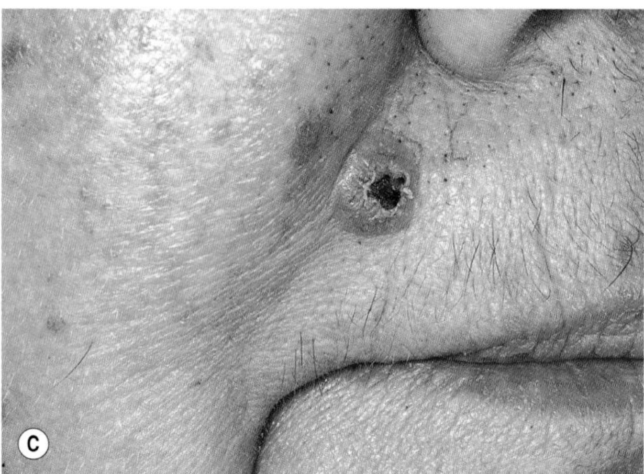

Central crusting occurs as the lesion enlarges. The appearance is similar to keratocanthoma.

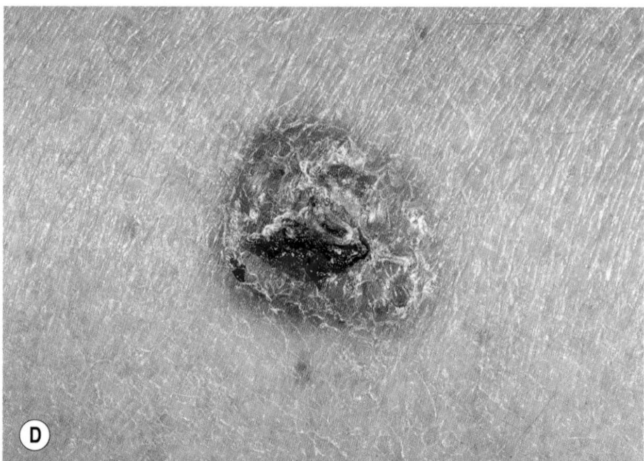

A dome-shaped papule covered with scale resembles an irritated seborrheic keratosis.

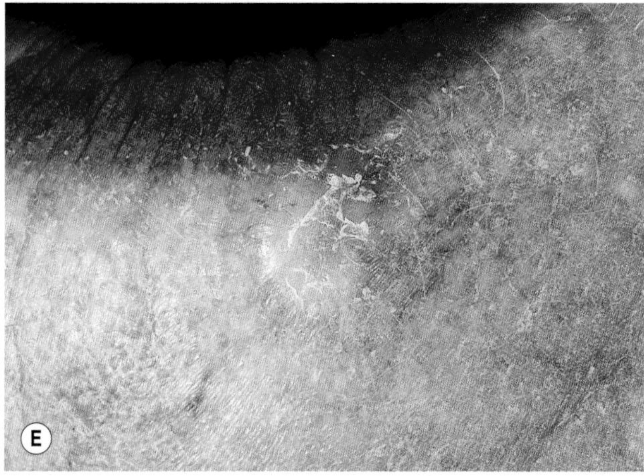

Tension on the surrounding skin accentuated this tiny translucent lesion with surface telangiectasia.

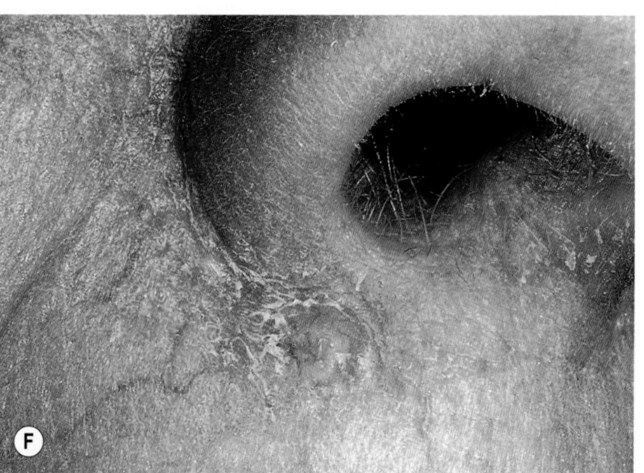

Small lesions can be missed on physical examination.

Figure 21-3

NODULAR BASAL CELL CARCINOMA

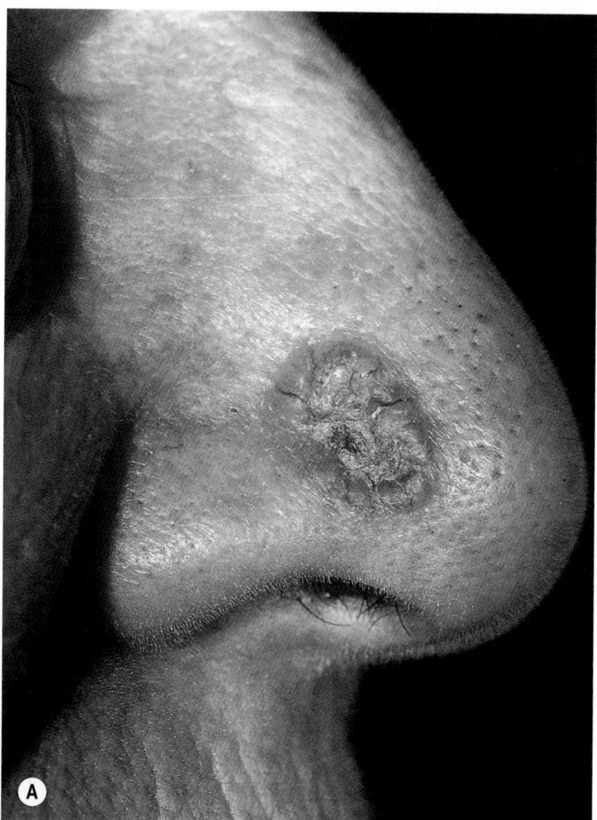

The center is ulcerated and is covered with a crust.

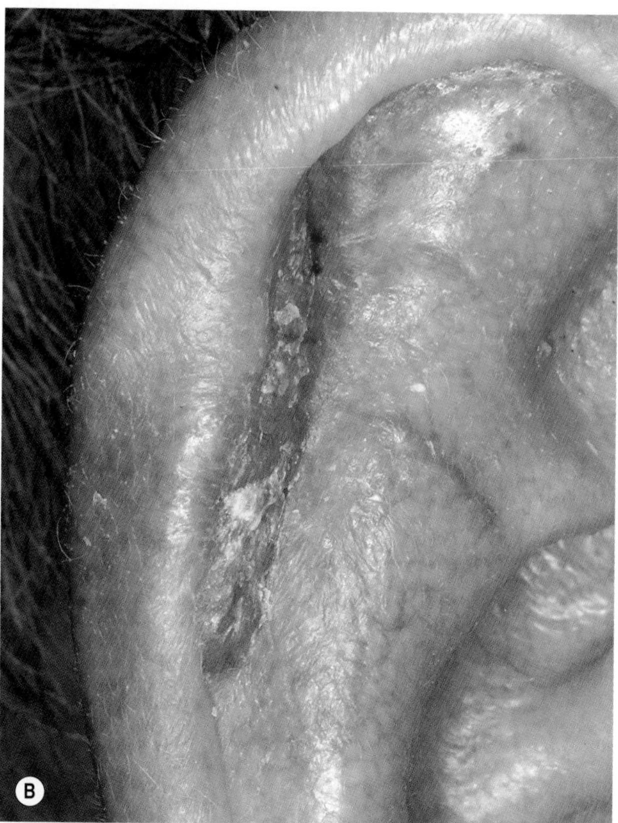

This lesion appeared to be inflammatory and was treated with topical steroids. After repeated cycles of healing and ulceration, a biopsy proved the diagnosis.

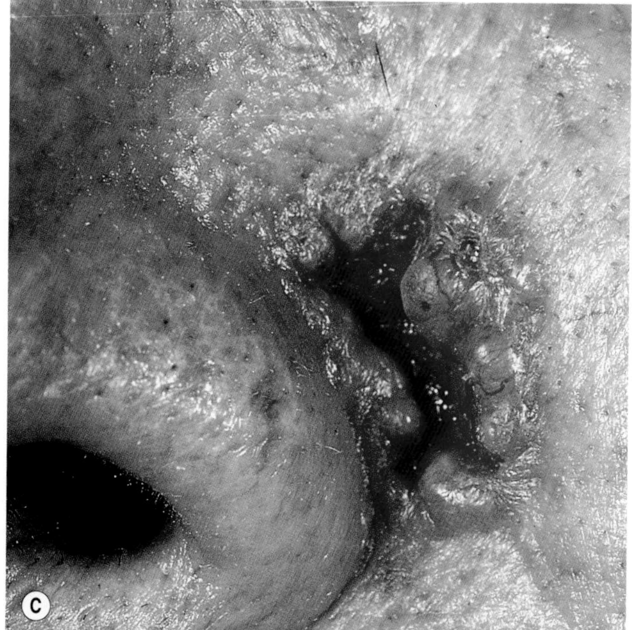

A deep ulcer is surrounded by a nodular tumor. In the past this type of lesion was referred to as a rodent ulcer.

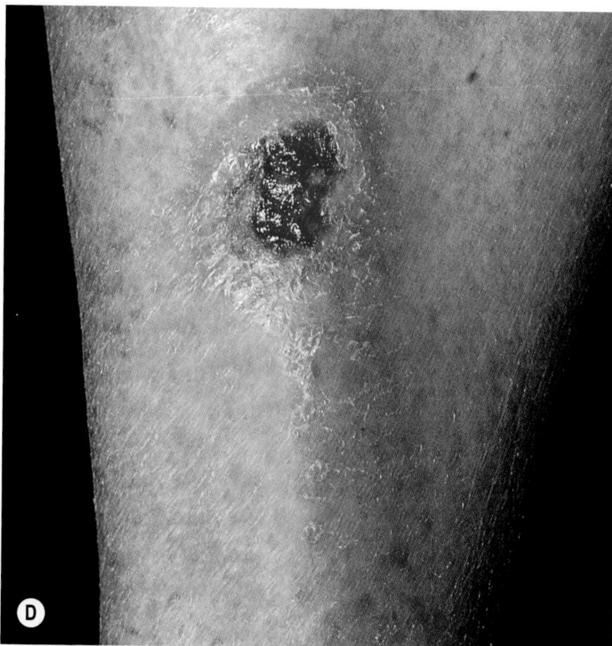

Lesions can appear anywhere on the body. Suspect basal cell carcinoma when a small leg ulcer fails to heal after conventional therapy. Close examination reveals a nodular border.

Figure 21-4

PIGMENTED BASAL CELL CARCINOMA. BCCs may contain melanin that imparts a brown, black, or blue color through all or part of the lesion. Clinically, the lesion resembles a melanoma or pigmented seborrheic keratosis, but close inspection reveals the characteristically elevated, pearly white, translucent border (Figure 21-5). Surface microscopy (see Chapter 22, Dermoscopy) may be used for more accurate diagnosis. Pigmented BCC must not have a pigment network and must have one or more of the following six positive features: large gray-blue ovoid nests, multiple gray-blue globules, maple leaf–like areas, spoke wheel areas, ulceration, and arborizing "treelike" telangiectasia. A biopsy confirms the diagnosis. The histologic pattern most frequently associated with pigment is the nodular pattern.

CYSTIC BASAL CELL CARCINOMA. This variant of nodular BCC appears as a smooth, round, cystic mass. Cystic BCC behaves like nodular BCC.

SCLEROSING OR MORPHEAFORM BASAL CELL CARCINOMA. Morpheaform BCC is an insidious tumor possessing innocuous surface characteristics that can mask its potential for deep, wide extension. The tumor is waxy, firm, flat-to-slightly raised, and either pale white or yellowish, and resembles localized scleroderma, thus the designation morpheaform (Figure 21-6). The borders are indistinct and blend with normal skin. Lesions may become depressed and firm, resembling a scar. The tissue is rigid and difficult or impossible to remove with a curette. Localization of this tumor by inspection or biopsy is impossible. The average subclinical extension beyond clinically delineated borders was 7.2 mm in one study. Treatment consists of wide excision or, preferably, Mohs' micrographic surgery.

PIGMENTED BASAL CELL CARCINOMA

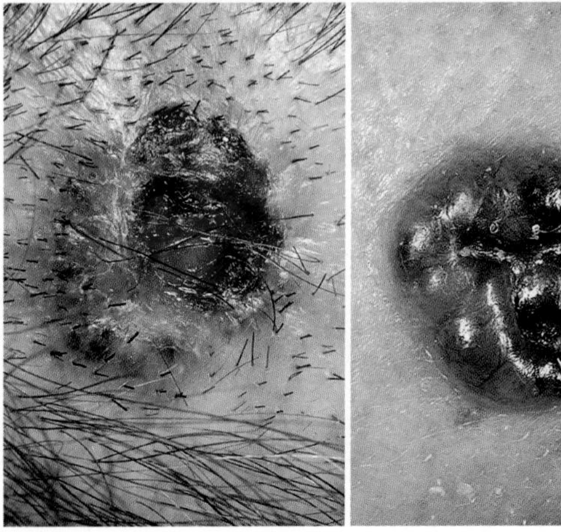

Figure 21-5 Variable amounts of melanin are seen in these special types of nodular basal cell carcinomas.

SCLEROSING BASAL CELL CARCINOMA

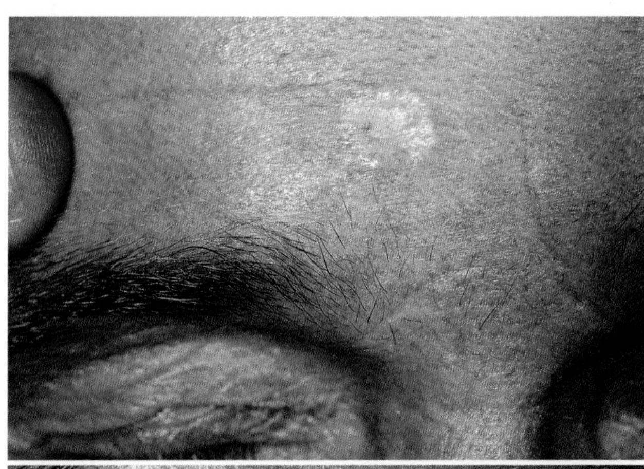

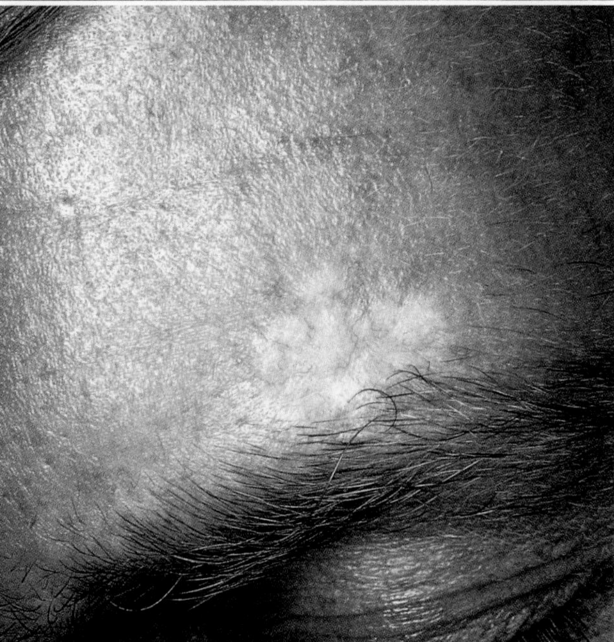

Figure 21-6 These hard, yellow masses may have ill-defined borders.

SUPERFICIAL BASAL CELL CARCINOMA. The least aggressive BCC is the superficial BCC. This tumor occurs most frequently on the trunk and extremities but may occur on the face. There may be one or more lesions. The tumor spreads peripherally, sometimes for several centimeters, and invades after considerable time. Slowly growing lesions may be present for years before patients seek help. The circumscribed, round-to-oval, red, scaling plaque resembles a plaque of eczema, psoriasis, extramammary Paget's disease, or Bowen's disease (Figure 21-7, *A–E*). However, careful inspection of the border shows its thin, raised, pearly white nature (see Figure 21-7, *E*). The characteristic features can also be appreciated by eliminating the redness with lateral finger pressure.

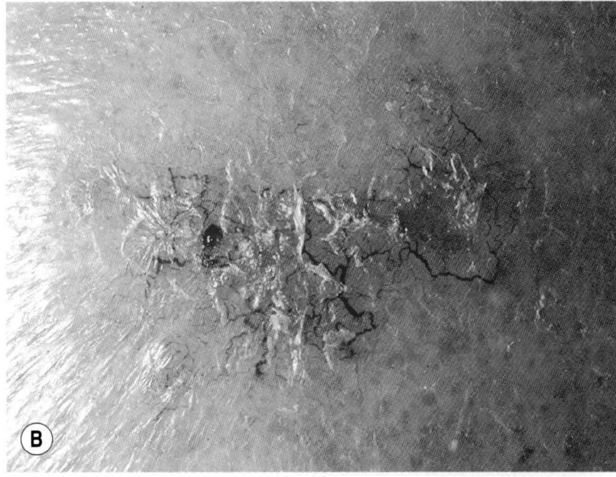

SUPERFICIAL BASAL CELL CARCINOMA

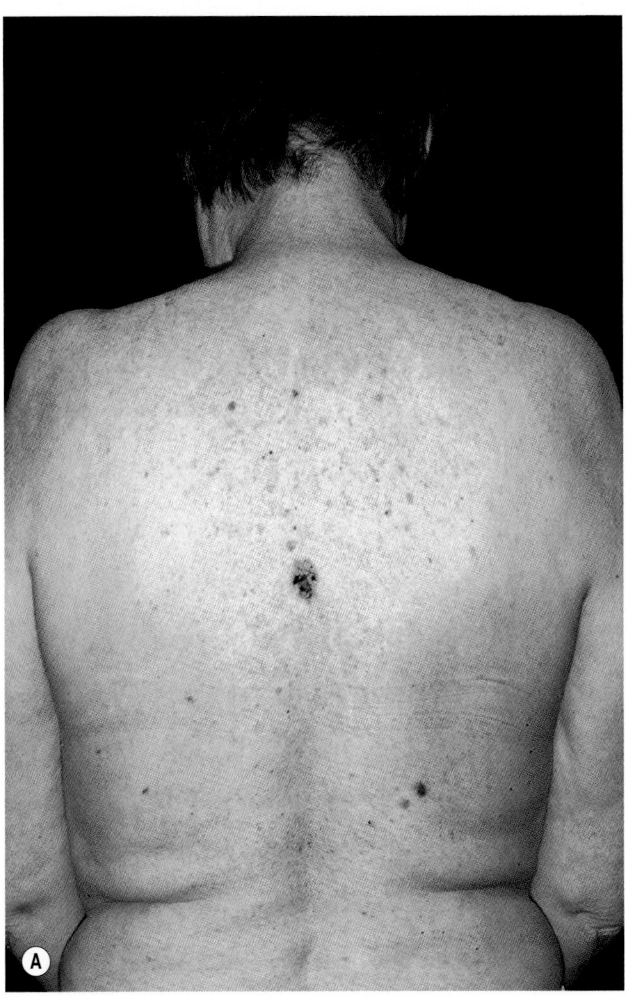

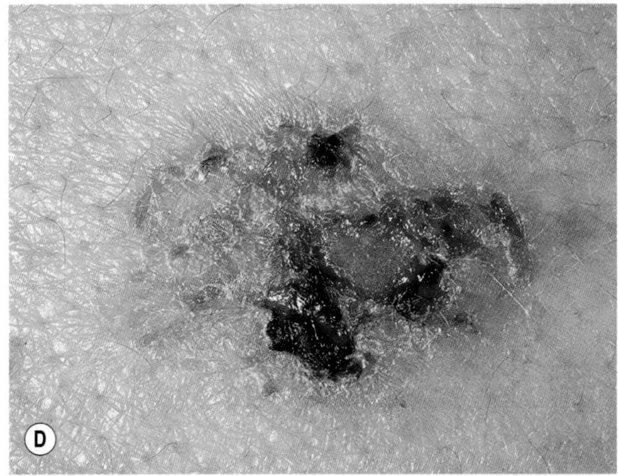

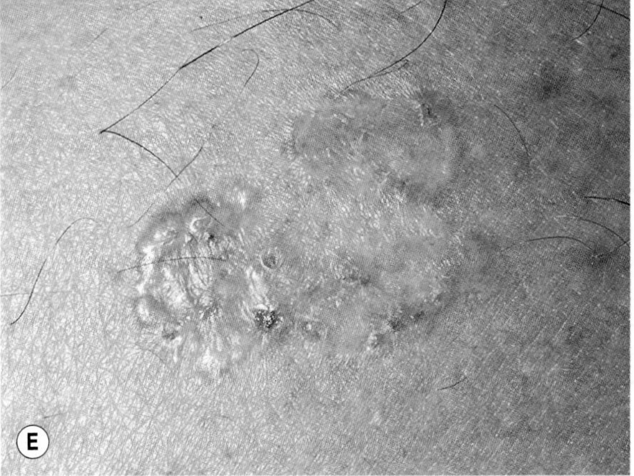

Figure 21-7 **A,** The trunk is the most common site. **B,** Telangiectasia may be prominent. **C,** Lesions resemble eczema or psoriasis. **D,** Crust and scale occur as the lesion enlarges. **E,** Tension on surrounding skin accentuates the raised border.

NEVOID BASAL CELL CARCINOMA SYNDROME (GORLIN-GOLTZ SYNDROME). This rare disease is inherited as an autosomal dominant trait with high penetrance and variable expressivity. The gene is located on chromosome 9q22.3-q31. It has the following major features: multiple BCCs appear at birth or in early childhood; numerous small pits on the palms and soles (Figure 21-8) (50% to 87%); epithelium-lined jaw cysts, which commonly cause symptoms (65% to 90%); ectopic calcification with lamellar calcification of falx cerebri (80%); and a variety of skeletal abnormalities, especially of the ribs, skull, and spine (70% to 75%). A characteristic facies is present in approximately 70% of patients. Physical findings include "coarse face" (54%), relative macrocephaly (50%), hypertelorism (42%), and frontal bossing (27%).

Numerous associated anomalies may be present (Box 21-1). There is great variation in the number and behavior of the nevoid BCC. The median number is eight. Although many patients have no BCCs or just a few, more than 1000 BCCs can be present. The first tumor occurs at a mean age of 23 years. Locally destructive tumors are not seen before puberty. Aggressive tumor behavior can occur after puberty, and all patients must be observed closely. Most of the highly invasive tumors involve embryonic cleft areas of the face. Development of multiple BCCs is enhanced by exposure to light and x-ray irradiation, but they also occur on unexposed surfaces. Multiple bilateral jaw cysts are the presenting complaint in approximately 50% of patients; a dentist, R.J. Gorlin, discovered the syndrome. The cysts appear during the first decade of life and displace the child's teeth, often in the premolar area. The first cyst occurs in 80% of patients by the age of 20 years. The number of cysts ranges from 1 to 28 (median, 3). They cause pain, drainage, and jaw swelling. The occurrence of multiple skeletal anomalies is highly suggestive and may be the earliest clue to the diagnosis of nevoid BCC syndrome in children. Complete or partial bridging of the sella turcica is present in 75% of patients. Splayed and bifurcated ribs occur in 40% of patients. Ovarian fibromas were diagnosed by ultrasound in 17% of patients at 30 years of age (mean).

The initial evaluation of patients suspected of having BCC syndrome should include the following: (1) family history; (2) dental consultations; and (3) radiographs of jaws, skull, chest, spinal column, and hands. Radiographs show calcification of the falx cerebri (65%) or tentorium cerebelli (20%); bridged sella (68%), bifid ribs (26%), and flame-shaped lucencies of the phalanges; and metacarpal and carpal bones of the hands (30%).

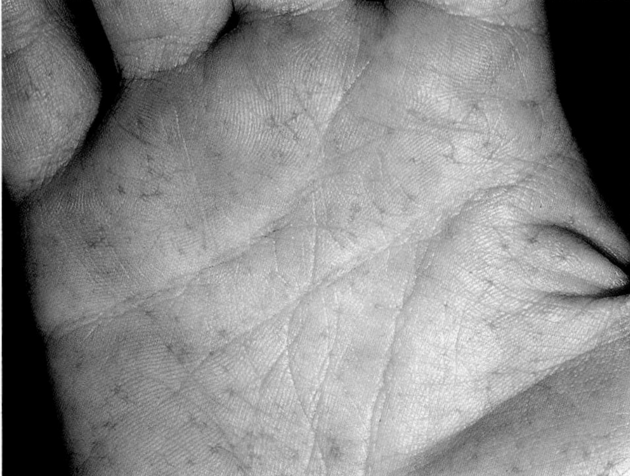

Figure 21-8 Nevoid basal cell carcinoma syndrome. Numerous small pits occur in the palms and soles.

Management and risk of recurrence

There are several factors to consider before choosing the best treatment modality. The most important are clinical presentation, cell type, tumor size, and location. Figure 21-9 presents a treatment algorithm for BCC.

CLINICAL TYPE. Nodular and superficial BCCs are the least aggressive and can be completely removed by electrodesiccation and curettage or by simple surgical excision.

Box 21-1 **Nevoid Basal Cell Carcinoma Syndrome**

Skin

Multiple nevoid basal cell carcinomas
Pits—palms and soles (50% to 65%)
Milia, cysts (epithelial and sebaceous)

Face and mouth

Multiple jaw cysts (65% to 90%)
- Presenting complaint in 50%

Characteristic facies (70%)
- Mandibular prognathism
- Broadening of the nasal root (25%)
- Frontal/temporoparietal bossing
- Ocular hypertelorism

Central nervous system

Lamellar calcification of falx cerebri (80%)
Bridging of the sella turcica (75%)
Mental retardation
Electroencephalographic abnormalities

Skeletal system anomalies (70% to 75%)

Rib anomalies (55%): bifurcation and splaying (40%), synostotic or partial agenesis, or rudimentary cervical ribs
Vertebrae (65%): kyphoscoliosis (50%), spina bifida occulta (40%)
Shortened metacarpals (usually fourth, fifth, or both) (28%)
Bone cysts—phalanges and other bones (46%)
Many others

Others

Lymphomesenteric cysts
Ovarian fibromas or cysts

Kimonis VE et al: *Am J Med Genet* 69:299, 1997. *PMID: 9096761*

HISTOLOGIC TYPE. The micronodular, infiltrative, and morpheaform BCCs have a higher incidence of positive tumor margins (18.6%, 26.5%, and 33.3%, respectively) after excision and have the greatest recurrence rate. Clinically, BCCs with these patterns have poorly defined borders and are not apparent during physical examination. They subtly extend into surrounding tissue and are easily missed by blind treatment techniques such as surgical excision. An average of 7.2 mm of subclinical tumor extension was found in morpheaform BCCs in one study, compared with 2.1 mm of extension in well-circumscribed nodular lesions. Routine pathologic examination of surgically excised BCCs may not detect a small nodule or strand of BCC on the other side of the excision margin. These tumors need more aggressive treatment with wide excision or microscopically controlled surgery.

TUMOR SIZE. In general, electrodesiccation and curettage afford excellent results for small (less than 1 cm) nodular BCCs located on the forehead or cheeks. Nodular BCCs on the forehead or cheeks that are larger and have well-defined margins should be excised and closed; electrosurgery for large tumors may result in large, unsightly scars. The margins of sclerosing BCCs cannot be determined by inspection, and either excision or, preferably, Mohs micrographic surgery should be performed. Superficial BCCs of any size can be adequately removed by electrosurgery or treated medically with imiquimod cream (Aldara).

LOCATION. Tumors around the nose, eye, and ear require special consideration. Lesions of the nose greater than 1 cm in diameter, lesions of the margin of the eyelid and the vermilion border of the lip, lesions involving cartilage, and sclerosing epitheliomas respond poorly to electrodesiccation and curettage. BCCs of the medial canthus are particularly dangerous. The skin rests close to bone and cartilage, and tumor cells initially invade and proceed to migrate undetected along periosteum or perichondrium. Healing occurs over inadequately treated tumors, and deep invasion and lateral extension can remain undetected, resulting in a tumor of massive proportions. Extension to the eye and brain is possible.

RISK OF RECURRENCE WITH ELECTRODESICCATION AND CURETTAGE (ED&C). Low-, intermediate-, and high-risk sites for recurrence following ED&C of primary BCC have been defined. The neck, trunk, and extremities are considered low-risk sites with a 5-year recurrence rate of 8.6%. The scalp, forehead, and temples are of intermediate risk with a 12.9% recurrence rate. High-risk sites, such as the nose, eyelids, chin, jaw, and ear, have a recurrence rate of 17.5%. To achieve a 95% cure rate using ED&C at middle-risk sites, lesions should measure less than 1 cm in diameter, and in high-risk areas a 95% cure rate using ED&C may be achieved by selecting lesions less than 6 mm in diameter.

RELATIVE RISK AND FOLLOW-UP. Patients treated for BCC should be observed periodically for 5 years or longer. Of patients with one BCC, a second BCC develops in 36% to 50% during the 5 years after treatment. In another series, another BCC developed in 41% of patients who had two or more previous skin cancers.

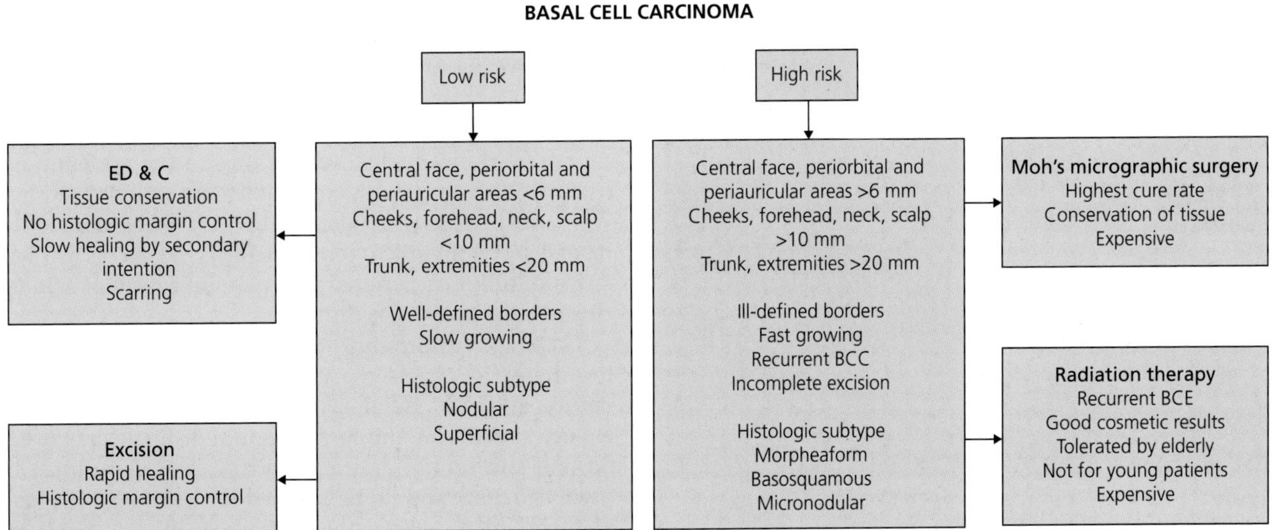

Figure 21-9 Adapted from Martinez JC, Otley CC: *MayoClin Proc* 76:1253, 2001. *PMID: 11761506*

Recurrent basal cell carcinoma

CLINICAL PRESENTATION

Inadequately treated BCC may recur. The tumor may be superficial in the scar tissue, on the border, or deep in the dermis or subcutaneous fat (Figure 21-10). The clinical presentation of recurrent BCC sometimes differs from the original tumor. A tumor that infiltrates scar tissue produces a subtle change in color and consistency that is easily missed. Erosions that appear spontaneously at the border or in the scar are suspicious. The characteristic pearly white border is often absent, but biopsy of the erosion with the curette can reveal the soft, amorphous, gelatinous tissue of BCC extending deep and laterally well beyond the border of the erosion. Deep recurrences show a normal or a brownish erythematous surface and can be confused with epidermal cysts.

Histologic picture, anatomic location, and size are factors in predicting recurrence.

HISTOLOGIC TYPE. Tumors of the morpheaform and basosquamous varieties have the greatest recurrence rate. BCCs that histologically show poor palisading or have a micronodular (islands of tumor) and/or infiltrating strand pattern without sclerotic stroma clinically have poorly defined borders and are not apparent during physical examination. They subtly extend into surrounding tissue and are easily missed by blind treatment techniques such as surgical excision. An average of 7.2 mm of subclinical tumor extension was found in morpheaform BCCs in one study, compared with 2.1 mm of extension in well-circumscribed nodular lesions. As mentioned previously, routine pathologic examination of surgically excised BCCs may not detect a small nodule or strand of BCC on the other side of the excision margin. These tumors need more aggressive treatment with wide excision or microscopically controlled surgery.

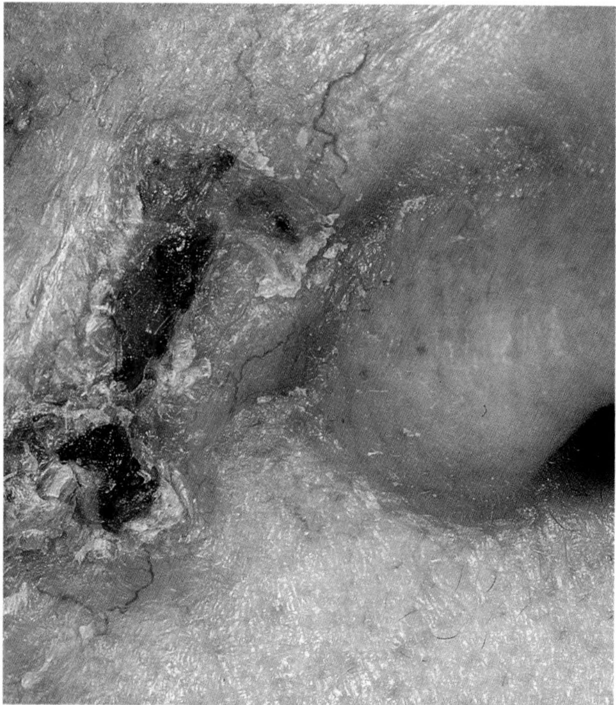

Figure 21-10 Recurrent basal cell carcinoma. A haphazard nodular tumor with telangiectasia surrounds and infiltrates under scar tissue.

LOCATION. Increasing diameter of the lesion and location of the lesion on various sites of the head, especially the nose and ear, are associated with an increased risk of recurrence, whereas location on the neck, trunk, limbs, or genitalia is associated with a decreased risk of recurrence with ED&C, radiation therapy, and surgical excision. BCCs on the nose or perinasal area may infiltrate along the perichondrium or penetrate into the embryonic fusion plane of the nasolabial fold, resulting in subclinical extension.

SIZE. The larger the tumor, the greater the chance of recurrence; increased subclinical extension is seen with larger tumors.

Treatment of basal cell carcinoma

The following section outlines various treatment modalities. Specific techniques are described in Chapter 27.

RECOMMENDED FOLLOW-UP EVALUATION. Patients with BCC may benefit from a once-yearly complete skin examination. Because the risk of a subsequent BCC decreases 3 years after an index tumor, the need for continued surveillance of patients with a BCC who have remained tumor-free after 3 years is probably limited.

BIOPSY. Biopsy alone of a small BCC often appears curative with no clinical evidence of residual tumor. Two thirds of clinically disease-free biopsy sites were shown to contain microscopic foci of BCC.

ELECTRODESICCATION AND CURETTAGE. ED&C is most beneficial for nodular BCCs less than 6 mm in diameter, regardless of anatomic site; selected larger BCCs, depending on their anatomic site; and superficial BCCs. It is not appropriate for morpheaform BCCs because margins cannot be clinically defined. Lesions on the nose and nasolabial folds may be treated if they are well-defined and very small; otherwise, these high-risk areas should be treated by Mohs micrographic surgery. ED&C is particularly useful for ear lesions, where mobilization of skin for closure after excision is difficult.

Curettage requires firm dermis on all sides and below the tumor to enable the curette to distinguish between dermis and soft tumor (Figure 21-11). If the tumor encroaches on the fat, the curette cannot distinguish between fat and soft tumor, and an alternate procedure must be used. Curettage should be avoided for lesions on the back and shoulders, where the dermis is thick, unless the BCCs are superficial and small. Proper technique requires vigorous curettage, usually two to three times; therefore lesions on the eyelid or lip area are treated by other methods. It is especially useful for lower extremity tumors, where tissue mobilization for excision may be difficult. Wounds created by electrosurgery ooze serum and accumulate crust during a 2- to 6-week healing period. The recurrence rate using ED&C performed by a fully trained dermatologist is 5.7%. The overall recurrence rate using surgical excision is 5.3%. The technique is explained in Chapter 27.

EXCISION SURGERY. Excision surgery is preferred for large tumors with well-defined borders on the cheeks, forehead, trunk, and legs. The cosmetic result is good and healing time is less than that required for electrosurgery. Excision with primary closure is technically difficult on the ears and nose. The advantage of feeling the tumor with a curette is lost and adequate margins must be taken. Lesions on the neck, trunk, and arms or legs have a 5-year cure rate of more than 99%. Excision of head lesions is less effective with increasing tumor size: the 5-year cure rate for lesions less than 6 mm in diameter is 97%; the rate is 92% for lesions that are 6 mm or larger.

Preoperative curettage. Preoperative curettage may assist the surgeon in better defining the tumor border and decreases the frequency of positive margins in the management of BCC. It offers a 24% reduction in surgical failure rates in the treatment of BCC. Curettage showed no benefit in the treatment of SCC. It is postulated that SCC differs from noninvasive BCC in that SCC invades as small nests in the absence of mucinous stroma and therefore does not loosen as readily from its surrounding matrix as does BCC. Thus, although preexcisional curettage of SCC does no harm, it may not improve surgical cure rates.

Incompletely resected basal cell carcinoma. Adequate excision, peripherally and in depth, is the key to surgical control, and the demonstration of tumor cells at the margins of excision is associated with recurrence rates of more than 30%. Data support the policy of immediate reexcision or Mohs micrographic surgery for all patients with incompletely excised BCCs rather than a "wait-and-see" policy after incomplete excision. Reexcision may not be necessary if the patient's life span is limited or if treatment of a possible recurrence would not be difficult.

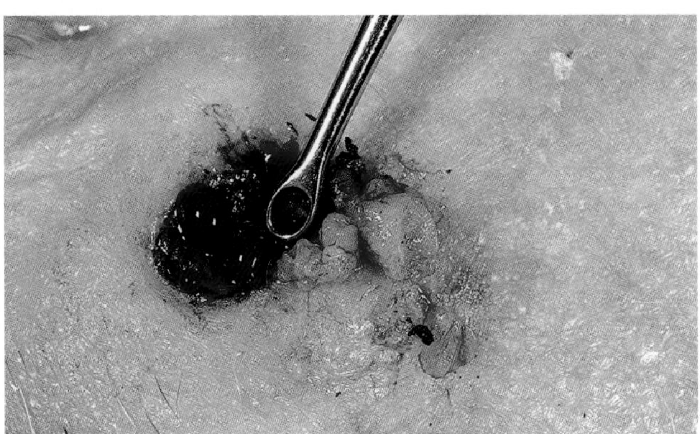

Figure 21-11 Nodular basal cell carcinoma. Curettage easily disrupts the poorly cohesive tumor.

MOHS' MICROGRAPHIC SURGERY. Mohs surgery is a microscopically controlled technique that may be used for all types and sizes of BCCs. The procedure is unnecessarily destructive for smaller lesions or for lesions with well-defined clinical margins, such as nodular or superficial multicentric BCCs.

Mohs surgery is the treatment of choice for most sclerosing BCCs and other BCCs with poorly defined clinical margins; for tumors in areas of potentially high recurrence (Box 21-2), such as the nose or eyelid; for very large primary tumors; and for large, recurrent BCCs. The technique is explained in Chapter 27.

RADIATION. Radiation is useful for elderly patients who cannot tolerate minor surgical procedures.

IMIQUIMOD 5% CREAM (ALDARA). Imiquimod is an immune response modifier that induces cytokines related to cell-mediated immune responses including interferon-alfa, interferon-gamma, and interleukin-12. Patient-administered imiquimod 5% cream used five to seven times per week for a period of 6 weeks effectively treated superficial BCC. Local skin reactions are common but well tolerated. The initial clearance rate at 12 weeks posttreatment is about 95%. The recurrence rate after 2 years is as high as 20%.

5-FLUOROURACIL. Five percent 5-fluorouracil (5-FU) cream is approved by the FDA for the treatment of superficial BCCs. Treat with 5% 5-FU cream twice daily for up to 12 weeks. Treatment is stopped sooner if the lesion is clinically resolved.

Box 21-2 **Indications for Mohs' Micrographic Surgery**

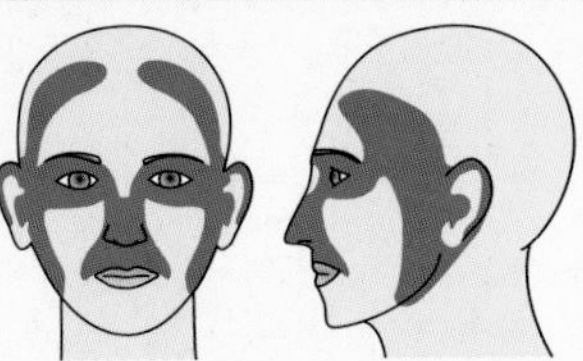

1. Extensive, recurrent skin cancers that have not responded to aggressive conventional surgical techniques or radiation
2. Unusually large primary skin cancers of long duration
3. Poorly differentiated squamous cell carcinoma
4. Morpheaform or fibrotic basal cell carcinoma
5. Tumors with poorly demarcated clinical borders
6. Tumors on the face in locations where deeper invasion of the skin along natural skin planes is possible or the extent of the tumor is difficult to define, such as eyelids, nasal alae, nasolabial folds, and circumauricular areas
7. Areas where maximum conservation of tumor-free tissue is important for preservation of function, such as the penis or finger

ACTINIC KERATOSIS

Actinic keratosis (AK) (solar keratosis) is a squamous cell carcinoma confined to the epidermis. The lesions are common, sun-induced, and increase in number with age. Most lesions remain superficial. Lesions that extend more deeply to involve the papillary and/or reticular dermis are termed squamous cell carcinoma (SCC).

The potential for change cannot be predicted by clinical signs or histologic characteristics. Thick lesions are worrisome. Patients with AKs need periodic evaluation and usually repetitive treatments to prevent the development of aggressive cancers. Individuals with light complexions are more susceptible than those with dark complexions. Years of sun exposure are required to induce sufficient damage to cause lesions. Actinic keratoses may undergo spontaneous remission if sunlight exposure is reduced, but new lesions may appear. Patients often present with lesions that were first noticed during the summer, suggesting that the lesions may become more active after sunlight exposure. Immunosuppression is a risk factor. SCC is up to 65 times as likely to develop in transplant patients as controls. Lesions appear 2 to 4 years after transplantation and increase in frequency.

PERSPECTIVE FOR THE PATIENT

An AK is an intraepidermal SCC. This definition is useful for the clinician and pathologist, but it confuses and worries the patient. The term actinic keratosis without the word cancer is appropriate for patients. Patients need to understand that these lesions can become thicker and change into invasive cancers but the chance of that happening is small. Periodic examinations, treatment, and preventive measures (e.g., sunscreens, clothing) are necessary.

CLINICAL PRESENTATION. Actinic keratoses begin as an area of increased vascularity, with the skin surface becoming slightly rough. Texture is the key to diagnosing early lesions. They are better recognized by palpation than by inspection. Very gradually an adherent, yellow, sharp scale forms. Removal of the scale may cause bleeding (Figures 21-12 and 21-13). Most lesions vary in size from 3 to 6 mm. The extent of disease varies from a single lesion to involvement of the entire forehead, balding scalp, or temples. AK can progress into thickened or hypertrophic lesions. Thickened lesions can progress to SCC and be clinically indistinguishable. Induration, inflammation, and oozing suggest degeneration into malignancy.

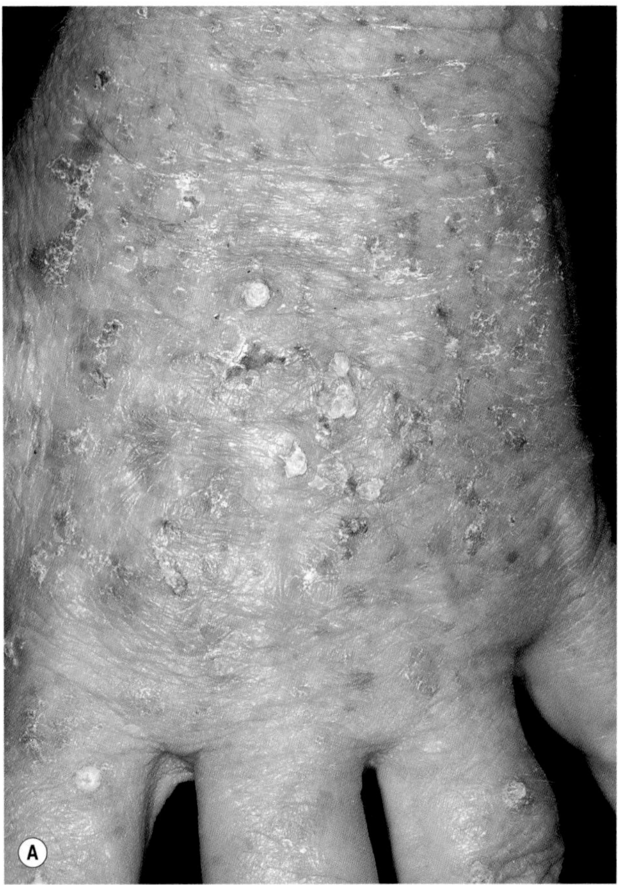

Several oval-to-round, red, indurated lesions with adherent scale.

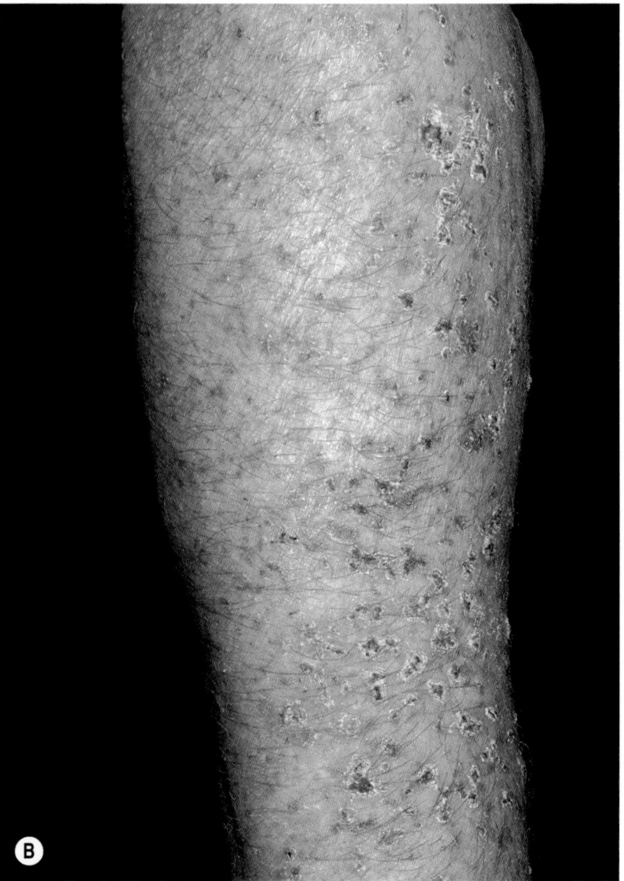

Lesions may appear in large numbers on exposed arms and legs.

Figure 21-12 Actinic keratosis. These are very extreme cases.

ACTINIC KERATOSIS

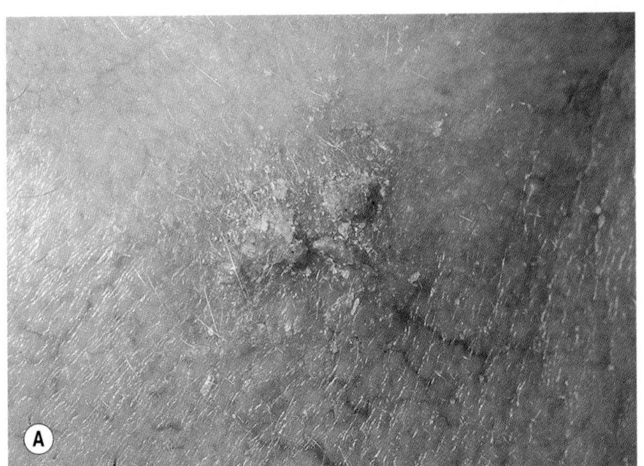

Classic lesion with sharp, adherent scale on a red base.

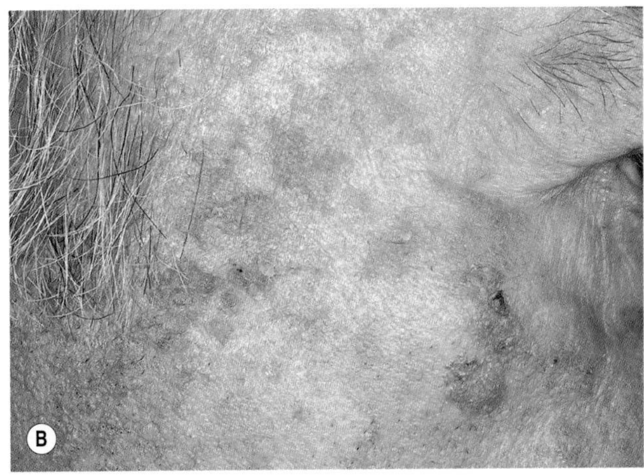

Many lesions may appear on the face. The surrounding skin is irregularly pigmented with dilated blood vessels.

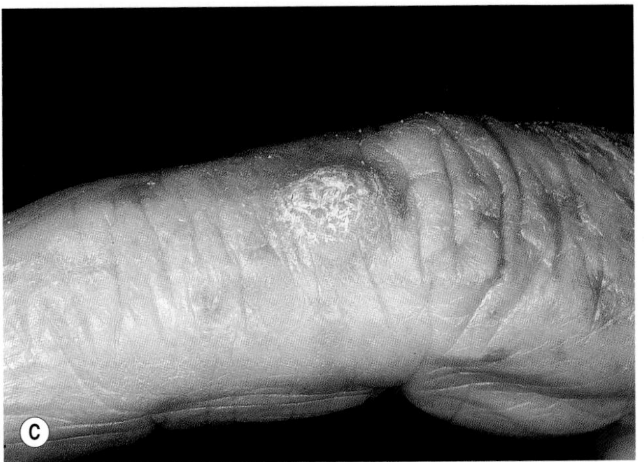

Thicker lesions may degenerate into squamous cell carcinoma.

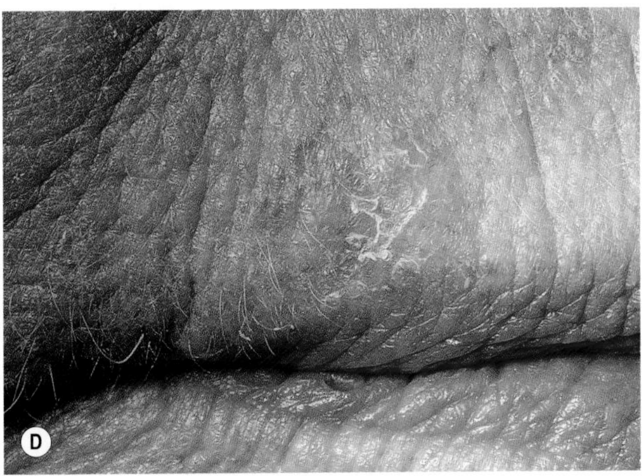

Keratoses on the lips may be deeper than they appear. Palpate to determine thickness.

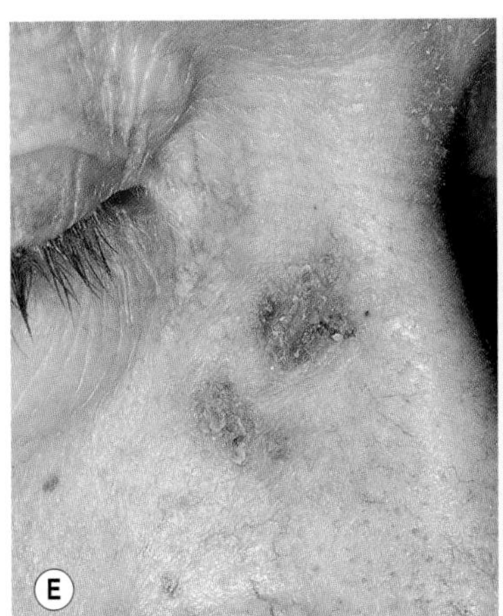

Large keratoses may have considerable depth.

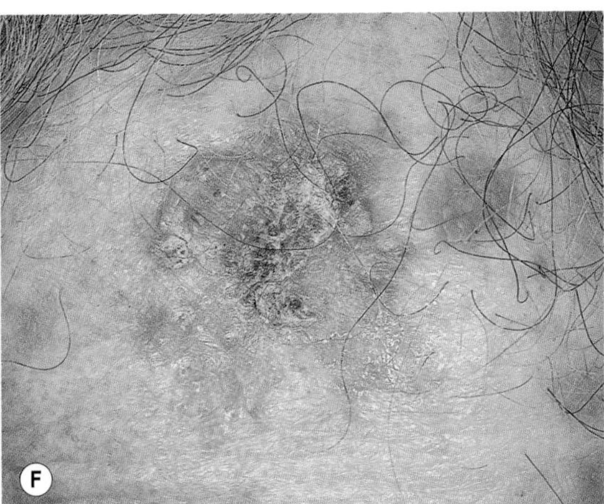

Very large lesions take months or years to form.

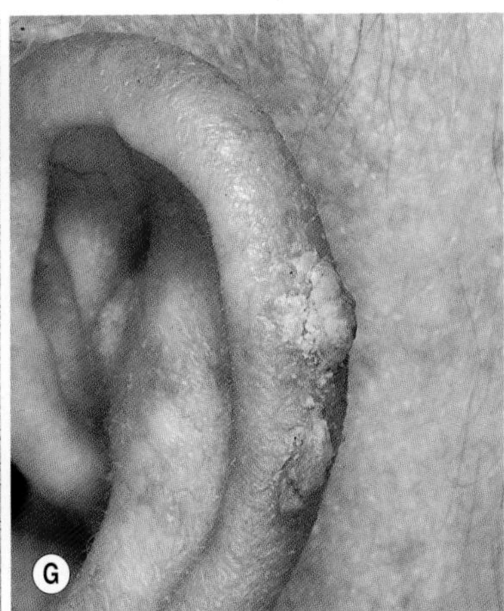

Squamous cell carcinoma has an identical appearance to actinic keratosis.

Figure 21-13

CLINICAL VARIANTS. Clinical variants include cutaneous horn, spreading pigmented AK, and actinic cheilitis. Cutaneous horn is a hypertrophic AK that accumulates keratin to become a conical hyperkeratotic protuberance. Pigmented AKs resemble a scaling lentigo, seborrheic keratosis, or melanoma (Figures 21-14 and 21-15). Lesions are very common and tend to be thick on the scalp (Figure 21-16). Actinic cheilitis is AK occurring on the lower lips. The lips are rough, scaly, and red, and may show fissuring, scaliness, and ulcerations. These findings can be seen in SCC of the lip (Figures 21-17 and 21-18). SCCs of the lip have approximately an 11% metastatic rate, which is higher than other cutaneous SCCs.

TRANSFORMATION INTO SQUAMOUS CELL CARCINOMA. After several years, a small percentage of lesions may increase in size and thickness, extend into the dermis, and become a risk for metastatic disease. A very low yearly transformation rate for single lesions can translate into a substantial lifetime risk of transformation for patients with several actinic keratoses. The average number of AKs per person is 7.7. The likelihood of an AK developing into a SCC is estimated to be 0.085% per lesion per year. Therefore SCC would develop at a rate of at least 10.2% over 10 years. Up to 60% of SCCs develop from actinic keratosis. Squamous cell carcinomas that evolve from actinic keratosis are not aggressive but may eventually metastasize.

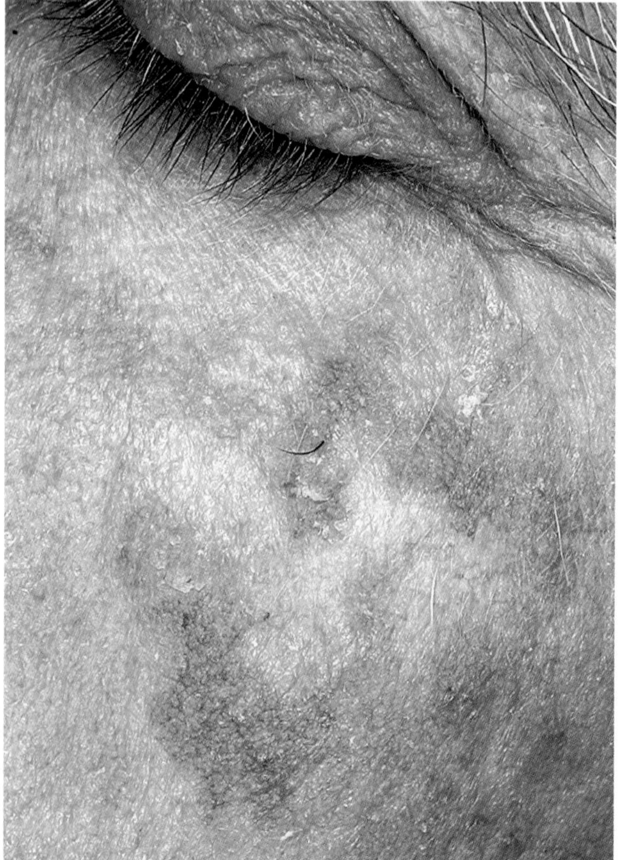

Figure 21-14 Pigmented actinic keratosis.

ACTINIC KERATOSIS VS. SQUAMOUS CELL CARCINOMA. There is no definite way to distinguish between an AK and a SCC without a biopsy. There is a continuum of clinical signs that makes distinction difficult. An increase in the thickness, redness, pain, ulceration, and size only suggests progression to SCC, but it is impossible to predict the point at which an individual AK will evolve into an invasive SCC. Lesions thought to be actinic keratoses or those not responding to treatment may actually be SCCs. Therefore treatment should be aggressive and patients monitored closely to prevent progression.

PATHOPHYSIOLOGY AND HISTOLOGY. Ultraviolet radiation initiates the process by inducing mutations in DNA, usually in the p53 tumor-suppressor gene in keratinocytes. Cells with dysfunctional p53 may, with additional exposure to UV radiation, be promoted to undergo an uncontrolled clonal cellular proliferation in the epidermis to produce an AK. Additional exposure to radiation may convert the AK into a SCC. Histologically, an AK consists of abnormal epithelial cells confined to the epidermis. The features of the cells are identical to those found in invasive SCC, including those that have metastasized. The cells have large pleomorphic nuclei and acidophilic cytoplasm (Figure 21-19). Some are in mitosis. They show signs of faulty cornification with dyskeratotic cells and parakeratosis. The term "squamous cell carcinoma in situ" is frequently used to describe a lesion with abnormal cells confined to the epidermis. The follicles are not involved, so there is no follicular plugging. Penetration through the dermoepidermal junction and into the dermis indicates the development of an invasive SCC.

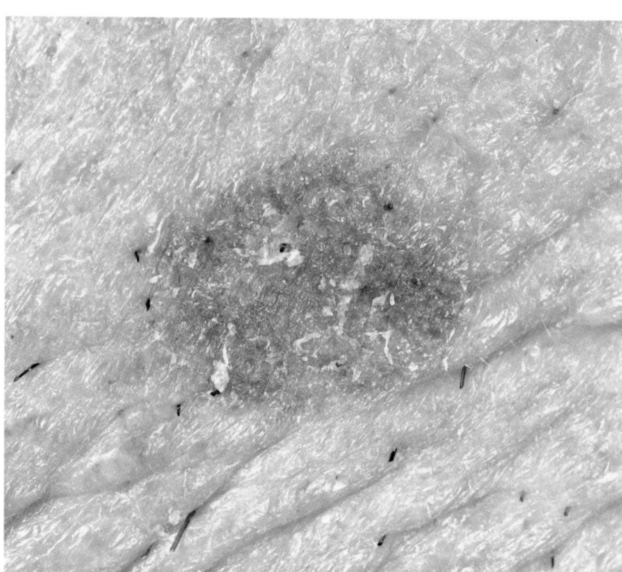

Figure 21-15 Pigmented actinic keratosis.

ACTINIC KERATOSIS

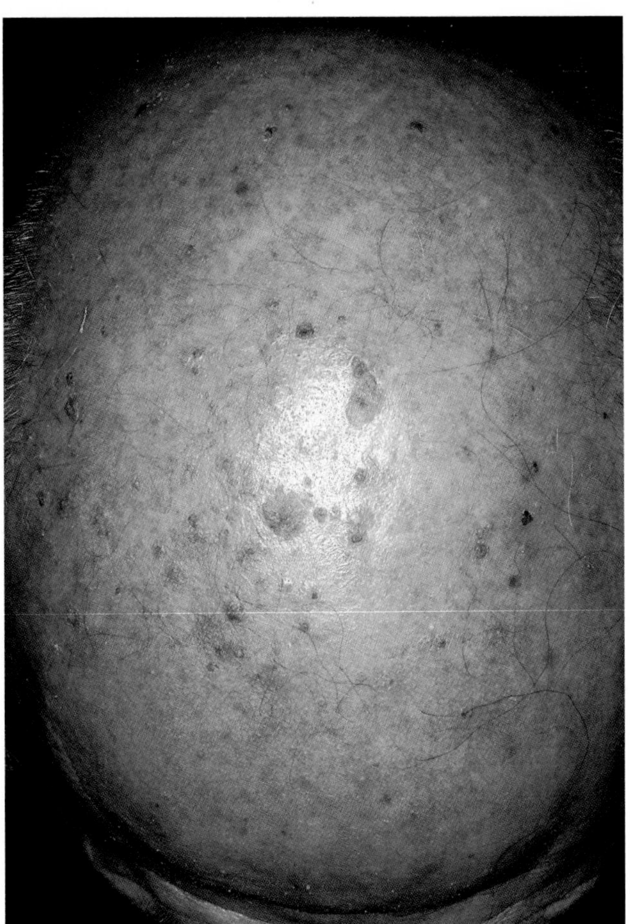

Figure 21-16 Actinic keratosis, scalp. Actinic keratosis is commonly found on the balding (or thin-hair) scalp. Cryotherapy is effective treatment. It is difficult to judge the depth of a lesion. Actinic keratosis may eventually invade and become squamous cell carcinomas. Repeatedly freezing the same recurrent lesion may miss a cancer. Curet or excise thicker lesions.

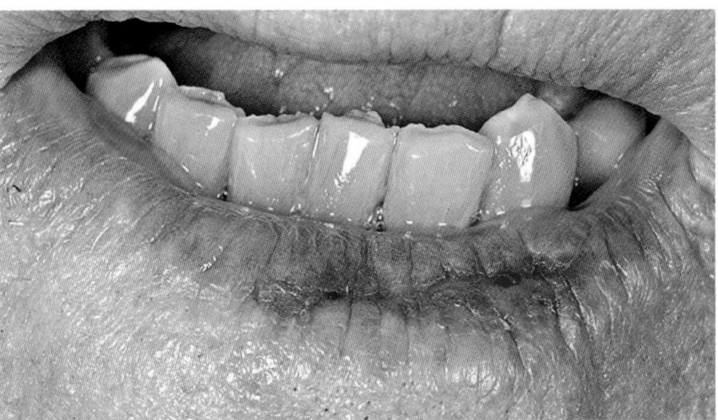

Figure 21-17 Broad superficial lesions may be present for months to years with little progression. These lesions respond to topical 5-fluorouracil.

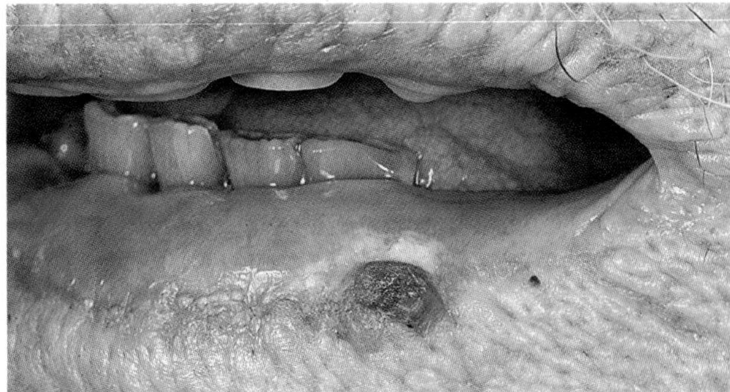

Figure 21-18 The depth of this lesion is difficult to judge by physical examination. Surgery is the most reliable treatment.

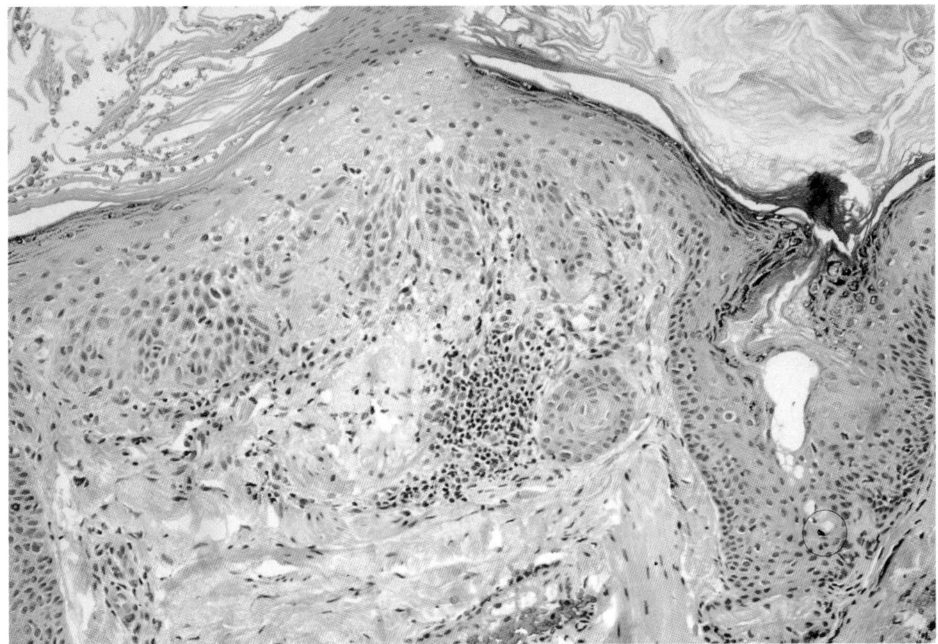

Figure 21-19 Keratin and crust are present on the surface. Atypical epithelial cells are confined to the epidermis and do not involve the follicular structure.

MANAGEMENT

Because actinic keratoses sometimes undergo spontaneous remission, definitive treatment may be delayed for patients with a few superficial lesions. Small lesions should be reexamined at a later date for spontaneous remission. Patients should make every effort to prevent further sun damage. This does not mean that patients must hibernate for a lifetime, but they should understand techniques to reduce sunlight exposure. There is a continuum and a progression from AK to SCC; therefore there is no way to reliably distinguish clinically between the two diagnoses. Because it can be impossible to distinguish between an AK and SCC, treatment of AK should be aggressive to stop the progression to SCC. All patients with AK should be examined carefully for BCCs.

CRYOTHERAPY. Cryotherapy is the treatment of choice for most isolated, superficial, AK. AK resides in the epithelium. Cryotherapy with liquid nitrogen causes the separation of the epidermis and dermis, resulting in a highly specific, nonscarring method of therapy for superficial lesions. Patients with darker complexions may develop hypopigmented areas after freezing, and treating multiple lesions on the faces of such patients may result in white-spotted faces. Topical 5-FU is the best alternative.

SURGICAL REMOVAL. Individual indurated lesions or those with thick crusts should be removed with minor surgical procedures. It is unnecessary to biopsy lesions less than 0.5 cm. Larger lesions or those occurring about or on the vermilion border of the lips should be examined. Electrodesiccation and curettage easily remove small, thicker lesions. The CO_2 laser may be superior to vermilionectomy for actinic cheilitis that is too extensive to be treated with topical 5-FU.

SUNSCREENS. Regular use of sunscreens prevents the development of solar keratoses. Sunscreens that contain a combination of ingredients to block both the UVA and the UVB spectrum of ultraviolet light are most effective. Sunscreens are best applied in the morning on days when sun exposure is anticipated. Sunscreens should be applied to the face, lower lip, ears, back of the neck, and backs of the hands and forearms. Hats should cover bald heads. The physician should explain that although sunscreens are used, additional lesions might occur, but that many superficial areas of involvement may actually improve.

TOPICAL CHEMOTHERAPY WITH 5-FLUOROURACIL. 5-FU is an effective topical treatment for superficial actinic keratosis. Thicker lesions, especially those on the scalp, may evolve into SCC and should be treated with more aggressive techniques. The agent is incorporated into rapidly dividing cells, resulting in cell death. Normal cells are less affected and clinically appear to be unaffected. Inflammation is induced during this process. Thick, indurated lesions become most inflamed and may best be managed by surgically removing them before instituting topical chemotherapy. The available preparations of 5-FU are listed in Table 21-2 and in the Formulary.

Table 21-2 Preparations for Treatment of Actinic Keratosis

Product	Active ingredient	Packaging
Carac	0.5% Fluorouracil	30 gm cream
Efudex	2% Fluorouracil	10 ml liquid
	5% Fluorouracil	10 ml liquid
	5% Fluorouracil	25 gm cream
Fluoroplex	1% Fluorouracil	30 ml solution
	1% Fluorouracil	30 gm cream
Aldara	5% Imiquimod	Cream—box of 12 or 24 packets

Patients should be cautioned about the various stages of inflammation encountered during treatment. Considerable discomfort may be experienced for 1 week or more during periods of intense inflammation. Pain can be minimized if only small areas are treated at one time; however, many patients wish to treat the full face instead of prolonging the unsightly erythema and crusting for weeks. Lesions on the back of the hands, arms, and lower legs require longer periods of treatment than those on the face (Table 21-3). Patients with a small number of lesions may be treated during the summer or winter. Patients with a large number of lesions who work outdoors are best treated in the winter. Pharmaceutical companies that manufacture 5-FU supply patient information sheets and videos with color photographs of the various stages of inflammation.

TREATMENT TECHNIQUE (5-FU) AND EXPECTED RESULTS

5-FU is available as a 0.5%, 1%, and 5% cream and a 1% and 2% solution. The 1% solution is helpful for the scalp with hair, and the 2% solution is used for individual lesions. Carac (5-FU 0.5% cream), a new formulation, is applied once daily for up to 4 weeks as tolerated. Irritation resolves within 2 weeks of cessation of treatment. Efudex or Fluoroplex is applied twice a day for 2 to 4 weeks. Applying 5-FU preparations two or three times a week is less effective. Significant irritation and discomfort are frequently encountered. Petrolatum may be applied between 5-FU applications to soothe raw, dry, and cracked areas. Oral pain medication (e.g., acetaminophen with codeine) controls pain at the peak of inflammation. Instruction handouts and videos supplied by 5-FU manufacturers are very helpful.

TOPICAL CHEMOTHERAPY WITH IMIQUIMOD. Imiquimod (Aldara) 5% cream is an immune response modifier approved for the treatment of genital warts.

ACTINIC KERATOSIS

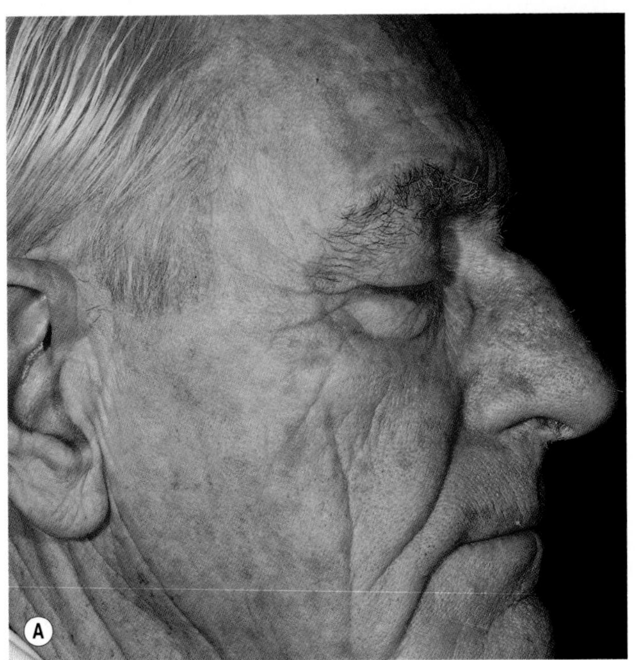

Diffuse involvement of the forehead. Lesions are superficial. Lesions on the cheek were not clinically apparent.

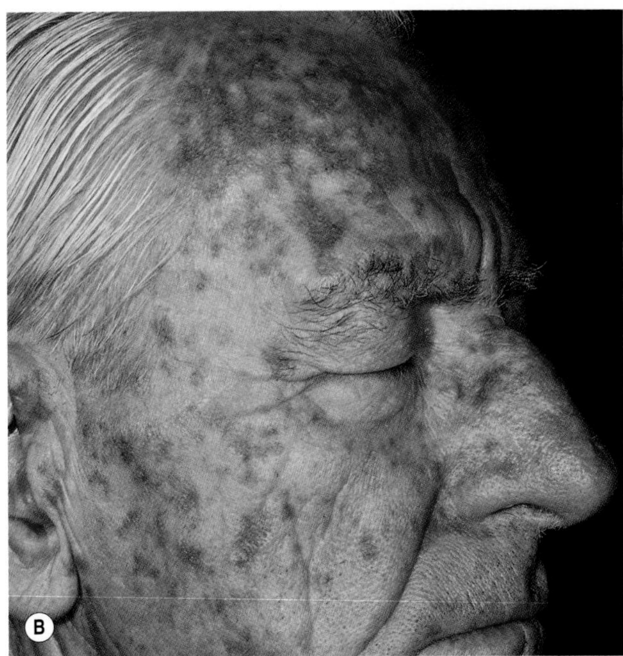

Maximum intensity of inflammation was reached 3 weeks after starting treatment. The medication has inflamed the cheek lesions that were not clinically apparent before.

Figure 21-20

Imiquimod applied three times a week for 16 weeks resulted in an 86.6% reduction in actinic keratosis. In the event of a local skin reaction, treatment may be reduced to two times per week. *PMID: 15837864*

INFLAMMATORY RESPONSE AND PHYSICIAN SUPERVISION. In the early inflammatory phase, erythema first appears in treated areas at predictable intervals (see Table 21-3). In the severe inflammatory phase (Figures 21-20, *B* and 21-21), erythema, edema, burning, stinging, and oozing reach maximum intensity at different intervals, depending on the site treated and the thickness of the lesions. In the lesion disintegration phase (Figure 21-22), erosion or ulceration, intense inflammation, discomfort, pain, crusting, eschar formation, and evidence of reepithelialization occur. When this phase is reached, treatment stops. Table 21-3 lists the approximate duration of treatment. Patients should be evaluated every 1 or 2 weeks during the treatment period. This irritating treatment is a major event for the patient. They are physically and mentally traumatized, and they will have many questions. Patients need close supervision, encouragement, and reassurance. They frequently call the office during treatment. The clinician must determine the endpoint of treatment and be prepared to manage excessive inflammation with wet compresses and group V to VI topical steroids. Infection responds to Bactroban ointment or oral antibiotics. Sunscreens can be irritating and should not be used during treatment. Sun exposure is avoided by using hats and clothing. Women may tolerate bland liquid makeup.

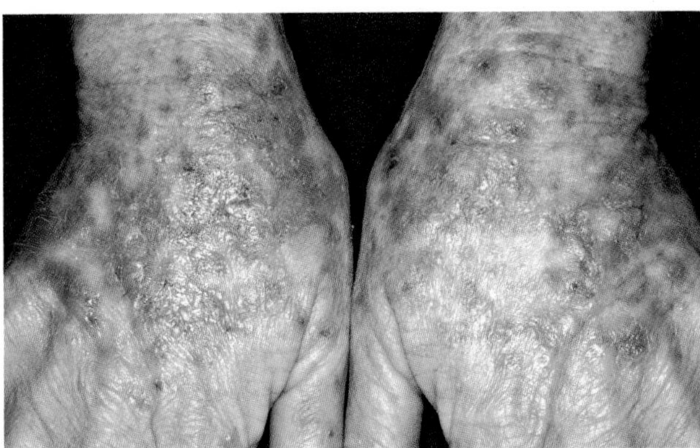

Figure 21-21 Lesions are intensely inflamed 3 weeks after starting 5-FU.

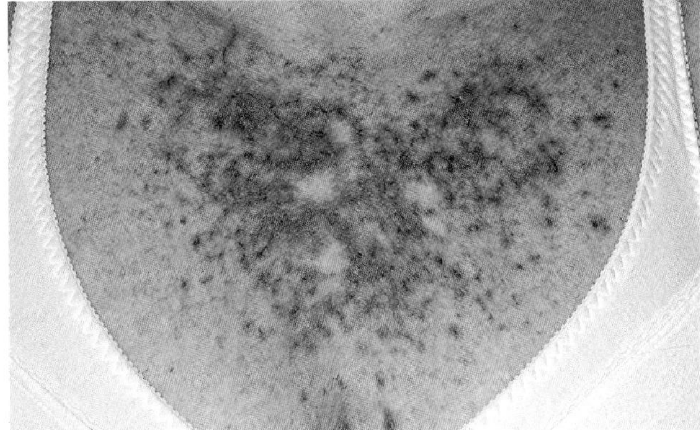

Figure 21-22 Lesion disintegration phase has been reached 4 weeks after starting 5-FU.

Table 21-3 Guidelines for Duration of 5-FU Therapy According to Site

Site	Early signs of inflammation (days)	Duration of treatment (weeks)
Face, lips	3-5	2-4
Scalp	4-7	3-5
Neck	4-7	2-4
Arms, hands, legs	10-14	4-8
Back	10-14	4-6
Chest	10-14	4-6

TOPICAL STEROIDS. Some authors suggest using topical steroids during the entire treatment period to suppress inflammation and decrease patient discomfort. This technique, however, may make it difficult to determine when therapy should be stopped.

ACTINIC KERATOSIS OF THE FACE. Patients with mild damage consisting of erythema and scaling can be treated with tretinoin cream 0.05% alone for several months. Small, superficial lesions that do not respond can then be treated with 5-FU or cryosurgery. Patients with many lesions can be pretreated with tretinoin cream applied once each day for 1 to 3 months. Pretreatment with tretinoin may improve the quality of the dermis and reduce subsequent treatment time with 5-FU. Tretinoin 0.025% cream should be prescribed for patients with sensitive skin. 5-FU may then be applied alone or in combination with tretinoin to complete the treatment program. Combination therapy may shorten the treatment period, but it produces more intense inflammation.

ACTINIC KERATOSES OF THE UPPER AND LOWER EXTREMITIES. These lesions are frequently multiple, hyperkeratotic, and distributed over a large area. Hyperkeratosis tends to limit penetration of topical 5-FU. Lesions on the extremities require longer treatment than those on the face. Lesions may be pretreated for 1 or 2 weeks or longer with twice daily applications of tretinoin 0.025% gel or 12% ammonium lactate to reduce hyperkeratosis, which interferes with 5-FU penetration. Plastic (Saran Wrap) occlusion is sometimes used to facilitate 5-FU penetration of thicker lesions.

ACTINIC CHEILITIS. Actinic cheilitis is treated effectively with 5-FU cream (Figure 21-23); however, pain and excessive crusting can make this a very unpleasant experience. Some authors suggest using 5% 5-FU cream three times a day for 14 to 18 days to obtain the optimal reaction in the shortest time. The objective is to reduce the morbidity to 2 weeks. Application of 5% lidocaine ointment relieves pain.

Cool compresses are applied several times each day if inflammation is intense. Group V topical steroids may be applied to red areas to suppress inflammation and pruritus. Appearance of a purulent exudate suggests infection; when this occurs, oral antistaphylococcal antibiotics or Bactroban ointment should be prescribed. In the healing phase, residual erythema and hyperpigmentation persist for several weeks.

CONTACT ALLERGY TO 5-FU. Contact allergy to 5-FU should be suspected if intense erythema and vesiculation occur (Figure 21-24). Patch testing is not reliable because many patients who are allergic to 5-FU do not show a positive patch test reaction.

PROGNOSIS. Patients should remain free of lesions for months and possibly years, but recurrences can be anticipated. Frequently, unsupervised patients inadequately treat their own newly evolving lesions, resulting in surface healing but untreated deeper abnormal cells. For this reason, no refills should be indicated on the initial prescription, and patients should be instructed to discard medication when treatment is finished.

TREATMENT WITH TOPICAL 5-FU

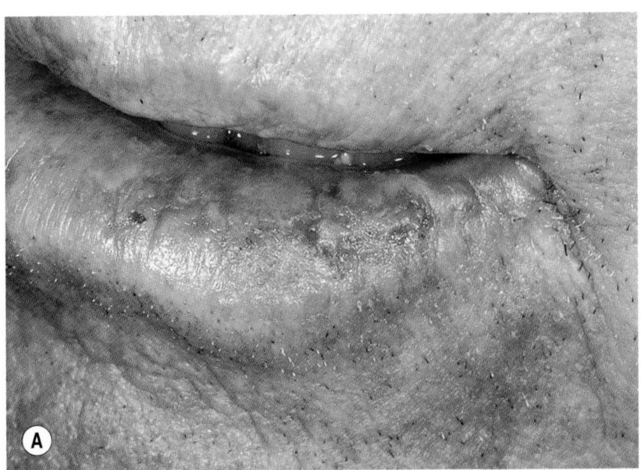

Before treatment. The lower lip is pinkish-white and smooth. The nonexposed upper lip is normal.

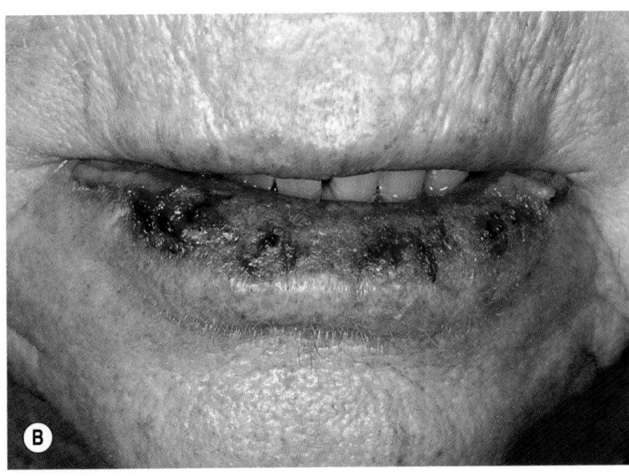

Two weeks after starting topical 5-FU. The entire lower lip is ulcerated.

Figure 21-23 Actinic cheilitis.

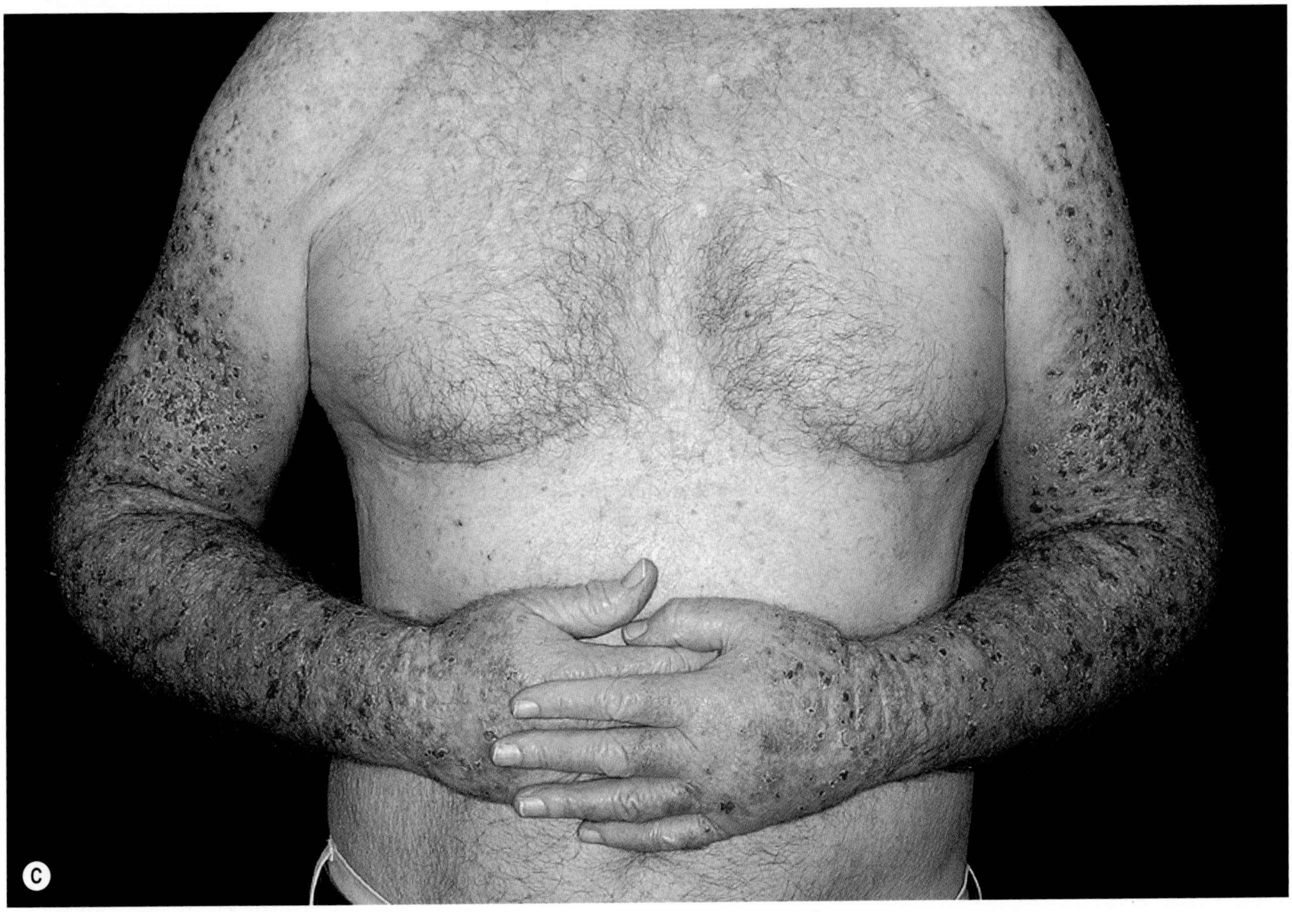

Figure 21-24 Contact dermatitis to 5-FU. Inflammation intensified more rapidly than expected. The patient continued to apply 5-FU because he understood that intense inflammation was to be expected. Examination showed vesiculation characteristic of contact dermatitis. Patch testing to the 5-FU cream proved the diagnosis.

SQUAMOUS CELL CARCINOMA IN SITU

Squamous cell carcinoma in situ (SCCIS) is a histologic diagnosis. Most pathologists reserve this term for a lesion with transepidermal keratinocyte atypia, indicating that the entire epidermis is filled with atypical keratinocytes. They use the term *actinic keratosis* (AK) for lesions in which atypical keratinocytes do no fill the epidermis. There is a trend to designate any lesion with intraepidermal atypia as SCCIS and then to specify the extent to which the cells extend from the basal layer and fill the epidermis. Some authors have suggested an atypia grading system similar to the system used to classify cervical pathology. This would notify the clinician as to the amount of atypical keratinocytes in the epidermis.

Clinically these findings can be seen in a number of lesions (Box 21-3), which have different prognoses and management options.

THE CLINICAL SPECTRUM. The diagnosis of AK is made by clinical examination. Early AK lesions are slightly elevated and have a sandpaper-like texture. Lesions may evolve into a keratotic papule with a red base. At this later time it is difficult to clinically differentiate where AK ends and where SCC begins. AK and in situ SCC have the same clinical and histologic features. AK is an SCC that is confined to the epidermis. AK can evolve into invasive SCC, but it is not possible to clinically recognize when this occurs.

HISTOLOGIC APPEARANCE. Histologically, AK is characterized by the presence of atypical keratinocytes at the basal cell layer of the epidermis, which in advanced lesions may extend into the entire epidermis (Figure 21-25). The histologic changes seen in the individual cells of AK and invasive SCC may be identical. Both show atypical keratinocytes with nuclear pleomorphism, disordered maturation, and increased numbers of mitotic figures. In early SCCIS atypical keratinocytes are confined to the basal and suprabasal layer of the lower one third of the epidermis. The follicular structure is uninvolved. As lesions progress, atypical keratinocytes extend into the lower two thirds of the epidermis. Buds of keratinocytes in the upper papillary dermis can often be found. The pathologic picture of SCCIS as defined by pathologists is reached when atypical keratinocytes extend to more than two thirds of the full thickness of the epidermis and involve the epithelia of the hair follicle. Buds of keratinocytes in the upper papillary dermis can also be found. A biopsy may not sample the entire lesion. One part of a lesion may have atypical cells confined to the basal layer while another may have atypical cells filling the entire thickness of the epidermis.

Box 21-3 Squamous Cell Carcinoma in Situ

- Actinic keratosis
- Bowen's disease
- Arsenical keratosis
- Bowenoid papulosis
- Erythroplasia of Queyrat

IMPLICATIONS FOR MANAGEMENT. There are no distinctive clinical criteria to differentiate some actinic keratoses from some squamous cell carcinomas. There is no biologic difference between AK and SCC. They represent a continuum of disease. A neoplastic-transformed keratinocyte is a SCC cell whether it resides in the epidermis or dermis. Actinic keratoses are composed of neoplastic keratinocytes confined to the epidermis. Therefore it is a SCC cell confined to a part of the epidermis and can be called an SCCIS. Most pathologists report a lesion with atypical keratinocytes confined to the lower one third or two thirds of the epidermis as an actinic keratosis. Lesions in which atypical keratinocytes fill the epidermis are termed SCC in situ. Some clinicians see the words squamous cell carcinoma in the term SCCIS and conclude that aggressive treatment is warranted. This practice can result in unnecessarily destructive treatment. Clinical judgment is required.

MANAGEMENT. It may not be good clinical practice to treat histologic SCCIS more aggressively than AK. Treat thin lesions with liquid nitrogen, topical 5-FU, or imiquimod. Do not freeze thicker lesions because the surface will be destroyed and malignant cells may be left at the base, which in time may evolve into SCC. Beware that lesions that appear thin may be discovered to be surprisingly deep after the decision is made to treat with desiccation and curettage. Treat thick lesions with desiccation and curettage or excision. Scalp actinic keratoses are often found to have thick scale that masks the depth of the lesion. Curettage is appropriate in these instances.

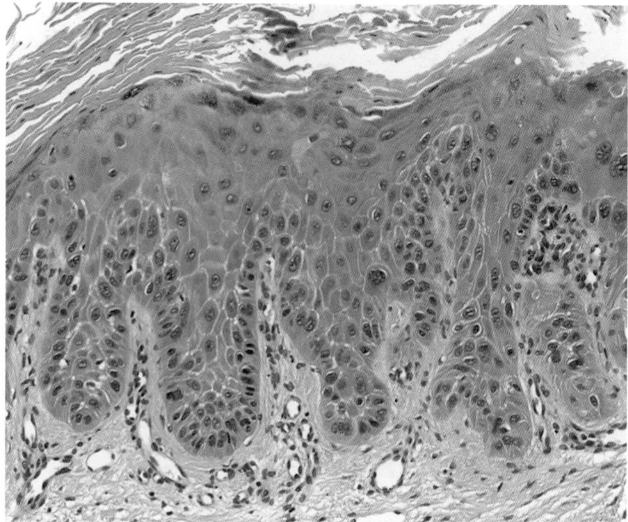

Figure 21-25 Squamous cell carcinoma in situ. Atypical keratinocytes extend to more than two thirds of the full thickness of the epidermis.

BOWEN'S DISEASE

Bowen's disease, also referred to as squamous cell carcinoma in situ, appears mainly on sun-exposed sites. SCCIS presenting on the mucous membranes of the glans penis, vulva, and oral mucosa is known as erythroplasia of Queyrat. Bowen's disease presents as a slowly growing, red, scaly patch. Lesions are found most often on the lower limbs of women and on the scalp and ears of men. Typical lesions are slightly elevated, red, scaly plaques with surface fissures and foci of pigmentation. The borders are well-defined (Figures 21-26 and 21-27), and lesions closely resemble psoriasis, chronic eczema, actinic keratosis, superficial basal cell carcinoma, seborrheic keratosis, and malignant melanoma. The plaque grows very slowly by lateral extension and may eventually, after several months or years, invade the dermis, producing induration and ulceration. When confined to the epidermis the atypical cells, in contrast to actinic keratosis, involve epidermal appendages, particularly the hair follicle (see Figure 21-27, *D*). In contrast to actinic keratosis, the basal cells in Bowen's disease are normal. Atypical cells are also found at the periphery of lesions in clinically uninvolved skin. Atypical cells in the epidermal lining of the hair follicle, although still confined to the epidermis, are deeper and more difficult to reach by treatment modalities such as topical 5-FU or electrosurgery, which only permit access to superficial areas.

Immunohistochemistry may sometimes be valuable in differentiating Paget's disease, superficial spreading melanoma, and Bowen's disease. The cause of Bowen's disease is unknown, but several patients with this disease were formerly treated with arsenic. There is no evidence that Bowen's disease is a skin marker for internal malignancy.

TREATMENT. Small lesions may be successfully treated with ED&C, cryosurgery, or excisional surgery. Larger lesions are treated with excisional surgery or 5-FU cream applied twice a day for 4 to 8 weeks. Treatment is discontinued when erosion and superficial necrosis occur. A large area surrounding the lesion should be treated in order to destroy the clinically inapparent disease. Some authors suggest plastic occlusion to enhance penetration to the hair follicle. A once-daily application of imiquimod 5% cream (Aldara) for up to 16 weeks is very effective; 93% of patients had no residual tumor present in their 6-week posttreatment biopsy specimens. Imiquimod is a topical immune response modifier that stimulates the production of interferon-alfa and other cytokines. It is inconveniently packaged in small foil envelopes. Express medication through a hole created with a pin to conserve medication. Bowen's disease has been successfully treated in renal transplant patients with 5% imiquimod and 5% 5-FU therapy.

Close follow-up of patients after treatment is required because recurrences are relatively common. Recurrence is related to follicular involvement and ill-defined lateral margins. If left untreated, development of invasive carcinoma is possible but uncommon.

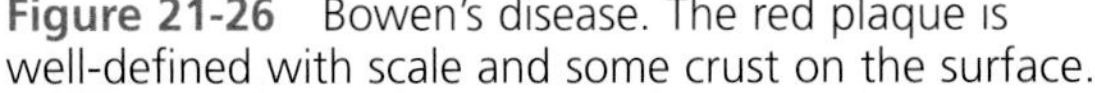

Figure 21-26 Bowen's disease. The red plaque is well-defined with scale and some crust on the surface.

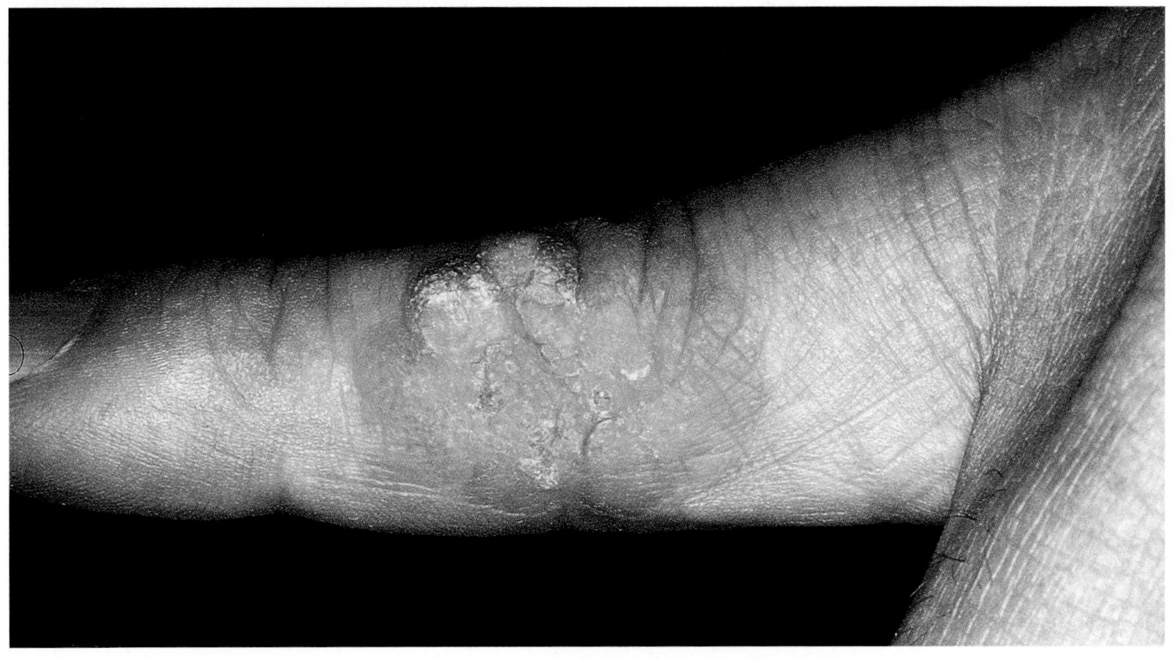

BOWEN'S DISEASE

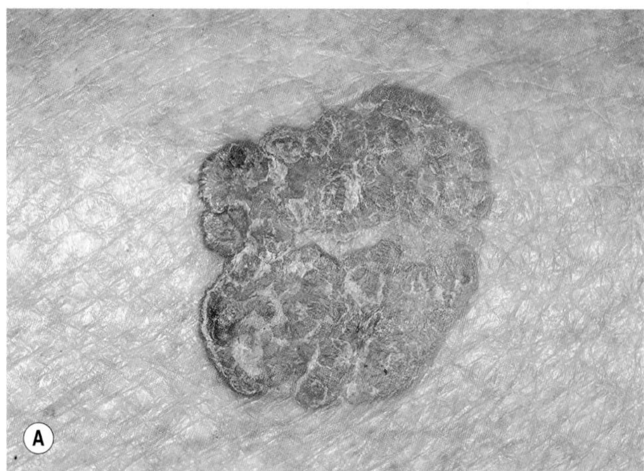

This sharply demarcated, erythematous plaque with an irregular border had been present for months. The surface was hyperkeratotic and crusted. Lesions can become fissured and ulcerated.

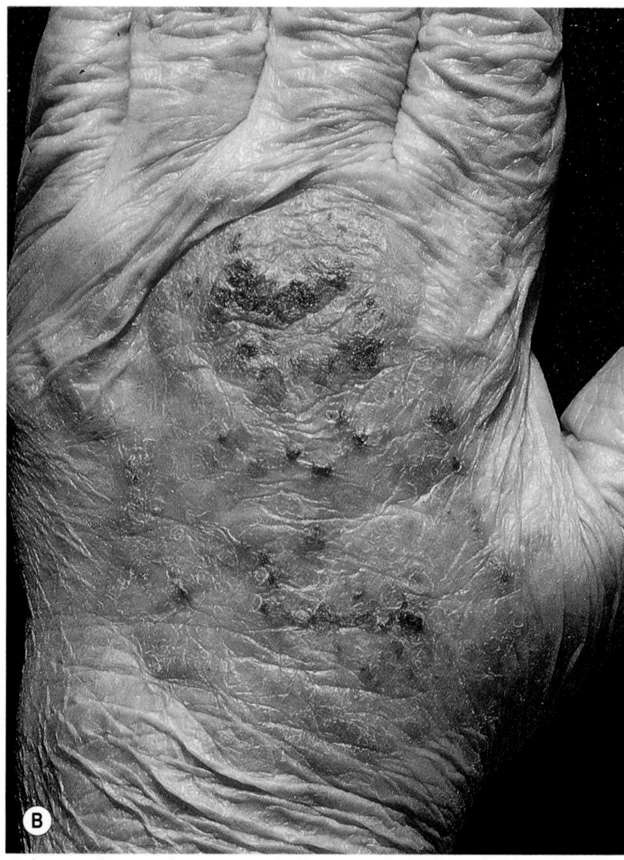

A large plaque that was misdiagnosed as tinea and psoriasis. Scale and crust form on a surface that intermittently oozes serum.

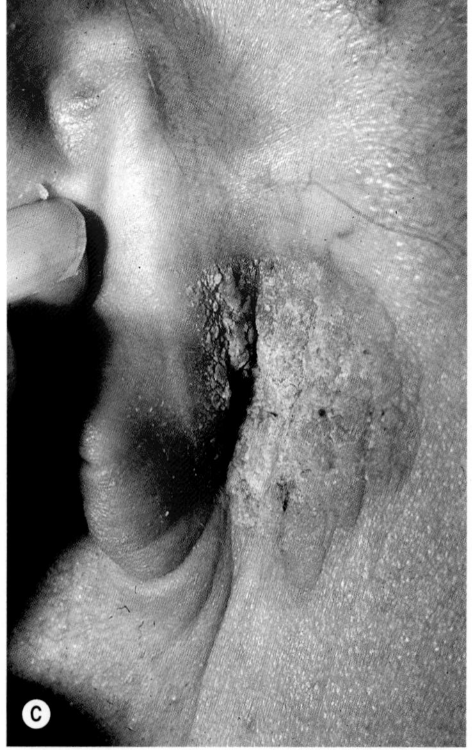

A broad thick lesion that may have degenerated into squamous cell carcinoma.

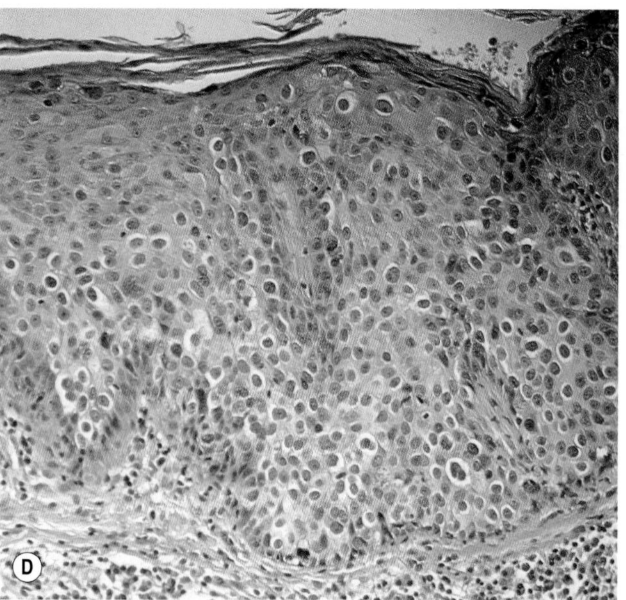

Atypical cells are present throughout the entire thickness of the epidermis. The dermoepidermal junction remains distinct and intact.

Figure 21-27

ERYTHROPLASIA OF QUEYRAT

Clinically and histologically, erythroplasia of Queyrat of the penis resembles Bowen's disease and is probably the same entity. It is a carcinoma in situ that mainly occurs on the glans penis, the prepuce, or the urethral meatus of elderly males. It appears exclusively under the foreskin of the uncircumcised penis and is a moist, slightly raised, well-defined, red, smooth or velvety plaque (Figure 21-28). A coinfection with human papillomavirus type 8 and carcinogenic genital human papillomavirus types have been demonstrated. Analogous to Bowen's disease of the skin, erythroplasia of Queyrat grows very slowly and has the potential for degeneration into squamous cell carcinoma. Similar lesions may occur on the vulva. 5-FU cream or imiquimod cream (Aldara) are treatment options. Recurrences are unlikely because the hair follicles that serve as foci for recurrence are absent on the penile mucosa. A 3- to 4-week course is usually required. Use of 5% lidocaine ointment is recommended for pain. Neodymium:YAG or carbon dioxide laser therapy provides excellent cosmetic and functional results. However, the high incidence of recurrence indicates the need for careful follow-up and patient self-examination. Erythroplasia involving the distal glans penis around the urethra and extending into the urethral meatus may require Mohs microscopically controlled surgery.

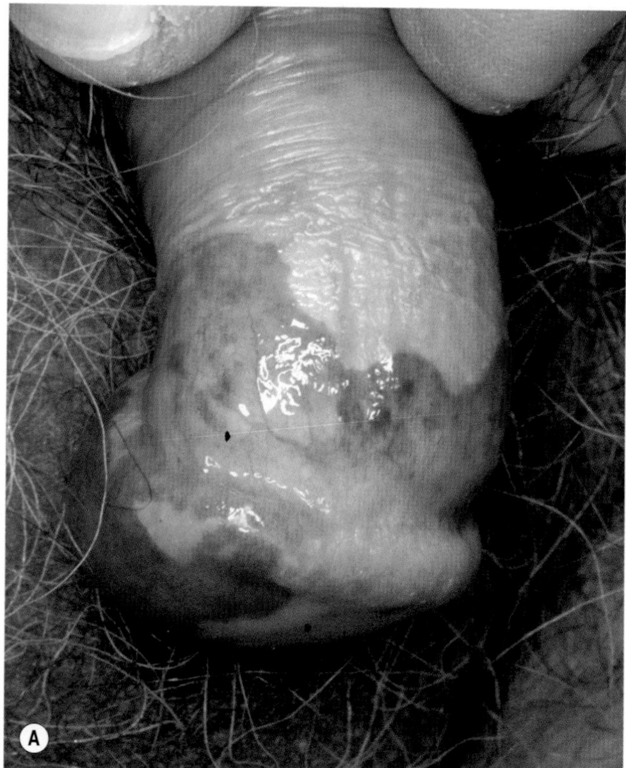

A moist, glistening, slightly raised plaque.

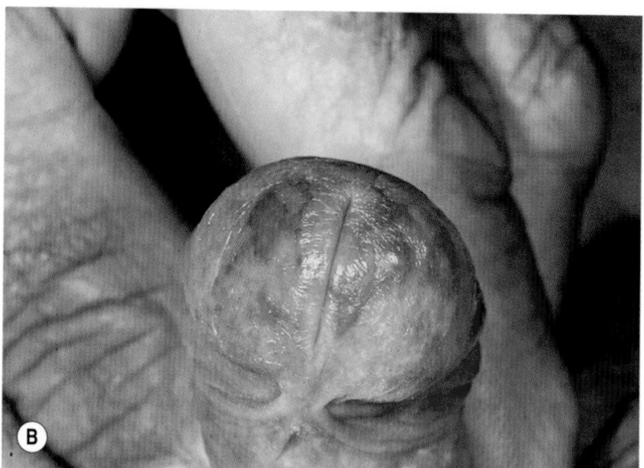

A minimally raised plaque with variable texture.

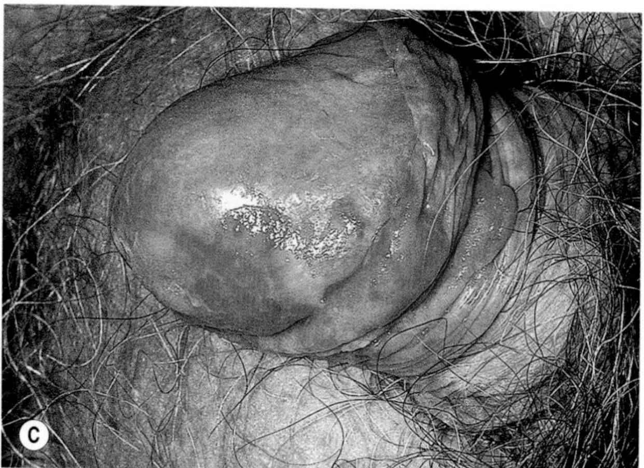

A broad lesion involving the glans and shaft. It occurs most often in uncircumcised men.

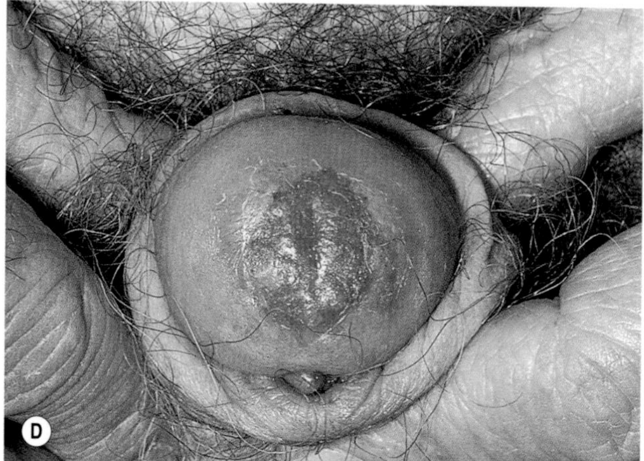

An early lesion surrounding the urethral meatus.

Figure 21-28 Erythroplasia of Queyrat.

ARSENICAL KERATOSES AND OTHER ARSENIC-RELATED SKIN DISEASES

Pentavalent, inorganic arsenic, dispensed years ago as Fowler's solution (potassium arsenite solution) for psoriasis and other diseases, may cause a number of problems. Arsenical keratoses are discrete, round, wartlike, or pointed keratotic lesions that appear 20 or more years after chronic arsenic ingestion (Figure 21-29). Arsenical keratoses may degenerate into squamous cell carcinoma. Lesions are most common on the palms and soles but may occur elsewhere. Bowen's disease, multiple basal cell carcinomas, and changes in pigmentation characterized by small, round, white macules ("raindrops on a hyperpigmented background") are additional findings in patients with chronic arsenic ingestion. A significant excess of bladder cancer mortality occurred in patients treated with Fowler's solution. Exposure to Chinese proprietary medicines containing inorganic arsenic poses a risk for the development of cutaneous and systemic malignancies.

Chronic arsenic toxicity from drinking well water polluted with arsenic has been reported. No treatment is necessary for arsenical keratosis unless signs of degeneration occur.

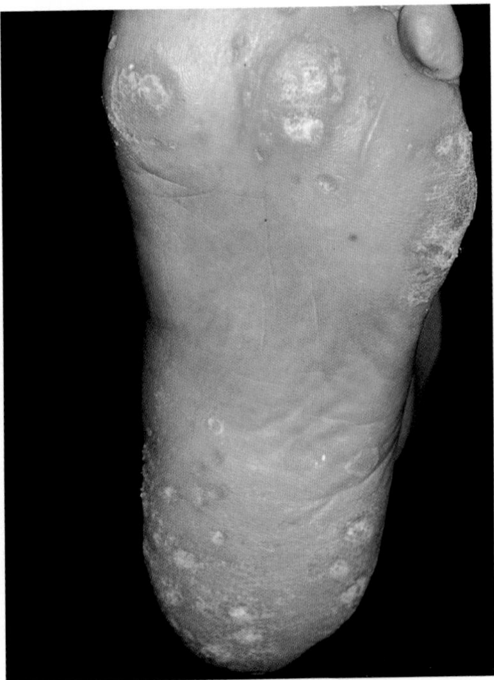

Figure 21-29 Arsenical keratoses. Discrete, wartlike, keratotic lesions occur on the palms and soles.

SQUAMOUS CELL CARCINOMA

Nonmelanoma skin cancer is the most common cancer in the United States. Approximately 80% of nonmelanoma skin cancers are BCC, and 20% are SCC. SCC is the second most common cancer among whites. Unlike BCCs, cutaneous SCCs are associated with a substantial risk of metastasis.

Squamous cell carcinoma arises in the epithelium and is common in the middle-aged and elderly population. SCCs are often separated into two major groups based on their malignant potential. Those arising in areas of prior radiation or thermal injury, in chronic draining sinuses, and in chronic ulcers are typically aggressive and have a high frequency of metastasis. SCCs originating in actinically damaged skin are less aggressive and less likely to metastasize.

ETIOLOGY AND RISK FACTORS. UVB radiation is important for the induction of SCC. Risk factors include exposure to sunlight during childhood, sunburns, ionizing radiation, light skin, hazel or blue eyes, blonde or red hair, outdoor occupations, freckling or facial telangiectasia, living in the South, and psoriasis treatment with oral psoralen and ultraviolet A radiation (PUVA). Arsenic, used in medications in the past and in drinking water, produces tumors and carcinoma in situ. Human papillomavirus types 6 and 11 are found in tumors of the genitalia and type 16 in periungual tumors. UVB radiation damages DNA (by inducing the formation of pyrimidine dimers) and its repair system and alters the immune system. UVB radiation induces mutation of p53 tumor-suppressor genes. These mutations are found in SCC. Keratinocytes undergo clonal expansion and form actinic keratosis. Uncontrolled proliferation of abnormal cells leads to SCCIS and invasive SCC.

Box 21-4 **Lesions from Which Squamous Cell Carcinoma Originates**

Actinic keratosis
Cutaneous horn
Bowen's disease
- Erythroplasia of Queyrat

Chemical exposure
- Arsenic (internal)
- Tar (external), except therapeutic tars

Leukoplakia
Lichen sclerosis (vulva)
Sites of chronic infection
- Chronic sinus tracts
- Osteomyelitis

Thermal burn scars (Marjolin's ulcer)
- Radiation-damaged skin

Cell-mediated immunity and immune function may be modulated by UVB radiation. Immunosuppression leads to a great increase in the risk of SCC. Renal transplant recipients have a 253-fold increase in the risk of SCC. Longer wavelength UVA radiation damages DNA and is also carcinogenic. SCC arises in skin that has been damaged by thermal burns or chronic inflammation. It also occurs from epidermal diseases of unknown origin, such as Bowen's disease (Box 21-4).

LOCATION. Like basal cell carcinoma, SCCs are most common in sun-exposed areas; however, the distribution is different. SCCs are common on the scalp, backs of the hands, and the superior surface of the pinna; BCC is rarely found on these sites.

INCIDENCE. In 1994 in the United States, the lifetime risk of SCC was 9% to 14% among men and 4% to 9% among women. The incidence is highest in lower latitudes such as the southern United States and Australia. The incidence increases rapidly with age and sun exposure and is approximately twice as high in men as in women. A sharp increase in incidence during the past 2 decades has been documented.

COMMON PRECURSOR LESIONS. Actinic keratosis is the most common precursor of SCC. AKs begin on sun-exposed skin as isolated or multiple, 2- to 6-mm, flat, pink, brown, rough lesions that are more easily felt than seen. Early lesions may involute. Lesions may persist for long periods without changing. A small number become thicker, accumulate scale, and evolve into SCC. Another form of SCCIS is Bowen's disease, which presents as sharply demarcated, erythematous, velvety, or scaly plaques on sun-exposed areas. The red, smooth plaques of Bowen's disease on the glans penis of uncircumcised men are called erythroplasia of Queyrat.

PATHOPHYSIOLOGY. Atypical squamous cells originate in the epidermis from keratinocytes and proliferate indefinitely. A flat, scaly lesion becomes an indurated SCC when cells penetrate the epidermal basement membrane and proliferate into the dermis.

CLINICAL MANIFESTATIONS. SCCs arising from actinic keratosis may have a thick, adherent scale. The tumor is soft and freely movable and may have a red, inflamed base. These lesions are most frequently observed on the bald scalp, forehead, ears, and backs of the hands (Figures 21-30 and 21-31). Cutaneous horns may begin as actinic keratosis and degenerate into SCC. SCCs originating on the lip (Figures 21-32 and 21-33) or from apparently normal skin are aggressive and metastasize to the regional lymph nodes and beyond.

Those SCCs beginning in actinically damaged skin, but not from actinic keratosis, appear as firm, movable, elevated masses with a sharply defined border and little surface scale. SCCs that arise in actinically damaged skin were previously thought to have a minimal potential for metastasis; however, such lesions may be aggressive.

KERATOACANTHOMAS VS. SQUAMOUS CELL CARCINOMA. Keratoacanthomas are sometimes difficult to differentiate from SCC. Keratoacanthomas appear suddenly and grow rapidly (see p. 790). They reach a certain size (usually 0.5 to 2.0 cm), stop growing, and then regress weeks to months later. They begin as red- to flesh-colored, dome-shaped papules with a smooth surface and a central crater filled with a keratinous plug. The pathologist sometimes has difficulty differentiating the benign keratoacanthoma from SCC. Tumors that cannot be classified are treated as SCCs.

METASTATIC POTENTIAL. The potential for SCCs to metastasize is related to the size, location, degree of differentiation, histologic evidence of perineural involvement, immunologic status, and depth of invasion (Table 21-4). SCC first metastasizes to regional lymph nodes in the majority of cases.

TUMOR SIZE AND DEPTH. In one study, no carcinoma less than 2 mm thick metastasized. Tumors between 2 and 6 mm thick with moderate differentiation and a depth of invasion that does not extend beyond the subcutis can be classified as low-risk carcinomas. The risk of metastasis is high for undifferentiated carcinomas greater than 6 mm thick that have infiltrated the musculature, the

Table 21-4 Influence of Tumor Variables on Local Recurrence and Metastasis of Squamous Cell Carcinoma

Factor	Local recurrence	Metastasis
Size		
<2 cm	7.4%	9.1%
≥2 cm	15.2%	30.3%
Depth		
<4 mm/Clark I to II	5.3%	6.7%
≥4 mm/Clark IV, V	17.2%	45.7%
Differentiation		
Well differentiated	13.6%	9.2%
Poorly differentiated	28.6%	32.8%
Site		
Sun-exposed	7.9%	5.2%
Ear	18.7%	11.0%
Lip	10.5%	13.7%
Scar carcinoma (non–sun-exposed)	N/A	37.9%
Previous treatment	23.3%	30.3%
Perineural involvement	47.2%	47.3%
Immunosuppression	N/A	12.9%

From Rowe DE, Carroll RJ, Day CL: *J Am Acad Dermatol* 26:976, 1992. *PMID: 1607418*

perichondrium, or the periosteum. Another study of SCCs on the trunk and extremities showed that, like melanoma, tumor behavior correlated best with the level of dermal invasion and the vertical tumor thickness. Tumors that recurred were at least 4 mm thick and involved the deep half of the dermis or deeper structures. All tumors that proved fatal were at least 10 mm thick. Investigators concluded that patients whose tumors penetrate through the dermis or exceed 8 mm in thickness are at high risk of recurrence or death.

LOCATION. Tumors on the scalp, forehead, ears, nose, and lips are at higher risk for metastases (Figure 21-34). Tumors developing at sites of chronic inflammation such as ulcers, scar tissue, and previous radiation sites also have higher rates of metastasis.

SQUAMOUS CELL CARCINOMA

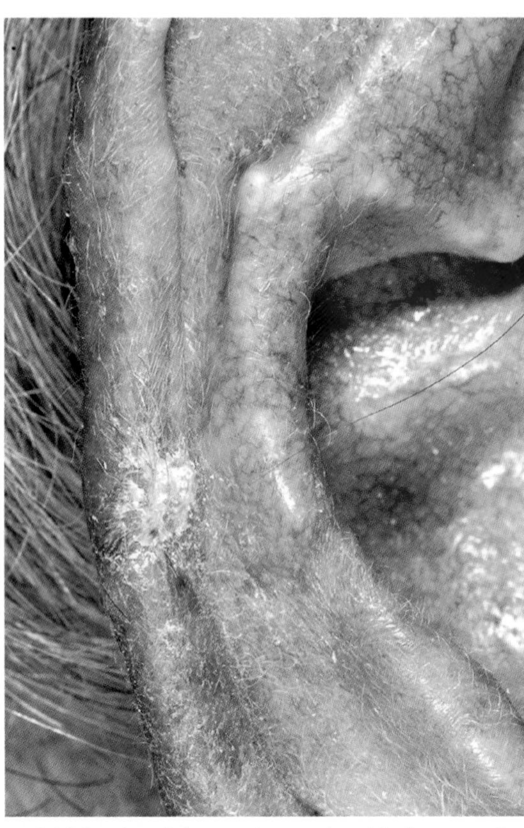

Figure 21-30 A red, keratotic papule with dense surface scale. Lesions may be misinterpreted as actinic keratosis. Cryotherapy may destroy the surface but leave deeper malignant cells untreated. Check draining lymph nodes.

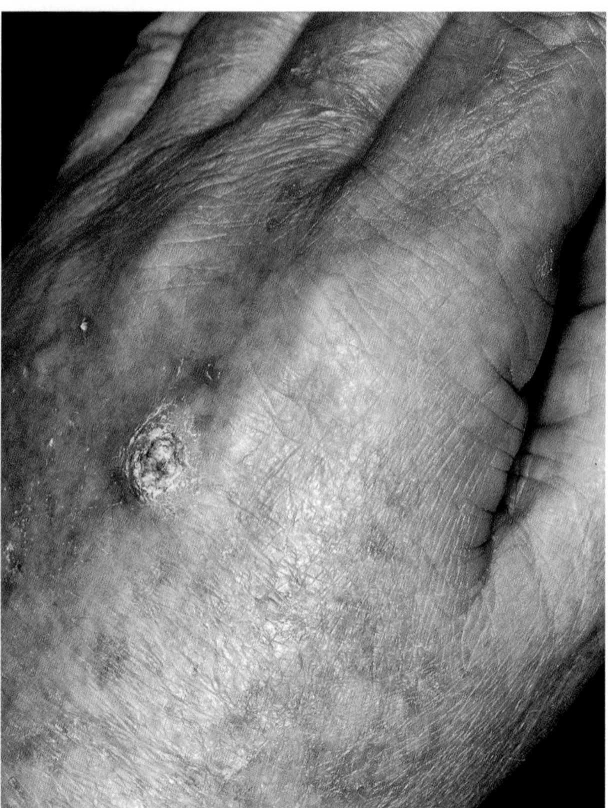

Figure 21-31 Nodular lesions may be painful. The lesion had been treated several times in the past with cryotherapy. It has been present for 2 years and demonstrated little progression in depth.

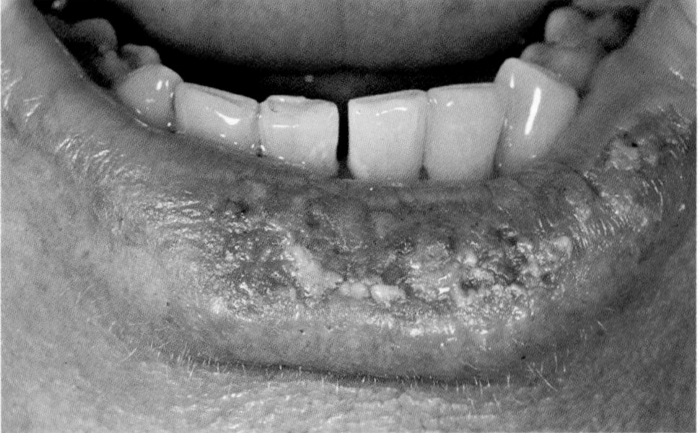

Figure 21-32 Several ulcerated lesions are present on the lower lip of this patient who has spent years working outdoors.

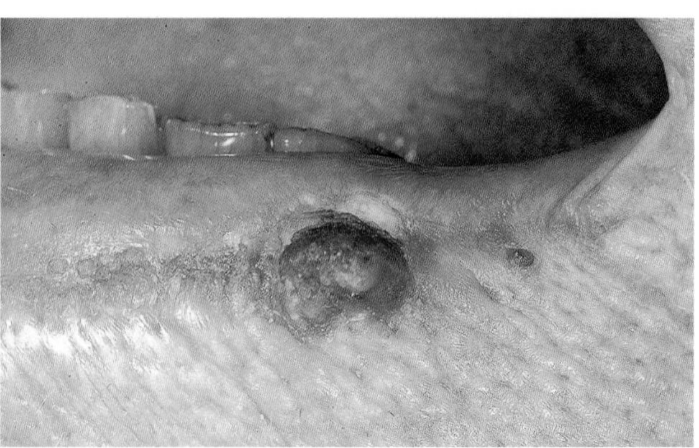

Figure 21-33 The sun-exposed lower lip is a common site. Palpation reveals a deep nodular mass.

MODE OF SPREAD. Cutaneous SCC may spread by (1) expansion and infiltration, (2) shelving or skating, (3) conduit spread, or (4) metastasis. SCC grows locally by expansion and infiltration. When the tumor reaches a hard surface (muscle, cartilage, bone), it may spread laterally (shelves or skates) under normal skin along facial or capsular planes, muscle, perichondrium, and periosteum. Shelving and skating occur in areas with little subcutaneous tissue, such as the scalp, ears, eyelids, nose, and upper lips. The spreading of a tumor along the nerve or vessel in the perineural or perivascular space is called conduit spread. This occurs in areas with major nerve trunks on the head and neck. Failure to recognize these three local modes of spread may result in an inadequate surgical procedure. Most SCCs are located on the head and neck. These metastasize, primarily by way of the lymphatics, initially to the superficial (first echelon) draining lymph nodes, and then spread to deeper (second echelon) nodes. Distant metastasis occurs by hematogenous dissemination, most commonly to the lungs, liver, brain, skin, or bone. SCCs originating on the lip (see Figures 21-32 and 21-33) and pinna metastasize in 10% to 20% of cases.

ORGAN TRANSPLANT RECIPIENTS AND IMMUNOSUPPRESSION

Host immune surveillance plays a role in determining the metastatic potential of SCC. Patients with lymphoproliferative disorders, renal transplant patients, and those undergoing chronic oral corticosteroid therapy are at high risk. Renal transplant recipients are at increased risk for skin cancer, most frequently SCC. SCCs are also more aggressive in renal transplant patients, in whom they are associated with a higher risk of metastasis than in the general population. HLA-B mismatching is significantly associated with the risk of SCC in renal transplant recipients, as is HLA-DR homozygosity.

The head and neck is the predominant site in male patients, and the trunk is the predominant site in female patients. The most common site in younger patients is the chest; in older patients, the face. The ear is a common site in male patients; no tumors were located there in female patients. The level of sun exposure is the most important factor in explaining distribution of SCC (Figure 21-35).

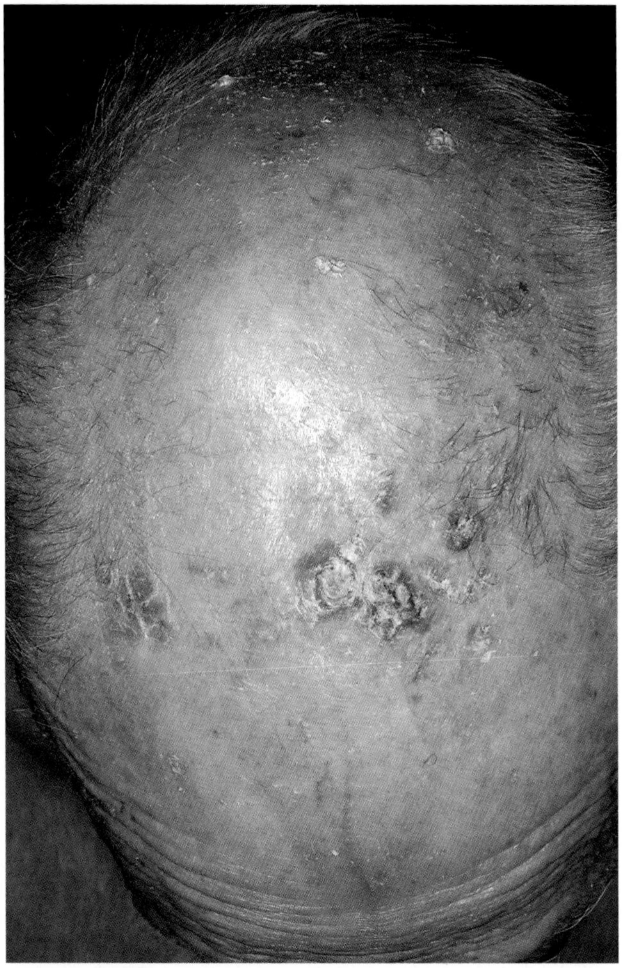

Figure 21-34 Squamous cell carcinoma on the scalp. It is often difficult to distinguish between actinic keratosis and squamous cell carcinoma. Excise or curet thicker lesions. Do not repeatedly freeze recurrent crusted scalp lesions.

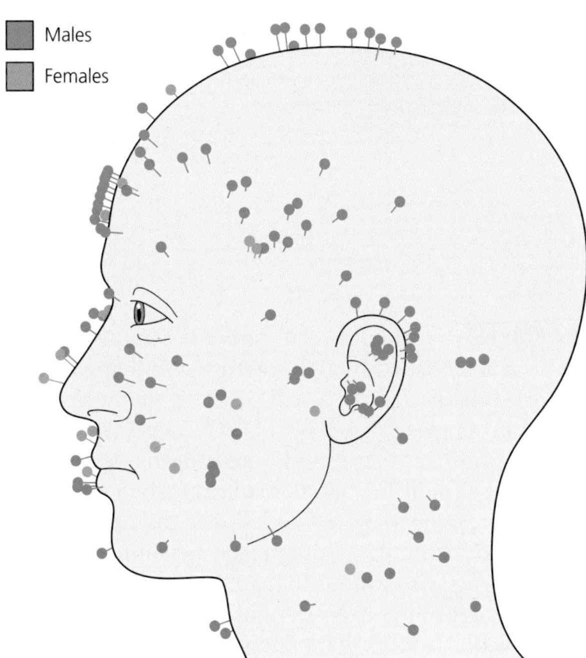

Figure 21-35 Distribution of squamous cell carcinomas in the head and neck region of organ transplant recipients (*Arch Dermatol* 141(4):447-451, 2005. *PMID: 15837862*)

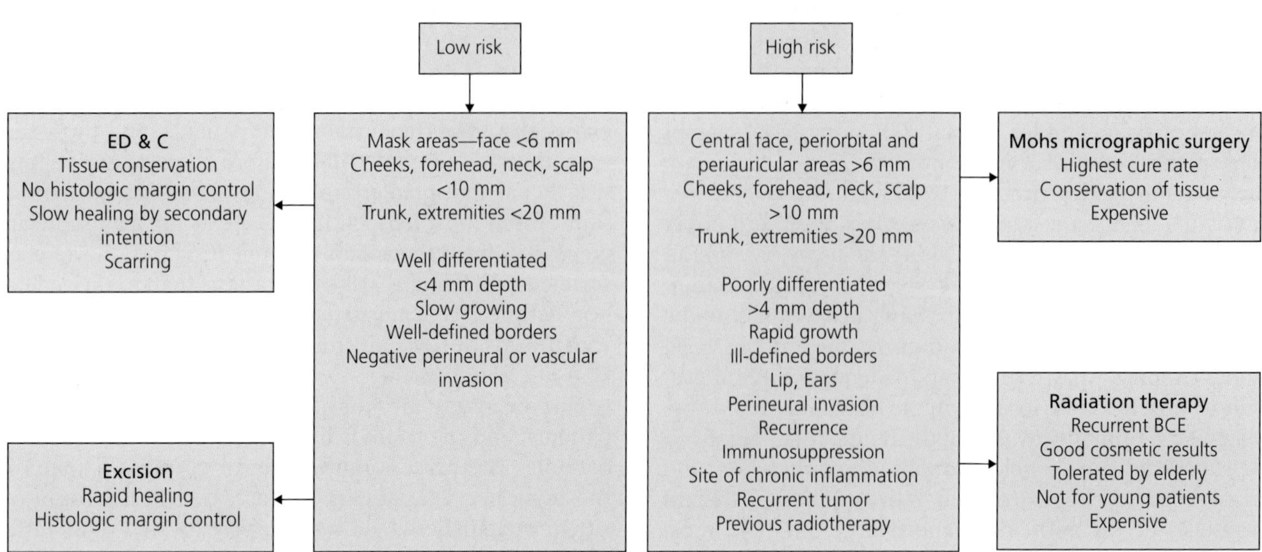

Figure 21-36 Adapted from Martinez JC, Otley CC: *MayoClin Proc* 76:1253, 2001. *PMID: 11761506*; Miller SJ: *Dermatol Surg* 26:289, 2000; Johnson TM, et al: *J Am Acad Dermatol* 26:467, 1992. *PMID: 1564155*

Table 21-5 Surgical Guidelines for Primary Squamous Cell Carcinoma

Size	Histologic grade	Anatomic location	Depth of invasion	Surgical margin
<2 cm	1	Low risk*	Dermis	4 mm
≥2 cm	2, 3, 4	High risk†	Subcutaneous tissue	6 mm

From Brodland DG, Zitelli JA: 27:241, 1992. *PMID: 1430364*
*Includes tumors less than 1 cm located in "high-risk" areas.
†Scalp, ears, eyelids, nose, and lips.

TREATMENT. Guidelines of care for cutaneous SCC have been established by the American Academy of Dermatology (Figure 21-36). Small SCCs evolving from actinic keratosis are treated by ED&C. Larger tumors or those on or near the vermilion border of the lips are best excised and should include the subcutaneous fat. Histologic microstaging may help to direct therapy. Tumors thinner than 4 mm can be managed by simple local removal. Patients with lesions that are between 4 and 8 mm thick or that exhibit deep dermal invasion should undergo excision. Tumors that penetrate through the dermis are staged by the surgeon and treated with several modalities including excisional and Mohs surgery, neck dissection, radiation therapy, and chemotherapy. Larger tumors or those about the nose and eyes require special consideration (see Box 21-2, p. 811). Surgical margins for excision of primary cutaneous SCCs have been proposed (Table 21-5).

When SCC metastasizes, it spreads first to local nodal groups. The combination of Mohs micrographic surgery and sentinel lymphadenectomy may be an option for management of SCCs at high risk for metastasis.

RECOMMENDED FOLLOW-UP EVALUATION. SCC patients may benefit from a once-yearly complete skin examination. Since the risk of subsequent SCCs increases with the number of previous SCCs, patients with multiple previous SCCs might merit more frequent examination.

LEUKOPLAKIA

Leukoplakia is the most common premalignant lesion of the oral mucosa. Leukoplakia is a clinical term used to describe a range of nonspecific white lesions, from slightly raised, white, translucent areas to dense, white, opaque lesions, with or without ulceration on the vermilion border of the lips (Figure 21-37), oral mucosa, or vulva. When a biopsy is taken, the term leukoplakia should be replaced by the diagnosis obtained histologically. Smoking is the most common cause of oral lesions, but chronic irritation from carious teeth or malaligned dentures and betel nut chewing (Taiwan) are also causes.

CLINICAL PRESENTATION. The most common sites of oral leukoplakia are the commissures and the buccal mucosa. Leukoplakias in the floor of the mouth more often present in smokers than in nonsmokers. Leukoplakias on the borders of the tongue are more common among nonsmokers than smokers. A particularly aggressive form of oral leukoplakia that begins with hyperkeratosis, spreads to become multifocal and verruciform in appearance, and later becomes malignant has been termed proliferative verrucous leukoplakia. Lesions are often bilateral and affect mandibular, alveolar, and buccal mucosa.

MALIGNANT DEGENERATION. SCC develops in 17% of all patients with leukoplakia. In one study of 500 patients with oral leukoplakia, there was SCC in 9.6% of cases and dysplasia in an additional 24%. One study found a 2.9% annual malignant transformation rate for patients with leukoplakia. Almost 50% of oral SCCs are associated with or preceded by leukoplakia. Leukoplakia on the floor of the mouth and the ventral surface of the tongue is associated with the highest risk of cancer.

Degeneration to carcinoma takes 1 to 20 years. Clinically, the patches are white, slightly elevated, usually well-defined plaques that show little tendency to extend peripherally.

DIFFERENTIAL DIAGNOSIS. The differential diagnosis includes candidiasis, lichen planus, habitual cheek biting, white sponge nevus, and secondary syphilis. A lesion unique to acquired immunodeficiency syndrome (AIDS), termed hairy leukoplakia, presents as an asymptomatic, slightly raised, poorly demarcated lesion with a corrugated or "hairy" surface composed of white papillary projections. It occurs principally on the lateral borders of the tongue. *Candida* organisms are frequently observed on the lesion surface. Human papillomavirus and Epstein-Barr virus have been identified in the lesions. Dyskeratosis congenita is a congenital multisystem disorder, characterized by skin pigmentation, dystrophic nails, and leukoplakia.

HISTOLOGIC CHARACTERISTICS. Histologic changes occur, varying from mild scaling and epidermal thickening with minimal inflammation to varying degrees of dysplasia or carcinoma in situ. The clinical appearance of leukoplakia does not generally correlate well with the histopathologic change; therefore biopsy should be performed for all cases to determine which lesions are precancerous. Small lesions may be biopsied and simply followed if the histology is benign. Plaques that histologically exhibit atypical features should be excised, electrodesiccated, destroyed with the laser, or frozen with liquid nitrogen.

PROGNOSIS. There are no reliable predictors of which leukoplakia lesions will develop into SCC. The increasing incidence of head and neck cancers emphasizes the importance of early identification of the oral white patches that will develop into carcinomas. The DNA content (ploidy) in cells of oral leukoplakia can be used to predict the risk of oral carcinoma. Cells in lesions are classified as diploid (normal), tetraploid (intermediate), or aneuploid (abnormal). A carcinoma developed in 3% of patients with diploid lesions, in 60% with tetraploid lesions, and in 84% with aneuploid lesions. The cumulative disease-free survival rate was 97% among the group with diploid lesions, 40% among the group with tetraploid lesions, and 16% among the group with aneuploid lesions. Ploidy is determined with a multistep procedure performed on paraffin-embedded tissue samples.

TREATMENT. Many lesions clear spontaneously or regress when cigarette or pipe smoking is stopped. If a young man with leukoplakic lesions stops using tobacco for 6 weeks, most of his leukoplakic lesions will resolve clinically. Long-term follow-up is desirable to check for recurrences.

Leukoplakia of the vulva and the lip can be successfully treated with 5-FU. Lip lesions are treated twice daily with applications of 1% 5-FU solution until erythema and erosions become marked in approximately 10 to 21 days. Discomfort is intense and can be relieved with cool compresses or topical lidocaine gel. Localized dysplastic oral leukoplakia is treated with surgical excision, electrosurgery, cryosurgery, or CO_2 laser evaporation. Tretinoin (Retin-A) gel shows only a limited effect in controlling oral leukoplakia.

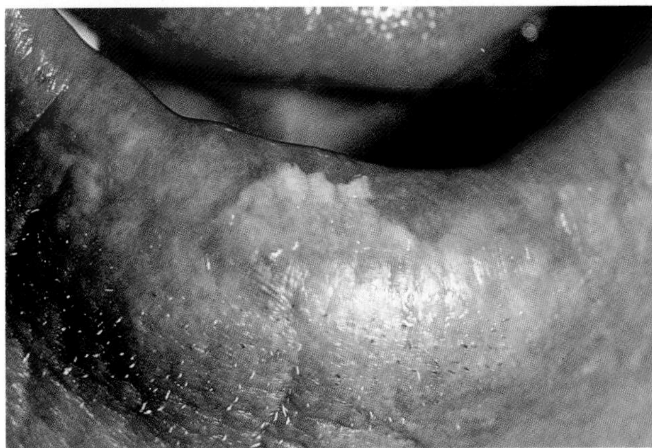

Figure 21-37 Leukoplakia. A thin, white plaque had been present on the lip for over 2 years. This patient smoked.

VERRUCOUS CARCINOMA

Verrucous carcinoma (VC) is a term encompassing three rare entities: oral florid papillomatosis (Figure 21-38), giant condylomata of Buschke-Löwenstein (perineum) (Figure 21-39), and epithelioma cuniculatum (plantar surface of the foot) (Figure 21-40). Verrucous carcinoma can occur at other sites. They typically develop at sites of chronic irritation and inflammation. The term verrucous carcinoma was coined to denote a locally aggressive, exophytic, low-grade squamous cell carcinoma with little metastatic potential. Verrucous carcinomas have been reported on many other skin surfaces. Verrucous carcinomas are probably caused by human papillomaviruses (HPVs) and are most often associated with HPV-6 and HPV-11. They are thought to represent an intermediate lesion in a pathologic continuum from condyloma to squamous cell carcinoma. All three entities have similar biologic potential and show bulky, exophytic, fungating growth, with a high degree of cellular differentiation histologically. A slowly growing tumor extends in surface area and locally compresses and displaces rather than infiltrating contiguous structures, and rarely metastasizes. Histologically, the tumor displays massive epidermal thickening with local invasion minus cellular atypia. In their early stages, all tumors may be mis-

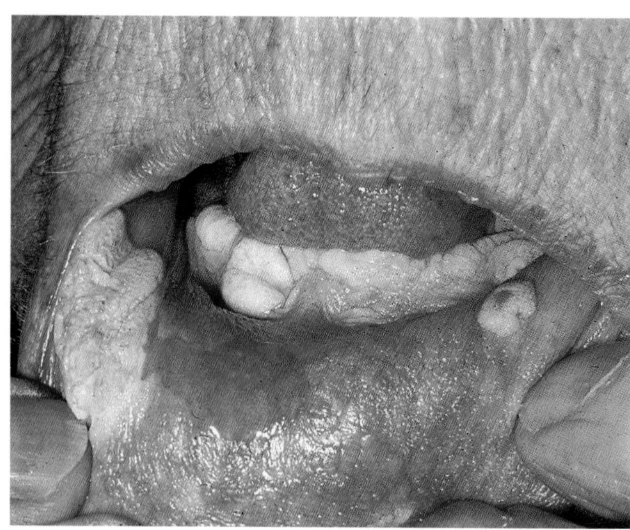

Figure 21-38 Oral florid papillomatosis. A white verrucous growth that may extend widely over the oral mucosa.

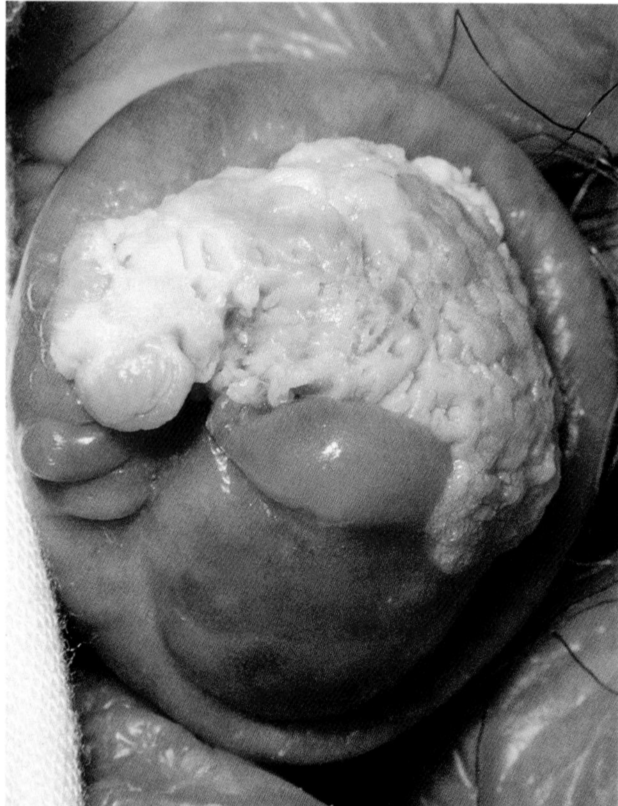

Figure 21-39 The giant condylomata of Buschke-Löwenstein occurs on the male and female genitalia. They initially appear as warts, but grow relentlessly despite multiple attempts at conservative topical and surgical treatment.

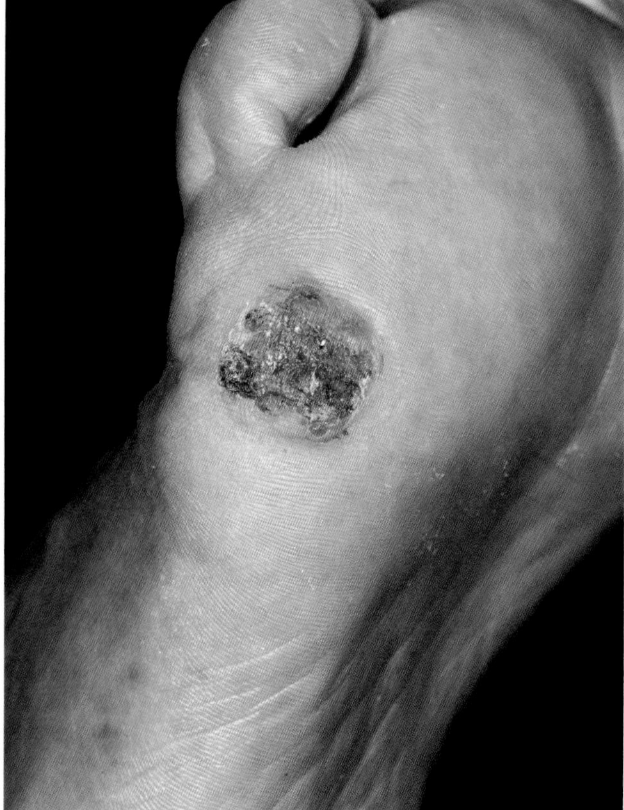

Figure 21-40 Epithelioma cuniculatum. A lesion was present for months and was suspected of being a plantar wart.

taken for warts. However, tumors are unresponsive to locally destructive procedures and slowly, over months or years, increase in size, become indurated, and deeply penetrate the dermis. Conservative local excision, Mohs microscopically controlled surgery, radiation therapy, CO_2 laser, systemic chemotherapy, and administration of acitretin and intralesional interferon-1 have all been advocated.

ORAL FLORID PAPILLOMATOSIS. The incidence of VC among oral carcinomas is 2% to 12%. These very rare tumors are most often reported in white men between 55 and 65 years of age. Tobacco chewing is a risk factor. Many patients have poor oral hygiene or dentures. Early lesions appear as white patches on a red base. Lesions develop into extensive gray-white, warty tumors with a deeply cleaved surface on the gingival mucosa and may extend to the entire oral mucosa and into the larynx and trachea (Figure 21-38). Local aggression with bone, muscle, and salivary gland invasion occurred in 53% of cases in one study. Multiple infections with low- and high-risk HPVs and their rapid replication during hyperkeratinization may participate in the histogenesis of oral VC. *PMID: 18580072*

White sponge nevus is autosomal dominant and is characterized by white lesions that appear from birth to adolescence.

BUSCHKE-LÖWENSTEIN TUMOR. This tumor, a carcinoma-like condylomata acuminata, is verrucous carcinoma of the anogenital mucosal surface (Figure 21-39). The incidence varies from 5% to 24% of all penile cancers. These tumors occur most commonly in uncircumcised men on the glans and prepuce and have the same clinical appearance on the vulva, vagina, cervix, and anorectum. Transformation into invasive carcinoma has been described.

VERRUCOUS CARCINOMA (EPITHELIOMA CUNICULATUM) PLANTARE. This tumor occurs in older men with a mean age of 60 (Figure 21-40). Exophytic tumors with ulceration and sinuses draining foul-smelling discharge cause pain and bleeding. This tumor mimics a variety of other skin lesions with its insidious onset. Plantar warts, ischemic ulcers, melanoma, and SCC must be considered.

PRIMARY CUTANEOUS LYMPHOMAS

A variety of T- and B-cell neoplasms can involve the skin, either primarily or secondarily (Table 21-6). The term *primary cutaneous lymphoma* refers to cutaneous T-cell lymphomas (CTCLs) and cutaneous B-cell lymphomas (CBCLs) that present in the skin with no evidence of extracutaneous disease at the time of diagnosis. After the gastrointestinal tract, the skin is the second most common site of extranodal non-Hodgkin's lymphoma, with an estimated annual incidence of 1:100,000.

Table 21-6 Relative Frequency and Disease-Specific 5-Year Survival of 1905 Primary Cutaneous Lymphomas Classified According to the WHO-EORTC Classification

WHO-EORTC classification	No.*
Cutaneous T-cell lymphoma	
Indolent clinical behavior	
Mycosis fungoides	800
Folliculotropic MF	86
Pagetoid reticulosis	14
Granulomatous slack skin	4
Primary cutaneous anaplastic large cell lymphoma	146
Lymphomatoid papulosis	236
Subcutaneous panniculitis-like T-cell lymphoma	18
Primary cutaneous CD4$^+$ small/medium pleomorphic T-cell lymphoma	39
Aggressive clinical behavior	
Sézary syndrome	52
Primary cutaneous NK/T-cell lymphoma, nasal-type	7
Primary cutaneous aggressive CD8$^+$ T-cell lymphoma	14
Primary cutaneous/T-cell lymphoma	13
Primary cutaneous peripheral T-cell lymphoma, unspecified	47
Cutaneous B-cell lymphoma	
Indolent clinical behavior	
Primary cutaneous marginal zone B-cell lymphoma	127
Primary cutaneous follicle center lymphoma	207
Intermediate clinical behavior	
Primary cutaneous diffuse large B-cell lymphoma, leg type	85
Primary cutaneous diffuse large B-cell lymphoma, other	4
Primary cutaneous intravascular large B-cell lymphoma	6

From Blood 105(10):3768-3785, 2005; Epub 2005 Feb 3. *PMID: 15692063*

*Data are based on 1905 patients with a primary cutaneous lymphoma registered at the Dutch and Austrian Cutaneous Lymphoma Group between 1986 and 2002.

CUTANEOUS T-CELL LYMPHOMA

The term cutaneous T-cell lymphoma (CTCL) encompasses a broad group of lymphomatous neoplasms of helper T cells that present in the skin but later may involve lymph nodes, peripheral blood cells, and the viscera. They vary in histology, immunophenotype, and prognosis. CTCL has replaced Hodgkin's disease as the most common adult lymphoma. These diseases are rarely, if ever, curable and need chronic management.

MYCOSIS FUNGOIDES

Mycosis fungoides (MF) is the most common form of cutaneous T-cell lymphoma. It is a rare non-Hodgkin's lymphoma of unknown etiology. The incidence of CTCLs from 1973 to 2002 was 6.4 cases per million. Mycosis fungoides accounts for 72% of CTCLs; Sézary syndrome accounts for 2.5%. The incidence of CTCL is 50% greater in black people than in white people. Men are affected twice as often as women, and incidence increases greatly with age. Childhood cases of mycosis fungoides are reported.

COURSE OF MF. The disease starts insidiously in young adults. A persistent eruption in young adults should be evaluated for possible CTCL. The immunocompetence of CTCL patients varies and this affects their clinical course and response to therapy. The skin lesions evolve from flat patches to thin plaques and tumors. The disease progresses to systemic involvement as the cells lose their affinity for the epidermis, alter their surface expression, and expand within the dermis, peripheral blood, and lymph nodes. The disease has an excellent prognosis in the initial stage when it is confined to the skin. The disease is fatal once systemic spread has occurred. The staging of the disease is based on the degree of skin involvement. For limited patch-or-plaque mycosis fungoides, treatment is skin-directed therapy, which can target the malignant T cells and the Langerhans cells.

MOLECULAR THEORY OF ORIGIN. CTCL is a malignancy of a single clone of CD4-positive T cells. Each patient develops a unique clone of malignant cells with unique surface receptors. The disease advances with the development of progressively more aggressive subclones. Initially, Langerhans cells carry antigens from the skin to peripheral lymph nodes, where they present the antigens to CD4-positive T cells and convert them to cutaneous T-cell lymphoma cells (CTCL cells). The T cells acquire cutaneous lymphoid antigen (CLA) on their surfaces, which acts as a skin-selective homing receptor. CLA permits adherence of the T cell to dermal blood vessels, giving the cells the ability to infiltrate the skin. A unique feature of early-stage CTCL is epidermotropism, in which malignant cells are found in the proximity of the epidermis, where the cellular growth environment is conducive to their proliferation. A second set of antigenic peptides permits immunologic attack against the malignant cells through the use of photopheresis.

MALIGNANT T CELLS. The malignant cells function as T cells but they have a propensity to home to the skin, to be activated and persist in an activated state, and later to achieve clonal dominance and accumulate in the skin, lymph nodes, and peripheral blood. Sézary syndrome is a more aggressive form of cutaneous T-cell lymphoma in which the skin is diffusely affected and malignant cells are found in the peripheral blood. Many other forms of T-cell lymphoma exist (see Table 21-6), which are all characterized by expansions of malignant T cells within the skin.

SKIN-HOMING CAPACITY OF MALIGNANT CELLS AND CLONES. Malignant lymphocytes home to the skin through interactions with dermal capillary endothelial cells (Figure 21-41). Circulating lymphoma cells extravasate through endothelial cells and into the dermis. The lymphoma cells, which now have an affinity for epidermal cells, cluster around Langerhans cells, forming Pautrier's microabscesses. The epidermal malignant lymphocytes belong to a malignant clone and are present in small numbers in the dermal infiltrate. Over time the malignant cells may lose their dependence on the skin environment, alter their surface expression, and expand within the dermis, peripheral blood, and lymph nodes.

DIAGNOSIS. The diagnosis is made by recognizing the clinical characteristics of the various stages of the disease and is supported by laboratory studies (Table 21-7). Multiple biopsies at different sites are useful. It is important to biopsy suspected lesions early enough so that potentially curative treatment can be initiated. Immunophenotypic and gene rearrangement studies can confirm clinical suspicion when histology is equivocal. Evaluation for systemic involvement includes examination of peripheral blood for Sézary cells and biopsy of palpable lymph nodes.

DISEASE PROGRESSION. There are four phases in the evolution of the disease: pre-MF, patch (flat, scaly, red, sometimes pruritic), plaque, and tumor. Most patients with patches or plaques do not have disease progression. Lesions from the last three phases may be present simultaneously. Erythroderma may occur at any time. There are many clinical variants. Lymphadenopathy may develop at any stage. Survival time is less than 3 years once the tumor phase begins. Despite the new laboratory diagnostic methods, recognition of the physical signs of the disease by the clinician and routine histology are still the most sensitive methods of detection.

DIAGNOSIS OF EARLY DISEASE. Early mycosis fungoides can be confused with eczema. A four-point scoring system was developed to aid the diagnosis of early disease (Table 21-7).

CLINICAL CRITERIA

A description of the clinical criteria findings of early disease are presented in Box 21-5.

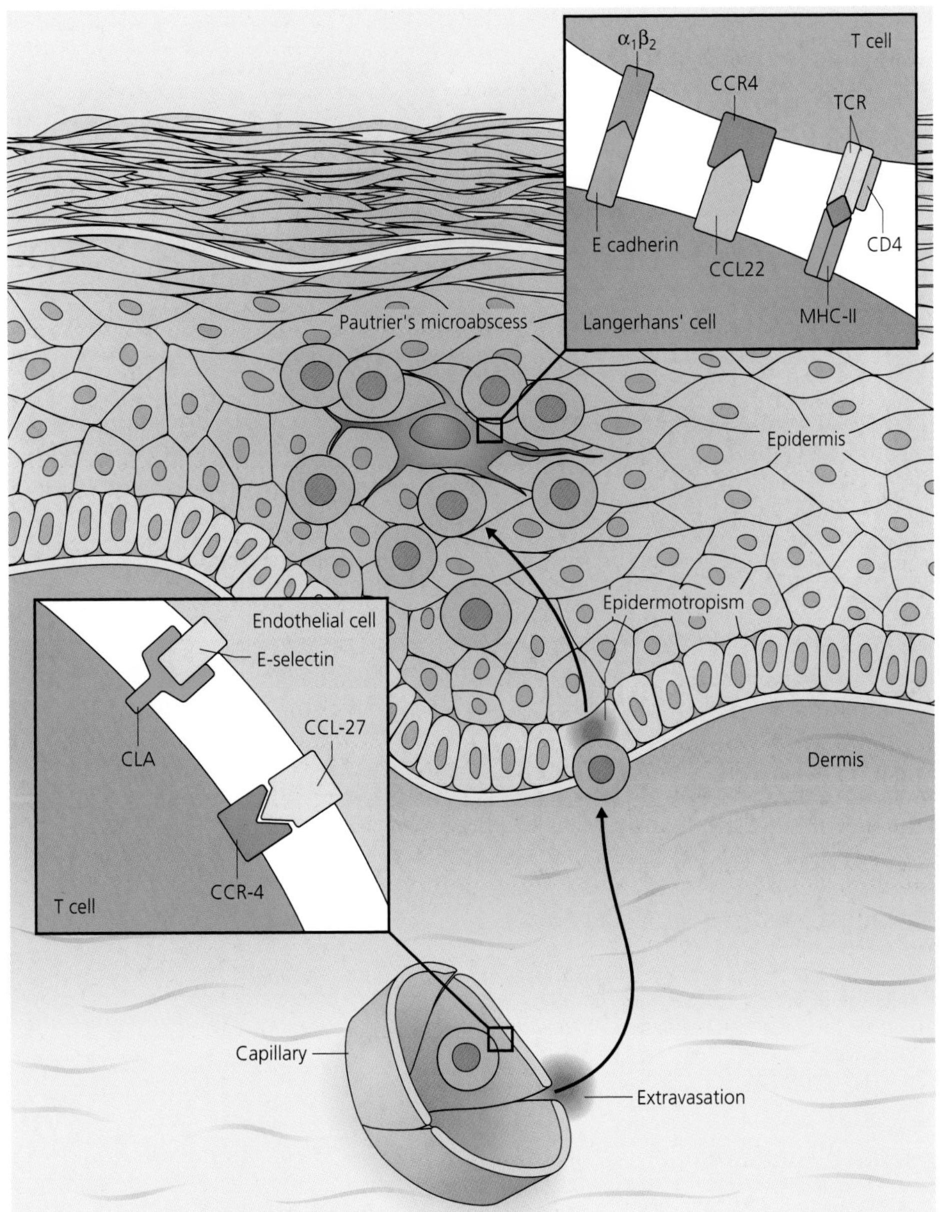

Figure 21-41 Mycosis fungoides is a cancer of skin-homing T cells. In cutaneous T-cell lymphoma, cells home to the skin by interacting with dermal capillary endothelial cells and extravasate into the dermis. From there, the lymphoma cells display an affinity for epidermal cells and cluster around Langerhans' cells, forming Pautrier's microabscesses, which can be observed on histologic examination. Girardi M et al: *N Engl J Med* 350(19):1978-1988, 2004. *PMID: 15128898*

Box 21-5 **Criteria Description: Early Mycosis Fungoides**

A. HISTORY

Persistent disease

Lesions increase in size and number over time. They incompletely clear with topical corticosteroids and recur when therapy is discontinued, or they continue to develop in untreated areas. Drug eruptions may do the same and a trial of discontinuation of the drug may be indicated.

B. MORPHOLOGY OF LESIONS

Patch-phase MF lesions vary in size (>5 cm in diameter), shape, and color. Untreated lesions expand slowly to form well-demarcated lesions that may coalesce or undergo spontaneous clearing. Progression and regression produce irregularly shaped lesions. Poikiloderma is the local juxtaposition of mottled pigmentation, telangiectasia, and epidermal atrophy (cigarette paper wrinkling) interspersed with slight infiltration. Persistent poikilodermatous patches on non–sun-exposed skin, particularly the buttocks, should be considered MF until proven otherwise by biopsy.

C. NUMBER OF LESIONS

Most patients present with multiple lesions and several sites of involvement. Disorders that might be confused with unilesional MF are nummular eczema, lichen simplex chronicus, erythema chronicum migrans, and tinea corporis.

D. DISTRIBUTION OF LESIONS

Lesions often initially develop on relatively non–sun-exposed skin, such as the trunk below the waistline ("bathing suit" distribution), flanks, breasts, inner thighs, inner arms, and periaxillary areas.

Table 21-7 Algorithm for Diagnosis of Early Mycosis Fungoides (MF)*

(A total of 4 points is required for the diagnosis of MF based on any combination of points from the clinical, histopathologic, molecular biologic, and immunopathologic criteria.)

Criteria	Scoring system
Clinical	
Basic Persistent and/or progressive patches/thin plaques	2 points for basic criteria and two additional criteria
Additional 1. Non–sun-exposed location 2. Size/shape variation 3. Poikiloderma	1 point for basic criteria and one additional criterion
Histopathology	
Basic Superficial lymphoid infiltrate	2 points for basic criteria and two additional criteria
Additional 1. Epidermotropism without spongiosis 2. Lymphoid atypia†	1 point for basic criteria and one additional criterion
Molecular biologic (T-cell receptor gene rearrangement analysis)	
1. T-cell clonal pattern must be detected by PCR-based analysis of T-cell receptor gene (TCR) rearrangements‡	1 point for clonality
Immunopathologic (Immunophenotyping)§	
1. <50% $CD2^+$, $CD3^+$, and/or $CD5^+$ T cells 2. <10% $CD7^+$ T cells 3. Epidermal/dermal discordance of CD2, CD3, CD5, or CD7‖	1 point for one or more criteria

Adapted from *J Am Acad Dermatol* 53(6):1053-1063, 2005. *PMID: 16310068*
*Proposed by The International Society for Cutaneous Lymphoma (ISCL).
†Lymphoid atypia is defined as cells with enlarged hyperchromatic nuclei and irregular or cerebriform nuclear contours.
‡Contact lab to determine specimen required (e.g., fresh-frozen tissue, formalin-fixed paraffin block).
§Contact lab to determine specimen required (e.g., 5-mm punch biopsy submitted in tissue culture medium not frozen or fixed).
‖T-cell antigen deficiency confined to the epidermis.

HISTOPATHOLOGIC CRITERIA

Biopsy specimens must have a superficial lymphoid infiltrate. Epidermotropism without spongiosis and lymphoid atypia each qualify as 1 point.

Atypical lymphoid cells are present that are slightly larger than normal lymphocytes and have hyperchromatic, irregularly contoured (convoluted) nuclei. Such cells have been termed "mycosis cells," "Lutzner cells," or "Sézary cells."

The histologic diagnosis of MF is difficult because many subtle changes, most of which may be present to some degree in many inflammatory and neoplastic cutaneous conditions, may be present. An initial punch biopsy will confirm the lymphoid nature of a lesion. Then early MF must be distinguished from inflammatory disorders.

The pathologist looks for a number of features: Pautrier's microabscesses (atypical lymphocytes in collections within the epidermis), haloed lymphocytes (caused by retraction artifact surrounding intraepidermal lymphocytes), exocytosis (presence of lymphocytes in the epidermis), hyperconvoluted intraepidermal lymphocytes, and lymphocytes aligned within the basal layer ("string of pearls").

Multiple biopsies from a variety of lesions may be required. Stop all topical treatments and systemic immunosuppressants at least 2 to 4 weeks before performing a biopsy.

MOLECULAR BIOLOGIC CRITERIA

A dominant T-cell clonal pattern must be detected by polymerase chain reaction (PCR)-based analysis of T-cell receptor gene rearrangements. This is worth 1 point.

Clonal proliferation from a single lymphocyte is a feature of malignancy. Populations of neoplastic lymphocytes contain the same gene rearrangement. Clonal rearrangement of T-cell receptor (TCR) genes can be demonstrated in lesional tissue in most cases. Populations of reactive lymphocytes contain a mixture of gene rearrangements. One recommended method utilizes DNA extracted from fresh-frozen tissue and PCR-based clonality analysis of T-cell receptor γ gene rearrangements. PCR can be used to monitor the response to therapy by detecting the presence or absence of the malignant clone in the skin or blood.

IMMUNOPATHOLOGIC CRITERIA

This process is used to identify cells based on the types of antigens or markers on the surface of the cell. Studies on paraffin or frozen sections using a panel of antibodies to cell surface or cytoplasmic molecules will demonstrate loss of one or more T-cell-associated antigens (such as CD2, CD3, CD4, CD5, CD7, CD26) by the neoplastic T cells. Loss of CD7 expression is not a reliable marker. Any one of three features must be present to generate 1 point: loss of T-cell antigens with less than 50% of T cells expressing CD2, CD3, and/or CD5; less than 10% of T cells expressing CD7; or epidermal/dermal discordance for expression of CD2, CD3, CD5, and/or CD7.

STAGING PROCEDURES. A baseline workup includes physical examination. Document the presence of lymphadenopathy and hepatosplenomegaly. Obtain a complete blood cell count (review the buffy coat smear for Sézary cells), biopsy with gene rearrangement analysis, perform flow cytometric studies of the blood to detect a circulating malignant clone, and obtain computed tomographic scans of the chest, abdomen, and pelvis.

STAGING. Staging at initial diagnosis is helpful in guiding treatment and it has prognostic value. Most cancers are staged by the TNM system. The T stage describes the tumor, N the nodal status, and M the presence or absence of metastasis. A modified staging classification describes new prognostic subsets (Box 21-6).

PROGNOSIS. Patients with T1 disease have the same life expectancy as age-matched individuals. Patients with T2 disease have a median survival of about 10 to 12 years and a 25% risk of progressing to more advanced disease. Patients with only tumors or erythroderma have a median survival of 4 to 5 years. Nodal enlargement may not suggest pathologic involvement. The presence of increased numbers of $CD8^+$ T cells in the skin is a good prognostic factor. Imaging with CT is performed for T3-4 disease to assess visceral and nodal involvement. Positron emission tomography (PET) scanning can increase the sensitivity of detection of affected lymph nodes.

Box 21-6 **Staging by TNM Classification to Define Mycosis**

The American Joint Committee on Cancer (AJCC) Fungoides

TNM(B) definitions

Primary tumor (T)

T1: Limited patch/plaque (<10% of skin surface involved)
T2: Generalized patch/plaque (≥10% of skin surface involved)
T3: Cutaneous tumors (one or more)
T4: Generalized erythroderma (with or without patches, plaques, or tumors)
[NOTE: Pathology of T1-T4 is diagnostic of cutaneous T-cell lymphoma (CTCL). When characteristics of more than one T-type tumor exist, both are recorded and the highest is used for staging, for example, T4(3).]

Regional lymph nodes (N)

N0: Lymph nodes clinically uninvolved; the pathology is negative for CTCL
N1: Lymph nodes clinically enlarged, histologically uninvolved; the pathology is negative for CTCL
N2: Lymph nodes clinically unenlarged, histologically involved; the pathology is positive for CTCL
N3: Lymph nodes enlarged and histologically involved; the pathology is positive for CTCL

Distant metastasis (M)

M0: No visceral disease
M1: Visceral disease present
The TNM classification includes a subcategory for patients with CTCL:

Blood involvement (B)

B0: No circulating atypical cells (<1000 Sézary cells [$CD4^+/CD7^-$]/ml)
B1: Circulating atypical cells (≥1000 Sézary cells [$CD4^+/CD7^-$]/ml)
B2: Leukemic involvement defined by absolute Sézary cell count ≥1000 cells per µL, CD4/CD8 ratio ≥10 by flow cytometry, aberrant expression of normal T-cell markers, molecular evidence of clonality, or chromosomal abnormality in a T-cell clone

TNM stage groupings

Stage IA
T1, N0, M0
Stage IB
T2, N0, M0
Stage IIA
T1-T2, N1, M0
Stage IIB
T3, N0-N1, M0
Stage IIIA
T4, N0, M0
Stage IIIB
T4, N1, M0
Stage IVA
T1-T4, N2, M0
T1-T4, N3, M0
Stage IVB
T1-T4, N0, M1
T1-T4, N1, M1
T1-T4, N2, M1
T1-T4, N3, M1

CLINICAL PRESENTATIONS

Pre-MF. The pre-MF phase is the first phase in which the diagnosis is suspected, but it cannot be made by clinical or histologic criteria. This premycotic phase persists for months or years and is suspected when inflammation persists and recurs after repeated courses of topical steroids. Spontaneous remissions occur. Nonspecific pruritic eruptions or pruritus alone may be the only manifestation. A red, scaly, eczematous-like or psoriasis-like eruption and an atrophic, mottled, telangiectatic eruption, referred to as large-patch parapsoriasis or poikiloderma vasculare atrophicans, may occur. These two latter dermatoses possess characteristic features that allow one to predict with a greater degree of certainty that the evolution of typical MF may occur. These dermatoses can be present for as long as 35 years before the plaques and tumors of MF develop.

Eczematous form. The eczematous form presents with persistent, nonspecific, flat, red, itchy, eczematous areas that resemble asteatotic eczema or atopic dermatitis, except that the lesions tend to remain fixed in location and size, and the margins are sharply delineated (Figures 21-42 and 21-43).

The poikilodermatous-parapsoriasis lesion. Lesions of parapsoriasis en plaques are sharply circumscribed and have a faint erythema and sometimes a yellowish cast, a fine scale, and a slightly wrinkled surface. On the trunk and limbs, the lesions are usually 1 to 5 cm and round, oval, or fingerlike (digitate dermatosis). On the buttocks and thighs, where they occur more commonly, lesions present as patches as large as 15 cm. Patients with long-standing parapsoriasis-like lesions that are resistant to conventional treatment require careful monitoring for the possible development of cutaneous lymphoma (Figure 21-44).

Poikiloderma vasculare atrophicans is a term used to describe lesions that have telangiectasia; "cigarette-paper" skin with fine, wrinkly atrophy; and mottled pigmentation (Figures 21-45 and 21-46). The appearance of poikilodermatous changes is an ominous sign. The terms parapsoriasis variegata or parapsoriasis lichenoides are used to describe variants of these lesions that present with a netlike or reticulated pattern.

Histologic examination of early patch lesions shows a superficial bandlike or lichenoid infiltrate, mainly consisting of lymphocytes and histiocytes. Atypical cells with small- to medium-sized, highly indented (cerebriform), and sometimes hyperchromatic nuclei are few, and mostly confined to the epidermis (epidermotropism). They colonize the basal layer of the epidermis either as single, often haloed cells or in a linear configuration.

Patch stage. The disease enters the patch stage when histologic changes are characteristic of MF. The morphology of the lesion does not necessarily change.

Plaque stage. The plaque stage is entered gradually when dusky red-to-brown, sometimes scaly areas become elevated above the surrounding uninvolved skin because of acanthosis (thickening of the epidermis). Plaques can arise from uninvolved skin. Itching becomes more persistent and intense and may be intolerable. The plaques vary in shape with round, oval, arciform, or serpiginous patterns, occasionally with central clearing. The extent of involvement varies from a few isolated areas to a major portion of the skin (Figures 21-47 to 21-49). Infiltration of the entire skin produces a thickened red hide with scale (exfoliative dermatitis) or without scale (erythroderma). MF may begin as exfoliative erythroderma. Infiltration and plaques in hairy areas may produce alopecia.

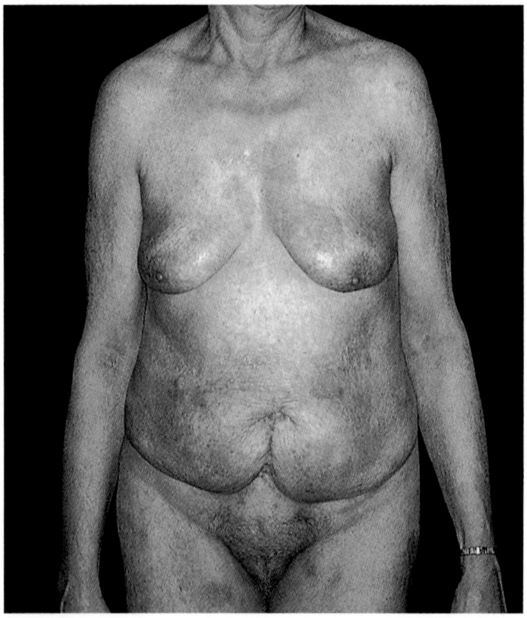

Figure 21-42 The eczematous or patch phase presents with red macules that have a fine scale. Lesions may be multiple. Itching is variable. Lesions are hypopigmented or hyperpigmented in dark-skinned individuals. Patches slowly evolve into plaques.

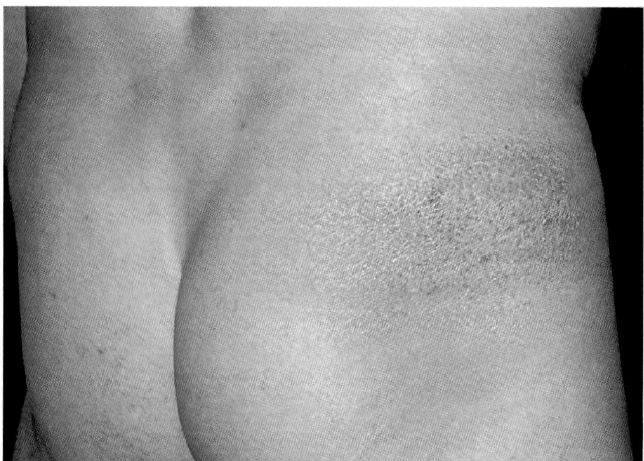

Figure 21-43 Patches may affect any area but they are found most often in sun-protected locations such as the buttocks and lower trunk. Early lesions look like nummular eczema. They tend to remain fixed in location for months.

POIKILODERMATOUS-PARAPSORIASIS LESIONS

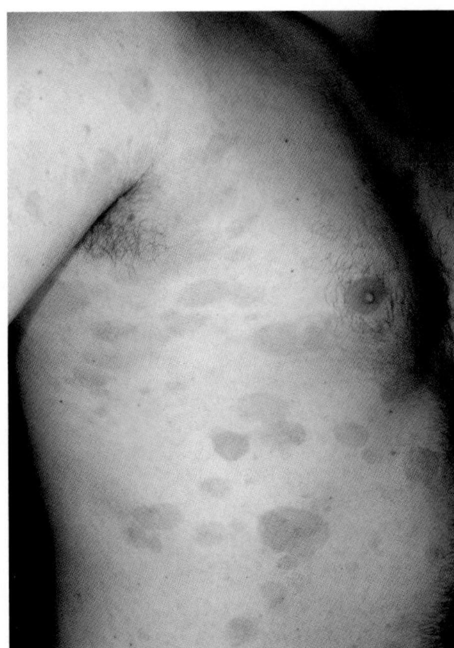

Figure 21-44 Parapsoriasis (small plaque). Lesions are well-circumscribed, slightly scaly, light yellow, oval superficial plaques that are concentrated on the trunk. A digitate pattern that follows the dermatome is characteristic. This form of the disease rarely degenerates into lymphoma. Parapsoriasis with larger irregular plaques has the potential to progress to cutaneous T-cell lymphoma.

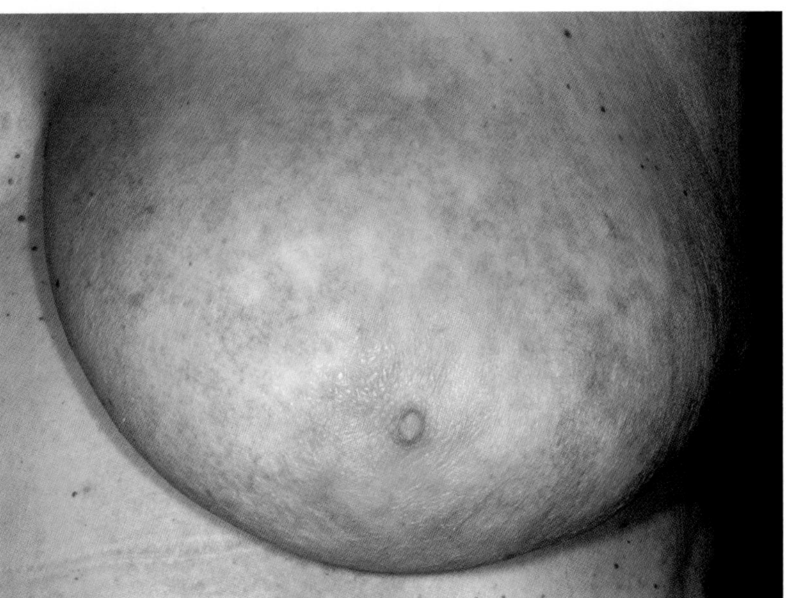

Figure 21-45 Poikilodermic lesions. The skin is atrophic, wrinkled, dry, and dyspigmented with telangiectasias.

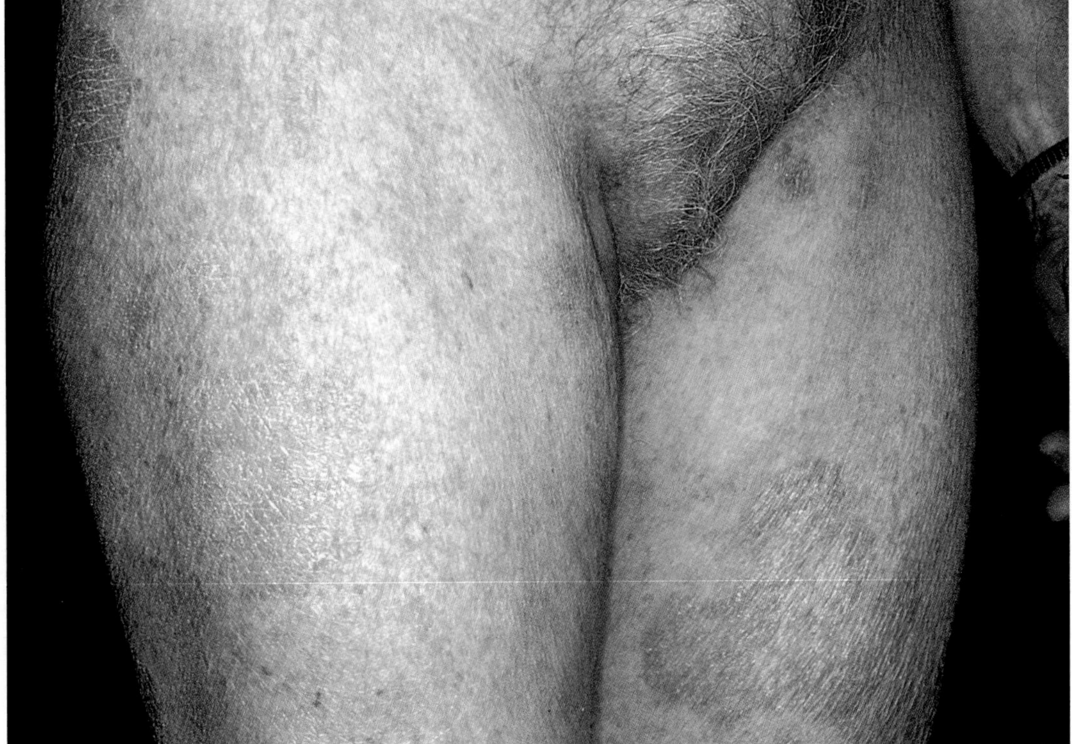

Figure 21-46 Mycosis fungoides (poikiloderma vasculare atrophicans). Red-brown hyperpigmented plaques with an atrophic, wrinkled surface tend to remain fixed in location.

MYCOSIS FUNGOIDES PLAQUE STAGE

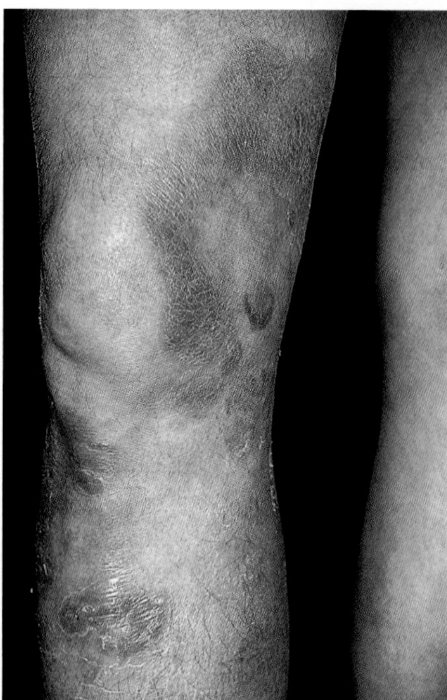

Figure 21-47 Early plaques have a fine scaling surface. The well-demarcated, erythematous lesions slowly evolve into tumors.

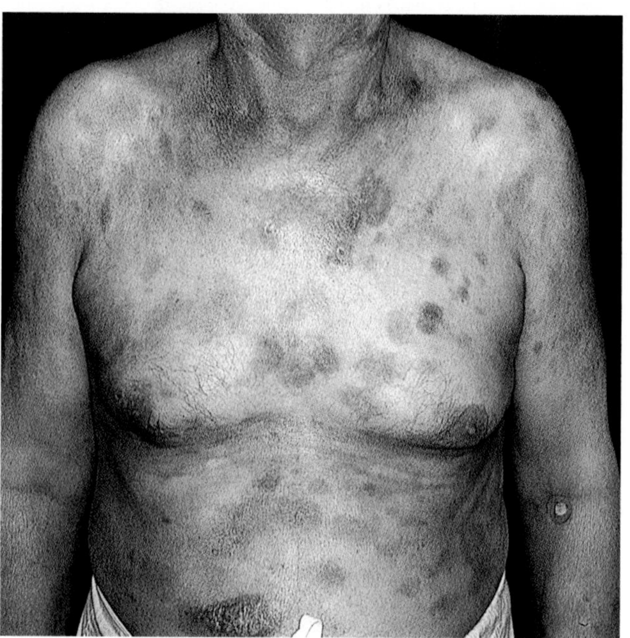

Figure 21-48 Annular or serpiginous plaques may be numerous. Central clearing may occur. Itching may be intense at this stage.

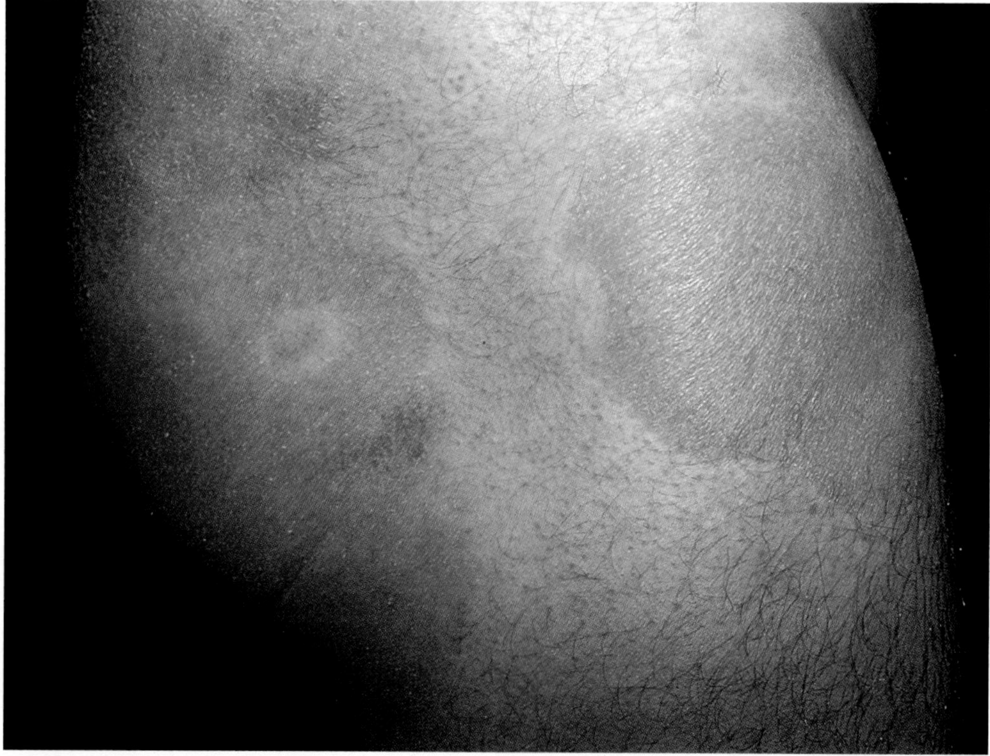

Figure 21-49 Large plaques have slowly evolved from stable macular, scaling, eczematous-appearing lesions.

Histologically, epidermotropism is more pronounced than in the patches. The presence of intraepidermal collections of atypical cells (Pautrier's microabscesses) is observed in only a minority of cases. With progression to tumor stage, the dermal infiltrates become more diffuse and epidermotropism may be lost. The infiltrate becomes mixed (lymphocytes, eosinophils, and plasma cells) as the plaque stage progresses. The tumor cells increase in number and size, showing variable proportions of small, medium-sized, and large cerebriform cells, blast cells with prominent nuclei, and intermediate forms. Transformation to a diffuse large-cell lymphoma that may be either $CD30^-$ or $CD30^+$ may occur and is often associated with a poor prognosis.

Tumor stage. Tumors develop from preexisting plaques or erythroderma, or they may originate from red or normal skin. Itching may decrease in intensity. Tumors vary in size, some becoming huge or mushroom-shaped (thus the term mycosis fungoides, which has been in use for 150 years) (Figures 21-50 to 21-52). Necrosis and ulceration of plaques and tumors are common.

In the early stages, the disease remains confined to the skin. Superficial lymphadenopathy may be detected in the plaque stage, and deep lymphadenopathy with visceral metastasis, such as to the spleen, lungs, or gastrointestinal tract, may occur during the tumor stage.

TUMOR STAGE

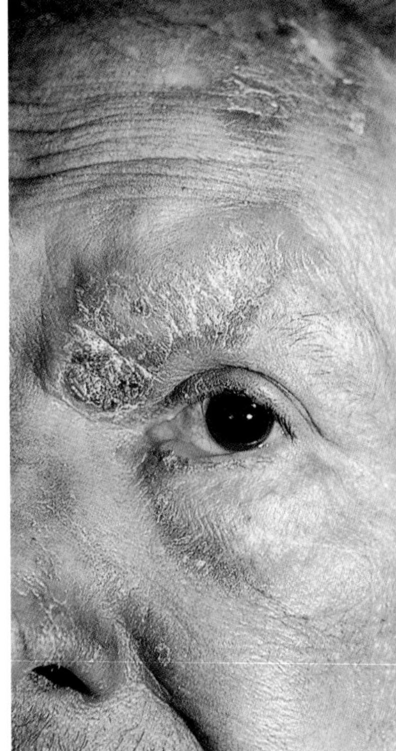

Figure 21-50 Tumors are ulcerated and exophytic. They resemble a mycotic infection; thus the archaic term mycosis fungoides.

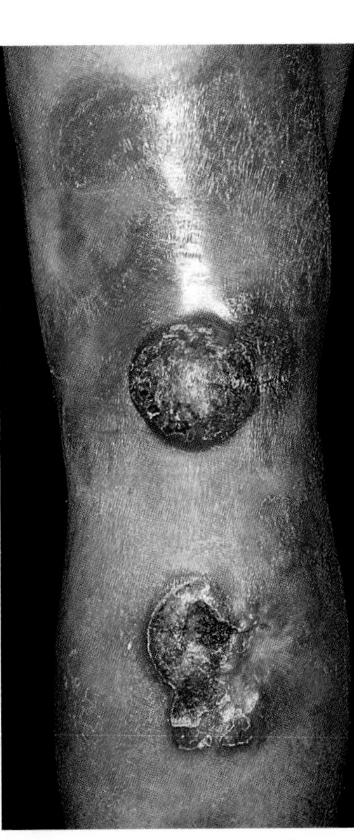

Figure 21-51 Red-violet, dome-shaped tumors may be exophytic or ulcerated.

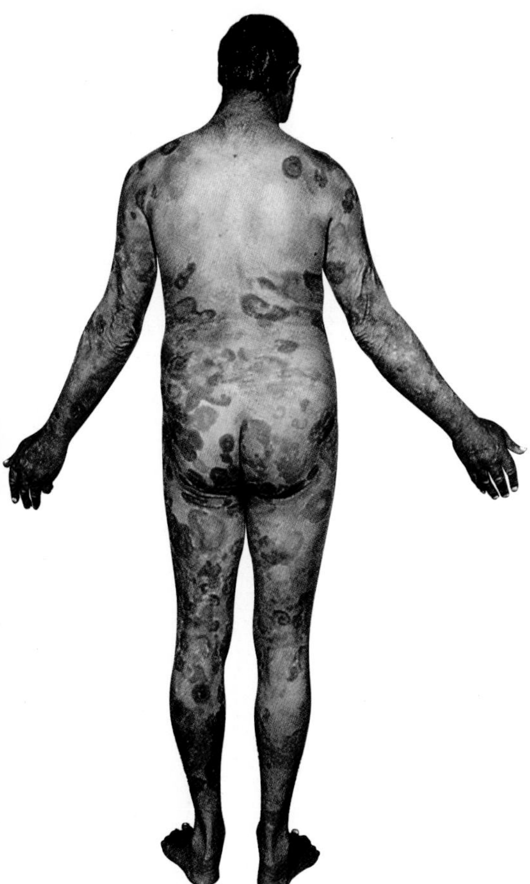

Figure 21-52 Widespread tumors have an annular and serpiginous pattern with central clearing.

SÉZARY SYNDROME

Sézary syndrome (SS), the leukemic form of MF, is an aggressive lymphoma (Figure 21-53). The estimated 5-year survival rate is 11%. SS consists of the triad of erythroderma, lymphadenopathy, and cerebriform lymphocytes (Sézary cells) in the peripheral blood, lymph nodes, and skin. Patients may have generalized pruritus, exfoliative dermatitis and thickening of the skin, ectropion, alopecia, and thickening of the palms and soles. The erythema may wax and wane during the day, or it may disappear and be replaced by plaques and tumors. Evidence supporting the diagnosis includes Sézary cells comprising more than 5% to 20% of circulating lymphocytes or more than $1000/mm^3$, an expanded population of $CD4^+/CD7^-$ circulating lymphocytes by flow cytometry, an elevated CD4/CD8 ratio, or a clonal *TCR* gene rearrangement. Skin biopsy may reveal features resembling those found in the early stages of classic MF. Circulating cells with hyperconvoluted nuclei (Sézary cells) appear to be identical to those found in the skin infiltrates of MF (Figure 21-54).

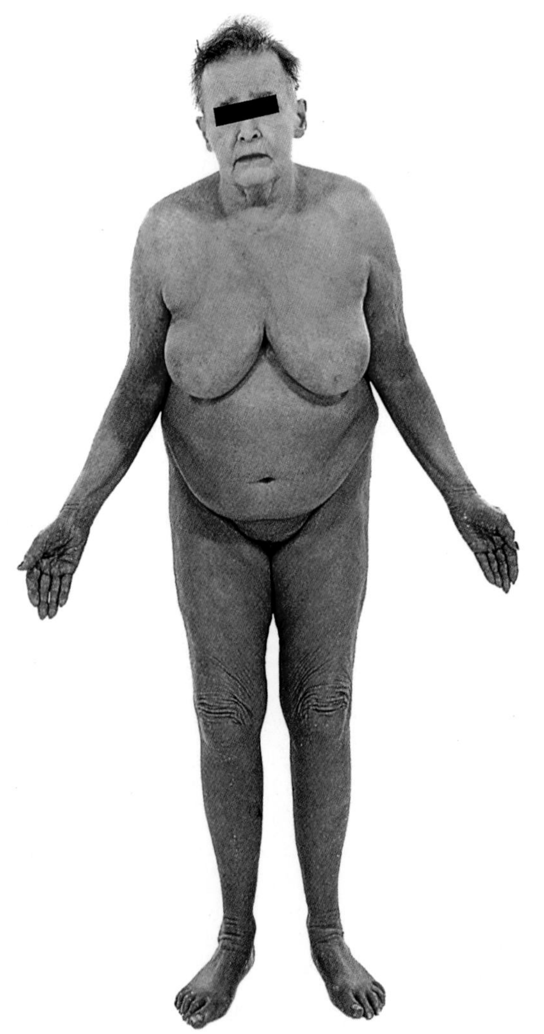

Figure 21-53 Sézary syndrome. Generalized erythroderma with scaling and thickening of the palms and soles.

TREATMENT. See Boxes 21-7 to 21-9 for treatment regimens for MF/SS. See *National Comprehensive Cancer Network Clinical Practice Guidelines in Oncology* (www.nccn.org) for a complete discussion of treatment of all stages of cutaneous T-cell lymphoma. For limited patch-or-plaque mycosis fungoides, the treatment of choice is often a skin-directed therapy, which potentially can simultaneously target both the malignant T cells and the stimulating Langerhans cells.

These types of treatments produce remissions, but long-term remissions are uncommon. Treatment is considered palliative for most patients, though major symptomatic improvement is regularly achieved.

Some experts think that the disease can be cured with aggressive treatment when the disease is confined to the skin. Stable, localized, non–plaque disease may last for years. Because of the efficacy of topical nitrogen mustard, PUVA, and electron beam therapy in inducing and maintaining remissions, we now rarely see rapid evolution of the disease in patients whose CTCL is diagnosed early. Patients with clinical stage IA mycosis fungoides who are treated do not have an altered life expectancy. Less than 10% progress to more advanced stages and few die from the disease. Therapy for CTCL is dependent on the clinical stage. The goal of therapy is to achieve and maintain a remission or obtain palliation in advanced cases. Clinically visible disease should be treated. Patients in remission should be observed indefinitely. Maintenance therapy is routine at some centers.

Topical nitrogen mustard. Topical application of mechlorethamine has produced regression of cutaneous lesions, with particular efficacy in early stages of disease. The overall complete remission rate is related to skin stage; 50% to 80% of TNM classification T1 and 25% to 75% of T2 patients have complete responses. Treatments are usually continued for 2 to 3 years. Continuous 5-year disease-free survival may be possible in as many as 33% of

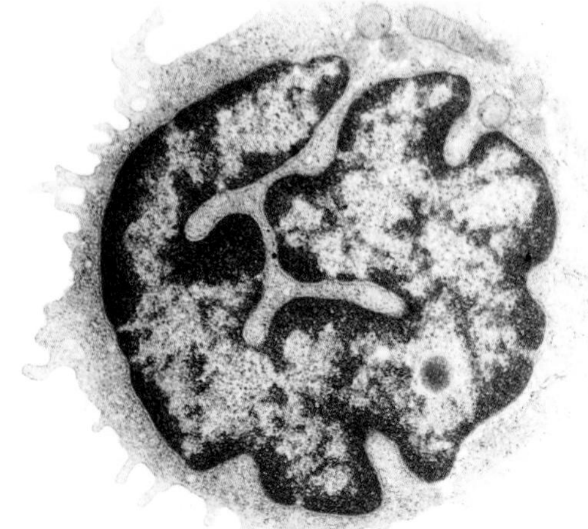

Figure 21-54 Sézary cells. Nuclei are hyperconvoluted.

T1 patients. Topical mechlorethamine is a cost-effective and convenient therapy for patients with limited patch and plaque mycosis fungoides. Topical nitrogen mustard (10-mg vial) has been used for more than 20 years. There is no systemic absorption (laboratory monitoring not required). An aqueous solution (10 to 20 mg/dl) is prepared by the patient or an ointment (10 to 20 mg of mechlorethamine [HN2]/100 gm of Aquaphor) is prepared by the pharmacist. Solution is applied once daily with a cloth or brush to the entire body surface except the groin. Areas of disease activity may become inflamed. After several weeks, treatment is limited to the affected area. Slow responders are treated two times daily or with higher concentrations (30 to 40 mg/dl). Application is continued until complete clearance. A 2- to 6-month trial of daily application of solution (either lesional or total body surface) or a 6- to 12-month trial is suggested. This is followed by maintenance therapy (average 6 months). Acute or delayed hypersensitivity reactions (5% with ointment, >30% with aqueous) occur. Desensitization is then accomplished, and treatment is resumed. Complete responses were achieved in 80%, 68%, and 61% of patients in stages IA, IB, and IIA of the disease, respectively. Topical carmustine (BCNU) is also effective, but systemic absorption occurs. Telangiectasias may develop where the drug is applied. Although the response rate to total skin electron beam therapy was superior to that of topical mechlorethamine, the long-term survival results were similar. Keep medication refrigerated. Medication is available from several pharmacists, including Crown Drugs (Philadelphia, Pa) or the Yale Medical Center Pharmacy (New Haven, Conn).

Topical corticosteroids. Topical corticosteroids, especially class I compounds, are an effective treatment for patch-stage mycosis fungoides. Corticosteroids produced total response rates of 94% (complete response, 63%) in T1 disease, which is comparable to the results seen with topical chemotherapy. The complete response rate decreased to 25% in T2 disease. Most patients were treated with clobetasol propionate emollient cream.

Bexarotene. Bexarotene 1% retinoid gel (Targretin) has an overall response rate of 44% to 63% (complete response, 8% to 21%) in patients with refractory stage IA-IIA CTCL. The predominant side effect is mild to moderate local irritation or rash. The medication is very expensive.

PUVA and UVB. Therapeutic trials with PUVA have shown a 62% to 90% complete remission rate with early cutaneous stages achieving the best responses. Continued maintenance therapy with PUVA at more protracted intervals is generally required to prolong remission duration. PUVA combined with interferon alpha-2a is associated with a high response rate. CTCL often begins in sun-shielded regions, such as the buttocks and inferior surface of the breasts. This suggests that sun exposure to the trunk and extremities alters the environment of certain regions of the skin so that CTCL cells find those sites inhospitable. This may explain why UVB or PUVA therapy can maintain

Box 21-7 **Treatment Option Overview for Mycosis Fungoides and Sézary Syndrome**

- Topical corticosteroids
- Topical chemotherapy with mechlorethamine (nitrogen mustard) or carmustine (BCNU)
- Psoralen and ultraviolet A radiation (PUVA)
- Ultraviolet B radiation (UVB)
- Total skin electron beam radiation therapy (TSEBT)
- Radiation of symptomatic skin lesions
- Interferon-alfa alone or in combination with topical therapy
- Single-agent and multiagent chemotherapy
- Bexarotene (topical gel or oral); retinoids
- Denileukin diftitox
- Combined modality treatment

Adapted from National Cancer Institute: http://www.cancer.gov.

Box 21-8 **Mycosis Fungoides/Sézary Syndrome: Treatment for Stages I and II***

- Psoralen and ultraviolet A radiation (PUVA)
- Total-skin electron-beam radiation therapy (TSEBT)
- Topical mechlorethamine (nitrogen mustard)
- Local electron-beam radiation or orthovoltage radiation therapy may be used to palliate areas of bulky or symptomatic skin disease
- Interferon-alpha alone or in combination with topical therapy
- Bexarotene, an oral or topical retinoid
- Oral methotrexate
- Pegylated liposomal doxorubicin
- Vorinostat, an oral histone deacetylase inhibitor

Adapted from: National Cancer Institute. www.cancer.gov
*Treatment can produce complete resolution of skin lesions in stage I. With therapy, survival is same as controls.

Box 21-9 **Mycosis Fungoides/Sézary Syndrome: Treatment for Stages III and IV**

- Psoralen and ultraviolet A radiation (PUVA)
- Total skin electron-beam radiation
- Local electron-beam radiation or orthovoltage radiation
- Fludarabine, 2-chlorodeoxyadenosine, pentostatin
- Interferon-alpha alone or in combination with topical therapy
- Denileukin diftitox (interleukin-2 fusion toxin)
- Systemic chemotherapy (single agent or combination) Extra-corporeal photochemotherapy
- Topical mechlorethamine (nitrogen mustard)
- Bexarotene, an oral or topical retinoid
- Pegylated liposomal doxorubicin
- Vorinostat, an oral histone deacetylase inhibitor

Adapted from: National Cancer Institute. http://www.cancer.gov

a patient in remission. PUVA is very effective in the limited, "thin," plaque stage of CTCL. High rates of remission are induced within 2 to 6 months with a regimen of two or three treatments per week, increasing the dosage of UVA by 0.5 J/cm^2 in alternate treatments, as tolerated. The dosage is held constant, and then slowly tapered to once per week, once per 2 weeks, once per month, once every other month for 6 months, and then once every 3 months for an indefinite period. Total response rates of 95% (complete response in 79% of T1 cases, 59% of T2 cases) are reported. Duration of remission averaged 3.6 years with maintenance PUVA at least once per month. Complete remission occurs faster compared with topical therapy.

Traditional broad-band UVB phototherapy (280 to 320 nm) has been associated with an 83% total and complete response rate in T1 disease. However, long-wave UVA penetrates deeper into the dermal infiltrates than UVB. "Shadowed" areas (e.g., scalp, perineum, axillae, skinfolds, soles) may not receive adequate exposure. The combination of interferon and PUVA showed high complete remissions in preliminary studies.

Total skin electron beam therapy (TSEBT). Electron radiation of appropriate energies will penetrate only to the dermis, and thus the skin alone can be treated without systemic effects. This therapy requires considerable technical expertise to deliver, can result in short- and long-term cutaneous toxic effects, and is not widely available. Based on the long-term survival of these early-stage patients, electron-beam radiation therapy is sometimes used with curative intent. Long-term disease-free survival can be achieved in patients with unilesional mycosis fungoides treated with local radiation therapy. Management of stage IB/IIA (generalized patch/plaque, T2) disease is with HN2, PUVA, TSEBT, and UVB. TSEBT should be considered as initial therapy for patients with aggressive disease or extensive thick plaques, or for patients who fail HN2 or PUVA. TSEB therapy is the most reliable method for inducing complete remission in generalized patches, plaques, and tumors. Complete response rates of up to 98% for limited plaques and 36% for tumors are reported. The majority of patients have a relapse within 5 years. After attaining complete remission with TSEBT, some physicians initiate adjuvant therapy, most commonly topical nitrogen mustard. Adjuvant HN2 or oral PUVA should be administered for at least 6 months after a complete response to TSEBT. A total of ≈36 Gy is given over ≈10 weeks with a 1-week split after 18 to 20 Gy. "Shadowed" areas need supplemental treatment. Adverse effects are erythema, desquamation, alopecia, loss of nails, and inability to sweat.

Extracorporeal photopheresis. Extracorporeal photopheresis is useful for treating Sézary syndrome and the erythrodermic phase of MF. It is also effective alone or in combination with adjunctive therapy for extensive patch or plaque disease and some tumor-stage disease. Remissions longer than 3 years have been achieved in some patients. Photopheresis involves long-wave radiation (UVA) of leukocytes taken from the patient who has ingested 8-methoxypsoralen, with subsequent reinfusion of the leukocytes to the patient. The treatment is given on 2 consecutive days every month for 6 months. Patients who have a CD4/CD8 ratio of less than or equal to 5 do better than those with few or no CD8$^+$ cells in their skin.

ADVANCED DISEASE. Individual tumors respond to orthovoltage x-irradiation. All of the treatments for advanced disease may be initially successful in inducing remissions, but none appears to prolong survival. Many new agents are being tested. Anti-T-monoclonal antibodies and recombinant fusion proteins (denileukin diftitox; trade name Ontak) may prove useful for extracutaneous disease.

LYMPHOMATOID PAPULOSIS. Lymphomatoid papulosis (LyP) is a rare disease in which the skin lesions have a neoplastic-like histology, but the clinical course is benign and chronic. It is a self-healing papulonecrotic or papulonodular skin disease with histologic features suggestive of a (CD30$^+$) malignant lymphoma. LyP usually occurs in adults and is characterized by the papular, papulonecrotic, and/or nodular skin lesions at different stages of development, predominantly on the trunk and limbs. Individual skin lesions disappear within 3 to 12 weeks, and may leave scars. Disease duration varies from several months to more than 40 years. In up to 20% of patients LyP may be preceded by, associated with, or followed by another type of malignant (cutaneous) lymphoma, generally mycosis fungoides, cutaneous anaplastic large cell lymphoma, or Hodgkin's lymphoma. The histologic picture is extremely variable.

LyP has an excellent prognosis. There is no cure. Low-dose oral methotrexate (5 to 20 mg/week) is the most effective therapy. Patients with few and nonscarring lesions may elect not to treat their disease. *PMID: 15692063*

PAGET'S DISEASE OF THE BREAST

Paget's disease of the breast is a special form of ductal carcinoma, which arises in the main excretory ducts of the breast and extends to the skin from invasion of the epidermis of the nipple, areola, and surrounding skin by malignant cells originating from the underlying ductal carcinoma. An underlying carcinoma of the breast may be palpated, but in approximately 40% of cases, the cancer is clinically impalpable and radiologically undetectable.

CLINICAL PRESENTATION. The disease begins insidiously in one breast with a small area of erythema on the nipple that drains serous fluid and forms a crust (Figures 21-55 and 21-56). The inflammation is usually attributed to trauma, and partial healing comforts the patient. Patients equate lumps rather than inflammatory changes with cancer and, consequently, the disease continues. Malignant cells migrate through the epidermis, and the disease becomes initially apparent on the areola and, at a much later date (1 year or more), on the surrounding skin (see Figure 21-55). The process appears eczematous, but the plaque is indurated and has sharp margins, which remain relatively fixed for weeks. Ulceration is a late finding. Paget's disease of the male nipple is very rare and is more aggressive than in females.

DIAGNOSIS. Clinically and histologically, the process is very similar to Bowen's disease; however, Bowen's disease of the nipple is very rare. A crucial point to note is that Paget's disease of the breast is a rare, unilateral disease, whereas eczematous inflammation of the nipples is common and almost invariably bilateral. Cytologic diagnosis can be made from nipple scrape smears. A biopsy may be studied with conventional stains and immunohistochemistry (Figure 21-57). Compared to conventional mucin histochemistry using diastase periodic-acid-Schiff with and without Alcian blue, immunocytochemical techniques are more reliable for distinguishing Paget's disease from superficial spreading malignant melanoma and from primary intraepidermal carcinoma.

TREATMENT. Treatment is surgical with adjuvant therapy being dictated by the stage and nature of the underlying tumor. Modified radical mastectomy is the standard of care with breast conservation appropriate in a select group of patients with Paget's disease. This select group includes patients who are diagnosed with nipple-areola changes alone without evidence of a palpable mass or mammographic abnormality. In this group of patients, breast conservation offers local recurrence rates comparable to rates in patients with invasive or noninvasive cancers. In patients diagnosed with associated palpable masses or mammographic abnormalities suggestive of cancer, the recurrence rates are higher and mastectomy is warranted. *PMID: 14990209*

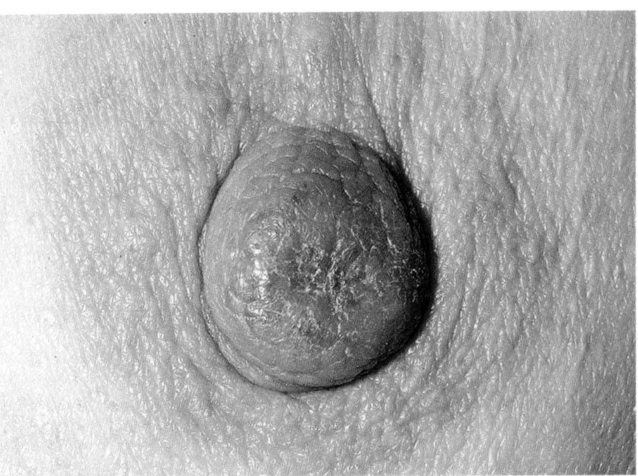

Figure 21-55 Paget's disease. Early lesions are subtle and present with erythema, scale, and crust. They may ooze serum. A diagnosis of irritation or eczema may be suspected. The infiltrating process spreads to the areola and beyond.

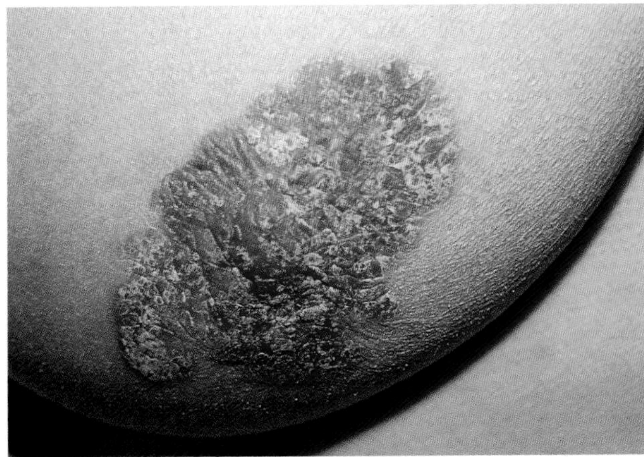

Figure 21-56 A red, scaling plaque drains serous fluid and forms a crust. The lesion appears eczematous but, unlike eczema, is unilateral.

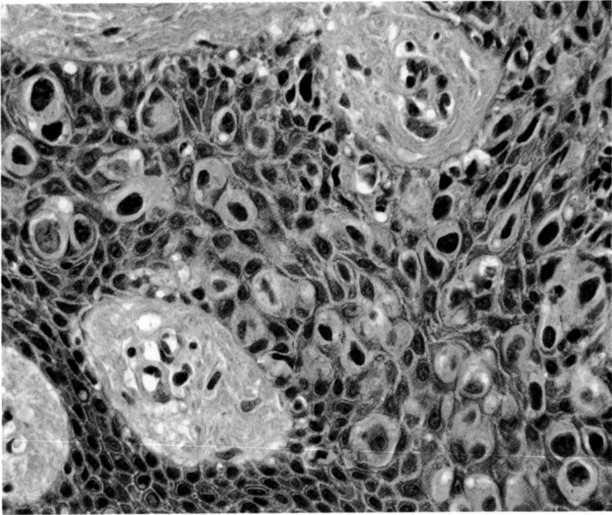

Figure 21-57 Paget's disease. Paget cells are situated above the basal layer in contrast to melanoma cells that are found in the basal layer. Ovoid tumor cells are present in all layers of the epidermis. The cells contain pale-staining cytoplasm and large-hyperchromatic nuclei.

EXTRAMAMMARY PAGET'S DISEASE

Extramammary Paget's disease (EMPD) is a rare cutaneous adenocarcinoma that occurs on apocrine-rich skin in elderly women more often than in men. The most commonly affected site is the labia majora. Two thirds of cases occur on the vulva and one third on the perianal skin; 14% occur on the male genitalia (scrotum). Only 2% of cases are found in the axillae, eyelids, external ear canals, truncal skin, and mucosal surfaces.

ASSOCIATION WITH UNDERLYING MALIGNANCY. Several subtypes are reported: primary cutaneous disease, primary skin disease with secondary contiguous or lymphatic metastases, secondary EMPD arising from an underlying adnexal carcinoma, and EMPD in association with visceral malignancies. Search for a contiguous, underlying, or distant malignancy. The most common related cancers are rectal, genitourinary (including bladder, renal, and prostate), uterine, breast, hepatic, pancreatic, and adnexal (e.g., porocarcinoma) carcinomas. When an underlying malignancy is present, up to 50% of lesions have already metastasized. Lymphatic or visceral metastatic disease may occur. This is possible if the pagetoid cells are not confined to the epidermis. The risk of adjacent adnexal carcinoma is 4% in vulvar EMPD and 7% in perianal EMPD. The risk of an associated internal malignancy is 14% in perianal disease and 20% in vulvar disease. The 5-year survival of patients with invasive EMPD is 72%. Patients with another tumor before EMPD and patients with another tumor after EMPD have a worse prognosis.

CLINICAL PRESENTATION. The disease in males and females appears as a unilateral, well-demarcated, weeping, and eczematous or erythematous plaque or plaques, averaging 6 to 12 cm in diameter; they are most frequently observed on the labia majora (Figure 21-58) and scrotum (Figure 21-59). Multicentric and vague margins may extend beyond the clinically detectable lesion. This leads to high rates of recurrent disease. The most common presenting symptom is long-standing pruritus. Persistent itching and burning are common. The course is unpredictable, ranging from indolent disease to aggressive malignancy. Several dermatoses can mimic EMPD. Lichen sclerosus et atrophicus, lichen simplex chronicus, leukoplakia, Bowen's disease, or chronic yeast infections are in the differential diagnosis.

HISTOLOGIC CHARACTERISTICS. Intraepithelial clusters of large round cells with oval vesicular nuclei and increased pale-staining cytoplasm are present. Paget's cells may develop from apocrine cells. Histologically, Paget's disease resembles Bowen's disease and superficial spreading melanoma. Immunoperoxidase stains are helpful in establishing the diagnosis and in excluding conditions that resemble Paget's disease.

MANAGEMENT. Conventional surgical excision or Mohs micrographic surgery, followed optionally by radiation therapy, is the treatment for regionally confined disease. There are several case reports documenting the successful treatment of extramammary Paget's disease with imiquimod cream. Perform a physical examination to search for internal malignancy.

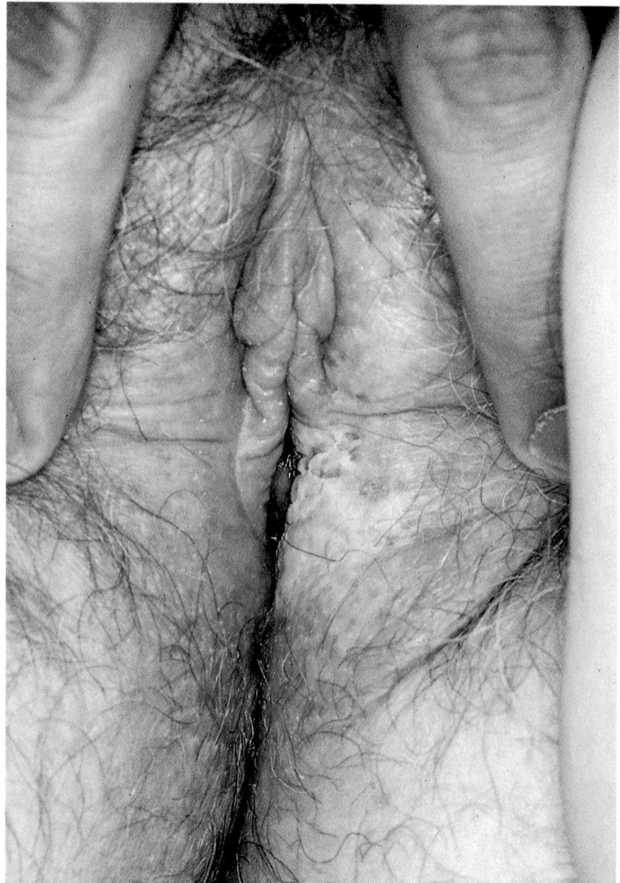

Figure 21-58 Extramammary Paget's disease. A white, eroded plaque with ill-defined borders on the labia.

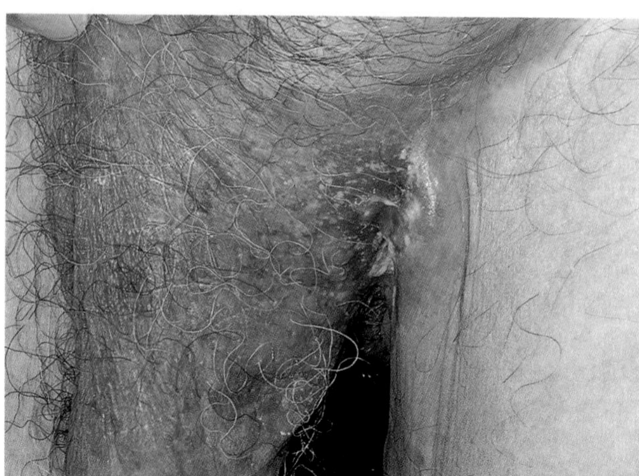

Figure 21-59 Extramammary Paget's disease. Three biopsies were taken before malignant cells were demonstrated at the periphery of this chronic ulcer at the base of the scrotum.

CUTANEOUS METASTASIS

The incidence of cutaneous metastasis in patients with malignancy is approximately 2% to 10%. Cutaneous metastases may be the first sign of extranodal metastatic disease, particularly in patients with melanoma, breast cancer, or mucosal cancers of the head and neck. In a series of papers, Brownstein and Helwig stated several aspects of cutaneous metastasis. They determined the incidence and relative importance of the gender of the patient, the location of the metastatic growth, the morphology of the metastatic lesion, and the histologic features of the metastatic lesion in identifying the site of the primary tumor. The incidence of some of these features is summarized in Figure 21-60. The most helpful information for localizing the primary tumor is the gender of the patient and the location of the skin tumor.

MORPHOLOGIC CHARACTERISTICS. The most common representation of cutaneous metastasis is an aggregate of discrete, firm, nontender, skin-colored nodules that appear suddenly, grow rapidly, attain a certain size (often 2 cm), and remain stationary (Figure 21-61). Accurate clinical diagnosis is rare; the lesions are most frequently diagnosed as cysts or benign fibrous tumors. In several instances, the clinical picture is that of a vascular tumor such as a pyogenic granuloma, hemangioma, or Kaposi's sarcoma (Figure 21-62). The periumbilical Sister Mary Joseph's nodule heralds an underlying gastric tumor.

The second most common pattern of cutaneous metastasis is inflammation with erythema, edema, warmth (Figures 21-63 and 21-64), and tenderness. The primary tumor is usually in the breast, and malignant cells spread to the subepidermal lymphatic vessels, where they create obstruction. The initial diagnosis is frequently a bacterial infection, such as erysipelas or cellulitis. The patient is, however, afebrile and appears to be healthy.

The third and least common pattern simulates a cicatricial condition and resembles discoid lupus erythematosus or morphea. Asymptomatic sclerodermoid plaques, sometimes associated with hair loss (alopecia neoplastica), are most frequently located on the scalp and are caused by metastasis from breast cancer in women and lung or kidney tumors in men. Carcinoma en cuirasse is seen with breast cancer and appears as a hard, infiltrated plaque with a leathery appearance that results from fibrosis and lymph stasis.

HISTOLOGIC CHARACTERISTICS. In general, the histologic features of primary and metastatic tumors are similar, but metastatic tumors are often less differentiated. Frequently, biopsy specimens are not interpreted as originating from a distant site. Adenocarcinoma metastatic to the skin is most often secondary to cancer of the large intestine, lung, or breast. Squamous cell carcinoma metastatic to the skin customarily originates from the oral cavity, lung, or esophagus. Undifferentiated lesions usually originate from the breast or lungs.

MODE OF SPREAD. Tumors that invade veins, such as carcinoma of the kidney and lung, frequently present as cutaneous metastasis occurring in diverse skin sites distant from the primary tumor. Cancers that invade lymphatics, such as carcinoma of the breast and squamous cell carcinoma of the oral cavity, appear late in the course of the disease and may invade skin overlying the primary tumor.

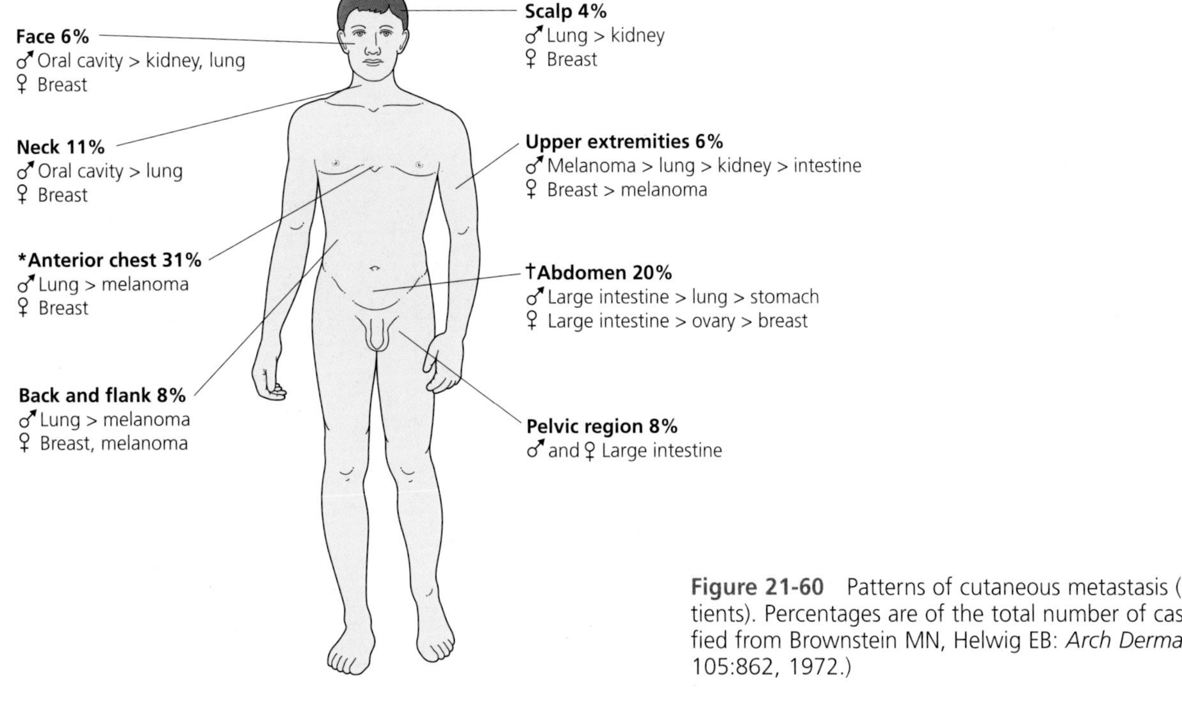

Figure 21-60 Patterns of cutaneous metastasis (724 patients). Percentages are of the total number of cases. (Modified from Brownstein MN, Helwig EB: *Arch Dermatol* 105:862, 1972.)

CUTANEOUS METASTASIS

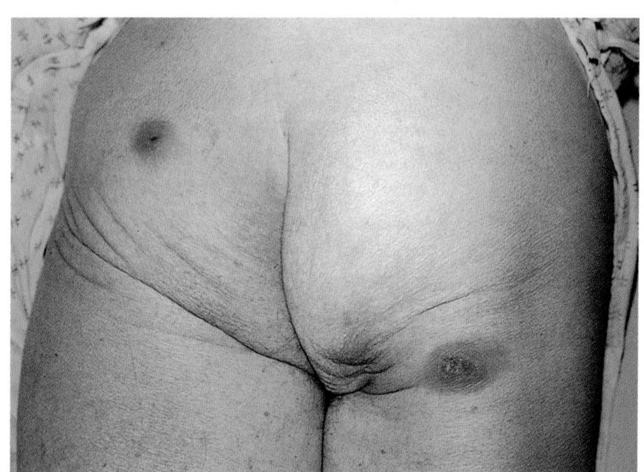

Figure 21-61 Metastatic carcinoma. The nodules had remained fixed in size after an initial rapid growth.

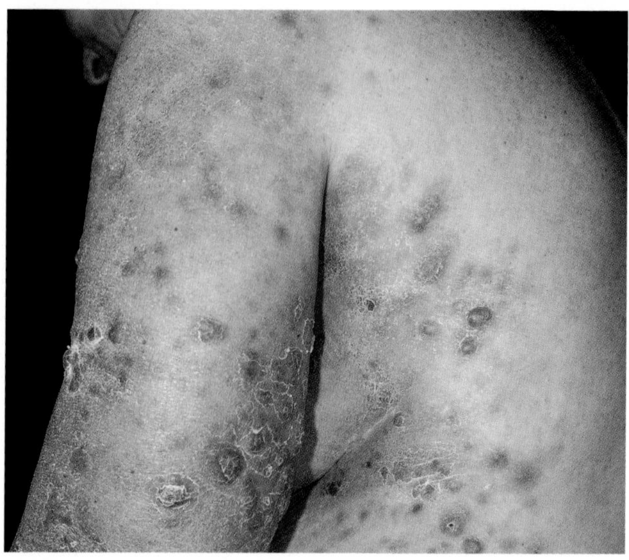

Figure 21-62 Metastatic carcinoma of the breast. Nodules appear vascular and resemble Kaposi's sarcoma.

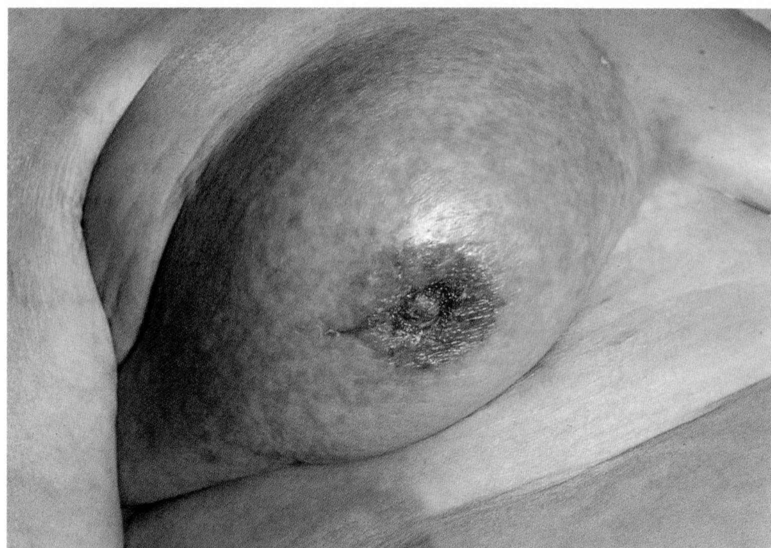

Figure 21-63 Inflammatory cutaneous metastasis with erythema, edema, and crusting.

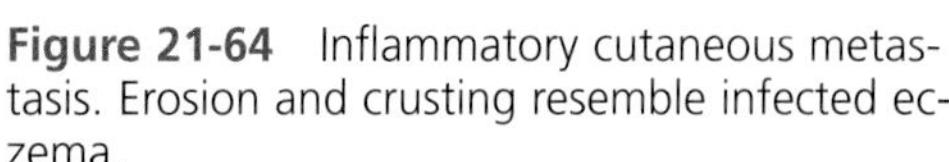

Figure 21-64 Inflammatory cutaneous metastasis. Erosion and crusting resemble infected eczema.

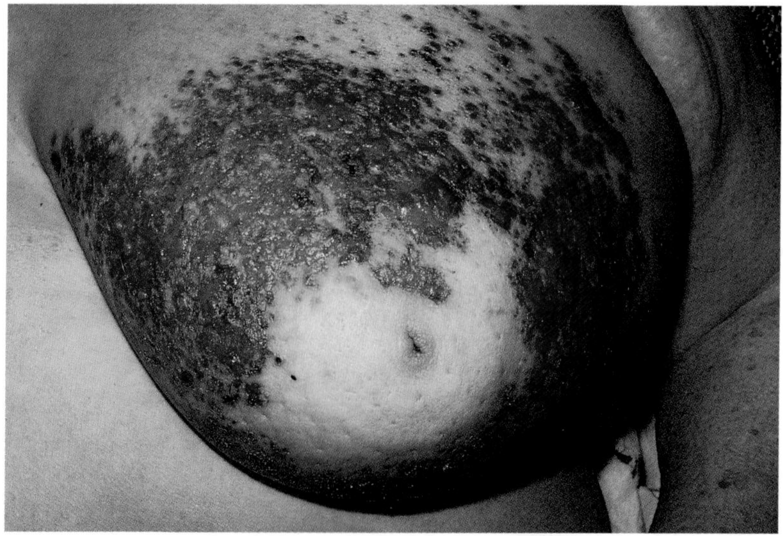

Chapter 22

Nevi and Malignant Melanoma

CHAPTER CONTENTS

- **Melanocytic nevi**
  - Common moles
  - Special forms
  - Atypical nevi
- **Malignant melanoma**
  - Superficial spreading melanoma
  - Nodular melanoma
  - Lentigo maligna melanoma
  - Acral-lentiginous melanoma
  - Benign lesions that resemble melanoma
- **Management of melanoma**
  - Biopsy
  - Surgical therapy
  - Initial diagnostic workup
  - Follow-up examinations
- **Staging and prognosis**
- **Treatment of lentigo maligna**
- **Dermoscopy**

MELANOCYTIC NEVI

Nevi, or moles, are benign tumors composed of nevus cells that are derived from melanocytes. Many myths surround moles, for example, that hairs should not be plucked from moles or that moles should not be removed or disturbed.

NEVUS CELLS. The nevus cell differs from melanocytes. The nevus cell is larger, lacks dendrites, has more abundant cytoplasm, and contains coarse granules. Nevus cells aggregate in groups (nests) or proliferate in a non-nested pattern in the basal region at the dermoepidermal junction. Nevus cells in the dermis are classified into types A (epithelioid), B (lymphocytoid), and C (neuroid). Through a process of maturation and downward migration, type A epidermal nevus cells develop into type B cells and then into type C dermal nevus cells.

INCIDENCE AND EVOLUTION. Moles are so common that they appear on virtually every person. They are present in 1% of newborns and increase in incidence throughout infancy and childhood. The incidence peaks in the fourth to fifth decades. Nevi then diminish in number with advancing age.

Size and pigmentation may increase at puberty and during pregnancy. Nevi may occur anywhere on the cutaneous surface. There is a strong correlation between sun exposure and the number of nevi. Acquired nevi on the buttocks or female breast are unusual.

NEVI VS. MELANOMA. Nevi exist in a variety of characteristic forms that must be recognized to distinguish them from malignant melanoma. Except for certain types, such as large congenital nevi and atypical moles, most nevi have a very low malignant potential.

Nevi vary in size, shape, surface characteristics, and color. The important fact to remember is that each individual nevus tends to remain uniform in color and shape. Although various shades of brown and black may be present in a single lesion, the colors are distributed over the surface in a uniform pattern.

Melanomas consist of malignant pigment cells that grow and extend with little constraint through the epidermis and into the dermis. Such unrestricted growth produces a lesion with a haphazard or disorganized appearance, which varies in shape, color, and surface characteristics. The characteristics of uniformity cannot always be relied on to differentiate benign from malignant lesions because very early melanomas may appear quite uniform, having a round or oval shape with a uniform brown color.

EXAMINATION WITH A HAND LENS AND DERMOSCOPE. Careful inspection of suspicious lesions with a powerful hand lens and dermoscope will reveal a number of features that cannot be appreciated with the naked eye. Dermoscopy is discussed at the end of the chapter.

Common moles

Nevi may be classified as acquired or congenital, but a clinical classification based on appearance and conventional nomenclature is used here. Common acquired nevi appear after 6 months of age. They enlarge and increase in number through the third and fourth decades and then slowly disappear. Most are less than 5 mm in diameter. Fifty-five percent of adults have between 10 and 45 nevi greater than 2 mm in diameter. Nevi tend to be concentrated on sun-exposed sites.

CLASSIFICATION. Common moles are subdivided into three types—junction, compound, and dermal—based on the location of the nevus cells in the skin (Figure 22-1). The three types represent sequential developmental stages in the life history of a mole. During childhood, nevi begin as flat junction nevi in which the nevus cells are located at the dermoepidermal junction. They evolve into compound nevi when some of the cells migrate into the dermis. Migration of all of the nevus cells into the dermis results in a dermal nevus. Dermal nevi usually form only in adults, but this evolution does not consistently occur. Nevi with cells confined to the dermoepidermal junction area tend to be flat, whereas those with cells confined to the dermis are usually elevated.

JUNCTION NEVI. Junction nevi are flat (macular) or slightly elevated, and they are light brown to brown-black with uniform pigmentation that may be slightly irregular (Figure 22-2). The surface is smooth and flat to slightly elevated, and the border is round or oval and symmetric. Most lesions are hairless. Junction nevi vary in size from 0.1 to 0.6 cm; some are larger. Junction nevi may change into compound nevi after childhood, but they remain as junction nevi on palms, soles, and genitalia. Junction nevi are rare at birth and generally develop after the age of 2 years. Degeneration into melanoma is very rare.

COMPOUND NEVI. Compound nevi are slightly elevated and flesh-colored or brown. They are elevated and smooth or warty and become more elevated with increasing age (Figure 22-3). They are uniformly round, oval, and symmetric. Hair may be present. If a white halo appears at the periphery of the lesion, it is referred to as a halo nevus.

DERMAL NEVI. Dermal nevi are brown or black, but may become lighter or flesh-colored with age. Lesions vary in size from a few millimeters to a centimeter. The variety of shapes reflects the evolutionary process in which moles extend downward with age and nevus cells degenerate and become replaced with fat and fibrous tissue.

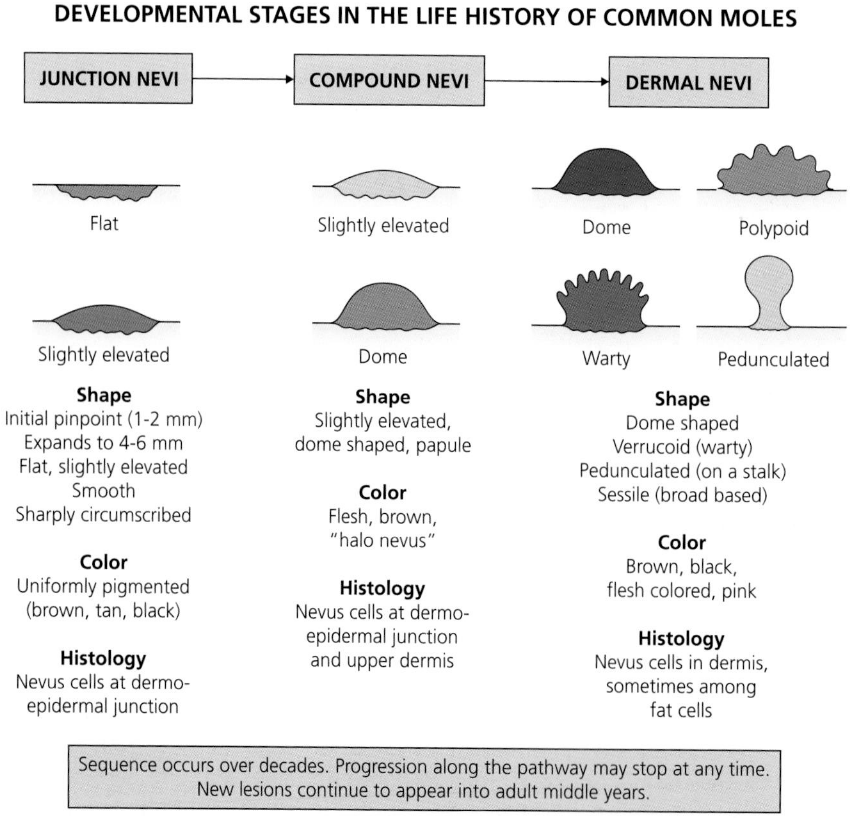

DEVELOPMENTAL STAGES IN THE LIFE HISTORY OF COMMON MOLES

JUNCTION NEVI → COMPOUND NEVI → DERMAL NEVI

JUNCTION NEVI	COMPOUND NEVI	DERMAL NEVI
Flat Slightly elevated	Slightly elevated Dome	Dome Polypoid Warty Pedunculated
Shape Initial pinpoint (1-2 mm) Expands to 4-6 mm Flat, slightly elevated Smooth Sharply circumscribed	**Shape** Slightly elevated, dome shaped, papule	**Shape** Dome shaped Verrucoid (warty) Pedunculated (on a stalk) Sessile (broad based)
Color Uniformly pigmented (brown, tan, black)	**Color** Flesh, brown, "halo nevus"	**Color** Brown, black, flesh colored, pink
Histology Nevus cells at dermo-epidermal junction	**Histology** Nevus cells at dermo-epidermal junction and upper dermis	**Histology** Nevus cells in dermis, sometimes among fat cells

Sequence occurs over decades. Progression along the pathway may stop at any time. New lesions continue to appear into adult middle years.

Figure 22-1

MELANOCYTIC NEVI

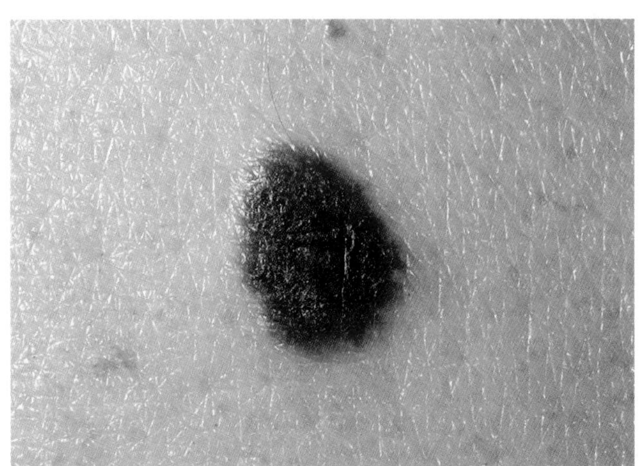

Figure 22-2 Junction nevus. The lesion is slightly raised, dark, and uniform.

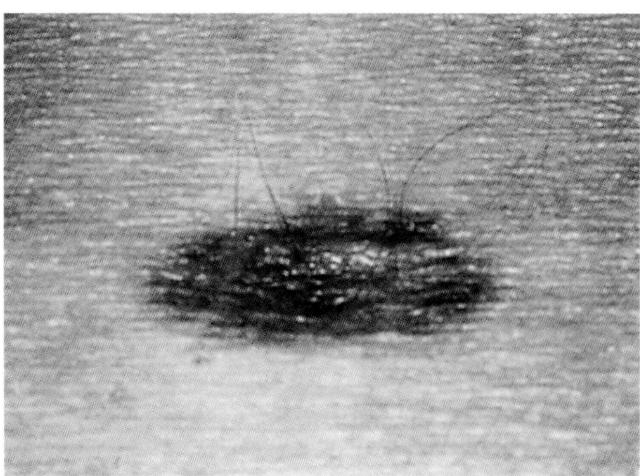

Figure 22-3 Compound nevus. The surface is covered with uniform brown-black dots.

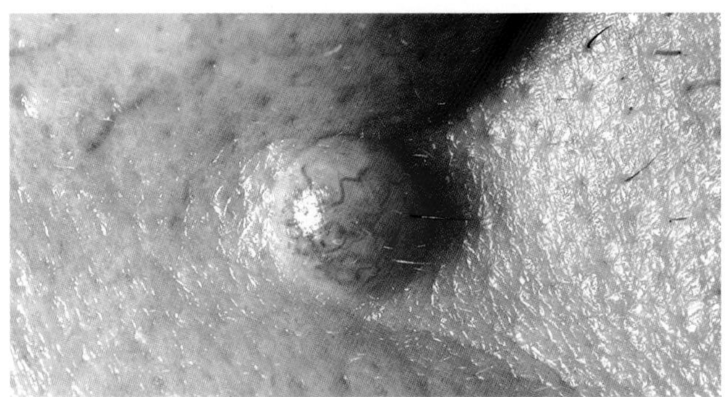

Figure 22-4 Dermal nevus. Flesh colored with surface vessels; resembles basal cell carcinoma.

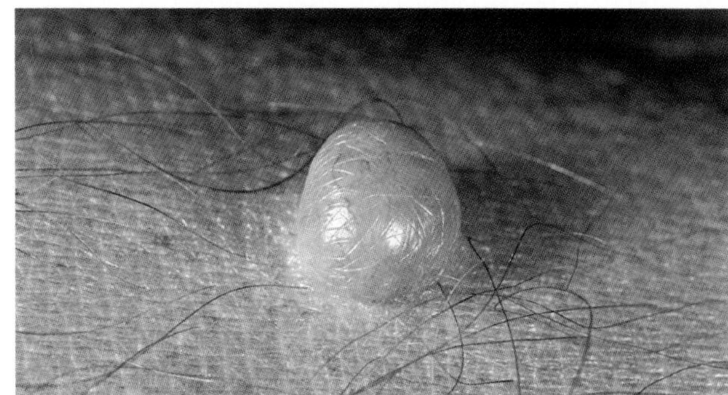

Figure 22-5 Dermal nevus. Dome shaped.

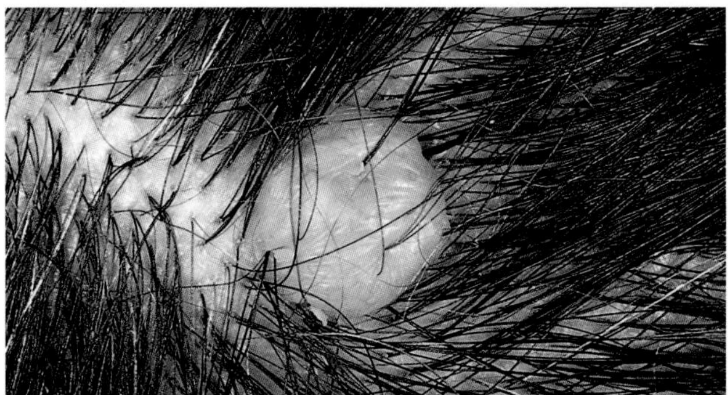

Figure 22-6 Dermal nevus. Flesh colored and dome shaped.

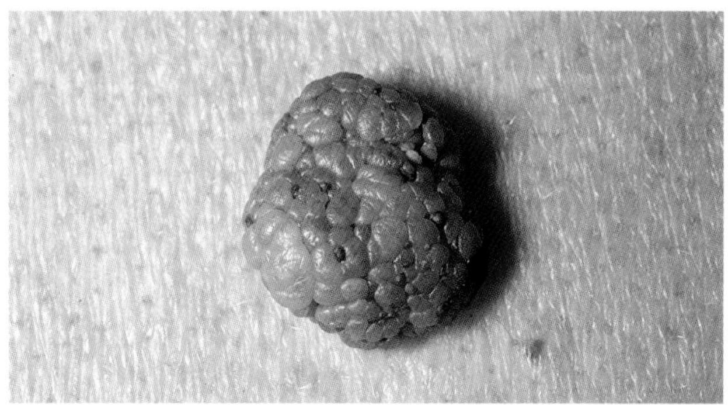

Figure 22-7 Dermal nevus. Warty (verrucous) surface.

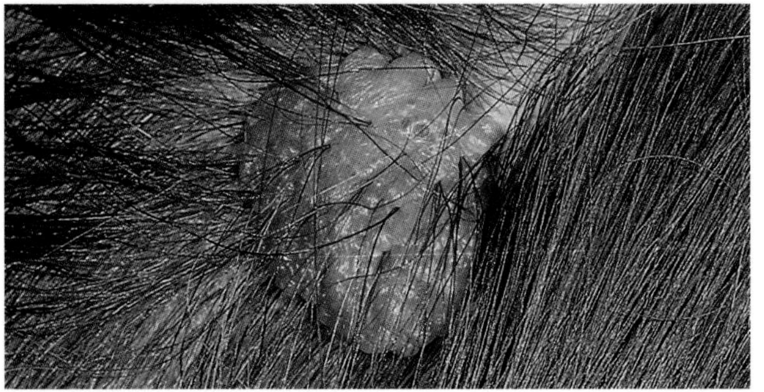

Figure 22-8 Dermal nevus. Polypoid.

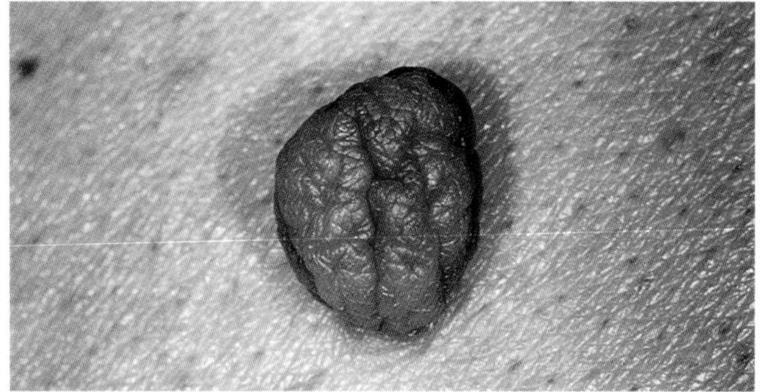

Figure 22-9 Dermal nevus. Pedunculated with a soft, flabby, wrinkled surface.

Dome-shaped lesions are the most common (Figures 22-4 through 22-6). They generally appear on the face and are symmetric, with a smooth surface. They may be white or translucent, with telangiectatic vessels on the surface mimicking basal cell carcinoma. The structure may be warty (Figure 22-7) or polypoid (Figure 22-8). Pedunculated lesions with a narrow stalk are located on the trunk, neck, axillae, and groin. They may appear as a soft, flabby, wrinkled sack (Figure 22-9).

Elevated nevi are exposed and are prone to trauma from clothing and other stimuli, often causing them to bleed and inflame, making some patients to suspect malignancy. A white border may appear, creating a halo nevus. Degeneration to melanoma is very rare, but dermal nevi may resemble nodular melanoma; therefore knowledge of duration and a history of recent change is important.

MANAGEMENT

SUSPICIOUS LESIONS. Any pigmented lesion suspected of being malignant should be biopsied or referred for a second opinion. Suspicious lesions should be completely removed by excisional biopsy down to and including subcutaneous tissue.

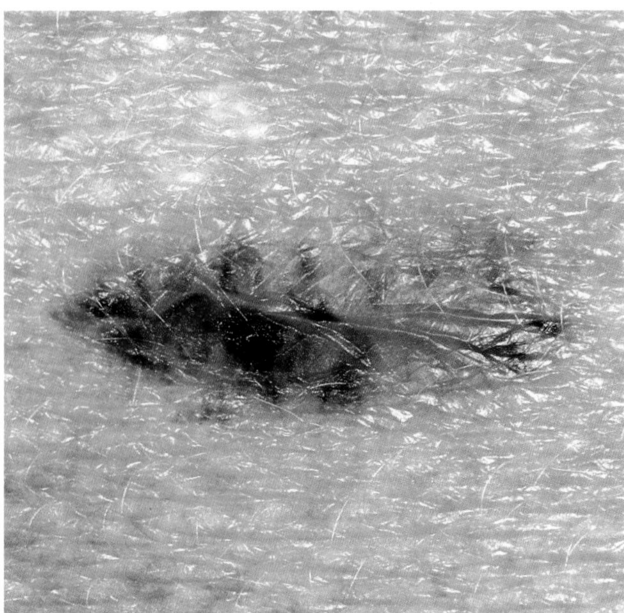

Figure 22-10 Recurrent, previously excised nevi (pseudomelanoma). Brown, macular pigmentation may appear in the scar of an incompletely removed nevus.

NEVI. Patients frequently request removal of nevi for cosmetic purposes. It is good practice to biopsy all pigmented lesions; therefore total removal by electrocautery should be avoided. Nevi are removed either by shave excision or by simple excision and closure with sutures. Most common nevi are small and shave excision is adequate.

RECURRENT PREVIOUSLY EXCISED NEVI (PSEUDOMELANOMA). Weeks to months after incomplete removal of a nevus, brown macular pigmentation may appear in the scar (Figure 22-10). Some nevus cells remain with shave excision and partial repigmentation is possible. Residual pigmentation may be removed with electrocautery or cryosurgery. An unusual histologic picture resembling melanoma (pseudomelanoma) may follow partial removal of nevi. If the repigmented area is excised, the pathologist should be notified that the submitted tissue was acquired from a previously treated area. Histologically, the melanocytes appear atypical but are confined to the epidermis, and there is no lateral spread of individual melanocytes as is seen in melanoma.

NEVI WITH SMALL DARK SPOTS. A small percentage of small dark spots within melanocytic nevi are due to melanoma. These roundish areas of brown or black hyperpigmentation measure 3 mm or less in diameter and are located peripherally. Biopsy specimens of nevi with small dark dots should be sectioned to ensure histologic examination of this focus of hyperpigmentation.

Special forms

Special forms of pigmented lesions include congenital nevus, halo nevus, speckled lentiginous nevus, Becker's nevus, benign juvenile melanoma (Spitz nevus), blue nevus, labial melanotic macules, and atypical nevi (dysplastic nevi, Clark nevi).

CONGENITAL MELANOCYTIC NEVI. It is estimated that between 1% and 6% of the population have a congenital melanocytic nevus (CMN). Congenital melanocytic nevi (birthmarks) are present at birth and vary in size from a few millimeters to several centimeters, covering wide areas of the trunk, extremity, or face. Some lesions first become apparent during infancy. Not all pigmented lesions present at birth are congenital nevi; café-au-lait spots may also be present at birth. The largest lesions are referred to as giant hairy nevi. Giant congenital nevi on the trunk are referred to as bathing trunk nevi. Congenital nevi may contain hair; if present, it is usually coarse. Such nevi are uniformly pigmented, with various shades of brown or black predominating, but red or pink may be a minor or sometimes predominant color. Most are flat at birth but become thicker during childhood, and the surface becomes verrucous and sometimes nodular.

Size. CMNs are arbitrarily divided into groups according to their size in infancy: small (<1.5 cm in diameter), medium (1.5 to 19.9 cm in diameter), and large (>20 cm in diameter). Most grow in proportion to the growth of the child. CMNs on the head will increase in size by a factor of 1.5 and on the rest of the body by a factor of 3.

Histologic characteristics. Nevus cells occur (1) in the lower two thirds of the dermis, occasionally extending into the subcutis; (2) between collagen bundles distributed as single cells or cells in single file, or both; and (3) in the lower two thirds of the reticular dermis or subcutis associated with appendages, nerves, and vessels. Some congenital nevi do not have these microscopic features. Large congenital nevi usually do have the classic microscopic findings of congenital nevi, whereas small congenital nevi most often do not show these classic features. Medium-sized congenital nevi may or may not show these classic microscopic features.

Malignant potential. Melanoma can develop in any CMN and the risk may correlate with the size of the nevus. The malignant potential of congenital nevi may be dependent on the histologic pattern of the lesion rather than the clinical size. Small congenital nevi frequently lack melanocytes in the deeper dermis. The increased risk of melanoma formation in large congenital nevi may be a result of transformation of cells residing deep in the dermis. Melanomas may develop in large CMNs before puberty; melanomas in small and medium CMNs generally develop at or after puberty.

SMALL CONGENITAL MELANOCYTIC NEVI. The incidence of malignant degeneration in small congenital nevi (<1.5 cm in diameter) is extremely low and prophylactic removal is not essential (Figure 22-11). Almost all melanomas arising in small congenital nevi are of the epidermal variety. Therefore clinical observation will detect malignant changes in small CMNs. If small CMNs are to be excised, delaying this procedure until just before puberty would be appropriate because small congenital nevi do not undergo malignant transformation in prepubertal age groups.

MEDIUM-SIZED CONGENITAL MELANOCYTIC NEVI. The risk of the occurrence of malignant melanoma in medium-sized (1.5 to 19.9 cm in diameter) congenital melanocytic nevi is the subject of controversy (Figures 22-12 and 22-13). Universally accepted recommendations regarding the management of such lesions have not been made. A short-term follow-up study showed no increased risk for malignant melanoma arising in banal-appearing medium-sized lesions or that prophylactic excision of all such lesions is mandatory. Lifelong medical observation seems a reasonable alternative for many medium-sized CMNs.

Another approach would be to perform a punch or small incisional biopsy. If the histologic pattern is that of an acquired nevus (superficial variant of congenital nevi), then the malignant potential is extremely low, and any malignant transformation would most likely be of the epidermal variety, which would be detectable by clinical observation. If the histologic pattern is that of the deeper dermal tumor, then a significant risk may be present; prophylactic excision at the earliest stage possible would be indicated.

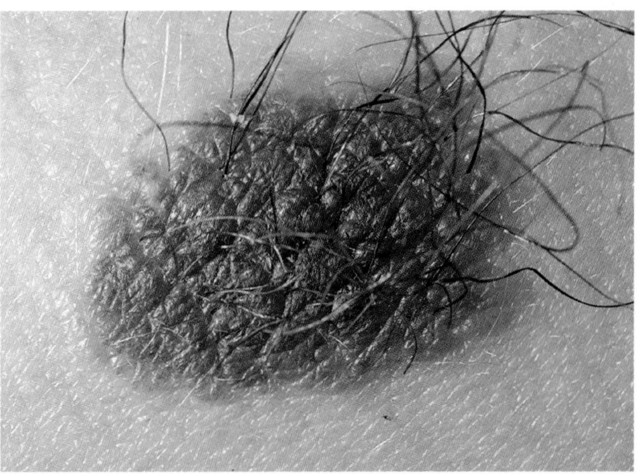

Figure 22-11 A small congenital nevus has a uniform cobblestone surface and is covered with hair.

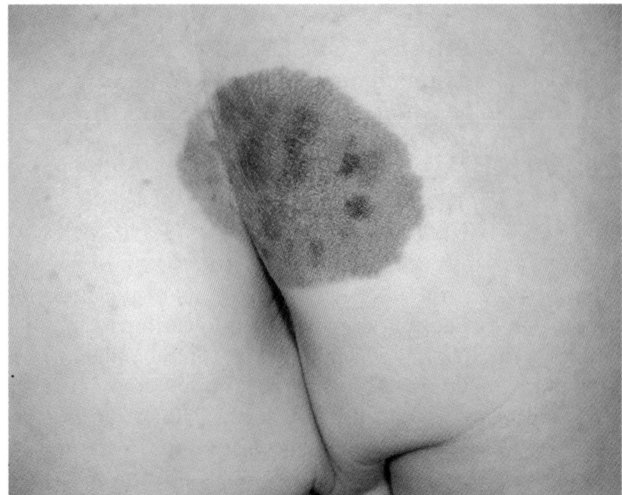

Figure 22-12 Medium-sized congenital nevus. Pigmentation is variable and nonuniform, but a biopsy showed all such areas were benign.

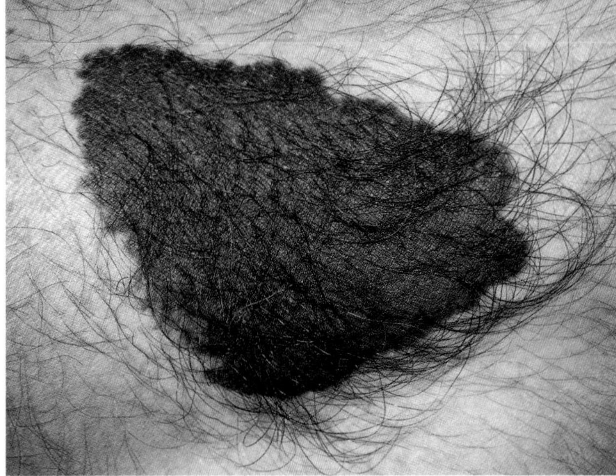

Figure 22-13 Medium-sized congenital nevus. The border is irregular and appears notched, but that characteristic is maintained in a uniform manner around the entire border.

LARGE CONGENITAL MELANOCYTIC NEVI. Large congenital melanocytic nevi (comprising ≥5% body surface area in preadolescents and >20 cm in adolescents and adults) may undergo malignant transformation (Figures 22-14 and 22-15). The incidence ranges from 1.8% to 7.1%. Approximately half of the melanomas occur by 3 to 5 years of age. Therefore large, thick lesions should be removed as soon as possible. Large CMNs lighten with time and most nodules occur before the age of 2 years. There is an initial darkening with a subsequent significant lightening with age accompanied by increased surface irregularities, nodules, and hair growth. The most common anatomic site is the trunk. Most are associated with satellite congenital nevi, which can be extensive and involve a variety of sites. As many as two thirds of melanomas developing in giant CMNs have nonepidermal origins and are deeper in the dermis or lower subcutaneous tissue. Therefore clinical observation will fail to detect most malignant transformations in these patients.

DERMOSCOPY OF CONGENITAL MELANOCYTIC NEVI. The most commonly observed dermoscopic features are globules (79.7%), reticular networks (70.3%), hypertrichosis (68.9%), milia-like cysts (52.7%), and perifollicular hypopigmentation (32.4%). *PMID: 17709659*

NEUROCUTANEOUS MELANOCYTOSIS (NCM). Patients with large CMNs are at risk for NCM, where the leptomeninges contain excessive amounts of melanocytes and melanin. Central nervous system melanomas may occur from malignant degeneration of these melanocytes. Benign proliferation of melanocytes in the leptomeninges may result in complications or death. Patients at greatest risk for developing NCM are those with large CMNs found on the back, head, or neck. Large CMNs of the trunk are associated with a symptomatic NCM occurrence of 4.8%, and an overall mortality from NCM and cutaneous melanoma of 2.3%. If symptomatic NCM developed in those with truncal nevi, however, the occurrence of death rises to 34%. *PMID: 16635656* Patients with >20 satellite melanocytic nevi are at greatest risk of developing NCM. Most patients with large CMNs have multiple satellite nevi but no melanoma has ever been reported in satellite nevi.

MANAGEMENT OF CONGENITAL MELANOCYTIC NEVI. Risk assessment and treatment options are considered for each patient. Medical and psychosocial concerns need to be discussed. Management goals are to decrease the risk for developing melanoma by surgical removal and producing good cosmetic results. Removal of a small CMN, with a low risk for developing melanoma, may result in a disfiguring scar and would not be acceptable. Removal of a large, thick CMN that leaves a large, dense scar may be acceptable. Timing of surgery is a consideration. The best surgical scars result from surgery performed early in life; however, it may be best to delay surgery until after age 2 when the full extent of the nevus is evident. Very large lesions may require multiple procedures. CMNs should be removed down to the fascial layer.

PROPHYLACTIC TREATMENT. Prophylactic removal is considered for thick lesions in which it is difficult to detect melanoma. Dense nevi with a wrinkled (rugous) surface have the greatest risk. Growths that appear in covered areas (e.g., scalp, medial buttocks, perianal, genital areas) that are difficult to examine and follow are considered for early excision.

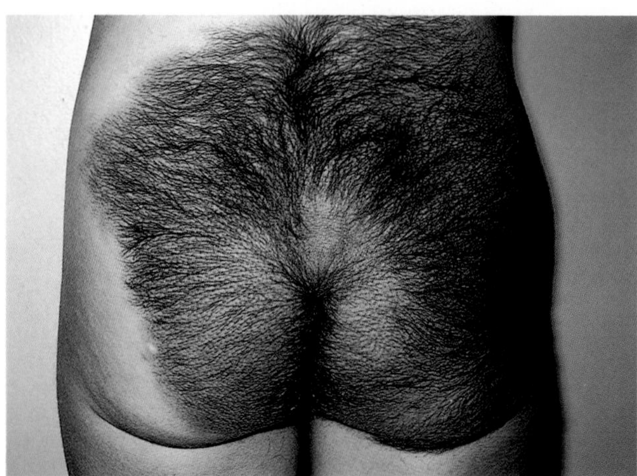

Figure 22-14 Large congenital hairy nevus.

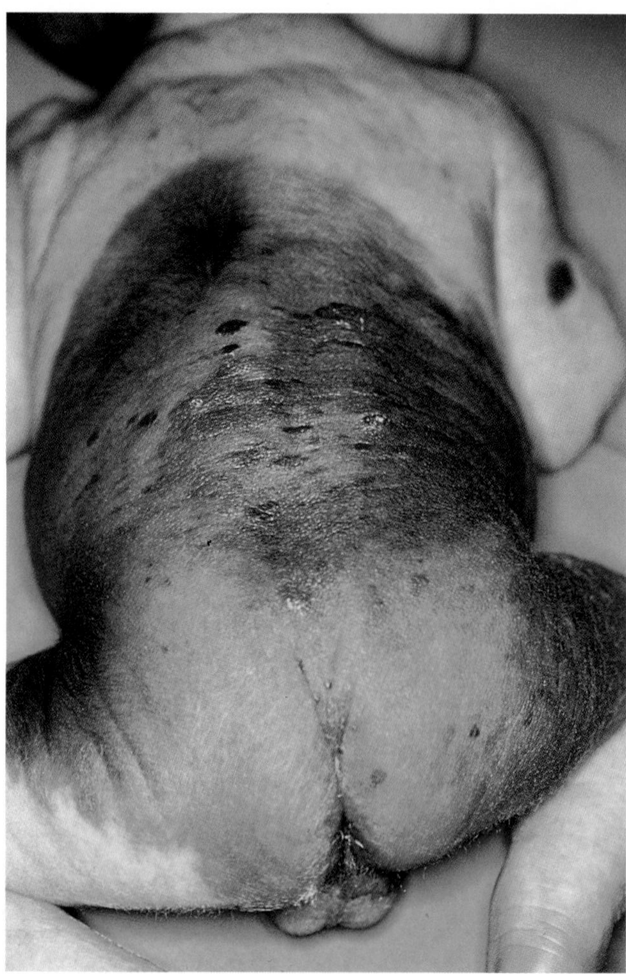

Figure 22-15 Giant congenital nevus (bathing trunk nevus).

SPECKLED LENTIGINOUS NEVUS. Speckled lentiginous nevus (nevus spilus) is a common hairless, oval or irregularly shaped brown lesion that is dotted with darker brown-to-black spots. They may appear at any age. Lesions can appear at birth or in early infancy as lightly colored café-au-lait macules. Pigmented macules and papules then develop over a period of months to years. Lesions may be very large. It has been suggested that speckled lentiginous nevus is a subtype of congenital melanocytic nevus. The brown area is usually flat, and the black dots may be slightly elevated and contain typical nevus cells (Figure 22-16). The spots range from 1 to 3 mm in diameter and may be lentigines, junctional, compound, or intradermal nevi. The background hyperpigmentation histologically has the features of a lentigo or café-au-lait macule. There is considerable variation in size, ranging from 1 to 20 cm. The anatomic position or time of onset is not related to sun exposure. Transformation into melanoma is rare. The risk of transformation may be similar to that for classic congenital nevi of similar size. Examine lesions periodically and educate the patient regarding the clinical signs of melanoma. Routine excision is not necessary. Biopsy suspicious areas. Speckled lentiginous nevus is flat and necessitates excision and closure if the patient desires removal. Lasers have been used to treat both the background hyperpigmentation and the speckles of speckled lentiginous nevi.

SPECKLED LENTIGINOUS NEVUS

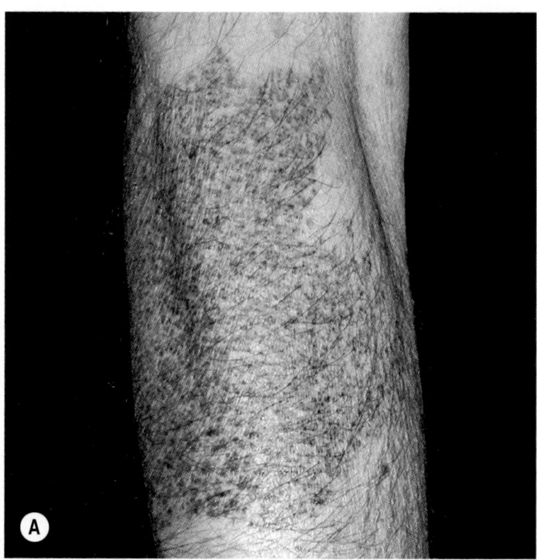

A large, brown, macular lesion resembling a café-au-lait spot. Tiny black papules are uniformly distributed over the surface.

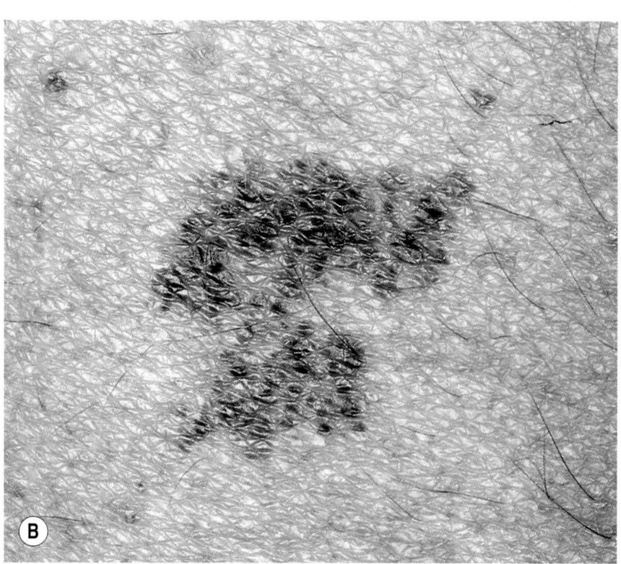

The macular pigmentation is less prominent than in the lesion illustrated in **A.**

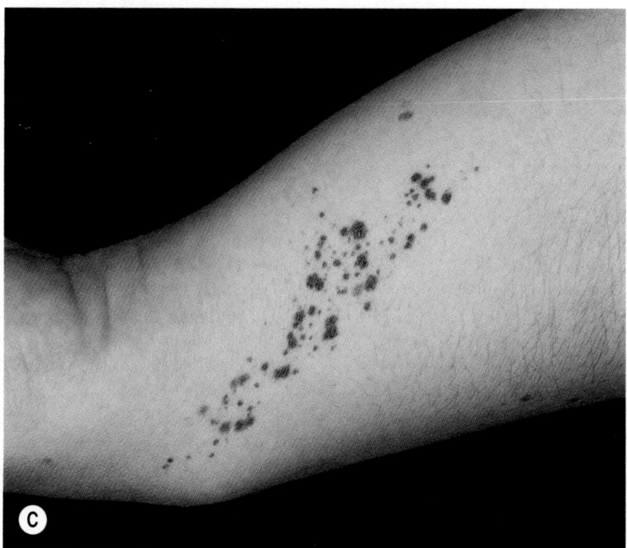

The macular pigmentation is almost entirely absent. The multiple papules containing nevus cells predominate.

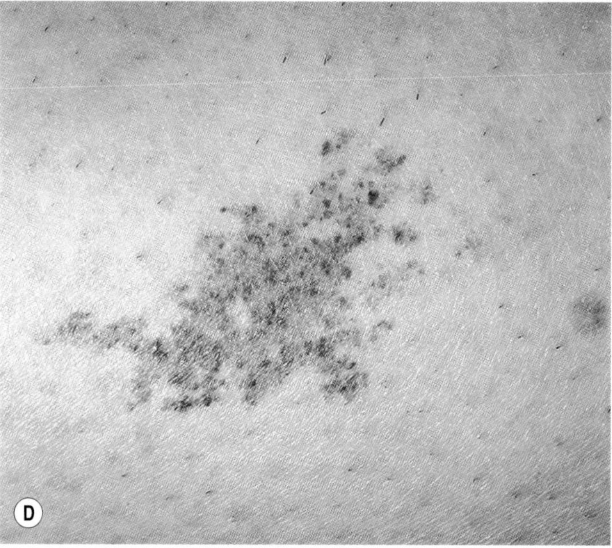

Macular pigmentation is variable.

Figure 22-16

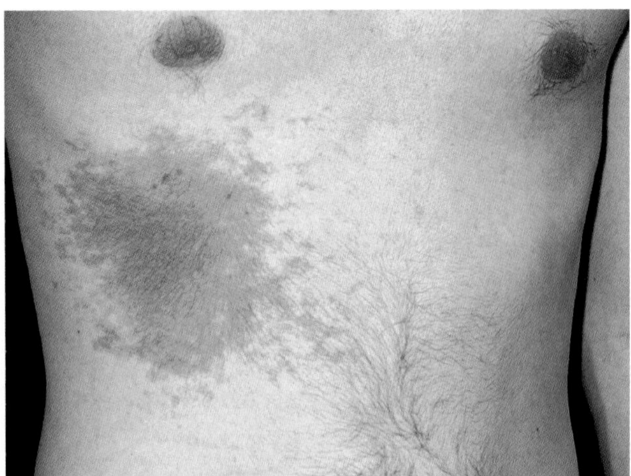

Figure 22-17 Becker's nevus. This irregular lesion contains no hair. It has been stable in size for years.

BECKER'S NEVUS. Becker's nevus is not a nevocellular nevus because it lacks nevus cells. The lesion is a developmental anomaly consisting of either a brown macule (Figure 22-17), a patch of hair (Figure 22-18), or both (Figure 22-19). Nonhairy lesions may later develop hair. The lesions appear in adolescent men on the shoulder, submammary area, and upper and lower back; they rarely appear on the lower limbs. Becker's nevus varies in size and may enlarge to cover the entire upper arm or shoulder. The border is irregular and sharply demarcated. Malignancy has never been reported.

Becker's nevus syndrome is the presence of an epithelial nevus showing hyperpigmentation, increased hairiness, and hamartomatous augmentation of smooth muscle fibers as well as other developmental defects such as ipsilateral hypoplasia of the breast and skeletal anomalies, including scoliosis, spina bifida occulta, or ipsilateral hypoplasia of a limb. The Becker's nevus syndrome usually occurs sporadically.

Dermoscopic features of Becker's nevus include network, focal hypopigmentation, skin furrow hypopigmentation, hair follicles, perifollicular hypopigmentation, and vessels.

Becker's nevus is usually too large to remove by excision. The hair may be shaved or permanently removed. Laser removal of hair and pigmentation is reported.

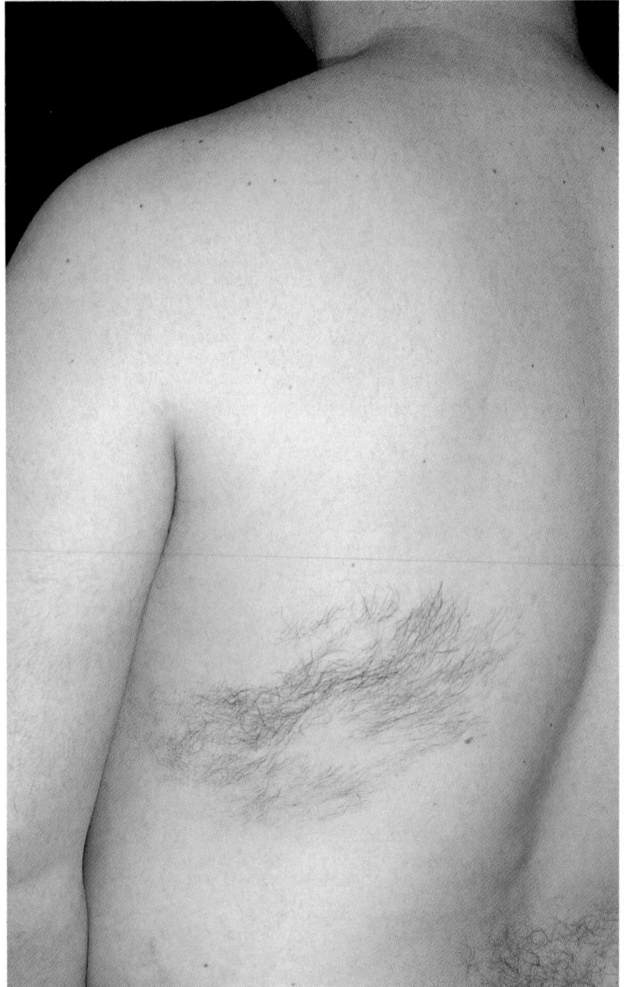

Figure 22-18 Becker's nevus. This lesion contains no pigmentation.

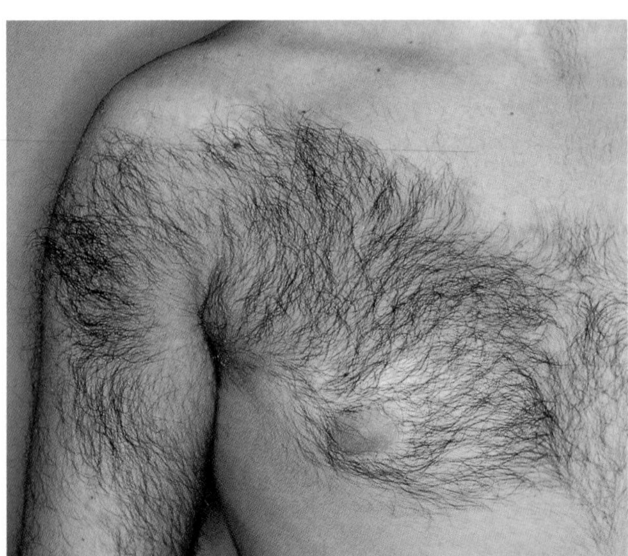

Figure 22-19 Becker's nevus. A typical lesion with macular pigmentation and hair.

HALO NEVI. A compound or dermal nevus that develops a white border is called a halo nevus. The incidence in the population is estimated to be 1%. Halo nevi are found most commonly in children. The average age of onset is 15 years. The depigmented halo is symmetric and round or oval with a sharply demarcated border (Figure 22-20). There are no melanocytes in the halo area. Halo nevi have the dermoscopic features of benign melanocytic nevi, with globular and/or homogeneous patterns that are typically observed in children and young adults. Halo nevi structural patterns remain unchanged over time. Patients with Turner's syndrome (short stature, gonadal dysgenesis, webbed neck, cubitus valgus, and lymphedema at birth) have a halo nevus prevalence of 18%. *PMID: 15337976*

HISTOLOGIC CHARACTERISTICS. T lymphocytes at the site of depigmentation suggest that these cells participate in the halo phenomenon. Most halo nevi are located on the trunk; they never occur on palms and soles. They may occur as an isolated phenomenon, or several nevi may spontaneously develop halos. Halos may repigment with time, or the nevus may disappear. Repigmentation often takes place over months or years; however, it does not always occur. Repigmentation does not follow removal of the nevus. The incidence of vitiligo may be increased in patients with halo nevi. A halo may rarely develop around malignant melanoma, but in such instances it is usually not symmetric.

Removal of a halo nevus is unnecessary unless the nevus has atypical features. Parental concern over this impressive change is often reason for a conservative excision. In such cases, the mole part of a halo nevus may be removed by shave, excision, or laser.

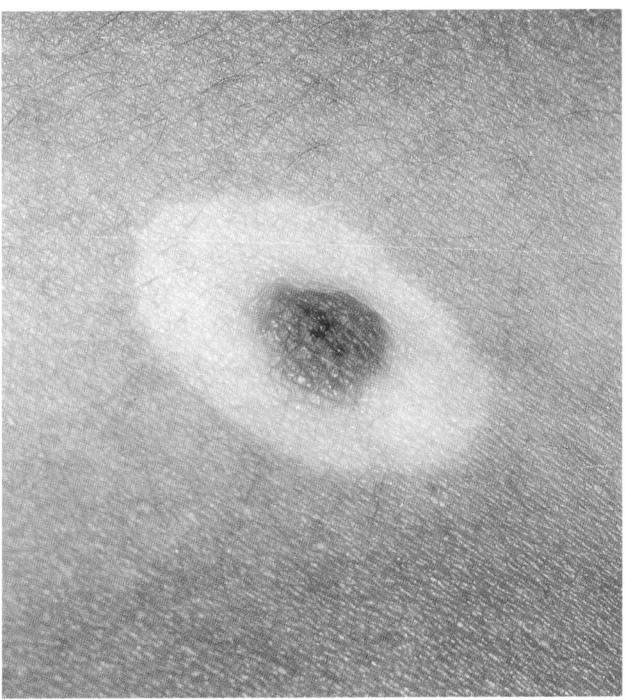

Figure 22-20 Halo nevus. A sharply defined, white halo surrounds this compound nevus.

SPITZ NEVUS. Spitz nevus (benign juvenile melanoma) is most common in children but does appear in adults. The term melanoma is used because the clinical and histologic appearance is similar to that of melanoma. They are hairless, red or reddish-brown, dome-shaped papules or nodules with a smooth (Figure 22-21) or warty surface; they vary in size from 0.3 to 1.5 cm. The color is caused by increased vascularity, and bleeding sometimes follows trauma. Spitz nevi are usually solitary but may be multiple. They appear suddenly and, contrary to slowly evolving common moles, patients can sometimes date their onset. The Spitz nevus should be removed for microscopic examination. Histologic differentiation from melanoma is sometimes difficult. Dermoscopy of Spitz nevus shows (1) a starburst pattern, characterized by a prominent, black to blue diffuse pigmentation and pseudopods regularly distributed at the periphery in a radiate pattern; and (2) a globular pattern, typified by a discrete, brown to gray-blue pigmentation and a peripheral rim of large brown globules, often extending throughout the entire lesion.

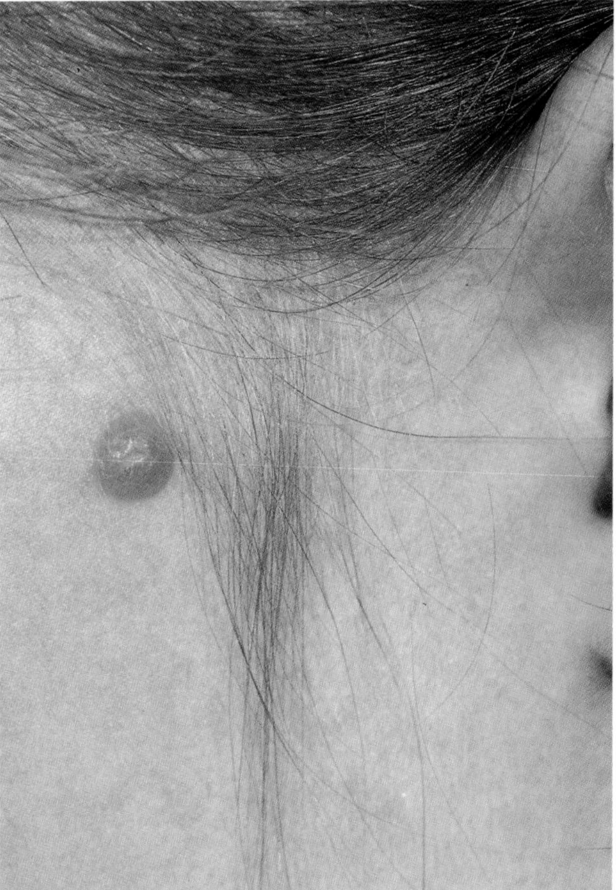

Figure 22-21 Benign juvenile melanoma (Spitz nevus). A reddish, dome-shaped nodule that generally appears in children.

BLUE NEVUS. The blue nevus is a slightly elevated, round, regular nevus, usually less than 0.5 cm, and contains large amounts of pigment located in the dermis (Figure 22-22). The brown pigment absorbs the longer wavelengths of light and scatters blue light (Tyndall effect). The blue nevus appears in childhood and is most common on the extremities and dorsum of the hands. A rare variant, the cellular blue nevus, is larger (usually greater than 1 cm) and nodular and is frequently located on the buttocks.

Melanomas are reported as arising in association with a common or cellular blue nevus and arising de novo and resembling cellular blue nevi. Blue nevi may be removed for cosmetic purposes.

LABIAL MELANOTIC MACULE. Brown macules on the lower lip are relatively common, especially in young adult women (Figure 22-23). Histologically, they resemble freckles and not lentigo, but unlike freckles, they do not darken with sun exposure. They are benign. Cryotherapy or laser surgery is used for patients who request treatment.

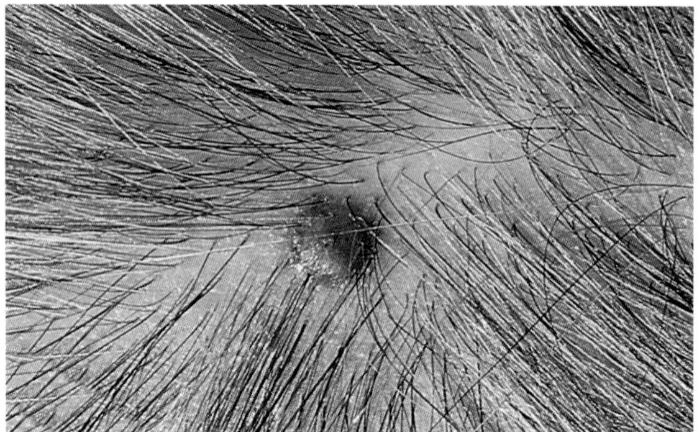

Figure 22-22 Blue nevus. Most lesions are small and round.

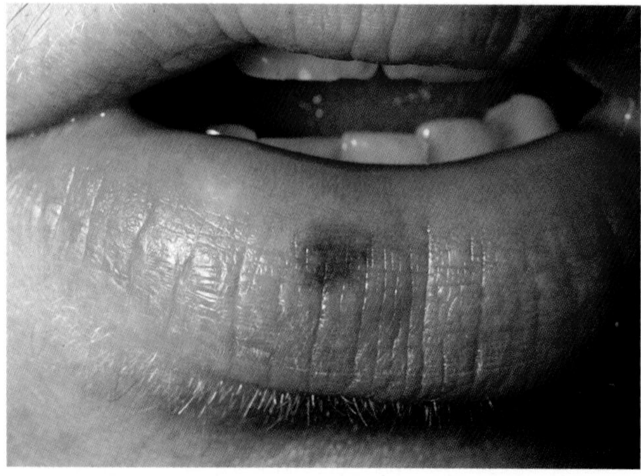

Figure 22-23 Labial melanotic macule. These common lesions worry the patient who suspects melanoma. They are benign.

Atypical nevi

Atypical nevi, also referred to as dysplastic nevi or Clark nevi, may be inherited in a familial pattern or occur sporadically. They are usually larger than 5 mm in diameter and are either flat or flat with a raised center ("fried-egg lesion") (Table 22-1). They are darkly or irregularly pigmented with shades of brown and pink and usually have irregular or indistinct borders. Dysplastic nevi are common, with a prevalence rate of about 5%. Dysplastic nevi differ from common acquired nevi by (1) beginning to appear near puberty instead of in childhood and (2) continuing to develop past the fourth decade. Atypical nevi are a "marker" for patients at an increased risk for development of melanoma and a precursor lesion to melanoma. No data are available to assess what effect prophylactic removal has on decreasing the risk for future development of melanoma.

FAMILIAL MELANOMA AND MELANOMA PRECURSORS. Cutaneous melanoma may occur as isolated, so-called sporadic cases; in association with multiple atypical nevi; or in familial clusters, in which case it is referred to as the atypical mole syndrome (AMS), formerly known as dysplastic nevus syndrome. In the late 1970s the dysplastic nevus (DN) or atypical mole (AM) was identified in melanoma-prone families. It was then determined that AMs are cutaneous markers that identify specific family members who are at increased risk for melanoma. The AM may also be the single most important precursor lesion of melanoma. These nevi may occur in persons from melanoma-prone families and in persons who lack both a family history and a personal history of melanoma.

ATYPICAL MOLE SYNDROME AND FAMILIAL MELANOMA. Numerous families with multiple melanoma patients have been reported. These patients usually develop melanoma at a young age, have a predisposition to multiple primary melanomas, and have the tendency to develop thin, superficial-spreading melanomas. Large, unusual-looking moles were initially recognized as a precursor to melanoma in patients with familial cutaneous melanoma. This syndrome was named B-K mole syndrome from two of the probands, and the precursor nevi were designated as B-K moles and later referred to as dysplastic nevi (DN). The syndrome is now called the atypical mole syndrome (AMS). Recent estimates suggest that approximately 32,000 persons in the United States have familial AMS with familial melanoma, accounting for approximately 5.5% of all melanomas diagnosed in this country. Hereditary malignant melanoma and atypical moles represent pleiotropic effects of a mendelian autosomal dominant gene with high penetrance.

One study showed that the hereditary cutaneous malignant melanoma/AMS does not predispose to other cancers.

DEFINITION. The National Institutes of Health (NIH) Consensus Conference on Diagnosis and Treatment of Early Melanoma has defined the familial atypical mole and melanoma syndrome as (1) the occurrence of malignant melanoma in one or more first- or second-degree relatives; (2) a large number of melanocytic nevi (MN), often more than 50, some of which are atypical and often variable in size; and (3) melanocytic nevi that demonstrate certain histologic features. AMS probably represents a spectrum. At one end all members of a kindred have atypical moles (AMs) and some have malignant melanoma (MM). At the other end are persons with one AM without a personal or family history of MM.

ASSOCIATION WITH MELANOMA. Patients with AMS, familial or sporadic, are at significant risk for developing melanoma. Atypical moles have been observed in 8% of patients with nonfamilial (sporadic) melanoma, and the transformation into superficial-spreading melanoma has been photographically documented. Family members without atypical moles do not show any apparent increase in melanoma risk. The frequency of sporadic AMS in the general population is unknown.

Atypical moles are found on the skin of 90% of patients with hereditary melanomas, and more than 50% of melanomas in this group are associated histologically with and probably evolve from atypical moles. The lifetime risk of developing cutaneous melanoma among the white population in the United States is approximately 0.8%; that is, 1 in 125 persons who have AMS and no family members with the disease have a 6% risk of developing melanoma. Persons who have AMS and a history of melanoma have a 10% risk of getting a second melanoma; persons who have AMS and have a family member with melanoma have a 15% risk. The lifetime risk of melanoma approaches 100% for those people with AMS from families with two or more first-degree relatives who have cutaneous melanoma.

Among atypical mole-bearing family members, those patients with melanoma have very large numbers of nevi more frequently than patients with AMS without melanoma. Family members with AMS have more nevi than do patients who have only common acquired types of nevi.

Classification of atypical melanocytic nevi

CLINICAL CLASSIFICATION

The clinical diagnosis of atypical melanocytic nevi is established when at least three of the following characteristics are present:

- Diameter greater than 5 mm
- Ill-defined borders
- Irregular margin
- Varying shades in the lesion
- Presence of papular and macular components

Table 22-1 Differences between Atypical Moles and Common Nevi

Characteristics	Atypical moles	Common nevi
Distribution	Back most common, upper and lower limbs, sun-protected areas, female breasts, scalp, buttocks, groin	Usually sun-exposed areas; most above the waist
Number	Less than 10 to greater than 100	10 to 40
Age at onset	Appear as normal nevi at age 2 to 6 years; increase in number and size at puberty; new nevi appear throughout life	Absent at birth; appear at age 2 to 6; grow vertically in uniform manner throughout life; several may appear at puberty
Size	Usually greater than 5 mm and commonly greater than 10 mm	Usually less than 6 mm
Shape and contour	Irregular border; flat (macular) areas; margin fades into surrounding skin; always has a macular component	Round, symmetric, uniformly macular or papular smooth border
Color	Variable within a single lesion; brown, black, red, pink	Uniform tan, brown, black; darken during pregnancy or at adolescence; become lighter with age
Histologic characteristics	Persistent lentiginous melanocytic hyperplasia; melanocytic nuclear atypia;* lamellar fibroplasias; concentric eosinophilic fibroplasias; sparse, patchy lymphocytic infiltration	Nevus cells at dermoepidermal junction and/or in dermis

*May not be essential to make diagnosis.

CLINICAL FEATURES OF ATYPICAL MOLES

MORPHOLOGY. These unusual nevi differ in a number of important ways from typical acquired pigmented nevi or moles (see Table 22-1). Atypical moles are larger than common moles. They have a mixture of colors, including tan, brown, pink, and black. The border is irregular and indistinct and often fades into the surrounding skin. The surface is complex and variable, with both macular and papular components (Figure 22-24). A characteristic presentation is a pigmented papule surrounded by a macular collar of pigmentation ("fried-egg lesion") (Figure 22-25). In one study, the total number of nevi and macular components were the only useful features to predict histologic melanocytic dysplasia. However, "fried-egg lesions" often do not display histologic melanocytic dysplasia. In contrast, the absence of a macular component in melanocytic nevi in a person with fewer than 13 total body nevi accurately predicts the absence of melanocytic dysplasia on histologic examination.

SURFACE CHARACTERISTICS. The surface characteristics of atypical nevi are distinctive and can be appreciated with a hand lens and dermoscope (see Figure 22-46).

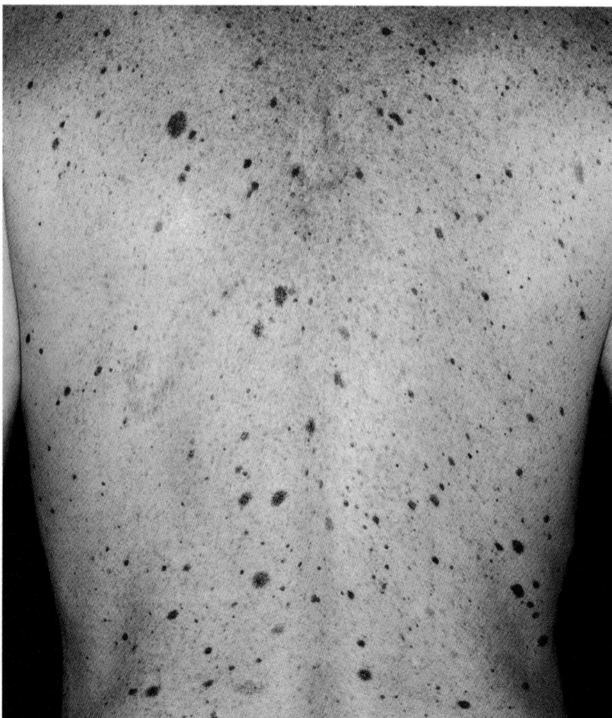

Figure 22-24 Atypical nevi. There are numerous large nevi present. Superficial spreading melanomas have been removed from the upper back and the midline on the left side (note scars). Nevi are larger than 1 cm and irregularly pigmented.

DEVELOPMENT AND DISTRIBUTION. Atypical moles (AMs) are not present at birth, but begin to appear in the mid-childhood years as typical common moles. The appearance changes at puberty, and newer lesions continue to appear well after the age of 40. Common moles occur most often on sun-exposed areas. AMs occur in those locations and at unusual sites such as the scalp, buttocks, and breast. The predilection sites for melanoma in familial AMs patients of both genders correspond with the distribution of nevi; in males, nevi and melanoma counts are higher on the back; in females, both the back and the lower extremities are affected. These findings strongly suggest an association between nevus distribution and melanoma occurrence and site in familial AMs.

HISTOLOGIC CHARACTERISTICS. The NIH Consensus Conference listed the histologic criteria as follows: architectural disorder with asymmetry, subepidermal (concentric eosinophilic and/or lamellar) fibroplasia, and lentiginous melanocytic hyperplasia with spindle or epithelioid melanocytes aggregating in nests of variable size and forming bridges between adjacent rete ridges. Melanocytic atypia may be present to a variable degree. In addition, there may be dermal infiltration with lymphocytes, as well as the "shoulder" phenomenon (intraepidermal melanocytes extending singly or in nests beyond the main dermal component).

MANAGEMENT. Recommendations for treatment of patients with AMs have been given in the National Institutes of Health Consensus Development Conference statement, October 24 to 26, 1983. These, along with other recommendations, are given in Box 22-1.

Box 22-1 **Recommendations for the Management of AMs**

- Examine total cutaneous surface every 3 to 12 months, beginning around puberty.
- Use hair-blower for scalp examination.
- Consider total cutaneous photographs as baseline.
- Excise lesions suspected to be melanoma.
- Educate patient on self-examination of skin.
- Recommend sun avoidance and/or protection.
- Suggest screening of blood relatives for AM and MM.
- Suggest regular ophthalmologic examinations for ocular nevi and ocular melanoma.

ATYPICAL MOLES

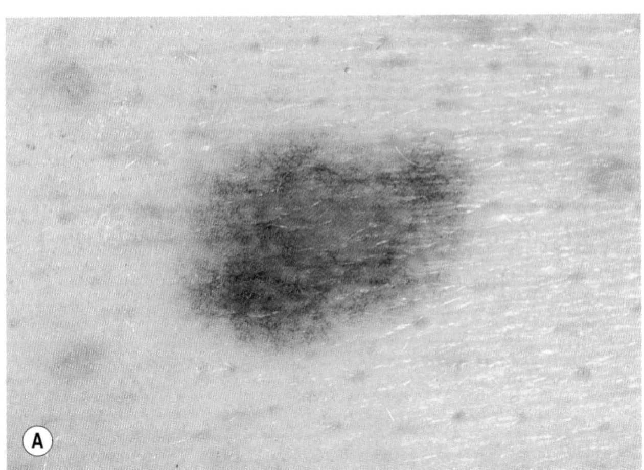
Macular, variable pigmentation, ill-defined borders.

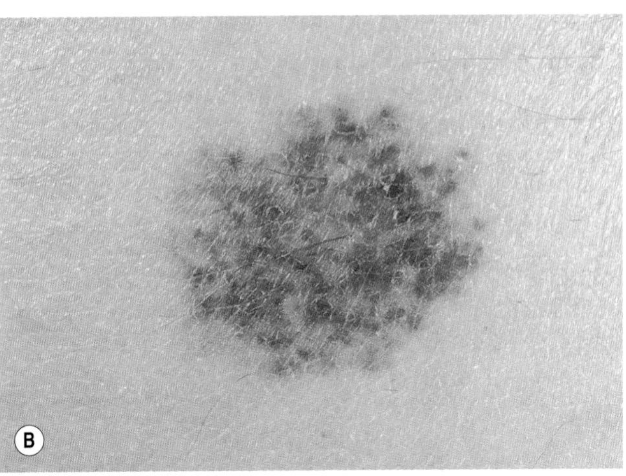
Macular, complex pigmentation, notched border.

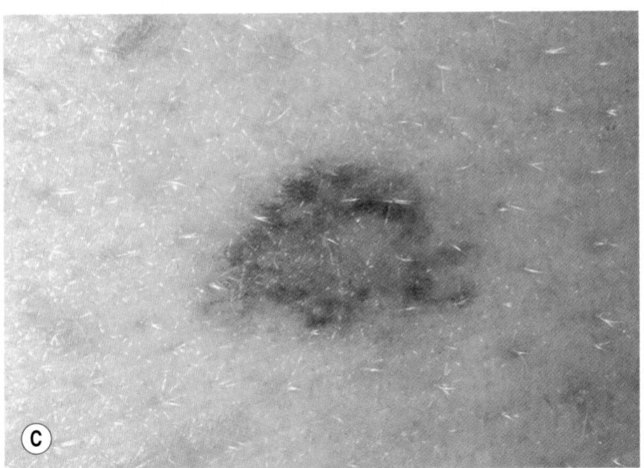
Macular, variable pigmentation, fades at border.

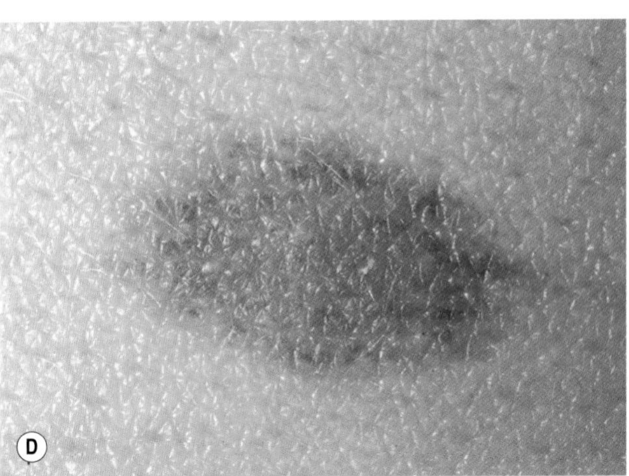
Papular, large lesion.

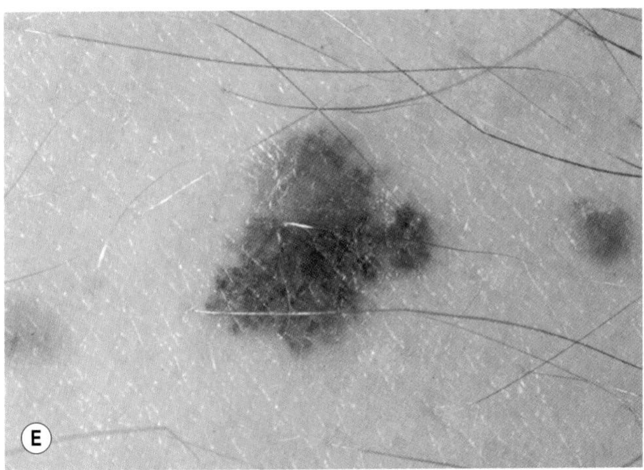
Macular, papular, variable pigmentation, irregular border.

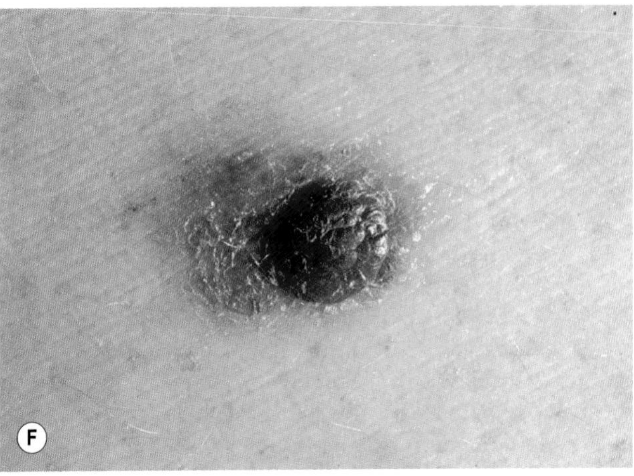
"Fried-egg lesion," raised with dark center, macular periphery, pigmentation fades at border.

Figure 22-25

MALIGNANT MELANOMA

Malignant melanoma is a malignancy of melanocytes that occurs in the skin, eyes, ears, gastrointestinal tract, leptomeninges, and oral and genital mucous membranes. One of the most dangerous tumors, melanoma has the ability to metastasize to any organ, including the brain and heart.

EPIDEMIOLOGY. In the United States, melanoma is the fifth most common cancer in men and the sixth most common cancer in women. A total of 62,000 cases of melanoma were diagnosed in the United States in 2006.

The incidence of malignant melanoma is increasing rapidly worldwide. Currently, 1 in 63 Americans will develop melanoma during their lifetime; the risk was 1 in 1500 in 1935. The highest incidence is in Australia and New Zealand. The median age at diagnosis is 57 years, and the median age at death is 67 years. Males are approximately 1.5 times more likely to develop melanoma than females. The most common areas are the back for men and the arms and legs for women.

Whites have a 10-fold greater risk of developing cutaneous melanoma than blacks, Asians, or Hispanics. Whites and blacks have a similar risk of developing plantar melanoma. Noncutaneous melanomas (e.g., mucosal) are more common in non-white populations.

RISK FOR MELANOMA. The risk factors for melanoma are listed in Table 22-2.

Table 22-2 Risk Factors for Developing Cutaneous Melanoma

Risk status	Relative risk (%)*
Greatly increased risk	
Personal history of atypical moles, family history of melanoma, and greater than 75-100 moles	35
Previous nonmelanoma skin cancer	17
Congenital nevus (giant, >20 cm)	15-5
History of melanoma	9-10
Family history of melanoma in parent, sibling, or children	8
Immunosuppression	8-6
Moderately increased risk	
Clinically atypical nevi (2-9)	7.3-4.9; no family history of melanoma/sporadic atypical nevi
Large number of nevi	
51-100	5.0-3.0
26-50	4.4-1.8
Chronic tanning with UVA (PUVA treatments [>250] for psoriasis)	5.4
Modestly increased risk	
Repeated blistering sunburns	
3	3.8
2	1.7
Freckling	3.0
Fair skin, inability to tan	2.6
Red or blond hair	2.2
Clinically atypical nevus (1)	2.3

Adapted from Robinson JK: *Dermatol Nurs* 12:397, 2000.
*The relative risk is the degree of increased risk for persons with the risk factor(s) as compared with persons without the risk factor. If the relative risk is 1, there is no increased risk.

ULTRAVIOLET RADIATION EXPOSURE. Increased exposure to ultraviolet (UV) radiation is considered to be a factor for the increased incidence of melanoma. Sunburns are a risk factor for melanoma. Sunburns are primarily due to UVB (280 to 320 nm) radiation. Melanomas are also increased in people exposed to ultraviolet A (UVA) radiation. High doses of UVA radiation are received in sun beds and with exposure to psoralen and UVA (PUVA) therapy.

PUVA and risk of melanoma. Oral methoxsalen (psoralen) and ultraviolet A radiation (PUVA) is effective therapy for psoriasis and other skin conditions. It is carcinogenic. An increased risk of melanoma is observed beginning 15 years after first exposure to oral methoxsalen (psoralen) and ultraviolet A radiation (PUVA). This risk is greater in patients exposed to high doses of PUVA, appears to be increasing with the passage of time, and should be considered in determining the risks and benefits of this therapy.

RISK AND SUN EXPOSURE. Increased recreational sun exposure and alterations of the upper atmosphere by pollutants that result in increased radiation may be the two most important factors in the disproportionate rise in the incidence of melanoma. People who suntan poorly or sunburn easily or who have had multiple or severe sunburns have a twofold to threefold increased risk for developing cutaneous melanoma. Individuals with recreational and vacation sun exposure who experience acute episodic exposures to sunlight may be at greater risk than those with constant occupational sun exposure. Continuous UV radiation exposure, either in adult life or during adolescence, seems to play a protective role in melanoma risk. Those with outdoor occupations have been found to have a lower risk of acquiring melanoma. Intermittent exposure is associated with significant risk increases of melanoma. It is postulated that sunlight causes cutaneous immunosuppression.

SUNSCREEN EFFECTIVENESS. Chemical sunscreens block UVB but are less effective at blocking UVA, which comprises 90% to 95% of ultraviolet energy in the solar

Table 22-3 Signs Suggesting Malignancy in Pigmented Lesions

Sign		Implication
Changes in color		
Sudden darkening; brown, black		Increased number of tumor cells, the density of which varies within the lesion, creating irregular pigmentation
Spread of color into previously normal skin		Tumor cells migrating through epidermis at various speeds and in different directions (horizontal growth phase)
Red		Vasodilation and inflammation
White		Areas of regression or inflammation
Blue		Pigment deep in dermis, sign of increasing depth of tumor
Changes in characteristics of border		
Irregular outline		Malignant cells migrating horizontally at different rates
Satellite pigmentation		Cells migrating beyond confines of primary tumor
Development of depigmented halo		Destruction of melanocytes by possible immunologic reaction and inflammation
Changes in surface characteristics		
Scaliness	Bleeding	
Erosion	Ulceration	
Oozing	Elevation	
Crusting	Loss of normal skin lines	
Development of symptoms		
Pruritus	Pain	
Tenderness		

spectrum. Sunscreens prevent erythema and sunburn, but inhibit accommodation of the skin to sunlight; therefore their use may permit excessive exposure of the skin to UVA. Laboratory data suggest that melanoma is promoted by UVA; therefore UVB sunscreens might not be effective in preventing melanoma. Sunscreen use may give people a false sense of security and encourage excessive exposure. Wearing hats and protective clothing and avoiding sunbathing are more protective than chemical sunscreens. For white, freckled children, the use of a broad-spectrum sunscreen with a high sun protection factor attenuates the development of nevi and, by deduction, decreases the risk of developing a melanoma. Sunscreens that contain zinc oxide or titanium dioxide reflect light and are referred to as physical rather than chemical sunscreens. These compounds effectively block UVA light.

ABCDs OF MALIGNANT MELANOMA RECOGNITION. The goal is to recognize melanomas at the earliest stage. Compared to common acquired melanocytic nevi, malignant melanomas tend to have Asymmetry, Border irregularity, Color variation, and Diameter enlargement. Changes in shape and color are important early signs and should always arouse suspicion. Ulceration and bleeding are late signs; hope of cure diminishes greatly if the diagnosis has not been made before such changes occur. The specific signs that appear during the evolution of each type of melanoma are listed and illustrated on the following pages. A list of all possible changes at all stages of development is given in Table 22-3.

CHARACTERISTICS OF BENIGN MOLES. Moles evolve and change during life. All of the changes occur over long periods of time and are nearly imperceptible. Circumferential enlargement occurs in common nevi of children. Benign acquired nevi progress from lentigo simplex, to flat pigmented junctional nevi, to elevated pigmented compound nevi, to more elevated skin-colored intradermal nevi over decades. Intradermal nevi continue to elevate as collagen is laid down over nests of nevus cells in the upper dermis. Therefore the distance between the dermoepidermal junction and the top of the underlying intradermal nevus increases with age.

Benign moles have a more uniform tan, brown, or black color. The border is regular and the lesion is roughly symmetric; if the lesion could be folded in half, the two halves would superimpose. Most acquired benign moles are 6 mm or less in diameter and appear early in life.

RECENT CHANGE IN A MOLE. The patient's description of a change in a mole may be the earliest sign of melanoma. Changing color; developing erythematous or hyperpigmented halos; increasing diameter, height, or asymmetry of borders; or changing surface characteristics as well as pruritus, pain, bleeding, ulceration, or tenderness all suggest evolution into melanoma.

PRECURSOR LESIONS

Acquired melanocytic nevi. People with an increased number of benign melanocytic nevi have an increased risk for the development of melanoma. The number at which point the risk becomes significant varies from person to person, depending on factors such as family history and sun exposure. Because 80% of all patients have up to 50 benign nevi, a practical "cut-off" number of nevi over which patients might be at an increased risk for the development of melanoma would be 50. The relative risk for these patients has ranged from 3 to 15 when compared with the relative risk for patients with either no nevi or fewer than five nevi.

Atypical nevi. Atypical nevi may be observed in persons with or without melanoma and may be inherited in a familial pattern or occur sporadically. They are usually larger than 5 mm in diameter and are either flat or flat with a raised center ("fried-egg lesion"). They are darkly or irregularly pigmented with shades of brown and pink and usually have irregular or indistinct borders. Patients with atypical nevi outside of the familial melanoma setting have an increased risk for the development of melanoma but the rate is much lower. One clinically atypical nevus was associated with a 2-fold increased risk for the development of melanoma, whereas 10 or more atypical nevi conferred a 12-fold increased risk over patients without atypical nevi.

Congenital nevi. The malignant potential of congenital nevi is dependent on size and histologic pattern (see p. 851).

FOUR MAJOR CLINICAL-HISTOPATHOLOGIC SUBTYPES

Melanoma either begins de novo or develops from a preexisting lesion, such as a congenital or atypical mole. A classification into several different types was devised after observing that the microscopic anatomy of the tumor at the periphery of the elevated tumor mass was variable and possessed characteristic patterns that could be correlated with distinctive clinical presentations. The proposed types are superficial spreading melanoma (SSM), lentigo maligna melanoma (LMM), nodular melanoma (NM), and acral-lentiginous melanoma (ALM).

Many, but not all, pathologists recognize these various clinicopathologic types of melanoma. Some melanomas do not conform to this clinicopathologic classification and may be labeled exclusively as malignant melanoma. Malignant melanoma may be a single entity that has various clinical and histologic forms varying with the degree of differentiation of the tumor cell. The potential for a melanocyte to degenerate and become neoplastic is probably influenced by a number of factors, including degree of skin pigmentation, heredity, immunologic status, quantity of solar radiation, gender of the individual, and anatomic position on the body.

GROWTH CHARACTERISTICS. Once a melanocyte becomes neoplastic, constraints on its localization are removed, and it may leave its assigned position at the basal layer of the epidermis. A well-differentiated malignant melanocyte retains its affinity for the epidermis and may grow slowly horizontally, only to be restrained or eliminated in some areas by a still-competent immunologic system. Years of slow growth and regression by a number of such cells on the face produce the LMM.

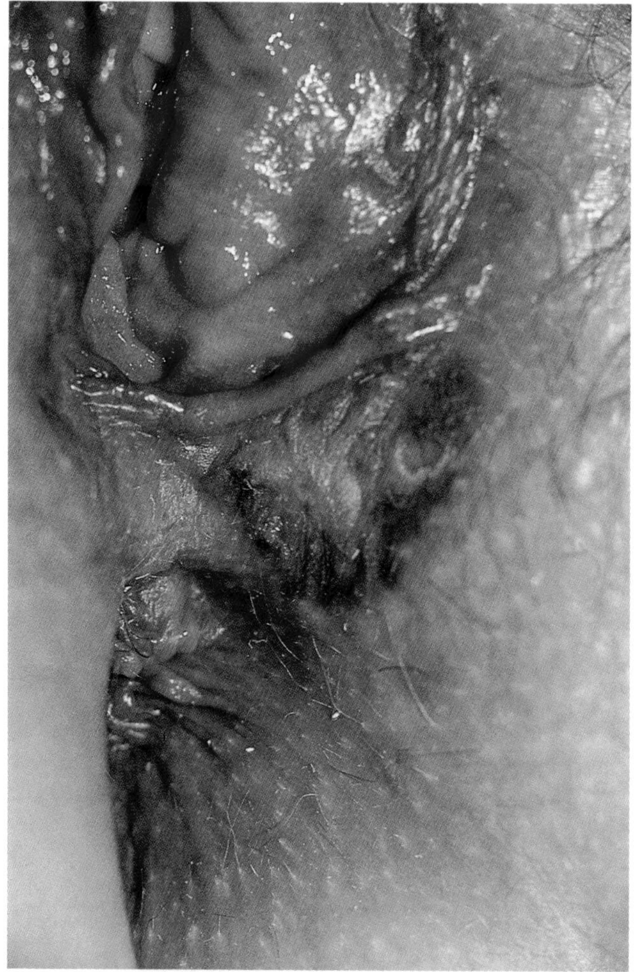

Figure 22-26 Superficial spreading melanoma. Modesty prevented the patient from asking the physician about this lesion on the vulva, which had been present for 2 years. Fortunately, it was discovered during a complete examination of the skin.

A more immature group of cells would be more aggressive and extend and regress at a faster rate, stimulating new vessel formation and inflammation. Such biologic behavior could be expected to produce the SSM. Melanomas in which the cells are extending laterally are considered to be in the horizontal (radial) growth phase. This phase may endure for months or years.

A poorly differentiated cell knows no bounds, has no affinity for the epidermis, and grows both horizontally and vertically, producing a mass or NM. Melanomas in which cells have begun to grow vertically into the dermis and form a mass are considered to be in the vertical growth phase. The validity of the type classification has yet to be settled; however, it does enable one to understand the growth and evolution of malignant melanoma; and therefore is an aid to making an early diagnosis. The various types of melanomas have specific characteristics.

Superficial spreading melanoma

Superficial spreading melanoma (SSM) (Box 22-2) is most common in middle age, from the fourth to fifth decade. It develops anywhere on the body, but most frequently on the upper back of both genders and on the legs of women (Figures 22-26 to 22-30). SSM begins in a nonspecific manner and then changes shape by radial spread and regression (see Figure 22-28). The random migration of cells, along with the process of regression, results in lesions with an endless variety of shapes and sizes. The shape is bizarre if left untreated for years. The hallmark of SSM is the haphazard combination of many colors, but it may be uniformly brown or black. Colors may become more diverse as time proceeds. A dull red color is frequently observed, which may occupy a small area or may dominate the lesion. The precursor radial growth phase may last for months or for more than 10 years. Nodules appear when the lesion is approximately 2.5 cm in diameter.

Box 22-2 **Superficial Spreading Melanoma**
70% of melanomas
Diameter >6 mm
Located on trunk in men and women and the legs in women
Irregular asymmetric borders
Begins as flat or elevated brown lesion
Evolves into black, blue, red, white colors

Figure 22-27 Distribution of superficial spreading melanoma of the skin in men and women. (From *Causes and effects of changes in stratospheric ozone,* Washington, DC, National Academy Press. Courtesy New York University Melanoma Cooperative Group and the National Academy Press.)

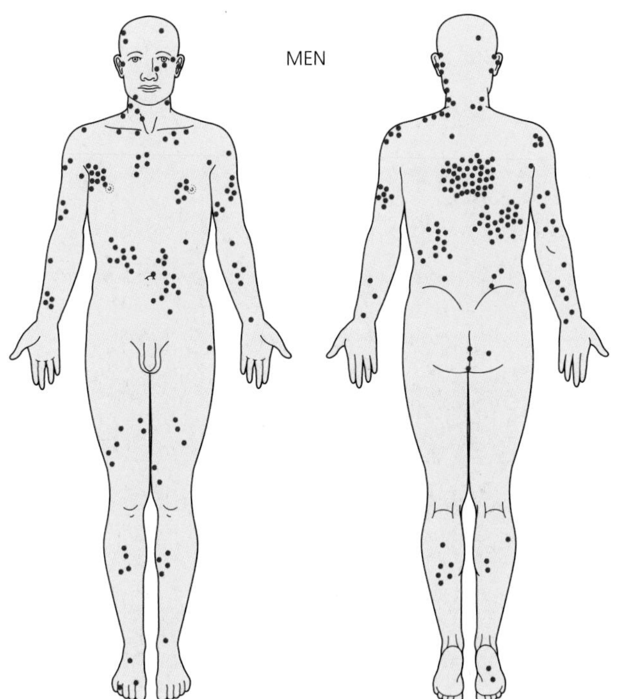

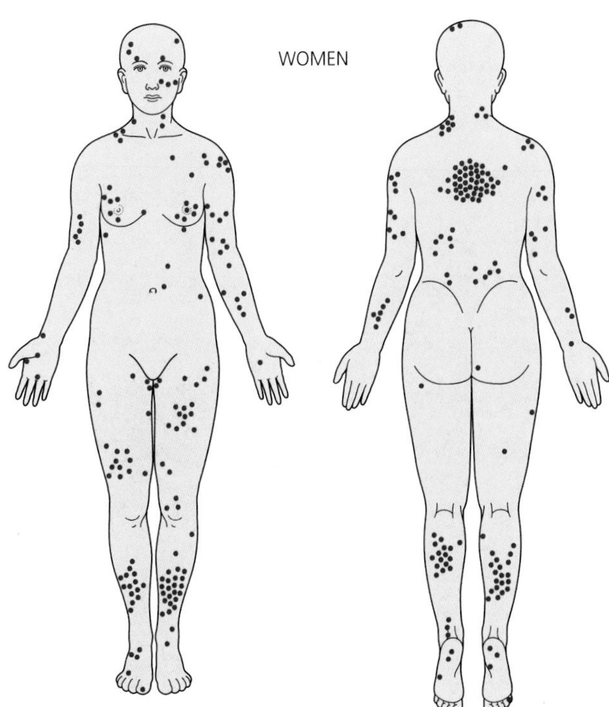

SUPERFICIAL SPREADING MELANOMAS

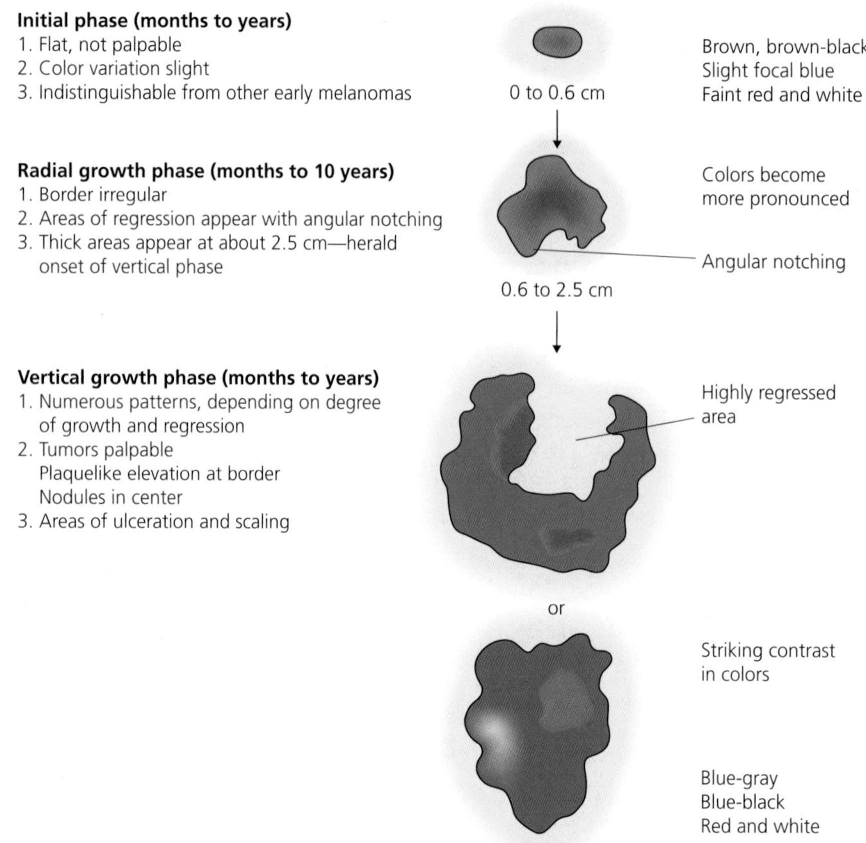

Figure 22-28 Superficial spreading melanomas in all stages of development. The small early lesions have irregular borders, irregular pigmentation, and small white areas indicating regression. The largest tumors show an accentuation of all of these features.

SUPERFICIAL SPREADING MELANOMAS

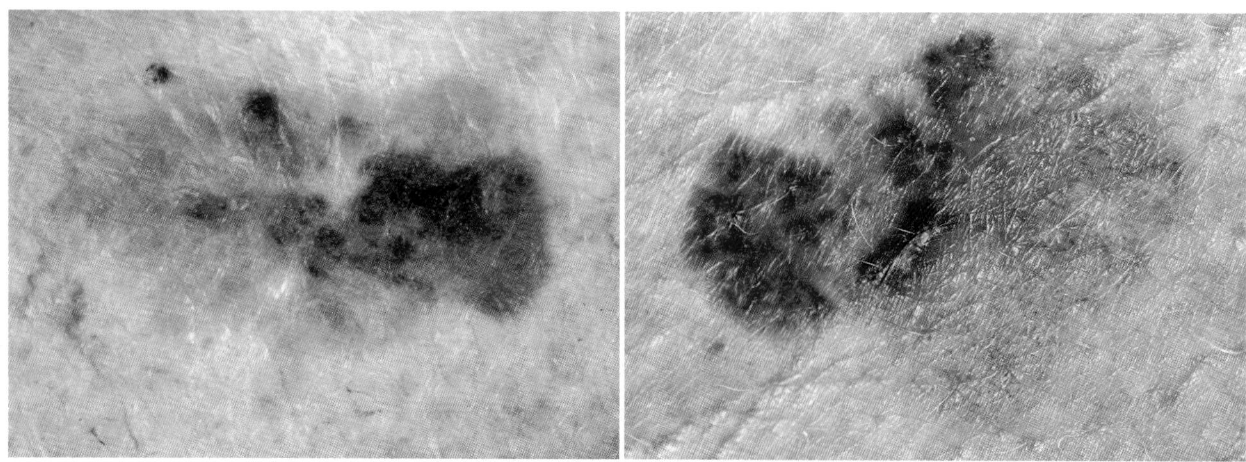

Figure 22-29

SUPERFICIAL SPREADING MELANOMAS

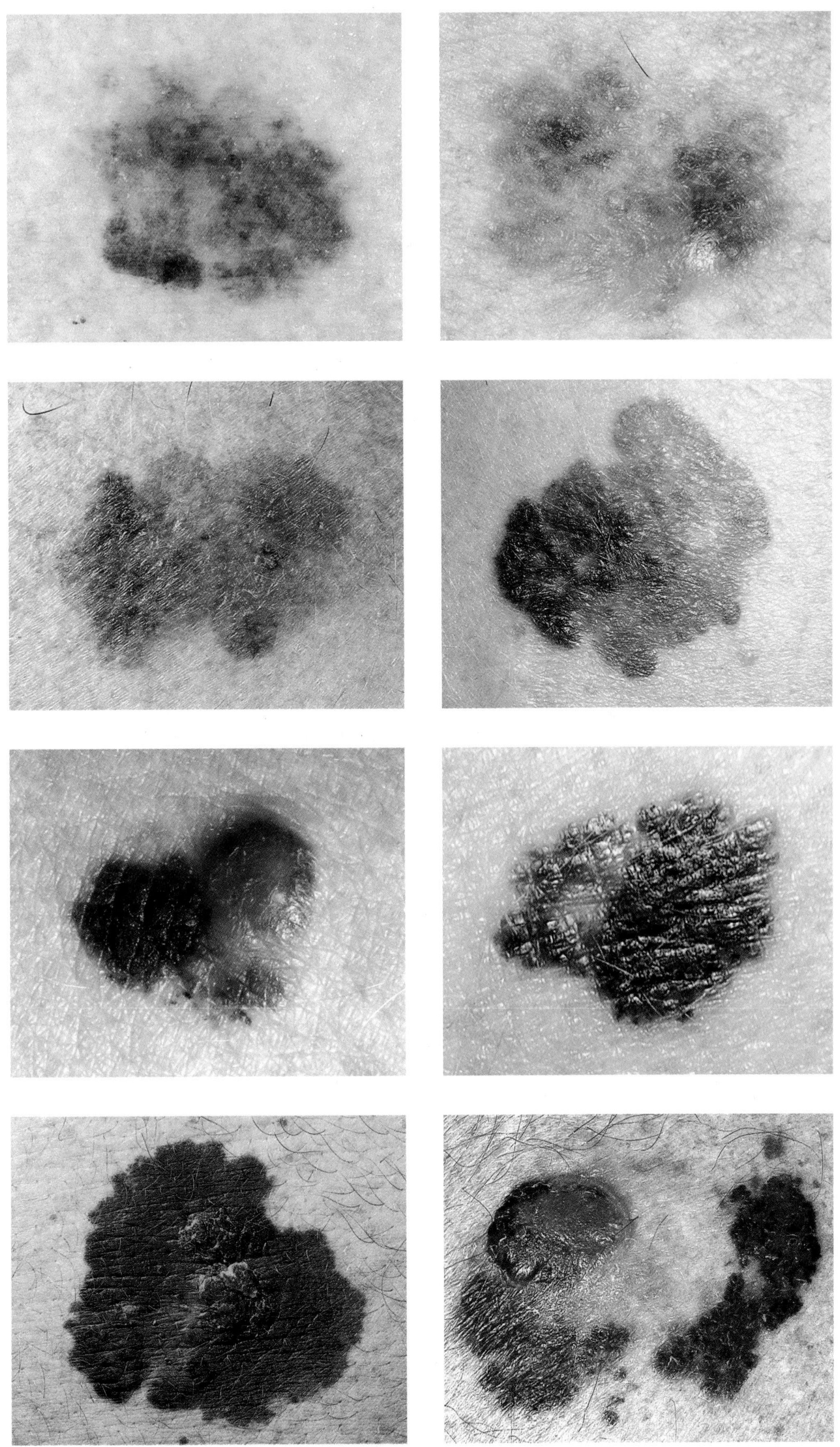

Figure 22-30

Nodular melanoma

Nodular melanoma (NM) (Figures 22-31 and 22-32, Box 22-3) occurs most often in the fifth or sixth decade. It is more frequent in males than females, with a ratio of 2:1. It is found anywhere on the body. NM is most commonly dark brown, red-brown, or red-black and is dome-shaped, polypoid, or pedunculated. It is occasionally amelanotic (flesh-colored) and resembles flesh-colored dermal nevi or basal cell carcinoma. These amelanotic melanomas represent 1.8% to 8.1% of all melanomas. NM is the type of melanoma most frequently misdiagnosed because it resembles a blood blister, hemangioma, dermal nevus, seborrheic keratosis, or dermatofibroma (see Figure 22-32).

Box 22-3 **Nodular Melanoma**
15% to 20% of melanomas
Located on trunk and legs
Rapid growth: weeks, months
Brown-to-black papule or nodule
Ulcerates and bleeds

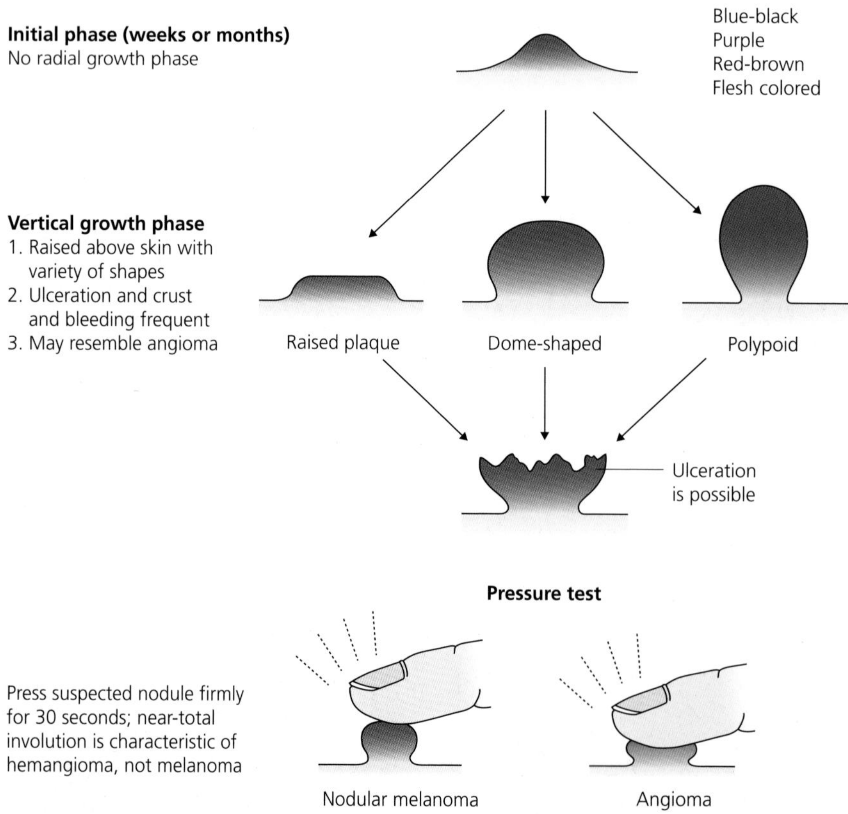

Figure 22-31 There are raised plaque, dome-shaped, and polypoid lesions. Some appear to be originating from nevi. A halo has developed around one of the plaque-shaped melanomas.

NODULAR MELANOMAS

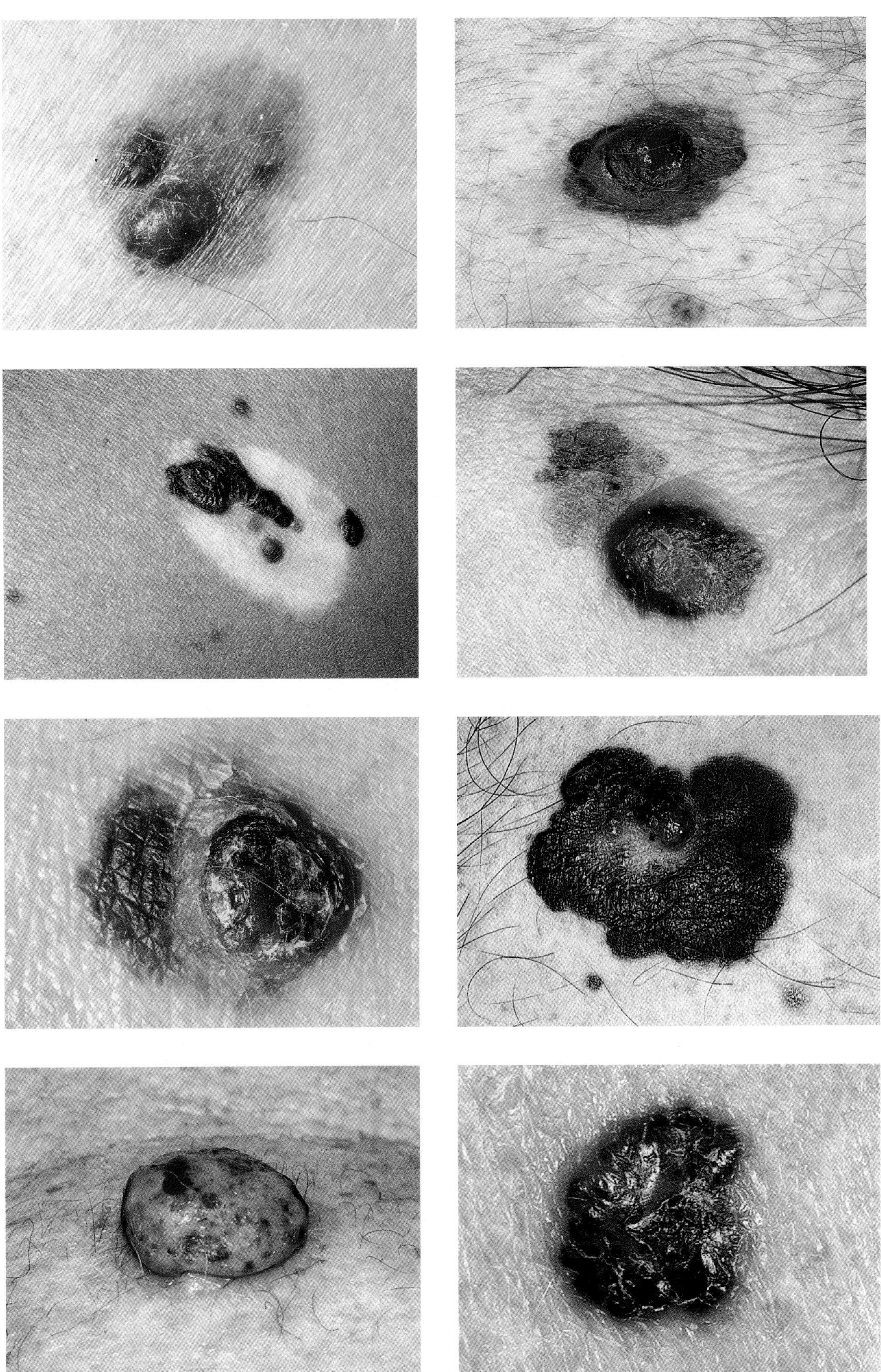

Figure 22-32

Lentigo maligna melanoma

Lentigo maligna melanoma (LMM) (Figures 22-33 and 22-34, Box 22-4) usually presents in the sixth or seventh decade. Most are located on the face, but 10% are on other exposed sites, such as the arms and legs. The radial growth phase is called lentigo maligna (LM) or Hutchinson's freckle. The radial growth phase may last for years and never develop a vertical growth phase. The risk of progression of LM to LMM varies with age, but is lower than commonly believed. For a patient aged 45 years with LM, the estimated risk of developing LMM by age 75 is 3.3%. Estimated lifetime risk of transformation to melanoma is 4.7%. For a patient aged 65 years with LM, the risk of developing LMM is 1.2%, and the lifetime risk of transformation to melanoma is 2.2%. These risk estimates apply to patients in whom LM is discovered incidentally.

LMM may have a complex pattern. Years of migration and regression can produce lesions with a shape more varied and bizarre than that of SSM. The color is more uniform than SSM, but red and white may later occur. Tumors are generally in the center of the lesion, away from the border. LMM may ulcerate or undergo changes similar to other lesions when they enter the tumor stage. Nodules are usually single and generally appear when the lesion has assumed a size of 5 to 7 cm but may occur in much smaller lesions. LMM does not have a better prognosis than other forms of melanoma; as with other types of melanoma, the prognosis depends on tumor thickness.

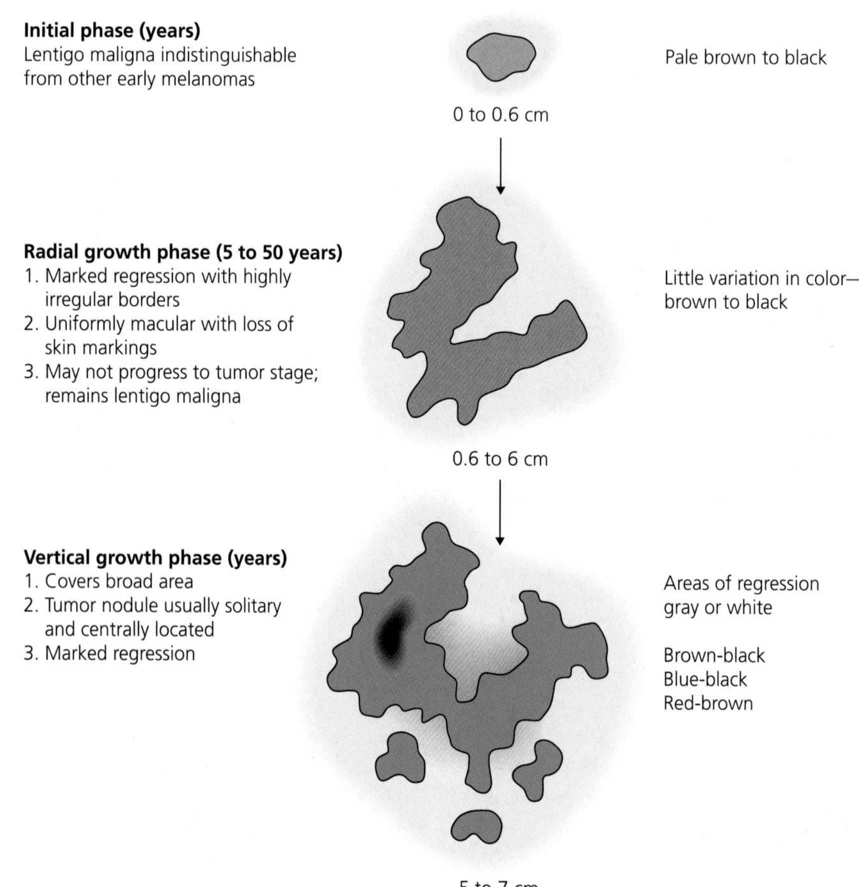

Figure 22-33 The lesions grow slowly and regress for several years, forming highly irregular borders. The color remains brown or black until the tumor stage is reached.

LENTIGO MALIGNA MELANOMA

Box 22-4 **Lentigo Maligna Melanoma**
4% to 15% of melanomas
Located on head, neck, and arms (sun-damaged skin)
Average age 65 years
Slow growth: 5 to 20 years
Arises in <10% of intraepithelial precursor lesions (lentigo maligna)
Precursor lesion is usually large (3 to 6 cm diameter)
Precursor lesion exists for 10 to 15 years
Brown-to-black macular pigmentation
Raised blue-black nodules

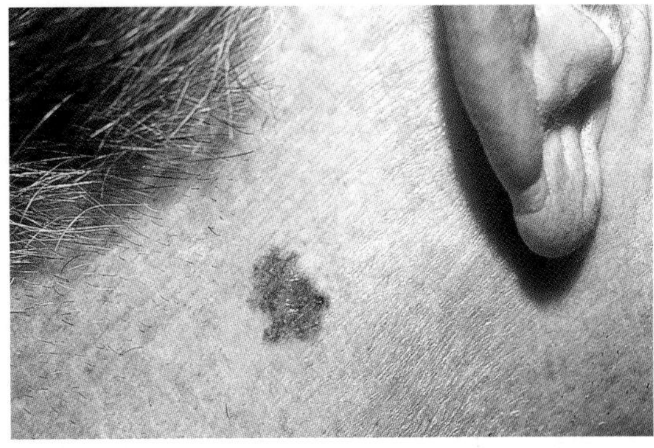

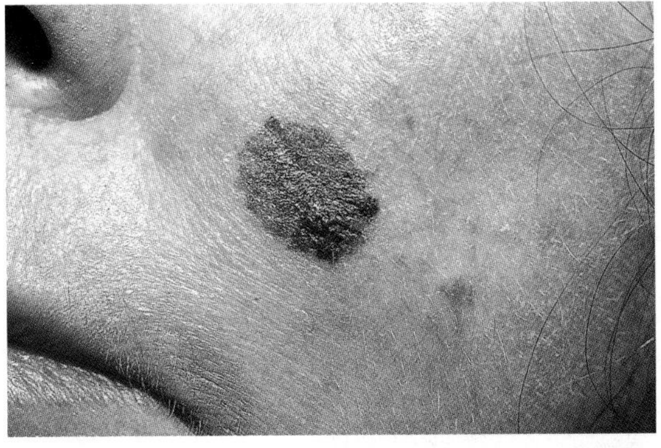

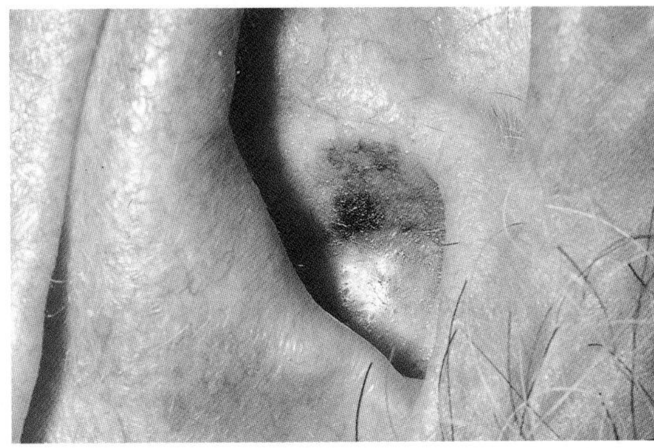

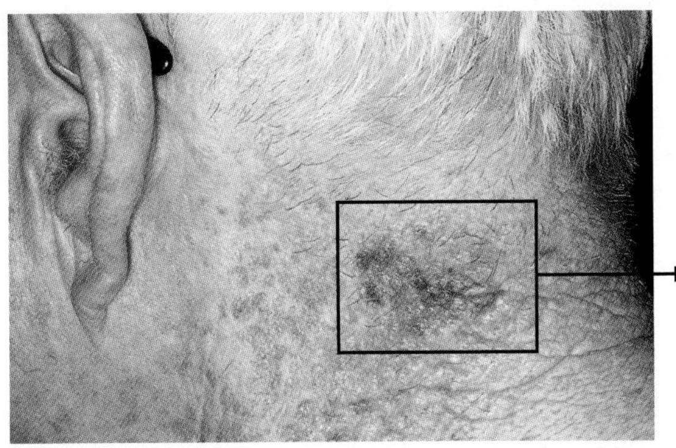

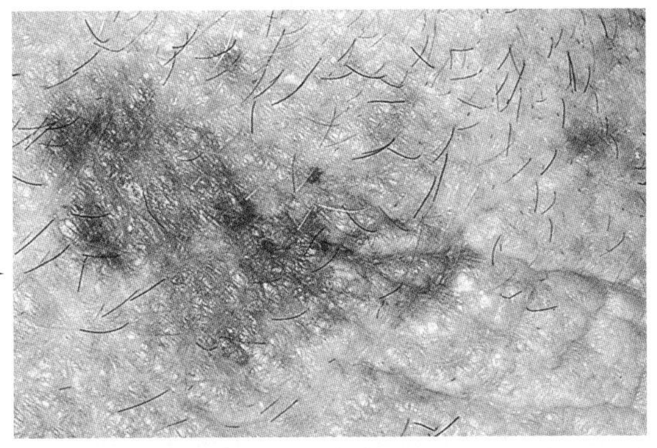

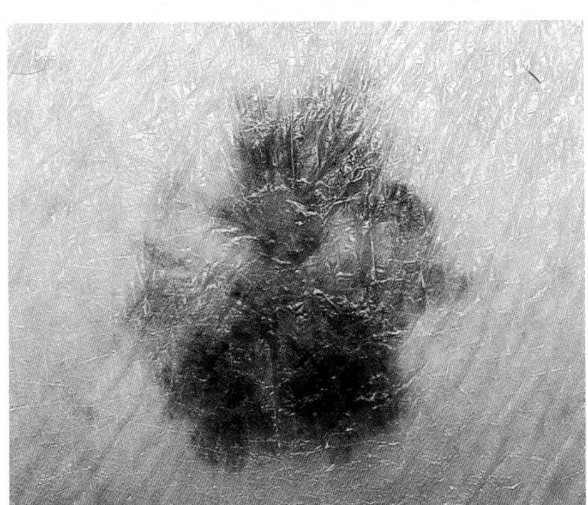

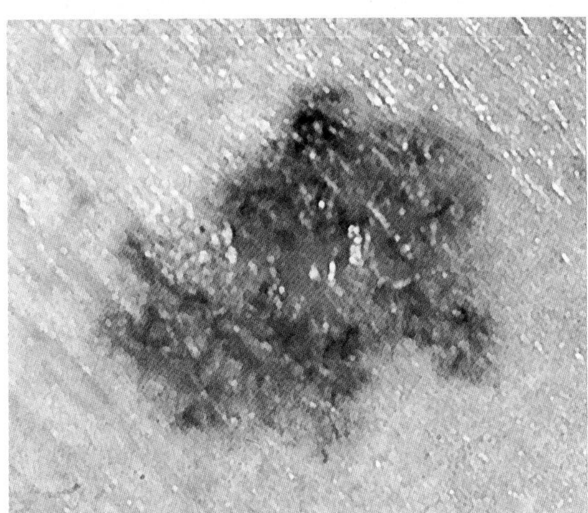

Figure 22-34

Acral-lentiginous melanoma

Acral-lentiginous melanoma (ALM) (Figures 22-35 to 22-38, Box 22-5) appears on the palms, soles, terminal phalanges, and mucous membranes. Similar in clinical presentation to LM and LMM, ALM has the same colors and tendency to remain flat. Like LM, plantar melanomas may remain latent for a number of years, making patients with these lesions good candidates for therapeutic cures if detected early. ALM is most frequent in blacks and Asians. The sole of the foot is the most prevalent site of malignant melanoma in non-whites. Small areas of elevation may be associated with deep invasion; the tumor is very aggressive and metastasizes early. The sudden appearance of a pigmented band originating at the proximal nailfold (Hutchinson's sign) is suggestive of acral-lentiginous melanoma (see Figure 22-36). Acquired melanocytic lesions on the sole larger than 7 mm in maximum diameter should be examined histologically.

Box 22-5 **Acral-Lentiginous Melanoma**
2% to 8% of melanomas in whites
30% to 75% of melanomas in blacks, Asians, and Hispanics
Located on palms, soles
Under nail plate: Hutchinson's sign (pigment spreads to proximal and lateral nailfolds)

RARE TYPES. The following melanoma variants account for less than 2% of melanomas: melanoma arising from congenital nevus, mucosal (lentiginous) melanoma, ocular melanoma, malignant blue nevus, amelanotic melanoma (no pigment), and desmoplastic/neurotropic melanoma (markedly fibrotic stroma).

ACRAL-LENTIGINOUS MELANOMA

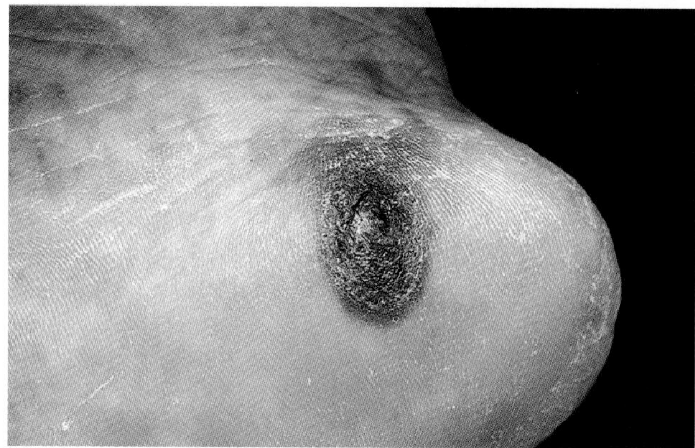

Figure 22-35 A large, dark, flat lesion.

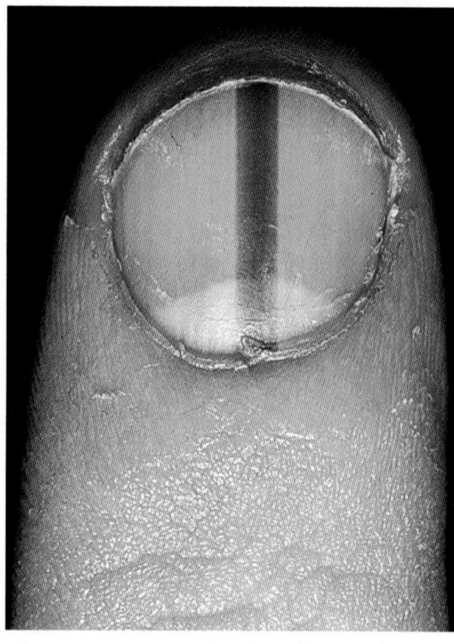

Figure 22-36 The sudden appearance of a pigmented band at the proximal nailfold is suggestive of melanoma.

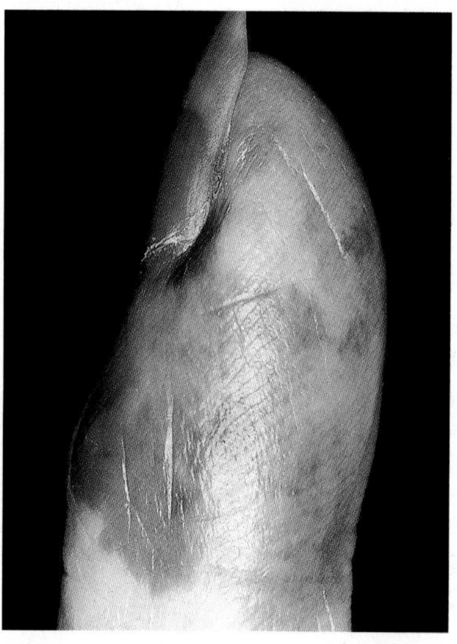

Figure 22-37 Periungual spread of pigmentation from a melanoma to the proximal and lateral nailfolds is called Hutchinson's sign.

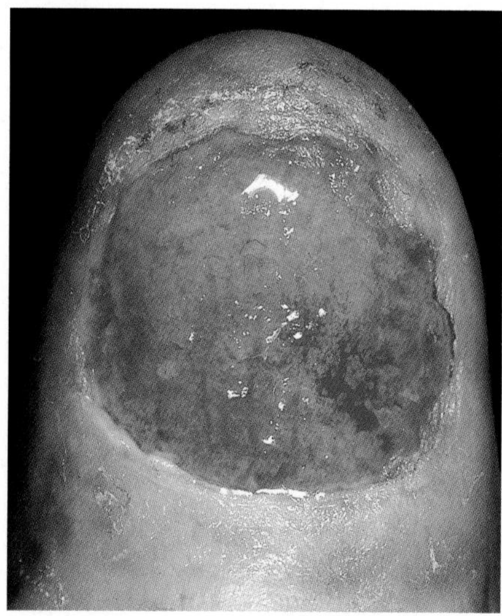

Figure 22-38 Melanoma involving the entire nail bed.

Benign lesions that resemble melanoma

Typical nevi or other lesions, such as those of seborrheic keratosis, angiomas, and dermatofibromas, may have features that suggest melanoma. Biopsy specimens of these lesions should be obtained (Figures 22-39 to 22-42).

LESION EXAMINATION

OBSERVATION PLUS MAGNIFICATION PLUS DERMOSCOPY. Several different lesions can be recognized by observation or magnification with a 10× ocular micrometer. The 10× ocular micrometer is a superior instrument for studying the surface characteristics of seborrheic keratosis, basal cell carcinoma, dermatofibroma, compound nevi, dermal nevi, halo nevi, and hemangiomas. Many lesions can be scanned quickly. The dermoscope (see Figure 22-46) is an invaluable instrument for examination of flat to slightly raised pigmented lesions such as atypical nevi and lesions suspected of being melanoma. Examining numerous seborrheic keratoses with a dermoscope is inefficient. The horn pearls and keratin structure are clearly appreciated with 10× ocular magnification.

SCREENING FOR MELANOMA. Most pigmented lesions can be diagnosed on the basis of clinical criteria. Examination of the surface with 10× magnification is highly recommended for the initial evaluation of all skin growths. However, there are many small lesions in which the distinction between a benign and malignant process cannot be made by observation and magnification. Dermoscopy is useful for the diagnosis of these doubtful skin lesions.

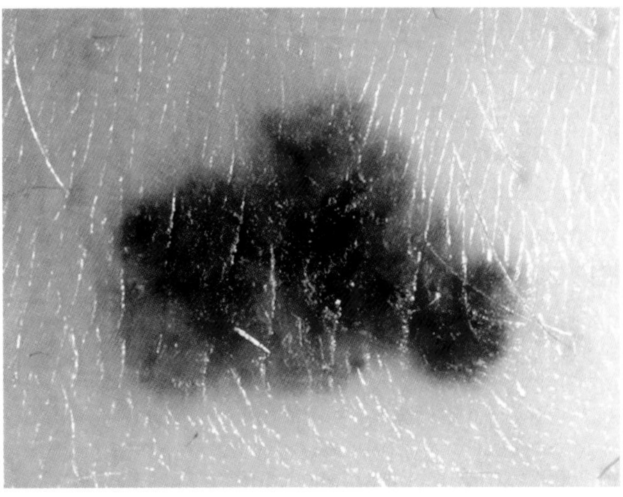

Figure 22-40 Melanoma mimic. Compound nevus with an irregular border.

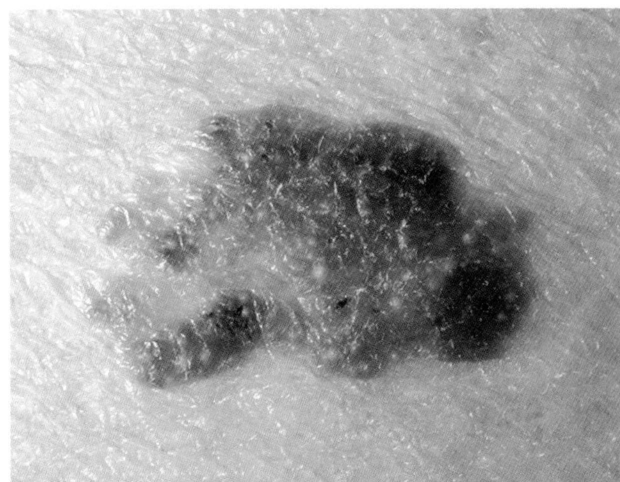

Figure 22-41 Melanoma mimic. Seborrheic keratosis with variable pigmentation and an irregular border. The horn pearls (typical of seborrheic keratosis) suggest that the lesion is benign.

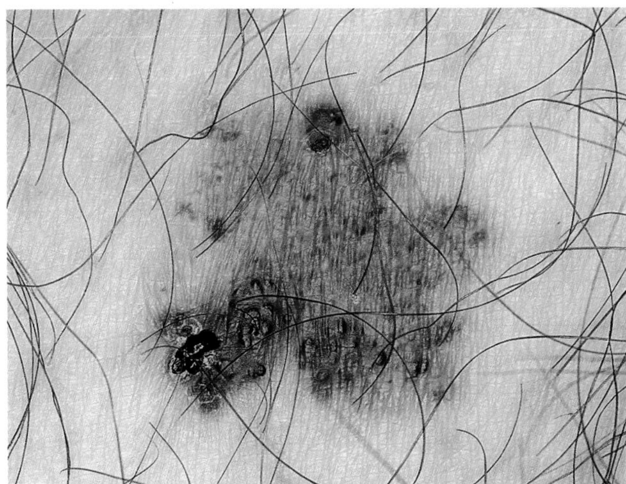

Figure 22-39 Melanoma mimic. Hemangioma with an irregular border and variable pigmentation.

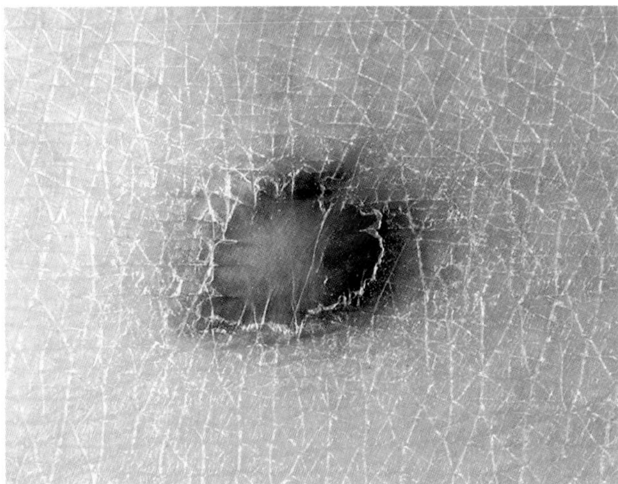

Figure 22-42 Melanoma mimic. Dermatofibroma with dark pigmentation at the border.

MANAGEMENT OF MELANOMA

The classification and management of melanomas are summarized in Tables 22-4 to 22-8.

Biopsy

Whenever possible, excise the lesion for diagnostic purposes using narrow margins (2 to 3 mm of normal skin). Wider margins (>1 cm) may disrupt cutaneous lymphatic flow and affect the ability to identify the sentinel node(s). Incisional biopsy does not adversely affect survival. A punch biopsy technique is appropriate when the suspicion for melanoma is low, when the lesion is large, or when it is impractical to perform an excision. Punch through the thickest part of the lesion. Perform a repeat biopsy if the initial biopsy specimen is inadequate for accurate histologic diagnosis or staging. Shave biopsies are discouraged because partial removal of the primary melanoma may not provide accurate Breslow depth measurement.

HISTOLOGIC FINDINGS AND PROGRESSION

Melanocytes progress through a series of steps toward malignant transformation (Figure 22-43). The first step is a proliferation of melanocytes to form nests along the basal layer to form a benign nevus.

The next step is the formation of a dysplastic nevus. Random cytologic atypia appears in the basement membrane area. Clinically, lesions increase in diameter, show variation in color and symmetry, and have irregular borders. Cells that degenerate to cancer (melanoma) loose the ability to remain localized. They enter the radial growth phase and proliferate intradermally. All cells have changed to atypical tumor cells. Cells penetrate into the papillary dermis singly or in small nests and the lesion becomes slightly raised. The vertical growth shows cells invading the papillary dermis and reticular dermis. Lentiginous melanoma initially have an in situ radial growth phase and in time may enter a vertical growth phase. Lateral intraepidermal extension of melanoma cells occurs in all subtypes except nodular melanoma.

RADIAL GROWTH PHASE TUMORS. Large and atypical melanocytes first proliferate in the epidermis above the epidermal basement membrane. They are arranged haphazardly at the dermal-epidermal junction, show upward (pagetoid) migration, and lack the biologic potential to metastasize. They then invade the papillary dermis (Clark level 2). Malignant cells confined above the epidermal basement membrane (in situ) or in the papillary dermis (microinvasive) are called radial growth phase melanomas. These are almost always less than 1 mm thick.

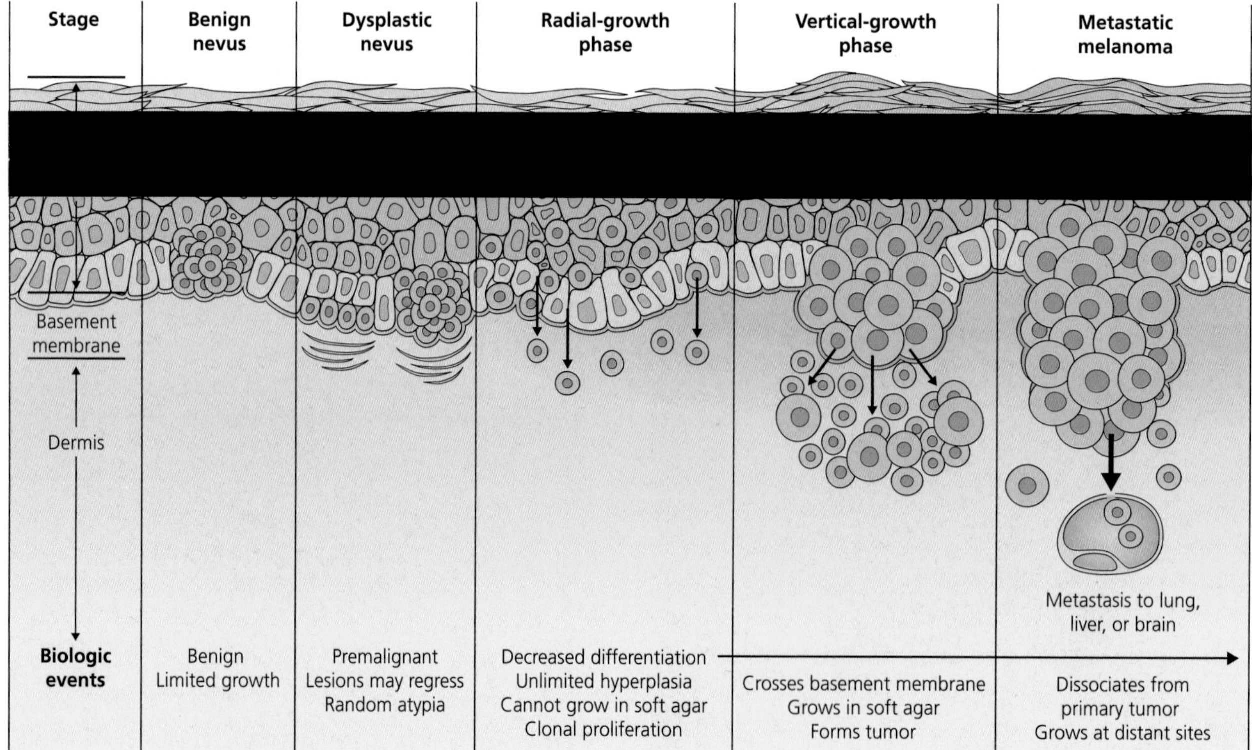

Figure 22-43 The proliferation of melanocytes in the process of forming nevi and subsequent development of dysplasia, hyperplasia, invasion, and metastasis.

VERTICAL GROWTH PHASE TUMORS. Tumors that have invaded the reticular dermis have entered the vertical growth phase. They have metastatic potential. There are mitoses and nuclear pleomorphism. Cells fail to maturate as the tumor extends downward into the dermis. Clark level 3 and 4 tumors are usually in the vertical growth phase.

TUMOR THICKNESS (BRESLOW MICROSTAGE). Tumor thickness, as defined by the Breslow depth, is the most important histologic determinant of prognosis. The tumor is step-sectioned (Figure 22-44). The section with the deepest level of penetration of tumor is used to measure thickness. An ocular micrometer is placed on the microscope. The pathologist measures the thickness of the tumor in millimeters from the top of the granular cell layer (or base of superficial ulceration) to the deepest part of the tumor. The report is given as Breslow level, followed by the depth reported in millimeters.

ULCERATION. The presence of ulceration microscopically, defined as the loss of epidermis overlying the melanoma, is the next most important histologic determinant of patient prognosis and should be used to upstage patients with melanoma when present.

TUMOR THICKNESS (CLARK LEVEL). Clark levels measure tumor invasion anatomically. The tumor depth is reported by anatomic site (e.g., epidermis, depth in dermis) and assigned a Clark level of invasion (see Figure 22-44). Clark levels appear to affect prognosis only in thinner (<1-mm depth) melanomas.

PATHOLOGY REPORT. The pathologist determines the tumor thickness in millimeters (Breslow level) and presence of ulceration.

Reporting of other histologic features is encouraged: Clark level, growth phase, tumor infiltrating lymphocytes, mitotic rate, regression, angiolymphatic invasion, microsatellitosis, neurotropism, and histologic subtype.

MITOTIC RATE. The mitotic rate per square millimeter in the dermal part of the tumor is reported. Although ulceration is considered the most important prognostic factor after Breslow thickness for localized cutaneous melanoma, many studies have shown that mitotic rate is a significant prognostic factor.

TUMOR-INFILTRATING LYMPHOCYTES. Tumor-infiltrating lymphocytes are defined as brisk, nonbrisk, and absent. An infiltrative lymphocytic response may indicate favorable survival.

HISTOLOGIC REGRESSION. Areas of epidermis and dermis that have no recognizable tumor and are flanked by areas of melanoma indicate regression. Many studies have found regression to be associated with a worse prognosis and decreased survival. Regression is thought to be particularly important in thin melanomas. Extensive regression can be found in patients with thin (<1 mm) melanomas associated with metastases.

ANGIOLYMPHATIC INVASION AND ANGIOTROPISM. Vascular invasion in nodular melanomas is associated with tumor thickness, histologic diameter, ulceration, lymph node involvement, and distant metastases. Angiotropism is a prognostic factor that predicts risk of metastasis.

Special stains. The pathologist may use immunohistochemical staining for lineage (S-100, homatropine methylbromide 45) or proliferation markers (proliferating cell nuclear antigen, Ki67) in difficult cases.

Figure 22-44 To obtain the Breslow microstage, an ocular micrometer mounted on the microscope is used. Measurement is made from the granular cell layer to the section with the deepest penetration of tumor. When ulceration is present at the surface, measurement starts at the ulcer base.

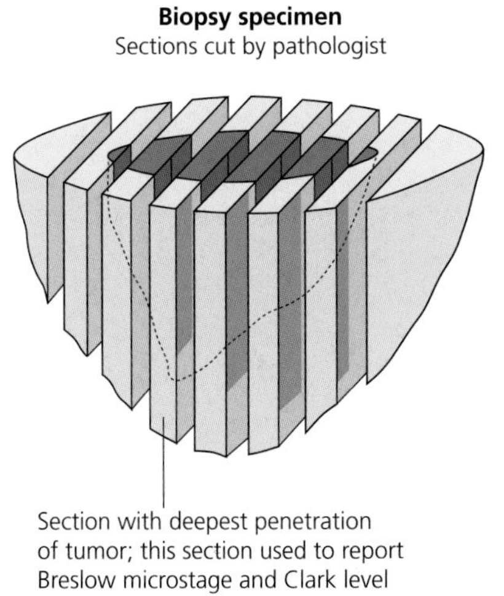

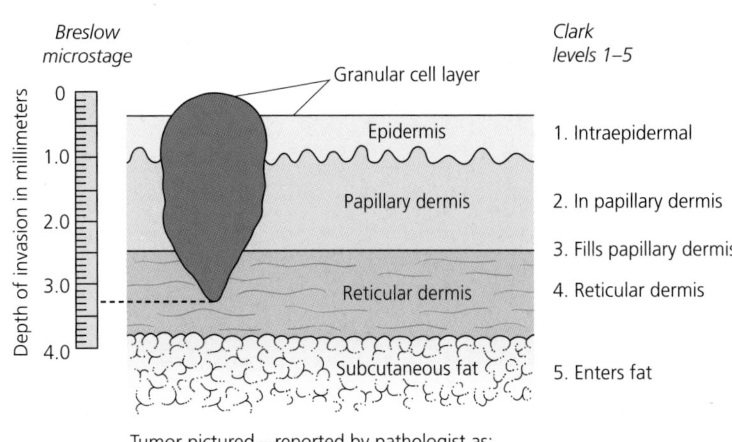

Surgical therapy

EXCISION AFTER BIOPSY (RESECTION MARGINS)

Complete surgical removal of the entire neoplasm must be accomplished with histologic verification of removal. Recommended surgical margins based on depth of the tumor (Breslow measurement) and diameter of the melanoma are listed in Table 22-4.

Compromises are necessary for lesions on the digits, head and neck, and face. Excising to deep fascia is not thought to be necessary for melanoma tumors confined to the upper levels of the skin. It does not improve local recurrence or survival rates. Wider cutaneous margins may be appropriate for large in situ tumors.

METASTATIC STAGING AND PROGNOSIS

The presence or absence of micrometastasis in the sentinel lymph node (SLN) is the most important prognostic factor for recurrence and the most powerful predictor of survival.

SENTINEL LYMPH NODE BIOPSY. The SLN is defined as the first node in the lymphatic basin that drains the lesion and is at the greatest risk for the development of metastasis. Although no survival benefit has been proven for the procedure, the staging information is useful in identifying patients who may benefit from further surgery or adjuvant therapy.

Indication. SLN biopsy is appropriate for melanomas deeper than 1.0 mm and for tumors 1 mm or less when histologic ulceration is present and/or classified as Clark level 4 or higher. The SLN biopsy is inappropriate for nonulcerated Clark level 2 or 3 melanomas 0.75 mm or less in depth and is uncertain in tumors 0.76 to 1.0 mm deep unless they are ulcerated or are Clark level 4 or higher.

Procedure. Preoperative radiographic mapping (lymphoscintigraphy) and vital blue dye injection around the primary melanoma or biopsy scar (at the time of wide local excision or reexcision) are performed to identify and remove the initial draining regional node(s). Some centers use technetium 99m-labeled radioisotope and a hand-held gamma probe. The sentinel node is examined for micrometastasis with histology and immunohistochemistry. A therapeutic lymph node dissection is performed if micrometastasis is present. Preceding diagnostic excisions of malignant melanoma with a maximum margin of 10 mm do not alter the lymphatic flow or interfere with accurately obtaining the SLN of the primary tumor.

There are several reasons to perform sentinel lymph node biopsy. It improves the accuracy of staging and provides valuable prognostic information to guide treatment decisions. It facilitates early therapeutic lymph node dissection for those patients with nodal metastases. SLN biopsy identifies patients who are candidates for adjuvant therapy with interferon alfa-2b and identifies homogeneous patient populations for entry into clinical trials of adjuvant therapy agents.

ELECTIVE LYMPH NODE DISSECTION. Patients with clinically enlarged lymph nodes and no evidence of distant disease should undergo a complete regional lymph node dissection. The value of elective lymph node dissection for other patients has not been defined. Randomized surgical trials fail to support a role for elective lymph node dissection in patients with clinically negative lymph nodes.

Initial diagnostic workup

Routine imaging studies including chest radiography and blood work have limited, if any, value in the initial workup of asymptomatic patients with primary cutaneous melanoma 4 mm or less in thickness. On the other hand, negative results may alleviate patient anxiety. Indications for initial imaging studies and blood work are most appropriately directed based on findings from a thorough medical history and thorough physical examination (Table 22-8).

STAGING AND PROGNOSIS

The melanoma staging criteria were updated with the publication of the 6th edition of the *AJCC Cancer Staging Manual* in 2002. Tables 22-5 and 22-6 describe the stages of melanoma and the median survival associated with each stage.

The AJCC staging criteria for melanoma are divided into four stages. Localized melanoma is classified under stage I and stage II. Stage III melanoma includes regional metastases, and stage IV distant metastases. Each stage uses the TNM (tumor, node, metastasis) classifications when determining stage of disease.

The histologic evaluation of melanoma provides critical staging information. The depth of invasion (Breslow level expressed in millimeters) is the most important histologic prognostic parameter in evaluating the primary tumor. The American Joint Committee on Cancer (AJCC) Melanoma Staging Committee studied 17,600 melanomas. Results of this evidence-based study were incorporated into the 2002 AJCC melanoma TNM staging classification. The 2002 AJCC staging system incorporates Breslow depth, Clark level, and ulceration. Tumor thickness and ulceration were the most powerful predictors of survival. The level of invasion (Clark level) had significance only in thin (≤1.0 mm) melanomas.

Staging for localized melanoma: Stages I and II

MELANOMA THICKNESS

The primary criteria for the T classification are tumor thickness (measured in millimeters) and the presence or absence of ulceration (determined histopathologically). Ten-year survival rates for each of the T categories in clinically staged patients are shown in Table 22-7. Stage groupings are used to determine follow-up examination intervals (Table 22-8). The sole difference in the definitions of clinical versus pathologic stage grouping is whether the regional lymph nodes are staged by clinical/radiologic examination or by pathologic examination (after partial or complete lymphadenectomy).

ULCERATION

Melanoma ulceration is defined as the absence of an intact epidermis overlying a major portion of the primary melanoma based on microscopic examination of the histologic sections. Melanoma ulceration heralds such a high risk for metastases that its presence upstages the prognosis of all such patients compared with patients who have melanomas of equivalent thickness without ulceration. Survival rates for patients with an ulcerated melanoma are proportionately lower than those for patients with a nonulcerated melanoma of equivalent T category but are similar to those of patients with a nonulcerated melanoma of the next highest T category.

PATHOLOGIC STAGING OF LYMPH NODES

The number of lymph nodes is the most important feature, followed by the tumor burden within the lymph node. If 1 node is involved, the classification is N1; if 2 to 3 nodes are involved, the classification is N2; and if 4 or more metastatic nodes, matted nodes, or in-transit metastases or satellites with metastatic node(s) are involved, the classification is N3.

Lymph nodes with disease identified by immunostains only and not seen with hematoxylin-eosin staining are considered N0. A special designation of N0 (immunohistochemically positive) is used.

MELANOMA—CLASSIFICATION AND STAGING

Table 22-4 Surgical Management of Melanoma

Tumor thickness (mm)	Radius of excision (cm)	Options for lymph nodes
In situ	0.3-0.5	Observation
<1.0	1	Selective sentinel lymph node biopsy, observation
1.1-2.0	1-2	Sentinel lymph node biopsy, observation
2.1-4.0	2	Elective lymph node dissection
>4.0	2	Sentinel lymph node biopsy, observation, elective lymph node dissection

From *Surg Clin North Am* 83(2):385-403, 2003. *PMID: 12744615*

Table 22-5 TNM Classification for Melanoma: American Joint Committee on Cancer, 2002

T classification	Thickness (mm)	Ulceration status
T1	1.0	a: without ulceration and level II/III b: with ulceration or level IV/V
T2	1.01–2.0	a: without ulceration b: with ulceration
T3	2.01–4.0	a: without ulceration b: with ulceration
T4	>4.0 mm	a: without ulceration b: with ulceration
N classification	**No. of metastatic nodes**	**Nodal metastatic mass**
N1	1	a: micrometastasis* b: macrometastasis†
N2	2–3	a: micrometastasis b: macrometastasis c: in-transit met(s)/satellite(s) without metastatic nodes
N3	4 or more metastatic nodes, or matted nodes, or in-transit metastasis/satellite(s) with metastatic node(s)	
M classification	**Site of metastasis**	**Serum lactate dehydrogenase (LDH) level**
M1a	Distant skin, subcutaneous, or nodal metastases	Normal LDH
M1b	Lung metastases	Normal LDH
M1c	All other visceral metastases Any distant metastasis	Normal LDH Elevated LDH

From *J Clin Oncol* 19(16):3635-3648, 2001; Final Version of the American Joint Committee on Cancer Staging System for Cutaneous Melanoma. *PMID: 11504745*

*Micrometastases are diagnosed after sentinel or elective lymphadenectomy.

†Macrometastases are defined as clinically detectable nodal metastases confirmed by therapeutic lymphadenectomy or when nodal metastasis exhibits gross extracapsular extension.

MELANOMA—CLASSIFICATION AND STAGING

Table 22-6 Melanoma Stage Definitions from Edition 6 of AJCC Cancer Staging Manual, 2002

Stage	Classification	Definition
Stage I: Stage I cancer is diagnosed in patients who have primary lesions that are 1 mm or less in thickness with no evidence of metastasis.		
Stage IA	T1a N0 M0	Primary lesions are 1 mm or less in thickness with no ulceration and do not invade reticular dermis or subcutaneous fat (Clark level <IV or V).
Stage IB	T1b or T2a N0 M0	Primary lesions are 1 mm or less in thickness and have ulceration or invasion to Clark level IV or V (T1b) or patients whose primary lesions are 1.01–2.0 mm in thickness without ulceration.
Stage II: Stage II cancer is diagnosed in patients who have thicker primary lesions, without evidence of metastasis.		
Stage IIA	T2b or T3a N0 M0	Primary lesions are 1.01–2.00 mm thick and have ulceration (T2b) or patients whose primary lesions are 2.01–4.00 mm thick without ulceration (T3a).
Stage IIB	T3b or T4a N0 M0	Primary lesions are 2.01–4.00 mm thick and have ulceration (T3b) or patients whose primary lesions are more than 4.00 mm thick without ulceration (T4a).
Stage IIC	T4b N0 M0	Primary lesions are more than 4.0 mm thick and have ulceration.
Stage III: Stage III cancer is diagnosed when the melanoma spreads to the regional lymph nodes and/or an in-transit or satellite metastasis is present.		
Stage IIIA	T1-4a N1a or N2a M0	Primary lesions are of any depth without ulceration and 1 to 3 nodes are involved with microscopic disease as discovered after a sentinel or elective lymphadenectomy.
Stage IIIB	T1-4b N1a or N2a M0, T1-4a N1b or N2b M0, or T1-4a/b N2c M0	Primary lesions are of any depth with ulceration and 1 to 3 nodes are involved with microscopic disease. ***or*** Patients whose primary lesions are of any depth without ulceration and who have 1 to 3 nodes involved with macroscopic disease as discovered on clinical examination and confirmed by therapeutic lymphadenectomy or when nodal metastasis displays gross extracapsular extension. ***or*** Patients whose primary lesions are of any depth with or without ulceration and who have in-transit or satellite metastasis without the presence of metastatic lymph nodes.
Stage IIIC	T1-4b N1b M0, T1-4b N2b M0, or any T N3 M0	Primary lesions are of any depth with ulceration and 1 to 3 lymph nodes are macroscopically involved (N1b or N2b). ***or*** Patients with any depth of tumor with or without ulceration and 4 or more metastatic nodes, matted nodes, or in-transit or satellite metastasis with the presence of metastatic node(s) (N3).
Stage IV: Stage IV cancer is diagnosed when the melanoma spreads to distant sites, including the skin, subcutaneous tissue, lymph nodes, and organs. The three levels of division of stage IV disease are based on the M status.		
M1a	(any T, N)	Any depth of tumor, with or without ulceration, with or without nodal involvement, and with distant metastasis limited to distant skin, subcutaneous tissue, or lymph nodes and a normal lactate dehydrogenase (LDH) level.
M1b	(any T, N)	Includes patients with these same criteria but who also have metastasis to the lungs and a normal LDH level.
M1c	(any T, N)	Includes patients with these same criteria but who also have metastasis to any other visceral sites and a normal LDH level or any patient with distant metastasis regardless of the site but with an elevated LDH level.

MELANOMA—CLASSIFICATION AND STAGING

Table 22-7 Survival Rates for Melanoma TNM and Staging Categories

Pathologic stage	TNM	Thickness (mm)	Ulceration	No. + nodes	Nodal size	Distant metastasis	SURVIVAL (%)			
							1-year	2-year	5-year	10-year
IA	T1a	1	No	0	—	—	99.7	99.0	95.3	87.9
IB	T1b	1	Yes or level IV, V	0	—	—	99.8	98.7	90.9	83.1
	T2a	1.01–2.0	No	0	—	—	99.5	97.3	89.0	79.2
IIA	T2b	1.01–2.0	Yes	0	—	—	98.2	92.9	77.4	64.4
	T3a	2.01–4.0	No	0	—	—	98.7	94.3	78.7	63.8
IIB	T3b	2.01–4.0	Yes	0	—	—	95.1	84.8	63.0	50.8
	T4a	>4.0	No	0	—	—	94.8	88.6	67.4	53.9
IIC	T4b	>4.0	Yes	0	—	—	89.9	70.7	45.1	32.3
IIIA	N1a	Any	No	1	Micro	—	95.9	88.0	69.5	63.0
	N2a	Any	No	2-3	Micro	—	93.0	82.7	63.3	56.9
IIIB	N1a	Any	Yes	1	Micro	—	93.3	75.0	52.8	37.8
	N2a	Any	Yes	2-3	Micro	—	92.0	81.0	49.6	35.9
	N1b	Any	No	1	Macro	—	88.5	78.5	59.0	47.7
	N2b	Any	No	2-3	Macro	—	76.8	65.6	46.3	39.2
IIIC	N1b	Any	Yes	1	Macro	—	77.9	54.2	29.0	24.4
	N2b	Any	Yes	2-3	Macro	—	74.3	44.1	24.0	15.0
	N3	Any	Any	4	Micro/ macro	—	71.0	49.8	26.7	18.4
IV	M1a	Any	Any	Any	Any	Skin, Sub-Q	59.3	36.7	18.8	15.7
	M1b	Any	Any	Any	Any	Lung	57.0	23.1	6.7	2.5
	M1c	Any	Any	Any	Any	Other visceral	40.6	23.6	9.5	6.0

From Balch CM: *J Clin Oncol* 19:3635, 2001.

Table 22-8 Follow-up Guidelines

Breslow depth (mm)	History and physical examination	Chest radiography (CXR)/laboratory studies
Stage I (A and B)	Every 3-4 mo for year 1, every 6 mo for year 2, and yearly thereafter up to year 5; yearly thereafter as clinically indicated	No
Stage II (A, B, C)	Every 3-4 mo for years 1-3, every 6 months for years 4 and 5, and yearly thereafter as clinically indicated	CBC, chemistry panel, and LDH
Stage III (A, B, and C)	Every 3-4 mo for years 1-3, every 6 mo for years 4 and 5, and yearly thereafter as clinically indicated	CBC, chemistry panel, LDH; imaging studies, as indicated
Stage IV	Every 3-4 mo	CBC, chemistry panel, LDH; imaging studies, as indicated

CBC, Complete blood count; *LDH,* lactate dehydrogenase.

Follow-up examinations

Follow patients to detect asymptomatic metastases and additional primary melanomas. Demonstrate self-examination of skin and lymph nodes. Routine physician examinations are performed at least annually. History and physical examination directs the need for laboratory tests and imaging studies.

An overview of the management of melanoma is shown in Figure 22-45.

Follow-up intervals

Patients with thicker tumors have elevated risk of recurrence in the early years after diagnosis and need to be followed more frequently (see Table 22-8).

Recurrence may develop after 10 years or more of a patient being disease free. Late recurrence may be local, and survival subsequent to treatment of these metastases is often protracted. Therefore patients with cutaneous melanoma should be observed for life.

Medical treatment

Adjuvant high-dose interferon-alfa produces increases in relapse-free survival rates and overall survival rates in selected patients (stages IIB, IIC, IIIA, IIIB, IIIC). Interferon alfa-2b therapy is used for patients with regional nodal and/or in-transit metastasis and for node-negative patients with primary melanomas deeper than 4 mm. The use of interferon alfa-2b therapy is uncertain in patients with ulcerated intermediate primary tumors (2.01 to 4.0 mm in depth) and inappropriate for node-negative patients with nonulcerated tumors less than 4.0 mm deep. Vaccines and biologic response modifiers show promise in prolonging survival.

TREATMENT OF LENTIGO MALIGNA

Lentigo maligna is found predominantly in areas of actinic damage where cosmetically unsatisfactory scars may result from conventional surgery. Cryosurgery is an efficient alternative to conventional surgery provided that patients are selected properly and extension of cryonecrosis is monitored. Several case reports and studies suggest that lentigo maligna responds to 5% imiquimod cream (Aldara).

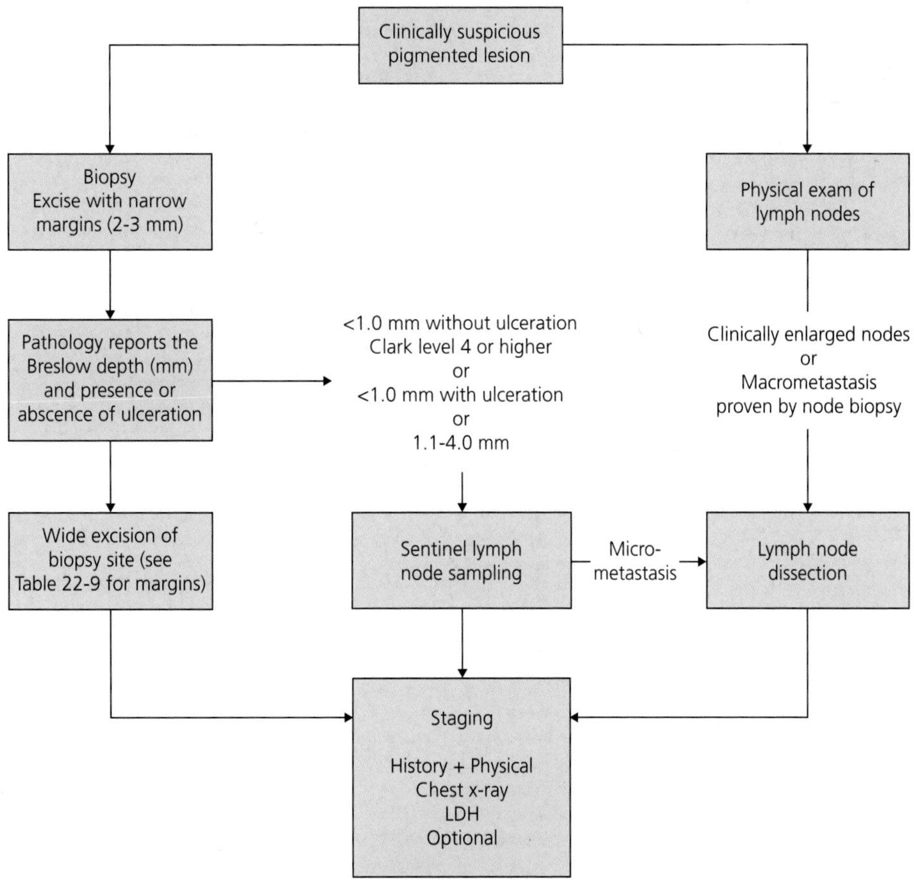

Figure 22-45

DERMOSCOPY

Dermoscopy (epiluminescent microscopy, magnified oil immersion diascopy) is a technique used to see a variety of patterns and structures in lesions that are not discernible to the naked eye (www.dermoscopy.org). Lotion or mineral oil may be applied to the surface of the lesion to make the epidermis more transparent. Examination with a 10× ocular micrometer, a microscope ocular eyepiece (held upside down), or a dermoscope (Figure 22-46) (available from surgical supply houses) reveals several features that are helpful in differentiating between benign and malignant pigmented lesions. The DermLite and DermoGenius are highly accurate oil-free pocket epiluminescent microscopes. A clear and deep view into pigmented lesions can be made in seconds with these instruments. Many lesions can be examined in a short time. Dermoscopy provides additional criteria for the diagnosis of melanoma.

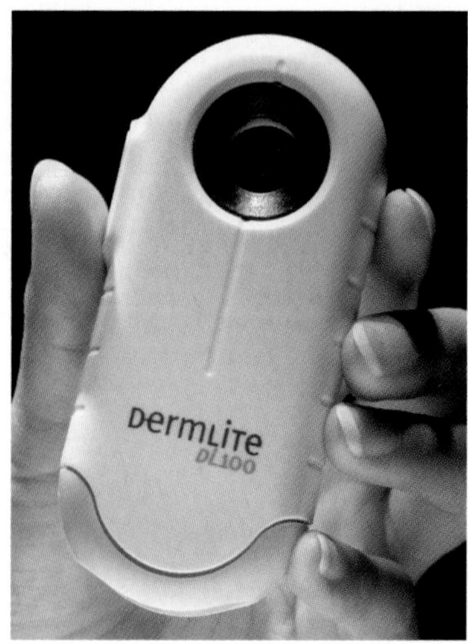

Figure 22-46 Dermoscope.

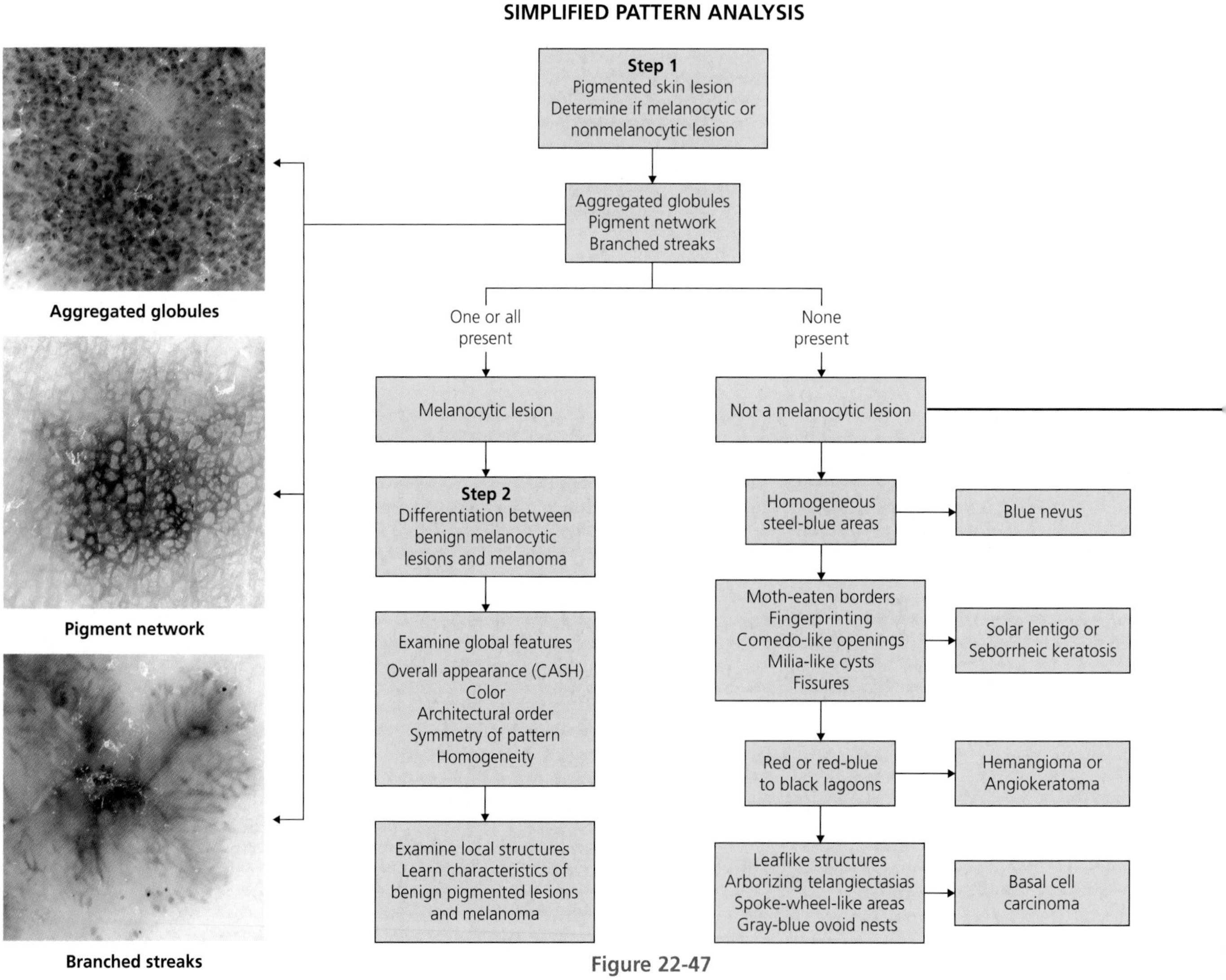

SIMPLIFIED PATTERN ANALYSIS

Step 1
Pigmented skin lesion
Determine if melanocytic or nonmelanocytic lesion

Aggregated globules
Pigment network
Branched streaks

One or all present → Melanocytic lesion

Step 2
Differentiation between benign melanocytic lesions and melanoma

Examine global features
Overall appearance (CASH)
Color
Architectural order
Symmetry of pattern
Homogeneity

Examine local structures
Learn characteristics of benign pigmented lesions and melanoma

None present → Not a melanocytic lesion

Homogeneous steel-blue areas → Blue nevus

Moth-eaten borders
Fingerprinting
Comedo-like openings
Milia-like cysts
Fissures → Solar lentigo or Seborrheic keratosis

Red or red-blue to black lagoons → Hemangioma or Angiokeratoma

Leaflike structures
Arborizing telangiectasias
Spoke-wheel-like areas
Gray-blue ovoid nests → Basal cell carcinoma

Aggregated globules

Pigment network

Branched streaks

Figure 22-47

DERMOSCOPIC CHARACTERISTICS OF BENIGN AND MALIGNANT MELANOCYTIC LESIONS. A standardized terminology for dermoscopy patterns was established in 1989. A number of diagnostic methods using these criteria have been devised. Pattern analysis is based on the assessment of numerous individual criteria. A simplified Pattern Analysis method is accurate and easy to learn and is felt to be more accurate than other simplified methods.

SIMPLIFIED PATTERN ANALYSIS

There are two steps in the process of pattern analysis (Figure 22-47). The first step is to decide whether the lesion is melanocytic or nonmelanocytic. Determine if aggregated globules, a pigment network, or branched streaks are present. If present the lesion is melanocytic (e.g., nevus, melanoma). If not look for structures characteristic of nonmelanocytic lesions. Learn characteristics of global features of pigmented lesions (Figure 22-48) and local structures of benign pigmented lesions and melanoma to make a diagnosis.

See Figures 22-47 and 22-48 along with Tables 22-9 to 22-15 for a thorough path to dermoscopy analysis.

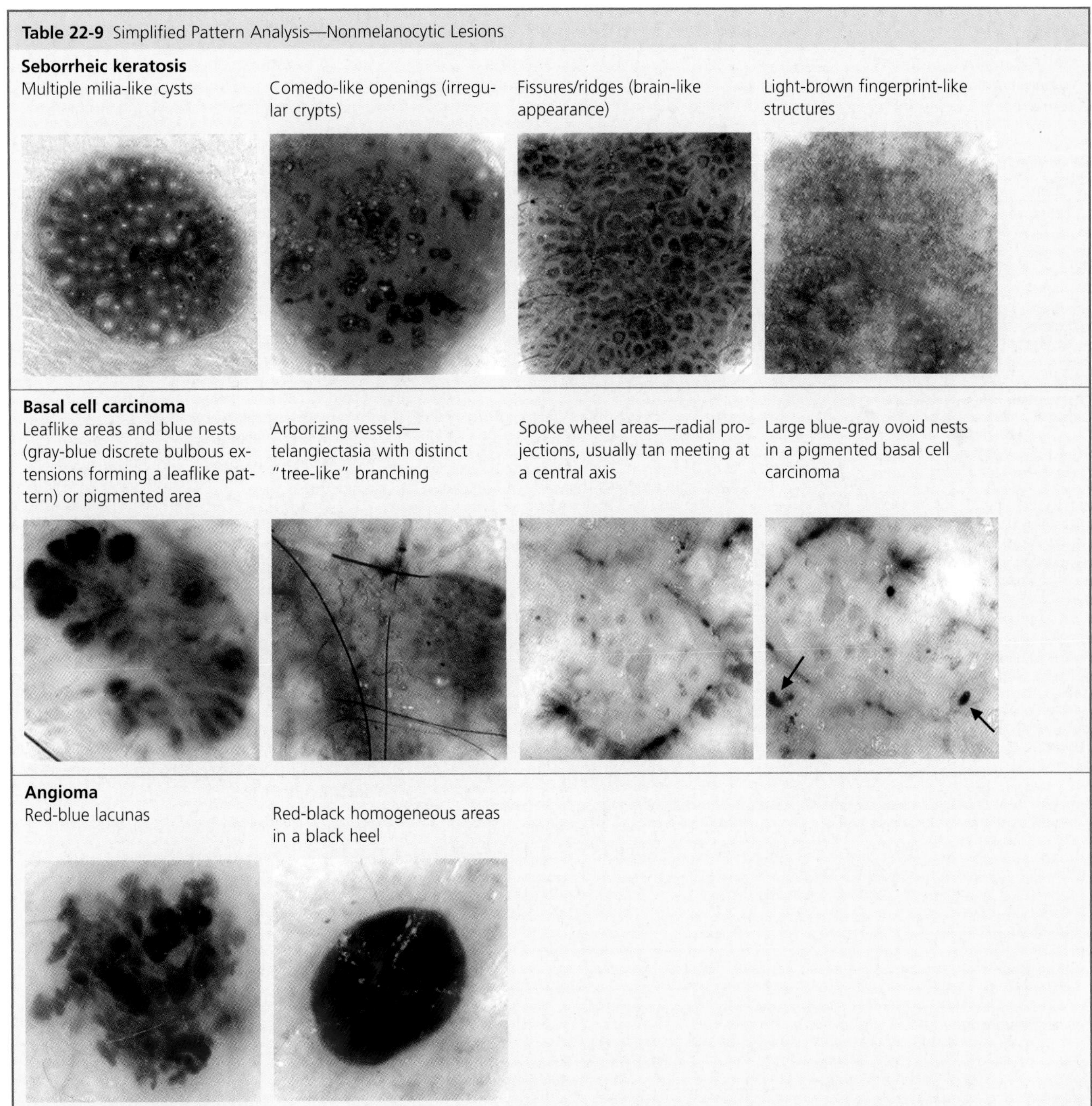

Table 22-9 Simplified Pattern Analysis—Nonmelanocytic Lesions

Seborrheic keratosis			
Multiple milia-like cysts	Comedo-like openings (irregular crypts)	Fissures/ridges (brain-like appearance)	Light-brown fingerprint-like structures
Basal cell carcinoma			
Leaflike areas and blue nests (gray-blue discrete bulbous extensions forming a leaflike pattern) or pigmented area	Arborizing vessels—telangiectasia with distinct "tree-like" branching	Spoke wheel areas—radial projections, usually tan meeting at a central axis	Large blue-gray ovoid nests in a pigmented basal cell carcinoma
Angioma			
Red-blue lacunas	Red-black homogeneous areas in a black heel		

Courtesy www.Dermoscopy.org.

DERMATOSCOPIC CHARACTERISTICS OF BENIGN PIGMENTED LESIONS. The dermatoscopic characteristics of benign melanocytic nevi are described in Table 22-10, and an example is shown in Figure 22-48.

THE PIGMENT NETWORK

The presence of a pigment network usually implies that the lesion is melanocytic. The pattern may be subtle or present only in a small area. The network of common lesions such as lentigo and junctional nevi fades and thins at the

Table 22-10 Dermoscopic Characteristics of Benign Pigmented Lesions

Lesion	History	Clinical presentation	Dermoscopy
Congenital melanocytic nevi	Present at birth or shortly after. Change over time; may enlarge and develop more hairs and new nodules.	Brown or black, smooth or pebbled texture, tan and dark, speckled background, increased terminal hairs	Globular or homogenous pattern. Globules of varying shapes, sizes, and numbers. Globules may have a dense "cobblestone" arrangement. There may be no pigment network. Milia-like cysts may be seen.
Melanocytic nevi (junctional nevi, compound nevi, dermal nevi)	Acquired in early childhood. Increase in number and size. Regress after third decade.	Begin as brown macules and can progress to dome-shaped, cerebriform, or pedunculated papules	Most have one or more of the following features: a network, globules, dots, streaks, and structureless areas. Structures usually are regular in shape and size and have a uniform distribution.
Junctional nevi	Become thicker during adolescence. Usually change color and sometimes develop hair.	Macular, light to dark brown, symmetric, and smoothly textured; center darker than periphery	Honeycomb-like network pattern—uniform and homogeneous distribution. Network often prominent in center and fades toward edges. Network in center is often obscured by heavy pigmentation. Small black dots and globules may be present.
Compound nevi	Become thicker during adolescence. Change color and sometimes develop hair.	Slightly raised or papillomatous; uniformly light to dark brown	Network pattern is less prominent. Central pigmentation is less intense. Globules (distributed uniformly) may be present. Large globules may form a cobblestone pattern.
Dermal nevi		Smooth or papillomatous surface; elevated, dome-shaped, sessile, or pedunculated papules or nodules that are light brown	No network or black dots. Red dots and lines correspond to dilated blood vessels. A few globules may be present. Globules may be angulated.
Spitz nevi	Mostly seen in children. Firm, round, 2- to 8-mm papules. Face is most common location.	Smooth, dome-shaped, variable telangiectases, and uniform color (usually pink or tan to dark brown)	1. Starburst pattern (50% of cases)—black-blue-whitish structureless center surrounded by a thickened network that ends abruptly at periphery. Pigmented streaks radiate from periphery. This resembles a bursting star. 2. Globular pattern (25% of cases)—uniform distribution of globules and dots throughout or globules at periphery surrounding a brown to blue-gray center.
Blue nevi		Dome-shaped papules; diffuse slate-gray to blue	Blue pigmentation distributed throughout. No globules, dots, or network (because pigment is located in dermis).
Halo nevi	Several may be present. Central nevus may disappear. Eventually halo may disappear.	Zone of hypopigmentation around melanocytic neoplasm	Central nevus is light-brown and structureless. Occasional dots and globules.
Lentigines and ephelides			Pigment networks, usually with relatively thin and lightly pigmented network lines.
"Ink spot" lentigines			Have a dark (nearly black) network that is irregular, with marked variation in line thickness.
Dermatofibromas			Usually have a flat ring of lightly pigmented network around a central hypopigmented papule.

Adapted from Rao BK, Wang SQ, Murphy FP: *Derm Clin* 19:269, 2001.

DERMOSCOPIC VIEWS OF NEVI

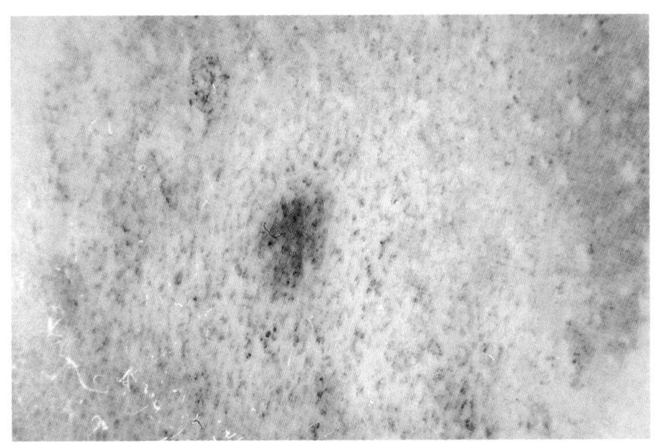

Congenital nevus

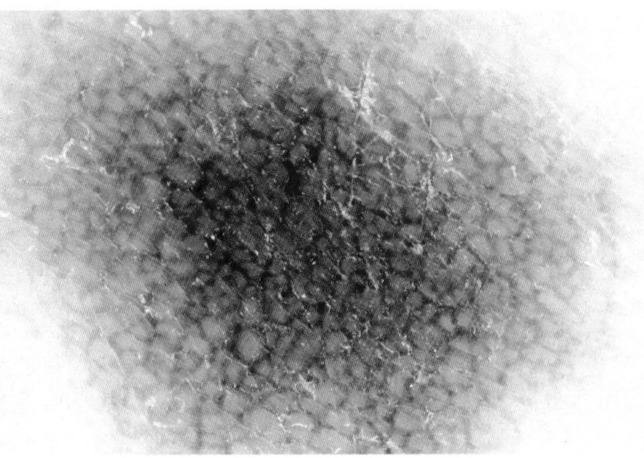

Junctional nevus

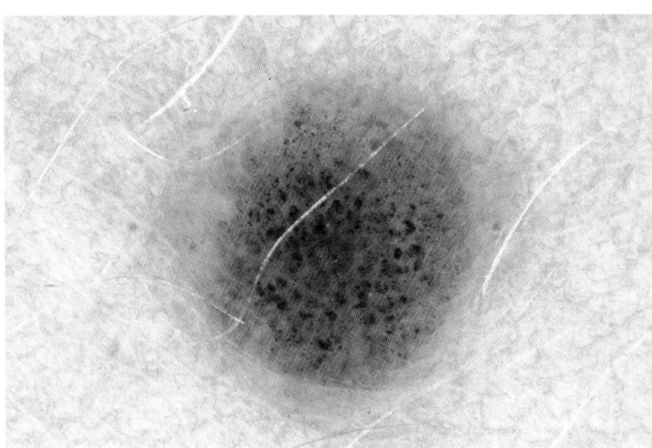

Compound nevus

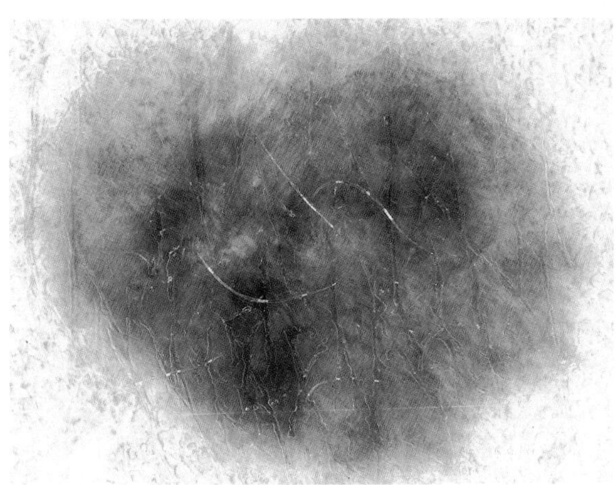

Blue nevus

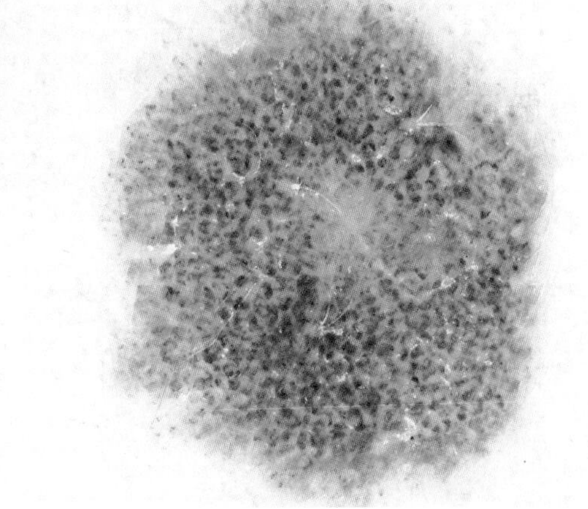

Halo nevus

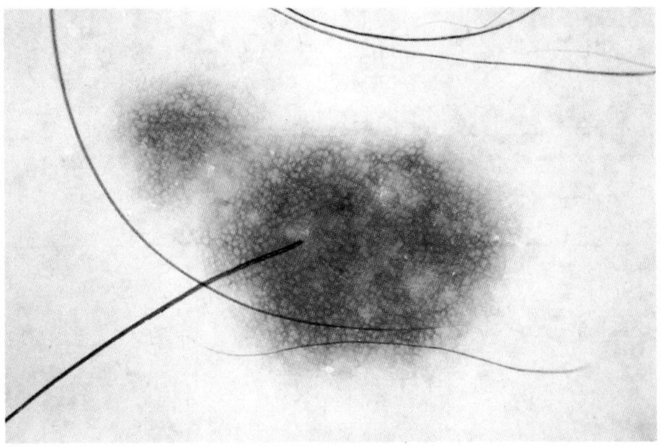

Lentigo

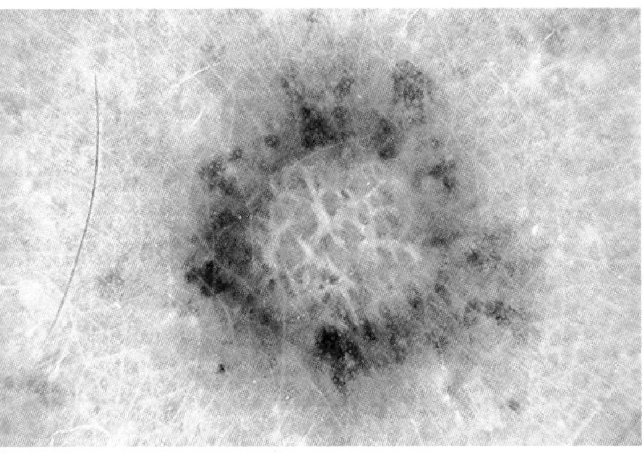

Dermatofibroma

Figure 22-48

Table 22-11 Diagnostic Criteria for Pattern Analysis

Diagnosis	Global patterns	Specific local features	Additional local features	Confounding features
Melanoma	Multicomponent, reticular, globular, parallel-ridge, unspecific	Atypical pigment network, irregular dots/globules, irregular streaks, blue-whitish veil, irregular pigmentation, regression structures, dotted or linear irregular vessels	Hypopigmented areas, hairpin vessels, red globules	Homogeneous or starburst pattern; typical pigment network, regular dots/globules, regular streaks, milia-like cysts
Clark nevus	Reticular, globular, homogeneous	Typical pigment network, regular dots/globules, regular diffuse or localized pigmentation, hypopigmented areas	Regular streaks, regression structures	Multicomponent pattern; atypical pigment network, irregular dots/globules, irregular streaks, irregular pigmentation, dotted vessels
Unna's and Miescher's nevi	Globular, cobblestone, reticular, homogeneous, unspecific	Regular dots/globules, exophytic papillary structures, typical pseudonetwork, comma vessels	Comedo-like openings, milia-like cysts	Multicomponent pattern; irregular pigmentation
Reed and Spitz nevi	Starburst, globular, multicomponent	Regular streaks, regular diffuse pigmentation, reticular blue-whitish veil, regular dots/globules	Dotted vessels, typical pigment network	Reticular pattern; atypical pigment network, irregular dots/globules, irregular streaks, irregular pigmentation
Recurrent nevus	Multicomponent, homogeneous, unspecific	Irregular pigmentation, irregular streaks, white areas	Atypical pigment network, irregular dots/globules	All local features mentioned in this row are commonly found in melanoma
Blue nevus	Homogeneous	Regular diffuse pigmentation	Hypopigmented areas	Irregular diffuse pigmentation, arborizing vessels
Congenital nevus	Multicomponent, cobblestone, globular, reticular	Regular dots/globules, typical pigment network, localized multifocal hypopigmentation, regular pigmentation	Milia-like cysts, comedo-like openings, exophytic papillary structures	Localized irregular pigmentation, regression structures
Combined nevus	Multicomponent, homogeneous, globular, reticular	Typical pigment network, regular dots/globules, localized regular pigmentation	Hypopigmented areas, exophytic papillary structures	Atypical pigment network, localized or diffuse irregular pigmentation
Lentigo	Reticular	Typical pigment network or pseudonetwork, regular diffuse pigmentation	Milia-like cysts, regular dots/globules	Atypical pigment network, irregular pigmentation
Labial and genital melanosis	Unspecific, parallel	Regular diffuse pigmentation, typical pigment network	Regular streaks	Atypical pigment network, irregular pigmentation
Basal cell carcinoma	Unspecific, multicomponent, globular	Leaflike areas, irregular blue-gray dots/globules, arborizing vessels	Milia-like cysts, hairpin vessels	Irregular gray-bluish pigmentation
Seborrheic keratosis	Unspecific, globular, reticular, homogeneous	Milia-like cysts, comedo-like openings, exophytic papillary structures, regular diffuse pigmentation, hairpin vessels	Typical pigment network, hypopigmented areas, dotted vessels, gyri and sulci, whitish-yellowish horn masses	Multicomponent pattern; irregular pigmentation, regression structures, irregular dots/globules
Vascular lesions	Lacunar, globular, homogeneous	Red lacunas, diffuse or localized structureless reddish-black to reddish-blue pigmentation	Parallel pattern, regular dots/globules, whitish-yellowish keratotic areas	Multicomponent pattern; irregular dots/globules, whitish veil
Dermatofibroma	Reticular, unspecific, multicomponent	Annular pigment network, central white patch	Localized pigmentation or crusting, regular dots/globules, erythema	Irregular white areas

Adapted from: www.dermoscopy.org and *Derm Clin* 19:269, 2001.

Table 22-12 Patterns Seen with Dermoscopy

Pattern	Diagnostic significance	Histology
Reticulated pattern or brown pigment "network"	Network of brownish lines over a tan background	Pigment in epidermal basal cells; it is regular or irregular, narrow or wide
Diffuse pigmentation or blotches	Irregularly shaped, dark brown or black areas of pigmentation of various sizes; some resemble "ink spots"	Areas where there is melanin in all levels of epidermis and/or upper dermis
Brown globules	Circular to oval pigmented structures	Nests of melanocytes or melanophages at dermoepidermal junction or in upper dermis
Black dots	Sharply circumscribed and round; various sizes but often very small	Focal collection of melanin in stratum corneum
Depigmented or hypopigmented areas	Zones of relatively lighter pigmentation	Patchy areas of epidermis that contain less melanin or a relatively thinned epidermis where telangiectasias are often noticeable
White areas	These areas have no pigment; areas of "regression" in melanomas	Zones with no melanin in epidermis and dermis; areas of fibroplasia and telangiectasias
Gray-blue areas	Irregular, confluent, gray-blue to whitish blue diffuse pigmentation	Fibrosis and melanophages or melanocytes of midreticular dermis location; melanin in deeper dermis causes blue hue
Radial streaming pseudopods	Linear brown to black streaks radiate from border of a pigmented lesion into surrounding skin; also seen in central areas of lightly pigmented melanomas; pseudopods are curved extensions	Radially arranged nests; confluent pigmented junctional nests at periphery
Milia-like cysts (pseudocysts)	White or black round structures imbedded in a seborrheic keratosis or papillomatous dermal nevus	Intraepidermal horn globules underneath surface
Comedo-like openings	White or black round structures protruding from surface of a seborrheic keratosis or papillomatous dermal nevus	Intraepidermal horn globules reaching surface; keratin plugs in adnexal ostia
Telangiectasia	Short red hairlike strands	Dilated vessels in papillary dermis
Red-blue areas	Red round globules	Dilated vascular spaces in papillary dermis in hemangiomas or angiokeratoma
Leaflike areas	Flecks of pigment in a pearly white papule	Pigmented clusters in a basal cell carcinoma
Central white scarlike patch + delicate pigment network at periphery	Dermatofibroma	Epidermal hyperplasia and pigment in basal layer

Adapted from Bahmer F et al: *J Am Acad Dermatol* 23:1159, 1990.

periphery. The typical honeycomb-like pattern of the pigment network on the trunk and proximal extremities results from pigmentation along the rete ridges. The pseudonetwork patterns on the face, palms, and soles result from junctional pigment outlining hair follicles, sebaceous glands, and eccrine ducts. Pigment on the palms and soles outlines linear skin markings along or across the skin furrows, resulting in a parallel, lattice, or fibrillar pattern. Growing melanomas distort the normal skin anatomy and cause variation in pigmentation patterns and structures. Networks in melanomas are variable. Thin melanomas and melanomas in situ may have only very subtle pigmentation changes. Subtle thickening and darkening of pigment network lines may be seen near the periphery in early lesions. As Breslow thickness increases, the pigment network tends to become more variable in thickness and color density. The lines become thick and dark. They also become darker near the periphery. These result from wide and shallow pigmented rete ridges. Pseudopods and radial streaming occur at the edge of a region of thickened, darkened network at the periphery.

Many lesions will lack classic dermoscopy features of melanoma. This ill-defined group of possible early melanomas will include many atypical nevi. Clinical judgment using all available information must be used to make the decision to excise or observe. Total number of lesions, history of melanoma, family history, body site, and surgical morbidity such as scarring are factors to consider before making the final management decision.

Table 22-13 Melanoma-Specific Dermoscopic Criteria for Pattern Analysis

	Definition	Histopathologic correlates
Atypical pigment network 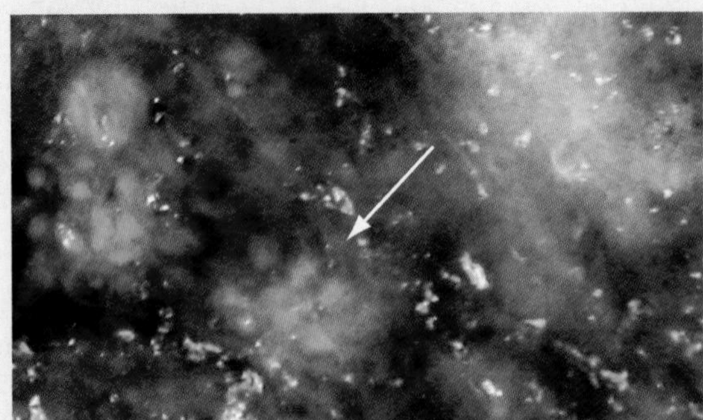	Black, brown, or gray network with irregular meshes and thick lines	Irregular and broadened rete ridges
Blue-whitish veil 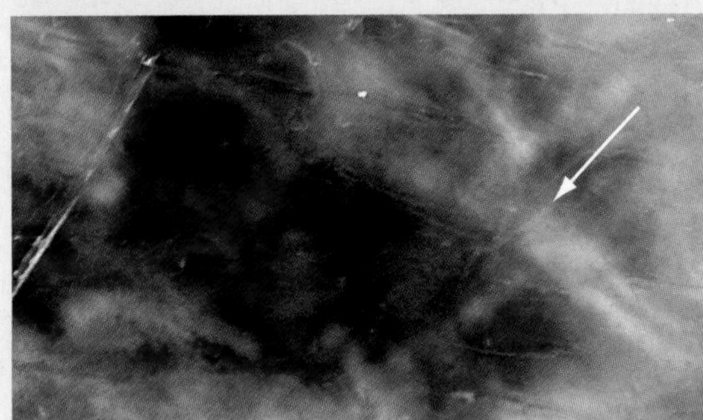	Irregular, confluent, gray-blue to whitish-blue diffuse pigmentation	Acanthotic epidermis with focal hypergranulosis above sheets of heavily pigmented melanocytes in the dermis
Atypical vascular pattern 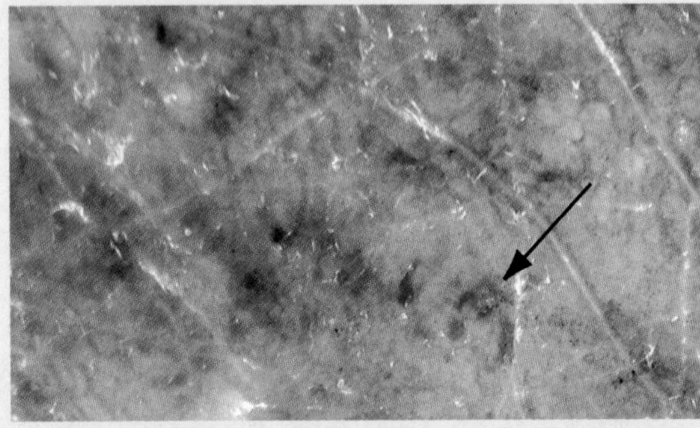	Linear-irregular or dotted vessels not clearly combined with regression structures	Neovascularization
Irregular streaks 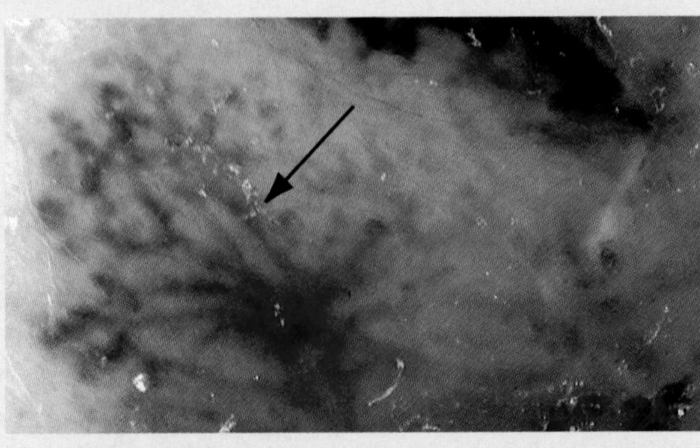	Irregular, more or less confluent, linear structures not clearly combined with pigment network lines	Confluent junctional nests of melanocytes

Adapted from Argenziano G et al: *Arch Dermatol* 134:1563, 1998; Consensus Net Meeting on Dermoscopy (CNMD), 2000 (under the auspices of the European Society of Dermato-Oncology). *PMID: 9875194*

Table 22-13 Melanoma-Specific Dermoscopic Criteria for Pattern Analysis—cont'd

	Definition	Histopathologic correlates
Irregular pigmentation 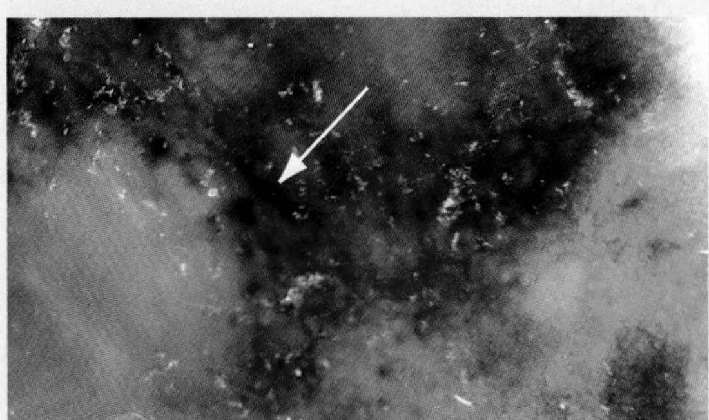	Black, brown, and/or gray pigmented areas with irregular shapes and distribution	Atypical melanocytes and melanin throughout the epidermis and/or upper dermis
Irregular dots/globules 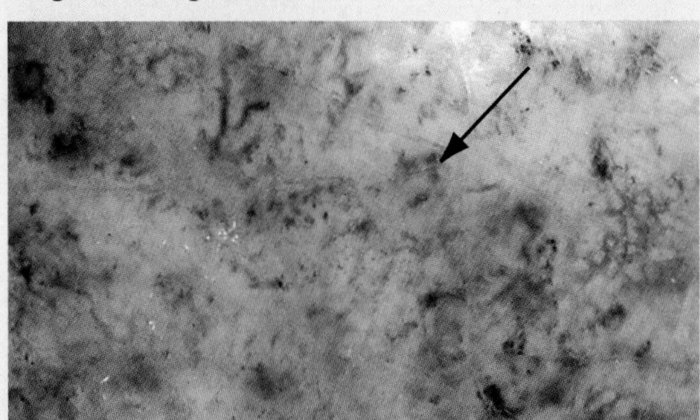	Black/brown, and/or gray round-to-oval, variously sized structures irregularly distributed within the lesion	Pigment aggregates within stratum corneum, epidermis, dermoepidermal junction, or papillary dermis
Regression structures 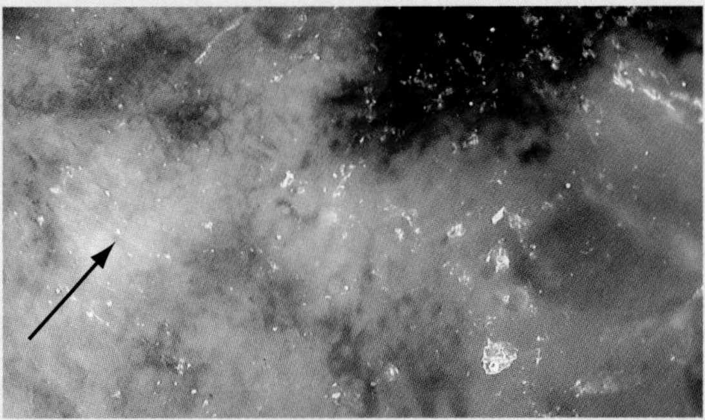	White areas (white scarlike areas) and blue areas (gray-blue dots) may be associated, thus featuring "blue-whitish" areas virtually indistinguishable from blue-whitish veil	Thickened papillary dermis with fibrosis and/or variable amounts of melanophages
Light brown structureless areas 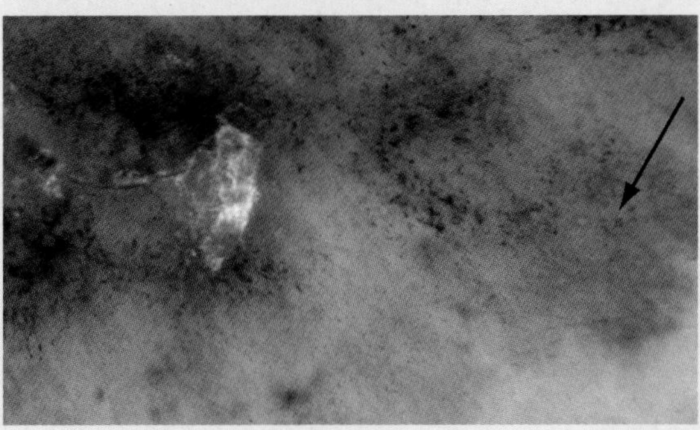	Structureless light brown to fawn-colored, peripherally arranged areas of variable size and shape that are larger than 10% of a lesion. The structureless areas tend to end abruptly at the edge of a lesion. These areas are found at periphery of thin melanoma.	Flattening of rete ridges and marked scattering of atypical melanocytes in upper epidermal layers in the absence of significant dermal changes

DERMOSCOPIC CLASSIFICATION OF ATYPICAL NEVI

STRUCTURAL FEATURES PLUS DISTRIBUTION OF PIGMENTATION. The following dermatoscopic classification allows characterization of the different dermatoscopic types of atypical nevi. Knowledge of these dermatoscopic types should reduce unnecessary surgery for benign melanocytic lesions (Figures 22-49 and 22-50).

Atypical nevi are classified according to structural features, that is, reticular, globular, or homogeneous patterns, or combinations of these types. The nevi are also characterized by distribution of pigmentation (see Tables 22-13 and 22-15).

CLASSIFICATION BY MAIN STRUCTURAL COMPONENTS

Nevi are first classified according to structural features: reticular pigment network, pigmented globules, and homogeneous pigmentation (see Table 22-14). When a clear predominance of one of these structural components is seen, the nevus is classified as reticular, globular, or homogeneous.

Table 22-14 Dermoscopic Types of Atypical Melanocytic Nevi—Structural Features

Type	Definition and predominant features
Clear predominance of one structural component	
Reticular	Pigment network
Globular	Numerous globules or dots
Homogeneous	Homogeneous brown pigmentation
Dominant presence of two structural components	
Reticular-globular	>3 meshes of pigment network with >3 globules of dots
Reticular-homogeneous	>3 meshes of pigment network with homogeneous brown pigmentation in at least one fourth of the lesion
Globular-homogeneous	>3 globules or dots with homogeneous brown pigmentation in at least one fourth of the lesion
Unclassified	No specific pattern

DERMOSCOPIC TYPES OF ATYPICAL MELANOCYTIC NEVI

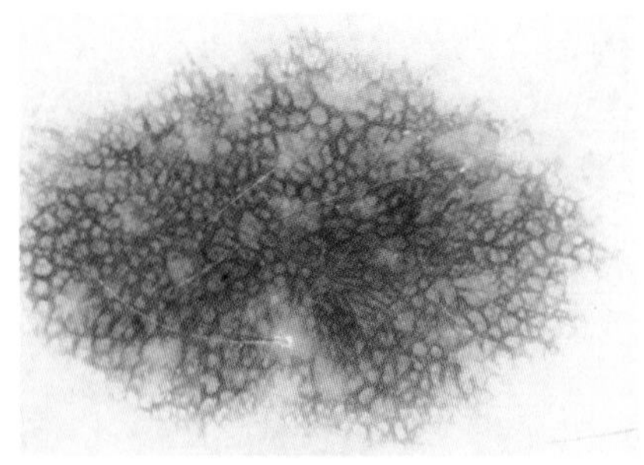
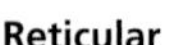
Reticular

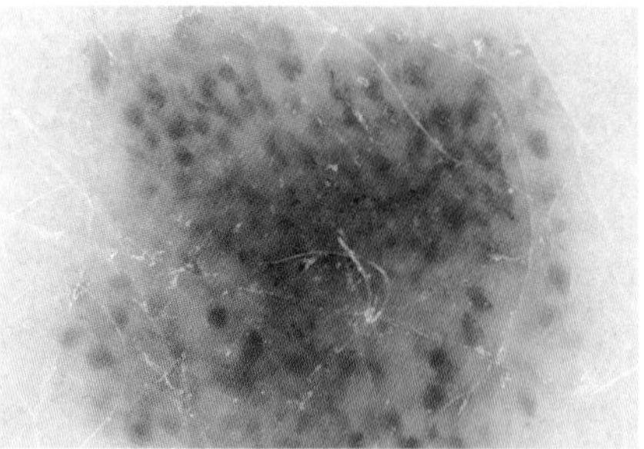
Globular

Homogeneous

Reticular-globular

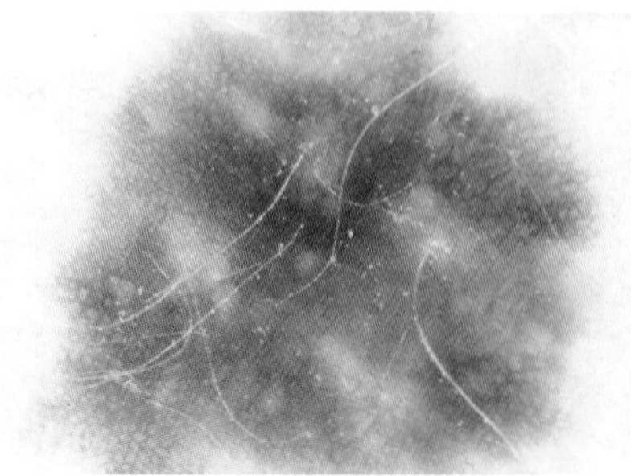
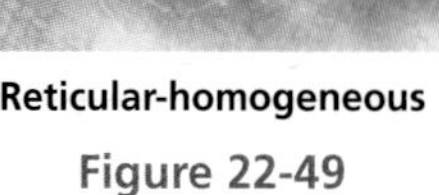
Reticular-homogeneous

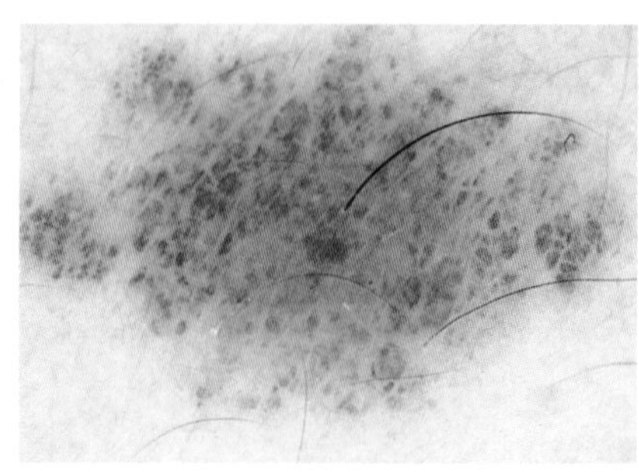
Globular-homogeneous

Figure 22-49

CLASSIFICATION BY COMBINATIONS OF STRUCTURAL COMPONENTS

In the case of the dominant presence of two structural components, the nevus is classified as reticular-globular, reticular-homogeneous, or globular-homogeneous (see Table 22-14). No single nevus shows all three structural components. The most common are the reticular type, followed by the reticular-homogeneous and globular-homogeneous types.

CLASSIFICATION BY DISTRIBUTION OF PIGMENTATION

The distribution of the pigmentation is then classified as central hyperpigmented or hypopigmented, eccentric peripheral hyperpigmented or hypopigmented, and multifocal hyperpigmented or hypopigmented (see Table 22-15). In cases where hyperpigmentation and hypopigmentation are present, classification is based on the predominant distribution of color.

Table 22-15 Dermoscopic Types of Atypical Melanocytic Nevi—Distribution of Pigmentation

Pigmentation	Definition
Central hyperpigmented	Hyperpigmented area (significantly darker than entire lesion) surrounded by fainter parts of lesion
Eccentric peripheral hyperpigmented	Hyperpigmented area (significantly darker than entire lesion) reaching one part of border of lesion
Central hypopigmented	Hypopigmented area (significantly fainter than entire lesion) surrounded by darker parts of lesion
Eccentric peripheral hypopigmented	Hypopigmented area (significantly fainter than entire lesion) reaching one part of border of lesion
Multifocal hyperpigmented and hypopigmented	Patchy distribution of hyperpigmented and hypopigmented areas

Adapted from Hofmann-Wellenhof R, Blum A, Wolf IH et al: *Arch Dermatol* 137:1575, 2001. *PMID: 11735707*

DERMOSCOPIC TYPES OF ATYPICAL MELANOCYTIC NEVI

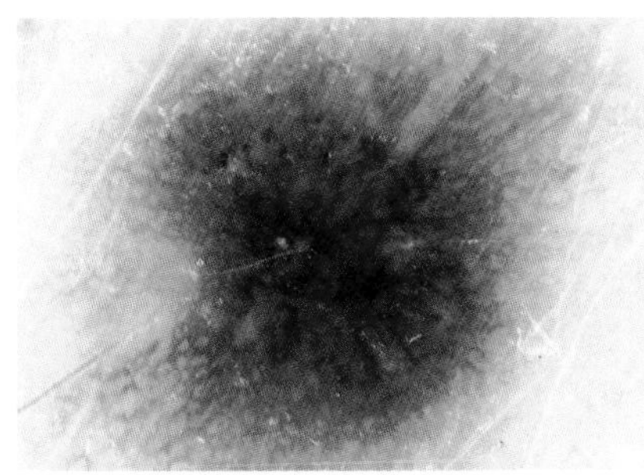

Central hyperpigmented

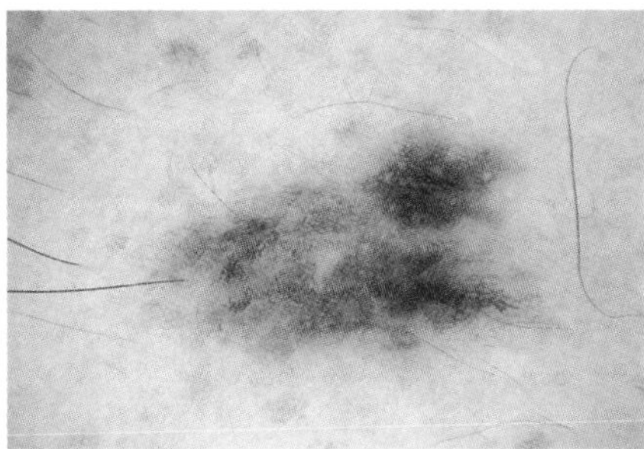

Eccentric peripheral hyperpigmented

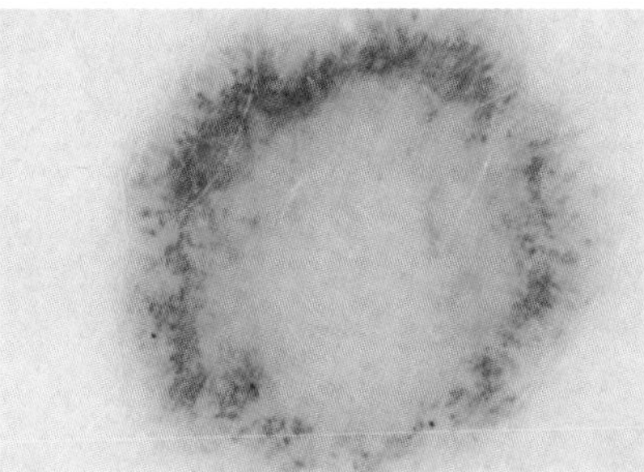

Central hypopigmented

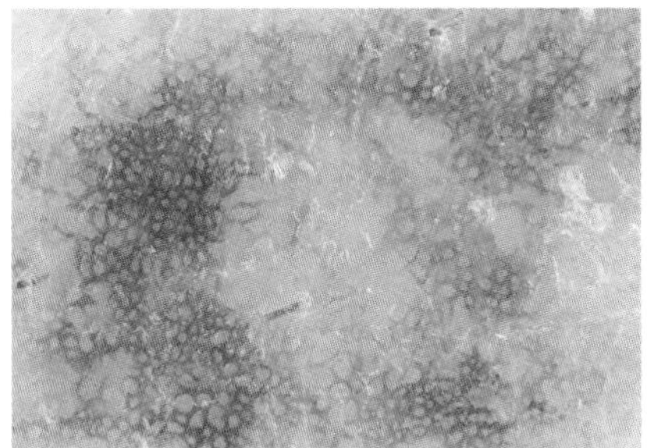

Central hypopigmented

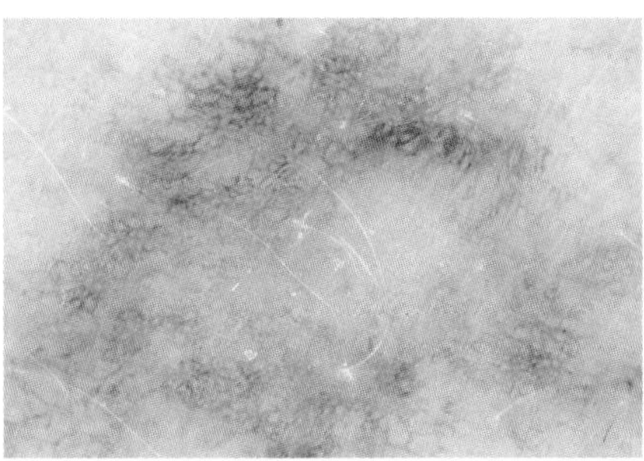

Eccentric peripheral hypopigmented

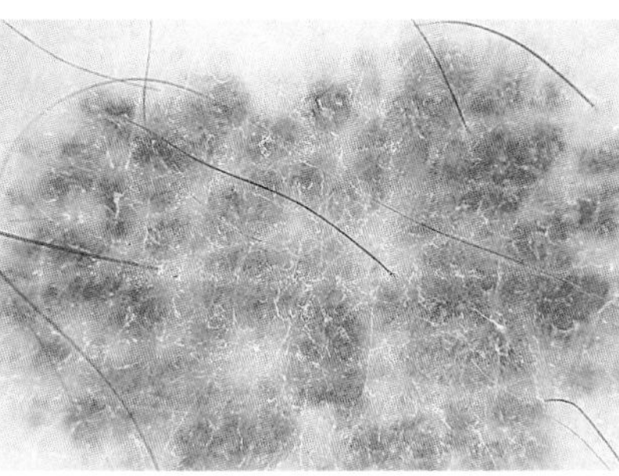

Multifocal hyperpigmented and hypopigmented

Figure 22-50

INTERPRETATION AND MANAGEMENT

Most individuals have one predominant type of nevus. A lesion that does not belong to the predominant type of nevus in a given patient should be considered an atypical lesion and therefore deserving of special attention.

Atypical nevi with the reticular pattern and uneven pigmentation are especially prone to overdiagnosis as melanoma. The most common heterogeneous distribution of pigmentation is multifocal hyperpigmentation or hypopigmentation, followed by central hypopigmentation and central hyperpigmentation. Eccentric peripheral hyperpigmentation is often found in malignant melanoma. Atypical nevi with eccentric peripheral hyperpigmentation should be regarded as the most relevant simulators of melanoma within the morphologic spectrum of atypical nevi. Therefore this type of nevus should be excised or monitored using digital dermoscopy at 3-month intervals. When the eccentric peripheral hyperpigmentation increases, excision of the lesion is necessary.

LIMITATIONS OF DERMOSCOPY

Dermoscopy may enhance the clinician's ability to diagnose melanoma. Knowledge and experience are required. Even experienced users may obtain a false sense of security in 20% or more cases of melanoma that lack classic dermoscopy features of melanoma. The dermoscopy feature most common in thin melanomas (Breslow thickness of <0.75 mm) is an irregular pigment network. Atypical nevi often have hyperpigmentation and bridging of the rete ridges, which give them a similar appearance by dermoscopy. Dermoscopy criteria for melanoma variants such as amelanotic melanomas, desmoplastic melanomas, lentigo maligna melanoma, or nevoid melanomas are lacking. A patient's report of change in a lesion is an important risk factor for melanoma. Approximately 10% of melanomas have no characteristic dermoscopy findings. The decision to perform a biopsy of a lesion of moderate to high clinical suspicion for melanoma before dermoscopy observation should not be changed by the lack of dermoscopy criteria for melanoma.

Chapter 23

Vascular Tumors and Malformations

CHAPTER CONTENTS

CONGENITAL VASCULAR LESIONS

A number of different congenital vascular lesions occur in the skin. Most represent developmental malformations and do not appear to be genetically determined. Vascular structures may be abnormal in size, abnormal in numbers, or both. These varied lesions have been referred to by many terms that have since been abandoned in favor of a simple classification, consisting of two groups, that is based on history and physical examination. The two major categories are hemangiomas and vascular malformations (Table 23-1 and Box 23-1).

Hemangiomas are vascular tumors composed of hyperplastic vascular endothelial cells that have the capacity for excessive proliferation but normally undergo eventual regression and involution. Vascular malformations are

Table 23-1 Congenital Vascular Lesions

	Hemangiomas of infancy	**Malformations**
Occurrence	40% present at birth Most occur in first year of life	99% present at birth
Location	Common on face, any area	Common on limbs, any area
Appearance	Well delineated Red (superficial) Blue (deep)	Poorly circumscribed
Course	Rapid neonatal growth Slow involution	No change in size Grows in proportion to child No involution May fluctuate in size with growth spurt at puberty
Vessel type	Predominantly arterial	Predominantly venous, but any combination of capillary, venous, arterial, and lymphatic components can occur
Histology	Proliferative phase: endothelial hyperplasia, increased number of mast cells Involutional phase: fibrosis, fatty infiltration, diminished cellularity, normal mast cell count	Normal endothelial cell turnover Normal mast cell count Flattened endothelium

Box 23-1 **Congenital Vascular Lesions**
Hemangiomas of infancy • Superficial (strawberry) • Deep (cavernous) • Mixed (involves dermis and subcutis) Malformations • Salmon patch • Nevus flammeus Syndromes • Sturge-Weber syndrome • Cobb syndrome • Klippel-Trénaunay syndrome • Maffucci's syndrome Other arteriovenous malformations

hamartomas of mature endothelial cells. Vascular malformations result from structural abnormalities of mature endothelial cells that are usually present at birth and do not undergo hyperplasia with rapid proliferation. They have a normal pattern of growth and enlarge proportionally as the child grows. They do not resolve spontaneously. The distinction between a port-wine stain and hemangioma of infancy may be difficult during the first few weeks of life.

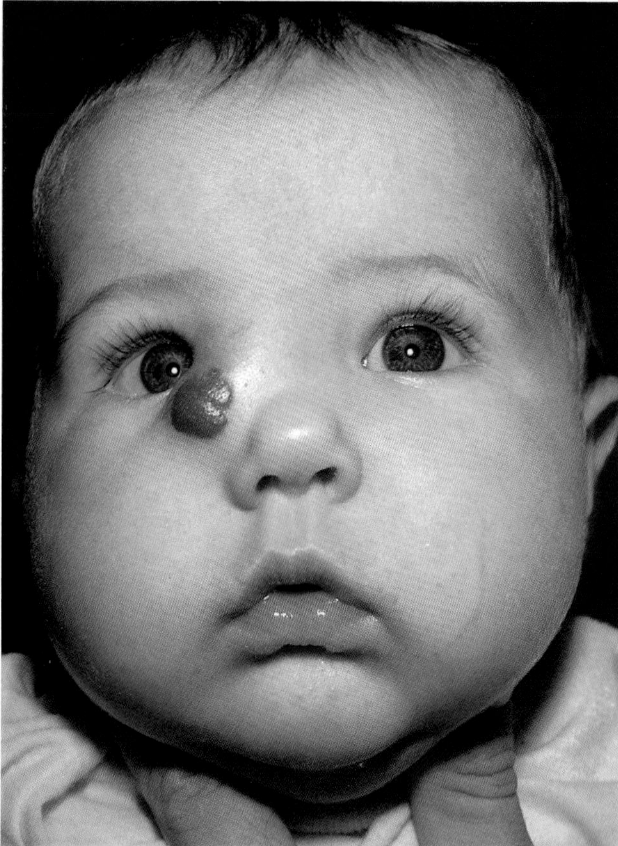

Figure 23-1 Hemangioma of infancy. Nodular lesions are superficial, deep, or mixed. This lesion has a superficial pedunculated and deep component.

Hemangiomas of infancy

Hemangiomas of infancy are benign neoplasms that result from rapid proliferation of endothelial cells. After an initial proliferating phase, many undergo complete regression with fibrosis. The color depends on its location. Hemangiomas involving the papillary dermis (superficial strawberry hemangiomas) are red; those in the reticular dermis and subcutaneous fat are blue or colorless (deep, cavernous hemangiomas) (Figure 23-1). All have the same vascular components and histopathology. Early hemangiomas are highly cellular, and numerous mast cells are present in the stroma. Lumina are more obvious and larger as the lesion matures. Vascular spaces may have features of capillaries, venules, and arterioles. Progressive interstitial fibrosis occurs during regression. Thrombocytopenic purpura and chronic consumption coagulopathy complicating very large hemangiomas is named Kasabach-Merritt syndrome.

SUPERFICIAL HEMANGIOMAS

Superficial (strawberry) hemangiomas may be present at birth but more often appear within the first 2 weeks of life in 1% to 3% of infants; the female-to-male ratio is 3:1. Many children have one, but 15% to 20% have several. Most are small, harmless birthmarks that proliferate for 8 to 18 months and then slowly regress over the next 5 to 8 years, leaving normal or slightly blemished skin. They consist of a collection of dilated vessels in the dermis surrounded by masses of proliferating endothelial cells. These cells are responsible for the unique growth characteristics. The lesions begin as nodular masses or as flat, ill-defined,

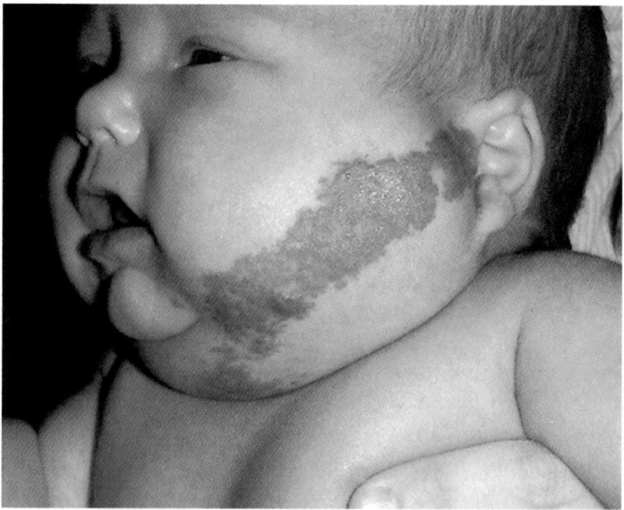

Figure 23-2 Hemangioma of infancy. A segmental lesion with plaquelike features and a dermatomal like distribution. This type often involves a broader anatomic area than localized round lesions.

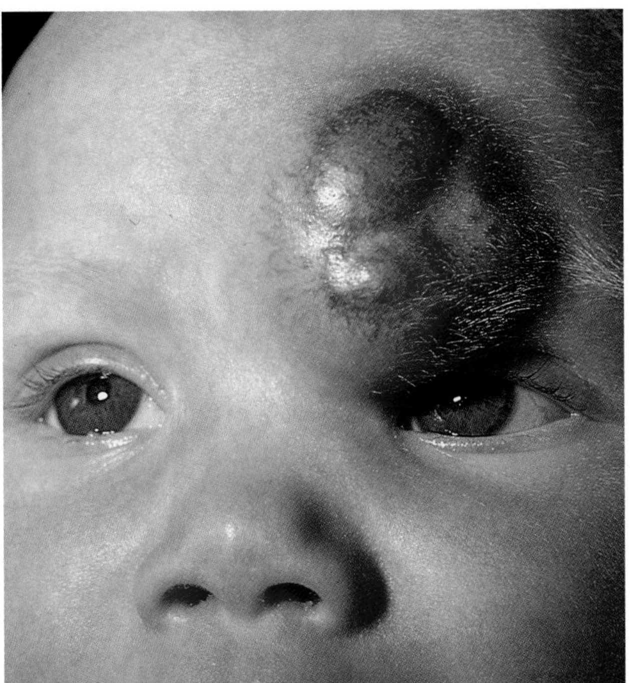

Figure 23-3 Strawberry hemangioma. A rapidly growing mass that is encroaching on the orbit.

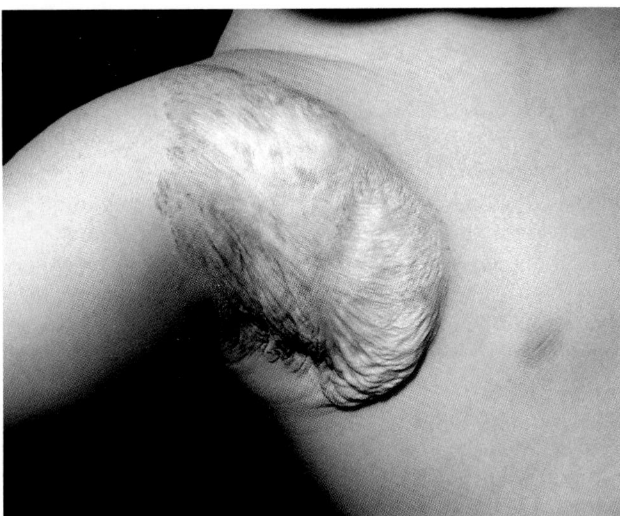

Figure 23-4 Hemangioma of infancy. Regression of a large deep lesion resulted in a flaccid wrinkled sac.

telangiectatic macules that are mistaken for bruises. Superficial hemangiomas grow rapidly for weeks or months, forming nodular, protuberant, compressible masses of a few millimeters to several centimeters. In rare instances the lesions may almost cover an entire limb. They are bright red with well-defined borders (Figure 23-2). Vital structures can be compressed, and rapidly growing areas (Figure 23-3) may ulcerate. Larger lesions (>6 cm) ulcerate more frequently.

Hemangiomas may block vision, interfere with feeding or respiration, or obstruct the external auditory canal. Recurrent bleeding may complicate ulceration. Most have a benign course. An inactive phase lasting several months is followed by fibrosis and involution. About 30% of lesions resolve by the third birthday, 50% by the fifth, and 70% by the seventh. The mass shrinks and fades in color during the scarring process. Involution begins in most cases by age 3; those present after ages 7 to 9 infrequently undergo further regression. Regression is characterized by normal-appearing skin (approximately 70% of cases) or by atrophy, scarring, telangiectasia, pigmentation changes, and deformity (Figure 23-4).

Location and risk. Hemangiomas of infancy in certain locations may be associated with other anomalies or have a risk of developing complications. Most complications arise during the proliferative growth phase (Table 23-2).

MANAGEMENT

Nonintervention. Lesions that are relatively small and indolent should remain untouched if they are to involute spontaneously. In most cases, the result is very satisfactory. Patients should be seen regularly to reassure their parents and to monitor growth (measurements, photographs). Small areas of bleeding and ulceration are treated with cool, wet compresses. Lesions with functional impairment, deep ulceration, or infection need treatment. Facial lesions that pose a cosmetic problem are also considered for treatment. Ultrasound, roentgenography, or magnetic resonance imaging is performed in infants with multiple cutaneous hemangiomas to rule out visceral involvement.

Treating ulcers and rapidly proliferating lesions. Ulceration is the most frequent complication. It usually occurs during the proliferation phase. It is more common in areas of trauma. Ulcerations are painful, may become infected, and heal with scarring. Ulceration is managed with local wound care, topical and systemic antibiotics, systemic and intralesional corticosteroids, flashlamp-pumped pulsed dye laser, interferon alfa-2a, and pain medication.

Local wound care. Compresses (saline, Burow's solution) reduce and absorb exudate and debride. Metronidazole gel or mupirocin ointment treats infection.

Petroleum jelly (Vaseline) impregnated gauze and barrier creams are used for ulceration around the anus and female genitalia. Occlusive dressings (e.g., polyurethane film dressing) act as a barrier, control pain, and encourage healing.

Table 23-2 Hemangiomas with Special Risks

Location	Complication and risk
Periorbital	Rapidly growing hemangiomas near orbits may cause refractive errors, astigmatism, strabismus, ptosis, and stimulus deprivation amblyopia if untreated. Permanent visual deficits may result from ocular compromise as short as 2 weeks.
Pelvic and perineal	Urogenital and anorectal anomalies such as hypospadias, anterior or vestibular anus, imperforate anus, and atrophy or absence of labia minora. Perineal hemangiomas are prone to ulceration and infection as a result of frictional and chemical trauma.
Lumbosacral	Underlying spinal anomalies—occult spinal dysraphism, tethered spinal cord, and lipomeningomyelocele. Ultrasound or magnetic resonance imaging for infants with a hemangioma overlying midline lumbosacral region.
Facial	Head and neck—most common location for hemangiomas of infancy, accounting for 60% of cases.
Lip, oropharynx, nasal tip, ears	May incompletely involute and may require surgical intervention to minimize residual scarring and deformity.
Preauricular	May be associated with hemangiomas involving parotid gland, but do not usually compromise facial nerve.
Diffuse facial	Tend to localize to segmental distributions within frontonasal, maxillary, or mandibular facial area. More likely to ulcerate. Increased incidence of visceral hemangiomas, most commonly involving liver, gastrointestinal tract, and brain.
PHACES syndrome	Large facial segmental hemangiomas in association with visceral hemangiomatosis meet criteria for PHACES syndrome (posterior fossa abnormality, hemangioma, arterial anomaly, cardiac defects, coarctation of the aorta, eye/ocular abnormality, sternal defect).
Beard distribution (preauricular, chin, lower lip, anterior neck)	Association with laryngeal or subglottic hemangiomas that may rapidly compromise airway during proliferative growth phase
Laryngeal and subglottic	May cause stridor, persistent cough, hoarseness, respiratory distress, or cyanosis; many infants will present with respiratory symptoms between 6 and 12 weeks of life. Radiographs, MRI scan, or laryngoscopic visualization defines extent.

Adapted from *Clin Pediatr (Phila)* 44(9):747-766, 2005. *PMID: 16327961*

Infection. Systemic antibiotics (first-generation cephalosporins) are used frequently.

Corticosteroids. Rapidly growing lesions or those that have the potential to interfere with vital structures such as the eyes, auditory canals, and airways or those that threaten permanent disfigurement should be treated initially with prednisone given in divided doses twice a day. The proliferative phase is inhibited and the hemangioma shrinks. Treatment should be maintained until cessation of growth or shrinkage of the hemangioma is accomplished. Most lesions stabilize and markedly regress in 2 to 4 weeks. Prednisone may then be given in a single, early-morning dose tapered on an alternate-day schedule for a few weeks and then discontinued. The pace of tapering depends on several factors (i.e., the age of the infant, the indication for treatment, any toxic effects, and any rebound growth). Administration of oral prednisone or prednisolone (2 to 3 mg/kg per day) given over a mean of 1.8 months before tapering had a response of 84% in stabilizing or shrinking most growing cutaneous hemangiomas.

Because nearly 40% of patients reported rebound with tapering, brief courses of 2 to 3 weeks' duration are probably inadequate. Occasionally, higher doses and longer treatment may be required. A second course of treatment is given for recurrences. Lesions that do not regress by late childhood may be evaluated for surgical excision.

Intralesional steroids. Intralesional steroids (triamcinolone 10 to 20 mg/ml, with a maximum injection of 3 to 5 mg/kg per procedure) are used for rapidly expanding and ulcerated lesions. Multiple injections into the tumor are used and the procedure may be repeated a few times at 4- to 8-week intervals. Periorbital hemangiomas have been associated with ophthalmic complications in 40% to 80% of cases. Strabismus and amblyopia are the most common. Intralesional steroids are frequently used by the ophthalmologist to treat lesions that do not respond to oral steroids (Box 23-2). In most cases, clinical response is noticed within 1 to 3 days. The first change is a blanching of the vascular pattern, followed by a rapid regression in the size of the mass. Involution is most rapid in the first or second week after treatment. Retinal occlusion is a potential risk. Surgery is used for lesions that do not respond to corticosteroids.

Box 23-2 **Guidelines for the Use of Intralesional Steroids in Periorbital Hemangiomas**

Evaluation

History and physical examination
Computed tomography scan
Avoidance of immunization with live virus vaccines
Short-acting, light, general anesthetics

Pharmacologic agent

Triamcinolone 10 to 20 mg/ml, with a maximum injection of 3 to 5 mg/kg per procedure

Procedure

Anterior approach to the eyelid is preferred
Multiple injection sites: 0.1-ml aliquot
Aspirate before injecting (27- or 30-gauge needle)
Digital pressure is then applied to avoid hematomas
Repeat up to three times at 8-week intervals or until regression has ceased

Lasers. The vascular-specific pulsed dye laser (flash-lamp-pumped) is the treatment of choice for superficial cutaneous hemangiomas at sites of potential functional impairment and on the face. The yellow laser light is absorbed by oxyhemoglobin. Short pulses are used so that only targeted vessels are heated without affecting surrounding tissue. Hemangiomas with a deep component do not respond because the effect of the pulsed dye laser (PDL) is limited by its depth of vascular injury (1.2 mm). Even totally superficial capillary hemangiomas that are greater than 3 to 4 mm in thickness respond slowly and incompletely after several treatments.

Early therapeutic intervention may not prevent proliferative growth of the deeper or subcutaneous component of the hemangioma. Guidelines for the recommendation of laser therapy include periorificial location and the potential for functional impairment, ulceration or location over an area of increased risk of ulceration (such as the diaper region), and anatomic areas where there is a concern for cosmetic disfigurement. Consider treatment of facial hemangiomas that do not regress by the school-age years to relieve the social burden on young patients. Pulsed dye lasers are also effective for removing residual telangiectasias associated with regression. At least 75% of patients can achieve 50% lesional lightening. Infants may be more responsive than adults. Generally, six treatment sessions are required; further treatments are often beneficial. Lesional reduction can be significant.

Pain is intolerable for infants and young children. Topical or general anesthesia is required. Immediate skin darkening is secondary to an intravascular coagulum. The blackening resolves in 1 or 2 weeks. The safety record is excellent. Scarring, fibrosis atrophy, cutaneous depression, and pigmentary changes develop in about 1% of patients.

There are no age restrictions for pulsed dye laser treatment; even premature infants have safely undergone therapy. Superficial coagulation with argon lasers and deeper coagulation with Nd:YAG lasers are associated with significant scarring and generally are not used.

Topical imiquimod. Imiquimod cream was used to treat infantile hemangiomas in the proliferative phase. The cream was applied three times per week for 4 weeks. Because of inflammation with erythema and crusting, a rest period of 2 weeks was given. A marked reduction of inflammation and size was observed. Treatment was restarted and continued for 2 more weeks. Complete regression was noted 4 weeks later.

Surgery. The pros and cons of a surgical approach must be considered because the scar may be worse than the results from spontaneous regression. Most hemangiomas are managed medically. Aesthetic correction may be delayed until after involution at the age of 8 to 10 years to correct residual scarring or to remove fibrofatty tissue. Early excisional surgery is indicated for function- or life-threatening hemangiomas where pharmacologic therapy is not effective or tolerated. Reevaluate at about age 4. Consider surgery of a hemangioma that is causing scarring or is involuting very slowly. Psychosocial issues are a concern. Surgery may produce a more normal appearance and preserve self-esteem. Early surgery is considered for children with very large or mixed (subcutaneous and cutaneous) head and neck cutaneous or mucosal hemangiomas where irreversible and unaesthetic scars are predictable.

Interferon alfa-2b. Interferon alfa-2b (an antiangiogenic protein) is an option for steroid-resistant, organ-interfering, and/or life-threatening giant hemangiomas. It slowly halts the growth of hemangiomas and may result in a higher rate of shrinkage than that seen with corticosteroids. Subcutaneous injections of 1 to 3 million units/m^2 per day of interferon alfa-2b during the first month and subsequently every 48 to 72 hours, depending on the evolution in each case, were used. Treatment lasts from 3 to 12 months. Volume reduction and remission of their complications occur. Therapy is generally well tolerated in children. Side effects include fever, neutropenia, and an increase in serum aminotransferase levels and neurotoxicity. Fever and malaise are treated with acetaminophen. The occurrence of spastic diplegia was reported in 5 of 26 children treated with interferon alfa-2a. The neurologic changes improved in two patients, but in the remaining three patients paralysis was permanent. Therefore most experts limit the use of interferon-alfa to those infants with life-threatening or severely function-threatening hemangiomas that have failed to respond to steroid therapy. Decreased urinary basic fibroblast growth factor (bFGF) levels correlated with hemangioma involution. Patients who receive interferon alfa-2b and prednisone seem to improve faster. Imaging studies and urinary (bFGF) levels are used to monitor treatment response.

DEEP HEMANGIOMAS

Deep (cavernous) hemangiomas are collections of dilated vessels deep in the dermis and subcutaneous tissue that are present at birth. Apparently localized and superficial venous lesions may coexist with venous ectasias and deep vein anomalies. Clinically they appear as pale, skin-colored, red, or blue masses that are ill-defined and rounded (Figure 23-5). Most are asymptomatic. Hyperhidrosis over the lesion is common, and often there are recurrent episodes of thrombophlebitis in or near the lesions. Like superficial hemangiomas, the lesions enlarge for several months, become stationary for an indefinite period, and undergo spontaneous resolution. They are managed like superficial hemangiomas.

KASABACH-MERRITT SYNDROME. Kasabach-Merritt syndrome is a variant of disseminated intravascular coagulation (DIC) in which platelets and clotting factors are locally consumed within a giant hemangioma (Table 23-3). This disorder is suspected when children with large hemangiomas present with pallor, petechiae, ecchymoses, easy bruising, prolonged bleeding from superficial abrasions, or rapid changes in the size or appearance of the hemangioma. There is thrombocytopenia, microangiopathic hemolytic anemia, and an acute or chronic consumption coagulopathy in association with a rapidly enlarging hemangioma (Figure 23-6). The cause of DIC is not known, but blood is static in the venous sinusoids, and both platelets and contact factors may be activated by the abnormal endothelium. Kasabach-Merritt syndrome occurs most often in young infants during the first few weeks of life, but it may occur in adults.

The majority of hemangiomas are very large and occur on the limbs or trunk. Prednisone 2 to 4 mg/kg/day is indicated when the hemangioma rapidly enlarges and the platelet count drops precipitously. The initial response is often inadequate, and combined steroid/radiation treatment is then indicated. Interferon (IFN)-alfa therapy is added and steroids are tapered if the addition of radiation fails.

HEMANGIOMAS ASSOCIATED WITH CONGENITAL ABNORMALITIES. The association of hemangiomas with congenital abnormalities is rare. Most of the vascular lesions associated with congenital malformations and syndromes are malformations, such as the port-wine stain, or other true vascular malformations and are not hemangiomas. A few malformation syndromes have an association with cutaneous hemangiomas. These include PHACE syndrome (**p**osterior fossa brain malformation, multiple **h**emangiomas, **a**rterial anomalies such as coarctation of the aorta, **c**ardiac defects, **e**ye abnormalities), midline abdominal and sternal defects in conjunction with facial hemangiomas, and spinal cord and vertebral abnormalities with sacral hemangiomas. Large facial hemangiomas (occupying at least one fourth to one half of the facial surface) may be linked to the Dandy-Walker malformation (cystic expansion of the fourth ventricle into the posterior cranial fossa) or other posterior fossa brain abnormalities (e.g., hypoplastic cerebellum, posterior fossa arachnoid cyst). Ophthalmologic disorders (choroidal hemangioma, microphthalmos, and strabismus) may also be present. Brain-imaging studies should be performed on all asymptomatic infants with extensive facial hemangiomas to assess for hydrocephalus and fourth-ventricle anomalies.

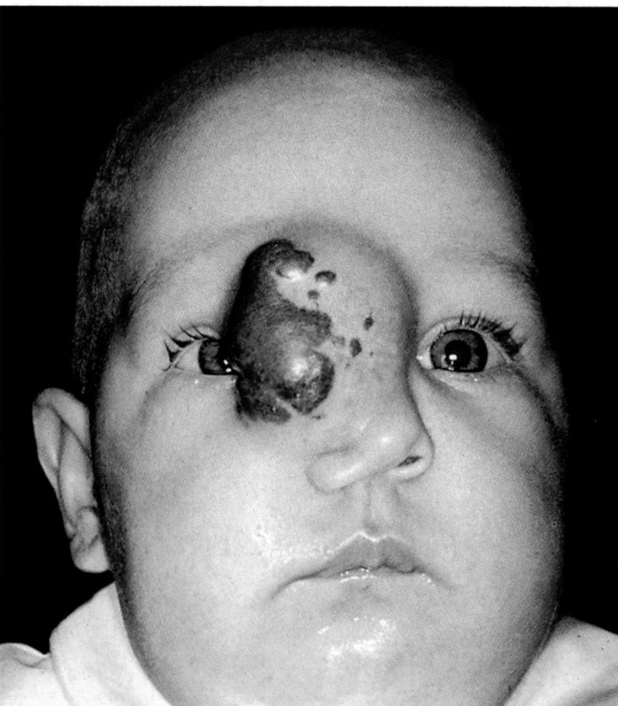

Figure 23-5 Cavernous hemangioma. Cavernous hemangioma is a collection of dilated vessels deep in the dermis and subcutaneous tissue that presents as a pale, skin-colored, red, or blue mass.

Table 23-3 Kasabach-Merritt Syndrome	
Associated vascular malformations	Kaposiform hemangioepithelioma, tuftedangioma, congenital hemangiopericytoma, lymphatic malformations
Hematologic manifestations	Thrombocytopenia, hemolytic anemia, coagulopathy
Risks	Severe thrombocytopenia with life-threatening bleeding, local invasion by vascular lesion into vital organs of surrounding tissues Infections caused by skin breakdown can lead to sepsis
Treatment	Combination therapy—corticosteroids, chemotherapy, antiplatelet medications, transfusions

Adapted from *Clin Pediatr (Phila)* 44(9):747-766, 2005.
PMID: 16327961

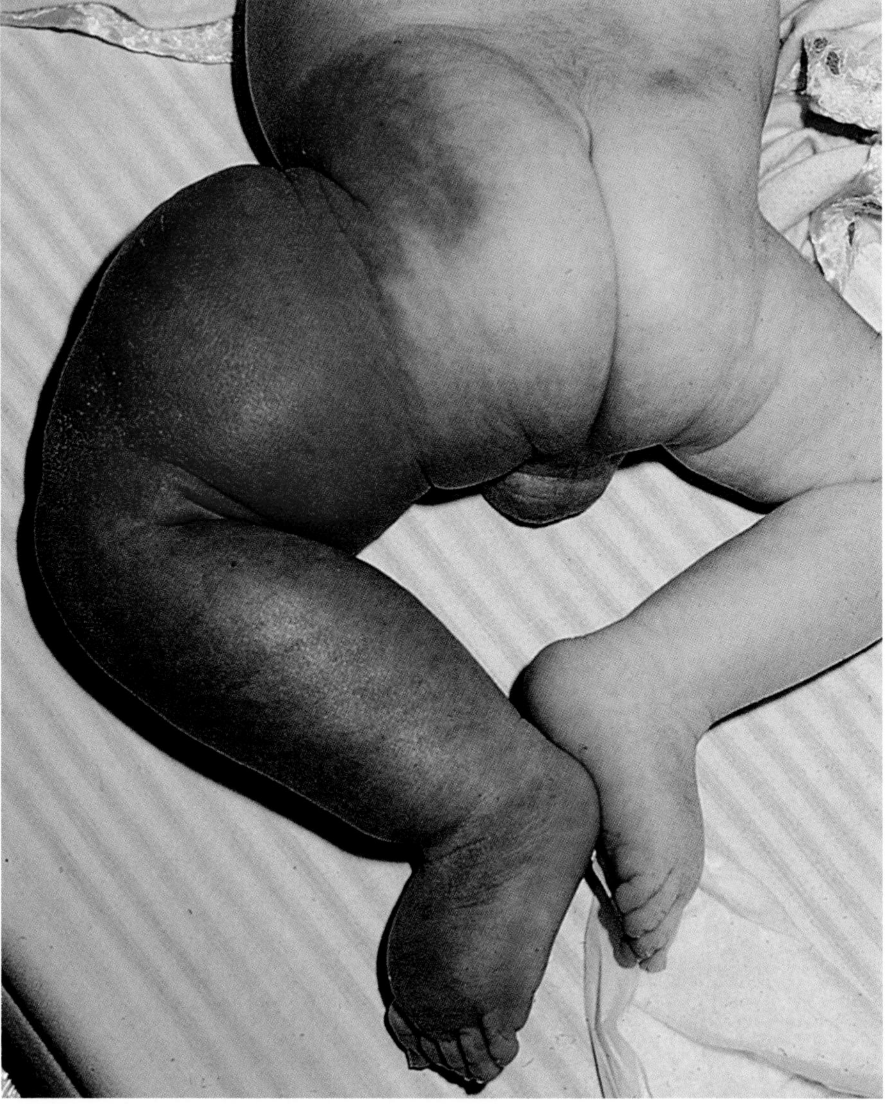

Figure 23-6 Kasabach-Merritt syndrome. Thrombocytopenia, microangiopathic hemolytic anemia, and an acute or chronic consumption coagulopathy occur in association with a rapidly enlarging hemangioma. (Courtesy Nancy B. Esterly, MD.)

Malformations

Vascular malformations are anomalies that result from inborn errors of vascular morphogenesis. They are congenital (present at birth). There is no cellular proliferation in enlarging vascular malformations. They expand with the child's growth because of progressive ectasia resulting from changes in blood or lymphatic flow and pressure.

NEVUS FLAMMEUS (PORT-WINE STAINS)

A nevus flammeus is a congenital vascular malformation that commonly involves the face and neck of newborns, although lesions have been described in nearly all sites, including mucous membranes. The lesion is a vascular ectasia rather than a proliferative process. It results from progressive vascular dilatation of preexisting blood vessels. There is a decrease in nerve fibers associated with the ectatic blood vessels, and it is postulated that the lesion results from a neural deficiency of sympathetic innervation of the blood vessels.

In most cases these distinctive lesions are developmental anomalies that are not genetically transmitted. They are present at birth in 0.1% to 0.3% of infants. Port-wine stains are a significant cosmetic problem that does not fade with age. These lesions are usually unilateral; they frequently occur on the face, but they also can appear anywhere on the body (Figures 23-7 to 23-11). They may be a few millimeters in diameter or may cover an entire limb. Size remains stable throughout life. Nevus flammeus appears at birth as a flat, irregular, red-to-purple patch. Initially the lesions are smooth, but later they may become papular, simulating a cobblestone surface (see Figure 23-10). Two thirds of all patients develop nodularity or hypertrophy by the fifth decade of life. Unlike the salmon patch, nevus flammeus tends to darken with age. The entire depth of the dermis contains numerous dilated capillaries. Approximately 10% of all patients with facial port-wine stains have glaucoma without leptomeningeal involvement. Ipsilateral glaucoma is frequent when nevus flammeus involves both the ophthalmologic and the maxillary divisions of the trigeminal nerve, but it is unlikely when the face is affected in either one of the upper divisions of the fifth cranial nerve or solely below the eye. Dilated conjunctival vessels are common when the lids are involved, but this finding is not correlated with the presence or absence of glaucoma.

SYSTEMIC SYNDROMES. Nevus flammeus may be a component of neurocutaneous syndromes (Table 23-4), such as Sturge-Weber syndrome (nevus flammeus of the trigeminal area) (see Figure 23-13) or Klippel-Trénaunay-Weber syndrome. When it occurs over the midline of the back, nevus flammeus may be associated with an underlying spinal cord arteriovenous malformation.

VASCULAR MALFORMATIONS

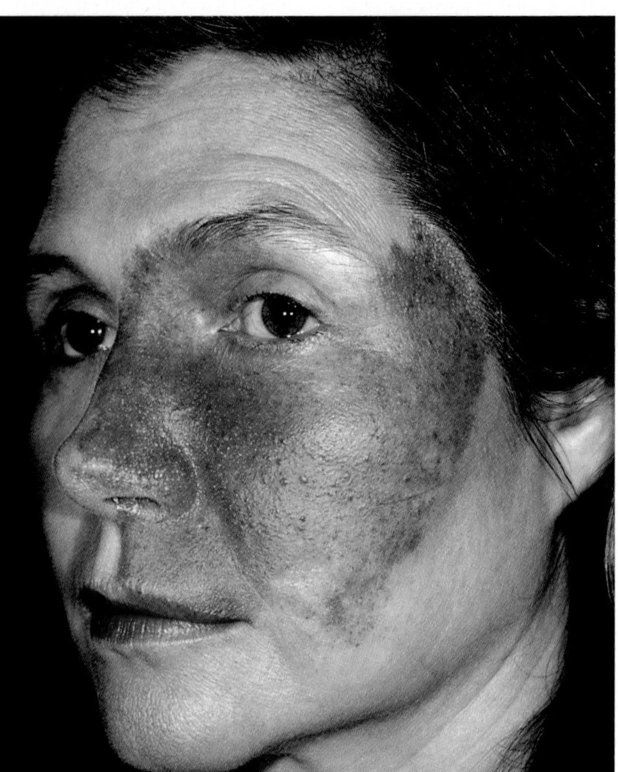

Figure 23-7 Nevus flammeus. The face is the most frequently involved site. Lesions become thicker and darker in color with advancing age.

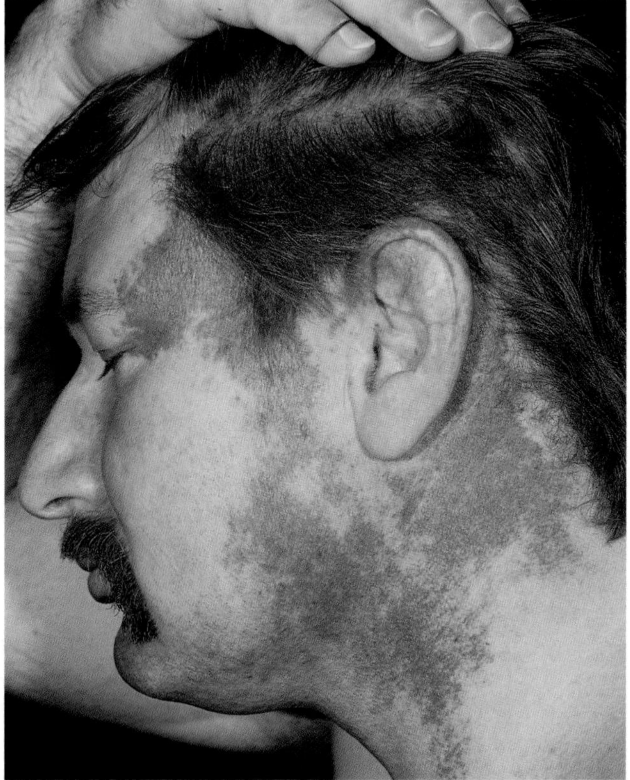

Figure 23-8 Nevus flammeus. An extensive lesion with a relatively smooth surface.

VASCULAR MALFORMATIONS

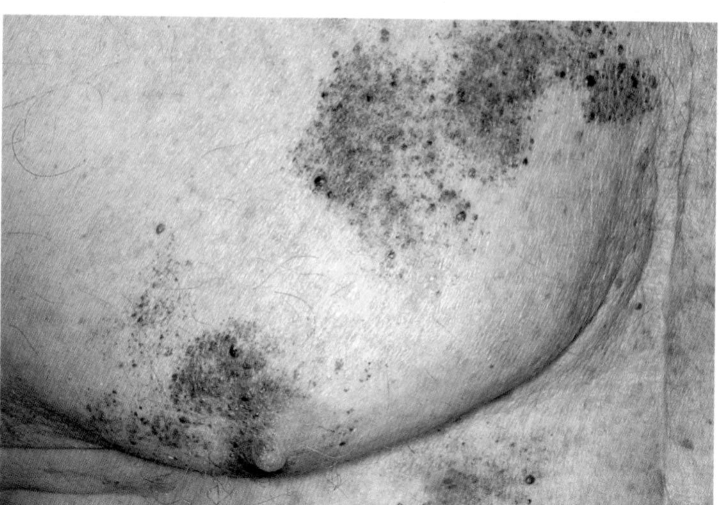

Figure 23-9 Nevus flammeus. The surface of lesions varies from smooth to papular. This lesion has a distinctive purple-studded papular surface.

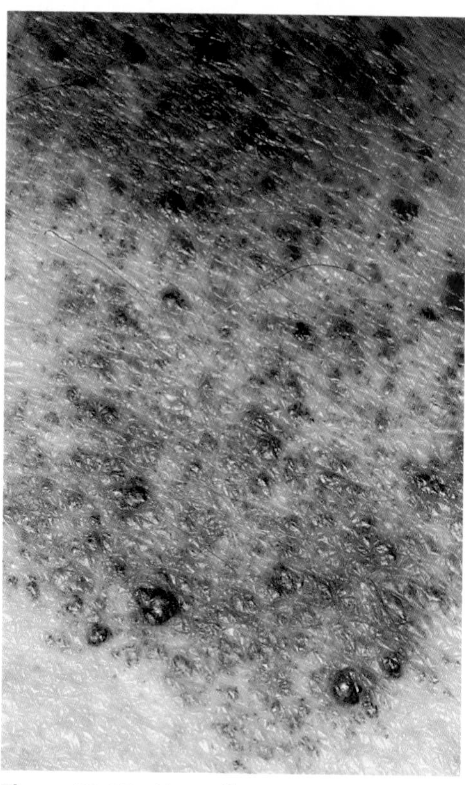

Figure 23-10 Nevus flammeus. Lesions may become studded with papules and develop a cobblestonelike appearance.

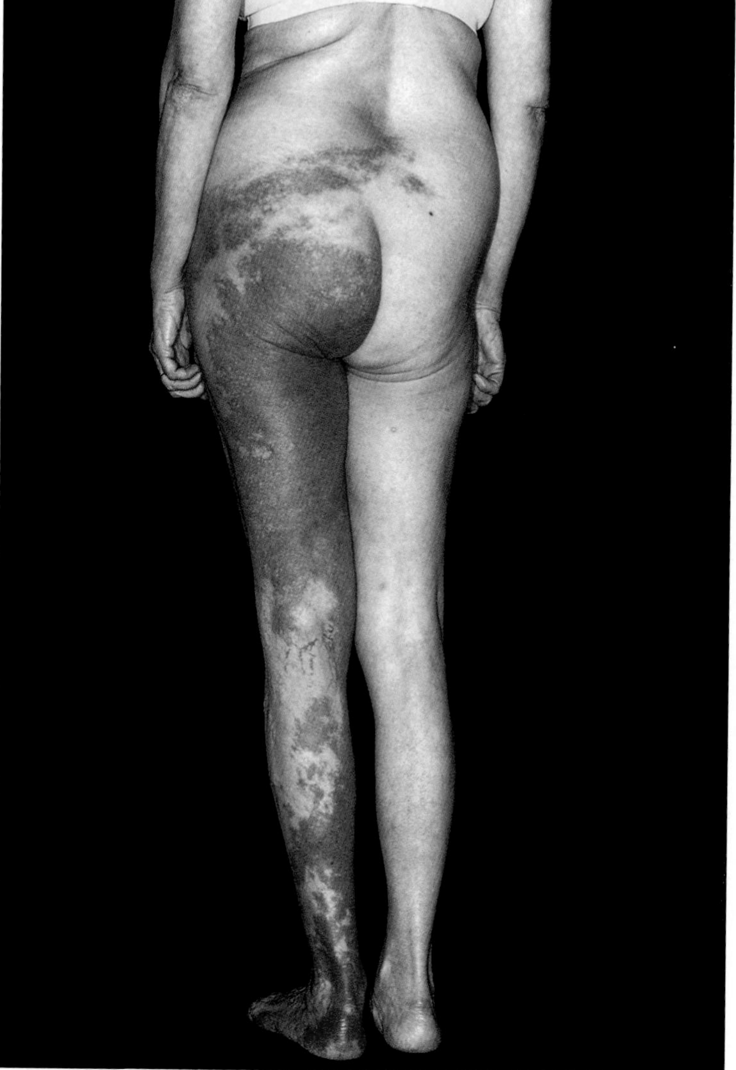

Figure 23-11 Nevus flammeus covering the entire lower limb. The affected limb is 2 inches longer than the normal side.

Table 23-4 Neurocutaneous Syndromes with Vascular Abnormalities

	Cobb syndrome	Sturge-Weber syndrome	Osler-Weber-Rendu syndrome
Synonym	Cutaneomeningospinal angiomatosis	Encephalotrigeminal angiomatosis	Hereditary hemorrhagic telangiectasia
Inheritance	Not familial	Dominant partial trisomy or not familial	Autosomal dominant
Gender distribution	More in males	Equal	Equal
Age of onset	Childhood or adolescence	Two thirds present with hemangioma at birth	Childhood
Skin lesion	Port-wine stain or angiokeratomas in dermatomal distribution corresponding within segment or two of area of spinal cord involvement*	Ipsilateral capillary angioma or port-wine stain in distribution of superior and middle branches of trigeminal nerve;* associated cavernous changes may occur No consistent relationship between extent of skin lesion and degree of meningeal involvement	Telangiectasia (skin and mucous membranes)*
CNS findings	Arteriovenous or venous angioma of spinal cord* Neurologic signs of cord compression or anoxia	Angioma of meninges* Intracranial gyriform calcifications Mental retardation (60%)* Epilepsy (usually focal)* Hemiparesis contralateral to skin lesions* Visual impairment (50% of patients have one or more various eye abnormalities)*	Angiomas in brain or spinal cord with signs of localized tumor
Associated findings	Angioma of vertebrae Renal angioma Kyphoscoliosis	Renal angioma Coarctation of aorta High, arched palate Abnormally developed ears	Pulmonary arteriovenous anastomoses Hemorrhage from lesions in mouth, GI tract, and GU tract and associated anemia
Diagnostic aids	Lateral spine x-ray film Computed tomography Magnetic resonance imaging	EEG Computed tomography Magnetic resonance imaging	Computed tomography Magnetic resonance imaging
Treatment	Surgical removal of spinal cord angioma if possible	Anticonvulsants Surgical removal of intracranial lesion if possible Cosmetic procedures for skin lesions	Cautery of bleeding lesions

*Major component of this syndrome.
CNS, Central nervous system; *EEG,* electroencephalogram; *GI,* gastrointestinal; *GU,* genitourinary.

Fabry-Anderson disease	Ataxia telangiectasia	von Hippel-Lindau disease
Angiokeratoma corporis diffusum	Cephalo-oculocutaneous telangiectasia	Angiomatosis retinae et cerebelli syndrome
Recessive trait (X chromosome)	Autosomal recessive	Autosomal dominant
Males tend to full syndrome: angiokeratomas; extremity pain; high blood pressure; cardiomegaly; albuminuria; hypohidrosis	Equal	Equal
Childhood	Childhood	Adult
Small, clustered angiokeratomas (symmetric, mucosal, increased over bony prominences) Palmar mottling	Telangiectasia (increased in sun-exposed areas) Inelasticity	Port-wine stains in some; most with no cutaneous lesions Café-au-lait spots
Cerebral vascular accidents Neuronal glycolipid deposition (peripheral neuritis)	Progressive cerebellar ataxia (voluntary movements)* Ocular telangiectasia (spread from canthal fold)* Peculiar eye movements (nystagmus, poor control)* Retarded Slow dysarthric speech Decreased tendon reflexes	Cerebellar hemangioblastoma and cyst* Spinal hemangioblastoma (rarely) Retinal hemangiomas (tangle of vessels away from disc)*
Stooped posture Slender limbs; thin, weak muscles Dilated, tortuous conjunctival and retinal vessels Varicose veins and stasis edema Scant facial hair Hypogonadism	Sinopulmonary infections* Hypoplastic or absent thymus Small spleen Retarded growth Malignancies (reticulum cell sarcoma, Hodgkin's disease, lymphosarcoma, gastric carcinoma)	Pheochromocytoma Pancreatic cysts Hepatic angiomas Renal hypernephromas (20%) Polycythema (erythropoietic substance from tumor)
Urinary glycolipids (ceramide trihexoside) Slit lamp Biopsy—renal or marrow (lipid deposits)	Diminished or absent IgA Increased serum alpha-fetoprotein	Hemogram (polycythemia) Urinalysis, excretory urograms Computed tomography Magnetic resonance imaging
Symptomatic	Control infections Plasma infusions (IgA) Thymus transplant Transfer factor	Supportive

Sturge-Weber syndrome. Sturge-Weber syndrome (SWS) is a congenital neurocutaneous disorder with a facial capillary malformation (port-wine stain), abnormal blood vessels of the brain (leptomeningeal angioma), or abnormal blood vessels in the eye predisposing to glaucoma. Variants exist where only one of these three structures is involved with the vascular malformation. These patients may develop seizures, headaches and migraines, strokelike episodes, focal neurologic impairments, visual problems, and cognitive deficits. SWS occurs sporadically and is congenital. No patterns of inheritance have been identified. Sturge-Weber syndrome (Box 23-3) consists of a large facial nevus flammeus in the distribution of the ophthalmologic division of the trigeminal nerve (forehead, eye, and maxillary area) and ipsilateral leptomeningeal angiomatosis (Figures 23-12, 23-14 and 23-15). Bilateral nevus flammeus occurs in 40% of patients. Epilepsy and mental retardation occur in many patients. Glaucoma, buphthalmos, and blindness are present in 30% to 60% of cases. Patients who do not have nevus flammeus on the areas served by branches V1 and V2 of the trigeminal nerve have no signs or symptoms of eye and/or central nervous system (CNS) involvement (see Figure 23-13). Nevus flammeus of the eyelids, bilateral distribution of the birthmark, and unilateral nevus flammeus involving all three branches of the trigeminal nerve are associated with a significantly higher likelihood of having eye and/or CNS complications. Twenty-four percent of those with bilateral trigeminal nerve nevus flammeus have eye and/or CNS involvement, compared with 6% of those with unilateral lesions. All those who have eye and/or CNS complications have port-wine stain involvement of the eyelids; in 91% both upper and lower eyelids are involved, whereas in 9% only the lower eyelid is involved. None of those with upper eyelid nevus flammeus alone have eye and/or CNS complications. In summary, patients with nevus flammeus of the eyelids, bilateral lesions, and unilateral lesions involving all three divisions of the trigeminal nerve should be studied for glaucoma or for CNS lesions.

Box 23-3 **Sturge-Weber Syndrome (Encephalotrigeminal Angiomatosis)**

Vascular malformations of the central nervous system and the face (port-wine stain or nevus flammeus) in a V1 trigeminal nerve distribution

Port-wine stain (capillary malformation)

- Involves the ophthalmic branch of the trigeminal nerve, in particular the upper eyelid and supraorbital region
- May extend into the maxillary (V2) and mandibular (V3) regions
- May have associated soft tissue and bony overgrowth
- May be hidden in the scalp or mouth
- May be absent in the forme fruste of Sturge-Weber syndrome

Leptomeningeal malformation

- Usually ipsilateral to port-wine stain
- Capillary and venous anomalies
- No correlation between the size of facial and CNS malformations
- Characteristic computed tomography/magnetic resonance imaging findings may allow diagnosis in patients before onset of CNS manifestations

CNS manifestations

- Seizures
- Mental retardation
- Contralateral hemiplegia or hemisensory deficits
- Contralateral homonymous hemianopsia (impaired vision in half of the visual field)

Ocular involvement

- Ipsilateral to the port-wine stain
- Can be seen with V1 or V2 involvement
- Glaucoma
- Buphthalmos (enlargement of the ocular globe)
- Vascular malformations of the conjunctiva, episclera, choroid, and retina

From Mirowski GW et al: *J Am Acad Dermatol* 41:772, 1999. *PMID: 10534644*

Klippel-Trénaunay syndrome. The syndrome is characterized by the triad of capillary and venous malformations, venous varicosity, and hyperplasia of soft tissue—and possibly bone—in the affected area. If in addition there is an arteriovenous fistula, the term Park-Weber syndrome is used. The lower limb is the most commonly involved area.

TREATMENT. A nevus flammeus (port-wine stain) has the potential to cause lasting detrimental psychologic effects.

Lasers. Laser therapy is effective for midline lesions in adults and children. Centrofacial lesions and lesions involving maxillary areas in adults and children respond less favorably than lesions located elsewhere on the head and neck.

Individuals are treated as outpatients; patients under 12 years of age usually require some form of sedation or anesthesia, since the procedure is painful and cooperation during the procedure is necessary.

Cosmetics. The cosmetic appearance of some patients with nevus flammeus can be significantly improved by using the tinted waterproof makeup Covermark. Covermark is sold on the Internet (www.covermark.com). Dermablend is a similar product that is generally available in department stores or at www.dermablend.com.

SALMON PATCHES

Salmon patches (stork bite, angel's kiss) are actually variants of nevus flammeus; they are present in approximately 40% to 70% of newborns. They are red, irregular, macular patches resulting from dilation of dermal capillaries. The most common site is on the nape of the neck (Figure 23-16), where the lesion is referred to as a stork bite. They are often inconspicuous and covered by hair. Salmon patches on the face fade within 1 year, but those on the nape may persist for life.

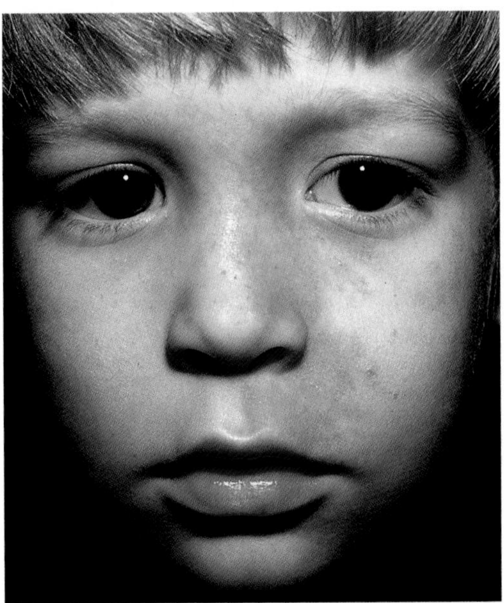

Figure 23-12 There is partial involvement of V1. The risk for Sturge-Weber is low.

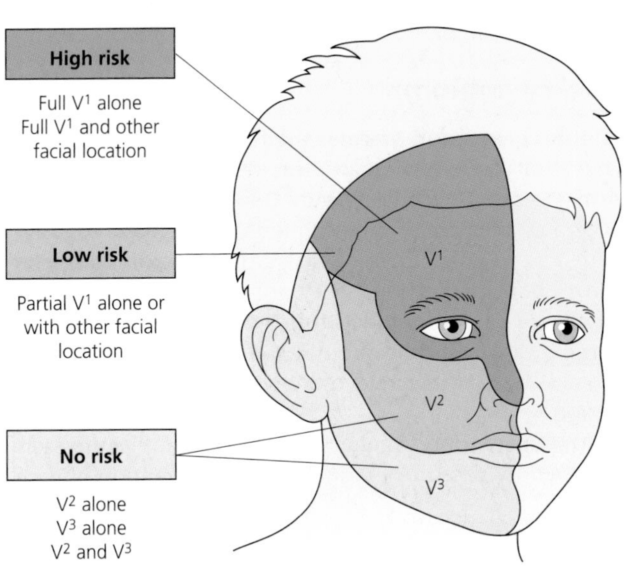

Figure 23-13 Facial port-wine stains and risk of Sturge-Weber syndrome.(Adapted from Enjolvas O, Riche MC, Merland JJ: *Pediatrics* 76:48, 1985.)

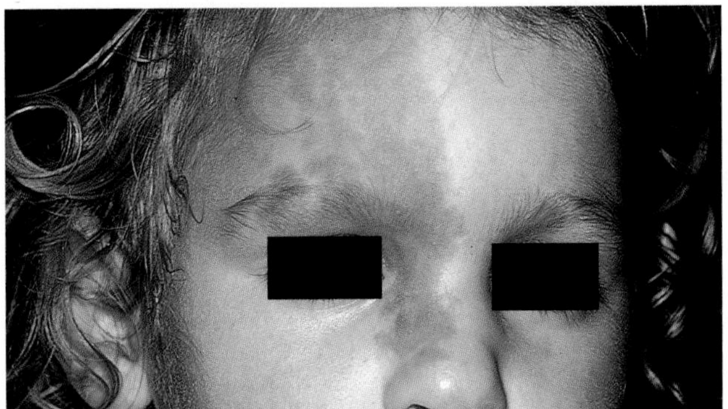

Figure 23-14 Sturge-Weber syndrome. Involvement of the entire V1 area puts the patient at high risk of having Sturge-Weber syndrome.

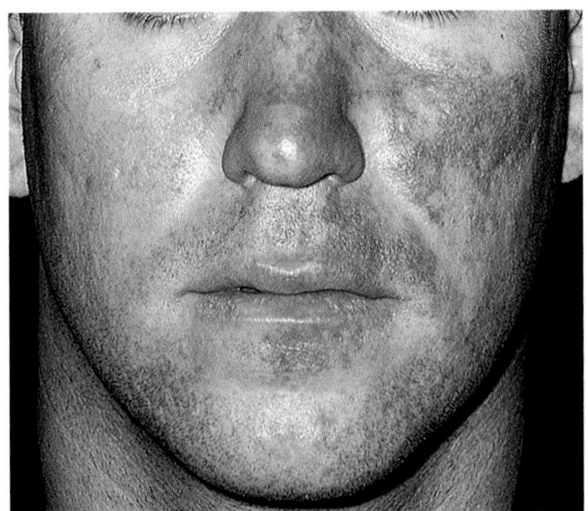

Figure 23-15 Port-wine stain involving V2. There were no CNS or ocular findings of Sturge-Weber syndrome.

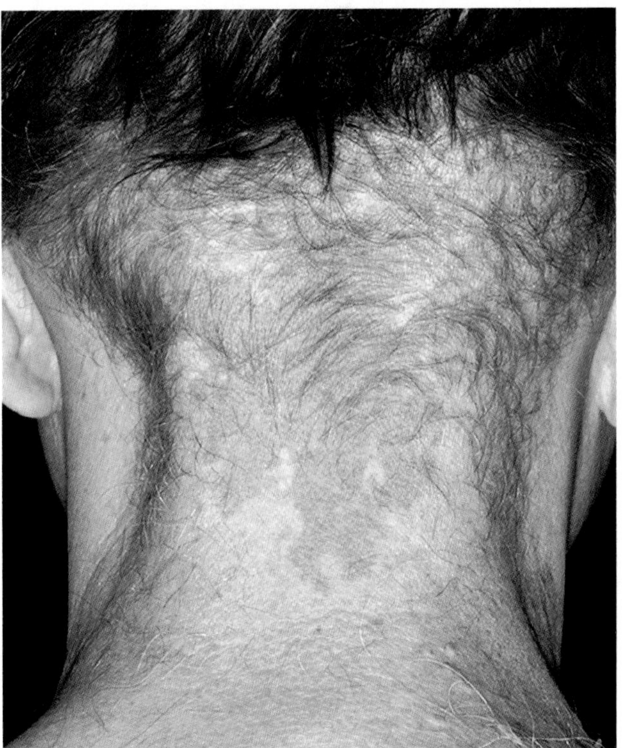

Figure 23-16 Salmon patch (stork bite). A variant of nevus flammeus found in many individuals on the nape of the neck.

ACQUIRED VASCULAR LESIONS

Cherry angioma

The most common vascular malformation is the benign cherry or senile angioma. These 0.5- to 5-mm, smooth, firm, deep red papules (Figure 23-17) occur in virtually everyone after age 30 and numerically increase with age. Patients recognize them as new growths, prompting concerns about malignancy. They are most common on the trunk and vary in number from a few to hundreds. Some pregnant women show an increased number of cherry angiomas during pregnancy that involute in the postpartum period.

Trauma produces slight bleeding. The papules are easily removed by scissor excision or electrodesiccation and curettage.

Angiokeratomas

Angiokeratomas are lesions characterized by dilation of the superficial dermal blood vessels and hyperkeratosis of the overlying epidermis. The term is applied to four different vascular malformations. The most common are angiokeratomas of the scrotum (Fordyce spots) or vulva (Figure 23-18) characterized by multiple, 2- to 3-mm, red-to-purple papules that occasionally bleed with trauma. The onset is between the ages of 20 and 50 years. Increased venous pressure may be implicated, such as occurs with pregnancy and hemorrhoids. If desired, removal is performed by simple scissor excision or electrodesiccation and curettage. The other forms of angiokeratomas are rare. They consist of red-brown-black, hyperkeratotic plaques varying in size and distribution. Numerous cutaneous angiokeratomas (angiokeratoma corporis diffusum) are part of Fabry-Anderson disease (see Table 23-4).

Figure 23-17 Cherry angioma. Multiple small, red papules commonly occur on the trunk.

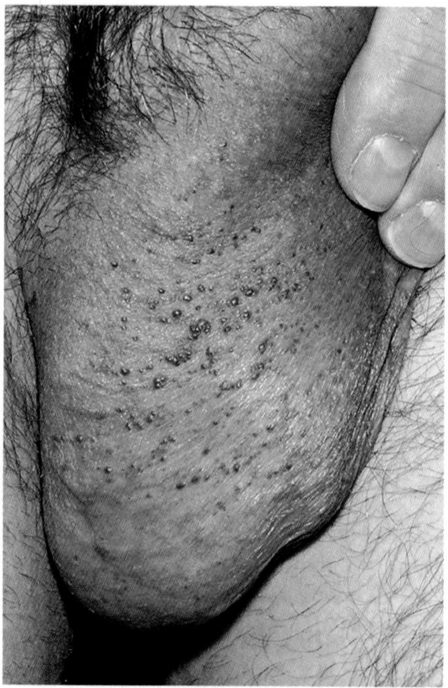

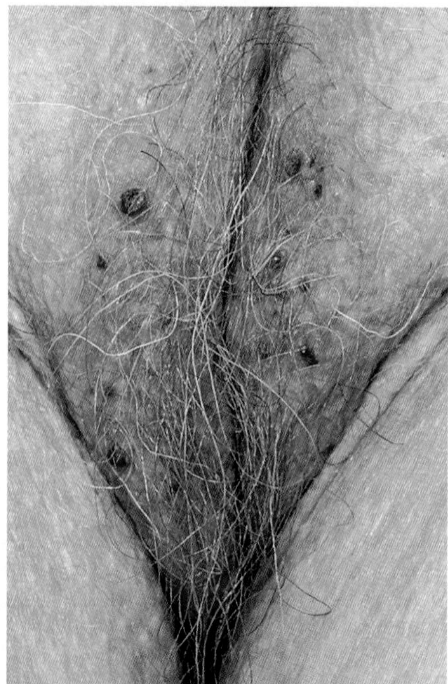

Figure 23-18 Angiokeratomas (Fordyce spots). Multiple red-to-purple papules consisting of multiple small blood vessels.

Venous lake

Venous lakes are dark blue, slightly elevated, 0.2- to 1-cm, dome-shaped lesions composed of a dilated, blood-filled vascular channel. They are common on sun-exposed surfaces of the vermilion border of the lip (Figure 23-19, *A*), the face, and the ears (Figure 23-19, *B*). Lesions resemble melanoma, but firm compression forces the blood out and proves they are vascular. They occasionally bleed following trauma and can be removed by electrodesiccation or with lasers.

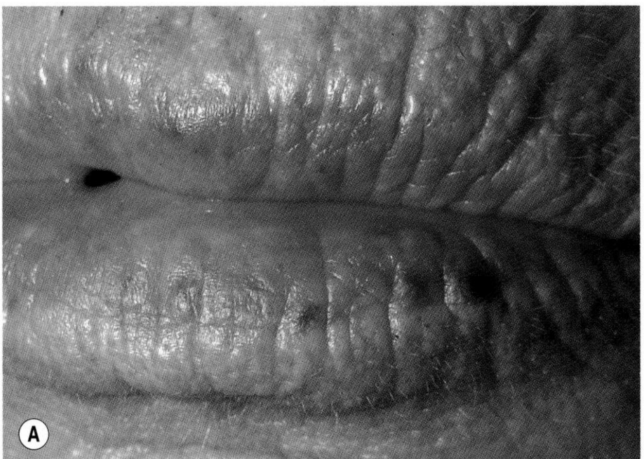

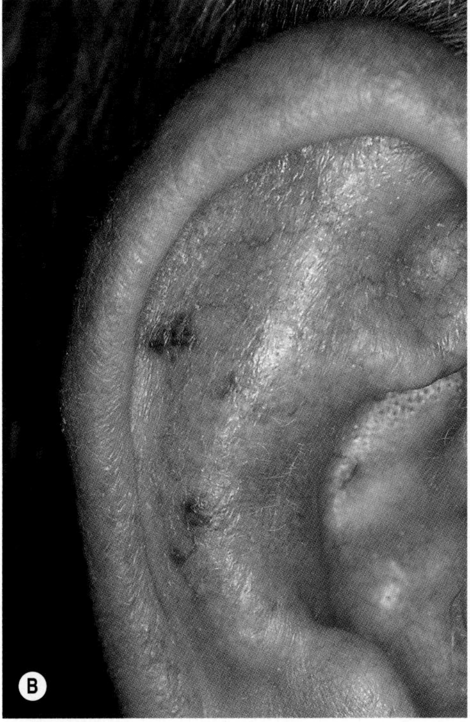

Figure 23-19 Venous lake. Dark blue papules caused by dilation of venules found on the vermilion border of the lower lips, ears, neck, and face. Several lesions may be present. Compression forces the blood out and flattens the lesion, proving that it is not a melanoma. Actinic damage is probably the cause.

Lymphangioma circumscriptum

These uncommon but distinctive hamartomatous malformations consist of dilated lymph channels, which may be filled with serosanguineous fluid, that communicate with deeper lymph channels. The appearance of the lesions has been compared to a mass of frog's eggs ("frog spawn"). They consist of tiny to 5-mm, grouped, translucent or hemorrhagic vesicles on a dull red or brown base (Figure 23-20). Some lesions contain a mixture of vascular and lymph channels. Lesions may appear in the setting of postmastectomy lymphedema as a result of lymphatic damage following surgery and radiation. This is referred to as secondary lymphangioma (lymphangiectasis).

The malformations consist of a collection of subcutaneous lymphatic cisterns with a thick muscle coat that communicates through dilated channels lined with lymphatic endothelium with the superficial vesicles. There is no communication between the cysts and the adjacent normal lymphatics. The contraction of the muscle coat may force fluid to the surface and create the vesicles. The depth and extent of involvement cannot be adequately estimated from the cutaneous examination. Magnetic resonance imaging has been used to demonstrate accurately the true extent of involvement.

TREATMENT. Treatment is indicated for cosmetic reasons and to prevent leakage of fluid and recurrent infection. The lesions recur unless the deep communicating cisterns are removed or destroyed. Small groups of surface vessels can be destroyed by electrosurgery. Surgical removal of the subcutaneous cisterns, leaving sufficient skin for primary closure, results in acceptable cure rates. Residual skin vesicles separated from their underlying cysts regress. Surface lymphatic vessels are vaporized, and communicating channels to deeper cisterns are sealed with the CO_2 laser, which, unlike the argon laser, is not color dependent for vaporization.

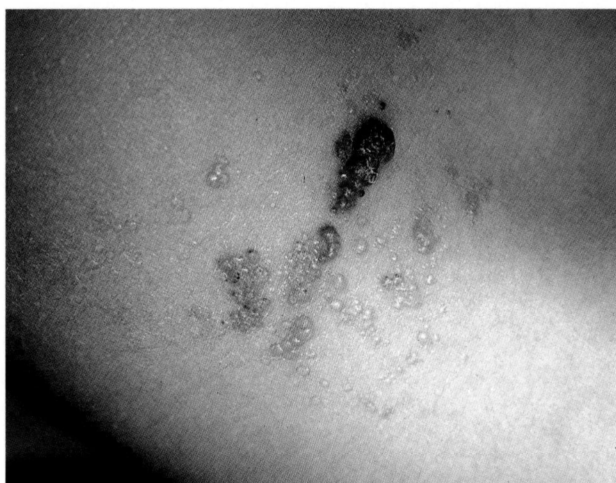

Figure 23-20 Lymphangioma circumscriptum with dilated lymph channels. Appearance has been compared to a mass of frog's eggs ("frog spawn"). Lesions are filled with clear or blood-tinged fluid.

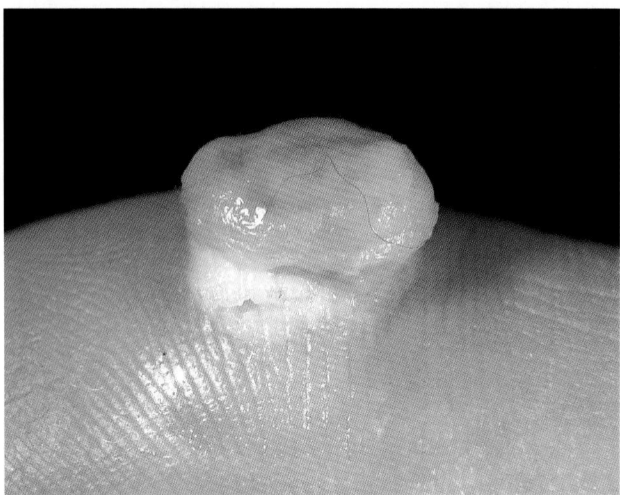

Figure 23-21 Pyogenic granulomas have either a glistening yellow or red surface. The base of this lesion contains a collarette of white scale.

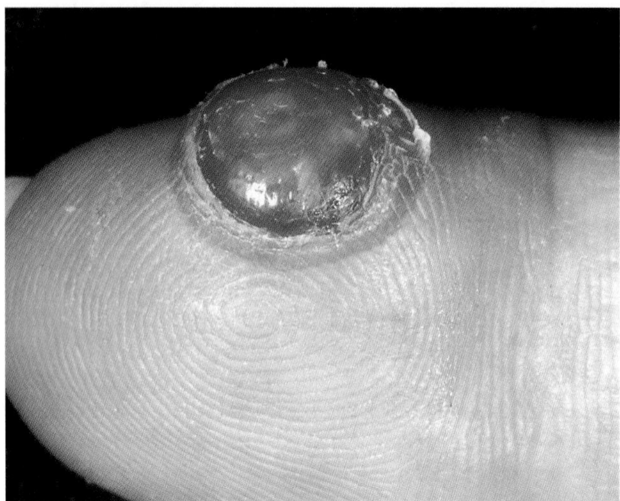

Figure 23-22 Pyogenic granuloma. A dome-shaped tumor with a moist, fragile surface. The lesion may bleed profusely with the slightest trauma.

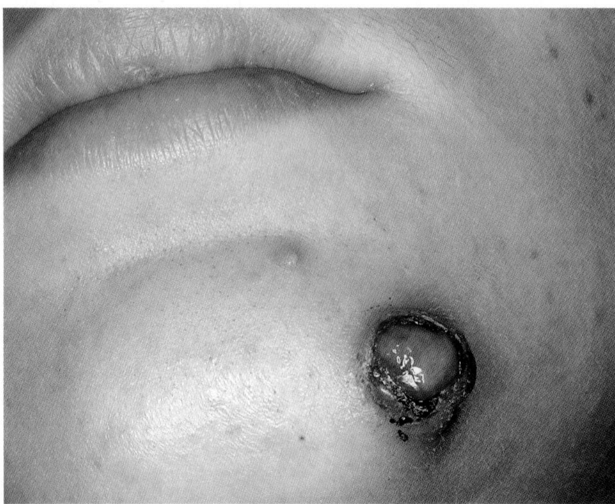

Figure 23-23 Pyogenic granuloma. Most lesions are small. The major complaint is profuse and prolonged bleeding.

Pyogenic granuloma (lobular capillary hemangioma)

Pyogenic granuloma is a benign acquired vascular lesion of the skin and mucous membranes that is common in children and young adults. It often appears as a response to an injury or hormonal factors. Pyogenic granuloma may develop in cysts of acne patients treated with isotretinoin. The base of the lesion is often surrounded by a collarette of scale (Figure 23-21). Lesions are small (less than 1 cm), rapidly growing, yellow-to-bright-red, dome-shaped (Figures 23-22 and 23-23), fragile protrusions that have a glistening, moist-to-scaly surface. They are most commonly seen on the head and neck region and on the extremities, especially the fingers. Pyogenic granuloma occurs in pregnant women (pregnancy epulis) and is found primarily in the gingiva. The word epulis is used to describe a localized growth on the gingiva.

The slightest trauma causes bleeding that is difficult to control. The dermis is composed of a mass of capillaries. Pyogenic suggests an infectious origin, but the lesion is neither a hemangioma nor a neoplasm. It is an inflammatory and hyperplastic condition, better interpreted as a florid expression of granulation tissue proliferation. Pyogenic granuloma–like lesions occur in patients with acquired immunodeficiency syndrome (AIDS) who develop cat-scratch disease (bacillary angiomatosis).

TREATMENT. Treatment consists of firm and thorough curettage of the base and border. Electrodesiccation is often necessary to eradicate the lesions completely and to control bleeding. Pyogenic granuloma recurs if the smallest piece of abnormal tissue remains. Multiple recurrent lesions are more common in adolescents or young adults, and they occur after attempts of electrodesiccation or surgical removal of the primary single lesion. Spontaneous resolution usually occurs within 6 months. Pregnancy epulis usually regresses following childbirth.

BACILLARY ANGIOMATOSIS

Bacillary angiomatosis is an infectious disease caused by two species of *Bartonella: B. quintana* and *B. henselae*. Cats may serve as a reservoir of the disease in some patients. A cat scratch or bite may transmit the bacteria. Homelessness, poverty, and alcoholism are risk factors for *B. quintana* infection, and unsanitary living conditions may predispose to ectoparasites that transmit the infection.

Skin lesions may be solitary or multiple, and some patients have a widespread eruption with innumerable lesions. The lesions begin as red-to-purple, pinpoint-size papules that increase in size to form nodules and tumors. Superficial lesions resemble pyogenic granuloma; deeper lesions appear as red subcutaneous nodules that may enlarge to several centimeters in diameter. Involvement of the oral and genital mucous membranes is also frequent. (See also Figure 15-42, p. 615).

Kaposi's sarcoma

Kaposi's sarcomas (KS), or multiple idiopathic hemorrhagic sarcomas, are vascular neoplasms that were rarely seen before the AIDS era. KS can be divided into five subsets on the basis of clinical and epidemiologic criteria (Table 23-5). The incidence of second malignancies (especially lymphoreticular neoplasms) is increased in classic Kaposi's sarcoma and in KS patients with AIDS. Both classic and AIDS-associated Kaposi's sarcomas are caused by human herpesvirus 8 (HHV-8).

PATHOGENESIS. Human herpesvirus 8 in the presence of host immunosuppression is the primary factor in the development of all forms of Kaposi's sarcoma. Serologic studies show that, unlike other human herpesviruses, Kaposi's sarcoma–associated herpesvirus is not ubiquitous. Like other human herpesviruses, most primary infections appear to be asymptomatic. The virus can be transmitted sexually and by other means. The virus has been found in saliva and semen of infected persons. The highest rates of infection are in central Africa. Homosexual men, regardless of their HIV serostatus, have an asymptomatic infection rate of almost 40%.

CLASSIC KAPOSI'S SARCOMA. The rare classic form generally appears on the hands, feet, or lower legs and progresses up the arms and legs. It begins as violaceous macules and papules and very slowly progresses to form plaques with multiple red-purple nodules (Figure 23-24).

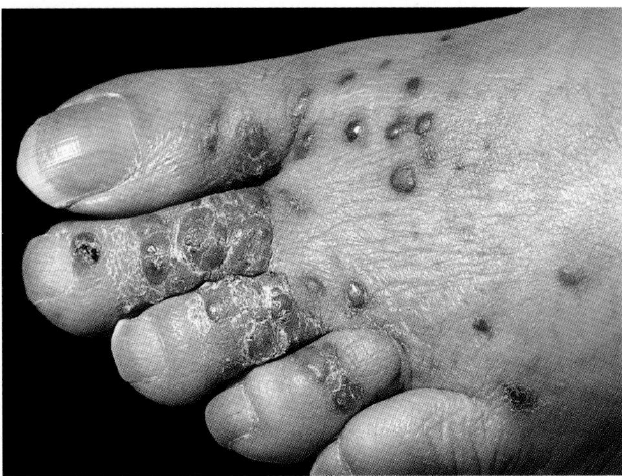

Figure 23-24 Kaposi's sarcoma. Most lesions are on the lower extremities. Shown here are plaques and tumors.

It occurs almost exclusively in elderly males of Jewish, Greek, or Italian descent. The male to female ratio is 15 to 1. Progression of this disease in the elderly is slow (years or decades) and, although lymph node and visceral involvement can occur, most of these patients die of unrelated causes. Immunocompetent asymptomatic patients with little progression can simply be observed. Excision or intralesional injection of interferon alfa-2b (1 million to 3 million units) is effective for single lesions.

Table 23-5 Clinical Features of Kaposi's Sarcoma

	Classic	African cutaneous	African lymphadenopathic	AIDS	Immunosuppressive
Epidemiology	Sporadic (endemic)	Endemic	Endemic	Endemic	Sporadic
Age (years)	50-70	<10, >20	<10	25-42	20-80
Mean age	68	35	<10	35	—
M:F ratio	3:1	10-15:1	1-2:1	Male, homosexual	10-17:1
Incidence	0.02	—	0.1-0.85*,†	40% -70%, up to 90%	—
% cancers diagnosed	0.06	—	9	—	—
Sites	Legs, feet	Extremities	Nodes	Head, neck, upper aspect of trunk	Variable
Lesion type	Nodular	Nodular, florid, infiltrating	Lymphadenopathic	Macules, plaques, nodules	Nodules
Node involvement	Rare	Uncommon, indolent	Expected	Common	Variable
Course	Indolent	Locally aggressive	Aggressive	Fulminant	Fulminant
Treatment response	Good	Good	Good initially	Poor	Variable

From Piette WW: *J Am Acad Dermatol* 16:855, 1987. *PMID: 3553249*
*Cases per 100,000 population.
†Representative incidence figures from Tanzania.

ENDEMIC AFRICAN KAPOSI'S SARCOMA. Kaposi's sarcoma in HIV-negative and HIV-positive patients is the most frequently occurring tumor in central Africa. It accounts for up to 50% of tumors reported in men in some countries. There are two forms: cutaneous and lymphatic. Both are rare in patients between 10 and 20 years of age. The cutaneous form typically occurs in men (median age, 41 years) with indolent disease and nodules or plaques on edematous limbs. Lymph node or systemic involvement is uncommon. The aggressive lymphadenopathic form is seen in children younger than 10 years of age. In eastern and southern Africa, KS makes up 25% to 50% of soft tissue sarcomas in children and 2% to 10% of all cancers in children. Cutaneous lesions may surface; the prognosis is poor. Endemic KS responds to local radiation therapy or chemotherapy. Complete (32%) and partial (54%) regression of cutaneous lesions was achieved with radiation therapy, which is the treatment of choice for this disease.

KAPOSI'S SARCOMA ASSOCIATED WITH IMMUNOSUPPRESSION. Kaposi's sarcoma develops in 0.1% to 5.3% of transplant recipients (especially in certain ethnic groups), of which 67% to 80% are men. The median interval from organ transplantation to the diagnosis of KS is 30 months. A primary herpesvirus 8 infection transmitted by the transplanted organs is a possible source. This type of KS is aggressive, involving lymph nodes, mucosa, and visceral organs in about half of patients, sometimes in the absence of skin lesions. Some tumors regress after therapy is withdrawn, and others respond to radiation and chemotherapy.

EPIDEMIC OR AIDS-RELATED KAPOSI'S SYNDROME. The incidence of KS in American men with AIDS has decreased dramatically since 1981. It is the most common tumor that occurs in patients infected with the human immunodeficiency virus. KS probably occurs as a multicentric rather than a metastatic disease in AIDS. Unlike the classic form, lesions are often multifocal and widespread when first detected. They are most commonly found on the trunk and the head and neck areas. Mucous membranes are involved. They initially form slightly raised, oval or elongated, poorly demarcated, rust-colored infiltrates. Rapid progression to red or purple nodules and plaques may follow (Figures 23-25 and 23-26). They may look like granulation tissue, stasis dermatitis, pyogenic granuloma, capillary hemangiomas, or trichophytic Majocchi's granuloma. More than half of the patients have generalized lymphadenopathy at the time of first examination. Eventually most patients develop extracutaneous disease (oral cavity, gastrointestinal [GI] tract, lungs, and lymph nodes) (see Chapter 11). It is important to treat cutaneous lesions for cosmetic purposes, because their presence is a constant reminder of a fatal disease. Limited cutaneous disease is treated with alitretinoin gel (Panretin), intralesional vinblastine, radiation therapy, laser therapy, or cryotherapy. Antiretroviral therapy helps resolve immunosuppression and slows progression or shrinks KS. The response is unpredictable and other treatments are required. The response to radiation therapy and chemotherapy is less than that seen in classic KS.

TREATMENT. AIDS-KS is not curable. KS treatments are not specific and rely on reconstitution of the immune system and systemic administration of cytotoxic agents. The goals are palliation of symptoms; shrinkage of tumors to alleviate edema, organ compromise, or psychologic stress; and prevention of disease progression. Local and systemic therapies are used. Observation is appropriate for immunocompetent asymptomatic patients with little progression of disease over a long period of time. In some cases the disease regresses spontaneously. In cases of iatrogenic KS, immunosuppressive agents should be reduced or discon-

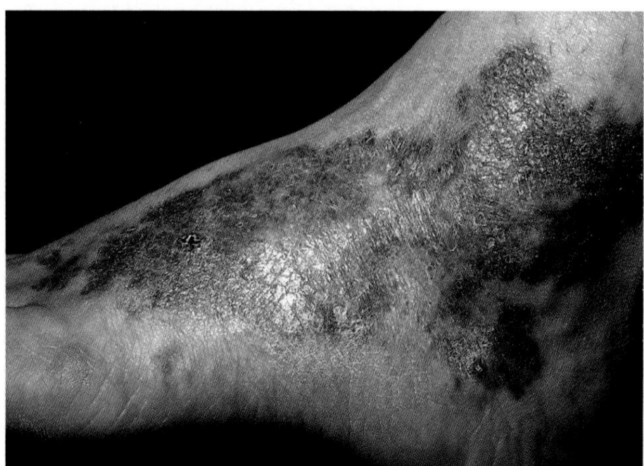

Figure 23-25 Kaposi's sarcoma—a broad superficial plaque.

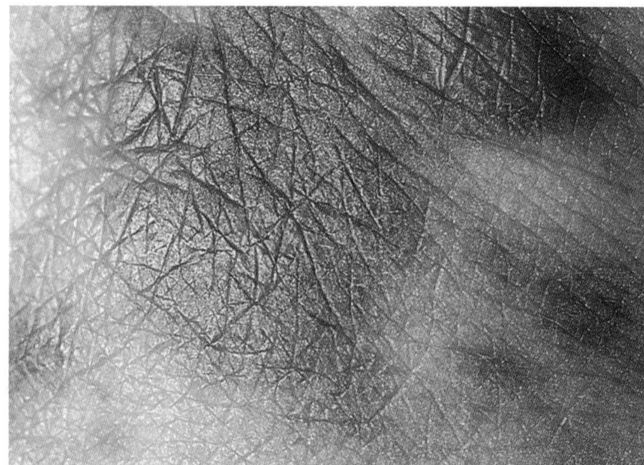

Figure 23-26 Kaposi's sarcoma. Early lesion consisting of violaceous macules and plaques.

tinued, if possible. Switching to sirolimus in organ transplant recipients has also been reported as efficacious. Classical KS usually progresses only slowly and does not always require chemotherapy. Antiretroviral therapy alone or in combination with chemotherapy (liposomal doxorubicin) is the mainstay of treating HIV-associated KS. After immunoreconstitution there is often complete remission of HIV-associated KS.

Staging (T1), CD4 cell count (<200 cells/μL), and positive HHV-8 DNA in plasma at the time of diagnosis predict evolution towards death or the need for chemotherapy. *PMID: 18520345*

Follow-up. Reevaluate every 6 to 12 months for HIV-associated disease. Examine the skin and mucous membranes, the lungs (chest x-ray), and the gastrointestinal tract (occult blood, sonography, perhaps endoscopy). In classical Kaposi's sarcoma lymph node ultrasonography and skin examination are usually sufficient.

Systemic therapy. Systemic therapies for AIDS-KS produce significant side effects. Systemic treatment for KS is indicated for patients with rapidly progressive mucocutaneous disease, causing lymphedema, ulceration, and pain, and for those with symptomatic visceral involvement and/or pulmonary involvement and debilitating KS-related symptoms. Regression of KS with highly active antiretroviral therapy (HAART) is well documented. It is often the only therapy needed in the early stages of the disease and/or for slowly proliferating disease. In patients with rapidly proliferating disease, the first-line therapy is chemotherapy with or without antiretroviral therapy followed by maintenance with HAART. Liposomal anthracyclines are the first choice for the treatment of advanced or rapidly proliferating AIDS-KS because they are more effective when used in combination with HAART. Paclitaxel is used after failure of first-line or subsequent systemic chemotherapy, and also as second-line therapy. Combination chemotherapy (doxorubicin, bleomycin, vincristine, vinblastine) is used when liposomal anthracyclines or paclitaxel is not available.

Surgery. Excision is appropriate for single lesions and resectable recurrences.

Radiation. Kaposi's sarcoma is a radiosensitive tumor. Radiation therapy was the primary form of local therapy for KS before the AIDS epidemic. Response rates of greater than 80% were achieved. Radiation therapy is indicated for large tumor masses, especially those that interfere with normal function. The rate of regression of individual lesions following radiotherapy is 80% to 90%. A total dose of 20 to 30 Gy delivered in individual doses of 4 to 5 Gy is required. Lymph nodes are treated with a total target goal of 40 Gy (5 × 2 Gy/week).

Liquid nitrogen cryotherapy. Liquid nitrogen cryotherapy is easily applied as a primary therapy. A complete response is observed in 80% of treated Kaposi's sarcoma lesions. There is often persistent Kaposi's sarcoma in the deeper dermis under the treated site, but the cosmetic effect is excellent. Patients receive an average of three treatments per lesion. Treatment is repeated at 3-week intervals, allowing adequate healing time. One treatment consisted of two freeze-thaw cycles, with thaw times ranging from 11 to 60 seconds per cycle (range, 10 to 20 seconds for macular lesions and 30 to 60 seconds for papular lesions). Treatment is well tolerated. Blistering occurs frequently, but pain is limited. Secondary infection does not occur. Keep treated lesions covered until they heal, because blister fluid may contain HIV cells.

Intralesional chemotherapy. Intralesional chemotherapy is more effective than cryotherapy for nodular lesions greater than 1 cm in diameter. It is also useful for the treatment of symptomatic oral lesions. Postinflammatory hyperpigmentation may respond to cryotherapy or may be camouflaged with cosmetics. Vinblastine is prepared from stock solutions to the desired concentration. Vinblastine-containing syringes can be stored under refrigeration after preparation. Vinblastine 0.1 mg (0.5 ml of a 0.2 mg/ml solution) is injected per square centimeter of lesion. Oral lesions and larger cutaneous lesions respond best to 0.2 mg/cm^2. In this setting, increasing the concentration of vinblastine to 0.4 to 0.6 mg/ml is recommended to reduce the volume injected per square centimeter of lesion to 0.5 ml. A maximum total dose of 2 mg during clinic visits is recommended. After a healing interval of 3 weeks, each treated lesion may require an additional one to two injections for maximal response. Pain lasts for 1 to 2 days. Local anesthesia does not reduce the efficacy of treatment or the pain experienced by the patient.

Topical retinoids. Alitretinoin (Panretin) used for 12 to 16 weeks produced a response rate of 36%. Alitretinoin gel may be used for KS that is not severe enough to use systemic chemotherapy and for patients who have received systemic chemotherapy and want to treat lesions that remain.

Alitretinoin is not indicated when systemic anti-KS therapy is required (e.g., in patients with more than 10 cutaneous lesions in the prior month, symptomatic lymphedema, symptomatic pulmonary KS, or symptomatic visceral involvement).

RADIATION THERAPY

Interferon. Interferon results in relatively long-term response durations in patients with relatively preserved immune function. The response rate to interferon varies from 20% to 60%. Hepatic toxicity, constitutional symptoms, and myelosuppression limit its use.

Interferon results in response durations of up to 2 years. The time of response for interferon-alfa is 8 to 12 weeks. It is therefore not inappropriate for rapidly progressive KS. Combined treatment with interferon and chemotherapy agents may cause severe hematologic toxicity.

TELANGIECTASIAS

Telangiectasias are permanently dilated, small blood vessels consisting of venules, capillaries, or arterioles. The maximum diameter is 1 mm. Vessels appear as single strands, in groups as small macules, or with a central punctum. They accompany a variety of diseases and sometimes are clues to the underlying diagnosis (Box 23-4). Telangiectasias are usually only a cosmetic problem; they rarely bleed.

Spider angiomas

Spider angiomas (nevus araneus) form as arterioles (spider bodies), become more prominent near the surface of the skin, and radiate capillaries (spider legs) (Figure 23-27). They are present in 10% to 15% of normal adults and young children. Once formed, they tend to be permanent. Bleeding rarely occurs. The face, neck, upper part of the trunk, and arm are involved in adults. In children they are most often seen on the hands and fingers. They increase in number with liver disease and during pregnancy and are probably stimulated by higher-than-normal estrogen concentrations. Lesions usually disappear at the end of the pregnancy. Spider angiomas should be distinguished from the flat patches of tiny vessels of uniform size (telangiectatic mats) seen in scleroderma.

TREATMENT. Local anesthesia is optional in the following procedure for treatment. The blood is forced out of the spider by pressing firmly on the lesion; with continuous pressure, the finger is moved slightly to one side to expose the central arteriole, and the central arteriole is gently electrodesiccated. If the arteriole has been destroyed, the radiating capillaries may not fill. Incompletely destroyed lesions may recur. Vigorous desiccation may cause a pitted scar. Recurrences are uncommon. Lasers are also effective.

Box 23-4 **Classification of Telangiectasia**

Primary (cause unknown)

Ataxia telangiectasia
Generalized essential telangiectasia
Hemorrhagic hereditary telangiectasia (Osler-Weber-Rendu syndrome)
Spider angiomas
Unilateral nevoid telangiectasia syndrome

Secondary (part of known entity)

Actinically damaged skin
After laser or electrosurgery
After cryosurgery
Basal cell carcinoma
Collagen vascular disease
- Dermatomyositis
- Lupus erythematosus
- Scleroderma

Cushing's syndrome
Estrogen excess
- Cirrhosis
- Oral contraceptives
- Pregnancy

Metastatic carcinoma
Necrobiosis lipoidica diabeticorum
Poikilodermas
Pseudoxanthoma elasticum
Radiation therapy injury
Rosacea
Telangiectasia macularis eruptiva perstans (generalized cutaneous mastocytosis)
Topical steroid induced
Xeroderma pigmentosa

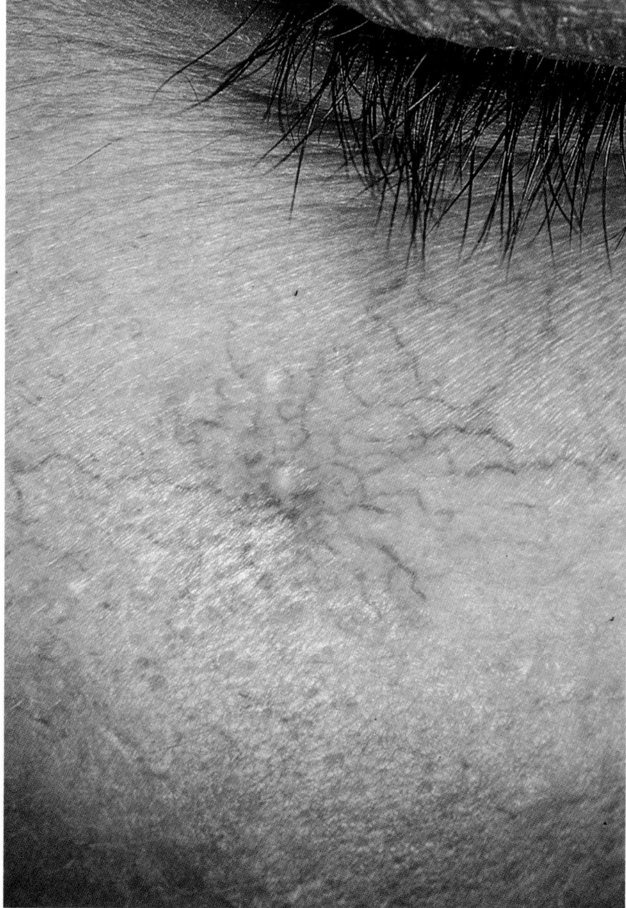

Figure 23-27 Spider angioma. Lesions appear in 10% to 15% of children and adults. Most patients have one or two lesions. They are found most commonly on the face, upper part of the trunk, and backs of the hands. Lesions may occur during pregnancy and resolve months after delivery. Suspect liver disease in patients with many lesions.

Hereditary hemorrhagic telangiectasia

Hereditary hemorrhagic telangiectasia (HHT) (Osler-Weber-Rendu syndrome) is an autosomal dominant disease characterized by epistaxis, cutaneous telangiectasias, and visceral arteriovenous malformations that affect many organs. The characteristic lesions begin as tiny, flat telangiectasias, with a few vessels radiating from a single point. Arterioles in the dermis become dilated and communicate directly with the venules without intervening capillaries. Engorged lesions are fragile and bleed easily with the slightest trauma. Few to numerous lesions occur, primarily on the lips, tongue (Figure 23-28), nasal mucosa, forearms, hands, fingers, palms and soles, under the nails, and throughout the gastrointestinal tract, but any skin area or internal organ may be involved. Epistaxis is the most common manifestation. It may require multiple transfusions and oral iron supplements. Recurrent epistaxis begins by the age of 10 years and becomes more severe in later decades. Although lesions may be prominent during childhood, they are most often so small and subtle that stretching the lip is required to accentuate them. By the third or fourth decade, telangiectasias become more apparent, and the diagnosis is easily made. HHT is the most common cause of pulmonary arteriovenous fistula; 5% to 15% of persons with HHT have pulmonary arteriovenous malformations. High-resolution helical computed tomographic scanning without the use of contrast material demonstrates the vessels. Chest radiography, arterial blood gas measurements, and finger oximetry are screening tests for suspected pulmonary arteriovenous malformations. Most lesions occur near the base of the lungs.

The distribution and clinical appearance of the telangiectasia in CREST syndrome (calcinosis, Raynaud's phenomenon, esophageal involvement, sclerodactyly, telangiectasia) and HHT are very similar.

Recurrent bleeding from nasal or gastrointestinal telangiectasia is fatal in a small number of cases. GI bleeding usually starts in the fifth or sixth decade.

Genetic testing. Genetic testing is complex and only performed at a few centers in the United States. Prenatal diagnosis for pregnancies at increased risk is possible by analysis of DNA extracted from fetal cells obtained by amniocentesis usually performed at about 15 to 18 weeks of gestation or by chorionic villus sampling (CVS) at about 10 to 12 weeks of gestation. The disease-causing allele of an affected family member must be identified before prenatal testing can be performed.

TREATMENT. Bleeding points are treated by electrocautery. Local hyperfibrinolysis has been demonstrated in lesions mediated by an increase in tissue plasminogen activator. This finding provides a basis for the use of antifibrinolytic drugs. Epistaxis improved and hemoglobin levels increased with tranexamic acid (1 gm four times daily), an antifibrinolytic drug that is 10 times as potent as aminocaproic acid and has a longer half-life. Intranasal tranexamic acid is also effective.

Scleroderma

The telangiectasias of CREST syndrome and scleroderma have a unique morphology. They occur as flat (macular), 0.5-cm, rectangular collections of uniform tiny vessels; these are the so-called telangiectatic mats (see Figure 17-30). These mats are most commonly found on the face, lips, palms, and backs of the hands. Telangiectasias may be present around the lips, tongue, and mucous membranes. Involvement of the oral mucosa also suggests Osler-Weber-Rendu syndrome.

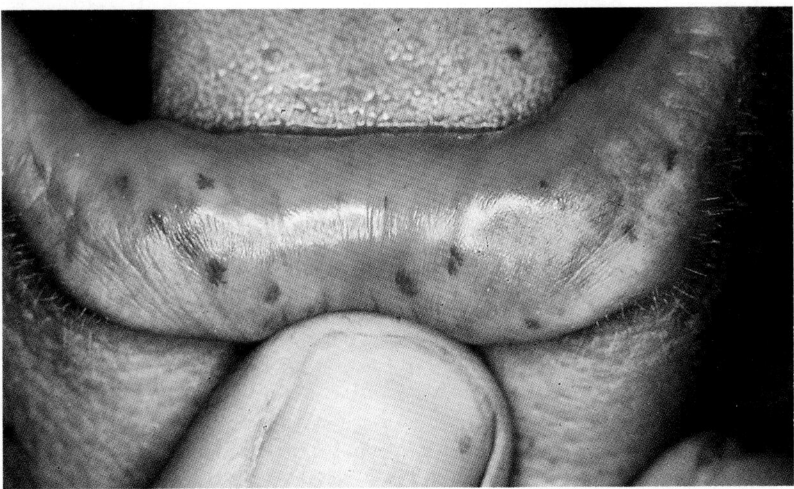

Figure 23-28 Hereditary hemorrhagic telangiectasia. Telangiectasias are found on the lips, oral mucosa, nasal mucosa, skin, and conjunctiva. Epistaxis is the most common manifestation of the disease. Blood transfusions may be required.

Unilateral nevoid telangiectasia syndrome

Numerous threadlike telangiectasias that appear in a unilateral dermatomal distribution are called unilateral superficial telangiectasias. There are acquired and congenital forms. The congenital form is more common in males. The acquired form begins with states of increasing estrogen blood levels: (1) at puberty in females, (2) during pregnancy (Figure 23-29), or (3) with alcoholic cirrhosis. In subsequent pregnancies the syndrome recurs once it has appeared, although it may appear for the first time during a second pregnancy. Most cases involve the trigeminal, C3, C4, or adjacent dermatomes. The distribution suggests an estrogen-sensitive nevoid anomaly. Telangiectasias may involve the oral and gastric mucosa. Lesions may clear as levels of estrogen decrease.

Pulsed dye laser, 585 nm, is an effective treatment, but the response is short-lived, with a 100% recurrence.

Generalized essential telangiectasia

Widespread idiopathic telangiectasia (generalized essential telangiectasia) is a rare disorder characterized by the development and gradual spreading of telangiectasias. It is seen primarily in women and is sometimes familial. The average age at onset is 38 years. For no apparent reason telangiectases start to appear in the lower extremities and progress steadily to involve the skin of the trunk, the arms, and the face (Figure 23-30). General health is not affected, and standard laboratory tests are normal. Conjunctival telangiectasias are rarely reported.

The telangiectasias slowly progress over years or decades and are not accompanied by associated systemic problems. Autosomal dominant transmission has been suggested. Lesions have been reported to resolve with tetracycline. Successful treatment with the 585-nm flashlamp-pumped pulsed dye laser has been reported.

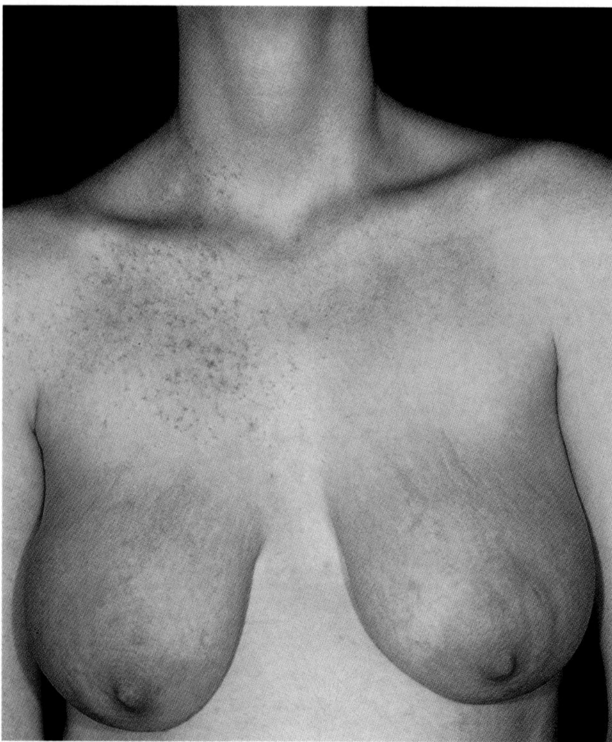

Figure 23-29 Unilateral nevoid telangiectasia syndrome. Telangiectasia appeared on the right chest and arm during pregnancy.

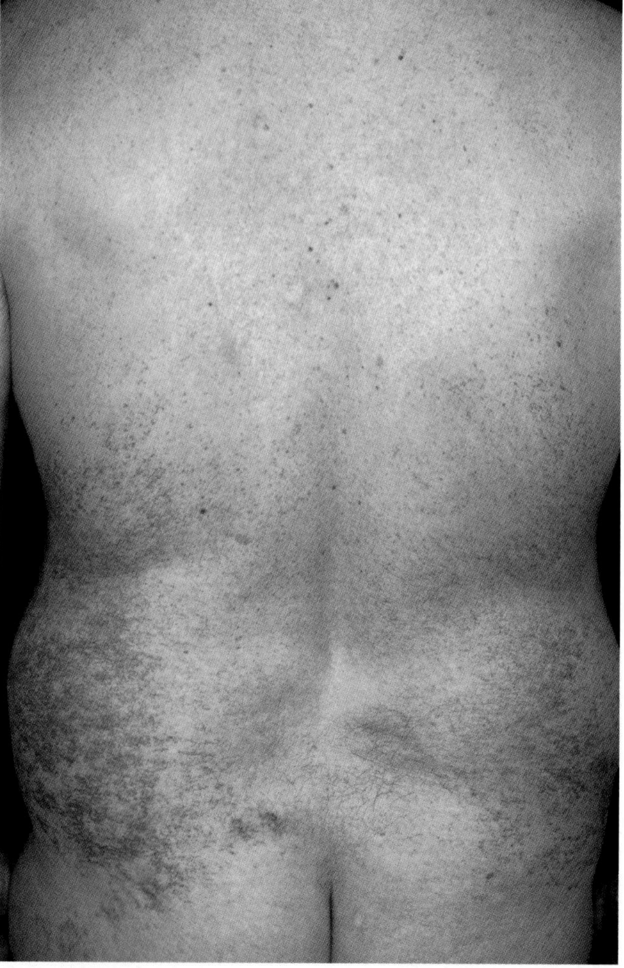

Figure 23-30 Generalized essential telangiectasia. The age of onset is usually in the fourth or fifth decade. The dilated blood vessels are capillary telangiectasias. They do not bleed.

Chapter 24

Hair Diseases

CHAPTER CONTENTS

Physicians are frequently confronted with hair-related problems. Most complaints are from patients with early-onset pattern baldness. The physician must be able to recognize this normal, inherited hair loss pattern so that detailed and expensive evaluations can be avoided. Other patients have complaints about abnormal hair growth; these diseases must be recognized and not dismissed as balding. The signs of hair loss or excess growth are at times subtle. The signs usually seen with cutaneous disease, such as inflammation, may be absent. A systematic approach to evaluation is essential.

ANATOMY

TYPES OF HAIR. There are three types of hair. Thick, pigmented hairs are called terminal hairs. Terminal hairs on the top of the head and in the beard, axillary, and pubic areas are influenced by androgens. Androgens are important in regulating hair growth. At puberty, androgens increase the size of follicles in the beard, chest, and limbs and decrease the size of follicles in the bitemporal region, which reshapes the hairline in men and many women.

Lanugo hairs are the fine hairs found on the fetus; similar fine hairs (peach fuzz) found on the adult are called vellus hairs. Vellus hair is short, fine, and relatively nonpigmented and covers much of the body. Hair on the rest of the body is independent of androgens.

HAIR STRUCTURE. The hair shaft is dead protein. It is formed by compact cells that are covered by a delicate cuticle composed of platelike scales. The living cells in the matrix multiply more rapidly than those in any other normal human tissue. They push up into the follicular canal, undergo dehydration, and form the hair shaft, which consists of a dense, hard mass of keratinized cells. Normal hairs have a pointed tip. The hair in the follicular canal forms a cylinder of uniform diameter. Short hairs with tapered tips either have short growth cycles or have experienced the recent onset of anagen.

The growing shaft is surrounded by several concentric layers (see Figure 24-2). The outermost glycogen-rich layer is called the outer root sheath. It is static and continuous with the epidermis. The inner root sheath (Henle's layer, Huxley's layer, and cuticle) is visible as a gelatinous mass when the hair is plucked. It protects and molds the growing hair but disintegrates before reaching the surface at the infundibulum.

The hair shaft that emerges has three layers—an outer cuticle, a cortex, and sometimes an inner medulla—all of which are composed of dead protein. The cuticle protects and holds the cortex cells together. Split ends result if the cuticle is damaged by brushing or chemical cosmetic treatments. The cortex cells in the growing hair shaft rapidly synthesize and accumulate proteins while in the lower regions of the hair follicle. Systemic diseases and drugs may interfere with the metabolism of these cells and reduce the hair shaft diameter. Pigment-containing melanosomes are acquired deep in the bulb matrix and are deposited in the cortical and medullary cells.

HAIR FOLLICLE. Humans have about 5 million hair follicles at birth. No follicles are formed after birth, but their size changes under the influence of androgens. The hair follicle is formed in the embryo by a club-shaped epidermal down-growth—the primary epithelial germ that is invaginated from below by a flame-shaped, capillary-containing dermal structure called the papilla of the hair follicle. The central cells of the down-growth form the hair matrix, the cells of which form the hair shaft and its surrounding structures. The matrix lies deep within the subcutaneous fat. The mature follicle contains a hair shaft, two surrounding sheaths, and a germinative bulb (Figure 24-1). The follicle is divided into three sections. The infundibulum extends from the surface to the sebaceous gland duct. The isthmus extends from the duct down to the insertion of the erector muscle. The inferior segment, which exists only during the growing (anagen) phase, extends from the muscle insertion to the base of the matrix. The matrix contains the cells that proliferate to form the hair shaft (Figure 24-2). The mitotic rate of the hair matrix is greater than that of any other organ. The cells begin to differentiate at the top of the bulb. The inner and outer root sheaths protect and mold the growing hair. The inner root sheath disintegrates at the duct of the sebaceous gland. Hair growth is greatly influenced by any stress or disease process that can alter mitotic activity.

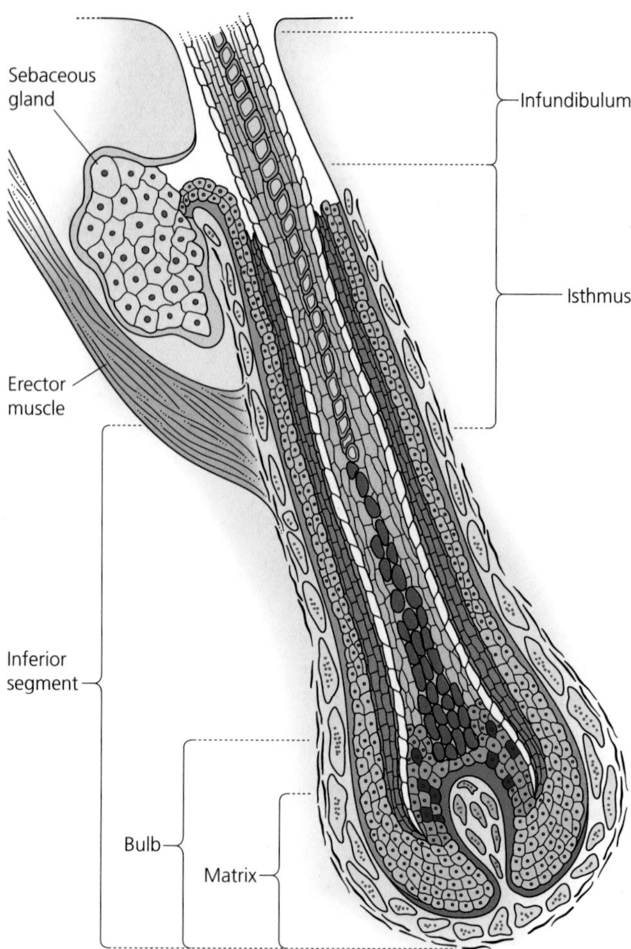

Figure 24-1 Hair follicle. Longitudinal section showing the three sections: the infundibulum, the isthmus, and the inferior segment.

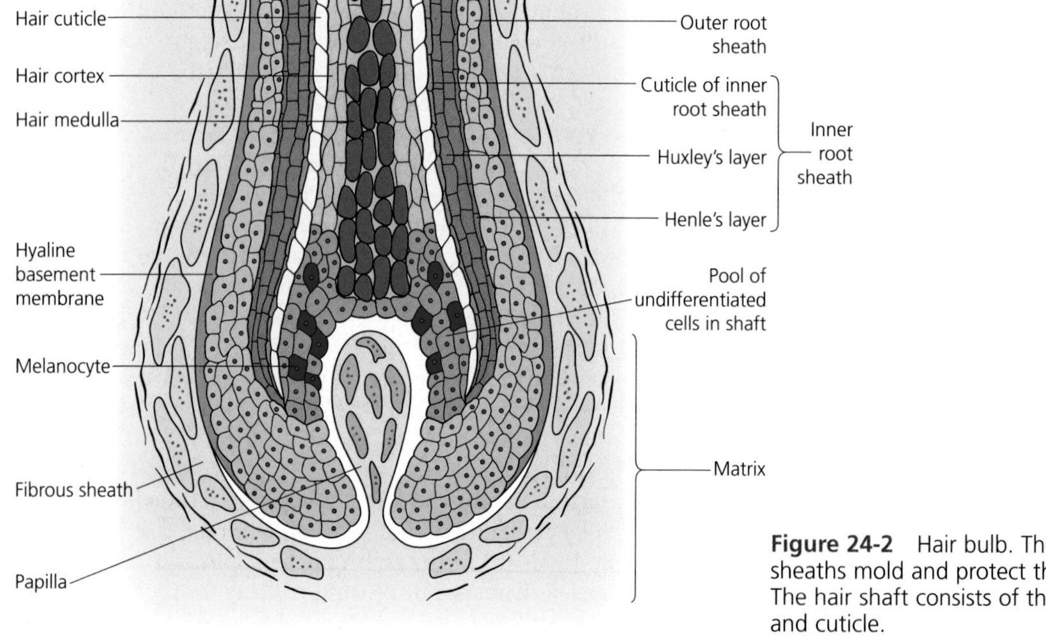

Figure 24-2 Hair bulb. The outer and inner root sheaths mold and protect the growing hair shaft. The hair shaft consists of the medulla, hair cortex, and cuticle.

PHYSIOLOGY

Cycling of hair follicles depends on the interaction of the follicular epithelium with the dermal papilla. The dermal papilla induces hair-follicle formation from the overlying epithelium at the onset of each new follicular cycle (Figure 24-3). The bulge consists of cells in the outer root sheath, which is located near the insertion of the arrector pili muscle. The dermal papilla interacts with germ cells in the hair-follicle bulge to regenerate the lower follicle. Stem cells in the bulge portion of the outer root migrate out of the follicle and regenerate the epidermis after injury.

Rapidly proliferating matrix cells in the hair bulb produce the hair shaft. The matrix cells differentiate, move upward, and are compressed and funneled into their final shape by the rigid inner root sheath. The shape (curvature) of the inner root sheath determines the shape of the hair. The bulk of the hair shaft is called the cortex. Pigment in the hair shaft is produced by melanocytes interspersed among the matrix cells. The volume of the dermal papilla determines the diameter of the hair shaft.

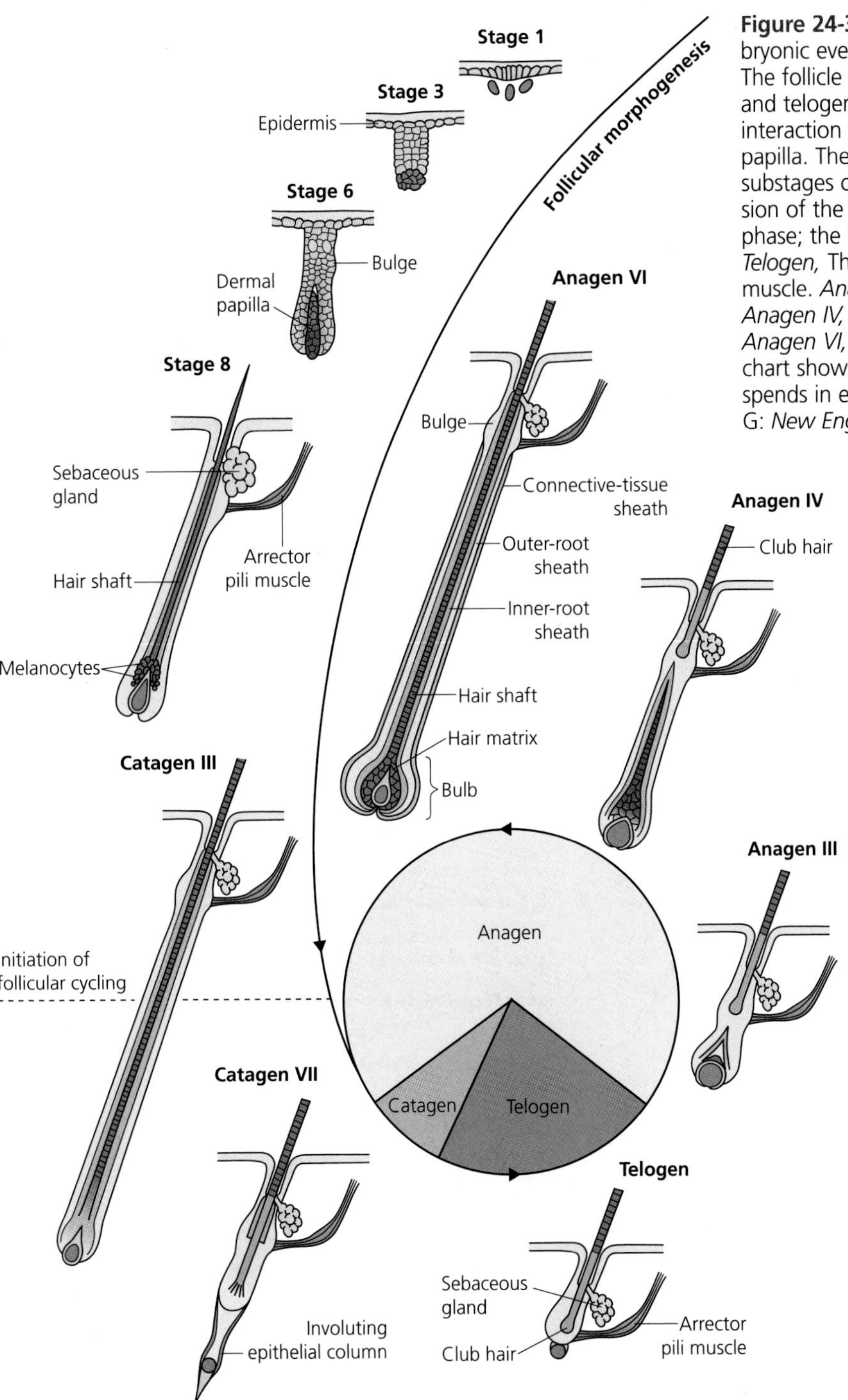

Figure 24-3 Stages 1, 3, 6, and 8 represent the embryonic events of the development of the hair follicle. The follicle then enters a three-stage (anagen, catagen, and telogen) growth cycle. The cycle depends on the interaction of the follicular epithelium and the dermal papilla. The Roman numerals indicate morphologic substages of anagen and catagen. *Catagen III,* Conclusion of the growth phase. *Catagen VII,* Transition phase; the inferior segment separates from the papilla. *Telogen,* The hair ascends to the level of the erector muscle. *Anagen III,* The growing cycle resumes. *Anagen IV,* The growing hair forces the club hair out. *Anagen VI,* The mature follicle is restored. The pie chart shows the proportion of time the hair follicle spends in each stage. (Adapted from Paus R, Cotsarelis G: *New Engl J Med* 341:491, 1999.) *PMID: 10441606*

HAIR GROWTH CYCLE

The average scalp has more than 100,000 hairs. The growth phase of scalp hair is approximately 1000 days (range, 2 to 6 years). Hair in other areas, such as the eyebrows and eyelashes, has a shorter growth phase (1 to 6 months). Scalp hair grows 0.3 to 0.4 mm/day, or approximately 6 inches a year.

Humans have a mosaic growth pattern; hair growth and loss are not cyclic or seasonal, as in some mammals, but occur at random, so that hair loss is continuous (see Figure 24-3). Each hair follicle perpetually goes through three stages in the hair growth cycle: catagen (transitional phase), telogen (resting phase), and anagen (growing phase) (Figure 24-4). Approximately 90% to 95% of hairs are in the anagen phase, and 5% to 10% are in the telogen phase. Up to 100 telogen hairs are lost each day from the head, and about the same number of follicles enter anagen. The duration of anagen determines the length of hair, and the volume of the hair bulb determines the diameter.

Anagen and telogen hairs from hair-plucked preparation are shown in Figure 24-5.

ANAGEN (GROWTH). The anagen or growth phase begins with resumption of mitotic activity in the hair bulb and dermal papilla. Interactions between the dermal papilla and the overlying follicular epithelium are required for the onset of anagen. The follicle grows down and meets the dermal papilla, recapitulating the embryonic events of development of the hair follicle. A new hair shaft forms and forces the tightly held club hair out. During anagen, hair grows at an average rate of 0.35 mm/day, or 1 cm in 28 days; this rate diminishes with age.

Hair follicles in different areas of the body produce hairs of different lengths. The length is proportional to the duration of the anagen cycle. Scalp hair remains in an active growing phase for an average of 2 to 6 years. The active growing phase is much shorter and the resting stage is longer for hair on the arms, legs, eyelashes, and eyebrows (30 to 45 days), which explains why these hairs remain short. Approximately 90% to 95% of scalp hairs are in an active growing phase at any one time. Continuous anagen occurs in some dogs (e.g., poodles) and in merino sheep; these animals do not lose or shed hair.

CATAGEN (INVOLUTION). Catagen is a process of involution that occurs with cell death in follicular keratinocytes. It is the phase of acute follicular regression that signals the end of anagen. Less than 1% of scalp hairs are in this 2- to 3-week transitional phase at any one time. Cell division in the hair matrix stops, and the resting, or catagen, stage begins. The outer root sheath degenerates and retracts around the widened lower portion of the hair shaft to become a club hair. The lower follicle shrinks away from the connective tissue papilla and ascends to the level of the insertion of the erector muscle. The dermal papilla condenses and moves upward, coming to rest underneath the hair-follicle bulge. The completion of catagen is marked by formation of the normal club hair.

TELOGEN (REST). All activity ceases and the structure rests during the telogen phase. The telogen phase in the scalp lasts for 2 to 3 months before the scalp follicles reenter the anagen stage and the cycle is repeated. The percentage of follicles in the telogen stage varies according to the body region. Approximately 5% to 10% of scalp hairs are in the telogen phase at any one time, and these follicles are randomly distributed. The telogen phase is much longer in eyebrow, eyelash, trunk, arm, and leg hair. Approximately 40% to 50% of follicles on the trunk are in the telogen phase. The inactive dead hair, or club hair, has a solid, hard, dry, white node at its proximal end; the white color is due to a lack of pigment. The club hair is firmly held in place and then ejected. A new anagen hair grows and replaces the shed telogen hair. Approximately 25 to 100 telogen hairs are shed each day; possibly twice this number are lost on the days the hair is shampooed. Seasonal shedding occurs in other animals but is random in humans.

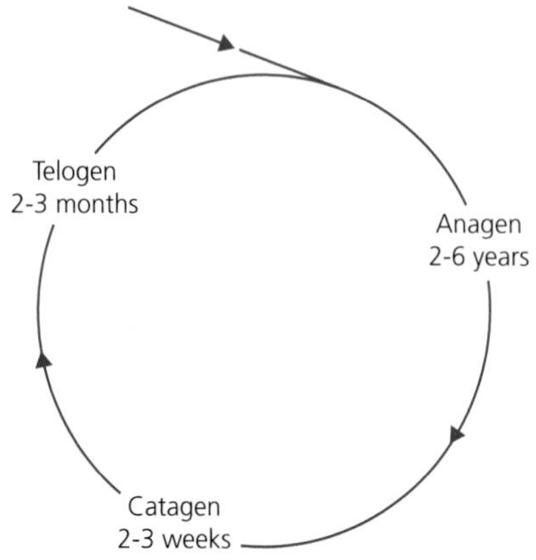

Figure 24-4 Hair growth cycle—scalp.

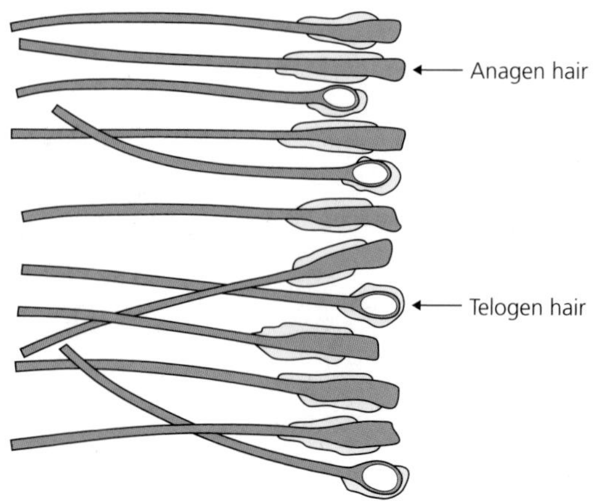

Figure 24-5 Hair pluck preparation showing anagen and telogen hairs.

EVALUATION OF HAIR LOSS

The causes of hair loss (alopecia) are numerous. Most hair problems seen by the practitioner are due to changes in hair-follicle cycling. Scarring alopecias are due to other causes. A classification is used here that is based primarily on distribution and scarring (i.e., localized [patchy] vs. generalized and scarring vs. nonscarring). A systematic approach for evaluation of hair loss is outlined in Box 24-1 and Table 24-1. The evaluation of the woman who complains that "My hair is falling out in large amounts" is presented in Figure 24-6.

DIAGNOSIS OF HAIR DISEASE

HISTORY. Inquire about drugs, severe diet restriction, vitamin A supplementation, and thyroid symptoms. Determine the time of onset and the duration of hair loss. Abrupt-onset telogen effluvium is most often related to a specific event. Gradual or imperceptible onsets are more complicated and involve possible shortened anagen, as well as a differential diagnosis that includes alopecia areata, androgenetic alopecia, and diffuse primary scarring alopecias.

PHYSICAL EXAMINATION. Examine the scalp surface and hair shafts. Microscopically examine hair ends and hair shaft diameters. Hair density may be reduced by 50% before hair thinning becomes clinically apparent; therefore observation is an inaccurate method of evaluating density and loss.

HAIR PULL TEST. For the hair pull test, obtain a sample 3 cm above the auricle. Tightly grasp 20 to 40 hairs firmly between the thumb and forefinger. Exert a slow, constant traction to slightly tent the scalp, and slide the fingers up the hair shafts. There should be fewer than six club hairs extracted. Repeat the count on the opposite side of the head and in two other areas. Examine the hair bulbs.

DAILY COUNTS. The patient collects hair lost in the first morning combing and includes those lost during washing for 14 days, saving them in clear plastic bags. The patient counts the hairs and records the number on the bags. Examine the hairs under the microscope to determine if the bulbs are anagen or telogen. Daily hair shed counts are not necessary if the pull test is positive. It is normal to lose up to 100 hairs daily and 200 to 250 hairs on the day of shampooing. If the hair is shampooed daily, the counts should be less than 100.

PART WIDTH. Make a coronal part with a comb over the vertex. Note the part width. Make a series of parallel parts over the vertex and visually compare the part diameter. Do the same over the occipital and temporal scalp. Visually compare the part diameters in the different anatomic scalp areas. Hair density is greatest in childhood and decreases progressively with age. The hair is less dense in the vertex in both genders, and thinning increases with age.

HAIR SHAFT EXAMINATION (CLIP TESTS). Grasp 25 to 30 hairs between the thumb and forefinger just at the scalp surface. Cut the hair between the fingers and the scalp. Hair just above the fingers is cut and discarded. Float the hairs onto a wet microscope slide and cover with another slide. Evaluate hair shaft diameter and structure. There are many rare diseases that produce shaft structural abnormalities such as pili torti in which the hair is twisted on its axis.

HAIR GROWTH WINDOW. Select an area where the hair fails to grow and an area that can be covered by the remaining hair. Cut the hair short; then shave a 2.0 cm^2 area. Occlude the area with an occlusive dressing and remove it in 1 week if trichotillomania is suspected. Normal growth is 2.5 mm in 1 week and 1 cm in 1 month. This test proves to the patient that the hair is growing.

HAIR PLUCK—TRICHOGRAM. This is a painful technique but is still used by some clinicians. Abruptly extract hairs from the scalp with a rubber-tipped needle holder. Cut the excess hair 1 cm from the roots, float the hairs onto a wet microscope slide or Petri dish, and examine with a hand lens (see Figure 24-5).

Telogen hairs have small, unpigmented, ovoid bulbs and do not contain an internal root sheath. Anagen hairs have larger, elongated, pigmented (if hair is pigmented) bulbs shaped like the end of a broom, surrounded by a gelatinous internal root sheath.

There are diseases in which hair fragments with absent bulbs are obtained during a hair pull. Processes that interfere with cell division cause the shaft to be poorly formed and therefore apt to break under tension. Alopecia areata, antimetabolite therapy, and small doses of ionizing radiation interrupt the mitotic activity in the cells that normally contribute to the growing hair.

Box 24-1 **Systematic Approach to Evaluation of Hair Loss**

History	**Diagnostic procedures**
Sudden vs. gradual loss	Hair pull test
Presence of systemic disease or high fever	Daily counts Part width
Recent psychologic or physical stress	Possible trichotillomania
Medication or chemical exposure	Potassium hydroxide examination for fungi
Examination	**Scalp biopsy**
Localized vs. generalized	**Hormone studies**
Scarring vs. nonscarring	
Inflammatory vs. noninflammatory	
Presence of follicular plugging	
Skin disease in other areas	

Table 24-1 A Simplified Tool for the Diagnosis of Alopecia (This scheme will diagnose 97% of cases of alopecia)

Disease	Scalp	Pattern	Pull test	Laboratory	Treatment
Diffuse loss (nonscarring)					
Telogen effluvium	Normal	Diffuse	Increased telogen	Disease specific	Disease specific
Diffuse alopecia areata	Normal	Irregularly diffuse	Increased telogen	—	Topical immunotherapy
Androgenetic alopecia (men)	Normal	Hamilton (Figure 24-7)	Negative	—	Minoxidil Finasteride 1 mg Surgery
Androgenetic alopecia (women)	Normal	Ludwig (Figure 24-8)	Negative	Testosterone DHEAs	Minoxidil Oral contraceptives Spironolactone
Systemic disease (thyroid, iron deficiency, systemic lupus erythematosus, dermatomyositis)	Normal in most	Diffuse	Normal or increased telogen	Thyroid function Iron/IBC ANA	Disease specific
Patchy loss (scarring)					
Discoid lupus erythematosus	Atrophy, dyspigmentation, follicular plugging	Patchy	Negative	Biopsy	Intralesional steroids Hydroxychloroquine
Lichen planopilaris	Hairs trapped in "islands"	Patchy	Negative	Biopsy Immunofluorescence	Intralesional steroids Hydroxychloroquine
Frontal fibrosing alopecia	Advancing edge perifollicular papules	Develops on frontal hairline, extends backwards	Negative	Biopsy Immunofluorescence	Same as lichen planopilaris
Pseudopelade	Scarring, noninflammatory	Moth-eaten pattern	Negative	Biopsy Immunofluorescence	Topical steroids Hydroxychloroquine
Central centrifugal cicatricial alopecia	Scarring in localized pattern	Patchy over crown	Negative	Biopsy	Avoid hair traction
Folliculitis decalvans	Pustules at periphery Bogginess	Patchy	Negative	Biopsy Immunofluorescence	Antibiotics
Dissecting cellulitis/folliculitis	Abscess formation	Diffuse	Negative	Biopsy, culture	Antibiotics
Acne keloid	Pustules and dense follicular papules	Occipital scalp	Negative	Biopsy, culture	Antibiotics
Tufted folliculitis	Many hairs arise from a giant follicle	Occipital scalp	Negative	Biopsy	Antibiotics
Patchy loss (nonscarring)					
Alopecia localized	Normal	Patchy + exclamation mark hairs	May be + at margins	KOH children	Intralesional steroids Minoxidil Anthralin
Tinea capitis	Scale or papules or pustules	Patchy	Hair breakage	KOH Fungal culture	Oral antifungal antibiotics
Traction alopecia	± Scarring	Patchy, marginal	Hair breakage	—	Avoid
Trichotillomania	± Scarring, normal	Patchy with stubble	Usually negative	—	Fluoxetine, others Psychotherapy
Syphilis	Normal	Moth-eaten	Increased telogen	RPR	Penicillin
Hair breakage	Normal	Patchy or marginal	Broken hairs	—	—

EVALUATION OF HAIR LOSS

"My hair is falling out in large amounts"

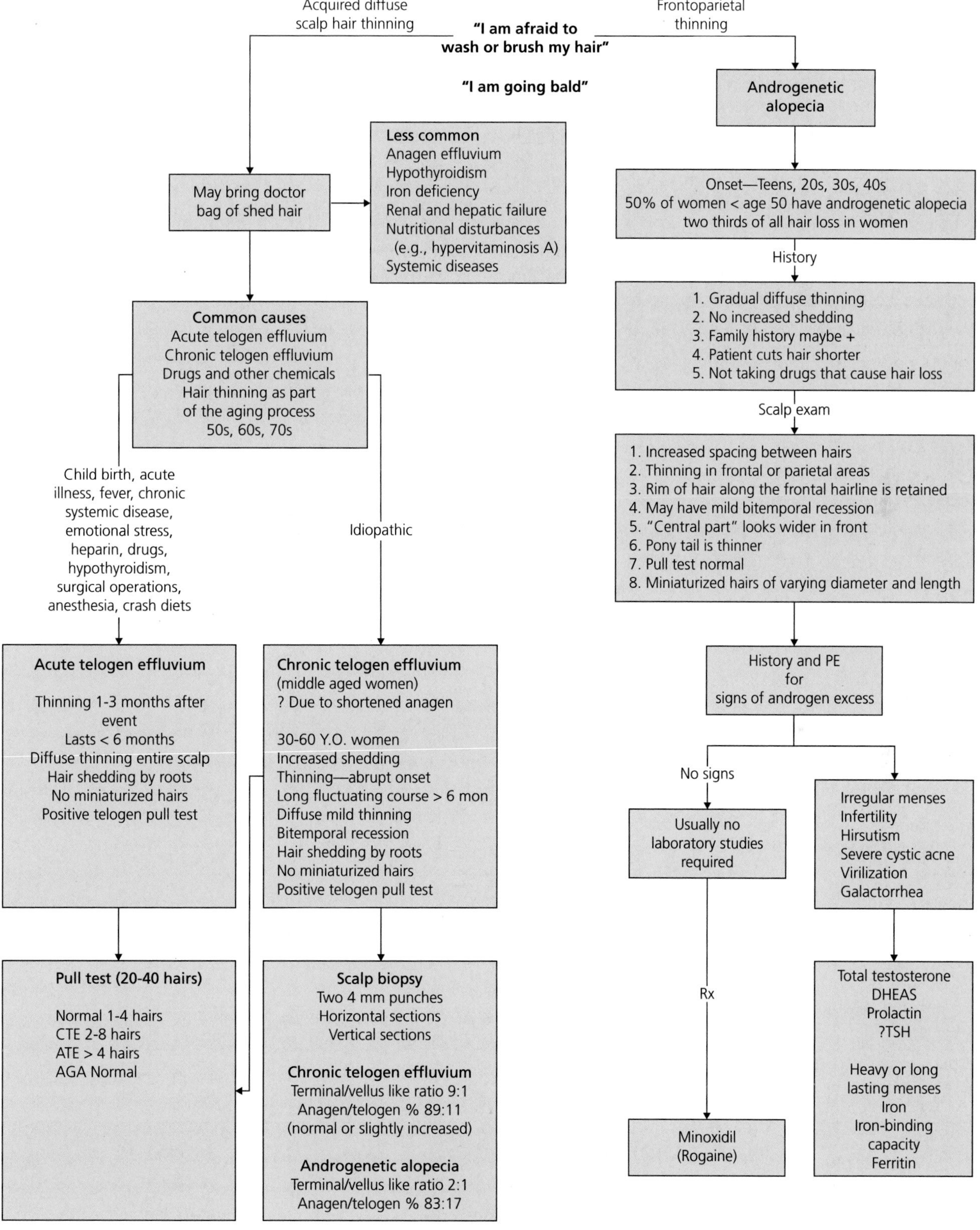

Figure 24-6

GENERALIZED HAIR LOSS

Diffuse hair loss (Box 24-2 and Table 24-2) usually occurs without inflammation or scarring. The loss affects hairs throughout the scalp in a more or less uniform pattern. The hair pull test is important for differential diagnosis.

TELOGEN EFFLUVIUM. A number of events have been documented that prematurely terminate anagen and cause an abnormally high number of normal hairs to enter the resting, or telogen, phase (see Box 24-2). The follicle is not diseased but has had its biologic clock reset and undergoes a normal involutional process. Usually no more than 50% of the patient's hair is affected. Scarring and inflammation are absent. Resting hairs on the scalp are retained for approximately 100 days before they are lost; therefore telogen hair loss should occur approximately 3 months after the event that terminated normal hair growth.

Kligman explained this process and identified the various precipitating events (see Box 24-2). The most common causes are briefly discussed here. High fever from any cause may result in a sudden diffuse loss of club hairs 2 to 3 months later. Hair loss begins abruptly and lasts for approximately 4 weeks. Hair pluck tests show telogen counts that vary from 30% to 60%. Full recovery can be expected.

Severe emotional and physical traumas have been documented to cause diffuse hair loss. Hair loss has been reported to occur 2 weeks after severe psychologic or physical trauma, but because that is too short a time for the induction of the telogen phase, the loss must have occurred by another mechanism. Some individuals may experience increased shedding caused by idiopathic shortening of anagen (a short anagen syndrome). They have increased shedding and decreased hair length. For every 50% reduction in the duration of anagen, there is a corresponding doubling of follicles in telogen.

Box 24-2 **Hair Loss**

GENERALIZED*

Telogen effluvium
- Acute blood loss
- Childbirth
- Crash diets (inadequate protein)

Drugs
- Coumarin
- Heparin
- Propranolol
- Vitamin A

High fever
Hypothyroidism and hyperthyroidisms
Physical stress (e.g., surgery)
Physiologic (e.g., neonate)
Psychologic stress
Severe illness (e.g., systemic lupus erythematosis)

Anagen effluvium

Cancer chemotherapeutic agents
Poisoning
- Thallium (rat poison)
- Arsenic

Radiation therapy

Generalized patchy

Secondary syphilis: "moth eaten" alopecia

LOCALIZED†

Androgenetic alopecia
- Male pattern
- Female pattern

Hirsutism
Alopecia areata
Trichotillomania
Traction alopecia
Scarring alopecia
- Developmental defects: aplasia cutis

Physical injury: burns, pressure
Infection
- Fungal: kerion
- Bacterial: folliculitis, furuncle
- Viral: herpes zoster

Neoplasms
- Metastatic carcinoma
- Sclerosing basal cell carcinoma

Others
- Lupus erythematosus
- Lichen planus
- Cicatricial pemphigoid
- Scleroderma

*Diffuse, uniform loss, but many hairs left randomly distributed in area of loss.
†Most or all hair missing from involved area.

Table 24-2 Features Differentiating Telogen Effluvium and Anagen Effluvium

Clinical presentation	Telogen	Anagen
Onset of shedding after insult	2-4 months	1-4 weeks
Percent of hair loss	20-50	80-90
Type of hair loss	Normal club (white bulb)	Anagen hair (pigmented bulb)
Hair shaft	Normal	Narrowed or fractured

CHRONIC TELOGEN EFFLUVIUM. Chronic telogen effluvium (CTE) refers to a diffuse hair loss all over the scalp and persists for more than 8 months. Patients present with hair loss with increased shedding and thinning of abrupt onset and fluctuating course. There is diffuse thinning all over the scalp, frequently accompanied by bitemporal recession. CTE usually affects 30- to 60-year-old women. It may be distinguished from classic acute telogen effluvium by its long fluctuating course and from androgenetic alopecia by its clinical and histologic findings. CTE lasts from 6 months to 7 years. The long, fluctuating course is different than that seen in acute telogen effluvium. The presence of 20% to 30% telogen hairs and 15% to 35% dystrophic hairs on the trichogram (plucked hair) confirms the diagnosis. A biopsy can support the diagnosis but is usually not necessary. CTE is distinguished from androgenetic alopecia by distribution and trichogram and a biopsy is usually unnecessary.

Men are treated with 5% minoxidil solution. Premenopausal women are prescribed 5% minoxidil solution plus cyproterone acetate (not available in the United States), 50 mg, from day 5 to day 15 of their menstrual cycle, always taken together with ethinyl estradiol, 0.035 mg/day. Postmenopausal women are treated with 5% minoxidil solution plus cyproterone acetate, 50 mg/day. Alternatives to cyproterone acetate, 50 mg/day, could be spironolactone, 50 to 100 mg/day.

Biopsies confirm the diagnosis but are usually not necessary. Two 4-mm punch biopsy specimens are taken from the mid or posterior parietal scalp. Specimens are sectioned horizontally and vertically. The findings are shown in Figure 24-6, p. 919.

POSTPARTUM HAIR LOSS. The percentage of follicles in telogen progressively decreases during pregnancy, particularly during the last trimester. Diffuse but primarily frontotemporal hair loss occurs in a significant number of women 1 to 4 months after childbirth. The loss can be quite significant, but recovery occurs in less than 1 year. Hair growth usually returns to the prepregnancy state.

DRUGS. Cytotoxic drugs that directly affect hair matrix cell proliferation cause profound hair loss, inducing an anagen effluvium. A large number of drugs probably cause telogen effluvia. These are listed in Box 24-3.

Box 24-3 **Drugs Probably Associated with Telogen Effluvium**

Acitretin	Danazol
Aminosalicylic acid	Enalapril
Amphetamines	Levodopa
Bromocriptine	Lithium
Captopril	Metoprolol
Carbamazepine	Propranolol
Cimetidine	Pyridostigmine
Coumadin	Trimethadione

ANAGEN EFFLUVIUM. Anagen effluvium (see Box 24-2 and Table 24-2) is the abrupt loss of hair from follicles that are in their growing phase. An abrupt insult to the metabolic and follicular reproductive apparatus must be delivered to create such an event. Cancer chemotherapeutic agents and radiation therapy are capable of such an insult. The rapidly dividing cells of the matrix and cortex are affected. The insult causes a change in the rate of hair growth but does not convert the follicle to a different growth phase, as occurs in telogen effluvium. High concentrations of antimetabolites or radiation bring the entire metabolic process to an abrupt halt, and the entire hair and hair root are shed intact. The only hairs left are those in the telogen phase. These are dead, wedged into the hair canal, and unaffected by any acute event. The stem cells of the hair follicles are spared because of their slow cycling, and they generate a new hair bulb. Insults of less intensity slow the mitotic rate of the bulb and cortex cells, causing bulb deformity and narrowing of the lower hair shaft. Narrow, weakened hair shafts are easily broken and shed without bulbs. Since 90% of scalp hairs are in the anagen phase, a large number of hairs can be affected. Patients with 10% to 20% of their hair remaining after an insult almost certainly have had an anagen effluvium. Minoxidil 2% topical has no benefit in the prevention of chemotherapy-induced alopecia.

LOOSE ANAGEN HAIR SYNDROME. The loose anagen hair syndrome (LAS) is a rare sporadic or familial hair disorder that affects children but may be seen in adults. The female to male ratio is 6:1. LAS is due to a defective anchorage of the hair shaft to the follicle that results in easily and painlessly pluckable hair.

LAS may result from premature keratinization of the inner root sheath that produces an impaired adhesion between the cuticle of the inner root sheath and the cuticle of the hair shaft.

The typical patient with LAS is a young girl with short blond hair that does not grow long, but LAS can affect children with dark hair. The signs are reduced hair length, increased hair shedding, and altered hair texture. They may have sparse hair that does not grow long and have patches of dull, unruly hair. Others just have increased hair shedding. The child needs few haircuts, and the hair is difficult to manage. Examination shows diffuse thinning and irregular bald patches attributable to traumatic painless extraction of hair tufts. Hair is dull, unruly, or matted. Up to 300 hairs are shed daily. Most cases are isolated, but it can occur in hereditary or developmental disorders including coloboma, Noonan's syndrome, and hypohidrotic ectodermal dysplasia.

Microscopic examination shows anagen hair without sheath. The bulb is often misshapen, and its proximal portion often shows a visible ruffled cuticle. The pull test in children with LAS shows more than 3 and often more than 10 loose anagen hairs. The pull test in normal children shows one or two loose anagen hairs. The trichogram shows at least 70% loose anagen hairs. Most patients improve with age.

LOCALIZED HAIR LOSS

Androgenetic alopecia in men (male pattern baldness)

Baldness in men is not a disease, but rather a physiologic reaction induced by androgens in genetically predisposed men. The pattern of inheritance is probably polygenic. Thinning of the hair begins between the ages of 12 and 40 years, and about half the population expresses this trait before the age of 50.

HAMILTON PATTERNS. The progression and various patterns of hair loss are classified by the Hamilton male baldness classification system (Figure 24-7). Triangular frontotemporal recession occurs normally in most young men (type I) and women after puberty. The first signs of balding are increased frontotemporal recession accompanied by midfrontal recession (type II). Hair loss in a round area on the vertex follows, and the density of hair decreases, sometimes rapidly, over the top of the scalp (types III through VII).

PATHOPHYSIOLOGY. Androgenetic alopecia is due to the progressive shortening of successive anagen cycles. There are two populations of scalp follicles: androgen-sensitive follicles on the top and androgen-independent follicles on the sides and back of the scalp. In genetically predisposed individuals, and under the influence of androgens, predisposed follicles are gradually miniaturized, and large, pigmented hairs (terminal hairs) are replaced by thin, depigmented hairs (vellus hairs).

Inflammation surrounds the bulge area of the outer root sheath. The inflammation may damage the follicle stem cells, which results in a decrease in hair-follicle density. Hair follicles are still present, but removing androgens or treatment with minoxidil or finasteride does not result in the conversion of miniaturized follicles back to terminal ones.

Skin androgen metabolism. Testosterone is converted to the more potent dihydrotestosterone by 5α-reductase. Skin cells contain 5α-reductase (types I and II). The type I enzyme is found in sebaceous glands, and the type II enzyme is found in hair follicles and the prostate gland. Testosterone and dihydrotestosterone act on androgen receptors in the dermal papilla. They increase the size of hair follicles in androgen-dependent areas such as the beard area during adolescence, but later in life dihydrotestosterone binds to the follicle androgen receptor and activates transformation of large, terminal follicles to miniaturized follicles. The duration of anagen shortens with successive hair cycles, and the follicles become smaller, producing shorter, finer hairs. Androgenetic alopecia does not develop in men with a congenital absence of 5α-reductase type II. Finasteride, which inhibits 5α-reductase type II, slows or reverses the progression of androgenetic alopecia.

TREATMENT. The desire for treatment varies. Some men accept the inevitable; others find baldness intolerable. Topical treatment (minoxidil), oral treatment (finasteride), and several surgical procedures are available. The drugs can enlarge existing hairs and retard thinning in the vertex and the frontal regions. They have no benefit for men who are bald or those with bitemporal recession without hair. Benefits are seen in 6 to 12 months. Treatment must be continued indefinitely. If treatment is stopped, benefits are lost within 6 to 12 months, and hair density will be the same as before treatment. Patients who begin balding at an early age are most distressed and are tempted to consult non-

Figure 24-7 Hamilton classification of male pattern baldness.

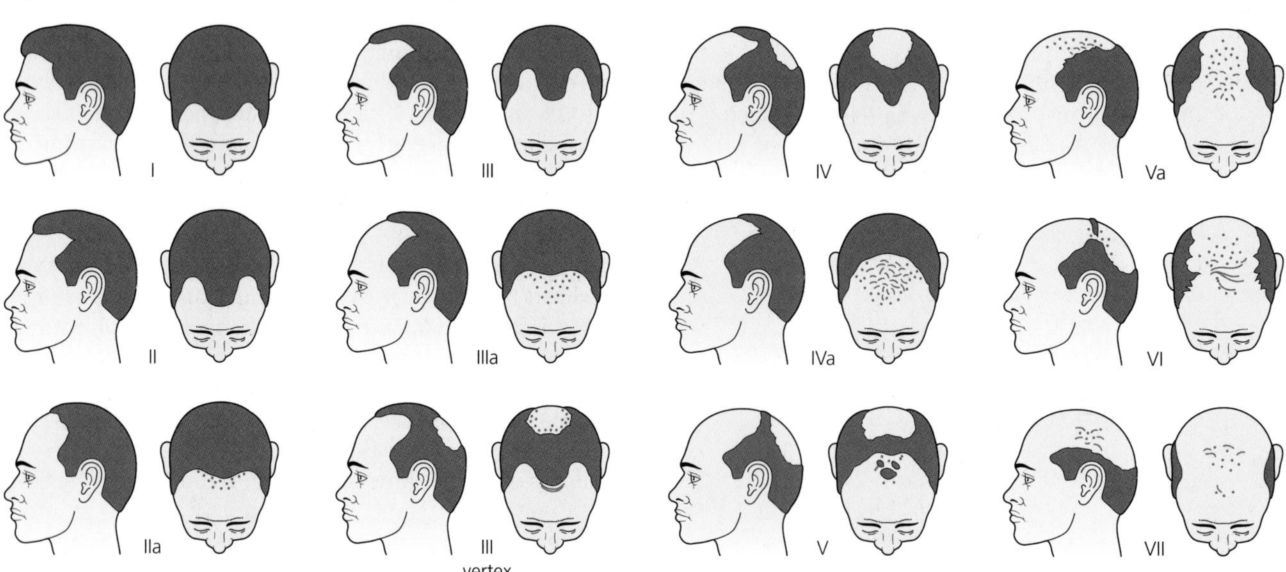

physician "experts" at hair clinics. These clinics offer a variety of topical preparations, none of which has any value. Selected patients may be referred for hair transplants, plastic surgical rotation flaps, or wigs.

Minoxidil. Minoxidil was developed to treat hypertension. It increases the duration of anagen, causes follicles at rest to grow, and enlarges miniaturized follicles. These effects occur in only a minority of patients. Minoxidil 2% (Rogaine) and 5% (Extra Strength Rogaine) are available over-the-counter in a solution or foam preparation. Generic brands of the 2% solution are available. One milliliter of solution is applied twice daily and spread lightly with a finger. An applicator conveniently and effectively applies the medication. Minoxidil increases nonvellus hairs. Spontaneous reversal to the pretreatment state occurs in 1 to 3 months after stopping treatment. Ideal candidates are men younger than 30 years of age who have been losing hair for less than 5 years. The solutions produce a modest increase in hair on scalps of young men and women with mild to moderate hair loss, with continuous twice daily application for years to maintain the effect. In men with androgenetic alopecia, 5% topical minoxidil was clearly superior to 2% topical minoxidil in increasing hair regrowth, and the magnitude of its effect was marked (45% more hair regrowth than 2% topical minoxidil at week 48). *PMID: 12196747*

One 48-week study in women showed that 5% topical minoxidil was superior to 2% topical minoxidil in the patient assessment of treatment benefit. Application of 2% topical minoxidil in this study showed that differences in patient assessment of hair growth at week 48 were not significantly different from placebo. *PMID: 15034503* A 48-week study in men found a mean increase in hairs per square centimeter of 12.7 with 2% minoxidil, and 18.5 with 5% minoxidil. One study found that topical use of 2% minoxidil caused small but statistically significant increases in left ventricular end-diastolic volume, cardiac output, and left ventricular mass. Dizziness and tachycardia have been reported with 2% solution. Local irritation, itching, dryness, and erythema may occur and are likely attributable to the vehicle of alcohol and propylene glycol. The medication is applied to a dry scalp twice a day. The hair should not be wet for at least 1 hour afterward. About one third of these patients grow hair that is long enough to be cut or combed. Hair growth is evident in 8 to 12 months. Minoxidil may stop or retard the progression of male pattern baldness. In one large study of long-term use almost all patients gradually avoided continuing the treatment. The causes of discontinuation in the majority of patients were the insignificant cosmetic effect and an aversion to this topical treatment method. *PMID: 17917938*

Finasteride. Finasteride (Propecia 1 mg) taken daily is an effective oral therapy for androgenetic alopecia in men. Some physicians prescribe finasteride (Proscar 5 mg) and instruct patients to split the 5-mg tablet with a pill splitter into four equal parts. The cost savings is considerable.

Androgenetic alopecia (male pattern hair loss) is caused by androgen-dependent miniaturization of scalp hair follicles, with scalp dihydrotestosterone (DHT) level implicated as a contributing cause. Finasteride blocks 5α-reductase type II, which inhibits the conversion of testosterone to dihydrotestosterone and decreases serum and cutaneous dihydrotestosterone concentrations. This slows further hair loss, inhibits androgen-dependent miniaturization of hair follicles, and improves hair growth and hair weight in men with androgenetic alopecia.

In men with male pattern hair loss, finasteride 1 mg/day slowed the progression of hair loss and increased hair growth in clinical trials over 2 years. Therapy leads to slowing of further hair loss.

Efficacy is evident within 3 months of therapy. The drug produces progressive increases in hair counts at 6 and 12 months. Finasteride treatment for 4 years leads to sustained improvement in hair weight. Hair weight increased to a larger extent than hair count. *PMID: 16781295* Finasteride is effective in men with vertex male pattern hair loss and hair loss in the anterior/mid area of the scalp. It may not be effective for men who are older than 60 years of age because type 2 5α-reductase activity in the scalp may not be as high as in younger men.

In postmenopausal women with androgenetic alopecia, finasteride 1 mg/day taken for 12 months did not increase hair growth or slow the progression of hair thinning. Finasteride is contraindicated in women who are or may potentially be pregnant because of the risk that inhibition of conversion of fetal testosterone to DHT could impair virilization of a male fetus. Approximately 20% to 30% of men do not respond. Treatment must be continued indefinitely.

SIDE EFFECTS. In clinical trials 4.2% of men reported side effects related to sexual dysfunction, which resolved both after discontinuation and spontaneously in many men who chose to remain on drug treatment. A later study showed that sexual side effects are much less common than reported in clinical trials. The sexual function of all patients remained stable during treatment with 1 mg of finasteride. *PMID: 15262698* No other significant adverse effects related to finasteride treatment were observed. In men aged 40 to 60 years, 1 mg/day of finasteride for 48 weeks lowers serum prostate-specific antigen concentration. *PMID: 17196507* Finasteride is beneficial in women with hirsutism, but the drug should be used cautiously in women because of its potential feminizing effects on male fetuses.

MINOXIDIL VS. FINASTERIDE. A study showed that 2% minoxidil produced faster initial improvement in mid-frontal/vertex alopecia areata (AA) in up to one third of treated patients, whereas finasteride produced marginally better results with increasing duration of treatment. Both agents were equally effective in stopping the progression of AA. *PMID: 12975174*

HAIR TRANSPLANTS. Hair transplants have been used successfully for years to permanently restore hair. Age is not a determining factor. Androgen-independent hairs from the lateral and posterior areas of the scalp are used. The surgeon must have a sense of aesthetics to properly design the anterior hairline. There are many techniques used for harvesting and implanting the graphs. The techniques are constantly changing and improving.

SCALP REDUCTION AND FLAPS. An anterior-posterior elliptic excision of bald vertex scalp with primary closure can provide an instant hair effect. The procedure can be repeated every 4 weeks until hair margins converge or scalp tissue becomes too thin. Grafts or flaps may be used later to fill any remaining void. Alternately, several types of flaps can be designed by the creative surgeon to fill voids.

HAIR WEAVES. Hair weaves have been refined by the HAIRCLUB (www.hairclub.com) in the United States. They create a matrix of crisscrossing, transparent fibers, fitted and shaped to the client's thinning area. The matrix is porous, allowing the scalp to "breathe." New hair is added to the matrix strand by strand to re-create the pattern and hair flow of the client's own hair. The matrix is then fused to the client's remaining growing hair using a medical adhesive called polyfuse. The client returns to HAIRCLUB for haircuts and to replace the Polyfuse every 5 weeks. Clients are generally satisfied with the process and prefer it to a wig.

Adrenal androgenic female pattern alopecia

Chronic, progressive, diffuse hair loss in women in their 20s and 30s is a frequently encountered complaint. These women, who usually have a normal menstrual cycle and lack any abnormalities on physical examination, have been classified as having "male pattern baldness," a genetic trait, and have been dismissed without further evaluation. Recent studies have shown that some of these women have increased levels of the serum adrenal androgen dehydroepiandrosterone sulfate (DHEA-S) and a distinct pattern of central scalp alopecia, which has been called adrenal androgenic female pattern alopecia.

Male pattern baldness results in a gradual regression of the hair on the central scalp and gradual frontotemporal recession, as well as a gradual decrease in hair shaft diameter in the areas of hair loss. In contrast, most women with diffuse alopecia experience a gradual loss of hair on the central scalp, with retention of the normal hairline without frontotemporal recession. There are a variety of anagen hair diameters. With advancing age, the central thinning becomes more pronounced; in contrast to male pattern baldness, a fringe of hair along the frontal hairline persists (Figure 24-8). In exceptional cases, a course similar to that in men is seen, with deep frontotemporal recession.

LABORATORY FINDINGS. The laboratory investigation of female patients with diffuse alopecia with both female and male patterns is outlined in Table 24-3. Laboratory evaluation for some androgenetic alopecia patients should initially include determination of the serum DHEA-S and total serum testosterone (T) levels, testosterone-estradiol–binding globulin (TeBG) level for the T/TeBG ratio, and serum prolactin levels.

TREATMENT. In a 48-week study of 381 women with female pattern hair loss, 5% topical minoxidil applied twice a day demonstrated statistical superiority over the 2% topical minoxidil group in the patient assessment of treatment benefit. Application of 2% topical minoxidil showed that differences in patient assessment of hair growth at week 48 were not significantly different from placebo. *PMID: 15034503*

Table 24-3 Laboratory Values for Evaluation of Diffuse Female Alopecia

Laboratory parameter	Female pattern alopecia	Female pattern alopecia with hirsutism	Male pattern alopecia (frontotemporal recession)
DHEA-S	Normal or elevated	Normal or elevated	Elevated
T	Normal	Normal or elevated	Elevated
TeBG	Normal	Decreased or normal	Decreased or normal
T/TeBG prolactin*	Normal	Elevated	Elevated

DHEA-S, dehydroepiandrosterone sulfate; *T*, total serum testosterone; *TeBG*, testosterone-estradiol–binding globulin; *T/TeBG*, androgenic index.
*If elevated, suspect pituitary disease (e.g., pituitary prolactin secreting adenoma).

FEMALE PATTERN—ALOPECIA

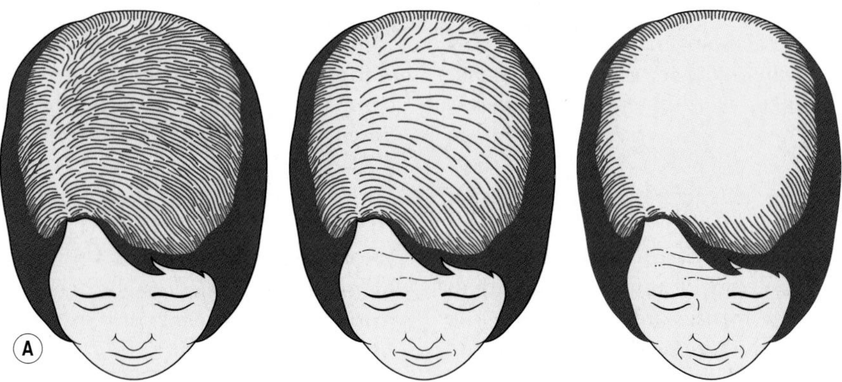

Ludwig pattern. Evolution of the female type of androgenetic alopecia.

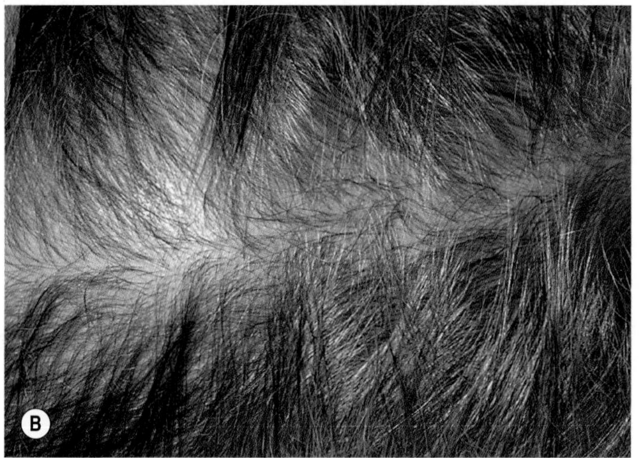

Widening of the hair part is an initial change.

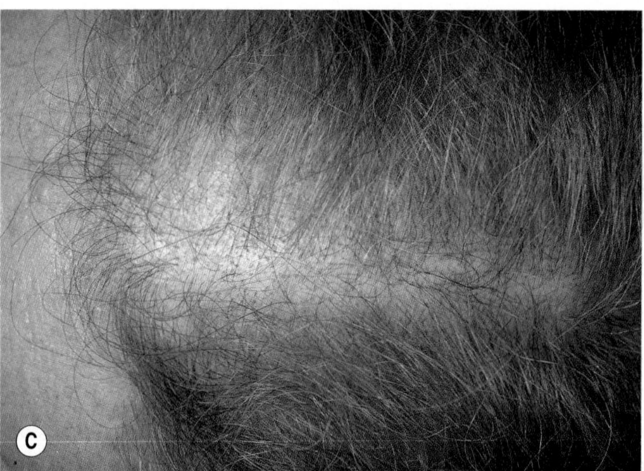

More extensive widening of the hair part.

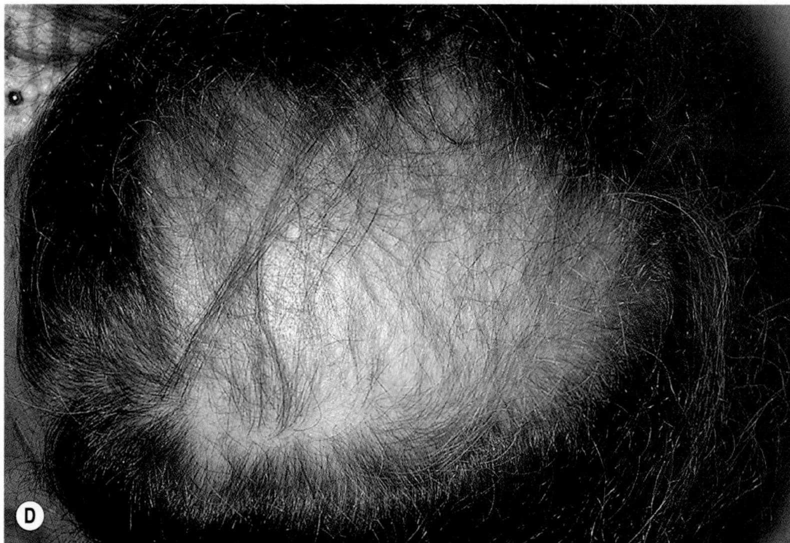

Diffuse hair loss over the crown. The frontal hair line is preserved.

Figure 24-8

Hirsutism

Hirsutism is defined as excessive terminal hair that appears in a male pattern (i.e., sexual hair) in women. Hirsutism affects 5% to 10% of women. The differential diagnosis is shown in Box 24-4.

IDIOPATHIC HIRSUTISM. Hirsute patients with normal ovulatory function and circulating androgen levels have idiopathic hirsutism (IH). A history of regular menses is not sufficient to exclude ovulatory dysfunction, since up to 40% of hirsute women with menses are anovulatory. The excessive body hair is due to increased sensitivity of the pilosebaceous unit to normal plasma levels of androgen. These women may have increased numbers of androgen receptors and increased 5α-reductase activity. These patients respond to antiandrogen or 5α-reductase inhibitor therapy (finasteride). Less than 20% of all hirsute women have IH.

VIRILIZATION. Virilization is the combination of hirsutism plus other signs of masculinization, such as deepening of the voice and temporal balding (Box 24-5). Virilization may be the sign of an ovarian or adrenal tumor. Virilization is associated with markedly increased androgen production by the ovaries or adrenal glands (or both) and markedly increased levels of plasma androgens.

BODY HAIR. The number of hairs per unit area is determined by genetic factors. Mediterranean men and women have more body hairs per unit area than Asians. Hair follicles cover the entire body except for the lips, palms, and soles. There are two types of hair follicles: vellus and terminal. Most women have some terminal hair in the so-called male sexual pattern around the areolae and extending from the pubis in the midline of the abdomen. In women, excess androgen production stimulates vellus hairs to develop into long, coarse, pigmented terminal hairs in most areas of the body except the scalp, where terminal hairs are converted to vellus hairs, resulting in balding. Women in whom hirsutism develops after puberty, especially if accompanied by signs of virilization such as infrequent or absent menses, have an abnormal condition and require further evaluation.

HIRSUTISM IS NOT HYPERTRICHOSIS. Hypertrichosis is excessive hair growth in a nonsexual pattern stimulated by medications such as glucocorticoids, phenytoins, minoxidil, or cyclosporine; or it exists as a result of heredity.

GENERAL GUIDELINES. Test for elevated androgen levels in women with moderate or severe hirsutism or hirsutism of any degree when it is sudden in onset, rapidly progressive, or associated with other abnormalities such as menstrual dysfunction, obesity, or clitorimegaly. Polycystic ovary syndrome (PCOS) is the most likely diagnosis in a woman with moderate or severe hirsutism and elevated testosterone level. Women who desire treatment are treated with oral medication or hair removal methods such as lasers or photoepilation. Oral contraceptives are first-line drugs. Add an antiandrogen after 6 months if the response is poor. Antiandrogen monotherapy is used only with adequate contraception. Insulin-lowering drugs are not recommended.

Over 80% of patients with hirsutism have PCOS whereas about 10% have idiopathic hirsutism or nonspecific functional hyperandrogenism. Less than 10% have other disorders listed in Box 24-4 as specific identifiable disorders.

Box 24-4 **Etiology and Differential Diagnosis for a Patient Presenting with Hirsutism**

- Ferriman-Gallwey scale
  - Score of 8 to 15—mild hirsutism
  - 50% have idiopathic condition*
  - 50% have elevated androgen levels
- Hyperandrogenism
  - Polycystic ovary syndrome—most cases
  - Nonclassic congenital adrenal hyperplasia—2%
  - Androgen-secreting tumors—0.2%; 50% are malignant
- Primary presenting symptoms (not hirsutism)
  - Cushing's syndrome†
  - Hyperprolactinemia
  - Acromegaly
  - Thyroid dysfunction
  - Hyperandrogenism, insulin resistance + acanthosis nigricans†
  - Mild, idiopathic hyperandrogenism—8%

*Hirsutism in a patient with normal androgen levels and normal ovarian function (normo-ovulation and no polycystic ovaries on ultrasound).
†If clinical findings are highly suggestive of these rare disorders, further biochemical testing might be needed.

Box 24-5 **Hirsutism and Virilization—Clinical Findings in Women**

Hirsutism: Excessive hair growth in women in 9 key androgen-sensitive anatomic sites:

- Face
- Chest
- Areola
- Linea alba
- Lower back
- Upper back
- Buttocks
- Inner thigh
- External genitalia

Virilization: The combination of hirsutism plus:

- Acne and increased sebum production
- Clitoral hypertrophy
- Decrease in breast size
- Deepening of the voice
- Frontotemporal balding
- Increased muscle mass
- Infrequent or absent menses
- Heightened libido
- Hirsutism
- Malodorous perspiration

PATHOGENESIS OF HIRSUTISM. The growth of sexual hair is dependent on the presence of androgens. Androgens induce vellus follicles in sex-specific areas to develop into terminal hairs, which are larger and more heavily pigmented. Hirsutism is caused by increased androgen production and/or an increased sensitivity of the hair follicles to androgens. Vellus hair is transformed irreversibly to terminal hair in androgen-sensitive areas of the skin. Race and ethnicity are important factors. Asian women have less dense hair than white women.

Testosterone is the major circulating androgen. It is produced by the ovaries and adrenal glands. Testosterone levels are highest in the early morning. Measuring plasma-free testosterone level is more sensitive than total testosterone level in detecting excess androgen production.

DOCUMENTING HIRSUTISM. The presence of hirsutism is determined by the modified Ferriman-Gallwey scoring system (mFG) for hirsutism. This grades the hair growth between 0 (absence of terminal hairs) and 4 (extensive terminal hair growth) at nine different body sites (upper lip, chin, chest, upper and lower back, upper and lower abdomen, arm, and thigh) (Figure 24-9).

Less than 5% of black or white women of reproductive age have a total score in excess of 7. In a white or a black woman, hirsutism is said to be present when the mFG score is 6 to 8.

Medications that cause hirsutism include anabolic or androgenic steroids and valproic acid. If hirsutism is moderate or severe or if mild hirsutism is accompanied by features that suggest an underlying disorder, elevated androgen levels should be ruled out. Disorders to consider are neoplasm and endocrinopathies (PCOS is the most common). Measure plasma testosterone level in the early morning on days 4 to 10 of the menstrual cycle. Plasma total testosterone level should be rechecked along with free testosterone level if the plasma total testosterone level is normal in the presence of risk factors or progression of hirsutism on therapy. Simultaneous assay of 17-hydroxyprogesterone level may be indicated in subjects at high risk for congenital adrenal hyperplasia.

HISTORY AND PHYSICAL EXAMINATION. The prepubertal onset of hirsutism with progression over years suggests functional disorders such as PCOS. Rapid progression of excess terminal hair growth and signs of virilization are indications of an ovarian or adrenal androgen-producing tumor (Box 24-6).

Determine the existence of hirsutism. Unwanted hair growth may just represent an increased ethnic and genetic predisposition for facial hair growth. It is important to establish that the excess hair is terminal and not vellus and that a male pattern distribution exists.

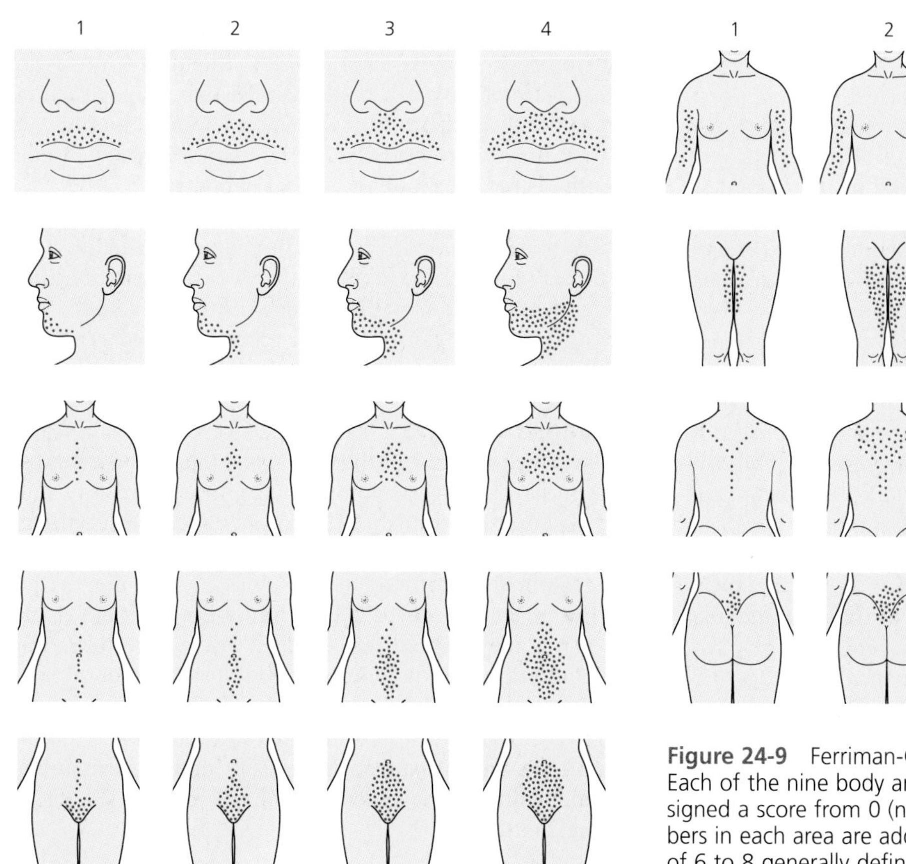

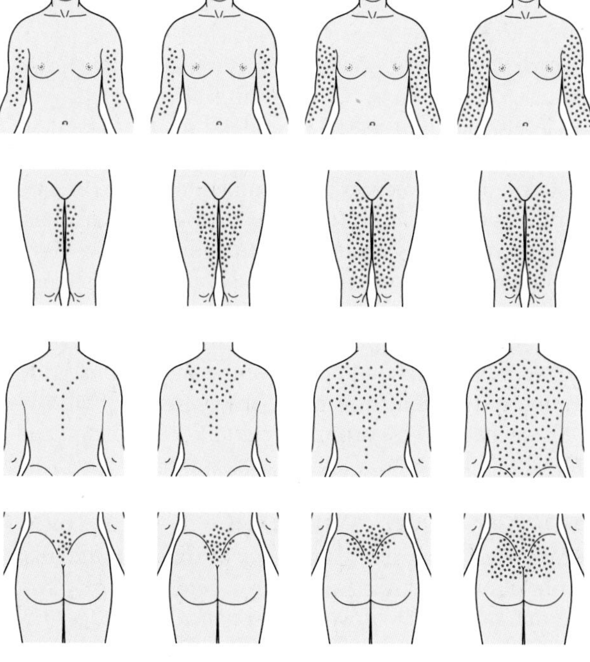

Figure 24-9 Ferriman-Gallwey hirsutism scoring system. Each of the nine body areas most sensitive to androgen is assigned a score from 0 (no hair) to 4 (frankly virile). The numbers in each area are added to obtain the total score. A score of 6 to 8 generally defines hirsutism.

Box 24-6 History and Physical Examination for a Patient Presenting with Hirsutism

History

- Time course of hair growth
- Other androgenic symptoms
- Menstrual and reproductive history
- Symptoms of virilization*
- Changes in weight
- Changes in the size of the patient's extremities, changes in head size, or changes in body contour
- Medications (e.g., androgenic drugs, skin irritants)
- Psychosocial issues
- Family history (particularly androgen excess disorders and/or type 2 diabetes)

Physical examination

- Standard scoring of the excess body hair (modified Ferriman-Gallwey score)
- Blood pressure
- Anthropometric measurements
- Skin: signs of acne, androgenetic alopecia, or acanthosis nigricans
- Signs of virilization*
- Thyroid
- Evidence of galactorrhea
- Adrenal or ovarian masses
- Features of Cushing's syndrome or of acromegaly

*Clinical features of virilization include hirsutism, acne, androgenetic alopecia, clitorimegaly, deepening of the voice, increased muscle mass, breast atrophy, and amenorrhea.

Box 24-7 Initial Investigations in a Patient Presenting with Hirsutism

Exclusion of related disorders
- Basal or stimulated 17-hydroxyprogesterone levels
- TSH levels
- Prolactin levels

Determination of biochemical hyperandrogenemia
- Total and free testosterone levels, dehydroepiandrosterone sulfate levels
- Free androgen index (calculated as the ratio of total testosterone divided by SHBG and multiplied by 100)

Confirmation of ovulatory function
- Progesterone levels on days 20 to 22
- Pelvic ultrasonography

SHBG, sex hormone binding globulin.

Laboratory evaluation. Initial investigations are shown in Box 24-7. Pelvic ultrasonography and 17-hydroxyprogesterone levels may be ordered to exclude related disorders. Thyroid-stimulating hormone (TSH) and prolactin levels are ordered if oligomenorrhea or amenorrhea is present. Determine androgen levels for moderate to severe hirsutism or in those with hirsutism and menstrual dysfunction. Basal levels of total testosterone >6.9 nmol/l (>200 ng/dl) and of dehydroepiandrosterone sulfate >18.9 nmol/l (>7000 ng/ml) suggest an ovarian or adrenal androgen-producing tumor. Patients with these tumors have the sudden onset and rapid progression of hirsutism and the presence of virilization. For a detailed algorithm see *PMID: 16354894* and *18252793*.

POLYCYSTIC OVARY SYNDROME. Polycystic ovary syndrome (PCOS) is the most frequent cause of anovulatory infertility and hirsutism. It is a heterogeneous syndrome that affects 6% of women of reproductive age. The etiology is unknown. The onset is in the peripubertal years. There is insulin resistance, androgen excess, and abnormal gonadotropin secretion. There are signs and symptoms of elevated androgen levels, menstrual irregularity, and amenorrhea.

A genetic defect may cause an increase in the concentrations of intraovarian androgens and stop ovulation. The polycystic ovary forms when an anovulatory state exists. Bilaterally enlarged polycystic ovaries develop, defined by the presence of more than eight follicles per ovary, with the follicles less than 10 mm in diameter. These findings are seen on ultrasound examinations in more than 90% of women with PCOS, but they are also present in up to 25% of normal women. Serum testosterone and luteinizing hormone (LH) levels are elevated in most affected women. Women present with menstrual irregularities, infertility, and androgen excess symptoms of hirsutism and acne. Some women have normal cycles. Virilizing signs such as clitorimegaly, deepening of the voice, temporal balding, or masculinization of body habitus are almost always absent. Obesity is present in up to 70% of patients.

PCOS is associated with hyperinsulinemia, insulin resistance, an increased risk for type 2 diabetes mellitus, acanthosis nigricans, lipid abnormalities, and hypertension. Hyperinsulinemia may be the cause of the overproduction of ovarian androgens. The risk of endometrial cancer is three times higher than in normal women.

Diagnosis of PCOS. In the absence of pregnancy and when amenorrhea or oligomenorrhea has persisted for 6 months or longer without a diagnosis, a history and physical examination should be undertaken, with particular attention to patterns of hair distribution and a search for acanthosis nigricans.

The diagnosis of PCOS is primarily clinical (Figure 24-10). Many women have elevated levels of testosterone, LH, and fasting insulin and reduced levels of sex hormone–binding globulin. Conditions to exclude in the diagnosis of polycystic ovary syndrome are listed in Table 24-4.

Patients with hirsutism and PCOS should have an assessment and management of all risk factors shown in Figure 24-10.

POLYCYSTIC OVARY SYNDROME

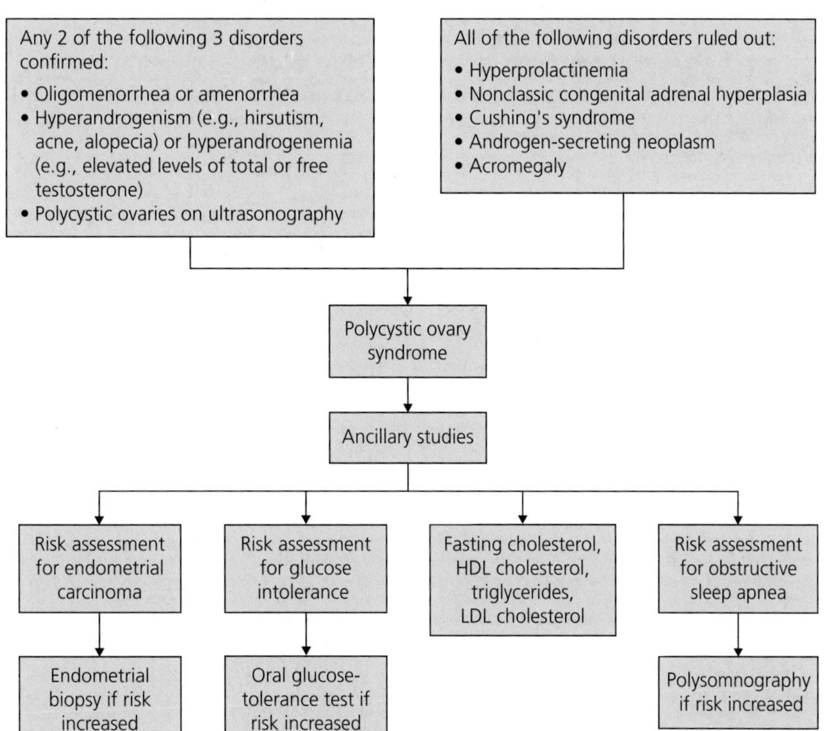

Figure 24-10

Table 24-4 Conditions for Exclusion in the Diagnosis of Polycystic Ovary Syndrome

Condition	Hyperandrogenemia, hyperandrogenism, or both	Oligomenorrhea or amenorrhea	DISTINGUISHING FEATURES: Clinical	DISTINGUISHING FEATURES: Hormonal or biochemical
Nonclassic congenital adrenal hyperplasia caused by deficiency of 21-hydroxylase	Yes	Not often	Family history of infertility, hirsutism, or both; common in Ashkenazi Jews	Elevated (basal) level of 17-hydroxyprogesterone in morning or on stimulation
Cushing's syndrome	Yes	Yes	Hypertension, striae, easy bruising	Elevated 24-hr urinary free cortisol level
Hyperprolactinemia or prolactinoma	None or mild	Yes	Galactorrhea	Elevated plasma prolactin level
Primary hypothyroidism	None or mild	May be present	Goiter may be present	Elevated plasma thyrotropin and subnormal plasma thyroxine levels; prolactin level may also be increased
Acromegaly	None or mild	Often	Acral enlargement, coarse features, prognathism	Increased plasma insulin-like growth factor I
Premature ovarian failure	None	Yes	May be associated with other autoimmune endocrinopathies	Elevated plasma follicle-stimulating hormone level and normal or subnormal estradiol level
Simple obesity	Often	Not often	Diagnosed by exclusion	None
Virilizing adrenal or ovarian neoplasm	Yes	Yes	Clitorimegaly, extreme hirsutism, or male pattern alopecia	Extremely elevated plasma androgen level
Drug-related condition*	Often	Variably	Evidence provided by history	None

From *New Engl J Med* 352(12):1223-1226, 2005. *PMID: 15788499*

*A drug-related condition is a condition attributable to the use of androgens, valproic acid, cyclosporine, or other drugs.

Treatment of PCOS. Weight reduction, diet, and exercise are essential. Low-dose oral contraceptive pills prevent endometrial hyperplasia and cancer and treat hirsutism and acne. Antiandrogens may be combined with oral contraceptive pills for the treatment of hirsutism (see hirsutism treatment in the following section).

HIRSUTISM TREATMENT (GENERAL GUIDELINES)

Hirsutism in obese patients. Hirsutism improves with weight loss. Women with hirsutism have anxiety and depression related to their appearance and this needs to be addressed. A decrease in hair with therapy may require 6 to 24 months. Women with PCOS may have anovulatory infertility, type 2 diabetes, and an increased risk of cardiovascular disease and of endometrial cancer. Impaired glucose tolerance or type 2 diabetes is observed in up to 40% of patients with PCOS.

Oral medications. See Box 24-8 for a listing of oral medications used to treat hirsutism. Oral contraceptives are the first-line treatment for patients with hirsutism and PCOS. They control hyperandrogenic skin changes, regulate menstrual cycles, and provide contraception. Oral contraceptives that contain antiandrogenic progestins (cyproterone acetate and drospirenone) may be preferred.

Antiandrogens may also be used as first-line treatment. These have teratogenic potential and may be used with oral contraceptives. The four antiandrogens listed in Box 24-8 are equally effective. The combination of oral contraceptives and antiandrogens provides contraception, reduces the risk of irregular menstrual bleeding, and suppresses androgen levels by a different mechanism.

Liver function tests are performed before taking oral contraceptives and antiandrogens. Kidney function and serum potassium levels are measured when spironolactone is used, especially in patients with diabetes or hypertension.

Glucocorticoids and long-acting gonadotropin-releasing hormone analogs are used as second-line therapy in patients with severe hirsutism who do not respond to antiandrogens.

Box 24-8 **Oral Medications for Hirsutism***

Oral contraceptives

Antiandrogens

Cyproterone acetate 50-100 mg/day on menstrual cycle days 5-15, with ethinyl estradiol 20-35 mcg on days 5-25

Spironolactone 100-200 mg/day [given in divided doses (twice daily)]

Finasteride 2.5-5 mg/day

Flutamide 250-500 mg/day (high dose), 62.5 to <250 mg (low dose)

Glucocorticoids

Hydrocortisone 10-20 mg twice daily

Prednisone† 2.5-5 mg nightly or alternate days

Dexamethasone 0.25-0.50 mg nightly

Long-acting gonadotropin-releasing hormone analogs

Combination therapy

*At least 6 months of treatment are needed for a response.

†Prednisone is preferable to dexamethasone because the dose can be more finely titrated to avoid side effects.

Treatment (specific medications). Treatment consists of pharmacologic therapy or direct hair removal, or both. Hirsutism is caused by increased levels of circulating androgens and the response of the hair follicle to local androgens. Treatment options include either (1) drugs that target androgen production and action or (2) lasers and intense pulsed light (IPL) therapy, or both.

COSMETIC MEASURES. Cosmetic measures to manage hirsutism include shaving, chemical depilatory agents to dissolve the hair, and epilation methods, such as plucking or waxing. Scarring, folliculitis, and hyperpigmentation may occur with plucking or waxing. Bleaching with products containing hydrogen peroxide and sulfates masks dark hair. Bleaching can cause irritation.

Eflornithine cream. Topical eflornithine (Vaniqa) is an irreversible inhibitor of ornithine decarboxylase, an enzyme that catalyzes the rate-limiting step for follicular polyamine synthesis, which is necessary for hair growth. The topical preparation reduces the rate of hair growth. Results take about 6 to 8 weeks, but hair regrows once the cream is stopped.

Photoepilation. Light-source-assisted hair reduction (photoepilation) is effective. Methods include lasers and nonlaser light sources, such as intense pulsed light (IPL) therapy.

Vellus hair follicles may remain and can be converted into terminal hairs when androgen excess is present and explains why many women experience hair regrowth. These techniques are particularly effective in the hands of experienced therapists who are aggressive enough to produce lasting results. Eflornithine cream during treatment may produce a more rapid response. Cost is a significant limiting factor for many patients. Different skin types require different approaches (Table 24-5). These techniques are more effective than electrolysis.

Table 24-5 Selection of Photoepilation Methods—Laser and Intense Pulsed Light (IPL) Therapy

Skin/hair color	Choice of photoepilation device
Light skin/dark hair	Relatively short wavelength
Dark skin/dark hair	Relatively long wavelength or IPL
Light/white hair	IPL + radiofrequency

Adapted from *J Clin Endocrinol Metab* 93(4):1105-1120, 2008. Epub 2008 Feb 5. *PMID: 18252793*

PHARMACOLOGIC THERAPY. Most women are treated with oral contraceptives. Antiandrogens have teratogenic potential. Therefore antiandrogen monotherapy is avoided unless contraception is used. Reducing insulin levels pharmacologically attenuates both hyperinsulinemia and hyperandrogenemia. However, drugs such as metformin have been shown to be less effective than antiandrogens.

Oral contraceptive monotherapy. Oral contraceptives contain a synthetic estrogen, ethinyl estradiol, in combination with a progestin. Most of these progestins are derived from testosterone and exhibit mild degrees of androgenicity. Other progestins, including cyproterone acetate (CPA) and drospirenone, are structurally unrelated to testosterone and function as androgen receptor antagonists. Oral contraceptives reduce hyperandrogenism by suppression of LH secretion (and therefore ovarian androgen secretion) and stimulation of hepatic production of sex hormone binding globulin (SHGB) (thereby increasing androgen binding in serum and reducing serum free androgen concentrations). The evidence from studies supporting the effectiveness of oral contraceptives is weak.

Antiandrogen monotherapy. Spironolactone is an aldosterone antagonist that exhibits dose-dependent competitive inhibition of the androgen receptor and inhibition of 5α-reductase activity. Studies show that spironolactone 100 mg/day can significantly lower the Ferriman-Gallwey scores. Spironolactone's effects are dose dependent. Spironolactone is well tolerated but has a dose-dependent association with menstrual irregularity unless an oral contraceptive is also used. Hyperkalemia is rare. It may cause diuresis, postural hypotension, and dizziness early in treatment. Antiandrogens may cause fetal male pseudohermaphroditism if used in pregnancy.

Cyproterone acetate (CPA). CPA is not available in the United States. CPA is a progestogenic compound with antiandrogen activity that inhibits the androgen receptor and 5α-reductase activity. It suppresses serum gonadotropin and androgen levels. Because of its long half-life, CPA is usually administered in a reverse sequential way. Doses of ethinyl estradiol (20 to 50 mcg/day) are given for 3 weeks (days 5 to 25) to assure normal menstrual cycling, and CPA is administered for the first 10 days (days 5 to 15) of the cycle. Doses of 50 to 100 mg/day of CPA are often prescribed until the maximal effect is obtained, and then lower doses (such as 5 mg/day) are prescribed for maintenance. CPA is also available as an oral contraceptive at lower daily doses of 2 mg of CPA with 35 mcg of ethinyl estradiol. CPA is generally well tolerated, but there are dose-dependent metabolic effects similar to those of higher doses of oral contraceptives.

Finasteride. Finasteride is second-line therapy. Spironolactone is the preferred drug. Finasteride inhibits type 2 5α-reductase activity. Enhanced 5α-reductase activity in hirsutism probably involves both type 1 and type 2 5α-reductase enzymes. Therefore finasteride produces only a partial inhibitory effect. There are no major adverse effects. Spironolactone 100 mg per day may be more effective than finasteride 5 mg per day with more prolonged treatment. The optimum dose of finasteride has not been determined; 5 mg of finasteride is the most commonly used dose but 7.5 mg may be more effective. Doses of 2.5 and 5 mg may be equally effective.

Flutamide. Flutamide is second-line therapy. It is not used for the routine management of hirsutism. The potential for hepatotoxicity and its high cost limit its value. Flutamide is a pure antiandrogen with a dose-response inhibition of the androgen receptor. Doses ranging from 250 to 750 mg/day are similar in efficacy to spironolactone 100 mg/day and finasteride 5 mg/day. The most frequently used dose is 500 mg/day; 250 mg/day may be just as effective. Hepatic toxicity resulting in liver failure and death is reported. The effect may be dose related; no hepatotoxicity was observed in adolescent girls and women receiving flutamide 62.5 to 250 mg/day or in young women receiving up to 375 mg/day. Therefore the lowest effective dose should be used, and the patient should be monitored.

Glucocorticoid therapy. Glucocorticoids are not first-line therapy. They have a potential for significant adverse effects and are less effective than antiandrogens. Low dosages of glucocorticoids reduce adrenal androgen secretion without significantly inhibiting cortisol secretion. Unfortunately, suppression of serum testosterone concentration is not optimal. Glucocorticoids are used to suppress adrenal androgens in women with classic congenital adrenal hyperplasia caused by 21-hydroxylase deficiency (CYP21A2). In these patients, glucocorticoids help prevent hirsutism. In women with the nonclassic form of CYP21A2 deficiency, glucocorticoids produce ovulation induction, but their role in the management of hirsutism is less clear.

Gonadotropin-releasing hormone (GnRH) analogs. GnRH agonist therapy is second-line therapy. It has no therapeutic advantages when compared with oral contraceptives and antiandrogens. It is expensive and complicated to use.

Alopecia areata

Alopecia areata (AA) is a common asymptomatic disease characterized by the rapid onset of total hair loss in a sharply defined, usually round, area. The diagnosis is made by observation. Any hair-bearing surface may be affected. The cause is unknown. An interaction between genetic and environmental factors may trigger the disease. Alopecia areata is a partial loss of scalp hair, alopecia totalis is 100% loss of scalp hair, and alopecia universalis is 100% loss of hair on the scalp and body.

PREVALENCE

The incidence of AA in the United States is 0.1% to 0.2% of the population. Sixty percent of patients present with their first patch before 20 years of age. Familial incidence is 37% in patients who had their first patch by 30 years of age and 7.1% in patients who had their first patch after 30 years of age.

CLINICAL PRESENTATION. A wide spectrum of involvement is seen. Most patients report the sudden occurrence of one to several 1- to 4-cm areas of hair loss on the scalp that can be easily concealed by covering with adjacent hair. The skin is smooth and white or may have short stubs of hair. The hair shaft in AA is poorly formed and breaks on reaching the surface (Figure 24-11). Some patients complain of itching, tenderness, or a burning sensation before the patches appear.

AA appears to progress as a wave of follicles prematurely enters telogen. The event weakens or narrows the hair shaft, which continues to grow before the telogen phase is complete. Most weakened hairs fracture when they reach the surface. The affected hairs that are often found retained at the periphery of a lesion have a normal upper shaft and a narrowed base—"exclamation point" hair.

Regrowth begins in 1 to 3 months and may be followed by loss in the same or other areas. The new hair is usually of the same color and texture, but it may be fine and white. Occasionally the white color remains. The eyelashes, beard (Figure 24-12), and, rarely, other parts of the body may be involved. Total hair loss of the scalp (alopecia totalis), seen most frequently in young people, may be accompanied by cycles of growth and loss, but the prognosis for long-term regrowth is poor. Total body hair loss (alopecia universalis) is very rare.

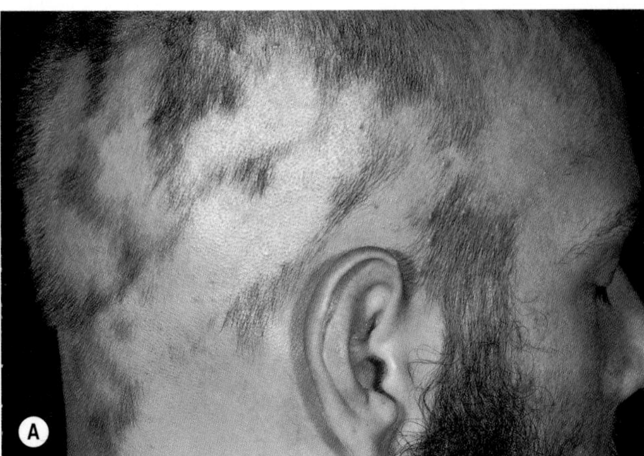

Multiple round and oval patches of hair loss.

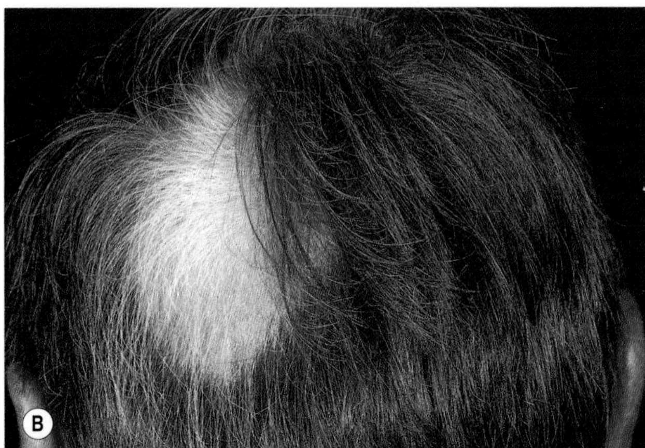

The regrown hair is white.

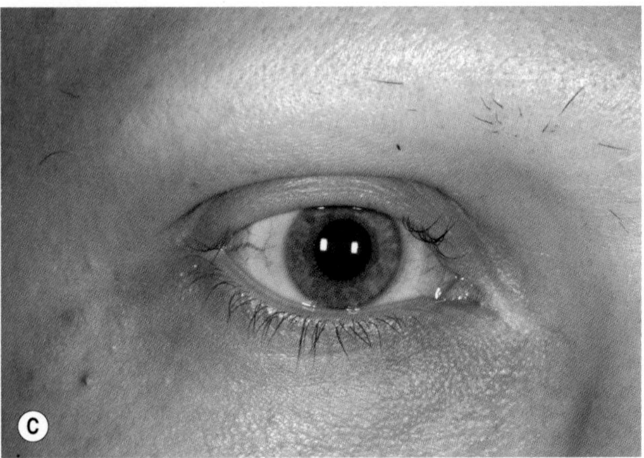

Loss of eyelashes and eyebrows is a common finding.

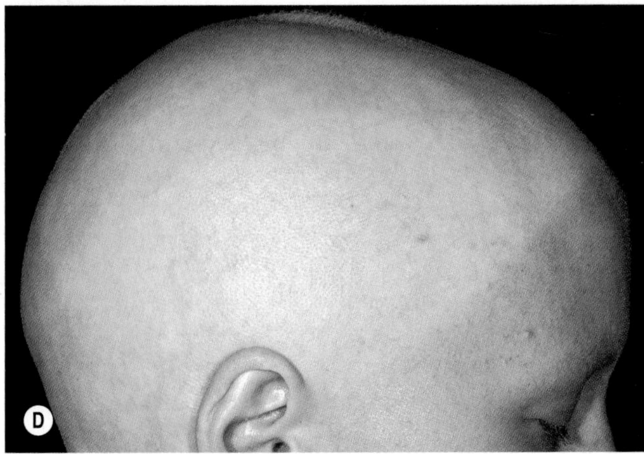

Alopecia totalis. The hair has regrown for short periods. The prognosis for normal regrowth is poor.

Figure 24-11 Alopecia areata.

PSYCHOLOGIC IMPLICATIONS. Hair plays an important role in one's appearance and self-image, and sudden hair loss in a bizarre pattern is psychologically painful. It affects the quality of life and limits social freedom. Those affected equate partial hair loss with balding and fear total hair loss. The appearance is striking, and people stare. AA is devastating for image-conscious teenagers. Patients make attempts to hide bald spots by covering them with adjacent long hairs. Those with extensive loss who cannot adequately camouflage the spots may go into hiding or obtain a wig. A network of support groups across the country is available to help people cope with fears, loneliness, and concerns. The National Alopecia Areata Foundation (www.naaf.com), provides informational brochures, newsletters, research, updates, sources of scalp prostheses, videotapes for schoolchildren, and locations of support groups and holds an annual conference to help patients cope with the condition. The physician can provide continuing support for this difficult problem.

NAIL CHANGES. Nail dystrophy may be associated with AA. The incidence is 10% to 66%. Pitting with an irregular pattern, or in organized transverse or longitudinal rows and longitudinal striations, may result in a sandpaper appearance seen in one or all of the nails of some patients with AA (Figure 24-13). Dystrophy precedes, coincides with, or occurs after resolution of AA.

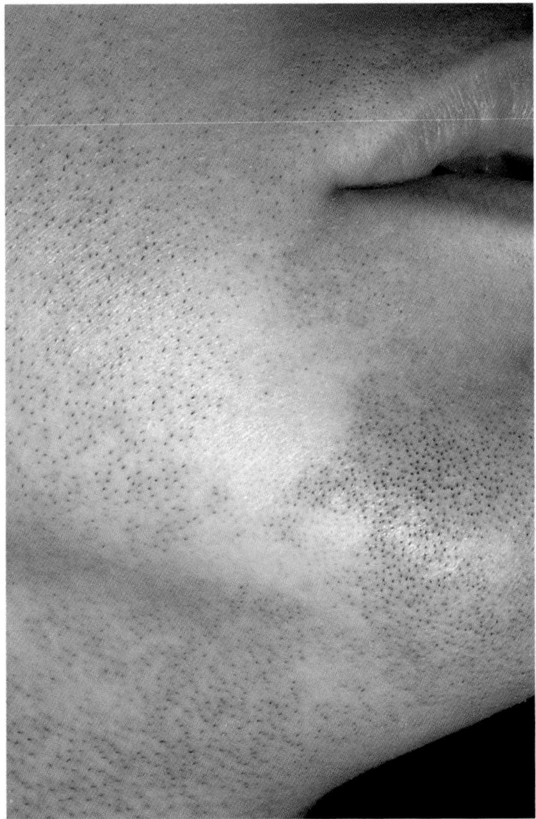

Figure 24-12 Alopecia areata. The beard area is the second most common area to be affected.

PROGNOSIS. The course is unpredictable; recovery may be complete or partial. Several episodes of loss and regrowth are typical. The prognosis for total permanent regrowth in cases with limited involvement is excellent. Most patients entirely regrow hair within 1 year without treatment; 10% develop chronic disease and may never regrow hair. Patients with a family history of AA, young age at onset, immune diseases, nail dystrophy, atopy, and extensive hair loss have a poor prognosis.

DIFFERENTIAL DIAGNOSIS. The differential diagnosis includes trichotillomania and telogen effluvium. In trichotillomania there are short and broken hairs. A 4-mm punch biopsy may be required. Hair loss occurs over the entire scalp with telogen effluvium. The "moth-eaten" or diffuse alopecia of secondary syphilis may be confused with AA.

ETIOLOGY. The etiology is unknown. Genetic factors are important. There is a higher incidence of a family history in patients with AA. Stress is frequently cited. One study concludes that there is little evidence that emotional stress plays a significant role in the pathogenesis of AA.

IMMUNOLOGIC FACTORS. AA may be an autoimmune disease mediated by T lymphocytes directed to hair follicles. There are associations between AA and autoimmune disorders. An incidence of 8% to 11.8% in the frequency of thyroid disease has been reported. AA patients have an increased prevalence of antithyroid and thyroid microsomal antibodies. AA patients have a fourfold greater incidence of vitiligo. The significance of these findings is unknown.

PATHOLOGY. A peribulbar lymphocytic infiltrate ("swarm of bees") with no scarring is characteristic. The acute follicular inflammation attacks the hair bulb in the subcutaneous fat. This inflammation terminates the anagen stage, forcing the follicle into catagen. Since the bulge area is spared, a new hair bulb and shaft grow at the start of the anagen stage, once the inflammation has subsided or has been controlled with glucocorticoids.

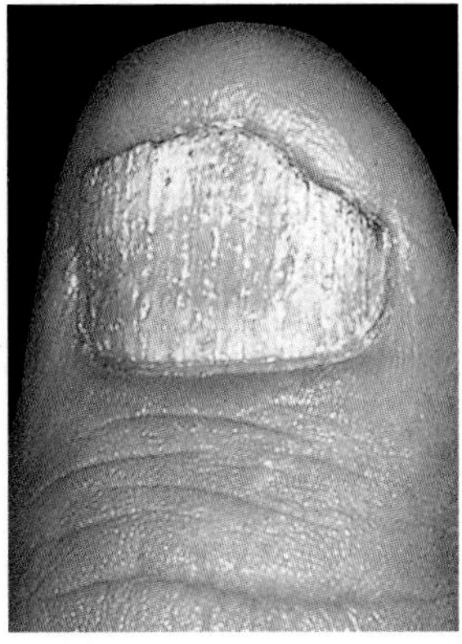

Figure 24-13 Shallow pitting of the nail occurs in some patients with alopecia areata.

TREATMENT. Treatments control but do not cure, and do not prevent the spread of AA. Treatments according to age and severity are listed in Boxes 24-9 and 24-10.

Observation. The majority of patients with a few small areas of hair loss can be assured that the prognosis for regrowth is excellent. If there is great anxiety or if bald areas cannot be concealed, then intralesional injections should be considered.

Topical steroids. Topical steroids are of little value.

Intralesional injections. Intralesional corticosteroid injections are first-line therapy for patients with less than 50% of scalp involvement. Regrowth is seen in 4 to 8 weeks. Repeat injections every 4 to 6 weeks. Atrophy occurs with larger volumes and concentrations of triamcinolone and with injections that are too superficial. Children younger than 10 years may not tolerate the pain. Stop treatment if there is no response after 6 months of treatment. Intralesional steroid injections do not alter the course of the disease, and the hair may once again be shed.

Minoxidil (topical solution). Minoxidil (Rogaine 5% solution) must be applied twice daily. The 5% concentration is more effective. The response is variable. Hair regrowth occurs in 20% to 45% of patients with 20% to 99% scalp involvement. The response is slow and requires months of treatment. Initial hair regrowth is usually seen after 12 weeks. Minoxidil does not change the course of the disease, and continual use is required to sustain growth. Anthralin or betamethasone dipropionate enhances the efficacy of minoxidil solution. Anthralin is applied 2 hours after the second minoxidil application. Betamethasone dipropionate cream is applied twice daily, 30 minutes after each use of minoxidil. These treatments are not effective for alopecia totalis/universalis.

Anthralin. Anthralin results in regrowth in 20% to 25% of patients. Irritation is not necessary, and short-contact therapy is effective. Side effects include irritation, scaling, folliculitis, and regional lymphadenopathy. Protect treated skin from sun exposure. Anthralin temporarily stains the skin. It may have a nonspecific immunomodulating effect. The treatment is safe and may be considered for refractory cases. Combination therapy with 5% minoxidil plus 0.5% anthralin is more effective than when either drug is used as a single agent. New hair growth is seen within 3 months. Anthralin is a good choice for children.

Topical immunotherapy. Topical immunotherapy with contact sensitizers is the most effective treatment for chronic, severe AA. The mechanism is not clear, but it probably has an immunomodulating effect. Dinitrochlorobenzene (DNCB), diphenylcyclopropenone (DPCP), and squaric acid dibutylester (SADBE) have been used. The success rate in the most experienced hands is approximately 60% in patients with 25% to 99% scalp involvement. This is not routine therapy and is not available in some teaching centers.

Box 24-9 **Treatment for Patients with Alopecia Areata According to Age and Severity of Condition**

Patients <10 years of age

5% topical minoxidil solution, topical glucocorticoid, or both
Anthralin (short contact)*

Patients >10 years of age

<50% of scalp affected
- Intralesional glucocorticoid, 5% topical minoxidil solution, or both, with or without topical glucocorticoid
- Anthralin (short contact)*

>50% of scalp affected
- 5% topical minoxidil solution, with or without topical glucocorticoid
- Topical immunotherapy
- Anthralin (short contact)*
- Oral glucocorticoid
- Scalp prosthesis

Eyebrows and beard affected

Intralesional glucocorticoid, 5% topical minoxidil solution, or both

From Price VH: *New Engl J Med* 341, 1999. *PMID: 10577120*
*Anthralin is left on the scalp for 20 to 60 minutes.

Systemic corticosteroids. Systemic corticosteroids are effective but rarely used. The side effects, high relapse rate, long treatment periods, and inability to change prognosis limit their use. Young adult patients with active disease affecting more than 50% of the scalp are the best candidates. Poor long-term outcome of severe alopecia areata in children treated with high-dose pulse corticosteroid therapy has been reported. *PMID: 1827946* A 6-week taper of prednisone resulted in 25% regrowth in 30% to 47% of patients with mild to extensive AA, alopecia totalis, or alopecia universalis, with predictable and transient side effects. Patients with recent-onset AA (1 year) and a bald surface of greater than 30% of the scalp were given 250 mg of methylprednisolone intravenously twice a day on 3 successive days. Another study using the same dosages supports these findings. *PMID: 18205838* The course of the ongoing episode of AA was stopped in eight patients. At the 6-month follow-up, a regrowth on 80% to 100% of the bald surfaces was observed in six patients.

Cyclosporine. Oral cyclosporine is effective for treatment of AA. However, the side effects, high recurrence rate, and long treatment periods limit the use of this drug.

Hair weaves and wigs. See treatment section under androgenetic alopecia in men. High-quality wigs are available.

Box 24-10 **Suggested Methods of Treatment for Alopecia Areata**

Intralesional glucocorticoid

All sites

The preferred compound is triamcinolone acetonide (10 mg/ml), administered with a 3-ml syringe with a 30-gauge 1½-inch-long needle. Concentrations of 2.5 to 8 mg/ml may also be used; 2.5 mg/ml is used for the beard area and eyebrows. Inject 0.1 ml or less into the mid-dermis at multiple sites 1 cm apart; do not raise wheal or inject into subcutaneous tissue. Repeat every 4 to 6 weeks; if atrophy of the skin occurs, do not reinject affected site until atrophy resolves. Optional topical anesthesia may be used: apply a mixture of 2.5% lidocaine and 2.5% prilocaine (EMLA cream) in a thick layer to intact skin and cover with occlusive dressing for 1 hour before injections are given; remove cream immediately before injections.

Scalp

The maximal dose is 20 mg per visit. When more than 50% of scalp is affected, inject only selected sites.

Eyebrows

The maximal dose is 1.25 mg per visit injected into the mid-dermis of each brow at five or six sites (for a total of 2.5 mg to both brows).

Beard

The maximal dose is 7.5 mg per visit.

5% Topical minoxidil solution

Scalp and beard

The maximal dose is 1 ml per application. Apply twice daily to affected sites. Spread solution with fingers. Wash hands afterward. This treatment is not effective for patients with total (100%) loss of scalp hair.

Eyebrows

Using a finger, apply two applications to each eyebrow twice daily using a mirror to ensure precise placement. Hold a cotton ball over the eye for protection. Wash hands afterward.

Anthralin (short contact)*

Apply 0.5% to 1% anthralin cream to affected scalp once daily; leave on 20 to 30 minutes daily for 2 weeks, and then 45 minutes daily for 2 weeks, up to a maximum of 1 hour daily. Wash hands afterward, and avoid getting anthralin in the eyes.

Remove from scalp with mineral oil; then wash off with soap and water. Do not use on brows or beard. Some patients tolerate overnight application.

Topical glucocorticoid

Apply twice daily.

Topical immunotherapy

Use diphencyprone or squaric acid dibutylester to induce contact sensitization. For initial sensitization, apply 2% solution of selected contact allergen in acetone to a 4 cm^2 area on one side of the scalp. After initial sensitization, apply diluted solution of contact allergen weekly to same half of scalp in two coats. For both the sensitizing application and subsequent weekly applications, the patient washes off the allergen after 48 hours. Adjust concentration of allergen according to the response to the previous week's treatment. Desired responses include mild itching, erythema, and scaling.

Concentrations of allergen that elicit responses range from 0.0001%, 0.001%, 0.01%, 0.025%, 0.05%, 0.1%, 0.25%, 0.5%, and 1.0% to 2.0%. After hair growth is established on the treated side (in 3 to 12 months), then both sides of the scalp are treated. Apply contact sensitizer with wooden applicator tipped with generous amount of cotton (the physician or nurse applying weekly treatment must wear gloves). To minimize side effects it is recommended that the allergen be applied in a physician's office and not be given to the patient for use at home.

Oral glucocorticoids

Active, extensive, or rapidly spreading alopecia areata

For patients weighing >60 kg the recommended treatment is 40 mg of oral prednisone daily for 1 week; then 35 mg daily for 1 week; 30 mg daily for 1 week; 25 mg daily for 1 week; 20 mg daily for 3 days; 15 mg daily for 3 days; 10 mg daily for 3 days; and 5 mg daily for 3 days. Prednisone may be used with 5% topical minoxidil solution twice daily and intralesional triamcinolone acetonide injections, given as previously described, every 4 to 6 weeks. Topical therapy should be continued twice daily with or without intralesional injections every 4 to 6 weeks after prednisone is tapered.

Active, less extensive alopecia areata

Twenty milligrams of oral prednisone should be given daily or every other day; dose should be tapered slowly by increments of 1 mg after the condition is stable.

*Anthralin is left on the scalp for 20 to 60 minutes.

Adapted from Price VH: *New Engl J Med* 341, 1999. *PMID: 10498493*

Trichotillomania

Trichotillomania (TTM) is a chronic impulse control disorder characterized by repetitive hair-pulling, resulting in alopecia. Others feel it should be classified more appropriately as a disorder on the obsessive-compulsive spectrum.

There is increased tension immediately before pulling or when attempting to resist the behavior. Feelings of pleasure, gratification, or relief from pulling out the hair are characteristic.

PREVALENCE. Prevalence rates range from 0.6% to 13%. This conscious or subconscious habit or tic is most commonly performed by young children, adolescents, and women. Many children have a benign, self-limited form of hair pulling. The average age of onset is 11 to 13 years. The female to male ratio is 2.5:1. Increased prevalence has been documented in adults with anxiety and with affective disorders.

DERMATOLOGIC MANIFESTATIONS. Hair is twisted around the finger and pulled or rubbed until extracted or broken. The favorite site is the easily reached frontoparietal region of the scalp, but any scalp area or the eyebrows and eyelashes may be attacked (Figure 24-14). The affected area has an irregular angulated border, and the density of hair is greatly reduced; but the site is never bald, as in alopecia areata. Several short, broken hairs of varying lengths are randomly distributed in the involved site. Hair that grows beyond 0.5 to 1 cm can be grasped by small fingers and extracted (Figures 24-15 and 24-16).

PSYCHIATRIC MANIFESTATIONS. The symptom may first manifest during inactive periods in the classroom, while watching television, or in bed while waiting to fall asleep. Parents seldom notice the behavior. In many children trichotillomania is triggered by hospitalizations or medical interventions, problems at home, or difficulties at school. Cases also occur with severe sibling rivalry, a disturbed parent-child relationship, and mental retardation. Comorbidity with mood and anxiety disorders and in patients with a primary depressive illness increases in incidence, with trichotillomania arising in adolescence and adulthood. Some psychiatrists classify it as an obsessive-compulsive disorder in adults.

The course is chronic, with remissions and exacerbations. Patients can spend 1 to 3 hours per day pulling hair, resulting in severe hair loss, suffering, and loss of productive social and work relationships. Shame is a prominent component. Hair pullers fear discovery and avoid health care visits and worry about being critically judged. Psychologic suffering is intense.

DIAGNOSIS. The diagnostic criteria are listed in Box 24-11. First, the patient should be asked if he or she manipulates the hair. Parents or teachers may be aware of the habit. A potassium hydroxide and Wood's light examination rules out noninflammatory tinea capitis. Areas of alopecia areata are completely devoid of hair. In questionable cases, a hair pluck can be performed from the diseased areas; in trichotillomania, it shows no telogen hair roots. Nearly 100% of the hairs are in the active-growing, anagen phase. The absence of telogen hairs is the reason no hair is released on gentle hair traction. Skin biopsy specimens (4- or 5-mm punch extending into the subcutaneous tissue) show normal hairs, absence of hairs in follicles, and no infiltration of leukocytes. Catagen hairs are present in 74%, pigment casts in 61%, and traumatized hair bulbs in 21% of patients; these findings are most evident in areas affected for less than 8 weeks.

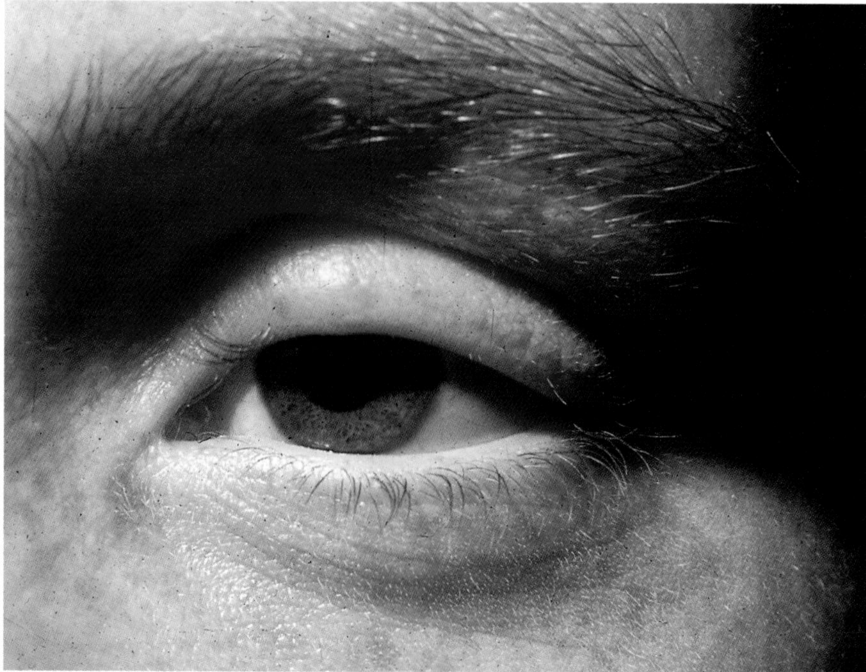

Figure 24-14 Trichotillomania. Extraction of the eyelashes may produce a clinical presentation that is identical to alopecia areata.

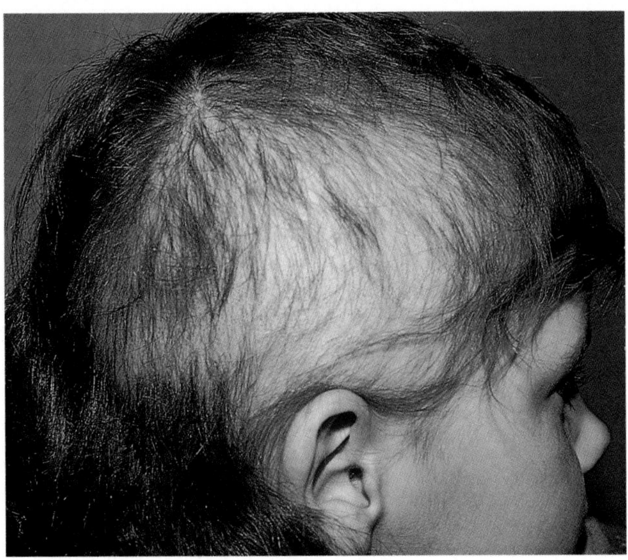

Figure 24-15 Hair has been manually extracted from a wide area of the scalp. There is no inflammation or scarring.

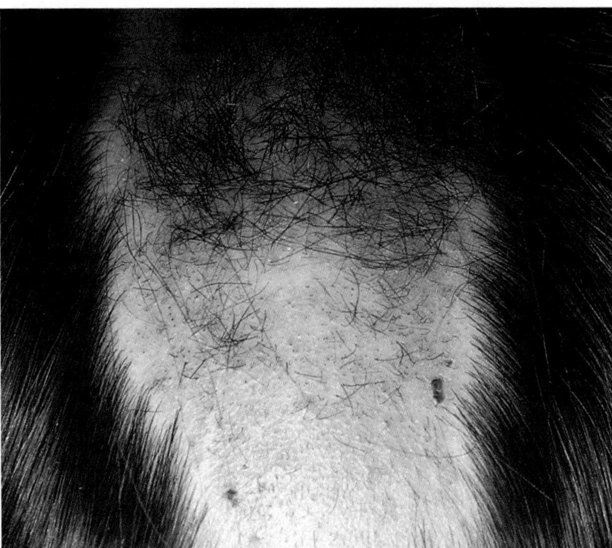

Figure 24-16 Several short hairs are randomly distributed in the involved site.

TREATMENT. A summary of treatment strategies is listed in Box 24-12. Many patients are psychologically stable and require only a discussion of the problem with an understanding physician or parent. Many of these cases resolve spontaneously. Advise parents to divert the child's attention when hair is being pulled and to be accepting and supportive rather than judgmental or punitive. Patients with extensive involvement or those who persist in the habit should undergo psychiatric evaluation. The relative effectiveness and long-term benefits of behavioral and drug treatments are not established. A meta-analysis demonstrated that habit-reversal therapy was superior to pharmacotherapy with clomipramine. Clomipramine was more efficacious than placebo, while there was no evidence to demonstrate that selective serotonin reuptake inhibitors (SSRIs) are more efficacious than placebo in the treatment of trichotillomania. *PMID: 17727824* Many other oral medications have been tried. For more information visit the Trichotillomania Learning Center at www.trich.org.

Traction (cosmetic) alopecia

Prolonged tension created by certain hairstyles (such as braids or ponytails), hair rollers, and hot hair–straightening combs may result in temporary or, rarely, permanent hair loss in an area corresponding exactly to the stressed hair. The scalp may appear normal or may show evidence of inflammation or scarring.

Box 24-11 **Diagnostic Criteria for Trichotillomania**

1. There is an increasing level of tension immediately before hair pulling or during attempts to avoid pulling.
2. There is a sensation of relief, pleasure, or gratification during hair pulling.
3. The pulling is not better explained by a general medical condition or other mental disorder.
4. Significant distress or impairment in occupational, social, or other areas of functioning is experienced as a result of the pulling.

From *Psychiatr Clin North Am* 29(2):487-501, 2006. *PMID: 16650719*

Box 24-12 **Guidelines for the Treatment of Trichotillomania**

- Establish adequate physician-patient relationship to improve insight, acknowledgment of disease, and compliance with treatment.
- Evaluate all sites of pulling.
- Assess motivation for treatment.
- Inquire about trichophagia.
- Consider psychiatric referral.
- Evaluate and treat comorbid conditions (e.g., skin picking, mood disorders, anxiety disorders).
- Guide patient to educational and support groups.
- Evaluate for habit-reversal therapy.
- Institute modified habit reversal.
- Evaluate pharmacotherapy: clomipramine (evaluating the adverse effects of clomipramine).
- Consider introducing posthypnotic suggestions.
- Institute relapse-prevention strategies.

Modified from Koran LM: Trichotillomania. In *Obsessive-compulsive and related disorders in adults. A comprehensive clinical guide* (p 185), Cambridge, U.K., 1999, University Press.

Scarring alopecia

The classification of scarring alopecia is confusing. The cicatricial or scarring alopecias cause destruction of follicles and result in irreversible hair loss. They occur with either destruction of the follicle or scarring of the reticular dermis. Scarring alopecias are classified as primary or secondary. In primary scarring alopecias (Box 24-13), the follicle is the target of inflammation. In secondary scarring alopecias (Box 24-14), the follicle is destroyed by a nonfollicular process. In primary scarring alopecias, the inflammation is either primarily lymphocytic or neutrophilic. All parts of the follicle can be involved, but the bulge area of the follicle, where the arrector pili muscles insert, is the primary target of the inflammatory process. This bulge contains the stem cells for regeneration of the lower follicle during normal follicular cycling. The end stage is smooth skin with no follicular orifices. The primary cause may be related to sebaceous glands.

Box 24-13 **Primary Scarring Alopecia (Classification based on Clinical Presentation and Histology)**

Initially lymphocytic

Chronic cutaneous lupus erythematosus
Lichen planopilaris
- Classic lichen planopilaris
- Frontal fibrosing alopecia
- Lassueur-Graham-Little syndrome (LPP and LP and spinous lesions)
- Pseudopelade (Brocq)

Central centrifugal cicatricial alopecia (follicular degeneration syndrome, hotcomb alopecia)

Neutrophilic

Folliculitis decalvans
Dissecting cellulitis/folliculitis

Mixed

Acne keloid
- Tufted folliculitis

Acne necrotica
Erosive pustular dermatosis

Adapted from Cicatricial alopecia: clinico-pathological findings and treatment, *Clin Dermatol* 19(2):211-225, 2001. *PMID: 11397600*

Box 24-14 **Secondary Scarring Alopecia**

Inherited and congenital disorders

Aplasia cutis, chondrodysplasia punctata, cutis verticis gyrata, Darier's disease, eccrine hamartoma, epidermal nevi, epidermolysis bullosa, hair follicle hamartoma, hypotrichosis congenita, ichthyosis (sex-linked recessive), incontinentia pigmenti, keratosis pilaris spinulosa decalvans, neurofibromatosis, polyostotic fibrous dysplasia, porokeratosis of Mibelli, scarring follicular keratosis

Physical/chemical agents

Chemical burns, insect bites, mechanical trauma or laceration, radiation dermatitis, thermal burns

Sclerosing disorders

Lichen sclerosis et atrophicus, morphea, scleroderma, scleroderma en coup de sabre and facial hemiatrophy, sclerodermoid porphyria cutanea tarda

Dermal granulomatous infiltrations

Actinic granuloma; amyloidosis; infections caused by fungi, protozoa, syphilis, tuberculosis, viruses, etc.; Miescher's granuloma; necrobiosis lipoidica; sarcoidosis

Dermal neoplastic infiltrations

Adnexal tumors, basal cell carcinoma, dematofibrosarcoma protuberans, lymphoma, melanoma, metastatic carcinoma, squamous cell carcinoma, etc.

Adapted from Cicatricial alopecia: clinico-pathological findings and treatment, *Clin Dermatol* 19(2):211-225, 2001. *PMID: 11397600*

CENTRAL CENTRIFUGAL SCARRING ALOPECIA (FOLLICULAR DEGENERATION SYNDROME). This disease is common and occurs most often in blacks. Scarring alopecia is most prominent on the crown (Box 24-15). There is migration of the hair shafts through the outer root sheath. The inner root sheath disappears very low in the follicle below the isthmus. Premature desquamation of the inner root sheath is found in inflamed and noninflamed follicles and in the "normal" scalp. There is a spectrum of severity from slowly progressive (over decades) and relatively noninflammatory disease to rapidly progressive (over years) and highly inflammatory disease. Patients with highly inflammatory disease would have been described as having folliculitis decalvans. The end stage may be described as pseudopelade.

Box 24-15 **Central Centrifugal Scarring Alopecia (Follicular Degeneration Syndrome, Hotcomb Alopecia)**

- Middle-aged black females, some black males
- Some have history of hotcomb usage
- Scarring alopecia starts on the vertex, spreads forwards and outwards and gradually assumes the central, elongated configuration of female pattern alopecia; most active disease at the periphery; eventual burnout
- Lymphocytic inflammation
- Premature disintegration of the inner root sheath
- Release of hair fragments into the dermis, causing granulomatous inflammation
- Differential diagnosis—discoid lupus erythematosus, lichen planopilaris, folliculitis decalvans, pseudopelade, tufted folliculitis
- Treatment—minimal hair grooming; no oily scalp preparations, traction, heat, chemicals, straighteners, perming, or dyeing; treat with topical or intralesional steroids, topical minoxidil

CHRONIC CUTANEOUS LUPUS ERYTHEMATOSUS

Chronic cutaneous lupus erythematosus (discoid lupus erythematosus) is a common cause of scarring alopecia (see p. 683) (Box 24-16). Women are more often affected. Early discrete bald patches look like pseudopelade or lichen planopilaris. Late lesions are more pronounced and clinically diagnostic. The combination of diffuse scaling, erythema, telangiectases, and mottled hyperpigmentation within areas of scarring is highly characteristic. Follicular plugging and epidermal atrophy occur (Figures 24-17 and 24-18). With time, plugged follicles disappear, and the skin becomes smooth, atrophic, and scarred. Biopsy of early lesions shows follicular inflammatory changes; late lesions show scarring in the reticular dermis. Treatment includes intralesional steroids and antimalarials (hydroxychloroquine).

Box 24-16 Chronic Cutaneous Lupus Erythematosus

- Young to middle-aged women
- Lesions on sun-exposed areas—face, ears, scalp
- Well-circumscribed, erythematous, scaly plaques
- Follicular plugging, telangiectasia, atrophy, and dyspigmentation
- Early, active lesions may be sensitive and pruritic
- Developed lesion—scaly crust with follicular spines (carpet tack scale attached to the undersurface)
- No active border like lichen planopilaris and others
- Patches without visible inflammation may resemble alopecia areata or pseudopelade
- Interface alteration at dermoepidermal junction
- Lymphocytic infiltrates—perifollicular + between follicles, around superficial and deep blood vessels, and in and around eccrine glands
- Diagnosis is difficult at fibrosis stage
- Immunofluorescence—IgG, IgM, or complement deposits in a band at epidermal-dermal junction
- Treat with topical clobetasol propionate once or twice daily; intralesional triamcinolone acetonide suspension 10 mg/ml repeated every 4 to 6 weeks (very effective); imiquimod cream (*PMID: 17142214*); tacrolimus ointment 0.1%
- Oral corticosteroids such as prednisone 10 to 20 mg daily in morning, and later reduce to alternate-day therapy with a gradually reducing dosage for multiple itchy lesions
- Use hydroxychloroquine sulfate, retinoids (isotretinoin, acitretin), azathioprine, and cyclosporine for more extensive disease

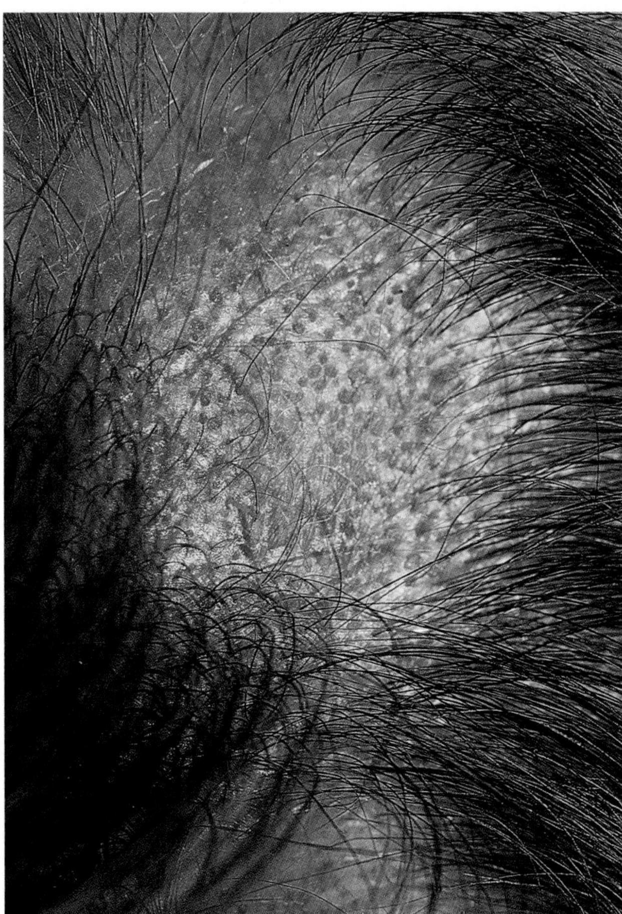

Figure 24-17 Discoid lupus erythematosus. Red, scaly plaques that evolve to irregular atrophic hypopigmented or hyperpigmented plaques. Scales fill dilated hair follicles and form "carpet tack scale."

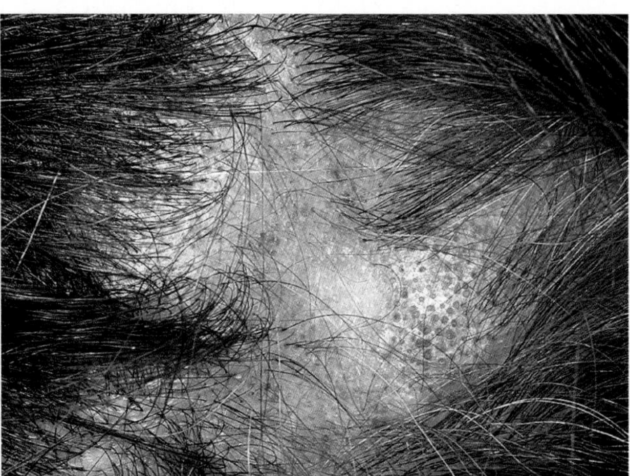

Figure 24-18 Discoid lupus erythematosus. Lesions eventually form smooth atrophic scars as seen in the middle of this lesion.

LICHEN PLANOPILARIS (Figure 24-19)

Follicular lichen planus of the scalp (lichen planopilaris [LPP]) is more common in women. There are several clinical presentations (Box 24-17). Typical lesions present with erythema and perifollicular scaling or as scattered foci of partial hair loss. It may be insidious or fulminate. The frontal-central scalp and crown are most commonly involved. Large areas of the scalp may be involved. Lesions are most active at the expanding border. LPP is more active at the periphery of the plaque than is discoid lupus erythematosus. Other skin and mucosal lesions of lichen planus may be present. Patients complain of pain, stinging, or burning in active areas. Others have a large area of central scarring alopecia on the crown, so-called central centrifugal cicatricial alopecia (CCCA) (see p. 938). This is discussed in a later section of this chapter. Histologic verification is required for diagnosis. Biopsy of early lesions shows lichenoid interface inflammation involving only the follicles and the perifollicular dermis. Immunofluorescence in active stages shows cytoid body staining by anti-IgM and anti-IgA.

LPP is difficult to treat. Superpotent topical steroids, intralesional steroids, and short courses of oral steroids are common first-line treatments. Doxycycline and tetracycline (*PMID: 17467854*) have been tried for their antiinflammatory effects. Hydroxychloroquine, isotretinoin, dapsone, thalidomide, and cyclosporine have all been tried.

Figure 24-19 Lichen planopilaris. Patchy alopecia, hyperkeratotic follicular papules. Spectrum of findings ranging from pure follicular involvement without evidence of scarring to cicatricial alopecia of the scalp.

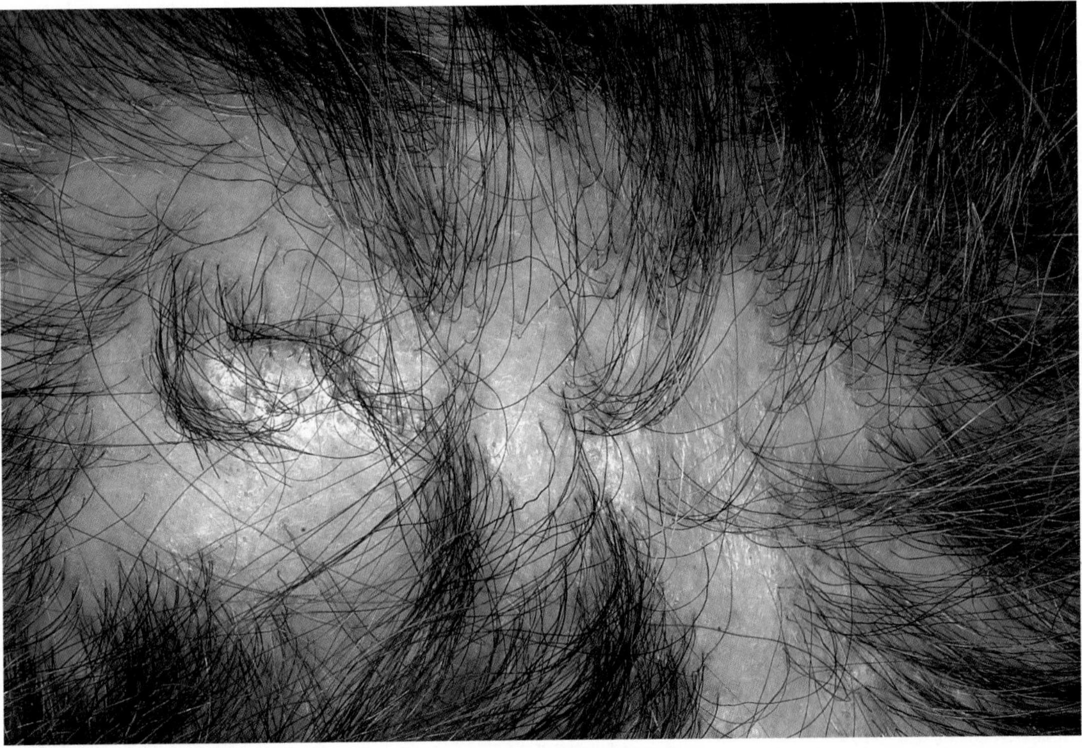

Box 24-17 **Classic Lichen Planopilaris**

- Adult women
- Lesions show a centrifugal pattern centered on the vertex, but can occur all over the scalp
- Spinous, hyperkeratotic, follicular papules with perifollicular erythema
- Smooth, atrophic, polygonal-shaped patches of alopecia with activity at the margins of the lesions that are spreading outwards; leaving central scarring behind is typical
- Lichenoid dermatitis at the dermoepidermal junction
- Concentric lamellar fibrosis around follicles in advanced lesions
- Immunofluorescence is positive in 50% of patients; highlights cytoid bodies with IgG, IgA, IgM, or C3
- Differential diagnosis—lupus erythematosus, pseudopelade, and folliculitis decalvans
- Treat with clobetasol propionate topical steroid
- Intralesional triamcinolone acetonide suspension 10 mg/ml for active lesions
- Oral agent: tetracycline *PMID: 17467854*
- Other oral agents—corticosteroids, long-term hydroxychloroquine sulfate, tetracycline, azathioprine, and cyclosporine

LICHEN PLANOPILARIS WITH FRONTAL SCLEROSING ALOPECIA

Frontal fibrosing alopecia (FFA) is felt to be a variant of LPP. Postmenopausal women present with a scarring process that develops on the frontal hairline and then gradually extends backwards. There may be associated eyebrow loss. The advancing edge of the area of alopecia may demonstrate minute perifollicular papules at the bases of terminal hairs. Biopsy findings are that of LPP.

Box 24-18 **Classic Pseudopelade of Brocq (Nonspecific Cicatricial Alopecia)**

- A noninflammatory, progressive scarring alopecia of unknown origin
- Original patch is usually on the crown
- Occurs primarily in young to middle-aged women
- Lesions are round or oval; several may coalesce to form irregular, bald, slightly depressed patches
- No areas of folliculitis; hairs at periphery are easily extracted
- Patches spread slowly over decades or progression is rapid
- May become bald in a few years
- Biopsy hair-bearing skin at the edge of a scarred plaque
- Lymphocytic infiltrates occur around follicular infundibulum and mid follicles in early lesions
- Differential diagnosis—lupus erythematosus, lichen planopilaris, folliculitis decalvans, follicular degeneration syndrome; may have originated as these diseases but with time have burned out and lost their diagnostic clinical and histologic features
- Treatment resistant to topical steroids, 5% minoxidil, intradermal steroids; oral medications usually ineffective

PSEUDOPELADE (Figure 24-20)

Pseudopelade is an archaic term that designates a rare, slowly progressive cicatricial alopecia without clinically evident folliculitis (Box 24-18). The disease process spreads centrifugally from the crown. It does not describe any one disease entity but may represent the end stage of various forms of scarring alopecia. Pseudopelade of Brocq was a term originally used to describe white adult males with asymptomatic, irregularly shaped, widely distributed clusters of hairless patches that are at times atrophic. Periods of disease progression are followed by dormant periods.

Figure 24-20 Pseudopelade. Asymptomatic, flesh-colored, bald area is present over the parietal scalp. Lesions coalesce to form irregular, atrophic, bald patches with a "footprints in the snow" appearance. Atrophy rather than scarring is present.

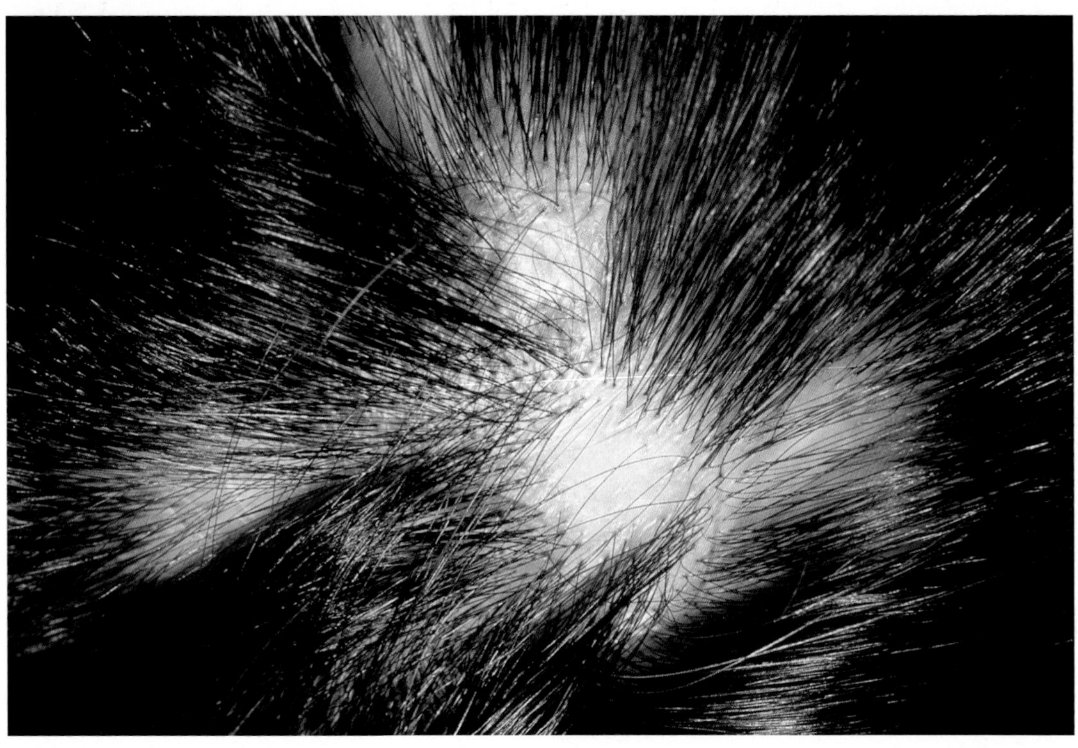

FOLLICULITIS DECALVANS (Figures 24-21 and 24-22)

Folliculitis decalvans is a chronic pustular eruption of the scalp resulting in patchy permanent alopecia (Box 24-19). Late-stage lesions show wide areas of scarring with active pustular lesions at the margins. The etiology is unknown. Chronic bacterial folliculitis or altered host immune responses are proposed mechanisms. *Staphylococcus aureus* may be cultured from pustular lesions. Biopsy specimens of early lesions show follicular neutrophilic abscesses in the infundibula or upper or mid levels of the follicle. Late lesions show dermal lymphocytes, destruction of follicles, and dermal scarring. Systemic and topical antibiotics (mupirocin) and daily bactericidal antibiotic treatment of the nasal vestibules to eliminate the carrier state of *Staphylococcus* may help. One, two, or three 10-week courses of a combination of 300 mg of rifampicin and 300 mg of clindamycin twice daily for 10 weeks arrested the disease. Dapsone 100 mg per day was effective. Some patients have areas of tufted folliculitis. Tufted hair folliculitis (a possible variant of folliculitis decalvans) is characterized by follicular fusion in which multiple hair tufts emerge from a single dilated follicular orifice. These two entities may form part of a spectrum of a single disease.

Box 24-19 **Folliculitis Decalvans**

- Occurs in adults and runs a very long course
- Crops of pustules surround multiple expanding oval areas of alopecia
- Episodes of folliculitis can occur for years, causing tufted folliculitis in some cases
- Sometimes found in beard, pubic and axillary areas, inner thighs
- Initial neutrophilic infiltration
- Moderate perifollicular dermal fibrosis
- Differential diagnosis—bacteria, fungal, or viral folliculitis; follicular degeneration syndrome; and acne necrotica
- Treatment—culture pustules; povidone-iodine shampoo, topical antibiotics (Cleocin or mupirocin); topical steroids sometimes effective; oral antibiotics: tetracycline, minocycline, cephalosporins, ciprofloxacin; rifampin with clindamycin, or sulfamethoxazole/trimethoprim; oral corticosteroids

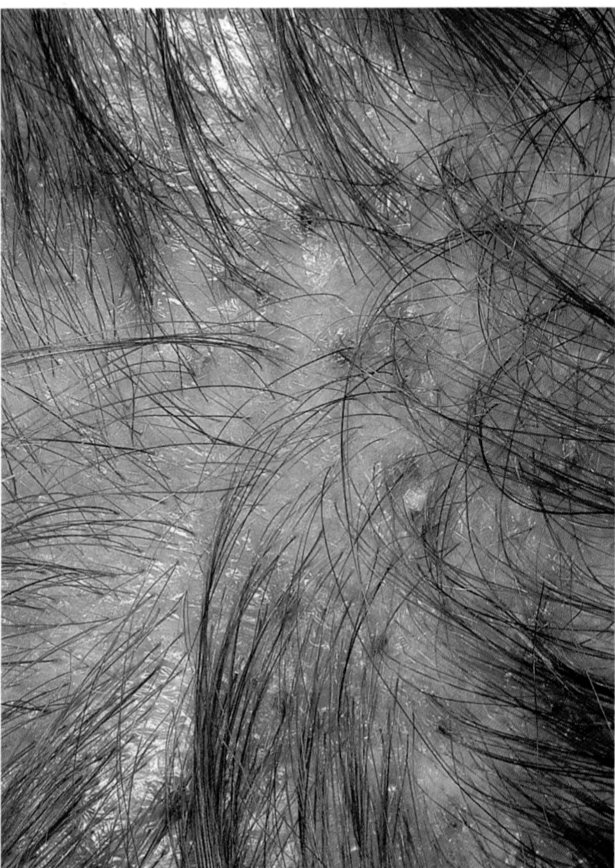

Figure 24-21 Folliculitis decalvans. Well-defined irregular-to-oval atrophic plaques of alopecia with follicular pustules at the advancing margins.

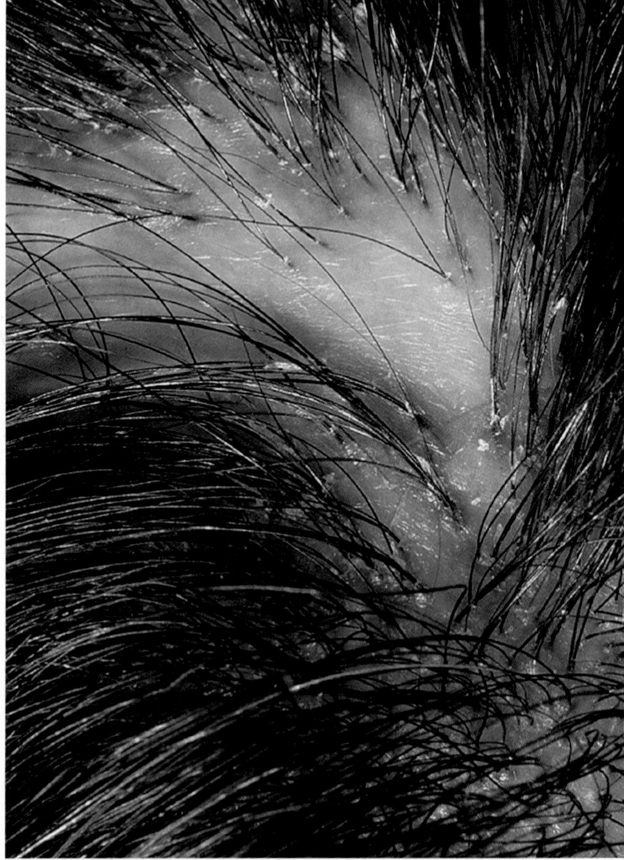

Figure 24-22 Folliculitis decalvans. Chronic folliculitis leads to progressive scarring.

Box 24-20 Dissecting Cellulitis

- Young black men
- Presents as follicular rupture with abscess formation
- Painful fluctuant draining scalp nodules form extensive interconnected abscesses with sinus tracts
- Scarring is extensive
- Part of the follicular occlusion triad (dissecting folliculitis, acne conglobata, hidradenitis suppurative)
- Neutrophilic, lymphohistiocytic, granulomatous inflammation
- Fibrosis in dermis and in subcutis
- Differential diagnosis—folliculitis decalvans, acne keloid, fungal kerion
- Treatment—early cases: tetracycline, doxycycline, minocycline, cephalosporins, ciprofloxacin; advanced cases: isotretinoin, oral corticosteroids, dapsone; drainage of large abscesses

DISSECTING CELLULITIS (Figures 24-23 and 24-24)

This rare disease most often affects young black men (Box 24-20). Multiple inflammatory nodules are concentrated on the crown, vertex, and occiput. They evolve into coalescing, boggy, fluctuant, oval, and linear ridges that eventually discharge purulent material. There may be little or no pain. The presence of hair follicles appears to be essential for disease progression. Eventually, dense dermal fibrosis, sinus tract formation, hypertrophic scarring, and permanent hair loss occur. The "follicular occlusion triad" consists of dissecting folliculitis, hidradenitis suppurativa, and acne conglobata. Isotretinoin is effective.

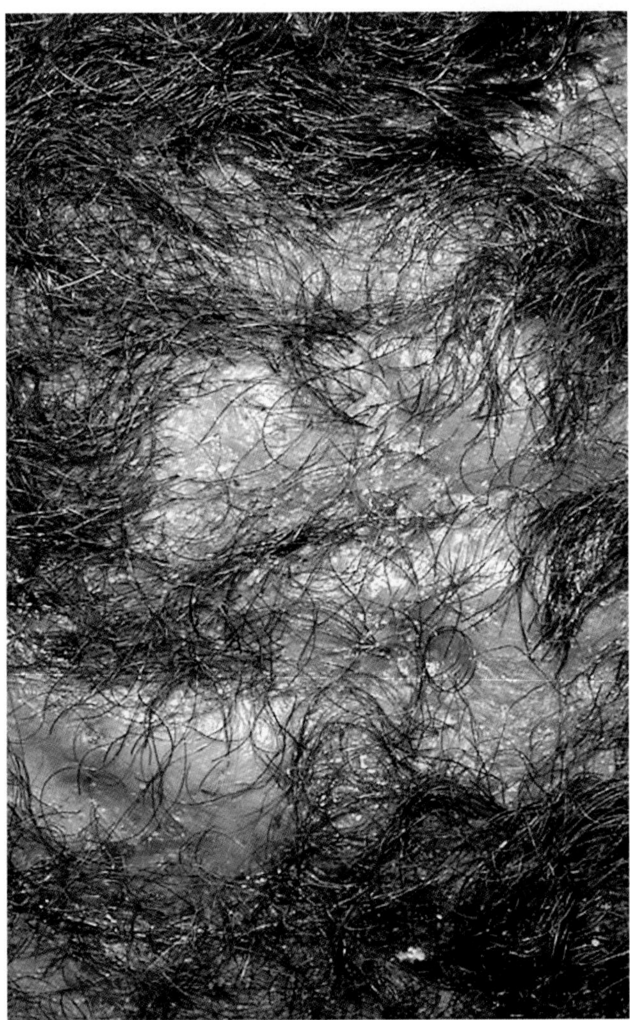

Figure 24-23 Dissecting cellulitis. Superficial and deep intercommunicating abscesses and widespread scarring alopecia.

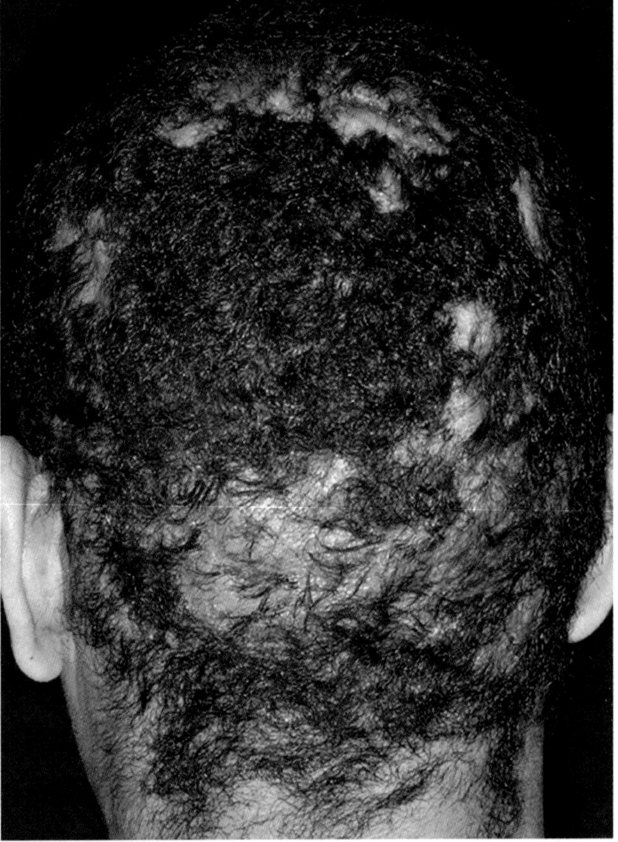

Figure 24-24 Dissecting cellulitis. End stage is extensive thick scarring alopecia.

ACNE KELOIDALIS

Acne keloidalis usually affects young black men. Small, follicular papules with occasional pustules occur on the occipital scalp and posterior neck (Box 24-21). They coalesce into firm papules and become thick and elevated (Figures 24-25 and 24-26; also see Figures 9-24 and 9-25 on p. 355). Abscesses and sinuses with pus may develop. There may not be any symptoms, or there may be mild burning or itching. Histologically, there is inflammation, fibroplasia, and disappearance of sebaceous glands. Treatment is discussed on p. 355.

Box 24-21 Acne Keloid (Acne Keloidalis Nuchae)

- Young black, men on the occipital scalp and neck; much less common in whites
- Presents as follicular papules or pustules progressing to fibrosis papules and extensive keloidal plaques that lack hair
- Inflammation is initially neutrophilic
- Differential diagnosis—folliculitis decalvans; acne necrotica; dissecting folliculitis; bacterial, fungal, or viral folliculitis
- Treatment—povidone-iodine shampoo, topical antibiotics (clindamycin, mupirocin); oral antibiotics (doxycycline, minocycline, cephalexin, sulfamethoxazole/trimethoprim); many weeks of suppression with oral antibiotics may be necessary; topical and intralesional steroids may help; excisional surgery may be necessary in advanced cases

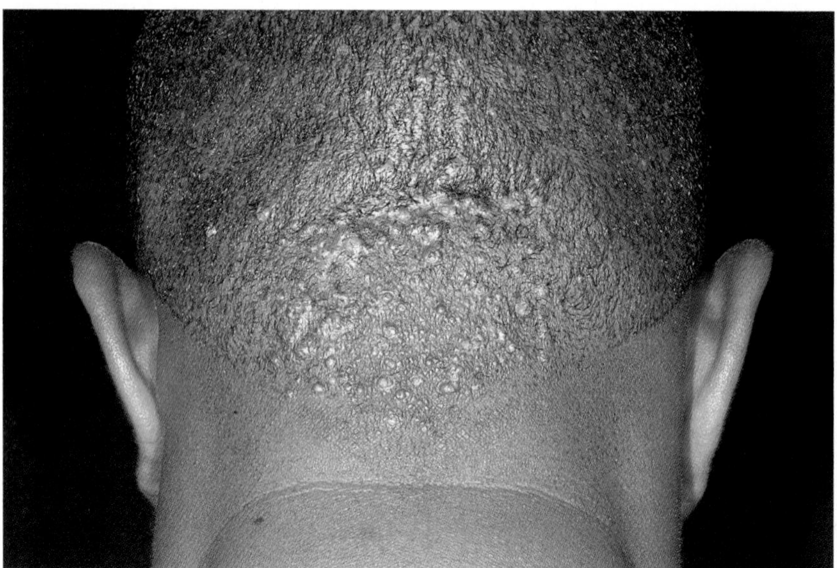

Figure 24-25 Acne keloidalis. Follicular papules and pustules are concentrated on the back of the scalp above the hairline.

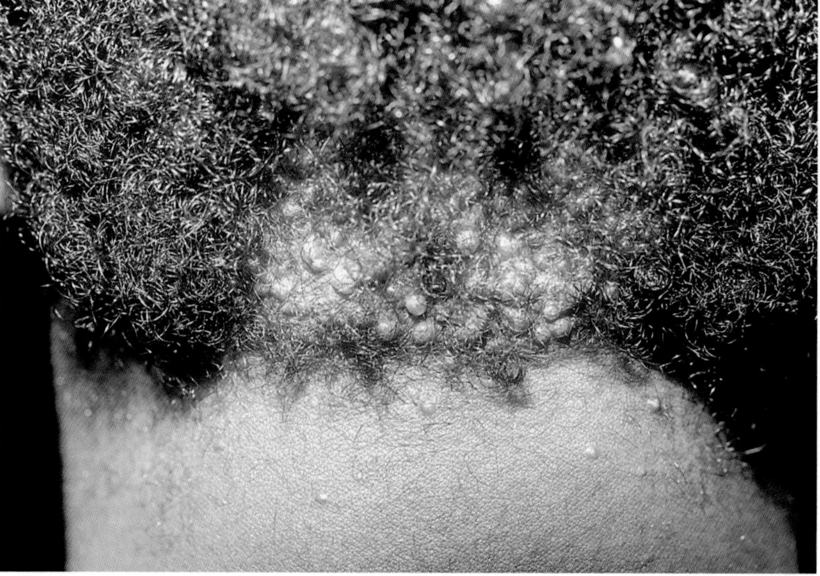

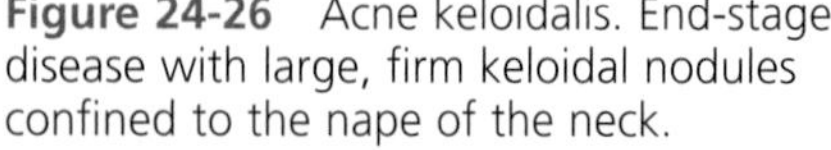

Figure 24-26 Acne keloidalis. End-stage disease with large, firm keloidal nodules confined to the nape of the neck.

Box 24-22 Tufted Folliculitis

- A number of hairs emerging from a single follicular orifice may be seen in any scarring folliculitis; this is called tufted folliculitis
- Three to ten hairs arise from a giant follicle
- Controversial whether tufted folliculitis is an entity or is secondary to other forms of scarring alopecia (lichen planopilaris, discoid lupus erythematosus, folliculitis decalvans)
- Follicular rupture and abscess formation
- Fibrosis around upper and mid follicles
- Neutrophils present around upper follicles
- Differential diagnosis—discoid lupus erythematosus, lichen planopilaris, pseudopelade, folliculitis decalvans, dissecting folliculitis, Lassueur-Graham-Little syndrome, follicular degeneration syndrome
- Treatment—same as that for folliculitis decalvans

TUFTED FOLLICULITIS (Figures 24-27 and 24-28). Tufted folliculitis (TF) may not be a specific disease but an end stage of other diseases such as folliculitis decalvans or acne keloid (Box 24-22). Patients present with an inflamed scalp with pustules from which *S. aureus* can be cultured. It leads to patches of scarring alopecia within which multiple hair tufts emerge from dilated follicular orifices. Tufted folliculitis can be differentiated from folliculitis decalvans only by finding several hair tufts scattered within patches of scarring alopecia.

Tufting of hair is caused by clustering of adjacent follicular units attributable to a fibrosing process and to retention of telogen hairs within the involved follicular units.

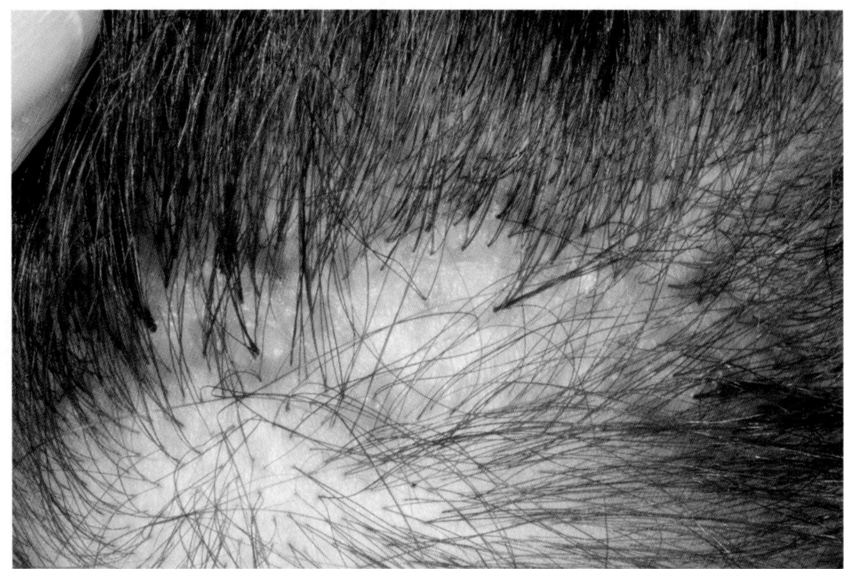

Figure 24-27 Tufted folliculitis. Initial inflammatory folliculitis stage may be any one of several scarring alopecia variants (folliculitis decalvans, acne keloidalis, common staphylococcal folliculitis, and dissecting cellulitis that leads to tufts of hairs emerging from the same ostium.

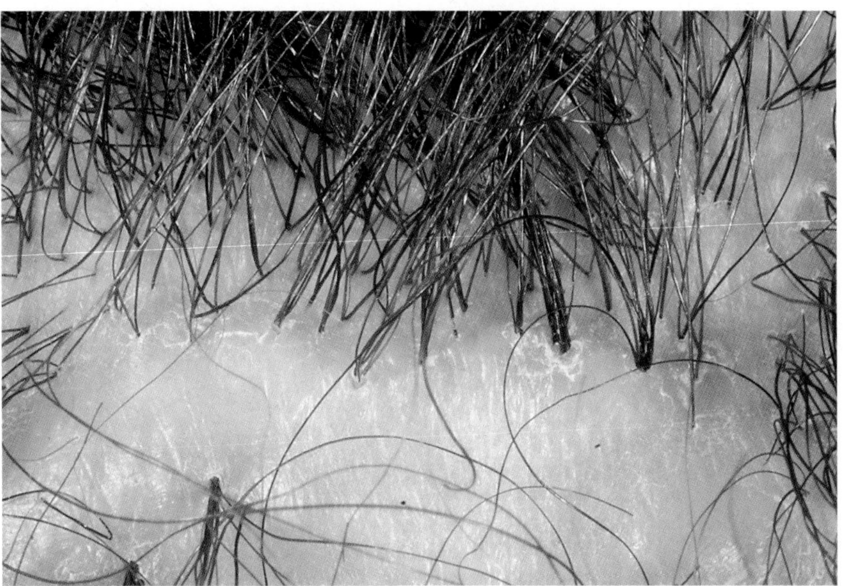

Figure 24-28 Tufted folliculitis. End-stage disease with several hairs (tufts) emerging from the same ostia.

ACNE NECROTICA

Acne necrotica is a severe form of scalp folliculitis. Papules and pustules evolve to form crusts leaving depressed scars. Acne necrotica may also appear on the face.

EROSIVE PUSTULAR DERMATOSIS

Erosive pustular dermatosis is a disease of unknown origin that occurs in the elderly and often in actinically damaged scalp skin. Lesions may follow trauma or destructive procedures for actinic keratoses. Patients present with red, pustular, crusted, and eroded plaques on the scalp (Figure 24-29). Removal of crusts reveals purulent material. The lesions progress slowly and heal with scarring alopecia. Then adjacent areas become affected. Biopsy shows patchy or diffuse inflammatory infiltrates with lymphocytes and plasma cells in the dermis. *PMID: 17637361* Potent topical steroids, topical tacrolimus ointment, calcipotriol (calcipotriene) cream, and isotretinoin (0.75 mg/kg/day) are some of the reported treatments. *PMID: 16205074*

TRICHOMYCOSIS

Trichomycosis is an asymptomatic infection of axillary or pubic hair caused by *Corynebacterium*. The hair shaft becomes coated with adherent yellow (occasionally red or black), firm concretions (Figure 24-30). Hyperhidrosis is often present. The hair is shaved, and hyperhidrosis is controlled with antiperspirants. Naftifine hydrochloride 1% cream (Naftin) is effective for superficial fungal infections and also has antibacterial properties. It is reportedly effective for trichomycosis.

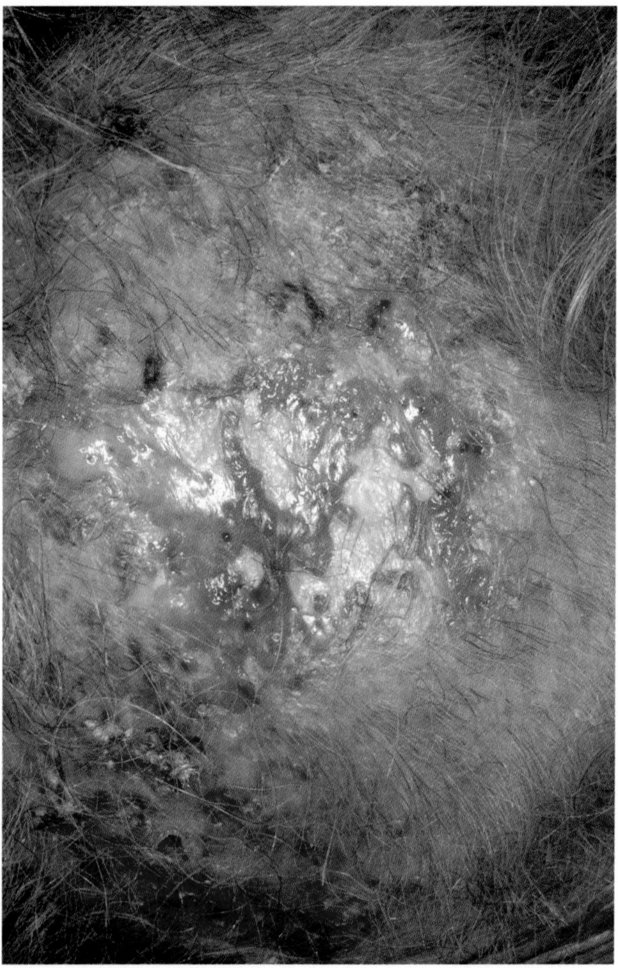

Figure 24-29 Erosive pustular dermatosis. Diffuse crusting associated with multiple pustular, exudative, and erosive lesions. The pustular lesions progressively merge.

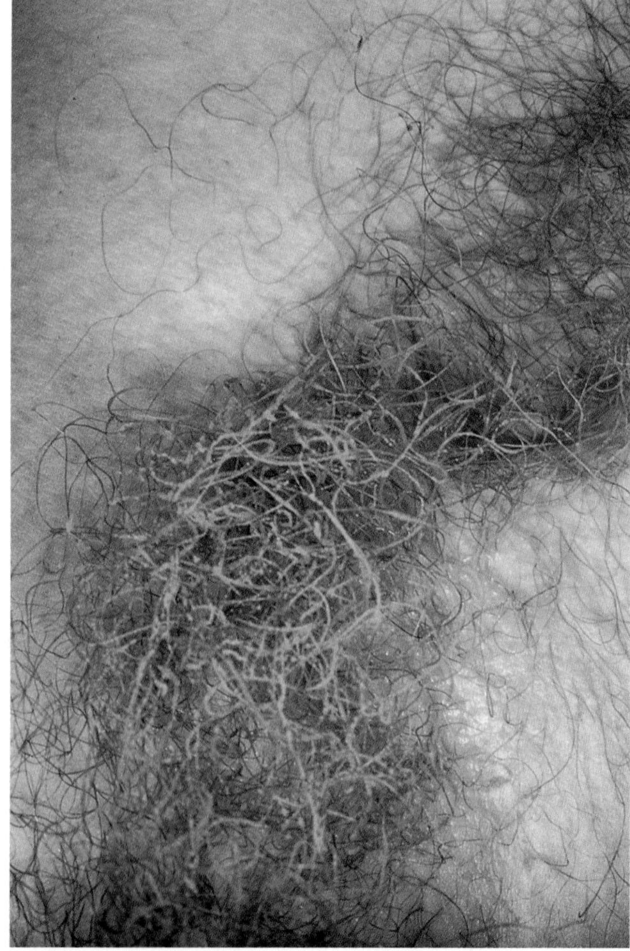

Figure 24-30 Trichomycosis axillaris. Yellow concretions are adherent to the axillary hair. These concretions are composed of a mass of diphtheroid organisms and not fungi.

Chapter 25

Nail Diseases

CHAPTER CONTENTS

- Anatomy and physiology
- Normal variations
- Nail disorders associated with skin disease
- Acquired disorders
  - Bacterial and viral infections
  - Fungal nail infections
  - Trauma
- The nail and internal disease
- Color and drug-induced changes
- Congenital anomalies
- Tumors

See pages 948-949 for photos of the most common nail disorders.

ANATOMY AND PHYSIOLOGY

ANATOMY. The nail unit consists of several components (Figure 25-1). The nail plate is hard, translucent, dead keratin. The nailfold includes the skin surrounding the lateral and proximal aspects of the nail plate. The proximal nailfold overlies the matrix. Its keratin layer extends onto the proximal nail plate to form the cuticle. Capillary loops at the tip of the proximal nailfold are normally small and inapparent, but they become distinct in diseases such as systemic lupus erythematosus and scleroderma. The proximal nailfold epithelium covers the proximal nail plate for a few millimeters and then makes a 180-degree turn and curves back into direct contact with the nail plate. It makes another 180-degree turn and becomes continuous with the nail matrix.

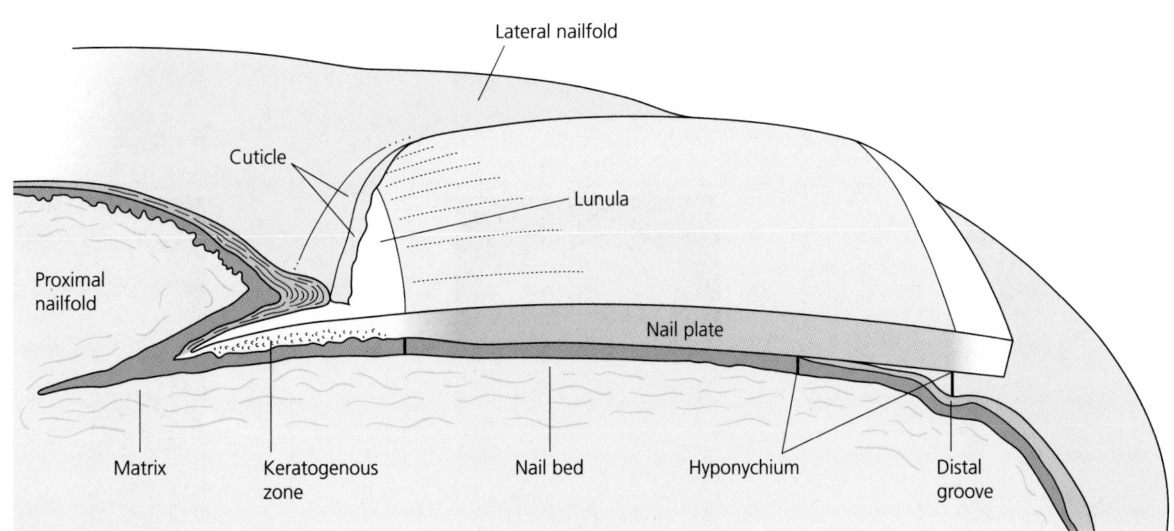

Figure 25-1 Diagrammatic drawing of an adult fingertip, showing nail structures through a longitudinal midline plane.

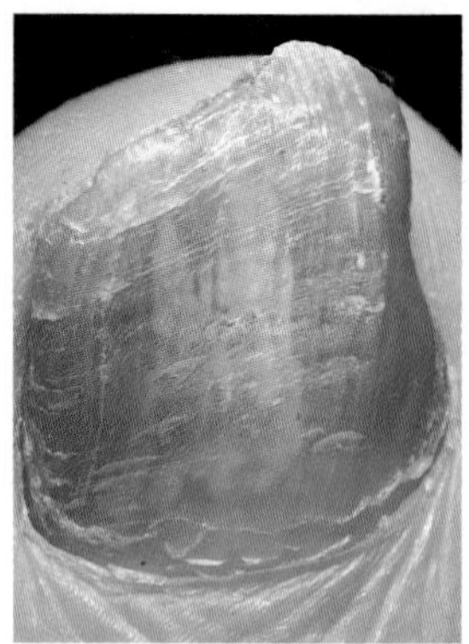
Distal subungual onychomycosis, pp. 957, 960

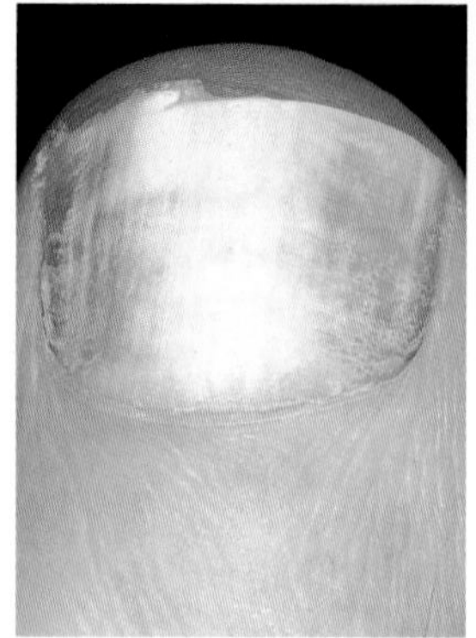
White superficial onychomycosis, p. 958

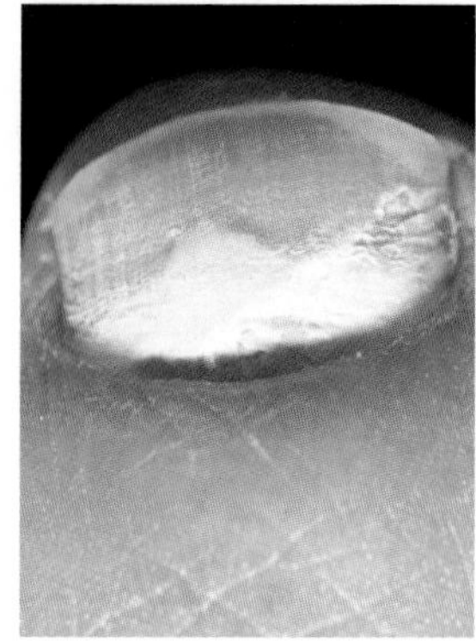
Proximal subungual onychomycosis, p. 958

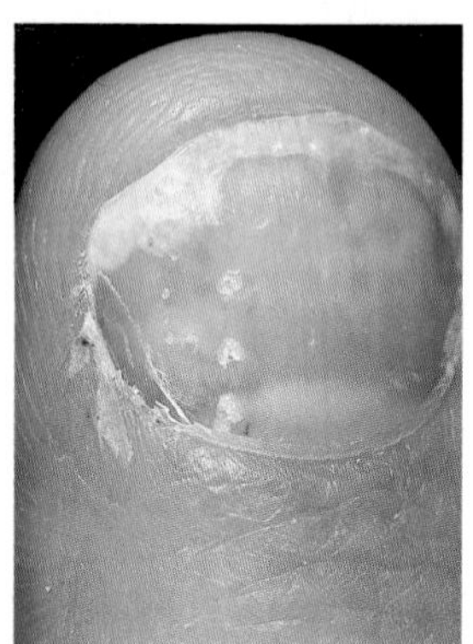
Psoriasis—pitting, pp. 275, 951

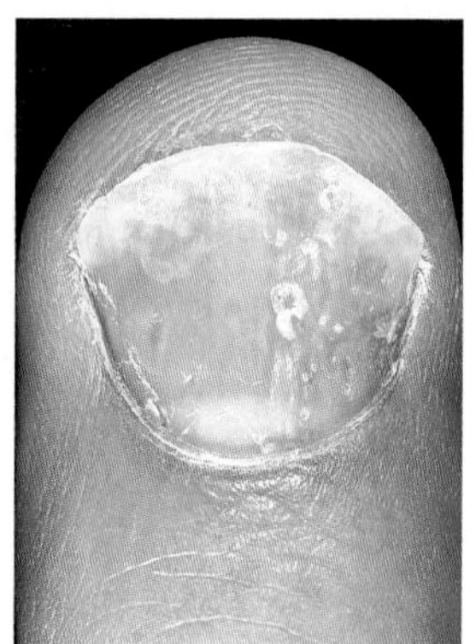
Psoriasis—onycholysis, pp. 275, 951

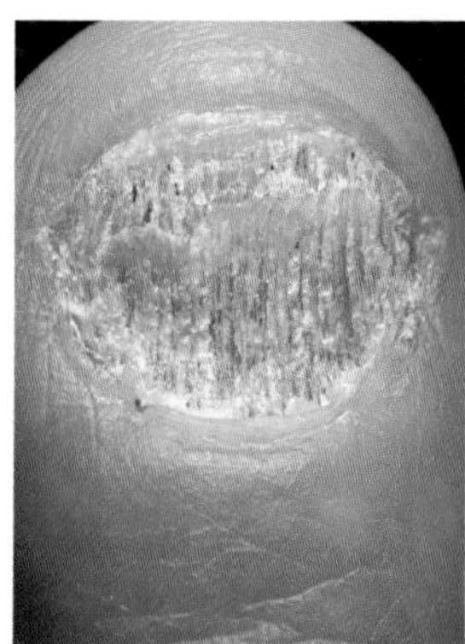
Psoriasis—plate alteration, pp. 275, 951

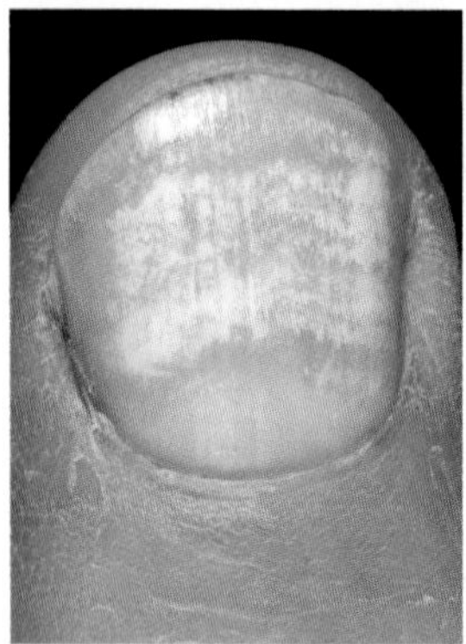
Leukonychia, p. 964

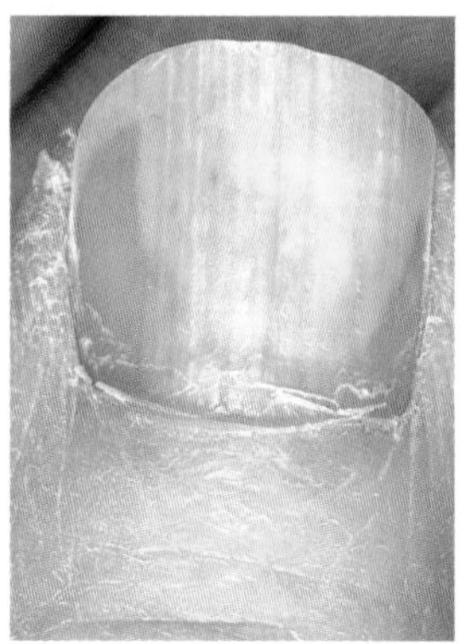
Onycholysis—secondary infection, p. 962

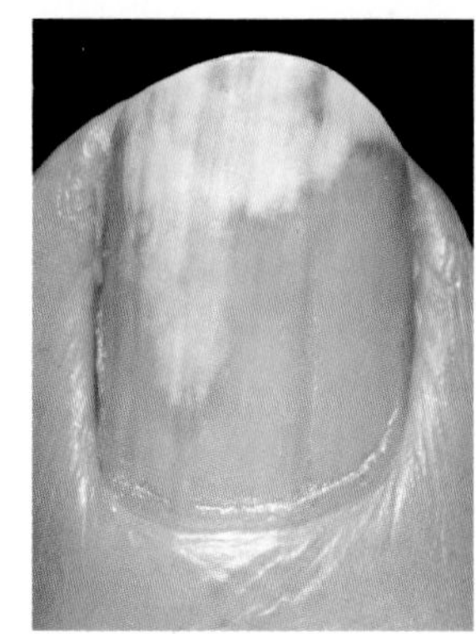
Onycholysis—trauma, p. 962

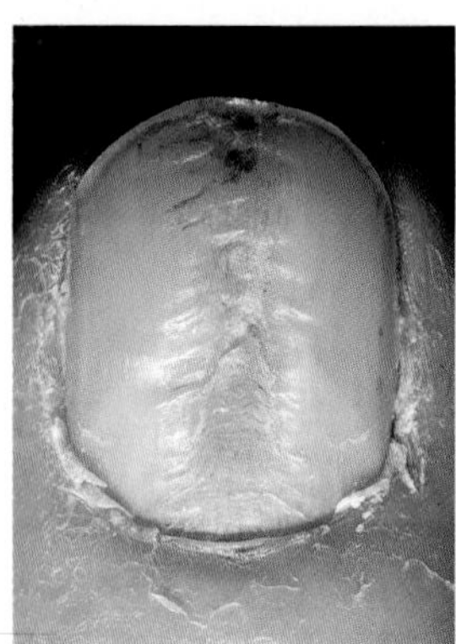
Habit-tic deformity, p. 965

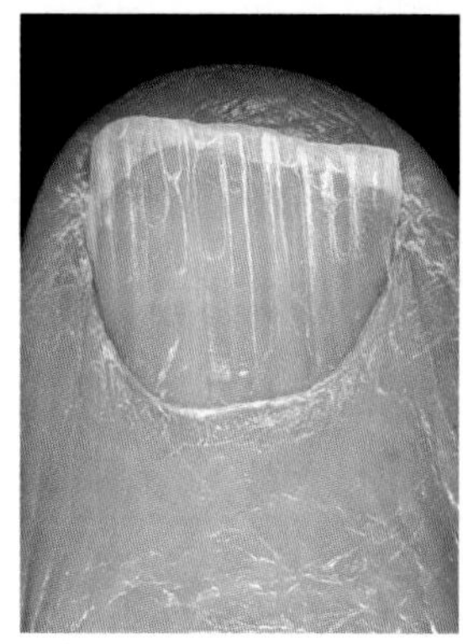
Ridging, p. 950

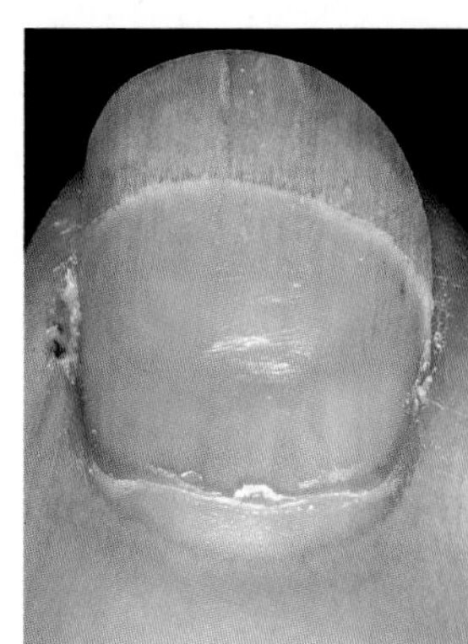
Beau's lines, p. 966

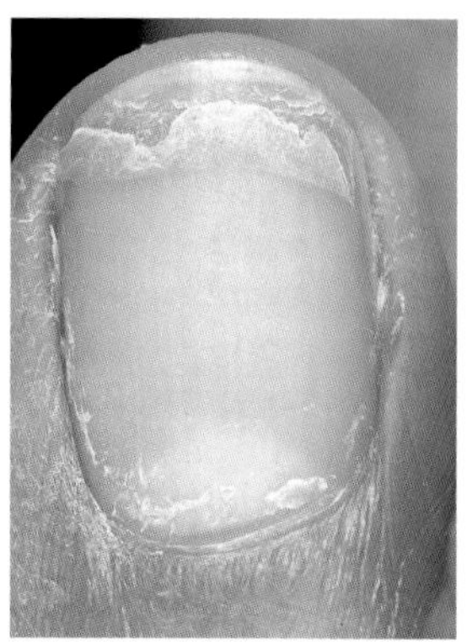
Distal splitting, p. 965

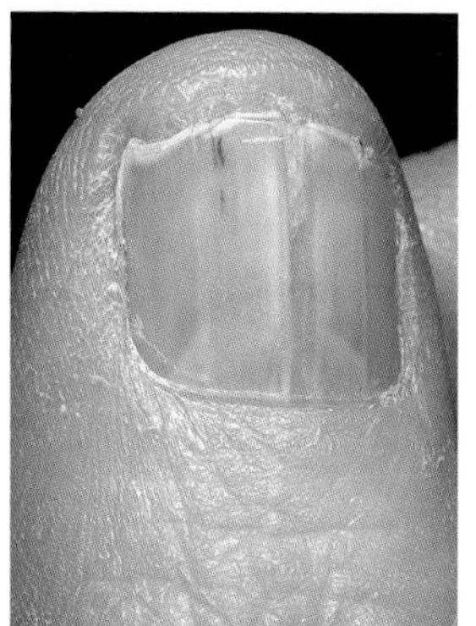
Darier's disease

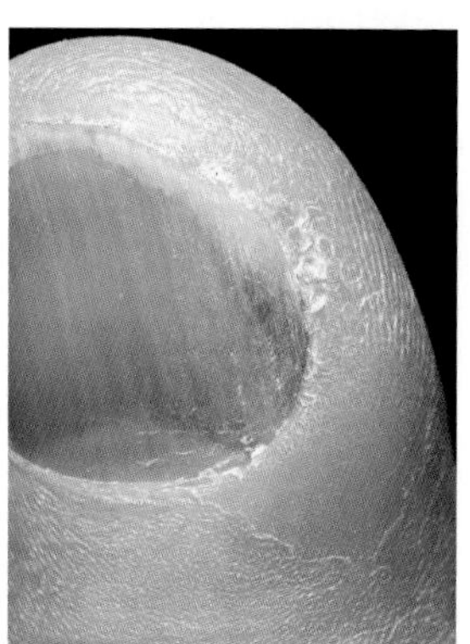
Acute paronychia, p. 953

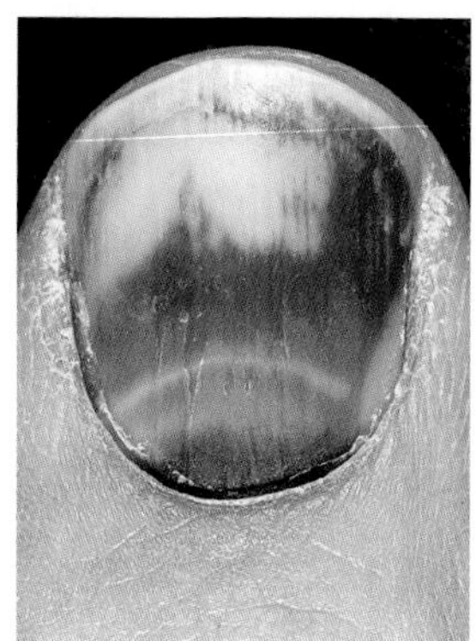
Trauma, p. 964

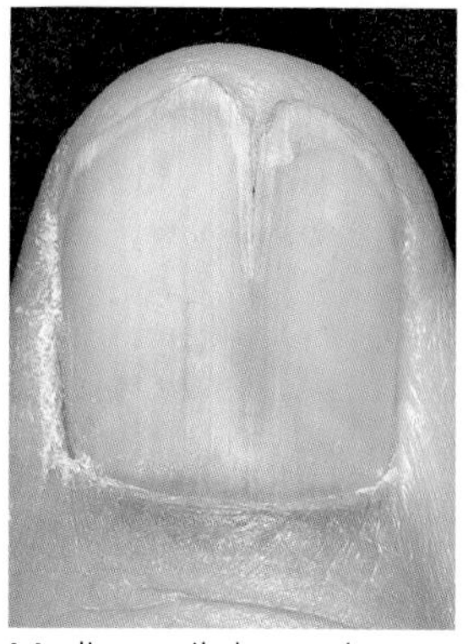
Median nail dystrophy, p. 966

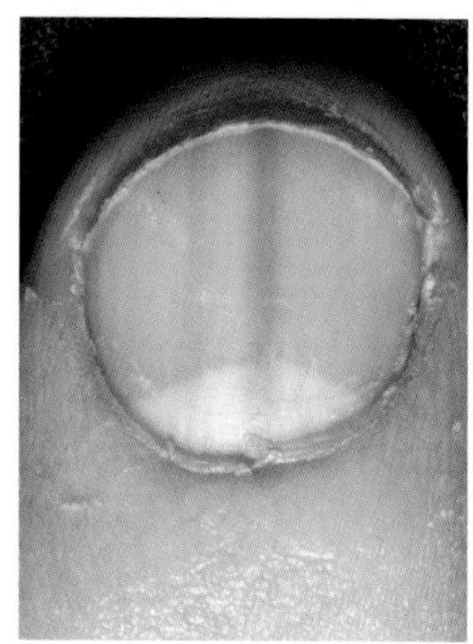
Pigmented band, pp. 870, 950

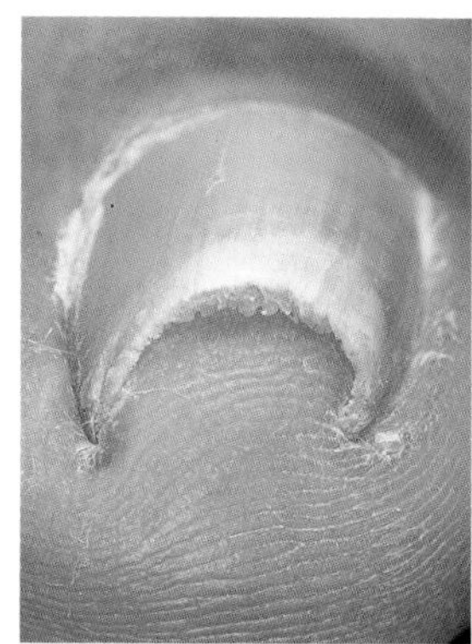
Pincer nail, p. 966

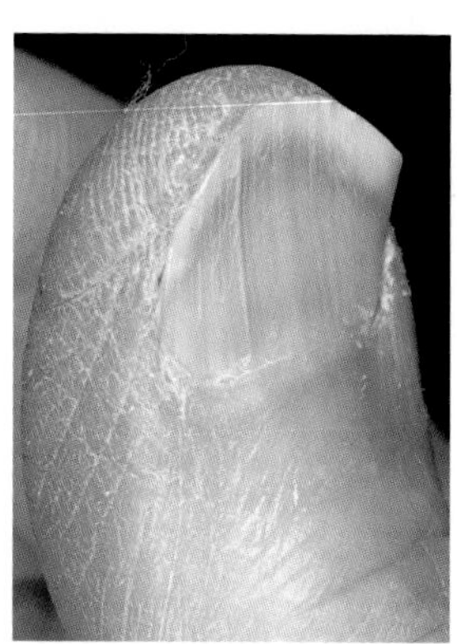
Spoon nails, p. 967

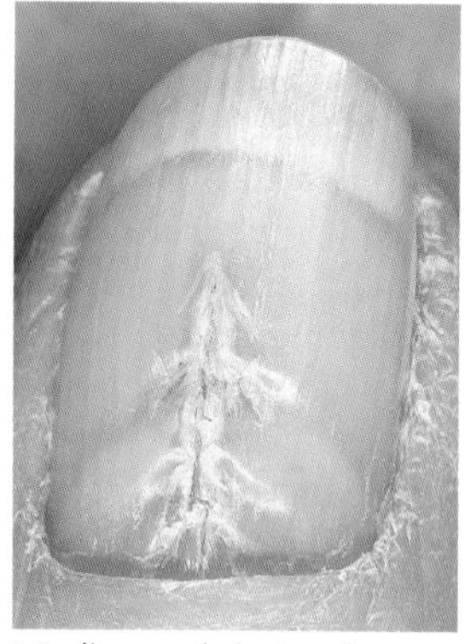
Median nail dystrophy, p. 966

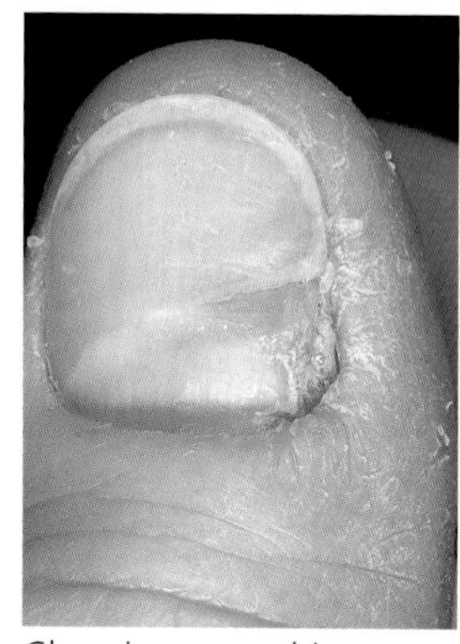
Chronic paronychia, p. 954

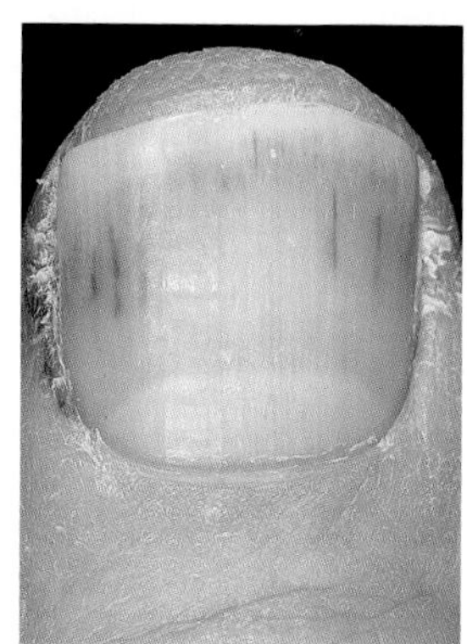
Splinter hemorrhages, p. 950

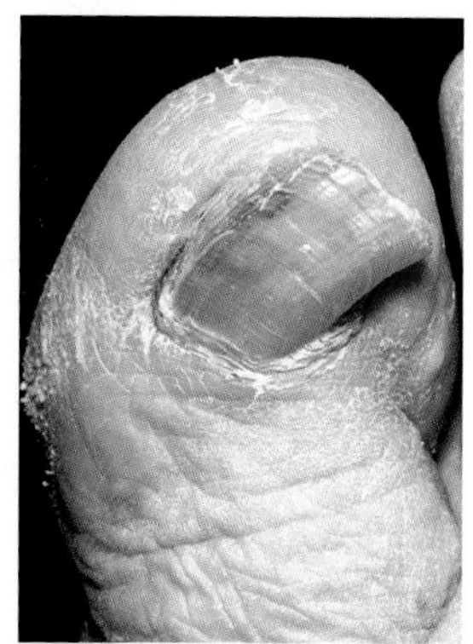
Plate hypertrophy, p. 964

The matrix epithelium synthesizes 90% of the nail plate. The lunula (white half-moon), which is visible through the nail plate, is the distal aspect of the nail matrix. It is continuous with the nail bed. The nail bed extends from the distal nail matrix to the hyponychium. As the nail streams distally, material is added to the undersurface of the nail, thickening it and making it densely adherent to the nail bed. The nail bed consists of parallel longitudinal ridges with small blood vessels at their base (Figure 25-2). Bleeding induced by trauma or vessel disease, such as lupus, occurs in the depths of these grooves, producing the splinter hemorrhage pattern viewed through the nail plate. The hyponychium is a short segment of skin lacking nail cover; it begins at the distal nail bed and terminates at the distal groove.

NAIL BIOPSY. Ungual biopsies are used to diagnose tumors, inflammatory disease, and infections. A punch or excisional biopsy technique is chosen, which provides a sufficient amount of tissue and produces a minimal amount of scarring. In practice these procedures are performed by some dermatologists and orthopedic hand surgeons. All of these techniques have recently been described. *PMID: 1740326*

GROWTH RATES. Nails grow continuously, but their growth rate decreases both with age and with poor circulation. Fingernails, which grow faster than toenails, grow at a rate of 0.5 to 2 mm per week. It takes approximately 5.5 months for a fingernail to grow from the matrix to the free edge and approximately 12 to 18 months for a toenail to be replaced. A reduction in the rate of matrix-cell division occurs during systemic diseases such as scarlet fever, causing thinning of the nail plate (Beau's lines).

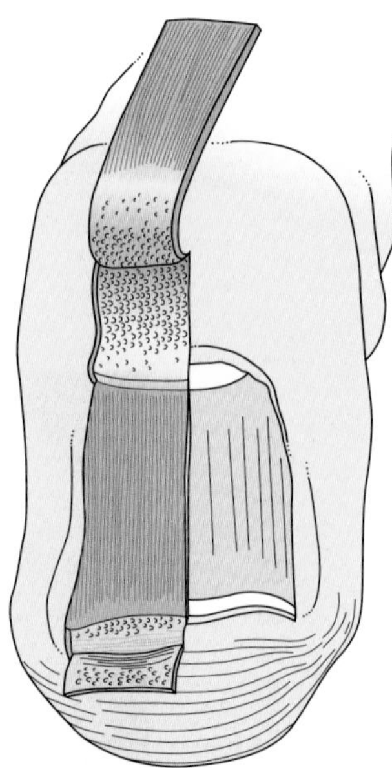

Figure 25-2 Dermal topography underlying nail unit. The nail bed consists of parallel longitudinal ridges with small blood vessels at their base. Anatomic pathology of splinter hemorrhages is obvious.

NORMAL VARIATIONS

The shape and opacity of the nail vary considerably among individuals. Aging may increase or decrease nail thickness. Longitudinal ridging (Figure 25-3) is common in aging, but this variant is occasionally observed among the young. Beading occurs at all ages but is more common in the elderly (Figure 25-4). The beads cover part or most of the plate surface and are arranged longitudinally. A pigmented band or bands occur in more than 90% of blacks (Figure 25-5). The sudden appearance of such a band in whites necessitates further investigation.

Nail structure can be altered by primary skin diseases, infections, trauma, internal diseases, congenital syndromes, and tumors. A more detailed discussion with illustrations of the most commonly encountered entities is presented in the following sections.

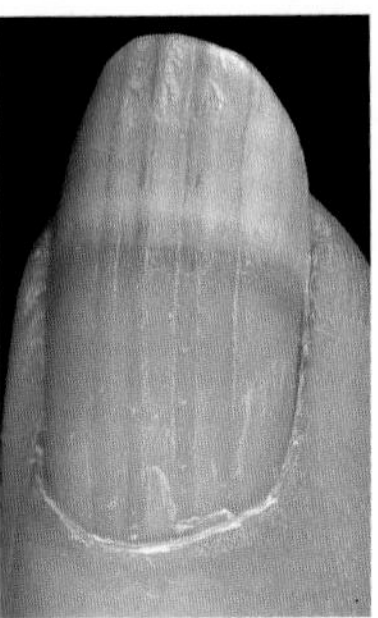

Figure 25-3 Longitudinal ridging. Parallel elevated nail ridges are a common aging change. This change does not indicate any deficiency.

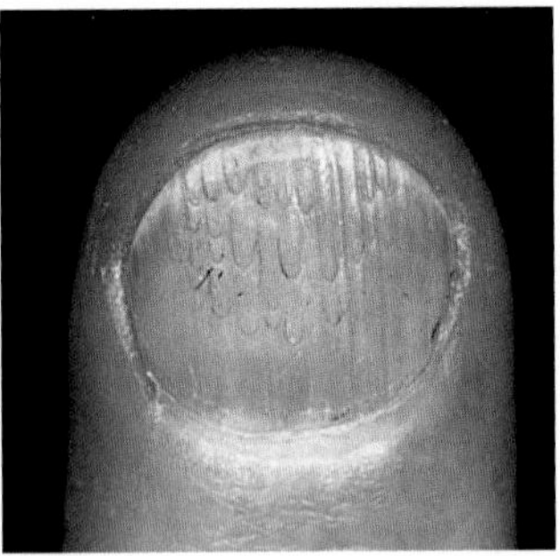

Figure 25-4 Longitudinal ridging and beading. A variant of normal, most commonly seen in the elderly.

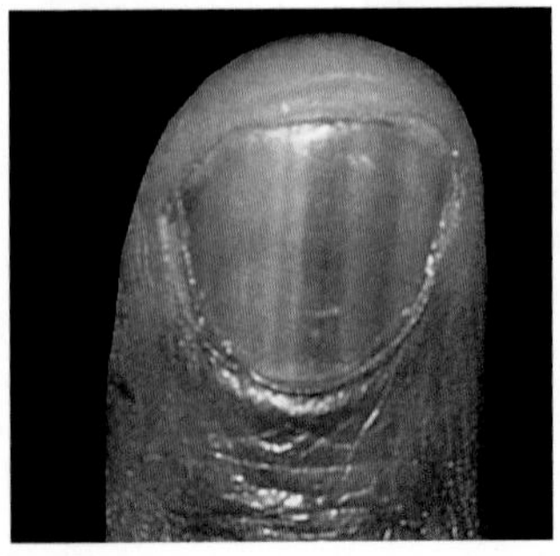

Figure 25-5 Pigmented bands occur as a normal finding in more than 90% of blacks.

NAIL DISORDERS ASSOCIATED WITH SKIN DISEASE

PSORIASIS. Nail changes are characteristic of psoriasis (see p. 275), and the nails of psoriasis patients should be examined. These changes offer supporting evidence for the diagnosis of psoriasis when skin changes are equivocal or absent.

The incidence of nail involvement in psoriasis varies from 10% to 50%. Nail involvement usually occurs simultaneously with skin disease but may occur as an isolated finding. Over 50% of patients suffer from pain, and many are restricted in their daily activities.

Onycholysis. Psoriasis of the hyponychium results in the accumulation of yellow, scaly debris that elevates the nail plate. The debris is commonly mistaken for nail fungus infection. Psoriasis of the nail bed causes separation of the nail from the nail bed. Unlike the uniform separation caused by pressure on the tips of long nails, the nail detaches in an irregular manner (Figure 25-6). The nail plate turns yellow, simulating a fungal infection. Separation begins at the distal groove or under the nail plate and may involve several nails.

Nail deformity. Extensive involvement of the nail matrix results in a nail losing its structural integrity, resulting in fragmentation and crumbling. Gross alteration of the nail plate surface and nail bed splinter hemorrhages are common (Figure 25-7).

Pitting. Pitting, or sharply defined ice pick–like depressions in the nail plate, is the most common finding (Figure 25-8). The number, distribution, patterns, and depth vary. Nail plate cells are shed in much the same way as psoriatic scale is shed, leaving a variable number of tiny, punched-out depressions on the nail plate surface. They emerge from under the cuticle and grow out with the nail. Many other cutaneous diseases may cause pitting (e.g., eczema, fungal infections, and alopecia areata), or it may occur as an isolated finding in a normal variation.

Oil spot lesion. Psoriasis of the nail bed may cause localized separation of the nail plate. Cellular debris and serum accumulate in this space. The brownish-yellow color (Figure 25-9) observed through the nail plate looks like a spot of oil.

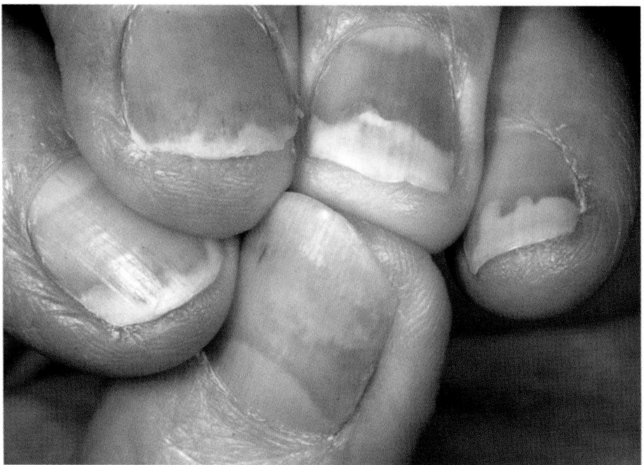

Figure 25-6 Psoriasis. Separation of the nail plate from the nail bed (onycholysis) may be present on several nails. Fungal infections have a similar appearance.

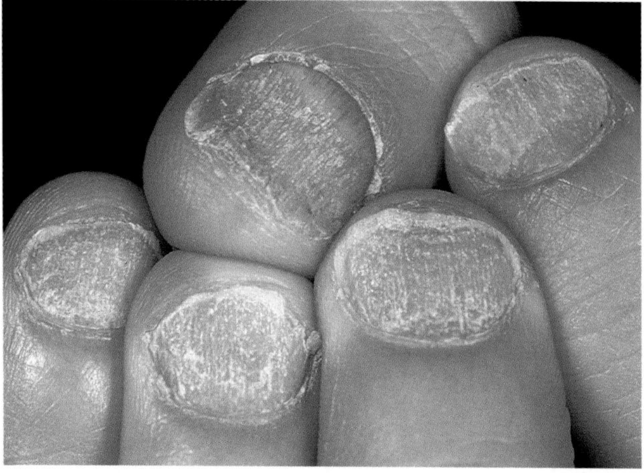

Figure 25-7 Psoriasis of the entire nail matrix causes grossly deformed nails.

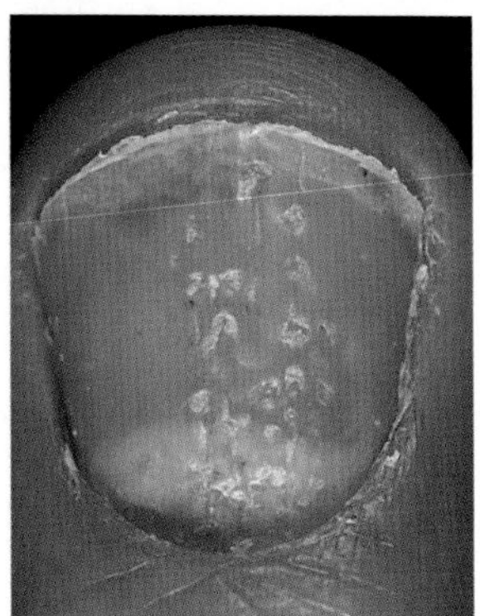

Figure 25-8 Psoriasis. Pitting is the most common nail change found in psoriasis.

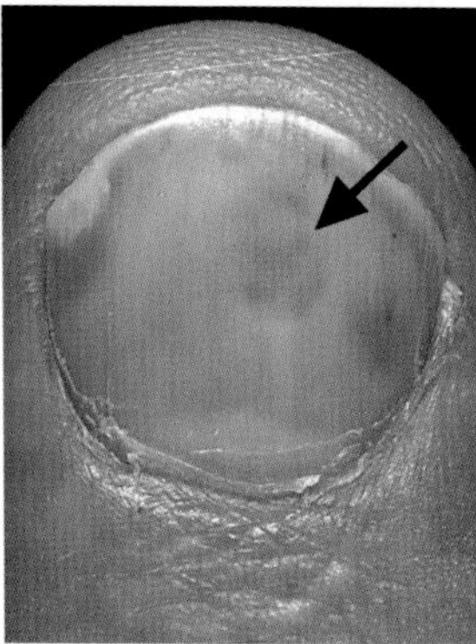

Figure 25-9 Psoriasis of the nail bed causes serum to leak under the nail plate and make an "oil spot."

TREATMENT

Nail psoriasis is difficult to treat, but may respond to different approaches used alone or together. PMID: 17572277 Relapse is common. Nails may improve when patients are treated with systemic agents such as cyclosporine, methotrexate, acitretin, or biologic agents.

TRIAMCINOLONE ACETONIDE. Intralesional injection at monthly intervals into the matrix with triamcinolone acetonide (Kenalog) (2.5 to 10 mg/ml) delivered with a 30-gauge needle is the standard treatment for psoriatic nail disease used by most dermatologists. A simplified protocol has been proposed. Triamcinolone acetonide (0.4 ml, 10 mg/ml) is injected, following ring block, at each of four periungual sites: two at the nail matrix and one in each lateral nailfold, directed medially towards the nail bed. This method is utilized to achieve delivery of the agent to both the nail matrix and the nail bed. If needed, a second set of injections is administered after 2 months. Subungual hyperkeratosis, ridging, and thickening respond well. Benefits are sustained for at least 9 months. Onycholysis and pitting are less responsive.

CALCIPOTRIOL. Calcipotriol cream or ointment once daily every weeknight and clobetasol once daily every weekend for 6 months followed by clobetasol twice weekly for the second 6 months reduce subungual hyperkeratosis. Calcipotriol ointment twice daily for up to 5 months is less effective. Calcipotriene 0.005% and betamethasone dipropionate 0.064% ointment (Taclonex ointment, Dovobet ointment) is a combination that may be effective with once-daily application to nails and nailfolds.

TAZAROTENE. Tazarotene 0.1% gel (Tazorac) is applied each evening for up to 24 weeks to fingernails. Medication can be used under occlusion or unoccluded. Tazarotene gel reduced onycholysis (in occluded and nonoccluded nails) and pitting (in occluded nails).

BIOLOGIC DRUGS. Case reports show rapid improvement of psoriatic nails with etanercept and infliximab. There is little merit in treating psoriatic nails with photochemotherapy (PUVA) or topical 5-fluorouracil (5-FU).

PUSTULAR PSORIASIS OF THE NAIL APPARATUS

Pustular psoriasis of the nail bed, matrix, or surrounding skin is common and may be painful. It has a chronic course and poor response to treatment. Severe cases are treated with systemic retinoids. Topical calcipotriol is effective in about 50% of patients with localized disorder and is also useful as maintenance therapy after retinoid treatment. Calcipotriene 0.005% and betamethasone dipropionate 0.064% ointment (Taclonex ointment, Dovobet ointment) is a combination that may be more effective than calcipotriene alone.

LICHEN PLANUS

Approximately 25% of patients with nail lichen planus (LP) have LP in other sites before or after the onset of nail lesions. Nail LP usually appears during the fifth or sixth decade of life. The matrix, nail bed, and nailfolds may be involved in producing a variety of changes, few of which are characteristic. Minimal inflammation of the matrix induces longitudinal grooving and ridging, which are the most common findings of LP of the nail. The development of severe and early destruction of the nail matrix with scarring characterizes a small subset of patients with nail LP. A pterygium, caused by adhesion of a depressed proximal nailfold to the scarred matrix, may occur after intense matrix inflammation (Figure 25-10). The nail plate distal to this focus is either absent or thinned out. In most cases, nail LP is self-limiting or promptly regresses with treatment. Permanent damage to the nail is uncommon, even in patients with diffuse involvement of the matrix. Matrix lesions may respond to intralesional triamcinolone acetonide (2.5 to 5 mg/ml) delivered with a 30-gauge needle every 3 or 4 weeks. Severe cases respond to prednisone (20 to 40 mg/day). This may require a long course of treatment in which the possible risks may outnumber the advantages. Onychomycosis may be confused clinically with lichen planus.

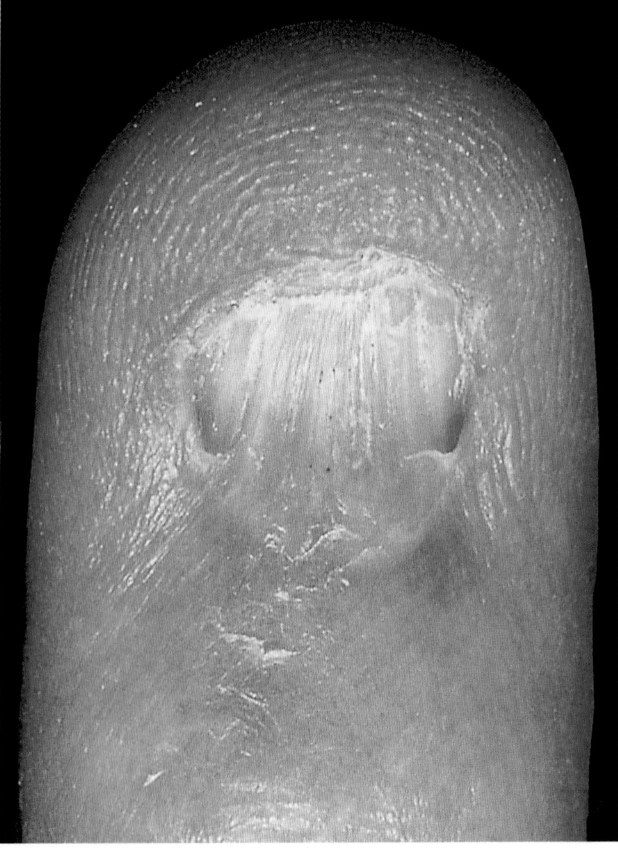

Figure 25-10 Lichen planus. Inflammation of the matrix results in adhesion of the proximal nailfold to the scarred matrix, a pterygium.

ACQUIRED DISORDERS

Bacterial and viral infections

ACUTE PARONYCHIA. The rapid onset of painful, bright red swelling of the proximal and lateral nailfold may occur spontaneously or may follow trauma or manipulation (Figures 25-11 and 25-12). Superficial infections present with an accumulation of purulent material behind the cuticle (see Figure 25-12). The small abscess is drained by inserting a 23- or 21-gauge needle tip or similar instrument between the proximal nailfold and the nail plate and lifting the nailfold with the tip of the needle (see Figure 25-13). Pain is abruptly relieved as the purulent material drains. There is no need for anesthesia or daily dressing. A diffuse, painful swelling suggests deeper infection, and cases that do not respond to antistaphylococcal antibiotics may require deep incision. Acute paronychia rarely evolves into chronic paronychia.

Treatment. Treatment of acute paronychia is determined by the degree of inflammation. If an abscess has not formed, the use of warm water compresses may be effective. The combination of a topical antibiotic (mupirocin or bacitracin/neomycin/polymyxin B) and a group II or III corticosteroid such as betamethasone dipropionate cream is safe and effective for treatment of uncomplicated acute bacterial paronychia and seems to offer advantages compared with topical antibiotics alone. Persistent lesions are treated with oral antistaphylococcal antibiotics and/or deep surgical drainage.

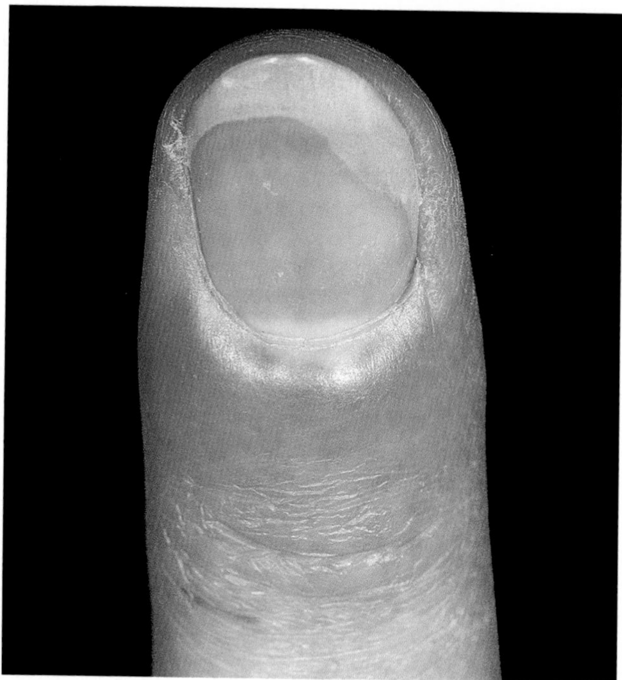

Figure 25-11 Acute paronychia. Erythema and purulent material occur at the proximal nailfold.

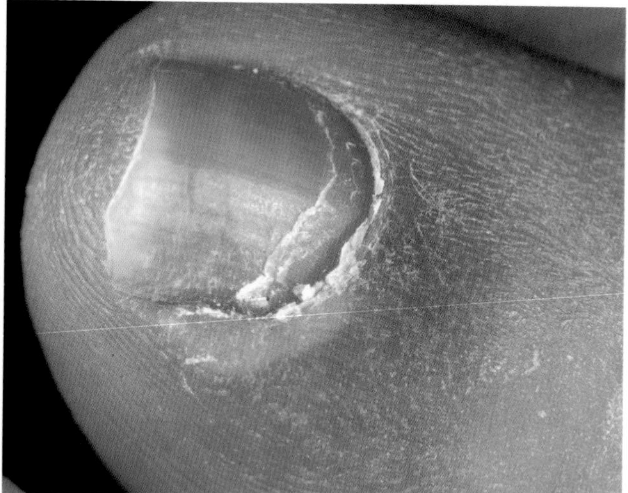

Figure 25-12 Acute paronychia. Acute pain and swelling of the lateral nailfold may follow any form of trauma (biting, sucking, chemical irritants).

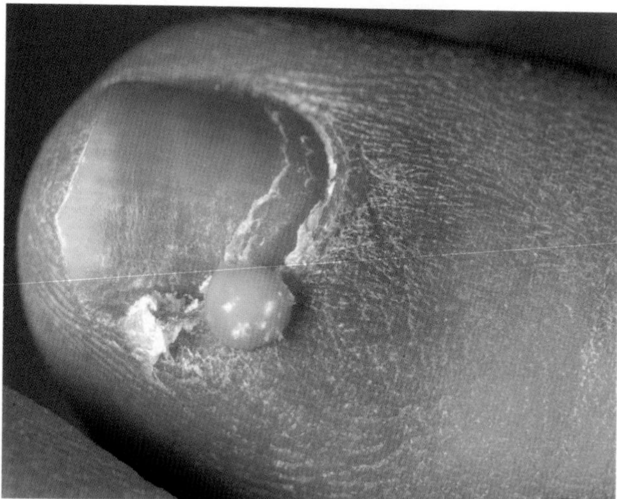

Figure 25-13 Acute paronychia. Elevation of the lateral nailfold releases a large amount of purulent material. Pain is relieved immediately. Flush the cavity with normal saline.

CHRONIC PARONYCHIA. Chronic paronychia is not a yeast infection, but rather an inflammation of the proximal and lateral nailfolds. Chronic paronychia evolves slowly and presents initially with tenderness and mild swelling about the proximal and lateral nailfolds (Figure 25-14). Significant contact irritant exposure is a major cause. Individuals whose hands are repeatedly exposed to moisture (e.g., bakers, dishwashers, and dentists) are at greatest risk. Manipulation of the cuticle accelerates the process. Typically, many or all fingers are involved simultaneously. The cuticle separates from the nail plate, leaving the space between the proximal nailfold and the nail plate exposed to infection. Many organisms, both pathogens and contaminants, thrive in this warm, moist intertriginous space. The skin about the nail becomes pale red, tender or painful, and swollen. Occasionally a small quantity of pus can be expressed from under the proximal nailfold. A culture of this material may grow *Candida* or gram-positive and gram-negative organisms. *Candida* is probably just a colonizer of the proximal nailfold rather than a direct cause of the disease. It disappears when the physiologic barrier is restored. The nail plate is not infected and maintains its integrity, although its surface becomes brown and rippled. There is no subungual thickening such as that present in some fungal infections. Proximal separation of the nail plate from the matrix area may occur as a consequence of nail matrix damage. The nail plate may sometimes present a green discoloration of its lateral margins as a result of *Pseudomonas aeruginosa* colonization. The process is chronic and responds very slowly to treatment. Psoriasis of the fingers may present in a similar form (Figure 25-15).

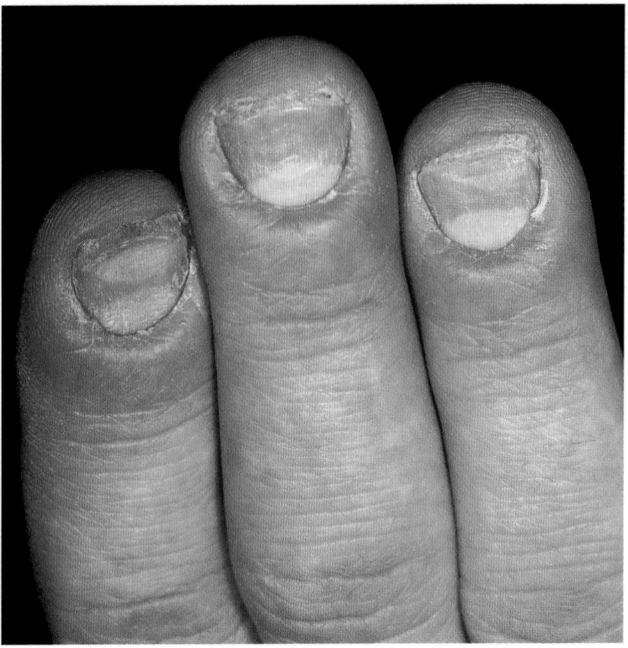

Figure 25-14 Chronic paronychia. Erythema and swelling of the nailfolds. The cuticle is absent. Chronic inflammation has caused horizontal ridging of the nails.

Figure 25-15 Psoriasis of the proximal and lateral nailfolds and nail matrix produces erythema, swelling, and nail plate distortion. Differentiation from chronic paronychia may be difficult. Nail pits suggest psoriasis.

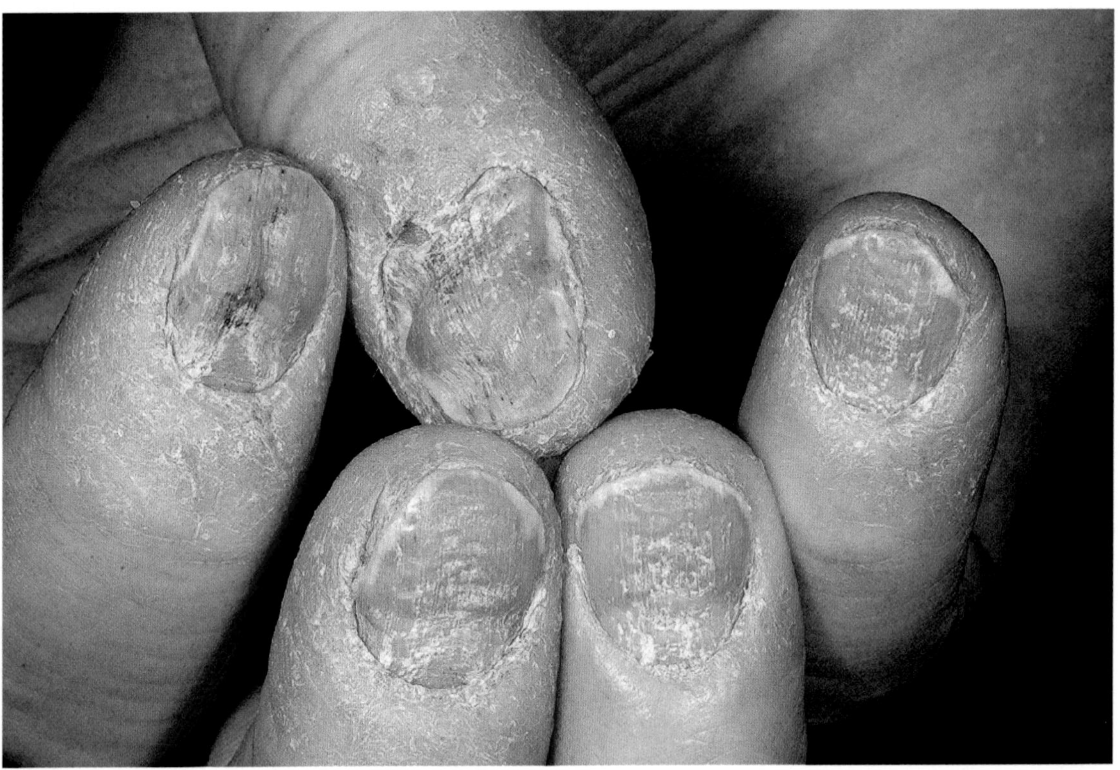

Treatment. Resolution of chronic paronychia depends on avoiding exposure to contact irritants and on treatment of underlying inflammation and infection. Every attempt must be made to keep the proximal nailfold dry. Patients should refrain from washing dishes and from washing their own hair. Rubber or plastic gloves are of some value, but moisture accumulates in them with prolonged use. The hands stay dry if a cotton glove is worn under the rubber glove. Controlling inflammation is the primary goal. Topical steroid creams (group V) applied twice daily for up to 3 weeks are more effective than systemic antifungals. Oral antibiotics do not penetrate this distal site in sufficient concentration, and the variety of organisms is too numerous to respond to a single oral agent. Treatments to keep the space between the nail plate and proximal nailfold may help. Place fungoid tincture (miconazole), ciclopirox (olamine) topical suspension or one or two drops of 3% thymol in 70% ethanol (compounded by a pharmacist) at the proximal nailfold and wait for this liquid to flow by capillary action into the space created by the absent cuticle. Slight elevation of the proximal nailfold with a flat toothpick facilitates penetration. This should be repeated two or three times a day for weeks, until the cuticle is re-formed. The cuticle may never re-form in patients with long-standing inflammation. Fluconazole (200 mg/day) for 1 to 4 weeks may control chronic inflammation. Short courses of fluconazole may have to be repeated as the infection recurs.

DRUG-INDUCED PARONYCHIA. The protease inhibitors lamivudine and indinavir, used to treat human immunodeficiency virus, have been reported to cause paronychia and ingrown toenails in about 4% of patients receiving these drugs. Pyogenic granuloma–like lesions, staphylococcal superinfection, onycholysis, and severe skin dryness may also be present. The nails of the great toes are usually affected. The lesions appear 2 to 12 months after starting treatment. Complete regression of skin manifestations occurs within 9 to 12 weeks after the drugs are withdrawn. Inhibition of endogenous proteases may explain the initial hypertrophy of the nailfold and the subsequent development of pyogenic granuloma–like lesions.

PSEUDOMONAS INFECTION. Repeated exposure to soap and water causes maceration of the hyponychium and softening of the nail plate. Separation of the nail plate (onycholysis) exposes a damp, macerated space between the nail plate and the nail bed, which is a fertile site for the growth of *Pseudomonas*. The nail plate assumes a green-black color (Figure 25-16). There is little discomfort or inflammation. This presentation may be confused with subungual hematoma (see Figure 25-32), but the absence of pain with *Pseudomonas* infection establishes the diagnosis. Apply a few drops of a mixture of one part chlorine bleach/four parts water under the nail three times a day. Vinegar (acetic acid) may also be used.

HERPETIC WHITLOW. In the past, dentists and nurses were at risk of acquiring herpes simplex virus (HSV) infection of the fingertip. Young adults are typically affected by HSV-2. HSV-1 infection of the hand occurs in children as a result of autoinoculation following herpetic gingivostomatitis. The risk has greatly diminished with the use of gloves. The appearance and course of the disease resemble those at other body sites, except that there is extreme pain from the swollen fingertips (Figure 25-17). Lymphangitis and lymphadenitis, secondary to HSV infection of the hand, are possible complications, particularly with HSV-2 infection. Herpes simplex virus infection in AIDS patients is characterized by atypical presentations and unusual locations. Herpetic finger infections in these patients may rapidly progress to the complete destruction of nail structures.

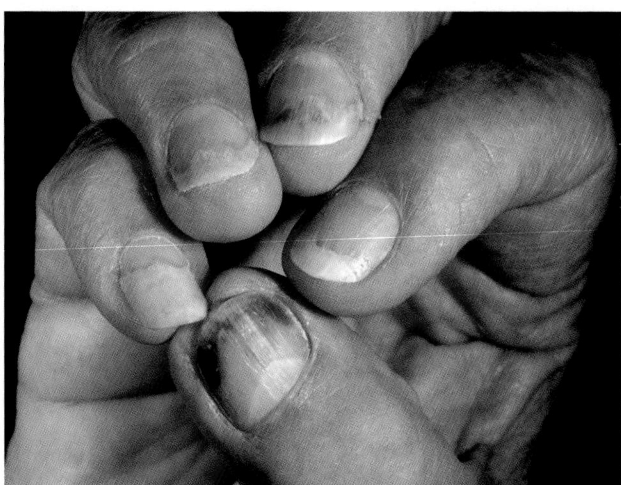

Figure 25-16 *Pseudomonas* colonized the space between the nail and the nail plate after onycholysis occurred, imparting a green color to the nail plate.

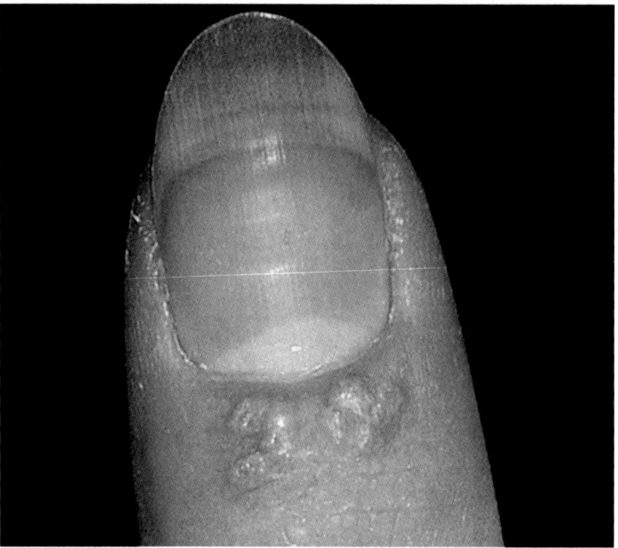

Figure 25-17 Herpes simplex of the finger (herpetic whitlow). Inoculation followed examination of a patient's mouth.

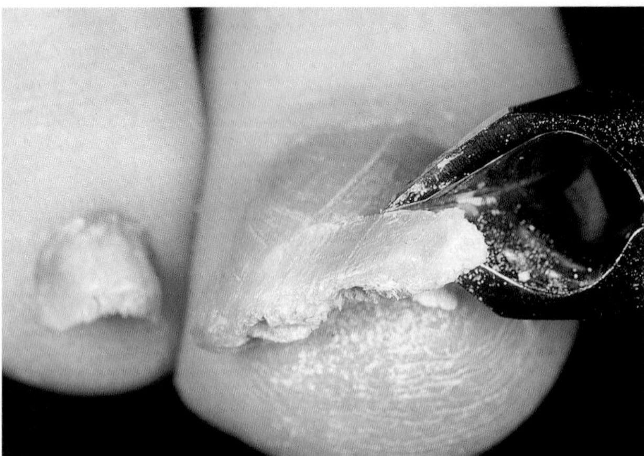

Figure 25-18 Clip the nail plate to relieve pain and expose subungual material for KOH examination and to obtain a nail sample for histology for evaluation of onychomycosis.

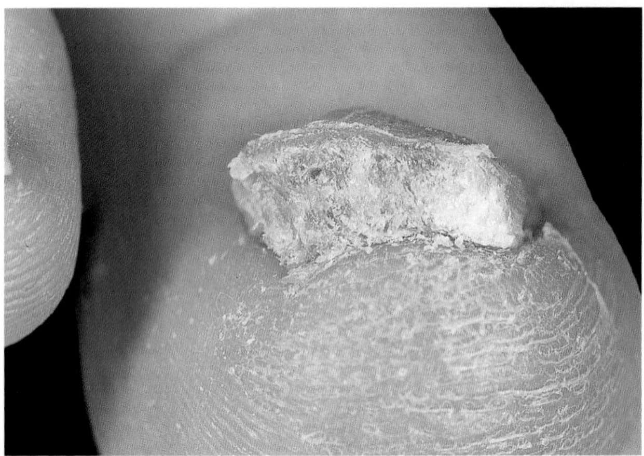

Figure 25-19 Subungual debris has been exposed for sampling. Reduce thick nails with an anvil cutter to relieve shoe pressure.

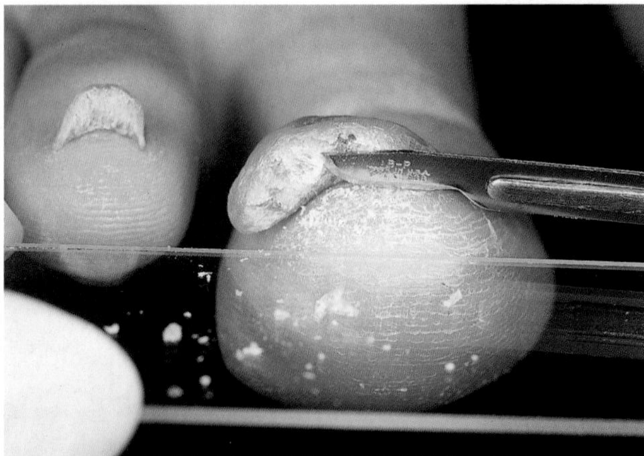

Figure 25-20 Remove subungual debris for KOH fungal examination.

Fungal nail infections

Tinea of the nails is also called tinea unguium. Dermatophytes *Trichophyton rubrum* and *Trichophyton mentagrophytes* are responsible for most fingernail and toenail infections. Certain nondermatophyte nail pathogens (e.g., *Scytalidium dimidiatum* and *Scytalidium hyalinum*) may also cause infection. Other nondermatophyte nail pathogens (certain species of *Acremonium, Alternaria, Aspergillus, Fusarium, Onychocola,* and *Scopulariopsis*) may cause infection. *Candida albicans* can occasionally be a pathogen in fingernail disease. Multiple pathogens may be present in a single nail. Nail infection may occur simultaneously with hand or foot tinea or may occur as an isolated phenomenon. Onychomycosis is estimated to affect approximately 2% to 13% of the population of North America and Europe. The disease may also occur in children. Trauma predisposes to infection. There is a tendency to label any process involving the nail plate as a fungal infection, but many other cutaneous diseases can change the structure of the nail. Fifty percent of thick nails are not infected with fungus. Many patients with nail disease have psoriasis and are not infected with fungus. Differential diagnosis is discussed at the end of this section.

TINEA VS. PSORIASIS. Differentiation of fungal infection from dystrophic changes resulting from psoriasis or other causes is difficult. Potassium hydroxide (KOH) preparations, culture, and, occasionally, nail unit biopsy specimens are used. These tests are time-consuming and may yield false-negative results. Histologic examination of distal nail clipping specimens by routine histology and periodic acid-Schiff (PAS) staining is an accurate and simple method for differentiating onychomycosis from nail psoriasis (Figure 25-18). It is equal to culture and superior to KOH preparation in leading to the correct diagnosis of dermatophyte infection.

LABORATORY DIAGNOSIS. The diagnosis of fungal nail infection may be established with both a potassium hydroxide (KOH) examination and a culture, and occasionally a nail biopsy. Physicians without the facilities to perform a KOH or culture may obtain these services from local or specialty laboratories, such as the University Center for Medical Mycology, Department of Dermatology, www.medicalmycology.org. These specialty laboratories provide convenient containers for specimen collection. Mayo Medical Laboratories provides a similar service (www.mayomedicallaboratories.com). Confirm the species of fungus before starting oral antifungal treatment. When performing cultures, obtain crumbling debris from under several nails and at different parts (proximal and distal areas of infection) of the infected nail (Figure 25-19). Collect subungual debris from under the distal edge of the nail with a curette. Sample the nail surface with a curette or scrape it with a #15 scalpel blade (Figure 25-20). Fungi are found in the nail plate and in the cornified cells of the nail bed. Hyphae that are present in the nail plate may not be viable; therefore sample the cornified cells of the nail bed if possible.

Nail biopsy. Many clinicians initiate therapy after confirming the presence of hyphae in a nail biopsy specimen. The potassium hydroxide test is the most cost-effective diagnostic method but a nail biopsy using nail clipping for histology is more sensitive. Submit the nail clipping in the same formalin solution used for skin biopsies. The laboratory will stain sections of the nail with periodic acid-Schiff, which stains fungal hyphae. The fungal species cannot be identified with this method.

Nail collection techniques for culture. First swab the nail plate with alcohol to remove bacteria. Fragments of nail plate and nail bed scrapings are inoculated onto Sabouraud's medium with and without antibiotics to identify the fungal species. Use fresh Sabouraud's with antibiotics. Antibiotics degrade in old media and do not effectively suppress bacterial contaminants. The dermatophyte test medium contains the antibiotic cycloheximide and phenol red as a pH indicator. Dermatophytes release alkaline metabolites that turn the medium from yellow to red in 7 to 14 days. Some nondermatophytes, such as *Scopulariopsis, Aspergillus, Penicillium,* black molds, and yeast, may cause a color change and give a false-positive reaction. The nail plate and hard debris can be adequately softened for direct examination by leaving the fragments, along with several drops of potassium hydroxide, in a watch glass covered with a Petri dish for 24 hours. (See Chapter 13 on fungal infections for details of the KOH examination.)

PATTERNS OF INFECTION. There are four distinct patterns of nail infection. Several patterns of infection may occur simultaneously in the nail plate. *T. rubrum* and *T. mentagrophytes* invade the nail plate more frequently than *T. violaceum* or *T. tonsurans*. *Aspergillus, Cephalosporium, Fusarium,* and *Scopulariopsis,* generally considered contaminants or nonpathogens, have been isolated from infected nails. They may be found in any pattern of nail infection, especially distal subungual onychomycosis and white superficial onychomycosis. The contaminants do not respond to griseofulvin or the newer oral antifungal agents. The four patterns of nail infection are illustrated in Figure 25-21.

Distal subungual onychomycosis. Distal subungual onychomycosis (Figures 25-22 and 25-23) is the most common pattern of nail invasion. Fungi invade the hyponychium, the distal area of the nail bed. The distal nail plate turns yellow or white as an accumulation of hyperkeratotic debris causes the nail to rise and separate from the underlying bed. Fungus grows in the substance of the plate, causing it to crumble and fragment. A large mass composed of thick nail plate and underlying debris may cause discomfort with footwear.

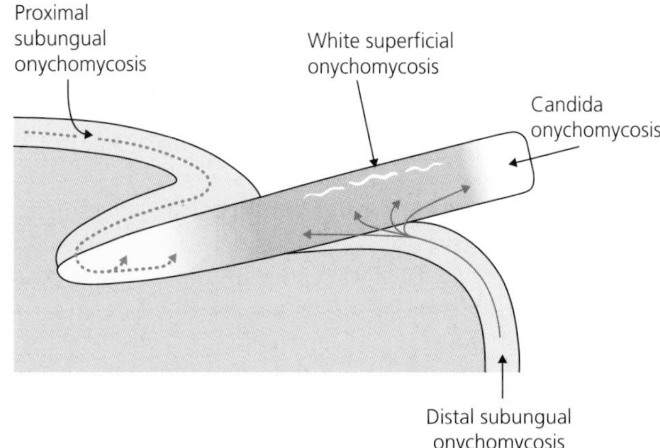

Figure 25-21 Four types of onychomycosis showing different entry points by infecting organisms.

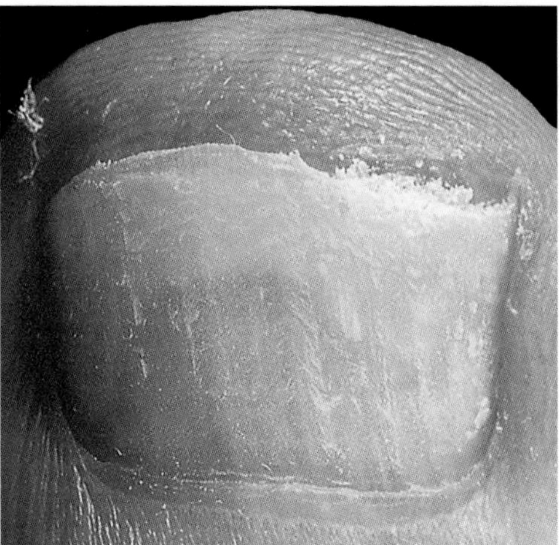

Figure 25-22 Distal subungual onychomycosis. Early changes showing subungual debris at the distal end of the nail plate.

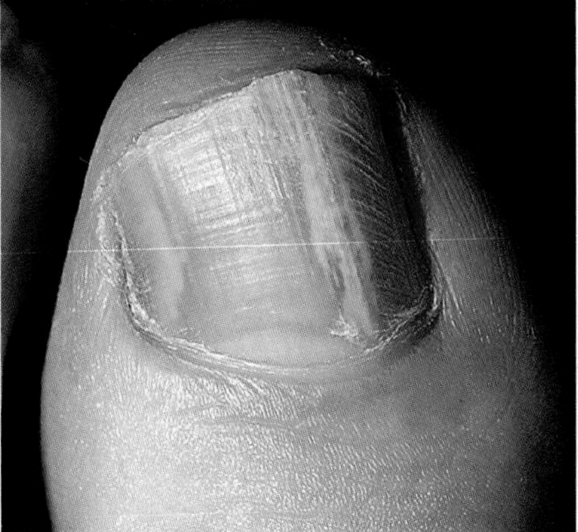

Figure 25-23 Distal subungual onychomycosis. The infection has progressed proximally to form a linear channel. Channeling is a highly characteristic feature of a fungal infection.

White superficial onychomycosis. This is caused by surface invasion of the nail plate, most often by *T. mentagrophytes.* The surface of the nail is soft, dry, and powdery and can easily be scraped away (Figure 25-24). The nail plate is not thickened and remains adherent to the nail bed.

Proximal subungual onychomycosis. Microorganisms enter the posterior nailfold-cuticle area, migrate to the underlying matrix, and finally invade the nail plate from below. Infection occurs within the substance of the nail plate, but the surface remains intact. Hyperkeratotic debris accumulates and causes the nail to separate (Figure 25-25). Transverse white bands begin at the proximal nail plate and are carried distally with outward growth of the nail plate. *T. rubrum* is the most common cause. This is the most common pattern seen in patients with AIDS.

Candida onychomycosis. Nail plate infection caused by *C. albicans* is seen almost exclusively in chronic mucocutaneous candidiasis. It generally involves all of the fingernails. The nail plate thickens and turns yellow-brown.

There are many other patterns of infection. Linear, yellow or dark brown streaks appear at the distal end and grow proximally in some patterns. In others, some or all of the nail plate may appear yellow; in these areas, the nail can be separated from the underlying bed.

DIFFERENTIAL DIAGNOSIS. Psoriasis is most commonly confused with onychomycosis, and the two diseases may coexist. More confusion exists, since psoriatic nail disease may present as an isolated phenomenon without other cutaneous signs. The single distinguishing feature of psoriasis, pitting of the nail plate surface, is not a feature of fungal infection. Leukonychia, the occurrence of white spots or bands that appear proximally and proceed out with the nail, is probably caused by minor trauma and may be confused with proximal subungual onychomycosis. Eczema or habitual picking of the proximal nailfold induces the nail plate to be wavy and ridged, but its substance remains intact and hard. Numerous, less common nail diseases may be confused with tinea unguium.

GENETIC PREDISPOSITION. *Trichophyton rubrum* onychomycosis frequently occurs in several members of the same family in different generations. The infection is rare in persons marrying into infected families. Predisposed individuals may acquire *T. rubrum* infection in childhood from their infected parents. The infection remains asymptomatic and localized to the plantar region. Nail invasion begins in adult life, possibly from nail trauma.

QUALITY-OF-LIFE ISSUES. Onychomycosis physically and psychologically affects patients' lives. It is capable of having a negative effect on quality of life via social stigma and disrupting daily activities. The problems are embarrassment, functional problems at work, reduction in social activities, fear of spreading the infection to others, and a significant incidence of pain. Onychomycosis can interfere with standing, walking, and exercising. Associated physical impairments can result in paresthesia, pain, discomfort, and loss of manual dexterity. Patients may also suffer from loss of self-esteem and social interaction. Insurance companies consider this disease a *cosmetic nuisance* and are reluctant to pay for treatment unless the patient is physically impaired by the disease.

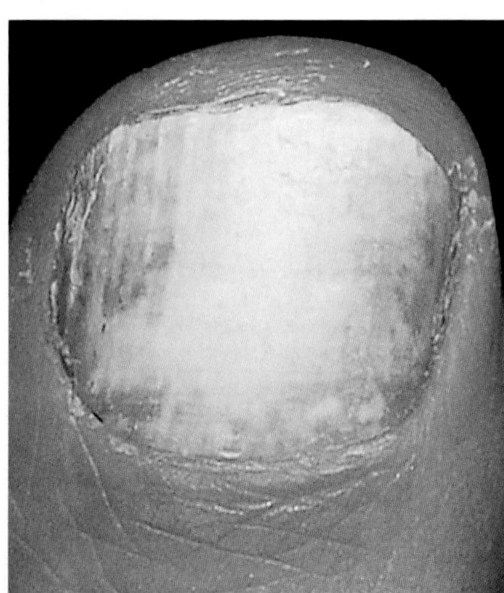

Figure 25-24 White superficial onychomycosis. The surface is soft, dry, and powdery and can easily be scraped away. The nail plate is not thickened and does not separate from the nail bed.

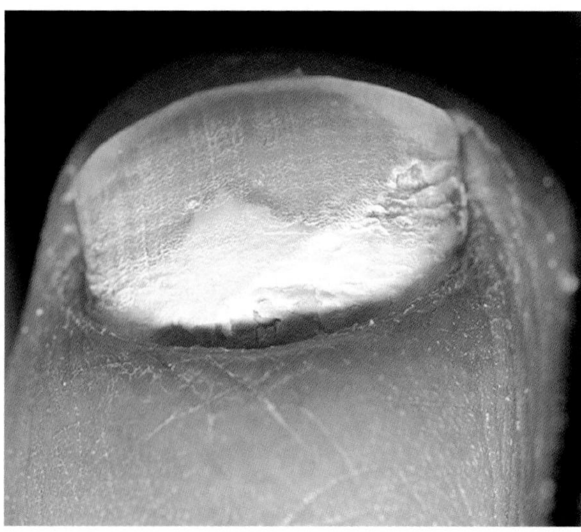

Figure 25-25 Proximal subungual onychomycosis. Fungal invasion of the proximal plate produces leukonychia. Infection may involve the entire thickness of the proximal plate.

TREATMENT

ORAL AGENTS: TERBINAFINE, ITRACONAZOLE, FLUCONAZOLE. These drugs penetrate keratinizing tissue. The levels reached in the nail plate exceed those in plasma. Therapeutic levels persist in the nails for at least 1 month after discontinuation of therapy. Terbinafine has higher cure rates and a slower relapse rate. Itraconazole can influence the level of many drugs. Terbinafine is relatively free of interactions. Table 25-1 discusses recommended dosages.

Continuous terbinafine. Continuous treatment with terbinafine is the optimal therapy for onychomycosis. Continuous terbinafine (250 mg/day for 12 weeks) is significantly more effective than intermittent itraconazole (400 mg/day for 1 week every 4 weeks for 12 weeks) in the treatment of toenail onychomycosis. Continuous terbinafine is more effective than intermittent terbinafine regimens and is just as safe. *PMID: 16467022*

Griseofulvin is less effective than the newer antifungal agents. Periodic debridement of infected nail during the course of treatment may increase the cure rate.

PROGNOSTIC FACTORS. A variety of clinical signs present at the initial clinical evaluation indicate a poor overall prognosis for ultimate cure of onychomycosis (see p. 960).

RESPONSE TO TREATMENT. Cure of all 10 toenails may be unattainable. A nail plate with a normal appearance is not always attainable after a successful therapeutic onychomycosis regimen. Some residual change is likely after chronic infection. Successful eradication of the fungus may leave the nail abnormal and the residual changes may be unrelated to infection or a result of damage to the nail unit from long-standing disease (e.g., onycholysis). Clinical and mycologic criteria are important to ascertain both the diagnosis and the resolution of onychomycosis. In severe cases of onychomycosis, up to 10% of the nail surface is likely to remain abnormal in appearance even when mycology indicates a cure of fungal infection.

It takes 12 to 18 months for a newly formed toenail plate and 4 to 6 months for a fingernail to replace a diseased nail. Immediately after completion of therapy the nail usually does not appear to be clear of infection. A proximal area of normal-appearing nail, representing newly formed nail plate that is devoid of infection, may be present. Visible clearance of the infection will occur after the process of nail plate turnover is complete. If onychomycosis is suggested based on clinical observation, diagnostic laboratory tests should be performed. If these produce negative findings, they should be repeated. Clinical manifestations of other nail disorders—such as psoriasis, neoplasms, and lichen planus—may mimic those of onychomycosis but can be diagnosed by nail-unit biopsy.

PREVENTING RECURRENCE. Preventing recurrence of tinea pedis may prevent recurrence of onychomycosis. Prolonged use of a topical antifungal agent applied around the toes, after clinical response of onychomycosis to an oral agent, may prevent nail reinfection. Use of a topical antifungal cream for 1 year after clinical cure of onychomycosis has prevented reinfection in the 12-month follow-up period. A twice weekly application of terbinafine cream in the nail area, between the toes and on the soles, would be a reasonable prevention program. Trauma to the tips of nails from tight-fitting shoes may be the single most important event for encouraging hyphae invasion in the region of the hyponychium that leads to distal subungual onychomycosis.

Table 25-1 Oral Antifungal Agents for Treating Tinea of the Nails

Antifungal agent	Indication	Dosage	Monitoring	Mycologic cure rate (%)
Terbinafine	First-line therapy for dermatophytic infections (most cases of onychomycosis)	Continuous: terbinafine 250 mg/day (12 wk for toenail infection, 6 wk for fingernail infection)	CBC, LFT at baseline and every 4-6 weeks during therapy	70-88
		Pulse dosing: terbinafine 500 mg/day × 1 wk per mo × 3 mo	No recommendation	58.7
Itraconazole	Alternative first-line therapy of dermatophytic infections Preferred therapy for nondermatophytic and candidal infections	200 mg daily for 6 weeks (fingernails) and for 12 weeks (toenails)	LFT at baseline and every 4-6 weeks during therapy	45.8-63
		Pulse dosing: 200 mg bid for first week of each month; fingernails, 2-3 pulses; toenails, 3-4 pulses	None	38.3
Fluconazole	First-line therapy for candidal infections but also active against dermatophytes	One 150-mg dose each week for 9 months	None	47

Adapted from Finch JJ, Warshaw EM: Toenail onychomycosis: current and future treatment options, *Dermatol Ther* 20(1):31-46, 2007 (doi:10.1111/j.1529-8019.2007.00109.x). *PMID: 17403258*

POOR PROGNOSTIC FACTORS FOR CURE OF ONYCHOMYCOSIS

1. Areas of nail involvement >50%
2. Significant lateral disease
3. Subungual hyperkeratosis >2 mm
4. White/yellow or orange/brown streaks in the nail
5. Total dystrophic onychomycosis (with matrix involvement)
6. Nonresponsive organisms (e.g., *Scytalidium* mold)
7. Patients with immunosuppression
8. Diminished peripheral circulation

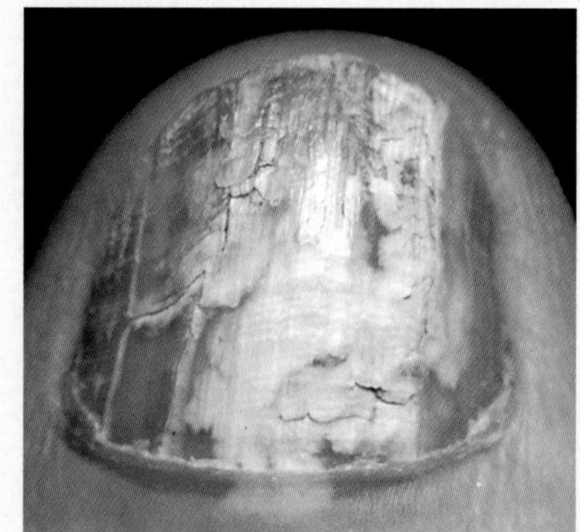

Areas of nail involvement >50%

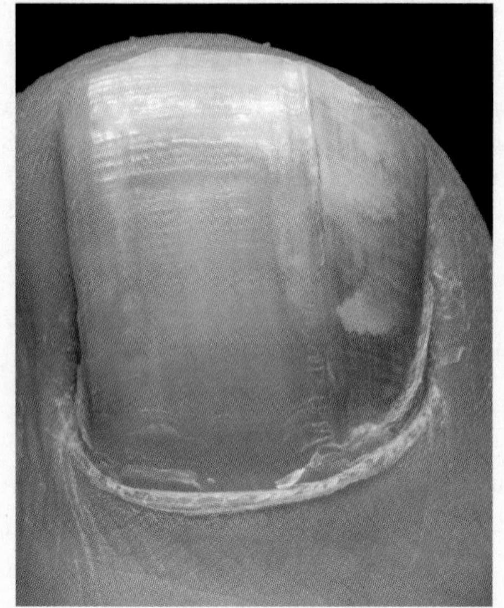

Significant lateral disease

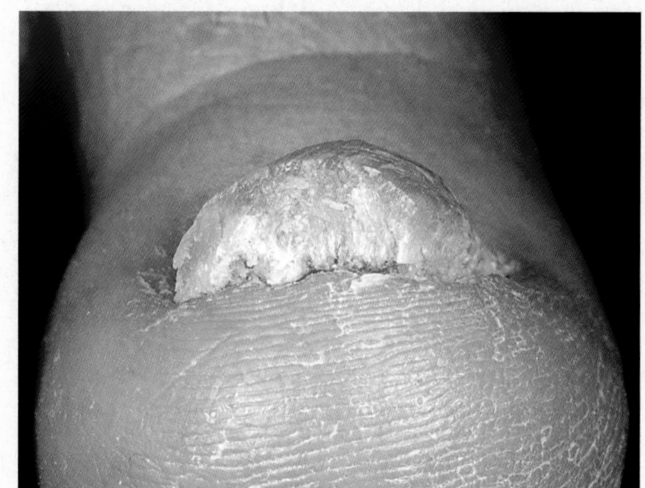

Subungual keratosis >2 mm

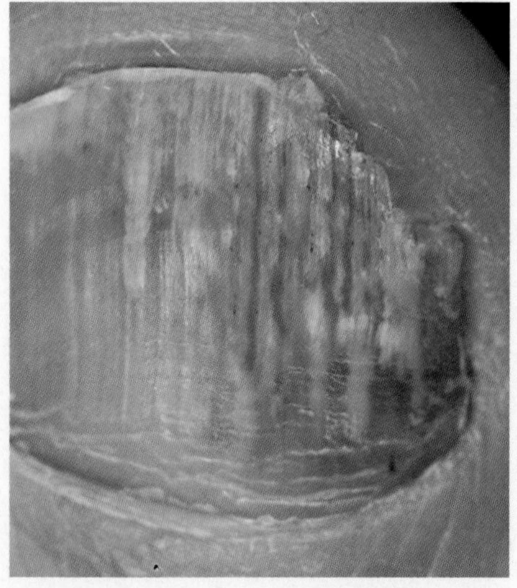

White-yellow or orange-brown streaks

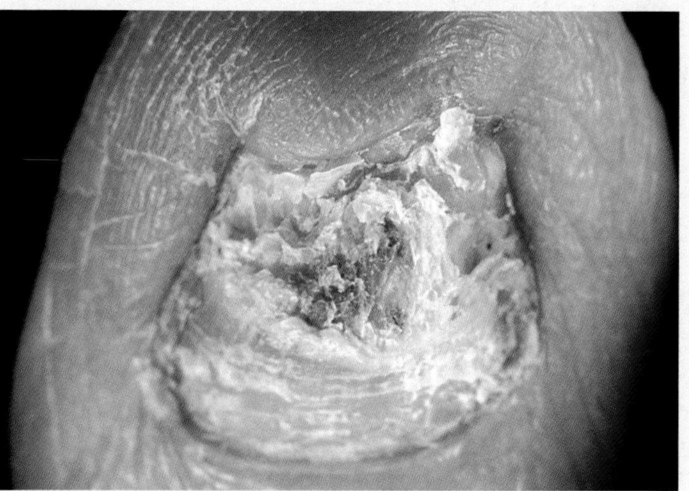

Total dystrophic onychomycosis

Adapted from *J Am Acad Dermatol* 56(6):939, 2007. *PMID: 17307276*

Shoes or boots that create a confined, damp, and warm atmosphere facilitate the development of fungal infection. Protect feet in communal showers. Medicated powders applied directly to the toe webs and soles (not poured into shoes) will help maintain a dry environment but will probably not prevent recurrence.

DRUG INTERACTIONS. Itraconazole has an affinity for cytochrome P-450 enzymes and therefore has the potential for interactions. Terbinafine is not metabolized through this system and has little potential for drug-drug interactions. Drug interactions are usually less severe with fluconazole than with itraconazole.

LABORATORY MONITORING. Many physicians check liver function and complete blood counts before and at 6 weeks during treatment with terbinafine. Laboratory tests are not required during pulse dosing of itraconazole.

SAFETY OF ORAL AGENTS. Terbinafine and itraconazole are available in a generic from at a considerable savings. Patients have the impression that they cause many side effects, especially liver disease. These drugs have been used in Europe and the United States for several years. They have a very low incidence of serious side effects.

RECURRENCE RATES. Studies of terbinafine and itraconazole demonstrated that at 5 years, 23% of terbinafine-treated patients and 53% of itraconazole-treated patients experienced a relapse or reinfection, after achieving mycologic cure at 1 year. At 5-year follow-up, 13% of the itraconazole group and 46% of the terbinafine group remained disease-free. Another study showed that 11% of terbinafine responders showed evidence of relapse 18 to 21 months after cessation of treatment. *PMID: 17403258* Patients treated with itraconazole or terbinafine who experience recurrence of onychomycosis can be retreated with response rates similar to those of the initial course.

MECHANICAL REDUCTION OF INFECTED NAIL PLATE. A nail clipper with pliers handles may be used to remove substantial amounts of hard, thick debris. One should insert the pointed tip of the instrument as far down as possible between the diseased nail and the nail bed. Adherent thick nail plate can be reduced by sanding or cutting the surface layers with the clippers. Removal of the infected nail may accelerate resolution of the infection.

SURGICAL REMOVAL. Painful or extremely infected nails (usually the nail of the first toe) can be removed by a simple surgical procedure.

NONSURGICAL AVULSION OF NAIL DYSTROPHIES. If nails are very thick at baseline, consider occlusion with 40% urea cream under tape in addition to oral therapy. Symptomatic dystrophic nails may be painlessly removed with a urea compound (Figure 25-26). The technique has its greatest application in removing hypertrophic mycotic nails and can be used to treat other hypertrophic nail conditions of the nail plate, such as psoriatic nails. The procedure also facilitates subsequent treatment with topical antifungal agents. The technique removes only grossly diseased or dystrophic nails, not normal nails. Forty percent urea gel or cream is commercially available or by prescription.

Cloth adhesive tape is used to cover the normal skin surrounding the affected nail plate, which has been pretreated with tincture of benzoin. The urea cream is generously applied directly to the nail surface and covered with a piece of plastic wrap. This in turn is covered with a finger that is cut from a plastic glove and held in place with adhesive tape. Patients are instructed to keep the area completely dry with the aid of plastic gloves or booties.

An alternate technique uses adhesive felt (moleskin) and waterproof, stretchable tape (Blenderm). A nail-shaped hole is cut in a piece of moleskin, and the moleskin is applied, sticky surface down, on the dorsal aspect of the toe so that just the nail is exposed through the hole. The well is filled with the urea cream and covered with Blenderm tape. The patient returns to the physician in 7 to 10 days. At that time the treated nails are removed, when possible, either by lifting the entire nail plate from the nail bed or by cutting the abnormal portions with a nail cutter. This is followed by light curettage until a clinically normal nail is reached at all margins.

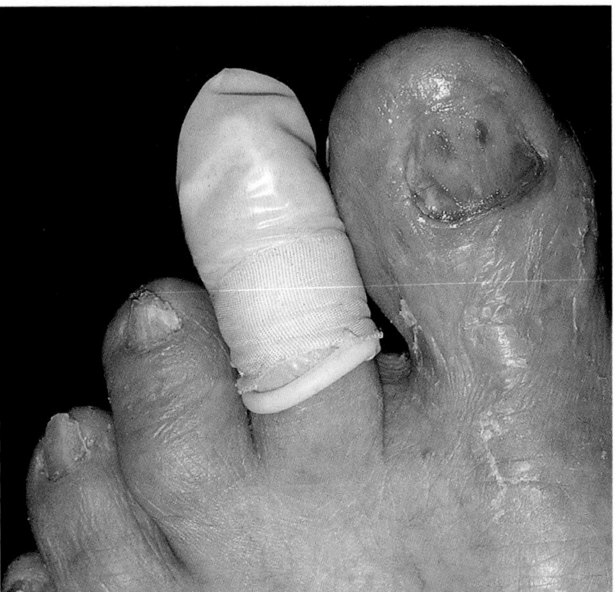

Figure 25-26 Nonsurgical avulsion of nail dystrophies. A 40% urea medication is occluded to remove infected nail plate.

Trauma

ONYCHOLYSIS

Onycholysis, the painless separation of the nail from the nail bed, is common. Separation usually begins at the distal groove and progresses irregularly and proximally, causing part or most of the plate to become separated. The nonadherent portion of the nail is opaque with a white (Figure 25-27), yellow (Figures 25-28 and 25-29), or green tinge. The causes of onycholysis include psoriasis, trauma, *Candida* or *Pseudomonas* infections, internal drugs, PUVA photochemotherapy, contact with chemicals, maceration from prolonged immersion, and allergic contact dermatitis (e.g., to nail hardener and adhesives). Onycholysis is known to be associated with thyroid disease (especially hyperthyroidism). Consider screening patients with unexplained onycholysis for asymptomatic thyroid disease.

When other signs of skin disease are absent, onycholysis is most frequently seen in women with long fingernails. With normal activity, the extended nail inadvertently strikes objects and acts as a lever to pry the nail from the nail bed. Forcing a stylus between the nail plate and bed while manicuring can cause separation.

TREATMENT. All of the separated nail is removed, and the fingers are kept dry. Removing the separated nail eliminates the lever, and dryness discourages infection. One should not cover the cut nails; occlusion promotes maceration. Any form of manipulation should be discouraged. Avoid exposure to contact irritants. Yeast commonly grows in the space between the nail and nail bed. Use liquid topical agents that can flow under the nail such as fungoid tincture that contains miconazole. Use oral fluconazole (Diflucan) for resistant cases. A short course of fluconazole (e.g., 150 mg daily for 5 to 7 days) may have to be repeated as the nail grows out.

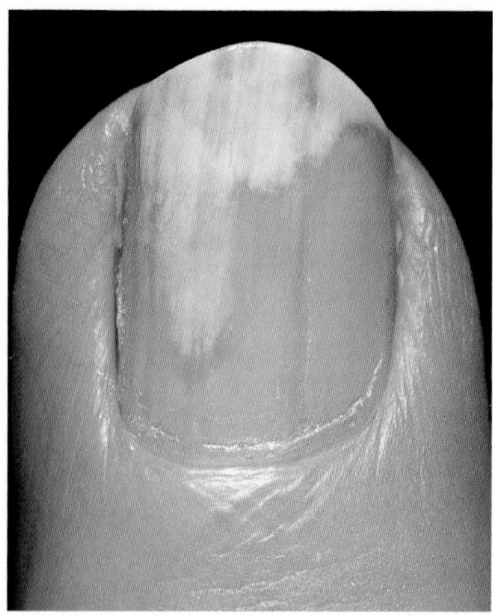

Figure 25-27 Onycholysis. Separation of the nail plate starts at the distal groove. Minor trauma to long fingernails is the most common cause.

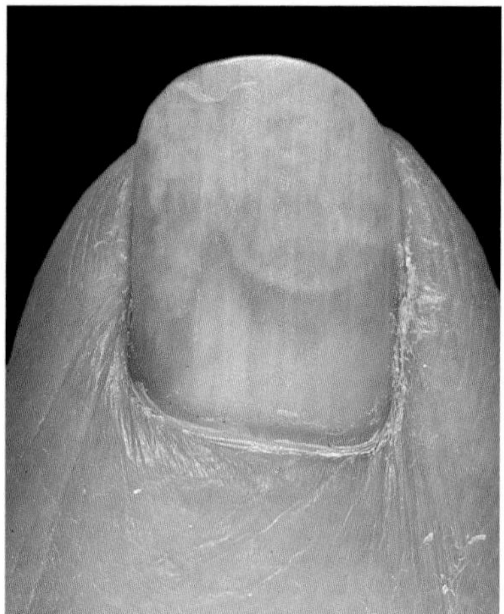

Figure 25-28 Onycholysis. The yellow color may indicate a secondary *Candida* infection. Psoriasis and tinea have a similar appearance.

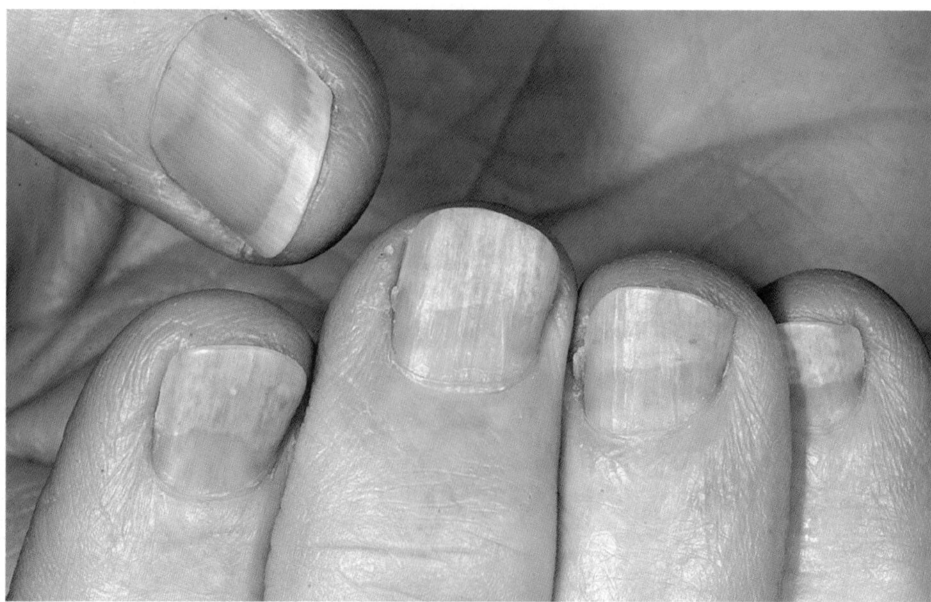

Figure 25-29 Onycholysis. Involvement of many nails simultaneously is the typical presentation.

PHOTOONYCHOLYSIS. Onycholysis may be precipitated by exposure to ultraviolet radiation. Photoonycholysis may occur with the use of tetracycline antibiotics and cytotoxic drugs. Nail changes with the taxanes, primarily docetaxel, are reported in up to 30% to 40% of patients. Prolonged weekly exposure to paclitaxel, other taxanes, and anthracyclines causes onycholysis in some patients, which may be precipitated by exposure to sunlight. Patients receiving these drugs should protect their nails from sunlight. The reaction does not warrant discontinuation of therapy.

NAIL AND CUTICLE BITING

Nail biting is a nervous habit that usually begins in childhood and lasts for years. One or all nails may be chewed as far as the lunula. The nail plate is chiseled and bitten from the nail bed by the teeth. Nail growth occurs during periods of physical activity, but periods of physical inactivity seem to promote zealous nail biting. Thin strips of skin on the lateral and proximal nailfold may also be stripped (Figure 25-30).

Patients are aware of their habit but seem powerless to control it. In one study mild aversion such as painting the nail plate with a distasteful preparation such as Nail Cure (Purepac) or Sally Hansen Nail Biter resulted in significant improvements in nail length. A second effective method of habit reversal is to have patients perform a competing response whenever they have the urge to nail bite or find themselves biting their nails.

NAIL PLATE EXCORIATION

Digging or excoriating the nail plate is much less common than biting. This destructive practice may result in gross deformity of the nail plate.

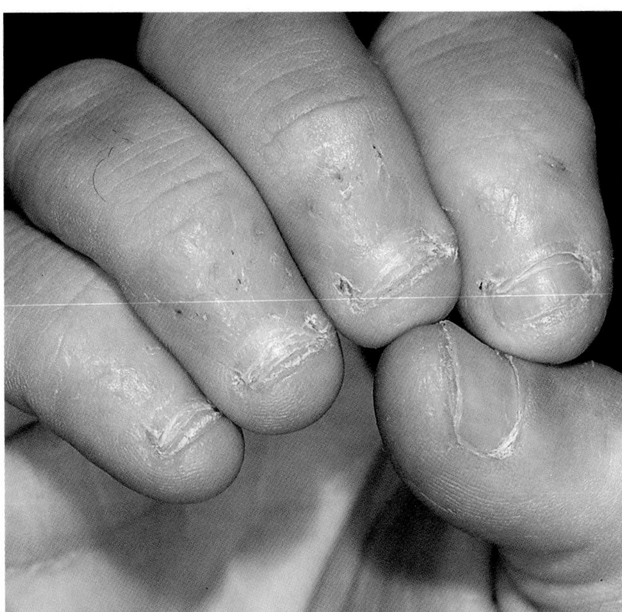

Figure 25-30 Nail, cuticle, and finger biting.

HANGNAIL

Triangular strips of skin may separate from the lateral nailfolds, particularly during the winter months. Attempts at removal may cause pain and extension of the tear into the dermis. Separated skin should be cut before extension occurs. Constant lubrication of the fingertips with skin creams (e.g., Aquaphor ointment) and avoidance of repeated hand immersion in water are beneficial.

INGROWN TOENAIL

Ingrown fingernails and toenails are common; the large toe is most frequently affected. The nail pierces the lateral nailfold and enters the dermis, where it acts as a foreign body. The first signs are pain and swelling. The area of penetration becomes purulent and edematous as exuberant granulation tissue grows alongside the penetrating nail (Figure 25-31). Ingrown nails are caused by lateral pressure of poorly fitting shoes, improper or excessive trimming of the lateral nail plate, or trauma.

TREATMENT

Ingrown nail without inflammation. Separate the distal anterior tip and lateral edges of an ingrown toenail from the adjacent soft tissue with a wisp of absorbent cotton coated with collodion. This gives immediate relief of pain and provides a firm runway for further growth of the nail. The collodion fixes the cotton in place, waterproofs the area, and permits bathing. The cotton insert may need reinsertion in 3 to 6 weeks. Cotton without collodion may be used, but it may have to be replaced frequently. This method is not applicable to patients with infected acute inflammation of the lateral nailfold.

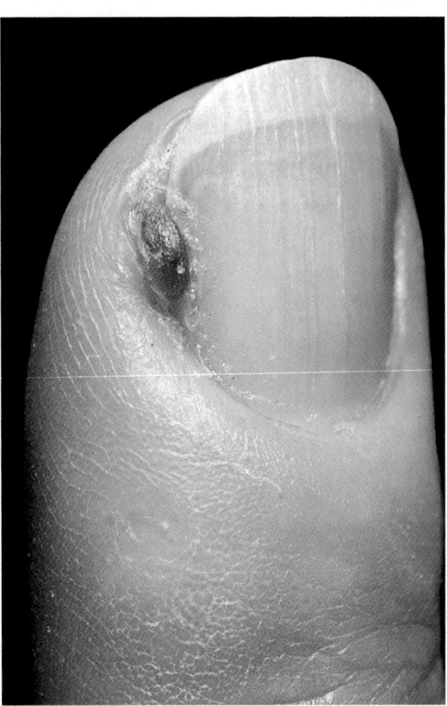

Figure 25-31 An ingrown nail has stimulated the formation of granulation tissue.

Ingrown nail with inflammation. The lateral nailfold is infiltrated with 1% or 2% lidocaine (Xylocaine). Nail-splitting scissors are inserted under the ingrown nail parallel to the lateral nailfold. The tip is inserted toward the matrix until resistance is met, and the wedge-shaped nail is then cut and removed. Granulation tissue is reduced with a silver nitrate application or removed with a curette. For a few days, the inflamed site is treated with a water or Burow's cool, wet compress until the swelling and inflammation have subsided. Shoes should be worn that allow the toes to fall naturally, without compression. The new nail is forced up and over the lateral nailfold by inserting cotton under the lateral nail margin and allowing it to remain in place for days or weeks.

Recurrent ingrown nail. Patients with recurrent ingrown nails may require the use of liquid phenol for permanent destruction of the lateral portions of the nail matrix. The use of oral antibiotics as an adjunctive therapy in treating ingrown toenails does not play a role in decreasing the healing time or postprocedure morbidity.

SUBUNGUAL HEMATOMA

Subungual hematoma (Figure 25-32) may be caused by trauma to the nail plate, which causes immediate bleeding and pain. The quantity of blood may be sufficient to cause separation and loss of the nail plate. The traditional method of puncturing the nail with a red-hot paperclip tip remains the quickest and most effective method of draining the blood. Alternatively, a carbon dioxide laser can be used to melt the nail at the center of the discolored area and decompress the hematoma. No anesthesia is required with this procedure. Trephining the nail with a hand drill, dental drill, or a fine-point scalpel blade can be painful because of the pressure required to puncture the nail. Often digital nerve block is necessary when drilling methods are used. Trauma to the proximal nailfold causes hemorrhage that may not be apparent for days. The nail plate may emerge from the nailfold with bloodstains that remain until the nail grows out. Young children with subungual hematoma may be victims of child abuse.

NAIL HYPERTROPHY

Gross thickening of the nail plate may occur with tight-fitting shoes or other forms of chronic trauma. The nail plate is brown, very thick, and points to one side (Figure 25-33). Shoes compress the nail plate against the toe and cause pain. The substance of the nail plate may be reduced with sandpaper or a file, or the nail can be removed and the nail matrix permanently destroyed with phenol so that the nail will not regrow.

WHITE SPOTS OR BANDS

White spots (leukonychia punctata) in the nail plate, a very common finding, possibly result from cuticle manipulation or other mild forms of trauma (Figure 25-34). The spots or bands may appear at the lunula or may appear spontaneously in the nail plate and subsequently disappear or grow with the nail. Psoriasis of the mid-nail matrix can also produce this change.

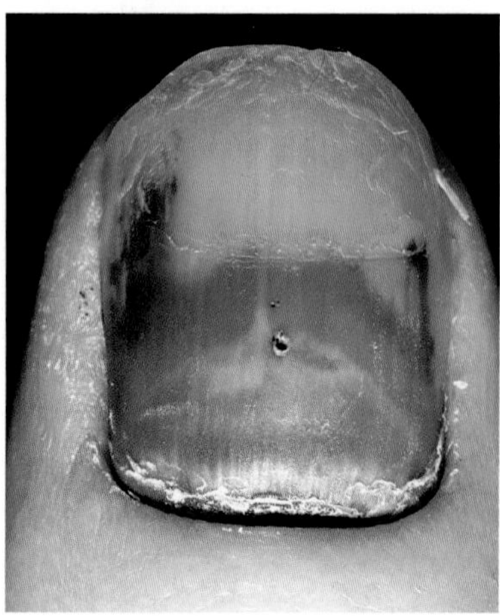

Figure 25-32 Subungual hematoma. A *Proteus* or *Pseudomonas* infection might be suspected if there were no history of trauma.

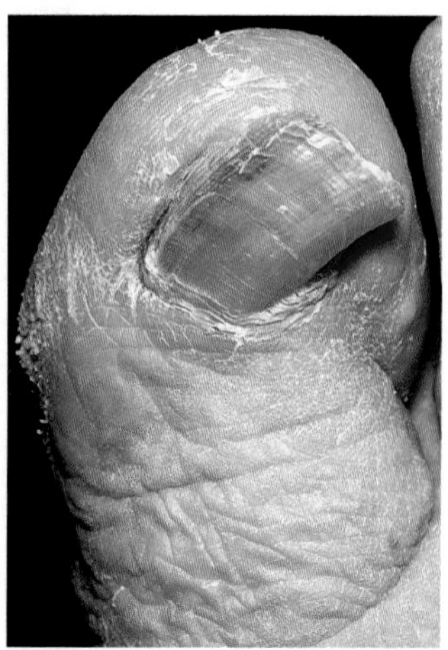

Figure 25-33 Nail hypertrophy. The nail plate becomes thick and distorted, often causing discomfort when shoes are worn.

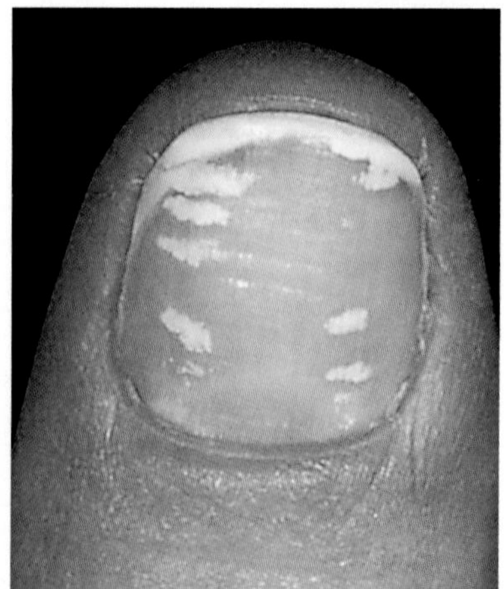

Figure 25-34 White spots (leukonychia punctata). A common finding often mistaken for a fungal infection.

DISTAL PLATE SPLITTING (BRITTLE NAILS)

The splitting into layers or peeling of the distal nail plate may resemble or be analogous to the scaling of dry skin (Figure 25-35). This nail change is found in approximately 20% of the adult population. Repeated water immersion and the frequent use of nail polish removers increase the incidence of brittle nails, particularly in women. Local measures to rehydrate the nail plate should be initiated. A moisturizer may be applied after the nails have been soaked in water. Protection with rubber-over-cotton gloves and application of heavy lubricants (e.g., Aquaphor ointment) directly to the nail plate provide improvement. The moisturizing agent may be applied under occlusion with a white cotton glove or sock. Nail enamel may slow the evaporation of water from the nail plate. It should be removed and reapplied no more than once a week. A number of nail conditioning products (e.g., Elon nail products) are available from Dartmouth pharmaceuticals online (www.ilovemynails.com) and in pharmacies. Patients with brittle nails who receive the B-complex vitamin biotin (2.5 mg/day) may improve and have up to a 25% increase in nail plate thickness. A 10-mg dose of silicon daily, a useful form of which is choline-stabilized orthosilicic acid, has a similar effect.

HABIT-TIC DEFORMITY

Habit-tic deformity is a common finding and is caused by biting or picking a section of the proximal nailfold of the thumb with the index fingernail. Although the condition is most common to the thumbnails, all nails can be affected. The lesion is often noted as an incidental finding in a patient seeking treatment for another cutaneous disease. The resulting defect consists of a longitudinal band of horizontal grooves that often have a yellow discoloration. The band extends from the proximal nailfold to the tip of the nail (Figure 25-36). This should not be confused with the nail rippling that occurs with chronic paronychia or chronic eczematous inflammation of the proximal nailfold. The ripples of chronic inflammation appear as rounded waves (Figure 25-37), in contrast to the closely spaced, sharp grooves produced by continual manipulation.

The method of formation is demonstrated for the patient. Some patients are not aware of their habit, and others who admit to nail picking may not realize that they have created the defect. Patients who discontinue manipulation are able to grow relatively normal nails; there are those, however, who find it impossible to stop.

From a psychiatric perspective, it is often unclear how to classify habit-tic disorders. The heterogeneity of behaviors complicates the diagnostic process. In some cases it might be classified as obsessive-compulsive disorder. In other cases, the behavior is automatic, bearing similarities to the impulse control disorder trichotillomania, which may be related to obsessive-compulsive disorders. Obsessive-compulsive disorder sometimes responds to the serotonin reuptake inhibitor fluoxetine (Prozac), and patients with habit-tic deformity may respond to this medication.

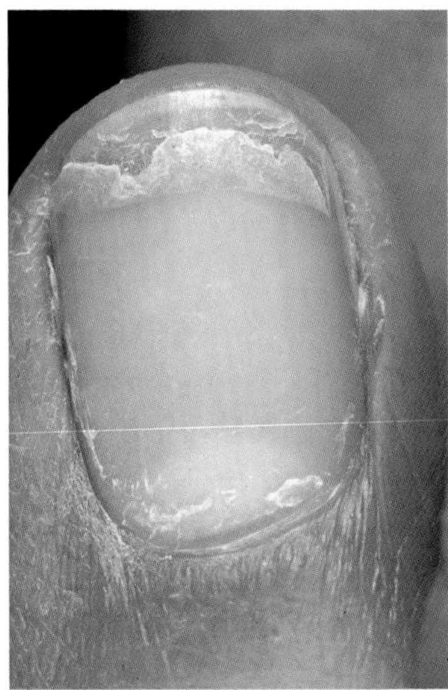

Figure 25-35 Distal nail splitting. The nail splits into layers or the distal nail plate peels, a change analogous to the scaling of dry skin.

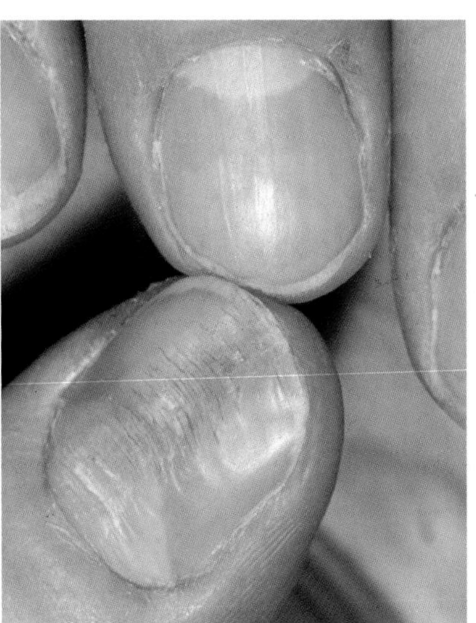

Figure 25-36 Habit-tic deformity. A common finding on the thumbs caused by picking the proximal nailfold with the index finger.

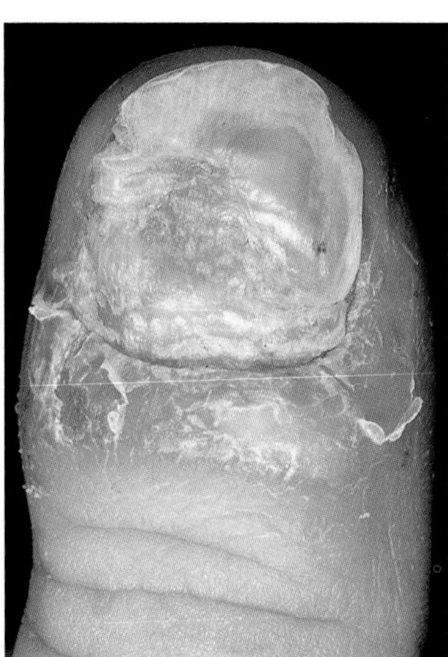

Figure 25-37 Nail rippling caused by chronic inflammation of the proximal nailfold. A normal nail grows once the eczema has been controlled.

MEDIAN NAIL DYSTROPHY

Median nail dystrophy is a distinctive nail plate change of unknown origin. A longitudinal split appears in the center of the nail plate. Several fine cracks project from the line laterally, giving the appearance of a fir tree. The thumb is most often affected (Figure 25-38). There is no treatment, and after a few months or years the nail can be expected to return to normal. Recurrences are possible.

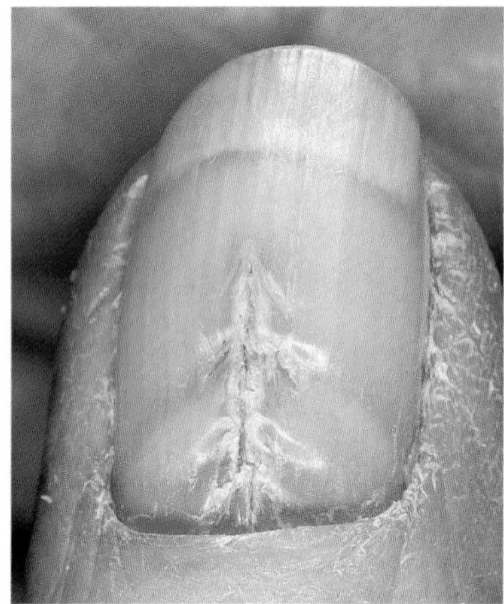

Figure 25-38 Median nail dystrophy.

PINCER NAILS (CURVATURE)

Inward folding of the lateral edges of the nail results in a tube- or pincer-shaped nail (Figure 25-39). The nail bed is drawn up into the tube and may become painful. The toenails are more commonly involved than the fingernails. Shoe compression is thought to cause pincer nails, but the etiology is uncertain. If pain is significant, surgical removal of the nail or reconstruction of the nail unit is required.

THE NAIL AND INTERNAL DISEASE

BEAU'S LINES

Beau's lines are transverse depressions of all of the nails that appear at the base of the lunula weeks after a stressful event has temporarily interrupted nail formation (Figure 25-40). The lines progress distally with normal nail growth and eventually disappear at the free edge. They develop in response to many diseases, such as syphilis, uncontrolled diabetes mellitus, myocarditis, peripheral vascular disease, and zinc deficiency, and to illnesses accompanied by high fevers, such as scarlet fever, measles, mumps, hand-foot-and-mouth disease, and pneumonia, and to chemotherapeutic agents.

YELLOW NAIL SYNDROME

Yellow nail syndrome is a rare acquired condition defined by the presence of yellow nails associated with lymphedema and/or chronic respiratory manifestations. Chronic respiratory manifestations include pleural effusions, bronchiectasis, chronic sinusitis, and recurrent pneumonias. The spontaneous appearance of yellow nails occurs before, during, or after certain respiratory diseases and in diseases associated with lymphedema. Patients note that nail growth slows and appears to stop. The nail plate may become excessively curved, and it turns dark yellow (Figure 25-41). The surface remains smooth or acquires transverse ridges, indicating variations in the growth rate; nails grow at less than half the normal rate. Partial or total separation of the nail plate may occur. The nails show an increased curvature about the long axis, the cuticles and lunulae are lost, and usually all the nails are involved. The nails grow very slowly, at a rate of 0.1 to 0.25 mm/week, compared with 0.5 to 2 mm/week for normal adult fingernails. Nails that grow slowly often become thicker. The lymphatic impairment associated with yellow nail syndrome appears to

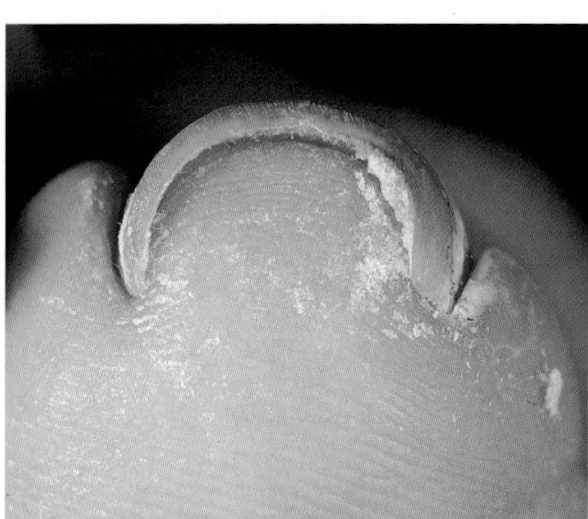

Figure 25-39 Pincer nails (overcurvature). Inward folding of the lateral edges of the nail results in a tube- or pincer-shaped nail.

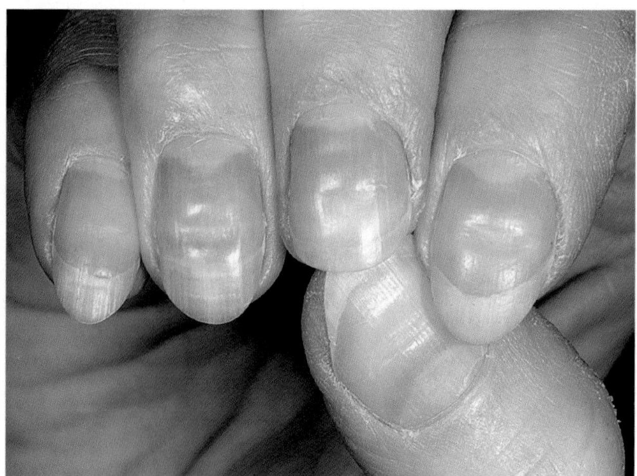

Figure 25-40 Beau's lines. A transverse depression of the nail plate that occurs several weeks after certain illnesses.

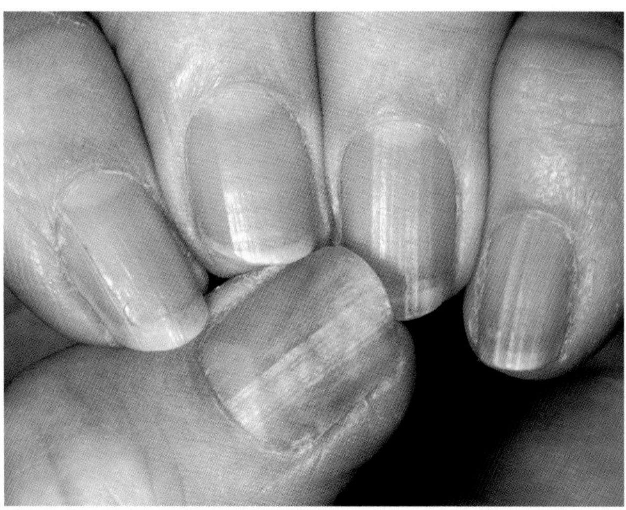

Figure 25-41 Yellow nail syndrome.

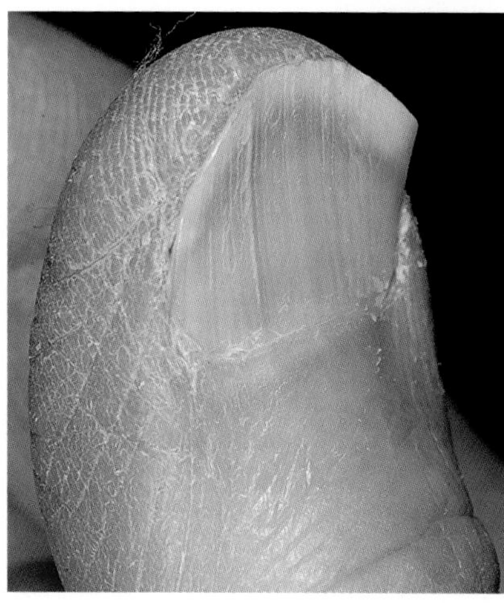

Figure 25-42 Spoon nails (koilonychia). Most cases are a variant of normal.

be secondary, and predominantly functional in nature, rather than as a result of structural changes. Yellowish nail pigmentation has been reported in patients with AIDS. The nails may spontaneously improve, even when the associated disease does not improve. Oral vitamin E in dosages of up to 800 international units/day for up to 18 months may help. Yellow nails that were treated with a 5% vitamin E solution (containing DL-α-tocopherol in dimethyl sulfoxide), two drops twice a day to the nail plate, showed marked clinical improvement and an increase in nail growth rate. Yellow nails improve in about half of patients, often without specific therapy.

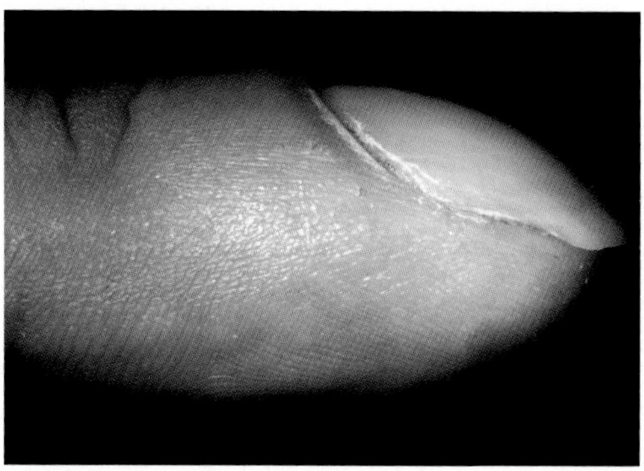

Figure 25-43 Finger clubbing. The distal phalanges are enlarged to a rounded, bulbous shape. The nail enlarges and becomes curved, hard, and thickened.

SPOON NAILS

Lateral elevation and central depression of the nail plate cause the nail to be spoon shaped; this is called koilonychia (Figure 25-42). Spoon nails are seen in normal children and may persist a lifetime without any associated abnormalities. The spontaneous onset of spoon nails has been reported to occur with iron deficiency anemia and in 50% of patients with idiopathic hemochromatosis. The nail reverts to normal when the anemia is corrected.

FINGER CLUBBING

Finger clubbing (Hippocratic nails) is a distinct feature associated with a number of diseases, but it may occur as a normal variant. Clubbing is painless unless associated with pulmonary hypertrophic osteoarthropathy, and then there is periarticular pain and swelling, most often in the wrists, ankles, knees, and elbows (Figure 25-43).

The features of clubbing occur in stages. The first is periungual erythema and a softening of the nail bed, giving a spongy sensation on palpation. The proximal nailfold feels as though it is floating on the underlying tissue. Next there is an increase in the normal 160-degree angle between the nail bed and the proximal nailfold. Lovibond (Lovibond's angle) showed that when viewed from the lateral aspect, an angle of greater than 180 degrees made by the nail as it exits the proximal nailfold can differentiate true clubbing from other conditions, such as nail curving and paronychia.

An increase in the depth of the distal phalanges is the last change. The distal phalanges of the fingers and toes are enlarged to a rounded, bulbous shape. The nail enlarges and becomes curved, hard, and thickened. The process usually takes years.

Vascular endothelial growth factor may play a central role in the development of clubbing. It is a platelet-derived factor induced by hypoxia and is produced by diverse malignancies.

All patients with cyanotic congenital heart disease have clubbing. In North America, 80% of acquired clubbing is associated with pulmonary disease. Clubbing is associated with a variety of lung diseases, cardiovascular disease, cirrhosis, colitis, and thyroid disease. One third of patients with lung cancer have evidence of clubbing. The changes are permanent. *PMID: 17976417*

TERRY'S NAILS

Terry's nails are white or light pink but retain a 0.5- to 3-mm normal, pink, distal band (Figure 25-44). The findings are associated with cirrhosis, chronic congestive heart failure, adult-onset diabetes mellitus, and age. It has been speculated that Terry's nails are a part of aging and that associated diseases "age" the nail. These changes are not associated with hypoalbuminemia or anemia.

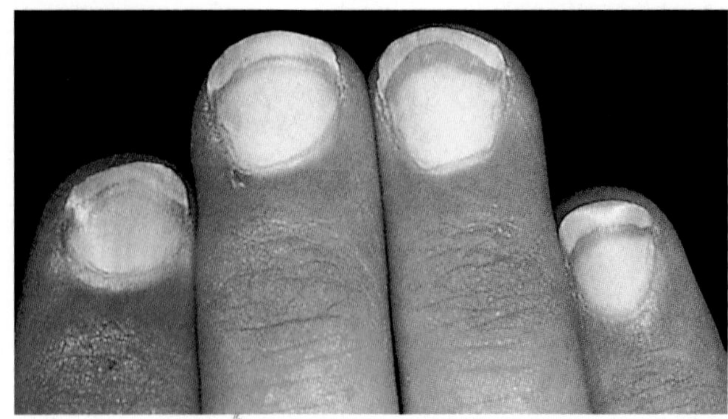

Figure 25-44 Terry's nails. The nail bed is white with only a narrow zone of pink at the distal end.

Table 25-2 Color Changes of Nails

Etiology	Pattern of color change
Brown nails	
Antimalarial drugs	Diffuse blue, brown
Cancer chemotherapeutic agents (Table 25-4)	Transverse black bands
Hyperbilirubinemia	Diffuse brown
Junctional nevi	Longitudinal brown bands
Malnutrition	Diffuse brown or black bands
Melanocyte stimulating hormone oversecretion Addison's disease Cushing's disease (after adrenalectomy) Pituitary tumor	Longitudinal brown bands
Melanoma	Longitudinal bands, may increase with width (Hutchinson's sign)
Normal finding in more than 90% of blacks	Longitudinal brown bands
Photographic developer	Diffuse brown
Green nails	
Pseudomonas	Green streaks and patches
Yellow nails	
Yellow-nail syndrome	Diffuse yellow
Onycholysis	Distal nail separation
Blue nails (blacks)	
Zidovudine treatment for AIDS	Diffuse blue
Antimalarial drugs	Diffuse blue
Minocycline	Diffuse blue
Wilson's disease	Diffuse blue
Hemorrhage	Irregular

COLOR AND DRUG-INDUCED CHANGES

Changes in nail color may result from a color change in the nail plate or in the nail bed. Several articles list changes associated with nail pigmentation. Some of these changes are listed in Tables 25-2 and 25-3. Cancer chemotherapeutic drugs have been associated with a variety of changes in the nail unit.

CONGENITAL ANOMALIES

Numerous congenital syndromes involve nail changes. The most widely understood syndromes all have autosomal dominant inheritance patterns.

Among other signs of pachyonychia congenita, there are yellow, very thick nail beds with elevated nails, palmar and plantar hyperkeratosis, and white keratotic thickening of the tongue. Some patients have erupted teeth at birth. In nail-patella syndrome, there are defective short nails and small or absent patella, in addition to other signs.

Table 25-3 White Nail or Nail Bed Changes

Disease	Clinical appearance
Anemia	Diffuse white
Arsenic	Mees' lines: transverse white lines
Cirrhosis	Terry's nails: most of nail, zone of pink at distal end (Figure 25-44)
Congenital leukonychia (autosomal dominant; variety of patterns)	Syndrome of leukonychia, knuckle pads, deafness; isolated finding; partial white
Darier's disease	Longitudinal white streaks
Half-and-half nail	Proximal white, distal pink; azotemia
High fevers (some diseases)	Transverse white lines
Hypoalbuminemia	Muehrcke's lines: stationary paired transverse bands
Hypocalcemia	Variable white
Malnutrition	Diffuse white
Pellagra	Diffuse milky white
Punctate leukonychia	Common white spots
Tinea and yeast	Variable patterns
Thallium toxicity (rat poison)	Variable white
Trauma	Repeated manicure: transverse striations
Zinc deficiency	Diffuse white

TUMORS

A limited number of tumors have been reported to occur about and under the nails (Table 25-4).

WARTS. The most common periungual growth is the periungual wart. It is discussed in Chapter 12. Warts are most common in children who bite their nails. Warts on the lateral nailfold and on the fingertip may extend deeply under the nail (Figure 25-45). A longitudinal nail groove may result from warts situated over the nail matrix. Warts are epidermal growths, but, if massive, they can erode the underlying bony matrix by displacement.

DIGITAL MUCOUS CYSTS. Digital mucous cysts (focal mucinosis) are not true cysts but rather a focal collection of mucin lacking a cystic lining. These soft, dome-shaped, translucent, pink-white structures occur on the dorsal surface of the distal phalanx of the middle-aged and the elderly (Figure 25-46). These structures contain a clear, viscous, jellylike substance that exudes if the cyst is incised. There are two types. The cysts on the proximal nailfold are

Table 25-4 Nail-Unit Tumors

Diagnosis	Clinical findings
Malignant	
Squamous cell carcinoma	Verrucous lesion, onycholysis, or subungual growth; nail plate destruction
Bowen's disease	Hyperkeratosis and onycholysis
Melanoma	Longitudinal brown subungual band; pigmented macule extending onto periungual skin (Hutchinson's sign); mass below nail; loss of nail plate; ulceration
Benign	
Myxoid cyst	Dome-shaped, translucent, proximal nailfold
Acquired digital fibrokeratoma	Looks like a garlic clove with outer skin stripped off; usually projects from proximal nail groove
Glomus tumor	Red or blue suffusion beneath nail plate; pressure blanches capillaries and causes pain
Giant cell tumor of tendon sheath	Arises from synovial lining cells associated with distal interphalangeal joint synovia and tendons; firm and deeply fixed to underlying fibrous tissue; does not arise on nail unit
Exostosis	Painful, bony growth; x-ray film confirms diagnosis
Warts	May occur on any surface about nail; spread by nail biting
Keratoacanthoma	Rapidly growing mass, central crust
Pyogenic granuloma	Red, vascular excrescence often devoid of an epithelial cover; profuse bleeding with slight trauma

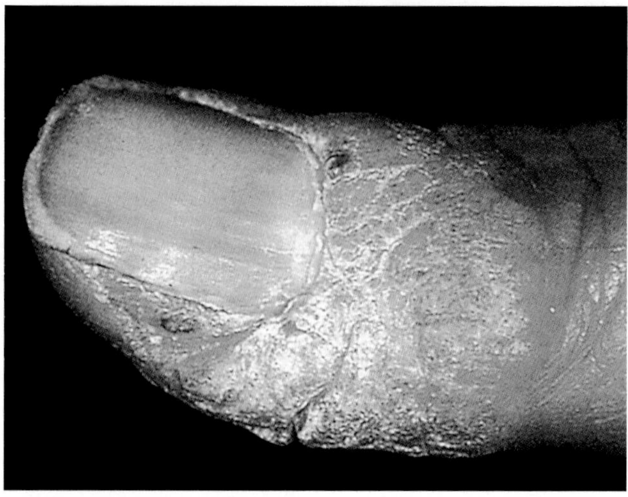

Figure 25-45 Periungual wart.

DIGITAL MUCOUS CYST

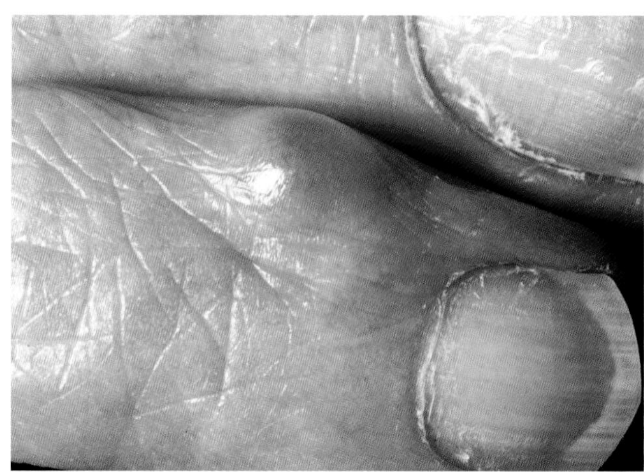

Digital mucous cyst, intact.

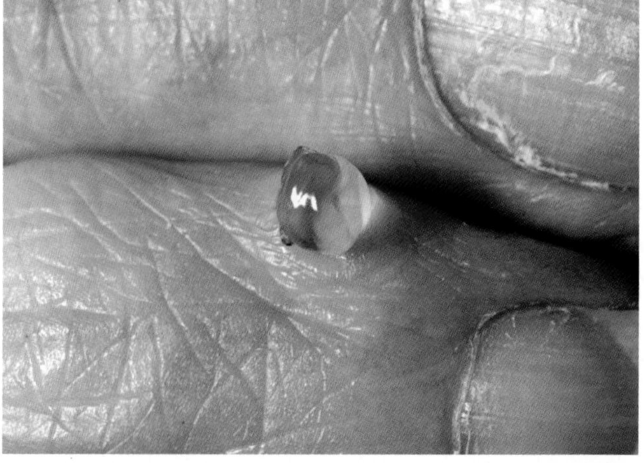

Incision with a #11 surgical blade. A clear, sometimes blood-tinged, viscous, jellylike substance exudes when the cyst is incised.

Figure 25-46

not connected to the joint space or tendon sheath. They result from localized fibroblast proliferation. Compression of the nail matrix cells induces a longitudinal nail groove. The cysts located on the dorsal-lateral finger at the distal interphalangeal (DIP) joint are probably caused by herniation of tendon sheaths or joint linings and are related to ganglion and synovial cysts.

Simple surgical excision, intralesional steroid injections, and unroofing of the cyst followed by electrodesiccation and curettage have a high recurrence rate.

Excision of the lesion with its pedicle and associated portions of the joint capsule affords a high cure rate but may result in subsequent partial loss of motion.

Cryosurgery. Cryosurgery using either the open-spray or the cryoprobe technique yields a cure rate of up to 75%. A local anesthetic is injected before treatment. The roof of the cyst is removed with scissors and the gelatinous material is expelled to facilitate freezing of the base of the lesion. Either a flat cryoprobe of approximately the same size as the cyst or a direct intermittent open spray to the center of the lesion is applied. The freeze time is 30 to 40 seconds when the cryoprobe technique is used and 20 to 30 seconds when the open-spray technique is used. The treated site becomes edematous and exudative, and a bulla develops in most cases. Healing is complete in 4 to 6 weeks. Lesions can be retreated if necessary.

Multiple punctures. A high cure rate may be achieved with the simple technique of repeated punctures and expression of the cyst contents (Figure 25-46, *B*). Cysts that resisted multiple needlings are usually reduced to small, asymptomatic nodules. Without anesthesia, the cyst is punctured with a medium-sized hypodermic needle (26 gauge) to a depth of 3 to 5 mm. The clear contents, sometimes tinged with blood, are squeezed out by fingertip pressure. The patient is given a supply of needles to repeat the procedure at home if the cyst recurs. From 1 to 10 needlings result in a cure or in an asymptomatic lesion.

Carbon dioxide laser. Carbon dioxide laser vaporization performed under local anesthesia resulted in complete remission in four out of six patients. No side effects of therapy occurred.

PYOGENIC GRANULOMA. Pyogenic granuloma occasionally occurs in the lateral nailfold. This benign mass of vascular tissue is removed with thorough electrodesiccation and curettage (Figure 25-47 and see p. 906). Recurrences are common if any residual tissue is left. Periungual malignant melanoma can mimic pyogenic granuloma.

PYOGENIC GRANULOMA

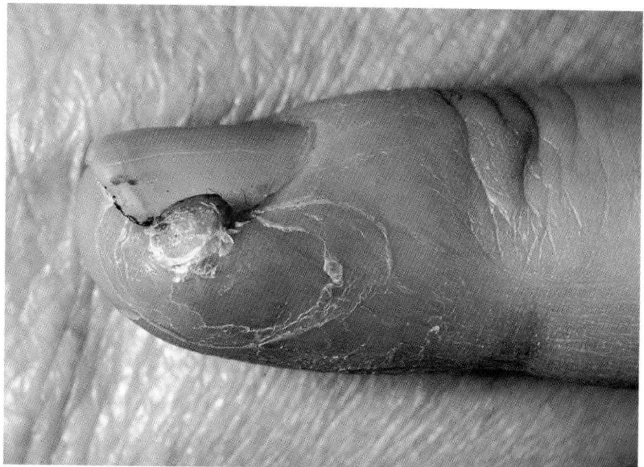

Lesions may form at the lateral nailfold and be caused by an ingrown nail.

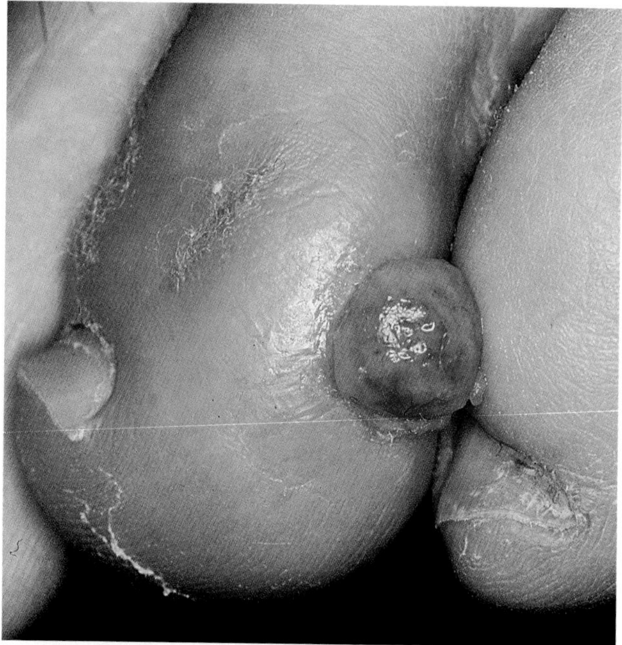

A pedunculated nodule with a smooth, glistening surface. The surface frequently becomes crusted, eroded, or ulcerated. Minor trauma may produce considerable bleeding.

Figure 25-47

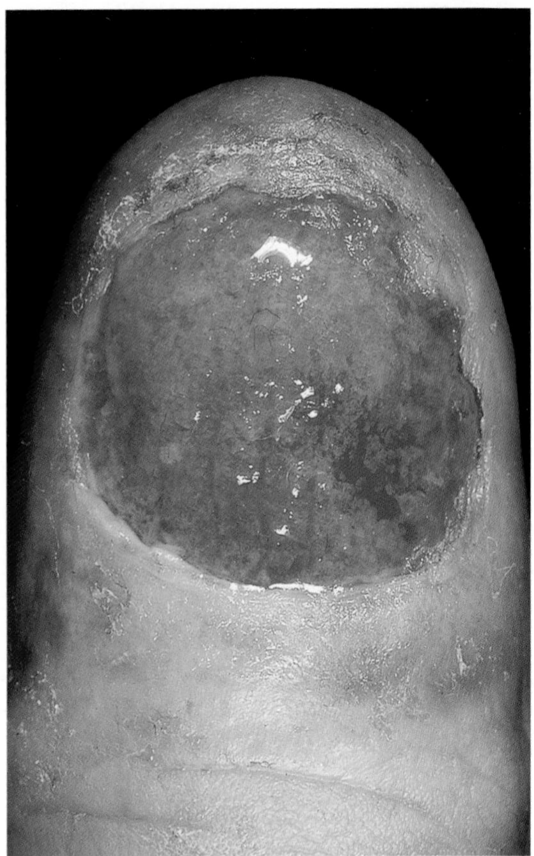

Figure 25-48 Melanoma involving the entire nail bed. This is a rare presentation.

NEVI AND MELANOMA. Junctional nevi can appear in the nail matrix and produce a brown pigmented band. Brown longitudinal bands are common in blacks (see Figure 25-5) but rare in whites. Melanoma of the nail region, or melanotic whitlow, although rare, is a distinctive lesion (Figures 25-48 and 25-49). Most are classified as acral lentiginous melanomas. The growth is usually painless and slow, and it can occur anywhere around or under the nail. The lesion may present as a pigmented band that increases in width. There has not been enough experience to make specific recommendations concerning the management of pigmented bands in whites. The spontaneous appearance of such a band is noteworthy to most physicians, who promptly require a biopsy. Benign subungual nevi are rare in whites, so subungual nevoid lesions should be regarded as malignant until proved otherwise. Nail matrix biopsy of longitudinal melanonychia is accomplished by shave, punch, or excision. Biopsies of possible subungual melanomas should be carried out by surgeons regularly doing such procedures. *PMID: 17437887*

Melanocytes in normal nail matrices are distributed in the basal layer and in the lower half of the epithelium. Therefore malignant melanoma of the nail matrix can arise from melanocytes situated in the squamous epithelium above the basal layer.

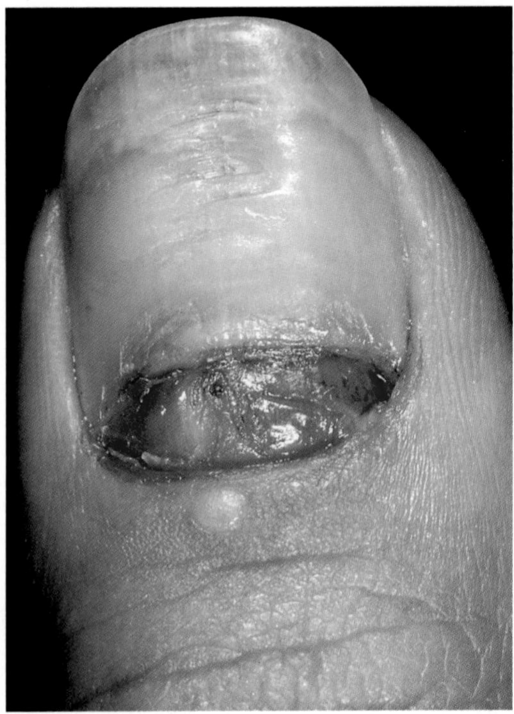

Figure 25-49 Melanoma arising from the nail matrix.

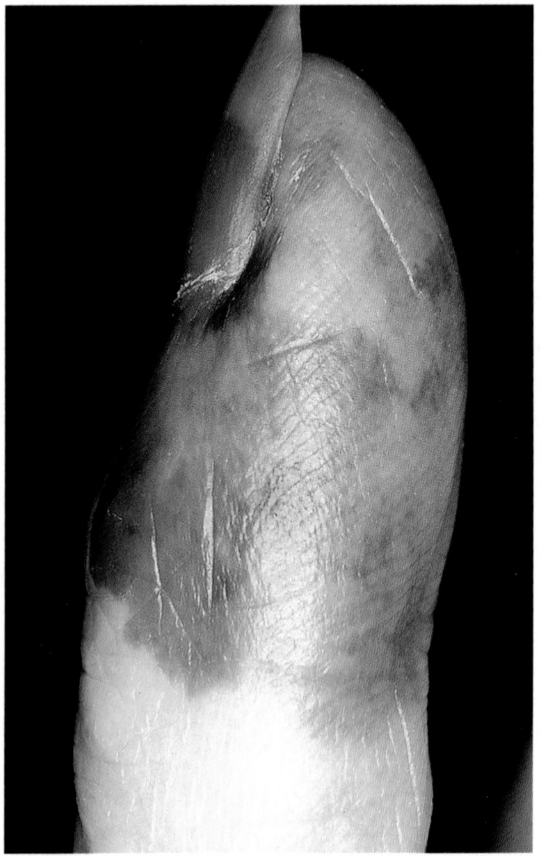

Figure 25-50 Hutchinson's sign. Extension of pigmentation onto the nailfolds is a classic sign of subungual melanoma.

ABCDEF CRITERIA. The most salient features of subungual melanoma can be summarized according to the newly devised criteria that may be categorized under the first letters of the alphabet, namely, ABCDEF of subungual melanoma. In this system *A* stands for age (peak incidence being in the fifth to seventh decades of life) and for African Americans, Asians, and Native Americans, in whom subungual melanoma accounts for up to one third of all melanoma cases. *B* designates brown to black and with breadth of 3 mm or more and variegated borders. *C* stands for change in the nail band or lack of change in the nail morphology despite, presumably, adequate treatment. *D* indicates the digit most commonly involved. *E* stands for extension of the pigment onto the proximal and/or lateral nailfold (i.e., Hutchinson's sign), and *F* designates family or personal history of dysplastic nevus or melanoma.

Hutchinson's sign. Hutchinson's sign, periungual extension of brown-black pigmentation from longitudinal melanonychia onto the proximal and lateral nailfolds, is an important indicator of subungual melanoma (Figure 25-50). Periungual hyperpigmentation also occurs in Bowen's disease of the nail unit. Hyperpigmentation of the nail bed and matrix may reflect through the "transparent" nailfolds simulating Hutchinson's sign. Conditions that mimic Hutchinson's sign are listed in Box 25-1.

Box 25-2 lists nail pigment changes that should be biopsied. Biopsy techniques are described on PMID: 1740326

LONGITUDINAL PIGMENTATION OF THE NAIL (Figure 25-51). This is a common finding with multiple possible causes. History (time of onset, duration, medications) and exam (diameter, color) are important. Dermoscopy is also valuable. The most frequent causes of longitudinal nail pigmentation are listed in Box 25-3.

Dermoscopy. Dermoscopy allows visual inspection through the stratum corneum and nail plate and provides magnification. The distal free edge of the nail plate is also examined. Proximal nail matrix pigment appears in the upper nail plate and pigment produced in the distal nail matrix appears in the lower part of the nail plate. The site to biopsy is derived from this information. An alternate method is to obtain a nail clipping and stain it with Fontana-Masson stain. The pathologist examines the distal edge and records the location of the pigment.

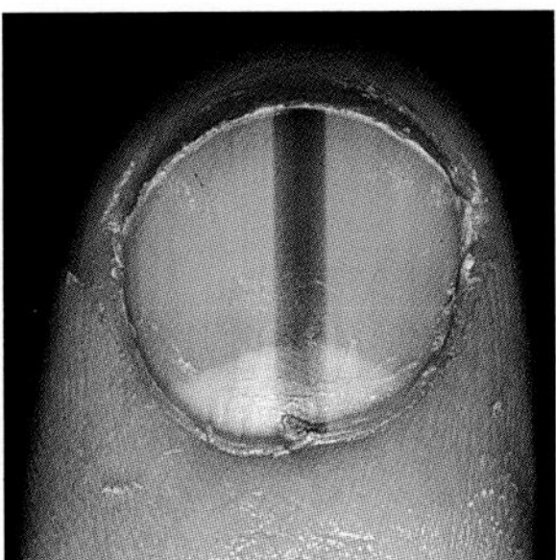

Figure 25-51 Longitudinal pigmentation.

Box 25-1 **Conditions That May Produce a Pseudo-Hutchinson's Sign**

Addison's disease
AIDS
Bowen's disease
Drug-induced pigmentation
Laugier's sign
Malnutrition
Nail matrix nevi (heavily pigmented)
Peutz-Jeghers syndrome
Racial pigmentations (phototypes V and VI)
Radiation therapy
Trauma

From *J Am Acad Dermatol* 56(5):835-847, 2007. Epub 2007 Feb 22. Review. PMID: 17320240

Box 25-2 **Nail Pigment Changes That Should Be Biopsied***

1. Isolated pigmented band on a single digit that develops during fourth to sixth decade of life; although melanoma can be seen in children, it is a very rare event
2. Nail pigmentation that develops abruptly in a previously normal nail plate
3. Pigmentation that suddenly becomes darker or larger, or pigment becomes blurred near nail matrix
4. Acquired pigmentation of thumb, index finger, or large toe
5. Pigment that develops after a history of digital trauma and in which subungual hematoma has been ruled out
6. Any acquired lesion in patients with a personal history of melanoma
7. If pigmentation is associated with nail dystrophy including partial nail destruction or absence of nail plate
8. If pigmentation of periungual skin (including lateral nailfolds) is found to be present (Hutchinson's sign); this includes pigment of cuticle or hyponychium

Adapted from *J Am Acad Dermatol* 56(5):835-847, 2007. Epub 2007 Feb 22. Review. PMID: 17320240
*Any lesion with an irregular dermoscopy pattern should be biopsied.

Box 25-3 **Most Frequent Causes of Longitudinal Melanonychia**

Drug- and radiation-induced LM
Endocrine LM (Addison's disease)
LM associated with HIV infection
LM associated with inflammatory nail disorders
Nutritional LM (vitamin B_{12} or folate deficiency)
Traumatic LM
Ethnic (racial) LM
Nevi of nail matrix
Melanoma of nail matrix

Adapted from *J Am Acad Dermatol* 56(5):835-847, 2007. Epub 2007 Feb 22. Review. PMID: 17320240
LM, Longitudinal melanonychia.

Chapter 26

Cutaneous Manifestations of Internal Disease

CHAPTER CONTENTS

Certain cutaneous diseases are frequently associated with internal disease. The skin disease itself may be inconsequential, but its presence should prompt investigation of possible related internal disorders. A selected group of such diseases is discussed in this chapter. Pigmentary skin changes associated with internal diseases are also discussed in Chapter 19.

CUTANEOUS MANIFESTATIONS OF DIABETES MELLITUS

Approximately 30% of patients with diabetes mellitus develop a skin disorder sometime during the course of disease. A list of these disorders follows:

- *Candida* infections (mouth, genital)
- Carotenodermia (yellow skin)
- Diabetic bullae
- Diabetic dermopathy (shin spots)
- Diabetic thick skin
- Erythema (face, lower legs, feet)
- External otitis
- Finger pebbles
- Foot ulcers
- Acanthosis nigricans (insulin resistance syndromes)
- Gas gangrene (nonclostridial)
- Granuloma annulare (localized or generalized)
- Insulin lipodystrophy
- Necrobiosis lipoidica
- Yellow nails
- Perforating disorders
- Eruptive xanthomas

Necrobiosis lipoidica

Necrobiosis lipoidica (NL) is a disease of unknown origin, but more than 50% of the patients with NL are generally insulin dependent. The average age at onset is 30 years. It is frequently associated with diabetes. More than 75% of patients with NL either have or will develop diabetes mellitus. However, it is seen in only 0.3% to 0.7% of the entire diabetic population. The skin lesions may appear years before the onset of diabetes, and most patients with diabetes do not develop NL. The disease may occur at any age, but it most commonly appears in the third and fourth decades. Most of the patients are females, and in most cases the lesions are confined to the anterior surfaces of the lower legs (Figure 26-1).

NECROBIOSIS LIPOIDICA

Erythematous violaceous plaques on the anterior surfaces of the lower legs.

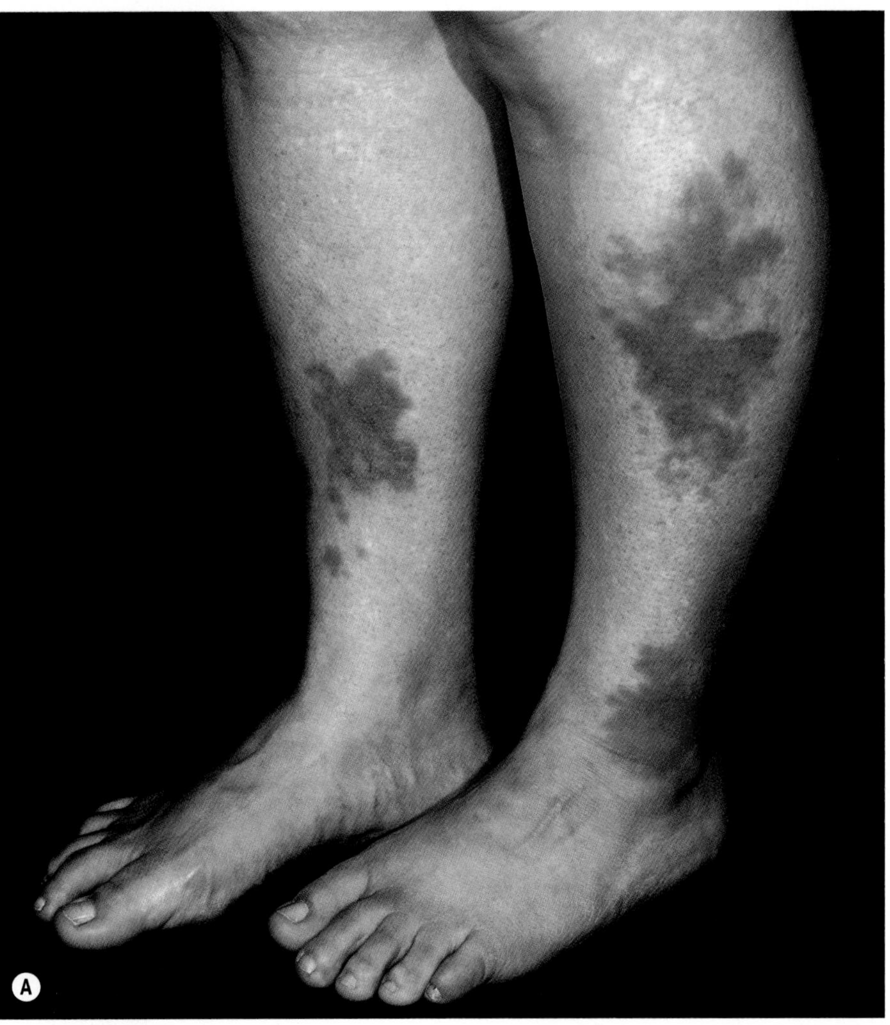

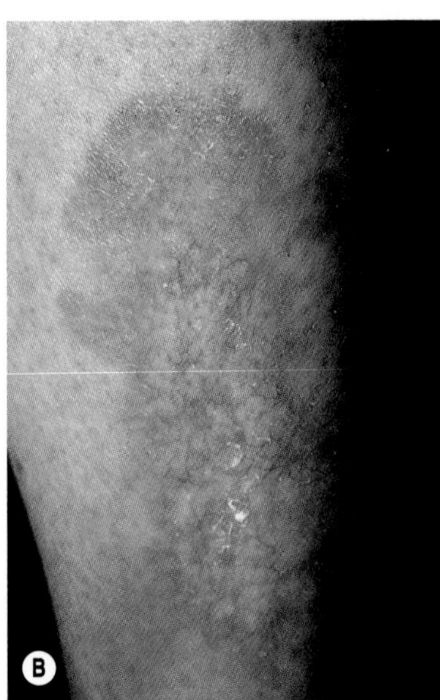

The central area is waxy yellow with prominent telangiectasia.

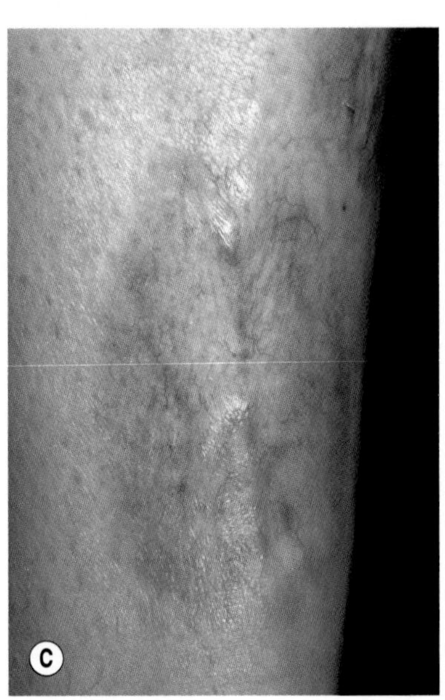

End-stage disease with atrophy and telangiectasia.

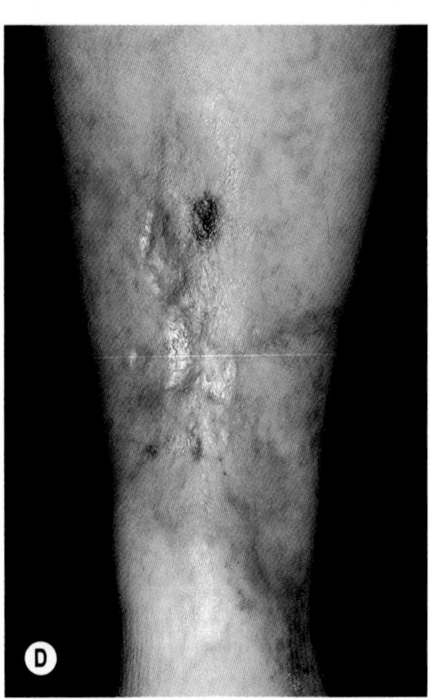

Severe disease with dense fibrosis and ulceration.

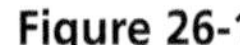

Figure 26-1

The eruption begins as an oval, violaceous patch and expands slowly. The advancing border is red, and the central area turns yellow-brown. The central area atrophies and has a waxy surface; telangiectasias become prominent (Figure 26-1, *B* and *C*). Ulceration occurs, particularly following trauma, in 13% of cases (Figure 26-1, *D*). In many instances the clinical presentation is so characteristic that biopsy is not required.

TREATMENT. Currently, there are no evidence-based guidelines for the treatment of necrobiosis lipoidica.

Topical and intralesional steroids. Topical and intralesional steroids arrest inflammation but promote further atrophy. Clobetasol propionate under occlusion has successfully treated thick plaques. Intralesional injections effectively control small areas of NL, but the concentration of triamcinolone acetonide (10 mg/ml) should be diluted with saline or Xylocaine to 2.5 mg/ml to avoid atrophy.

Systemic corticosteroids. A 3- to 5-week course of systemic corticosteroids may arrest the disease; however, restitution of atrophic skin lesions is not achieved. Ulceration of NL can at times be successfully treated with oral prednisolone.

Pentoxifylline. Pentoxifylline (Trental) 400 mg three times a day is reported to result in significant improvement after 1 month of treatment. Ulcerating NL is reported to respond within 8 weeks of administration of 400 mg of pentoxifylline twice a day. Pentoxifylline is thought to decrease blood viscosity by increasing fibrinolysis and red blood cell deformability and also to inhibit platelet aggregation.

Aspirin and dipyridamole. Low-dose aspirin and dipyridamole are thought to inhibit platelet aggregation, but reports concerning their efficacy in healing ulcers in plaques of NL are conflicting. The recommended treatment is aspirin 3.5 mg/kg every 48 hours, which for the average patient is 325 gm daily (one tablet); or dipyridamole (Persantine) (25-, 50-, or 75-mg tablets) 2 to 3 mg/kg/day, which for the average patient is 150 to 200 mg daily in divided doses. For effective control of ulceration, platelet-inhibition therapy must be used for a minimum of 3 to 7 months. Recommended treatment schedules should be followed because there is evidence that higher dosages can decrease treatment effectiveness.

Other treatments. Cyclosporine, tacrolimus ointment 0.1%, etanercept, mycophenolate mofetil, fumaric acid esters, photochemotherapy with topical PUVA, chloroquine (200 mg/day), hydroxychloroquine (400 mg/day), inflixamab, and thalidomide (150 mg/day) are reported to be effective.

Skin grafting. Skin grafting is effective for extensive disease.

Granuloma annulare

There are conflicting reports about the association of granuloma annulare (GA) with diabetes mellitus. Most patients with the localized form of granuloma annulare do not have clinical or laboratory evidence of diabetes. The association between disseminated granuloma annulare and diabetes has been established, but the frequency is unknown. In a retrospective study 12% of patients with GA had diabetes mellitus. Those patients suffered significantly more often from chronic relapsing GA than nondiabetic patients. Granuloma annulare can be associated with HIV and can present at all stages of HIV infection. Generalized GA is the most common clinical pattern in HIV infection.

CLINICAL PRESENTATION. Granuloma annulare is characterized by a ring of small, firm, flesh-colored or red papules. The localized form, most common in young adult females, is most frequently found on the lateral or dorsal surfaces of the hands and feet (Figure 26-2). The disease begins with an asymptomatic, flesh-colored papule that undergoes central involution. Over months, a ring of papules slowly increases in diameter to 0.5 to 5 cm (Figure 26-3). The duration of the disease is highly variable. Many lesions undergo spontaneous involution without scarring, whereas others last for years. The familial occurrence of GA is uncommon but has been noted in siblings, twins, and successive generations.

Disseminated GA occurs in adults and appears with numerous flesh-colored or erythematous papules, some of which form annular rings. The papules may be accentuated in sun-exposed areas. The course is variable; many lesions persist for years.

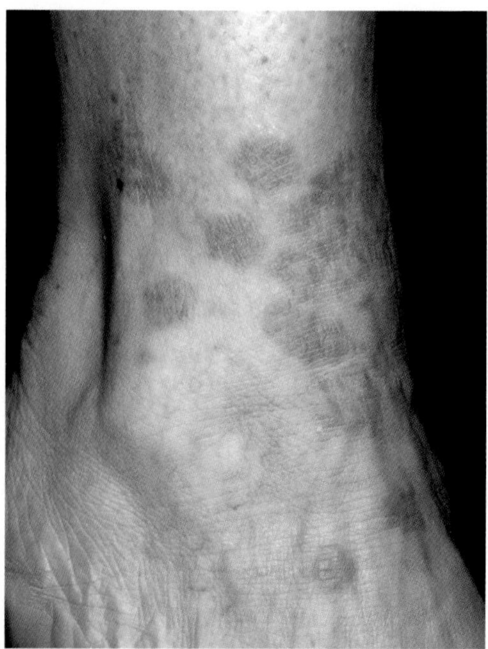

Figure 26-2 Granuloma annulare. The dorsal surfaces of the hands and feet and the extensor aspects of the arms and legs are the most common sites. Lesions are either papular or broad superficial plaques.

Generalized perforating GA is characterized by 1- to 4-mm umbilicated papules on the extremities and is most commonly seen in children and young adults. Biopsy shows transepithelial elimination of degenerating collagen fibers. GA occurred during anti–tumor necrosis factor (anti-TNF) therapy (4.5% of 119 patients) (infliximab adalimumab, etanercept) for rheumatoid arthritis. *PMID: 17728330* Patients who develop GA usually heal, remain remarkably healthy, and do not ordinarily develop other odd diseases. *PMID: 17638746*

Subcutaneous GA occurs in children. Painless subcutaneous nodules in the lower anterior tibial region or foot and in the scalp, typically in the occiput, are the most common presenting features. The mean age at presentation is 3.9 years. Diagnosis requires an excisional biopsy. Lesions may recur after excision. Lesions may resolve spontaneously and recur after excision. No record of progression to systemic illness is reported.

DIAGNOSIS. The clinical presentation is characteristic, and biopsy may not be required. The histology shows collagen degeneration, a feature similar to that seen in necrobiosis lipoidica.

TREATMENT. Localized lesions are asymptomatic and are best left untreated. Those patients troubled by appearance may be treated with intralesional injections of triamcinolone acetonide (2.5 to 5 mg/ml). The solution should be injected only into the elevated border. Topical steroids have little effect. Localized lesions have responded to imiquimod cream. Disseminated GA has been reported to respond to dapsone, isotretinoin, etretinate, hydroxychloroquine, niacinamide (1.5 gm/day), fumaric acid esters, hydroxyurea, narrow-band ultraviolet B therapy, and psoralen and ultraviolet A therapy (PUVA). Four patients with disseminated GA were treated with a cycle of cyclosporine therapy for 6 weeks. Cyclosporine was started at a dose of 4 mg/kg/day for 4 weeks, and subsequently reduced by 0.5 mg/kg/day every 2 weeks. The lesions resolved within 3 weeks and there were no relapses. *PMID: 16831309*

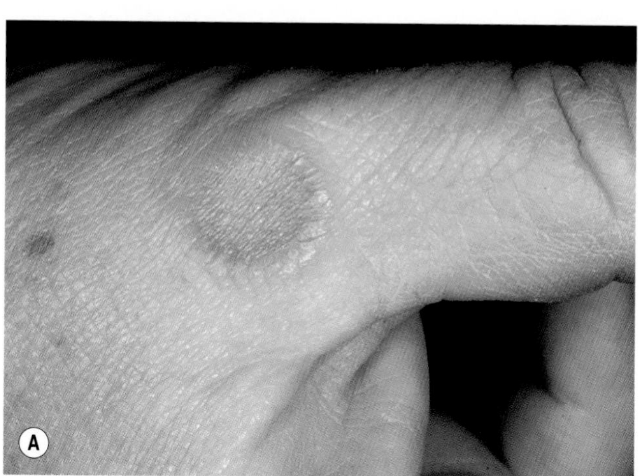

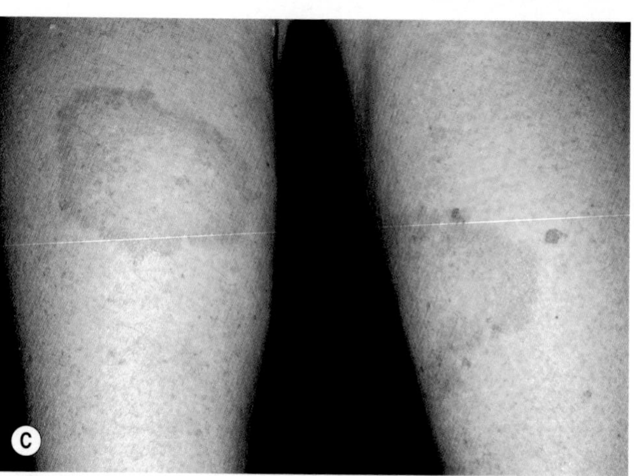

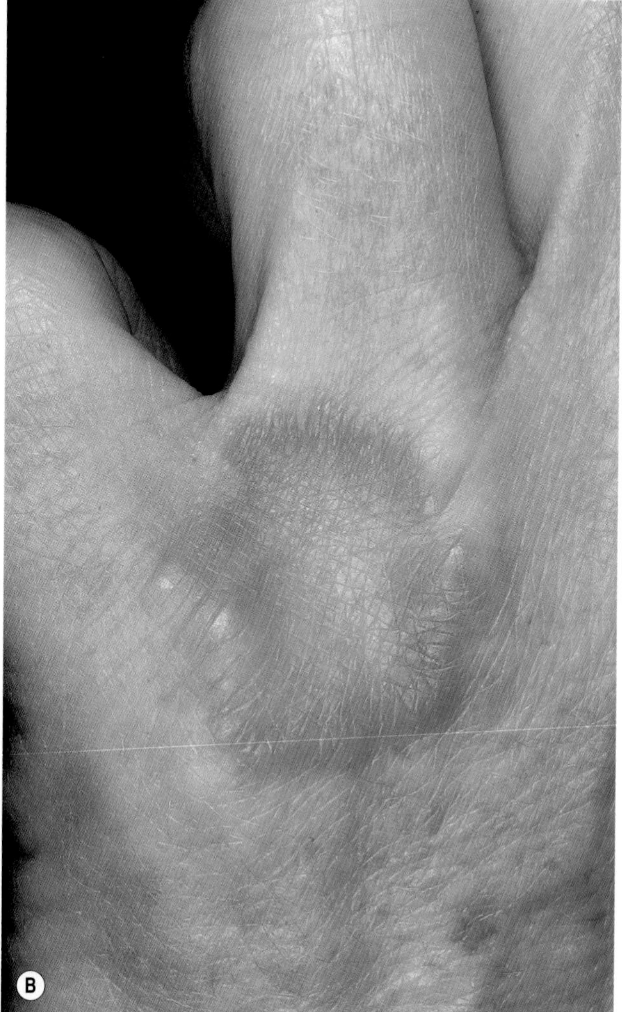

Figure 26-3 Granuloma annulare. **A,** A ring of flesh-colored to red papules slowly expands. **B,** The border is either papular or smooth, and the center is depressed. **C,** Round and annular lesions can extend over wide areas.

ACANTHOSIS NIGRICANS

Acanthosis nigricans (AN) is a nonspecific reaction pattern that may accompany obesity; diabetes; excess corticosteroids; pineal tumors; other endocrine disorders (Box 26-1); multiple genetic variants; drugs such as nicotinic acid, estrogens, and corticosteroids; and adenocarcinoma. AN is classified into malignant and benign forms (Box 26-2).

CLINICAL CHARACTERISTICS. In all cases the disease presents with symmetric, brown thickening of the skin. In time the skin may become quite thickened as the lesion develops a leathery, warty, or papillomatous surface (Figure 26-4). The lesions range in severity from slight discoloration of a small area to extensive involvement of wide areas. The most common site of involvement is the axilla (Figure 26-5), but the changes may be observed in the flexural areas of the posterior neck (Figure 26-6) and groin,

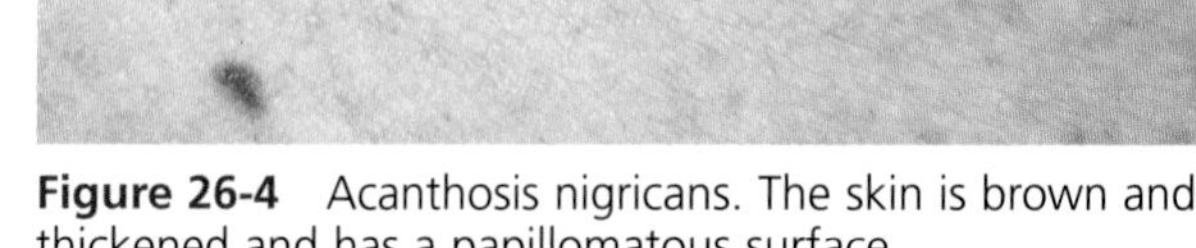

Figure 26-4 Acanthosis nigricans. The skin is brown and thickened and has a papillomatous surface.

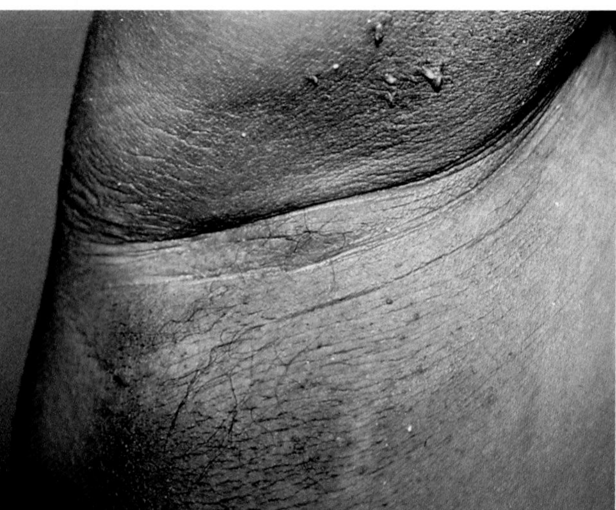

Figure 26-5 Acanthosis nigricans. The axilla is the most common site of involvement. The skin is thickened and hyperpigmented.

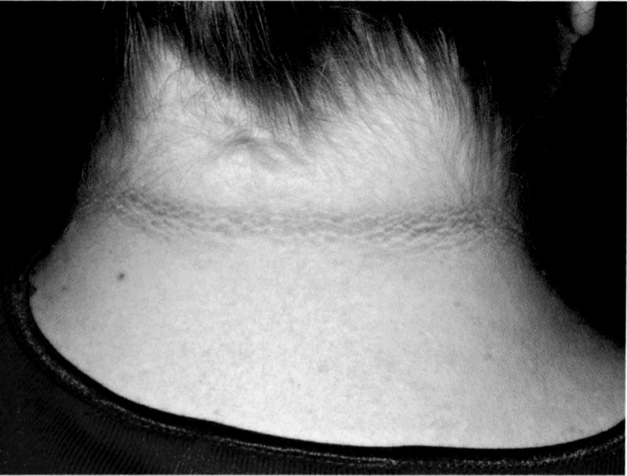

Figure 26-6 Acanthosis nigricans of the neck. The patient was obese.

Box 26-1 **Endocrine Syndromes with Acanthosis Nigricans (Most Have Insulin Resistance + Hyperinsulinemia + AN)**

- Insulin-resistant states
  - Type A syndrome
  - Type B syndrome
  - Lipoatrophic diabetes
  - Leprechaunism
  - Acral hypertrophy syndrome
  - Pinealoma
  - Pineal hyperplasia syndrome
- Hyperandrogenic states
  - Type A and B syndromes
  - Polycystic ovary disease
  - Ovarian hyperthecosis
  - Stromal luteoma
  - Ovarian dermoid cysts
- Acromegaly
- Cushing's disease
- Pituitary basophilism
- Obesity
- Hypothyroidism
- Addison's disease
- Hypogonadal syndrome with insulin resistance
- Prader-Willi syndrome
- Alström syndrome

Adapted from Lowella EE, Fenske NA: *J Am Acad Dermatol* 34:892, 1996. *PMID: 8621823*

Box 26-2 **Classification of Acanthosis Nigricans**

Benign

- Obesity related
- Hereditary (many syndromes)
- Endocrine syndromes

Malignant

along the belt line, over the dorsal surfaces of the fingers, in the mouth, and around the areolae of the breasts (Figure 26-7) and umbilicus. During the disease process, there is papillary hypertrophy, hyperkeratosis, and an increased number of melanocytes in the epidermis.

BENIGN ACANTHOSIS NIGRICANS. The majority of cases are idiopathic and are associated with obesity; this process is referred to as pseudoacanthosis nigricans. Most patients with AN have either clinical or subclinical insulin resistance. There is a high prevalence of AN in obese adults. There is a positive correlation between the development of AN and the severity of the obesity. AN is a common finding in overweight youth. Nearly 40% of Native American teenagers, 13% of blacks, 6% of Hispanics, and less than 1% of white, non-Hispanic children between the ages of 10 and 19 have AN. AN identifies a subgroup within an ethnic group that has the highest insulin concentration, the most severe insulin resistance, and the highest risk for the development of type 2 diabetes.

The interaction between excessive amounts of circulating insulin with insulin-like growth factor receptors on keratinocytes may lead to the development of acanthosis nigricans.

In rare instances AN may occur as an autosomal dominant trait with no obesity, associated endocrinopathies, or congenital abnormalities; it may appear at birth or during childhood and is accentuated at puberty.

DRUG-INDUCED ACANTHOSIS NIGRICANS. Drug-induced acanthosis nigricans has occurred with the use of nicotinic acid and, rarely, with other agents.

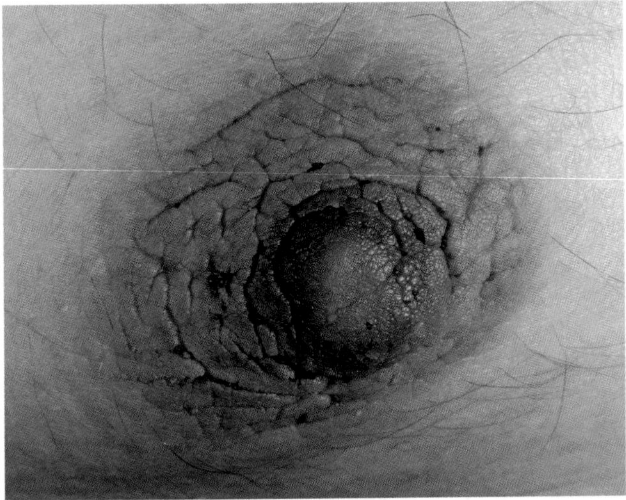

Figure 26-7 Acanthosis nigricans. The areola may be affected.

ENDOCRINE SYNDROMES WITH ACANTHOSIS NIGRICANS. In a large and heterogeneous group of conditions, insulin action at the cellular level is markedly reduced (see Box 26-1). AN appears to represent a cutaneous marker of tissue insulin resistance, irrespective of its cause (antibodies to the insulin receptor or congenital or acquired defects of receptor or postreceptor function). These patients may not require insulin therapy, and many do not have diabetes. For patients without diabetes, insulin resistance is established by the documentation of high levels of circulating insulin or by the observation of an impaired response to exogenous insulin. Prolonged hypersecretion of insulin may lead to pancreatic exhaustion, glucose intolerance, and type 2 diabetes.

Two syndromes of insulin resistance and AN are of special interest. Type A syndrome, also called the HAIR-AN syndrome, is characterized by hyperandrogenemia (HA), extreme insulin resistance (IR), and acanthosis nigricans (AN) occurring in the absence of obesity or lipoatrophy. It is distinguished from type B insulin resistance by a lack of antibodies to the insulin receptor or other evidence of autoimmune disease. It is familial and affects mainly black women who have the onset of AN in infancy or childhood.

TREATMENT. Lesions are usually asymptomatic and do not require treatment. Reducing thicker lesions in areas of maceration may decrease odor and promote comfort. A 12% ammonium lactate cream, applied as needed, may soften lesions. Retinoic acid (Retin-A cream or gel) applied each day, or less often if irritation occurs, is effective.

MALIGNANT ACANTHOSIS NIGRICANS. The cases of greatest concern are those originating in nonobese adult patients. These cases may result from secretion of tumor products with insulin-like activity or transforming growth factor alpha, which stimulates keratinocytes to proliferate. These patients must be evaluated for internal malignancy. The stomach is the most common site for the tumor, but cancer in several other areas has been reported. Malignant AN has a different clinical appearance. Lesions develop rapidly and tend to be more severe and extensive. Hyperpigmentation is prominent and is not limited to the hyperkeratotic areas. Mucous membrane involvement and thickening of the palms and soles occur more frequently. Itching is common. The presence of AN in conjunction with tripe palms and the sign of Leser-Trélat is highly suggestive of an internal malignancy. In approximately one third of patients, the skin lesions precede the clinical manifestations of cancer, and in several cases they have disappeared with successful removal of the tumor. A recurrence of acanthosis nigricans may mark the recurrence or metastasis of the previously treated cancer. In patients with malignant acanthosis, chemotherapy may relieve many of the distressing cutaneous symptoms.

XANTHOMAS AND DYSLIPOPROTEINEMIA

The plasma lipids and lipoprotein levels are under the control of a number of genetic and environmental influences. Abnormalities in a number of these lipids or subfractions result in dyslipoproteinemias and xanthomas. Xanthomas are lipid deposits in the skin and tendons that occur secondary to a lipid abnormality. These localized deposits are yellow and are frequently very firm. Although certain types of xanthomas are characteristic of certain lipid abnormalities, none is absolutely specific because the same form of xanthomas occurs in many different diseases; further investigation is always required. The molecular defect of various lipid disorders is now known; however, the classification and diagnosis are still based on history and clinical presentation (Table 26-1).

PATHOPHYSIOLOGY. The liver secretes lipoproteins, which are particles composed of various combinations of cholesterol and triglycerides. These particles are made water soluble to facilitate transport to peripheral tissues by polar phospholipids and 12 different specific proteins termed apolipoproteins. The apolipoproteins also serve as cofactors for plasma enzymes and interact with cell surface receptors. Lipoproteins are divided into five major classes: chylomicrons, very-low-density lipoproteins (VLDL), intermediate-density lipoproteins (IDL), low-density lipoproteins (LDL), and high-density lipoproteins (HDL). LDL and HDL have each been divided into two subfractions.

CLASSIFICATION: PRIMARY VS. SECONDARY HYPERLIPOPROTEINEMIA. Dyslipoproteinemias are categorized as primary or secondary. Primary conditions (Table 26-2) are genetically determined and were grouped by Fredrickson into five or six types on the basis of specific lipoprotein elevations. This classification recognizes elevations of chylomicrons (type I), VLDL or pre-beta lipoproteins (type IV), "broad beta" disease (or type III hyperlipoproteinemia), beta lipoproteins (LDL) (type II), and elevations of both chylomicrons and VLDL (type V). In addition, the combined elevations in pre-beta (VLDL) and beta (LDL) lipoproteins were recognized as type IIb hyperlipoproteinemia. This older classification still provides a useful conceptual framework. It does not, however, include HDL cholesterol nor does it differentiate severe monogenic

Table 26-1 Xanthomas

Type	Clinical characteristics	Associated lipid abnormality
Xanthelasma	Inner or outer canthus; plane or papular	No lipid abnormality; increased frequency of apo E-ND phenotype and hyperapobetalipoproteinemia; type II*
Eruptive	Crops of discrete yellow papules on an erythematous base on buttocks, extensor aspects of elbows and knees; lesions clear when triglycerides return to normal	Indicative of hypertriglyceridemia and seen with types I, II, IV, and rarely III and diabetes mellitus
Plane	Palms and palmar creases, eyelids, face, neck, chest	Biliary cirrhosis; type III; reported in types II, IV
Tuberous	Lipid deposits in dermis and subcutaneous tissue; plaquelike or nodular; frequently found on elbows or knees	Hypertriglyceridemia (familial or acquired); types II and III; biliary cirrhosis
Tendinous	Nodules involving elbows, knees, Achilles tendon, and dorsum of hands and feet	Indicates hypercholesterolemia; type II, occasionally type III

*There are five types of familial hyperlipidemia.

Table 26-2 Primary Dyslipidemia (Genetic Dyslipidemias)

Phenotype	Lipoprotein at increased concentration	Cholesterol concentration	Triglyceride concentration	Dermatologic lesion(s)
I	Chylomicrons	+	++++	Eruptive xanthomas
IIa	LDL	++++	+	Tendon, tuberous, and intertriginous xanthomas; xanthelasma, plane
IIb	VLDL and LDL	++++	++	Tendon, tuberous, and intertriginous xanthomas; xanthelasma, plane
III	IDL	+++	+++	Tuberoeruptive, tuberous, plane (palmar creases)
IV	VLDL	+	+++	Eruptive xanthomas
V	Chylomicrons and VLDL	++	++++	Eruptive xanthomas

lipoprotein disorders from the more common polygenic disorders. The World Health Organization has classified lipoprotein disorders on the basis of arbitrary cut-points, but the traditional classification will be used in this text.

Secondary hyperlipoproteinemias occur as a result of another disease process that can induce symptoms (Box 26-3), lipoprotein changes, and xanthomas that mimic the primary syndromes. Diagnosis should be made as follows:

1. Determine the type of xanthoma.
2. Measure fasting blood levels of cholesterol, triglycerides, and HDL, VLDL, and LDL.
3. Rule out secondary diseases (see Box 26-3). The diagnosis of primary hyperlipoproteinemia is one of exclusion.
   a. Thyroid, liver, renal function tests
   b. Glucose tolerance tests
   c. Complete blood count (CBC); serum and urine immunoelectrophoresis
   d. Chest x-ray film, bone marrow aspiration
   e. Antinuclear antibodies (ANAs) testing

XANTHELASMA AND PLANE XANTHOMAS. Plane xanthomas occur in several areas of the body and are flat or slightly elevated (Figures 26-8 and 26-9). Xanthelasma is the most common form (see Figure 26-8). Xanthelasma can be associated with familial hypercholesterolemia, phenotype IIa or IIb, but 50% of the patients have normal cholesterol levels. Longevity studies have shown that xanthelasma, with or without hypercholesterolemia, is a risk factor for death from atherosclerotic disease. Further study of these patients with normal levels of cholesterol and triglycerides often reveals an elevated LDL and VLDL and decreased HDL. This profile is found for patients who have a high risk of atherosclerotic cardiovascular disease. Premature carotid atherosclerosis is observed in some patients with normolipidemic and hyperlipidemic xanthelasma. Patients with xanthelasma should be considered to have an increased risk of cardiovascular disease independent to the level of plasma lipids. It may be that all patients with xanthelasma have an increased risk for atherosclerosis.

Trichloroacetic acid (TCA) is commonly used for cosmetic treatment. Papulonodular lesions required an average of two applications with 100% TCA, three with 70% TCA, and four with 50% TCA. Flat plaques responded to an average of one, two, and three sittings with 100%, 70%,

Box 26-3 **Acquired Disorders of Lipoprotein Metabolism**

Hypercholesterolemia
Nephrotic syndrome
Hypothyroidism
Dysgammaglobulinemia
Acute intermittent porphyria
Obstructive liver disease

Combined hyperlipidemia
Nephrotic syndrome
Hypothyroidism
Glucocorticoid excess/Cushing's disease
Diuretics
Uncontrolled diabetes
Alcohol
Estrogens
β-Adrenergic blocking agents
Isotretinoin (13-*cis*-retinoic acid)

Hypertriglyceridemia
Diabetes mellitus
Uremia
Sepsis
Obesity
Systemic lupus erythematosus
Dysgammaglobulinemia
Glycogen storage disease, type I
Lipodystrophy
Drugs
Alcohol
Estrogens
β-adrenergic blocking agents
Isoretinoin (13-*cis*-retinoic acid)

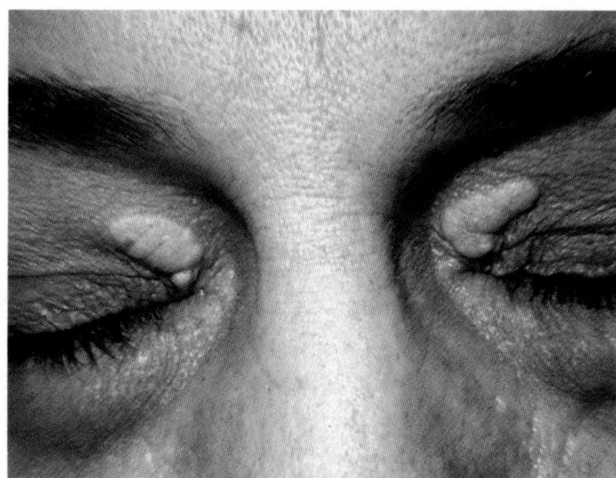

Figure 26-8 Xanthelasma. Lesions are usually located on the medial side of the lids.

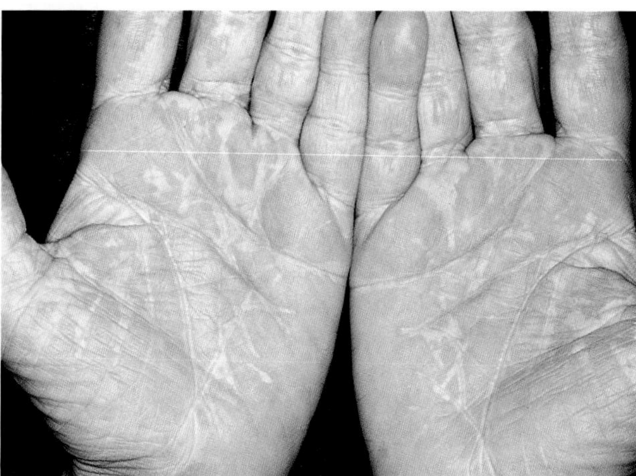

Figure 26-9 Plane xanthomas (macular) of the palms are characteristic of type III dysbetalipoproteinemia.

ERUPTIVE XANTHOMAS

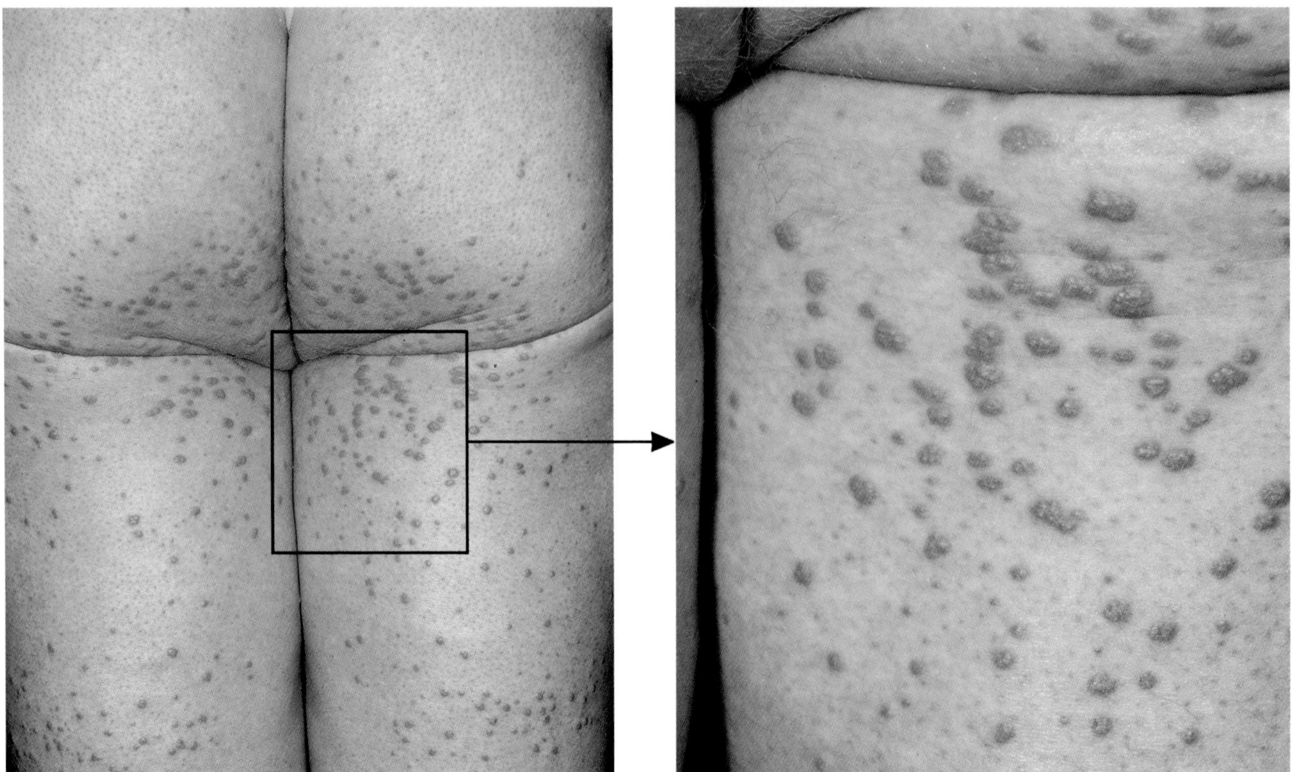

Figure 26-10 Eruptive xanthomas are found on the buttocks, shoulders, and the extensor surfaces of the extremities. The red-yellow papules erupt abruptly and may resolve in a few weeks. Pruritus is common. They are a sign of hypertriglyceridemia and appear in secondary hyperlipidemias (e.g., diabetes).

and 50% TCA, respectively. Macular lesions responded to only one application of all strengths of TCA applied. Hypopigmentation is the most common side effect, followed by hyperpigmentation. Scarring is a minor problem. *PMID: 16467024*

ERUPTIVE XANTHOMAS. These are yellow, 1- to 4-mm papules with a red halo around the base. They appear suddenly in crops on extensor surfaces of the arms, legs, and buttocks and over pressure points (Figure 26-10). Lesions clear rapidly when serum lipid levels are lowered.

TUBEROUS XANTHOMAS. These are slowly evolving yellow papules, nodules, or tumors that occur on the knees, elbows, and extensor surfaces of the body and the palms (Figure 26-11).

TENDINOUS XANTHOMAS. These smooth, deeply situated nodules are attached to tendons, ligaments, and fascia. They are most often found on the Achilles tendons and the dorsal aspects of the fingers.

REGRESSION OF XANTHOMAS. Certain xanthomas disappear with treatment. The eruptive and palmar xanthomas can regress rapidly. The eruptive type of tuberous xanthomas can disappear. Tendinous xanthomatous lesions tend to persist.

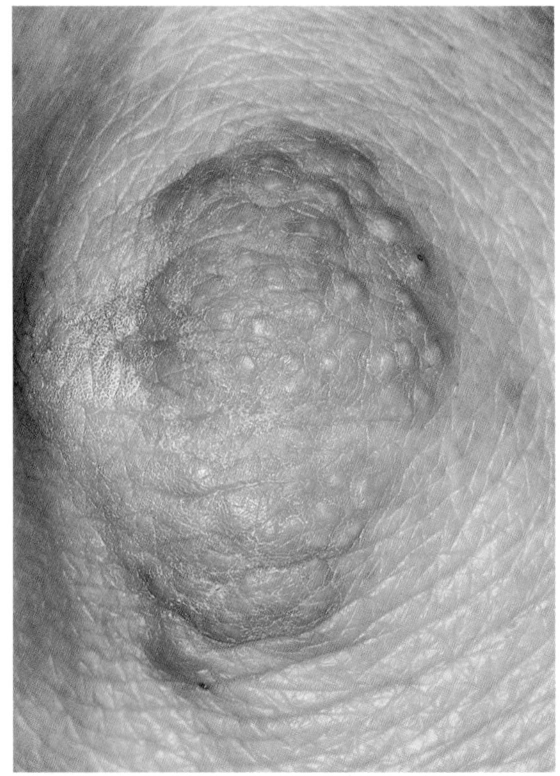

Figure 26-11 Tuberous xanthomas are painless, red-yellow nodules that develop in pressure areas.

NEUROFIBROMATOSIS

The neurofibromatoses comprise at least two autosomal dominant disorders with an incidence of approximately 1 in 3000. These diseases have tumors surrounding nerves. Neurofibromatosis 1 (NF1) is the most common and is characterized by congenital lesions of the skin, central nervous system, bone, and endocrine glands. The cardinal features of the disorder are café-au-lait spots, axillary freckling, cutaneous neurofibromas, and iris hamartomas (Lisch nodules). Common complications include learning disability, scoliosis, and optic gliomas. Neurofibromatosis 2 (NF2) is characterized by bilateral acoustic neuromas and other nerve tumors. Skin and other systemic manifestations are minimal or absent. Café-au-lait macules, freckling, and neurofibromas localized to a segment of the body are called segmental neurofibromatosis (NF5). The *NF1* gene is located on chromosome 17 and the *NF2* gene is found on chromosome 22.

NEUROFIBROMATOSIS 1. NF1 is a disorder of neural crest–derived cells characterized by the presence of café-au-lait spots, multiple neurofibromas, and Lisch nodules (pigmented iris hamartomas); there are several other less common features. There is considerable variation of manifestations within the same family. It occurs in approximately one of every 3500 births and affects both genders with equal frequency and severity. Neurofibromatosis is one of the most common mutations in humans; at least half of the cases represent new mutations.

CLINICAL MANIFESTATIONS

Café-au-lait spots. Café-au-lait spots are light-colored to brown macules (see Chapter 19). The criteria for establishing the diagnosis with reference to the number and size of café-au-lait spots are listed in Box 26-4. The spots are present in virtually every patient with neurofibromatosis, usually at birth, but they may not appear for months. Their size and number increase with age (Figure 26-12, *A*). Intertriginous freckling, a pathognomonic sign, may occur in the axillae, inframammary region, and groin (Figure 26-12, *B*). Café-au-lait macules alone are not absolutely diagnostic of NF1, regardless of their size and number.

Box 26-4 **Diagnostic Criteria for Neurofibromatosis 1 (NF1)**

Six or more café-au-lait macules
  1.5 cm in postpubertal individuals
  0.5 cm in prepubertal individuals
Two or more neurofibromas of any type ***or***
One or more plexiform neurofibromas
Freckling of axillae or inguinal area
Bilateral optic gliomas
Two or more Lisch nodules
Sphenoid wing dysplasia ***or***
Congenital bowing ***or***
Thinning of the long bone cortex (with or without pseudoarthrosis)
First-degree relative with NF1 by these criteria
  NF1 diagnosis: Two or more features

Adapted from National Institutes of Health Consensus Development Conference: Neurofibromatosis. Conference statement, *Arch Neurol* 45:576, 1988.

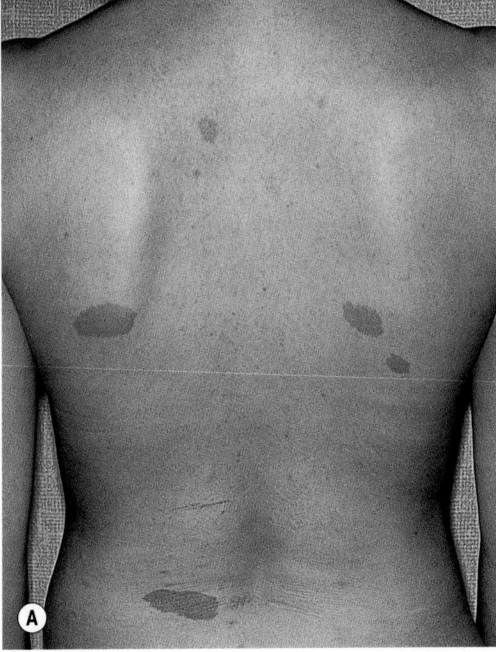

Café-au-lait spots vary in size and have a smooth border.

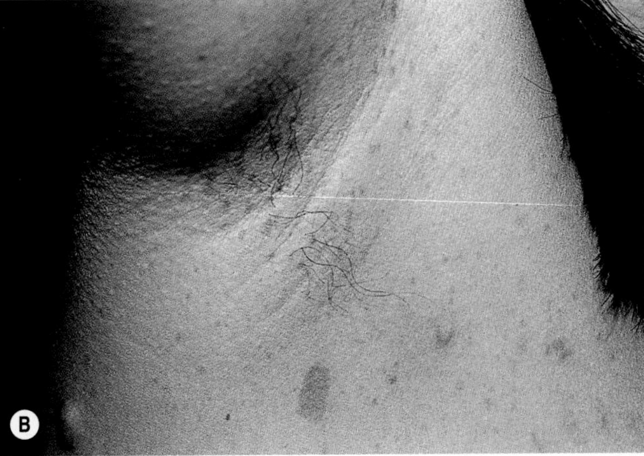

Axillary freckling (Crowe's sign) is a pathognomonic sign.

Figure 26-12 von Recklinghausen's neurofibromatosis.

PRESUMPTIVE EVIDENCE OF NEUROFIBROMATOSIS

- Six or more café-au-lait macules over 5 mm in greatest diameter if prepubertal
- Six or more café-au-lait macules over 15 mm in greatest diameter if postpubertal

NEUROFIBROMAS. Tumors are usually not present in childhood, but they begin to appear at puberty. Tumors increase in both number and size as the patient ages. Some patients have only a few small tumors, whereas others develop hundreds over the entire body surface, including the palms and soles (Figure 26-13).

There are three different types of cutaneous tumors. The most common is sessile or pedunculated. Early tumors are soft, dome-shaped papules or nodules that have a distinctive violaceous hue. Digital pressure on the soft tumor causes invagination or "button-holing." When the soft tumors attain a certain size, they bend and hang or become pendulous. The plexiform neuroma is an elongated tumor that occurs along the course of peripheral nerves. Elephantiasis neuromatosa is a term used to describe a diffuse tumor of nerve trunks that extends into surrounding tissues, causing gross deformity. This form of neuroma produced the facial deformity in Joseph Merrick of London, England, the man who was described in the play and movie *The Elephant Man*. Most tumors are benign, but malignant degeneration to a neurofibrosarcoma or malignant schwannoma has been reported in approximately 2% of cases; it rarely occurs before age 40.

LISCH NODULES. Lisch nodules (LNs) are pigmented, melanocytic, iris hamartomas (Figure 26-14). They increase in number with age and are asymptomatic. The prevalence of LNs and neurofibromas according to age is shown in Figure 26-15. All adults with neurofibromatosis who are 21 years of age or older have LNs. LNs have never been seen in the absence of neurofibromatosis. They are never the only clinical sign of NF1. They are more likely to be present in younger patients than are neurofibromas (see Figure 26-15) and therefore help to make the diagnosis in younger patients. No association has been found between LNs and overall clinical severity. They are markers for the von Recklinghausen's neurofibromatosis gene; they may be present in immediate relatives who have no cutaneous or other specific signs of the disease. LNs may be seen without the aid of instruments, but slit-lamp examination is essential for differentiation from iris freckles or nevi. Iris freckles are flat and have a lacework structure, whereas LNs are raised, round, dome-shaped, brown papules that are present in both eyes.

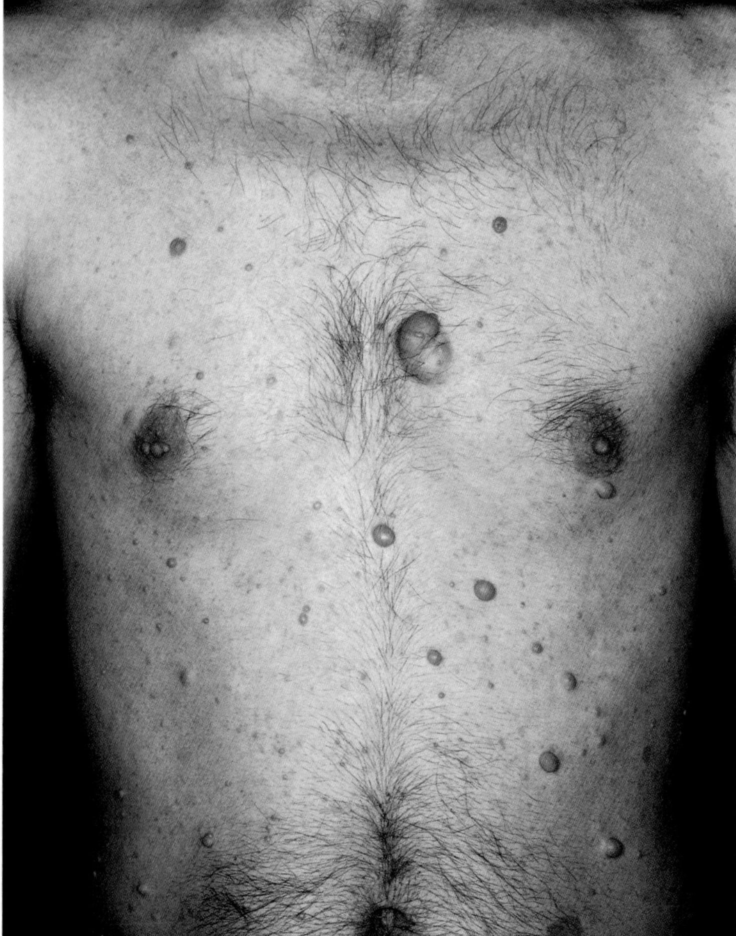

Figure 26-13 von Recklinghausen's neurofibromatosis. Adult patient with hundreds of neurofibromas.

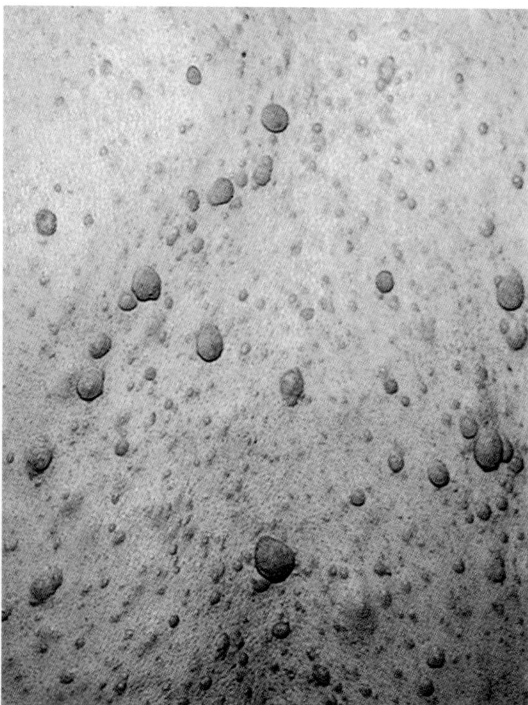

SYSTEMIC MANIFESTATIONS. Neurofibromatosis has a broad spectrum of systemic manifestations; the most important are listed in Box 26-5.

NATURAL HISTORY. Survival rates are significantly impaired for relatives with neurofibromatosis, are worse in probands, and are worst in female probands. Malignant neoplasms or benign central nervous system tumors occur in 45% of probands. Compared with the general population, male relatives with neurofibromatosis have the same rate of neoplasms, whereas female relatives have a nearly twofold higher rate. Nervous system tumors are disproportionately represented.

DIAGNOSIS. NF1 is considered to be present in an individual with two of the criteria listed in Box 26-4, provided no other disease accounts for the findings.

NF1 should be suspected in children with a large head circumference (above the 97th percentile for age) and one of the following: a mild cognitive impairment, a learning disability, or a selective visual-spatial impairment.

LISCH NODULES

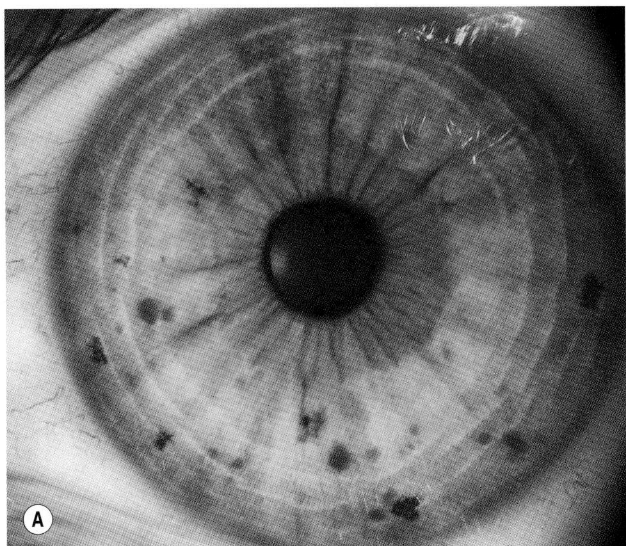

Pigmented iris hamartomas are present in more than 60% of patients with neurofibromatosis who are 7 years of age or older.

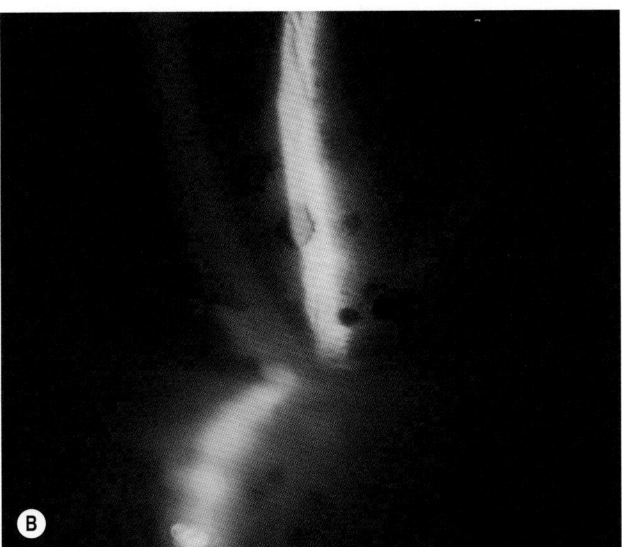

Slit-lamp examination is essential for differentiation from iris freckles. Iris freckles are flat and have a lace-work structure; Lisch nodules are raised, round, fluffy, and light brown. (Courtesy Lucian Szmyd, MD.)

Figure 26-14 von Recklinghausen's neurofibromatosis.

Box 26-5 **Systemic Manifestations of Neurofibromatosis**
Central nervous system tumors
Optic gliomas
Astrocytomas, acoustic neuromas, meningiomas, neurilemmomas
Constipation
Headache
Intellectual handicap
Kyphoscoliosis
Macrocephaly
Malignant disease
Neurofibrosarcoma
Malignant schwannoma
Neuroblastoma
Wilms' tumors
Rhabdomyosarcoma
Leukemia
Pheochromocytomas
Premature or delayed puberty
Pseudoarthrosis (tibia, radius)
Seizures
Speech impediment
Short stature

From Riccardi VM: *New Engl J Med* 305:1617, 1981. *PMID: 6796886*

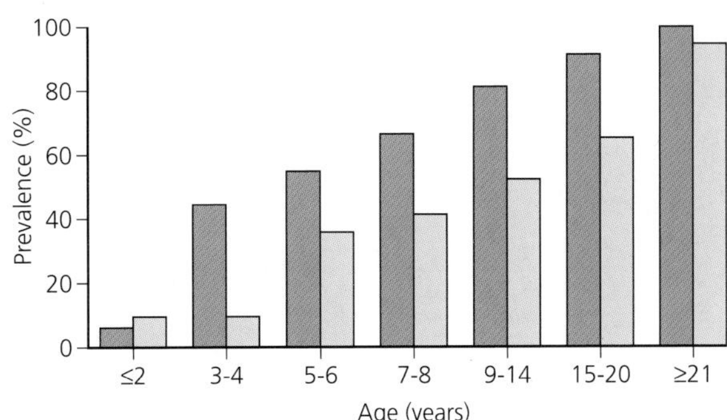

Figure 26-15 Prevalence of Lisch nodules (dark blue bars) and neurofibromas (light blue bars) in 167 patients with neurofibromatosis 1, according to age. (Modified from Lubs ML et al: *New Engl J Med* 324:1264, 1991.) *PMID: 1901624*

SEGMENTAL NEUROFIBROMATOSIS (NF5). Segmental neurofibromatosis (neurofibromatosis type 5) is a rare disorder characterized by café-au-lait macules and neurofibromas, or only neurofibromas, limited to one region of the body (Figure 26-16). Segmental neurofibromatosis has only been described in about 100 patients. The median age at onset is 28 years. The neurofibromas most commonly occupied either a cervical or a thoracic dermatome and were unilateral. Café-au-lait macules were present in 26% of patients. Axillary freckling occurs in only 10% of patients. Most patients with segmental neurofibromatosis (93%) do not have a family history of neurofibromatosis. The lesions are strictly unilateral and noninherited in most cases; however, in a few patients, the disease becomes generalized. These patients should be examined for LNs and other signs of neurofibromatosis.

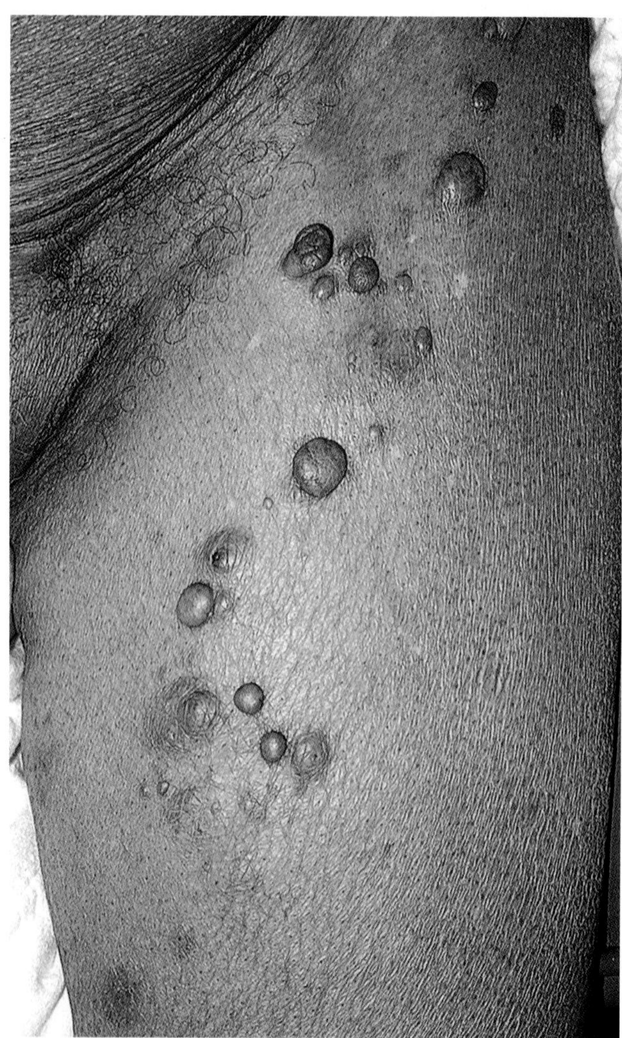

Figure 26-16 Segmental neurofibromatosis (NF5). Tumors are restricted to a segment of skin.

GENETIC COUNSELING. The patient's offspring, both male and female, have a 50% chance of inheriting this autosomal dominant disease. The penetrance is virtually 100%, but the expressivity is extremely variable. The severity of the disease is highest in those born to an affected mother. Fifty percent of cases are new mutations in which the parents are unaffected. All family members and relatives should be examined for the triad of Lisch iris nodules, solitary neurofibromas, and café-au-lait spots.

The LN is a reliable indicator of NF1; slit-lamp examination is important to establish the diagnosis. All people older than 20 years who have NF1 also have LNs. Therefore minimally affected and unaffected parents and adult siblings can be identified. If the diagnosis is in doubt and a child has no LNs, the examination should be repeated periodically. LNs often appear before neurofibromas. Adult siblings and adult children of affected persons can be counseled that their risk of having affected children is the same (approximately 1 in 3500) as that of the parents of patients with sporadic cases if all three elements of the triad are absent. Patients who have a segmental pattern of neurofibromatosis should be counseled that genetic transmission of their trait, though rare, is possible.

MANAGEMENT. There are more than 60 neurofibromatosis clinics in the United States. These clinics are usually based at teaching centers where a group of specialists provides a team approach to management. Internet resources are available.

Cutaneous tumors may be excised. The patient must be followed closely to detect malignant degeneration of neurofibromas. Genetic counseling is of utmost importance. Periodic complete evaluations are required to detect the numerous possible internal manifestations. Magnetic resonance imaging with gadolinium enhancement is the primary neuroimaging modality used for diagnosis, management, and screening of family members.

TUBEROUS SCLEROSIS

Tuberous sclerosis (epiloia) is an autosomal dominant disease of variable penetrance that is characterized by multiple hamartomas of the skin, central nervous system, kidneys, heart, retina, and other organs. The skin lesions (adenoma sebaceum, shagreen patch, white macules, or periungual fibromas) are reliable markers of the disease. Tuberous sclerosis (TS) affects at least 1 in 6000 people; two thirds of cases occur sporadically; one third are familial. Mildly affected individuals may be undiagnosed. The triad of epilepsy, angiofibromas (adenoma sebaceum), and mental retardation (the Vogt triad) that is typically associated with tuberous sclerosis is present in only 25% of patients. Mental retardation may be present in less than 50% of patients.

Box 26-6 **Revised Diagnostic Criteria for Tuberous Sclerosis Complex (TSC)***

Major features

1. Facial angiofibromas or forehead plaque
2. Nontraumatic ungual or periungual fibroma
3. Hypomelanotic macules (more than three)
4. Shagreen patch (connective tissue nevus)
5. Multiple retinal nodular hamartomas
6. Cortical tuber (a)
7. Subependymal nodule
8. Subependymal giant cell astrocytoma
9. Cardiac rhabdomyoma, single or multiple
10. Lymphangiomyomatosis (b)
11. Renal angiomyolipoma (b)

Minor features

1. Multiple randomly distributed pits in dental enamel
2. Hamartomatous rectal polyps (c)
3. Bone cysts (d)
4. Cerebral white matter migration lines (a, d, e)
5. Gingival fibromas
6. Nonrenal hamartoma (c)
7. Retinal achromic patch
8. "Confetti" skin lesions
9. Multiple renal cysts (c)

Definite TSC: Either two major features or one major feature with two minor features

Probable TSC: One major feature and one minor feature

Possible TSC: Either one major feature or two or more minor features

(a) When cerebral cortical dysplasia and cerebral white matter migration tracts occur together, they should be counted as one rather than two features of TSC.

(b) When both lymphangiomyomatosis and renal angiomyolipomas are present, other features of TSC should be present before a definitive diagnosis is assigned.

(c) Histologic confirmation is suggested.

(d) Radiographic confirmation is sufficient.

(e) One panel member recommended that three or more radial migration lines constitute a major feature.

*From the 1998 Tuberous Sclerosis Alliance Consensus Conference and National Institutes of Health Consensus Conference: Tuberous sclerosis complex, *Arch Neurol* 57(5):662, 2000.

DIAGNOSTIC CRITERIA. In July 1998 the Tuberous Sclerosis Alliance (www.tsalliance.org), then known as the National Tuberous Sclerosis Association, convened a consensus conference and developed a revised scheme for TS diagnostic criteria (Box 26-6).

The new diagnostic criteria eliminated any single finding as specifically distinctive or characteristic of the disease. Originally, cortical tubers were believed to be pathognomonic. Evidence now suggests that radiographic brain imaging and histologic studies are unable to distinguish these tubers from isolated cortical dysplasia. Two other types of brain lesions—subependymal giant cell astrocytomas and subependymal nodules—can be distinguished from cortical tubers and from each other. The two subependymal lesions have a histologic and radiographic appearance that differs from the cortical tuber, whereas the giant cell astrocytoma is the only one that tends to enlarge. It is important to distinguish between the three different brain lesions for identification and monitoring purposes. Dermatologic manifestations are especially important in diagnosing TS.

CLINICAL MANIFESTATIONS. The time course of tuberous sclerosis lesions is illustrated in Figure 26-17.

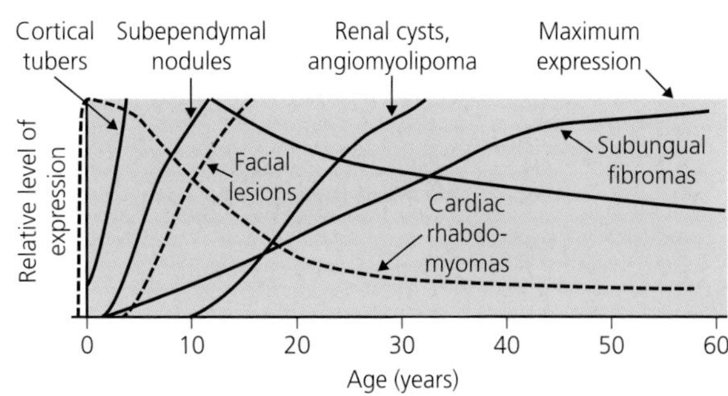

Figure 26-17

Adenoma sebaceum. Adenoma sebaceum is the most common cutaneous manifestation of tuberous sclerosis. The lesions consist of smooth, firm, 1- to 5-mm, yellow-pink papules with fine telangiectasia (Figure 26-18). Their color and location suggest an origin from sebaceous glands, but these growths are benign hamartomas composed of fibrous and vascular tissue (angiofibromas). The angiofibromas are located on the nasolabial folds, cheeks, chin, and, occasionally, on the forehead, scalp, and ears. The number varies from a few inconspicuous lesions to dense clusters of papules. They are rare at birth but may begin to appear by ages 2 to 3 years and proliferate during puberty. They may be mistaken for multiple trichoepitheliomas, an autosomal dominant condition that appears on the central face. A secondary feature, the "forehead plaque," is a large angiofibroma. Patients with the autosomal dominant disorder multiple endocrine neoplasia type 1 (MEN1) can develop multiple angiofibromas and several other types of cutaneous tumors in addition to tumors of pituitary, parathyroid, and enteropancreatic endocrine tissues.

Shagreen patch. The shagreen patch is highly characteristic of tuberous sclerosis and occurs in as many as 80% of patients; it occurs in early childhood and may be the first sign of disease. The lesion varies in size from 1 to 10 cm. There is usually one lesion, but several may be present. They are soft, flesh-colored to yellow plaques with an irregular surface that has been likened to pigskin (Figure 26-19). The lesion consists of dermal connective tissue and appears most commonly in the lumbosacral region.

Whitish macules and white tufts of hair. Hypomelanotic macules (oval, ash-leaf shaped, stippled, or "confetti shaped") are randomly distributed with a concentration on the arms, legs, and trunk. They are the earliest sign of tuberous sclerosis (Figure 26-20). They are present in 40% to 90% of patients with the disease and number from 1 to 32 in affected individuals. The white macules are present at birth and increase in number and size throughout life. They vary from 0.5 to 12 cm in diameter. The "confetti" macules are the rarest of the three types and consist of numerous 1- to 3-mm macules. Wood's light examination can be used to accentuate the white macules and is particularly useful for examining patients with light skin. A biopsy shows melanocytes, thus excluding the diagnosis of vitiligo. Hypopigmented macules, present at birth, are not invariably associated with tuberous sclerosis, but their presence is an indication for further study. It is essential that the diagnosis be established as soon as possible so that parents can obtain genetic counseling. A tuft of white hair with no depigmentation of the scalp skin underlying the white tuft has been reported as an early sign of tuberous sclerosis.

Periungual fibromas. Periungual fibromas appear at or after puberty in approximately 50% of cases. They are smooth, flesh-colored, conical projections that emerge from the nailfolds of the toenails and fingernails (Figure 26-21).

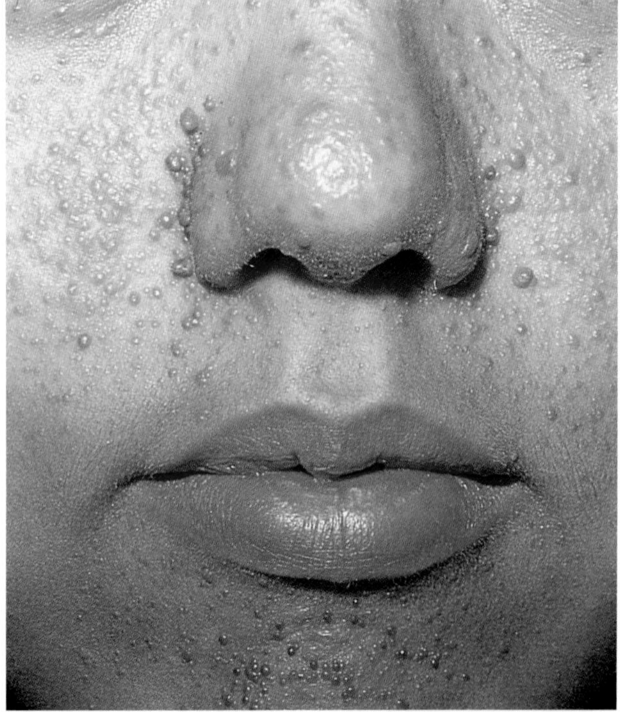

Figure 26-18 Adenoma sebaceum appears during childhood or early adolescence. These angiofibromas first appear as flat, pink macules and later become papular. Lesions may bleed easily.

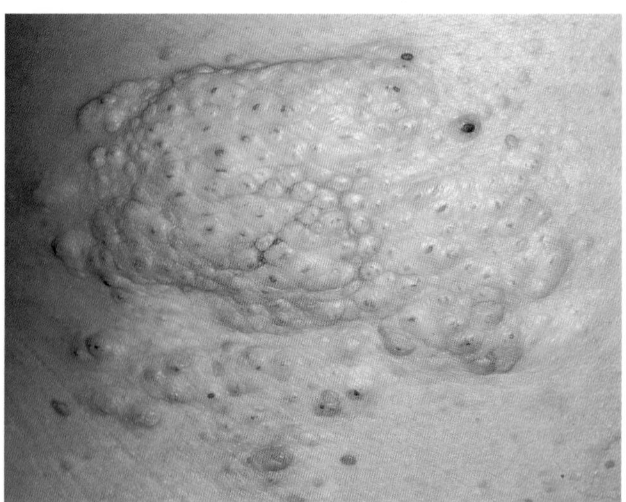

Figure 26-19 Shagreen patch is most commonly found in the lumbosacral region. The patch appears in childhood or early adolescence.

SYSTEMIC MANIFESTATIONS. Mental retardation occurs in less than 50% of cases. Subependymal nodules and cortical and white matter tubers are characteristic of tuberous sclerosis. Sclerotic patches (tubers) consisting of astrocytes and giant cells are scattered throughout the cortical gray matter. Calcium is deposited in tubers and may be detected shortly after birth by computed tomography (CT) scan, magnetic resonance imaging (MRI), or x-ray films and is found in 90% of affected children. Brain lesions cause seizures in more than 90% of patients. Benign tumors consisting of vascular fibrous tissue and fat and smooth muscle are found in numerous organs, including the kidneys, liver, and gastrointestinal tract. Gray or yellow retinal plaques occur in 25% of cases. The incidence of enamel pitting in the adult is 100%. A dental disclosing solution swabbed on dry teeth exposes the pits.

GENETIC COUNSELING. TS belongs to the family of tumor-suppressor-gene syndromes. These genes normally function as cellular "brakes." When they lose their function (as a result of mutations), uncontrolled proliferation and tumor formation occur. Affected patients typically have one inactivating mutation in either the *TSC1* or the *TSC2* gene in all germ-line and somatic cells. The patient's offspring, both male and female, have a 50% chance of inheriting this autosomal dominant disease. The penetrance is high, but expressivity is variable. Patients with normal parents acquire the disease from a new mutation.

Approximately 50% of tuberous sclerosis complex (TSC) families show genetic linkage to *TSC1* and 50% to *TSC2*. Among sporadic TSC cases, mutations in *TSC2* are more frequent and often accompanied by more severe neurologic deficits. Intellectual disability is significantly more frequent in *TSC2* sporadic cases than in *TSC1* sporadic cases. The *TSC1* (chromosome 9) and *TSC2* (chromosome 16) genes encode distinct proteins, hamartin and tuberin, respectively, that are widely expressed in the brain. Mosaicism is the phenomenon in which a fraction of, rather than all, germ-line and somatic cells contain a mutation of chromosomal abnormality. It occurs in all genetic disorders in which spontaneous mutations occur. Because of this phenomenon, some patients' mutation may not be detected with present methods of testing. The failure to detect mosaicism has important implications for genetic counseling.

The Tuberous Sclerosis Alliance provides information and support for physicians, patients, and families (www.tsalliance.org).

DIAGNOSIS AND MANAGEMENT. The diagnosis of tuberous sclerosis must be sought in infants with white macules, white hair tufts, or other cutaneous signs. The diagnosis may be established by demonstrating brain calcifications that may occur in early infancy. Brain lesions in tuberous sclerosis are of three kinds: cortical tubers, white matter abnormalities, and subependymal nodules. CT imaging demonstrates calcified subependymal nodules. MR imaging demonstrates more clearly cortical and white matter lesions than CT imaging. A positive scan result is often obtainable before the calcifications are present on skull x-ray films and even before the pathognomonic cutaneous findings appear.

Facial angiofibromas may be surgically removed for cosmetic purposes by electrosurgery, cryosurgery, dermabrasion, or lasers.

DIAGNOSTIC STUDIES. In newly diagnosed patients, testing helps to confirm the diagnosis and to identify complications. For patients with an established diagnosis, studies can identify treatable complications. Tests sometimes provide evidence of disease in asymptomatic relatives of children with tuberous sclerosis complex. Affected relatives who have abnormal tests usually have at least subtle findings.

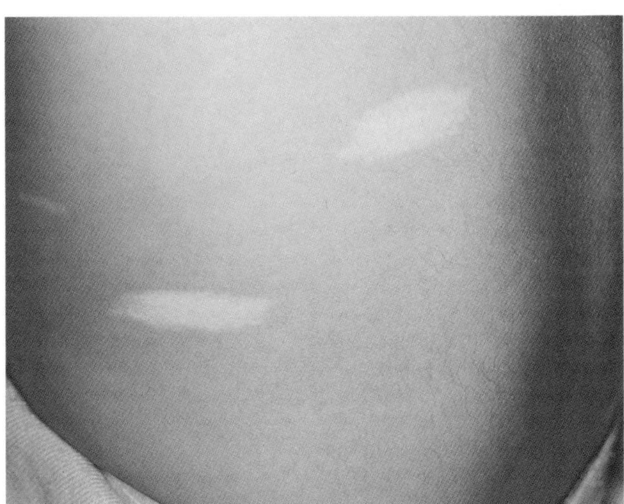

Figure 26-20 Ash-leaf macules (hypomelanotic macules) are often present at birth.

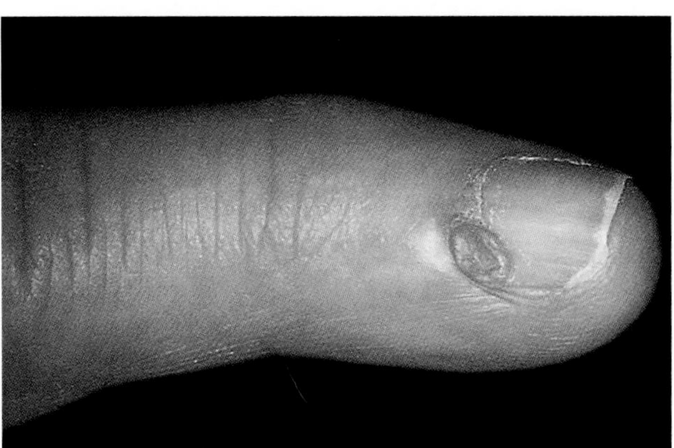

Figure 26-21 Tuberous sclerosis. Periungual fibromas.

INTERNAL CANCER AND SKIN DISEASE

The skin can be associated with internal malignancy in a variety of ways. The skin lesions may be a marker for an inherited syndrome (i.e., the genodermatoses), may represent a reaction to the tumor (the paraneoplastic syndromes) (Figure 26-23), may be caused by a carcinogen, may occur as a result of treatment, or may represent direct tumor extension or metastasis to the skin. These disease associations are listed in Tables 26-3 and 26-4.

Cutaneous paraneoplastic syndromes

Paraneoplastic syndromes (PNSs) are diseases that appear before or concurrently with an internal malignancy. They represent a remote or systemic effect of a neoplasm. There is a wide range of categories of PNSs, including endocrine, neurologic, hematologic, rheumatic, renal, and cutaneous. They may be the initial clue to the presence of an underlying neoplasm. The activity of a PNS can parallel the course of the tumor and thus be used as a marker of remission or recurrence. PNSs are estimated to occur in 7% to 15% of patients with cancer.

The cutaneous changes are thought to result from the production of biologically active hormones or growth factors, or antigen-antibody interactions induced by or produced by the tumor. Many of these syndromes, such as acanthosis nigricans, are proliferative skin disorders. Products secreted by the tumor, such as transforming growth factor alpha, may stimulate keratinocytes to proliferate.

FAMILIAL CANCER SYNDROMES

Many familial cancer syndromes have cutaneous signs that can help make a diagnosis. An overview of some of the familial cancer syndromes with cutaneous findings appears in Figure 26-24 and Table 26-4.

Oncologists or dermatologists may be the first to suspect a familial cancer syndrome when high-risk features are noted. These include a cluster of relatives within the patient's family who have the same or similar cancers, the development of cancer at a young age, or the presentation of more than one tumor or a second primary tumor. Many familial cancer syndromes have skin signs. These syndromes may occur as the result of a new mutation and present without a family history. The most common are hereditary breast and ovarian cancers, hereditary nonpolyposis colon cancer, and familial adenomatous polyposis. There are many other familial cancer syndromes, many of which have cutaneous signs. Patients suspected of having a familial cancer syndrome are referred to a genetic counselor or a clinical geneticist. Visit Mendelian Inheritance in Man (www.ncbi.nlm.nih.gov/omim/) for details of all familial syndromes.

Text continued on p. 996.

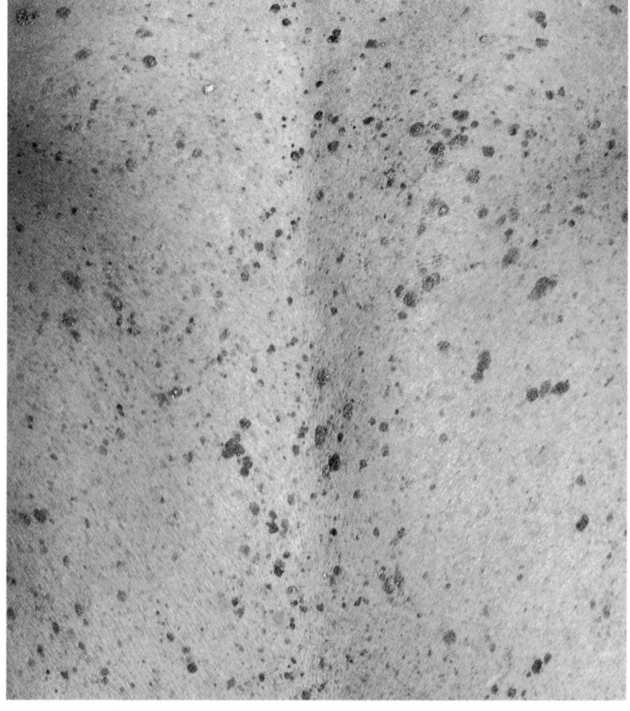

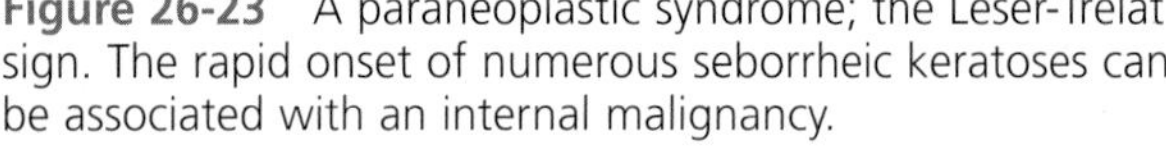

Figure 26-23 A paraneoplastic syndrome; the Leser-Trélat sign. The rapid onset of numerous seborrheic keratoses can be associated with an internal malignancy.

FAMILIAL MULTIPLE CANCER SYNDROMES
AUTOSOMAL DOMINANT 'CANCER FAMILY SYNDROMES'

Cowden's disease
(Multiple hamartoma syndrome)

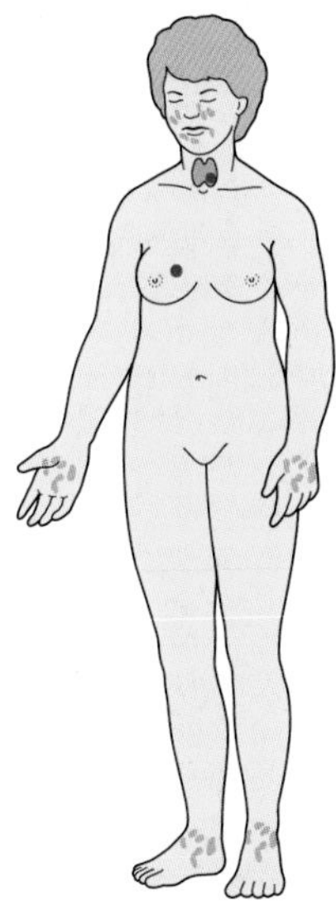

Females

Mucocutaneous lesions
- Facial papules
- Oral papules
- Hand keratosis

Breast lesions
- Cancer
- Fibrocystic

Thyroid
- Goiter
- Carcinoma

Muir-Torre syndrome

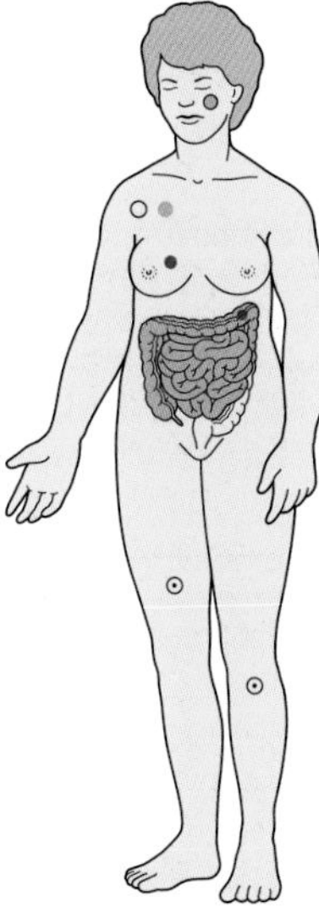

Males = females

Skin tumors
- Sebaceous gland (at least 1)

Keratoacanthomas

Internal tumors
- Colorectal
- Genitourinary
- Breast

Gardner's syndrome
(Familial adenomatous polyposis with extraintestinal manifestations)

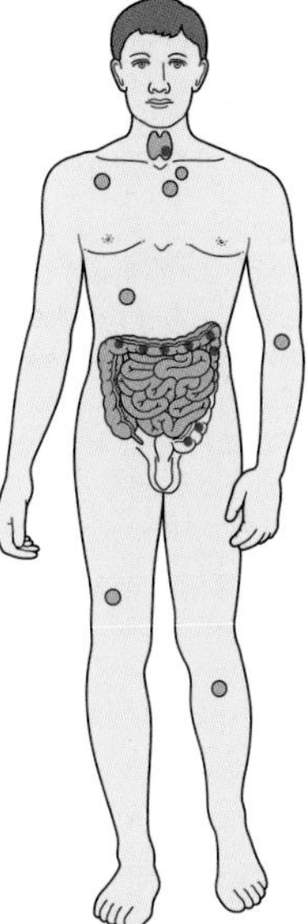

Males = females

Skin signs
- Epidermal cysts

Osteomas (palpable)
- Skull
- Jaw

Pigmented ocular fundus lesions

Colon
- Polyps > 100
- Adenocarcinoma

Thyroid carcinoma

• Solid tumors

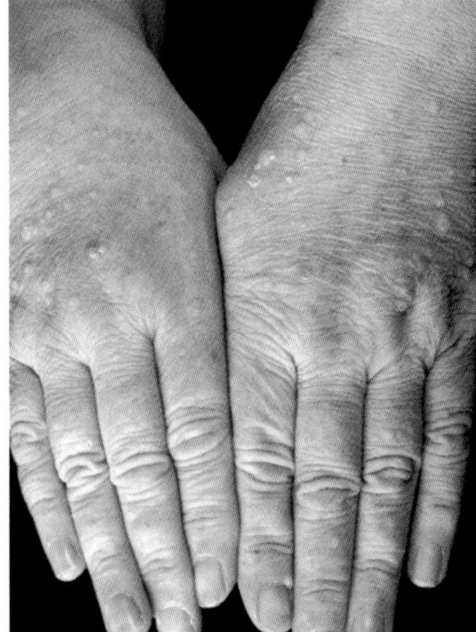

Acral keratosis

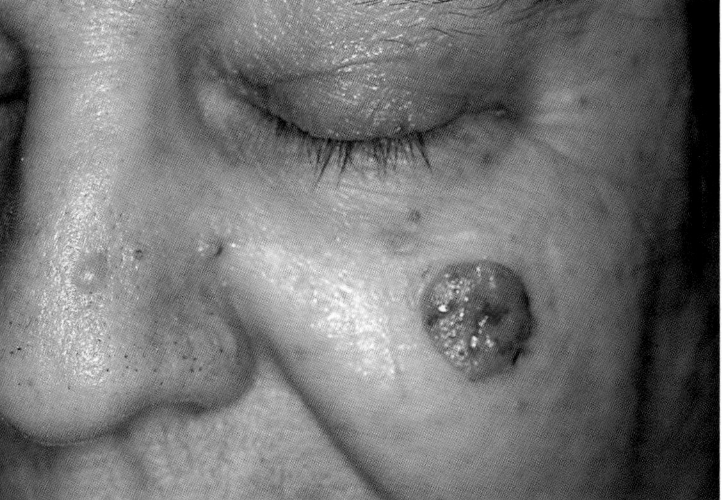

Sebaceous carcinoma

Figure 26-24

Table 26-3 Cutaneous Lesions and Internal Malignancy—Paraneoplastic Syndromes (Sorted Alphabetically)

Syndrome	Clinical presentation	Malignancy
Ataxia telangiectasia	Cerebellar ataxia, telangiectasia (e.g., pinna, bulbar conjunctiva)	Reticulum cell sarcoma, Hodgkin's lymphoma, gastric
Alopecia mucinosa	Patch of follicular papules and boggy infiltrate, face, trunk, scalp	Mycosis fungoides
Amyloidosis	Macroglossia; smooth tongue; shiny, translucent, waxy papules on eyelids, nasolabial folds, lips, and intertriginous areas; "pinch purpura"—skin bleeds with trauma	Multiple myeloma
Acanthosis nigricans	Adult onset in absence of obesity, endocrinopathy, and family history; hyperkeratotic, hyperpigmented skin folds in flexural areas (neck, axillae, antecubital fossa, breast, groin)	Abdominal cancer, other adenocarcinomas
Bazex's syndrome (acrokeratosis paraneoplastica)	Three stages: (1) psoriasiform lesions, tips of fingers and toes; (2) keratoderma, hands and feet; (3) lesions extend locally and new lesions appear on knees, legs, thighs, arms	Carcinoma of esophagus, tongue, lower lip, upper lobes of lungs
Bloom syndrome	Erythema face ("butterfly area"), stunted growth	Acute leukemia
Carcinoid syndrome	Episodes of flushing (face, neck, chest), dyspnea, asthma, diarrhea, murmur of pulmonary stenosis and insufficiency Dermatitis same as skin findings of pellagra: starts as an erythematous phototoxic eruption on sun-exposed regions; bullae appear and heal with hyperpigmentation	Serotonin-containing tumor of body parts such as appendix, small intestine, bronchus (i.e., usually one that has already metastasized to liver) Elevated urinary levels of 5-hydroxyindoleacetic acid
Cowden disease (multiple hamartoma syndrome)	Warty papules on face, hands, mouth	Breast, thyroid
Dermatomyositis (adult)	Heliotrope erythema eyelids, bluish-red plaques on knuckles (i.e., Gottron's sign), scaling violaceous plaques over elbows and knees; involvement of skin over back and shoulders (i.e., shawl sign); dilated capillary loops in cuticles, myopathy	Ovarian, cervical, lung, and pancreatic, gastric carcinomas, non-Hodgkin's lymphoma
Erythema gyratum repens	Rapidly moving waxy bands of erythema with serpiginous outline and "wood grain" pattern	Breast, lung, stomach, bladder, prostate Transitional cell carcinoma of kidney
Florid cutaneous papillomatosis	Pruritic papules that are indistinguishable from common viral warts; lesions first appear on dorsal aspects of hands and wrists and then spread to trunk and occasionally to face	Gastric adenocarcinoma and other intraabdominal cancers Cancers of breasts, lungs, lymph nodes
Gardner's syndrome	Epidermal cysts, cutaneous osteomas and fibromas, polyps in small and large intestine	Adenocarcinoma of colon
Glucagonoma syndrome	Migratory necrolytic erythema in intertriginous and dependent areas, elevated serum glucagon levels	Glucagon-secreting alpha cell tumor of pancreas
Hypertrichosis lanuginosa acquisita (acquired)	Lanugo-type (i.e., fetal) hair (malignant down) near eyebrows and on forehead, ears, nose; some patients have extensive involvement and hair is easily pulled out	Solid tumors of lung (both small and nonsmall cancers), colorectal tumors, breast malignancies
Hypertrophic osteoarthropathy and digital clubbing	Digital clubbing and periostitis with polyarthralgia	Peripheral non–small-cell lung cancer most common
Ichthyosis (acquired)	Generalized scaling, rhomboidal scales, prominent on trunk and extremities, spares flexural area	Hodgkin's disease; other lymphoproliferative malignancies; cancer of lung, breast, cervix
Kaposi's sarcoma	Red papular and nodular neoplasms most common on lower legs	Internal organ Kaposi's sarcoma, high incidence of other cancers
Leser-Trélat sign	Sudden appearance (3-6 months) and rapid increase in size and number of seborrheic keratoses; some cases arise in presence of chemotherapeutic agents such as cytarabine, and seborrheic keratoses become inflamed	Adenocarcinomas of stomach, lungs, colon, rectum, breasts
Melanosis (generalized)	Generalized cutaneous melanosis	Metastatic melanoma

Table 26-3 Cutaneous Lesions and Internal Malignancy—Paraneoplastic Syndromes (Sorted Alphabetically)—cont'd

Syndrome	Clinical presentation	Malignancy
Metastases to skin	Metastasis to any cutaneous site	Variety of tumors
Muir-Torre syndrome	Multiple sebaceous adenomas	Visceral carcinomas
Multicentric reticulohistiocytosis	Reddish-brown papular skin lesions in association with progressive development of severe destructive arthritis; lesions on face, hands, ears, and forearms; 50% have oral mucosal involvement	One third of cases associated with malignancy Cancers of breasts, lungs, muscles, gastrointestinal and genitourinary tracts, and hematologic system
Paget's disease (breast)	Eczematous crusted lesion of nipple, areola	Breast
Paget's disease (extramammary)	Eroded scaling plaques of vulva, scrotum, axillae, perianal, groin	Cervical cancer and adenocarcinoma of anus and rectum
Palmoplantar keratoderma (tylosis)	Skin thickening of palms and soles; leads to irregular, cobblestone appearance of skin	Breast, lung, gastric cancers, leukemias, lymphomas
Paraneoplastic pemphigus	Painful, intractable, erosive ulcerative stomatitis and polymorphic cutaneous eruption (erythema, papules, iris lesions, bullae, erosions)	Non-Hodgkin's lymphoma (80%), chronic lymphocytic leukemia, Castleman disease, thymoma, and Waldenström macroglobulinemia
Peutz-Jeghers syndrome	Pigmented macules on lips and oral mucosa, polyposis of small intestine	Adenocarcinoma of stomach, duodenum, colon
Pityriasis rotunda	Scaly, circular, hyperpigmented patches on trunk, buttocks, and thighs Lesions are 1-3 cm or larger May become confluent and polycyclic Scale is similar to that of ichthyosis vulgaris. Hyperpigmented in dark-skinned individuals and hypopigmented in light-skinned individuals	Hepatocellular and gastric carcinoma; leukemia, lymphoma, upper gastrointestinal carcinomas, prostate cancer
Sipple's syndrome	Multiple mucosal neuromas	Medullary carcinoma of thyroid, C-cell neoplasia, pheochromocytoma
Sweet's syndrome	Fever, neutrophilia, tender erythematous plaques on upper extremities and face and begin as tender, erythematous plaques or nodules Elevated erythrocyte sedimentation rate More common in women	Underlying cancer in 20% of cases; 80% of cases involve hematologic malignancies; acute myeloid leukemia is most common
Tripe palms	Rugose, velvety palms Often occur simultaneously with other paraneoplastic syndromes Acanthosis nigricans occurs in 75% of cases of tripe palms	Gastrointestinal and lung malignancies most common; head and neck, genitourinary (ovarian) system
Trousseau's syndrome	An acquired hypercoagulability with recurrent superficial thrombophlebitis Thrombi occur in arterial or venous system Tender erythematous cords or nodules typically appear in subcutaneous fat over trunk or extremities	50% of cases associated with cancer; lung cancers, pancreatic cancer
Urticaria pigmentosa (disseminated maculopapular form)	Brown-red macules and papules that contain mast cells and urticate when traumatized	Hematologic malignancies
von Hippel-Lindau disease	Angiomas of skin, angiomatosis of cerebellum or medulla	Hypernephroma, pheochromocytoma
Von Recklinghausen's neurofibromatosis	Café-au-lait spots, white macules, multiple cutaneous neuromas, internal neuromas	Malignant neurilemmoma, astrocytoma, pheochromocytoma
Wiskott-Aldrich syndrome	Eczematous lesions in atopic dermatitis distribution	Reticuloendothelial malignancy

Table 26-4 Some Familial Cancer Syndromes with Cutaneous Findings

Presenting cancer	Skin lesion	Age of onset of skin lesions	Distribution	Syndrome	OMIM*	Risk of other malignancy	Other features
Colorectal	Sebaceous carcinoma or adenoma; keratoacanthoma	5th-6th decades	Facial, mainly meibomian glands	Muir-Torre phenotype of HNPCC	120435	Endometrial cancer; ovarian cancer; tumors within HNPCC spectrum	Can precede development of visceral tumors
Colorectal; CNS; hematologic	Café-au-lait macules	Childhood	Generalized; trunk	Biallelic mutations in mismatch repair genes	120435	Early-onset cancers	Family members might be heterozygous, risks similar to HNPCC
Bowel polyps	Mucocutaneous pigmentation	Childhood	Centrofacial; oral mucosa; perianal	Peutz-Jeghers syndrome	175200/ 602216	Cancer of colon, stomach, pancreas; breast cancer; ovarian cancer; SCTAT	Gynecomastia; intussusception
Colorectal cancer with polyps	Epidermoid cysts; fibromas; lipomas; pilomatricomas	Adulthood	Mainly facial	Familial adenomatous polyposis (Gardner's syndrome)	175100	Colorectal cancer; small-bowel cancer; CNS tumors; hepatoblastoma; thyroid cancer	Many colonic polyps; osteomas; supernumerary teeth
Renal cancer (chromophobe renal-cell cancer, hybrid chromophobe-oncocytomas)	Triad of lesions including fibrofolliculomas, trichodiscomas, and acrochordons	3rd decade	Face; neck; upper trunk	Birt-Hogg-Dubé syndrome	135150	Renal cancer; colonic polyps; colorectal cancer	Pulmonary cysts; pneumothorax
Renal-cell carcinoma (type II papillary renal cancer)	Cutaneous leiomyomas	3rd decade	Face; extensor surfaces of extremities; back	Hereditary leiomyomatosis renal-cell carcinoma	605839	Uterine fibroids and leiomyosarcoma; cutaneous leiomyosarcoma	Lesions are painful in cold weather
Renal-cell carcinoma	Angiofibromas; ash-leaf macules; shagreen patch; fibroma	Childhood	Centrofacial; back; subungual	Tuberous sclerosis	191100	Angiomyolipomas; renal-cell carcinoma; astrocytoma	CNS seizures
Optic glioma; meningioma; astrocytoma	Café-au-lait macules; neurofibromas; freckling in axillae or groin	Childhood	Trunk	Neurofibromatosis type 1	162200	Neurofibrosarcoma; glioma; rhabdomyosarcoma; pheochromocytoma; duodenal carcinoid	Lisch nodules on eyes; pseudoarthrosis tibia; macrocephaly

Adapted from *Lancet Oncol* 9(5):462-472, 2008. *PMID: 18452857*

*OMIM is the Online Mendelian Inheritance in Man (www.ncbi.nlm.nih.gov/omim/).

HPNCC, hereditary nonpolyposis colorectal cancer; *LAMB,* lentigines, atrial myxomas, blue nevus; *NAME,* nevus, atrial myxoma, ephilides; *SCTAT,* sex-cord tumors with annular tubules; *VIPoma,* vasoactive intestinal peptide tumor.

Table 26-4 Some Familial Cancer Syndromes with Cutaneous Findings—cont'd

Presenting cancer	Skin lesion	Age of onset of skin lesions	Distribution	Syndrome	OMIM*	Risk of other malignancy	Other features
Prolactinoma	Angiofibromas; collagenomas; café-au-lait macules; subcutaneous lipoma	Early adulthood	Angiofibroma: face; other lesions: neck, arms, trunk	Multiple endocrine neoplasia 1	131100	Pancreatic islet, parathyroid, and adrenal cortex adenomas (i.e., glucagonoma, insulinoma, and VIPoma)	Primary hyperparathyroidism in 3rd decade is first sign; Cushing's syndrome; acromegaly; hypogonadism; Zollinger-Ellison syndrome
Medullary thyroid cancer; pheochromocytoma; primary parathyroid hyperplasia	Cutaneous lichen amyloidosis	Pruritus from infancy Cutaneous lichen amyloidosis precedes medullary thyroid cancer	Interscapular	Multiple endocrine neoplasia 2A	171400	Medullary thyroid cancer usually precedes pheochromocytoma by 10 years Pheochromocytoma usually adrenal and bilateral	Primary hyperparathyroidism
Medullary thyroid cancer; pheochromocytoma	Pedunculated nodules; mucosal neuromas; corneal neuromas; flushing	Pruritus from infancy Cutaneous lichen amyloidosis precedes medullary thyroid cancer	Eyelids; cornea	Multiple endocrine neoplasia 2B (Wagenmann-Frobese syndrome)	162300	Aggressive thyroid cancer with early onset and early metastases	Marfanoid body habitus; coarse facial features; developmental delay
Breast cancer; follicular thyroid cancer; endometrial cancer	Facial trichilemmomas; acral keratoses; papillomatosis of oral mucosa	Pruritus from infancy Cutaneous lichen amyloidosis precedes medullary thyroid cancer	Face; palmar, plantar, oral mucosa	Cowden syndrome (*PTEN* hamartoma tumor syndrome)	158350	Ovarian cancer; prostate cancer; transitional-cell bladder cancer; glioblastoma multiforme; colon cancer	Macrocephaly; Lhermitte-Duclos disease; facial phenotype; skeletal anomalies
Atrial myxoma; primary pigmented adrenocortical nodular hypoplasia; psammomatous melanotic schwannomas	Pigmentation; lentigines; blue nevus; cutaneous myxomas	Early adulthood	Centrofacial and genital pigmentation	Carney complex (LAMB or NAME syndrome)	160980	Pituitary tumors	Primary pigmented adrenocortical nodular Cushing's hypoplasia causes syndrome and acromegaly
Basal-cell carcinoma	Acrochordons; palmar/plantar pits; epidermal cysts; nevi	Childhood, but more likely in late teens and early adulthood	Basal-cell carcinoma: face; nevi: generalized	Nevoid basal-cell carcinoma syndrome (Gorlin's syndrome)	109400	Medulloblastoma	Coarse face; skeletal anomalies; odontogenic keratocytes of jaw

Cowden disease (multiple hamartoma syndrome)

Cowden disease (multiple hamartoma syndrome) is a multisystem disease inherited as an autosomal dominant trait with incomplete penetrance and variable expression.

The incidence is estimated to be 1 in 200,000. It is characterized by multiple hamartomas of ectodermal, endodermal, and mesodermal origin and a high incidence of malignant tumors of the breast and/or thyroid gland. The mucocutaneous manifestations are the most characteristic feature and are the key to diagnosis. The diagnostic criteria for Cowden disease are listed in Box 26-7.

Box 26-7 **Cowden Disease Diagnostic Criteria**

Pathognomonic criteria

Mucocutaneous lesions

- Multiple facial trichilemmomas
- Mucosal lesions
- Acral keratoses

Major criteria

Breast cancer
Thyroid cancer, especially follicular thyroid carcinoma
Macroencephaly
Hamartomatous outgrowths of cerebellum (Lhermitte-Duclos disease)

Minor criteria

Thyroid lesions (e.g., adenoma or goiter)
Mental retardation (IQ 75)
Hamartomatous intestinal polyps
Fibrocystic disease of the breast
Lipomas
Fibromas
Genitourinary tumors or malformations

Operational diagnosis for individual

(1) Mucocutaneous lesions alone if
  a. Six facial papules with three trichilemmomas
  b. Cutaneous facial papules and oral mucosal papillomatosis
  c. Oral mucosal papillomatosis and acral keratoses
  d. Six or more palmar/plantar keratoses
  or
(2) Two major criteria, but one must include macrocephaly or Lhermitte-Duclos disease
  or
(3) One major and three minor criteria
  or
(4) Four minor criteria

Adapted from Lindor NM, Greene MH: *J Natl Cancer Inst* 90:1059, 1998; and Tsao H: *J Am Acad Dermatol* 42:939, 2000. *PMID: 10827397*

MUCOCUTANEOUS LESIONS. Facial papules and oral mucosal papillomatosis are the most sensitive indicators of the disease. The asymptomatic cutaneous lesions are usually noticed at age 20, and no further progression of lesions is seen after the age of 30. The principal cutaneous lesion is a papule that may be smooth or keratotic. Cutaneous facial papules are of two types: lichenoid, flesh-colored, flat-topped papules are found in the centrofacial and periorificial areas; and flesh-colored, elongated, verrucoid, papillomatous lesions are found clustered around the mouth (Figure 26-25), nose, eyes, and on the ears. The majority of these lesions are trichilemmomas. The differential diagnosis of these facial papules includes Darier's disease and adenoma sebaceum found in tuberous sclerosis. Acral keratoses are located primarily on the dorsum of the hands and feet. They resemble flat warts (i.e., they are flesh-colored, flat-topped papules 1 to 4 mm in diameter). Palmoplantar keratoses are isolated, pinpoint-to-pea-sized, translucent, hard papules that may show a central depression.

The oral lesions are white, smooth-surfaced papules, 1 to 3 mm in diameter, that often coalesce, giving a cobblestone appearance. They are located primarily on the gingival, labial, and palatal surfaces.

BREAST LESIONS. Breast lesions are the most important and potentially serious abnormality of Cowden disease. Ductal adenocarcinoma occurs in more than 30% of patients, and fibrocystic disease occurs in 60% of patients. The median age of diagnosis of breast cancer is 41 years. All women with Cowden disease should be considered for prophylactic bilateral total mastectomy by their third decade of life.

THYROID GLAND LESIONS. Palpable enlargement (goiter and adenoma) is the most frequently reported internal abnormality of Cowden disease. Carcinoma is reported in several cases.

A wide variety of other abnormalities and malignancies have been reported, but the incidence is low.

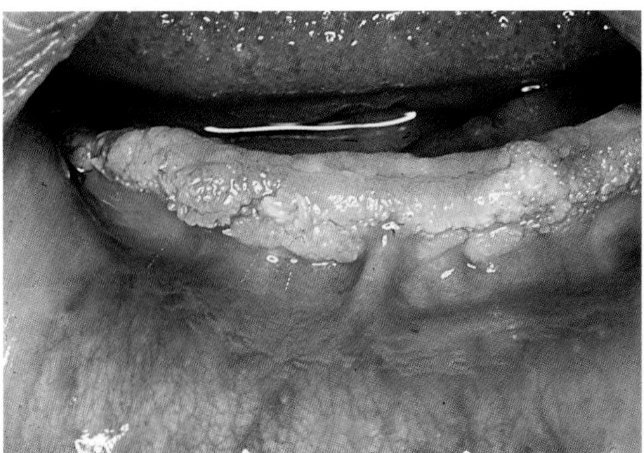

Figure 26-25 Cowden disease. White oral papules often coalesce.

Muir-Torre syndrome

Muir-Torre syndrome (MTS) is a rare autosomal dominant genodermatosis characterized by at least one sebaceous gland tumor and a minimum of one internal malignancy. The common presentation is the presence of sebaceous tumors along with a low-grade visceral malignancy. The presence of sebaceous tumors warrants a search for an internal malignancy. This syndrome is now considered a subtype of the more common hereditary nonpolyposis colorectal cancer (HNPCC) syndrome. MTS and HNPCC syndrome are associated with *hMSH2* gene mutations.

SKIN TUMORS. Sebaceous tumors appear before the internal malignancy in 22% of patients concurrently in 6% of patients, and after the internal malignancy in 56% of patients. The sebaceous gland tumors (adenoma, sebaceoma, epithelioma, or carcinoma) usually occur on the trunk, face, and scalp (Figure 26-26). They vary from small, asymptomatic papules or nodules that resemble cysts or benign tumors to waxy papules. The syndrome may occur in individuals with a single sebaceous gland tumor. Some benign sebaceous neoplasms in MTS might have a high potential for malignant transformation or may be well-differentiated sebaceous carcinomas with low-grade malignancy, mimicking sebaceous adenoma/sebaceoma.

Single or multiple keratoacanthomas occur in approximately 20% of patients. The median age for the appearance of the skin lesions is 53 years (range, 23 to 89 years). Sebaceous gland tumors in the general population are rare. A tumor diagnosed as a sebaceous adenoma, sebaceous epithelioma, or sebaceous carcinoma should alert the clinician to the possibility of visceral cancer both in the patient and in family members. Sebaceous hyperplasia commonly seen on the face is not associated with malignancy.

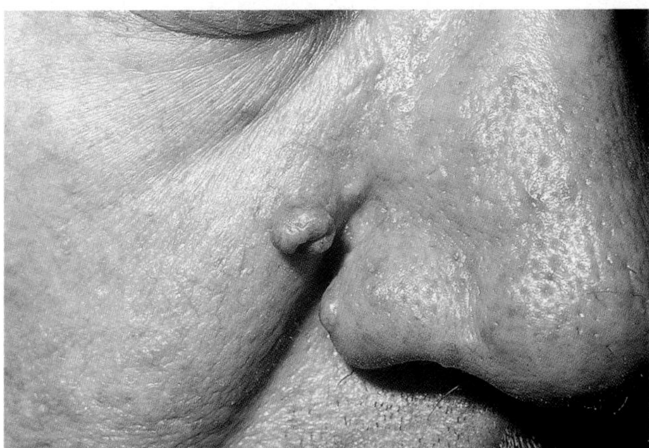

Figure 26-26 Muir-Torre syndrome. A sebaceous adenoma is the most characteristic marker of the disease.

INTERNAL TUMORS. The most commonly associated neoplasms are colorectal (47%); 58% of these tumors occur proximal to or at the splenic flexure.

MTS patients have a genetic predilection to hereditary nonpolyposis colorectal cancer (HNPCC). There are at least eight other major cancer susceptibility syndromes that infer an increased risk for colorectal cancer and/or colorectal polyposis. Therefore the differential diagnosis of hereditary colorectal cancer can be complex. Genitourinary tumors (21%), breast carcinomas (12%), and hematologic disorders (9%) are also common. Fifty-three percent of patients develop one cancer, 37% develop two to three cancers, and 10% develop four to nine cancers. Cutaneous lesions occur before or concurrent with the diagnosis of the initial cancer in 63% of patients. The median age for the detection of the initial visceral neoplasm is 53 years (range, 23 to 89 years). A few cases have been associated with polyps in the colon, but widespread gastrointestinal polyposis is rare. There is a relatively low potential for malignancy in both cutaneous and internal tumors, but metastasis from internal malignancies does occur, particularly from colon cancer.

EPIDEMIOLOGY. Muir-Torre syndrome may appear de novo, but there is often a variable family history of cutaneous and/or internal tumors. Males and females are equally affected. This may be one of the four subtypes of cancer family syndrome characterized by a genetically determined (autosomal dominant) predisposition to multiple visceral malignancies that arise at an early age and pursue a relatively benign course. As in cancer family syndrome, colon cancers in Muir-Torre syndrome are often more proximal to the splenic flexure than in the general populace.

MANAGEMENT. Regular follow-up and searches for new malignancy and also evaluation and monitoring of family members are necessary. Patients and their families should be counseled about genetic predisposition.

TREATMENT. The combination of interferon with isotretinoin or isotretinoin alone may prevent tumor development.

Gardner's syndrome

Gardner's syndrome (familial adenomatous polyposis with extraintestinal manifestations) is an autosomal dominantly transmitted disease with a similar penetrance in both genders of nearly 100%. It consists of intestinal polyposis, epidermal cysts, multiple osteomas, mesenteric fibromas, desmoid tumors, pigmented ocular fundus lesions, unerupted teeth, and odontomas. The incidence is approximately 1 of 8300 to 1 of 16,000 births. The adenomatous polyposis coli *(APC)* gene on chromosome 5q21 is altered by point mutations in the germ line of Gardner's syndrome patients. The identification of these genes should aid in the counseling of patients with genetic predispositions to colorectal cancer.

CUTANEOUS SIGNS. Polyposis is a nearly constant feature, but epidermal cysts occur in approximately 35% of cases. Epidermal cysts are frequently the presenting complaint and appear most often on the head and neck, but they frequently also occur in areas such as the legs, where epidermal cysts are rarely found. Gardner's syndrome should be considered in patients with epidermal cysts in unusual areas. The cysts can occur in childhood, but the average age at onset is 13 years. They range from a few to many lesions and can be small or large enough to distort normal structures. Osteomas can be recognized clinically and radiographically in childhood. They most commonly appear on the head and neck and can be seen and felt.

Osteomas. Multiple osteomas, especially of the skull and jaws, are found in a number of affected and at-risk relatives. In some, these "markers" are found early in life, before the appearance of colonic polyps. Radiography of the jaws may serve as a valuable tool for the early detection of carriers of Gardner's syndrome.

Pigmented ocular fundus lesions. Pigmented ocular fundus lesions are a reliable clinical marker for the disease and are found in 90% of patients and 47% of relatives who are at a 50% risk for Gardner's syndrome. The presence of bilateral lesions, multiple lesions (more than four), or both is a specific and sensitive clinical marker for the syndrome. The lesions are discrete, darkly pigmented, and round, oval, or kidney shaped; they range in size from 0.1 to 1 (or more) optic-disc diameters. A total of 1 to 30 lesions may be present.

Thyroid carcinoma. Carcinoma of the thyroid gland is frequently reported in these patients. It has the following characteristics: female predominance (89%), youth (average 23.6 years; range, 16 to 40 years), papillary form (88%), and multicentricity (70%).

Colonic polyps and cancer. Colonic polyps can be detected before the patient reaches puberty. They are usually asymptomatic, number greater than 100, and invariably progress to adenocarcinoma. Sulindac reduces the number and size of colorectal adenomas in patients with familial adenomatous polyposis, but its effect is incomplete, and it is unlikely to replace colectomy as primary therapy. Gardner's syndrome patients who undergo aggressive bowel surgery when polyps are detected can have a normal life span. All family members should be examined. Genetic counseling is essential for this autosomal dominantly inherited disease.

Birt-Hogg-Dubé syndrome and renal carcinoma

Birt-Hogg-Dubé syndrome (BHD) is an autosomal dominant genodermatosis of unknown incidence characterized by skin fibrofolliculomas, an increased risk of spontaneous pneumothorax, and renal and possibly other tumors. The fibrofolliculomas tend to appear in the third or fourth decade of life. Trichodiscomas and other cutaneous tumors (angiofibromas) have been reported. Clinical features are variable. Some patients have numerous papules and others have none (Figure 26-27).

Fibrofolliculomas and trichodiscomas are benign hair follicle hamartomas, which usually present as many small asymptomatic skin-colored papules on the face, neck, scalp, and upper trunk.

The prevalence of spontaneous pneumothorax and renal tumors is low. Various other extracutaneous tumors are reported. Colorectal cancer is not part of this syndrome. BHD should be suspected in patients with few or even without fibrofolliculomas and/or trichodiscomas who may present with (familial) renal tumors (hybrid oncocytic tumor, chromophobe renal cell carcinoma, clear cell tumors, oncocytoma) and/or spontaneous pneumothorax. Older age and male gender increase the risk for renal tumors. Chromophobe renal cell carcinomas are locally invasive but rarely metastasize. Tumors less than 3 cm are observed, whereas tumors larger than 3 cm are treated with nephron-sparing procedures including partial nephrectomy. The risk of spontaneous pneumothorax is inversely associated with age. Between 15% and 30% of BHD-affected patients develop renal cancers. Patients develop renal tumors in their 20s or 30s and often present with multiple, bilateral renal cancers.

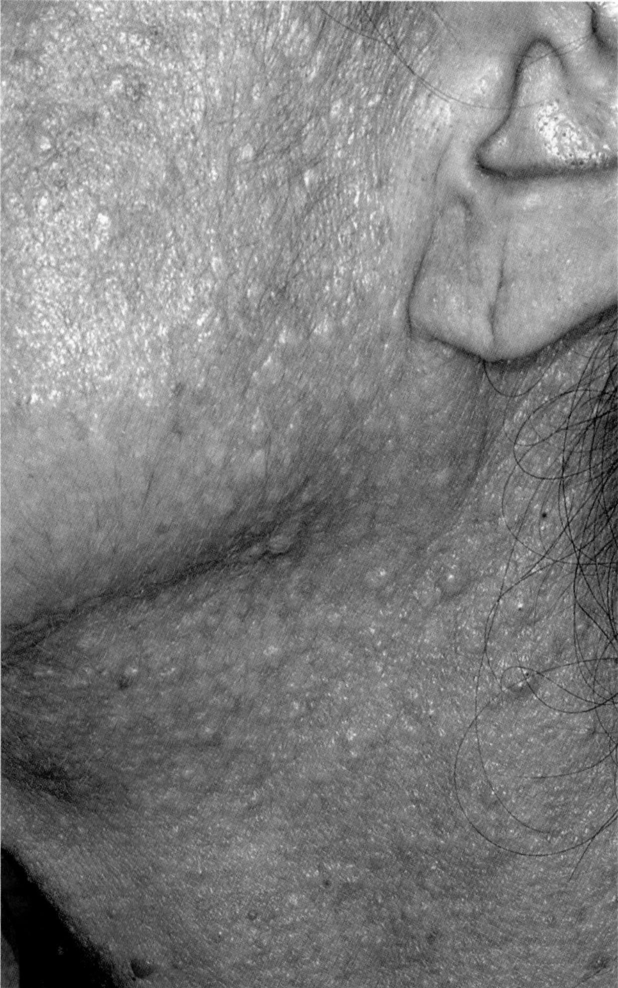

Figure 26-27 Birt-Hogg-Dube syndrome. Multiple, small, skin-colored, dome-shaped papules distributed over the face, neck, and upper trunk.

Index

A

Page references followed by a *f,t,* or *b* indicate figures, tables, or boxes, respectively. Entries preceded by [online icon] can be found online.

B

C

D

E

F

G

H

I

J

K

L

M

O

R

S

T

U

X

Y

Z

CORTICOSTEROIDS (TOPICAL)*

Group	Brand name	%	Generic name	(gm; unless noted)
I	Clobex shampoo	0.05	Clobetasol propionate	4 oz
	Clobex spray			2 oz, 4.25 oz
	Clobex lotion			4 oz
	Condran tape		Flurandrenolide	3×24, 3×80 roll
	Cormax cream	0.05	Clobetasol propionate	15, 30, 45
	Cormax ointment	0.05		15, 30, 45
	Cormax scalp solution	0.05		50 ml
	Ultravate cream	0.05	Halobetasol propionate	15, 50
	Ultravate ointment	0.05		15, 50
	Diprolene lotion	0.05	Augmented betamethasone dipropionate	30 ml, 60 ml
	Diprolene ointment	0.05		15, 50
	Diprolene gel	0.05		15, 50
	Olux foam	0.05	Clobetasol propionate	50, 100 gm can
	Olux-E			50, 100 gm can
	Psorcon ointment	0.05	Diflorasone diacetate	15, 30, 60
	Temovate-E cream	0.05	Clobetasol propionate	15, 30, 60
	Temovate ointment	0.05	Clobetasol propionate	15, 30, 45
	Temovate gel	0.05	Clobetasol propionate	15, 30, 60
	Vanos cream	0.1	Fluocinonide	30, 60, 120
II	Cyclocort ointment	0.1	Amcinonide	15, 60
	Diprolene AF cream	0.05	Augmented betamethasone dipropionate	15, 50
	Diprosone ointment	0.05	Betamethasone dipropionate	15, 45
	Diprosone aerosol	0.1	Betamethasone dipropionate	85
	Elocon ointment	0.1		
	Halog cream	0.1	Halcinonide	15, 30, 60
	Halog ointment	0.1		15, 30, 60
	Halog solution	0.1		20, 60 ml
	Halog-E cream	0.1		30, 60
	Kenalog ointment	0.5	Triamcinolone acetonide	15
	Lidex cream	0.05	Fluocinonide	15, 30, 60
	Lidex-E	0.05	Fluocinonide	15, 30, 60
	Lidex gel	0.05		15, 30, 60
	Lidex ointment	0.05		30, 60
	Lidex solution	0.05		20, 60 ml
	Psorcon cream	0.05	Diflorasone diacetate	15, 30, 60
	Topicort cream	0.25	Desoximetasone	15, 60
	Topicort gel	0.05		15, 60
	Topicort ointment	0.25		15, 60
III	Kenalog cream	0.5	Triamcinolone acetonide	15
	Betatrex cream	0.1	Betamethasone valerate	45
	Cutivate ointment	0.005	Fluticasone propionate	15, 30, 60
	Cyclocort lotion	0.1	Amcinonide	60 ml
	Cyclocort cream	0.1	Amcinonide	30, 60
	Diprosone cream	0.05	Betamethasone dipropionate	15, 45
	Diprosone lotion	0.05	Betamethasone dipropionate	20, 60 ml
	Elocon ointment	0.1	Mometasone furoate	15, 45
	Kenalog cream	0.5	Triamcinolone acetonide	20
	Kenalog paste	0.5	Triamcinolone acetonide	5